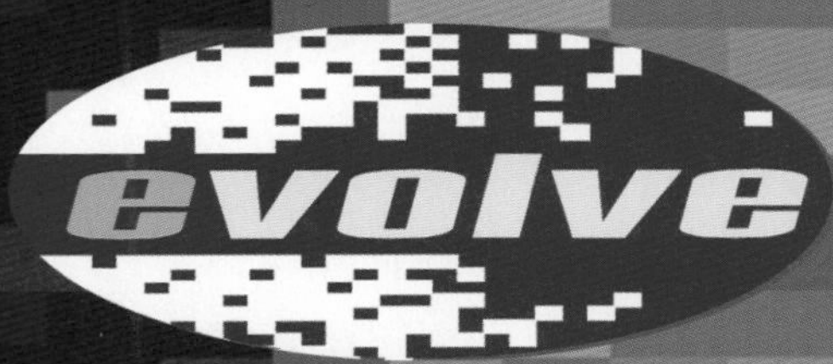

The Latest Evolution in Learning.

Evolve provides online access to free learning resources and activities designed specifically for the textbook you are using in your class. The resources will provide you with information that enhances the material covered in the book and much more.

Visit the Web address listed below to start your learning evolution today!

LOGIN: http://evolve.elsevier.com/Darby/Hygiene

Evolve Student Learning Resources for Darby and Walsh, *Dental Hygiene Theory and Practice*, 2nd Edition offers the following features:

- **Web Links**
  To connect you to Internet information on relevant and related topics.
- **Content Updates**
  Updated information will be posted as needed to keep you current on the latest research.
- **Competency-based Evaluation Forms**
  To help you evaluate your skills on performing the procedures in the text.
- **References and Suggested Readings**
  To support the research in each chapter and provide you with resources for additional information on related topics.

Think outside the book...evolve.

Dental Hygiene Theory and Practice

2nd Edition

Dental Hygiene Theory and Practice

2nd Edition

Michele Leonardi Darby, BSDH, MS
Eminent Scholar, University Professor, and Graduate Program Director,
Gene W. Hirschfeld School of Dental Hygiene,
College of Health Sciences,
Old Dominion University,
Norfolk, Virginia

Margaret M. Walsh, RDH, MS, MA, EdD
Professor,
Department of Preventive and Restorative Dental Sciences,
School of Dentistry,
University of California–San Francisco,
San Francisco, California

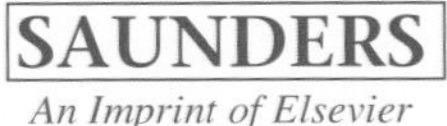

SAUNDERS
An Imprint of Elsevier

11830 Westline Industrial Drive
St. Louis, Missouri 63146

NOTICE

Dental hygiene is an ever-changing field. Standard safety precautions must be followed, but as new research and clinical experience broaden our knowledge, changes in treatment and drug therapy may become necessary or appropriate. Readers are advised to check the most current product information provided by the manufacturer of each drug to be administered to verify the recommended dose, the method and duration of administration, and contraindications. It is the responsibility of the licensed prescriber, relying on experience and knowledge of the patient, to determine dosages and the best treatment for each individual patient. Neither the publisher nor the author assumes any liability for any injury and/or damage to persons or property arising from this publication.

Previous edition copyrighted 1995.

ISBN-13: 978–0–7216–9162–6
ISBN-10: 0–7216–9162–5

Acquisitions Editor: Shirley Kuhn
Developmental Editor: Helaine Tobin
Publishing Services Manager: Pat Joiner
Project Manager: Gena Magouirk
Designer: Jonel Sofian

Printed in China

Last digit is the print number: 9 8 7 6 5

Contributors

Esther Andrews, CDA, RDA, RDH, MA
Impressions, Study Casts, and Oral Stents
Adjunct Professor,
Periodontics Department,
College of Dentistry,
University of Illinois–Chicago;
Lecturer,
Dental Hygiene Program,
Kennedy-King College,
Chicago, Illinois

Gerry J. Barker, RDH, BS, MA
Persons with Cancer
Professor and Coordinator of Oncology Education,
Department of Dental Public Health and Behavioral Science,
School of Dentistry,
University of Missouri–Kansas City,
Kansas City, Missouri

Deborah Bauman, BSDH, MS
Persons with Diabetes Mellitus
Associate Professor,
Gene W. Hirschfeld School of Dental Hygiene,
College of Health Sciences,
Old Dominion University,
Norfolk, Virginia

Marilyn Beck, RDH, BSDH, MEd
Root Morphology and Instrumentation Implications
Associate Professor Emeritus,
Department of Dental Hygiene,
College of Health Sciences,
Marquette University,
Milwaukee, Wisconsin

Helene Bednarsh, RDH, MPH
Infection Control
Boston Public Health Commission,
Boston, Massachusetts

Denise M. Bowen, RDH, MS
Mechanical Plaque Control: Toothbrushes and Toothbrushing
Professor,
Department of Dental Hygiene,
Idaho State University,
Pocatello, Idaho

Lee Ann Branscome Simmons, BSDH, MS
Persons with Orthodontic Appliances
Instructor,
Dental Hygiene Program,
Delaware Technical and Community College,
Wilmington, Delaware

Kim Krust Bray, RDH, MS
Periodontal Chemotherapy
Associate Professor and Director,
Graduate and Degree Completion Studies,
Division of Dental Hygiene,
School of Dentistry,
University of Missouri–Kansas City,
Kansas City, Missouri

Ginger B. Mann, BSDH, MS
Persons with Mental Retardation
Adjunct Faculty,
University of North Carolina,
Chapel Hill, North Carolina

Cheryl A. Cameron, RDH, PhD, JD
Restorative Therapy
Associate Vice Provost and Professor of Dental Public Health Sciences,
School of Dentistry,
University of Washington,
Seattle, Washington

Bonnie J. Craig, DipDH, RDH, MEd
Persons with Fixed and Removable Dentures
Associate Professor and Director,
Bachelor of Dental Science Program in Dental Hygiene,
Faculty of Dentistry,
University of British Columbia,
Vancouver, British Columbia, Canada

Eve Cuny, BS, MS
Infection Control
Director of Environmental Health and Safety and Assistant Professor,
Pathology and Medicine,
School of Dentistry,
University of the Pacific,
San Francisco, California

Michele Leonardi Darby, BSDH, MS
The Evolving Profession of Dental Hygiene;
Human Needs Theory and Dental Hygiene Care;
Cross-cultural Practice;
Dental Hygiene Diagnosis
Eminent Scholar, University Professor, and Graduate Program Director,
Gene W. Hirschfeld School of Dental Hygiene,
College of Health Sciences,
Old Dominion University,
Norfolk, Virginia

Lori Drummer, CDA, RDH, MEd
Ergonomics
Dental Hygiene Program Coordinator,
College of Lake County,
Grayslake, Illinois;
Adjunct Faculty,
Dental Hygiene Program,
College of DuPage,
Glen Ellyn, Illinois

Kathy J. Eklund, RDH, MPH
Infection Control
Associate Professor and Director of Infection Control and Occupational Health,
The Forsyth Institute,
Boston, Massachusetts

Joan Gugino Ellison, RDH, MS
Persons with Respiratory Diseases
Instructor,
Dental Hygiene Program,
Harrisburg Area Community College,
Harrisburg, Pennsylvania

Gwen Essex-Lancaster, RDH, MS
Oral Hygiene Assessment: Soft Deposits, Plaque Biofilm, Calculus, and Stain;
Local Anesthesia
Assistant Clinical Professor,
Department of Preventive and Restorative Dental Sciences,
Division of Dental Hygiene,
School of Dentistry,
University of California–San Francisco,
San Francisco, California

Maureen E. Fannon, RDH, MS
Pit and Fissure Sealants
Adjunct Professor,
Periodontics Department,
University of Illinois–Chicago;
Lecturer,
Dental Hygiene Program,
Kennedy-King College,
Chicago, Illinois

Margaret J. Fehrenbach, RDH, MS
Extraoral and Intraoral Clinical Assessment
Oral Biologist, Educational Consultant, and Dental Hygiene Practioner,
Seattle, Washington;
Adjunct Faculty,
Marquette University,
Milwaukee, Wisconsin

Jacquelyn Fried, RDH, BA, MS
Tobacco Cessation
Acting Chair and Associate Professor,
Degree Completion Program,
Department of Dental Hygiene,
University of Maryland Dental School,
Baltimore, Maryland

Joan I. Gluch, RDH, PhD
The Older Adult
Adjunct Associate Professor and Director,
Community Health,
School of Dental Medicine,
University of Pennsylvania,
Philadelphia, Pennsylvania

Marylou E. Gutmann, RDH, BS, MA
Extrinsic and Intrinsic Stains and their Management
Professor and Graduate Program Director,
Caruth School of Dental Hygiene,
Baylor College of Dentistry,
A Component of the Texas A & M University System Health Science Center,
Dallas, Texas

Renee Hannebrink, RDH, MS
Local Anesthesia
Dental Hygiene Practitioner,
Los Altos Hills, California

Kathleen O. Hodges, RDH, BS, MS
Nonsurgical, Supportive, and Mechanized Periodontal Therapies
Associate Professor and Senior Clinical Coordinator,
Department of Dental Hygiene,
Idaho State University,
Pocatello, Idaho

Ruth Hull, BSDH, MS
Behavioral Management of Pain and Anxiety
Clinical Research Associate,
Pharmaceutical Product Development, Inc.,
Wilmington, North Carolina

Juliana J. Kim, BSDH, MS
Dentinal Hypersensitivity Management
Director,
Professional Relations, Domestic and International,
Philips Oral Healthcare,
Snoqualmie, Washington

Sandra M. Kramer, RDH, MA
Practice Management;
Professional Development
Private Practioner, Educator, and Consultant,
Kensington, California

Stacy Long, RDH, BS, MS
Nutritional Counseling
Senior Project Manager,
Clinical Operations,
PPD Development,
Austin, Texas

Laura Lee MacDonald, DH, BScD(DH), MEd
Concepts of Health and Wellness
Associate Professor,
School of Dental Hygiene,
University of Manitoba,
Winnipeg, Manitoba, Canada

Richard B. McCoy, DDS, MS
Restorative Therapy
Acting Chair,
Department of Restorative Dentistry,
School of Dentistry,
University of Washington,
Seattle, Washington

Jeanne Maloney, RDH, MS
Fluorides and Chlorhexidine
Former Director,
Department of Dental Hygiene,
University of New Haven,
New Haven, Connecticut

Anne Miller, RDH, MS
Fluorides and Chlorhexidine
Formerly with Oral B Laboratories,
Lindenhurst, Illinois

Cara Miyasaki-Ching, RDHEF, MS
Personal, Dental, and Health Histories;
Vital Signs
Director,
Dental Assisting Program;
Instructor,
Dental Hygiene Program,
Foothill College,
Los Altos Hills, California

Laura Mueller-Joseph, RDH, MS, EdD
Persons with Cardiovascular Disease
Associate Professor,
Dental Hygiene Department,
Farmingdale State University of New York,
Farmingdale, New York

Brenda Parton Maddox, RDH, MS
Mechanical Plaque Control: Interdental Care and Supplemental Aids
Department Head,
Dental Hygiene,
Wake Technical Community College,
Raleigh, North Carolina

Maria Perno Goldie, RDH, MS
Women's Health
Adjunct Faculty,
Department of Preventive and Restorative Dental Sciences,
Division of Dental Hygiene,
School of Dentistry,
University of California–San Francisco,
San Francisco, California

Dorothy A. Perry, RDH, PhD
Acute Gingival and Periodontal Conditions, Lesions of Endodontic Origin, and Avulsed Teeth;
Persons with HIV Infection
Assistant Dean for Curricular Affairs and Associate Professor,
Department of Preventive and Restorative Dental Sciences,
Division of Dental Hygiene,
School of Dentistry,
University of California–San Francisco,
San Francisco, California

Janice Pimlott, DipDH, BScD, MSc
Assessment of the Dentition
Professor,
Dental Hygiene Program;
Director,
Interprofessional Initiative,
University of Alberta,
Edmonton, Alberta, Canada

Sandra K. Rich, RDH, MPH, PhD
Behavioral Foundations for the Dental Hygiene Process
Associate Professor,
School of Dentistry,
University of Southern California,
Los Angeles, California

Dorothy Rowe, RDH, MS, PhD
Persons with Neurologic and Sensory Disabilities
Associate Professor,
Department of Preventive and Restorative Dental Sciences,
School of Dentistry,
University of California–San Franscisco,
San Franscisco, California

Kathleen M. Schlotthauer, RDH, MS
Persons with Alcohol and Substance Abuse Problems
Associate Professor,
Dental Hygiene Program,
Harrisburg Area Community College,
Harrisburg, Pennsylvania

Michelle L. Sensat, BSDH, MS
Persons with Autoimmune Diseases
Assistant Professor and Preclinical Coordinator,
Department of Dental Hygiene,
College of Dentistry,
University of Nebraska,
Lincoln, Nebraska

Karen M. Shattuck, RDH, BSDH, MS
Dental Hygiene Care Plan
Professor and Clinical Coordinator,
Dental Hygiene Department,
Hudson Valley Community College,
Troy, New York

Ann Eshenaur Spolarich, RDH, PhD
Pharmacologic History;
Persons with Disabilities
Independent Research Consultant,
National Health Educator,
Phoenix, Arizona

Peggy T. Tsutsui, RDH, MS
Instruments and Instrumentation Theory
Associate Professor and Program Director,
Department of Dental Hygiene,
School of Dentistry,
University of Southern California,
Los Angeles, California

Susan Lynn Tolle, BSDH, MS
Periodontal and Risk Assessment
Professor and Director of Clinical Affairs,
Gene W. Hirschfeld School of Dental Hygiene,
Old Dominion University,
Norfolk, Virginia

Lynn Utecht, RDH, MA, MD
Managing Medical Emergencies
Head,
Department of Dermatology,
US Naval Hospital,
Rota, Spain

Margaret M. Walsh, RDH, MS, MA, EdD
The Evolving Profession of Dental Hygiene;
Human Needs Theory and Dental Hygiene Care;
Nitrous Oxide–Oxygen Analgesia
Professor,
Department of Preventive and Restorative Dental Sciences,
School of Dentistry,
University of California–San Francisco,
San Francisco, California

Lee E. Wentworth, MS, PhD
Persons with Neurologic and Sensory Disabilities
Associate Professor,
Department of Anatomy,
School of Medicine;
Department of Stomatology,
School of Dentistry,
University of California–San Francisco,
San Francisco, California

Karen B. Williams, RDH, MS, PhD
Persons with Eating Disorders
Professor and Director of the Clinical Research Center,
School of Dentistry,
University of Missouri–Kansas City,
Kansas City, Missouri

Judy Yamamoto, RDH, MS
Pit and Fissure Sealants
Associate Clinical Professor,
Department of Preventive and Restorative Dental Sciences,
Division of Dental Hygiene,
University of California–San Francisco,
San Francisco, California

Vivian Young-McDonald, RDH, BS
Persons with Osseointegrated Dental Implants
Implant Coordinator,
Oral and Maxillofacial Surgery Private Practice,
Piedmont, California

Sandra Z. Zagar, RDH, BS, MSA
Persons with Alcohol and Substance Abuse Problems
Assistant Professor and Senior Clinical Coordinator,
Dental Hygiene Program,
Harrisburg Area Community College,
Harrisburg, Pennsylvania

Pamela Zarkowski, BSDH, MPH, JD
Legal and Ethical Decision Making
Professor and Associate Dean for Academic Administration,
School of Dentistry,
University of Detroit Mercy,
Detroit, Michigan

Nancy Zinser, RDH, MS, PhD
Dentinal Hypersensitivity Management
Professor and Chair,
Department of Dental Health Services,
Palm Beach Community College,
Lake Worth, Florida

Reviewers

Josette L. Beach, RDH, MS
Portland Community College,
Portland, Oregon

Ann Brunick, RDH, MS
Chairperson,
Department of Dental Hygiene,
University of South Dakota,
Vermillion, South Dakota

Jean Byrnes-Ziegler, RDH, MS
Associate Professor,
Dental Hygiene Program Director,
Harcum College,
Bryn Mawr, Pennsylvania

Deborah L. Carl, RDH, MEd
University of Southern Indiana,
Evansville, Indiana

Marilyn Cortell, RDH, MS
Full-time Assistant Professor,
New York City Technical College;
Adjunct Faculty,
New York University,
Brooklyn, New York

Cheryl H. DeVore, RDH, MS, JD
College of Dentistry,
Ohio State University,
Columbus, Ohio

Ann Overton Dickinson, RDH, MS
St. Louis Community College–Forest Park,
St. Louis, Missouri

Lori J. Drummer, CDA, RDH, MEd
Dental Hygiene Program Coordinator,
College of Lake County,
Grayslake, Illinois;
Adjunct Faculty,
Dental Hygiene Program,
College of DuPage,
Glen Ellyn, Illinois

Patricia Anne Frese, RDH, BS, MEd
University of Cincinnati/Raymond Walter College,
Cincinnati, Ohio

Judith A. Hall, RDH, BS
Delaware Technical and Community College,
Wilmington, Delaware

Rita Jablon, CDA, RDH, LDH, BGS
Indiana University Northwest,
Gary, Indiana

Mary E. Jorstad, RDH, BS, MA
Lake Land College,
Mattoon, Illinois

Darnyl King, RDH, AS, BA, MS
Georgia Perimeter College,
Dunwoody, Georgia

Deborah S. Manne, RDH, RN, MSN, OCN
Clinical Assistant Professor,
School of Dentistry,
University of Missouri–Kansas City,
Kansas City, Missouri

Stacy B. Marshall, RDH, MSEd, DMD
Darton College,
Albany, New York

Barrie A. Montrose, RDH, MDPH
Hudson Valley Community College,
Troy, New York

Patricia J. Nunn, RDH, MS
Professor and Chair,
Department of Dental Hygiene,
College of Dentistry,
University of Oklahoma,
Oklahoma City, Oklahoma

M. Elaine Parker, RDH, MS, PhD
Department of Dental Hygiene,
Dental School,
University of Maryland,
Baltimore, Maryland

Juanita Robinson, CDA, EFDA, LDH, MSEd
Dental Education,
Indiana University Northwest,
Gary, Indiana

Judith E. Romano, RDH, BS, MA
Hudson Valley Community College,
Troy, New York

Mary Jo Cosgrove Saxe, RDH, MHA
Pennsylvania College of Technology,
Williamsport, Pennsylvania

Karen Shattuck, RDH, BSDH, MS
Professor and Clinical Coordinator,
Dental Hygiene Department,
Hudson Valley Community College,
Troy, New York

Kathi R. Shepherd, RDH, MS
Department of Periodontology and Dental Hygiene,
University of Detroit Mercy,
Detroit, Michigan

Dawn R. Smith, BSDH, MS
College of Dentistry,
Howard University,
Washington, District of Columbia

Diane Hardiman Smith, RDH, EdM
Instructor,
Dental Hygiene Program,
Portland Community College,
Portland, Oregon

Danielle A. Victoriano, RDH, BS
Clinical Instructor,
Program in Dental Hygiene,
School of Dentistry,
Health Sciences Center,
Louisiana State University,
New Orleans, Louisiana

Stephanie E. Wall, RDH, MS, MEd
Private Practice,
Los Angeles, California

Virginia Medina Wagner, CDA, RDH, BHS
Adjunct Faculty,
Tallahassee Community College,
Tallahassee, Florida

Jane Weiner, RDH
NOVA Southeast College of Dental Medicine,
Ft. Lauderdale, Florida

Mary Ellen Young, BS, RDH
Lake Washington Technical College,
Kirkland, Washington

To my parents for their continued guidance and love.
To my husband, Dennis, and our children, Devan and Blake, for making everything worthwhile.
MLD

To the memory of my parents, who gave me so much love and support over the years,
and to Jerry and T.J., for their patience, love, and encouragement.
MMW

This work is dedicated to Linda E. DeVore, RDH, MA for her outstanding leadership in advancing the dental hygiene profession.

PREFACE

EVIDENCE-BASED KNOWLEDGE—THE FOUNDATION OF DENTAL HYGIENE

Dental Hygiene Theory and Practice, ed 2 is for students and professionals who are interested in the use of evidence-based knowledge to guide decision making in practice. Societal values and healthcare reforms forecast the need for dental hygienists able to assess situations, access information, make evidence-based decisions, and collaborate with dentists and other health professionals in providing quality healthcare. Research evidence provides a framework for making decisions, solving problems, explaining phenomena, and predicting outcomes that enables the practitioner to continually reevaluate and advance service to society.

This book prepares dental hygienists to view their profession with pride, understand its territory and scope, and influence its advancement. The book uses the process of care guided by a client's human needs to operationalize the roles of the dental hygienist as practitioner, client advocate, manager, researcher, oral health promoter, and change agent.

Dental Hygiene Theory and Practice, ed 2 is predicated on four key assumptions:

- Oral health and systemic health are inextricably linked.
- Both theory and research serve as the basis for decision making in all dental hygiene roles.
- Dental hygienists are responsible and accountable for the services they provide and for the professional judgments and decisions they render.
- Accountability requires a systematic approach to practice, and this approach is the dental hygiene process.

Given these assumptions, society has a right to access care from individuals who are competent in making dental hygiene assessments, diagnoses, and care plans; providing interventions; and evaluating clinical outcomes.

HUMAN NEEDS THEORY

Human needs theory serves as a unifying theme in this book. Dental hygiene promotes oral and systemic health through the fulfillment of human needs. Human needs are universal, transcend all cultures, and are applicable to both individuals and groups. Human need fulfillment contributes to the quality of life of the individual, community, nation, and world. These facts were recognized by the World Health Organization when, in 1984, it redefined health as "the extent to which an individual or group is able, on the one hand, to realize aspirations and satisfy needs and, on the other hand, to change and cope with the environment." Because dental hygiene care assists individuals in their attainment of human needs, it is an essential component of the healthcare system, it enhances quality of life, and it is valued in today's wellness-oriented society.

TERMINOLOGY

An effort was made to use the most current terms, e.g., terms from the American Academy of Periodontology Classification of Periodontal Diseases and Conditions, American Dental Association insurance codes and definitions, *diabetes mellitus type 1* and *type 2,* and *plaque biofilm.* Progressing through the book, the reader may quickly notice that the term *client* is used more frequently than *patient.* We are sensitive to the responses that the term *client* may evoke. However, we deliberately chose the term *client* because it is broader in scope than the term *patient* and can refer to a group as well as an individual. Given that the focus of dental hygiene is to prevent oral disease and promote wellness, the term *client* recognizes that not all of those for whom we provide care are in need of "treatment" for a disease. Last, the term *client* acknowledges the autonomy of the recipient of care, since individuals who seek dental hygiene care generally choose to do so in partnership with the dental hygienist.

TEXTBOOK FORMAT

Dental Hygiene Theory and Practice, ed 2 is organized into eight major sections:

- Section 1: *Conceptual Foundations for Dental Hygiene (5 chapters)*
- Section 2: *Preparation for the Client Appointment (3 chapters)*
- Section 3: *Dental Hygiene Assessments (7 chapters)*
- Section 4: *Dental Hygiene Diagnosis, Care Plan, and Evaluation (2 chapters)*
- Section 5: *Implementation (14 chapters)*
- Section 6: *Pain and Anxiety Control* (4 chapters)
- Section 7: *Dental Hygiene Care for Individuals with Special Needs (16 chapters)*
- Section 8: *Practice Management (3 chapters)*

In terms of format, chapters include:

- **Objectives** to guide the teacher and the learner in developing competencies.
- **Key Terms** to focus the reader on the language of the profession and the important concepts that this language conveys.
- **Evidence-based explanations** of the subject.
- **Procedures** with detailed steps and rationales to ensure that the learner understands the reason underlying each step in the attainment of clinical competencies.
- **Client Education Issues** to remind the learner that there is more than just flossing and toothbrushing in educating a person about his or her oral and systemic health.
- **Legal, Ethical, and Safety Issues** that highlight areas in need of management to protect the health and welfare of both client and practitioner.
- **Key Concepts** that summarize the main points of the chapter at a glance.
- **Critical Thinking Exercises** that provide opportunities for independent thought, problem solving, and critical thinking.

Recognizing that this book may be used throughout North America, we have included, where appropriate, information that reflects the practice of dental hygiene in Canada.

Section 1: Conceptual Foundations for Dental Hygiene describes the evolving profession of dental hygiene, introduces human needs theory and the process of dental hygiene care, and provides the behavioral science and communication theory used by successful dental hygienists in human interactions. The dental hygiene process provides the framework for delivering quality care to all types of clients in a variety of settings and serves as the core of professional practice. Given dental hygiene's focus on oral disease prevention and health promotion, an entire chapter is devoted to health and wellness. Moreover, since we live in a global society and culture influences health, disease, behavior, beliefs and lifestyle, a chapter on cross-cultural practice is included in this section.

Section 2: Preparation for the Client Appointment describes guidelines for infection control in dental hygiene care and strategies for adapting to guidelines as they change. One chapter is devoted to the management of medical emergencies and another to the application of ergonomic principles to prevent repetitive strain injuries in practitioners.

Section 3: Dental Hygiene Assessments includes chapters that delineate the competencies of the dental hygienist in assessment of a client's general, dental, and periodontal health and risk status.

Section 4: Dental Hygiene Diagnosis, Care Plan, and Evaluation defines the dental hygiene diagnosis, distinguishing it from a dental diagnosis and illustrating how a dental hygiene diagnosis is made. This section also details the value of including client goals in the care plan and demonstrates how evaluation is used to document outcomes of care. With evaluation, the dental hygienist is accountable for care provided and can be confident that interventions made a positive difference in the individual's systemic and oral health status.

Section 5: Implementation presents numerous evidence-based interventions that comprise dental hygiene care. Specific clinical procedures, in table format, facilitate competency development in a variety of services, including personal oral care, instrumentation and root morphology, stain management, nonsurgical periodontal therapy, periodontal chemotherapy, caries risk assessment and management, tobacco cessation, supportive diagnostic aids, and restorative therapy.

Section 6: Pain and Anxiety Control covers both the behavioral and pharmacologic management of the client via anxiety-reducing protocols and administration of desensitizing agents, intraoral local anesthetics, and nitrous oxide–oxygen analgesia. Pain and anxiety control is essential for quality dental hygiene care across clients' lifespans.

Section 7: Dental Hygiene Care for Individuals with Special Needs recognizes that dental hygienists care for a growing number of individuals with diseases or disabilities that affect their daily living, self-care, and ability to access healthcare. Special needs clients that dental hygienists are likely to encounter have been given chapter status to assure competence in this area of practice.

Section 8: Practice Management provides the capstone for the dental hygienist who is interested in developing competencies in leadership, practice management, and legal and ethical decision making.

Glossary

A comprehensive glossary defines terms quickly and easily for the busy reader and reflects contemporary usage of terms as found in current literature.

Comprehensive Index

The detailed index makes finding information quick and easy.

SUGGESTED USE OF THIS LEARNING PACKAGE

OBJECTIVES AND KEY TERMS. All of us appreciate direction. At the start of each chapter, the reader should review the Objectives and the Key Terms as a way of previewing the most critical content in the chapter. When the reader encounters information within the chapter that is previewed in the Objectives and Key Terms, the reader should make special note of it. This information is highlighted again in the Key Concepts at the end of each chapter. In this learning sequence, significant information is made readily apparent to the learner, and learning is reinforced.

SCENARIOS AND CASE STUDIES. Scenarios and case studies are found throughout the textbook to challenge the reader in new situations. These learning strategies integrate complex information that requires the dental hygienist to assess, diagnose, plan care, and evaluate the outcome of care. In essence, scenarios and case studies provide simulated experience in evidence-based decision making and stimulate the cognitive processes of the dental hygienist in preparation for real practice situations. Scenarios and case studies can be assigned by the instructor as homework, used for developing individual and group problem solving skills, or used as a basis for class discussion or review by a study group.

CRITICAL THINKING EXERCISES. Exercises have been designed to encourage active learning, critical thinking, and professional judgment. These exercises can be assigned by the instructor as homework, used for developing individual and group problem solving skills, or used as a basis for class discussion or review by a study group.

PROCEDURES. Over 50 procedures provide step-by-step descriptions of core clinical procedures that must be mastered to achieve clinical competence. These descriptions also contain information about the materials and equipment necessary to carry out the procedures and rationales to ensure that the hygienist comprehends the science underlying each step of the procedure to make competence easier to achieve. These procedures are also on the text website and can be downloaded for use as *Competency-based Evaluation Forms* for use in laboratory, preclinical, or clinical settings. Once downloaded, these forms can be used for self-evaluation, peer evaluation, instructor evaluation, and/or reevaluation.

LEGAL, ETHICAL, AND SAFETY ISSUES. The dental hygienist's expertise in oral disease prevention and risk assessment, therapy, and health promotion and wellness has assumed value to the public. In return, the public is holding the dental hygienist accountable for a defined scope of practice. The dental hygienist must be alert to potential ethical dilemmas and legal risks. These issues can serve as topics for in-class discussions and role-playing opportunities.

CLIENT EDUCATION ISSUES. Competence in educating clients requires oral communication skills, sensitivity, and empathy. Moreover, it requires knowing what to say to the client. Client education topics are highlighted at the end of each chapter to suggest potential issues to focus dental hygienist–client discussions. These issues can serve as topics for in-class discussions and role-playing opportunities.

Textbook Website (with Downloadable Resources)

A website, found at http://evolve.elsevier.com/Darby/hygiene/, has been developed to support the content of the book and to enhance the faculty's instructional repertoire and student learning. The website includes:

TEST QUESTIONS BANK. With the current emphasis on student and curricular learning outcomes, competence, and assessment of learning, a bank of over 800 test questions can easily become part of an educator's overall assessment plan. These questions available on the website can be used independently by students or integrated into benchmark examinations that verify student knowledge at various points throughout the curriculum. With so many questions available, along with supporting rationales for the correct answers, questions can be selected and integrated into an annual comprehensive exam to prepare students for the National Board Dental Hygiene Examination.

ELECTRONIC IMAGE COLLECTION. An electronic image collection can be downloaded for PowerPoint presentations, handouts, and examinations.

WEBSITE LINKS. Website information and resources are posted on the website by chapter to connect students and faculty to Internet information on relevant and related topics. These are website resources that the dental hygienist will use in practice.

COMPETENCY-BASED EVALUATION FORMS. Procedures from the textbook have been modified into *Competency-based Evaluation Forms* and posted on the text website. These can be downloaded for use in laboratory, preclinical, or clinical settings. Once downloaded, these forms can be used for self-evaluation, peer evaluation, instructor evaluation, and/or reevaluation.

REFERENCES AND SUGGESTED READINGS. References and suggested readings for each chapter can be accessed readily from the website. These relevant citations can be used to support evidence-based decisions or as a start to a search of the literature for a written paper, research project, oral presentation, or table clinic assignment or simply for those who need to know more.

TEACHING AND LEARNING TIPS. Suggestions for overcoming instructional challenges and optimizing learning opportunities will be posted on an ongoing basis by faculty who are experts in teaching dental hygiene concepts and competencies.

CONTENT UPDATES. Periodic content updates are posted as research evidence changes the way dental hygienists practice. This feature serves as a mechanism for the contributors and editors to update the content of the book prior to subsequent editions.

Acknowledgments

We would like to express our sincere appreciation to all the contributors who helped make *Dental Hygiene Theory and Practice, ed 2* a reality, including the original contributors. Very special thanks are extended to the faculty and staff of the Gene W. Hirschfeld School of Dental Hygiene, Old Dominion University and to the faculty and staff of the Division of Dental Hygiene at the University of California–San Francisco, who made it possible for us to complete this book despite the demands of continuing responsibilities. Appreciation is extended to the American Dental Hygienists' Association and the American Dental Association. We also acknowledge the authors and publishers who granted permission to use concepts, quotes, photographs, figures, and tables. Several individuals who contributed content reviews of selected areas and/or photographs and diagrams should be acknowledged: Jane Eisen, DDS, ORALSCAN Laboratories, Inc.; Jerry Rollins, University of California– San Francisco; Cynthia Fong, DENTSPLY; Edward Green, DDS, Edward J. Taggart, DDS, Margaret Ash, DDS, and Sarah Talamantes RDH, University of California–San Francisco, School of Dentistry; Connie Drisko, RDH, DDS, University of Louisville, Kentucky, School of Dentistry; Thomas Flynn, DMD, University of Connecticut; Bruce Barker, DDS, University of Missouri–Kansas City School of Dentistry; James R. Clark, University of Washington School of Dentistry, Department of Orthodontics; Ann Gabrick, MSW, LSCSW, Eating Disorders Unit, Baptist Medical Center, Kansas City, Missouri; Robert Cowan, DDS, Advanced Education General Dentistry, University of Missouri–Kansas City School of Dentistry; Greg Mann; Theresa J. Kellerman; M.J. McDonald; M.A. Conover; Paul Hains, Down syndrome client, University of North Carolina School of Dentistry; Linda Ross Santiago, RDH, Diablo Valley College, Pleasant Hill, California; James R. Winkler, DDS, School of Dental Medicine, Clinic of Periodontology and Fixed Prosthodontics, University of Berne; Kathleen Muzzin, Caruth School of Dental Hygiene, Baylor College of Dentistry, Texas A & M University System; Kenneth Marinak, DDS, Gene W. Hirschfeld School of Dental Hygiene, Old Dominion University, Norfolk, Virginia; Philip R. Melnick, DMD University of California–Los Angeles, School of Dentistry; Dr. Christopher Wyatt and Dr. R.W. Priddy, Faculty of Dentistry, University of British Columbia, Vancouver, Canada; Jon B. Suzuki, DDS, PhD, MBA, School of Dental Medicine, University of Pittsburgh, Pittsburgh, PA; F.T. McIver, DDS, Department of Pediatric Dentistry, University of North Carolina School of Dentistry; Bob Perry from Oral-B Laboratories; Victoria Vick, RDH, formerly with Procter & Gamble; GlaxoSmithKline; Schick Technologies; Nordent, Inc.; ADEC, Inc.; DENTSPLY International Professional Division and the Preventive Division; Electro Medical Systems; Osprey Communications; Colgate Oral Pharmaceuticals; Premier Dental Products Company; Hu-Friedy Dental Manufacturing Company, Inc.; Tony Riso Company; Florida Probe Corporation; Basseler USA; Hartzell & Sons; Bausch and Lomb; DentalView, Inc.; Tech Poll Studios, Inc.; Singer Professional Services, Inc.; 3i-Implant Innovations; the QUE Corporation; and Waterpik Technologies.

Appreciation is extended to Venkat Varkala and Joanna Hill for assistance in organizing and typing manuscript and Marye J. McClanahan for assistance in organizing and question development.

Since the work of those who contributed to the first edition remains central to this revision, we want to gratefully acknowledge the work of Barbara Heckman, Margaret Tan, Ann Flynn Scarff, Glenn Gordon, Merry Greig Cosgrove, Mari-Anne L. Low, Pamela Parker Brangan, Deanne Shuman, Beth McKinney, and Linda G. Kraemer.

Our special thanks go to the staff at Elsevier Science, particularly Shirley Kuhn, Editor for Health-Related Professions; Helaine Tobin, Senior Developmental Editor; Kathleen Macciocca, Senior Editorial Assistant; Jeanne Allison, Developmental Editor; and Gena Magouirk, Project Manager, for shepherding the manuscript throughout the publication process. We are indebted to Dr. Helen Yura Petro for her mentorship and generosity in sharing time and knowledge, without which the human needs conceptual model for dental hygiene would never have become a reality. Without the contributions of these outstanding individuals, the book would not have been possible.

As with any new text, we shall be grateful to readers who have suggestions for additions or revisions or who are interested in sharing their responses with us.

Michele Leonardi Darby
Margaret M. Walsh

CONTENTS

Dental Hygiene Theory and Practice

2nd Edition

SECTION 1

Conceptual Foundations for Dental Hygiene

CHAPTER 1

THE EVOLVING PROFESSION OF DENTAL HYGIENE

OBJECTIVES

Mastery of the content in this chapter will enable the reader to:

- Define the discipline of dental hygiene
- Define dental hygienist
- Define the dental hygiene process of care
- Discuss the historical development of professional dental hygiene
- Explain the paradigm for the discipline of dental hygiene
- Define conceptual model and describe two that relate to dental hygiene
- Describe the six roles of the dental hygienist
- Explain the purpose of standards of practice
- Explain the purpose of practice acts and licensure
- Identify at least two professional dental hygiene organizations

KEY TERMS

American Dental Hygienists' Association
Canadian Dental Hygienists' Association
Change agent
Client
Clinical Practice Standards for Dental Hygienists in Canada
Clinician
Collaborative practice model
Conceptual model
Consumer advocate
Dental hygiene
Dental hygiene actions
Dental hygiene practice standards
Dental hygiene process
Dental hygienist
Environment
Health/oral health
Human needs conceptual model
International Dental Hygienists' Federation
Manager
National Dental Hygienists' Association
Occupational model
Oral health educator
Paradigm
Professional model
Researcher
Evidence-based practice

WHAT IS DENTAL HYGIENE?

Dental hygiene is the study of preventive oral healthcare, including the management of behaviors to prevent oral disease and to promote health.

WHO IS THE DENTAL HYGIENIST?

The *dental hygienist* is a licensed oral healthcare professional who integrates the roles of clinician, educator, consumer advocate, manager, change agent, and researcher to prevent oral disease and to promote health.

The dental hygienist uses the *dental hygiene process* as a systematic approach to dental hygiene care. The key behaviors in the dental hygiene process include:

- Assessment
- Diagnosis
- Planning
- Implementation
- Evaluation

A brief definition of the five steps of the dental hygiene process of care follows.

STEPS OF THE DENTAL HYGIENE PROCESS OF CARE

Steps	Definition
Assessment	The systematic collection of data to identify client problems, needs, and strengths
Diagnosis	The identification of client oral health problems that dental hygiene interventions can improve
Planning	The establishment of goals and selection of dental hygiene interventions that can move the client closer to optimal oral health
Implementation	The process of carrying out the dental hygiene care plan designed to meet the assessed needs of the client
Evaluation	The measurement of the extent to which the client has achieved the goals specified in the plan of care

The dental hygiene process is the foundation of professional dental hygiene practice and provides a framework for delivering quality dental hygiene care to all types of clients in any environment. The dental hygiene process requires decision making and assumes that dental hygienists are responsible for identifying and resolving client problems within the scope of dental hygiene practice.

To create an overall picture of the profession of dental hygiene, the remainder of this chapter will introduce the history of dental hygiene, the paradigm for the discipline of dental hygiene, conceptual models of dental hygiene, guidelines for practice, and professional organizations for dental hygienists.

HISTORY OF DENTAL HYGIENE

Nineteenth Century to the Twentieth Century[1]

In *A Practical Guide to the Management of the Teeth,* published in 1819, Levi Spear Parmly emphasized the importance of daily preventive oral health behavior (toothbrushing, flossing, and use of a dentifrice) to preserve the teeth and gingiva from oral disease. At that time, some dentists were beginning to recognize the value of preventive therapies for the public. In 1845 the editors of the *American Journal of Dental Science* published an editorial criticizing dentistry's neglect of preventive oral healthcare and its focus on mechanical dentistry and surgery. By the twentieth century more dentists wanted to provide preventive oral healthcare to patients but had time to perform only the dental procedures for which they were trained.

Dr. Alfred C. Fones, a leader in the oral hygiene movement, recognized that teaching children appropriate oral health behaviors was critical to the prevention of dental disease over the life span. Fones developed a plan to operationalize this concept in the Bridgeport, Connecticut, public schools by preparing women to implement the program.[2] These women were to provide children with prophylactic dental care and instruction in toothbrushing, flossing, nutrition, and general hygiene. Dr. Fones' concept of women working as preventive specialists was the root of the evolution of the dental hygiene profession of today. He opened the first school of dental hygiene in 1913. As the "father of dental hygiene," Fones presented a theory of dental hygiene that emphasized the role of the dental hygienist as a health educator of the public. In 1934, he wrote:

> It is primarily to this important work of public education that the dental hygienist is called. She must regard herself as the channel through which dentistry's knowledge of mouth hygiene is to be disseminated. The greatest service she can perform is the persistent education of the public in mouth hygiene and the allied branches of general health.[3]

Fones emphasized the educational and public health aspects of dental hygiene. He did not like the then commonly used term "dental nurse" because of its association with disease. He used the term "hygienist" to describe "one who is versed in the science of health and prevention of disease."[4] Eventually, the term "dental hygienist" took hold.

Table 1–1 gives a chronology of some of the key events that shaped the evolution of the emerging profession of dental hygiene. Although the practice of dental hygiene has changed markedly over the last century, the changes have been slow and have varied significantly throughout various geographic locations both nationally and internationally. Nevertheless, the foundation of dental hygiene practice has been oral health promotion and disease prevention to facilitate consumers' self-care, arrest the disease process, and decrease the incidence of oral disease. These key elements have led dental hygienists to be recognized today as the preventive oral health specialists in the Western healthcare system.

DENTAL HYGIENE'S PARADIGM

A *paradigm* is a widely accepted worldview of a discipline that shapes the direction and methods of its practitioners, educators, administrators, and researchers.[5] A discipline's paradigm comprises:

- Major concepts selected for study by the discipline
- Statements about the major concepts that define them in a global manner.

A paradigm specifies the unique perspective of each discipline and is the first level of distinction between disciplines.[6,7] In a discipline, the body of knowledge

Text continues on p. 7.

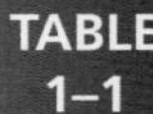

HISTORICAL POINTS OF INTEREST IN THE EVOLUTION OF DENTAL HYGIENE

Date	Event
1843	Beginning of the oral hygiene movement
1870	Professor Andrew McLain of the New Orleans Dental College published "Prophylaxis, or Prevention of Dental Decay," in which he advanced the concept of oral cleanliness, preventive measures, and diet. He was also the first to use the term "prophylaxis."
1888	Southern Dental Association resolved that a person should be employed to visit public and private schools to instruct children in the proper care of the teeth.
1898	Dr. M.L. Rhein employed a young woman whom he called a dental nurse to perform prophylactic and educational services in his office.
1902	Dr. Cyrus Mansfield Wright of Cincinnati, Ohio, was probably the first to suggest that women be trained to clean teeth and that their profession be considered a subspecialty of dentistry; advocated 1 year of college study.
1902	F.W. Low advocated a new profession of women who would go from house to house to clean and polish teeth; he called the profession odonticure.
1903	Dr. Thaddeus P. Hyatt of New York City promoted the value of educating the public concerning mouth hygiene among his colleagues and encouraged the acceptance of the dental hygienist; known as the "father of preventive dentistry."
1905	Dr. W. George Ebersole, founder of the Mouth Hygiene Association, began using a dental nurse in his office to perform prophylactic and educational services.
1906	Dr. Alfred C. Fones trained his assistant, Mrs. Irene Newman, to provide prophylactic procedures in his practice; acknowledged that training would eventually occur in colleges; considered the founder of dental hygiene.
1907	The first dental law to allow prophylactic treatment by a specially trained person, other than a dentist, was accepted in the state of Connecticut. With this law, it became illegal for Connecticut dentists to employ unlicensed assistants to perform prophylactic procedures in their offices.
1910	The Ohio College of Dental Surgery began offering a course for dental nurses. The program was discontinued in 1914 because of the strong opposition by Ohio dentists.
1913	The term "dental hygienist" was coined.
1913	Dr. Alfred C. Fones started the first courses for dental hygienists at his carriage house in Bridgeport, Connecticut.
1914	Dr. H.S. Seip, president of the Pennsylvania Dental Association, advocated licensing of the dental nurse.
1914	27 women became the first graduates of Dr. Fones' program.
1914	Fones' 5-year Bridgeport demonstration project in the public schools was initiated to have dental hygienists provide prophylactic treatment, classroom talks and lectures, and education for parents; the project proved the success of the dental hygienist in education and dental disease prevention.
1914	Colorado College of Dental Surgery initiated a dental nurse program; this became a dental hygiene program in 1920.
1915	Connecticut and Massachusetts dental laws outlined the scope of dental hygiene practice.
1916	Rochester Dental Dispensary initiated a dental hygiene education program.
1916	Forsyth Dental Infirmary initiated a dental hygiene education program.
1916	New York State enacted legislation defining dental hygiene practice.
1916	Columbia University became the first school of dental hygiene to develop specific educational requirements.
1917	Emma Crabbe was employed by Yale and Towen Company of Stamford, Connecticut to provide prophylactic treatment to its employees.
1917	First dental hygiene license issued to Irene Newman in Connecticut.
1918	University of California initiates a 1-year dental hygiene program in San Francisco.
1919	The University of Minnesota instituted the first 2-year education program in dental hygiene.
1920-1925	Dental hygiene education programs started at the University of Michigan, Temple University, University of Pennsylvania, Northwestern University, and Marquette University.
1922	American Dental Association adopted a model dental hygiene practice act to be used by the states.
1923	First meeting of the American Dental Hygienists' Association held in Cleveland, Ohio; Winifred A. Hart elected as its first president.
1925	American Dental Hygienists' Association adopted a constitution and by-laws.
1926	American Dental Hygienists' Association drafted the Code of Ethics.
1927	American Dental Hygienists' Association inaugurated the *Journal of the American Dental Hygienists' Association;* the name was changed to *Dental Hygiene* in 1972 and to *Journal of Dental Hygiene* in 1988.
1931	16 dental hygiene education programs were in existence.
1932	American Dental Association established the Committee on Dental Hygiene to collect data on dental hygiene education and practice.
1932	National Dental Hygienists' Association established by African American dental hygienists.
1937	American Dental Association established the Council on Dental Education to oversee education programs in dentistry and dental hygiene.
1939	University of Michigan offered a baccalaureate degree program in dental hygiene.
1940	American Dental Hygienists' Association recommended that dental hygiene education programs be 2 years in length.
1941	University of California in San Francisco initiates a baccalaureate degree in dental hygiene.
1946-1953	United States Public Health Service initiated research studies to measure the effectiveness of the expanded use of dental assistants and dental hygienists; Forsyth Dental Clinic initiated a research project to evaluate the feasibility of dental hygienists restoring primary teeth.
1947	American Dental Association Council on Dental Education required that all dental hygiene programs be *at least* 2 years in length and proposed curriculum standard.

TABLE 1–1 HISTORICAL POINTS OF INTEREST IN THE EVOLUTION OF DENTAL HYGIENE—CONT'D

Date	Event
1947	Francis Stolle, in a paper presented at the third Congress of Dental Education and Licensure in Chicago, stated that dental hygiene education should be a university discipline with full credit toward a BS or BA degree.
1950	Full-time dental hygienist hired by the Canadian Department of National Health and Welfare in Ottawa.
1950	Establishment of an accreditation committee on dental hygiene education by the Canadian Dental Association.
1951	American Dental Association Council on Dental Education recommended that dental hygienists receive expanded training ("expanded duties"); it also began accrediting dental hygiene education programs.
1951	University of Toronto established the first dental hygiene education program in Canada.
1954	Dental hygiene licensure available in all 50 states, the District of Columbia, and Puerto Rico.
1958	The National Honor Society of Dental Hygiene, Sigma Phi Alpha, was established.
1960-1965	Graduate education leading to the master's degree initiated at Columbia University, the University of Iowa, and the University of Michigan.
1962	National Dental Hygiene Board Examination was developed and immediately recognized by 25 states.
1963	University of Manitoba established the School of Dental Hygiene.
1963	Vocational Education Act of 1963 contributed to the growth of dental hygiene programs in technical schools and community colleges.
1965	15,400 dental hygienists employed in the United States.
1965	Dental Hygiene Educators Conference held to establish student competencies, define responsibilities of dental hygienists, and develop an educator's network.
1966	Allied Health Professions Personnel Training Act provided capitation grants to dental hygiene programs.
1967	National Advisory Commission on Health Manpower identified need for additional allied health professionals.
1968	Health Manpower Act provided funds for the education of health professionals.
1968	Administration of the first Northeast Regional Board Examination.
1968	Canadian Department of National Health and Welfare convened the Ad Hoc Committee on Dental Auxiliaries; this committee's report was significant in developing expanded services for dental hygienists in Canada.
1968	University of British Columbia established the Program of Dental Hygiene; terminated the program in 1986; established baccalaureate degree completion program in 1992.
1970	First International Symposium on Dental Hygiene, sponsored by the American Dental Hygienists' Association, held in Italy.
1970	*Curriculum Essentials* document published by the American Dental Hygienists' Association.
1970	Commissioning of baccalaureate-trained dental hygienists as officers in the United States Army.
1970	Training in Expanded Auxiliary Management (TEAM) projects funded to study the feasibility of teaching registered dental hygienists to perform expanded services under dentist supervision.
1970	International Liaison Committee on Dental Hygiene was founded and included representatives of dental hygiene associations from Canada, Japan, the Netherlands, Norway, Sweden, the United Kingdom, and the United States.
1970	Studies conducted at Forsyth Dental Clinic, the University of Pennsylvania, the University of Iowa, and Howard University reported that graduate dental hygienists could be trained to successfully perform expanded services; several projects were stopped because of local dentist opposition.
1971	University of Montreal established the baccalaureate degree program in dental hygiene.
1971	Second International Symposium on Dental Hygiene held in Switzerland.
1971	Dental hygienists became involved in Dental Auxiliary Utilization (DAU) Demonstration Projects in North Carolina, Iowa, Alabama, Kentucky, Florida, Maryland, Missouri, and Ohio.
1972	Third International Symposium on Dental Hygiene held in the United Kingdom.
1972	Dental hygiene education programs established at six colleges: d'Enseignement general et professional in Quebec; another established at CEGEP John Abbot in 1973.
1973	Fourth International Symposium on Dental Hygiene held in the Netherlands.
1974	Canadian Dental Association sponsored the Conference on Dental Auxiliaries held at Banff, Alberta; issues discussed included the role of auxiliaries, guidelines for implementing change, and problems experienced by dental hygienists and dental assistants (e.g., lack of career mobility, levels of supervision, mechanisms for quality assurance, need for representation on policy-making bodies, and continuing education).
1975	The Professional Corporation of Dental Hygienists of Quebec, with the endorsement of the Quebec government, transformed dental hygiene into an autonomous, self-regulating profession.
1975	Fifth International Symposium on Dental Hygiene held in Japan.
1976	Linda Krol, in California, became the first dental hygienist to own and manage a dental hygiene practice.
1977	Sixth International Symposium on Dental Hygiene held in Sweden.
1977	University of Toronto established a baccalaureate degree completion program in dental hygiene.
1978	Hygienists Political Action Committee established.
1979	Two decades of rapid expansion resulted in 201 dental hygiene programs in the United States.
1979	University of Montreal established a baccalaureate degree completion program.
1979	73,500 licensed dental hygienists in the United States.
1980	Canadian Dental Hygienists' Association presented 14 recommendations to the commission on the review of health services in Canada; recommendations addressed research in dental care delivery, the regulation and supervision of dental hygienists, the need for practice standards and quality assurance mechanisms, improvements in dental hygiene education and accreditation, and a larger role for dental hygienists.
1980	By this time, 33 states had dental hygiene representation on boards of dental examiners.

Table continued on following page

TABLE 1–1 HISTORICAL POINTS OF INTEREST IN THE EVOLUTION OF DENTAL HYGIENE—CONT'D

Date	Event
1980	11 states required mandatory continuing education for dental hygiene licensure.
1980	Federal Trade Commission proposed that state restrictions requiring dentist supervision of dental hygienists be nullified.
1980	American Dental Hygienists' Association adopted policy that a dental hygienist may own a dental hygiene practice.
1981	American Dental Hygienists' Association membership exceeded 22,000.
1981	Eighth International Symposium on Dental Hygiene held in the United Kingdom.
1982	First Conference on Dental Hygiene Research, sponsored by the Working Group on the Practice of Dental Hygiene's Subcommittee on Research and the University of Manitoba, held in Winnipeg, Manitoba.
1983	The State of Washington established a Dental Hygiene Examining Committee to license dental hygienists, and a Dental Hygiene Practice Act to govern the practice of dental hygiene.
1983	Ninth International Symposium on Dental Hygiene held in the United States (Philadelphia).
1984	Legislation permitting unsupervised dental hygiene practice in nursing homes, hospitals, institutional settings, and public health facilities was passed in the state of Washington.
1985	American Dental Hygienists' Association published *Standards of Applied Dental Hygiene Practice.*
1986	American Dental Hygienists' Association adopted policy supporting the baccalaureate degree as the minimum entry-level credential for practice.
1986	Legislation was passed in Colorado permitting unsupervised dental hygiene practice (independent dental hygiene practice) in all settings; this excluded root planing and radiographic services.
1986	Health Manpower Pilot Project (HMPP #139), sponsored by the University of California at Northridge and accepted by California Office of Statewide Health Planning and Development, was designed to study safety and access to dental hygiene care in unsupervised settings; California Dental Association attempted to stop the project with lawsuits.
1986	International Dental Hygienists' Federation was founded during the Tenth International Symposium on Dental Hygiene in Oslo, Norway.
1986	Colleges d'Enseignement general et professionnel's (CEGEP) in Hull and Chicoutimi, Quebec, established dental hygiene programs.
1987	Ontario dental hygienists were granted self-governing status.
1988	American Dental Hygienists' Association published *Prospectus on Dental Hygiene* to project a future course for the profession.
1988	The Canadian Working Group on the Practice of Dental Hygiene published *Clinical Standards for Dental Hygienists in Canada.*
1989	Eleventh International Symposium on Dental Hygiene held in Ottawa, Ontario.
1990	State dental associations in Georgia, Montana, Pennsylvania, South Carolina, South Dakota, Tennessee, and Virginia considered preceptorship as a dental hygiene training option.
1990	The Academy of General Dentistry's legislature rescinded its existing policy on formal accredited education as the only route for training dental hygienists.
1991	The American Dental Hygienists' Association engaged in strategic planning aimed at the goal of professionalization of dental hygiene.
1991	Legislatures of Ontario passed the Regulated Health Professions Act. This legislation established the College of Dental Hygienists of Ontario, the regulatory body for the provinces' dental hygienists. (Dental hygienists in the three Canadian provinces of Quebec, Alberta, and Ontario are now self-governing.)
1992	Twelfth International Symposium on Dental Hygiene held in The Hague, the Netherlands.
1992	The American Dental Hygienists' Association House of Delegates adopted a definition and theoretical paradigm for the professional discipline of dental hygiene.
1993	The American Dental Hygienists' Association adopted framework for a new code of ethics.
1994	Arkansas, Idaho, Michigan, Mississippi, Missouri, North Carolina, South Carolina, and Virginia acquired mandatory continuing education for licensure renewal.
1994	Rhode Island changed law to allow general supervision.
1994-2001	The expansion of dental hygiene practice acts in Canada and in some states in the United States to permit forms of unsupervised dental hygiene practice.
1995	A third Dental Hygiene Research Conference was held in Minneapolis with participants from Israel, Sweden, and Canada.
1995	Arizona and Texas adopted continuing education as a requirement for licensure renewal.
1995	Minnesota law was changed to allow dental hygienists to administer nitrous oxide.
1995	Minnesota, Nebraska, and South Carolina allowed dental hygienists to administer local anesthesia.
1995	Nevada law was changed to allow dental hygienists to provide care under general supervision.
1996	North Dakota allowed dental hygienists to practice under general supervision.
1996	ADHA issued a position paper on polishing procedures.
1996	ADHA went online with a website that can be accessed at http://www.adha.org
1996	Vermont law changed to require continuing education as part of licensure renewal.
1997	Alaska and Colorado allowed dental hygienists to administer nitrous oxide.
1997	Dental hygienists in Maine were allowed to administer local anesthesia.
1997	Qualifying dental hygienists in Oregon could obtain a limited access permit to initiate services for patients in nursing homes, adult foster homes, residential care facilities, adult congregate care facilities, and mental health residential programs.
1998	ADHA worked to make sure dental benefits were included in the State Children's Health Insurance Program (SCHIP).
1998	ADHA issued a position paper on oral prophylaxis.
1998	Iowa, Louisiana, and Wisconsin allowed dental hygienists to administer local anesthesia.
1998	Kansas, Ohio, and Tennessee allowed dental hygienists to practice under general supervision.

TABLE 1–1 HISTORICAL POINTS OF INTEREST IN THE EVOLUTION OF DENTAL HYGIENE—CONT'D

Date	Event
1998	Nevada allowed dental hygienists who obtain special authority from the dental board to perform services in a health facility, school, or other board-designated setting without supervision.
1998	Dental hygienists endorsed as RDHAP (registered dental hygienist in alternative practice) could provide services to patients who brought them a prescription from a dentist or physician at residences for the homebound, schools, residential facilities, institutions, and in dental health professional shortage areas.
1999	Louisiana and Pennsylvania required continuing education as a requirement for licensure renewal.
1999	Illinois dental hygienists were allowed to administer nitrous oxide.
1999	New Mexico dental hygienists were allowed to practice in collaborative practices that were based on written agreement between the dental hygienist and one or more consulting dentists.
1999	Iowa dental hygienists obtained self-regulation through a dental hygiene committee.
1999	Connecticut dental hygienists with 2 years experience were allowed to practice without supervision in institutions, public health facilities, group homes, and schools.
2000	Dental hygienists in Tennessee were allowed to administer nitrous oxide.
2000	Dental hygienists in Illinois were allowed to administer local anesthesia.
2000	ADHA held the Fourth National Research Conference on Evidence-Based Research.
2000	To increase access to care, self-regulation was adopted for dental hygienists in Iowa.
2001	Iowa allowed dental hygienists to administer nitrous oxide.
2001	New York allowed dental hygienists to administer nitrous oxide.
2001	Missouri dental hygienists with 3 years experience were allowed to provide services such as prophylaxis, placement of sealants, and application of fluorides, without supervision, to Medicaid-eligible children.
2001	Missouri dental hygienists were permitted to be Medicaid providers.
2001	Colorado dental hygienists were permitted to be Medicaid providers.
2001	Minnesota dental hygienists obtained limited authorization to be employed or retained by a healthcare facility to perform dental hygiene services without the patient first being examined by a licensed dentist.
2001	Maine dental hygienists were allowed to practice in public or private schools, hospitals, or other nontraditional practices under public health supervision status.

Adapted in part from Motley W: *History of the American Dental Hygienists' Association, 1923–1982,* Chicago, 1986, American Dental Hygienists' Association.

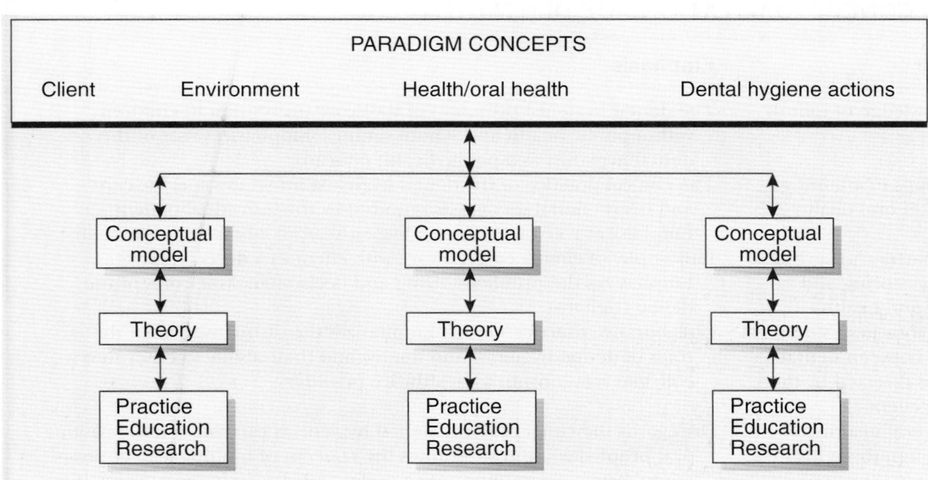

FIGURE 1–1 ✦ Dental hygiene theory development framework. *(From American Dental Hygienists Association: Proceedings of the 69th Annual Session, House of Delegates, Denver, June 1993.)*

progresses from a single paradigm to multiple conceptual models and multiple theories derived from each model[8] (Figure 1–1). The four major concepts of the paradigm for the discipline of dental hygiene, as defined by the American Dental Hygienists' Association,[9] are described in the table on the following page.

These four paradigm concepts identify the phenomena central to the discipline of dental hygiene in an abstract global manner. They can be defined, developed, and expanded in numerous ways by the development of conceptual models of dental hygiene.

CONCEPTUAL MODELS OF DENTAL HYGIENE

Conceptual models are important for dental hygiene because they provide philosophical and practical perspectives on the care dental hygienists deliver. A *conceptual model* can be thought of as a school of thought within a discipline. There can be as many conceptual models as there are scholars who can think them up. Conceptual models explain dental hygiene from different perspectives. For example, one model might explain dental

FOUR MAJOR CONCEPTS OF THE DENTAL HYGIENE PARADIGM

Concepts	Definition
Client	The recipient of dental hygiene care; includes persons, families, groups, and communities of all ages, genders, and sociocultural and economic states
Environment	Factors other than dental hygiene actions that affect the client's attainment of optimal oral health. These include economic, psychologic, cultural, physical, legal, educational, ethical, and geographic factors.
Health/Oral health	The client's state of being that exists on a continuum from optimal wellness to illness and fluctuates over time as the result of biologic, psychologic, spiritual, and developmental factors. Oral health and overall health are interrelated because each influences the other.
Dental hygiene actions	Interventions that a dental hygienist can initiate to promote oral wellness and to prevent or control oral disease. These actions involve cognitive, affective, and psychomotor performances and may be provided in independent, interdependent, and collaborative relationships with the client and the healthcare team.

hygiene as a public health–oriented practice, another as an auxiliary occupation, still another as a collaborative profession, or another as an independent profession. One model builder may use terms such as "auxiliary," "dependence," "supervision," "dental care," and "duties," whereas another may stress "professionalism," "independent decision making," and the "process of care." Terms and beliefs are defined according to the focus of the particular conceptual model.

Table 1–2 describes, in chronologic order, the general focus of several conceptual models of dental hygiene, some of which will be discussed in more detail in the following sections.

Occupational Model versus the Professional Model

Table 1–3 compares some of the basic propositions of the occupational model of dental hygiene with those of the professional model of dental hygiene. The *occupational model*[9] views dental hygiene as technology based. According to this model, the dental hygienist is a dental *auxiliary* who implements treatment plans and carries out isolated duties as directed by the supervising dentist. This conceptual model emphasizes the provision of oral prophylaxis in the dental office (defined as oral hygiene

TABLE 1–2 SUMMARY OF SELECTED CONCEPTUALIZATIONS OF DENTAL HYGIENE

Theorists	Goal of Dental Hygiene	Emphasis
Fones, 1934	To channel dentistry's knowledge of mouth hygiene to the public	The dental hygienist promotes oral disease prevention in children within public health and school settings. Emphasizes role of the dental hygienist as a public health educator
Wilkins and McCullough, 1959, 1964	To aid individuals and groups in attaining and maintaining optimum oral health	The clinical practice of the dental hygienist integrates specific care and instructional services as required by the individual patient. Emphasizes role of the dental hygienist as an auxiliary to the dentist
Woodall, 1980, 1985, 1989, 1993	To involve the client as a partner in care as a necessary condition for restoring and maintaining the client's oral health	Philosophy of client-centered care with client as a decision maker. Emphasizes the problem-solving and decision-making roles of the dental hygienist
Darby, 1983	To promote and maintain the client's oral health via collaboration between dental hygienists and dentists as directed by the oral health needs of the client	Collaborative practice model. Emphasizes the distinctiveness of the roles of dental hygienist and dentist and their ability to enter into a collegial relationship as healthcare providers
Walsh and Robertson, 1985	To promote and maintain oral health and to control oral disease through three distinct professional, mechanical oral hygiene interventions	Disregards the concept of the dental hygienist's carrying out the routine oral prophylaxis and substitutes the concept of multiple categories of dental hygiene care: preventive oral prophylaxis, therapeutic scaling and root planing, and periodontal maintenance care
Wilkins, 1989	To aid individuals and groups in attaining and maintaining optimal oral health, with the hygienist as a cotherapist with dentist	Emphasizes the preventive, educational, and therapeutic role of the dental hygienist as both an auxiliary and a co-therapist with the dentist
Darby, 1990	To facilitate the client's attainment of total self-care	Client demonstrates a self-care deficit. Dental hygiene care is necessary when the client is unable to fulfill self-care needs because of developmental, social, psychological, financial, physical, or mental reasons.
Darby and Walsh, 1991	To assist individuals in meeting their human needs through the use of interventions aimed at meeting deficits in human needs related to the performance of oral health behaviors that will lead to optimal oral wellness over the life span	Human needs theory suggested as a conceptual framework for the dental hygiene process. Requires dental hygienists to be aware of basic human needs and identifies 8 human needs related to dental hygiene care; encourages dental hygiene diagnoses based on deficits in these 8 human needs related to dental hygiene care; and aims dental hygiene interventions at eliminating these deficits

instruction, thorough calculus removal, and coronal polishing) as the primary duty delegated to the dental hygienist by the dentist under direct supervision. Expertise, evaluation of the effect of dental hygiene care on oral health and disease, and decision making are not stressed.

Under the occupational model, the focus of assessment is to gather data for the dentist to use in determining the dental diagnosis and treatment plan, part of which will be implemented by the dental hygienist. This model conveys the idea that the dental hygienist, as an auxiliary person, is accountable to the supervising dentist, who is then accountable to the client.

In contrast, the *professional model*[9] perceives dental hygiene to be knowledge based. This model conveys the view that dental hygienists use a *process of care* to assess needs, diagnose oral hygiene problems, and plan, implement, and evaluate dental hygiene care. According to this model the dental hygienist is responsible for making decisions about dental hygiene care and is accountable to the client. Each of these conceptual models has a unique perspective on dental hygiene that will guide dental hygiene education and clinical practice in very different ways.

Collaborative Practice Model

Collaboration occurs when individuals with differing strengths work together as equal partners to achieve better results than each could achieve working alone. The *collaborative practice model*[10] assumes that dentists and dental hygienists work together as colleagues, each offering professional expertise for the goal of providing optimum oral healthcare to the public. Although both professions can and should work together to improve the oral health status of the public, each has a specific role that complements and augments the effectiveness of the other. The collaborative practice model emphasizes the distinct roles of dental hygienist and dentist and their ability to enter into a collegial relationship as healthcare providers. In this model, the dentist and the dental hygienist are in a co-therapist relationship. In a collaborative practice, dental hygienists are viewed as experts in their field, are consulted about appropriate dental hygiene interventions, are expected to make clinical dental hygiene decisions, and are given freedom in planning, implementing, and evaluating the dental hygiene component of the overall care plan.

Human Needs Conceptual Model

The *human needs conceptual model*[11] of dental hygiene defines the paradigm concepts of client, environment, health/oral health, and dental hygiene actions in terms of human needs theory. The primary concern of this model is for the whole person who either has oral disease or may develop it, rather than for the oral disease itself, and for the role of the environment and dental hygiene actions in meeting human needs related to health. This conceptual model provides a comprehensive and humanistic approach to dental hygiene care and is explained in detail in Chapter 2.

TABLE 1–3 SAMPLE PROPOSITIONS FROM TWO CONCEPTUAL MODELS OF DENTAL HYGIENE

Occupational	Professional
Hygienist implements preventive treatment plans developed by dentist	Hygienist implements self-generated preventive care regimens
Secondary care providers	Primary care providers
Hygienist carries out isolated duties as indicated by supervising dentist	Hygienist uses process of care to assess needs, plan and implement care, and evaluate client
Hygienist is an auxiliary of dentistry	Hygienist is a professional who collaborates with the dentist and other health professionals
Hygienist is responsible for less complex, easier oral healthcare services	Hygienist is responsible for services that include some of the more difficult techniques to master in oral healthcare
Hygiene care involves an oral prophylaxis every 6 months at a 30- to 45-min appointment	Hygiene care involves multiple interventions that may require multiple appointments and appointment lengths
Hygienist is responsible for less valued services, leaving the dentist time for important services	Hygienist is responsible for preventive and oral maintenance care, which is highly valued by today's wellness-oriented consumer
Unsupervised dental hygiene practice reduces the quality of oral healthcare and increases client risks	Unsupervised dental hygiene practice increases public access to oral hygiene care and lowers healthcare costs
Dentistry is responsible for making decisions about dental hygienists	The dental hygiene profession is responsible for making decisions about dental hygienists
Dental hygienists are accountable to the dentist	Dental hygienists are accountable to the client (consumer)
Client is passive because the dentist is responsible for the client's oral health	Client is active because clients are responsible for their own oral health
Hygienist fulfills role through the function of a clinician	Hygienist fulfills role through functions of clinician, educator/health promoter, manager, change agent, consumer advocate, and researcher
Dental hygiene is technically based	Dental hygiene is knowledge based

ROLES OF THE DENTAL HYGIENIST

In 1984 the American Dental Hygienists' Association sponsored a conference to articulate the evolving functional roles of dental hygienists. Outcomes of that conference offered a comprehensive view of the dental hygienist as a licensed professional member of the healthcare team who serves as a clinician, oral health educator, manager, consumer advocate, change agent, and researcher (Table 1–4). These roles and functions are used by all clinical dental hygienists in most practice settings. Although most dental hygienists are clinical practitioners, others have pursued nonclinical careers by going into business for themselves (e.g., dental staff placement agencies, private continuing education companies, consulting firms), or working in public health, private industry, academia, or with other government agencies. Regardless of the career path, all dental hygienists function in the roles described in the following sections and in Table 1–4.

Dental Hygiene Clinician

The role of the dental hygiene *clinician* includes the assessment of signs of health and disease in the oral cavity; identification of the dental hygiene problem (dental hygiene diagnosis); and the planning, implementation, and evaluation of dental hygiene care. The responsibilities of the dental hygiene clinician are defined in the following box and include providing preventive, therapeutic, and educational services.

As a clinician, the dental hygienist helps the client set oral health goals and collaborates with the client to meet those goals. The dental hygiene clinician makes decisions independently or in collaboration with the client and family, the dentist, or other healthcare professionals.

In the United States and Canada, clinical dental hygienists usually provide dental hygiene care in collaboration with a general dentist or a dental specialist in a private dental practice. Other clinical hygienists have chosen to provide dental hygiene care in public health facilities, the armed forces, corporate dental clinics, research institutions, and extended care facilities (Table 1–4).

> **Responsibilities of the Dental Hygiene Clinician**
>
> **Preventive**
> Methods employed to prevent oral disease and promote health (e.g., applying topical fluoride to teeth)
>
> **Therapeutic**
> Methods employed to arrest or control oral disease (e.g., scaling and root planing periodontally involved teeth)
>
> **Educational**
> Methods employed in both preventive and therapeutic aspects of clinical dental hygiene care to explain concepts regarding oral disease and health, to demonstrate self-care techniques, to reinforce learning, to evaluate understanding, and to determine ability to perform desired behaviors (e.g., teaching toothbrushing and flossing)

Educator/Oral Health Promoter

Trends in society have underscored the importance of the role of the dental hygienist as an *oral health educator.* Trends toward consumerism, self-care, disease prevention, and healthy lifestyles mean that clients want and need extensive information from the dental hygienist to promote oral health and prevent oral disease. Dental hygienists assume the role of educator when clients have learning needs.

In the teacher–client relationship the dental hygienist explains concepts regarding oral health and disease, demonstrates self-care procedures, determines client understanding, reinforces learning or desired behavior, and evaluates the client's progress in learning. If a client has good oral health, teaching focuses on the continuation of present oral health practices. In contrast, a client with active disease is taught about the disease process, the dental and dental hygiene care required to control the disease, and the client behaviors required to restore and maintain health. Sometimes teaching is unplanned and informal, as when the dental hygienist responds to a client's question about an oral health issue in casual conversation. Other educational activities may be planned and more formal, as when the dental hygienist teaches an oral cancer patient to use high-concentration fluoride gel on a daily basis at home, or is called on to provide continuing education for dental office staff development.

Teaching is involved in the full range of dental hygiene activities directed toward helping the client achieve oral wellness. The role of oral health educator involves effectively communicating not only with clients, but also with dentists and other healthcare professionals. This educator role is critical in meeting the oral health and human needs of individuals, families, and communities. Practice acts in most legal jurisdictions specify oral health education as a responsibility of the dental hygienist.

Dental hygiene educators who teach in settings other than private practice work primarily in:

- ✦ Schools of dental hygiene and dentistry
- ✦ Public school systems
- ✦ Public health departments

A faculty member in a school of dental hygiene prepares students for careers as professional dental hygienists. Dental hygiene faculty members are responsible for teaching current dental hygiene theory and practice, advancing dental hygiene knowledge through research, and providing public service. Schools of dentistry often employ a dental hygienist to teach periodontal and preventive oral health concepts and skills to predoctoral

Text continues on p.13.

TABLE 1–4 SIX INTERRELATED ROLES OF THE PROFESSIONAL DENTAL HYGIENIST

Roles/Settings	Responsibilities Include but are Not Limited to:
Clinician Managed care programs Hospitals Community health projects Extended care facilities Clinical practice (e.g., private practice, group practice, independent practice, armed forces)	Uses the dental hygiene process of care (assesses, diagnoses, plans, implements, and evaluates) to prevent or control oral diseases Integrates all other roles to promote wellness, prevent illness, maintain health, and facilitate coping Provides care to clients based on knowledge and skill with consideration for human needs Accepts the consumer as a partner in providing preventive and therapeutic oral healthcare, which includes: Assessing the consumer's oral health status Developing comprehensive oral health profiles based on health histories; clinical examination and the individual's knowledge, attitudinal, and behavioral characteristics that serve as the basis for referral and for the provision and evaluation of therapeutic and preventive professional care Planning for care and disease prevention or control Prioritizing oral health needs of consumers and making referrals to appropriate treatment centers Performing dental hygiene diagnoses and making appropriate referrals Determining which treatment needs are within scope of training and abilities, providing care, and assessing client responses and care outcomes Implementing appropriate clinical services Adapting oral health prevention, care, and education programs to the existing knowledge, values, and behaviors of diverse consumers Designing systems to monitor oral health prevention, care, and education programs to ensure that services are effective Evaluating the effectiveness of the consumer's self-care and dental hygiene care in attaining or maintaining oral health Interpreting current theory and research and applying evidence-based findings to oral healthcare Identifying group dynamics and communication patterns and, where necessary, developing behavioral intervention strategies to promote effective healthcare delivery Works in collaboration with other healthcare professionals to provide dental hygiene care to a general or specific group of people for the purpose of promoting health and preventing disease Provides care with full knowledge of and adherence to moral, ethical, and legal responsibilities
Educator/Oral Health Promoter Public health programs Public school programs Faculty in dental schools and dental hygiene schools Clinical and managed care programs Staff development in healthcare agencies	Utilizes educational theory and methods to analyze oral health needs Develops oral health promotion strategies Promotes concepts of prevention in community-based programs designed for specific population groups Designs and produces instructional materials and media for the consumer Uses communication theory, marketing strategies, and computer skills Conducts research Conducts health promotion (e.g., health screenings, risk appraisal, behavior modification classes, educational programs, and wellness programs) Has a clinical dental hygiene background exhibiting practice skills and theoretical knowledge Applies educational theory and the teaching–learning process (e.g., assessing the health knowledge and oral health status of individuals and groups; planning health education; transmitting current concepts, facts, and theories of health promotion and disease prevention to individuals and groups; and evaluating educational outcomes) Analyzes health needs and behavioral characteristics of specific population groups Marshals political, organizational, and economic support to make health plans and policies operational Develops health promotion strategies and healthcare programs that are attractive and relevant to the social and cultural values of the targeted population and that are based on scientifically accurate information Manages resources and delivers programs that are cost-effective and utilized by the targeted population Works independently or in collaboration with other health professionals to provide health education for the purpose of influencing behavior in a manner that promotes health Evaluates health education and health promotion strategies in healthcare programs through appropriate methods Uses communication and interpersonal skills to meet learning needs of clients Promotes, and recruits for, the profession of dental hygiene
Administrator/Manager Health promotion programs Disease prevention programs Educational institutions Clinical practices Managed care programs Community health agencies Armed forces Oral healthcare industry	Evaluates and modifies programs of oral health education or oral healthcare Utilizes data collection, persuasion, and protocol skills to justify initiation and development of health promotion or healthcare Organizes services for consumers Communicates objectives of the program to consumers, health professionals, and agency personnel Identifies, gathers, and procures necessary resources for program operation Applies organizational skills in formulating policies and procedures and in carrying out operational aspects of the program Manages human and material resources effectively

Table continued on following page

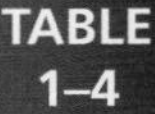

TABLE 1–4 SIX INTERRELATED ROLES OF THE PROFESSIONAL DENTAL HYGIENIST—CONT'D

Roles/Settings	Responsibilities Include but are Not Limited to:
	Evaluates program quality in relation to predetermined goals, perceived needs of the population served, and cost-effectiveness to meet national standards Modifies the program on the basis of evaluation results Delegates some responsibility and supervises other personnel Coordinates activities of others in the healthcare team Provides staff development training
Client Advocate Public dental programs Consumer groups Dental referral systems Periodontal disease screening centers Individual and group self-care programs Clinical practice settings	Influences legislators, health agencies, and other organizations on existing health problems and available resources to resolve problems Protects human and legal rights based on the belief that clients have the right to make their own decisions about health and life Uses strategies to influence those who control access to oral healthcare (e.g., legislators, health agency personnel, organizations, general public) for the purpose of obtaining health services for individuals and groups Represents individuals or groups in procurement of needed oral health services and assists them in obtaining services Develops networking systems to bring existing health problems and available resources together to resolve problems Monitors the quality of professional services and consumer self-care programs Addresses the growing concern for quality of care while ensuring cost containment Advises consumers on the relative worth of payment mechanisms, commercial products, political issues affecting oral health, and criteria for evaluating professional services Uses screening, referral, and persuasive skills to bring people into healthcare delivery systems Applies legal, financial, and informational leverage to protect oral healthcare for consumers Assists clients in obtaining the best possible care in the situation with informed consent and knowledge of alternatives Supports clients in the decisions they make (e.g., actively reassures clients that it is their decision and they have a right to make it without giving in to outside pressures)
Change Agent Lobbyist for legislative changes in healthcare Hospitals Community health agencies Client care coordinator in healthcare facility Entrepreneur Coordinator of oral healthcare services for persons with disabilities Nursing home services director State dental health program administration Community project coordinator	Implements processes and evaluates the success of programs that promote (change) health for clients Promotes the need for innovation and change in healthcare Uses current knowledge and interpersonal skills Works with individuals, organizations, agencies, and social institutions that have authority for, or influence on, dental hygiene education, health, and practice Creates an atmosphere conducive to the dynamics of change and selects mechanisms that are compatible with the target of change Promotes public's well-being and attainment of dental hygiene's oral health goals for society Uses appropriate areas of influence to promote health for individuals, families, or communities Systematically develops career alternatives and develops roles for hygienists, including these activities to fulfill this responsibility: Analyzing of barriers to gaining employment Removing resistance Changing attitudes, beliefs, and values of dental hygienists and potential employers Instructing students in essential knowledge and skills Placing graduates in a variety of career settings Creating change through the legislative process Utilizes the steps in the process of change Influences legislators, health agencies, and other organizations to solve existing health problems
Researcher Research institutions, higher education, oral healthcare industry, clinical practice	Interprets and applies findings and solves problems Develops a knowledge base for dental hygiene to extend the boundaries of the profession's body of knowledge Contributes to creation of new knowledge to benefit society Data collection and evaluation to develop new modalities of service Conducts research for the purpose of improving client care Applies the scientific method in: Selecting therapeutic and preventive modalities and educational concepts and methods Evaluating the effectiveness of selected procedures, materials, and methods Modifying oral healthcare or education on the basis of findings Interprets and evaluates research findings and applies findings to practice Uses principles of problem solving in clinical and nonclinical work efforts Participates in studies to determine the validity of procedures, materials, or education Contributes to the theoretical and scientific knowledge base for dental hygiene practice, through communication of findings

dental students in classroom, laboratory, and clinical settings. Such dental hygiene educator positions require at least a baccalaureate degree, and usually require a graduate degree in dental hygiene, public health, education, or some related basic or behavioral science discipline.

Dental hygiene educators in public health departments develop oral health educational materials and protocols for service programs, such as fluoride rinse programs for elementary school children, dental screenings, and special programs for Native Americans. Moreover, public health dental hygienists also provide classroom oral health education instruction to students, parents, and teachers (Table 1–4).

Manager

In various settings in which dental hygiene care is provided, the dental hygienist acts as manager or administrator. A *manager* is a person whose official position is to guide and direct the work of others. Responsibilities commonly associated with a manager include:

- ✦ Planning
- ✦ Decision making
- ✦ Organizing
- ✦ Staffing
- ✦ Directing
- ✦ Controlling

Dental hygienists use management skills when they understand the administrative structure of the employment setting and use this structure to achieve organizational goals. The dental hygienist as manager is knowledgeable about the line of authority, responsibilities of various co-workers, and channels of communication; is able to use and contribute to organizational policies and procedures; and values human and material resources. Other managerial strategies are used in the management of client periodontal care, for example, setting care priorities, eliminating causative factors, deciding on appropriate continuing care intervals and self-care measures, and providing general client management.

Dental hygiene administrators may direct professional educational programs for dental hygienists and other related health professions, serve as deans and associate deans of schools of allied health, serve as associate deans of schools of dentistry, or administer statewide dental programs. These dental hygiene administrators also are employed in upper level and middle management positions in federal, state, and local health departments, and in private companies that market oral healthcare products. The minimum educational requirement is a graduate degree in dental hygiene or a related field. Many academic administrative positions require that the dental hygienist have a doctoral degree (Table 1–4).

Client Advocate

Client advocate refers to the dental hygienist's role in protecting and supporting clients' rights and well-being. Historically, the patient was kept in a subordinate position within the healthcare setting. The issuance of such landmark legislation as the 1967 Freedom of Information Act and the 1974 Privacy Act led to an attitude of openness and broadened expectations about the rights of the consumer. Consumers demand their right to participate actively in their own healthcare and seek ways of exercising this right.

As an advocate, the dental hygienist believes that clients have the right to make their own decisions about healthcare after they have been provided with the information necessary to make an informed choice. The dental hygienist facilitates client decision making by providing clients with the information they need and by interpreting what the clients' rights are in a given situation. Dental hygienists may interpret findings for clients, identify other variables and alternatives to consider, involve others in the decision making process (dentist, physician, family), and help clients assess the options.

Moreover, the dental hygienist helps maintain a safe environment for clients and takes steps to prevent injury and to protect clients from possible adverse effects of treatment measures. Confirming that a client does not have an allergy to a local anesthetic and checking to see whether a client has taken prescribed prophylactic antibiotics prior to dental hygiene care are examples of the dental hygienist's client advocacy role. Clients frequently need information and assistance in negotiating the many complexities in today's healthcare system. The dental hygienist, serving in the role of advocate, can provide clients with the information they need to make intelligent choices about their oral healthcare. Once a client has arrived at a healthcare decision, the dental hygienist demonstrates respect for the client's decision (Table 1–4).

Change Agent

Change is the process of altering, modifying, or transforming an idea, event, individual, family, group, or community. The rapidity of societal, scientific, and technologic change has created a need for dental hygienists who can manage change.

The dental hygienist as *change agent* focuses on a systematic approach to creating change. See Roles of the Dental Hygienist as Change Agent, which describes four change agent roles of the dental hygienist and lists the phases of the change process.

If change agents view change as being evolutionary rather than revolutionary, the chances of a successful change are greater and the effects longer lasting. Incremental changes, guided by a master plan, are more likely to be achieved[13] (Table 1–4).

Researcher

The education that students receive today is not expected to sustain a lifelong career. Throughout a professional career, the dental hygienist uses research skills to remain current in the art and science of dental hygiene. In any employment setting and role the dental hygienist must be able to question, be creative, and think analytically to

Roles of the Dental Hygienist as Change Agent[12]

Catalyst
The energizing force to get things started

Solution Giver
Has definite ideas for solving a problem, but is not married to his or her own ideas. Adopts the objective stance that the idea and not the person is subject to rejection. This objective posture gives ideas a greater chance for survival as the seed for change is planted.

Resource Linker
Helps individuals and groups find and make the best use of resources, which may be people with the time, expertise, money, or motivation to help solve a particular problem

Process Helper
Understands the change process (See Phases of the Planned Change Process)

Phases of the Planned Change Process[12]

Assessment Phase
When dissatisfaction is identified

Planning Phase
When an accurate diagnosis of the problem is made and objectives are formulated; includes examining alternative strategies and goals, establishing specific goals, and agreeing to act. At this point, there may be a question regarding what might have to be given up by those involved, and anxiety and resistance may surface. During this stage it is very important to have the support of the group and identify sources of power within the group to support the change. Such support is essential if change is to occur.

Implementation Phase
Initiation of the actual change effort

Evaluation Phase
An ongoing process to determine the success or failure of the change. Success of the change is measured by how well the original ineffectiveness is relieved and functional efficiency is achieved.

Termination Phase
Occurs after the change has been accepted and is an integral part of the operation. During this phase, hygienists gradually reduce their role, remaining available for support in emergencies.

systematically solve problems and improve oral health. Whether the goal is evaluating a new therapeutic intervention or evaluating client progress, all professional behaviors require the analytic skills of a researcher.

A profession's research efforts are closely linked with its service role and accountability to the public. Therefore, dental hygiene practice can be only as good as the research that supports it. The *researcher* tests assumptions underlying dental hygiene practice and investigates dental hygiene problems to improve oral healthcare and the practice of dental hygiene. The dental hygiene researcher may be employed in an academic setting; in a federal, state, or local health agency; in a research institution (e.g., National Institute of Dental Research); or in private industry. The minimal educational requirement is a graduate degree in dental hygiene or a related field, with a doctoral degree preferred.

GUIDELINES FOR DENTAL HYGIENE CARE

The professional standards of practice and practice acts and licensure provide important guidelines for dental hygiene care. Each will be discussed briefly in the following sections.

Standards of Practice

STANDARDS IN THE UNITED STATES. In 1979 the ADHA created the Commission for Assurance of Competence and established the Task Force to Develop Standards of Practice in 1980. These actions demonstrated the profession's willingness to assume responsibility for the quality of care that its members provide. By 1982, the *dental hygiene practice standards* were established, however they are now going through a review process so that they reflect comtemporary practice. Standards serve the profession and society in the following ways:

- Define the activities of dental hygienists that are unique to dental hygiene
- Provide consumers, employers, and colleagues with guidelines as to what constitutes quality dental hygiene care
- Provide guidelines for establishing goals for clinical dental hygiene education
- Serve as the foundation for competence assurance and continued professional development

Standards of practice should be based on current scientific evidence, which is the synthesis of findings from relevant research studies that have investigated the same question or phenomena.[14]

Evidence-based standards can then be used as part of the clinical decision-making process that also includes the practitioner's experience and judgment, the clinical circumstances, and the client's preferences and values (Figure 1–2).[15]

STANDARDS IN CANADA. Practice standards evolved somewhat differently in Canada. In 1981 the Working Group on the Practice of Dental Hygiene was established by the Department of National Health and Welfare. As part of their charge to undertake a comprehensive review of dental hygiene in Canada, the Working Group recommended the establishment of the Advisory Committee on the Development of Clinical Practice

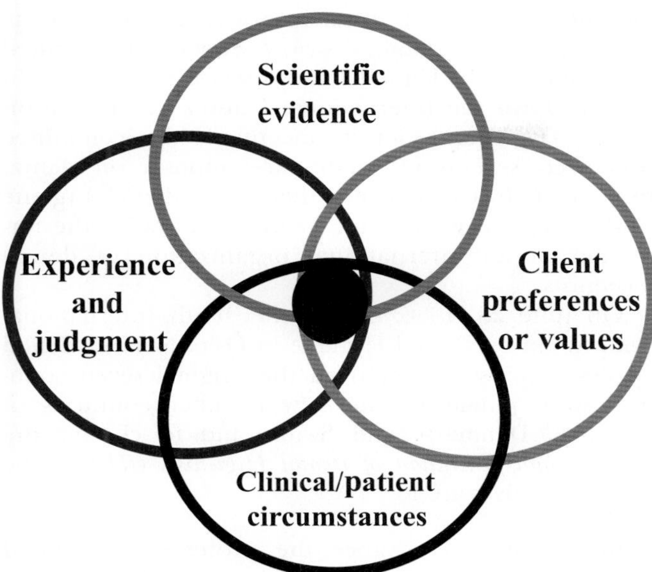

FIGURE 1–2 ✦ Evidence-based decision-making process. *(From Forrest JL, Miller SA: National Center for Dental Hygiene Research, 2001.)*

Standards for Dental Hygienists. In 1983 a project to develop clinical dental hygiene practice criteria and standards was initiated. These standards were modeled after the methodology used by the Manitoba Association of Registered Nurses in the Standards of Nursing Care[16] and were evaluated for content validity by dental hygiene practitioners, the Canadian Dental Hygienists' Association, and the Professional Corporation of Dental Hygienists of Quebec.

The *Clinical Practice Standards for Dental Hygienists in Canada* serve as a landmark event in dental hygiene's professional growth and development in Canada. According to the Canadian Dental Hygienists' Association, the standards "ensure that the highest level of dental hygiene care possible is provided to the Canadian public (quality of care) and that dental hygiene practitioners are capable of performing their roles in a competent manner . . . . dental hygienists have the professional responsibility to read and employ the published clinical practice standards in their work setting."[16]

Both U.S. and Canadian dental hygienists have used the dental hygiene process as the underlying structure in their standards of practice.

Practice Acts and Licensure

Dental practice acts are laws established in each state (United States) or province (Canada) to regulate the practice of dentistry and dental hygiene. Locales such as Washington State, Alberta, Ontario, and Quebec have separate practice acts for dental hygiene. Although the laws that regulate dental hygiene practice vary with each licensing jurisdiction, each reflects common elements. In general, the practice act does the following:

- Establishes criteria for the education, licensure, and relicensure of dental hygienists
- Defines the legal scope of dental hygiene practice
- Protects the public by making the practice of dental hygiene by uncredentialed and unlicensed persons illegal
- Creates a board empowered with legal authority to oversee the policies and procedures affecting the practice of dental hygiene in that jurisdiction

The board in each jurisdiction is given legal authority to design and administer licensing examinations to graduates of approved schools of dental hygiene. Individuals who pass the licensing examination earn a license to practice dental hygiene as it is defined in that jurisdiction. The license can be denied, revoked, or suspended for a variety of reasons, such as incompetence, negligence, chemical dependency, illegal practice, and criminal misconduct.

PROFESSIONAL DENTAL HYGIENE ORGANIZATIONS

Professional organizations exist to collectively represent the views of a profession and to influence resolution of issues relevant to education, practice, and research in that profession. Professional organizations have an enormous effect on dental hygiene because they address issues of professional growth, education, access to care, research and theory development, quality assurance, manpower, legislation, and collaboration with other professionals. Although many organizations exist, only the major ones are discussed in this chapter.

American Dental Hygienists' Association

The *American Dental Hygienists' Association (ADHA)* is a national organization of approximately 35,000 dental hygienists. The mission of the ADHA is to advance the art and science of dental hygiene by increasing the public's awareness of and ensuring access to quality oral healthcare; promoting the highest standard of dental hygiene education, licensure, and practice; and representing and promoting the interests of dental hygienists.

The goals of the ADHA are to:

- Maximize the utilization of the services of dental hygienists and to continue consumer advocacy in the healthcare delivery system
- Promote the dental hygienist as a primary care provider of preventive and therapeutic services
- Promote the self-regulation of dental hygiene education, licensure, and practice
- Serve as the authoritative resource on all issues related to dental hygiene
- Promote research relevant to dental hygiene
- Increase membership and participation in the ADHA
- Provide for a viable financial base

Founded in 1923, the ADHA has a tri-level structure by which individual members are automatically part of local (component), state (constituent), and national levels of governance. The official publications of the ADHA include the *Journal of Dental Hygiene, Access,* and *Education Update.* The House of Delegates is its legislative body, which is composed of voting members who represent each constituent based on a proportional formula. The Board of Trustees, presided over by the organization's elected president, consists of voting members (president, president-elect, vice-president, treasurer, immediate past president, and 13 district trustees) and nonvoting, ex officio members (executive director and editorial director). The ADHA plays a major role in issues that deal with legislation, access to care, education, practice, research, public relations, and health policy. The ADHA offers a variety of both tangible and intangible benefits and should be supported by professional and student dental hygienists in the United States.

National Dental Hygienists' Association

In 1932, the *National Dental Hygienists' Association (NDHA)* was founded by African American dental hygienists to address the needs and special problems of minority dental hygienists. The purposes of the NDHA are to:

- Cultivate and promote the art and science of dental hygiene
- Improve individual and community dental health
- Maintain the professional status of dental hygienists
- Encourage mutual support and goodwill among minority professionals
- Expand continuing education and employment opportunities
- Facilitate student recruitment and scholarship

The NDHA has members in most states and offers annual scholarships to minority students and a courtesy membership to new graduates for one year. It holds an annual convention in conjunction with the National Dental Association and publishes a newsletter.

Canadian Dental Hygienists' Association

The *Canadian Dental Hygienists' Association (CDHA),* officially founded in 1965, is the national association for registered dental hygienists in Canada. With a structure similar to that of the ADHA, the CDHA has provincial organizations supported by local components. The CDHA publishes *The Probe* as its official journal and has played a prominent role in developing continuing education, formal dental hygiene education, portability of licensure, and dental hygiene research and theory. The ADHA and CDHA have worked together to achieve many common goals. It should be supported by professional and student dental hygienists in Canada.

International Federation of Dental Hygienists

As the dental hygiene profession grew worldwide, forward-thinking representatives of national dental hygiene organizations from seven countries (Canada, Japan, the Netherlands, Norway, Sweden, the United Kingdom, and the United States) met for the first time in 1970 to form the International Liaison Committee on Dental Hygiene. From its inception, the committee organized several international symposia on dental hygiene to focus on issues that affect dental hygiene worldwide, and worked for many years toward the formation of an international organization of dental hygienists.

On June 28, 1986, during the Tenth International Symposium on Dental Hygiene in Oslo, Norway, dental hygiene representatives from the original seven countries were joined by the new member countries of Australia, Denmark, and Switzerland to charter the *International Federation of Dental Hygienists (IFDH).* The IFDH objectives are to:

- Represent and advance the profession of dental hygiene on a nongovernmental, worldwide basis
- Promote and coordinate the exchange of knowledge and information about the profession and its education and practice
- Raise the public's level of awareness of the preventability of oral disease through proven regimens
- Foster the exchange of dental hygiene human resources

The IFDH recognizes that the need for dental hygiene is universal and that dental hygiene services should be unrestricted by consideration of nationality, sex, race, creed, color, politics, or social status. The IFDH provides a formal network by which dental hygienists worldwide can promote collegiality among nations, commitment to maintaining universal standards of dental hygiene care and education, and access to quality oral healthcare.

DENTAL HYGIENE IN TRANSITION

Dental hygiene continues to change in response to the needs and demands of a global society. The world at large is in transition. Political and economic systems are being redefined, demographics are changing, and science and technology are extending the parameters of human life. The changing world exerts social, political, cultural, and economic influences on the emerging profession of dental hygiene.

Dental hygiene continues to evolve as society in general and healthcare in particular continue to change. Since its inception in the early twentieth century, the dental hygiene profession has evolved from being satisfied with an auxiliary status to the expectation of self-regulation, professional autonomy, and decision making in dental hygiene practice to increase access to quality care for the public and to take its place within the context of a true profession (Figure 1–3).

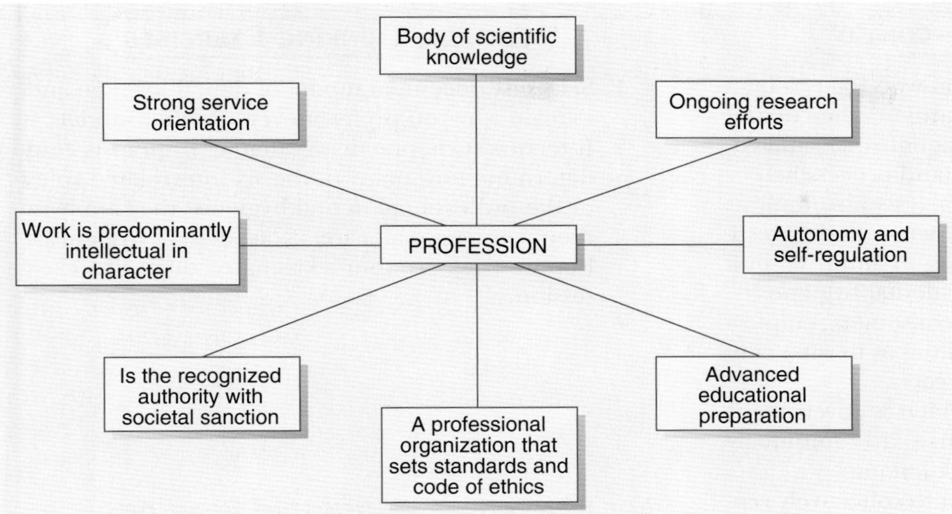

FIGURE 1–3 ✦ Characteristics of a true profession.

Client Education Issues

✦ The profession of dental hygiene emphasizes the prevention of oral disease and the client's role in controlling factors that cause disease.

Legal, Ethical, and Safety Issues

✦ Dental hygienists must be licensed in the jurisdiction in which they practice.

Key Concepts

- ✦ Dental hygiene is the study of preventive oral healthcare including the management of behaviors to prevent oral disease and promote health.
- ✦ The dental hygienist is a licensed oral healthcare professional who integrates the roles of clinician, educator, consumer advocate, manager, change agent, and researcher to support total health through the prevention of oral disease and the promotion of health.
- ✦ The dental hygiene process includes assessment, diagnosis, planning, implementation, and evaluation. It is the foundation of professional dental hygiene practice and provides a model for organizing and providing dental hygiene care in a variety of settings.
- ✦ A paradigm specifies the unique perspective of each discipline and is the first level of distinction between disciplines.
- ✦ The paradigm for the discipline of dental hygiene consists of the following four major concepts: client, environment, health and oral health, and dental hygiene actions.
- ✦ A conceptual model can be thought of as a school of thought within a discipline. There can be as many conceptual models as there are scholars who can think them up.
- ✦ The occupational model views dental hygiene as technology based. The professional model perceives dental hygiene to be knowledge based.
- ✦ The collaborative practice model assumes that dentists and dental hygienists work together as colleagues, each offering professional expertise for the goal of providing optimum oral healthcare to the public.
- ✦ The human needs conceptual model of dental hygiene defines the paradigm concepts of client, environment, health/oral health, and dental hygiene actions in terms of human needs theory.
- ✦ The dental hygiene clinician provides preventive, therapeutic, and educational services and makes decisions independently or in collaboration with the client and family, the dentist, or other healthcare professionals.
- ✦ Dental hygienists assume the role of oral health educator when clients have learning needs.
- ✦ Dental hygienists use management skills when they understand the administrative structure of the employment setting and use this structure to achieve organizational goals.
- ✦ Consumer advocacy refers to the dental hygienist's role in protecting and supporting clients' rights and well-being.

KEY CONCEPTS—CONT'D

- A change agent is an individual who focuses on a systematic approach to change. The dental hygienist acts in four change agent roles: analyst, solution giver, resource linker, and process helper
- The dental hygiene researcher tests assumptions underlying dental hygiene practice and investigates dental hygiene problems to improve oral healthcare and the practice of dental hygiene.
- Standards of practice provide consumers, employers, and colleagues with guidelines as to what constitutes quality dental hygiene care.
- Licensure is the process by which a government agency certifies that individuals are minimally qualified to practice in its jurisdiction.
- Professional organizations exist to collectively represent the views of a profession and to influence resolution of issues relevant to that profession.

CRITICAL THINKING EXERCISES

1. Select a conceptual model of dental hygiene and explain why you prefer it over all other models.
2. Interview two practicing dental hygienists and determine how many of the six interrelated roles of the professional dental hygienist they apply in their professional careers as dental hygienists. Report back to your classmates during a class session.

For References, Suggested Readings, and Related Websites, visit
http://evolve.elsevier.com/Darby/hygiene/

CHAPTER 2

Human Needs Theory and Dental Hygiene Care

OBJECTIVES

Mastery of the content in this chapter will enable the reader to:

- Describe Maslow's hierarchy of needs theory
- Identify and define the four central paradigm concepts for the dental hygiene human needs conceptual model
- Discuss the relationship of human needs theory to the dental hygiene process
- Define the eight human needs related to dental hygiene care
- For each of the eight human needs, identify at least one related deficit and plan a dental hygiene intervention to meet the unmet need.

KEY TERMS

Biologically sound and functional dentition
Client
Conceptualization and problem solving
Dental hygiene actions
Environment
Freedom from pain
Freedom from stress
Health
Human need
Human needs theory
Love and belonging needs
Oral health
Physiologic needs
Protection from health risks
Responsibility for oral health
Safety needs
Self-actualization
Self-esteem needs
Skin and mucous membrane integrity of the head and neck
Wholesome facial image

Dental hygiene care focuses on the promotion of oral health and the prevention of oral disease over the human life span. To this end, the dental hygienist is concerned with the whole person, applying specific knowledge about the client's emotions, values, family, culture, and environment as well as general knowledge about the body systems. Clients are viewed as being actively involved in the process of dental hygiene care, because ultimately it is they who must use self-care and seek professional care to obtain and maintain oral wellness.

Human needs theory can assist dental hygienists to understand the relationship between human need fulfillment and human behavior when providing dental hygiene care. A *human need* is defined as a tension in a person's system. This tension may express itself in some goal-directed behavior that continues until the goal is reached. Human needs theory explains that need fulfillment dominates human activity, and behavior is organized in relation to unsatisfied needs. Moreover, unsatisfied needs serve as motivators that can be used to guide the client toward optimal oral wellness.

Before discussing the human needs conceptual model of dental hygiene[1,2] it is necessary to review basic human needs theory. Although many human needs theorists have provided the theoretical substance for understanding human needs and the motivation inherent in meeting these needs, Maslow's work is highlighted here as a basis for discussing human needs theory in dental hygiene.

MASLOW'S HIERARCHY OF NEEDS

Abraham Maslow identified and assigned priorities to basic human needs. According to his theory, certain human needs are more basic than others; that is, some needs must be met before individuals turn their attention to meeting other needs.[3] Maslow prioritized human needs in a hierarchy of five categories based on their power and strength to motivate behavior (Figure 2–1). The hierarchy is arranged with the most imperative needs at the bottom and the least imperative at the top. On the most basic, or first, level of human needs are *physiologic needs,* such as the need for food, fluids, sleep, and exercise. According to Maslow's theory, a person is dominated by physiologic needs; if these needs are not reasonably satisfied, all other categories of needs in the hierarchy may seem irrelevant or be relegated to low priority.

On the second level are *safety needs,* including the need for both physical and psychological security. Safety needs include the need for stability, protection, structure, and freedom from fear and anxiety. In times of danger, the need to ensure safety and protection becomes paramount. Every other need becomes less important. Loss of parental protection, war, and being confronted with new tasks, strangers, or illness all are threats to the need for safety.[4]

On the third level are *love and belonging needs.* They include the need for affectionate relationships and the need for a place within one's culture, group, or family. Love and belonging needs are expressed in the desire for tenderness, affection, contact, intimacy, togetherness, and face-to-face encounters. Love needs involve both giving and receiving love. Love and belonging needs also are expressed in the need to overcome feelings of alienation, aloneness, or strangeness brought on by the scattering of family, friends, and significant others.[4]

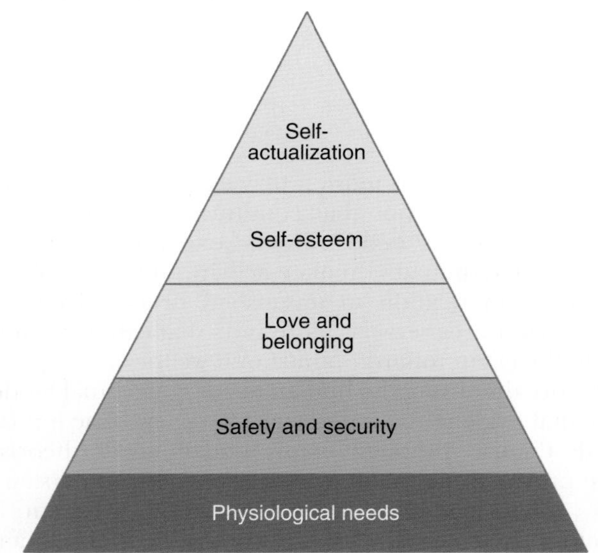

FIGURE 2–1 ✦ Maslow's hierarchy of needs. *(Modified from Potter PA, Perry AG:* Fundamentals of Nursing, *ed 3, St Louis, 1993, Mosby.)*

On the fourth level of Maslow's hierarchy are *self-esteem needs* such as the feeling of confidence, usefulness, achievement, and self-worth. Esteem needs include the need for a stable, firmly based, wholesome self-evaluation; the need for respect and esteem of self as well as esteem from others; a desire for strength, mastery, and competitiveness; and a need for feeling confident, independent, and freed. Deprivation of these needs results in feelings of inferiority, helplessness, and discouragement. Fulfillment of esteem needs results in feelings of capability and a willingness to be a contributor to society.[4]

The final level of the hierarchy is the need for what Maslow calls *self-actualization,* a state in which each person is fully achieving his or her potential and is able to solve problems and cope realistically with life's situations.[4]

Maslow points out that those individuals in whom a certain need has always been met or satisfied are best equipped to withstand deprivation of that need at some future time. Individuals whose needs have not been met in the past respond differently to current need deprivation than the does person who has never been deprived.[4]

Maslow's hierarchy of needs is a theoretical model; that is, the priorities given human needs generally are true of people, but not necessarily of all individuals. For example, a woman who attempts to meet her self-esteem needs by working 18 hours at a time may ignore physiologic needs for adequate sleep and nutrition because her need for self-esteem takes priority. Eventually, however, this woman may be forced to give more attention to her physiologic needs if she can no longer function as usual because she has been weakened by inadequate nutrition and rest. Thus, the hierarchy of needs can still be applied to individuals who seem to have different priorities.

HUMAN NEEDS CONCEPTUAL MODEL OF DENTAL HYGIENE

The human needs conceptual model of dental hygiene has been selected as a theoretical framework for dental hygiene care because:

- ✦ Human needs theory transcends all ages, cultures, genders, and nationalities
- ✦ Human needs theory was recognized by the World Health Organization when it redefined *health* as "the extent to which an individual or group is able, on the one hand, to realize aspirations and satisfy needs and, on the other hand, to change and cope with the environment"
- ✦ Human need fulfillment contributes to the quality of life of individuals, communities, nations, and the world
- ✦ Human need fulfillment emphasizes a client-centered, humanistic approach to dental hygiene care
- ✦ Human needs theory connects the oral cavity with the total person
- ✦ Unsatisfied needs can motivate human behavior and guide the client toward oral wellness

In the human needs conceptual model of dental hygiene, basic human needs theory is utilized to explain the four major concepts of the dental hygiene paradigm: client, environment, health and oral health, and dental hygiene actions. The resultant definitions of the four major concepts provide the theoretical framework for the dental hygiene process and the context within which dental hygiene care is provided. The relationship of human needs theory to the four major paradigm concepts is described in the following sections.

Concept 1: Client

In the human needs conceptual model of dental hygiene, a *client* is viewed as a biologic, psychological, spiritual, social, cultural, and intellectual human being who is an integrated, organized whole and whose behavior is motivated by fulfillment of his or her human needs. Figure 2–2 shows a model for this concept. This model indicates that to meet their human needs and thereby to restore their sense of wholeness as human beings, individuals respond holistically to life situations as integrated beings. Individuals are also unique beings because the nature of their experience is theirs alone. In many circumstances they have the power to choose their way of life, and their choices give meaning to their existence.[2,4] The client can be an individual, a family, or a group and is viewed as having eight human needs that are especially related to dental hygiene care.

Concept 2: Environment

Environment is the milieu in which the client and dental hygienist find themselves. The environment affects the client and the dental hygienist, and the client and dental hygienist are capable of influencing the environment. In the human needs conceptual model of dental hygiene the concept of environment is defined to include dimensions such as society, climate, geography, politics, economics, education, socioethnocultural factors, significant others, the family, the community, the state, the nation, and the world. These dimensions are viewed as influencing the manner, mode, and level of human need fulfillment for the person, family, and community. The model for the concept of environment in the human needs conceptual model of dental hygiene is shown in Figure 2–3.

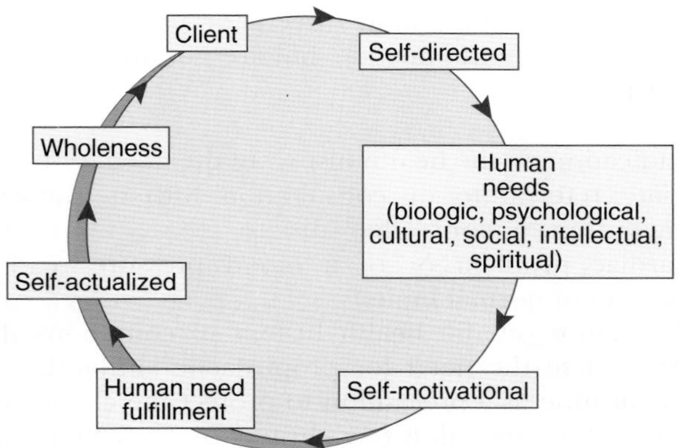

FIGURE 2–2 ✦ The concept of client in the human needs conceptual model of dental hygiene. *(Modified from Yura H, Walsh M:* The nursing process, *ed 5, Norwalk, Conn, 1988, Appleton & Lange.)*

Concept 3: Health and Oral Health

In the human needs conceptual model of dental hygiene the concept of *health* is viewed as a relative condition; it is a state of well-being with both objective and subjective aspects that exists on a continuum from maximal wellness to maximal illness (Figure 2–4). The higher the level of human need fulfillment, the higher the state of wellness for the individual. An individual's health may change along this continuum under the influence of biologic, psychological, spiritual, social, and cultural factors that are interrelated and fluctuate over time.[2,4] Maximal wellness is achieved with maximal fulfillment of human needs; maximal illness occurs with minimal or absent human need fulfillment. Along the health continuum,

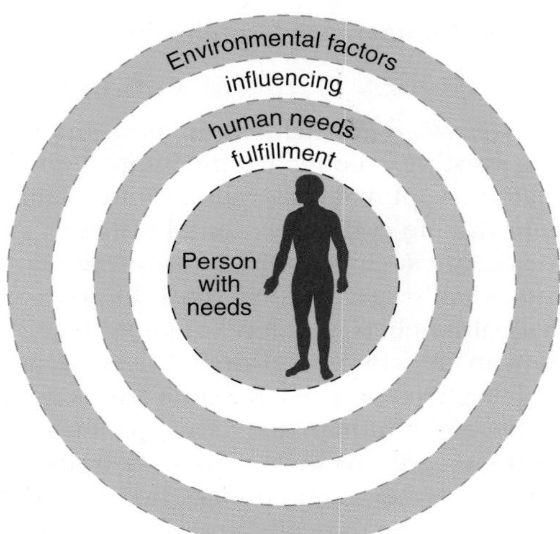

FIGURE 2–3 ✦ The concept of environment in the human needs conceptual model of dental hygiene. *(Modified from Yura H, Walsh M:* The nursing process, *ed 5, Norwalk, Conn, 1988, Appleton & Lange.)*

+ HEALTH/ORAL HEALTH CONTINUUM -
Wellness ..... Health/oral health ..... Illness....... Death
Oral wellness .... Oral disease
Human need fulfillment .... Deficits in human need fulfillment

FIGURE 2–4 ✦ The concept of health and oral health in the human needs conceptual model of dental hygiene. *(Modified from Yura H, Walsh M:* The nursing process, *ed 5, Norwalk, Conn, 1988, Appleton & Lange.)*

there are degrees of wellness and illness that are associated with varying levels of human need fulfillment.

Although oral health per se involves the orofacial complex, it exists in a biologic interrelationship with the entire body and is therefore influenced by the same factors as general health. Oral health can affect general health through oral infections and impaired masticatory function; conversely, the oral tissues are often sensitive indicators of the general health of the individual.[5] Many systemic diseases produce oral changes that may be part of the primary disease process (e.g., oral cancer) or a complication of it (e.g., candidiasis [yeast infection] resulting from antibiotic therapy for a systemic problem). Because the oral cavity is analogous to other body cavities, its health status is governed by the same physical and chemical laws and physiologic principles, and affected by the same social, cultural, psychological, and spiritual factors as other body cavities.[5,6] For that reason, oral health as well as general health is associated with human need fulfillment. Viewed through the conceptual framework of human needs theory, *oral health* is defined as the oral condition that results from the interaction of individuals with their environment, under varying levels of human need fulfillment.

Concept 4: Dental Hygiene Actions

Dental hygiene actions are defined as those interventions aimed at assisting clients in meeting their human needs related to optimal oral wellness and quality of life throughout the life cycle. The dental hygienist's actions take into account such client and environmental factors as the individual's age, gender, roles, lifestyle, culture, attitudes, health beliefs, and level of knowledge.

Inherent in the concept of dental hygiene actions is the dental hygiene process. Baseline assessment as to whether the eight human needs especially related to dental hygiene care are met provides a framework for dental hygienists to make dental hygiene diagnoses based on unmet human needs, and then to plan, implement, and evaluate dental hygiene actions. The model for the concept of dental hygiene actions is shown in Figure 2–5.

DENTAL HYGIENE'S EIGHT HUMAN NEEDS

The eight human needs listed in Table 2–1 relate to physical, emotional, intellectual, social, and cultural dimensions of the client that are inherent in dental hygiene care. Figure 17–3 (Chapter 17) provides a tool for assessing the eight human needs related to dental hygiene care and for using them to make dental hygiene diagnoses, to set goals, and to plan and evaluate dental hygiene interventions designed to meet the identified unmet needs. Through the dental hygiene process, the dental hygienist contributes to the fulfillment of these human needs in the client. The eight human needs related to dental hygiene care are described in the following sections.

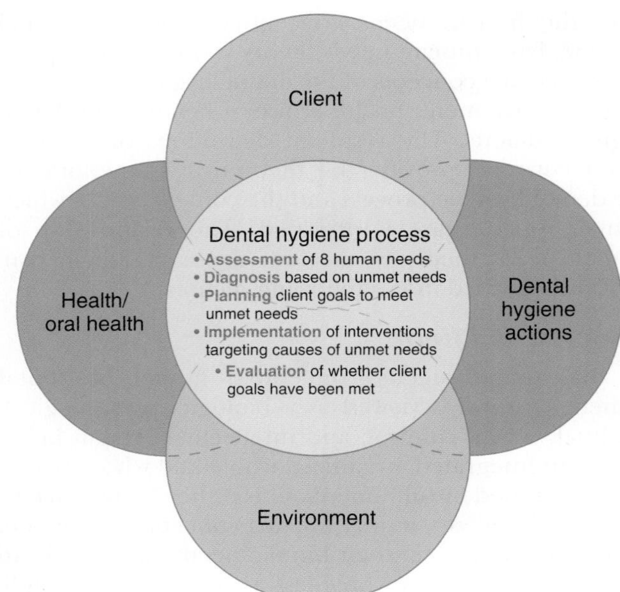

FIGURE 2–5 ✦ The concept of dental hygiene actions in the human needs conceptual model of dental hygiene as it relates to the dental hygiene process. *(Modified from Yura H, Walsh M:* The nursing process, *ed 5, Norwalk, Conn, 1988, Appleton & Lange.)*

Protection from Health Risks

Protection from health risks is the need to avoid medical contraindications related to dental hygiene care to be free from harm or danger involving the integrity of the body structure and environment around the person. Generally, the need for protection from health risks encompasses the need to be in a state of good general health through efficient functioning of body organs and systems, or under the active care of a physician in a controlled state of general health that provides for adequate function of body organs and systems.

ASSESSMENT. To assess this human need, the dental hygienist obtains information related to the client's general health by careful evaluation of the client's verbal and nonverbal behavior during the health history taking, as well as by clinical examination (see Chapter 9). Indications that the client's need for protection from health risks is unmet include, but are not limited to, the following:

- ✦ Indication on the health history of the need for immediate referral to or consultation with a physician regarding uncontrolled disease (e.g., signs of a cardiac problem or of a blood pressure reading outside of normal limits)
- ✦ Indication on the health history of conditions that necessitate the need for prophylactic antibiotic premedication as a precaution to protect the client from bacterial endocarditis (e.g., history of a heart murmur, prosthetic joint replacement, or mitral valve prolapse)
- ✦ Evidence of a health condition with the potential to become a medical emergency

TABLE 2–1 HUMAN NEEDS RELATED TO DENTAL HYGIENE CARE

Human Needs	Some Dental Hygiene Actions/Implications
Protection from Health Risks The need to avoid medical contraindications related to dental hygiene care.	Antibiotic premedication for the prevention of bacterial endocarditis Consult with physician regarding a client whose blood pressure is outside of normal limits Discuss modification of care plan with client to address safety factors
Freedom from Stress The need to feel safe and to be free from fear and emotional discomfort in the oral healthcare environment, and to receive appreciation, attention, and respect	Offer nitrous-oxide-oxygen to reduce apprehension Initiate and/or refer to a program for control of oral habits, substance abuse, chemical dependency, stress; if oral pain is reported, initiate pain control immediately and, if appropriate, refer client to dentist for immediate care
Wholesome Facial Image The need to feel satisfied with one's oral-facial features and breath	Refer for orthodontic consultation Make bleaching trays for tooth whitening Polish teeth to remove extrinsic stains Focus on positive attributes and features (i.e., compliment client on some aspect of his or her appearance) Encourage the client to seek other support systems to share feelings about body changes Be sensitive to client's feelings of insecurity, fears of rejection, or loss of self-worth Be aware of your own feelings
Skin and Mucous Membrane Integrity of Head and Neck The need to have an intact and functioning covering of the person's head and neck area, including the oral mucous membranes and gingivae, which defend against harmful microbes, provide sensory information, resist injurious substances and trauma, and reflect adequate nutrition	Observe and record findings about all skin and mucous membranes in and around the oral cavity Recognize, care for, and follow-up on specific lesions significant to the general and oral health of the client Dental hygiene strategies: Plaque control instruction Therapeutic scaling and root planing Referral to other healthcare providers Subgingival irrigation with antimicrobial solution Oral cancer examination Recognize signs of inadequate nutrition and initiate change
Biologically Sound Dentition The need for intact teeth and restorations that defend against harmful microbes, provide for adequate function, and reflect appropriate nutrition and diet	Continuously evaluate client's dentition Refer for dental exam Polish amalgam restorations
Conceptualization and Problem Solving The need to grasp ideas and abstractions to make sound judgments about one's oral health	Explain rationale and details of methods recommended for the prevention and control of oral diseases Measure the client's oral health knowledge Appeal to the client's need for conceptualization and problem solving Promote self-evaluation of oral cavity and head and neck by the client
Freedom from Head and Neck Pain The need to be exempt from physical discomfort in the head and neck area	Initiate pain control strategies (i.e., reassurance, utilization of desensitizing agents, instrumentation techniques with care and gentleness, administration of topical anesthesia, local anesthetics and nitrous oxide–oxygen analgesia) Utilize appropriate supragingival and subgingival instrumentation procedures and techniques
Responsibility for Oral Health The need for accountability for one's oral health as a result of interaction between one's motivation, physical capability, and social environment	Initiate behavior patterns to maintain oral wellness and measure the client's oral health behaviors Appeal to the client's sense of self-care and the client's active participation in formulating objectives for dental hygiene care Facilitate decision making by the client

Adapted from Yura H, Walsh M: *The nursing process,* ed 5, Norwalk, Conn., 1988, Appleton & Lange.

IMPLICATIONS FOR DENTAL HYGIENE CARE. The need for stable general health significantly affects all dental hygiene care provided and its expected outcomes. If the dental hygienist has any questions regarding the client's general health status and its influence on dental hygiene care, the client's physician should be consulted before dental hygiene care is provided and clients with no physician of record should be referred to one for examination. Initially obtaining information about the client's general health and updating it at each dental hygiene care appointment are essential to ensuring that the client's need for protection from health risks is met.

Clients also may reveal lifestyle practices that place them at risk for oral injury, oral infection, or oral cancer. For example, the potential for oral injury may exist in an adolescent who plays contact sports without the benefit of an athletic mouth protector. A client taking an immunosuppressant drug may be at risk for oral infection, and the person who uses spit tobacco (smokeless tobacco) has a risk for oral cancer. All of these individuals have an unmet human need for protection from health risks that can be met through comprehensive dental hygiene care.

Freedom from Stress

The need for *freedom from stress* is the human need to feel safe and to be free from fear and emotional discomfort in the oral health care environment and to receive appreciation, attention, and respect from others.

ASSESSMENT. Fulfillment of this need can be assessed by evaluating the client's verbal and nonverbal behavior, as well as by careful examination of the face and oral cavity for signs of stress. Nonverbal behavior is evaluated by careful observation of the client upon reception, during history taking, and throughout the provision of dental hygiene care. For example, indications that the client's need for freedom from stress is unmet include, but are not limited to, the client's self-report or display of at least one of the following:

- Fear or anxiety
- Concern about:
  - previous negative dental experiences
  - cost of care
  - current care to be provided
  - infection control
  - radiation exposure
  - mercury toxicity
  - fluoride toxicity
- Oral habits related to stress (e.g., bruxism, nailbiting, thumbsucking)
- Substance abuse
- The client's expression of dissatisfaction with the dental hygienist or dental hygiene care throughout any phase of the dental hygiene process of care
- Excessive perspiration (sweaty palms or beads of perspiration on forehead) or crying

IMPLICATIONS FOR DENTAL HYGIENE CARE. To some clients, the dental hygiene appointment itself may signal threat or danger and may trigger stress and anxiety. Being confronted with strangers, uncontrollable objects (e.g., dental hygiene instruments), loss of parental protection (for children), and the risk (however minute) of contracting an infectious or life-threatening disease such as acquired immunodeficiency syndrome (AIDS) all are threats to the need for freedom from stress.

If stress is apparent at the beginning of or during the dental hygiene appointment, the dental hygienist initiates stress control interventions immediately, if appropriate, or refers the client to the dentist for immediate care. Ways in which the dental hygienist can provide stress control for clients are listed under Stress and Anxiety Control Interventions. For example, the dental hygienist may discuss with the client previous negative experiences related to dental or dental hygiene care and reassure the client that every effort will be made to provide care in as comfortable and safe a manner as possible. Planned care and its rationale should be discussed in detail, as should the methods taken to ensure the client's freedom from stress. (Also, see Chapter 32 on behavioral management of pain and anxiety.)

To help satisfy the client's human need for freedom from stress, the hygienist should answer all questions as completely as possible. For instance, clients often ask about safety factors associated with radiation, infection control, mercury-containing dental restorations (amalgam), water fluoridation, and fluoride therapy. The client must be reassured about the safety of these procedures and provided with factual knowledge about the rationales for their use. Informing the client about current research findings is frequently a strategy for meeting the client's freedom from stress need in the oral healthcare environment. Of course, current standards of care to ensure the client's safety and protection always should be followed.

In general, to meet the client's need for freedom from stress, the dental hygienist is sensitive to the client's

Stress and Anxiety Control Interventions

Demonstrating humanistic behaviors such as compassion, warmth, empathy, acceptance of feelings, sensitivity, respect for privacy, listening, helping, demonstrating, and touching
Providing the client with a sense of control (e.g., always ask permission, explain procedures, make care predictable, and stop when the client requests a break)
Encouraging client involvement and participation in care
Obtaining informed consent
Communicating openly and honestly
Planning short appointments and scheduling them in the early morning
Using nitrous oxide–oxygen analgesia unless contraindicated
Conversing with the client throughout the appointment, regularly asking how the client is doing
Using the tell-show-do approach
Reinforcing client successes in treatment

verbal and nonverbal cues, practices humanistic behavior during professional interactions, communicates with empathy, and provides positive reinforcement of desired behavior. At all times the dental hygienist demonstrates, through behavior, the unique worth of each client as a human being and ensures that the client's dignity is supported. It is particularly critical for the dental hygienist to be aware of and to exhibit respect for diversity in cultural and ethnic groups and the health beliefs, values, and behaviors associated with them.

Freedom from Pain

The need for *freedom from pain* is the human need to be exempt from physical discomfort in the head and neck area.[5] This human need is a strong motivator for clients to perform behavior that will lead to its fulfillment.

ASSESSMENT. Fulfillment of this need can be assessed by evaluating the client's verbal and nonverbal behavior, as well as by careful examination of the face and oral cavity for signs of physical discomfort. Verbal behavior is evaluated by inquiring about the client's reason for seeking dental hygiene care and by collecting data during history taking and during the intraoral and extraoral examinations. Nonverbal behavior is evaluated by careful observation of the client upon reception, during history taking, and throughout the provision of dental hygiene care. For example, when the need for freedom from pain is fulfilled, the client:

- ✦ Reports comfort and no systemic pain, no medication is being taken for pain, and no extra- or intraoral pain or sensitivity is found upon examination
- ✦ Displays ease of movement, relaxed face, hands, and legs
- ✦ Speaks without hesitation or breaks in sentences
- ✦ Evidences no excessive perspiration (no sweaty palms or beads of perspiration on forehead) and no crying

Specific indications that the client's need for freedom from pain is *unmet* include, but are not limited to, the client's self-report or display of at least one of the following:

- ✦ Extraoral or intraoral pain or sensitivity
- ✦ Discomfort or pain during dental hygiene care

IMPLICATIONS FOR DENTAL HYGIENE CARE. If physical pain is apparent at the beginning of or during the dental hygiene appointment, the dental hygienist should initiate pain control interventions immediately, if appropriate, or should refer the client to the dentist for immediate care. Ways in which the dental hygienist can provide pain control for clients are discussed in Chapters 34 and 35. Because the mouth is very sensitive, dental hygienists need to perform instrumentation techniques as carefully and as gently as possible, especially when treating a client who is not anesthetized.

Wholesome Facial Image

The need for a *wholesome facial image* is the need to feel satisfied with one's own oral-facial features and breath. Facial image is determined by each individual's perception of his or her physical characteristics and the interpretation of how that image is perceived by others. Self-concept both influences and is influenced by each person's view of his or her own physical characteristics.[5,6]

Facial image is influenced by normal and abnormal physical changes and by cultural and societal attitudes and values. For example, normal developmental changes such as growth and aging affect a person's facial image. Cultural values lead Surma women in Ethiopia to wear lip plates as a sign of physical beauty. In the United States, society emphasizes youth, beauty, and wholeness, a fact that is apparent in television programs, movies, and advertisements. Thus, these cultural attitudes and values affect how people perceive their physical bodies, because body image is a combination of the ideal and the real.[6]

Pain Control Interventions

Providing the client with a sense of control (e.g., always ask permission, explain procedures, and make care predictable)
Reassuring the client that the dental hygiene care procedure will be made as comfortable as possible
Adjusting the chair so that the client with back trouble is comfortable
Applying topical desensitizing agents to sensitive roots
Performing instrumentation techniques with as much care and gentleness as possible
Using topical and local anesthetic agents, if indicated, to block the transmission of painful stimuli during dental hygiene care
Depositing a few drops of anesthetic solution and waiting for 5 seconds before advancing the needle during intraoral administration of local anesthetic agent
Administering nitrous oxide–oxygen analgesia to control a client's apprehension and to help him or her relax, if indicated
Taking the client seriously when concern is expressed
With regard to supragingival and subgingival instrumentation, the dental hygienist should:
- Adapt instrument blades to the tooth to prevent tissue laceration
- Keep the working-end tip of the instrument in contact with the tooth so that it is not in soft tissue
- Refrain from resting the mouth mirror on the floor of the client's mouth
- Run the hand piece at moderate speed
- Keep the tip of the ultrasonic scaler and the rubber cup in constant and gentle motion when using them to prevent heat from building up on the tooth

People generally do not adapt quickly to changes in the physical body. For example, people who experience normal aging often report that they do not feel different, but when they look in the mirror they are surprised by their aged facial characteristics.[6] Facial disfigurement due to disease, trauma, or surgery is an obvious stressor affecting body image. For example, tooth loss is a stressor that affects facial image through a change in personal appearance.[6]

The importance of a change in appearance is determined partly by individual perceptions of the alteration and by personal estimations of how others perceive that alteration. For example, if someone associates possession of natural teeth with femininity or masculinity, loss of teeth may be a very significant alteration, one that may threaten the person's sexuality or sense of self. Similarly, clients with dentures, a cleft lip, or facial disfigurement after surgical treatment of oral cancer may reduce social contacts out of fear of people's reactions to them.[7] Such clients may feel isolated, excluded, stigmatized, or helpless. Their feeling of social isolation may be based in reality, because people may avoid contact with them for fear of causing embarrassment or offense. Thus, body image stressors can negatively alter the client's body image, which in turn may negatively alter the client's self-concept and behavior.[7]

Indications that the client's need for a wholesome facial image is fulfilled include such evidence as the client's statement of satisfaction with his or her appearance, being neatly groomed, and making an effort to bring out the best of facial assets with careful makeup and attention to hairstyle. The dental hygienist must be careful to assess wholesome facial image in terms of the client's culture and not from an ethnocentric perspective (see Chapter 5).

ASSESSMENT. The dental hygienist bases the assessment of the client's need for a wholesome facial image on information obtained from the health, dental, personal, and cultural histories; perceptions resulting from direct observation of the client; and inferences from casual conversation with the client. For example, the satisfaction a client has with the general appearance of the teeth, mouth, and facial profile can be determined by asking specific questions such as, "Is anything about your teeth bothering you?" or "Is there anything about your mouth that concerns you?" Similar questions may elicit responses indicating dissatisfaction with such conditions as extrinsic stain, calculus, receding gums, bleeding gums, a discolored restoration, or malaligned teeth. Indications that the client's need for a wholesome facial image is *unmet* include, but are not limited to, the client's self-report of dissatisfaction with the appearance of the teeth, gingivae, facial profile, or breath. Such unmet needs have implications for dental hygiene care and for referral to other health professionals for additional care.

IMPLICATIONS FOR DENTAL HYGIENE CARE. Tooth loss, malaligned teeth, oral cancer, and facial disfigurement are examples of facial image stressors related to the oral cavity that dental hygiene clients may experience. The dental hygienist should listen to the doubts about treatment outcomes expressed by clients undergoing treatment related to these stressors, and provide information and reassurance as needed. Complimenting such clients on some aspect of their appearance assists them to focus on positive attributes and features. For some clients, encouragement to seek other support systems to share feelings about body changes may be helpful in assisting them to reinforce accomplishments, strengths, and positive attributes.[7]

Facial image stressors affect self-concept and motivate behavior, including oral health behavior. The dental hygienist's acceptance of a client with an altered self-concept due to facial image stressors may be the factor that stimulates positive rehabilitative results. For example, for clients whose physical appearance has changed drastically from head and neck cancer surgery and who must adapt to a new body image, being accepted by the dental hygienist as a human being who has ideas, feelings, and values and who is worthy and whole despite illness or physical alterations is important and can provide an example for the client and his or her family that affirms the client's self-worth. The client's feelings of insecurity, fears of rejection, or loss of self-worth can be lessened through sensitive, knowledgeable dental hygiene care.

Being in touch with one's own feelings and expectations about clients undergoing such facial image stressors is extremely important, because a dental hygienist's reaction to a client's illness or physical alteration can have a significant impact on the client's self-concept and the outcome of care. A client with low self-esteem because of altered facial image may be particularly sensitive to the way the dental hygienist involves the client in his or her own care. A dental hygienist with mixed feelings about the client's physical alteration may be hesitant in making suggestions, thus inadvertently implying that the client might be unable to follow suggestions, or may insist that the client assume too much responsibility for his or her own care, thus causing anxiety and frustration. In either case the client's self-esteem and facial image may be additionally threatened rather than strengthened. If, however, the dental hygienist demonstrates confidence in the client's abilities and is confident in his or her personal feelings about and expectations of the client, then the client's sense of wholesome facial image, as well as self-worth, will be reinforced.[7]

Skin and Mucous Membrane Integrity of the Head and Neck

The need for *skin and mucous membrane integrity of the head and neck* is defined as the need for an intact and functioning covering of the person's head and neck area, including the oral mucous membranes and periodontium. These defend against harmful microbes, provide sensory information, resist injurious substances and trauma, and reflect adequate nutrition.

ASSESSMENT. Assessment of this human need occurs initially by careful observation of the client's face, head, and neck area as part of an overall appraisal of the client upon reception and seating, and by careful examination of the oral cavity and adjacent structures and the periodontium prior to planning and implementing dental hygiene care (see Chapters 12 and 15).

With regard to dental hygiene care, indications that this human need is *unmet* include, but are not limited to, the following:

- ✦ The presence of extraoral and intraoral lesions, tenderness, or swelling
- ✦ Gingival inflammation
- ✦ Bleeding on probing
- ✦ Probing depths or attachment loss greater than 4 mm
- ✦ Presence of xerostomia (dry mouth), with accompanying oral mucous membranes that are not uniform in color
- ✦ Presence of extraoral or intraoral manifestations of nutritional deficiencies
- ✦ Evidence of an eating disorder (e.g., trauma around the mouth from implements used to induce vomiting)

IMPLICATIONS FOR DENTAL HYGIENE CARE. The dental hygienist has the responsibility to observe all skin and mucous membranes in and about the oral cavity, including the periodontium, and to record and call to the attention of the dentist and the client those areas that evidence disease. A variety of skin and oral mucosal lesions may be observed that may or may not be symptomatic. Recognition, treatment, and follow-up of specific lesions may be of great significance to the general and oral health of the client. Routine extraoral and intraoral examination of clients at the initial appointment and each maintenance care appointment provides an excellent opportunity to control oral disease by early recognition of lesions that can then receive treatment and follow-up care. At least annually, clients should be screened to detect potentially cancerous lesions. Moreover, it may be necessary for the dental hygienist to postpone a current appointment because of a client's need for urgent medical consultation or because of evidence of infectious lesions, such as herpes labialis.

Because periodontal disease is epidemic in the United States and elsewhere, the human need for skin and mucous membrane integrity of the head and neck is usually *unmet* in clients seeking dental hygiene care. In periodontal disease, the sulcular, or pocket, epithelium becomes ulcerated and bleeds readily on gentle probing. Because the epithelium is not intact, harmful microbes enter the periodontal tissues. Exudate may appear at the entrance to the pocket or may be expressed from the pocket. Under these circumstances, dental hygiene strategies to meet the human need for skin and mucous membrane integrity of the head and neck include the following:

- ✦ Providing bacterial plaque control instruction
- ✦ Performing scaling with or without a coronal polish
- ✦ Performing root planing, and possibly subgingival irrigation with antimicrobial agents
- ✦ Referral to the general dentist or the periodontist for specialty care

Dental hygienists use their extraoral and intraoral examination and interviewing skills to identify nutritional problems and provide sound counseling or appropriate referral. Dental hygienists are in an excellent position to recognize signs of poor nutrition and to take steps to initiate change. Regular contact with continued-care clients at 3-, 4-, or 6-month intervals enables dental hygienists to make observations of the clients' physical status, food intake, and response to dental hygiene care. Dental hygienists should inform dentists of observations that indicate nutritional problems and should incorporate approaches to solving the problem in their care plans. When malnutrition or a serious eating disorder such as anorexia nervosa or bulimia nervosa is suspected, referral of the client for medical evaluation is a priority (see Chapter 47).

Biologically Sound and Functional Dentition

The human need for a *biologically sound and functional dentition* refers to the need for intact teeth and restorations that defend against harmful microbes, provide for adequate functioning and esthetics, and reflect appropriate nutrition and diet.

ASSESSMENT. Assessment of this need is ongoing throughout the dental hygiene care appointment, but initially occurs while the hygienist is taking a careful dental history and carefully observing the client's dentition as part of a thorough examination of the oral cavity and adjacent structures preliminary to dental hygiene care. Indications that the client's need for a biologically sound dentition is *unmet* include, but are not limited to, the following:

- ✦ Difficulty in chewing
- ✦ Defective restorations
- ✦ Teeth with signs of dental caries, abrasion, or erosion
- ✦ Missing teeth
- ✦ Ill-fitting prosthetic appliances
- ✦ Teeth with calculus, bacterial plaque, or extrinsic stain
- ✦ Rampant caries
- ✦ Report of high daily sugar intake
- ✦ Evidence of an eating disorder (e.g., erosion of teeth, particularly on the lingual and incisal surfaces of maxillary anterior teeth and the occlusal and palatal surfaces of maxillary molars)

IMPLICATIONS FOR DENTAL HYGIENE CARE. Complete examinations with accurate documentation by records and chartings are basic to all healthcare. The dental hygienist is an advocate for a sound, functional dentition. Therefore, the dental hygienist documents existing conditions of the teeth, including restorations, all deviations from normal, and missing teeth.

A bitewing radiographic survey may assist with charting signs of posterior interproximal dental caries. All teeth with signs of disease and all functional problems should be called to the immediate attention of the dentist. Referral to the dentist, application of topical fluoride and sealants, and recommendation fluoride therapy at home are the interventions most frequently used by dental hygienists to ensure that the client's need for a biologically sound dentition is met.

Nutritional assessment also is particularly important for clients who may be at risk for nutritional problems related to tooth loss, ill-fitting dentures, dental caries, and periodontal diseases. A complete nutritional assessment includes collecting data from observation and from a dietary history (see Chapter 28).

Conceptualization and Problem Solving

The human need for *conceptualization and problem solving* refers to the need to understand ideas and abstractions to make sound judgments about one's oral health.[5] The need for conceptualization related to dental hygiene care is considered to be met if the client understands the rationale for recommended oral hygiene interventions; participates in setting goals for oral healthcare; has no questions about professional dental hygiene care or dental treatment; and has no questions about the etiology of the oral problem, its relationship to oral diseases, and the importance of the solution suggested to solve the problem.

ASSESSMENT. This need is assessed by listening to clients' responses while counseling them about the causes of oral diseases, ways to prevent and control disease, and contraindications to care. Indications that this need is *unmet* include, but are not limited to, the following:

- ✦ Evidence that the client does not understand what bacterial plaque is, its relationship to oral disease, or the importance of daily plaque control or other preventive self-care or professional procedures
- ✦ Evidence that the client has questions, misconceptions, or a lack of knowledge about salient issues related to recommended dental or dental hygiene care

IMPLICATIONS FOR DENTAL HYGIENE CARE. In counseling clients, dental hygienists need to present the rationale and details of methods recommended for the prevention and control of oral diseases. For example, to help a client conceptualize what bacterial plaque is, where it needs to be disturbed, and its relationship to periodontal disease, the dental hygienist may:

- ✦ Use a disclosing tablet to point out the location of plaque in a client's own mouth and relate it to the inflammatory response of the tissues
- ✦ Sketch on a pad of paper the location of plaque on the cervical third of teeth and relate it graphically to periodontal destruction in the client's mouth
- ✦ Use already prepared materials to show where plaque accumulates around the neck of the tooth and in the sulcus and its effect on periodontal tissues

It is important for the dental hygienist to question the client about or have the client demonstrate use of any explained plaque control device to clarify whether or not the client has understood the concepts presented.

Responsibility for Oral Health

The need for *responsibility for oral health* refers to the need for accountability for one's oral health as a result of interaction between one's motivation, physical capability, and social environment.

ASSESSMENT. This need is assessed from data collected in the client's health, dental, personal, and cultural histories and from direct observation of whether or not the client performs adequate daily oral self-care and seeks adequate professional care to prevent and control oral diseases. Indications that this need is *unmet* include, but are not limited to, the following deficits related to the client:

- ✦ Inadequate oral self-care
- ✦ In the case of small children, inadequate parental supervision of daily oral hygiene practices
- ✦ No dental exam within the last 2 years

IMPLICATIONS FOR DENTAL HYGIENE CARE. The dental hygienist should assess the client's oral health behaviors and suggest behavior patterns to the client (or to the parent when the client is a child) that should be initiated to obtain and maintain oral wellness. In providing client education the dental hygienist should appeal to the client's sense of self-determination and try to evoke the client's need for responsibility for oral health. The dental hygienist should encourage the client to participate in setting goals and objectives for dental hygiene care, and thus facilitate decision making by the client. Deficits in psychomotor skill development necessary for the client to properly manipulate the toothbrush, floss, or other oral hygiene tools for personal oral hygiene care must be addressed by the dental hygienist and the client. Recommendations for compensating for psychomotor skill deficits that might be related to degenerative disabilities also should be addressed.

A primary role of the dental hygienist is to motivate clients to adopt and maintain behavior patterns related to oral health. In this effort, the dental hygienist should view the client as being actively involved in the process of care. Using information from the client's history, oral examination, radiographs, and all other data collected during the initial assessment, the dental hygienist in collaboration with the client establishes goals for dental hygiene care. These goals must be related realistically to the client's individual needs, values, and ability level. Because each client has personal requirements for self-care, clients must participate in setting goals and must personally commit themselves to achieving them if oral disease control and prevention are to be successful over the life span.

SIMULTANEOUSLY MEETING NEEDS

Identification of the eight human needs related to dental hygiene care is a useful way for dental hygienists to evaluate and understand the needs of all clients and to achieve a client-centered practice. A client entering the oral healthcare environment may have one or more unmet needs, and dental hygiene care delivered within a human needs conceptual framework may address all of them simultaneously. Human needs theory provides a holistic and humanistic perspective for dental hygiene by addressing the client's needs in the physical, emotional, intellectual, and social dimensions, and defines the territory for the practice of client-centered dental hygiene. Applying this theory when interacting with clients, whether the client is an individual, a family, or a community, enhances the dental hygienist's relationship with the client and promotes the client's adoption of and adherence to the dental hygienist's professional recommendations.

Oral disease disrupts clients' ability to meet their human needs not simply in the physical dimension, but also in the emotional, intellectual, social, and cultural dimensions. Therefore, the dental hygienist plans and provides interventions for clients with diverse needs. The dental hygienist first assesses clients for unmet needs and then considers how dental hygiene care can best help them meet those needs. After identifying which of a client's human needs are unmet, the dental hygienist, in collaboration with the client, must set goals and establish priorities for providing care to fulfill these needs. Setting goals and establishing priorities, however, does not mean that the dental hygienist provides care for only one need at a time. In emergency situations, of course, physiologic needs take precedence, but even then the dental hygienist is aware of the client's other psychosocial needs. For example, when providing care for a client with painful gingivitis, whose human needs for skin and mucous membrane integrity of the head and neck and for freedom from pain require immediate attention, the dental hygienist also takes into consideration the client's need for freedom from stress and wholesome facial image. Often, one need may take priority and the dental hygienist must first be concerned with the highest priority need (such as helping the client cope with a fear of having his or her teeth scaled before helping the client restore the integrity of the gingival tissues). But equally often the dental hygienist simultaneously addresses needs such as assisting a client in meeting the need for responsibility for oral health while also helping the client achieve freedom from pain.

CLIENT EDUCATION ISSUES

- ✦ The dental hygienist explains modification to care required due to medical conditions so that the client is not put at risk for life-threatening disease.
- ✦ The dental hygienist discusses with the client previous negative experiences related to dental or dental hygiene care and reassures the client that every effort will be made to provide care as comfortably and safely as possible.
- ✦ For clients undergoing treatment related to facial image stressors, the dental hygienist listens to their doubts about treatment outcomes and provides information and reassurance as needed.
- ✦ In counseling clients, dental hygienists present the rationale and details of methods recommended for the prevention and control of oral diseases and ask questions to determine if the clients need clarification of concepts presented.
- ✦ In providing client education, the dental hygienist appeals to the clients' sense of self-determination and tries to evoke their need for responsibility for oral health.
- ✦ The dental hygienist encourages clients to participate in setting goals and objectives for dental hygiene care, and thus facilitates decision making by the client.

LEGAL, ETHICAL, AND SAFETY ISSUES

- ✦ The dental hygienist discusses all procedures with clients, obtains informed consent, and encourages their participation in the dental hygiene care plan.
- ✦ It may be necessary for the dental hygienist to postpone a current appointment because of a client's need for urgent medical consultation or because of evidence of infectious lesions such as herpes labialis.
- ✦ Medical contraindications must be addressed prior to any intraoral instrumentation associated with dental hygiene care.

Key Concepts

- Dental hygiene care focuses on the promotion of oral health and the prevention of oral disease over the human life span.
- The dental hygienist is concerned with the whole person, applying specific knowledge about the client's emotions, values, family, culture, and environment as well as general knowledge about the body systems.
- Clients are viewed as active participants in the process of dental hygiene care because the ultimate responsibility to use self-care and seek professional care to obtain and maintain oral wellness is theirs.
- The human needs conceptual model of dental hygiene provides a framework for dental hygiene care. It focuses on the client and has eight human needs as its basic units of assessment. Baseline assessment as to whether or not the eight human needs are met provides a framework for dental hygienists to make dental hygiene diagnoses based on unmet needs, and then to plan, implement, and evaluate dental hygiene care.

Critical Thinking Exercises

Given the following scenario, use the dental hygiene human needs conceptual model to list the human needs that are in deficit and to plan dental hygiene interventions to meet the identified human need deficits.

Scenario: Devan Sacks, age 12, is a new client in the dental practice and has been scheduled for dental hygiene care. Devan is in the seventh grade and is one of the star players on the girls soccer team. She is accompanied by her mother, Margaret (age 32), and her sister Bridget (age 10). After completing health, dental, and personal histories, the dental hygienist initiates the assessment phase of the dental hygiene process of care, including a baseline assessment of human needs related to dental hygiene care, a complete dental and periodontal assessment, and dental hygiene education and skill level assessment. Significant findings include 6-mm probing depths around tooth numbers 19 and 30, and 4- to 5-mm pockets around tooth numbers 22 to 27. Oral hygiene was generally poor. Client has a knowledge deficit regarding bacterial plaque, periodontal disease process, and status of the oral cavity.

For References, Suggested Readings, and Related Websites, visit
http://evolve.elsevier.com/Darby/hygiene/

CHAPTER 3

Concepts of Health and Wellness

OBJECTIVES

Mastery of the content in this chapter will enable the reader to:

- Discuss the concept of health
- Describe the healthcare paradigms: disease treatment–oriented, disease prevention–oriented, and health promotion–oriented
- Discuss a healthcare model associated with each of the paradigms
- Differentiate between the three levels of prevention—primary, secondary, and tertiary—and provide an oral health example for each
- Describe health promotion strategies the dental hygienist might employ to facilitate client oral health: oral health marketing, health education, collaboration, use of mass media, community organization, advocacy, and legislation

KEY TERMS

Advocacy
Agent-host-environment model
Collaboration
Community organization
Disease prevention paradigm
Health
Health education
Health field concept
Health promotion framework
Health promotion paradigm
Healthy public policy
Macrosocial health education
Medical model
Microsocial health education
Oral health–related quality of life model
Primary prevention
Secondary prevention
Social marketing
Tertiary prevention
Treatment of disease paradigm
Wellness movement

WHAT ARE HEALTH AND WELLNESS?

Dental hygienists are advocates of personal and professional oral healthcare for the prevention of oral disease and the promotion of health. Effective dental hygiene care involves thinking holistically about the client, envisioning the totality of the body, the mind, and the spirit; perceiving how the client relates to the community; and understanding which factors influence client health. Consider the following:

SCENARIO 1

George Fountaine is 30 years old and has just been diagnosed with multiple sclerosis. He is actively involved in his profession as a computer programmer for the high school curriculum. He is committed to fitness and leads a generally healthy lifestyle. George nurtures his self-awareness through spiritual activity. Despite the prognosis associated with multiple sclerosis, he does not feel impending doom in his life, but rather a challenge, a learning experience, an opportunity to offer himself to those around him. George is healthy and well. He is able to meet his human needs.

SCENARIO 2

Sherry Gillmore and her husband have two sons, both of whom are doing very well in school and in their extracurricular activities. Prior to marriage and a family, she had a career teaching English as a second language (ESL). When her sons were in elementary school she stayed home to raise them, but now that they are in high school she would like to find employment with an ESL program. Her husband has been transferred to a rural community that is predominantly white and middle class white. There are no ESL programs in or around the vicinity. She feels distraught at the potential inability to fulfill her desire to continue her work with the ESL community, a passion she has never lost. Physically she is in good shape, but emotionally she is very unhappy and in turmoil. She is not well. Her human needs are going unmet.

Do you agree with the concluding statements of these two scenarios? What constitutes a healthy state? What does it mean to be well? Exploring these questions helps dental hygienists to conceptualize their role in healthcare and their view of the health of their clients.

HEALTH

Health is more than merely the absence of disease or infirmity. Health is a state of physical, mental, and social well-being and is directly related to human need fulfillment. The World Health Organization has defined health as "the extent to which an individual or group is able, on the one hand, to realize aspirations and satisfy needs, and on the other hand, to change and cope with the environment."[1] This concept of health recognizes the ongoing role of human need fulfillment. Because the conceptualization of health guides the provision of healthcare by practitioners and healthcare systems, various paradigms of health and healthcare systems will be reviewed.

PARADIGMS AND MODELS OF HEALTHCARE

Three major paradigms or conceptual frameworks of healthcare are evident in today's healthcare system. They are as follows:

- ✦ Disease treatment
- ✦ Disease prevention
- ✦ Health promotion

These paradigms are defined by the intent and approach each takes to achieving health. Although they are not mutually exclusive, each one has its own emphasis or focus (Table 3–1).

Treatment of Disease Paradigm

The *treatment of disease paradigm* is based on the definition of health as "the absence of disease." Represented by the *medical model,* the treatment of disease paradigm views the art and science of medicine as the fount from which all improvements in health flow. This paradigm equates the level of healthcare with the quality of medicine[2] and promotes passive treatment-based healthcare. In healthcare systems based on this paradigm:

- ✦ Little is done in terms of identifying the cause of the disease and thwarting its occurrence through prevention.
- ✦ There is heavy reliance on the physician to cure the disease with little effort or responsibility required from the diseased person.
- ✦ There is little accountability from sectors other than the healthcare system that also influence the health of the public, such as industry, housing, environment, culture, and lifestyle.

TABLE 3–1 PARADIGMS AND ASSOCIATED MODELS OF HEALTH

Paradigm	Model of Health or Health Behavior
Treatment oriented	Medical model
Prevention oriented	Agent-host-environment model
	Health field concept
Health promotion oriented	Oral health–related quality of life model
	Human needs model of dental hygiene
	Health promotion framework

Treatment-based healthcare systems around the world have been criticized for incurring escalating costs, requiring a multitude of professional manpower (with emphasis on the most expensive: the physician), and reacting to health problems rather than solving them. A general perception of this traditional paradigm for healthcare is that it makes for an uncontrollable healthcare system unsupportable by finite human, material, and financial resources.

In the treatment of disease paradigm, the provision of dental hygiene care includes the following: the dental hygienist performs periodontal debridement, the "patient" is scheduled for another appointment, periodontal debridement is performed, and the cycle repeats itself. Little if any attention is given to the cause of the condition, the condition is simply treated. This approach to care perpetuates a reliance on the dental hygienist for the achievement and maintenance of periodontal health.

Disease Prevention Paradigm

The *disease prevention paradigm* emphasizes the importance of identifying the causative agent of disease and avoiding it. Models representing this paradigm are the agent-host-environment model[3] and the health field concept.[4]

AGENT-HOST-ENVIRONMENT MODEL. The *agent-host-environment model* conceptualizes disease as the result of an imbalance in one or all of three factors: the agent (e.g., bacteria), the host (e.g., the person), and the environment. Examples of the application of this model are water fluoridation to develop caries-resistant tooth surfaces and the incorporation of oral health education as a component of school health curricula.

The agent-host-environment model also identifies three levels of preventive measures: primary, secondary, and tertiary (Table 3–2). *Primary prevention* consists of interventions to prevent the onset of disease or injury. This level is a major focus of dental hygiene practice. Examples of such dental hygiene actions include school-based education programs that encourage abstinence from tobacco use, recommending the use of dental floss for preventing periodontal diseases, and mouthguard fabrication for preventing sport-related injury.

Secondary prevention consists of interventions designed to stop or minimize the progression of early disease while the person is generally asymptomatic. Examples of such dental hygiene actions include chairside oral hygiene instruction for an individual with mild gingivitis, recommending daily fluoride gel for persons with caries activity, and applying desensitizing agents for dentinal hypersensitivity.

Tertiary prevention consists of interventions to prevent disability and to improve or restore function and prevent further deterioration. Performance of nonsurgical periodontal therapy to increase periodontal attachment is an example of a dental hygiene action in the area of tertiary prevention.

HEALTH FIELD CONCEPT. The *health field concept* (Figure 3–1) attributes the health status of the individual and the community to interaction between four elements:

- ✦ Human biology, which is the basic biology of an individual resulting in both physical and mental aspects of health, such as diabetes
- ✦ Environment, which encompasses everything external to the body and over which the individual has little or no control, such as natural disasters and industrial pollution
- ✦ Lifestyle, which includes all decisions made by individuals that affect their health and over which they, more or less, have control, such as smoking, diet, exercise, excessive alcohol consumption, and wearing seatbelts
- ✦ Healthcare organization, which encompasses the quantity, quality, and administration of the healthcare system, such as the healthcare paradigm applied, the availability of hospital beds, oral health services provided, the purchase of magnetic resonance imaging (MRI) technology, and the monies to finance research

The health field concept provides a comprehensive, systematic framework to analyze the cause of disease. It presents a new perspective on health that was not addressed in the treatment of disease paradigm. The health field concept maps out the significant influence on health of the underlying elements of lifestyle, environment, biology, and the healthcare organization. It demands unification of all participants in decisions that affect health: health professionals, the scientific community, governments, the business sector, and the people themselves. Consider the following scenario:

TABLE 3–2 MODES OF ORAL HEALTH INTERVENTION FOR THE THREE LEVELS OF PREVENTION

Level	Mode	Activity
Primary	Health promotion	Chairside oral hygiene instruction Classroom education Workshops for caregivers
	Specific protection	Athletic mouth protectors Water fluoridation Self-applied and professionally applied oral health products Pit and fissure sealants (no caries activity)
Secondary	Early detection and early treatment	Detecting disease as a result of oral screening programs, self-examination, or professional examinations Pit and fissure sealants (given incipient caries) Oral physiotherapeutic aids for periodontal pockets
Tertiary	Treatment and rehabilitation	Surgical and nonsurgical periodontal therapy Restorative, prosthodontic, and reconstructive therapy

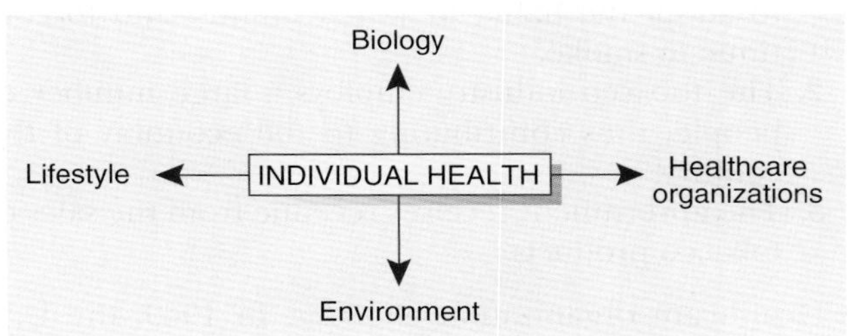

FIGURE 3–1 ✦ Health field concept. *(A new perspective on the health of Canadians: A working document, Health Canada, 1974.© Reproduced with the permission of the Minister of Public Works and Government Services, Canada, 2003.)*

SCENARIO 3

Mary Marks, a young mother of two children who wants to pursue her premarriage career but finds job opportunities limited, smokes 20 cigarettes per day. Don, her dental hygienist, recommends that she consider joining the tobacco-use cessation program that he is offering through the dental practice. He encourages her to do so because she is at risk for oral cancer and other negative health effects as a result of her smoking. Mary says, "I know I should quit. I realize that I should because it is likely killing me. I just can't even consider doing it right now."

This scenario provides a good example for an oral health application of the health field concept. According to this model, blaming Mary for putting herself at risk for cancer is an oversimplification. Rather, the four elements of human biology, environment, lifestyle, and healthcare organization should be included in counseling Mary since they influence Mary's tobacco-use habit in the following ways:

- Human biologic element: Mary is physically and psychologically addicted to tobacco.
- Lifestyle element: It was not until the 1960s that society began to be informed that tobacco use had negative health effects. By this time, it was the socially acceptable thing to do. Smoking was the norm; the nonsmoker was in the minority. Today, although the message is clear, Mary still chooses to use tobacco. The evidence for this choice appears to be related in part to the psychosocial gratification of tobacco use as part of her lifestyle.
- Environmental element: Relevant environmental elements are:
    1. Tobacco companies present appealing and tantalizing advertisements in household magazines, on billboards, and through other media. The advertising imagery presented is designed to entice people to adopt the habit, to switch brands, and to continue to smoke.
    2. The tobacco industry employs a large number of people, thus contributing to the economy of the country.
    3. The government receives revenue from the sales of tobacco products.
- Healthcare organization element: In 1969, the U.S. Surgeon General stated that smoking is a health hazard. Initially, much of the healthcare response was focused on the treatment of tobacco-related diseases instead of the prevention of the tobacco-use habit. Even though significant healthcare dollars are spent on the treatment of such diseases, additional funding for tobacco cessation programs is required to help many tobacco users overcome their addiction. Recognizing and discussing these elements with Mary provide a more comprehensive analysis of her problem and may motivate her to think more objectively about finding solutions for her tobacco use.

Health Promotion Paradigm

The *health promotion paradigm,* also referred to as the *wellness movement,* focuses on creating environments that enable people to increase control over and improve their current and future health.[5,6] This paradigm centers on the population as a whole and less so on the individual. All in the community (individuals, healthcare organizations, and government) are seen as responsible for the creation of environments that predispose and enable people to achieve health and realize their aspirations. Several forces or trends that initiated the wellness movement include consumer consciousness regarding health, the healthcare cost crisis, mind and body awareness, and industry's responsiveness and initiatives (e.g., work site health promotion programs) to reduce absenteeism and high turnover rates and to improve employee morale.

Health promotion calls for:

- Building public policy
- Strengthening community action through empowerment of communities to assume ownership and control of their own destinies)
- Development of personal skills and reorientation of health services

In the health promotion paradigm, health is seen as a community or societal responsibility versus an individual one, and social structure is seen as a critical component of health and well-being.[7]

Models or approaches to healthcare that represent the health promotion paradigm are the human needs model of dental hygiene, the oral health–related quality of life model,[8] and the health promotion framework model.[6] Each of these models considers the impact that (oral) health has on individual and societal well-being and quality of life. The human needs model of dental hygiene is discussed in depth in Chapter 2. The other two models are discussed in the following sections.

ORAL HEALTH–RELATED QUALITY OF LIFE MODEL. The *oral health–related quality of life model,* developed by dental hygiene scholars at the University of Missouri at Kansas City, postulates that the continuum of health and disease is influenced by environmental, sociocultural, and economic influences that are either modifiable or nonmodifiable risk factors (Figure 3–2). These influences, along with people's beliefs and response to variables that have an impact on their life, affect their perceptions of quality of life.

HEALTH PROMOTION FRAMEWORK. *The health promotion framework* evolved from the health field concept. The framework is aimed at achieving health for all by accepting specific challenges, identifying mechanisms, and implementing health promotion strategies to meet these challenges (Figure 3–3).

HEALTH PROMOTION: A CHALLENGE TO THE HEALTH PROFESSIONS

Achieving health for all is a challenge for health professionals, one that can be met by the strategies of health promotion: marketing, health education, collaboration, mass media, community organization, advocacy, and legislation (Figure 3–4). Dental hygienists can engage in each of these activities, thereby actively participating in the challenge as change agents, client advocates, and educators/oral health promoters.

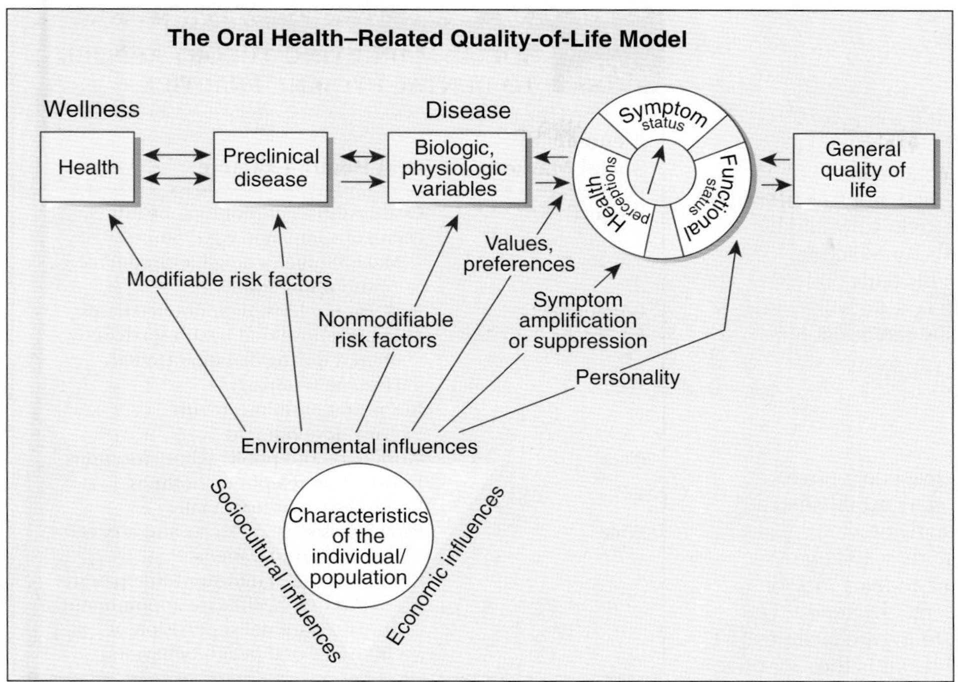

FIGURE 3–2 ✦ Oral health–related quality of life. *(From Williams K et al: Oral health–related quality of life: A model for dental hygiene,* Journal of Dental Hygiene *72(2):19, 1998.)*

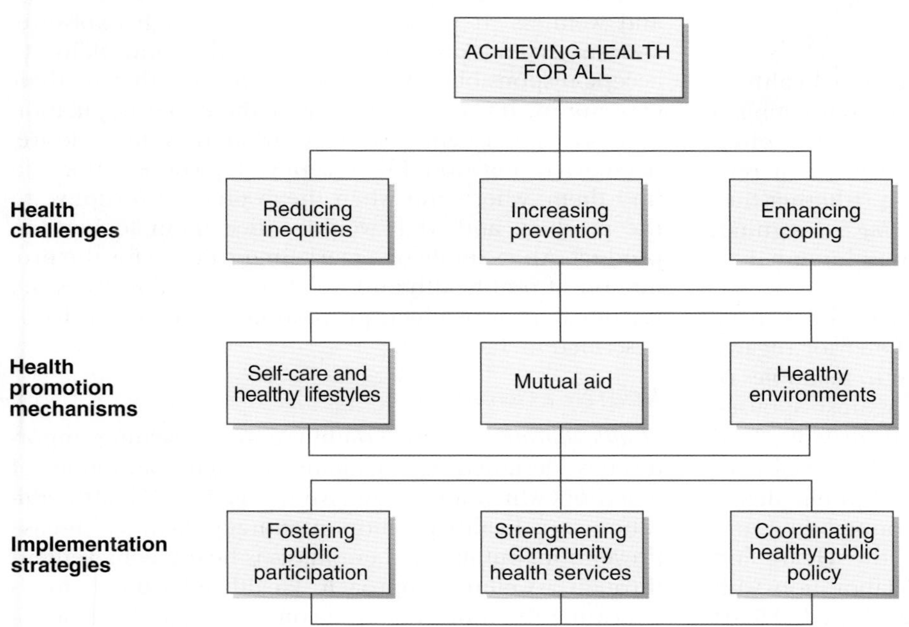

FIGURE 3–3 ✦ Health promotion framework. *(Adapted from* Achieving health for all: A framework for health promotion, *Health Canada, 1986. © Reproduced with the permission of the Minister of Public Works and Government Services, Canada, 2003.)*

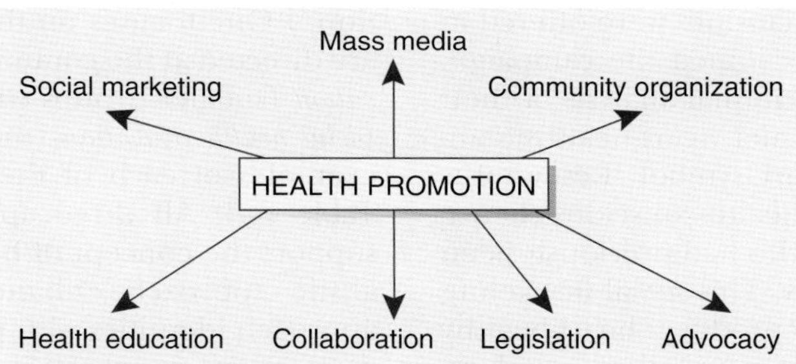

FIGURE 3–4 ✦ Health promotion strategies.

Marketing

SCENARIO 4

Harriet Green has been practicing dental hygiene for 20 years. Mr. Smith, a long-standing client, fell and broke his hip. He cannot attend his regular dental hygiene appointment. Harriet pays him a home visit, not to perform any periodontal debridement (because to do so would be in violation of her scope of practice in the jurisdiction where she resides), but to assist him in his daily oral healthcare. She helps him to determine how he will manage daily toothbrushing and how she can assist him.

SCENARIO 5

Bruce Front has been practicing dental hygiene for five years. Within two years of his graduation he established a mobile dental hygiene service and currently provides dental hygiene care to residents in more than 13 large Canadian facilities, one of which is home to Mary Jackson. He realized the need and demand for dental hygiene services for the elderly residing in long-term care facilities and marketed his services to them. The result is the provision of regular dental hygiene care that otherwise was not provided by the oral health profession community.

Both Harriet and Bruce are marketing oral health to their surrounding community. They are marketing a concept to society: the concept of dental hygienists offering a full range of services to clients within their own homes. What Bruce and Harriet are doing (whether they realize it or not) is part of *social marketing*:[9] designing, implementing, and controlling programs intended to influence hygienists' social acceptability.

Generally, nonprofit organizations like health associations tackle social marketing to change behavior regarding social practices not conducive to health. Examples of such marketing include campaigning against spouse-, child-, and elder-abuse; drinking and driving; and tobacco and substance abuse. For successful social marketing, the organization must have a good public image consisting of credibility, integrity, accountability, and goodwill for the public. For example, the Heart and Stroke Foundation of Manitoba, in collaboration with numerous Manitoba restaurants, developed Heart Smart, a program that enabled people to enjoy the pleasures of dining out but avoiding meals laden with cholesterol and calories. Heart-healthy cuisines were offered in many restaurants that voluntarily joined the campaign. Restaurateurs welcomed the nutritional analysis of their menus. Those menu items that met heart-healthy standards were signified with a heart symbol. Restaurants could profitably offer a menu to health-conscious clients, adding new patrons from those who had previously been limited in healthy food selections. This social marketing campaign identified a tangible product, heart-healthy menu choices, and facilitated informed choice making about dietary intake.

TABLE 3–3 SOCIAL MARKETING THEORY APPLIED TO DENTAL HYGIENE PRACTICE

Elements of Social Marketing	Oral Health Example
Product	Oral health as part of total health Name of campaign, e.g., "Smile" Make "Smile" a tangible product, e.g., with photographs
Promotion	Radio and television announcements Free preventive oral health services offered during National Dental Hygiene Campaign Bus poster announcements Website development
Place	Workplace and public school locations Information telephone hotlines Booth display at local mall
Price	Psychic costs (client's fear and anxiety) Monetary considerations Resource costs (childcare while parent attends oral healthcare appointment, time for parental supervision of children's oral health behaviors)

Social marketing is essential for promoting health and wellness. It persuades people, through exposure, awareness, and provision of knowledge and skills, to accept responsibility for their health and that of their community. It is essential to know the target population of a social marketing strategy: what they like, desire, need; what they would be receptive to; where you would find them; where and when they would be receptive to the product; and what would entice them to buy the product. An example of a marketing strategy for the promotion of oral health and well-being that illustrates the relationship of product, promotion, place, and price is described in Table 3–3.

Health Education

Health education is "any combination of learning opportunities designed to facilitate voluntary adoption of behaviors which are conducive to health."[10] Health education as a health promotion strategy includes disease prevention, but its main emphasis is health achievement through a wellness approach. Health education entails educating the individual, the community, and the political sector of the community.

There are three approaches to oral health education.[11] One focuses on the individual and the other two are directed at the community level: *microsocial health education* (smaller groups within a community) and *macrosocial health education* (the community at large). Several examples of each of these approaches are outlined in Table 3–4. All three approaches to health education support the concept of health promotion. The individualistic approach enhances self-help, the microsocial approach identifies with people helping people, and the macrosocial approach considers the creation of public policy.

TABLE 3–4 APPROACHES TO ORAL HEALTH EDUCATION

Approach	Activities
Individualistic	One-to-one oral health instruction regarding the relationship between bacterial plaque, periodontal diseases, and systemic disease
Microsocial	Town meeting regarding the initiation of community water fluoridation
	Caregivers oral health education workshop
Macrosocial	Informative letters to legislators or ministers of parliament or congress regarding need for universal oral healthcare coverage
	Lobbying for self-regulation of dental hygiene to achieve universal access to quality dental hygiene care

Modified from Locker D: Approaches to dental health education. In: *Preventative dental services,* ed 2, Ottawa, 1988, Health and Welfare Canada.

Collaboration

Collaboration is an important element of healthcare. The health professional who collaborates with others—including other health professionals and other individuals and groups that influence health—is the health professional who realizes that health is a holistic achievement.

SCENARIO 6

Harriet takes Mr. Smith's blood pressure, as she routinely does, and finds that despite his medication to control his hypertension, his blood pressure is higher than normal. She asks Mr. Smith if he would like her to call his physician. She does so, and the physician schedules Mr. Smith for an appointment in a week's time. Harriet wonders about Mr. Smith's diet, realizing that he lives alone and has no one to help him prepare his food while his hip is healing. She suggests that a home-care agency come in every day with a prepared hot meal. He thinks that would be a marvelous idea; in fact, the social worker at the hospital had suggested this and he just hadn't followed through on it.

Harriet is demonstrating collaboration with other health professionals by:

- ✦ Being aware of a client's holistic health to enhance the person's capacity to adopt preventive and promotional practices
- ✦ Interacting with other disciplines to avoid territorial boundaries over disease, which limit the opportunity to enhance a client's self-care, mutual aid, and coping ability

In the spirit of collaboration, health professionals provide clients with information on health-promoting resources and programs in the community, such as smoking cessation programs, cardiovascular fitness programs, fat-free cooking programs, and various support groups.

Collaboration also must occur among decision makers and society outside of the healthcare arena to create healthy environments. An illustration of this collaboration would be mandating elder-abuse as a reportable condition. If dental hygienists' head and neck examinations lead them to suspect that clients are being abused, they are required to report their suspicions to the respective authority. Society does not tolerate abuse, and healthcare professions are in the position of possibly detecting abuse. Government bodies (on behalf of the people) require action to be taken to help the victims of abuse.

Collaboration fuels the health promotion mission by encouraging discussion among healthcare providers, promoting linkages between them, and creating enabling environments for the achievement of health. Primary care nursing centers in Canada are just such environments. They offer opportunities for dental hygienists and nurses to collaborate.[12] These centers primarily provide accessible, affordable, quality healthcare services to people who typically are under-serviced. This population group tends to experience oral health problems. Integrating a dental hygiene service into these centers assists these clients in achieving oral health (see Suggestions for Dental Hygiene Collaboration with Primary Care Nursing Centers).

Mass Media

SCENARIO 7

The www.umanitoba.ca/outreach/wisdomtooth is launched! Since 1996 when Maryanne and Marie created the site, it has had over 50,000 hits. People are accessing oral health information via cyberspace. Originating as an undergraduate student project, "wisdom tooth" remains a site because of the dedication and commitment of Maryanne and Marie, who are practicing dental hygienists volunteering their services as webmasters of the site. The site is acclaimed for its creativity and quality of information. Having received the Yahoo Pick of the Week award just three weeks after its launch date, it has since been copyrighted (translated) by the University of Brazil so that Web users in Brazil can access the information. Links to other health sites make the "wisdom tooth" a wealthy resource for the health consumer. Periodic assessments of the site indicate that it is a well-used source of oral health information for people around the world and that the demand for this service is high; people want to be informed about oral health care.[13]

Maryanne, Marie, and their fellow colleagues are reaching large numbers of people with oral health messages through cyberspace. Scenario 6 is an example of the use of mass media to increase public awareness and knowledge of oral health and quality of life.

Nonprofit organizations such as the American Dental Hygienists' Association, the Canadian Dental Hygienists' Association, and local professional associations collaborate with corporate sponsors to promote oral health via mass media. This collaboration is mutually beneficial to both groups. Nonprofit organizations can use mass media

Suggestions for Dental Hygiene Collaboration with Primary Care Nursing Centers

Nursing Center Staff In-service Topics

Relationship of alcohol and tobacco use to oral cancer
Oral cancer self-examination techniques
Management of xerostomia
Fluorides throughout the life span
Identification of gingival infection
Recognition of oral lesions
Athletic mouth protectors

Other Collaborative Efforts

Identify referral sources for dental treatment in public and private delivery systems
Facilitate establishment of referral networks
Volunteer as an oral health consultant
Participate in oral health screenings
Establish dental hygiene student community service sites at primary care nursing centers
Guest lecture in nursing education programs

From Fellona M, DeVore L: Oral health services in primary care nursing centers: Opportunities for dental hygiene and nursing collaboration, *Journal of Dental Hygiene* 73(2):69, 1999.

such as commercial television and radio rather than relying on public service announcements, which have smaller audiences and are often less flashy and attractive because of smaller budgets. The corporate sponsor of such programs benefits in that it becomes linked with a credible source, and hence its own credibility is increased. Examples of other mass media activities that dental hygienists can engage in to promote oral health are:

- ✦ Serving as contributing health editors to household magazines
- ✦ Holding press conferences during local, state, or national dental hygiene gatherings
- ✦ Performing radio and television spots

Community Organization

Community organization aims at developing the skills, abilities, and understandings of groups of people for the purpose of self-led improvement. If a group is to be used effectively as a medium for change, those people who are to be changed and those who are exerting influence for the change must have a sense of belonging to the same group.

An example of community organization occurred at the Tsewultan Health Center at Cowichan Tribes, British Columbia. A dental hygienist was hired as an oral health consultant to work with the community in achieving three objectives: 1) to decrease the rate of tooth decay in the community by 50% for 5-year-olds; 2) to increase the percentage of dental visits by the citizens of the community to at least once a year; and 3) to decrease the number of children requiring general anesthetic to treat decay by 10% per year. The dental hygienist initially spent time in the community, establishing a presence at many of the community events. This enabled her to build a trusting relationship with the citizens—a critical step in facilitating the objectives. She listened to residents' perceptions of their oral health needs and how they could be met. Eventually, the community: 1) developed a library of audiovisual materials at the health center (collaborating with the local school library to purchase 201 children's books on dental topics); 2) routinely offered training sessions for staff at the center; and 3) reestablished a fluoride supplement program. Most recently, a dental health center was opened on the reserve. This initiative illustrates the principles of community organization of working for and with the people.

Advocacy, Legislation, and Public Policy

SCENARIO 8

The dental practice that employs Harriet is situated in a predominantly Hispanic neighborhood. The practice has surveyed the neighborhood and knows that only about half of the 5-year-olds have had an oral health screening, referral, and follow-up. Harriet initiates a petition to hire dental hygienists to perform oral screening in the community school. She confers with her dental hygiene colleagues, the mayor of the community, and the parent council of the school, all of whom sign a petition to be taken to the regulatory body.

Harriet advocates for regulatory changes for her profession. Advocacy and legislation go hand-in-hand in that advocacy is generally the precursor to legislation. *Advocacy*, in this context, is the education of decision makers to provide the essential political support for changes, whereas *legislation* makes these behaviors mandatory. Examples of public policy for health instigated through advocacy and legislation include the requirement that smokers must extinguish their cigarettes before entering public places, that traffic stop signs must be placed at street intersections, and that schoolchildren must be immunized against numerous childhood diseases prior to attending school.

A *healthy public policy* considers its health implications.[13] Such a policy considers the health impact as of equal importance as the primary goal of that policy.

The Dental Hygienist's Role in Health Promotion

Dental hygienists are preventive oral healthcare specialists with responsibility to:

- ✦ Promote oral health as being integral to overall health
- ✦ Prevent oral disease
- ✦ Reduce inequities among population groups (e.g., increasing access to dental hygiene care)

These responsibilities can be achieved by employing the strategies of health promotion to foster public participation, strengthen community health service, and influence healthy public policy. The responsibility of dental hygienists, and all health professionals, is to serve as a resource to the community and sometimes as a "mover and shaker" to ensure healthy environments.[14]

FOSTERING PUBLIC PARTICIPATION. Fostering public participation requires helping people assert control over factors that affect their health to enable them to act in ways that preserve or improve their health. For example, oral health is an important component of prenatal education, tobacco cessation programs, workshops for caregivers and nurses' aides, and school health curricula. Whether individually or through dental hygiene associations, dental hygienists have a responsibility to foster public participation in influencing public policy to ensure that oral health issues are presented as part of these and other programs. Strategies dental hygienists can use include serving on school boards, parent–teacher associations, boards of institutional facilities, and governmental health promotion task forces. Such participation will help to increase awareness of the significance of oral health to general health and to quality of life.

STRENGTHENING COMMUNITY SERVICES. Dental hygienists work as change agents and consumer advocates to lead the public in their demands for access to quality community oral healthcare. The elderly in long-term care facilities and daycare centers, institutionalized individuals with mental and physical impairments, and other high-risk groups such as immigrants and Native Americans/Inuit, have limited access to oral disease prevention and oral health promotion services. When oral healthcare is provided to these disadvantaged groups it often is treatment oriented. To increase access to prevention and health promotion–oriented care dental hygienists can use strategies such as organizing public forums to provide the rationale and incentive for the public to lobby community councils, legislators, and higher government for these services.

INFLUENCING HEALTHY PUBLIC POLICY. As consumer advocates and change agents, dental hygienists provide leadership in the development of public policies related to oral health. For example, dental hygienists help to ensure that national, state, and local health surveys include oral health–related assessments to accurately document need so that public policy can be based on accurate research. Dental hygienists also work to convince decision makers to support oral health–promotion policy. Issues dental hygienists may advocate for include:

- ✦ Cost-effectiveness of employing dental hygienists in a variety of nontraditional settings (e.g., schools, institutions, work sites)
- ✦ Community-based annual oral cancer screenings
- ✦ Oral health education in school curricula
- ✦ School-based fluoride rinse programs
- ✦ Elimination of nutritionally unsound foods in school cafeterias
- ✦ Community water fluoridation
- ✦ Pit and fissure sealants and fluoride rinses for the prevention of dental caries in children
- ✦ Control of tobacco marketing and advertising practices that target youth

Achieving health for all is the mission of health promotion.

CLIENT EDUCATION ISSUES

- ✦ Health is determined by the individual and community.
- ✦ The health care system offers three approaches to care: treatment of disease, disease prevention, and health promotion.
- ✦ Individuals and communities can assert control over factors that affect their health.
- ✦ Health professionals are facilitators of health for all.
- ✦ The dental hygienist is a valuable resource that clients can use to achieve and maintain their health.

LEGAL, ETHICAL, AND SAFETY ISSUES

- ✦ It is the client's right to be treated in an environment of respect and unconditional regard.
- ✦ The client's autonomy is maintained at all times.
- ✦ Dental hygiene interventions are offered within the scope of dental hygiene practice and within the jurisdiction where the dental hygienist resides.

Key Concepts

- Health is the extent to which an individual or group is able to realize and satisfy its needs and to change and cope with the environment.
- Quality of life is affected by oral disease and oral conditions.
- Dental hygienists have an important role to play in promoting oral health as integral to overall health, preventing oral disease, and reducing inequities among population groups.
- Three approaches to healthcare are evident in today's health care system: treatment of disease, disease prevention, and health promotion. The dental hygienist is focused on the latter two approaches, but also participates in the treatment of oral disease.
- The agent-host-environment model of disease prevention identifies three levels of prevention: primary, secondary, and tertiary.
- The human field concept attributes health status to biology, environment, lifestyle, and healthcare organization. This model has led to the reordering of public health policies.
- Health promotion is any activity that enhances health; such actions enable people to make healthy choices and create healthy environments. Strategies include marketing, health education, collaboration, mass media use, community organization, and advocacy and legislation.
- The dental hygiene profession collaborates with individuals, groups and other health professionals to prevent oral disease and promote health.
- To reach clients who may not have access to dental hygiene care, the dental hygiene profession employs marketing principles.
- Dental hygienists engage in health education when they provide oral hygiene instructions to a client during an individual dental hygiene appointment, present an oral health session to caregivers of residents in a long-term care facility, or are involved in the creation of policy for mouthguards to be worn during all contact sports.
- The use of mass media provides the opportunity to reach a large number of people with a health message that may lead to the adoption of a healthy behavior.
- Community organization is a health promotion activity in which the dental hygienist may participate to assist in the creation of healthy environments.
- Advocacy and legislation often go hand-in-hand to bring about healthy public policy.
- The dental hygiene profession, like all health professions, is challenged to facilitate the worldwide mission to achieve health (oral health) for all.

Critical Thinking Exercises

1. Create a visual conceptual model of how you perceive health. Work in groups to define health and develop a drawing that reflects that definition. Share your definition and conceptual model of health with the rest of the class.
2. Interview a health-related organization regarding its mission, goal and objectives, population served, success of the programming, and the role the dental hygiene profession might play in collaborating with the group. Be familiar with the concept of and assess the organization fulfillment of health promotion. Prepare an oral presentation for your classmates and provide them with literature (pamphlets, posters) obtained from the organization.

For References, Suggested Readings, and Related Websites, visit
http://evolve.elsevier.com/Darby/hygiene/

CHAPTER 4

BEHAVIORAL FOUNDATIONS FOR THE DENTAL HYGIENE PROCESS

OBJECTIVES

Mastery of the content in this chapter will enable the reader to:

- Relate the importance of communication to the profession of dental hygiene
- List the basic components of the communication process
- List factors that affect interpersonal communication
- Describe the CARE principle
- List types of nonverbal behavior
- Discuss therapeutic communication techniques
- Discuss nontherapeutic communication techniques
- Identify major theories of motivation
- Identify communication techniques appropriate throughout the life span

KEY TERMS

Andragogy
Attribution theory
CARE principle
Closed-ended question
Contextual factors
Empathy
Interpersonal communication
Intonation
Locus of control
Message
Motivation
Nontherapeutic communication
Nonverbal communication
Open-ended questions
Pedagogy
Receiver
Self-efficacy
Self-efficacy theory
Sender
Therapeutic communication
Verbal communication

Effective communication with the client is essential for providing optimal dental hygiene care (Table 4–1). For example, during the assessment phase of the dental hygiene process, the hygienist needs to communicate effectively with the client to obtain and validate information concerning medical, dental, and personal/social histories, and oral health status and behaviors. Communication skills also influence client adherence to preventive and other therapeutic recommendations. When rapport, confidence, and trust are present, a client is more likely to share confidential information and to follow specific oral healthcare recommendations. If dental hygienists possess technical skills and knowledge but are unable to communicate effectively with clients, they may fail to reach important goals related to client oral health, comfort, and long-term behavioral change.

BASIC ELEMENTS OF THE COMMUNICATION PROCESS

Sender, Message, and Receiver

Interpersonal communication is the process by which a person sends a message to another person with the intention of evoking a response. The basic elements of communication[1] are shown in Figure 4–1. The *sender* is the person who constructs a message to initiate the interpersonal communication. The message construction process is known as encoding. The *message* itself contains information the sender wishes to transmit. It must be in a format of symbols that are understandable to the other person. It should be clearly organized and well expressed and may be composed of both verbal and nonverbal

TABLE 4–1 MODES OF COMMUNICATION IN THE DENTAL HYGIENE PROCESS

Dental Hygiene Process	Modes of Communication
Assessment	
Gathering information related to the current status of client	Interviewing for health, dental, and sociocultural histories, details of oral hygiene behaviors Intraoral and extraoral examinations (using visual, tactile, olfactory, and auditory methods) Observing nonverbal behavior
Dental Hygiene Diagnosis	
Identifying human need deficits that require dental hygiene care	Written analysis and assessment of findings Discussion with collaborating dentist Discussion with other healthcare providers, e.g., physician of record Discussion of oral health findings with client
Planning	
Determining appropriate dental hygiene interventions and referrals	Discussion with client to set goals and to determine methods of implementing dental hygiene care and an oral hygiene regimen Discussion with collaborating dentist and other members of the health team Written documentation of plan; obtaining informed consent
Implementation	
Providing dental hygiene care	Interacting with client during the delivery of dental hygiene interventions Oral health teaching Written documentation of services rendered
Evaluation	
Evaluating outcomes of dental hygiene care	Obtaining verbal and nonverbal feedback from client Recording results of previous dental hygiene care including oral health education Documentation of treatment outcomes

Adapted from Potter PA, Perry AG: *Fundamentals of nursing: Concepts, process, and practice,* ed 3, St Louis, 1993, Mosby.

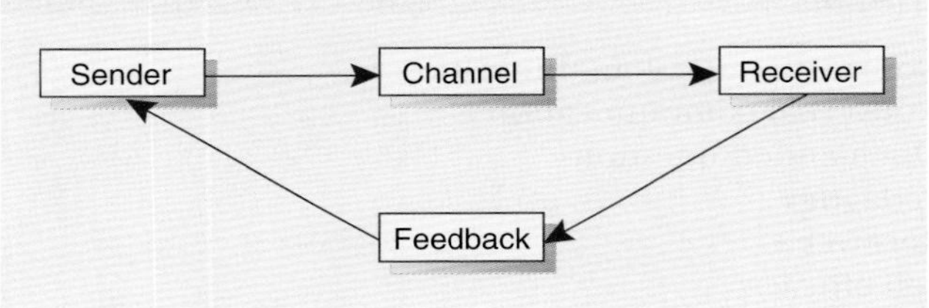

FIGURE 4–1 ✦ Basic communication model.

content. The message is sent via a channel that involves visual, auditory, and tactile senses. For example, facial expression uses a visual channel, spoken words use an auditory channel, and touch uses a tactile channel. The *receiver* is the person who accepts the message and deciphers its meaning, a process known as decoding. The receiver must share a common language with the sender to decode the message accurately. Communication is most effective when the receiver and the sender accurately perceive the meaning of one another's messages.

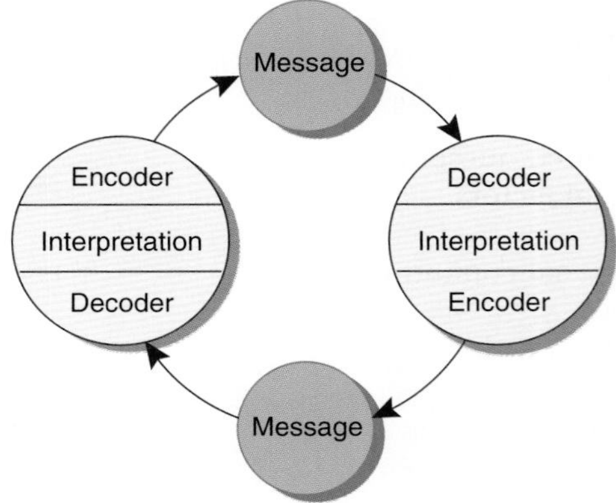

FIGURE 4–2 ✦ Wilbur Schramm feedback model. *(Adapted from Schramm W: How communication works. In Schramm W, ed:* The process and effects of mass communication, *Urbana, Ill, 1955, University of Illinois Press.)*

Feedback

The dynamic process of communication does not generally stop with one encoded and decoded message. The receiver is prompted to respond and provides a feedback message. The receiver then becomes the sender and the cycle repeats itself. The feedback model of communication illustrates how each person has an encoding and a decoding role in the communication process (Figure 4–2). In a social situation, both persons assume equal responsibilities to seek openness and clarification. In the dental hygienist–client relationship, however, the dental hygienist assumes primary responsibility. Dental hygienists need to seek verbal and nonverbal feedback to make sure good communication has occurred. Message transmission is influenced by the sender's and receiver's physical and developmental status, perceptions, values, emotions, knowledge, sociocultural background, roles, and environment. These factors are discussed in the following section.

FACTORS THAT AFFECT INTERPERSONAL COMMUNICATION

Many contextual factors influence interpersonal communication. *Contextual factors* include the environment, the internal factors of the sender and receiver, the nature of their relationship, the situation prompting communication, and the sociocultural factors present that influence interpretation of the message (see Contextual Factors Influencing Communication).[1]

Environmental Factors

The physical surroundings in which communication takes place influence the communication process. For example, people are more likely to communicate effectively in an environment that is comfortable. Factors such as lighting, heating, ventilation, and acoustics may affect the communication process. In the oral healthcare setting, confidentiality may be important if clients are revealing sensitive information about their health. A bustling environment may pose annoying distractions that could block communication.

Internal and Relationship Factors

A person's perceptions, knowledge, values, emotions, and level of need fulfillment influence the way messages are sent and received.[1]

PERCEPTIONS. Perceptions can vary greatly from person to person. One individual's analysis of a situation may differ entirely from another's, even though all basic elements are the same. As an example, it is possible for a dental hygienist to take a very aggressive approach to oral health education. The hygienist may communicate strong demands for client response and loud, clear warnings about the progression of disease if recommendations are not followed. Some clients may perceive the dental hygienist as an authority figure they can respect and respond to very favorably. Others, however, may be offended, perceive the dental hygienist as "pushy" and judgmental, and have a generally adverse reaction to the hygienist's attempts to influence their behavior or health.

Perceptions are formed based on past experience and are difficult to change. If clients had previous contact with a dental hygienist who communicated respect and warmth, they would be more likely to respond well to the hygienist's attempt to resolve a health issue that has become more pressing. When a hygienist takes an aggressive stance with a new client, however, the risk of blocked communication from the client's negative perception of the dental hygienist is great.

VALUES. Values are personal beliefs that may have moral and ethical implications. Whatever we consider important in our lives influences the way we communicate our ideas and feelings. Each individual has a unique set of values that has been shaped by personal experiences. The hygienist can influence the communication process by exercising tolerance and understanding for the wide differences of opinion that exist.

Not all clients value oral health. Individuals have reasons, both known and unknown, for holding their respective values. A person from an impoverished background may have to prioritize values to survive. Oral health and education may not be highly valued when

Contextual Factors Influencing Communication

Psychophysiologic Context

The internal factors influencing communication:

- ✦ Physiologic status (e.g., pain, hunger)
- ✦ Emotional status (e.g., anxiety, anger)
- ✦ Growth and development status (e.g., age)
- ✦ Unmet needs (e.g., emotional stress, physical pain)
- ✦ Attitudes, values, and beliefs (e.g., meaning of oral health)
- ✦ Perceptions and personality (e.g., optimist/pessimist, introvert/extrovert)
- ✦ Self-concept and self-esteem (e.g., positive or negative)

Situational Context

The reason for the communication:

- ✦ Information exchange
- ✦ Goal achievement
- ✦ Problem resolution
- ✦ Expression of feelings

Relational Context

The nature of the relationship between the participants:

- ✦ Social, helping, or working relationship
- ✦ Level of trust between participants
- ✦ Level of self-disclosure between participants
- ✦ Shared history of participants
- ✦ Balance of power and control

Environmental Context

The physical surroundings in which communication takes place:

- ✦ Privacy level
- ✦ Noise level
- ✦ Comfort and safety level
- ✦ Distraction level

Cultural Context

The sociocultural elements that affect the interaction:

- ✦ Educational level of participants
- ✦ Language and self-expression patterns
- ✦ Customs and expectations

Adapted from Potter PA, Perry AG: *Fundamentals of nursing,* ed 5, St Louis, 2001, Mosby.

food, shelter, and clothing are not readily available. On high school campuses, a sugar-free diet may not be valued when candy and soft-drink machines beckon. Water fluoridation may not be valued by people who have been deluged with information from antifluoridationists.

Values can be changed, but experts suggest that they are slow to form and to change. For value change to occur in the oral healthcare environment,[1] oral healthcare professionals must:

- Be aware of their own values and how they affect the choices they make in planning and implementing oral health behavior change programs
- Understand the client's values through careful observation and analysis of behavior
- Avoid imposing their values on a client who has a different set of values

Sometimes client values related to oral health and disease can be changed by education. The methods used to obtain change and the degree of success are dependent on how wide the gap is between the desired value and the client's current value.

EMOTIONS. Do not underestimate the influence of emotions in everyday communication. Emotions are strong feelings people have about other people, places, and things in their environment. Fear, wonder, love, sorrow, and shame are examples of a few strong human emotions that touch all individuals at some time in their lives.

Hygienists who are empathetic may become emotionally involved in their clients' lives. Dental hygiene clients may have serious general health problems that are causing them grief and suffering. The hygienist should be compassionate, but must act professionally throughout the process of care.

In contrast, emotions that are rooted in the hygienist's own personal life should not interfere with client care. For example, the following is an interesting hypothetical situation:[1]

SCENARIO 1

A young hygienist has had an argument with her husband before coming to work. Her husband is just out of law school and establishing his practice. The hygienist's income is needed for the family's survival. Her husband has proposed that they begin having children. The hygienist knows that she and her husband would have difficulty rearing a family now, particularly since she would soon have to take a leave from work.

The hygienist goes to work angered by her husband's lack of understanding. The first client she sees is a 24-year-old mother of three who is divorced and living on welfare. The hygienist cannot allow herself to transfer her anger at her husband to the client's situation. This would prevent her from understanding this client as an individual. If the hygienist is to communicate effectively with the client, she must be aware of her emotions.

KNOWLEDGE. Communication can be hindered when levels of knowledge differ between the participants. Recipients of oral healthcare may be highly educated but have an area of expertise quite outside the realm of oral health. A highly technical vocabulary is inappropriate with a client unless terms are carefully explained. Most clients have no need to distinguish between the mesials and distals of their teeth. This terminology, however, is essential in professional communication and is commonplace for members of the oral healthcare team. If the dental hygienist uses language the client cannot understand, or "talks down" to the client, the hygienist loses that client's attention and cooperation and lessens the chances that goals will be achieved. The effective dental hygienist monitors client feedback to guide the appropriate level of language usage.

Sociocultural Background

Sociocultural differences are important in social interaction and communication. A dental hygienist who has a broad understanding of cultural diversity is better prepared to communicate with clients from varying backgrounds (see Chapter 5).

FORMS OF COMMUNICATION

Interpersonal communication is never static, but rather is a dynamic, ongoing process. Messages may be verbal or nonverbal. In nonprofessional communication people rarely analyze the meaning of every gesture or word. In the professional role, however, the dental hygienist must use critical thinking to focus on each aspect of communication to ensure that interactions are purposeful and effective.

Verbal Communication

Using the spoken word to convey a message is *verbal communication.* The most important aspects of verbal communication are vocabulary, intonation, clarity, and brevity.[1]

VOCABULARY. For communication to be successful, sender and receiver must be able to translate each other's words. Dental jargon sounds like a foreign language to most clients and should be used only with other oral healthcare professionals. Technical terms should be simplified to an appropriate level to enable clients to know what the dental hygienist is saying. If clients do not understand, they often will tune out and a total breakdown of communication will result. By using simple, common language devoid of all superfluous terminology, the hygienist will be easily understood and is more likely to send accurate, straightforward, meaningful information. When dental hygienists provide care to clients who speak a different language, an interpreter usually is needed.

INTONATION. *Intonation* is the modulation of the voice. The whisper of confidentiality, the rising crescendo of anger, and the dull tones of despair are examples of how tone of voice dramatically affect's a message's meaning.[2] The dental hygienist must be aware of voice tone to avoid sending unintended messages. Moreover, clients' voice tone often provides valuable information about their emotional state.

CLARITY. Communication is enhanced when messages sent are simple, brief, and direct. Speaking slowly, enunciating clearly, providing examples to make explanations easier to understand, and repeating the most important part of the message all help to achieve clarity. Using short sentences and familiar words to express ideas simply enhances clarity. For example, asking "Where is your pain?" is better than saying "Please point out to me the location of your discomfort."[1]

Nonverbal Communication

Nonverbal communication is the use of body language rather than words to transmit a message. Effective nonverbal communication complements and strengthens the message conveyed by verbal communication so that the receiver is less likely to misinterpret the message.

Nonverbal communication includes body movement such as facial expression, eye behavior, gestures, posture and gait, and touch. Because body language is hard to control, it often reveals true feelings. However, it takes practice, concentration, and sensitivity to others for the dental hygienist to become an astute observer of body language. For example, there probably is something wrong with a client who says she is "fine," but is wringing her hands. Dental hygienists also should be aware of their own body language to avoid sending mixed messages to clients. Saying "It's good to see you" while wearing a frown does not establish trust and may cause anxiety. To facilitate communication, various aspects of body language are discussed in the following sections.

FACIAL EXPRESSION. The most expressive part of the body is the face. Facial expression often reveals thoughts and feelings and conveys emotions such as anger, fear, sadness, surprise, happiness, and disgust. Clients closely watch the facial expression of the dental hygienist. A dental hygienist may frown when she or he is concentrating, and a client may interpret the facial expression as anger or disgust. Although it is hard to control facial expressions, the dental hygienist should avoid showing shock or disgust in the client's presence.

EYE BEHAVIOR. Eye behavior can be discussed separately from facial features and body movements, but obviously the messages being sent depend on all behaviors collectively. Generally, in Western culture we are told to make eye contact with people as we speak to them. Eye contact is often made before the first spoken word. Thus, it is the first message sent when two people meet. The eye can convey trust, interest, or attention. Eye contact is avoided when we feel uncomfortable and maintained steadily when we are taking an offensive as opposed to a defensive approach to someone.

Along with the muscles of the forehead and the eyebrows, the eyes are extremely expressive. Raising an eyebrow can imply a question. Raising both eyebrows may indicate shock or surprise. Narrowed eyes may suggest skepticism, whereas widely open eyes show amazement.

A dental hygienist works in close proximity to a client's eyes and should always monitor them for nonverbal messages that convey pain or discomfort. Additionally, the dental hygienist's eyes are likely to be watched by the client for signs of approval, disapproval, kindness, or displeasure. A face mask hides most of the hygienist's face; therefore, eyes become an even more important source of expression and communication.

GESTURES. *Gesture* usually refers to movement by the arms, hands, head, or possibly the whole body. These movements may reveal much about a person's feelings. For example, a client's hands clenching the arm of the dental unit is a cue that he or she is experiencing pain or stress.

POSTURE AND GAIT. Posture and body movement may be considered another category of gesture. The way a person moves can tell us whether that person is comfortable or uncomfortable, bold or timid. A shift in posture can be an indication of a changing emotional state. Movement toward someone suggests trust and liking. Movement away sends a negative message. The speed at which people move can mean something definite. A slow movement suggests uncertainty; a rapid movement can indicate eagerness, playfulness, or possibly impatience. Posture is affected by a person's size and overall physical appearance. An erect posture and a sharp, snappy step can do much to draw respect to a person of any size.

TOUCH. Touching is one of the most sensitive means of communication and is most closely related to the human need for freedom from stress. Touch can be reassuring in some contexts. A hand gently placed on a shoulder may mean more to a client than any verbal expression of support (Figure 4–3). It is important to note, however, that people have different attitudes toward being touched. Some are not accustomed to it and may cringe or pull away as the hygienist attempts to comfort them. Touch should be used discriminately to avoid misinterpretation.

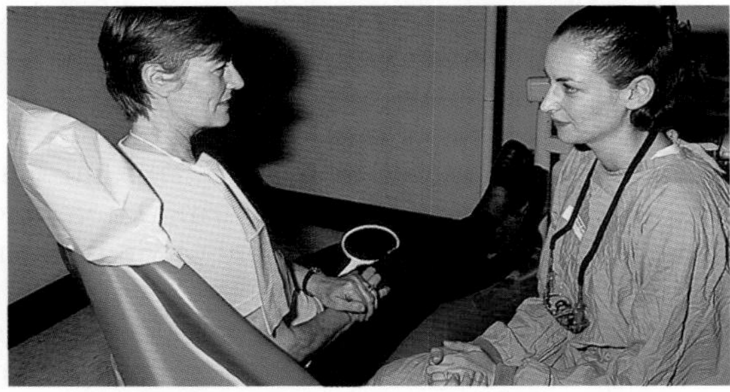

FIGURE 4–3 ✦ Dental hygienist using eye contact to communicate reassurance.

The nature of the dental hygiene process of care requires touching clients. The way in which the hygienist touches the client can communicate feelings about the client and the practice of dental hygiene. Rough, jerking movements may send a message of careless indifference, resulting in uncooperative behavior from a client. Accidental touching, such as bumping a person's nose or hitting his or her front teeth with the mouth mirror, also can carry a negative message such as carelessness or haste. A professional, careful approach to touching is appreciated and respected by clients.

PROFESSIONAL DENTAL HYGIENE RELATIONSHIPS

The dental hygienist applies knowledge, understanding of human needs, communication, and a commitment to ethical behavior to create professional relationships with clients. Having a philosophy based on caring and respect for others helps the dental hygienist to establish helping relationships with clients.

The *CARE principle* is used as a simple mnemonic or memory-assisting technique to identify aspects of care important to effective dental hygienist–client helping relationships:

CARE

C = Comfort
A = Acceptance
R = Responsiveness
E = Empathy

Comfort

Comfort in the mnemonic refers to the hygienist's ability to deal with embarrassing or emotionally painful topics related to a client's health; to be aware of the client's physical and emotional response during dental hygiene care; and to provide verbal support to a client who fears oral healthcare procedures. Aspects of dental hygiene practice related to client comfort and communication include effectively addressing a client's loss of teeth and need to wear a prosthetic appliance, a client's inability to seek oral healthcare because of financial difficulties, a client's fear of injections, and clients' discomfort from having their personal space "invaded" during care.

Personal space is invisible and travels with a person. *Territoriality* refers to the need to maintain and defend one's right to this personal space. During interpersonal communication individuals maintain varying distances between each other depending on their culture, their relationship, and the circumstance. Touching the head and neck area is usually reserved for intimate relationships such as between lovers or a parent and a child. When personal space is violated people often become defensive and communication becomes ineffective. Because dental hygienists work within the client's intimate zone of personal space, it is important to convey professional confidence, gentleness, and respect when doing so. Examples of these actions are listed in Zones of Personal Space and Touch.

To meet the client's human need for freedom from stress, the hygienist strives to keep the client's comfort a top priority.

Acceptance

Acceptance refers to the dental hygienist's ability to accept clients as the people they are without allowing any judgment of the clients' attitudes or feelings to interfere with communication. For example, a client may appear unwilling to assume responsibility for his or her health, and may be critical or untrusting. The client's poor oral health may seem to be self-imposed and related to an unhealthy lifestyle. But the client's appearance and attitudes may have deep cultural roots that are unfamiliar to the hygienist. The dental hygienist must develop an attitude of acceptance toward individuals whose values and sociocultural backgrounds seem unusual or foreign.

Responsiveness

Responsiveness in a healthcare provider is the ability to reply to messages at the very moment they are sent. It requires sensitive alertness to cues that something more

Zones of Personal Space and Touch

Zones of Personal Space

Intimate zone (0 to 18 inches)
- ✦ Performing physical assessment
- ✦ Placing and removing dental napkin or radiation shield
- ✦ Performing intraoral procedures

Personal zone (18 inches to 4 feet)
- ✦ Sitting next to the client's chair
- ✦ Taking the client's health, dental, and personal/social history
- ✦ Providing oral hygiene education to an individual client

Social zone (4 to 12 feet)
- ✦ Sitting at a conference table
- ✦ Conducting a tobacco-cessation support group

Public zone (12 feet and greater)
- ✦ Speaking at a community forum
- ✦ Testifying at a legislative hearing
- ✦ Lecturing to a class of students

Zones of Touch

Social zone (permission not needed)
- ✦ Hands, arms, shoulders, back

Consent and vulnerable zone (permission and special care needed)
- ✦ Mouth, neck, head, face

Adapted from Potter PA, Perry AG: *Fundamentals of nursing,* ed 5, St Louis, 2001, Mosby.

needs to be said. When a client arrives for a dental hygiene appointment and mentions oral discomfort, the comment should be pursued immediately. Scaling and root planing might have been scheduled, but other problems may be an immediate priority and supersede the planned care.

Empathy

Empathy is said to result when we place ourselves in another's "shoes." Empathy means perceiving clients as they see themselves, sensing their hurt or pleasure as they sense it, accepting their feelings, and communicating this understanding of their reality.[1]

In expressing empathy the dental hygienist communicates understanding the importance of the feelings behind a client's statements. Empathy statements are neutral and nonjudgmental. They can be used to establish trust in difficult situations. For example, the dental hygienist might say to an angry client who has lost mobility after a stroke, "It must be very frustrating to know what you want and not be able to do it." This perception of clients' viewpoints helps the dental hygienist to better understand them, their reaction to dental hygiene care, and their capabilities for taking responsibility for their own health.

THERAPEUTIC COMMUNICATION TECHNIQUES

Dental hygiene practice is based on helping relationships. In such relationships the dental hygienist assumes the role of professional helper. The dental hygienist uses therapeutic communication to promote a psychological climate that facilitates positive change and growth.

Therapeutic communication is a process of sending and receiving messages between a client and a healthcare provider that assists the client to make decisions and reach goals related to comfort and health. No single communication technique works with all clients. One individual may be encouraged to express feelings when the dental hygienist is silent, whereas another may need coaxing with active questioning. Practice and experience, based on a strong theoretical foundation, are required for choosing communication techniques to use in different situations. See Therapeutic Communication Techniques for some techniques that can be applied by the dental hygienist.[1]

Therapeutic Communication Techniques

Silence
Attentive listening
Humor
Conveying acceptance
Related questions
Paraphrasing
Clarifying
Focusing
Stating observations
Offering information
Summarizing

Silence

Silence can be used effectively in communication because it provides an opportunity for the senders and receivers of messages to gather and reorganize their thoughts and feelings. During silent moments, nonverbal messages such as loss of eye contact or a wrinkled brow can be sent. Remaining silent may be uncomfortable, but adhering patiently to silence demonstrates the hygienist's willingness to listen and encourages clients to share their thoughts. Skill and timing are required to use silence effectively. The tendency for some is to want to break the silence too soon. Poor timing can prematurely interrupt clients' efforts in choosing words and frustrate their attempts to communicate.

The nature of dental hygiene care often precludes talking by the client. A common complaint, usually shared good-naturedly among clients, is that their dental hygienist asks them questions when the hygienist's hands are in their mouths! This typical scenario is unfair to the client. Common courtesy dictates that immediately upon asking a question, the hygienist removes hands, instruments, and saliva ejectors from the client's mouth to allow the client an opportunity to respond through speaking, not just grunting.

Listening Attentively

Caring involves an interpersonal interaction that is much more than two persons talking back and forth. In a caring relationship, the dental hygienist establishes trust, opens lines of communication, and listens to what the client has to say. Listening attentively is key because it conveys to clients that they have the hygienist's full attention and interest. Listening to the meaning of what a client says helps create a mutual relationship.

The dental hygienist indicates interest by appearing natural and relaxed and facing the client with good eye contact. Whatever the services being rendered, the client should remain the center of attention, with the hygienist's ears available to evaluate and respond. Interpersonal attending skills shown in Table 4–2 facilitate active listening and communication.

Conveying Acceptance

Conveying acceptance requires a tolerant, nonjudgmental attitude toward clients. An open, accepting approach is needed to foster a helping relationship between hygienist and client. Care should be taken to avoid nonverbal behavior that may be offensive or that may prevent free-flowing communication. Gestures such as frowning, rolling eyes upward, or shaking the head may communicate disagreement or disapproval to the client. The dental hygienist should show willingness to listen to the client's viewpoint and provide feedback that indicates understanding and acceptance of the person.

TABLE 4–2 CHECKLIST OF INTERPERSONAL ATTENDING

Skill Area	Criteria
Eye contact	Listener consistently focuses on the face and eyes of the speaker
Body orientation	Listener orients shoulders and legs toward the speaker
Posture	Listener maintains slight forward lean, arms maintained in a relaxed position
Silence	Listener avoids interrupting the speaker, uses periods of silence to facilitate continued communication
Following cues	Listener uses verbal and nonverbal cues to facilitate communication and indicate interest and attention
Distance	Listener maintains distance of 3 to 4 feet from speaker
Distractions	Listener avoids distracting behaviors such as pencil tapping, looking at a clock, and extraneous movements

Modified from Geboy MJ: *Communication and behavior management in dentistry,* Baltimore, 1985, Williams & Wilkins.

Humor

Humor can help decrease client anxiety and embarrassment. Humor is a communication technique that should be used comfortably and naturally with clients of all ages and stages of development (Figure 4–4). The therapeutic advantages of humor and laughter have been documented. Laughter decreases serum control levels, increases immune activity, and stimulates endorphin release from the hypothalamus. In so doing, it relieves stress-related tension and pain. Cousins described the role of humor in his recovery from two life-threatening illnesses.[3] His experience suggests that laughter and positive emotions are vital to the success of any medical treatment as well as to life in general.

Healthcare personnel and facilities can be perceived as frightening by clients of all ages. Humor as a technique of communication can put people at ease. Even a simple smile can help establish a warm social bond. In her book *Communication in Health Care,* Collins states, "humor has childlike qualities of playfulness. If one can be playful, one still has vestiges of youth and vigor."[4] The unexpected, the incongruous, the pun, and the exaggeration or understatement are examples of humor that can be effective with both younger and older clients.

Asking Questions

One of the most critical and valuable tools in the dental hygienists' arsenal of communication skills is the art of questioning. Although there are many types of questions, there are only two basic forms: closed-ended questions, which are directive, and open-ended questions, which are nondirective.

CLOSED-ENDED QUESTIONS. *Closed-ended questions* require narrow answers to specific queries. The answer to

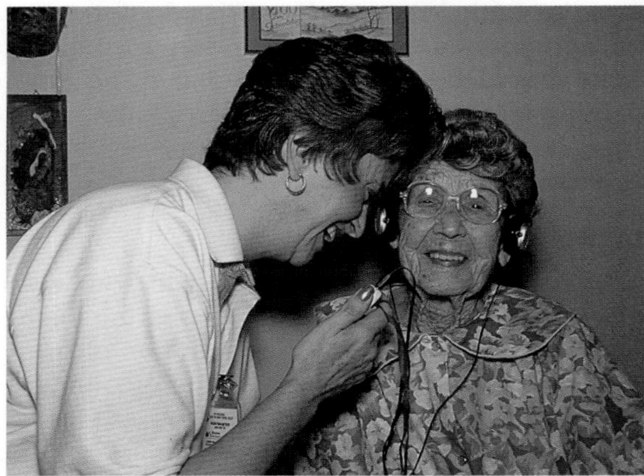

FIGURE 4–4 ✦ Sharing a joke or laughing with clients can assist in reducing stress and support a therapeutic relationship.

these questions is usually "yes" or "no" or some other brief answer. An example is, "Do you want to bleach your teeth?"

OPEN-ENDED QUESTIONS. *Open-ended questions* are generally used to elicit a wide range of responses on a broad topic. Open-ended questions usually:

- Cannot be answered by a single word or a simple "yes" or "no"
- Begin with *what, how,* or *why*
- Do not lead the client toward a specific direction
- Increase dialogue by drawing out the client's feelings or opinions

Open-ended questions are usually more effective than questions that require a simple "yes" or "no" answer. Open-ended questioning allows clients to elaborate and show their genuine feelings by bringing up whatever they think is important (see Examples of Open-ended Questions and Subcategories of Open-ended Questions that Enhance Communication). Skillful questioning by the dental hygienist promotes communication.

Paraphrasing

Paraphrasing means restating or summarizing what the client has just said. Through paraphrasing the client receives a signal that his or her message has been received and understood and is prompted to continue a communication effort by providing further information. The client may say, "I don't understand how I could have periodontal disease. My teeth and gums feel fine. I have absolutely no pain." The hygienist could paraphrase the statement by saying, "You're not convinced that you have

Examples of Open-ended Questions

How do you feel about your oral health?
What are you currently doing each day to care for your teeth?
Why do you feel you will never be able to floss regularly?

periodontal disease or any gum problems because you have no discomfort?" The client may respond, "Right, I just can't believe anything is wrong with my mouth." By actively listening and paraphrasing, the dental hygienist's response allows further analysis of the problem and opens the conversation for communication and problem solving.

The dental hygienist must actively listen and analyze messages received, however, so that the paraphrase is not only an accurate account of what the client actually says, but also of what the client feels. For example, if a client is sending verbal or nonverbal messages of anger or frustration about being told to floss more, the dental hygienist could say, "It sounds like this situation has really upset you and that you are frustrated with me for not recognizing your efforts." This response encourages clients to communicate further about health problems. Passive listening or silence on the part of the dental hygienist, with no attempt to decode the message, could result in an uncomfortable impasse in the communication process.

Clarifying

At times the message sent by the client may be vague. When clarification is needed, the discussion should be temporarily stopped until confusing or conflicting statements have been understood. For example, consider the following scenario in which a client has come to the oral care environment for oral prophylaxis.

SCENARIO 2

Client: My mother had pyorrhea and lost all her teeth at a young age. I'm sure it's hereditary. I can only hope to stall it off.

Hygienist: Mrs. Thompson, are you having some problem with your teeth or gums now?

In responding this way the hygienist is trying to get clarification. The client's rush of words seems to be related to her own problems, but the hygienist cannot be sure until the client states it clearly (see Subcategories of Open-ended Questions that Enhance Communication). In addition, the hygienist should be aware that statements made to the client may need clarification. In order to fulfill their human need for conceptualization and problem solving, clients need to understand why they are asked to comply with a specific home care regimen. In the following example, the dental hygienist has completed therapeutic scaling and root planing on the mandibular left quadrant, which has been anesthetized.

SCENARIO 3

Hygienist: Mr. Johnson, after you leave, try not to chew on your left side for awhile.

Client: Do you mean today or for several days?

Hygienist: Oh no, I just mean for a few hours.

Client: What might happen if I do chew on that side? Will it hurt my teeth or gums?

Hygienist: Oh no, I was referring to your anesthesia. I'm afraid you might bite your cheeks or tongue if you chew on that side since everything is numb. The numbness should be completely gone by about 5:00 P.M.

The more specific the hygienist can be, the clearer the message to the client.

Focusing

Sometimes when clients discuss health-related issues the messages become redundant or rambling. Important information may not surface because the client is off on a tangent. Dental hygienists ask questions to clarify when they are unsure of what the client is talking about. In focusing, however, the hygienist knows what the client is talking about, but is having trouble keeping the client on the subject so that data gathering and assessment can be completed. In such cases, the dental hygienist encourages verbalization, but steers the discussion back on track as a technique to improve communication. Rather than asking a question, a gentle command may be in order,

SUBCATEGORIES OF OPEN-ENDED QUESTIONS THAT ENHANCE COMMUNICATION

Type	Purpose	Example
Clarifying questions	To seek verification of the content and/or feeling of your client's message	If I am hearing correctly, your major concerns are . . .. Is that so? From what you are telling me, I get the impression you are frustrated, or am I misreading your feelings?
Developmental questions	To draw out a broad response on a narrow topic	Would you please elaborate on that point? Can you give me an example of what you mean by that?
Directive questions	To change the conversation from one topic to another	What was the other issue you wanted to discuss with me?
Third-party questions	To probe indirectly by relating to a client how others feel about a situation and then asking the client to give an opinion or reaction	A lot of people feel our fees are reasonable. What's your opinion?
Testing questions	To assess a client's level of agreement or disagreement about a specific issue	How does that strike you? Do you think you could live with that?

such as "Please point to the tooth that seems to be causing your discomfort," or "Show me exactly what you do when you floss your back teeth."

Stating Observations

Clients may be unaware of the nonverbal messages they are sending. When a client is asked, "How are you, Mrs. Jones?" as a friendly greeting, she may respond, "Oh, just fine." Her appearance, gait, and mannerisms may indicate something different. She may look slightly unkempt, walk with a slow shuffle, and display generally unenthusiastic gestures and facial expressions. When nonverbal cues conflict with the verbal message, stating a simple straightforward observation may open the lines of communication. The hygienist may say, "You appear very tired, Mrs. Jones." This is likely to cause the person to volunteer more information about how she feels without need for further questioning, focusing, or clarifying.

To promote positive communication, however, the dental hygienist must use respectful language. The client may feel sensitive about how observations are worded. Saying you look "tired" is different from saying you look "haggard," which could embarrass or anger a person. Other observations that can soften a client's response are stating that teeth are crowded rather than crooked, that a troublesome tongue is muscular not fat, and that gingiva is pigmented not discolored.

Offering Information

Providing clients with detailed information facilitates communication. Although providing information may not be enough to motivate people to change health behaviors, clients have a right to receive information based on the hygienist's expertise so that they can make health-related decisions based on that information. In any setting, a dental hygienist maintains a professional obligation to provide health information to all clients, not just to individuals who request information.

Summarizing

Summarizing points discussed at a regularly scheduled appointment focuses attention on the major points of the communicative interaction. For example, the dental hygienist may conclude the appointment with, "Today we discussed the purpose of therapeutic scaling and root planing and the periodontal disease process, and we practiced flossing technique. Remember, you decided to floss daily and to try to slip the floss carefully down below the gum line." If the client is coming in for multiple appointments to receive quadrant or sextant scaling and root planing, the discussion from the previous appointment should be summarized before proceeding with new information. Documentation within the client's chart at each appointment should reflect topics discussed at each appointment as related to the client's goals.

The summary serves as a review of the key aspects of the information presented so that the client can ask for clarification. Adding new information in the summary may confuse the client; however, a comment about what will be discussed at the next appointment is appropriate. Such a statement might be, "At your next appointment, we will talk about use of the Perio Aid and continue discussion of the periodontal disease process."

FACTORS THAT INHIBIT COMMUNICATION

The dental hygienist may unintentionally impede communication. Nontherapeutic communication is a process of sending and receiving messages that does not help clients make decisions or reach goals related to their comfort and health (see Factors that Inhibit Communication). These nontherapeutic communication techniques should be avoided by the dental hygienist because they inhibit communication.[1]

Giving an Opinion

A helping relationship should foster the clients' ability to make their own decisions about health. A hygienist may be tempted to offer an opinion, which may weaken the clients' autonomy and jeopardize their need for responsibility for oral health. Clients may volunteer personal information about themselves and may ask for the hygienist's opinion. It is best in such a situation to acknowledge the individual's feelings, but to avoid the transfer of decision making from client to hygienist. The following scenario is a hypothetical situation presenting two possible responses by the dental hygienist in an interaction with a client.

SCENARIO 4

Hygienist: Mrs. Smith, you look troubled today.

Client: Well, actually, I'm feeling quite down in the dumps. Yesterday was my birthday and I didn't hear a word from my daughter. I'm sure you wouldn't do such a thing to your mother!

Hygienist: (Response #1) Heavens, no! How terribly inconsiderate of her.

The hygienist might have answered differently:

Hygienist: (Response #2) You seem to feel really disappointed. I'm sorry you're so distressed.

The latter response by the dental hygienist recognizes feelings without expressing an opinion that could make the client feel worse by confirming a doubt she has about her daughter, as in the first response.

Factors that Inhibit Communication

Giving an opinion
Offering false reassurance
Being defensive
Showing approval or disapproval
Asking why
Changing the subject inappropriately

Offering False Reassurance

Hygienists may at times offer reassurance when it is not well grounded. It is natural to want to alleviate the client's anxiety and fear, but reassurance may promise something that cannot occur. For example, the dental hygienist should not promise clients that they will experience no discomfort in an anticipated dental treatment. Although the dental hygienist may feel confident that the oral surgeon or periodontist is competent and kind, discomfort may be unavoidable. A person who is distraught about having periodontal disease should not be told, "There's nothing to worry about. You'll be fine." Indeed, depending on the amount of bone loss present and disease susceptibility of the client, the periodontist may not be able to control the disease, even with extensive therapy. The following scenario illustrates how the dental hygienist can listen and acknowledge a client's feelings without offering false assurance that the problem is a simple one.

SCENARIO 5

Mrs. Frank, a 75-year-old woman, has been told by the dentist that her remaining teeth are hopeless and must be extracted for a full denture placement. The hygienist enters the room as the dentist leaves.

Mrs. Frank: I can't believe this is happening to me. I don't deserve it. I've tried to take good care of my teeth. I'm so distressed. Oh, I'm sorry, I know you don't want to hear about my problems.

Hygienist: Mrs. Frank, I am interested in your feelings about this.

Being Defensive

When clients criticize services or personnel, it is easy for the hygienist to become defensive. A defensive posture may threaten the relationship between dental hygienist and client by communicating to clients that they do not have a right to express their opinions.

SCENARIO 6

Mr. Tucker has been a regular client in the dental practice for many years. At the last appointment, the dental hygienist noted a 2-mm circumscribed white lesion in the retromolar area. Mr. Tucker was a former smoker, and the dentist referred him to an oral surgeon for consultation and possible biopsy of the lesion. The following describes the hygienist–client interaction when Mr. Tucker returns for his periodontal maintenance appointment.

Client: I hope I don't have to see Dr. Herman today.

Hygienist: What's wrong, Mr. Tucker? Dr. Herman usually sees you after your periodontal maintenance care.

Client: He sent me to the oral surgeon and it was a complete waste of my time.

Hygienist: Of course it wasn't. Dr. Herman is an excellent dentist.

Client: You may think so but he didn't send you for a biopsy for no reason.

Hygienist: Mr. Tucker, that lesion looked very unusual. I'm sure Dr. Herman made a good decision in sending you.

In the preceding scenario the dental hygienist's response ignores the client's real feelings and hurts future rapport and communication with him. The hygienist should use the therapeutic communication techniques of active listening to verify what the client has to say and to learn why he is upset or angry. Active listening does not mean that the dental hygienist agrees with what is being said, but rather conveys interest in what the client is saying. This latter approach is illustrated in the following scenario.

SCENARIO 7

Client: I hope I don't have to see Dr. Herman today.

Hygienist: You sound upset. Can you tell me something about it?

Client: I just don't think he should have sent me to that oral surgeon.

Hygienist: You think the visit there was unnecessary?

Client: Yes, I didn't mind the biopsy, the results were negative, but first, I got lost trying to find the place, then I couldn't find a parking place, then they made me wait for 2 hours and, finally, they charged me a fortune for the procedure. Actually, I didn't mind the cost as much as the inconvenience.

Some care in listening led to discovery of the source of the client's anger, which was the inconvenience of a particular oral surgeon's location, parking, and office procedures. By avoiding defensiveness and applying active listening and paraphrasing, the hygienist allowed Mr. Tucker to vent his anger. Therefore, communication was facilitated, not blocked.

Showing Approval or Disapproval

Showing either approval or disapproval in certain situations can be detrimental to the communication process. Excessive praise may imply to the client that the hygienist thinks the behavior being praised is the only acceptable one. Often, clients may reveal information about themselves because they are seeking a way to express their feelings; they are not necessarily looking for approval or disapproval from the dental hygienist. In the following scenario, the hygienist's response cannot be interpreted as neutral.

SCENARIO 8

Client: I've been walking to my dental appointments for years. My daughter offered to drive me today and I accepted. She feels the walk has become too much for me.

Hygienist: I'm so glad you didn't walk over. You definitely made the right decision. Your daughter should drive you to your appointments from now on.

The discussion in Scenario 8 is likely to stop with the dental hygienist's statements. The client probably sees the hygienist's viewpoint as supportive of her daughter's. Perhaps the woman is better off having her daughter drive her. It is also possible that she is capable of walking, likes the exercise, and enjoys the independence of getting to her own appointments. The dental hygienist's strong statements of approval may inhibit further communication.

Behaviors that communicate disapproval cause clients to feel rejected, and their desire to interact further with the dental hygienist may be weakened. Disapproving statements may be issued by a dental hygienist who is not thinking carefully about how the client may react. The following scenario exemplifies a dental hygienist's response that communicates hasty disapproval.

SCENARIO 9

Client: I've been working so hard at flossing! I only missed two or three times last week.

Hygienist: Two or three days without flossing! You'll have to do better than that. Your inflammation will not improve at that rate.

Instead of this response the dental hygienist might have said, "You're making progress. Tell me more about your activities on those three days when you weren't able to floss. Perhaps together we could find a better way of integrating flossing into your lifestyle."

Asking Why

When people are puzzled by another's behavior, the natural reaction is to ask "why?" When the dental hygienists discover that clients have not been following recommendations, they may feel a natural inclination to ask why this has occurred. Clients may interpret such a question as an accusation. They may feel resentment, leading to withdrawal and a lack of motivation to communicate further with the dental hygienist.

Efforts to search for reasons why the client has not practiced the oral healthcare behaviors as recommended can be facilitated by simply rephrasing a probing "why" question. For example, rather than saying, "Why haven't you used the oral irrigator?" the hygienist might say, "You haven't used the oral irrigator. Is something wrong?" For anxious clients, rather than asking, "Why are you upset?" the hygienist might say, "You seem upset. Would you like to talk about it?

Changing the Subject Inappropriately

Changing the subject abruptly shows a lack of empathy and could be interpreted as rude. In addition, it prevents the client from discussing an issue that may have important implications for care. The following is a sample client–dental hygienist interaction.

SCENARIO 10

Hygienist: Hello, Mrs. Johnson. How are you today?

Client: Not too well. My gums are really sore.

Hygienist: Well, let's get you going. We have a lot to do today.

The dental hygienist's response shows insensitivity and an unwillingness to discuss Mrs. Johnson's complaint. It is possible that the client has a periodontal or periapical abscess or some other serious problem. The dental hygienist is remiss in ignoring the client's attempt to communicate a problem. Communication has been stalled and the client's oral health jeopardized. The client should be given an opportunity to elaborate on the message she is trying to send.

THEORIES OF MOTIVATION

Influencing people to comply with or adhere to regimens for oral hygiene care is one of the major challenges facing a dental hygienist. Compliance with oral hygiene recommendations can be interrupted by lapses or temporary slips back to one's former behavior. Occasional lapses are normal and may not necessarily threaten oral health.[5] But the complete breakdown of an individual's bacterial plaque control program must be prevented. The possibility of lapsing should be discussed with the clients so that they understand that occasional slips do not have to result in a total relapse to their previous status.

In the communication process a dental hygienist is constantly striving to influence the client's motivation to perform oral health behaviors. *Motivation* can be defined as the impulse that leads an individual to action. Many theories of motivation have been formulated and can be appropriately applied to client motivation in the healthcare environment.

Self-efficacy Theory

Self-efficacy, also known as self-confidence, is the belief in one's ability to perform specific behaviors.[6] *Self-efficacy theory* maintains that self-confidence about being able to perform a behavior has a strong influence on the ability to perform that behavior. Based on self-efficacy theory, motivation to brush and floss should be stronger when clients feel confident that they know how to floss and have the skill to do so. An important role of the dental hygienist is to help clients acquire this confidence by training them to perform personal oral hygiene skills and by providing them with ongoing support and encouragement.

Moreover, when others in the client's environment, especially those seen as similar to the client, have performed a particular task well and attested to their own successes, the client is led to think, "If they can do it, I can too." Thus, knowledge of the successes of peers in their endeavors to improve health behavior can strongly influence the client's feeling of self-efficacy to accomplish similar tasks.

Anxiety is a physiologic state that can result in negative self-appraisal. Repeated failure creates anxiety and can result in a disintegration of motivation. Past learning experiences that have been negative and resulted in failure yield feelings of inadequacy and fear of future failure. This lack of self-confidence can cause people to avoid activities that they believe will result in failure. This need to avoid failure may prevent a client from any attempt to incorporate new oral health behaviors into a daily effort.

Attribution Theory

Attributions are the explanations individuals give for their performance.[2] *Attribution theory* is a cognitive theory that emphasizes the importance of content of thoughts. What people attribute to their success or failure determines their feelings about themselves, their predictions of success at accomplishing the task, and the probability that they will try harder or not as hard at a task in the future. For example, when people attribute their failure to low ability, they feel depressed, predict that they will fail again, and use less effort in the future. Therefore, attributions affect expectations of success, emotional (affective) reactions, and persistence at future tasks.

If people attribute their success at performing a task to effort, they may feel pleased because effort is something they can control. They will predict that they can succeed in the future if they continue to exert effort and, in fact, will exert more effort in the future.

Moreover, when people perceive their effort to be a stable personality characteristic, they are more likely to feel positive about their successes and increase their effort and persistence in the future. For example, dental hygienists can encourage clients to view their effort-making as a stable characteristic by saying to them, "You are a hard-working person," rather than, "You really worked hard that time." Likewise, clients can be encouraged to think of themselves as conscientious individuals who are concerned about their health on a long-term basis.

The most problematic cycle in education is when learners attribute their lack of success to low ability. This leads to disillusionment and lack of effort toward future tasks. Ability is not within an individual's control. Unlike effort, it is not something that can be manipulated at will.

In addition, in academic settings with children it has been demonstrated that those students with low self-concepts and little confidence in their ability do not easily change their views of themselves. If the student does succeed at a task, the success is a surprise and the student tends to attribute it to luck or task ease.[7] Only with extreme patience and persistence can a teacher help students change effort attributions to change a negative self-concept to a positive one.

Locus of Control

Some clients may blame someone or something else for their poor performance in maintaining oral health. These people believe that external aspects of their environment have control over their failure (or their successes). The counterpart to these individuals is those who believe they hold their fates in their own hands and are responsible for their own actions. They are focused on the internal aspects of themselves and how they can influence their environment.

Psychologists categorize such internal and external personality dispositions under the construct *locus of control*. Much of the research in this area stems from the social learning theory of Rotter.[8] He developed a 23-item internal-external locus of control scale for classification of individuals. Three examples of items on Rotter's scale follow. The respondent reads each statement and selects the statement he or she most agrees with.

1a. Many times I feel that I have little influence over the things that happen to me. (external)
1b. It is impossible for me to believe that chance or luck plays an important role in my life. (internal)
2a. Getting a good job depends mainly on being in the right place at the right time. (external)
2b. Becoming a success is a matter of hard work; luck has little or nothing to do with it. (internal)
3a. Without the right breaks one cannot be an effective leader. (external)
3b. Capable people who fail to become leaders have not taken advantage of their opportunities. (internal)

Individuals classified as having an external locus of control believe that events are caused by factors beyond their control. They may believe that luck, task difficulty, or powerful others determine their future. Individuals classified as having an internal locus of control believe that an outcome is contingent on their own behavior or relatively permanent characteristics such as ability.

Table 4–3 indicates how locus of control can be used to understand client oral health behavior. It suggests some helpful strategies for communicating with clients who fit the locus of control descriptions.[9] Comments by clients that are similar to those suggested in the table can help the dental hygienist determine the client's orientation. Clients who function from an external locus of control often appear to be willing and agreeable, but are unlikely to adhere to recommendations. They may ultimately blame the clinician when their oral hygiene regimen fails. The challenge is for the clinician to redirect clients' perceptions of how effective they can be in achieving health goals by providing feedback that affirms their efficacy. In doing so, the hygienist helps clients to meet their need for responsibility for oral health.

Those individuals who are internally controlled are autonomous people who may follow good oral hygiene practices regardless of the clinician's influence. Some research has shown, however, that clients who are strongly internally controlled may sometimes comply less with professional recommendations. This lack of compliance

TABLE 4–3 INDICATORS OF INTERNAL AND EXTERNAL LOCI OF CONTROL

Internal Locus of Control	External Locus of Control
OWNERSHIP OF SITUATION	
"My teeth are very bad because I never took very good care of them."	"I've always had soft teeth."
"I should have found a dentist who could really help me."	"The dentist I went to didn't care."
"What can I do to keep my teeth?"	"Just take them all out. I know they'll go sooner or later."
NEED FOR INVOLVEMENT IN TREATMENT	
"Now, what will this series of treatments do for me in the long run? And let me see if I have the reasoning clearly understood."	"Just do what you need to do to fix me up."
REACTION TO PROFESSIONAL RECOMMENDATION	
"I'll try it out and see how it works."	"I'll do whatever you say. My teeth will be clean whenever you see me."

From *The Compendium of Continuing Education in Dentistry.* Woodall IR: Patient motivation and locus of control, *Compendium of Continuing Education in Dentistry* 6(suppl 6):147, 1985.

can be attributed to their often sharp consumer sense; they consider the health professional's advice as just another opinion in the broad range of information they constantly seek. They may challenge advice, listen silently, ignore recommendations, or try popular home remedies. They are skeptical but, on the whole, are highly desirable as clients because they are generally responsible, self-motivated individuals who will probably practice preventive measures.

COMMUNICATION, TEACHING, AND LEARNING THROUGH THE LIFE SPAN

The communication and the teaching and learning processes can be integrated in and applied through the life span. *Andragogy* is the term applied to the art and science of helping the older person learn, whereas *pedagogy* is the art and science of teaching children. Pedagogy assumes that the learners are young, dependent recipients of knowledge and that subject matter has been arbitrarily decided on by a teacher who is preparing them for their future. The teacher is the authority in this model and little regard is given to how learners feel about the material or to their contribution in the process. Andragogy, on the other hand, assumes that the initiative to learn comes from the learner who is viewed as entering the learning process with a background of prior knowledge and experience. The teacher is a facilitator who learns along with the student, who in turn benefits from the teacher's contribution. The adult learner has a diverse history of experiences and is, in general, independent and self-directed. Pedagogy assumes that the child learner is moving toward becoming a fully matured human being, whereas andragogy assumes that the learner has arrived at this point.[7] The purpose of this section is to address considerations for communication with persons throughout the life span. Table 4–4 summarizes the key developmental characteristics at different age levels over the life span and those communication techniques appropriate at each level.

PRESCHOOL AND YOUNGER SCHOOL-AGE CHILDREN

Communicating with children requires an understanding of the influence of growth and development on language, thought processes, and motor skills. Children begin development with simple, concrete language and thinking and move toward the more complex and abstract. Communication techniques and teaching methods also can increase in complexity as the child grows older.

Nonverbal communication is more important with preschoolers than it is with the school-age child whose communication is better developed. The preschooler learns through play and enjoys a gamelike atmosphere. Hence, dentists often call the dental engine their "whistle" or the "buzzy bee," and hygienists often refer to their polishing cup as the "whirly bird" and the saliva ejector as "Mr. Thirsty." Imaginary names help lighten the healthcare experience for small children. Oral health professionals are advised to use simple, short sentences, familiar words, and concrete explanations.

The Guidance-Cooperation Model

Five principles for communicating with young children are suggested in the guidance-cooperation model.[10] Because the model is neither permissive nor coercive, it is ideally suited for the preschool or young school-age child. Under this model, health professionals are placed in a parental role whereby the child is expected to respect and cooperate with them. The principles inherent to the guidance-cooperative model follow.

TELL THE CHILD THE GROUND RULES BEFORE AND DURING TREATMENT. Let the child know exactly what is expected of him or her. A comment such as, "You must do exactly as I ask and please keep your hands in your lap like my other helpers," will prepare the child to meet expectations. Structuring time so the child also knows what to expect may be useful. For fluoride treatments, a timer should be set and made visible so the child knows how long it will be before the trays will come out of his or her mouth.

PRAISE ALL COOPERATIVE BEHAVIOR When the child responds to a directive such as "open wide," praise him or her with, "That's good! Thank you!" When the child is

TABLE 4–4 TECHNIQUES FOR COMMUNICATING WITH CLIENTS THROUGH THE LIFE SPAN

Level	Developmental Characteristics	Communication Techniques
Preschoolers	Beginning use of symbols and language; egocentric, focused on self; concrete in thinking and language	Allow child to use his or her five senses to explore oral healthcare environment (handle a mirror, feel a prophy cup, taste and smell fluoride, etc.) Use simple language and concrete, thorough explanations of exactly what is going to happen Let child see and feel cup "going around" or compressed air before putting in his or her mouth
School-age children	Less egocentric; shift to abstract thought emerges, but much thought still concrete	Demonstrate equipment, allow child to question, give simple explanations of procedures
Adolescents	Concrete thinking evolves to more complex abstraction; can formulate alternative hypotheses in problem solving; may revert to childish manner at times; usually enjoy adult attention	Allow self-expression and avoid being judgmental Give thorough, detailed answers to questions Be attentive
Adults	Broad individual differences in values, experiences, and attitudes; self-directed and independent in comparison to children; have assumed certain family and social roles, periods of stability and change	Appropriately applied therapeutic communication techniques: maintaining silence, listening attentively, conveying acceptance, asking related questions, paraphrasing, clarifying, focusing, stating observations, offering information, summarizing, reflective responding
Older adults	May have sensory loss of hearing, vision; may have high level of anxiety; may be willing to comply with recommendations, but forgetful	Approach with respect, speak clearly and slowly Give time to formulate answers to questions and to elaborate Be attentive to nonverbal communication

Modified from Potter PA, Perry AG: *Fundamentals of nursing: Concepts, process, and practice,* ed 3, St Louis, 1993, Mosby.

sitting quietly, remember to praise him or her for cooperation. It is a mistake to ignore behavior until it is a problem.

KEEP YOUR COOL. Ignore negative behavior such as whining if it is not interfering with the healthcare. Showing anger will only make matters worse. Showing displeasure and using a calm voice for statements such as "I get upset (or unhappy, etc.) when you . . .," is likely to get the point across more successfully.

USE VOICE CONTROL. A sudden change in volume can gain attention from a child who is being uncooperative. Modulate voice tone and volume as soon as the child begins to respond.

ALLOW THE CHILD TO PLAY A ROLE. Let the child make some structured choices. For example, ask "Would you like strawberry or grape flavored fluoride today?" Most younger children enjoy the role of "helper" and are happy to hold mirrors, papers, and pencils, and to receive praise for their good work.

AVOID ATTEMPTING TO TALK A CHILD INTO COOPERATION. Do not give lengthy rationales for the necessity of procedures. Rather, acknowledge the child's feelings by making statements such as, "I understand that you don't like the fluoride treatment; however, we must do it to make your teeth stronger. I understand that you would rather be outside playing, but we need to polish your teeth now." Then firmly request the child's attention and cooperation and proceed with the service.

Both the preschool and school-age child are eager to learn and explore but may have fears about the oral healthcare environment, personnel, and treatment. Studies have shown that dental fears begin in childhood, and making early oral care a positive experience is necessary if the dental hygienist is interested in the client's long-term attitude toward oral health.[4] Rapport must be established as a foundation for cooperation and trust. The best teaching approaches for younger children follow behavioral rather than cognitive theory. Positive reinforcement used as immediate feedback, short instructional segments with simplified language and content that is concrete rather than abstract, close monitoring of progress, and encouragement for independence in the practice of oral hygiene skills are all indicated.

OLDER SCHOOL-AGE CHILDREN AND ADOLESCENTS

Adolescence is not a single stage of development. The rate at which children progress through adolescence and the psychological states that accompany the changes can vary considerably from one child to another.[4] In early adolescence (about 13 to 15 years old), children may rather suddenly demonstrate an ambivalence toward parents and other adults, manifested by questioning of adult values and authority. By late adolescence (18 years and older) much of the ambivalence is gone and values that characterize the adult years have fully emerged. Friendship patterns in early and mid-adolescence are usually intense as the child begins to

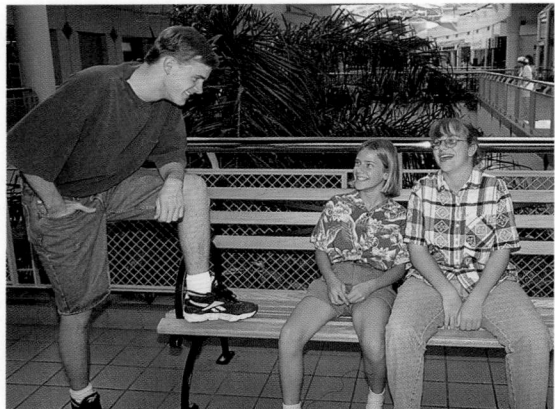

FIGURE 4–5 ✦ Interacting with peers helps to establish independence.

explore companionship outside the family and become established as an independent person (Figure 4–5).

Some common complaints from the adolescent's point of view can sensitize health professionals for positive interactions with this group of young people. First, a frequently voiced complaint of adolescents is that adults do not listen to them. They seem to feel that adults are in too much of a hurry, appear to be looking for certain answers, or listen only to what they want to hear. A second complaint is that too often a conversation turns into unsolicited advice or a mini-lecture. A young person, asked to describe specific experiences in dentistry, related the following[11]:

> My dentist bugged me a lot. He would become angry if I felt pain. He pushed my hair around and lectured constantly about young people and their hair.

Other less-common complaints from adolescents are that they are patronized, that they do not understand questions being asked, and finally that adults lack humor.

Dental hygienists should consider carefully these complaints and practice behaviors that enhance communication with adolescents. Being attentive and allowing the adolescent time to talk enhances rapport and communication. Some rapport-building questions at the beginning of the appointment may relate to family, school, personal interests, or career intentions. It is useful to have some knowledge of the contemporary interests of adolescents, which may include trends in music, sports, and fashion. They want a sense of being understood and do not want to be judged or lectured.

Adolescents have a strong human need for responsibility. An astute dental hygienist can use these unfulfilled needs to motivate the adolescent client to adopt oral self-care behaviors. This educational approach, based on human needs theory, can enhance adolescents' sense of personal responsibility toward the care of their mouths. In order that adolescents do not feel singled out, a dental hygienist might say, "We encourage all of our adult clients to floss daily. This is because we know it works. We've seen the results." Teenagers do not feel patronized or confused if questions and advice are offered in a sincere, straightforward manner.

ADULTS

Havinghurst delineated three developmental stages for adults and listed common adult concerns at each stage.[12] Although communication techniques may not differ greatly for the adult stages, knowledge of general differences in characteristics between age groups can enlighten the hygienist about typical concerns of clients at different periods of adulthood. An awareness of how priorities in life change for adults as they develop can help the hygienist identify learning needs and "teachable moments" for different clients. The Havinghurst adult stages have been summarized according to early adulthood, middle age, and late maturity. The dental hygienist should be aware, without asking personal questions, that young adults may be trying to institute oral hygiene self-care behaviors while adjusting to major life stresses such as bringing up young children, managing a home, or starting a demanding career. Adults in the middle years may be more settled in careers and have less responsibility for child care, but may be heavily involved in social responsibilities, adjusting to their personal physical

Havinghurst's Description of the Adult Developmental Stages

Early Adulthood

Selecting a mate
Learning to live with a marriage partner
Starting a family
Bringing up young children
Managing a home
Getting started in an occupation
Taking on civic responsibilities
Finding a congenial social group

Middle Age

Achieving adulthood and social responsibilities
Establishing and maintaining an economic standard of living
Assisting one's children to become adults
Developing durable leisure-time activities
Relating to one's marriage partner as a person
Accepting and adjusting to physical change
Adjusting to one's aging parent

Late Maturity

Adjusting to decreasing physical strength and to death
Adjusting to retirement and to reduced income
Adjusting to death of one's marriage partner
Establishing an explicit affiliation with one's age group
Meeting social and civic obligations
Establishing satisfactory physical living arrangements in light of physical infirmities

Modified from Darkenwald GG, Merriam SB: *Adult education: Foundations of practice,* New York, 1982, Harper & Row.

changes, or the demands of caring for aging parents. Older adults may be adjusting to decreasing physical strength, a chronic health problem, retirement, or death of a spouse.

Communication approaches appropriate for adults are the therapeutic communication techniques discussed previously in this chapter. In utilizing the techniques, it is important for the dental hygienist to be familiar with the adult developmental stages and aware of what demands may be preventing adults of the different stages from easily making oral healthcare behavior changes.

Modern adult learning theory has been supported by some basic assumptions (see Assumptions Related to Adult Learners). Keeping these assumptions in mind facilitates communication with adults who become "learners" as dental hygienists become "teachers" in the healthcare setting. These assumptions can enhance the dental hygiene educator's approach to teaching adults.

OLDER ADULTS

The elderly population is a highly diversified group (Figure 4–6). The wide variations in health and psychological states dictate the necessity of careful assessment of each individual[13] (see Chapter 48).

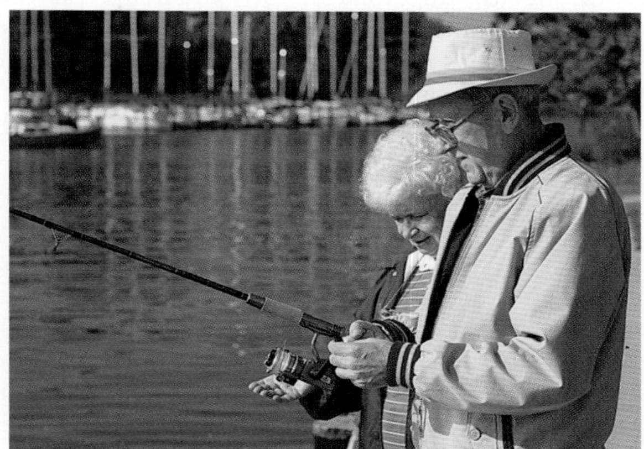

FIGURE 4–6 ✦ A retired couple enjoying fishing together.

Assumptions Related to Adult Learners

Adults are motivated to learn as they experience needs and interests that learning will satisfy; therefore, these are the appropriate starting points for organizing adult learning activities.
Adults are more likely than children or adolescents to acknowledge their needs readily. Mature adults know from past experience how to recognize needs and are motivated to seek information (education) to satisfy these needs.

Adults' orientation to learning is life-centered; therefore, the appropriate units for organizing adult learning are life situations, not subjects.
Adults are used to learning from everyday events rather than from books and formal lectures. They respond well to anecdotes about other clients' experiences with oral hygiene regimens because they identify with those individuals and their experiences. The dental hygienist may remark, "I have heard such good testimonials from my clients who have begun to floss regularly. They say their mouths feel so much healthier and do not feel really clean unless they floss every day." This statement is likely to have more impact on the client than simply providing information on the subject of flossing.

Experience is the richest resource for adults' learning; therefore, the core methodology of adult education is the analysis of experience.
When adults return for their maintenance care, the dental hygienist should help them analyze their experiences in trying to institute new self-care procedures. For example, if clients are experiencing difficulty in flossing technique or in incorporating flossing into a busy schedule, they should be encouraged to discuss the problems and receive help from the dental hygienist in developing solutions.

Adults have a deep need to be self-directing; therefore, the role of the teacher is to engage in a process of mutual inquiry with them rather than to transmit his or her knowledge to them and then evaluate their conformity to it.
The dental hygienist engages adults in discussions that lead to problem solving with their participation. The hygienist does not dictate solutions or expect adults to follow rules of oral hygiene that they have had no part in developing.

Individual differences among people increase with age; therefore, adult education must make optimal provision for differences in style, time, place, and pace of learning.
The dental hygienist expects people to differ widely in their responses to a particular educational methodology. Although adults are similar in that learning for them is life-centered, their individual histories of life experiences differ greatly.

Client Education Issues

- The dental hygienist and the client are in a partnership to maintain optimal oral hygiene health for the client.
- The dental hygienist provides the most accurate oral health information and feedback on the client's healthcare options, but respects the client's wishes regarding healthcare decisions.
- The dental hygienist strives to consider cultural and age-appropriate needs of the client in all health education efforts.

Legal, Ethical, and Safety Issues

- Clients have the right to accept or reject the dental hygiene care plan and still retain the respect of the dental hygienist.
- It is important to meet the client's need for conceptualization and understanding of health information to promote health literacy and informed oral healthcare decisions.
- The client has the right to personalized, up-to-date, evidence-based recommendations and care from the dental hygienist.

Key Concepts

- Communication during the dental hygiene process of care is a dynamic interaction between the dental hygienist and the client that involves both verbal and nonverbal components.
- Factors that may affect the communication process include internal factors of the client and the dental hygienist (e.g., perceptions, values, emotions, and knowledge), the nature of their relationship, the situation prompting communication, and the environment.
- Some communication approaches are therapeutic and helpful in assisting clients to make decisions and attain goals related to their comfort and health. Other approaches are nontherapeutic and unsuccessful in helping clients make decisions and attain goals related to their comfort and health.
- Communication techniques used by the dental hygiene clinician must be flexible to relate to the full range of client ages through the life span.

Critical Thinking Exercises

- Identify therapeutic and nontherapeutic communication techniques by name as two people role-play the following client–oral healthcare educator sessions.

1. In the first session, the "client" should improvise a story of frustration with his or her current oral hygiene regimen by explaining that a heavy workload, family responsibilities, or other interference make it difficult to maintain a good home care regimen. While glancing at a list of the possible responses as a prompt, the "educator" will try to respond with only therapeutic comments. Classroom listeners should try to determine which specific categories of therapeutic communication fit the educator's comments.
2. This time as the "educator" glances at the list of possible responses he or she will try to answer with mostly nontherapeutic responses. Classroom listeners should try to determine which specific categories of nontherapeutic communication fit the educator's comments.

For References, Suggested Readings, and Related Websites, visit
http://evolve.elsevier.com/Darby/hygiene/

CHAPTER 5

CROSS-CULTURAL PRACTICE

OBJECTIVES

Mastery of the content in this chapter will enable the reader to:

- Distinguish among the concepts of race, ethnicity, ethnic group, culture, and subculture
- Apply knowledge of culture to healthcare delivery
- Describe the importance of cultural health beliefs as related to dental hygiene care
- Identify cultural barriers to oral healthcare
- Identify some health-related beliefs and practices of various ethnic and religious groups

KEY TERMS

Cross-cultural competence
Cross-cultural dental hygiene
Culture
Ethnicity
Ethnocentrism
Eye contact
First-world countries
Gesticulation
Holism
Humanism
Implementation
Manner of speaking
Nonverbal communication
Physical contact
Poverty
Race
Second-world countries
Socioeconomic status
Stereotyping
Subculture
Third-world countries
Verbal communication
Zones of territory

National borders are disappearing in international trade, culture, health, education, and communication. North America continues to experience an influx of immigrants from all over the world; American icons such as McDonald's and Microsoft expand globally. "American-made" automobiles may be assembled in the United States by a Japanese-owned company using parts manufactured in a number of other countries, international students compete to study in American universities, and some companies require intercultural communication as basic training for new employees. Daily, people experience terrorism; rain forest destruction; pollution of the groundwater, bays, and oceans; global warming; and the production and distribution of illegal drugs. Clearly, each nation's policies articulate with all others. As the nations of the world become more racially and ethnically diverse, human efforts to find a common ground among all of mankind escalate. In a global society, dental hygienists must have *cross-cultural competence,* the ability to integrate current knowledge of oral healthcare with the ways of multiple cultures.

CROSS-CULTURAL DENTAL HYGIENE

Nations of the world are grouped according to levels of economic development:

- First-world countries are economically developed and capitalistic countries such as the United States,

Canada, South Korea, Switzerland, South Africa, and Germany.

- Second-world countries include the economically developed socialist countries such as Russia, Ukraine, and Moldova.
- Third-world countries are those countries that are still developing such as Afghanistan, Sudan, Somalia, and Latin America.

Access to care is a major issue in first-world countries; development of the healthcare infrastructure (hospitals and clinics, supplies and equipment, system for paying healthcare personnel) is a major challenge for second-world countries; third-world countries have no formal system of healthcare or public health, other than home remedies (Figure 5–1). By 2050, about 50% of the U.S. population is expected to be Asian, non-Hispanic black, Hispanic, and American Indian (Table 5–1). Non-Hispanic blacks, Hispanics, American Indians, and Alaskan Natives have the poorest oral and general health of any of the racial and ethnic groups in the United States. Dental hygienists who understand local cultures and culturally influenced healthcare practices are able to communicate with, educate, and motivate diverse people to achieve health. Furthermore, strategies for improving the health status of racial and ethnic minorities are prominent features of *Healthy People 2010*, the goal-setting health agenda developed by the U.S. Department of Health and Human Services.[1] Therefore, the ability to apply knowledge of culture in healthcare delivery is a competency gaining prominence in the health professions.

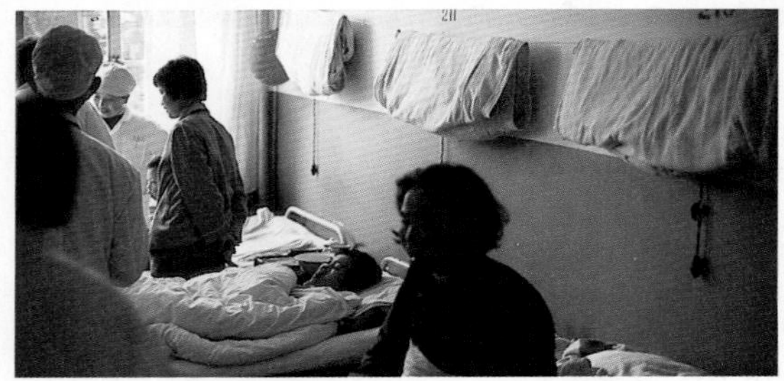

FIGURE 5–1 ✦ Patients at a hospital in a second world country.

Cross-cultural dental hygiene is the effective integration of the client's socioethnocultural background into the process of care. Cross-cultural dental hygiene encompasses the social, political, ethnic, religious, and economic realities that people experience in culturally diverse human interactions and environments. Cultural diversity is evident in different societal rules, languages, foods, dress, daily cultural practices, motivational factors, beliefs, values, and health behaviors. These factors influence human need fulfillment of the client. Therefore, they must be recognized and integrated into professional care if preventive and therapeutic goals are to be achieved.

Culture plays an integral role in dental hygiene care because oral health and wellness, disease, and illness are culturally determined. Conceptual differences exist between the client and the healthcare provider from different cultures. The human needs model provides a framework for implementing the dental hygiene process with culturally diverse clients. Human needs transcend all cultures; culture pervades all human interactions, and human needs have a culturally based etiology. Dental hygienists know how to assess clients but may not know how to interpret data when the client comes from a different culture. Furthermore, planning of interventions and the implementation of the care plan are further complicated by culture. Oral health therapy and promotion strategies must be delivered in relation to the cultural environment of the client. For example, a client's food preferences may result in an erroneous dental hygiene diagnosis of a need for a biologically sound and functional dentition; different cultural definitions of human attractiveness may be misdiagnosed as a need for a wholesome facial image; or language differences may be interpreted as a need for conceptualization and understanding. The client's home care products used

TABLE 5–1 DIVERSITY OF THE POPULATION OF THE UNITED STATES AS OF 2000

Race	Number	Percent of Total Population
Total population	281,421,906	100.0
Hispanic or Latino	35,305,818	12.5
Not Hispanic or Latino	246,116,088	87.5
One race	274,595,678	97.6
White	211,460,626	75.1
African American	34,658,190	12.3
American Indian and Alaska Native	2,475,956	0.9
Asian	10,242,998	3.6
Native Hawaiian and other Pacific Islander	398,835	0.1
Other	15,359,073	5.5
Two or more races	6,826,228	2.4

Data exceed total and 100% owing to rounding.
From US Census Bureau, Census 2000 Redistributing (Public Law 94–171) Summary File, Tables PL1 and PL2.

(or preferred) may result in a dental hygiene diagnosis of a need for prevention from health risks because of the practitioner's belief that the product causes oral harm or injury.

Dental hygiene care is culturally influenced. Although most Western therapies are based on research evidence, the vast majority of the world populations are non-Western. The techniques we use and the client behaviors we promote may be interpreted as good, bad, or indifferent, according to the cultural values of the client. Likewise, a dental hygienist may fail to recognize the client's cultural frame of reference and erroneously label the client as difficult, unmotivated, uncooperative, noncommunicative, or noncompliant. Western, non-Western, and third-world healthcare practices may be viewed as functional or dysfunctional, depending on the cultural system of origin. For example, the practice of putting a loved one in a nursing home may be viewed by some cultures as an appropriate action for providing the best possible care on a 24-hour basis, but other cultures would perceive this practice as barbaric or inhumane.

Concepts in Cross-cultural Dental Hygiene

Consideration of individual value systems and lifestyles should be included in the care plan for each client. For a dental hygienist to provide quality care to a client of different ethnic or cultural background, effective intercultural communication must take place. Effective intercultural communication means that each person involved in the transaction is able to understand the other from his unique cultural perspective.

HUMANISM AND HOLISM. Dental hygienists must understand basic dimensions of culture and their influence on human need, motivation, health promotion, and oral disease and healthcare. The dental hygienist may be at a disadvantage when the client is from a different race or ethnic group, speaks a different language, or is of a different socioeconomic status. Cultural differences create barriers to communication, decrease trust, and raise anxiety levels for both dental hygienist and client. Dental hygienists who are able to incorporate cultural perspectives into practice augment their effectiveness.

"*Humanism* attests to the dignity and worth of all individuals through concern for and understanding of their network of attitudes, values, behavior patterns, and way of life."[2] All humans have basic needs. Humanism recognizes the right of all humans to have their needs satisfied, but this is not a universally embraced principle. Although the United States promotes human rights, other governments and cultures may value country, religion, dictators, pride, or family over individual human rights.

Holism means that an individual is more than the total sum of parts; practitioners who are holistic show concern for and interest in all dimensions of the individual.[2] An individual is a biopsychosocial and spiritual being who brings uniqueness in race, culture, ethnicity, attitudes, beliefs, knowledge, and experience. These factors interact to constitute the individual. This interaction of factors causes clients and dental hygienists to have differing worldviews and interpretations about health and disease. A comparison of Western and non-Western views of the individual (Table 5–2) provides some insight into how culture can influence attitudes and behaviors. Evidence-based dental hygiene care is predicated on the beliefs of humanism and holism. The holistic philosophy as applied to healthcare has particular relevance in a multicultural environment. If applied, its tenets make the care setting a welcome place for individuals who might otherwise feel disconnected or disenfranchised (see Characteristics and Beliefs Inherent to Holistic Healthcare).

TABLE 5–2 MAJOR DIFFERENCES BETWEEN WESTERN AND NON-WESTERN VIEWS OF THE INDIVIDUAL, SOCIETY, AND HEALTH AND DISEASE

Western Values	Non-Western Values
Freedom of choice	Group decision making
Uniqueness of the individual	Group commonality
Independence	Compliance
Interdependence	Harmony
Competition	Cooperation
Nonconformity	Conformity
Expression of feelings	Control of one's feelings
Fulfillment of individual needs	Fulfillment of the needs of the group
Body is divided into organ systems with identifiable functions; dichotomous body and mind	Body is viewed as a union of flesh and soul
Body is viewed objectively, and is relatively immune to nonsomatic influences	Disease occurs as a result of disharmony or an imbalance of life forces

From Ho D: Psychological implications of collectivism: With special references to the Chinese case and Maoist dialects. In Eckensberber L, Lonner W, Poortinga Y, eds: *Cross-cultural contributions to psychology*, Amsterdam, 1979, Swets and Zeitlinger.

RACE AND ETHNICITY. *Race* refers to the classification of human beings based on physical characteristics such as skin color, stature, eye color, hair color and texture, facial characteristics, and general body characteristics, all of which are hereditary. Most people recognize three races—white (Caucasian), black (Negroid), and yellow (Mongoloid)—which overlap each other. There are more similarities than differences among the racial groups.

Ethnicity refers to the unique cultural and social heritage and traditions of minority groups within the primary racial divisions that reflect distinct customs, language, diet, work habits, religious beliefs, and methods of dealing with illness and death. People who share similarities in heritage and tradition, passed on from generation to generation, are said to be members of the same *ethnic group*. Ethnic groups share common factors: language, dialect, nationality, music, folklore, food preferences, geographic location, and a sense of uniqueness. Examples of ethnic groups include Japanese, Italian, Polish, Haitian, Kuwaiti, and Hispanic, just to name a few. Religious beliefs also constitute an important component of ethnicity. *Religion* is one's belief in a supernatural power, the creator and ruler of the universe. Religious beliefs shape values, ethics, morals, and behaviors. Some religious beliefs influence health beliefs and practices. For example, some religions teach practices related to hygiene and cleanliness, eating habits, dressing habits, and food preparation requirements (Table 5–3).

CULTURE AND SUBCULTURE. *Culture* is "the sum total of human behavior or social characteristics peculiar to a specific group and passed from generation to generation

Characteristics and Beliefs Inherent to Holistic Healthcare

Search for patterns and causes as well as symptoms
Emphasis is on the integrated whole person
Concern with human values
Caring is a component of healing
Pain is an indicator of disharmony
Mind is a co-equal factor in all illness
Prevention is synonymous with wholeness
Minimal intervention is advocated
Body is a dynamic system and field of energy
Client is autonomous
The professional is the therapeutic partner
Body and mind are interrelated
Value on qualitative information

Modified from Ferguson M: *The Aquarian conspiracy: Personal and social transformation in the 1980s,* Los Angeles, 1980, Putnam.

TABLE 5–3 GUIDE TO WORKING WITH PEOPLE OF VARIOUS RELIGIOUS GROUPS*

Religious Group	Basic Beliefs and Concepts	Healthcare Practices and Beliefs
Christian Scientists	Metaphysical approach to religion, sickness, and healing Prayer and religious counsel will heal the sick Sickness is mentally originated and can be cured through proper mental processes Body is its own laboratory Healing is private, abstract, and highly intellectual	Healing done by certified practitioner employing three dimensions of therapeutic treatment: Affirmation/Denial/Argument tries to destroy sick person's belief in suffering Absolute Consciousness of Good tries to convince sick person that he or she is well Impersonal Treatment practitioner focuses on own thoughts to free afflicted person Accept drugless practices, i.e., osteopaths and chiropractors, and natural methods, such as dietary regulation and manipulation of the body
Eastern Orthodox	God did not create humans in God's image; however, humans have the potential to become like God in terms of goodness Do not believe in original sin of Adam—rather humans choose to imitate Adam	Humans need the spirit of God for healing to occur Caring for the sick has a special place in the church Praying for the sick is a very involved process Sick are encouraged to seek scientific medical cures
Evangelists	Belief in: Authentic and authoritative Holy Scriptures The life, teachings, death, and resurrection of Christ and eternal life *Deliverance Evangelists:* Believe Holy Spirit has given them power of divine healing	Healing occurs by God in only some situations; God heals all through different people, modalities, and techniques
Jews	Ten commandments are a holy contract Modern contracts govern areas of personal and human behavior in an attempt to embody the spirit of ten commandments Reverence for life Emphasis on family and education Traditional Jewish kosher	Emphasis on cleanliness Circumcision performed to prevent disease Person responsible for avoiding threats to personal health

Table continued on following page

TABLE 5–3 GUIDE TO WORKING WITH PEOPLE OF VARIOUS RELIGIOUS GROUPS*—CONT'D

Religious Group	Basic Beliefs and Concepts	Healthcare Practices and Beliefs
Mormons (similar to conservative Protestants)	Two personages of God (Father and Son) have flesh and bone bodies; Holy Spirit does not Salvation comes through atonement of Christ and obedience of laws of Gospel	Holy handkerchief (faith healing method) and laying on of hands Seek scientific relief for illness and poverty
Native American Church or Peyotists (American Indians)	Belief in Great Spirit and Christian Trinity Earth is our mother to be treated with respect All people are brothers and sisters Abstinence from alcohol Peyote is consumed to have closer contact with God. Ritual is performed under guidance of "road chief"	Peyote is medicine (cactus found in Indian territory) Through prayer and communion with God, sins are forgiven and illness is cured
Pentecostalism (composed of Evangelists and Fundamentalists)	Concerned with holiness (state of mind and spiritual purity), literal interpretation of the Bible, and renewal of Pentecostal experiences, i.e., speaking in tongues	Belief in divine healing, prophecy, and working miracles
Spiritualism (Hispanics, Africans, African Americans, American Indians)	Visible world includes invisible world inhabited by good and evil spirits who influence human behaviors Spirits become visible through mediums Mediums share same ethnicity, cultural language, and social class as their followers	Mediums treat emotional and physical illness, whole person concept Powers of mediums derived from supernatural
Protestantism	Four principles of Protestantism Resolution to live by faith Freedom to initiate new life Openness to truth revealed in scientific and nonscientific ways Vocation in the world (caring for sick and poor)	Four principles of Protestantism lend themselves to faith healing as well as modern Western medicine
Islam (some people from Middle East, Northern Africa, Pakistan, India, Bosnia, Macedonia, Montenegro, Serbia)	Five obligations of all Muslims: Profession of faith in Allah Pray five times daily in the direction of Mecca Give alms to the poor Fast during the holy month of Ramadan Once in a lifetime, make a pilgrimage to Mecca (Hajj) Faith in the will of Allah *Qur'an* provides a guide to living Life is lived in harmony with the commands of Allah Pork and alcohol are forbidden; Halal meat can be consumed Traditional Muslims may follow Purdah: women are covered from head to foot in a burqua. Some women may simply wear a head cover.	Believe in the science of modern medicine Emphasize cleanliness, including mouth cleanliness Sewak or miswak from a plant (Salvadore Persica) may be used to clean mouth. Sewak is part of a religious ritual Prayer and recitation stimulate the body Ramadan is a way of reducing stress on the digestive system Healthcare sought primarily from the mullah or Iman Hakim is a Muslim practitioner who combines religious rituals for health Use herbs and natural religious ritual for treating illness Man knows Allah through illness Mohammed wrote about the process of cleaning one's teeth as an act that is pleasing to Allah May be treated by a same-gender healthcare provider; may require a same-gender interpreter

*Religion affects healthcare practices, beliefs, and interactions with healthcare providers. It is important to remember that not all people from a given religious group will act in a standard manner. Great variability exists within cultural groups based on socioeconomic status, level of education, and overall life experiences. This chart is not meant to be generalized to all people within a specific religion, but rather to serve as a beginning guide.
Data from Henderson G: *Understanding indigenous and foreign cultures,* Springfield, Ill, 1989, Charles C Thomas; and www.crescentlife.com.

or from one to another within the group."[2] Culture includes the rules of behavior each person learns to adapt successfully to life within a particular group and includes beliefs, values, traditions, experiences, customs, rituals, and language.

People who speak different languages perceive the world differently. Language systems that are different should not be viewed as deficient. In fact, dental hygienists who speak standard English should know that other cultures may find it difficult to comprehend because standard English:

- Lacks certain language sounds
- Has language sounds for which other sounds may serve as substitutes
- Doubles and drawls some of its vowel sounds in sequences that are difficult for non-Americans to imitate

- Requires several ways to indicate tense, gender, and plurality
- Does not mark negatives sufficiently for words to make optimally strong negative statements

Although cultures share commonalities in lifestyles and basic beliefs, significant differences exist in subcultural attitudes, interests, goals, and dialects. "A *subculture* is formed by a group of persons who have developed interests or goals different from the primary culture, based on such things as occupation (Hollywood culture), gender (gay culture), age (youth culture), social class (middle class), or religion (fundamentalism)."[2] Dental hygienists can be viewed as members of a subculture (dental hygiene) with unique philosophical attitudes, practices, beliefs, and values. Within American society, we are familiar with the culture of poverty, the drug culture, Yuppie culture, generation X, and "bag people" (street people). Members of subcultures have lifestyles, behaviors, and language significantly different from those of the general population. Some would consider these lifestyles to be unusual, different, or deviant from the predominant culture. For example, there may be people from the Polish ethnic group who are Catholic or Jewish, with subcultures that span several socioeconomic levels to the culture of poverty, gay culture, or the drug culture.

STEREOTYPING. *Stereotyping* is the erroneous behavior of assuming that people possess certain characteristics or traits simply because they are members of a particular group. Stereotyping fails to recognize the uniqueness of the individual and prevents us from perceiving the situation accurately and without bias. Stereotyping clouds our perceptions and makes us less effective as professionals and human beings. Although stereotyping can provide a comfortable foundation for an individual in a strange environment with new people, an accurate assessment should always be made of another human being.

Taking the time to learn about people is an important step toward eliminating old stereotypical thinking. Learning about other cultures, languages, customs, religions, and practices also enables the dental hygienist to accept and value culturally diverse people as individuals with unique human needs. Getting in touch with our own cultural base is important if improvement is to occur in the way we relate to people. Periodically, it is good to participate in a little self-assessment to monitor stereotypical thinking. For example, one can observe strangers, and develop personal assumptions about the way they look, dress, behave, or speak. Once strangers become acquaintances, personal assumptions can then be compared to the realities of who they are and what they are truly like.

ETHNOCENTRISM. Believing that one's culture is superior to that of others is *ethnocentrism.* People who are ethnocentric use their own cultures as the standard of excellence against which people from other cultures are judged. Ethnocentric behavior is characterized as judgmental, condescending, insulting, and narrow-minded. Dental hygienists who are ethnocentric may belittle clients whose oral health practices may be rooted in culture rather than research evidence. They may convey the feeling that their way is the right way and that the client is ignorant or uneducated. It is easy to fall prey to this type of thinking if we are blind to ethnocentrism in our own behavior. Ethnocentrism makes it difficult for many healthcare providers to care for clients from minority groups. It may lead to subtle discrimination in the workplace, employee turnover, and loss of clients.

Melting Pot versus Salad Bowl

Some social theorists advanced the proposition that people of different cultures in the United States assimilate into the mainstream white Anglo-Saxon Protestant culture. The theory of the melting pot explains that people give up their previous cultural identity in favor of the predominant culture of the society in which they find themselves. Such intermingling of cultural diversity is thought to result in a blended culture with liberty, equality, and justice for everyone.

The melting pot theory has given way to the salad bowl approach to explaining cultural assimilation. The salad bowl theory recognizes cultural diversity as separate and unique components that remain heterogeneous within society. As it relates to health, the salad bowl theory recognizes that culture influences the health status, beliefs, and behaviors of individuals, and that healthcare providers and managers thus must be prepared to accommodate these differences. Treatment, educational programs, and client–provider interactions must be culturally appropriate. Some work settings proactively encourage cultural awareness through employee-training programs that identify cultural biases and facilitate positive attitudes and behaviors such as valuing diversity and team building.

INCOME AS A DETERMINANT OF HEALTH

Culture of Poverty and Its Relationship to Health

Socioeconomic status is defined by a person's income, occupation, and level of education. In the United States and Canada, society is made up of a large middle socioeconomic group and smaller upper and lower socioeconomic groups. Socioeconomic status permeates every aspect of a person's life. It affects where one lives, how one spends money, how one uses free time, where one receives healthcare, how one pays for that healthcare, and, ultimately, one's general and oral health status.

Although poverty is universal, its definition is culturally determined. *Poverty* is relative based on the standards prevailing in the community. Poverty in one community might be regarded as wealth in another. The U.S. Bureau of the Census[3] reports that 32.3 million persons, or 11.8% of the population, live below the official government poverty level as defined by financial income. The poverty definition here is from the U.S. Office of Management and Budget and consists of a set of money income thresholds that vary by family size and composition. Families or individuals with income below their appropriate thresholds are classified below the poverty level (Table 5–4). Of the people living in poverty in the United States, the majority are children in female-headed households, hence the phrase the *feminization of poverty.* Moreover, many of the homeless are single-mother family units. Factors contributing to the feminization of poverty include teenage pregnancy, pregnancy out of marriage, divorce, abandonment, and female longevity. African Americans and Hispanics also are over-represented in the segment of the population classified as poor, making up 36% and 30%, respectively, of those in poverty. Poverty is the key predictor of poor oral health. Children with the most advanced oral disease are found within minority, poor, homeless, and migrant populations and those with HIV.[4] Poverty is a culture, and as a culture it is passed on from generation to generation. This can be observed in people on the welfare rolls, in the urban and rural poor, and in migrant workers who seem to be in an ongoing cycle of poverty. Persons living in poverty are likely to manifest the following:

- Unemployment
- Dependence on government assistance for survival
- External locus of control (e.g., fatalism, lack of control)
- Abuse of drugs, alcohol
- A live-for-today mentality
- Inability to set, or work toward, future goals
- Feelings of despair
- Loss of self-esteem and self-respect
- Lack of respect for others

These characteristics in clients affect the process of care. For example, the unemployed may need care but choose not to enter the healthcare setting because of financial barriers and no health insurance. Those who are eligible for government-funded healthcare may find that oral care is not covered or that healthcare providers are unwilling to accept them as clients. In some cultures, a fatalistic attitude might translate into a "no matter what I do, I'll lose my teeth anyway" attitude. Those who are chemically dependent have difficulty seeing other human needs as a priority. Those with a present-oriented philosophy may not seek care until the need has become an emergency; they find the future benefits derived from preventive behavior irrelevant. In addition, feelings of despair and loss of self-worth mean that personal healthcare is of little consequence.

In this manner, poverty continues to be a major barrier to healthcare that prevents individuals from meeting their basic human need for general and oral health. Other barriers to healthcare associated with poverty are disenfranchisement, lack of transportation, no health insurance, homelessness, seasonal work, prejudice, language difficulties, inadequate levels of education, general lack of understanding of the healthcare system and how it works (the subculture of healthcare), and a lack of healthcare personnel from the individual's own culture. Given these barriers, it is easier to understand why poor people might resort to self-therapy, home or herbal remedies, or the services of a folk or faith healer, all of which are more accessible, less expensive, and more familiar than the modern healthcare system.

Impoverished environments directly influence the health status of people who reside there. Low-income

TABLE 5–4 POVERTY THRESHOLDS IN 1999 BY SIZE OF FAMILY AND NUMBER OF RELATED CHILDREN UNDER 18 YEARS

Size of Family Unit	Weighted Average Threshold	Related Children under 18 Years: None	One	Two	Three	Four	Five	Six	Seven	Eight
One person (unrelated individual)	8,501									
Under 65 years	8,667	8,667								
65 years and over	7,990	7,990								
Two people	10,869									
Householder under 65 years	11,214	11,156	11,483							
Householder 65 years and over	10,075	10,070	11,440							
Three people	13,290	13,032	13,410	13,423						
Four people	17,029	17,184	17,465	16,895	16,954					
Five people	20,127	20,723	21,024	20,380	19,882	19,578				
Six people	22,727	23,835	23,930	23,436	22,964	22,261	21,845			
Seven people	25,912	27,425	27,596	27,006	26,595	25,828	24,934	23,953		
Eight people	28,967	30,673	30,944	30,387	29,899	29,206	28,327	27,412	27,180	
Nine people or more	34,417	36,897	37,076	36,583	36,169	35,489	34,554	33,708	33,499	32,208

From US Bureau of the Census: *Current Population Survey,* 2000.

housing is usually associated with isolation from the community; poor maintenance; inadequate heat, light, water, electricity, and ventilation; crowded living conditions; infestation; and lead poisoning. The frustrations experienced from inadequate housing and high-density living translate into high rates of crime, physical and emotional abuse, stress, psychological problems, alienation, and transmission of infectious diseases. According to *Healthy People 2010,* poor people get sick more often, experience greater complications with their illnesses, take longer to recover, and are less likely to regain their previous level of functioning, as compared with people from higher-income groups.[1] Individuals in poverty do not readily take advantage of preventive health services, nor do they perceive the long-term benefits of these services.[1]

Canada's experience with making healthcare accessible to all people presents an interesting model of the effects of poverty on health. In 1968, Canada initiated a national health insurance program to provide healthcare to people without regard to financial resources, age, ethnic origin, or creed. More than three decades later, health remains directly related to people's economic status.

Wealth and Its Relationship to Health

Wealth is usually associated with high levels of education, prestige, self-esteem, power, and internal locus of control. The wealthy are able to afford clean, comfortable housing, recreational activities, quality diets, and, of course, access to the healthcare system. Because of their higher levels of education, financially secure individuals are not intimidated by the healthcare system. They are able to verbalize their concerns, assert their needs, determine their level of participation in care, be critical healthcare consumers, and seek second opinions. Because the wealthy are typically employed, they benefit from third-party payment systems to finance large portions of their healthcare bills. People in the upper socioeconomic levels of society live longer and experience less disability than do those from low-income groups[1]

COMMUNICATING IN A CROSS-CULTURAL ENVIRONMENT

Members of different cultures actually live in different worlds. Lack of sensitivity to a client's cultural needs, preferences, and beliefs often creates barriers that lead to termination of the client–provider relationship. Communication within a culture is at best uncertain; communication between persons from different cultures is a complex and arduous task. A dental hygienist initiates communication by exhibiting a positive and empathetic attitude while attempting to establish some initial areas of commonality (e.g., parenthood, children, marriage). Customs, beliefs, and practices indigenous to various cultural groups can be found at this book's website at http://evolve.elsevier.com/Darby/hygiene/ in Website Information and Resources. Knowledge from these and similar sites can enhance cross-cultural competence.

Verbal Communication

A healthcare provider's ability in *verbal communication* with culturally diverse people facilitates care. Variations exist in the typical way members of diverse cultures think and communicate thoughts.

- ✦ *Polychronic* is a term to describe individuals who do many things at the same time, who are repetitive in their speech, and who place a low value on time. Latino, African, Arab, and Asian cultures are polychronic. Dental hygiene interventions that require action on the part of the client at specific time intervals may be difficult for individuals from these cultures.
- ✦ *Monochronic* refers to cultures whose members are linear in their thinking, sequential in behavior, and clock- and work-oriented. Western European cultures are characterized as being monochronic.

The language of a culture portrays the identity of the individual within that culture. A culture's view of the individual in society can be gleaned from the language used. European languages (and English) denote the individual as a private, singular entity who has importance, as exemplified by the pronoun "I." In Asian or African culture the self has a strong group identity (Figure 5–2). In Japanese, the first person pronoun is expressed differently, depending on the situation (e.g., whether the interaction is with a male or female, private or public, or written or oral).

Manner of Speaking

According to Western culture, an emotional speaker is viewed as assertive, self-assured, and tough-minded; a calm, objective speaker is seen as trustworthy, honest, and people oriented. Intensity of expression varies among different groups. For example, Asians respect silence and are hesitant toward spontaneity. Culturally sensitive dental hygienists intentionally modify their *manner of speaking* to facilitate positive interactions.

Nonverbal Communication

Culture is important in determining the meaning and interpretation of *nonverbal communication.* Various ethnic groups possess culturally acceptable gestures, etiquette,

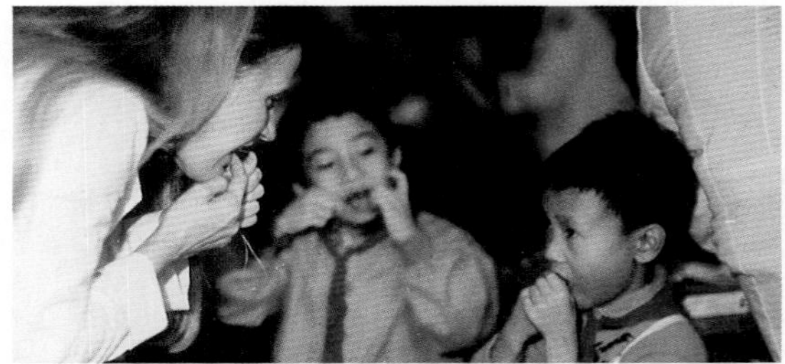

FIGURE 5–2 ✦ Group of Chinese school children learning to floss with the dental hygienist.

eye contact, physical contact, and methods of effective listening.

GESTICULATION. *Gesticulations* are signals made with the body that communicate emotions. Facial expressions can be used to communicate with or deceive other people. Culturally, a smile can mean very different things. The Japanese or Chinese may smile when they are embarrassed, not when they are happy.

Facial expressions of emotion are universal. There is cultural variability, however, in the rules for displaying these gestures. In most parts of the world, shaking the head from left to right means "no," but tossing the head to the side means "no" to some Arabs and in parts of Bulgaria, Greece, Turkey, and Bosnia-Herzegovina. Asian Indians may point with their chins. A slap on the back might denote friendliness among Anglo-Saxon whites, but is considered insulting to Asians. The sign for hitchhiking in America is vulgar when used in Australia.

ZONES OF TERRITORY. Each culture defines appropriate distances that are maintained between people in various situations. In other words, custom determines intimate, personal, social, and public distances or space kept between people. Therefore, human territoriality is culturally influenced, and a dental hygienist interested in making clients comfortable during healthcare encounters must do so in a multicultural context. For example, depending on the culture, the appropriate *zone of territory* may be based on the degree of respect, authority, and friendship between the individuals communicating. People of high status in European cultures maintain a larger social distance than do people in the United States.

Religious beliefs may also affect a person's zone of comfort. Muslims may refuse healthcare from a provider who is not of the same gender. Some followers of Islam cannot take courses or work in close proximity with persons from a different gender. When persons invade the prescribed territory, clients may communicate their discomfort through their behavior and actively attempt to readjust to more comfortable territory.

In the role of educator and clinician, dental hygienists invade the spatial zones of clients. This spatial closeness can be uncomfortable for people of any culture. In general, people from Anglo countries require larger zones of territory than those from non-Anglo countries. Americans tend to readjust their zones during interactions with people from countries that accept closer contact (contact culture), for example, Latin Americans, Africans, Arabs, and southern Europeans. Noncontact cultures include Americans, Asians, Pakistanis, Asian Indians, and northern Europeans. Germanic and Russian people tend to keep a distance and smile conservatively; Asians keep a proper distance and smile frequently. A dental hygienist must consider the client's culturally determined need for territoriality and attempt to explain procedures in detail to alert the person to necessary close encounters.

EYE CONTACT. In North America and some third-world countries, staring or continuously looking at another person is considered rude. Culture dictates looking at a person to establish eye contact, but then looking away to avoid staring. Indirect eye contact is acceptable and preferable within the Native American culture. Lack of eye contact may be interpreted as disinterest in England, Australia, Canada, or Saudi Arabia, and as polite behavior in some Far East countries.

PHYSICAL CONTACT. The dental hygienist's roles of clinician and educator require physical contact and touching of the client. Touch can convey acceptance or rejection, warmth or coldness, and positive or negative feelings.[5–8] Touching can communicate pleasure, empathy, closeness, and a desire to help. A sensitive touch can relieve tension and anxiety and instill confidence and courage. However, ethnicity, race, age, and gender affect how touch is interpreted as well as its effects. Physical contact is acceptable when greeting members of the same gender in Asian, Arab, Latin American, and Mediterranean countries. In the Far East, touching an older person is a sign of disrespect unless the person initiates the touching. Think about the custom of Iranian men and women kissing both sides of each other's faces as a gesture of friendship and greeting. When working with Hispanic, African, or African American clients, the dental hygienist should:

- ✦ Avoid forcing eye contact because it may be interpreted as disrespect
- ✦ Maintain close physical proximity
- ✦ Avoid unnecessary bodily touching

In some third-world countries people of the same gender maintain close contact, but people of opposite genders rarely touch. Traditional Japanese, Chinese, and Arab men and women seldom touch in public. Yet in China, it is common to see two women walking along the street arm-in-arm.

DENTAL HYGIENE PROCESS IN A CROSS-CULTURAL ENVIRONMENT

It is unlikely that a dental hygienist of one culture will be able to perceive, understand, and evaluate all the factors influencing clients from another culture unless cultural sensitivity is developed. In a global society, dental hygienists cannot afford to function ethnocentrically. The human needs model offers guidance in providing dental hygiene services in a cross-cultural environment. The client-centered focus of the model and the universality of human needs enable the dental hygienist to use the model during all phases of care, recognizing that culture is a significant variable affecting and defining human needs. The central concepts of the model (client, environment, health and oral health, and dental hygiene actions) can be considered from the viewpoint of the client, that is, how the client sees himself or herself, views

Guidelines for Cross-cultural Dental Hygiene

Approach each client (individual, family, community) as a valued individual with unique characteristics and experiences.

Be sensitive about asking intimate health history questions through an interpreter.

Get in touch with your own unique characteristics and life experiences. Sensitize yourself on how cultural factors have influenced your personal beliefs, attitudes, behaviors, practices, and values.

Identify biases and prejudices in your own life, their origins and their effects on interpersonal communication, that impact on your effectiveness as a healthcare provider, educator, manager, researcher, consumer advocate, and change agent.

Become a lifelong student of other cultures, particularly the cultures in your community

Assess clients' culturally related practices, attitudes, values, and beliefs as part of the process of care.

Display an accepting, nonjudgmental demeanor when presented with diverse beliefs and practices.

Reflect knowledge and recognition of the client's cultural practices throughout interactions.

Incorporate culturally relevant variables into client care.

Encourage clients to continue cultural health practices that can bring no harm; provide support, understanding, and time when trying to change potentially harmful cultural health practices.

Determine whether the dental hygiene care plan is in harmony with the client's cultural values; modify when conflict occurs.

Consider dietary practices. Provide nutritional counseling within the framework of the client's culture.

Develop collegial relationships with health professionals from various ethnic and minority groups as a way of promoting cultural exchange that ultimately improves care.

the environment, defines health and oral health, approaches dental hygiene care, or values oral health. Knowledge of the client's perceptions of reality influences the overall goals of dental hygiene care. The dental hygiene practitioner recognizes that the care of clients from different cultures or ethnic groups takes more time than does caring for clients from similar cultures. Longer time should be scheduled to accommodate the need for translation, repetition, clarification, and socialization to dental hygiene care. Additional guidelines for cross-cultural dental hygiene are listed in Guidelines for Cross-cultural Dental Hygiene.

Assessment, Diagnosis, and Care Planning

The culturally competent dental hygienist understands that values and experiences shape everyone's perceptions, beliefs, and attitudes. Most dental hygiene data collection tools direct the hygienist to gather information about the client's health, but only perceptive understanding of the values and beliefs of the culture, ethnic group, or subculture yields a true measure of the client's realities. Therefore, assessing clients to produce culture-specific information is essential.

An ethnic/cultural assessment guide is presented in Table 5–5. This guide need not be a separate form but may be incorporated into existing data collection documents, interactions, and procedures. The dental hygiene diagnosis should identify the client's human need(s) that can be fulfilled through dental hygiene care, the cause (due to or related to), the evidence for the diagnosis, and related cultural factors. (See Chapter 16 for information on the dental hygiene diagnosis.) With this detailed focus, an individualized care plan can be developed and appropriate interventions selected. Using a nonjudgmental approach, the dental hygienist assesses the client's level of acculturation, English language skills, cultural health practices, and home remedies. Factors such as language comprehension, number of years in the country, dietary preferences, and attitudes about the predominant culture can provide important cues for assessing the influence of the client's culture (Table 5–6). Some clients may be consistently late for appointments because they are less future oriented and more interested in the activity in which they were previously engaged. A dental hygienist, insensitive to the time orientation of such cultures, may erroneously attribute this action to a low value placed on oral health or to anxiety about obtaining dental hygiene care. The dental hygienist able to demonstrate acceptance of diversity can establish trust with the client and provide effective care.

Implementation

Dental hygiene interventions, whether educational, technical, or interpersonal, must be congruent with local cultural values. The client's values and needs guide the selection of preventive and therapeutic strategies and interventions. In an unpublished paper, McKinney[9] related an experience of a dental hygienist that occurred in Liberia, Africa. A Liberian girl was brought to a clinic by her family for oral care. The dental hygienist found that the child's oral and systemic health status was poor. Surprisingly, the dental hygienist's oral hygiene recommendations (i.e., cleaning the teeth, gums, and tongue with a toothbrush, sponge, or gauze) were met with refusal. The young girl's family believed that she was cursed and that any items placed in her mouth would become a danger to the other family members who might touch them. Even the dental hygienist's suggestion to bury the used gauze was unacceptable because the ground would also become cursed. The family wanted the dental hygienist to cure the girl, that is, to eliminate the curse. Within the cultural context, the only acceptable dental hygiene intervention was for the girl to use

TABLE 5–5 DENTAL HYGIENE CULTURAL ASSESSMENT

Culturally Relevant Categories	Key Questions to Ask the Client or to Consider
Ethnic origin	Ethnic identification of the client? Place of birth? Place of childhood?
Race or racial mix	Racial background?
Domiciliary history	Where the client lived and where the client now lives? How long in this country?
Valued habits, customs, behavior	Client's habits, customs, values, and beliefs about health, oral health, healthcare providers, and the healthcare system? How the client values courtesy, family, work, gender roles? How the client expresses emotion, stress, pain, spirituality, fear?
Communication	Client's communication style, e.g., manner of speaking, language spoken, need for interpreter, reading skill, method of showing respect or deference, eye contact, gesticulations, zone of territory?
Health beliefs and practices	Healing systems and practices used by the client (wearing of chains, using certain herbs or potions, voodoo, prayer, curandero, herbalist, etc.)? Explanation of disease and illness in the client's culture (fatalism, punishment from God, germ theory, evil spirits, imbalance between yin and yang, etc.) How the client determines seriousness of a health problem; when to seek care and from whom?
Nutritional factors	Any culturally/religiously determined food preferences and restrictions? Are particular foods used to treat illness or to achieve a desired characteristic, e.g., strength?
Sociologic factors	What impact does economic status have on health and disease, living conditions, lifestyle, ability to obtain healthcare? What effect does the person's home have on access to care? What effect does level of education have on health status and ability to obtain healthcare? Does the family (or significant others) participate in the dental hygiene care? Does the family or significant others practice preventive health behaviors? Are there key institutions in the client's life that can influence health behavior, e.g., family, school, mosque, church, NAACP, Tribal Council, etc.?
Psychological factors	How does the client respond to the healthcare system, e.g., anxiety, distrust, fear, loss of dignity, nonadherence, avoidance? How does the culture perceive attractiveness? How does the client relate to people/institutions/environments from other cultures?
Physical characteristics	What is within normal limits for individuals within this ethnic group, e.g., skin color, gingival color, facial characteristics? What variations in growth and development patterns exist within the cultural groups? What socioenvironmental, systemic, and oral diseases are prevalent within this cultural/ethnic/racial group? Are there any diseases to which individuals in this cultural/racial/ethnic group are resistant?

Modified from Bloch B: Bloch's ethnic/cultural assessment guide. In Orgue MS, Bloch B, Monroy LA, eds: *Ethnic nursing care: A multicultural approach,* St Louis, 1983, Mosby; US Department of Health and Human Services: *Oral health in America: A report of the Surgeon General,* Rockville, Md, 2000, US Department of Health and Human Services, National Institute of Dental and Craniofacial Research, National Institutes of Health.

her own finger to clean her mouth. The family graciously accepted several bottles of a commercial mouthrinse, as if these bottles contained a magical potion.

In Sri Lanka "[o]ral hygiene exercises are performed in Sunday schools run by the monks to propagate the teachings of Buddha. The religious leadership provided in the village gives the needed credibility to the program, and the villagers adhere strictly to the oral hygiene practices taught by the monks because of the respect they command in the villages."[10] Islamic tenets convey the idea that prayers from a clean mouth are received more favorably.[11]

These vignettes underscore the need to understand different cultures if client oral health is to be achieved. As long as cultural beliefs or practices cause no harm, the dental hygienist can determine their importance to the client and recognize that their continued practice might assist in maintaining an effective client–provider relationship (Figure 5–3). Even when the behavior is ineffective, the client's comfort with and belief in its effectiveness can lend strength and support in a situation in which the person might otherwise feel alienated and out of touch. Website Information and Resources at http://evolve.elsevier.com/Darby/hygiene/ provides resources for understanding people within various

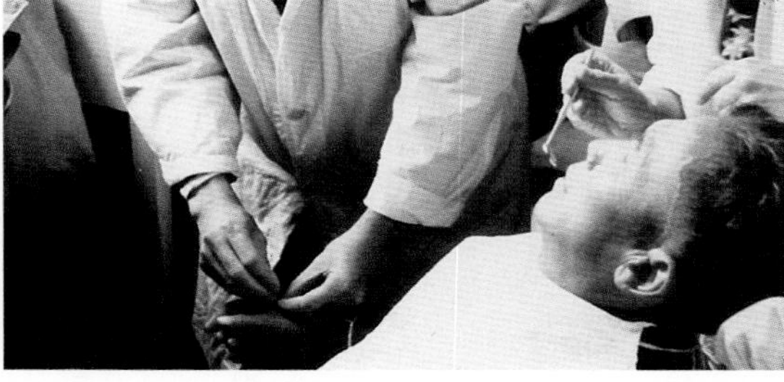

FIGURE 5–3 ✦ Asian man receiving acupuncture for pain control prior to dental treatment.

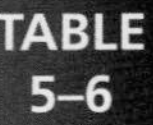

GUIDE TO WORKING WITH PEOPLE OF VARIOUS CULTURAL GROUPS*

Cultural Group	Basic Beliefs and Concepts	Healthcare Practices, Beliefs, Common Health Problems, and Remedies
African Americans	Life is a process rather than a state No division between physical, emotional, and spiritual needs Present oriented Frequently very religious Strong religious and community group support networks	Health occurs when there is harmony with nature; illness is disharmony Belief in both white magic and black magic Living and dead things influence health Employ faith healers, root doctors, and spiritualists to cast out evil spirits and demons Voodoo can cause or prevent malevolent forces Illness can be prevented by avoiding people who carry evil spirits, eating a good diet, and prayer *Common health problems:* Hypertension, cardiovascular disease, sickle cell disease, lactose-enzyme deficiency, obesity, diabetes, chemical and alcohol abuse, HIV May use home remedies or folk healing *Remedies:* Bangles: thin silver bracelets that let evil out and prevent it from entering the body; sound of bangles frightens evil spirits Talismans: drawn symbols that are worn or carried to ward off sickness Asafoetida: known as "incense of the devil," rubbed on to ward off colds and evil Snake: dehydrated, ground to a powder, and mixed with water; applied to skin lesions
Hispanics/Latin Americans (Spaniards, Cubans, Mexicans, Central and South Americans)	*Curanderos, espiritista, partera, senora*: folk healers, some of whom use the premise of humoral pathology *Humoral pathology*: Basic functions of body are regulated by body fluids (humors) defined by temperature and wetness: Blood (hot and wet) Phlegm (cold and wet) Black bile (cold and dry) Yellow bile (hot and dry) "Evil eye" is harmful magic Strong influence of the Catholic Church and family Flexible sense of time Respect for tradition Belief in bad magic, spells, and other harmful magic	Good health means balance among four humors Health is the result of good luck or reward from God Can maintain health and avoid disease via a balance among four humors Foods are classified as hot or cold unrelated to their temperature; hot and cold food must be eaten or avoided at certain times Illness is caused by an improper diet of hot and cold foods, dislocation of body parts, the supernatural, or envy (*envidia*) from others Illness can be prevented by proper diet, wearing of amulets, use of candles, prayer, avoiding too much success and harmful people Illness is the result of bad luck, punishment from God, or an imbalance among four humors *Common health problems:* Diabetes, poor nutrition, obesity, oral disease, hypertension, cardiovascular disease, hepatitis C, parasites, lactose-enzyme deficiency, HIV, coccidioidomycosis Expectations of the family to care for the young and the elderly *Remedies:* Burning candles to ward off evil spirits Amulets worn to ward off evil and as a protection against the evil eye *Manzanilla* (chamomile), an herb used to treat stomach disorders, anxiety, and insomnia
Asian/Pacific Islanders (Chinese, Hawaiians, Filipinos, Koreans, Japanese, Southeast Asians, e.g., Laotians, Cambodians, Hmong, Vietnamese)	The body is a gift that must be cared for and maintained Seldom complain about pain Strong family ties Preference for humility, modesty, self-control Respect for authority and tradition	Health is a state of harmony among body, mind, spirit, and nature (Taoism) Illness is caused by an upset in the balance (among body, mind, spirit, and nature) or by the weather, overexertion, or prolonged sitting Illness can be prevented by proper diet, exercise, avoiding temperature changes, and taking certain remedies May be disturbed by loss of blood, since they consider it to be body's life force May refuse surgery because they believe the body should remain intact *Common health problems:* Diabetes, tuberculosis, lactose-enzyme deficiency, malnutrition, hypertension, communicable diseases, cancer (esophageal, stomach, liver), coccidioidomycosis, and suicide

Table continued on following page

TABLE 5–6 GUIDE TO WORKING WITH PEOPLE OF VARIOUS CULTURAL GROUPS*—CONT'D

Cultural Group	Basic Beliefs and Concepts	Healthcare Practices, Beliefs, Common Health Problems, and Remedies
Asian/Pacific Islanders —cont'd		*Common health problems—cont'd* May use acumassage, acupressure, and acupuncture (Figure 5–3) Use of soy sauce may be a concern during nutritional counseling for individuals with high blood pressure *Remedies:* Jen Shen Lu Jung Wan: tonic taken to strengthen the entire system Thousand Year Eggs: old, uncooked eggs eaten daily for good health Huo Li Jian Mei Su: pills taken to maintain youth, health, and beauty Tiger Balm: all-purpose salve to relieve minor aches and pain Ginseng root: most famous all-purpose Chinese and Korean medicine Acupuncture—use of metal needles at certain points in the body to treat disease and control pain
Native Americans and Alaskan Natives	Both nature and the body must be treated with respect Great respect for elders Value placed on working together Present oriented Accumulation of wealth and goods is frowned on	Health is the result of total harmony with nature Prevention of illness is achieved through harmony of the body, mind, and spirit Illness can be associated with evil spirits, displeasing the holy people, disturbing nature, misusing a sacred ceremony Illness is the result of disharmony among the body, mind, spirit, and nature Large extended families who expect to be included in the healthcare process *Common health problems:* Alcoholism, suicide, obesity, tuberculosis, poor nutrition, oral disease, diabetes, hypertension, sexually transmitted diseases, accidents, and gallbladder disease *Remedies:* Sandpainting by medicine man Mask: to hide from evil spirits Sweet grass: burned as a rite of purification Thunderbird: a charm worn for protection and good luck Estafiata: leaves used to treat stomach ailments Use of herbs, ceremonies, fasting, meditation, heat, and massage
Whites	Youth valued over age Punctuality, physical attractiveness, competitiveness, cleanliness, achievement valued Control of emotion Emphasis on the nuclear family versus the extended family	Health is viewed as freedom from illness and disease; illness is the presence of disease symptoms, pain, disability, malformations llness may be the result of punishment from God, breaking religious rules, drafts, climate *Common health problems:* Cardiovascular disease, obesity, diabetes, gastrointestinal disease, cancer, suicide, chemical substance abuse *Remedies:* Varied because of the influence of multiple European cultures, e.g., Malocchio—horn-shaped amulet used by Italians to ward off the "evil eye"
Asian Indian	May follow Hinduism, Christianity, Sikhism, Islam, Zoroastrianism Modesty is highly valued Arranged marriages still common Elders and education highly valued Primary body forces (dosha): Vata, Pitta, Kapha	Balance of the dosha yields health May prefer same-gender healthcare provider Indian system of medicine known as Ayurveda emphasizes prevention and herbs The belief that pain and suffering are the result of karma may make symptom control difficult *Common health problems:* Malaria (in South India), cardiovascular disease, tuberculosis, pneumonia, rheumatic heart disease, nutritional deficits, cigarette smoking, dental caries, periodontal disease, sickle cell anemia, and communicable diseases *Remedies:* Herbal remedies of Ayurveda Yoga

TABLE 5–6 GUIDE TO WORKING WITH PEOPLE OF VARIOUS CULTURAL GROUPS*—CONT'D

Cultural Group	Basic Beliefs and Concepts	Healthcare Practices, Beliefs, Common Health Problems, and Remedies
Third world	Use of "magic" for good and evil throughout culture Believe in the "here" world and "nether" world Avoid certain people, cold air, and evil eyes Distrust in nature Faithful to punitive god Suspicious of other people Distrust friends, relatives, and strangers *Major Themes:* World is hostile and dangerous Individuals are vulnerable to attack from external sources Must depend on outside help to stay alive	Protective and evil magic determine illness, come from supernatural Spells and sacrifices will bring back health Will use healers from more than one healthcare system Good health centers on personal rather than scientific behaviors Explain emotional and physical illness in terms of imbalance between individual and physical, social, and spiritual life *Common health problems:* Malnutrition, high maternal and infant mortality, parasitic diseases *Remedies:* Herbs and home remedies
West Indies	Little value placed on time Present oriented Belief in voodoo	Obeah (witchcraft, black magic) power is very strong: scientific proof of sticking needles into people without bleeding or pain and frightening victims to death *Common health problems:* Malnutrition, hypertension, lactose intolerance, high maternal and infant mortality, parasitic diseases, sickle cell anemia, cancer (esophageal and stomach), coccidioidomycosis *Remedies:* Folk medicine, traditional healer (rootworker)

It is important to remember that not all people from a given culture will act in a standard manner. Great variability exists within cultural groups based on socioeconomic status, level of education, and overall life experiences. This chart is not meant to be generalized to all people within a specific culture, but rather to serve as a beginning guide

Data from Henderson G: *Understanding indigenous and foreign cultures*, Springfield, Ill, 1989, Charles C Thomas; and Spector RE: *Cultural diversity in health and illness*, ed 2, Norwalk, Conn, 1985, Appleton-Century-Crofts.

cultures. Obviously, not all people within a culture will subscribe to these beliefs. However, this can serve as a starting point for understanding peoples of diverse cultures.

Evaluation

In cross-cultural situations the evaluation phase of the dental hygiene process calls for an awareness of the client's cultural perspectives of what constitutes success. Frequent solicitation of the client's perspectives, level of understanding, psychomotor skill development, and self-care practices is particularly important. Evaluation should determine whether dental hygiene services are meeting the client's needs. Urging clients to talk about their oral health practices and status helps with cross-cultural communication. Validation occurs from feedback from the client and family (significant others) that the client's needs are being met.

FUTURE OF CROSS-CULTURAL DENTAL HYGIENE

Educational programs (undergraduate, graduate, and continuing education) are creating opportunities for international experiences for practitioners, students, and faculty and providing internships to develop cross-cultural competence. Programs leading to the baccalaureate degree and beyond possess foreign language requirements to enable dental hygienists to communicate outside their native language. Some are adding international and multicultural content to courses and developing student exchange and study abroad opportunities. Dental hygiene student organizations sponsor and promote activities that raise awareness about the diversity of the population while simultaneously developing competence in cross-cultural environments.

Dental hygienists work abroad for foreign dentists or multinational companies in global markets. International dental hygiene employment opportunities encompass both the profit and the nonprofit sectors, for example, private practice, the oral health products industry, higher education, the World Health Organization, Operation Smile International, Physicians for Peace, and other international service agencies.

CLIENT EDUCATION ISSUES

- ✦ Explain self-care and professional-care therapies for the control of oral diseases with the client's culture in mind.
- ✦ Provide nutritional counseling with knowledge of the client's culture and food preferences (see Chapter 28).

Legal, Ethical, and Safety Issues

- When language is a barrier, use an interpreter to enhance and validate communication.
- Investigate culturally based therapies to ensure their safety. Document in the client's chart the client's use of culturally based therapies and the client's response to professional care, instructions, and recommendations.
- Provide home care instructions supplemented with pictures and written instructions to enhance communication and compliance.
- Work to establish a trusting relationship as one strategy for maximizing compliance and minimizing risk of litigation.

Key Concepts

- Cross-cultural dental hygiene encompasses the social, political, ethnic, religious, and economic realities that people experience in culturally diverse interactions and environments.
- Culture plays an integral role in dental hygiene care because oral wellness, disease, and illness are culturally determined.
- Consideration of individual value systems and lifestyle should be part of the assessment and care plan for each client.
- Humanism recognizes the worth of all individuals through concern for and understanding of their network of attitudes, values, behavior patterns, and way of life.
- An individual is a biopsychosocial and spiritual being who brings uniqueness in race, culture, ethnicity, attitudes, beliefs, knowledge, and experience. This uniqueness affects the client's acceptance and response to care.
- One goal of cross-cultural dental hygiene is to make the oral healthcare setting a welcoming place for individuals who might otherwise feel disconnected or disenfranchised.
- Race refers to one of three classifications of human beings based on physical characteristics; ethnicity refers to unique cultural practices that reflect distinct customs, language, and social values. There are more similarities among racial groups than there are differences
- Culture is the rules of behavior learned in order for a person to adapt successfully to life within a particular group; it includes beliefs, traditions, experiences, customs, rituals, and language.
- People who speak different languages perceive the world differently.
- Stereotyping is the erroneous behavior of assuming that people posses certain characteristics simply because they are members of a particular group.
- Ethnocentrism is the erroneous belief that one's culture is superior to that of another.
- Socioeconomic status affects where one lives, how one spends money, where one receives healthcare, and ultimately, one's general and oral health status.
- Poverty is a key predictor of poor oral health.

Critical Thinking Exercises

1. Using the most current census data available on the Internet, identify the diverse cultural groups that reside in your community. (Hint: start your search at www.census.gov). Using the websites in Website Information and Resources at http://evolve.elsevier.com/Darby/hygiene/ and other links that you find, research their predominant healthcare practices and beliefs. What behaviors should you avoid when interacting with members of these cultural groups? What behaviors should you incorporate into your interactions to improve health outcomes?
2. Think about the clients you have treated. Share an experience in which you may have initially stereotyped the client, and then changed your thinking about that client. What personal assumptions did you initially make about the person? What factors did you base these initial assumptions on? What caused you to change your thinking?
3. Together with your peers, plan a social event. Have everyone bring a food to share with the group. As you enjoy the food, classify it according to the *U.S. Food Guide Pyramid.*
4. Chose a second-world or third-world country that you are interested in. Use the Internet to identify the oral and general health status of the people there.

For References, Suggested Readings, and Related Websites, visit
http://evolve.elsevier.com/Darby/hygiene/

SECTION 2

Preparation for the Client Appointment

CHAPTER 6

INFECTION CONTROL

OBJECTIVES

Mastery of the content in this chapter will enable the reader to:

- ✦ Assess risk of disease transmission in oral healthcare and plan appropriate control measures
- ✦ Interpret emerging guidelines for infection control
- ✦ Identify infectious diseases that pose a risk of transmission in oral healthcare
- ✦ Apply active and passive mechanisms of infectious disease transmission prevention
- ✦ Select appropriate protective attire for use during dental hygiene client care
- ✦ Prepare the dental environment prior to and after client care

KEY TERMS

Autoclave
Biologic indicator (spore test)
Chemical indicator
Chemical vapor sterilization
Critical instruments
Cross-contamination
Dermatitis
Disinfection/disinfectants
Dry-heat sterilization
e-antigen
Environmental Protection Agency (EPA)
Exposures
Fomites
Germicidal
Germicide
Immunizations
Infectious agent
Noncritical instruments
Nosocomial infection
Occupational Safety and Health Administration (OSHA)
Personal protective equipment (PPE)
Portal of entry
Post-exposure management
Semicritical instruments
Seroconversion
Standard of care
Standard precautions
Sterilization
Susceptible host
TB Mantoux test
Transmission-based precautions
Tuberculosis
Universal precautions
Work restrictions

BASIC INFECTION CONTROL CONCEPTS

Infection control refers to a comprehensive and systematic program that, when applied, prevents the transmission of infectious agents among persons who are in direct or indirect contact with the healthcare environment. The goal of infection control is to create and maintain a safe clinical environment to eliminate the potential for disease transmission from clinician to client, client to clinician, or client to client. Infection control is based on the premise that transmission occurs when an *infectious agent* has a *portal of entry* to a susceptible host (Table 6–1).

Although the challenge remains to meet the comprehensive needs of diverse clients, the premise of universal precautions goes beyond the individual to eliminate the potential for transfer of disease-causing microorganisms during the delivery of oral health services. Infection

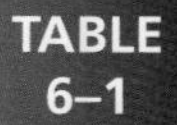

TABLE 6–1 PORTALS OF EXIT/ENTRY, MODES OF TRANSMISSION, AND POTENTIAL PATHOLOGY

Mode of Transmission	Potential Pathology
Portal of Exit/Entry: Skin and Mucous Membranes	
Any break in the integrity of the skin and mucous membranes (ocular mucosa) can lead to an infection	
DIRECT INOCULATION TO TISSUE SURFACE	
Infectious blood or serum onto mucosal surfaces/breaks in skin	HIV
Blood, saliva, tears, semen	HBV
Lesion exudate, saliva	Herpes
Portal of Exit/Entry: Oral Cavity	
Mucous membranes of the oral cavity are susceptible to infection; portal for ingestion	
DIRECT INOCULATION TO TISSUE SURFACE	
Pharyngeal secretions (infected droplet contact)	Pneumonia, TB
Exudate from oral lesion	Herpes, syphilis
Crevicular exudate	Abscesses
Saliva and blood	CMV, mononucleosis
INOCULATION INTO CIRCULATORY SYSTEM	
Blood	HIV, HDV, HCV
Blood, saliva, tears, semen	HBV
INGESTION OF PATHOGENS	
Saliva	Mumps, hand-foot-and-mouth disease
Portal of Exit/Entry: Gastrointestinal Tract	
Bowel elimination and vomiting are portals of exit for pathogens	
Fecal-oral	HIV
Portal of Exit/Entry: Respiratory Tract	
Pathogens residing in the respiratory tract can be released from the body when the person sneezes, coughs, talks, or even breathes. The microorganisms exit via the mouth and nose	
INFECTED DROPLET CONTACT: INHALATION, INGESTION, DIRECT INOCULATION	
Nasopharyngeal secretions	Flu, common cold, whooping cough, candidiasis, opportunistic *Pneumocystis carinii*
Pharyngeal secretions	TB
Nasopharyngeal secretions, blood, saliva, vesicle exudate	Measles, rubeola, rubella
PORTAL OF EXIT/ENTRY: GENITOURINARY SYSTEM	
Pathogens exit via male's urethral meatus or female's vaginal canal or enter through surface breaks in the skin and mucosa	
DIRECT INOCULATION TO TISSUE SURFACE	
Lesion exudate, saliva	Herpes
Lesion exudate, blood, pharyngeal secretions	Gonococcal infections
Lesion exudate	Syphilis
INOCULATION INTO CIRCULATORY SYSTEM	
Blood, semen, vaginal secretions, and breast milk	HIV
Blood, semen, saliva, tears	HBV, HDV, HCV
Portal of Exit/Entry: Blood	
A break in the skin by needle, instrument, or traumatic wound; burn or dermatitis; nonintact skin provides portals of exit/entry	
INOCULATION INTO CIRCULATORY SYSTEM	
Blood (also transmitted by semen, vaginal secretions, breast milk)	HIV
Blood (also transmitted by saliva, semen, tears)	HBV, HDV, HCV
DIRECT INOCULATION TO TISSUE SURFACE	
Blood, saliva	CMV, infectious mononucleosis

HIV, Human immunodeficiency virus; *HBV*, hepatitis B virus; *TB*, tuberculosis; *CMV*, cytomegalovirus; *HDV*, hepatitis D virus; *HCV*, hepatitis C virus.
Courtesy Barbara L. Heckman, RDH, MS.

control, via the principle of universal precautions, must be applied and consistently delivered to all clients.

Human needs theory relates directly to universal precautions:

- ✦ First, the universality of human needs transcends all ages, cultures, nationalities, genders, sexual orientation, behaviors, and the like. Universal precautions, the practice of infection control, are universally applied regardless of the individual being treated.
- ✦ Second, there is a link between human needs and health as defined by the World Health Organization. The World Health Organization defines health as "The extent to which an individual or group is able,

on the one hand, to realize aspirations and satisfy needs and, on the other hand, to change and cope with the environment." Infection control is truly the ability to change and cope with the environment.

- Third, of all the human needs, infection control is most applicable to protection from health risks. Although infection control practices cannot reduce unintended harm from the care itself, it can prevent unintended harm to the dental hygienist, the client, and other staff. The need for protection from health risks begins with the client. Protection from health risks centers traditionally on the client health history, but universal precautions do not depend on the health history, since clients may not always be aware of their health risks or emerging health concerns. Universal precautions treat all clients as potentially harboring disease-producing organisms and apply evidence-based protocols to reduce the potential harm associated with these organisms. The hygienist uses the patient's health history to make decisions about appropriate interventions. With infection control, the hygienist considers the procedures and the behaviors indicated to reduce the risk of disease transmission. Infection control encompasses behaviors and practices to meet this need.
- Fourth, another human need related to universal precautions is freedom from anxiety and stress. People need to feel safe in an oral healthcare environment. Part of this safety comes from the immediate recognition that infection control principles are being applied.
- Fifth, many human needs are fulfilled by a variety of client services and policies, but the need for conceptualization and understanding underlies every behavior relative to client care and must be monitored and measured. There must be evidence of the use of sound and appropriate infection control practices, and rationales must be explained before any care is delivered. From the onset, clients need to realize that their safety is paramount; this instills the belief that subsequent care is the most appropriate, as well.

Infection control also begins with assessment of the overall environment in which care is delivered and how to ensure it is free from biohazards. Dental hygienists conduct infection control assessment based on the intended procedures to be delivered:

- How will the client be treated, and what are the infection control implications associated with this procedure?
- How will the client understand the infection control practices and take comfort in their use?
- What specific infection control protocols are necessary to protect the client, clinician, staff, and their significant others from inadvertent disease transmission?

A model of infection control parallels the model of dental hygiene care. For example, clients must understand the selection and use of infection control procedures and the protective outcomes. However, the infection control model differs from the traditional client care model in that it focuses on tasks and procedures and not the client.

Scrutinizing each individual client health history will not determine the degree of risk for disease transmission. Dental procedures generate widely variant amounts of body fluids, and the dental instruments used vary in their tendency to release body fluids. Therefore, infection control is procedurally based, not client based. The cognitive goals in the infection control model relate to the explanation of infection control, the protective intent of infection control, and its benchmark status as a standard of care. Effective goals in the infection control model are designed to change a client's attitude in a positive manner and reduce fear or anxiety associated with dental hygiene care. The client must see infection control as protective, not punitive.

CDC and OSHA

Two agencies of the U.S. government play key roles in infection control. Guidelines and regulations developed by both of these agencies have established national standards for infection control.

- The *Centers for Disease Control and Prevention (CDC)* is one of eight federal public health agencies within the U.S. Department of Health and Human Services. Its mission is to promote health and quality of life by preventing and controlling disease, injury, and disability.
- The *Occupational Safety and Health Administration (OSHA)*, within the U.S. Department of Labor, serves to protect persons by ensuring a safe and healthy workplace.

Standards of Care

Standard of care refers to the level of care that a reasonably prudent practitioner would exercise. It is not a maximum standard or an ultimate level of quality, rather it is the minimum level that should be achieved in all aspects of client care. Infection control regulations, evidence-based guidelines, government agencies, licensing boards, and expert opinion are relied on to determine the standard of care for asepsis. The standard of care is limited because it does not promote excellence nor does it encourage performance improvement. In summary, the standard of care is a benchmark to ensure that the practice is providing the level of care that the client should receive from a reasonably prudent practitioner.

Dental healthcare workers adopt the principles, not just the practice, of infection control. As stakeholders in the creation of a safe clinical environment, their own human needs for conceptualization, understanding, freedom from fear and anxiety, and freedom from health risks must be met. Dental healthcare workers take actions to become and remain healthy. This begins with an assessment of personal health status and protection from disease (Figure 6–1).

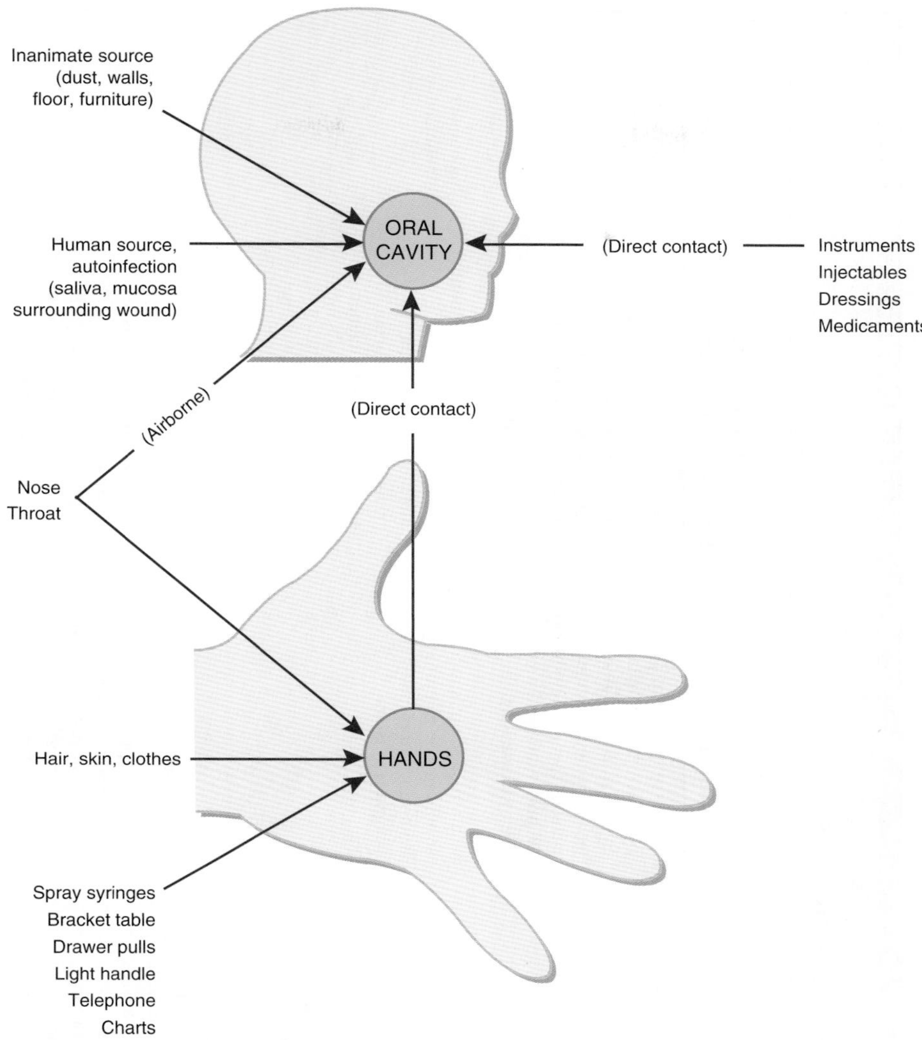

FIGURE 6–1 ✦ Vehicles of transmission of pathogens. *(Courtesy Johnson & Johnson.)*

STRATEGIES TO PREVENT DISEASE TRANSMISSION

Vaccinations

In addition to standard childhood vaccination schedules, additional *immunizations* are recommended for healthcare workers (Table 6–2). Healthcare workers in specific geographic locations or with underlying medical conditions may need immunizations that are not routinely recommended for healthcare workers in general. The healthcare worker's physician is consulted regarding the need for additional vaccinations.

Immunization for diphtheria, pertussis, and tetanus (DPT) is administered to all children in the United States and most other countries. Of these, only tetanus requires a booster. Adults do not need to receive a tetanus booster more than once every ten years. Additional vaccines recommended for all healthcare workers include hepatitis B, influenza, measles, mumps, rubella, and varicella. Several of these were probably administered during the worker's childhood and do not require boosters. Natural immunity through prior infection also is possible and would eliminate the need for vaccination. Pneumococcal vaccine is recommended for all adults age 65 or greater.

Work Restrictions

Work restrictions are recommended by the U.S. Public Health Service for healthcare workers with certain infections and following exposure to some diseases. These precautions are intended to protect the client. Many of these infections are preventable with vaccines, and all healthcare workers should be aware of the importance of receiving appropriate vaccinations early in their professional education to protect themselves and their clients. Individuals diagnosed with diphtheria should be excluded from duty until the illness resolves. Workers with mumps or measles should be excluded during the acute illness phase, as well as after exposure and during the incubation phase if not immunized. If diagnosed with hepatitis A, dental healthcare workers should

TABLE 6–2 RECOMMENDED IMMUNIZATIONS FOR HEALTHCARE PROVIDERS

Vaccine-Preventable Diseases	Immune Status Determination Prior to Vaccination	Vaccine of Choice	Contraindications	Postvaccination Side Effects/Complications	Boosters
Mumps	Persons born before 1956 are generally considered to be immune	Measles, mumps, and rubella (MMR) (live virus); one dose SC, any time from 15 months of age	Immunocompromised persons; persons with anaphylactic hypersensitivity to neomycin, gelatin, or eggs; pregnant persons (pregnancy should be prevented for 3 months after vaccination)	Adverse clinical reactions are rare. Other than reports of burning and/or stinging of short duration at the injection site, infrequent reactions are malaise, sore throat, headache, fever, and rash	No booster required
Measles (rubeola)	Persons born before 1956 are generally considered to be immune	MMR combined or measles vaccine (live virus vaccine); if person was vaccinated between 1963 and 1967 with killed measles vaccine, should be reimmunized with live virus vaccine; if susceptible, nonpregnant, and exposed, may be protected if immunized within 72 hours of exposure. One dose SC, with 2nd dose in 1 month	Live attenuated virus vaccine should not be given to immunocompromised or pregnant persons	5–15% of the vaccine recipients develop symptoms of attenuated measles; a transient rash may occur with about 5% of vaccines	No booster required
German measles (rubella)	Universal immunization, especially for unimmunized women of childbearing age if no laboratory evidence of immunity. If not immunized, provider could transmit rubella to associates and clients, some of whom might be pregnant (rubella is associated with serious birth defects)	Live attenuated rubella virus prepared in human cell cultures. Rubella vaccine may be given at any age. MMR combination may be used, since administration of vaccine to persons already immune is not deleterious. One dose SC.	Immunocompromised persons; persons with anaphylactic hypersensitivity to neomycin or eggs; pregnant persons (pregnancy must be prevented for 3 months after vaccination because of risk of infecting fetus)	Infrequent complications in healthy persons; may experience joint pain (40%); rarely will arthralgias persist for up to 10 days	No booster required

Tetanus and diphtheria (Td)	Essentially no natural immunity to tetanus toxoid; even individuals with a previous history of tetanus should receive immunization	Tetanus-diphtheria (adult); vaccine series requires 2 doses of Td toxoids 4–8 weeks apart, followed by a third dose 6–12 months after the second	Individuals with a history of neurologic or hypersensitivity reaction after previous dose; pregnancy	Some individuals have had neurological or hypersensitivity reactions; if boosters are given at a greater frequency than the recommended 10-year interval, tetanus toxoid can cause severe local pain and swelling	Td booster every 10 years
Poliomyelitis (enhanced-potency inactivated polio-virus [E-IPV] or live oral polio-virus [OPV])	Immunization recommended for all; oral poliovirus vaccine (OPV) if younger than 18 years of age, or *any age* if direct contact with a case of polio; otherwise inactivated poliovaccine (E-IPV) for persons older than 18 years of age	Oral, attenuated OPV (live attenuated virus) requires two doses 2–8 weeks apart, followed by a third dose 6–12 months after the second; IPV requires two doses 4–6 weeks apart, followed by a third dose 6–12 months after the second	OPV: immunocompromised persons or those with immunocompromised family members; persons with hypersensitivity to neomycin	OPV: persons older than 18 years of age are at slightly increased risk for vaccine-associated paralysis; virus may be shed after OPV, inadvertently exposing immunocompromised contacts to live vaccine virus	OPV or E-IPV boosters are recommended only for persons who have had direct contact exposure with oral secretions or feces of a person with poliomyelitis
Influenza (inactivated whole-virus and split virus-vaccine)	Virus content of vaccine is revised annually to include the new strains expected to be prevalent; the multitude of influenza viruses precludes attaining immunity to all	Influenza vaccine formulated annually after season's particular virus identified; yearly fall immunization recommended	Anaphylactic hypersensitivity to eggs	Local tenderness at injection site for 1 or 2 days (33%); malaise and low-grade fever for up to 2 days (infrequent) (viruses in vaccine not infectious, will not cause influenza); hypersensitivity (rare)	Temporary immunity requires annual reimmunization with vaccine incorporating new strains of virus
Hepatitis B recombinant DNA	Vaccines recommend for anyone over 15 months of age	Two doses IM 4 weeks apart; third dose 5 months after second	Individuals with a history of anaphylactic reaction to baker's yeast		Booster recommended when blood titer is low

Courtesy Barbara L. Heckman, RDH, MS.

refrain from direct client contact and avoid handling food others will eat. If suffering from an upper respiratory infection, the worker should avoid contact with clients who are high-risk due to being medically compromised. Workers suffering from active herpes zoster (shingles) may continue to work unrestricted, but should cover lesions to protect against exposure to blood and body fluids on non-intact skin.

A special set of precautions exists for healthcare workers who are carriers of hepatitis B. Recognizing that a special subcategory of hepatitis carrier exists, the e-antigen carrier, the CDC recommends that e-antigen–positive individuals consult with an expert review panel to determine what precautions may be necessary to safely treat clients. The *e antigen* is associated with a higher risk of transmission from healthcare worker to client in spite of universal precautions. Any healthcare worker who is a hepatitis B carrier should consult with a physician to determine status and explore options for treatment and concerns for client safety.

Universal Precautions

Universal precautions are the practices by which healthcare workers follow the same infection control protocols for all clients, regardless of the clients' infectious status or health history. Many individuals may be infected with the human immunodeficiency virus (HIV), hepatitis B virus (HBV), or other bloodborne disease not identified through the health history interview. Certain precautions are known to prevent the transmission of these viruses and should be applied during the care of all clients. These precautions protect both the healthcare worker and the client from disease transmission. More recent guidelines, known as standard precautions, address infections that are not necessarily bloodborne.

Standard Precautions

Standard precautions are a synthesis of the major features of universal precautions and body substance isolation precautions, and apply to:

- ✦ Blood
- ✦ Other bodily fluids, secretions, and excretions except sweat (BBF) regardless of whether or not they contain visible blood
- ✦ Non-intact skin
- ✦ Mucous membranes

Therefore, standard precautions apply to blood and all moist body substances. These guidelines are "first tier" in the prevention of *nosocomial infections* (infections acquired in the hospital and other medical care settings). Although these guidelines have replaced universal precautions in hospital settings, they have little application to most dental offices and clinics.

Isolation precautions had been developed to address the need to tailor infection control precautions to the various epidemiologic features of individual diseases. These precautions are updated and improved over time, as knowledge of disease transmission and prevention evolves.

Transmission-based Precautions

Transmission-based precautions are designed for clients documented as or suspected to be infected or colonized with highly transmissible or epidemiologically important pathogens. These are used when standard precautions may not be adequate to interrupt transmission in hospitals. As with standard precautions, these were developed for the treatment of patients in a hospital and are not applicable to oral healthcare settings.

Health History

Health history assessment is part of comprehensive oral healthcare. However, prior to the *Centers for Disease Control Blood-borne Pathogens Standard Recommendations* of various precautions to be followed, the importance of detecting clients with infectious diseases was paramount, especially for those with the highly transmissible hepatitis B virus. After dentistry accepted strict infection control guidelines and the concept of universal precautions, as regulated by OSHA, this goal carried far less importance in disease transmission. Since all clients are regarded as potentially infectious, the approach has been simplified.

The two major exceptions are the patient with untreated, active *tuberculosis* (TB) and the immunocompromised patient. The active TB patient should not be treated for elective procedures, and emergency procedures should be undertaken following special precautions such as the use of laminar airflow, UV light, and HEPA filter masks (see Policy for Treatment of Dental Clients with Active or Suspected Infection with Tuberculosis). Immunocompromised patients may require special treatment to protect them from infection, such as the use of sterile irrigation and prophylactic antibiotic premedication. This must be determined on a case-by-case basis, not as a routine measure.

For protection of the dental healthcare workers, vaccinations should be considered for other highly transmissible infectious diseases such as influenza.

Mycobacterium Tuberculosis Testing

Two types of skin tests are available to assist in the diagnosis of tuberculosis. The *TB tine test* is commonly used to screen infants and children and is not highly accurate. The *TB Mantoux test* consists of an intradermal injection of purified protein derivative into the forearm. The area is observed 48 hours after the injection for development of a wheal that is red, raised, and measures at least 10 mm across. For HIV-infected individuals a 5-mm wheal is considered positive due to the tendency to develop a less-reactive response if the immune system is compromised.

A positive skin test is an indication of infection with the bacterium, but is not an indication of active infection. In fact, the majority of individuals with a positive skin test do not have active tuberculosis. About 10% of infected individuals will develop active TB in their lifetime. About 5% develop the active disease shortly after exposure, and 5% will develop active disease later in life when their immune systems become compromised

Policy for Treatment of Dental Clients with Active or Suspected Infection with Tuberculosis

During initial health history and periodic updates ask clients about a history of TB disease and symptoms suggestive of TB. Symptoms include chronic cough, coughing blood, night sweats, and weight loss. *Note:* positive TB skin test without symptoms *does not indicate active infection* in most cases.

Clients with history and symptoms suggestive of active TB should be promptly referred to a physician for evaluation for possible infectiousness.

Elective dental treatment should be postponed until a physician confirms, using recognized diagnostic evaluations, that the client does not have active TB.

If urgent dental care must be provided for a client who has, or is suspected of having, active TB infection, TB isolation practices must be implemented. Treatment provided should be limited to the minimum necessary to relieve the client's immediate pain. Generally, referral to a medical center with proper isolation rooms will be required. Respiratory protection (HEPA filter masks) must be worn by dental care providers when performing procedures on these patients. The respirators must be fit tested prior to each use.

Dental healthcare workers with persistent cough and other symptoms suggestive of active TB should be evaluated promptly. The individual should not return to work until a diagnosis of TB has been excluded or until the individual is on therapy and a determination has been made that the worker is not infectious.

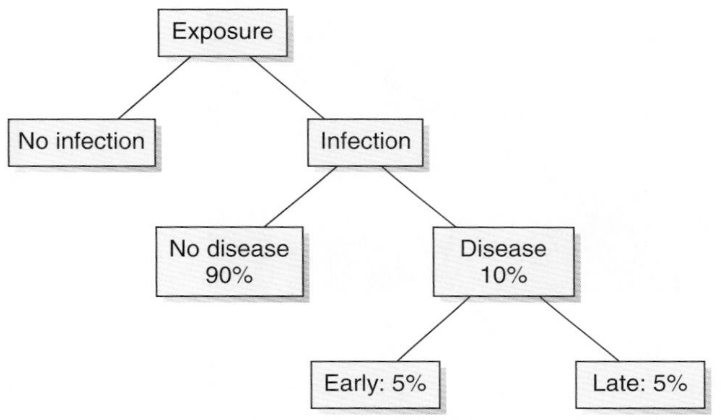

FIGURE 6–2 ✦ Progression following tuberculosis exposure.

(Figure 6–2). Most people who experience a positive skin test are placed on preventive chemotherapy for six months. The standard drug for prevention of active infection is isoniazid. This same medication is used in combination with other medications (e.g., rifampin, pyrazinamide) to treat active infection. Rare cases of tuberculosis do not respond to traditional therapy. These cases, referred to as drug-resistant tuberculosis, often result in death of the infected individual.

Engineering Controls (Figure 6–3)

Engineering controls are devices or equipment that reduce or eliminate a hazard. In the context of healthcare, this usually refers to:

- ✦ Devices that provide protective guarding of sharp instruments such as needles or scalpels
- ✦ Devices that replace sharp items such as needles with systems that do not contain a sharp surface
- ✦ Devices that eliminate worker exposure to sharp items; examples include sharps containers or needle covers with built-in retraction.

Engineering controls should be considered when it is reasonable to believe that the control measure will reduce the potential for exposure to a client's blood or body fluids. OSHA requires the use of sharps with engineered sharps injury protection when available and when found to provide superior protection compared with the standard devices. Examples include syringes with retractable needles or needle guards, scalpels with retractable blades or blade guards, and other devices that render the sharp safer through blunting, encapsulation, guarding, or destruction.

Work Practice Controls

Work practice controls reduce or eliminate a hazard by changing the way a task is performed. Figure 6–4 shows improper positioning of fingers, placing the dental hygienist at risk. Proper client positioning may reduce the hygienist's exposure to droplets generated during certain procedures. Use of a high-speed evacuator while spraying a client's mouth with air and water will reduce the amount of droplet splash if low-speed suction or no suction is used. Using an ultrasonic cleaner to decontaminate used dental instruments prior to sterilization is another example of work practice controls (Procedure 6–1).

Personal Protective Equipment

The term *personal protective equipment* refers to garments and other attire worn with the intent to protect the worker from exposure that cannot be controlled through the use of engineering, administrative, or work practice controls. In relationship to infection control, the exposure is to blood and other body fluids from clients. The attire selected should protect the worker from exposure to the skin, clothing, eyes, mouth, and other mucous membranes during the normal course of his or her duties (Figure 6–12).

The selection of attire must be based on the nature if the procedure, that is, how much blood and saliva can reasonably be anticipated for a given procedure, rather than on the health status of the client receiving treatment.

Text continued on page 88

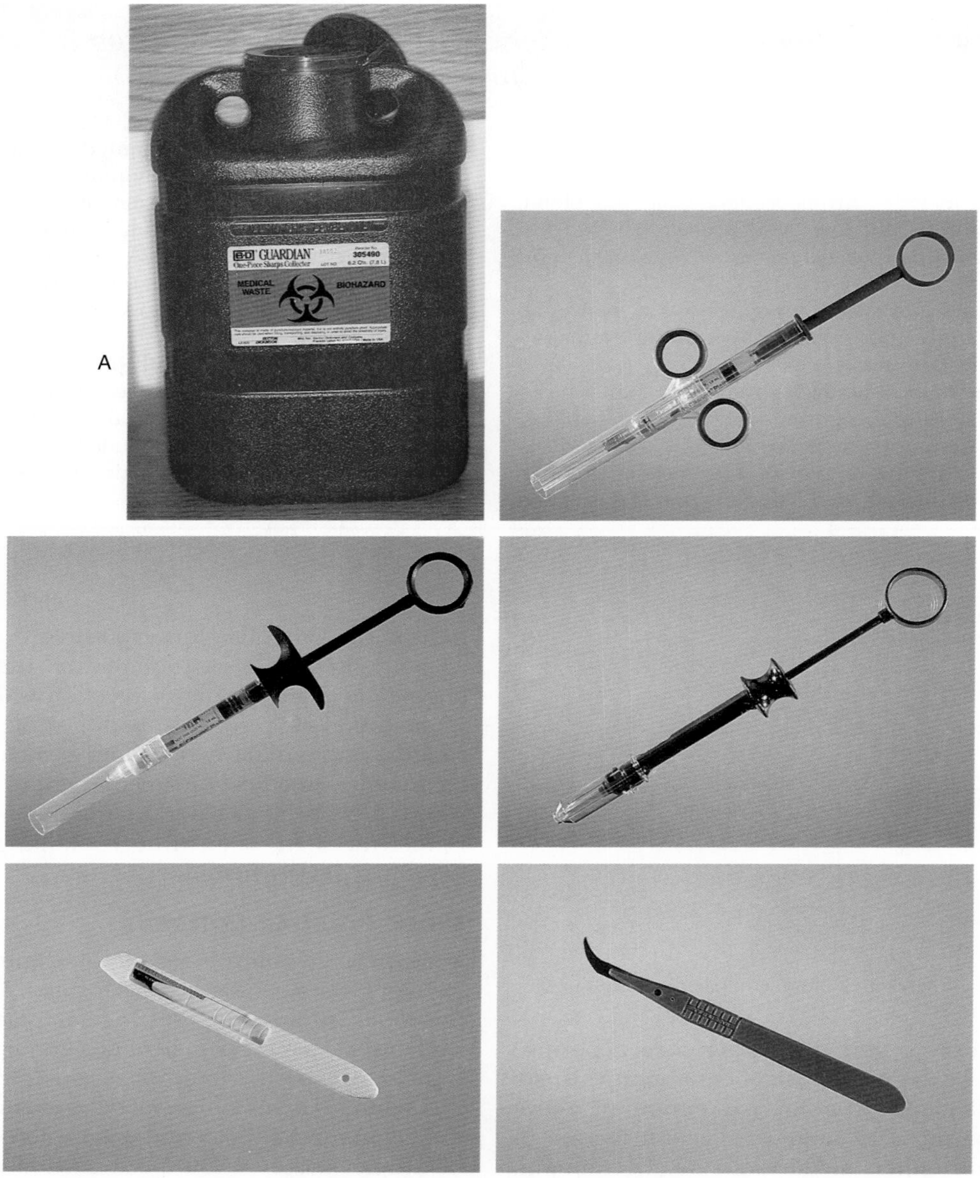

A B C D E F

FIGURE 6–3 ✦ Some devices that eliminate healthcare worker exposure to sharps. A, Sharps container with biohazard label warning. B, Disposable dental safety syringe. C, Reusable dental safety syringe with disposable needle. D, Disposable dental safety needle. E, Safety scalpel with retractable blade. F, Disposable scalpel with blade. *(A courtesy Barbara L. Heckman, RDH, MS.)*

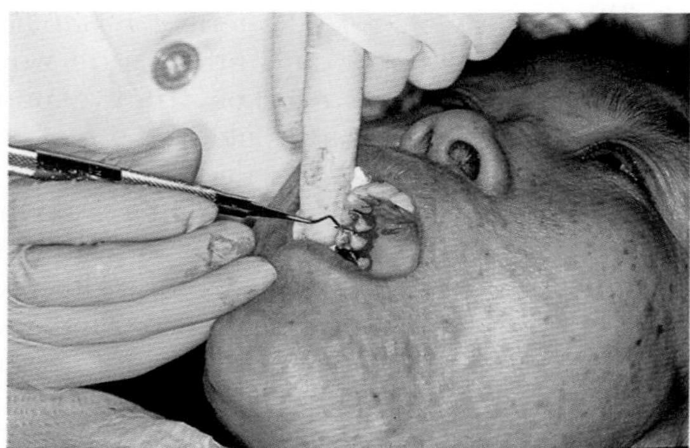

FIGURE 6–4 ✦ Example of improper positioning of operator's fingers, placing the dental hygienist at risk of a puncture wound.

Procedure 6–1 DECONTAMINATING INSTRUMENTS WITH AN ULTRASONIC CLEANER

EQUIPMENT

Nitrile gloves
Ultrasonic cleaning unit
Cleaning solution
Contaminated instruments
Instrument cassette
Face mask and protective eyewear

STEPS	RATIONALE
1. Wear heavy-duty, puncture-resistant nitrile gloves and protective eyewear when processing contaminated equipment. Although wearing a mask to protect the mucous membranes of the nose and oral mucosa is not emphasized as much in the literature on instrument recirculation, such a precaution provides additional protection in the event of exposure to contaminated aerosol spatter associated with some steps in instrument processing.	Heavy-duty, puncture-resistant gloves greatly minimize risk of exposure incidents involving contaminated reusable sharps. Protective eyewear and masks prevent exposure of mucous membranes to spatter and aerosols generated in instrument recirculation area.
2. Prepare the ultrasonic equipment solution according to the manufacturer's directions to ensure proper dilutions. Maintain the tank solution level at least three quarters full ($1\frac{1}{2}$ inches from the top of the holding tank) (Figure 6–5)	Specifically formulated high-quality detergent selection and proper dilution ensure optimal bioburden removal. Maintain solution at the proper level to ensure that all items being decontaminated are completely submerged.
3. Decant the holding solution into the drain of the sink while water is running, before the instrument container is moved from the containment area to the decontamination area (Figure 6–6). After the presoaking solution is removed, rinse the instruments in the basket or cassette with cool water. Drain off the excess water for additional contaminant reduction prior to immersing the basket or cassette into the ultrasonic solution in the holding tank (Figure 6–7)	The contaminated holding solution is diluted for disposal, since the presoaking solution may be different from the ultrasonic solution. Instruments are rinsed with cool water to remove residual holding solution and some of the softened bioburden. Drain off excess water to prevent dilution of ultrasonic cleaning agent.

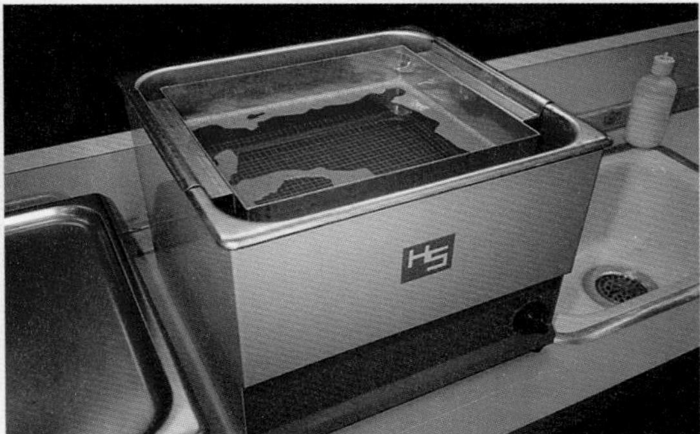

FIGURE 6–5 ✦ Ultrasonic cleaning unit.

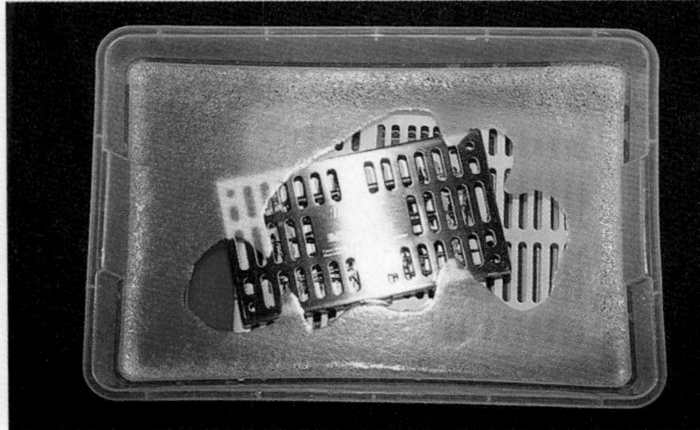

FIGURE 6–6 ✦ Decant holding solution into sink.

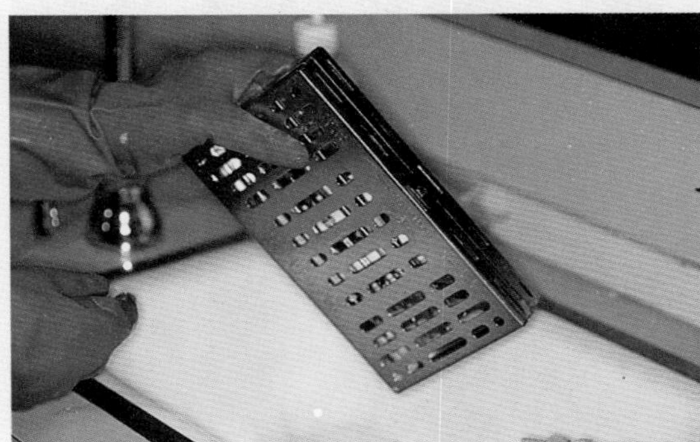

FIGURE 6–7 ✦ Drain excess water.

Continued on following page

Procedure 6–1 DECONTAMINATING INSTRUMENTS WITH AN ULTRASONIC CLEANER—CONT'D

STEPS	RATIONALE
4. After immersion of the instrument container, cover the tank with the lid and set the cleaning time for 6 to 10 minutes or until no visible debris remains (Figures 6–8 and 6–9). The number of instruments that will fit in the instrument basket depends on the size of the ultrasonic unit, which is usually related to the volume of care and number of dental and dental hygiene care providers. A small ultrasonic cleaner can effectively accommodate 8 to 10 instruments. When cassettes are used for transport from presoaking through ultrasonic cleaning to sterilization, the length of time for cleaning needs to be increased to 15 minutes to ensure effective decontamination.	Cover tank with lid whenever it is cleaning to prevent generated aerosols from escaping. Overloading the unit inhibits the ability of the unit's billions of tiny bubbles to collapse and create the turbulence necessary to effectively clean the surface of all instruments. Time required for effective cleaning may vary, depending on the amount or type of material or instruments and energy of the unit.
5. During the ultrasonic cleaning, a well-fitting cover must remain on the equipment to prevent contaminated aerosols from escaping into the atmosphere of the instrument recirculation center.	Cover tank with lid during operation to prevent generated contaminated aerosols from escaping.
6. When the timed cleaning cycle has ended, slowly and carefully lift up the basket, allowing excess solution to drain off the instruments into the tank to maintain the level of solution (Figure 6–10). Transfer the basket to an adjacent sink and rinse instruments thoroughly under running water (Figure 6–11). Drain instruments, inspect them, and set them aside for drying and advancement to the packaging area.	Following ultrasonic cleaning, both instruments and solution are contaminated and, therefore, require careful protected handling.

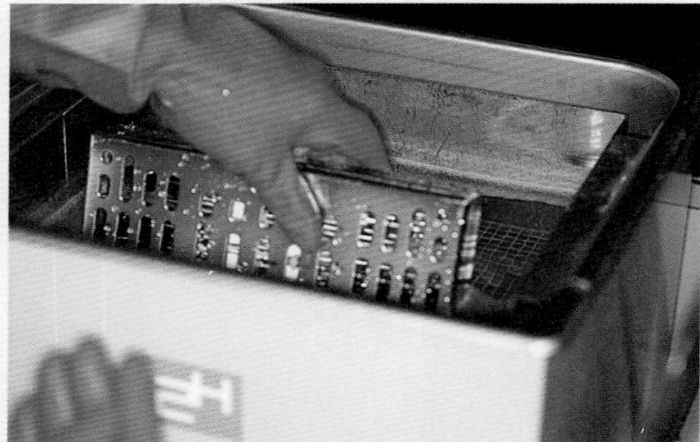

FIGURE 6–8 ✦ Immerse instrument cassette into ultrasonic cleaner solution.

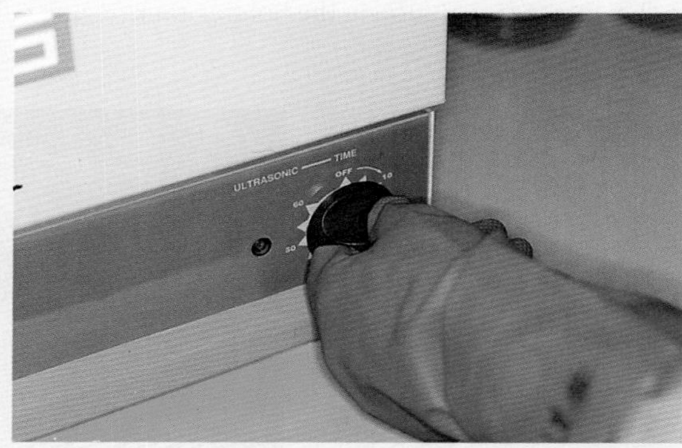

FIGURE 6–9 ✦ Set ultrasonic cleaning unit timer.

FIGURE 6–10 ✦ Lift basket to drain excess solution.

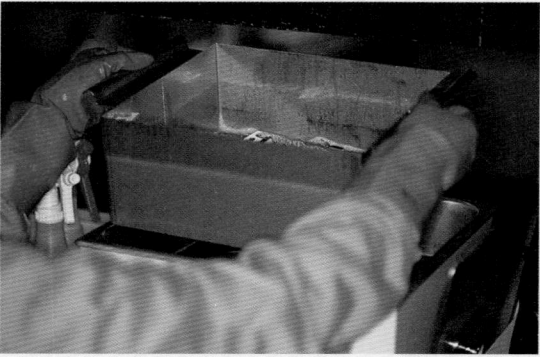

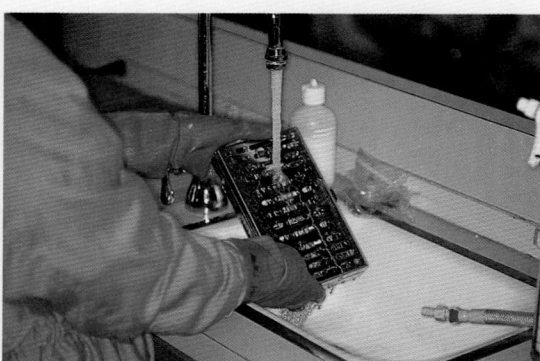

FIGURE 6–11 ✦ Rinse instrument cassette.

Procedure 6–1 DECONTAMINATING INSTRUMENTS WITH AN ULTRASONIC CLEANER—CONT'D

STEPS	RATIONALE
7. Carefully dry the instruments with a disposable towel to reduce the chance of instrument corrosion. Convection ovens may be used for drying instruments on trays or cassettes as an alternative to hand-drying. Non–stainless steel instruments require the additional protection of a rust inhibitor (sodium nitrite dip or spray) when steam sterilization is the method of renewal.	Wet carbon steel instruments and burs will rust (sodium nitrite spray will reduce rusting of items).
8. If instrument is accidentally dropped into ultrasonic chamber, retrieve it with tongs or forceps.	Instruments and solution are contaminated; avoid direct contact, and decrease risk of cuts and punctures.
9. Change the solution when it is visibly soiled, but at least once a day.	Maximize effectiveness of solution as a cleaning agent (blood solvent, bioburden penetration, rust inhibition).
10. Drain, rinse, and disinfect (spray-wipe-spray) the ultrasonic cleaning unit at the end of each day.	The tank and solution become contaminated with use.
11. Test the ultrasonic unit monthly to evaluate its operation and cleaning efficiency. An aluminum foil test may be useful to evaluate the ability of the ultrasonic unit to produce the high-frequency sound waves. The sound waves create the millions of tiny bubbles that collapse and create the cavitation, or scrubbing, action. Place a piece of aluminum foil in the ultrasonic solution and turn on the unit for the standard time. After the cycle is finished, remove foil and inspect for evidence of pitting on the aluminum foil surface. The pitting should be evident if the equipment is generating the high-frequency sound waves necessary to create an effective scrubbing action.	Inability of ultrasonic unit to generate high-frequency sound waves prevents effective scrubbing action and therefore may require longer processing, equipment repair or replacement, or increased risk of cuts or punctures due to need for hand scrubbing.

NOTE: Instrument basket/cassette, instruments, and solution are not sterilized or disinfected and must be treated as contaminated *until* they have been sterilized.
Courtesy Barbara L. Heckman, RDH, MS.

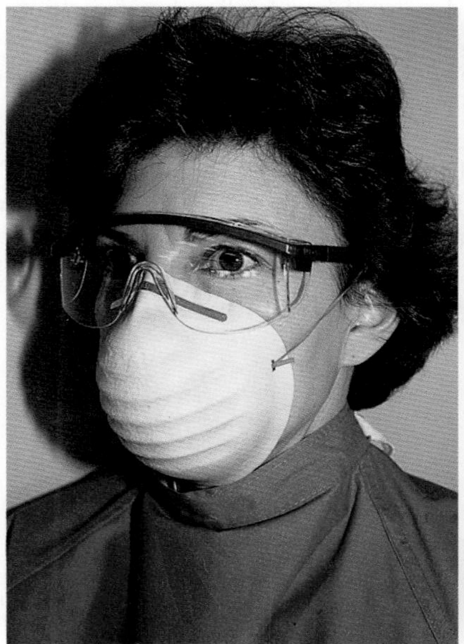

A

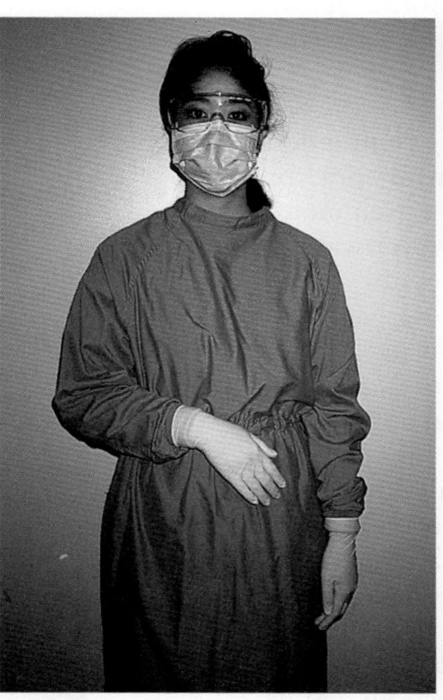

B

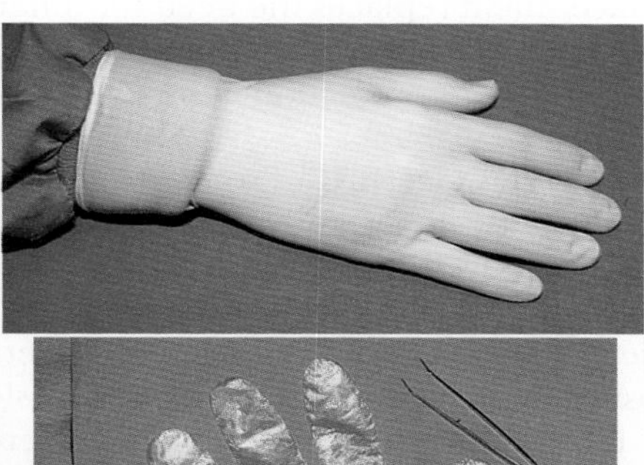

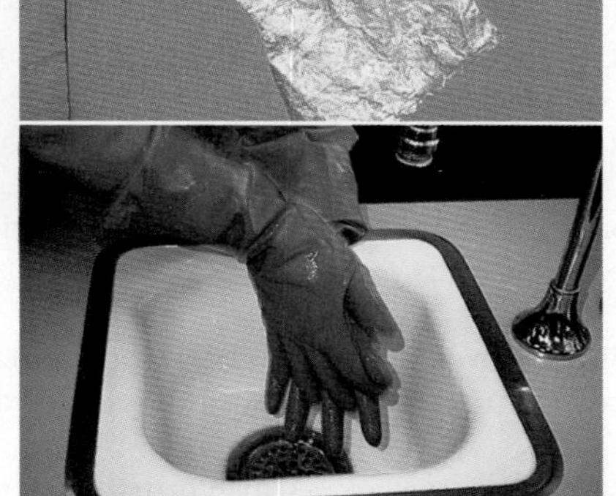

C

FIGURE 6–12 ✦ Personal protective equipment. A, Eyewear and facemask. B, Barrier gown. C, Gloves (surgical gloves, nitrile gloves, over-gloves). *(Courtesy Barbara L. Heckman, RDH, MS.)*

EYE PROTECTION. Eye protection should be worn whenever splashing, spatter, or spray of body fluids may be anticipated. Examples of such procedures include, but are not limited to, scaling and root planing, extrinsic stain removal with a rubber cup and slow-speed handpiece, spraying air and water, and the use of ultrasonic scalers. Glasses alone do not provide adequate eye protection. When selecting eyewear, look for confirmation that American National Standards Institute (ANSI) standards are used. These standards indicate appropriate protection for impact and fluids.

Goggles, glasses with side shields, or a face shield should be worn when the client care situation merits the use of eye protection (e.g., any intraoral procedure). Healthcare workers who wear prescription eyeglasses should consult an eyecare professional about having side shields fit to their glasses, or purchase goggles or face shields that fit over the prescription eyewear (Figure 6–12, *A*).

MASKS. Masks should be worn under the same circumstances that warrant the use of eye protection (Figure 6–12, *A*). Procedure or surgical masks protect the dental healthcare worker's mucous membranes and airway from exposure to body fluids that may be contained in the spray and spatter generated during dental procedures.

Masks are selected based on comfort, how well the periphery of the mask conforms to the contours of the face, and the level of filtration the mask provides. In general, a mask rated as *surgical* will have a filtration rating superior to masks rated as procedure masks.

A face shield replaces the need for other forms of protective eyewear only. Face shields do not provide the same respiratory protection as a mask.

PROTECTIVE CLOTHING. Protective clothing is intended to shield both intact and nonintact skin from spray or splash of body fluids during the course of treatment. Additionally, the protective clothing must provide a barrier to protect work clothes or street clothes from exposure. In most dental settings, a long-sleeved lab coat that falls below the knees is considered adequate. However, during exposure-prone procedures, such as surgical procedures, a more fluid-resistant material may be indicated. Protective clothing should be removed prior to leaving the work area, such as during lunch and other breaks. OSHA restricts healthcare workers from taking their own protective attire home for laundering. It is the employer's responsibility to arrange for laundering or use of disposable garments, in addition to providing adequate protective attire (Figure 6–12, *B*). (Clothing and paper that can absorb and transmit infectious agents are referred to as *fomites.*)

GLOVES. Gloves used in dental and dental hygiene procedures (Figure 6–12, *C*) fall into three categories:

- *Medical exam gloves* are nonsterile gloves that are available in a variety of sizes, materials, powdered and unpowdered, and either ambidextrous or right/left hand specific.
- *Surgical gloves,* individually packaged in pairs, are sterile until the package is opened or breached. These gloves are usually reserved for use in connection with dental surgical procedures.
- *Overgloves* are nonsterile, loosely fitting gloves that are worn over surgical gloves in order to avoid the cross-contamination of surgical gloves.
- *Nitrile gloves,* also know as *heavy-duty gloves,* are used during cleaning and disinfection procedures prior to and after client care.

HAND PROTECTION. An increase in the use of latex products has resulted in skin problems and allergic reactions. There has been an increase in reports of both allergic and nonallergic *dermatitis* among healthcare workers, and a small percentage of healthcare workers have a potentially life-threatening allergy to the proteins found in latex. Fortunately, the majority of reported problems are associated with nonallergic contact dermatitis. It is important to seek the advice of a qualified medical practitioner when experiencing dermal problems related to the use of medical gloves (Figure 6–13).

Handwashing is the most important behavior in the prevention of disease transmission (Procedure 6–2). However, frequent handwashing and the use of gloves may contribute to the development of nonallergic dermatitis, and it is important for dental healthcare workers to practice protective hand care. Practices that reduce the risk of dermatitis include:

- Thorough drying of hands after handwashing and before donning gloves
- Use of powder-free gloves (or low amounts of powder)
- Frequent use of lubricating hand lotions
- Use of cool water when washing hands
- Protecting hands from chapping and drying during cold weather
- Protecting hands from cuts and scratches when performing household chores

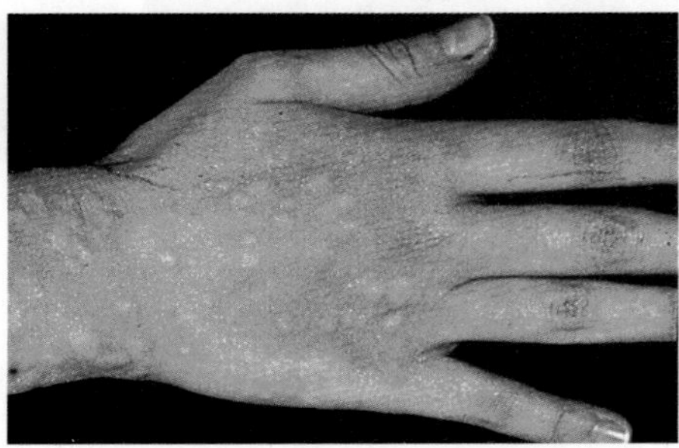

FIGURE 6–13 ✦ Nonallergic dermatitis from wearing latex gloves.

Procedure 6–2 HANDWASHING

EQUIPMENT
Liquid antimicrobial soap
Sink with running water
Personal protective equipment
Orangewood stick

STEPS	RATIONALE
1. Use sink with cool to lukewarm running water, liquid germicidal soap, and paper towels	Facilitates removal of organisms; paper towels are one-time-use disposable item
2. Remove jewelry from hands and forearms	Harbors microorganisms and perforates gloves, thereby compromising glove protection
3. Keep fingernails short and filed	Harbors dirt, sediment, secretions, and associated microorganisms; perforates gloves and impinges on client's mucosa
4. Inspect surface of hands for cuts or abrasions, sores, or hangnails in skin or cuticles	Harbors high concentrations of microorganisms; may serve as portals of exit, increasing a client's exposure to infection, or as portals of entry, increasing dental hygienist's risk of acquiring an infection. If hands exhibit exudative lesions or weeping dermatitis, CDC recommends refraining from direct/indirect contact with blood and saliva
5. Keep hands and protective clothing away from sink surface; if hands touch sink during handwashing, repeat process	Benefits of handwashing negated by touching inside sink, a contaminated area. Reaching over a sink increases risk of touching contaminated edge with hands or clothing
6. Control water flow and temperature, depending on the sink design, by pressing foot pedals with foot, pushing knee pedals with knee, turning on hand-operated faucets by covering faucets with a paper towel or by using elbow (Figure 6–14, *A*)	When hands contact a faucet, they are contaminated. Organisms spread easily from hands to faucet
7. Avoid splashing water against protective clothing	Microorganisms travel and grow in moisture
8. Regulate temperature of water at cool to lukewarm	Hot water opens pores, causing irritation, removes of protective skin oils, and increases skin's sensitivity to soap; cool water closes pores
9. Wet hands and lower arms thoroughly under running water. Keep hands and forearms lower than elbows during washing (Figure 6–14, *B*)	Hands are the most contaminated parts to be washed. Water should flow from the least to the most contaminated area
10. Apply liquid germicidal agent to hands, nails, and forearms and lather hands. Use foot-controlled soap dispenser or a barrier such as a paper towel between hand and soap container for dispensing liquid germicide	Germicidal soap minimizes microbial flora on epithelium and enhances further reduction as soap is used multiple times throughout the day. Residual effect is due to agent substantivity creating an antimicrobial barrier against many common skin contaminants. Rubbing hands together mechanically loosens and removes dirt and transient bacteria. *Bar soap is not recommended; when it becomes jelly-like it permits growth of microorganisms*
11. Wash hands using plenty of lather and friction for 2 minutes. Interlace the fingers and thumbs and rub the palms and back of hands with a circular motion	Friction loosens dirt and bacteria. Tests to evaluate handwashing found that thumb and fingertips were frequently missed. Interlacing fingers and thumbs ensures that all surfaces are cleaned

A
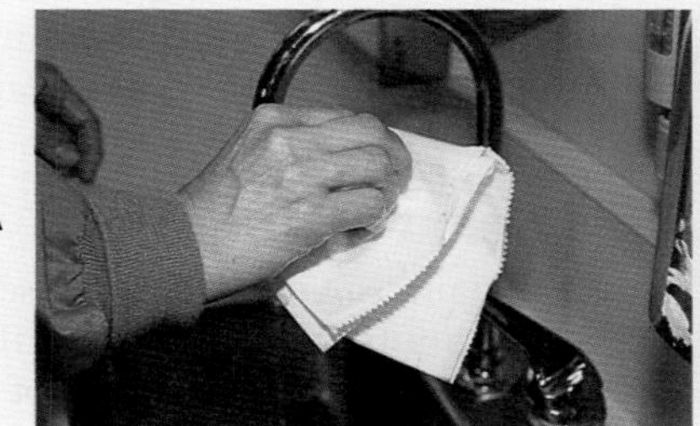

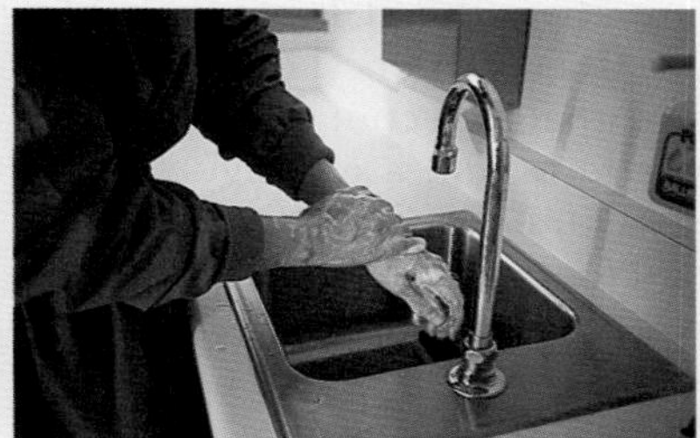
B

FIGURE 6–14

Continued on following page

Procedure 6–2 HANDWASHING—CONT'D

STEPS	RATIONALE
12. If areas underlying fingernails are soiled, clean them with a plastic or wood (orangewood) stick. Do not tear or cut the skin under or around the nail. An alternative is to use a sterile scrub brush but not more frequently than once a day	Blood, saliva, and plaque can contaminate the dental hygienist's hands. Fingernails are a common area for blood impaction if a glove is compromised. Blood under the fingernails is not easily removed by handwashing techniques. Skin is a natural barrier to be preserved; minimize brush use on hands to prevent dermatitis
13. Rinse hands and wrists thoroughly for 10 seconds, keeping hands down and elbows up (Figure 6–14, *C*)	Always rinse from least contaminated to most contaminated area
14. Dry hands thoroughly, wiping from the fingers down to the wrists and forearms (Fig 6–14, *D*)	Avoids recontamination of fingers. Drying hands prevents chapping and roughened skin that is susceptible to infection. Facilitates donning of gloves
15. Discard paper towel in proper receptacle	Prevents transfer of microorganisms. Avoid contaminating clean hands by touching receptacle
16. Turn off water with foot control or knee pedals. To turn off a hand-operated faucet, use a clean, dry paper towel.	Wet towel and wet hands allow the transfer of pathogens by capillary action
17. Keep hands and cuticles lubricated with hand moisturizer	Dry, chapped skin cracks easily, creating a portal of entry for infection

C

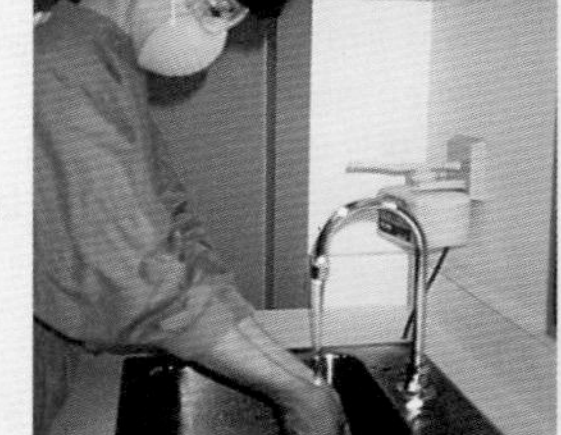

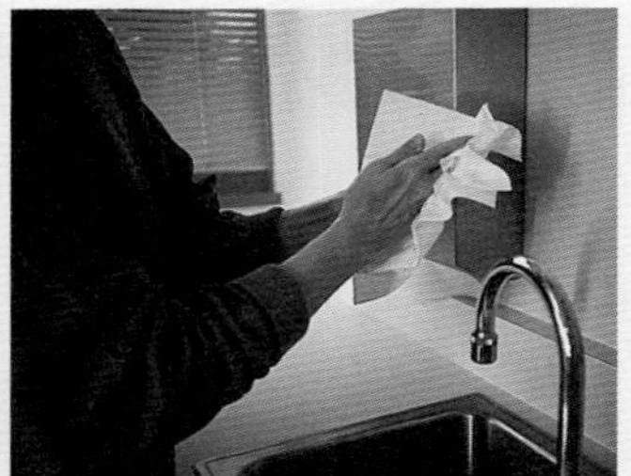

D

FIGURE 6–14, CONT'D.

Modified from Potter PA, Perry AG: *Fundamentals of nursing,* ed 5, St Louis, 2001, Mosby. Courtesy Barbara L. Heckman, RDH, MS.

TREATMENT AREA PREPARATION AND CLEAN-UP

The healthcare environment must be managed to prevent cross-contamination. Most items and surface areas in the dental care environment cannot be sterilized (Figure 6–15). Therefore, these must be cleaned and disinfected with an EPA-registered disinfectant or covered with a plastic barrier. Many items and surfaces that are touched with the gloved hands of the worker during dental treatment are difficult to adequately clean and disinfect. These include switches, knobs, hoses, brackets, and many other items used in the delivery of care. Therefore the use of impervious barriers should be considered for all items that may become contaminated with blood during dental procedures and are designed in a manner that makes removal of the blood difficult before disinfecting. Items targeted for surface cleaning and disinfection include, but are not limited to:

- ✦ Dental chair
- ✦ Operator chair
- ✦ Dental unit
- ✦ Dental light
- ✦ X-ray unit
- ✦ Countertops
- ✦ Air/water syringe handle and tubing
- ✦ Cabinets and knobs
- ✦ Pencils, pens, face mirror, safety glasses
- ✦ Dental unit and tubing
- ✦ Saliva ejector holder and tubing
- ✦ Bracket tables
- ✦ Portable equipment (e.g., ultrasonic cleaner and scaler)

Steps for cleaning and disinfection are presented in Procedure 6–3. It is during the cleaning and disinfection procedure that water lines coming from the dental unit are flushed to decrease the bacterial burden that accumulates on their narrow walls.

Equipment Sterilization

An important aspect of clinical asepsis is the sterilization of instruments and equipment when appropriate. *Sterilization* is the destruction of all living organisms, including highly resistant bacterial spores (Table 6–3). By applying this high level of destruction, the practitioner ensures to the greatest degree possible that all pathogenic

DESIGNATED USE AREAS WITHIN THE DENTAL HYGIENE CARE ENVIRONMENT

Area I (Contaminated Zone)—The Bracket Table/Instrument Tray or Cassette
Items within this area are used frequently during dental hygiene care and come into direct contact with mucous membranes and/or body fluids.

Area II (Contaminated Zone)—The Top of the Instrument Cabinet or Power Module
Items within this area are frequently used during dental hygiene care but will be contaminated (e.g., the suction tip, air/water tip, handpiece, and attachments).

Area III (Contaminated Zone)—The Adjacent Countertop Area Closest to the Client's Oral Cavity
Items placed in this area will eventually become contaminated because of the proximity to the source of contamination; apparatus that cannot be cleaned and disinfected properly such as ultrasonic scaling equipment must be protected with a barrier.

Area IV (Noncontaminated Zone)—The Remaining Area of the Countertop
Dental hygiene care items that cannot be sterilized or disinfected and therefore must not be contaminated (e.g., bulk materials such as topical fluoride, plaque control materials, records, forms, and pens) must be covered when not in use and should not be touched without the use of a barrier, such as an overglove.

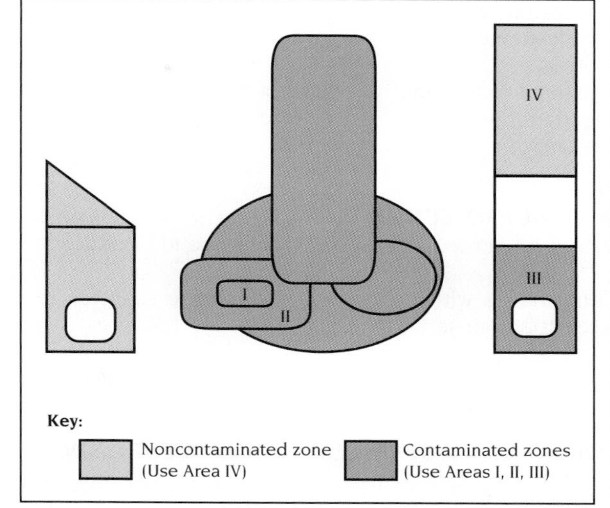

Adapted from Cottone JA et al. : Recommended clinical guidelines for infection control in dental education institution, *Journal of Dental Education* 55(9):621, 1991. Illustration adapted from Ino J, Miyasaki S, University of California, San Francisco, School of Dentistry, Clinic of Manual Infection Control Protocol, 1987. Courtesy Barbara L. Heckman, RDH, MS.

FIGURE 6–15 ✦ Designated use areas within the dental hygiene care environment.

TABLE 6–3

COMPARISON OF STERILIZATION METHODS

Method	Standard Sterilizing Conditions	Advantages	Precautions	Spore Testing
Steam autoclave	20 min at 121° C (250° F) (15 psi)	Time efficient Good penetration Sterilize water-based liquid	Do not use closed containers May damage plastic and rubber items Non–stainless steel metal items corrode Use of hard water may leave deposits	*Bacillus stearothermophilus* strips, vials, or ampules
Unsaturated chemical vapor	20 min at 132° C (270° F) (20–40 psi)	Time efficient No corrosion Items dry quickly after cycle	Do not use closed containers May damage plastic and rubber items Must use special solution Pre-dry instruments or dip them in special solution Provide adequate ventilation Cannot sterilize liquids	*Bacillus stearothermophilus* Strips
Dry heat oven	60–120 min at 160° C (320° F)	No corrosion Can use closed containers Large capacity per cost Items are dry after cycle	Longer sterilization time Cannot sterilize liquids May damage plastic and rubber items Do not open door before end of cycle Pre-dry instruments Cannot sterilize liquids	*Bacillus subtilis* strips
Rapid heat transfer	12 min at 191° C (375° F) (for wrapped items) 6 min at 191° C (375° F) (for unwrapped items)	No corrosion Short cycle Items are dry after cycle	May damage plastic and rubber items Do not open door before end of cycle Small capacity per cost Unwrapped items quickly contaminated after cycle	*Bacillus subtilis* strips
Ethylene oxide	10–16 hr at 61° C (110° F)	No corrosion Ideal for items damaged by heat and/or moisture	Long turnaround time Requires poststerilization aeration Insufficient aeration can cause tissue irritation Requires spark shield to prevent potential for explosion Requires adequate ventilation because of gas toxicity	*Bacillus subtilis* strips or vials

Courtesy Barbara L. Heckman, RDH, MS.

Procedure 6–3 TREATMENT AREA PREPARATION AND CLEAN-UP

EQUIPMENT

Personal protective equipment
Heavy-duty (nitrile) gloves
Chlorhexidine gluconate soap
Paper towels
EPA-registered disinfectant in a spray bottle
Plastic barriers
Chlorine bleach

STEPS	RATIONALE
A. PERSONAL PROTECTION	
1. Wear mask, protective eyewear, facemask, and clinic gown.	Prevents exposure of mucous membrane and skin to spatter and aerosol generation
2. Lather hands with chlorhexidine gluconate soap for 15 seconds and rinse.	Minimizes microbial flora on the epithelium and substantivity enhances further reduction as soap is used throughout the day
3. Don heavy-duty rubber gloves. Mix EPA disinfectant (Figure 6–16, *A*)	Minimizes risk of exposure incidents involving contaminated surfaces
B. ENVIRONMENTAL SURFACE AND EQUIPMENT DISINFECTION AND PREPARATION	
1. For dental units with external water container, discard chlorine bleach solution (1 part chlorine bleach to 10 parts water) in external water container. Rinse container and fill with water; move master toggle to on position. (Bottle will be pressurized to 40 psi, which may take up to 60 seconds.)	Ensures that external water container on some units has been disinfected
2. Flush each water line (water syringe and hand piece) for 3 minutes (Figure 6–16, *B*).	Controls accumulation of biofilms in the waterlines
3. Preclean all surfaces and equipment with iodophor mixed at the beginning of each day. Totally saturate surface with spray followed by vigorous wiping with paper towel. Holding paper towels behind appropriate surfaces reduces overspray.	Ensures that bioburden is removed prior to disinfection of surfaces and equipment
4. Disinfect precleaned surfaces by again spraying disinfecting agent thoroughly over surfaces. Allow surfaces to remain wet for 10 minutes. Wipe remaining wet areas (Figure 6–16, *C*).	Disinfectant needs 10 minutes to decrease microorganisms to a safe level (minimum time required to kill TB); spray delivery penetrates crevices
5. Use a sequence for cleaning and disinfecting.	Increases likelihood of comprehensive cleaning and disinfecting; decreases potential of cross-contamination from areas that cannot be sterilized

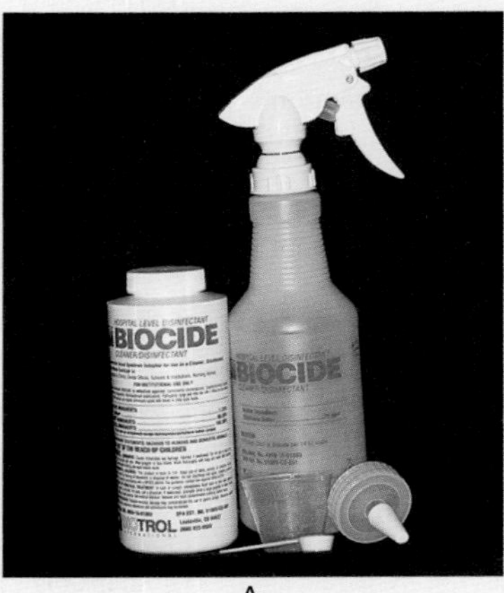

A

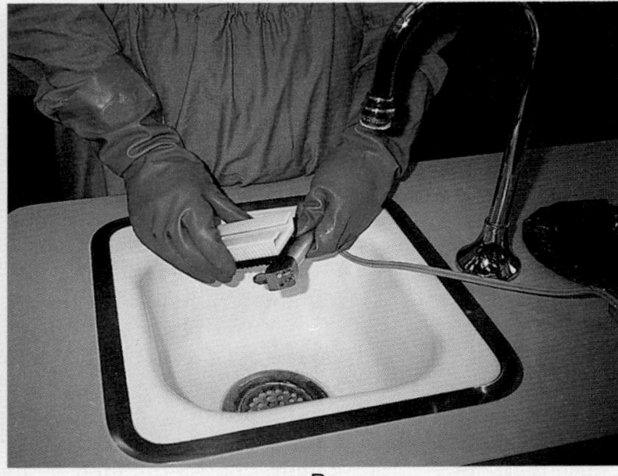
B

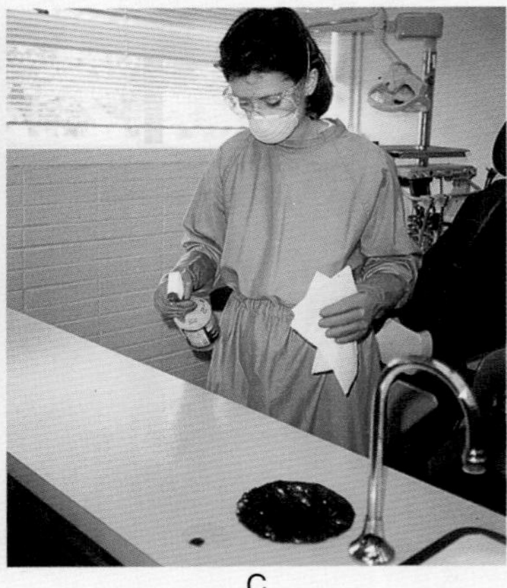
C

FIGURE 6–16 ✦ A, Bottles of intermediate-level disinfectant and EPA-registered, tuberculocidal, hospital-grade disinfectant. B, Air-water syringe water lines being flushed. C, Heavy-duty nitrile-gloved hands performing initial cleaning step of environmental disinfection. *(Courtesy Barbara L. Heckman, RDH, MS.)*

Procedure 6–3 TREATMENT AREA PREPARATION AND CLEAN-UP—CONT'D

STEPS	RATIONALE
6. Wash heavy-duty rubber gloves with handsoap, dry and remove. Spray with disinfectant prior to storage (Figure 6–16, *D*).	Reduces surface contaminants on gloves
7. After removal of heavy-duty rubber gloves, wash hands for another 15 seconds. Thoroughly rinse and dry hands	Reduces microorganisms on hands with each washing
8. Place disposable air/water syringe tip and saliva ejector insert and cover with barriers.	Prevents disease transmission from surfaces not sterilizable
9. Place protective barrier coverings on chair, bracket table, ultrasonic scaling unit, light handles, cords.	Prevents disease transmission from surfaces not sterilizable
10. Provide protective eyewear and antimicrobial mouthrinse for client.	Protects client's eyes during care and decreases oral contaminants
C. INFECTION CONTROL DURING THE APPOINTMENT (LEAVING AND RETURNING TO TREATMENT AREA)	
1. Rinse contaminated hand glove for minimum of 15 seconds. DO NOT use soap since soap can break down latex in gloves.	Decreases contaminant and debris on gloves
2. Dry gloves thoroughly using clean paper towel.	Decreases microorganism growth and makes overglove placement easier
3. Place overglove on top of hand glove.	Provides a barrier to the glove surface that is used in the client's mouth
4. Remove overglove prior to reentering client's mouth.	Overglove is contaminated
5. Change hand gloves after each client , or if glove tears or discolors.	Decreases chances of cross-contamination between clients and to self
D. INFECTION CONTROL BETWEEN CLIENTS	
1. Use a new mask for each client (change mask hourly on the same client).	Decreases chance of cross-contamination between clients and self; moist mask is no longer an effective filter.
2. Remove mask only by the elastic or cloth tie strings; never touch mask itself.	Decreases chance of cross-contamination
3. Remove and dispose of all barriers with exception of the cord covers that are disinfected.	Decreases chance of cross-contamination
4. Bleed water lines (syringe) for 30 seconds.	Minimizes buildup of biofilms
5. Wearing heavy-duty rubber gloves, disinfect all items as described above. Three-minute drying time required.	Less time required because effects are enhanced by multiple use of disinfectant throughout day
E. HANDWASHING BETWEEN CLIENTS OR AT THE END OF THE DAY	
1. Wash gloves with soap *prior to* removal.	Reduce contamination prior to waste disposal in trash bin
2. Following glove removal, using chlorhexidine gluconate soap and water, wash ungloved hands for 30 seconds.	Gloved hands promote growth of microorganisms; bioburden on hands must be reduced and rinsed away

D

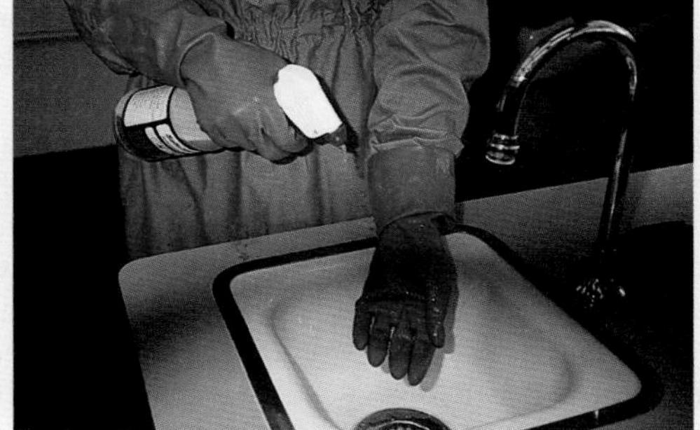

FIGURE 6–16, CONT'D ✦ D, Spraying nitrile gloves with environmental surface disinfectant. *(Courtesy Barbara L. Heckman, RDH, MS.)*

Continued on following page

Procedure 6–3 TREATMENT AREA PREPARATION AND CLEAN-UP—CONT'D

STEPS	RATIONALE
F. INFECTION CONTROL AT END OF PERIOD OF INSTRUMENT RECIRCULATION	
1. Wear heavy-duty rubber gloves, mask, clinic gown, and glasses throughout procedure.	Prevents exposure of mucous membrane and skin to spatter and aerosol generation
2. Place contaminated instruments in cassette and close cassette. Cassette is carried to the designated contaminated space in sterilization area.	Contaminated instruments are kept in an area designated "contaminated"
3. Prior to disinfection: a. Remove contaminated barriers b. Clean headpiece and mechanized scaler; insert with soap and water and prepare for sterilization. Write date on bag c. Clean suction filter d. Flush saliva ejector and high-speed suction with evacuation cleaner e. Run disinfectant (chlorine bleach solution [1 part chlorine bleach to 10 parts water]) through water system at end of day f. Clean sink and cuspidor cone with a chlorine cleanser	Bioburden must be removed from all surfaces prior to disinfection
4. Clean and disinfect all surfaces not covered by barriers; allow EPA-registered disinfectant to remain on surfaces for 10 minutes.	Spray-wipe-spray technique used as before
5. Clean and disinfect clinician's safety glasses, name tag, and badge.	These items are exposed to spatter and aerosol contaminants
6. Secure unit. Discard remaining EPA disinfectant.	Good management practice to use an equipment close-down procedure
7. Dispose of all waste in trash bags.	Designated trash bags facilitate proper waste management and disposal
8. Remove and place clinic gown with care in biohazard laundry container.	Facilitates proper laundering of contaminated gowns
9. Use evidence-based infection control protocols consistently. Update protocols regularly.	Increases likelihood that protocols will be carried out consistently

Modified from the infection control process evaluation form used at the School of Dental Hygiene, Old Dominion University, Norfolk, Virginia.

organisms are destroyed. The intent of instrument and equipment sterilization is not to establish a sterile environment in which dentistry may be performed. Indeed, such an environment would be impossible to establish. Rather, the sterilization process is intended to ensure the destruction of all organisms that have been introduced to an item during use on a client and to ensure that a thoroughly clean and safe device is provided for each client.

INSTRUMENT CLASSIFICATION. Dental instruments fall into three broad categories for determining the minimum level of management between clients. They are critical, semicritical, and noncritical.

- *Critical instruments* are instruments that penetrate soft tissue or bone. Therefore, critical instruments must be heat sterilized between each use or disposable items may be used. If disposable items (such as scalpels) are used, they must be discarded after each use, and not reprocessed for use on another client. Examples include periodontal probes, explorers, scaling and root planing instruments, and tip insert of an ultrasonic scaling unit (Figure 6–17).

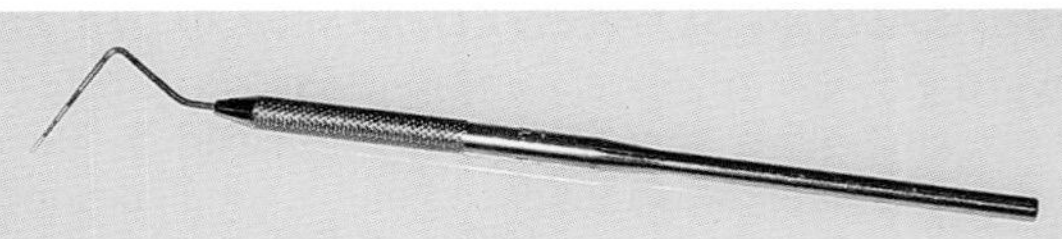

FIGURE 6–17 ✦ Example of critical equipment: periodontal probe. *(Courtesy Barbara L. Heckman, RDH, MS.)*

- *Semi-critical instruments* are not intended to penetrate soft tissue or bone, but come into contact with oral fluids. Examples include mouth mirrors, ultrasonic scaling handpieces, impression trays, and oral photography retractors (Figure 6–18). These instruments should also be heat sterilized between each use. If heat sterilization is not feasible due to heat sensitivity of the device or instrument , a high-level germicide may be used to reprocess the item. These *germicides* are chemical disinfectants that provide sterilization under certain conditions. Chemical germicides are not as reliable as heat sterilization methods, and *should not* be relied on if a heat sterilization alternative is available.
- *Noncritical instruments and devices* are those items that come into contact only with intact skin. Examples

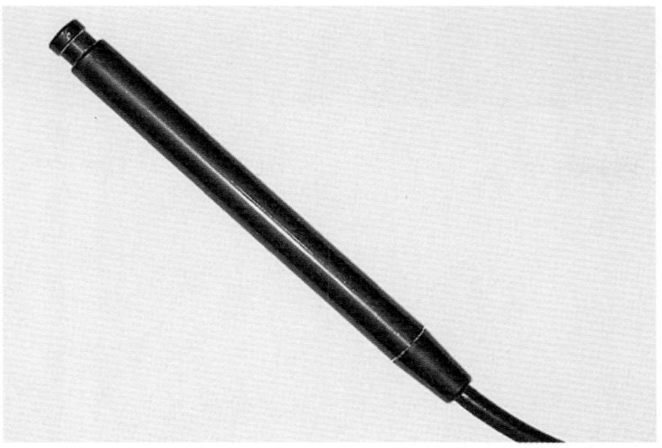

FIGURE 6–18 ✦ Example of semicritical equipment: ultrasonic scaler handpiece. *(Courtesy Barbara L. Heckman, RDH, MS.)*

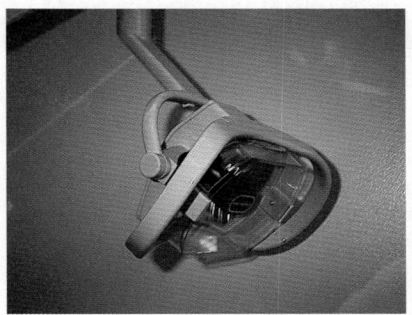

FIGURE 6–19 ✦ Example of noncritical equipment: dental light handle. *(Courtesy Barbara L. Heckman, RDH, MS.)*

TABLE 6–4 LEVELS OF DISINFECTION AND ASSOCIATED GERMICIDAL ACTION

Level	Capability	Essential Criterion	Examples
High	Inactivates resistant bacterial spores and other less-resistant microbial forms, such as bacteria (tubercle bacillus, vegetative bacteria), fungi, and viruses (lipid and medium-sized, and nonlipid and small)	Ability to kill bacterial spores required for a high-level classification; with extended exposure times, high-level disinfectants capable of sterilization (6–10 hours); EPA-registered "disinfectant/sterilant" indicated on the product label	2.0–3.2% glutaraldehyde preparations (immersion glutaraldehydes) and ethylene oxide
Intermediate	May not be able to inactivate bacterial endospores; there are differences among intermediate disinfectants in their ability to inactivate small, nonlipid viruses; as a group, will kill other microbial forms, including the second most resistant microorganism, *Mycobacterium tuberculosis*	Ability to kill *M. tuberculosis;* for the dental environment an intermediate-level disinfectant should be EPA-registered as tuberculocidal, hospital-grade (kills three species of basic test bacteria: *Staphylococcus aureus, Salmonella typhimurium,* and *Pseudomonas aeruginosa)* with appropriate virucidal activity	Formaldehyde, chlorine compounds, iodophor, alcohols, complex (synthetic) phenols
Low	Has the narrowest antimicrobial range; may inactivate certain viruses and vegetative bacteria	Will not kill tubercle bacilli, nonlipid viruses, or fungi; unacceptable for disinfection of items and equipment classified as critical or semicritical	Quaternary ammonium compounds, simple phenols an detergents

Courtesy Barbara L. Heckman, RDH, MS.

include an x-ray head, light handles, high- and low-volume evacuators, tubing for handpieces, instrument trays, countertops, and chair surfaces (Figure 6–19). These items may be decontaminated with an EPA-registered disinfectant (Table 6–4).

HEAT METHODS OF STERILIZATION. Sterilization is the destruction of all living microbial forms. Heat sterilization methods are the most time efficient and offer the highest level of verification through the use of a biologic or enzyme indicator. It is important to determine the method of sterilization that provides a safe and effective outcome for the type of devices being sterilized.

All heat methods must be employed using an FDA-approved sterilization device, and following the manufacturer's instructions for cycle time, temperature, and other parameters that may affect the final result. For satisfactory results, instruments must be thoroughly cleaned of all debris before being placed into appropriate packaging and sterilized. Three major types of heat sterilization are available:

- ✦ *Autoclave,* the most common method of heat sterilization in the dental office, uses steam in a pressurized chamber (usually 121° C for 20 minutes) to sterilize heat-stable instruments and devices. Water is placed into a chamber that dispenses the amount needed to provide steam for the process. Most autoclaves require several minutes to achieve the temperature necessary to begin the sterilization process. Additional time is needed to allow depressurization of the chamber once the cycle has been completed (Procedure 6–4).
- ✦ An unsaturated *chemical vapor sterilizer* uses a process similar to that of the autoclave; however, in place of steam, a chemical vapor is generated under pressure (see Guidelines for Assuring Performance of Unsaturated Chemical Vapor Sterilizers).

Procedure 6–4 USE OF THE STEAM AUTOCLAVE

EQUIPMENT

Autoclave
Packaging material
Indicator tape
Slow-change chemical indicator
Biologic monitor
Nitrile gloves
Insulated gloves

STEPS	RATIONALE
1. Check operating conditions (cycle time, temperature and pressure gauges) daily (Figure 6–20)	Suboptimal operating conditions cause sterilization failures (insufficient time or temperature to kill)
2. Keep operations manual in an accessible location within the noncontaminated zone of the re-circulation center for ease of reference (Figure 6–21). Review manual periodically.	Operation of sterilizing equipment varies; most sterilization failures are due to errors in following operation instructions
3. Use distilled or deionized water instead of water from community supply.	Hard water leaves deposits on instruments
4. Select packaging materials designed for use in a steam autoclave (plastic tubing, poly film paper pouches, open metal or glass containers) (Figure 6–22).	Packaging material not designed for steam autoclave prevents sterilizing agent (steam) from penetrating to instruments inside

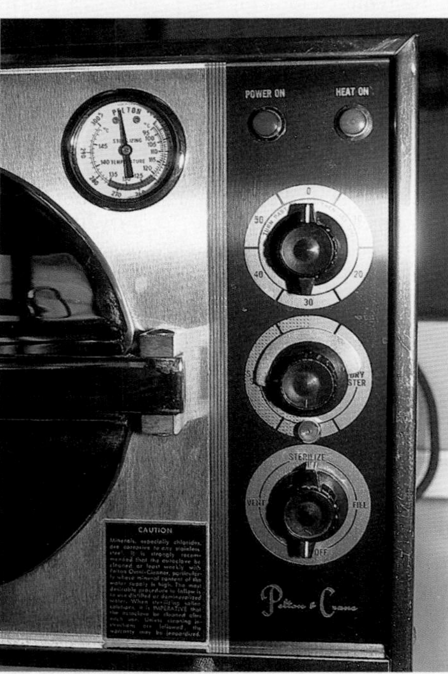

FIGURE 6–20 ✦ Close-up of autoclave showing gauges.

OMNI-CLAVE® STERILIZER
Solid State Models
OCM, OCR, OCR+ (ASME MODEL)

INSTALLATION

Remove and discard screws and washers securing Omni-Clave to shipping pallet. Attach feet to Omni-Clave (using screws provided) and insert rubber tips. COUNTER SURFACE **MUST** BE LEVEL TO ENSURE PROPER OPERATION AND TO PROLONG THE LIFE OF THE UNIT. Extra washers are provided to use on feet screws for uneven surfaces. Omni-Clave is designed for use **only** on alternating current. POSITION FUNCTION KNOB TO OFF POSITION BEFORE PLUGGING IN UNIT. Plug line cord into power outlet, ensuring unit is grounded by using three wire plug and a grounded receptacle. Fill reservoir (using distilled or demineralized water) within 2-1/2" (61.3cm) of top (approximately 2-1/2 quarts (2.4L) for OCM or 4-1/2 quarts (4.3L) for OCR and OCR+).

STEAM STERILIZING

LOAD—OCM and OCR safety door is opened by pushing on top of door handle while pulling handle up and sliding to right. OCR+ door is opened by pressing inward on door handle while rotating locking handle to right. Refer to paragraphs on **Preparation of Materials** and **Loading the Chamber** on back of this card.

FILL —Turn **lower** knob counterclockwise to **FILL.** When water level inside chamber covers fill plate, turn **lower** knob counterclockwise to **STERILIZE,** which stops flow of water. The fill plate is located on the tray rest in the bottom of the chamber (Figure 3). Close and lock door.

CAUTION: Temperature will now increase. Avoid contact that may cause injury.

SET —Rotate **middle** knob clockwise until it stops (indicator will point up). When temperature gauge indicates approximately ten degrees below desired setting, rotate middle knob counterclockwise until yellow **HEAT ON** light begins to flash. Allow temperature and pressure to stabilize (approximately five minutes), then make any final adjustments.

NOTE: Rotating middle knob clockwise increases (counterclockwise decreases) temperature and pressure.

Set timer knob to prescribed time period. Always rotate timer knob past 10 minute setting before setting time. Refer to chart on back for proper time-temperature relationship.

VENT—When bell rings (cycle complete), rotate lower knob counterclockwise to **VENT. After** pressure is discharged (pressure gauge should read zero), open door slightly.

DRY —Leaving door slightly open (1/2") (1.3cm), allow drying time of approximately five minutes. Leave knob in **VENT** position during drying time. This leaves the heating elements on and promotes drying and quick start up of next cycle.

WARNING: If door is NOT opened after venting or if autoclave is left unattended for longer than fifteen (15) minutes, dangerously high chamber temperatures will occur, creating a fire hazard.

UNLOAD—The trays may now be unloaded.

IMPORTANT:

1. Rotate upper timer knob beyond ten minutes before setting time.
2. Standby periods—if Omni-Clave is to be used within 15 minutes, leave door cracked with lower knob in **VENT** position. Otherwise, autoclave should be turned off to save energy and prevent chamber from reaching excessively high temperatures.
3. Add water to reservoir **only** when lower knob is in **VENT** or **POWER OFF** position. It is advisable to keep reservoir adequately filled.
4. At conclusion of all sterilizing for the day, turn lower knob to **POWER OFF.**
5. As soon as possible after bell rings at end of sterilizing cycle, turn to **VENT** position. This practice will prevent the autoclave from boiling dry.
6. Do not attempt to turn lower knob from **STERILIZE** to **FILL** or from **VENT** to **STERILIZE.** Stops are incorporated to prevent knob from being turned in this manner.
7. Safety valve is set for 35 psi (241.3 KPa).

DRY HEAT STERILIZING

LOAD—only two trays may be used on which to place instruments.

WARNING: Do NOT use cloth or any covering over items to be sterilized.

Properly position auxiliary dry heat door on autoclave by inserting upper portion inside chamber and then lower portion.

SET —Turn **lower** knob clockwise to **VENT.** While depressing **DRY HEAT INTERLOCK** button (below middle knob), rotate middle knob completely clockwise into **DRY STER** position until it stops.

CAUTION: Temperature will now increase. Avoid contact that may cause injury.

When thermometer on door reaches 320°F (160°C) (approximately 25 minutes), turn **TIMER** knob clockwise to desired setting.

VENT—When bell rings (cycle complete), rotate **middle** knob counterclockwise to **STEAM STER** which allows **DRY HEAT INTERLOCK** button to pop out. Rotate **lower** knob to **POWER OFF**, then remove auxiliary dry heat door.

UNLOAD—The trays may now be unloaded.

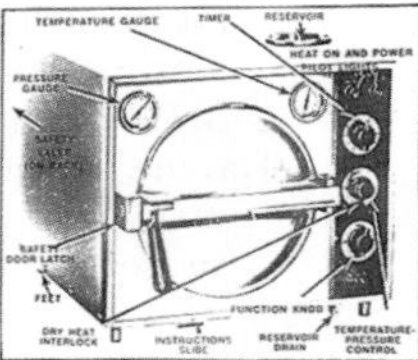

FIGURE 1—OCM AND OCR (SOLID STATE MODELS)

IMPORTANT:

1. Middle knob cannot be turned to **DRY STER** unless button is depressed. Button cannot be depressed unless lower knob is in **VENT** position.
2. When middle knob is in **DRY STER**, lower knob cannot be turned from **VENT** position.
3. The density of the load to be sterilized will determine the time required to reach sterilizing temperature of 320°F (160°C). Always distribute load loosely on trays.

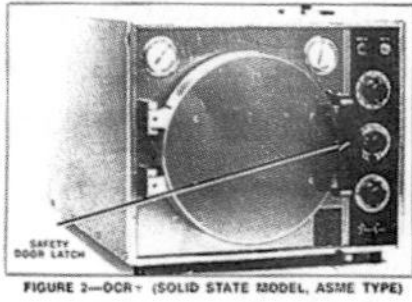

FIGURE 2—OCR+ (SOLID STATE MODEL, ASME TYPE)

FIGURE 6–21 ✦ Operations manual.

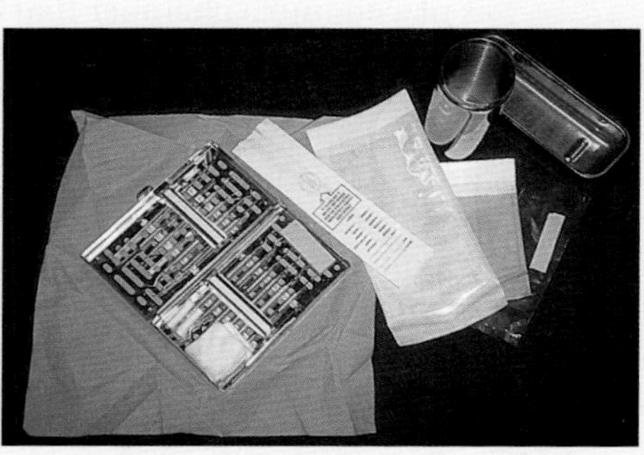

FIGURE 6–22 ✦ Various packaging materials.

Procedure 6–4 USE OF THE STEAM AUTOCLAVE—CONT'D

STEPS	RATIONALE
5. Avoid use of sealed or closed containers or aluminum foil for packaging materials.	Closed or impervious containers do not permit direct contact of steam with contacts
6. Package instruments securely without wrapping them too tightly.	Prevents formation of interior air pockets (inside packaging), which prevent penetration of sterilizing agent
7. Place no more than two layers of packs on each shelf. Upper layer is placed perpendicular and cross-wise to the one below; avoid package contact with chamber walls (Figure 6–23). Place opened containers on their sides.	Allows for thorough contact of steam with all chamber contents
8. Inspect all fittings and seals regularly, especially door gasket (see operations manuals for guidelines).	Ill-fitting seals and gaskets may inhibit proper sterilizing conditions (pressure and temperature)
9. Maintain equipment by washing internal surfaces weekly with mild detergent, and rinse well (Figure 6–24). Locate the discharge line and remove plug at the opening. Flush line with 3 to 4 quarts of hot water to clean screen/strainer.	Poor equipment maintenance may result in sterilization failure
10. Use indicator tape or markings on all packages (Figure 6–25). Place a slow-change chemical indicator into one item once a day; use a biologic monitor (spore test) once a week. Keep ongoing record of biologic monitoring results.	External indicator (rapid-change) tape identifies processed packages; slow-change indicators (internal packaging) assess instrument exposure to temperature and steam, time and temperature, or time; biologic monitoring verifies that the renewal process kills highly resistant bacterial spores (main guarantee of sterilization).
11. After autoclave cycle is complete and autoclave has been vented, open door and remove items from chamber wearing insulated gloves.	Prevents burns from steam and touching hot items

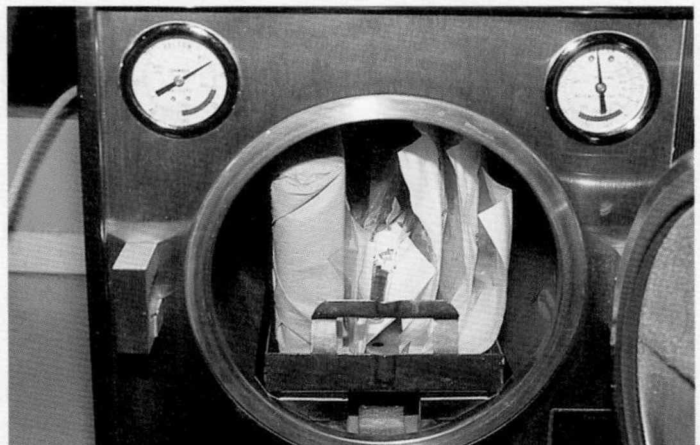

FIGURE 6–23 ✦ Packages loaded into autoclave.

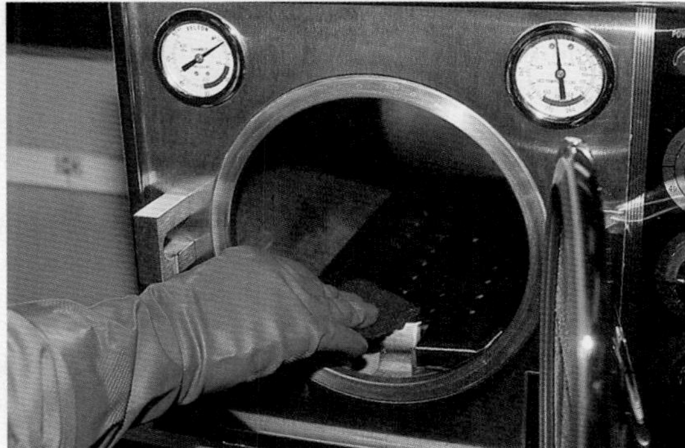

FIGURE 6–24 ✦ Nitrile-gloved hand washing interior of autoclave for maintenance care.

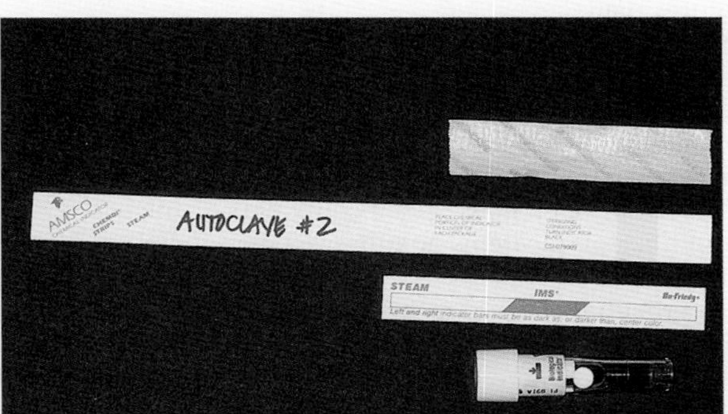

FIGURE 6–25 ✦ Postrenewal indicator tape, integrator, spore vial (top to bottom).

Courtesy Barbara L. Heckman, RDH, MS.

✦ *Dry-heat sterilization* uses high heat for a set period of time to achieve sterile results. Temperatures may reach as high as 350° F; therefore, some heat-sensitive items may not be placed in a dry-heat sterilizer (see Guidelines for Assuring Performance of Dry-heat Sterilizers)

CHEMICAL DISINFECTANTS AND STERILANTS. Several classes of chemical agents are available that will provide high-level disinfection and sterilization under given conditions. Varying degrees of corrosion and damage to certain materials may be anticipated if instruments or devices are in prolonged contact with the chemical agent (Table 6–5).

STERILITY ASSURANCE. Assurance that instruments have been thoroughly processed is obtained through a combination of methods. A *chemical indicator* allows the operator to determine that certain necessary parameters have been met. These indicators often are imbedded in pouches used to contain instruments during sterilization or are in the form of imbedded tape or indicator strips. Chemical indicators should be used with every packet of instruments as a signal to the user that the particular packet has been subjected to a heat sterilization process. The indicator is not an indication of effectiveness (Figure 6–26).

A more reliable method of verification exists in the use of *biologic indicators,* also called *spore tests* (Figure 6–27). Nonpathogenic spores that are especially resistant to the

Guidelines for Assuring Performance of Unsaturated Chemical Vapor Sterilizers

Check cycle time, temperature, and pressure gauges daily.

Keep the operations manual in an accessible location within the noncontaminated zone of the recirculation center for reference.

Use chemical solution prepared by the manufacturer and maintain an adequate level of solution for operation.

Select packaging materials designed for use in the chemical vapor sterilizer (paper, paper-plastic tubing, plastic—heat sealed is best). Perforated metal or plastic cassettes are to be wrapped in paper for processing and storage after sterilization. If glass or metal containers are used, their lids must be kept ajar.

Avoid use of sealed containers or aluminum foil for packaging materials.

Prevent the formation of interior air pockets by packaging instruments securely without wrapping so tightly that gas penetration is precluded.

Enhance gas access and penetration to instruments by dispersing packs and cassettes throughout the chamber to allow adequate space between items. Items should not touch. *Avoid overloading.*

Inspect all fittings and seals, especially the door gasket; refer to operations manual for adjustment or replacement procedures.

Maintain equipment by cleaning the unit weekly according to the manufacturer's recommendations.

Place indicator tape on all packages for clear identification of items processed (not an accurate predictor of sterilization). Place a slow-change chemical indicator into one item once a day and use a biologic monitor (spore test) once a week.

Data from Miller CH, Palenik CJ: Improving the performance of the office sterilizer, *Dental Asepsis Review* 11(1):1, 1990.

Guidelines for Assuring Performance of Dry Heat Sterilizers

Check operating conditions (cycle timing and operating temperature) daily.

Keep the operations manual in an accessible location within the recirculation center noncontaminated zone for ease of reference. Review manual periodically.

Use packaging materials specifically designed for dry heat sterilization (some plastic pouches or tubing, aluminum foil, closed or open glass/metal containers or trays).

Do *not* sterilize plastic items or adhesive tapes; there is potential for release of toxic gases.

Avoid overloading. Separate items on *all levels* by at least 0.5 inch. Cassettes or packages should be no more than two layers deep, with the top layer at a right angle to the bottom layer. Air circulation is essential.

Select an oven with an air circulation fan to provide more even heat distribution within the chamber.

Allow time for a warm-up period after the chamber has been loaded, prior to starting the sterilization cycle. Some ovens do this automatically; however, even these should be routinely monitored.

Do not interrupt the cycle by opening the door. The entire cycle *must be restarted* if such an interruption in sustaining the temperature occurs.

Maintain equipment by cleaning the unit with a mild detergent once a week. The unit should be rinsed well and allowed to air dry. Check the chamber and door insulation at this time.

Place a slow-change chemical indicator into one package or cassette once a day and use a biologic monitor (spore test) once a week.

Data from Miller CH, Palenik CJ: Improving the performance of the office sterilizer, *Dental Asepsis Review* 11(1):1, 1990.

sterilization process are imbedded on a strip or in a solution, which is then placed in the sterilizer with a load of instruments. The spore test strip is then incubated to determine whether the spores were indeed killed by the sterilization process.

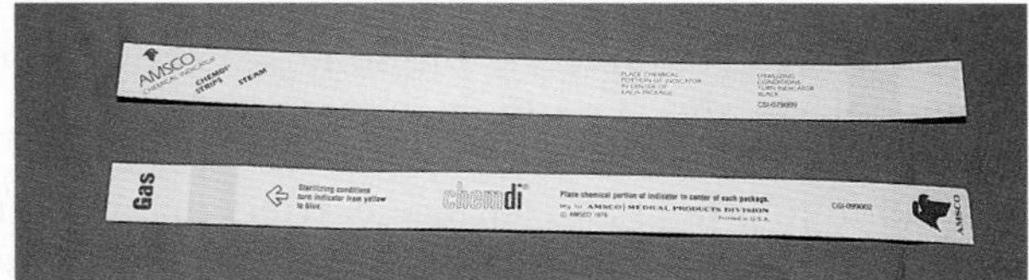

FIGURE 6–26 ✦ Chemical indicator strips. *(Courtesy Barbara L. Heckman, RDH, MS.)*

Bacillus stearothermophilus is a standard organism considered to be the spore most resistant to steam and chemical vapor sterilization. *Bacillus subtilis* is the spore most resistant to dry heat and ethylene oxide sterilization. For monitoring a combination of sterilization methods, dual species biologic indicators (containing both types of spores) would be an appropriate choice. Destruction of spores resistant to the specific sterilization methods indicates that all organisms, including the less hardy variety, have been eliminated. Spore testing should be done weekly to verify the proper functioning and operation of the sterilizer. Records of spore testing and their results should be kept in the dental office.

TABLE 6–5 CHARACTERISTICS OF CHEMICAL AGENTS FOR ENVIRONMENTAL SURFACE DISINFECTION

Agent	Action	Advantages	Disadvantages
Iodophors	Powerful germicidal action of iodine acts by iodination of proteins and subsequent formation of protein salts	EPA-registered and ADA-accepted Broad spectrum: bactericidal, tuberculocidal, and virucidal against hydrophilic and lipophilic viruses Biocidal activity within 5–10 minutes Economical Effective in dilute solution Few side effect reactions Surfactant carrier maintains surface moistness Residual biocidal action	Not a sterilant Unstable at high temperatures Dilution and contact time are critical Must be prepared daily to ensure tuberculocidal activity May discolor some surfaces Inactivated by hard water; distilled water recommended Inactivated by alcohol
Complex (synthetic) phenols	Phenolic compounds act as cytoplasmic poisons by penetrating and disrupting microbial cell walls, which results in denaturation of intracellular proteins	EPA-registered and ADA-accepted as both an immersion and a surface disinfectant Synergistic effect of combining two to three phenols Broad antimicrobial spectrum Tuberculocidal Useful on metal, glass, rubber, and plastic Less toxic and corrosive than glutaraldehyde Economical	Not sporicidal Must be prepared fresh daily Can degrade certain plastics and etch glass with prolonged exposure Film accumulation Skin and eye irritation
Chlorine compounds	Act primarily by oxidation; elemental chlorine is a potent germicide, killing most bacteria in 15–30 seconds	Some products are EPA-registered and ADA-accepted Rapid antimicrobial action Broad spectrum: bactericidal, uberculocidal, and virucidal; CDC has recommended sodium hypochlorite (diluted bleach 1:10 to 1:100) as an effective agent in destroying hepatitis B viruses) Economical Effective in dilute solution	Sporicidal only at high concentrations Cannot be reused (no reuse life) Must be prepared fresh daily Activity diminished by organic matter Unpleasant, persistent odor Irritating to skin and eyes Corrodes metals and damages clothing Degrades plastics and rubber
A class of glutaraldehyde surface disinfectants was developed in the mid-1980s, 0.25–0.50% glutaraldehyde, which is a derivation from the 2.0–3.2% glutaraldehyde used as immersion chemical sterilants/disinfectants	Glutaraldehydes have a broad antimicrobial spectrum and, at the lower concentration, have been EPA-approved as intermediate hospital surface disinfectants		May be sensitizing to the skin Vapor can irritate or injure eyes and nasal passages

Courtesy Barbara L. Heckman, RDH, MS.

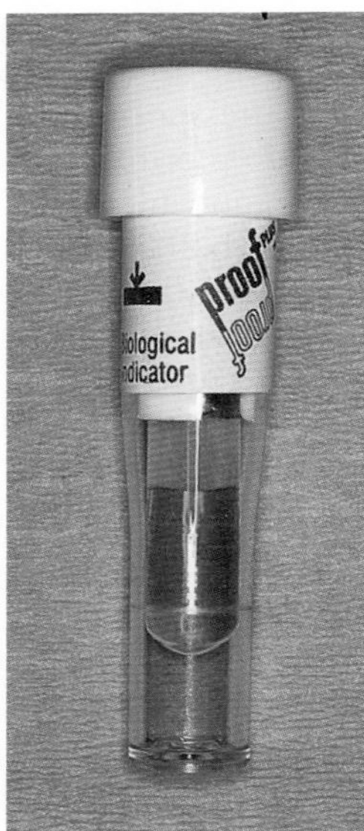

FIGURE 6–27 ✦ Spore test vial. *(Courtesy Barbara L. Heckman, RDH, MS.)*

DISINFECTION. *Disinfection* is the process of killing most but not all pathologic microorganisms. Disinfection of environmental surfaces in the dental operatory is standard practice for all areas contaminated during the dental procedures that were not protected with fluid-impervious barriers (Table 6–6). Contamination may result from droplets generated by devices such as the air/water syringe, handpieces, and sonic scalers, or from touching objects while wearing contaminated gloves.

BARRIERS. Equipment and surface barriers that provide protection against contamination with blood and body fluids are an effective means of environmental asepsis (Figure 6–28). The barriers must prevent contamination of the item being covered and must be handled carefully to avoid inadvertent contamination during use and removal. Barriers must be changed between each client. When properly used, barriers eliminate the need to disinfect the covered object between each client.

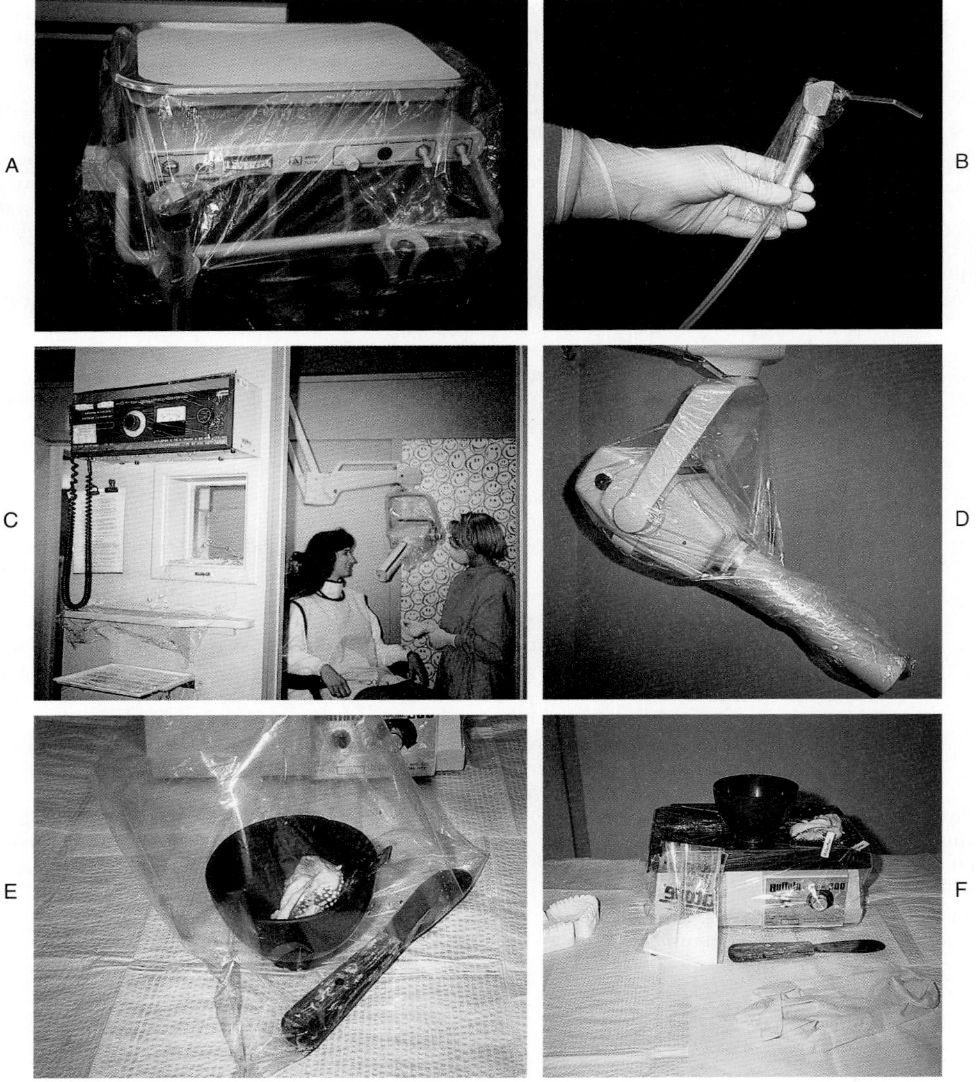

FIGURE 6–28 ✦ Barriers used to prevent contamination of nonsterilizable items. *(Courtesy Barbara L. Heckman, RDH, MS.)*

TABLE 6–6 STERILIZATION AND DISINFECTION OF DENTAL INSTRUMENTS, MATERIALS, AND SOME COMMONLY USED ITEMS*

	Steam Autoclave	Dry Heat Oven	Chemical Vapor	Ethylene Oxide	Chemical Disinfection/ Sterilization	Other Methods/Comments
Angle attachments*	+	+	+	++	+	
Burs						
Carbon steel	–	++	++	++	–	
Steel	+	++	++	++	+	
Tungsten-carbide	+	++	+	++	+	
Condensers	++	++	++	++	+	
Dappen dishes	++	+	+	++	+	
Endodontic instruments (broches, files, reamers)						Hot salt/glass bead sterilizer 10–15 seconds, 218°C (425°F)
Stainless steel handles	+	++	++	++	+	
Stainless with plastic handles	++	++	–	++	–	
Fluoride gel trays						
Heat-resistant plastic	++	– –	–	++	–	
Non–heat-resistant plastic	– –	– –	–	++	–	Discard (++)
Glass slabs	++	++	++	++	+	
Hand instruments						
Carbon steel	–	++	++	++	–	
	[Steam autoclave with chemical protection (1% sodium nitrite)]					
Stainless steel	++	++	++	++	+	
Handpieces*						Sterilizable preferably
Sterilizable*	(++)*	–	(+)*	++	– –	
Contra angles*	–	–	–	++	+	Combination synthetic phenolics or iodophors (–)
Nonsterilizable*	–	–	–	++	+	
Prophylaxis angles*	+	+	+	+	+	Discard (++)
Impression materials						Table 2
Impression trays						
Aluminum metal	++	+	++	++	–	
Chrome-plated	++	++	++	++	+	
Custom acrylic resin	– –	– –	– –	++	+	
Plastic	– –	– –	– –	++	+	Discard (++): preferred
Instruments in packs	++	+ Small packs	++	++ Small packs	– –	
Instrument tray set-ups						
Restorative or surgical	+ Size limit	+	+ Size limit	++ Size limit	– –	
Mirrors	–	++	++	++	+	
Needles						
Disposable	– –	– –	– –	– –	– –	Discard (++) Do not reuse
Nitrous oxide						
Nosepiece	(++)*	– –	(++)*	++	(+)*	
Hoses	(++)*	– –	(++)*	++	(+)*	
Orthodontic pliers						
High-quality stainless	++	++	++	++	+	
Low-quality stainless	–	++	++	++	–	
With plastic parts	– –	– –	– –	++	+	
Pluggers	++	++	++	++	+	
Polishing wheels and disks						
Garnet and cuttle	– –	–	–	++	– –	
Rag	++	–	+	++	– –	
Rubber	+	–	–	++	+	
Prostheses, removable	–	–	–	+	+	
Rubber dam equipment						
Carbon steel clamps	–	++	++	++	–	
Metal frames	++	++	++	++	+	
Plastic frames	–	–	–	++	+	
Punches	–	++	++	++	+	
Stainless steel clamps	++	++	++	++	+	

Table continued on following page

TABLE 6–6 STERILIZATION AND DISINFECTION OF DENTAL INSTRUMENTS, MATERIALS, AND SOME COMMONLY USED ITEMS*—CONT'D

	Steam Autoclave	Dry Heat Oven	Chemical Vapor	Ethylene Oxide	Chemical Disinfection/ Sterilization	Other Methods/Comments
Rubber items						
Prophylaxis cups	–	–	–	++	–	Discard (++)
Saliva evacuators, ejectors						
Low-melting plastic	–	–	–	++	+	Discard (++)
High-melting plastic	++	+	+	++	+	
Stones						
Diamond	+	++	++	++	+	
Polishing	++	+	++	++	–	
Sharpening	++	++	++	–	–	
Surgical instruments						
Stainless steel	++	++	++	++	+	
Ultrasonic scaling tips	+	– –	– –	++	+	
Water-air syringe tips	++	++	++	++	+	
X-ray equipment						
Plastic film folders	(++)*	– –	(+)*	++	+	
Collimating devices	–	– –	– –	++	+	

* As manufacturers use a variety of alloys and materials in these products, confirmation with the equipment manufacturers is recommended, especially for handpieces and the attachments.
++ Effective and preferred method.
+ Effective and acceptable method.
– Effective method, but risk of damage to materials.
– – Ineffective method with risk of damage to materials.
From American Dental Association Council on Dental Materials, Instruments, and Equipments; on Dental Practice; and on Dental Therapeutics: Infection control recommendations for the dental office and the dental laboratory: *Journal of the American Dental Association* 116:241, 1988.
Courtesy Barbara L. Heckman, RDH, MS.

CROSS-CONTAMINATION. *Cross-contamination* is the transfer of oral fluids and debris from a client to surfaces, equipment, materials, workers' hands, or another client. Because saliva is invisible yet capable of containing high numbers of bacterial and viral particles, cross-contamination is particularly problematic in oral healthcare. Pathogenic organisms, potentially present in a client's oral fluids, may survive on environmental surfaces for days, weeks, and even months if left untreated with a germicidal product.

Cross-contamination may be by direct or indirect means:

- ✦ *Direct cross-contamination* occurs when a worker fails to change gloves between clients, and when instruments are not properly cleaned and sterilized between uses. An example of direct cross-contamination is the use of a disposable dental product such as a saliva ejector on multiple clients.
- ✦ *Indirect cross-contamination* occurs when instruments, dental materials and their containers, equipment, or environmental surfaces are contaminated with a client's oral fluids, either through touch or spatter, and are not decontaminated before touched again or used in another client's mouth. Indirect cross-contamination occurs when a container of dental material is handled with contaminated gloves, is not disinfected, and then handled again with gloved hands when treating another client (Figure 6–29).

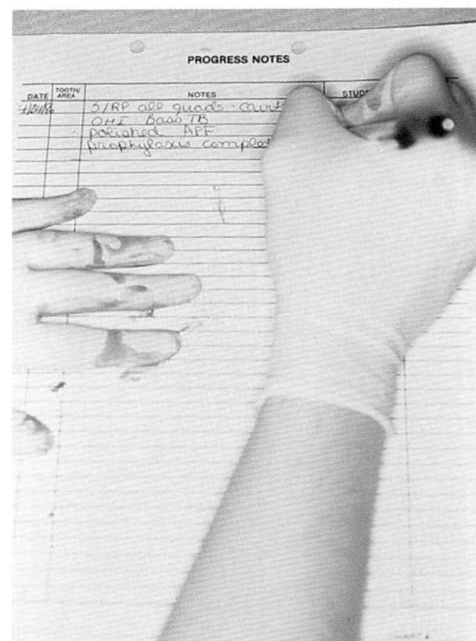

FIGURE 6–29 ✦ Indirect cross-contamination from a chart handled with a contaminated gloved hand.

Oral fluids introduced when working on the first client may be transferred to the gloves used for subsequent clients, placing them at risk for disease transmission. The result is that potentially pathogenic organisms present in the oral fluids may be transferred to a subsequent person. Also note skin exposure problem.

Exposure Prevention and Management

Dental healthcare workers are at risk for transmission of bloodborne pathogens. This risk is reduced by safe work practices, use of safe devices, use of personal protective equipment, awareness of personal health status, and attention to universal precautions. Most *exposures* are preventable. Programs for the prevention and management of injuries follow the public health doctrine of prevention:

- ✦ Primary prevention strives to prevent the injury in the first place.
- ✦ Secondary prevention strives to contain the injury.
- ✦ Tertiary prevention strives to return to a functional state of no exposure and prevent similar injuries from occurring again.

STEPS FOR RISK REDUCTION. *Primary prevention* involves all efforts to avoid injury during each facet of delivering oral healthcare services from setting up a treatment room, providing care, and post-treatment clean-up. Injuries may be prevented by use of engineering controls, work practice controls, personal protective equipment, and other methods of hazard abatement and risk reduction such as universal precautions. Therefore, the first step for risk reduction is to assess risks as environmental, administrative/procedural, and personal. After the risk is assessed it is important to determine if actions can be taken to remove or at least reduce risk by modifying policies, procedures, or practices. Risk assessment involves determining what is done, by whom, how it is done, and with what products and devices. Risk reduction then involves the selection of engineering or work practice controls appropriate to the anticipated procedures. Through all this, communication of hazards is most important and is accomplished by information on principles of injury prevention and management and training.

The ultimate lesson is that it is far better to prevent the exposure in the first place than to deal with the consequences of an exposure such as counseling, testing, and medical follow-up. The underlying theme of risk reduction is universal precautions. The use of universal precautions is based on exposure potential and is associated with specific procedures without regard to the known or perceived infectious status of a client. When OSHA determines risk, it is in regard to a specific job classification or task that has a measure of exposure potential. In practice, all employees are obligated to follow standards determined by OSHA; for students, it is prudent behavior and a safe standard of practice to follow OSHA requirements.

RISK REDUCTION PROTOCOLS. Wearing personal protective equipment (PPE) is one risk reduction protocol. When used appropriately, PPE act as a barrier between the clinician and the environment to prevent mucous membrane and skin exposure. PPE is task, not patient specific, and includes the wearing of gloves, face masks, protective eyewear, and protective attire.

Another risk reduction protocol relates to personal health status and vaccination history, particularly HBV vaccination. Vaccination provides excellent protection from infection after exposure to pathogenic organisms for which one has been vaccinated. Unfortunately, there are limited vaccine-preventable diseases and vaccines are not available for HCV or HIV.

Several risk reduction protocols center on the need to prevent percutaneous injuries:

- ✦ Use of medical devices with safety features designed to prevent injuries or by using safer techniques:
  - Never recap needles by hand
  - Never disengage needles from a reusable syringe
  - Use disposable needle systems
  - Dispose of needles/sharps in appropriate sharps disposal containers
- ✦ Avoidance of hand contact with sharps:
  - Never wipe instruments on gauze in a hand or wrapped around a finger; use a single-hand technique instead such as cotton rolls taped to an instrument tray or a commercial safe wipe device
  - Announce instrument passes to warn others of sharps and exposure potential
  - Create a neutral zone for sharps to avoid passing directly between healthcare workers
  - Use appropriate clean-up procedures to minimize hand contact with sharps

Work practice controls have some of the greatest impact on preventing bloodborne disease transmission. Given the types of exposures found in dental settings, over 90% are associated with needles or other sharp devices. The CDC determined that most occur outside the mouth and on the hands and fingers of the worker. Many of these are preventable with proper caution. With the use of safer devices along with the safe use of devices, about 80% of injuries could be prevented.

POSTEXPOSURE MANAGEMENT. When an injury occurs, the goal is to contain the injury as soon as possible to reduce the risk of transmission and seroconversion (secondary prevention). If an exposure occurs, immediate post-exposure management must be offered to the exposed worker. The circumstances, devices, degree, and severity of exposure must be reviewed. The client, if known, should be interviewed for any information he or she may provide on the bloodborne disease status or risk of infection.

The basic steps of post-exposure management are:

Step 1: Immediate first aid (no extraordinary measures). If an injury occurs there are basic first aid measures to immediately apply such as:

- ✦ Washing an area of percutaneous exposure
- ✦ Flushing nose, mouth, eyes, or skin with clean water, saline, or sterile irrigants

There is no scientific evidence that the use of antiseptics for wound care or bleeding the wound will reduce the risk of transmission of a bloodborne pathogen. The use of a caustic agent such as bleach is not recommended.

Step 2: Report the incident to a designated individual and complete an incident report form if required. This includes the source (client's name) and nature of the exposure (Figure 6–30).

Step 3: Designated individual should discuss the incident with the source client.

Step 4: Initiate referral to a healthcare professional capable of treating an exposed individual.

Step 5: Begin medical evaluation and follow-up in accordance with the most recent U.S. Public Health

Directions: Please fill in completely or place a check next to the appropriate response. (include acccidents, exposure to hazardous substance or disease.) This is to be completed by the supervisor. PLEASE PRINT.

1. Name:__________________
   Address:__________________
   City:_______ State:_________ Zip code:_________
   Social security number:____________
   School:_______________
2. Occurrence date & time:__________
3. Report date:______________________
4. Location of occurrence:
5. Activity involved (check all that apply):
   ____Lifting patient ____Transport patient
   ____Lifting other ____Transport equipmeny
   ____Invasive procedure/injection ____Equipment use/repair
   ____Other patient care ____Walking
   ____Non-work activity ____Hazardous substance/ infectious exposure
   Explain:____________________________________
   Other (explain):____________________________________
6. Type of injury (check all that apply):
   ____No apparent injury ____Foreign body
   ____Laceration/abrasion ____Strain/sprain
   ____Needlestick/instrument puncture:
   Needlestick/percutaneous injury (please identify) __________
   Type of fluid: ☐ Blood ☐ Saliva ☐ Blood mixed with saliva
   Amount of fluid:_____________________
   Depth of injury:_____________________
   Was fluid injected? ☐ Yes ☐ No
   ____Fracture ____Burn
   ____Amputation ____Bruise/crush
   ____Electrical shock ____Bite/scratch
   ____Splash/mucous membrane:
   Mucous membrane exposure (please identify):____________
   Estimated volume of material:____________________
   Duration of contact:________________________
   Was skin: ☐ Abraded? ☐ Chapped?
   ____Other (explain):__________________________________

FIGURE 6–30 ✦ Confidential incident report form used in postexposure management. *(Courtesy Gene W. Hirschfield School of Dental Hygiene, Old Dominion University, Norfolk, Va.)*

Service Guidelines. Medical follow-up should include counseling and testing as indicated and determined by the infection potential of the exposure. Testing may be for HIV, HBV, or HCV; testing may need to be repeated at certain intervals depending on physician's advice.

✦ HBV: Follow-up is determined by vaccination status. If the exposed person has not been vaccinated then this should be started. If the source individual has a history of HBV infection, hepatitis B immune globulin may also be recommended. Treatment

7. Part of body (check all that apply):

LEFT	RIGHT		LEFT	RIGHT	
____	____	Head	____	____	Elbow
____	____	Eye	____	____	Hand
____	____	Ear	____	____	Finger(s)
____	____	Face	____	____	Wrist
____	____	Neck	____	____	Leg
____	____	Chest	____	____	Groin
____	____	Abdomen	____	____	Knee
____	____	Back	____	____	Foot
____	____	Arm	____	____	Toe(s)
____	____	Shoulder	____	____	Ankle

8. Possible causes (check all that apply):

____Unclear as to policy/procedure ____Unaware of safety hazard

____Patient initiated occurrence ____Foreign material on floor

____Equipment defect/malfunction/ handling ____Improper body mechanics

____Poor illumination

9. Exposure source:____

☐ Source material contained HIV or other bloodborne pathogens

10. Supervisor notified at time of occurrence: ☐ Yes ☐ No

Name:____

11. Description of occurrence:____

____

____

12. Witnessed by (please print):

Name:______________________________ Telephone:____________

Name:______________________________ Telephone:____________

13. Measures taken to prevent reoccurrence: ______________________

____

____

14. Immediate treatment:

____No treatment necessary ____First aid

____Student health ____Refused treatment

____Emergency room ____Emergency care center

Hospital:____________________ Explain:______________________

FIGURE 6–30, CONT'D.

Figure continued on following page

15. Time lost: ☐ Yes ☐ No
Treatment facility:__________________________
Physician's name:__________________________

Briefly describe treatment:______________________________
____

OR

If incident is a blood or body fluid exposure, please adhere to Blood-Borne Pathogen Post-Exposure guidelines. Document only as directed.

16. Disposition:
____Returned to school
____Released to home
____Hospitalized Name of hospital:____________________
____Fatality
____Other (explain):______________________________________
____

17. Time lost: ☐ Yes ☐ No
Estimated absence:____________________

18. Signatures:

Student:________Date:_________________________ _________

Clinical supervisor/manager: ____________________Date:_________

Course supervisor: __________________________Date:_________

Comments:

Source patient:______________________

Name:____________________________

Address:__________________________

Phone number:______________________

FIGURE 6–30, CONT'D

should begin as soon as possible, preferably within 24 hours.

- HCV: There is no standard protocol at this writing; however, this is a rapidly evolving area and consultation with an infectious disease specialist is important.
- HIV: If post-exposure treatment is indicated, the course of treatment usually involves a 4-week regimen of one or more antiretroviral drugs, depending on the nature of the exposure. The basic regimen for an exposure with a recognized risk is for 2 drugs (zidovudine and 3TC), and the expanded regimen for exposures with an increased risk of HIV transmission is the basic regimen plus a protease inhibitor (indinavir or nelfinavir). Post-exposure management is an area of rapidly changing recommendations. It is important to seek the advice and care of an appropriate provider who is familiar with the current recommendations for testing and prophylaxis. In some instances, expert consultation may be advised, such as with pregnancy, known antiretroviral drug resistance in the source patient, or toxicity to the regimen. Exposure risk varies with the amount of blood, the titer of virus in the patient, and the severity of the exposure. Treatment should be initiated immediately, preferably within 2 hours. The goal is to prevent viral replication in the exposed worker, and there is biologic evidence that

this is possible. Post-exposure management by antiretroviral drugs may reduce the risk of infection by about 80%, but will not prevent all cases of infection. Post-exposure management may fail due to a resistant virus, an increased titer of virus, an increased dose of blood, or host factors.

Follow-up also involves counseling about signs and symptoms of infection, the importance of measures to not infect others, and the importance of seeking advice if illness occurs. For HCV, it may be necessary to monitor liver function and have tests for HCV antibody. Repeat testing may be recommended at 4 to 6 weeks. For HIV, baseline testing is part of the standard protocol and repeat testing may be indicated at 6 weeks, 12 weeks, and 6 months. If antiretroviral drugs are taken, the exposed person may need to have drug toxicity tests.

Most exposures do not lead to infection, and the risk of *seroconversion* may vary depending on the agent, the type of exposure, the amount of blood involved, and the amount of circulating virus in the source client. For HBV, the risk of infection ranges from 6% to 30% in persons not protected by vaccination or previous infection. Individuals who are hepatitis e–antigen positive are potentially more infectious and more likely to transmit diseases. The best protection is to be vaccinated against HBV. The number of healthcare workers infected occupationally has been greatly reduced due to the high rate of vaccination.

For HCV, the risk is about 1.8% on average for percutaneous exposures. There are no exact estimates on the number of healthcare workers occupationally infected with HCV. The average risk after a percutaneous exposure to HCV is about 0.3% or about 1 in 300. The risk after exposure to eyes, nose, or mouth is about 0.1% and the risk to skin is believed to be less than that unless the skin is damaged or compromised, in which case the risk would be higher. The number of healthcare workers occupationally infected is estimated as 54 through reports to the CDC; there are no dental healthcare workers in this estimate. However, there are about 134 healthcare workers whose infection may be occupational and there are 6 dental personnel in this estimate.

In *tertiary prevention*, the healthcare professional learns lessons from the exposure incident, restores those exposed to a state of no infection, and takes all steps to reduce future exposure risk. This consists of:

- ✦ Evaluating the circumstances of the exposure
- ✦ Reviewing policies, procedures, products, and practices
- ✦ Discussing appropriate modifications
- ✦ Determining how to communicate these to others

Maximum effort should be aimed at injury prevention.

Client Education Issues

- ✦ Explain infection control protocols used in the delivery of dental hygiene care and their underlying rationale.
- ✦ Explain that infection control is done to protect and *not* to keep an unnatural distance between the client and clinician.
- ✦ Discuss post-exposure protocols at the initial appointment in case of an exposure.

Legal, Ethical, and Safety Issues

- ✦ Using evidence-based infection control protocols is both an ethical and legal requirement for a dental hygienist.
- ✦ Evidence-based universal precautions are a standard of care. Practitioners who fail to render services using current standards of care place themselves at risk for both civil and criminal violations of the law.
- ✦ The reasonably prudent dental hygiene practitioner must stay current of changing infection control concepts, protocols, and governmental guidelines.
- ✦ It is unethical and illegal to refuse treatment to a client of record because that client has an infectious disease.

Key Concepts

- ✦ Sterilization and surface disinfection can be achieved by physical or chemical means based in the equipment, type of procedure, and level of risk of exposure.
- ✦ Handwashing is the most effective strategy in the prevention of infection and disease transmission.
- ✦ CDC recommendations for universal precautions indicate that healthcare workers use personal protective equipment when exposure to body fluids is likely.
- ✦ The basic tenet of universal precautions is that all clients should be viewed as potentially infected.
- ✦ Current infection control guidelines and recommendations are easily accessed via key Internet sites.
- ✦ Healthcare workers who adhere to infection control strategies reduce the risk of infection for themselves, their families, and their clients.

Critical Thinking Exercises

You have been hired by one of the most reputable dental practices in the community. On the second day of your employment, you accidentally insert a used hypodermic needle percutaneously into your thumb after administering a local anesthetic agent to your client. Because your client is a high-profile state legislator and you don't want to appear incompetent to your new employer or the client, you say nothing about the exposure incident. After three days of thinking about the situation, you report the incident to the office manager. Use the principles of post-exposure management to determine:

1. What steps should be taken by the office manager to protect the health and safety of the new dental hygienist?
2. What errors in judgment were made by the dental hygienist?
3. Explain the steps of the post-exposure management protocol that should have been taken by the dental hygienist.
4. What tertiary preventive strategies need to be initiated by the office manager for the practice?

For References, Suggested Readings, and Related Websites, visit
http://evolve.elsevier.com/Darby/hygiene/

CHAPTER 7

Managing Medical Emergencies

OBJECTIVES

Mastery of the content in this chapter will enable the reader to:

- Recognize persons at high risk for a medical emergency
- Describe protocols for performing CPR in adults, children, and infants
- State protocol for managing a victim with partial airway obstruction, with and without good air exchange, and complete airway obstruction
- Identify signs and symptoms of specific medical emergencies and appropriate treatment for each
- List basic equipment and drugs for managing medical emergencies in the oral care environment

KEY TERMS

Angina pectoris
Angioedema
Aura
Biologic death
Cardiac arrest
Clinical death
Diaphoresis
Gross negligence
Head-tilt/chin-lift maneuver
Medical alert box
Myocardial infarction
Polydipsia
Polyphagia
Polyuria
Syncope
Trendelenburg's position
Urticaria

ASSESSING RISK OF AN EMERGENCY

Prevention of and preparedness for potential emergencies are essential for protecting the client's health and safety. Client assessment, including observation of general physical status, vital signs, American Society of Anesthesiologists (ASA) physical status classification, and history of medical conditions with special attention to medication usage, reduces the likelihood of untoward reactions and potential emergencies (see Chapters 9, 10, and 11). Should a medical emergency arise, thorough knowledge of medical emergency protocols, well-trained office personnel, and availability of appropriate emergency equipment are vital in obtaining the best possible outcome. Comprehensive documentation of all assessment findings is made in the client's record and updated at each subsequent visit. In the event of an emergency, the hygienist stops all dental procedures and uses the steps found in Figure 7–1 to assess the situation.

Complex care plans, the use of oral and intravenous medications in the dental setting, the advancing mean age of the population presenting for care, and the increased number of medically compromised clients contribute to the potential for medical emergencies.

PREVENTING MEDICAL EMERGENCIES

Client assessment data are used to create a care plan that will reduce the likelihood of a medical complication. If a client is found to be at high risk the client's physician of record is consulted. Based on this consultation, the care plan can be modified or medications modified to avoid emergencies. Reduction of the stressful environment by careful appointment planning, good communication and client rapport, and dentist administration of antibiotics or anti-anxiety premedication can also improve clinical outcomes.

Most practices use health history forms that include a *medical alert box.* This blank box usually appears on the top corner of the health history form. If a client has a condition (allergy, hypertension, adrenal insufficiency, requirement for antibiotic premedication, etc.) that if unrecognized places the client at risk of a medical emergency, this condition should be written in red in the

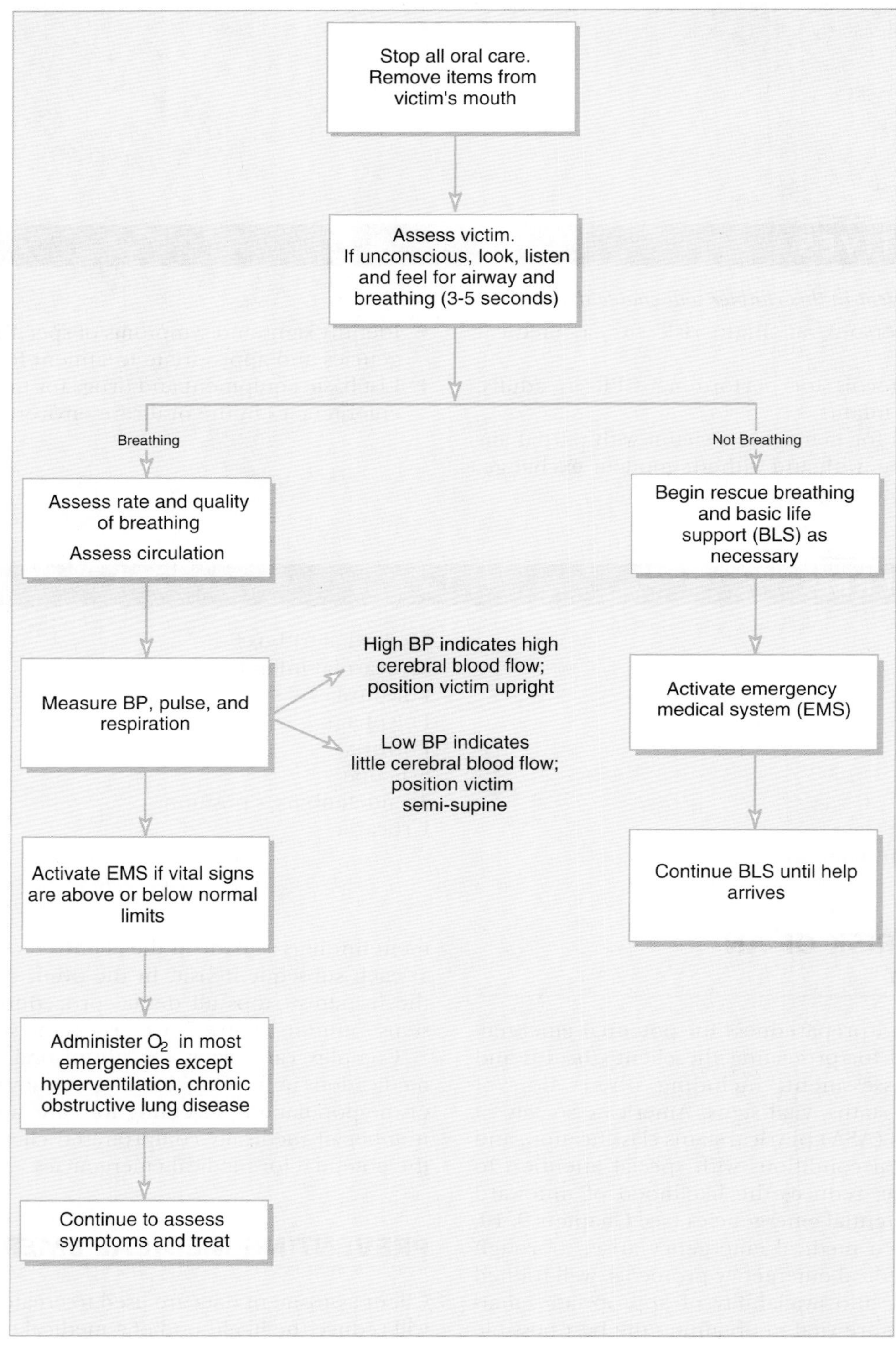

FIGURE 7–1 ✦ Dental hygiene actions taken in an emergency situation.

medical alert box clearly visible on the top of the health history form. The practitioner can then consider this condition as the care plan is developed and implemented.

CARDIAC ARREST

Signs and symptoms of *cardiac arrest* include absence of pulse, blood pressure, and respirations, and an ashen appearance. *Clinical death* is cessation of the heart and respiratory effort; it may be reversible with life support measures if initiated within 4 to 6 minutes. Life support measures include cardiopulmonary resuscitation (CPR), basic life support (BLS) and advanced cardiac life support (ACLS). *Biologic death* is permanent cellular damage, especially to the oxygen-sensitive brain cells, as a result of inadequate oxygen supply. Cardiac arrest may result from an acute reaction to medication, myocardial infarction, respiratory arrest, electric shock, drowning, trauma, asphyxiation, shock, or cardiac arrhythmia.

Office staff should conduct a cardiac arrest drill at least semiannually. Practicing a variety of scenarios will prepare the staff to respond rapidly and effectively in a real emergency. For basic life support protocol, see Procedure 7–1.

Procedure 7–1 BASIC LIFE SUPPORT FOR ADULT, INFANT, AND CHILD

EQUIPMENT

No special equipment required
If available, Ambu bag, CPR pocket mask

STEPS	RATIONALE
ONE PERSON	
1. Assess for unresponsiveness; ask questions and shake victim, "Are you OK?"; observe for spontaneous respirations; palpate carotid pulse.	Prevents injury from attempted resuscitation of a person who has not suffered a cardiac or respiratory arrest.
2. Activate the emergency medical system (EMS) usually by calling 911.	Activates mechanism for higher-level emergency personnel.
3. Place the victim supine on a firm surface (caution is needed if you suspect spinal injury). A backboard may be used.	External compression of the heart is facilitated; heart is compressed between the sternum and the hard surface.
4. Kneel at the level of the victim's shoulders.	Position allows performance of rescue breathing and chest compressions without moving knees.
5. Open victim's airway:	Maneuver opens the airway, moves the tongue or epiglottis as an airway obstruction.
a. Head-tilt/chin-lift maneuver (adults and children): place one hand on victim's forehead and apply firm, backward pressure with the palm to tilt the head back. Place fingers of other hand under the bony part of the jaw near the chin and lift to bring the chin forward and the teeth almost to occlusion, thus supporting the jaw and helping to tilt the head back (see figure below).	

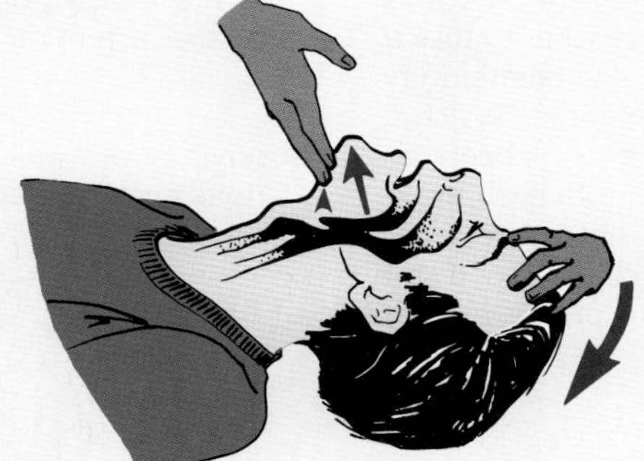

Head-tilt/chin-lift maneuver to open airway in adults and children. *(From Potter PA, Perry AG:* Fundamentals of nursing, *ed 5, St Louis, 2001, Mosby.)*

b. Jaw-thrust maneuver (adults and children): grasp angles of the victim's lower jaw and lift with both hands, thus displacing the mandible forward while tilting the head backward.	Safest first approach, without head-tilt, to opening the airway of the victim with suspected neck injury; can usually be accomplished without extending the neck.

Continued on following page

Procedure 7–1 BASIC LIFE SUPPORT FOR ADULT, INFANT, AND CHILD—CONT'D

STEPS	RATIONALE
6. Look, listen, and feel for breathing (3 to 5 seconds): a. Place your ear over victim's mouth and nose while maintaining an open airway. b. Look at victim's chest to check for rise and fall; listen and feel for breathing. If breathing, monitor vital signs until help arrives. If not breathing, begin rescue breathing.	Assesses the presence or absence of spontaneous breathing and the need to continue with rescue breathing.
7. Prepare for rescue breathing: a. For mouth-to-mouth resuscitation of an adult and child, pinch the victim's nose and occlude the mouth with yours. b. For an infant, place your mouth over the infant's nose and mouth (see figure to the right). (For mouth-to-mask resuscitation, place the heel and thumb of each hand on the borders of the mask to firmly seal margins, grasping the mandible with the index, middle, and ring fingers. Ventilate through the mouthpiece.)	Airtight seal is formed, and air is prevented from escaping from the nose. 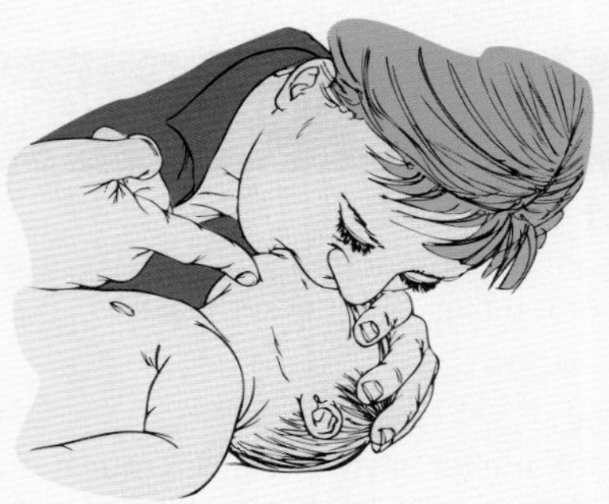 Airtight seal formed on infant's mouth. *(From Potter PA, Perry AG:* Fundamentals of nursing, *ed 5, St Louis, 2001, Mosby.)*
8. Perform rescue breathing: a. For mouth-to-mouth resuscitation of an adult, blow two slow breaths into the victim's mouth. Adequate time for the two breaths (1.5 to 2 seconds per breath for adult, 1 to 1.5 seconds per breath for infant or child) should be allowed to provide good chest expansion and decrease the possibility of gastric distention. If breaths go in and there is a pulse, continue rescue breathing at one breath every 5 seconds. Assess about every minute to determine if victim is breathing and if heart is beating. b. For mouth-to-mouth resuscitation of an infant or child, administer two slow breaths, 1 to 1.5 seconds per breath with a pause between for rescuer to take a breath. Continue rescue breathing at one breath every 3 seconds. Assess every minute to determine if victim is breathing on his or her own and if heart is beating.	In most adults, volume of 800 to 1200 ml is sufficient volume to make the chest rise. An excess of air volume and fast inspiratory flow rates are likely to cause pharyngeal pressures that exceed esophageal opening pressures, allowing air to enter the stomach and result in gastric distention, thereby increasing the risk of vomiting. Since an infant's air passages are smaller with resistance to flow quite high, it is difficult to make recommendations about the force or volume of the rescue breaths. Three factors to remember: (1) rescue breaths are the single most important maneuver in assisting a nonbreathing child; (2) an appropriate volume is one that makes the chest rise and fall; and (3) slow breaths provide an adequate volume at the lowest possible pressure, thereby reducing risk of gastric distention.
9. Observe for rise and fall of the chest wall with each respiration (see figure to the right). If lungs do not inflate, reposition the head and neck and try two more breaths. If still unsuccessful, suspect choking and proceed with obstructed airway procedures.	Observing chest wall movement ensures that artificial respirations enter the lungs.

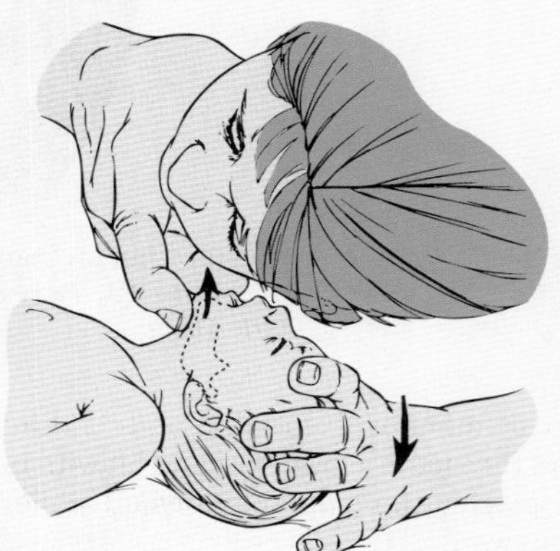

Listen and feel for breath and observe rise and fall of victim's chest. *(From Potter PA, Perry AG:* Fundamentals of nursing, *ed 5, St Louis, 2001, Mosby.)*

Procedure 7–1 BASIC LIFE SUPPORT FOR ADULT, INFANT, AND CHILD—CONT'D

STEPS	RATIONALE
10. Assess for presence of the carotid pulse; pulse check should take 5 to 10 seconds.	Carotid artery pulse will persist when the more peripheral pulses are no longer palpable.
a. Carotid pulse is most central and accessible in children over 1 year of age. However, in an infant, the short, chubby neck makes carotid difficult to palpate; brachial artery is recommended instead.	Performing external cardiac compressions on a victim who has a pulse may result in serious medical complications.
11. If the victim is pulseless, begin external cardiac compressions: **Adult:** a. Proper hand position (see illustration): (1) Using middle finger of the hand nearer the victim's legs, locate the margin of the rib cage on the side next to rescuer.	Properly performed external chest compressions can produce systolic blood pressure peaks of 60 to 80 mm Hg, but the diastolic pressure is low, with the mean blood pressure in the carotid arteries seldom exceeding 40 mm Hg. Blood flow through the carotid artery is only one fourth to one third of normal.
(2) Move fingers up the rib cage to the notch where the ribs meet the sternum. Place middle finger on notch, and index finger next to it, on the lower end of the sternum.	Proper hand position results in maximal compression of the heart between the sternum and the vertebrae. If compressions occur over the xiphoid process, the victim's liver can be lacerated.
(3) Place long axis of the heel of the hand (hand nearer victim's head) on the long axis of the sternum next to the index finger (see figure below).	Reduces risk of rib fracture during compressions.
(4) Remove first hand from notch; place on top of the hand on the sternum so that the hands are parallel to each other.	
(5) Either extend or interlace fingers, but keep fingers off the chest.	

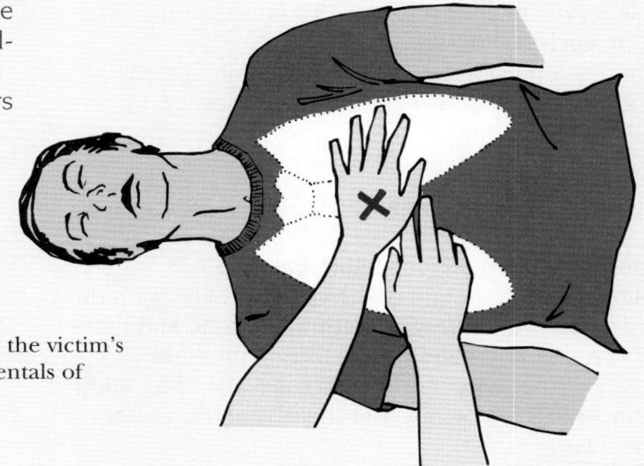

Correct position of the heel of the hand on the victim's sternum. *(From Potter PA, Perry AG:* Fundamentals of nursing, *ed 5, St Louis, 2001, Mosby.)*

STEPS	RATIONALE
b. Lock elbows, maintain arms straight and shoulders directly over the hands on victim's sternum (see illustration): (1) Compress chest 1.5 to 2 inches.	In this manner, each compression is straight down on the sternum.
(2) Compress chest 80 to 100 times per minute. After 2 ventilations, perform 15 external compressions with the mnemonic "one, and two, and three, and..." to 15.	Faster rate increases blood flow with an increased flow to the brain and heart. Faster rate also allows a pause for ventilation in two-rescuer CPR.
c. Ventilate lungs with two ventilations as in steps 7 and 8.	
d. Reassess victim after four cycles (2 ventilations, 15 compressions each cycle). If there is a pulse, continue rescue breathing at 1 breath every 5 seconds.	Determines return of pulse and respiration and the need to continue CPR.
Infant (1 to 12 months) a. Open airway by lifting the chin. Do not tilt the head back.	Overextension of the neck results in airway compromise.
b. Cover the infant's mouth and nose with your mouth and give 2 small, gentle breaths each 1 to 1.5 seconds long.	
c. Determine pulse by feeling for the brachial pulse located in the inner upper arm. If not present, initiate compressions.	Because of infant anatomy, the brachial pulse is easier to palpate.

Continued on following page

Procedure 7–1 BASIC LIFE SUPPORT FOR ADULT, INFANT, AND CHILD—CONT'D

STEPS	RATIONALE
d. Proper hand position (see figure below): (1) Draw an imaginary line between the nipples over the breastbone (sternum). (2) Place the index finger of the hand farther from the infant's head just under the intermammary line where it intersects the sternum (about one finger width below the nipple line).	Proper hand position results in maximal compression.

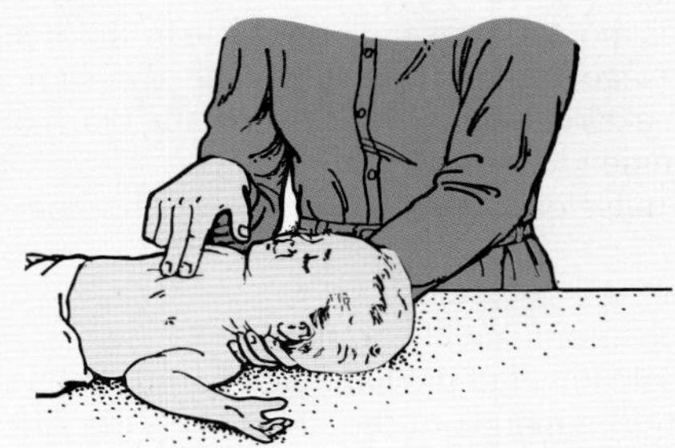

Correct position of the caregiver for compressions on infant's sternum. *(From Potter PA, Perry AG: Fundamentals of nursing, ed 5, St Louis, 2001, Mosby.)*

STEPS	RATIONALE
e. Using two fingers (middle and ring fingers), compress 0.5 to 1 inch. Give chest compressions at a rate of at least 100 times per minute.	Promotes adequate cardiac output.
f. Compression:ventilation ratio is 5:1, just as with child CPR. At the end of every fifth compression, a pause should be allowed for a ventilation (1 to 1.5 seconds). After one minute of repeated cycles, activate EMS.	
g. Reassess victim after 10 cycles (5 compressions, 1 ventilation each cycle).	Promotes adequate ventilation during CPR. Gets oxygen to the brain to prevent brain damage.
h. If you feel a pulse return, but no spontaneous breathing, give one breath every 3 seconds and discontinue chest compressions.	Determines return of pulse and respiration and the need to continue CPR.
Child (1 to 7 years) If you are alone, give one minute of CPR before activating EMS.	Gets oxygen to the brain to prevent brain damage.
a. Proper hand position (see figure below): (1) Locate lower margin of the victim's rib cage on the side next to the rescuer with the middle and index fingers on the hand nearer the victim's feet. (2) Follow the margin of the rib cage with the middle finger to the notch where the ribs and breastbone meet. (3) Place index finger next to middle finger. (4) Place heel of same hand next to index finger with long axis of the heel parallel to the sternum.	Proper position results in maximal compressions.
b. Compress sternum with one hand 1 to 1.5 inches at a rate of 100 times per minute.	Promotes adequate cardiac output.

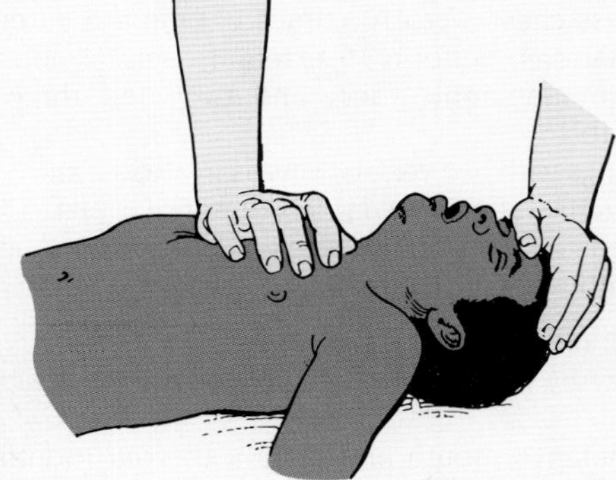

Correct position of the caregiver for compressions on child's sternum. *(From Potter PA, Perry AG: Fundamentals of nursing, ed 5, St Louis, 2001, Mosby.)*

STEPS	RATIONALE
c. At the end of every fifth compression, a pause should be allowed for ventilation (1 to 1.5 seconds).	Promotes adequate ventilation during CPR.
d. Reassess victim after 10 cycles (5 compressions, 1 ventilation each cycle).	Determines return of pulse and respiration and need to continue CPR.

Procedure 7–1 BASIC LIFE SUPPORT FOR ADULT, INFANT, AND CHILD—CONT'D

STEPS	RATIONALE
TWO PERSONS	
12. One person is positioned at the victim's side and performs ventilations and external cardiac compression while the other remains at the victim's head, maintains an open airway, and monitors the carotid pulse. The compression:ventilation ratio is 5:1 with a pause for ventilation (1.5 to 2 seconds). When the compressor becomes fatigued, the rescuers should exchange positions as soon as possible. This continues until help arrives or until the rescuers become exhausted	This continues until help arrives or until the rescuers become exhausted
13. After emergency care, document the situation on an incident report from and in the client's chart. Provide copy of incident report to emergency medical technician if victim is being transferred to a hospital.	Provides for continuity of care and protects operator from accusations of malpractice.

Adapted from *Basic life support for healthcare providers,* Dallas, 1997, American Heart Association; Potter PA, Perry AG: *Fundamentals of nursing,* ed 5, St Louis, 2001, Mosby.

OBSTRUCTED AIRWAY

An obstructed airway occurs when an object prevents the exchange of air in an individual. A foreign-body obstruction may occur:

- ✦ During eating (food particle blocks airway)
- ✦ During a dental procedure (aspiration of a dental instrument or piece of equipment),
- ✦ During resuscitation (aspiration of vomitus or blood)
- ✦ When unconscious (tongue falls backward, blocking pharynx)

If the victim has a partial airway obstruction with good air exchange and can cough forcefully, the hygienist should not interfere with attempts to dislodge the object but remain with the victim until it is dislodged or help arrives. Management of partial airway obstruction with poor air exchange and complete airway obstruction in the conscious and unconscious victim is discussed in Procedure 7–2.

OXYGEN ADMINISTRATION

During a medical emergency the body tissues may have an increased demand for oxygen or a diminished ability to receive or use oxygen, thus necessitating the administration of higher oxygen concentrations than exist in room air. Indications for oxygen administration include syncope, cardiac problems, and some respiratory difficulties. Oxygen should not be administered to a person experiencing an episode of hyperventilation. High levels of oxygen are contraindicated for individuals with chronic obstructive pulmonary diseases (COPD) such as emphysema (see Chapter 42).

The E cylinder is the recommended portable oxygen tank for in-office use. A clear facemask with tubing, nasal cannula, and a *positive-pressure apparatus (Ambu bag)* used to deliver the surrounding air to the victim are particularly valuable to prevent disease transmission between rescuer and victim. Competence in the use of the office oxygen system prior to an emergency is essential.

For a conscious client, a nasal cannula at a flow rate of 2 to 6 liters per minute or facemask at 8 to 12 liters per minute adequately delivers supplemental oxygen. The client should be allowed to breathe at his or her own rate while respiration rate and vital signs are monitored and medical assistance is summoned (see Chapter 10).

The unconscious client with adequate respiratory effort should receive the same type of oxygen administration, with careful observation should the respiratory effort diminish. An unconscious client without adequate respiratory effort should be placed in a supine position and the airway opened with the head-tilt/chin-lift maneuver (see Basic Life Support). The clinician then secures the mask over the client's face to cover the nose and mouth, starts the oxygen flow from the cylinder so that the flow inflates the positive-pressure bag, compresses the positive-pressure bag once every 3 to 5 seconds to inflate the victim's lungs, observes for chest movement and exhalation, repositions the victim's head if lungs are not adequately inflating, proceeds with the ABC assessment of BLS, and activates the EMS.

BASIC EMERGENCY DRUG KIT

The emergency drug kit should contain only drugs that the dental hygienist or dentist is trained to administer. Maintaining intravenous medications used for advanced life support in an emergency drug kit suggests that the need for these drugs is realized and can be administered competently. Maintaining an advanced emergency drug kit without the training to obtain intravenous access may subject the dental hygienist or dentist to liability claims.

Procedure 7–2 MANAGEMENT OF AN OBSTRUCTED AIRWAY

EQUIPMENT

No special equipment required

STEPS	RATIONALE
1. Treatment of an obstructed airway in a conscious victim is initiated only if there is a partial obstruction with poor air exchange or complete airway obstruction.	
a. Determine airway obstruction. If victim cannot speak or cough forcefully, initiate treatment.	In partial airway obstruction with good air exchange, the victim can cough forcefully; encourage spontaneous coughing and deep breathing. Monitor victim. No treatment is initiated unless air exchange becomes poor.
b. The rescuer is positioned behind the victim, wraps an arm around the victim's waist, places the thumb side of the fist between the victim's xiphoid and navel, supports the fist with the other hand, and presses the fist into the victim's abdomen with a brisk inward and upward motion. Each of these subdiaphragmatic abdominal thrusts (the Heimlich maneuver) should be distinct and repeated until the foreign body is removed or the victim loses consciousness.	Increased intraabdominal pressure from the Heimlich maneuver pushes up the diaphragm, which results in increased outflow of air from the lungs. The repeated abdominal thrust forces short bursts of air from the lungs. This dislodges the foreign body.
2. In an obese or pregnant victim, the rescuer is positioned behind the victim's chest. The thumb side of the fist is centered on the midsternum; the other hand is used to support the fist with backward motions administered until the foreign body is expelled or the victim loses consciousness.	Placement on midsternum avoids fracture of xiphoid and ribs and protects an unborn baby.
3. Treatment of obstructed airway in an unconscious person:	
a. Determine unconsciousness, summon help, and open the airway with head-tilt/chin-lift.	
b. Establish breathlessness and attempt ventilation.	
c. If ventilation is unsuccessful, reposition victim's head and attempt ventilation again. Activate EMS.	Always reposition if unable to ventilate because the tongue or soft tissue may be the cause of the airway obstruction.
d. If ventilation is still unsuccessful, kneel astride the victim and perform five abdominal thrusts by placing the heel of one hand just above the victim's navel and well below the xiphoid. Place the other hand over the first and press into the abdomen with distinct upward thrusts.	
e. For treatment of an obese or pregnant victim, kneel next to the victim and use the hand positions for CPR. Perform chest thrusts to expel the object.	
f. A finger sweep may be performed to remove a visualized foreign body in the victim's mouth.	Do not perform blind finger sweep in a child or infant as it may force the foreign body down further.
g. If obstruction is removed, ventilate the lungs twice and continue BLS as indicated.	
h. In an infant with a foreign body obstruction, a combination of back blows between the scapula and chest thrusts is recommended. Infant's head should be held lower than legs.	Allows gravity to help with the displacement of the obstruction.

TABLE 7–1 BASIC EMERGENCY DRUG KIT*

Drug/Route Administered	Action	Indication
Aromatic ammonia/inhaled	Chemical irritant	Syncope (fainting)
Epinephrine pen/subcutaneous	Cardiac stimulant and bronchodilator	Acute allergic reaction; acute bronchospasm (asthma)
Nitroglycerin/sublingual	Relaxes smooth muscle and dilates coronary arteries	Angina pectoris
Glucose/oral as sugar cubes, orange juice, or non-diet soft drink	Elevates blood sugar	Hypoglycemia
Bronchodilator/inhaled (albuterol, proventil, terbutaline)	Dilates bronchi in lungs	Bronchospasm/asthma
Antihistamine/oral (Benadryl)	Decreases the allergic response	Allergic reaction
Oxygen/inhaled	Increases oxygen to the brain	Respiratory distress

*Other medications may be included for use in advanced cardiac life support, but advanced training is needed to administer them.

The emergency kit should contain the basic drugs and items listed in Table 7–1.

MANAGEMENT OF SPECIFIC MEDICAL EMERGENCIES

Recognition of certain medical emergencies is essential for early intervention and appropriate treatment. When a medical emergency arises, the client's symptoms and vital signs need to be obtained rapidly. Guided by symptoms and vital signs, an assessment of the client's state of consciousness and neurological, respiratory, or cardiac status is performed. From this information, the type of emergency is identified and treatment rendered. Signs and symptoms of several conditions and the treatments for these disease processes are listed in Table 7–2. In all cases, the ABCs of BLS should be followed:

- ✦ **A**irway assessed and maintained
- ✦ **B**reathing assessed and maintained with ventilatory support provided as needed
- ✦ **C**irculation maintained, using CPR

Proper documentation of the emergency is required. The medical emergency incident report form in Figure 7–2 can be used for this purpose. A member of the oral care team should be assigned the responsibility to record information on the medical incident report form during the emergency situation. In the event that the victim is transferred to a hospital, a copy of the incident report and health history forms should accompany the victim.

TABLE 7–2 MANAGEMENT OF SPECIFIC MEDICAL EMERGENCIES

Condition	Signs/Symptoms	Management
Syncope	Sudden, transient loss of consciousness. The victim is pale and perspiring, may experience nausea and dizziness, pulse is weak, breathing shallow	Place in *Trendelenburg's position* (client's head lower than legs); maintain airway; monitor vital signs; administer oxygen; pass crushed ammonia capsule under victim's nose; place cool, damp cloth on forehead; reassure
Shock	Skin pale and clammy, change in mental status and eventual unconsciousness if untreated, drop in blood pressure, increase in pulse and respiratory rate	Position in Trendelenburg, maintain airway, monitor vital signs, administer oxygen, activate EMS and initiate BLS and transport to nearest emergency room; start large-bore IV (if trained)
Hyperventilation	Rapid or excessively deep respirations, light-headedness, dizziness, heart palpitations, tingling in extremities	Terminate procedure, reassure the client and encourage slow, deep breaths; may have client breath into a paper bag; *DO NOT administer oxygen.*
Asthma	Unproductive cough, shortness of breath, wheezing, anxiety, use of accessory muscles for breathing, cyanosis	Assist client to a position that facilitates breathing, administer client's own bronchodilator, administer oxygen, monitor vital signs, if necessary activate EMS and initiate BLS
Angina pectoris	Transient ischemia (lack of oxygenated blood) of the myocardium (heart muscle) manifested by crushing, burning, or squeezing chest pain, radiating to shoulder, arms, neck, or mandible lasting 2 to 15 minutes, shortness of breath, *diaphoresis* (sweating)	Terminate procedure, place client in comfortable position, monitor vital signs, administer oxygen, administer nitroglycerin if BP will tolerate; if pain is not relieved by rest and/or nitroglycerin (0.4 mg every five minutes for three doses), activate EMS and treat as a myocardial infarction

Table continued on following page

TABLE 7–2 MANAGEMENT OF SPECIFIC MEDICAL EMERGENCIES—CONT'D

Condition	Signs/Symptoms	Management
Myocardial infarction	Pain similar to angina pectoris but of longer duration and not relieved by rest and nitroglycerin; cold, clammy skin; nausea; anxiety; shortness of breath; weakness	Terminate procedure, place client in comfortable position, monitor vital signs, administer oxygen, activate EMS and initiate BLS as needed
Cardiac arrest	Ashen, gray, cold clammy skin; no pulse; no heart sounds; no respirations; unconscious	Activate EMS and initiate BLS
Congestive heart failure	Shortness of breath, weakness, cough, swelling of lower extremities, pink frothy sputum, distention of jugular veins	Terminate procedure, place chair back in upright position, administer oxygen, monitor vital signs, consult physician of record, activate EMS if necessary
Stroke or cerebrovascular accident (CVA)	The supply of oxygen to the brain cells is disrupted by ischemia, infarction, or hemorrhage of the cerebral blood vessels; sudden weakness of one side, difficulty of speech, temporary loss of vision, dizziness, change in mental status, nausea, severe headache, and/or convulsions	Terminate procedure, monitor vital signs, monitor airway, administer oxygen and initiate BLS as needed, activate EMS.
Generalized tonic-clonic (grand mal) seizure	*Aura* (change in taste, smell, or sight preceding seizure), loss of consciousness, sudden cry, involuntary tonic-clonic muscle contractions, altered breathing, and/or involuntary defecation or urination	Terminate procedure, lower dental chair and clear area of all sharp and dangerous objects, make no attempts to restrain the person; protect the head, assess and establish an airway, monitor vital signs, initiate BLS and activate EMS if needed—if stable, allow client to rest, arrange for medical follow-up, and arrange for assistance in leaving the dental facility
Nonconvulsive (petit mal) seizure	Sudden momentary loss of awareness without loss of postural tone, a blank stare, and a duration of several to 90 seconds, muscle twitches	Terminate procedure, observe closely, clear area of sharp objects, supportive care, may need physician evaluation
Adrenal crisis (cortisol deficiency)	Confusion, weakness, lethargy, respiratory depression, hypercalcemia, shock-like symptoms—weak, rapid pulse and low blood pressure— abdominal pain, loss of consciousness	Terminate procedure, activate EMS, place in Trendelenburg's position, monitor vital signs, administer oxygen, establish and maintain airway, initiate BLS as needed, transport to nearest emergency room
Hypoglycemia (hyperinsulinism)	Hunger, headache, cool moist skin, nausea, confusion, irritation, dizziness and weakness	Terminate procedure, administer oral sugar (sugar cubes, apple juice, orange juice, or sugar-containing soda), observation during recovery, if unconscious activate EMS and initiate BLS
Hyperglycemia (ketoacidosis)	*Polydipsia* (excessive thirst); *polyuria* (excessive urination); *polyphagia* (excessive hunger); labored respirations; nausea; dry, flushed skin; low blood pressure; weak rapid pulse; "fruity" breath odor followed by unconsciousness	Terminate procedure, activate EMS and support with BLS if necessary
Anaphylactic reaction	*Urticaria* (itchy wheals, also known as hives), *angioedema* (swelling of mucous membranes such as lips, tongue, larynx, pharynx), respiratory distress, wheezing, laryngeal edema, weak pulse, low blood pressure, may progress to unconsciousness and cardiovascular collapse	Terminate procedure; immediately activate EMS; establish and maintain airway; place in supine position; monitor vital signs; administer oxygen; initiate BLS as needed; if qualified, administer epinephrine
Reactions to local anesthesia	See Chapter 34 on local anesthesia *Toxicity from local anesthesia:* light-headedness, blurred vision and slurred speech, confusion, drowsiness, anxiety, tinnitus, bradycardia, tachypnea *Toxicity from vasopressor/vasoconstrictor:* anxiety, tachycardia, tachypnea, chest pain, dysrhythmias, cardiac arrest	Assess airway, breathing, circulation; initiate BLS as needed, administer oxygen, activate the EMS as needed.
Hemorrhage	Arterial is red in color and "spurts" Venous is darker in color and "oozes"	Compression over hemorrhage: for bleeding from a dental extraction or surgical site, pack the area with gauze and have the client bite down until bleeding stops; for nosebleeds, apply pressure to bleeding side, or pack the bleeding nostril with gauze; for severe bleeding, watch for signs of shock and activate the EMS

TABLE 7–2 MANAGEMENT OF SPECIFIC MEDICAL EMERGENCIES—CONT'D

Condition	Signs/Symptoms	Management
Foreign body in eye	Tearing, pain, and blinking of the eye	Pull the upper eyelid down over the lower lid, turn the lower eyelid down and examine. If particle is visible, remove it with moistened cotton-tip applicator, irrigate the eye; if particle cannot be easily removed, refer the client to a physician for prompt treatment
Chemical solution in eye	Tearing, pain, and blinking of the eye	Immediate copious irrigation with water and prompt evaluation by an ophthalmologist
Dislocated jaw	Pain and anxiety due to inability to return the mandible to the normal position, mouth remains open	Wrap thumbs in towels and place them on the occlusal surfaces of the mandibular teeth, fingers under the mandible; press down and back with the thumbs and pull up and forward with the fingers; mandible should slip into place
Avulsed tooth	Pain, swelling, bruising, empty socket	Tooth transported in victim's mouth, saline solution, milk, or wet wrap; tooth is placed into socket and secured as soon as possible (delay in replacement in socket results in poorer prognosis)
Broken instrument	Broken instrument	Dry area and examine for the tip, using gentle instrumentation to explore the area; use transillumination and radiographs as needed. Transport client to medical facility for chest radiograph if tip not recovered
Facial fracture	Pain, swelling, ecchymosis, deformity, crepitation on manipulation, limitation of movement, abnormal occlusion	Establish and maintain airway, support with bandage, transport to nearest emergency room
Fluoride poisoning (acute)	Nausea, abdominal pain, excessive salivation, vomiting, and diarrhea; in severe cases muscle cramping, bronchospasm, and cardiac arrest	Induce vomiting with ipecac syrup, then administer milk, monitor vital signs, activate EMS; initiate BLS as needed

Client name ______________________ Date ________ Time ________

Address ______________________ Home phone ________________

______________________ Work phone ________________

Incident described:

Vital signs

Time	BP	Pulse	Resp	Oxygen delivery	Medications administered

Treatment administered	Healthcare provider rendering care

Client response to treatment

____

Ambulance called (time)__________ Arrival time ________ Transported to __________

Emergency contact (time & name)______________________ Arrival time ________

Client driven home by ______________________ (relationship) Time __________

Follow-up phone call (time & name) ____________________ Time __________

Signature of attending dentist/physician ______________________________

FIGURE 7–2 ✦ Medical emergency incident report form.

Client Education Issues

- ✦ Explain the importance of having an accurate health history in the prevention of medical emergencies.
- ✦ Explain the importance of taking prescribed medications for the prevention of medical emergencies.
- ✦ Encourage clients to become CPR certified as a service to friends, families, and the community.
- ✦ Teach stress reduction strategies (see Chapter 32).
- ✦ Explain that complying with medication schedules, seeking regular preventive care, and reporting unusual symptoms immediately to a healthcare professional can prevent emergencies.

Legal, Ethical, and Safety Issues

- ✦ Taking a complete health, dental, and pharmacologic history is one step to reduce the risk of emergencies.
- ✦ Ensure that clients seek prompt medical care when signs and symptoms of potential disease are evident.
- ✦ Good Samaritan statutes generally provide immunity from civil prosecution to those rendering care in emergency situations. These statutes were enacted so that health professionals can render care to victims and be protected from lawsuits for negligent harm. These statutes vary from state to state, but gross negligence or willful misconduct is not covered in most jurisdictions. *Gross negligence* is the intentional failure to perform a task with reckless disregard of the consequences that affects the life of another, or a conscious act or omission that may result in grave injury. Under Good Samaritan statutes, services must be provided free of charge at the scene of an emergency (not within a healthcare environment). The definition of scene of an emergency remains open for debate; however, most courts exclude hospitals, dental offices, and other healthcare facilities. These statutes do not cover an emergency resulting from the actions of a provider during the course of treatment (see Chapter 54).
- ✦ The dental team should be trained to use all of the basic drugs contained in the emergency kit maintained with the dental practice setting.
- ✦ A medical emergency incident report form should be completed to document the situation, the victim's response and vital signs, treatment and medications administered, and emergency response time. A copy of this form, along with a copy of the client's health history form, should accompany the victim to the emergency room.
- ✦ Each member of the oral care team should have a specific role to play in the event of an emergency. These roles should be reviewed and practiced periodically.

Key Concepts

- ✦ Complete assessment of the client, including health, dental, and pharmacologic history and vital signs, is essential in the prevention of medical emergencies. Conditions that place a client at risk for a medical emergency should be written in red in the medical alert box of the health history form.
- ✦ Use stress reduction protocols to prevent anxiety-related emergencies (see Chapter 32).
- ✦ If a client is found to be at high risk, the client's physician should be consulted and the care plan and appointment schedule adjusted to avoid possible emergency situations.
- ✦ The office staff should be competent in using the emergency equipment and emergency drug kit, and should practice medical emergency drills using a variety of scenarios.
- ✦ When a medical emergency arises, rapid assessment of signs and symptoms along with vital signs will lead to the appropriate diagnosis and treatment. Document any client response that may lead to an emergency situation; document any client emergency.
- ✦ Complete a medical emergency report form to accompany the client to the hospital emergency room.

Critical Thinking Exercises

1. Syncope is one of the most common medical emergencies occurring in the dental setting. Discuss steps to prevent an episode of syncope in a client. Review the signs and symptoms of syncope and the management of this condition.
2. A client complains of squeezing chest pain and shortness of breath and exhibits significant diaphoresis. What condition(s) are you most concerned about? Discuss appropriate management for this client's condition. What could have been done to reduce the risk of this occurring?
3. Find the emergency drug kit in the healthcare facility. Identify each drug and item in the kit and its intended use. Check the expiration dates on all items. How is the emergency kit systematically updated to ensure currency of all items? How is the staff trained to ensure that all contents of the emergency kit can be used when necessary?
4. What is the emergency protocol in the healthcare facility? Does each member of the healthcare team have a clear role to play in the event of an emergency? Define these roles.
5. Role play the following emergency situations: cardiac arrest, insulin shock, diabetic coma, epileptic seizure, drug overdose, reaction to the local anesthetic agent, anaphylactic shock, obstructed airway, syncope.
6. Use the Internet to determine how symptoms may differ between a man and a woman experiencing cardiac arrest.
7. Use the Internet to find information on the automatic external defibrillator (AED). Explain its purpose and the procedure for use.

For References, Suggested Readings, and Related Websites, visit
http://evolve.elsevier.com/Darby/hygiene/

CHAPTER 8

ERGONOMICS

OBJECTIVES

Mastery of the content in this chapter will enable the reader to:

- ✦ Apply ergonomic principles in dental hygiene practice
- ✦ Discuss environmental factors leading to repetitive strain injuries (RSI)
- ✦ Describe modifications in the work environment that minimize the occurrence of RSI
- ✦ Modify client positioning based on ergonomic principles and client needs
- ✦ Relate proper grasp and instrument factors to ergonomic principles
- ✦ Relate proper hand stabilization to ergonomic principles
- ✦ Demonstrate neutral wrist, arm, elbow, and shoulder positions
- ✦ Discuss how appointment scheduling can reduce stress and RSI
- ✦ Demonstrate strengthening and stretching exercises and how each reduces RSI
- ✦ Describe common RSIs in terms of symptoms, risks, preventive measures, and treatment

KEY TERMS

Adhesive capsulitis (AC)
Carpal tunnel
Carpal tunnel syndrome (CTS)
Cervical disc disease
Cervical spondylolysis (CS)
Cubital tunnel syndrome
De Quervain's syndrome
Digital motion
Ergonomics
Extension (hyperextension)
Flexion of the tendons
Fulcrum (intraoral and extraoral)
Guyon's canal syndrome (GCS)
Lateral epicondylitis (LE)
Lumbar joint dysfunction (LJD)
Neutral positions
Phalen's test
Radial tunnel syndrome (RTS)
Repetitive strain injuries (RSI)
Synovial fluid
Tendon gliding exercise
Tension neck syndrome (TNS)
Thoracic outlet compression (TOC)
Tinel's test
Trapezius myalgia (TM)
Ulnar deviation

ERGONOMICS AND ITS PRINCIPLES

Ergonomics is the study of human performance and workplace design (Figure 8–1).

Ergonomists focus on a wide spectrum of workplace situations ranging from physical aspects of the environment to psychological threats to health (Table 8–1). Dental hygienists are at risk for *repetitive strain injuries (RSI),* musculoskeletal disorders involving the tendons, tendons sheaths, muscles, and nerves of the hands, wrists, arms, elbows, shoulders, neck, and back. When ergonomic principles are applied, a dental hygienist can practice comfortably and avert disability.[1–3] When ergonomic principles are ignored, RSIs may occur. Minimizing occupational risks in the workplace increases the likelihood of long-range health and wellness for the practitioner (Figure 8–2).

TABLE 8–1 ERGONOMISTS' PERSPECTIVES OF THE DENTAL HYGIENE WORKPLACE

Workplace Environment	Dental Hygiene Work Environment	Alterations to Dental Hygiene Practice	Repetitive Strain Injuries
Ergonomic design and layout	Layout and convenience of equipment placement in treatment area	Eliminate stretching for dental light and bracket table Reduce twisting motion of the back, shoulders, and elbow while reaching for dental hygiene instruments	Lumbar join dysfunction Carpal tunnel syndrome Thoracic outlet compression Tension neck syndrome Cervical spondylolysis Cervical disc disease Trapezius myalgia Rotator cuff tendonitis Rotator cuff tears Adhesive capsulitis Lateral epicondylitis Radial tunnel syndrome Cubital tunnel syndrome
Worker and equipment crossing point	Dull hand instruments Vibrations and stress from rotary instruments Improperly designed hand instruments	Maintain hand instruments Use principles of selective polishing Do not use handpieces with curly or retracting cords Use balanced instruments	Carpal tunnel syndrome Thoracic outlet compression Strained pronator muscle Guyon's canal syndrome Trigger finger nerve syndrome De Quervain's syndrome
Tasks and work to be performed	Repetitive movements and hand fatigue Clinician fatigue and stress on body	Change clinician positions Alternate instrument handle design and diameter Use proper client and clinician positioning	Lumbar joint dysfunction Carpal tunnel syndrome Thoracic outlet compression Tension neck syndrome Cervical spondylolysis Cervical disc disease Trapezius myalgia Strained pronator muscle Guyon's canal syndrome Trigger finger nerve syndrome De Quervain's syndrome
Psychological aspects and factors	Practice management and appointment scheduling	Alternate involved dental hygiene treatments with less-complicated maintenance appointments Increase continued-care intervals Lengthen appointment times	Lumbar joint dysfunction Carpal tunnel syndrome Thoracic outlet compression Tension neck syndrome Cervical spondylolysis Cervical disc disease Trapezius myalgia Rotator cuff tendonitis Rotator cuff tears Adhesive capsulitis Lateral epicondylitis Radial tunnel syndrome Cubital tunnel syndrome Strained pronator muscle Guyon's canal syndrome Trigger finger nerve syndrome De Quervain's syndrome

Environmental Factors

Flexibility of muscles and tendons is important for reducing the occurrence of RSI. Flexibility can be accomplished through physical exercise (discussed later in the chapter) and maintaining comfortable room temperatures. The colder the room, the less relaxed and flexible are muscles and tendons. Putting stress and strain on stiff muscles and tendons leads to RSI. Noise levels are another environmental factor to be considered. Relaxed atmospheres with minimal background noise contribute to a positive psychological state for clinician and clients.[3]

Equipment Factors

DENTAL UNIT. The treatment area consists of the dental unit and chair, the dental light, and the clinician's chair. The dental chair, a contoured chair for the client to sit in during dental care procedures, supports the client's head, torso, and feet. The dental chair also provides for easy maneuvering of the client via an articulating headrest, and foot and side power controls (Table 8–2). The dental light transmits illumination to maximize the clinician's view of the client's oral cavity. The dental unit contains essential treatment equipment such as the

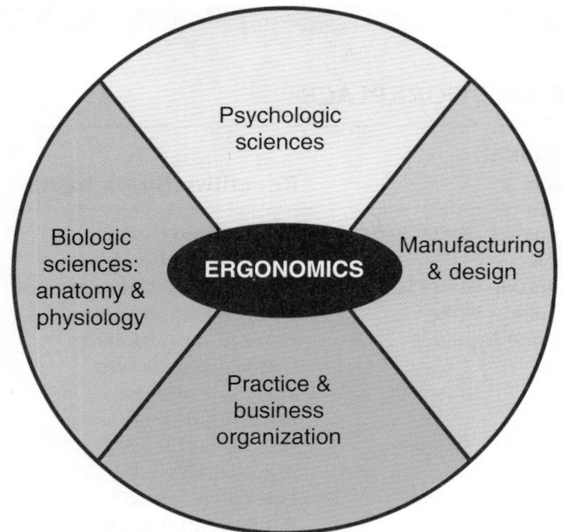

FIGURE 8–1 ✦ Multidimensional nature of ergonomics.

1. Environmental Factors
   - ✔ Comfortable temperature
   - ✔ Comfortable noise level
2. Equipment Factors
   - ✔ Properly designed clinician chair with freedom of movement
   - ✔ Properly designed dental chair
   - ✔ Bracket tray and dental light within reach
3. Positioning Factors
   - ✔ Proper clinician positioning
   - ✔ Proper client positioning
4. Performance Factors
   - ✔ Proper grasp and fulcrum
   - ✔ Maintained neutral wrist, elbow, and shoulder position
   - ✔ Maintained neck and back support
   - ✔ Proper wrist motion; limited digital motion and wrist extension and flexion
   - ✔ Appointment management
5. Instrument Factors
   - ✔ Properly maintain cutting edge
   - ✔ Use ergonomic handles
   - ✔ Variations in handle diameter and shape
   - ✔ Use balanced instruments
   - ✔ Use ultrasonic and sonic instruments
   - ✔ Avoid curly or retracting cords on motor-driven instruments and air/water syringes
   - ✔ Limit the use of instruments that cause vibrations
6. Exercises
   - ✔ Strengthening exercises
   - ✔ Chairside stretching exercises

FIGURE 8–2 ✦ Ergonomic checklist for dental hygienists.

TABLE 8–2 DENTAL CHAIR

Equipment	Description and Use
Contoured seat	The seat should provide comfort to a variety of clients (i.e., children, elderly) during treatment.
Lumbar support	A contoured design gives additional support to the torso and lumbar region.
Arm rests	These should support the client's arms comfortably and pivot for easy entering or leaving the dental chair
Foot or side power controls	These controls move the chair up or down and into a fully supine position. Provides numerous options to the clinician to access all areas of the client's mouth with minimal clinician back and neck strain. Side buttons require covering with disposable barriers to maintain asepsis. Foot controls provide the clinician with extra adaptability and range of motion.
360-degree rotation lever or foot control	Allows the dental chair to be rotated 360 degrees. This is beneficial when the dental chair must be moved to provide access for wheelchair-bound clients. This equipment also benefits the left-handed clinician to adjust the dental chair for proper clinician/client positioning.
Low base	This allows the dental chair to be placed closer to the floor, enabling the clinician to extend his or her arms when upper arm and body strength are needed during dental care.

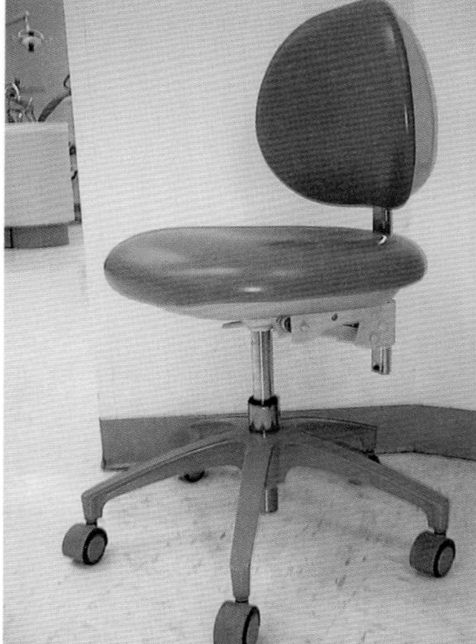

FIGURE 8–3 ✦ Traditional clinician's chair.

handpiece lines, water lines, air/water syringe, evacuation lines, and instrument tray(s). A cuspidor and cup filler also may be part of the dental unit (Table 8–3).

CLINICIAN'S CHAIR. The chair is one of the most important pieces of equipment for the delivery of care (Figure 8–3). It should have a broad, heavy base and be readily mobile, with a minimum of five free-rolling casters to maneuver around the client's head during care. The seat of the chair should allow for adequate body support and be adjusted easily for proper heights so the clinician's feet are flat on the floor with thighs parallel with the floor. New ergonomically designed chairs put the clinician in the proper position and lend total body support to

TABLE 8–3 DENTAL UNIT: PROMA DENTAL UNIT AND CLIENT CHAIR

Equipment	Description and Use
Dental chair (A)	Chair to support client during professional care
Dental light (I)	Overhead light transmitting illumination into the client's oral cavity for increased clinician visibility during dental care
Handpiece lines (B)	Attach the motor-driven handpiece from the power source to the dental unit; lines are electrical and air compressed
Water lines	Lines bring water to various parts of the dental unit including high-speed handpiece, three- way syringe, and cup filler
Three-way syringe (C)	Hand-held instrument attached to the dental unit provides air, water, or a combination of air and water; inserted in three-way syringe is an autoclavable or disposable tip
Evacuation lines (D)	High-speed and/or low-speed suction with autoclavable or disposable attachment tips
Instrument tray (F)	Movable stainless steel instrument tray usually attached to the dental light post
Cuspidor (G)	Movable cup or bowl utilized for expectoration by the client; many are equipped with a timed water flush system and may have a disposable paper lining
Cup filler (H)	Automatic water cup filler is activated by sensors when the disposable cup is empty

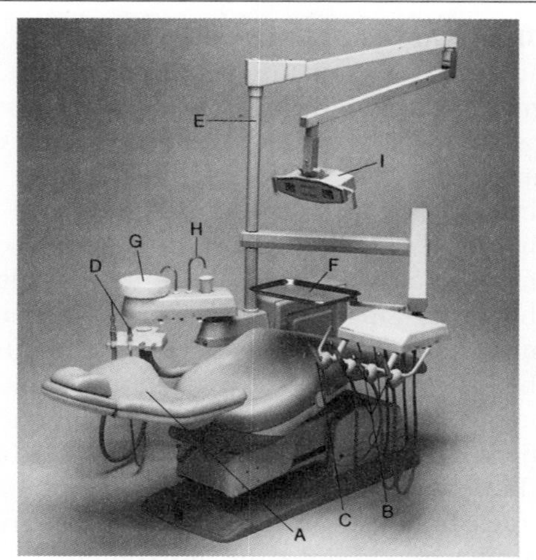

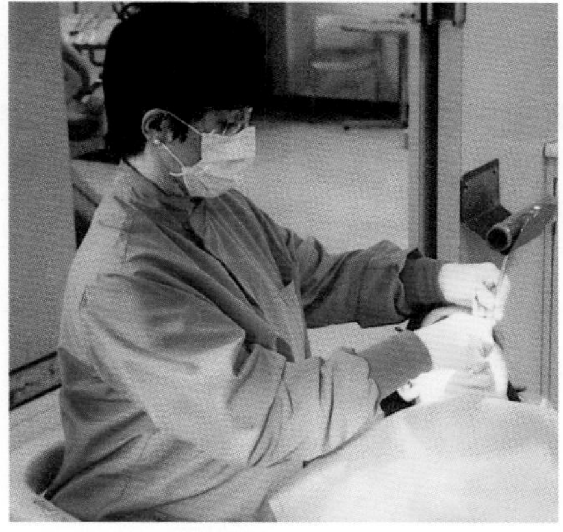

FIGURE 8–4 ✦ Neutral position of clinician. Note shoulders level and held in most relaxed position, elbows close to body, and forearms in same plane as wrists, hands, and client's mouth. *(Courtesy Nordent.)*

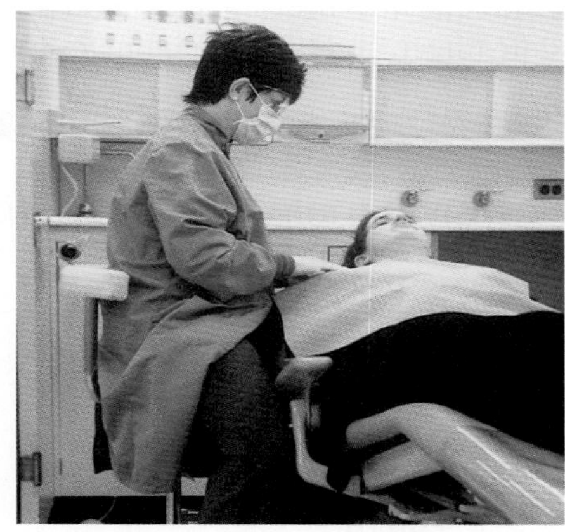

FIGURE 8–5 ✦ Clinician's stool positioned too high. *(Courtesy Nordent.)*

reduce strain on the spine, lower back, shoulders, and arms (Figure 8–4). Too high a chair position causes the body weight to be supported by the spine, back, and shoulders (Figure 8–5). Too low a position causes the clinician to slump and sit with a curved spine (Figure 8–6).

Cords on Powered Instruments.[3] Dental units are equipped with power-driven instruments and air/water syringes. These may be attached to the dental unit via:

- ✦ **Retractable cords:** Retract back into the dental unit to save space and avoid tangling
- ✦ **Curly cords:** Coiling characteristics allow cord to hang down a shortened distance and save space
- ✦ **Straight cords:** Straight, free-hanging cord

The retractable and curly power cords are encumbering and require constant pulling by the clinician. This

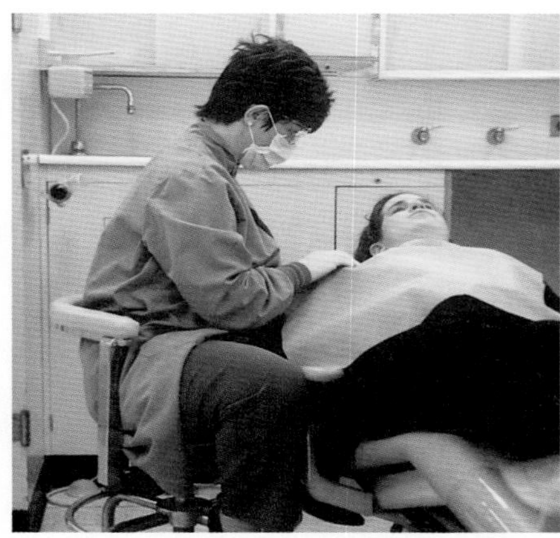

FIGURE 8–6 ✦ Clinician's stool positioned too low. *(Courtesy Nordent.)*

repetitive pulling motion increases fatigue and hand, arm, and shoulder muscle strain. A straight cord creates no tension while the clinician is using the motor-driven instrument.

Performance Factors

GRASP AND FULCRUM. Fundamentals of grasp include holding the instrument firmly, maintaining a secure grip, and maintaining control of the instrument without causing undue strain or fatigue to the clinician's hand, arms, and shoulders. The *modified pen grasp* is a three-finger grasp using the thumb, index finger, and middle finger. The pad of the thumb must be placed on the instrument handle and the joint bent slightly. The pad of the index finger should also be placed on the instrument handle, slightly superior to the thumb. The side of the middle finger is placed adjacent to the thumb below the index finger near the junction of the instrument handle and the functional shank of the instrument (Table 8–4). A space must be maintained between the index finger and thumb to facilitate freedom of movement when rolling the instrument into interproximal spaces and around line angles of the teeth during instrumentation. Rolling the instrument between the index finger, middle finger, and thumb eliminates turning and twisting of the wrist, which will lead to an RSI such as carpal tunnel syndrome.

Holding the instrument with all four fingers wrapped securely around the handle is the palm grasp. The thumb is placed on the handle pointed in the direction of the working end of the instrument. The modified pen grasp and palm grasp may be firm or light depending on the procedure being performed. Table 8–4 compares the procedure and instrument with the appropriate grasp. See Chapter 20 for a thorough discussion of instrument grasp.

FULCRUM AND HAND STABILIZATION. The *fulcrum* is the area on which the finger rests and against which it pushes while performing instrumentation. The fulcrum provides a basis for steadiness and control during stroke activation. Utilization of a proper fulcrum and hand stabilization reduces RSIs.

The *intraoral fulcrum* is established by resting the pad of the ring finger (fulcrum finger) inside the mouth against a tooth surface. The fulcrum finger usually is positioned on the occlusal incisal or facial surface of a tooth close to the working area or tooth being instrumented (Figure 20–8 and Table 8–5). The fulcrum finger must remain locked during instrument activation. A locked fulcrum

TABLE 8–4 GRASP, INSTRUMENT SELECTION, PROCEDURE, AND PRESSURE

Grasp	Instrument	Procedure	Pressure
Modified pen	Mouth mirror	Oral inspection	Light
		Tongue and cheek retraction	Light to firm
		Transillumination	Light
		Reflective illumination	Light
	Periodontal probe	Periodontal assessment	Light
		Measure pathology/lesions	Light
	Explorer	Caries examination	Firm
		Calculus detection	Light
	Curets	Plaque biofilm debridement	Light to firm
		Calculus removal	Firm
		Root debridement	Firm (lighten grasp as procedure is completed)
		Curettage	Light to firm
		Amalgam overhang removal	Firm
	Sickles	Calculus removal	Firm
		Amalgam overhang removal	Firm
	Hoes, files, etc.	Calculus removal	Firm
	Plastic instruments	Placing temporary fillings, periodontal pack, etc.	Light to firm
	Ultrasonic and sonic instruments	Calculus removal	Firm
		Plaque and endotoxin removal	Light to firm
		Orthodontic cement and bonding removal	Firm
		Overhang removal	Firm
	Porte polisher	Selective polishing procedures for all surfaces except maxillary anterior teeth-facial surfaces	Firm
	Slow-speed handpiece	Selective polishing procedures	Firm
		Amalgam polishing	Firm
		Sealant preparation	Firm
Palm	Curets, sickles, etc.	Instrument sharpening and maintenance	Firm
	Mouth mirror	Lip retraction with finger	Light
	Porte polisher	Selective polishing procedures on maxillary anterior teeth facials and maxillary posterior facial surfaces	Firm

allows the clinician to pivot on and gain strength from the fulcrum finger. Pivoting on the fulcrum finger helps to maintain a firm grasp, stability, and proper wrist motion. The middle and fulcrum fingers work together to add support during instrument activation. Splitting of the middle and fulcrum finger will cause decreased control, strength, and stability of the instrument. With decreased control, strength, and stability, the clinician will automatically tighten the grasp, contributing to RSI. Placing the fulcrum close to the working area is not always possible due to the client's inability to open the mouth wide, teeth alignment and position, pocket depth, or the angle of access. Utilization of a variety of intraoral fulcrums may be necessary. See Chapter 20's section on the fulcrum for a detailed explanation.

The *extraoral fulcrum,* positioned outside of the client's mouth, is utilized when instrumentation must be completed in deep periodontal pockets. It is accomplished by placing the broad side of the clinician's palm or back of the hand against an outside structure of the client's face

TABLE 8-5 FULCRUM FINGER PLACEMENT FOR DOMINANT HAND ON THE MANDIBULAR AND MAXILLARY ARCH

Area in Dental Arch	Facial/Right Handed	Lingual/Right Handed	Facial/Left Handed	Lingual/Left Handed
Mandibular right molar area	Occlusal surface of mandibular right 1st molar or premolars	Occlusal or occlusolingual line angle of mandibular right premolars	Occlusofacial line angle of mandibular right 1st molar or premolars	Occlusofacial surface of mandibular right 1st molar/premolars
Mandibular right premolar area	Incisal edge of mandibular right lateral or central incisor	Incisal edge of mandibular central incisors	Incisofacial edge of mandibular right anterior teeth	Incisofacial edge of mandibular right lateral incisors/canine
Mandibular left molar area	Occlusofacial line angle of mandibular left 1st molar/premolars	Occlusofacial line angle of mandibular left 1st molar/2nd premolar	Occlusal surface of mandibular left 1st molar/premolar	Occlusal or occlusolingual line angle of mandibular left 1st molar/premolars
Mandibular left premolar area	Incisofacial edge of mandibular left canine/lateral incisor	Incisofacial edge of mandibular left canine/lateral incisor	Incisal edge of mandibular anterior teeth	Incisal edge of mandibular anterior teeth
Mandibular right canine (distal)	Incisal edge of mandibular incisors	Incisal edge of mandibular central incisors	Incisal edge of mandibular incisors	Incisal edge of mandibular central incisors
Mandibular left canine (mesial)	Occlusofacial line angle of mandibular left 1st premolar/canine	Occlusofacial line angle of mandibular left 1st premolar or canine	Occlusofacial line angle of mandibular left 1st or 2nd premolar	Incisal edge of mandibular left canine
Mandibular left canine (distal)	Incisal edge of mandibular incisors	Incisofacial edge of mandibular central incisors	Incisal edge of mandibular incisors	Incisal edge of mandibular central incisors
Mandibular right canine (mesial)	Occlusofacial line angle of mandibular right premolars	Incisal edge of mandibular right canine	Occlusofacial line angle of mandibular right 1st premolar/canine	Occlusofacial line angle of mandibular right 1st premolar or canine
Maxillary right molar area	Occlusolingual line angle of maxillary right 1st molar/2nd premolar	Occlusolingual line angle of maxillary right molars	Occlusal surface of the tooth you are scaling or adjacent tooth	Occlusal surface of maxillary right 1st/2nd molar
Maxillary right premolar area	Incisolingual edge of maxillary right canine or premolars	Occlusolingual line angle of maxillary right 1st molar/premolars	Occlusal surface of the tooth you are scaling or adjacent tooth	Occlusal surface of maxillary right 1st premolar/2nd premolar
Maxillary left molar area	Occlusal surface of the tooth you are scaling or adjacent tooth	Occlusofacial line angle of maxillary left molars	Occlusolingual line angle of maxillary left 1st molar/2nd premolar	Occlusal surface of maxillary left molar area
Maxillary left premolar area	Occlusal surface of the tooth you are scaling or adjacent tooth	Occlusofacial line angle of maxillary left premolars	Incisolingual edge of maxillary canine or premolar	Occlusal surface of maxillary left premolar/molar area
Maxillary right canine (distal)	Incisofacial edge of maxillary incisors	Incisofacial edge of maxillary incisors	Incisolingual edge of maxillary right canine/lateral	Incisolingual edge of maxillary canine/lateral
Maxillary left canine (mesial)	Occlusofacial line angle of maxillary left premolars	Occlusofacial line angle of maxillary left 1st or 2nd premolar	Occlusal surface of maxillary left 1st premolar/canine	Occlusal surface of maxillary left premolars
Maxillary left canine (distal)	Incisolingual edge of maxillary left canine/lateral	Incisolingual edge of maxillary canine/lateral	Incisofacial edge of maxillary anterior teeth	Incisal edge of maxillary anterior teeth
Maxillary right canine (mesial)	Occlusal surface of maxillary right premolar/molar	Occlusolingual line angle of maxillary right premolars	Occlusofacial line angle of maxillary right premolar	Occlusolingual line angle of maxillary right premolars

such as the chin or cheek (Chapter 20, Figures 20–50 and 20–51). The benefits of using an extraoral fulcrum are:

- ✦ Easier accessibility to deep periodontal pockets
- ✦ Stability and control
- ✦ Additional options to instrument use in areas that are difficult to access
- ✦ Less twisting of the wrist during activation of maxillary posterior areas
- ✦ Decreased chance of RSI by offering the clinician less cumbersome or physically strenuous ways to instrument hard-to-reach areas of the client's mouth
- ✦ The action of the activation or pulling stroke is transmitted to the arm and shoulder and away from the wrist, decreasing the chance of RSIs to the nerves, tendons, and ligaments in the clinician's wrist and elbow

When no fulcrum is used, lateral pressure on the instrument during activation will cause the instrument to slip in the hand. To stabilize the instrument and gain control, the clinician will automatically tighten the grasp on the instrument. Tightening the grasp places stress on hand and arm muscles, tendons, and ligaments, leading to an increased occurrence of RSI.

WRIST MOTION DURING INSTRUMENT ACTIVATION.[2–4] Wrist motion and the fulcrum are related. Wrist motion is vital to the health of the clinician's hand, wrist, and forearm muscles, tendons, and ligaments. Pivoting on the fulcrum causes the hand, wrist, and forearm to move in one unified motion, often called "wrist rock." Failing to instrument using the unified motion causes the clinician to extend or flex the wrist (Figure 8–7, *A* and *B*). Continued flexion or extension of the wrist contributes to a variety of RSIs.

The use of digital motion during instrument activation is also a factor contributing to RSI. *Digital motion* is the push and pull motion of the instrument by utilizing the digits or fingers only. Muscle fatigue results quickly with digital motion, and a decrease in power and stability occurs.

APPOINTMENT MANAGEMENT.[3] Control of appointment procedures and time greatly reduces possible RSI. The dental hygienist should:

- ✦ Alternate new clients with continued clients
- ✦ Alternate root debridement and therapeutic scaling with maintenance appointments
- ✦ Alternate difficult appointments with less taxing ones
- ✦ Shorten continued-care intervals
- ✦ Allow for "buffer time" in the daily schedule

CLIENT-CLINICIAN POSITIONING FACTORS.[3,4]
Position of Client. Commonly used client positions include:

- ✦ Upright for interviewing and educating
- ✦ Semi-upright for treating persons with certain types of cardiovascular and respiratory diseases

A

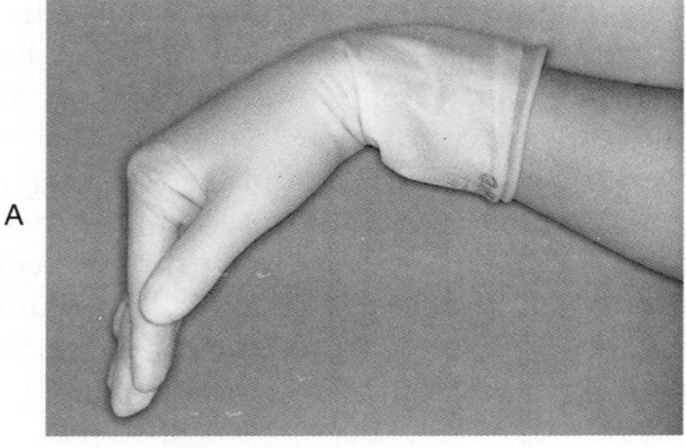

B

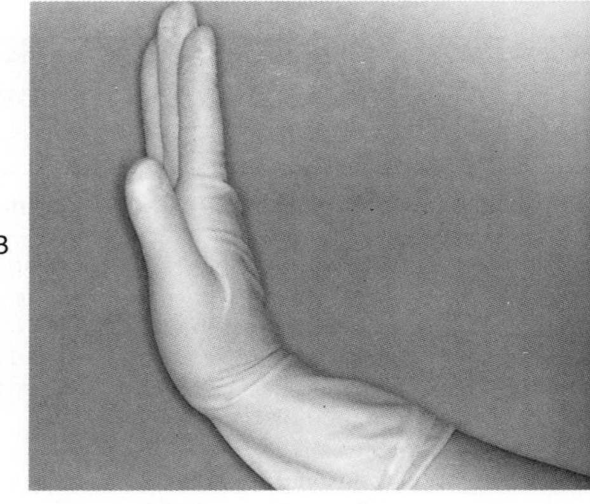

FIGURE 8–7 ✦ **A,** Flexion of the wrist. **B,** Extension of the wrist.

- ✦ Supine for treating most clients
- ✦ Trendelenburg for persons who are experiencing syncope

In the supine position, the client's mouth should be at about the height of the seated clinician's elbow. The distance from the client's mouth to the clinician's eyes should be about 14 to 16 inches. The headrest can be adjusted for maximum visibility on either the maxillary or mandibular arches. When treating the maxillary teeth, the maxilla should be perpendicular to the floor. When treating the mandibular teeth, the mandible should be parallel to the floor.

Clinician-client positioning is best explained using the face of a clock (Figure 8–8):

- ✦ The client's head is the center of the clock.
- ✦ The clinician moves around the face of the clock, positioning between the 8 o'clock and the 4 o'clock position.
- ✦ The right-handed clinician utilizes the range from 8 o'clock to 2 o'clock position. When teeth are out of alignment, the right-handed clinician may work in the 4 o'clock position.
- ✦ Left-handed clinicians work predominantly between the 10 o'clock and 4 o'clock positions with variations necessary at time to the 8 o'clock position.

Table 8–6 provides a reference for both right- and left-handed clinicians for accessing areas of the client's mouth. A variety of client positions are used during dental hygiene treatment (Figure 8–9).

TABLE 8–6 ACCESSIBLE AREAS OF THE CLIENT'S MOUTH

Right-Handed Clinician Clock Positions	Accessible Areas of the Client's Mouth	Left-Handed Clinician Clock Positions	Accessible Areas of the Client's Mouth
8 o'clock–9 o'clock	Mandibular right and left quadrants: all surfaces Maxillary right and left quadrants: all surfaces *Exception:* facial and lingual surfaces of maxillary and mandibular lingual teeth	3 o'clock–4 o'clock	Mandibular left and right quadrants: all surfaces Maxillary left and right quadrants: all surfaces *Exception:* facial and lingual surfaces of maxillary and mandibular anterior teeth
10 o'clock–2 o'clock	Mandibular right: mesial surfaces Mandibular anterior: all surfaces Mandibular left: posterior mesial surfaces	12 o'clock–2 o'clock	Mandibular right and left: mesial surfaces Mandibular anteriors: all surfaces
12 o'clock–2 o'clock	Mandibular left: posterior mesial surfaces from the facial approach Maxillary right: posterior distal and lingual surfaces	10 o'clock–12 o'clock	Mandibular right: mesial posterior surfaces from the facial approach Maxillary left: distal and lingual posterior surfaces
2 o'clock–4 o'clock	Mandibular right: distal of last tooth in the quadrant	8 o'clock–10 o'clock	Mandibular left: distal surfaces of last tooth in the quadrant

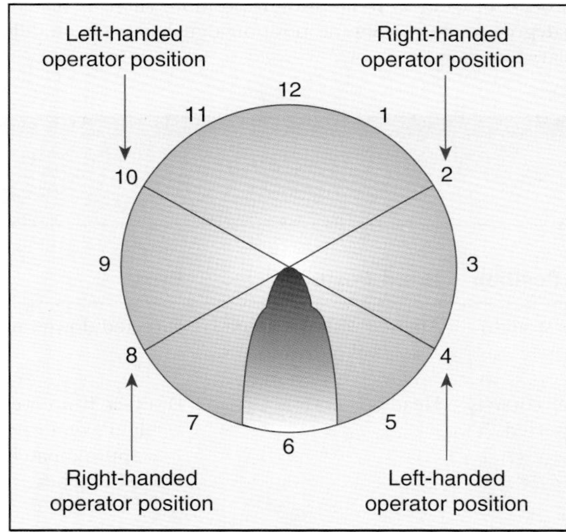

FIGURE 8–8 ✦ Possible clinician positions around the client. Right-handed clinician: 8 to 2 o'clock. Left-handed clinician: 4 to 10 o'clock.

Position of the Clinician. Clinician comfort and safety cannot be sacrificed for the client. Repetitively using incorrect clinician positioning causes stress and fatigue. Therefore, client positioning should allow the operator to perform intraoral procedures without increasing RSI. Table 8–7 lists the correct positioning of the arms, shoulders, legs, feet, back, head, and eyes of the clinician during care.

Wrist, Arm, Elbow, and Shoulder Position. Maintaining a neutral position of the wrist, arm, elbow, and shoulder reduces fatigue and injury to the clinician during care.[5] The *neutral positions* are basic to the prevention of occupational pain risks, particularly for those risks related to RSI.

Neutral positions include (Figure 8–4):

- **Shoulders:** Both shoulders level and held in their lowest, most relaxed position
- **Elbow:** Elbow held close to the clinician's body at a 90-degree angle
- **Arm:** Forearms held in the same plane as the wrist and hand
- **Wrist:** Wrist should never be bent; it is held straight

Back and Neck Support.[6] Adequate back and neck support reduces the occurrence of musculoskeletal injuries to the spine. Intervertebral discs in the spine resemble a jelly donut. When uneven pressure is put on an intervertebral disc, the effect is the same as if you pushed down on one side of a jelly donut: the contents of the disc or jelly donut are pushed out. Poor posture of the clinician results in uneven support of the spine and rupture of an intervertebral disc (Figure 8–6). Maintaining a straight back and neck and erect head, with feet flat on the floor and thighs parallel to the floor, properly supports the spine.

Instrument Factors

HAND INSTRUMENT CUTTING EDGE SHARPNESS.[1,3] Properly maintained sharp instruments are essential to the elimination of fatigue and stress on the hand, wrist, arm, and shoulders. Sharpening treatment instruments on a regular basis reduces mechanical stresses that cause RSI. The amount of force exerted is more likely to cause CTS than is the number of repetitions. Therefore, any instrument with a cutting edge should be kept as sharp as possible during the entire procedure. Instruments that are dull and not true to their original design cause the clinician to apply additional force, resulting in increased lateral pressure applied and a tightened grasp. Fatigue and repetitive stress on the clinician's body ensue.

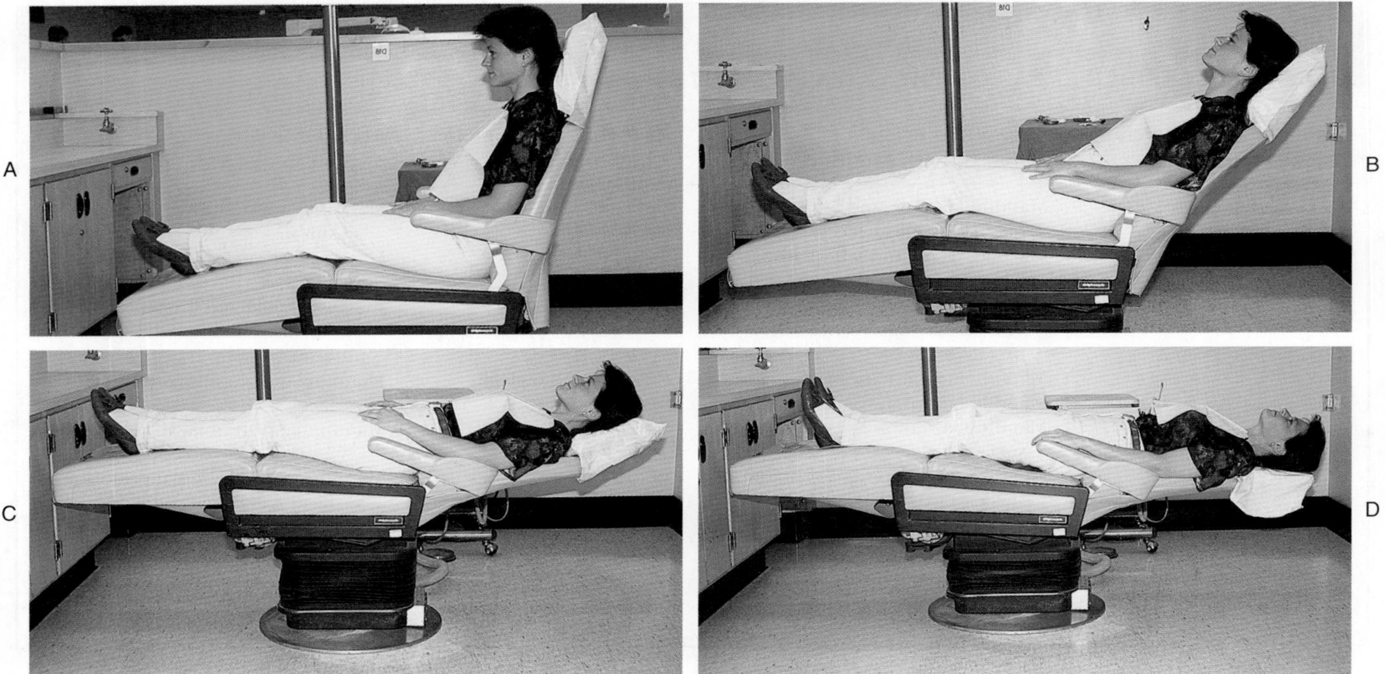

FIGURE 8–9 ✦ Basic client body positions used during the dental hygiene process of care. **A,** Basic upright position; client is seated in an 80-degree to 90-degree angle. **B,** Semi-upright position; client is seated in a 45-degree angle. **C,** Supine position that has been modified for mandibular instrumentation. **D,** Supine position that has been modified for maxillary insertion.

TABLE 8–7 CORRECT CLINICIAN POSITIONING

Feet/Legs/Thighs Position	Body Weight	Arms and Shoulder Position	Back Position	Head Position	Eyes
Feet flat on the floor	Centered on the seat of the clinician's stool	Shoulders are relaxed and inthe neutral position (parallel to the floor)	Back is straight	Aligned with the spine (sit tall in the clinician's stool)	Directed downward
Thighs parallel with the floor	Supported by the legs and thighs	Upper arms are relaxed	Lumbar curve is supported	Head is erect	Distance from eyes to client's oral cavity is approximately 14–16 inches
		Elbows are in the neutral position (close to the body)			

ERGONOMIC INSTRUMENT HANDLES.[3] Ergonomically designed instrument handles are larger in diameter and lighter in weight. Table 8–8 and Figure 8–10 compare instruments with standard handles and ergonomically designed handles. The function of the larger-diameter handles is to open the grasp just enough to dissipate the mechanical forces over a larger area of muscles. Instrument set-ups containing several styles of handles give the clinician the opportunity to rest different muscle groups while completing care. Alternating the use of different hand muscle groups decreases the occurrence of RSI.

BALANCED INSTRUMENTS. Instruments, both single- and double-ended, should be balanced. This means that the working end is centered over the long axis of the instrument handle. When the instrument is balanced, the lateral pressure placed on the instrument handle and shank during instrument activation will be aimed toward the working end (Figure 8–11). When an instrument is not balanced, the lateral pressure placed on the instrument when activated causes the instrument to turn slightly in the clinician's fingers. To compensate, the clinician will grasp the instrument handle tighter. Utilization of balanced instruments decreases the occurrence of RSI.

MECHANIZED INSTRUMENTS. Use of ultrasonic and sonic instruments reduces repetitive hand instrumentation motions to a great extent. Oral debridement procedures take numerous repetitive strokes and significant

TABLE 8–8 ERGONOMIC AND STANDARD INSTRUMENT HANDLES

Parameters	Ergonomic Design	Standard Design
Diameter (inches)	3/8″–7/16″	1/4″
Diameter (mm)	9.53 to 11.11	6.35
Shape	Round or hexagonal	Round or hexagonal
Construction	Hollow	Solid
Weight	Approx. 13.2 grams	Approx. 26.0 grams

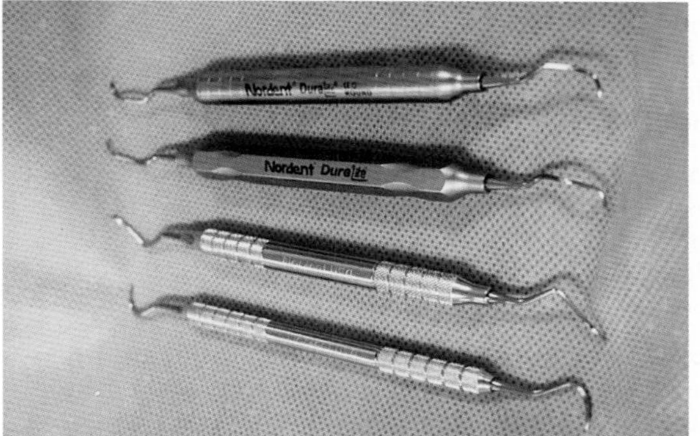

FIGURE 8–10 ✦ Variety of instrument handles. *(Courtesy Nordent.)*

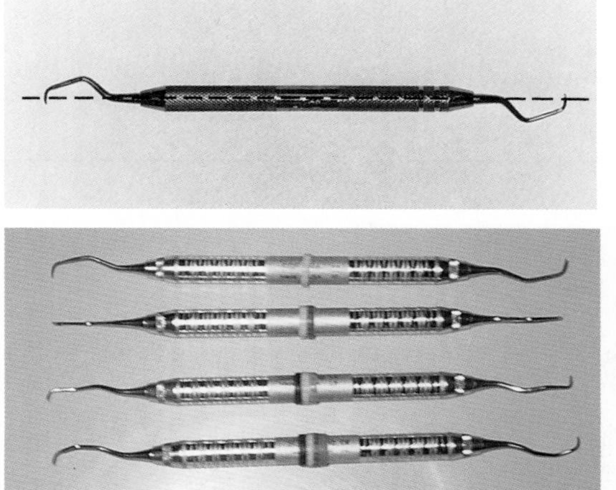

FIGURE 8–11 ✦ Balanced instrument. Note that when the working end is centered over the long axis of the handle, the instrument is balanced.

lateral pressure when using hand instrumentation techniques (see Chapter 23, section on mechanized instruments).

VIBRATING INSTRUMENTS.[1] Instruments causing vibrations, such as the motor-driven handpiece, cause fatigue and hand, arm, and shoulder muscle strain. Application of the principles of selective polishing limits the time the clinician uses an instrument that causes vibrations. A common RSI caused by vibratory instruments is Raynaud's syndrome, which results in blanching (often painful) fingers.

TABLE 8–9 STRENGTHENING EXERCISES

Strengthening Exercise	Improvements to the Body
Pelvic tilt	Lumbar spine
Hyperextension	Lumbar spine
Knee-to-chest	Lumbar spine
Sit-ups	Abdominal muscles and lumbar spine
Suspend from a bar	Lower back
Doorway stretch	Upper and lower back
Neck isometric	Cervical spine and neck
Rubber ball squeeze	Hand and fingers

PHYSICAL EXERCISE[6]

Strengthening Exercises

No one would consider working out in a gym or performing any kind of a strenuous activity without stretching and doing strengthening maneuvers first. However, oral care providers subject their bodies and muscles to strenuous activity every day without properly preparing their bodies for the workplace. Maintaining a healthy musculoskeletal system through daily exercise increases the professional's ability to work. Regular exercise:

- Improves strength and flexibility
- Improves lumbar spine, neck muscle, and lower back health
- Stretches and extends back muscles
- Strengthens abdominal muscles
- Strengthens finger, hand, and arm muscles

Strengthening exercises can be performed regularly to repair and maintain a healthy musculoskeletal system (Table 8–9 and Strengthening Exercises).

Chairside Stretching Exercises[6]

Stretching and warm-up exercises reduce muscle and joint soreness and injury. Warm-ups can also prepare the individual psychologically for activities involving skill and dexterity. It is recommended that the care provider stretch before work and periodically throughout the day by performing *tendon gliding exercises (TGE)* (Figure 8–12, *A* to *E*), that assist in the diffusion of *synovial fluid,* the lubricating fluid around the tendons in the hand and fingers:

- Hand and fingers are held straight, pointing upward
- Fingers are bent into a 90-degree angle from the hand
- Fingers are then closed into the hand
- Hand is arched back toward the top of the wrist
- Fingers are then further arched in the same direction
- Hold briefly and release
- Repeat four times

Strengthening Exercises

Pelvic tilt: Strengthen the lumbar spine
Lie on your back
Knees must be bent
Flatten and press the back into the floor
Hold briefly
Repeat

Hyperextension: Safeguard the lumbar curve
Lie on your stomach
Arch the body backward, in an upward direction
Hold briefly
Repeat

Knee-to-Chest: Stretch the lumbar spine
Lie on your back
Bring both knees to your chest
Hold briefly
Return to original position; avoid straightening the legs
Repeat

Sit-Ups: Strengthen the abdominal muscles
Lie on your back
Bend the knees
Support the neck
Gently raise the shoulders toward the knees
Hold briefly and return
Repeat

Suspend from a Bar: Relieve lower back pain
Firmly grasp the bar
Suspend your body from the bar; lift the feet slowly
Hold for a short time
Repeat

Doorway Stretch: Reverse poor posture
Stand in front of an open doorway
Place hands on either side of the doorframe
Gently allow your body to lean forward through the doorway
Hold briefly and return
Repeat

Neck Isometric: Stretch the cervical spine and relieve neck muscle strain
Grasp hands behind the head
Gently press your head back
Do not allow any backward movement
Hold briefly
Repeat

Rubber Ball Squeeze: Strengthen hand and finger muscles
Grasp a rubber ball firmly in your hand
Gently squeeze
Hold briefly
Repeat

Rubber Band Stretch: Strengthen hand and finger muscles
Extend a rubber band between the fingers of the hand
Gently stretch the rubber band until you feel resistance
Hold briefly
Release the rubber band
Repeat

A
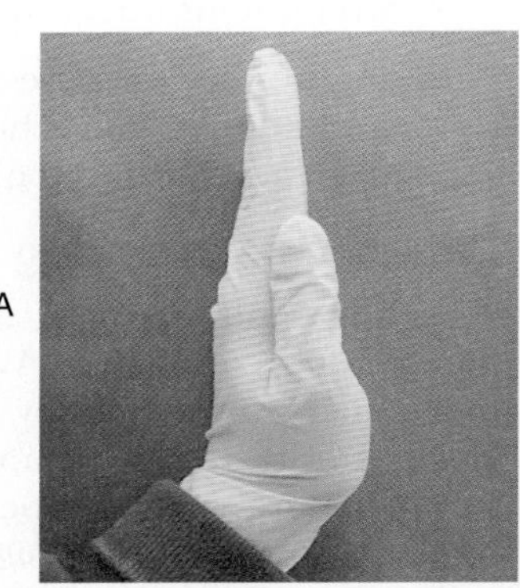

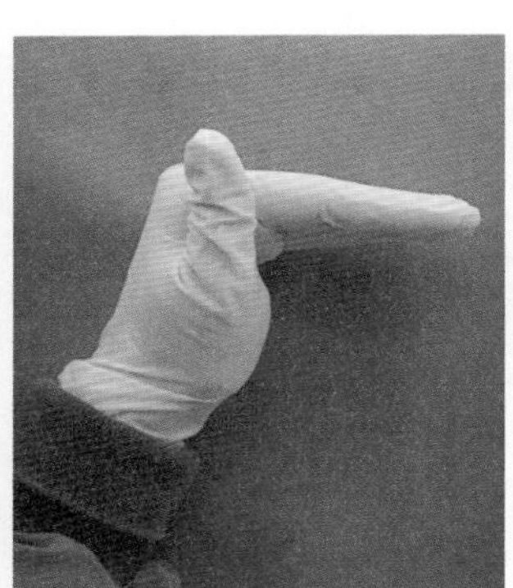
B

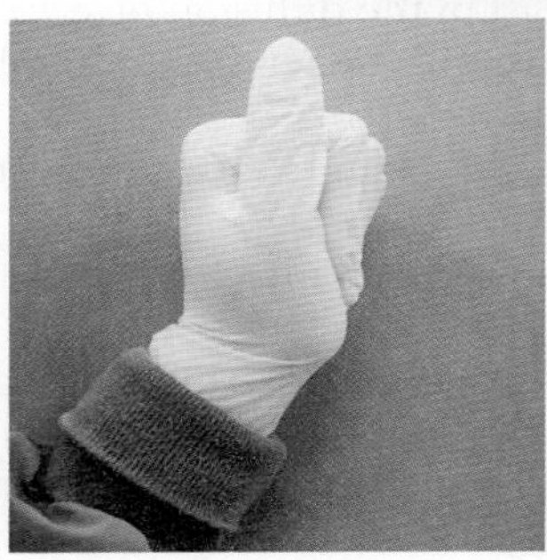
C

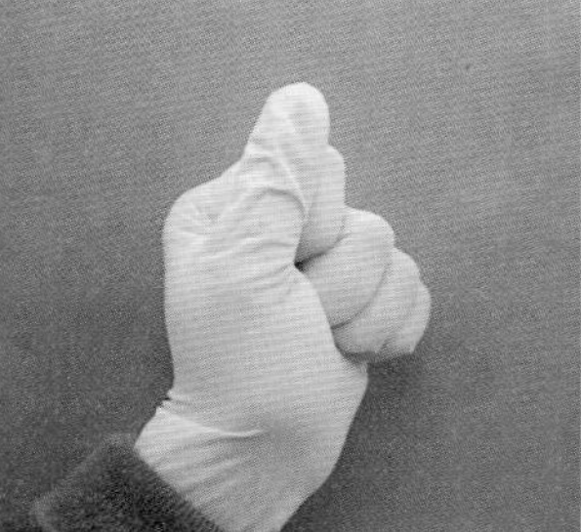
D

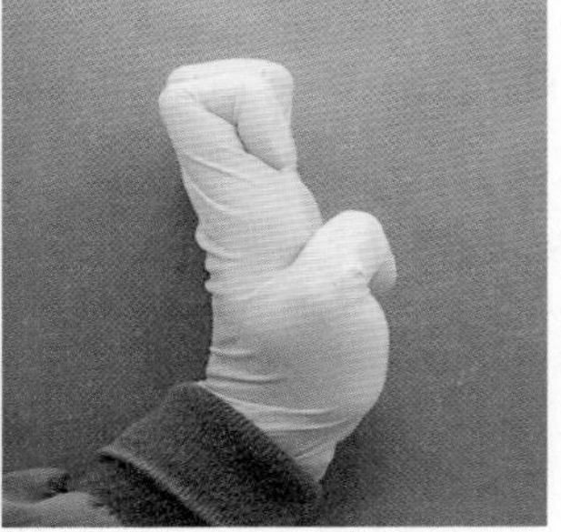
E

FIGURE 8–12 ✦ Tendon gliding exercises.

REPETITIVE STRAIN INJURIES (Table 8–10)

Hand, Wrist, and Finger Injuries

CARPAL TUNNEL SYNDROME.[2,4,7,8] *Carpal tunnel syndrome (CTS),* the most common RSI reported by dental hygienists, is:

- ✦ **Congenital:** Anatomic structure and development
- ✦ **Self-limiting:** Pregnancy
- ✦ **Systemic conditions:** Edema or arthritis
- ✦ **Nonmedical reasons:** Occupational or work-related

About 19 to 33% of dental hygienists report symptoms of CTS. CTS occurs when the median nerve becomes compressed within the carpal tunnel (Figure 8–13). The function of the median nerve is sensory and motor; it supplies sensation to the thumb, index finger, middle finger, and half of the ring finger. The nerve also supplies a branch to the muscles of the thumb called the thenar muscles.

The carpal bones of the wrist and the transverse carpal ligament form the carpal tunnel. The carpal bones and transverse carpal tunnel ligament form a furrow allowing the flexor tendons and the median nerve to pass through to the hand. Repetitive force and motion to the wrist cause inflammation and swelling of the tendons within the carpal tunnel. The enlarged tendons place undue pressure on the median nerve due to the swelling of the tendons and lack of space in the carpal tunnel. The pressure on the median nerve causes pain. Once the nerve is compressed, CTS begins. Repeated wrist flexion and hyperextension during instrumentation aggravate the tendons and cause swelling.

Symptoms. The earliest sign of CTS is numbness in the areas supplied by the median nerve. Additional signs and symptoms include:

- ✦ Pain in the hand, wrist, shoulder, neck, lower back
- ✦ Nocturnal pain in the hand(s) and forearm(s)
- ✦ Pain in the hand(s) while working
- ✦ Morning stiffness and numbness
- ✦ Daytime stiffness and numbness
- ✦ Loss of strength in hand(s); weakened grasp
- ✦ Cold fingers
- ✦ Increased fatigue in fingers, hand, wrist, forearm, shoulders
- ✦ Nerve dysfunction

Risk Factors. Repetition is the foremost risk factor causing CTS. Force, using vibrating instruments, mechanical stress, and cold temperatures can also initiate CTS. Holding the instruments tightly places additional force on the wrist and hand. Vibrating instruments, including slow-speed handpieces and ultrasonic scalers, have been identified as an independent risk factor for CTS.[2] Cold temperatures in the dental operatory decrease the flexibility of the clinician's finger, hand, arm, shoulder, neck, and back muscles. This inflexibility causes stiffness, making workplace performance stressful. Also, wearing gloves that are too tight can pinch the median nerve at the wrist.

TABLE 8–10 EFFECTS OF REPETITIVE STRAIN INJURIES

Common RSIs in Dental Hygiene	Area of the Body Affected
Carpal tunnel syndrome	Wrist, forearm, hand, fingers (index, middle, and 1/2 of ring fingers and thumb)
Thoracic outlet compression	Shoulder, arm, hand
Surgical glove–induced injury	Hand, fingers, wrist
Guyon's canal syndrome	Lower arm, wrist, fingers (1/2 of ring finger and little finger)
Strained pronator muscle	Elbow
Trigger finger nerve syndrome	Tendons in the fingers
De Quervain's syndrome	Base of the thumb
Tension neck syndrome	Neck, between shoulder blades, arm
Cervical spondylolysis	Neck, scapula and shoulders
Cervical disc disease	Neck and arm
Trapezius myalgia	Shoulders
Rotator cuff tendonitis	Shoulders
Rotator cuff tears	Shoulders
Adhesive capsulitis	Shoulders
Lumbar joint dysfunction	Spine
Lateral epicondylitis	Elbow and forearm
Radial tunnel syndrome	Elbow and forearm
Cubital tunnel syndrome	Elbow and forearm

Chairside Preventive Measures

- ✦ Maintain good operator posture: the client's mouth should be even with the clinician's elbow; the elbow should be held in the neutral position (90-degree angle created by the upper arm and forearm).
- ✦ Maintain proper position to support the clinician's body, thighs parallel to the floor and feet flat on the floor
- ✦ Neutral forearm and wrist position: avoid pinching the median nerve in the carpal tunnel
- ✦ Keep shoulders relaxed
- ✦ Use a unified motion (wrist, hand, forearm) during scaling and polishing; avoid flexion and extension of the wrist
- ✦ Avoid extremes in temperatures
- ✦ Avoid or limit exposure to vibrating instruments
- ✦ Avoid forceful pinching and gripping of instrument handles
- ✦ Wear properly fitting gloves
- ✦ Alternate clinician positions
- ✦ Perform tendon gliding exercises

Assessing Symptoms. CTS affects the median nerve, which supplies the thumb, index, middle, and half of the ring finger. If the symptoms are felt in the little finger and right half of the ring finger, CTS may not be the problem or the operator maybe suffering from CTS along with

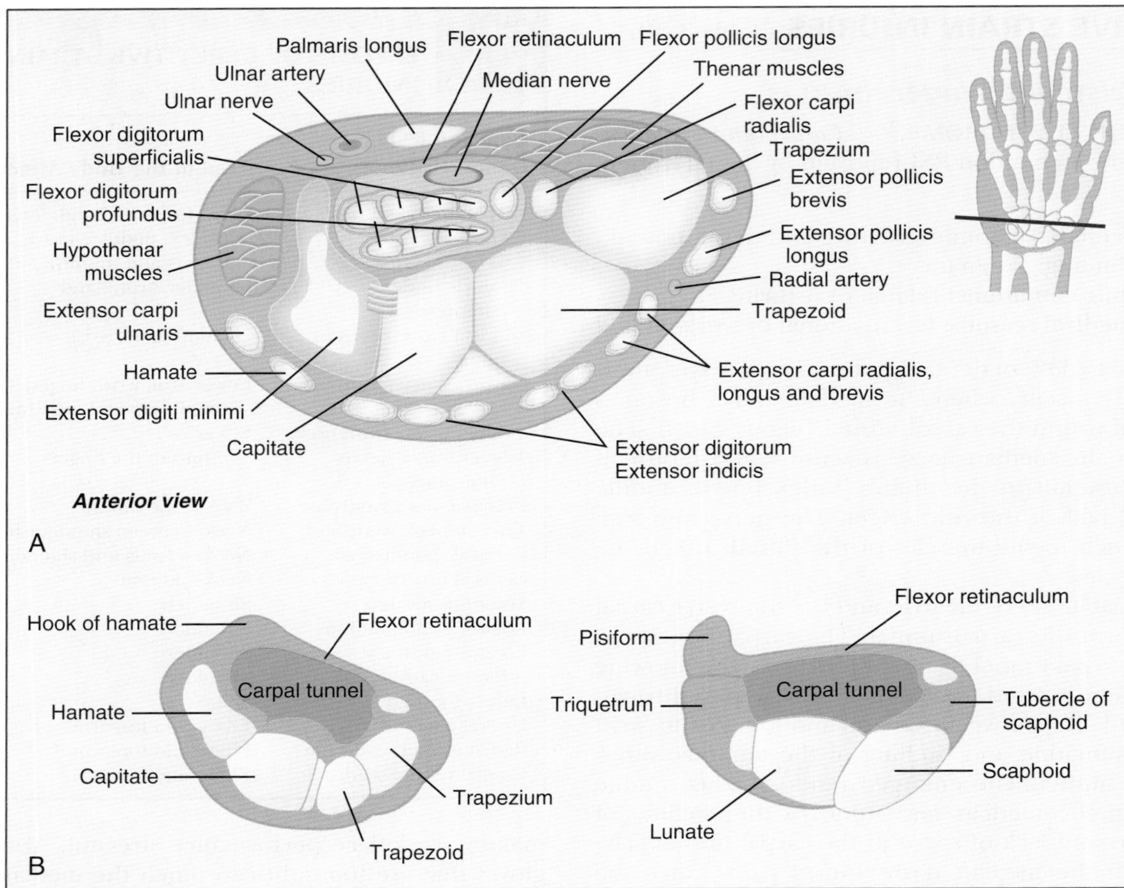

FIGURE 8–13 ✦ Carpal bones. The carpal bones form a trough through which the flexor tendons and median nerve traverse into the hand. **A,** Transverse section of the wrist and carpal tunnel. **B,** Diagram of transverse section through the carpal tunnel. *(Redrawn from Agur A:* Grant's atlas of anatomy, *ed 9, Baltimore, 1991, Williams & Wilkins.)*

another RSI. Two simple tests can be performed to indicate symptoms of CTS:[6]

- To perform *Phalen's test,* place the back of the hands against each other. Hold flexed wrists together at a 90-degree angle for one minute. Subjective sensory changes will be felt within one minute. These sensory changes indicate a positive test (Figure 8–14, *A*).
- *Tinel's sign* entails tapping of the median nerve at the ventral side of the wrist. If nerve compression is present, sensation is felt in the fingers. The sensation could range from a tingling feeling to an electrical type shooting pain (Figure 8–14, *B*).

Treatment. Conservative treatment includes corticosteroid injections to reduce inflammation of the tendons. *Iontophoresis,* an electrical current delivery system of corticosteroid, can also be utilized. The electrical current produces penetration of the corticosteroid through the skin into the carpal tunnel. This method is less painful, but not as effective as the injection of corticosteroid. CTS can also be treated with anti-inflammatory medications and vitamins (see Common Drug Therapies for CTS).

Common Drug Therapies for CTS

Antiinflammatory Drugs

Naproxen sodium 550 mg tablets
Prednisone 10 mg tablets
Motrin 800 mg tablets
Naprosyn 500 mg tablets
Aspirin 5 gr (325 mg) tablets
Indocin 50 mg capsules
Celebrex 200 mg capsules
Vioxx 25 mg tablets

Vitamins

B6

Wearing a wrist brace during the early stages of CTS helps to decrease symptoms by minimizing inflammation. The wrist is simply kept in the neutral position by the brace holding the carpal tunnel in the most open position, which allows the nerves and tendons to relax and heal.

Surgical treatment may be performed if conservative therapies fail. In surgery, the transverse carpal ligament is cut to relieve pressure on the median nerve. New surgical procedures for CTS use an endoscope or small

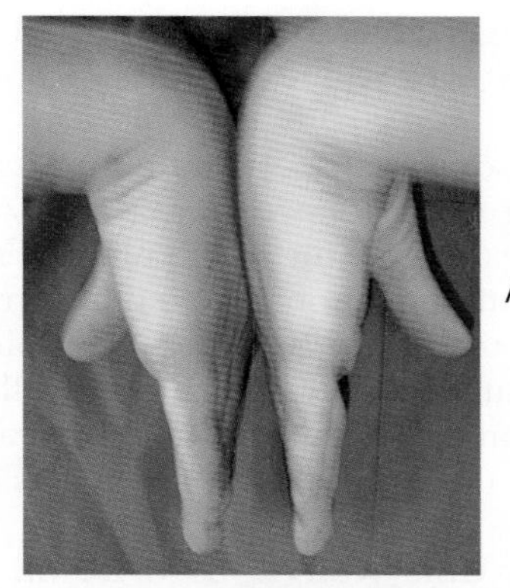

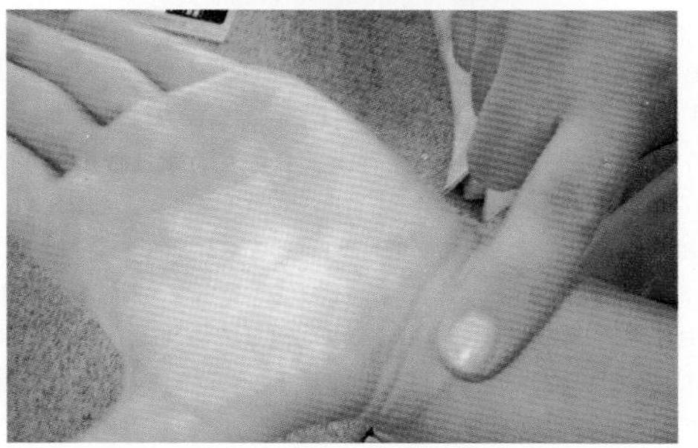

FIGURE 8–14 ✦ **A,** Phalen's test. **B,** Tinel's sign.

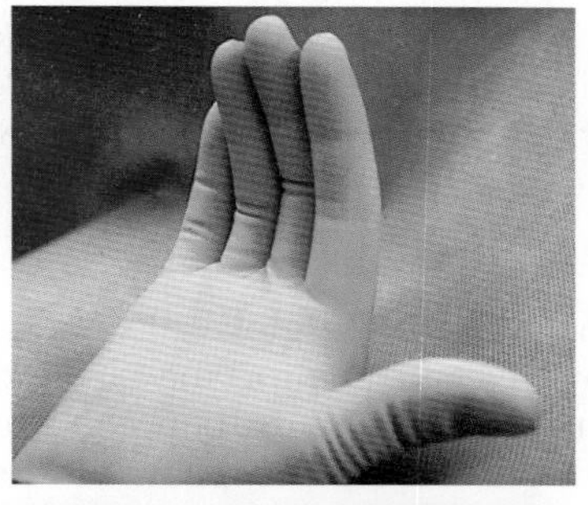

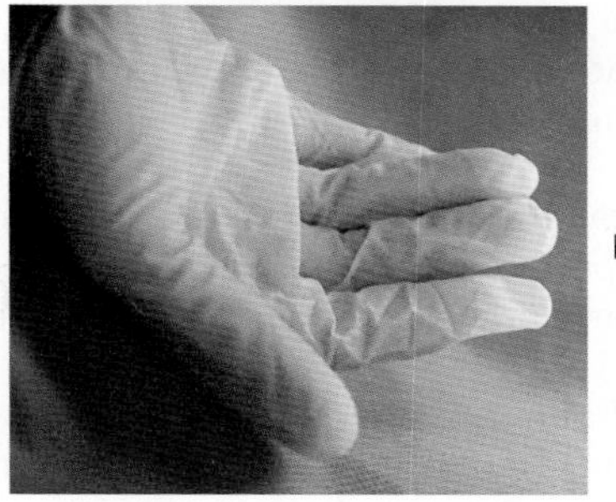

FIGURE 8–15 ✦ **A,** Glove is too tight. **B,** Glove is too loose.

fiber-optic camera and a procedure similar to the traditional surgery except that no incision is made in the palm. Rather, a small incision is made in the wrist. Healing time is decreased with the smaller incision.

THORACIC OUTLET COMPRESSION.[9] *Thoracic outlet compression (TOC)* is an RSI resulting in compression of the brachial artery and plexus nerve trunk at the thoracic outlet. TOC affects the hand, wrist, arm, and shoulder. Compression of the neurovascular bundle (brachial plexus, subclavian artery, and subclavian vein) results in decreased blood flow to the nerve functions of the arm. The compression occurs at the neck where the scalene muscles create an outlet or tunnel. The nerves and blood vessels run from the neck into the arm and hand.

Symptoms

- Numbness and tingling along the side of the arms and hands
- Neck and shoulder muscle spasms
- Weakness and clumsiness in the hand and fingers
- Coldness of the extremities
- Absence of radial pulse

Risk Factors. Poor posture is the main cause. Tilting of the head too much, hunching of the shoulders, and positioning the dental chair too high are all risk factors for TOC.

Chairside Preventive Measures

- Maintain proper clinician positions: head erect, back straight, shoulders in the neutral position
- Proper height of the dental chair and client positioning

Assessing Symptoms. Signs relate to both decreased motor function (nerve compression) and arterial symptoms (decreased blood flow).

Treatment. Initially, physical therapy, strengthening of the posterior trunk and shoulder muscles, and posture retraining exercises are recommended. If the recommended treatment fails, surgery may be required. The surgical procedure is directed at reducing the source of compression. Scar tissue or, in some cases, a congenital extra rib may be the cause of compression. An incision is made under the arm where the nerves and brachial plexus are located.

SURGICAL GLOVE INJURY.[1,3,10] Ill-fitting gloves can contribute to surgical glove injury (SGI). The glove should fit the hand and fingers snuggly but be neither too tight nor too loose from fingers to forearm (Figure 8–15, *A* and *B*).

Symptoms. SGI is commonly mistaken for CTS and TOC because so many of the symptoms are similar:

- Tingling in the fingers
- Cold extremities
- Loss of muscle control and hand strength
- Numbness or pain in fingers

Risk Factors. Wearing properly fitting gloves during dental care reduces RSI. When gloves are too tight, proper circulation to the clinician's hands and fingers is compromised. The wrist is also at risk if additional pressure is placed on the carpal tunnel by a glove that is too tight across the wrist. Wearing gloves that are too loose will cause the clinician to grasp the instrument handle tighter to compensate for the feeling of lack of control. Excess glove material at the fingertips hinders the clinician's ability to adequately roll the instrument in the fingers to adapt around line angles. The clinician will compensate by twisting the wrist or by flexing and hyperextending the wrist.

Chairside Preventive Measures

- Wear properly fitting gloves. Evaluate if the glove fits properly and comfortably around the fingertips, between the fingers, between the thumb and index finger, across the palm of the hand, and around the wrist.
- Do tendon gliding exercises and stretch the hand and fingers.

Assessing Symptoms. Gloves that do not fit properly cause SGI. If symptoms arrest when gloves are taken off or when different gloves are worn, SGI maybe determined.[1]

Treatment of Surgical Glove Injury. Simply wearing properly fitting gloves may be the only treatment necessary. If pressure to the wrist and compression of the median nerve in the carpal tunnel continue, treatment as seen in CTS cases may be necessary.

GUYON'S CANAL SYNDROME.[3,11] *Guyon's canal syndrome (GCS)* is caused by ulnar nerve entrapment at the wrist.[12,13] This syndrome differs from CTS in that the ulnar nerve does not pass through the carpal tunnel. The ulnar nerve passes through a tunnel formed by the pisiform and hamate bones and the ligaments that connect them.

Symptoms

- Numbness and tingling in the little finger and the right side of the ring finger
- Loss of strength in the lower forearm
- Loss of movement of the small muscles in the hand
- Clumsiness of the hand

Risk Factors. During instrumentation it is important to hold the little finger close to the fulcrum finger for stability and control. Maintaining this position of the two fingers avoids RSI. Holding the little finger a full span away from the hand and fulcrum finger causes nerve entrapment and symptoms of GCS.

Chairside Preventive Measures. Attention placed on hand and finger position during instrumentation reduces GCS and includes:

- Repositioning of the little finger while scaling and polishing
- Periodic hand stretches

Assessing Symptoms. During instrument adaptation and activation, symptoms will affect the little finger and half of the ring finger. If all digits are affected, GCS may not be problem or may be one of several problems.

Treatment. Conservative treatment includes hand strengthening exercises; wearing a hand/wrist splint at night to decrease pinching of the ulnar nerve, allowing a decrease in inflammation; and taking prescribed anti-inflammatory medications. If these therapies fail, surgery may be indicated. Surgical treatment will relieve ulnar nerve entrapment. During the surgical procedure, cutting of the roof of the Guyon's canal is completed.

TRIGGER FINGER NERVE SYNDROME.[3,14,15] Trigger finger nerve syndrome (TFNS or triggering) affects the movement of the tendons as the fingers and thumb *(flexion)* are bent and moved. The tendons are held in place on the bones by a series of ligaments called pulleys. Friction is reduced by a slippery coating called tenosynovium, allowing the tendons to glide easily through the tendon sheaths. When the tendons and tendon sheaths are inflamed and tenosynovium thickens, a nodule forms from the constant irritation of the tendon being pulled through the pulley. As the finger is flexed, the nodule passes under the ligament and becomes stuck. The finger cannot be extended back to its original position.

Symptoms. Inability to extend the fingers or thumb after they are flexed.

Risk Factors. Repetitive use of the fingers and hands causes overuse of the tendons in the fingers and thumb. Overuse often results from the fingers and thumb being flexed against resistance. Digital motion during instrumentation results in overuse of the finger and thumb tendons. Also, pinching the instrument handle causes the fingers and thumb to be flexed against resistance (Figure 8–16).

Chairside Preventive Measures. Minimizing finger motion and utilization of proper grasp, fulcrum, and unified motion of the hand, wrist, and forearm decrease the chance of TFNS.

- Maintain the appropriate modified pen grasp for the procedure.

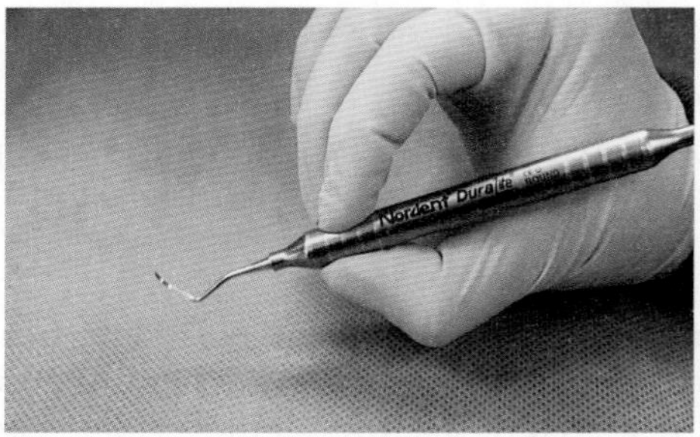

FIGURE 8–16 ✦ Pinched fingers on the instrument handle.

- ✦ Grasp the instrument handle using the pads of the fingers and thumb instead of pinching with the tips of the fingers.

Assessing Symptoms. When a nodule forms on the tendons of the fingers or thumb, a palpable click will be felt as the nodule snaps under the finger pulley.

Treatment. Initial treatment with corticosteroids may reduce the inflammation and shrink the nodule to relieve the triggering. In most cases, surgery is needed. A small incision is made in the palm of the hand to locate the pulley in question. Once the pulley is located, it is cut, eliminating the triggering and nodule involvement.

DE QUERVAIN'S SYNDROME.[3,12] *De Quervain's syndrome* is an inflammation of the tendons and tendon sheaths at the base of the thumb or the "anatomic snuff box." This condition occurs from repetitive motion combining hand twisting and forceful gripping along with prolonged work with the wrist held in ulnar deviation (Figure 8–17). Symptoms will occur when the pollicis longus and extensor pollicis longus tendons are unable to glide through the tunnel on the side of the wrist.

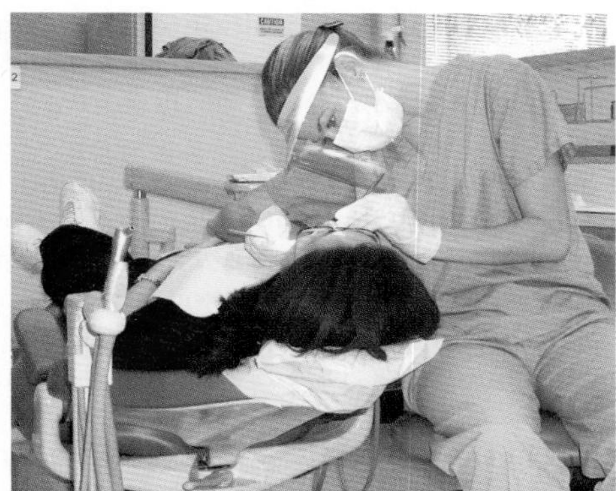

FIGURE 8–17 ✦ Wrist in ulnar deviation. *(Courtesy Sarah Talamantes Carter, University of California at San Francisco.)*

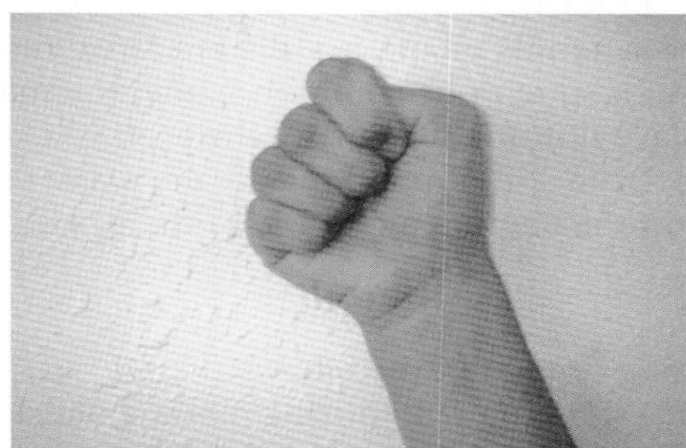

FIGURE 8–18 ✦ Finkelstein's test.

Symptoms

- ✦ Aching and weakness of the thumb (along the base)
- ✦ Pain migrating into the forearm.

Risk Factors. Repetitive ulnar deviation of the wrist while reaching for instruments or during instrumentation is the biggest risk factor causing De Quervain's syndrome. Twisting and bending the wrist in an ulnar direction (toward the little finger) and using a forceful grip on the instrument handle are also contributing risk factors.

Chairside Preventive Measures

- ✦ Avoid ulnar wrist deviation during instrumentation.
- ✦ Eliminate twisting of the wrist when reaching for dental instruments.
- ✦ Maintain a neutral wrist position and unified motion during dental care procedures.

Assessing Symptoms. *Finkelstein's test* is a simple way to assess symptoms[12] (Figure 8–18). This is accomplished by bending the thumb into the palm of the hand. Grasp the thumb with the four fingers. Place the wrist in the ulnar deviation position by bending the wrist toward the little finger. Pain over the tendons and tendon sheaths at the base of the thumb indicates possible De Quervain's syndrome.

Treatment. Milder cases may simply require rest, prescribed anti-inflammatory medication, immobilization of the wrist, a wrist splint, or ergonomic adjustments to the work environment. If the simple measures fail, corticosteroid injections and progressive physical and occupational therapy may be recommended. In severe or chronic cases, surgery may be in order. The surgical procedure involves relieving pressure on the tendon, allowing more space for that tendon.

Elbow and Forearm Injuries[1,13,16]

STRAINED PRONATOR MUSCLE (SPM). The muscle involved in SPM is an elongated, narrow pronator muscle in the forearm and flexor of the elbow joint. SPM is caused by compression of the median nerve as it passes under the pronator muscle. The pronator muscle wraps around the anterior aspect of the elbow.

Symptoms. Compression of the median nerve occurs, causing symptoms similar to those experienced by clinicians suffering with CTS.

Risk Factors. Repetitive and constant holding of the arms away from the body with the palm and thumb-side of the hand rotated downward during instrumentation is a risk factor. This position commonly occurs during instrumentation of the maxillary right posterior sextant. With the palm in a downward position, the clinician's arm must rotate and twist. Hyperextension of the wrist also occurs (Figure 8–7, *B*).

Chairside Preventive Measures

- ✦ Maintain neutral arm position: hold the arms close to the body

- Maintain neutral wrist position during dental care procedures
- Avoid rotation and twisting of the forearm

Assessing Symptoms. Since symptoms are similar to those of CTS, performing Phalen's and Tinel's test would rule out compression of the median nerve at the wrist (true CTS) because with this condition, compression occurs at the elbow. If the clinician is suffering from CTS symptoms but rules out true CTS, SPM maybe the cause.

Treatment. Therapy includes rest, anti-inflammatory medication, corticosteroid injections, environmental changes in the workplace, and repositioning of the clinician's body during instrumentation.

LATERAL EPICONDYLITIS.[1,17] *Lateral epicondylitis (LE),* also know as tennis elbow, is a degenerative disorder of the elbow. In spite of its common name, the majority of the cases are not due to sports injuries. It is a condition resulting from inflammation of the wrist extensor tendons on the lateral epicondyle of the elbow.

Symptoms

- Aching or pain in the elbow
- Sharp shooting pain during elbow extension

Risk Factors. Repetitive and constant use of a forceful grip or grasp, forceful wrist and elbow movement, and extension of the wrist during dental care procedures increase the risk of LE.

Chairside Preventive Measures

- Avoid wrist extension during dental care procedures
- Maintain proper neutral wrist position during instrumentation
- Utilize proper clinician positions, allowing neutral body positions to be maintained

Assessing Symptoms. The diagnosis of LE can be made with a physical examination. The examination includes palpation of the wrist extensor muscles at the lateral epicondyle of the elbow during resisted wrist extension. Pain during this exercise may indicate LE.

Treatment. Therapy includes rest, the use of anti-inflammatory medications, alterations in the work environment, a wrist splint to eliminate wrist extension, physical therapy, and corticosteroid injections.

RADIAL TUNNEL SYNDROME.[1,18] *Radial tunnel syndrome (RTS)* is a condition affecting the radial nerve as it is entrapped in the radial tunnel. The radial nerve allows the hand to be turned in a clockwise direction. The radial nerve starts at the side of the neck and travels through the armpit and down the arm to the hands and fingers. The radial nerve passes in front of the elbow through the radial tunnel.

Symptoms. Increased tenderness and pain at the lateral side of the elbow when the arm and elbow are being used may indicate RTS.

Chairside Preventive Measures. As with LE, maintaining proper wrist position and motion during care must be considered.

Assessing Symptoms. Unfortunately, RTS is often mistaken for LE. A history must be completed and assessed by the physician. Electrical tests should also be performed on the radial nerve.

Treatment. Therapy includes rest, anti-inflammatory medications, and possible surgery to relieve tension and pressure on the radial nerve. A small incision is made on the outside of the elbow near the area where the radial nerve travels into the forearm.

CUBITAL TUNNEL SYNDROME.[1,18] *Cubital tunnel syndrome* is a condition affecting the ulnar nerve as it crosses behind the elbow. As discussed earlier, the ulnar nerve controls the muscles in the right half of the ring finger and little finger of the hand. The ulnar nerve starts at the neck and runs through the armpit and down the arm to the hand and fingers. At the elbow the nerve crosses through a tunnel of muscle, ligament, and bone called the cubital tunnel. When the elbow is bent, the nerve is pulled up between bones, causing compression and entrapment of the ulnar nerve. When nerve compression occurs, impulses are slowed.

Symptoms

- Pain and numbness in the outer side of the ring finger and little finger
- Pain sometimes relieved when the elbow is straightened

Risk Factors. The clinician should avoid all prolonged gripping or grasping of instruments in the palm of the hand and holding the elbow in a flexed position during procedures.

Chairside Preventive Measures

- Maintain a neutral elbow position during procedures
- Alter instrument grasps; avoid prolonged use of palm grasp
- Avoid repetitive crossing of arms across the chest
- Avoid leaning on the elbow when sitting at a table

Assessing Symptoms. A simple test to assess if the pain and numbness in the fourth and fifth finger are being caused by ulnar nerve compression in the elbow is to simply straighten the elbow. Pain or numbness will usually disappear when the elbow is straight.

Treatment. Therapy consists of physical and occupational therapy, anti-inflammatory medications, and the use of an elbow extension splint. If the prescribed treatment fails, surgery may be required. The surgical procedure creates a new cubital tunnel for the ulnar nerve.

Shoulder Injuries[1,5]

TRAPEZIUS MYALGIA.[3,11,16] *Trapezius myalgia (TM)* is caused by static loading in the shoulder or stabilizing muscles over a long period of time. This condition is commonly found in workers in repetitive action occupations.

Symptoms. Pain and tenderness in the descending part of the trapezius muscle may indicate TM.

Risk Factors. Long dental procedures cause the clinician to remain in one position for too long. These periods of time cause static loading on muscles of the body, which are supporting the clinician's body weight.

Chairside Preventive Measures

- ✦ Manage appointment times: alternate long and short appointments
- ✦ Take stretching breaks during long procedures
- ✦ Change body positions
- ✦ Maintain proper clinician positions to ensure proper body support

Assessing Symptoms. Consistent pain and tenderness in the area of the trapezius muscle may indicate TM.

Treatment. Therapy consists of rest, physical therapy, massage, stretching exercises, and heat/ice regimens.

ROTATOR CUFF INJURIES. Rotator cuff injuries (RCI) include rotator cuff tendonitis and rotator cuff tears. Both affect the connective tissue in the shoulder and both are common causes for pain in the shoulder. The tendon most often affected is the supraspinatus tendon. Rotator cuff injuries are associated with repetitive motion and excessive, forceful exertion of the shoulder and arm.

Symptoms

- ✦ Pain when lifting the arm 60 to 90 degrees
- ✦ Functional impairment

Risk Factors. Static loading on the shoulder muscles and improper body support will lead to rotator cuff injuries.

Chairside Preventive Measures

- ✦ Avoid repetitive twisting and reaching for dental instruments
- ✦ Maintain neutral shoulder and arm positions
- ✦ Utilize proper clinician positions during dental care procedures

Assessing Symptoms. Constant pain in the shoulders and increased pain when raising the arms may indicate rotator cuff injuries. An MRI and further medical testing are frequently needed for accurate diagnosis.

Treatment. Therapy depends on the degree of injury. Once tears in the tendons occur, the treatment becomes complex. Active rehabilitation partnered with corticosteroid injections and anti-inflammatory medications may be required. If conservative therapy fails, surgery may be performed.

ADHESIVE CAPSULITIS.[1,11,13] *Adhesive capsulitis (AC),* also known as f*rozen shoulder,* results from immobility of the shoulder due to severe injury to the shoulder or repeated occurrences of rotator cuff tendonitis.

Symptoms. Symptoms are similar to symptoms for RCIs:

- ✦ Pain in the shoulder
- ✦ Limited range of motion of the shoulder

Risk Factors. Static loading and improper strain placed on the shoulder joint due to static loading increase the risk for AC.

Chairside Preventive Measures

- ✦ Avoid repetitive twisting and reaching for dental instruments
- ✦ Maintain proper shoulder and arm positions: neutral positions during dental care procedures
- ✦ Utilize proper clinician positions and movement during instrumentation

Assessing Symptoms. Limited range of motion and constant pain in the shoulder during lifting of the arms along with a history of rotator cuff tendonitis may indicate AC.

Treatment. Therapy includes physical therapy and rehabilitation, anti-inflammatory drug therapy, electrical stimulation, and heat/ice regimens. If therapy fails, a noninvasive treatment of forced shoulder movement may be required with the use of a general anesthetic.

Neck and Back Injuries

LUMBAR JOINT DYSFUNCTION.[3,11] *Lumbar joint dysfunction (LJD)* occurs from repetitive and continued twisting and rotating of the spine. When improper support of the clinician's spine is present during the performance of dental care, the intervertebral discs are put under tremendous pressure, possibly resulting in rupture or injury.

Symptoms. Discomfort and pain in the lumbar region of the spine may indicate LJD.

Risk Factors. Right-handed clinicians sitting in the 8 o'clock position (4 o'clock for left-handed clinicians) find accessing specific areas of the client's mouth easier. However, too much rotation of the midsection of the clinician's body while in this position will create strain on the lumbar curve. Care must be taken to avoid RSI while sitting in the 8 o'clock (4 o'clock) position.

Chairside Preventive Measures

- Avoid twisting the back and spine
- Properly support body weight
- Modify equipment placement to avoid twisting to reach dental instruments

Assessing Symptoms. Indications of LJD include constant lower back pain and limited movement of the back and spine.

Treatment. Therapy includes rest, workplace adjustments, physical therapy and occupational therapy, drug therapy, and possibly surgery.

TENSION NECK SYNDROME.[1] *Tension neck syndrome (TNS),* also called *tension myalgia,* involves the cervical muscles of the trapezius muscle.

Symptoms

- Pain or stiffness around the cervical spine in the neck
- Pain between the shoulder blades; pain may also radiate down the arms
- Muscle tightness and tenderness in the neck
- Palpable hardness in the neck
- Limited neck movement

Risk Factors. Risks include improper positioning of the clinician's head and neck during dental procedures. The head must be held erect. Bending the neck will result in a tremendous amount of pressure and stress on the cervical spine.

Chairside Preventive Measures

- Maintain proper clinician head and neck position to support neck and spine
- Maintain proper height of the dental chair and client position
- Support weight of the head properly over the entire spine, not just with the cervical portion of the spine
- Keep back straight during dental care procedures
- Periodic breaks and stretching exercises

Assessing Symptoms. If limited neck motion partnered with pain and discomfort are experienced, tension neck syndrome may be indicated.

Treatment. Treatment may include physical therapy, stretching exercises, and massage therapy. Ultrasonic and electrical muscle stimulation to increase blood flow may also be required.

CERVICAL SPONDYLOLYSIS AND CERVICAL DISC DISEASE.[1] *Cervical spondylolysis (CS)* and *cervical disc disease (CDD)* lead to degeneration of the cervical spine. These RSIs affect the neck, scapula, shoulders, and arms, causing osteoarthritis of the cervical spine and disc degeneration and herniation.

Symptoms

- Stiffness and limited motion of the neck
- Crepitus during active or passive movements of the neck
- Pain in the upper/middle cervical region of the spine
- Pain in the scapula of shoulder regions
- Muscle spasms

Risk Factors. Repeated stress and strain placed on the neck and cervical spine will result in RSI to these areas.

Chairside Preventive Measures

- Maintain proper clinician head and neck position during instrumentation to support neck and spine
- Properly seat clients for easy access to the mouth

Assessing Symptoms. Monitor the occurrence of pain during neck motion and crepitus in the cervical spine.

Treatment. Therapy includes posture retraining exercises to restore the normal curvature of the spine, strengthening exercises for the neck and back muscles, periods of rest, use of anti-inflammatory drugs, a cervical collar, and physical therapy.

CLIENT EDUCATION ISSUES

- Teach client that proper ergonomic positioning during appointments contributes to a successful therapeutic outcome.

LEGAL, ETHICAL, AND SAFETY ISSUES

- According to the professional code of ethics, dental hygienists have an ethical obligation to prevent disability and disease in themselves.
- Working while experiencing an untreated physical disability and pain may have ethical and legal implications if poor quality care is the outcome.

KEY CONCEPTS

- Using ergonomic principles in the workplace reduces the risk of RSI.
- Client positioning is dependent on the position of the clinician.
- Ergonomically designed equipment and proper positioning of both the clinician and client decrease the risk of RSI to the dental care provider.
- Fundamental grasp and hand stabilization during instrumentation reduce the occurrence of RSI to the clinician.
- Utilization of neutral wrist, arm, elbow, and shoulder positions will decrease the occurrence of RSI to the clinician.
- Instrument factors such as instrument maintenance, handle design, instrument manufacturing, and instrument choice affect the comfort and health of the clinician.
- Regular strengthening and stretching exercises increase the flexibility and strength of the body muscles and tendons, reducing the occurrence of RSI to the clinician.
- Knowledge of RSIs motivates practitioners to use ergonomic principles that prevent injury and long-term disability.
- Prevention of RSIs can be achieved if ergonomic principles are meticulously applied.
- If signs and symptoms of RSI occur, assessment of environment and workplace practices should be conducted and prompt medical attention must occur.

CRITICAL THINKING EXERCISES

Practice positioning a client in the dental chair. The clinician must be positioned for access and visibility to the client's mouth without compromising personal health and comfort.

1. Position the client in a semi-supine position. If no adjustments are made to the position of the clinician, what aspects of body dynamics are compromised? How can the clinician reposition and still follow ergonomic principles?
2. The client in the dental chair is a small child. If no adjustments are made to the position of the clinician, what aspects of body dynamics are compromised? How can the clinician reposition to follow ergonomic criteria? What alterations or adjustments can be made to the dental chair and/or position of the child in the dental chair so the clinician can follow ergonomic principles?
3. Place the client in the upright and Trendelenburg positions. When is the Trendelenburg position used?

For References, Suggested Readings, and Related Websites, visit
http://evolve.elsevier.com/Darby/hygiene/

SECTION 3

Dental Hygiene Assessments

CHAPTER 9

PERSONAL, DENTAL, AND HEALTH HISTORIES

OBJECTIVES

Mastery of the content in this chapter will enable the reader to:

- ✦ Systematically collect, analyze, and record information from a client's personal, dental, and health history
- ✦ Assess health status and risks, disease severity, and likelihood of a medical emergency via the health history interview
- ✦ Initiate appropriate referrals to minimize client health risks and practitioner's potential for litigation
- ✦ Recognize implications of client health status for dental hygiene care

KEY TERMS

ASA classification system
Back channeling
Chief complaint
Dental history
Dental hygienist–client relationship
Health history
Infective endocarditis (bacterial endocarditis)
Merck Manual of Diagnosis and Therapy
Open-ended questions
Personal history
Physicians' Desk Reference (PDR)
PDR Desk Reference Drug Interactions and Side Effects Index
PDR for Nonprescription Drugs
PDR for Herbal Medicine
Prophylactic antibiotic premedication
Total joint replacement
Vasopressor syncope

PURPOSE OF THE HEALTH HISTORY

A complete health history identifies a client's level of wellness (past and present) by collecting data about the physical, intellectual, emotional, and social dimensions of the client related to oral health and human needs (Figure 9–1). As the initial assessment phase of care, the history provides the foundation for all clinical decisions. Before dental hygiene procedures are implemented, a history is needed to determine the client's health status, contraindications to care, and necessity of a physician consultation. For example, periodontal instruments should not be used until the need for prophylactic antibiotic premeditation is determined. If a question occurs regarding the client's health status that cannot be answered by the dental hygienist or the dentist, then a physician consultation is mandatory prior to initiating care.

Dental hygiene care may complicate existing health conditions. Also, existing health conditions can influence the clinical outcomes, such as healing or oral disease progression. Because a client's health status is dynamic, the health history is updated at the beginning of each appointment. A health history wall plaque is available from the American Dental Association that reads "Please advise us of any changes in your medical history since your last visit." Posting the wall plaque in the reception area provides a gentle reminder of the importance of the health history.

Health history assessment enables the dental hygienist to:

- ✦ Establish baseline information about the client's personal, social, dental, and medical health status, including vital signs

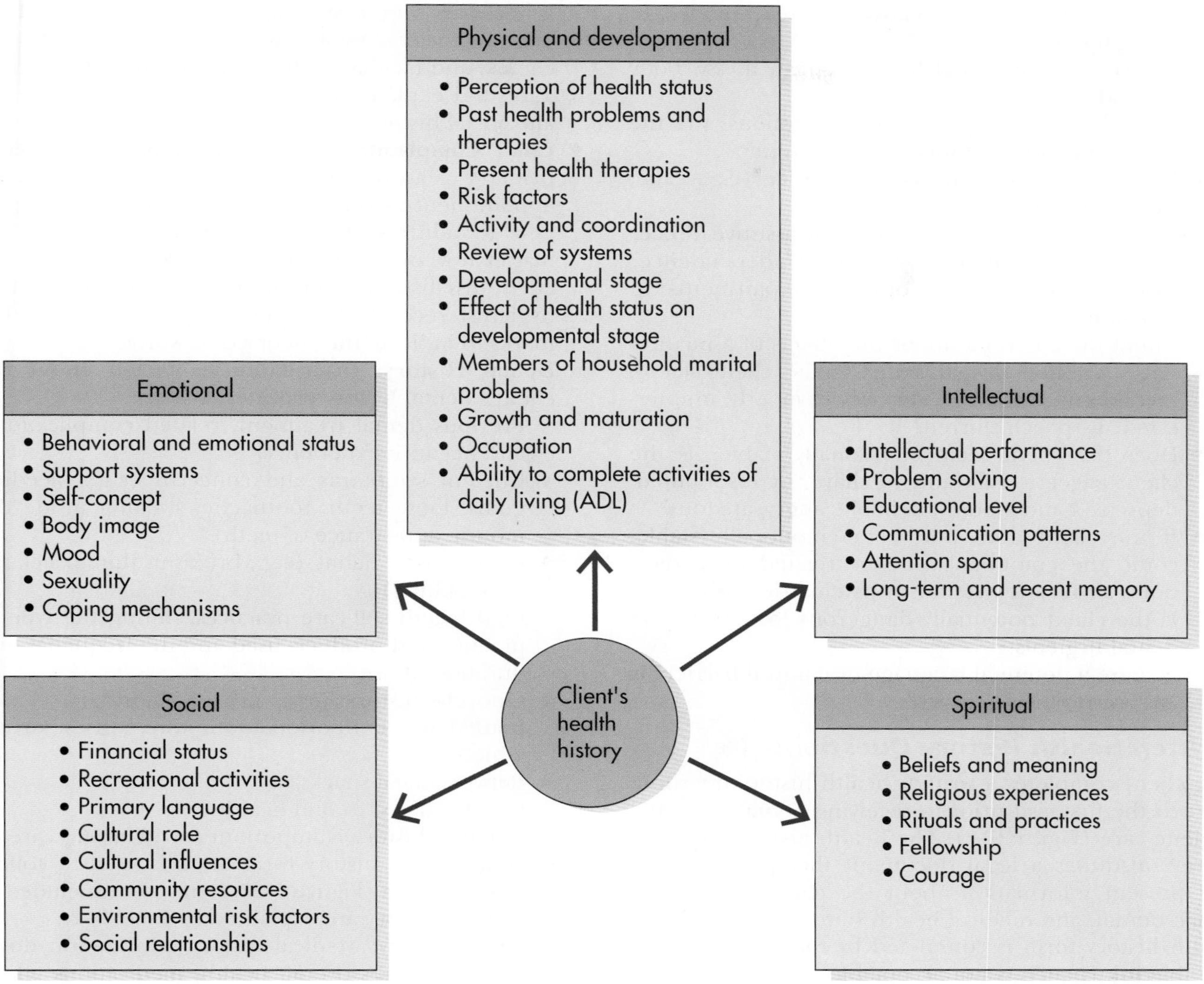

FIGURE 9–1 ✦ Dimensions of the health history.

- ✦ Assess overall physical and emotional health and nutritional status, including risk factors for disease
- ✦ Identify risk factors that necessitate precautions to ensure safe care and the prevention of medical emergencies:[1,2]
  - Diseases or medications that contraindicate care
  - Conditions that require special management prior to, during, or following care
  - Reactions to drugs or substances used in an oral care setting (e.g., latex or other sensitizing dental materials, anesthetic agents)
- ✦ Assist in the medical and dental diagnosis of various conditions and the identification of special physiologic states, such as pregnancy or menopause
- ✦ Identify conditions for which the client should be referred for medical evaluation
- ✦ Maintain legal documentation for managing client and practitioner risks and preventing potential litigation

HEALTH HISTORY ASSESSMENT

Obtaining a complete *health history* includes direct observation of the client, client completion of a written health history questionnaire, and a health history interview of the client.

Direct Observation

Assessment begins when the client enters the healthcare setting. Using direct observation, the dental hygienist mentally evaluates the following:

- ✦ What is the overall appearance of the client?
  - Emotional status: happy, depressed, fearful, agitated, intimidated
  - Physical gait: injuries, diseases, functional impairments, mobility
  - Color: pallor, ruddy, gray, yellow

Eyes: alert, bright, glassy, focused, reddened, pupil size

Dress and personal hygiene: neat, messy, body odors

- Does the client respond well to questions? Are the responses correct, applicable, coherent?
- Is the client using an assistive device (e.g., cane, walker, hearing aid)?
- How dependent is the client on the assistive device?
- Does the client prefer assistance or independence?
- Does the client have obvious impairments in function?
- Could the client be under the effects of a medication? Alcohol? Illegal drug? Is the client sleepy, incoherent, distracted, depressed, moody, uninterested? Is speech slurred?
- Does the client seem emotionally stable? Is the client eager to talk and to share, or disoriented, depressed and gloomy, irritable, angry, anxious?
- If the client does not seem emotionally stable, could the emotional state be related to medications, stroke, or systemic or psychiatric problems?
- Is the client potentially dangerous to self? To the dental hygienist?
- Is there a potential language or cultural barrier? Is an interpreter necessary?

Written Health History Questionnaire

The client completes a written health history questionnaire at the first visit prior to receiving dental or dental hygiene care (Figure 9–2). The health history questionnaire constitutes a legal document that provides past and present information about the client's personal/social, dental, and medical health status. Therefore, the health history form is completed by the client in nonerasable ink (pencil is not acceptable). The client signs the written health history form and any written comments concerning the health history to indicate accuracy. If the client is a minor (younger than 18 years of age), a parent or legal guardian should sign and date the health history form. The signature verifies accuracy of the information: a separate consent form with an appropriate client signature also grants permission for services to be rendered during the appointment (see Figure 54–3 in Chapter 54).

The client's health history is confidential and cannot be shared with others without the client's permission. Although many formats for the written health history questionnaire are available, all contain similar components:

- **Personal and Social History:** Personal and social information is factual demographic and lifestyle information about the client: the client's name, address, phone number (both home and business), date of birth, gender, marital status, occupation, cultural practices related to health and disease, referral source, types of insurance coverage, emergency contact, and previous dentist and current physician with addresses and phone numbers. Such information is necessary for conducting the business aspects of the dental practice, establishing a familiarity with new clients, and facilitating the provision of optimal care. Table 9–1 explains items to be included in a personal and social history.
- **Chief Complaint:** The *chief complaint* is the client's primary reason for seeking the oral healthcare appointment as verbalized by the client. It is important to address the client's primary concern, no matter how minor it is. Failure to do so can result in client dissatisfaction and noncompliance. The dental hygienist records the chief complaint in quotation marks to indicate the client's own words.
- **Dental History:** Information collected about the client's dental history provides data on:
  - Previous dental treatment, related complications, and negative experiences
  - Current symptoms and concerns (e.g., bleeding gums, loose teeth, toothache, swelling inside the mouth, appearance of teeth)
  - Current oral habits (e.g., bruxism, thumbsucking, cheek biting)
  - Oral health self-care practices, noting the type of practice and products used and the frequency and duration of use
  - Fluoride history (e.g., use of fluoridated water, bottled water, fluoride toothpaste, rinses, drops, tablets)
  - Between-meal snacks
  - Beliefs related to oral health
- The dental history is important for planning care. A separate dental history form often is used to collect this information (Figure 9–3). Items to be included in the dental history are explained in Table 9–2.
- **Medical History:** Medical history information documents the client's overall health, medications taken, risk factors for disease, allergies or unusual reactions, contraindications to care, undiagnosed conditions, and the need for physician consultation prior to oral health care. See Chapter 11 for detailed information about the pharmacologic history. Table 9–3 provides a comprehensive list of medical history items.

HEALTH HISTORY ORAL INTERVIEW

Although initially health history information is obtained using a structured written questionnaire, the dental hygienist uses the responses on the questionnaire as starting points for the client's health history interview. During the interview, the dental hygienist refines and broadens questions as needed to follow up on written responses so that the client's needs are correctly assessed. Tables 9–2 and 9–3 provide sample follow-up questions the dental hygienist verbally pursues during the health history oral interview.

- **Setting for the Interview:** The dental hygienist selects a place that is private enough to allow the client to

Medical Alert box

Date ___________

Name ______________________ Home Phone ( ) ______________ Bus Phone ( ) ______________

Address ______________________ e-mail address ______________

City ______________ State ______________ Zip Code ______________

Occupation ______________________ Social Security No. ______________

Date of Birth ____/____/____ Sex M F Height ______ Weight ______ Single ______ Married ______

Name of Spouse ______________ Emergency Contact & Relationship ______________ Phone ( ) ______________

If you are completing this form for another person, what is your relationship to that person.

____

Referred by ______________________________________

For the following questions, circle yes or no, or write in the appropriate response. Your answers are for our records and will be considered confidential. Please note that during initial visit, you will be asked some questions about your responses to this questionnaire and there may be additional questions concerning your health.

1. How would you rate your health? ☐ Good ☐ Fair ☐ Poor
2. Has there been any change in your general health within the past year?.......................... Yes No
   If yes explain ______________________
3. My last physical examination was on
   ______________________ (Attach last test results)
4. Are you under the care of a physician?.......................... Yes No
   If so, what is the condition being treated? ______________________
5. The name and address of my physician(s) is ______________________
   ____
6. Have you had any serious illness, operation, or been hospitalized in the past 5 years?.......................... Yes No
   If so, what was the illness or problem? ______________________
7. Have you had medical x rays in the last 5 years?.......................... Yes No
   If yes, explain. ______________________
8. Are you taking any medication(s) including non-precription and herbal medicine?.......................... Yes No
   If so, what medicines(s) are you taking? ______________________
9. Are you taking any of the following:
   a. Antibiotics or sulfa drugs b. Anticoagulants (blood thinners)
   c. High blood pressure medication d. Cortisone (steroids)
   e. Tranquilizers f. Aspirin
   g. Insulin, tolbutamide (Ornase) h. Digitalis or drugs for heart trouble
   i. Nitroglycerin j. Antihistamine k. Other
10. Taken any drug/medication in the past 6 months?.......................... Yes No
    If yes, why? ______________________
11. Do you have or have you had any of the following diseases or problems?
    a. Damaged heart valves or artificial heart valves, including heart murmur or rheumatic heart disease.......................... Yes No
    b. Cardiovascular disease (heart trouble, heart attack, angina, coronary occlusion, high blood pressure, arteriosclerosis, stroke.......................... Yes No
       1. Do you have chest pain upon exertion?.......................... Yes No
       2. Are you ever short of breath after mild exercise or when lying down?.......................... Yes No
       3. Do your ankles swell? .... Yes No
       4. Do you have inborn heart defects? .... Yes No
       5. Do you have a cardiac pacemaker?.......................... Yes No
       6. Have you taken fenfluramine/phentermine (fen-phen). Yes No
    c. Allergy.......................... Yes No
    d. Sinus trouble.......................... Yes No
    e. Asthma or hay fever.......................... Yes No
    f. Fainting spells or seizures.......................... Yes No
    g. Persistent diarrhea.......................... Yes No
    h. Diabetes.......................... Yes No
       1. Do you have to urinate (pass water) more than six times a day?.......................... Yes No
       2. Are you thirsty much of the time?.......................... Yes No
       3. Does your mouth frequently become dry?.......................... Yes No
       4. Have you had a recent weight gain or loss of more than 10 lbs? .... Yes No
       5. Are you slow at healing? .... Yes No
       6. Bruise easily?.......................... Yes No

FIGURE 9–2 ✦ Sample health history questionnaire. *(Modified from the American Dental Association and the Surgeon General's Report on Oral Health, 2000.)*

Figure continued on following page

i. AIDS or HIV infection.......................................Yes No
j. Thyroid problems.......................................Yes No
k. Respiratory problems, emphysema, bronchitis.......Yes No
l. Arthritis, rheumatism or painful swollen joints.......Yes No
m. Stomach ulcer or hyperacidity.......................................Yes No
n. Kidney trouble.......................................Yes No
o. Tuberculosis (Positive TB test, PPD test or chest x ray).......................................Yes No
p. Persistent cough or cough that produced blood.......Yes No
q. Persistent swollen glands in neck.......................................Yes No
r. Low blood pressure.......................................Yes No
s. Sexually transmitted disease (syphilis, gonorrhea, chlamydia etc).......................................Yes No
t. Epilepsy or other neurological disease.......................................Yes No
u. Mental health problems.......................................Yes No
v. Cancer.......................................Yes No
w. Problems of the immune system.......................................Yes No
x. Oral herpes/cold sores/ fever blisters.......................................Yes No
y. Mononucleosis.......................................Yes No
z. Neurologic disorder, e.g., cerebral palsy etc ....Yes No

12. Have you had abnormal bleeding?.......................................Yes No
a. Have you ever required a blood transfusion?...........Yes No
If yes, when ______

13. Do you have any blood disorder (anemia, bleeder, and leukemia)?.......................................Yes No

14. Have you ever had any treatment for a tumor or growth (surgery, radiation, or chemotherapy)?.......................................Yes No

15. Are you allergic or have you had a reaction to:
a. Local anesthetics.......................................Yes No
b. Penicillin or other antibiotics.......................................Yes No
c. Sulfa drugs.......................................Yes No
d. Barbiturates, sedatives or sleeping pills.......................................Yes No
e. Aspirin.......................................Yes No
f. Iodine.......................................Yes No
g. Codeine or other narcotics.......................................Yes No
h. Latex.......................................Yes No
i. Other.......................................Yes No

16. Have you had any serious trouble associated with previous dental treatment?.......................................Yes No

17. Do you have any disease, condition, or problem not listed above that you think I should know about?.......................................Yes No
If so, explain. ______

18. Are you wearing contact lenses?.......................................Yes No

19. Are you wearing removable dental appliances?.............Yes No

20. Do you use tobacco of any type?.......................................Yes No
If so, which type? ______
For how many years? ______
Are you a former tobacco user?.......................................Yes No
If so, which type? ______ For how many years ______
How much tobacco do/did you use a day? ______
If you stopped using tobacco products, how long ago did you stop? ______

21. Have you ever used alcoholic beverages?.......................................Yes No
How long ago did you stop using alcoholic beverages? ______
Do you currently use alcoholic beverages?.......................................Yes No
If so, which type? ______
Are you in recovery for alcoholism/ substance abuse? Yes No

22. Are you employed in any situation which exposes you regularly to x rays or other ionizing radiation?..............Yes No

For women only:

23. Are you pregnant?.......................................Yes No
If yes, due date? ______

24. Do you have any problems associated with your menstrual period?.......................................Yes No

25. Are you nursing?.......................................Yes No

26. Are you taking birth control pills?.......................................Yes No

27. Are you taking hormone replacements?.......................................Yes No

FIGURE 9–2, CONT'D.

be comfortable while providing personal information (e.g., the treatment room). The client is seated comfortably in an upright position in the dental chair and the dental hygienist is seated at eye level, about two feet from the client. During the interview, the dental hygienist is alone with the client unless the client is a child, in which case the parent or legal guardian is present. To ensure confidentiality and communicate respect, the health history interview should never be conducted in front of other clients or office staff. Clients respond best to a friendly, caring, nonjudgmental interviewer. Therefore, the hygienist must monitor personal verbal and nonverbal communication so the client feels accepted.

- **Objectives of the Interview:** Health history interviews achieve several objectives:
  - *To initiate the dental hygienist–client relationship.* The *dental hygienist–client relationship* is a partnership with a mutual concern—the client's well-being. The health history interview is the first step toward this trusting relationship so that interventions such as education and counseling can later occur.
  - *To provide the opportunity to observe the client's use of eye contact, nonverbal communication, and other body lan-*

TABLE 9–1 PERSONAL HISTORY ITEMS EXPLAINED

Items	Rationale	Implications for Professional Care
1. Name, address (home, business, email) telephone and fax numbers, gender, marital status, employer information, date	Conduct the business aspect of the practice. Assist in establishing rapport. Indicate when the form was last completed.	Address used to determine whether fluoride is present in the community water supply; however, client may drink water from another source. New health history forms should be updated at every appointment to gain better perspective of the client's health.
2. Date of birth	Indicate the client's age accurately. Asking "How old are you?" will not reflect the client's current age if a new health history is not completed every year. Assist in identifying oral conditions that are age related.	Young children should have morning appointments. Older people (>65 years) are prone to orthostatic hypotension; several pharmaceutical agents may also cause a client to be prone to orthostatic hypotension, e.g., antihypertensives, psychotherapeutics and Levodopa. Susceptible individuals should be raised to an upright position slowly with at least 2-3 pauses after lying supine. In terms of liability, a client who is a minor or legally incompetent will need a legal guardian to sign.
3. Height and weight	Calculate drug dosages. Assess obesity/overweight (risk for CVD, diabetes).	Maximum limitations to administer medications in the healthcare setting may need to be calculated. Use Maximum Dosage Charts for local anesthetic agents using the client's weight and considering age (less for very old or very young). Marked weight change may be a symptom of an underlying disease or disorder; physician referral may be needed.
4. Physical Activity	Determine commitment to health through regular exercise. Do you exercise on a regular basis?	Contributes to stress management. Used as an indicator of attitude toward one's health and potential for compliance.
5. Occupation/employment status of client's spouse, parent/guardian if client is a minor	Determine ethnologic risks for disease. Determine, in part, educational level. Determine potential financial barriers to care.	Appropriate assessment, planning, care, and evaluation will be necessary for the prevention or treatment of oral conditions related to client's occupation.
6. Previous dentist's name, address, and phone number	Determine where to obtain previous records or consultation on a pre-existing condition.	Client's previous records can be used as a reference to determine history of present acute/chronic oral conditions.
7. Physician's name, address, and phone number	Consult on disease, conditions, problems, or an emergency.	Physician's recommendations should be incorporated into the client's dental hygiene care plan.
8. Emergency contact	Communicate with a family member or friend regarding an emergency.	Contacted in the event of an emergency situation to escort client home or to hospital.
9. Referral source	Determine who should receive thank you acknowledgment.	Assist in establishing rapport with client and referral source. Referral source should be acknowledged and thanked.

guage, and to validate data obtained by observation with those obtained by written and verbal communication. For example, if the client reports no fear of dental care but appears anxious, the data conflict and more information needs to be gathered to form accurate conclusions.

- ✦ *To provide a mechanism by which the client can gain information as well.* If a positive dental hygienist–client relationship has been established the client will feel comfortable asking questions about treatments and trust the hygienist's responses and recommendations.

✦ **Interview Technique:** The health history interview involves three phases:

- ✦ *Orientation phase.* The dental hygienist opens the interview with introductions and spending a few minutes becoming acquainted with the client. Verbally asking the client's reason for the appointment clarifies the client's perception and identifies potential areas for education or community resources required to meet the client's expectations. Then the dental hygienist explains the need to ask additional questions about the client's health to ensure the provision of optimal care. This is an important time for the dental hygienist to foster trust and confidence with the client. Establishing a trusting relationship is important because during the health history interview the dental hygienist gathers information of a very personal nature. Before asking clients to share personal information, the dental hygienist assures clients that all information will be confidential.

Text continued on page 164

DENTAL HISTORY

Name ______________________________ Date ______________________________

Part I. Dental Experiences and Symptoms

1. What is the main reason for your visit?

____

2. When you look inside your mouth, do you know what to look for?

	Yes	**No**
Tooth Decay	☐	☐
Oral Cancer	☐	☐
Gum Disease	☐	☐
Cold Sores	☐	☐

3. Have you had dental x rays in the past 2 years?

☐ Yes Type ____________________ ☐ No

4. Have you had any complications or negative experiences associated with previous dental treatment?

☐ Yes Explain ____
☐ No

5. Generally, how have you felt about your previous dental appointments?

☐ Very anxious and afraid
☐ Somewhat anxious and afraid
☐ Don't care one way or the other
☐ Look forward to it

6. How much do you agree or disagree with this statement: oral health affects general health.

☐ Strongly agree ☐ Agree ☐ Disagree ☐ Strongly disagree

7. Are you experiencing any of the following symptoms?
(please check all that apply)

☐ Sensitive teeth
☐ Bleeding gums
☐ Bad breath
☐ Swelling inside mouth
☐ Sinus problems
☐ Sore jaw
☐ Difficulty chewing
☐ Burning sensation
☐ Tartar buildup
☐ Difficulty swallowing
☐ Toothache
☐ Filling fell out
☐ Abscess
☐ Yellowing teeth
☐ Sore gums
☐ Dry mouth
☐ Recession

8. Do you clench or grind your teeth in the daytime or at night?

☐ Yes ☐ No
If yes, do you wear a bite guard? __________ For how long? __________

9. In the past two years, have you been concerned about your breath or the appearance of your teeth or face?

(If yes, please check all that apply)

☐ Yellowing/graying teeth
☐ Stains
☐ Crowded, crooked teeth
☐ Spacing between teeth
☐ Gums
☐ Facial profile
☐ Bad breath

10. Have you experienced any injuries to your teeth, face and jaw?

☐ Yes Explain ____
☐ No

11. Have you experienced any of the following?

☐ Root planing
☐ Tooth extractions
☐ Dental implants
☐ Root canals
☐ Gum surgery
☐ Orthodontics/braces
☐ Head and neck radiation therapy
☐ Jaw surgery
☐ Severe pains of face/head
☐ Bad reaction to a local anesthetic
☐ Prolonged bleeding after dental treatment
☐ Other

FIGURE 9–3 ✦ Sample dental history questionnaire.

Part II. Oral Self Care

1. **Check the following you regularly use at home:**

☐ Soft toothbrush	☐ Dental floss	☐ Floss threader	☐ Fluoride rinse or gel
☐ Hard toothbrush	☐ Special brush	☐ Toothpick	☐ Fluorideted drops/tablets
☐ Medium toothbrush	☐ Floride toothpaste	☐ Mouthrinse	☐ Fluoridated water
☐ Oral irrigator	☐ Rubber tip	☐ Whitening products	☐ Fluoridated water at day care
☐ Denture adhesive	☐ Powered interdental cleaner		☐ Bottled water
☐ Denture cleaner	☐ Power brush		☐ Other ______________

2. **Check the type of toothpaste you use:**

☐ Fluoride	☐ Tartar control	☐ Gum benefit	☐ Multiple benefit
☐ Sensitivity protection	☐ Baking soda	☐ Peroxide	

3. **Estimate how long it takes you to clean your teeth and gums each time: Please indicate your best and most reliable estimate.**

   Brushing ____________ (time) Flossing ____________ (time)

4. **About how many times each day/week do you brush and floss?**

   brush about ________ times per day OR ________ times per week
   floss about ________ times per day OR ________ times per week

5. **Do you find it difficult to maintain an oral hygiene schedule due to your job or other reasons ?**

   ☐ Yes ☐ No

6. **Do any conditions make it difficult for you to adequately clean your teeth?**
   (If yes, please check all that apply)
   ☐ Hold a toothbrush ☐ Use dental floss ☐ Brush/floss for any length of time ☐ Poor vision

7. **Do you perform a monthly self-exam for oral cancer?** ☐ Yes ☐ No

Part III. Between-Meal Snacks

Please check which sweets and starches you eat between meals frequently

Food	Frequency	Food	Frequency
☐ Breath mints	________	☐ Canned/bottled beverages	________
☐ Cough drops	________	☐ Sugared liquids	________
☐ Chewing gum	________	☐ Chips	________
☐ Dried fruits	________	☐ Crackers	________
☐ Cookies	________	☐ Others	________

Part IV. Beliefs About Oral Health

1. **In your opinion, compared with the average person, how likely do you think you are to have cavities or other problems with your teeth and/or gums?**
   ☐ Much more likely ☐ About average ☐ Much less than average
   ☐ More than average ☐ Less than average

2. **How important is it for you to prevent cavities, gum problems, or other diseases of the mouth?**
   ☐ Very important ☐ Somewhat important ☐ Not at all important

3. **I believe that I have control over the condition of my mouth.** ☐ Yes ☐ No

4. **I believe that my oral health is**
   ☐ Excellent ☐ Good ☐ Fair ☐ Poor

Comments ____

____

FIGURE 9–3, CONT'D.

TABLE 9–2 DENTAL HISTORY ITEMS EXPLAINED

Item	Purpose	Relevant Questions	Implications for Professional Care
1. Chief complaint	Reveal why the client is seeking care	Is there a particular problem you are having with your teeth and mouth?	Must be addressed to client's satisfaction
2. Previous dental care	Indicate if the client seeks regular dental treatment; if recent oral radiographs should be requested Alert: oral radiographic exposure should be limited if radiographs taken recently	When was your last dental visit? Have you been treated by a specialist? Have you ever had braces, root canals, extractions, dental appliances, dental implants, or any other type of special care? What treatment was performed? Any problems?	Consider need for specialty care Specialized maintenance-care instructions for abutments, prosthesis, implants, etc.
3. Radiation history	Alert: limit oral radiographic exposure if client has been exposed to large amounts of recent radiation	What radiographs were taken? Have you had radiation therapy? When were radiographs taken? What was extent of radiation exposure?	Send for recent radiographs or consider taking current radiographs, if necessary Consider amount of radiation exposure from past dental and medical sources
4. Complications during dental treatment	Avoid similar complications	What type of complication occurred? How was it treated?	Complications often are a source of client dissatisfaction; avoid repeating the complication, if possible
5. Dental treatment anxiety	Identify clients prone to allergic reactions or to anxiety-related reactions such as syncope Alert: condition should be followed up with a physician consultation if cause of reaction is unknown Alert: need for sympathy, patience, short appointments, and possibly antianxiety agent, e.g., Valium or nitrous oxide–oxygen analgesia	What type of reaction occurred? What treatment was performed? What caused the reaction? Is client nervous about dental care? What causes the nervousness? What has been done to alleviate nervousness?	Unusual reactions caused by fear or anxiety should be investigated and stress reduction protocols initiated Consider physician consultation prior to care if allergic reaction is suspected from substance that may be part of the care plan Unreasonable fear or anxiety should be investigated and stress reduction protocols initiated
6. Client's perception of relationship between health and oral health	Assess client's understanding of systemic and oral health	Do your teeth affect your general health? In what way?	Educate client on link between oral and systemic health
7. Adverse oral symptoms reported by the client	Indicate conditions such as sensitivity, recession, bruxism, cracked tooth syndrome, undetected caries, sinus problems, periapical problems, eating disorders, improper self-care techniques	What causes the symptom? If cause is not known, ask the client about bruxing, sinus problems, self-care techniques	Avoid contacting sensitive teeth directly with the cold air/water syringe spray Recommend self-applied and professionally applied desensitizing agents
7a. Chewing ability	Indicate conditions such as ill-fitting dental appliances, missing teeth, dental caries	What causes this difficulty?	Refer to dentist for correction of problem Consider nutritional counseling until problem is resolved
7b. Periodontal health	Indicate conditions such as periodontal disease, blood disorder, leukemia, trauma, neoplasm, nutritional deficiency, immunosuppression	What causes your gums to bleed? How often does it occur? Mobile teeth? Bad taste in mouth? Receding gums?	Correlate etiology with health history condition; if no cause can be found, problem may be periodontal in nature
7c. Sores in mouth	Indicate condition such as herpes, recurrent aphthous ulcers, trauma, nutritional deficiency, immunosuppression Indicate a premalignant or malignant lesion or uncontrolled diabetes	Where and when did the sores occur? How long did they last? Is the cause known? What is the cause?	Take appropriate precautions for infectious lesions Determine differential diagnosis of lesion(s) and make appropriate referrals or consultations Client with poor healing or who cannot explain causal factors may need referral to an oral and maxillofacial surgeon

8. Oral habits	Alert: oral habits may be deleterious, e.g., cheek or lip biting, clenching, bruxism; holding items in teeth (pins, needles, paper clips, pipes) may cause abrasion; pushing gums with fingernail may cause recession; thumbsucking may contribute to malocclusion and a deep, narrow palatal vault	What type of habit? Frequency, duration, and intensity of habit?	Counsel client about habits detrimental to oral health
9. Client's satisfaction with teeth, face, and breath	Indicate conditions such as periodontal disease, blood disorder, trauma, leukemia, neoplasm, nutritional deficiency, immunosuppression	What causes the dissatisfaction? Any prior treatment? Bad breath?	Consider consultation with a dentist for cosmetic procedures or orthodontic therapy
10. Injury to teeth, face, and jaw	Identify clients with temporomandibular joint disorders, difficulty opening, problems with long appointments, malocclusion, or devitalized or ankylosed teeth	What type of injury? Any treatment? Any complications?	Refer to dentist for evaluation Short appointments indicated for clients who have difficulty opening mouth for long periods
11. Plaque control procedures	Indicate oral self-care behaviors Determine if a caregiver is required	Current toothbrushing procedure? Brush type(manual or powered; soft or hard)? Frequency of use? Replacement schedule? Dentifrice used? Additional cleansing devices and frequency of use? Mouthrinses and frequency of use?	Determine client need for additional education Determine extent of parent/caregiver supervision
12. Fluorides and dental sealants	Determine need for supplemental fluoride therapy Determine potential for dental fluorosis	Is fluoridated water regularly ingested? Bottled water? Bottled fruit juice? Fluoridated water while growing up? Date of last professional fluoride treatment? Fluoride mouthrinse use? Have you ever had dental sealants?	Determine need for client education
13. Sugar and beverage consumption	Identify source of stained teeth Alert: client may be prone to dental caries if drinking beverages with honey, sugar, or creamer substitute	What snacks do you usually eat? Frequency? What beverages do you usually drink? Frequency? How much is consumed? Is bottled water used? Is bottled fruit juice used?	Nutritional counseling indicated for caries risk related to sugar consumption Power toothbrush recommended to manage extrinsic stain
14. Beliefs about oral health	Identify client motivational strategies	How important is oral health in your life?	

TABLE 9–3 MEDICAL HISTORY ITEMS EXPLAINED

Item	Purpose	Relevant Questions	Implications for Professional Care
1. General Health			
1a. Estimation of client's general health	Determine how the client feels about his or her general health	How do you perceive your health? How much physical activity do you get daily?	Conflicting information from this question compared to information on the history may indicate that client is overly concerned about health and well-being or unable to understand seriousness of reported conditions. Modifications may be considered if client reveals a significant disability, medical or psychological condition.
1b. Reason for seeking dental hygiene or dental care	Reveal chief complaint in the client's own words	How important is your oral health to you? Type of problem, if any? Date of onset and type of symptoms?	Referral to specialist is warranted for conditions needing immediate attention.
1c. Date of last physical examination?	Reveal a significant medical problem Identify clients who do not obtain regular healthcare	What was it for? Any problems found? Was it with the same physician noted or was it with a specialist?	Careful planning modifications will need to be considered if client reveals a significant disability, medical or psychological condition. Many clients report infrequent visits to a physician; however, client may seek professional oral care one or more times a year. Dental hygienist plays role in assessment and identification of significant medical and oral conditions.
1d. Is the client currently under the care of a physician? If so, what for?	Indicate any surgery or anticipated surgery Determine if the client is seeking care from other physicians Determine if the client is at risk for a medical emergency from a condition	What is the nature of the condition? What type of treatment have you had or are you having? Any complications?	Recommended care modifications considered for a client with a medically compromising condition. Client may have several reported conditions and a separate physician for each; appropriate consulting physician should be determined. Stress reduction protocols implemented for clients with medical conditions that could be exacerbated by stress/anxiety from dental hygiene care.
1e. Have there been any changes in the client's health within the past year?	Identify an illness that may reflect on the client's oral care	What type of illness did you have? What treatment was involved? Were there any relapses or problems involved?	A recent change may indicate needed treatment modifications prior to or during care.
1f. Hospitalizations?	Determine if the client has a compromised health condition Alert for recurrence in oral cavity if hospitalized for cancer Identify local anesthesia precautions that may be needed if prior history of problems	What was reason for hospitalization? Did any problems occur? Were there any complications?	Existing or chronic medical conditions may indicate the need for modifications in care. Stress reduction protocols implemented for clients with medical conditions that could be exacerbated by stress/anxiety from dental hygiene care.
2. Nutrition and Diet			
2a. Has the client lost or gained more than 10 pounds in the last year?	Alert: marked change in weight may indicate an undiagnosed disease Determine undiagnosed condition, e.g., uncontrolled diabetes, AIDS, tuberculosis, anxiety, stress, carcinoma, heart failure, eating disorder, thyroid problems, GI problem(frequent nausea, diarrhea, heartburn, reflux disorder, lactose intolerance)	When did this occur? Cause? Did you change medication? Are you a vegetarian? Do you avoid certain foods? Do you skip meals? Diet (high or low protein, carbohydrate or fat; trendy diets such as grapefruit diet or Atkins diet)? Do you have any health problems that interfere with digestion or absorption of food?	Health history interview may indicate an undiagnosed condition; review history indicators (positive responses) with no known cause. Physician of record should be contacted if the client is unsure of cause of weight gain or weight loss.

2b. Dietary habits	Identify adequacy of client's diet	Have you ever had nutritional counseling? If so, from whom?	Dietary counseling may be indicated to promote healing after treatment.
3. Medications			
3a. Is the client taking any medications? List them.	Identify current medications being taken Avoid drug interactions with medications taken in the course of care Consider side effects of the drug	What type of current medications including prescription, over-the-counter, and nutritional supplements (e.g., vitamins, herbs, etc) are you taking? How long has the medication been taken?	Use *Physician's Desk Reference* to obtain information concerning medications the client is taking. Determine if client's medications are contraindicated or have possible interactions with drugs administered during dental hygiene care. Relate xerostomia, gingival enlargement, and postural hypotension to medications taken by the client or other underlying factors.
3b. Has the client taken any medications within the past year?	Reveal a prior condition or problem	What was the type of medication, dosage, and reason for its use? How long have you taken the medication?	Pharmacologic history could reveal a medical or psychological condition important to dental hygiene care, and indicate need for care modifications or physician referral.
3c. Is the client allergic to any medication?	Indicate medication that should not be prescribed in the course of dental or dental hygiene care	When was the allergy determined? What is the type of medication? What type of reaction occurred?	Dental hygienists' do not prescribe medications to the client; however, over-the-counter medications are available and often recommended by a dental staff member. If allergic, do not distribute the medication to the client.
3d. Has the client taken fen-phen (fenfluramine and phentermine) or dexfenfluramine or fenfluramine?	Determine the possible need for antibiotic premedication	When were the medications taken? How long did you take the medications? Have you had an echocardiogram to determine an adverse heart condition caused by the medications?	Physician consult indicated prior to care to determine need for antibiotic premedication.
3e. Has the client experienced an unusual reaction to penicillin, aspirin, sulfa drugs, or other medications?	Screen for idiosyncratic drug reactions or possibly unknown drug allergies Identify medications that should not be given to the client	What were the circumstances? What type of reaction did you have (e.g., allergic reaction, side effects, or psychogenic reaction)?	Avoid dispensing medication that may cause an allergic reaction or client discomfort.
3f. Hay fever/hives/skin rash	Alert to an unsuspected or undiagnosed drug or other allergy Alert: professional care should be deferred during periods when the client may experience an acute condition	When does the condition occur? What causes the condition? Any medications? Type?	Hives and skin rashes can be caused by allergens. Avoid administration or exposure to allergens, which may trigger an allergic episode.
3g. Is the client allergic to latex?	Prevent an allergic reaction	When did the allergy first occur? What type of reaction do you experience? Have you had allergy testing to determine the specific cause?	A client may be allergic to latex proteins or the powders used with latex gloves. Allergy testing may be indicated to determine the specific cause. When client has a latex allergy, avoid all latex items, e.g., rubber cup, latex gloves, local anesthetic agents with a latex diaphragm, rubber dam. If client has allergy to glove powder, use powderless gloves.
3h. Drug addiction	Alert: administering or giving narcotic medications or alcohol-containing products to a rehabilitated client may trigger a relapse Determine if liver dysfunction is present	When did the condition occur? What type of drug was involved? Is this currently a problem?	Avoid recommending/dispensing narcotic or alcohol-containing products to a rehabilitated client. Half-life of amide type local anesthetic agent may be prolonged in a person with liver dysfunction associated with drug addition thereby risking local anesthetic overdose; determine if liver dysfunction is present.

Table continued on following page

TABLE 9–3 MEDICAL HISTORY ITEMS EXPLAINED—CONT'D

Item	Purpose	Relevant Questions	Implications for Professional Care
4. Cardiovascular Conditions			
4a. Heart disease/heart failure/heart attack	Alert: prophylactic premedication may be required Identify clients who may need supplemental oxygen prior to dental hygiene care Identify clients who may be taking nitroglycerin, which needs to be readily accessible during treatment Identify clients for whom dental or dental hygiene care is contraindicated	What type of heart disease and when did it occur or when was it diagnosed? Hospitalized, and if so, how long and any complication? How severe was it? Any residual damage as a result of the heart attack? Any medication? Type? Any recurrences? Have you taken prophylactic antibiotic premedication for previous dental or dental hygiene care?	Physician consultation may be needed prior to care to determine need for antibiotic premedication. Stress reduction protocols implemented for clients with cardiac conditions that could be exacerbated by stress/anxiety from dental hygiene care. Assess degree of heart failure and determine ASA classification. Follow ASA classification for treatment modifications. May require physician consultation. Supplemental oxygen may be indicated for clients with significant heart damage. Physician consultation necessary for clients who report significant heart damage. Avoid treatment of clients who have had a heart attack within six months of the dental hygiene appointment.
4b. Pacemaker/intracardiac device (ICD)	Identify clients for whom electromagnetic interference is contraindicated Recognize that medical consultation may be needed prior to dental or dental hygiene care	When did you receive the ICD? Any complications?	Presence of pacemaker indicates a medically compromised heart condition that could require treatment modifications or stress reduction protocols. Most dental procedures are unlikely to interfere with a shielded pacemaker or ICD; these procedures include dental radiographs, dental drills, ultrasonic scalers and cleaners, and TENS, provided the equipment is not placed directly over the ICD implant site. Cover unshielded pacemaker with a lead apron to protect it from electrical interference.
4c. Heart murmur/mitral valve prolapse/rheumatic fever/rheumatic heart disease	Identify clients with cardiac malformations, which may result in endocarditis as a result of bacteremia caused by certain dental procedures	When was the condition diagnosed? Is the heart murmur organic, i.e., a congenital uncorrected cardiac malformation or a functional heart murmur? Have you previously taken prophylactic antibiotic premedication for previous dental or dental hygiene care?	Cardiologist or physician of record should be contacted if the client is unsure about premedication. Minimize number of appointments for those who take antibiotic premedication to prevent antibiotic resistance. During instructions, link need for good oral hygiene and oral health to minimize bacteremic exposures and risk of further heart disease.
4d. Chest pain/angina pectoris	Indicate undiagnosed angina Alert: minimize stress and use shorter appointments to prevent an anginal attack or myocardial infarct in the dental healthcare environment Identify need for good pain control Identify clients taking nifedipine, which can cause drug-influenced gingival enlargement	When was the onset of the condition? Type of angina? What causes the condition to occur? Were you under the care of a physician? Any medication(s), and how often is it taken?	Depending on client's ASA classification, supplemental oxygen and premedication with nitroglycerin 5 minutes before therapy may be indicated. Follow ASA classification treatment considerations. Clients with unstable angina or changes in the type of angina are considered *ASA IV status* and should not receive elective dental care unless upgraded to *ASA III status.*
4e. Swollen ankles	Identify conditions such as kidney disease, heart disease, an obstruction in the leg, anemia, and pregnancy (standing for long periods can cause this condition)	Do you know the cause of the condition? Are you under the care of a physician for the condition? Any medications? Type?	The cardiologist or physician of record should be consulted if there is no known cause of the condition. Careful drug administration indicated for client with kidney conditions due to impaired drug excretion.

Surgically Corrected Cardiovascular Lesions			
4f. Artificial heart valves	Identify need for prophylactic premedication Identify clients taking anticoagulants, which may cause gingival bleeding	When were the valves placed? Any complications? Any medications? Type?	Antibiotic premedication vital prior to dental procedures associated with significant bleeding. Minimize number of appointments for client who takes antibiotic premedication to prevent antibiotic resistance. During instructions, link need for good oral hygiene and oral health to minimize bacteremic exposures and further cardiac disease. Gingival bleeding in the absence of other indicators for periodontal disease may be caused by anticoagulant therapy.
4g. Cardiac bypass surgery	Identify persons who have had cardiac surgery	When was the bypass surgery performed? Complications? Medications?	Antibiotic premedication prior to dental hygiene care required up to 6 months post-bypass surgery. After 6 months post-bypass surgery, premedication not indicated.
4h. Hypertension (high blood pressure)	Identify need to assess blood pressure prior to dental and dental hygiene care Identify cause of xerostomia Reveal if the condition is a symptom of other disease states Identify who may experience postural hypotension when the dental chair is returned to the upright position	When was the condition diagnosed? Is the condition controlled? Are you currently seeking care from a physician for the condition? Any medications? Type?	Determine whether client is a candidate for elective dental or dental hygiene care following appropriate blood pressure recommendations. Client with known high blood pressure should have blood pressure taken prior to each appointment to determine if it is under control. Fluoride therapy, xylitol chewing gum, and saliva substitutes may be indicated for xerostomia caused by antihypertensive agents. Some antihypertensive agents can produce postural hypotension.
4i. Low blood pressure	Indicate underlying problem	Possible underlying pathology?	Client may be in shock, have infection, cancer, hemorrhage, fever, anemia, Addison's disease, a debilitating or wasting disease, or approaching death.
4j. Does the client use more than two pillows to sleep?	Indicate cardiovascular disease conditions (e.g., congestive heart failure)	Reason for using two pillows?	Client may be uncomfortable reclining in supine position.
5. Respiratory System			
5a. Lung disease	Identify who may be unable to recline fully in dental chair because of compromised breathing	When was the condition diagnosed? Type of lung disease? Any medications? Type? Problems lying in a supine position?	Raise back of chair for client with difficulty breathing in supine position. Physician consultation required prior to treatment for client with chronic signs and symptoms of lung condition. Keep in mind possible link between oral pathogens and respiratory infection.
5b. Persistent cough	Indicate respiratory problem due to smoking, infection, carcinoma, bronchitis, tuberculosis Alert: client may have compromised respiration	When did the condition start? Do you know the cause of the condition? Have you sought care from a physician for the condition? Any medications? Types?	Client who reports night sweats and coughing blood may have active tuberculosis and should have immediate physician referral prior to dental hygiene care. May be necessary to avoid aerosol production, e.g., use of mechanized instruments and air-abrasion system.
5c. Emphysema	Alert: nitrous oxide–oxygen analgesia is contraindicated for dental treatment	When was the condition diagnosed? Any medications? Type?	Continuous oxygen ventilation may be needed by client; avoid ignition of the oxygen source. Avoid use of nitrous oxide–oxygen analgesia.
5d. Bronchitis	Alert: client may have compromised respiration	When did the condition occur? Any medications? Type? Any recurrences?	Avoid aerosol production, e.g., use of mechanized instruments and air-abrasion system.

Table continued on following page

TABLE 9–3 MEDICAL HISTORY ITEMS EXPLAINED—CONT'D

Item	Purpose	Relevant Questions	Implications for Professional Care
5e. Tuberculosis	Alert: dental and dental hygiene treatment should be deferred if client is infectious (if on medication (usually isoniazid) for at least 2 weeks and not actively coughing, sneezing, or wheezing, the client is not infectious and can be treated); physician's clearance required	When was the condition diagnosed? Was a chest x-ray taken and what were the results? Any medications? Type?	Treatment postponed for client with active tuberculosis until physician's clearance is given.
5f. Asthma	Alert: stress may precipitate an attack; therefore, make the appointment as stress free as possible	When did the condition last occur? How often does it occur? If hospitalized, how long? When was the condition diagnosed? What causes the condition? Any medications? Type?	Have client bring bronchodilator to appointment. Nitrous oxide–oxygen analgesia can be administered to an anxious asthmatic client.
5g. Shortness of breath	Indicate conditions such as heart disease, obesity, emphysema, anemia, and asthma	When did the condition occur? What was the cause? Did you see a physician? Any medications? Type?	Refer client to physician prior to dental hygiene care if an undiagnosed condition is suspected. Physician consultation necessary if client has indicators of cardiovascular disease.
5h. Sinus problem	Identify clients prone to headaches or maxillary pain Identify who may have an allergy Alert: client may have problems breathing with a rubber dam	When does the condition occur? Any medications? Type?	Pain in maxillary teeth may be associated or possibly confused with sinus conditions Acute sinus problems during an appointment may indicate an acute allergic reaction to an allergen in the environment. Nitrous oxide–oxygen analgesia contraindicated with clients who cannot breathe nasally. Avoid blocking oral cavity if client's nasal passages are blocked.
6. Blood Conditions			
6a. Cerebrovascular accident (stroke)	Identify who may have physical impairments, be taking anticoagulants, and contraindicated dental and dental hygiene treatment Alert: alternative choices of local anesthetic agent may be indicated	When did condition occur? If hospitalized, how long? Complications? Recurrences? Any medications? Type? Any physical/mental/communication impairments? Any difficulty with oral hygiene? Do you measure your blood pressure regularly? Do you use special devices to carry out daily self-care behaviors?	Elective dental and dental hygiene care contraindicated for client who has had a stroke within 6 months of appointment. Anticoagulants (warfarin, heparin) may cause excessive bleeding during invasive dental/dental hygiene care. Physician consultation required prior to invasive procedure. Some clients may be required by the physician to refrain from taking anticoagulant medication for 1-4 days prior to care. Physical impairments may limit self-care behaviors and require modified oral hygiene aids. Avoid exposure to vasopressors (vasoconstrictors) in local anesthetic agents.
6b. Anemia	Identify risk for methemoglobinemia (a cyanosis-like state in susceptible individuals)	When was condition diagnosed? Any medications? Type? Any adverse reaction to local anesthetic agents?	Avoid administration of articaine and prilocaine local anesthetic agents or application of the topical agent benzocaine to prevent methemoglobinemia in susceptible individuals.
6c. Bruise easily	Reveal possible blood disorder Indicate need for medical consultation	When was condition noticed? Are you seeking care from a physician for the condition?	Bruising noted with accompanied fatigue, pallor, weight loss, fever, bone or joint pain, and repeated infections could indicate leukemia.

6d. Prolonged bleeding or blood disorder	Indicate blood disorder that causes prolonged bleeding. Indicate that client's physician may need to be consulted about prophylactic antibiotic premedication or problems with immunosuppression Reveal use of anticoagulants, NSAIDs, or aspirin Reveal condition that should be a consideration for invasive dental procedures	When did condition occur? How long was the bleeding? What were the circumstances? Are you seeking care from a physician for the condition? When was the condition diagnosed? Any medications? Type? Are you in remission?	Physician consultation prior to invasive dental procedures to determine if prolonged bleeding during the procedure will jeopardize client's health. A laboratory test to determine bleeding time may be indicated prior to the procedure. Avoid recommending aspirin or NSAIDs to control pain. Recognize clients on anticoagulant therapy.
6f. Hemophilia	Indicate need for medical consultation prior to any invasive procedure Identify clients at risk for increased bleeding	Any medication? Type? Any complications or problems?	Physician consultation prior to invasive dental procedures to determine if prolonged bleeding during the procedure will jeopardize client's health. Half-life of amide-type local anesthetic agents may be prolonged in clients with liver dysfunction associated with hemophilia, thereby risking local anesthesia overdose. Determine if liver dysfunction is present.
6g. Blood transfusion	Identify client who may have been exposed to hepatitis or human immunodeficiency virus (HIV)	When did the transfusion occur? What were the circumstances? Any problems or complications?	History of a blood transfusion followed by signs and symptoms of hepatitis or HIV infection may reveal an undiagnosed disease state. Physician consultation indicated prior to dental care.
7. Psychological Conditions			
7a. Fainting (syncope)	Indicate if client is fearful, anxious, or predisposed to fainting Reveal conditions such as transient ischemic attacks (prestroke), postural hypotension (orthostatic hypotension), and anemia Indicate need for humanistic behaviors during care	When did the condition occur? What was the cause? Any problems associated with it? How often has it occurred?	If cause is psychogenic, follow appropriate ASA stress reduction techniques. If fear and/or anxiety has specific cause (e.g., the local anesthetic syringe), avoid exposing client to the cause. Two to three chair adjustments should be performed when returning from supine position to upright position for client with history of orthostatic hypotension. Other medical conditions or causes should be further explored prior to care planning to determine if physician consultation is indicated or care plan modifications are indicated.
7b. Frequent headaches	Indicate chronic tension or other disease states Alert: common sign of cerebrovascular accident (CVA) includes mild to severe headaches	When does the condition occur? What type of headache? Any medications? Type?	Determine cause(s) of headaches and plan care accordingly. Physician consultation or immediate referral may be required for clients manifesting signs and symptoms of a TIA or CVA.
7c. Frequently exhausted	Indicate conditions that may be drug related, emotionally related, or indicate chronic fatigue syndrome or anemia Indicate inability to maintain daily self-care behaviors	When does the condition occur? What was the cause? Are you seeking care from a physician for the condition? Any medications? Type?	Determine cause(s) of the exhaustion and plan care accordingly. Physician medical consultation or immediate referral for diagnosis may be required. Consider alterations in oral self-care to minimize fatigue.
7d. Depressed/anxious/ psychiatric treatment	Indicate medications for emotional problems, drug-related conditions, need to limit stress, or inability to maintain self-care behaviors	Are you seeking care from a physician? Any medications? Type?	Review current medications to determine if drug interactions are contributing to emotional state. Follow ASA recommendations for anxious or fearful clients to minimize exacerbation of medical condition or cause a psychogenic emergency. Sedatives and tranquilizers predispose a client to postural hypotension. Emphasize positive behaviors and actions to build client's self-esteem. It may take three weeks or more for antianxiety agents to stabilize a client's emotional state.

Table continued on following page

TABLE 9–3 MEDICAL HISTORY ITEMS EXPLAINED—CONT'D

Item	Purpose	Relevant Questions	Implications for Professional Care
8. Mental/Emotional Illness	Identify emotional problems that may hinder healthcare	What is the diagnosed problem? How is problem managed?	Person may be drowsy or have xerostomia from medications such as antipsychotics, antianxiety, tranquilizers, antidepressants, antiparkinson. Compliance may be difficult. Client may overreact to stress.
9. Communicable Diseases			
9a. Herpes	Alert: dental and dental hygiene treatment is contraindicated with active oral lesions present	How long have you had the condition? Is it an oral condition? Does it recur? Causes of recurrence? When did it last recur?	Reschedule dental hygiene care for clients with active oral lesions. Counsel client concerning infectious states of a lesion and potential self-infection to other areas of the body or to other people via contact with the lesion. Recognize use of acyclovir or Abreva.
9b. Sexually transmitted diseases/infections (STDs or STIs)	Alert: dental and dental hygiene care is contraindicated if open oral sores are present	When was the condition diagnosed? What type of condition was it? Any medications? Type?	Visible signs of oral and pharyngeal lesion indicate need for immediate physician referral. Dental hygiene care should be deferred until clearance from physician is indicated. Recognize use of antibiotics.
9c. HIV infection/AIDS	Identify HIV-positive clients Identify inability to maintain self-care behaviors	Any recurrences? When were you diagnosed as HIV-positive? How is disease managed?	Recognize opportunistic infections and related problems such as candidiasis, mycobacterium avium complex, Kaposi's sarcoma, *Pneumocystis carinii* pneumonia, cytomegalovirus, neuropathy. Recognize use of protease inhibitors, antiviral drugs, and antiretroviral drugs. Antibiotic premedication is not usually required unless client's immune system is severely compromised.
9d. Tuberculosis (TB)	Identify clients with active TB	How was TB treated? Comply with treatment? Was physician clearance received?	Be alert to medications such as isoniazid, rifampin, pyrazinamide.
9e. Hepatitis/liver disease/jaundice	Identify who may have liver damage and bleeding problems Alert: client may be prone to drug toxicity reactions Reveal that client may have liver damage and be unable to metabolize drugs such as local anesthetics at a normal rate Reveal chronic carriers of the hepatitis B or C virus (antigen positive) Reveal conditions such as hepatitis infection	When did the condition occur? What was the cause? Any complications? Were you tested following infection to rule out a carrier state for hepatitis B?	Postpone care for client with active hepatitis A or E infections until a physician clearance is obtained. Client with liver damage or bleeding problems from a past hepatitis infection may need a physician consultation prior to treatment, especially if medications are to be given. Beware of impaired drug metabolism. Jaundice can be an indirect indication of hepatitis infection. Physician consultation or immediate referral for diagnosis may be required for clients with no specific etiology. Client with jaundice due to liver conditions will be medically compromised; physician consultation required prior to care, especially if medications are to be given during treatment. No treatment alterations required for jaundice that occurs at birth.
9f. Measles/chicken pox/scarlet fever/mumps	Facilitate diagnosis of enamel hypoplasia or pigmentation if high fevers were experienced	When did condition occur? Complications?	No alterations in dental hygiene care needed for usual childhood diseases with no complications.

10. Convulsions, Seizures, or Epilepsy	Alert: a client who indicates convulsions without a history of epilepsy may suggest undiagnosed epilepsy Alert: a client may have an epileptic seizure in the oral healthcare environment Identify clients taking an anticonvulsant Identify clients who may be taking valproic acid, which may cause increased bleeding, or phenytoin sodium (Dilantin), which may contribute to drug-influenced gingival enlargement. Also medications may cause drowsiness.	What type of seizures? Frequency? When was the last one? What signs signal the onset of a seizure? How long does it last? If hospitalized, how long? Medications taken? Seizures controlled by medications?	Epileptic seizures prevented by careful screening at the beginning of the appointment. Some seizures can be "triggered" by fatigue, recent alcohol consumption, exhaustion, psychological stress, flashing lights, and nitrous oxide–oxygen analgesia. Reschedule epileptic client who reports seizure-triggering factors. Stress-reduction protocol recommended for apprehensive epileptic clients. Medications may require alteration in care planning. Valproic acid requires bleeding time test prior to invasive procedures. Persons on Dilantin may have drug-influenced gingival enlargement.
11. Immunosuppression	Indicate a systemic disease, such as lupus or HIV/AIDS, or a person who has had an organ transplant Reveal clients with compromised healing Reveal clients with susceptibility to disease Identify need for prophylactic antibiotic premedication	What is the cause of the condition? When was the condition diagnosed? Any medications? Type?	Review client's current status for possible considerations in care planning. Possible prophylactic premedication with antibiotics may be necessary for clients reporting compromised healing or susceptibility to disease. Person on an immunosuppressant drug such as cyclosporine may have drug-influenced gingival enlargement. Prednisone and azathioprine also used to prevent rejection of transplant.
11a. Cortisone treatment	Alert: client may be immunosuppressed	What was the treatment for? When did the treatment occur? Complications?	Antibiotic premedication for immunosuppressed individuals may be indicated prior to dental hygiene care. Gingival inflammation may be suppressed.
11b. Kidney disease	Reveal who may have damaged kidneys and cannot excrete drugs normally Indicate possible need for antibiotic premedication	What type of kidney disease? When was the condition diagnosed? Any medications? Type? Are you unusually sensitive to drugs or medications? Type?	Client who has a kidney condition may need physician consultation prior to treatment for possible prophylactic antibiotic premedication or if medications are to be given during dental hygiene care.
12. Diabetes	Alert: dental hygiene appointment should be scheduled for soon after the client has had meal and prescribed insulin Alert: client may heal more slowly, be prone to infections, and need frequent maintenance Alert: risk for diabetes-related emergencies	When was condition diagnosed? Type of diabetes? Any medications? Type? Is diabetes controlled? How often is blood or urine glucose monitored? Do you have hypoglycemic episodes? How often?	ASA III or IV status may indicate need for antibiotics after extensive surgical procedures to minimize risk of postoperative infections. Avoid scheduling appointments during normal eating times. Use short-acting local anesthetic agents to allow client to eat, thereby raising blood glucose levels, if necessary. Client with a blood glucose level exceeding 240 mg/dl should be evaluated carefully before treatment. Physician consultation indicated for client with a blood glucose level exceeding 400 mg/dl.
12a. Frequent urination	Indicate disease states such as diabetes Indicate use of medications such as diuretics or substances in the diet	When did this condition occur? Are you aware of the cause of the condition? Have you sought care from a physician for the condition?	Client who reports increased hunger, thirst, and weight loss may have uncontrolled diabetes. Physician consultation indicated prior to dental hygiene care. Client taking diuretics may be predisposed to postural hypotension. Use caution when raising client from dental chair.
12b. Often thirsty	Indicate unsuspected conditions such as diabetes Indicate an underlying systemic or drug-related reason for xerostomia	When did condition occur? Are you aware of the cause of the condition? Have you sought care from a physician for the condition?	Client who reports increased hunger, thirst, and weight loss may have uncontrolled diabetes. Physician consultation indicated prior to dental hygiene care. Client taking diuretics may be predisposed to postural hypotension. Use caution when raising client from dental chair. Saliva substitutes and/or caries control interventions indicated for xerostomic conditions.

Table continued on following page

TABLE 9–3 MEDICAL HISTORY ITEMS EXPLAINED—CONT'D

Item	Purpose	Relevant Questions	Implications for Professional Care
13. Endocrine Diseases/ Imbalances	Identify persons experiencing hormonal disturbances or fluctuations, e.g., puberty, pregnancy, menopause, birth control medication, corticosteroids, thyroid disorders	Are you experiencing any hormonal problems?	Emphasize need for meticulous oral self-care. May need to monitor blood pressure. Recognize use of medications such as thyroid hormone, antithyroid, estrogen/progestin therapy, oral contraceptives, corticosteroids.
13a. Thyroid disease	Alert: hyperthyroid clients may be sensitive to heat, lose weight without dieting, be irritable or tense, and have an increased appetite Alert: hypothyroid clients may have recent weight gain and be unusually sensitive to cold temperatures Alert: untreated thyroid disease may lead to life-threatening situations	What type of thyroid disease? When was the condition diagnosed? Any medications? Type?	Postpone care for clinically hypothyroid or hyperthyroid clients. Immediate physician consultation indicated due to potential for life-threatening emergency. Use minimal amounts and small dosages of local anesthetic agent for controlled hyperthyroid client. Aspirate prior to each injection to avoid injection of anesthetic agent into bloodstream.
14. Cancer Treatment	Alert: risk of recurrence in the oral cavity; if treated with radiation to the head and neck region, there will be decreased healing and decreased secretion by the salivary glands Alert: avoid invasive surgery with clients who have compromised healing Identify clients who may need comprehensive fluoride therapy or salivary replacement therapy Identify clients receiving long-term therapy	Type of cancer diagnosed? When did the treatments occur? Is cancer in remission? Any medications? Type?	Render dental and dental hygiene care prior to cancer treatment (surgery, radiation therapy, chemotherapy). Recognize signs of oral cancer recurrence during oral assessments, e.g., lymphadenopathy. Avoid exposure to excess radiation after cancer radiation therapy. Antibiotic premedication and blood count may be indicated prior to dental hygiene care. Avoid tissue trauma following oral cancer treatment. Head and neck radiation destroys salivary glands; salivary replacement therapy and aggressive dental caries prevention is necessary. Need for customized fluoride mouth trays for head and neck cancer patient.
15. Gastrointestinal Diseases/Ulcers	Identify apprehensive clients Alert: client may have acute or chronic anxiety Identify who may be taking tranquilizers, antacids, antidiarrheals, antispasmodics, and laxatives	When was the condition diagnosed? Any medications? Type? Are you on a restricted diet?	Stress-reduction protocols implemented for clients with stress/anxiety from dental hygiene care. Sedatives and tranquilizers predispose client to postural hypotension. Instruct client in accordance with dietary requirements. Medications may cause xerostomia.
16. Sensory/Physical Disabilities			
16a. Eye disease (macular degeneration, glaucoma, blindness)	Identify clients who may have visual impairments	When was condition diagnosed? Type? Any surgery performed? Any medications?	May need modifications in oral self-care instructions. Adapt communication and education for the vision impaired.
16b. Hearing disorders	Identify clients who may have hearing impairments	When was condition diagnosed? Type? Any surgery performed? Any medications? Type?	May need modification in oral self-care instructions. Adapt communication and education for the hearing impaired.

16c. Physical disability	Identify clients with poor functional status	Type of condition? Limitations in movement/function? Type of assistive devices?	May need to perform wheelchair transfer. Medications may cause drowsiness and xerostomia. Need for barrier-free environment. Possible need for antibiotic premedication for prosthetic joint replacement.
16d. Swollen joints/arthritis	Identify clients who may have increased bleeding time from medications, such as aspirin and nonsteroidal antiinflammatory drugs Identify clients who may have difficulty moving, especially in the morning Alert: may need prophylactic antibiotic premedication	What joints are swollen? Temporomandibular joint affected? What causes the condition? Medications/treatment? Type?	Anticoagulant therapy may cause excessive bleeding during dental surgery. Physician consultation indicated prior to surgical procedure. Physical impairments may limit oral hygiene behaviors and require modified oral hygiene aids. Prophylactic antibiotic premedication may be needed prior to performing high-risk dental procedures on client with joint replacement. Client may be more comfortable at mid-morning or afternoon appointments. May need shorter appointments if having difficulty opening and closing mouth.
17. Substance Abuse			
Substance use/abuse (e.g., tobacco, alcohol consumption)	Alert: tissue changes associated with tobacco use, poor nutritional status, and poor healing, and the potential for noncompliance Alert: avoid alcohol-containing products such as mouthrinses for clients who are recovering alcoholics Identify clients with stain	What type of tobacco is used? How often and how much? How long has the tobacco been used? How often is alcohol ingested? How much is ingested? Have you ever tried to quit? If so, how? Would you like some help to stop your habit?	Avoid alcohol-containing products for clients receiving rehabilitation to stop substance abuse or history of abuse, or taking Antabuse. Alcohol consumption in clients with history of epilepsy predisposes them to seizures. Drug/alcohol rehabilitation programs may prohibit use of a vasopressor (vasoconstrictor) with local anesthetic administration. Provide tobacco cessation materials, assist with cessation effort, and arrange follow-up. Instructions on oral and systemic risks of substance abuse. High consumption of alcoholic beverages may contribute to alcoholism and xerostomia.
18. Pregnancy and Menopause			
18a. Is the client pregnant?	Alert: avoid elective treatment in the first trimester Alert: risk of preterm low–birth-weight babies in women with periodontal disease	How many months? Any complications? Parturition date?	Client may be uncomfortable in supine position, especially in later stages of pregnancy. Client may be prone to orthostatic hypotension. Avoid exposure to nitrous oxide–oxygen analgesia and medications during pregnancy. Avoid tetracycline antibiotic therapy to prevent intrinsic tooth staining in the offspring. Radiographs can be taken on pregnant women. Consider links between periodontal disease and low birth weight. Schedule frequent maintenance care.
18b. Is the client using birth control medications?	Alert: gingival bleeding problems might be partially related to hormonal balance Alert: some antibiotics may alter effectiveness of birth control medication	Name and type of medication? What is the treatment regimen?	Consider hormonal factors if excessive bleeding encountered. Consult with dentist or physician if client using birth control pills and taking antibiotic medication. Warn clients that antibiotics will decrease effectiveness of birth control medication. Maintain excellent oral hygiene.
18c. Is the client on hormone replacement therapy?	Alert: problems may be partially related to hormone balance	Name and type of medication? What is the treatment regimen?	Maintain excellent oral hygiene. Discuss cardiovascular disease risks for women on hormone replacement therapy.

Strategies for Effective Communication

Silence is helpful for making observations and provides the client with time to organize thoughts and present complete information to the interviewer.

Attentive listening demonstrates interest in the client's needs, concerns, and problems. Listening can be facilitated by maintaining eye contact, remaining relaxed, and using appropriate touch techniques.

Conveying acceptance demonstrates the interviewer's willingness to listen to the client's beliefs, values, and practices without being judgmental.

Related questions are planned. When asking these questions, the practitioner uses words and word patterns in the client's normal sociocultural context.

Paraphrasing provides an opportunity for the interviewer to validate information from the client without changing the meaning of the statement. Paraphrasing is the interviewer's formulation of what the client has said in more specific words.

Clarifying facilitates correct communication of information. It is achieved by asking the client to restate the information or by providing an example.

Focusing eliminates vagueness in communication, limits the area of discussion, and helps the interviewer direct attention to the pertinent aspects of a client's message.

Stating observations provides the client with feedback about how the interviewer observes behavior, action, facial expression, or activities.

Offering information allows the interviewer to clarify treatments, initiate health teaching, and identify and correct misconceptions.

Summarizing condenses the data into an organized review. It validates data because the client has the opportunity to confirm that they are correct. Summarizing indicates the end to a particular part of the interview.

From Potter PA, Perry AG: *Fundamentals of nursing*, ed 5, St Louis, 2001, Mosby.

- ✦ *Working phase.* The dental hygienist clarifies responses reported on the questionnaire using *open-ended questions* to obtain a response of more than a couple of words. For example, the dental hygienist may begin by saying, "Tell me about the chest pain you reported on the questionnaire." This technique leads to a discussion in which clients actively describe the issue in question. Using open-ended questions strengthens the dental hygienist–client relationship because it shows that the dental hygienist wants to invest time in hearing the client's thoughts. The use of eye contact and listening skills reinforces the dental hygienist's intent. The dental hygienist also uses *back channeling,* which includes active listening techniques such as "all right" or "uh-huh," which indicate the dental hygienist has heard what the client says. In addition, the dental hygienist uses communication strategies to facilitate communication (see Strategies for Effective Communication). Additional suggestions to enhance communication are in Chapter 4.
- ✦ *Termination phase.* The client is given a clue that the interview is coming to an end. For example, the dental hygienist may say, "We'll be finished with this in a minute," or "I have just one more question."

The health history is reviewed and updated at each appointment by documenting changes in the client's health since the last visit. After reviewing the health history with the client, the dental hygienist should date (month, day, and year) and sign the chart entries in nonerasable pen. Entries should be carefully written and legible; mistakes should be neatly lined out, initialed, and dated (if necessary). Because the client's chart is a legal record, mistakes should never be covered with correction fluid or made illegible. Positive (yes) answers to the health history questionnaire can be circled in red for easy visibility and fully documented with an explanatory comment. Changes are reviewed with the client and, as always, the client signs the documented information to verify accuracy.

DECISION MAKING AFTER OBTAINING THE HEALTH HISTORY

Several tools are used to interpret the data and determine the client's degree of medical risk.

American Society of Anesthesiologists' (ASA) Physical Status Classification System

The *ASA physical status classification system,* developed by the American Society of Anesthesiologists, rates the medical risk of a client who is to undergo local or general anesthesia for a surgical procedure. This system, which extends from ASA I–V, considers client anxiety and classifies medical risk (see ASA Physical Status Classification System to Determine Medical Risk).

Dental hygienists use the ASA classification system to determine whether treatment is safe for clients. A client who falls within the ASA IV status or greater should not receive treatment unless upgraded to the ASA III status. For example, clients with a history of uncontrolled diabetes should seek a medical consultation and possibly treatment from their physicians prior to dental hygiene care. If a client with an ASA IV status is in need of emergency care, then it would be best to treat the client in a hospital environment in case a life-threatening emergency occurs. Only palliative care is recommended for a client with an ASA V status.

ASA Physical Status Classification System to Determine Medical Risk

ASA I: A normal, healthy client without systemic disease.

ASA II: A client with a mild systemic disease (e.g., a healthy client with considerable anxiety; a healthy pregnant client; a client who has well-controlled Type II diabetes, well-controlled epilepsy, and/or well-controlled asthma).

ASA III: A client with severe systemic disease that limits activity but is not incapacitated (e.g., stable angina, exercise-induced asthma, postmyocardial infarct or cerebrovascular accident with no residual signs and symptoms more than 6 months before treatment).

ASA IV: A client with an incapacitating systemic disease that is a constant threat to life (e.g., unstable angina, myocardial infarction, or cerebrovascular accident within 6 months, uncontrolled epilepsy or uncontrolled diabetes).

ASA V: A moribund client not expected to survive 24 hours with or without an operation.

ASAE: Emergency operation. The 'E' preceeds the number to indicate the client's physical status, (e.g., *ASAE-III*).

Adapted from Malamed SF: *Medical emergencies in the dental office,* ed 5, St Louis, 2000, Mosby.

TABLE 9–4 SECTION DESCRIPTIONS FOR THE *PHYSICIANS' DESK REFERENCE**

Section Name	Color of Index	Purpose
1. *Manufacturer's Index* (e.g., Parke-Davis, Lederle, Procter & Gamble)	White	Provides name, addresses, and emergency phone numbers of the manufacturers whose products are listed in the *PDR*
2. *Product Name index* (e.g., Motrin, Procardia) • Refer to this section if the product name is known	Pink	Lists name given to the product by the manufacturer, also referred to as the brand name. These are in alphabetical order
3. *Product Category Index* (e.g., antiinflammatory agents) • Refer to this section if only the medical condition for the prescription is known	Blue	Lists products in the appropriate category for type of medication; represents the product's action in the body
4. *Generic and Chemical Name Index* (e.g., ibuprofen, nifedipine) • Refer to this section if only the generic or chemical name is known	Yellow	Lists products and their generic and chemical names
5. *Product Identification Section* Refer to this section when you have the drug in hand, but do not know the name of the drug	Full color	Provides color pictures of the products listed in sections 2 to 4
6. *Product Information Section* Refer to this section for detailed information about the drug and its actions	White	Drug descriptions divided into: • Clinical pharmacology (how the drug works) • Indications and contraindications • Warnings and precautions (side effects and drug interactions) • Adverse reactions (possible negative effects of the drug therapy)

*Consultation with the physician of record or a pharmacist is warranted if complete information cannot be found.

Stress and anxiety can cause medical emergencies such as *vasodepressor syncope* (fainting) and hyperventilation. Stress and anxiety can also exacerbate a client's medical condition, causing an emergency situation. Stress reduction protocols should be initiated to avoid an emergency. For information on stress reduction protocols, see Chapter 32.

USE OF *PDRs* AND *MERCK MANUAL*.[4,5] Before care, the dental hygienist investigates and documents medications currently taken by the client (see Chapter 11). Medications taken by the client can alter treatment outcomes, contraindicate medications for dental and dental hygiene care, or indicate the need for a medical consultation prior to initiating care. The *Physicians' Desk Reference (PDR),* an essential guide for dental hygiene practice, provides valuable information about prescription drug products.[5] For example, as shown in Figure 9–4, a drug's action, usage, contraindications, adverse reactions, warnings, and precautions are available and readily accessible in the *PDR.* The *PDR* also displays colored pictures of the dispensed form of medications, so a visual identification can be made when the client cannot verbally identify a medication. Sections of importance to the dental hygienist found in the *PDR* are described in Table 9–4. These sections are color-coded in the *PDR* for easy access by the practitioner.

Product information can be retrieved if the medication is identified in sections 2 to 4 of the *PDR.* Sections most commonly used are the Product Category Index (blue

CHROMAGEN® FORTE ℞
SOFT GELATIN CAPSULES

DESCRIPTION

CONTENTS : Each brown soft gelatin capsule contains: ferrous fumarate UPS, 460 mg (151mg elemental iron),ascorbic acid UPS, 60 mg, folic acid USP, 1 mg, cyanocobalamin USP, 10 mcg.
DISCUSSION: The amount of elemental iron and the absorption of the iron components of commercecial iron preparations vary widely. It is further established that certain "accessory components" may be included to enance absorption and utilization of iron. Chromagen® Forte Capsules are formulated to provide the essentisl factors for a complete, versatile hematinic.

ACTIONS

HIGH ELEMENTAL IRON CONENT: Ferrous fumarate, used in Chromagen® Forte Capsules, is a is an organic iron complex which has the highest elemental iron content of any hematinic salt-33%. This compares with 20% for ferrous sulfate (heptahydrate) and 13% for ferrous gluconate[1,2] Chromagen® Forte contains 151 mg of elemental iron.
MORE COMPLETE ABSORPTION: It has been repeatdly shown that ascorbic acid, when given in sufficient amounts, can increase the absorption of ferrous iron from the gastrointestinal tract.[3,4,5,6,7,8,9] The absorption-promoting effect is mainly due to the reducing action of ascorbic acid within the gastrointestinal lumen, which helps to protect or delay the formation of insoluble or less dissociated ferric compounds.[3]
PROMOTES MOVEMENT OF PLASMA IRON: Ascorbic acid also plays an important role in the movement of plasma iron to storage depots in the tissues.[10] The action, which leads to the transport of plasma iron to ferritin, presumably involves its reducing effect, converting transferrin iron from the ferric to the ferrous state[5] There is also evidence that ascorbic acid improves iron utilization, presumably as a further result of its reducing action,[6,9] and some evidence that it may have a direct effect upon erythropoiesis. Ascorbic acid is further alleged to enhance the conversion of folic acid to a more physiologically active form, folinic acid, which would make it even more important in the treatment of anemia since it would aid in the utilization of dietary folic acid.[11]
EXCELLENT ORAL TOLERATION: Ferrous fumarate is used in Chromagen® Forte Capsules because it is less likely to cause the gastric disturbances so ofen associated with oral iron therapy. Ferrous furnate has a low ionization constant and high solubility in the entire pH range of the gastrointestinal tract. It does not precipitate proteins or have the astringency of more ionizable forms of iron, and does not interfere with protolytic or diastatic activities of the digestive system. Because of excellent oral toleration, Chromagen® Forte Capsules can usuall be administered between meals when iron absorption is maximal.
FOLIC ACID SUPPLEMENTATION: The use of supplemental folic acid may be indicated in patients with increased requirements for this vitamin, such as iron deficiency anemia. Folic acid administration may reduce the risk of neural tube defects in the developing fetus.[12] Folic acid has also been shown to reduce circulating homocysteine levels in the blood[15,16] Folate as 5-methyltetrahydrofolate and B_{12} as methylcobalamin are involved in the remethylation reaction of homocysteine to methionine.[17,18] Elevated homocysteine plasma levels are associated with increased risk of preeclampsia, neural tube defects, myocardial infarction and arttherosclerosis.[19-23]

TOXICITY: Ferrous fumarate was found to be the least toxic of the three popular oral iron salts, with an oral LD_{50} of 630 mg/kg. In the same report, the LD_{50} of ferrous gluconate was reported to be 320 mg/kg and ferrous sulfate 230 mg/kg.[1,13]

INDICATIONS

For the treatment of all anemias responsive to oral iron therapy, such as hypochromic anemia associated with pregnancy, chronic or acute blood loss, dietary restriction, metabolic disease and post-surgical convalescence.

CONTRAINDICATIONS

Hemochromatosis and hemosiderosis are contraindications to iron therapy. Folic acid is contraindicated in patients with pernicious anemia **(see PRECAUTIONS).**

WARNING

Accidental overdose of iron-containing products is a leading cause of fatal poisoning in children under 6. Keep this product out of reach of children. In case ofaccidental overdose, call a doctor or poison center immediatly.

PRECAUTIONS

Folic acid should not be presccribed until the diagnosis of pernicious anemia has been eliminated, since it can alleviate the hematologic manifestations, while alowing neurological damage to continue undetected.[14]

ADVERSE REACTIONS

Average capsule doses in sensitive individuals or excessive dosage may cause nausea, skin rash, vomiting, diarrhea, precordial pain, or flushing of the face and extremities.

DOSAGE AND ADMINISTRATION

Usual adult dose is 1 soft gelatin capsule daily.

HOW SUPPLIED

Capsules: NDC 0281-0262-18, Unit Dose Box 100
CAUTION: Federal law prohibits dispensing witout prescription.

BIBLIOGRAPHY

[1]Berk, M.S. and Novich, M.A.: "Treatment of Iron, Deficiency Anemia With Ferrous Fumarate," Am. J. Obst. & Gynec., 203-206, 1962.[2]Shapleigh, J.B., and Montgonery, A.Am. Pract. & Dig. Treat. 10-461, 1959. [3]Brise, H, and Hallberg, L.: "Effect of Ascorbic Acid on Iron Absorption," Acta. Med. Scand. 171.376, 51-58, 1962. [4]New Drugs, p. 309, AMA, Chicago, 1966. [5]Mazur,A., Green, S. and Carleton, A,: "Mechanism of Plasma Iron Incorporation into Hepatic Ferritin," J. Bio. Chem. 3:595-603, 1960. [6]Greenberg, S.M. Tucker, A. E., Mathues, H and J.D. "Iron Absorption and Metabolism, I. Interrelationship of Ascorbic Acid and Vitamin E," J. Nutrition 63:19-31, 1957. [7]Moore, C.V. and Dubach, R. "Observations on the Absorption of Iron from Foods Tagged with Radioiron" Trans. assoc. Amer. Physic. 64:245, 1951. [8]Steinkamp, R. Dubach, R. and Moore, C.V.: "Studies in Iron Transportation and Metabolism," Arch. Int. Med. 95:181, 1955. [9]Gorten, M. K. and Breadley, J. E: "The Treatment of Nutritional Anemia in Infancy and Childhood with Oral Iron and Ascorbic Acid," J. Pediatrics, 45;1, 1954.[10]Mazur, A.: "Role of Ascorbic Acid in the Incorporation of Plasma Iron into Ferritin," Ann. N.Y. Acad. Sci, 92:223-229, 1961. [11]Cox, E.V. et al: "The Anemia of Scurvy," Amer. J. Med. 42: 220-227, 1967.[12]McEvoy, G.K, Ed.: AHFS Drug Information, p. 2667-2669, Am. Soc. Hosp. Pharm., Bethesda, 1996. [13]Berenbaum, M.C. et al.: Blood, 15:540, 1960. [14]Drug Information for the Health Care Professional", p.1365-1368, U.S. Pharmacopeial Conven., Rockville, 1995.[15]Franken DG, Boers GH, Blom HJ, Trijbels JM. "Effect of various regimens of vitamin B_6 and folic acid on mild hyperhomocysteinemia in vascular patients." J. Inheit. Metab. Dis. 1994;

FIGURE 9–4 ✦ Sample of information available in the *Physicians' Desk Reference. (Redrawn from* Physicians' desk reference, *ed 56, Montvale, NJ, 2002, Medical Economics Data.)*

pages) and Product Name Index (pink pages). After the medication is identified in a particular color-coded section, the reader is referred to the white pages of the Product Information Section to obtain extensive information about the particular medication. Boldfaced numbers in the *PDR* access either color photographs of the dispensed form of the drug or information concerning the medication.

The *PDR,* published yearly, reports new or revised information about prescription drug products. Other related publications include the *PDR Drug Interactions and Side Effects Index,* the *PDR for Nonprescription Drugs,* and the *PDR for Herbal Medicines.*

The *Merck Manual of Diagnosis and Therapy* is a standard reference handbook on diseases, including their etiology, signs and symptoms, diagnostic indicators, and treatment.[4] Essential facts about medical conditions identified in the health history can be found in the latest edition of the *Merck Manual.* Dental hygienists confronted with unfamiliar medical conditions will find readily available, concise descriptions of most diseases in this reference book.

Prophylactic Antibiotic Premedication[1,2]

Manipulation of mucosal tissues that results in bleeding during dental or dental hygiene procedures may cause a transient bacteremia. Although bacteremias rarely persist for more than 15 minutes, infectious microorganisms in the bloodstream may cause problems in at-risk individuals. Specifically, microbes may become lodged on damaged or abnormal areas of the heart valves, lining of the heart, and underlying connective tissue and cause *infective endocarditis* (a life-threatening infection of the lining of the heart and also the underlying connective tissue). A small number of clients with prosthetic total joint replacements is susceptible to an accumulation of bacteria in the area surrounding a joint replacement, which could result in an infection of the joint and loss of the joint replacement.

Prophylactic antibiotic premedication is the recommended administration of specific types of antibiotics 1 hour prior to the client's dental hygiene appointment to prevent infective endocarditis or prosthetic joint infection. Before initiating any dental hygiene care, prophylactic antibiotic premedication should be given to at-risk clients who are susceptible to infective endocarditis, prosthetic joint infection, or infection due to their immunocompromised status. Prophylactic antibiotic premedication also should be given to clients who may have difficulty resisting infections, that is, clients with unstable diabetes, persons undergoing anticancer chemotherapy, acute leukemia, renal transplantation, kidney dialysis, or persons taking immunosuppressive medications.

The client's periodontal health status may have a role in the risk of problems from bacteremias. Transient bacteremias can occur from day-to-day activities such as toothbrushing, flossing, and use of other interdental cleaners. Oral devices used inappropriately or in clients with poor oral hygiene and periodontal disease have produced bacteremias. Whether the bacteremia plays a role in the client's health is unknown; however, a healthy oral environment poses much less of a risk. Although good oral hygiene habits should be encouraged for all individuals, they are especially important for persons with conditions such as cardiovascular disease, recent joint replacements, pregnancy, diabetes, and immunosuppression, which place them at risk for more serious health complications.

INFECTIVE (BACTERIAL) ENDOCARDITIS. Because some dental procedures are more invasive than others, the type of procedure being performed and the risk of the client for infective endocarditis must be evaluated to determine whether the client is a candidate for prophylactic antibiotic premedication (Table 9–5). For example, taking oral radiographs on a client in a high-, moderate- or negligible-risk category does not indicate the need for prophylactic antibiotic premedication. However, it is recommended that a client receiving an oral prophylaxis who has had a previous episode of endocarditis should receive prophylactic premedication.

Each client should be individually evaluated regarding a recommendation for premedication. Overuse of antibiotics could result in antibiotic-resistant strains of bacteria, which would be detrimental to the client's long-term health.

The standard prophylactic regimen recommended by the American Heart Association is shown in Table 9–6.[1] One dose of the appropriate antibiotics 1 hour prior to the procedure is sufficient for the prevention of endocarditis. *Note that a history of cardiac surgery, in and of itself, is not an indication for premedication.*

TOTAL JOINT REPLACEMENT. Antibiotic premedication should not be routinely recommended for all clients with a total joint replacement (TJR), nor is it indicated for persons with surgically implanted pins, plates, or screws. Because some dental procedures are more invasive than others, the type of procedure being performed and the risk of the client for hematogenous total joint infection must be evaluated to determine whether the client is a candidate for prophylactic antibiotic premedication (Table 9–5). For example, a client who has had a TJR within the last two years who is scheduled for scaling and root planing will need antibiotic premedication. A client who had had a joint replacement over two years ago and has an appointment for oral impressions for bleaching stents will not need antibiotic premedication. If there is uncertainty concerning the client's joint replacement, the opinion of an orthopedic physician is indicated before dental hygiene care is initiated.

IMMUNOSUPPRESSED INDIVIDUALS. It is not possible to describe all conditions that may lead to decreased resistance to infection from a bacteremia; therefore, the immunosuppressed client's physician should be consulted concerning antibiotic premedication.

Antibiotic Premedication Dosage Regimen Guidelines

Each client should be evaluated individually for the need for prophylactic premedication. Tables 9–6 and 9–7 outline the current dosage regimens before dental hygiene care is initiated for clients at risk for infection, infective endocarditis, or late prosthetic joint infections. Table 9–8 discusses considerations for using antibiotics for clients at risk for infection.

Physician Consultation

The physician of record should be consulted if the client reveals a condition that may jeopardize safety during care. Medical consultations are recommended for:

- ✦ A condition that may need prophylactic antibiotic premedication
- ✦ Suspicion of an undiagnosed or uncontrolled condition
- ✦ Abnormal vital signs
- ✦ Precautionary treatment modifications (i.e., local anesthetics without vasoconstrictor)
- ✦ Persons with a history of fenfluramine/phentermine use (fen-phen)
- ✦ Persons taking a blood thinner (e.g., warfarin)

TABLE 9–5

ANTIBIOTIC PREMEDICATION GUIDELINES FOR PROFESSIONAL ORAL HEALTHCARE

Conditions	Prophylaxis Recommended*	Prophylaxis NOT Recommended
Dental procedures	Dental extractions Periodontal procedures including surgery, scaling and root planing, probing, and maintenance care (supportive periodontal therapy) Dental implant placement and reimplantation of avulsed teeth Endodontic (root canal) instrumentation or surgery only beyond the apex Subgingival placement of antibiotic fibers or strips Initial placement of orthodontic bands but not brackets Intraligamentary local anesthetic injections Every attempt should be made to complete procedures/services in as few appointments as possible Follow-up appointments should be scheduled at least 9 days apart if client is premedicated	Restorative dentistry* (operative and prosthodontic with or without retraction cord†) Local anesthetic injections (nonintraligamentary) Intracanal endodontic treatment; post placement and buildup Placement of rubber dams Postoperative suture removal Placement of removal prosthodontic or orthodontic appliances Taking of oral impressions Fluoride treatments Taking of oral radiographs Orthodontic appliance adjustment Shedding of primary teeth
Cardiac conditions	High-risk category Prosthetic cardiac valves, including bioprosthetic and homograft valves Previous bacterial endocarditis Complex cyanotic congenital heart disease (e.g., single ventricle states, transposition of the great arteries, tetralogy of Fallot) Surgically constructed systemic pulmonary shunts or conduits Moderate-risk category Most other congenital cardiac malformations (other than above and below) Acquired valvular dysfunction (e.g., rheumatic heart disease) Hypertrophic cardiomyopathy Mitral valve prolapse with valvular regurgitation and/or thickened leaflets	Negligible-risk category (no greater risk than the general population) – Isolated secundum atrial septal defect – Surgical repair of atrial septal defect, ventricular septal defect, or patent ductus arteriosus (without residua beyond 6 mo) – Previous coronary artery bypass graft surgery – Mitral valve prolapse without valvular regurgitation – Physiologic, functional, or innocent heart murmurs – Previous Kawasaki disease without valvular dysfunction – Previous rheumatic fever without valvular dysfunction – Cardiac pacemakers (intravascular and epicardial) and implanted defibrillators
Orthopedic conditions	Joint replacement clients – within the first two years of joint replacement – history of previous prosthetic joint infection – malnourishment – hemophilia – type 1 diabetes Joint replacement clients who are immunocompromised/immunosuppressed by: – any disease-, drug-, or radiation-induced immunosuppression – inflammatory arthropathics (rheumatoid arthritis, systemic lupus erythematosus)	*Not* routinely indicated for most clients with joint replacements or with plates, pins, or screws
Other conditions	Renal transplants/dialysis Immunosuppressive therapy (i.e., cyclosporine) Uncontrolled diabetes Sickle cell anemia Spina bifida (ventriculoarterial shunt)	

* Includes restoration of decayed teeth (fillings) and replacement of missing teeth
† Clinical judgment may indicate antibiotic use in selected circumstances that may cause significant bleeding
Adapted from Fitzgerald RH Jr et al: Advisory statement: Antibiotic prophylaxis for dental patients with total hip joint replacements, *Journal of the American Dental Association* 128(7):1004, 1997. Dajani AS et al: Prevention of bacterial endocarditis: Recommendations by the American Heart Association, *Journal of the American Medical Association* 277:22,1997. American Dental Association: American Academy of Orthopaedic Surgeons: Antibiotic prophylaxis for dental patients with total joint replacements, *Journal of the American Dental Association* 128(7):1004, 1997)

TABLE 9–6 AMERICAN HEART ASSOCIATION RECOMMENDATIONS FOR PROPHYLACTIC ANTIBIOTIC COVERAGE REGIMEN FOR SELECT DENTAL PROCEDURES IN ADULTS AND CHILDREN WITH HIGH AND MODERATE RISK FOR INFECTIVE ENDOCARDITIS

Situation	Agent	Child or Adult	Regimen*
Standard prophylaxis for persons not allergic to penicillin	Amoxicillin (oral)	Adult	2.0 g orally 1 hour before the procedure
		Child	50 mg/kg orally 1 hour before the procedure
Allergic to penicillin	Clindamycin (oral)	Adult	600 mg orally 1 hour before the procedure
		Child	20 mg/kg orally 1 hour before the procedure
	or		
	Cephalexin (oral)	Adult	2.0 g orally 1 hour before the procedure
	or cefadroxil (oral)	Child	50 mg/kg orally 1 hour before the procedure
	or		
	Azithromycin (oral) or	Adult	500 mg orally 1 hour before the procedure
	clarithromycin (oral)	Child	15 mg/kg orally 1 hour before the procedure
Unable to take oral medications	Ampicillin (intramuscularly or intravenously)	Adult	2.0 g within 30 minutes before the procedure
		Child	50 mg/kg within 30 minutes before the procedure
Allergic to penicillin and unable to take oral medications	Clindamycin (intravenously)	Adult	600 mg within 30 minutes before the procedure
		Child	20 mg/kg within 30 minutes before the procedure
	or		
	Cefazolin† (intramuscularly	Adult	1.0 g within 30 minutes before the procedure
	or intravenously)	Child	25 mg/kg within 30 minutes before the procedure

*Total children's dose should not exceed adult dose.
†Cephalosporins should not be used in individuals with allergic reactions to penicillins.
Adapted from Dajani AS et al: Prevention of bacterial endocarditis, *Journal of the American Medical Association* 277(22):1798, 1997.

TABLE 9–7 RECOMMENDED ANTIBIOTIC PROPHYLAXIS REGIMENS WITH TOTAL JOINT REPLACEMENTS*

Situation	Agent	Regimen
Patients not allergic to penicillin	Cephalexin, cephradine, or amoxicillin (oral)	2 g orally 1 hour prior to the dental procedure
Patients not allergic to penicillin and unable to take oral medications:	Cefazolin or ampicillin (intramuscularly or intravenously)	Cefazolin 1 g or ampicillin 2 g intramuscularly or intravenously 1 hour prior to the procedure
Patients allergic to penicillin	Clindamycin (oral)	600 milligrams orally 1 hour prior to the dental procedure
Patients allergic to penicillin and unable to take oral medications	Clindamycin (intravenously)	600 mg intravenously 1 hour prior to the procedure

* No second doses are recommended for any of these dosing regimens.
From the American Dental Association, American Academy of Orthopaedic Surgeons: Antibiotic prophylaxis for dental patients with total joint replacements, *Journal of the American Dental Association* 128(7):1004, 1997.

TABLE 9–8 DENTAL MANAGEMENT CONSIDERATIONS WHEN USING ANTIBIOTICS FOR CLIENTS AT RISK OF INFECTION

Management of At-risk Individuals	Management Rationale
1. Use prophylactic antibiotics only during the perioperative period (0.5–1 hour before treatment and no more than 6-8 hours after)	This reduces development of microbial resistance.
2. Establish and maintain the best oral health. Professional dental care is indicated on a regular basis. Aggressively treat acute orofacial infections. Educate the client.	Incidence and magnitude of bacteremias of oral origin are directly proportional to the degree of oral inflammation and infection.
3. Gentle rinsing with an antiseptic mouthrinse such as 0.12% chlorhexidine gluconate or povidone-iodine for 30 seconds prior to dental treatment.	Antiseptic mouthrinsing immediately before dental care may reduce the incidence and magnitude of bacteremia. Resistant microorganisms may result if the antiseptic is used in a sustained or frequently repeated manner.
4. Schedule appointments for procedures requiring antibiotic prophylaxis 9 to 14 days apart.	This reduces emergence of resistant microorganisms and allows repopulation of the usual antibiotic-susceptible flora.

Table continued on following page

TABLE 9–8 DENTAL MANAGEMENT CONSIDERATIONS WHEN USING ANTIBIOTICS FOR CLIENTS AT RISK OF INFECTION—CONT'D

Management of At-risk Individuals	Management Rationale
5. If appointments for procedures requiring antibiotic prophylaxis are scheduled less than 9 days apart or if a client is currently on a regimen antibiotic for other reasons, use an alternative regimen antibiotic.	This reduces emergence of resistant microorganisms.
6. A combination of procedures should be planned for a dental appointment in which the client is prophylaxed.	This reduces the number of times a client is premedicated, which lowers cost and decreases the likelihood of resistant microorganisms emerging.
7. Encourage full/partial denture wearers to have periodic oral exams and return to their provider if discomfort develops.	Ill-fitting removable oral prostheses can cause tissue ulceration with concomitant bacteremia of oral origin.
8. When unanticipated bleeding occurs, administer antibiotic prophylaxis within 2 hours following the procedure.	This provides effective prophylaxis when a client has not been premedicated and intraoral bleeding occurs. There is no prophylactic benefit if one administers antibiotic 4 or more hours after a procedure induces oral bleeding.

From Johnson TE et al: Management of patients needing antibiotic prophylaxis in a dental education setting, *Journal of Dental Education* 64(4):276, 2000.

TELEPHONE CONTACT. Immediate medical consultation by telephone with the physician of record and referral are indicated if the client reveals a condition that precludes dental hygiene care or needs urgent dental or medical attention. Telephone consultation with the client's physician should be documented in the client's dental record and followed up with a written consultation form (Figure 9–5).

WRITTEN REQUEST. When the dental hygienist requests information in writing from the client's physician, the request should be duplicated and a copy placed in the client's dental chart. Sample medical consultation forms are shown in Figure 9–6. For convenience, the medical consultation form can be on NCR-type paper or on the computer, which facilitates the duplication process. A formal written request for medical consultation is the preferred procedure.

REFERRAL. Clients should be referred for medical evaluation when an undiagnosed disease condition is suspected or when needed laboratory test results are not available.

Text continued on page 174

FOOTHILL COLLEGE
12345 El Monte Road, Los Altos Hills, CA 94022-4599
Dental Hygiene Care Facility Telephone #: (650) 949-7335 Fax #: (650) 949-7375

To:

From: Foothhill College Dental Hygiene Care Facility

Re: Confirmation of Phone Conversation

This is to confirm our phone conversation on ______________________ regarding our
(Date)

patient ______________________________.
(Patient's name)

According to our conversation, it is my understanding that: ______________________________

____

____

____

____

____

Please verify the conversation by completing the attached referral letter. Return the referral letter and the white copy of this letter to:

Foothill College Dental Hygiene Care Facility
12345 El Monte Road,
Los Altos Hills, CA 94022-4599

Thank you for your prompt attention to this matter.

______________________________ ______________________
(Dental hygiene student signature) (Date)

______________________________ ______________________
(Faculty signature) (Date)

white - return to Foothill College yellow - physician copy pink - FC patient chart

(3ref/9-95)

FIGURE 9–5 ✦ Sample medical telephone consultation form. *(From Foothill College, Dental Hygiene Program, Los Altos Hills, Calif.)*

FOOTHILL COLLEGE
12345 El Monte Road, Los Altos Hills, CA 94022-4599
Dental Hygiene Care Facility **Telephone #:** (650) 949-7335 **Fax #:** (650) 947-9788

To:

From: Foothill College Dental Hygiene Care Facility

Re: Need for Antibiotic Premedication

______________________ is being seen at the Foothill College Dental Hygiene Clinic. The treatment we are recommending involves scaling and root planing. This procedure involves the smoothing of the unattached surfaces of the teeth by removing calculus and/or cementum. It is performed with the use of a local anesthetic. The anesthetic of choice is ______________________. Since scaling and root planing procedures do contact the blood stream, causing a transient bacteremia, we are requesting this medical consultation prior to proceeding with dental hygiene treatment.

This patient's health history indicates: ______________________

Please evaluate this/these condition(s). Indicate your recommendations and/or contraindications for patient treatment by checking one of the following sections, and signing below. Please return the white copy to our clinic.

❑ Antibiotic premedication is necessary. If so, what regimen? (The patient must receive the prescription from you) ______________________

❑ Dental hygiene care should be postponed at this time because: ______________________

❑ No special considerations are required. Proceed with dental hygiene care.

❑ Other ______________________

______________________ (Dental hygiene student signature) ______________________ (Date)

______________________ (Faculty signature) ______________________ (Date)

______________________ (Physician signature) ______________________ (Date)

______________________ (Physician address, city, zip code) ______________________ (Physician's phone number)

white - return to Foothill College yellow - physician copy pink - FC patient's chart

(2premed/11-96)

FIGURE 9–6 ✦ Sample medical consultation form. *(From Foothill College, Dental Hygiene Program, Los Altos Hills, Calif.)*

FOOTHILL COLLEGE

12345 El Monte Road, Los Altos Hills, CA 94022-4599

Dental Hygiene Care Facility Telephone #:(650)949-7335 Fax #:(650) 947-9788

To:

From: Foothill College Dental Hygiene Care Facility

Re: Medical Clearance Prior to Dental Hygiene Treatment

______________________________ would like to receive dental hygiene treatment at the Foothill College Dental Hygiene Clinic. It is anticipated that the care may extend over a couple of months with a series of appointments of 3 1/2 hours duration. The treatment we are recommending involves scaling and root planing, which is the smoothing of the unattached surfaces of the teeth by removing calculus and/or cementum. This procedure is performed with the use of a local anesthetic, and the anesthetic of choice is ______________________________.

When there is any question regarding the patient's health status, it is our policy to obtain guidance from his/her physician prior to proceeding with dental hygiene care. This patient's health history indicates:

____

____

Please evaluate this health condition. Indicate your recommendations and/or contraindications for patient treatment by checking one of the following and signing below. Please return the white copy to our clinic.

❑ Postpone dental hygiene treatment at the present time because: ______________________________

____

❑ This patient's health status is not a contraindication for proceeding with dental hygiene treatment.

❑ Proceed with dental hygiene treatment including the following modifications: ________________

____

____

❑ Other ____

______________________________	______________________________
(Dental hygiene student signature)	(Date)
______________________________	______________________________
(Faculty signature)	(Date)
______________________________	______________________________
(Physician signature)	(Date)
______________________________	______________________________
(Physician address, city, zip code)	(Physician phone number)

white - return to Foothill College yellow - physician copy pink - FC patient chart

(7medcle/9-95)

FIGURE 9–6, CONT'D.

Client Education Issues

- Counsel clients predisposed to an emergency situation in the dental setting by utilizing the information on the clients' health history. For example, a client who has a history of diabetes mellitus should be counseled to eat and take his or her insulin, as normal, the day of an appointment.
- When a medical consultation is indicated, educate the client about the concerns of a suspected condition and the risks of proceeding with care without proper medical advice.
- Educate clients about the rationale for prophylactic antibiotic premedication.

Legal, Ethical, and Safety Issues

- The health history should be recorded in nonerasable pen only.
- The history form is completed by the client. Information can be added by the client and the dental hygienist while reviewing the health history form with the client. Emergency phone numbers and physician phone numbers should always be present on the form in the event that a medical emergency occurs and appropriate personnel can be notified.
- A *medical alert box,* a space at the top of the health history form, can be used to alert the practitioner to client conditions that require dental hygiene care modifications and to prevent health risks. Conditions should be written into the box in red.
- Mistakes or errors are carefully lined out, dated, and initialed. In some instances, explanations may be necessary to avoid confusion. For example, if at a later date, the client remembers an allergy to penicillin, the correction should be made and an explanation added, such as "client remembers an allergy to penicillin" (date and initial).
- Document the discussion that occurs during review of the written health history form. The hygienist should review the written comments with the client and the client should sign or initial.
- The health history form contains confidential information to be shared only with those involved directly with the client's treatment. The dental hygienist should check with state and local regulations concerning disclosure of the HIV/AIDS status of a client on the medical history form.
- Medical consultation or referrals should be written documents outlining the need for consultation or referral. One copy of the form is sent, faxed, or given to the client. One copy of the form is kept inside the client's chart to document the need for consultation or referral. When necessary, telephone consults should be documented in the client's chart, including details of the conversation and the name of the person spoken to at the physician's office.
- Signed informed consent forms should always be used.
- Care should be provided to a minor only after an appropriate signature is obtained from the parent or legal guardian on the minor's informed consent form.

Key Concepts

- The personal, dental, and health history form is a legal document that contains important information about the client's state of health.
- The dental hygienist–client relationship is a partnership, based on trust, that has the client's well-being as a mutual focus.
- The client completes the written health history questionnaires at the first visit. Then in an oral interview, the dental hygienist reviews, discusses, and verifies the information on the health history questionnaire. The health history is then reviewed at each appointment to document changes.
- The dental hygienist uses open-ended questions in the health history interview.
- The ASA Physical Status Classification system can be used to identify the medical risk of the client and can prevent medical emergencies from occurring.
- Stress reduction protocols control the risk of a medical emergency and create a satisfactory experience for the anxious client.
- The *PDR* is a key reference for identifying and determining drug actions, interactions, contraindications, adverse reactions, warnings, and precautions. The *Merck Manual* is a useful reference for information concerning diseases or medical conditions.
- In certain circumstances the client's physician should be consulted prior to dental hygiene care.

Key Concepts—cont'd

- Infective endocarditis can be a life-threatening state caused by high-risk dental procedures including scaling and root planing or other aspects of dental hygiene care. Clients susceptible to infective endocarditis should be carefully evaluated and referred to their physician or cardiologist if necessary to determine if prophylactic antibiotic premedication is needed.
- Clients with total joint replacements are susceptible to infections from high-risk dental procedures. Clients susceptible to joint infection should be carefully evaluated and referred to their physician or orthopedist if necessary to determine need for prophylactic antibiotic premedication.
- Immunosuppressed individuals may be susceptible to infections from high-risk dental procedures. Clients susceptible to life-threatening infections should be carefully evaluated and referred to their physician if necessary to determine need for prophylactic antibiotic premedication.
- Schedule appointments requiring prophylactic antibiotic premedication 9 to 14 days apart to reduce the emergence of resistant microorganisms.
- A client may have an undiagnosed disease that can be recognized by a comprehensive health history review. Because some clients may seek oral healthcare more often than medical care, the health history review and updates are monitors of a client's health and risk status.

Critical Thinking Exercises

Client Profile: Mr. Smith is a 35-year-old male client who currently is not married and is self-employed as a contractor.

Chief Complaint: "To get my teeth taken care of."

Dental History: Mr. Smith has not been to a dentist for over 10 years. A local endodontist referred him to the general dentist. The referral letter noted that Mr. Smith has a large abscess below the badly decayed tooth #30. The endodontist noted that Mr. Smith placed aspirin directly on the gingival tissues near #30, resulting in a chemical burn on the gingiva. Mr. Smith needs extensive restorative and nonsurgical periodontal care. Unfortunately, Mr. Smith has rescheduled his first appointment with the general dentist three times. Another appointment was scheduled for a full periodontal assessment with the dental hygienist. This appointment was also rescheduled several times by Mr. Smith, which delayed treatment for months.

Health History: Mr. Smith has a history of asthma and diabetes. His asthma is controlled with a bronchodilator (Albuterol); Type 1 diabetes is controlled by daily insulin and diet. His last asthma attack occurred recently at the endodontist's office, but was relieved by using the bronchodilator. Mr. Smith reports no problems with his diabetes and says that he is seeing a physician on a regular basis for the diabetes and the asthma. He is also taking medication (Procardia) to control high blood pressure. His vital signs recorded at the first office were within normal limits. He does not indicate any "yes" answers to questions concerning negative experiences in a dental office or nervousness about treatment.

Extraoral Examination: All within normal limits.

Supplemental Notes: Client arrives late for his 5:00 P.M. appointment. At 5:15 P.M. the dental hygienist escorts him to the treatment room to review the health and dental history. The hygienist notices that Mr. Smith appears to be nervous about dental treatment. Mr. Smith is "jumpy" and perspiring heavily. The health history is reviewed and no changes have occurred other than the recent asthma attack.

1. Before any dental hygiene assessments begin, what is the appropriate step in caring for Mr. Smith?
2. What is Mr. Smith's ASA classification?
3. What ASA protocols could apply to Mr. Smith?
4. What type of dialogue should occur with Mr. Smith to prevent a hypoglycemic episode before rendering dental hygiene care?
5. What type of behaviors are documented on the health history that might be suggestive of fear and anxiety?

For References, Suggested Readings, and Related Websites, visit
http://evolve.elsevier.com/Darby/hygiene/

CHAPTER 10

VITAL SIGNS

OBJECTIVES

Mastery of the content in this chapter will enable the reader to:

- Assess temperature, pulse, respiration, and blood pressure and record these vital signs measurements
- Initiate medical referrals for the health and safety of the client
- Minimize risk of a medical emergency via vital signs assessment
- Compare baseline measurements to current findings and communicate significant changes to the client and dentist

KEY TERMS

Auscultation
Auscultatory gap
Blood pressure
Bradycardia
Diastolic blood pressure
Hypertension
Hypotension
Korotkoff sounds
Manometer (mercury, aneroid, electronic)
Premature ventricular contractions (PVC)
Pulse
Radial pulse
Respiration
Sphygmomanometer (blood pressure cuff)
Stethoscope
Systolic blood pressure
Tachycardia
Temperature
Thermometer (mercury-in-glass, electronic, disposable, tympanic membrane)
Vital signs

VITAL SIGNS

Temperature, pulse, respiration rate, and blood pressure are indicators of health status referred to as *vital signs.* Measurement of vital signs provides baseline data on the client's state of health and assists with identifying undiagnosed medical problems (see Normal Values for Vital Signs in Children and Adults). Inspection, palpation, and *auscultation* (listening for sounds produced in the body either directly or with a stethoscope) are the basic techniques used to determine vital signs. Vital signs are part of the base data collected during assessment.

When to Take Vital Signs lists appropriate occasions for the dental hygienist to measure and record the client's vital signs.

Vital signs outside an acceptable range may indicate health problems, undiagnosed conditions, the need for referral to a physician, or the need to terminate dental hygiene care. In addition to illness, the temperature of the environment, physical exertion, diet, stress, improperly used equipment, and unreliable equipment can affect vital signs. The dental hygienist analyzes the vital signs to interpret their significance and make clinical decisions. If abnormal readings are obtained, the dental hygienist questions the client about possible causes and repeats vital sign measurement. When readings that exceed normal limits are validated, the dental hygienist communicates them to the client, dentist, and physician of record. The following practice guidelines assist in obtaining accurate vital signs:

NORMAL VALUES FOR VITAL SIGNS IN CHILDREN AND ADULTS

Age	Temperature	Pulse (Average and Range) (BPM)	Respirations (Average and Range) (RPM)	Blood Pressure (mm Hg)
1–3	37.7°C (rectal) 99.4°F	120 (80–140)	30 (20–40)	90/55–95/65
6–8	37°C (oral) 98°	100 (75–120)	20 (15–25)	95–105/57–65
10	37°C (oral)	70 (50–90)	19 (15–25)	102/62
Adolescents	37°C (oral)	70 (50–90)	18 (15–20)	110–120/65–80
Adults	37°C (oral) 97–98.6°F	80 (60–100)	16 (15–20)	120/80
Older adults (>70 years)	36°C (oral)	80 (60–100)	16 (15–20)	120–140/80–90

When to Take Vital Signs

During the client's initial visit (baseline readings)
Annually for a client who is within normal limits
Whenever a significant change occurs in the client's health history
At each appointment for a client with readings that exceed the normal limits but who is being currently monitored by a physician
Before the administration of a local anesthetic agent or nitrous oxide–oxygen analgesia
Before, during, and after surgical procedures
If the client reports symptoms that indicate a potential emergency situation or when a medical emergency is in progress

- ✦ Use properly working equipment designed for the size and age of the client (e.g., an adult-size blood pressure cuff should not be used for a child or obese person)
- ✦ Know the client's health and pharmacologic history; some illnesses, treatment(s), behaviors, and medications affect vital signs
- ✦ Minimize environmental factors that may affect vital signs (e.g., do not assess temperature in a warm, humid room)
- ✦ Use a systematic approach for each procedure
- ✦ Approach client in a calm, caring manner while demonstrating competence in vital sign measurement

BODY TEMPERATURE

Body temperature is regulated by the brain's hypothalamic area, which acts as the body's thermostat. The hypothalamus senses changes in temperature and sends impulses out to the body to correct them. For example, on a hot day the hypothalamus detects a rise in body temperature and sends signals to the skin to perspire and lower its temperature. In cold weather the hypothalamus detects a lowering of the body's temperature and signals the body to shiver, increasing body temperature.

TABLE 10–1 FACTORS THAT AFFECT BODY TEMPERATURE

Factors	Effects
Exercise	Increases body temperature
Hormonal influences	Decrease or increase body temperature
Before ovulation	Decrease body temperature below baseline
During ovulation	Increase body temperature to baseline or higher
Menopause	Periodically increase body temperature
Time variations	Temperature at minimum level
Early morning	Temperature is lowest
Daytime	Body temperature rises
Evening	Body temperature peaks
Stress (physical and emotional)	Increases body temperature
Warm environment	Increases body temperature
Cold environment	Decreases body temperature
Infection	Increases body temperature

No single temperature is normal for all people. The range of normal for body temperature is 96.0 to 99.5 degrees Fahrenheit (or 35.5 to 37.5 degrees Celsius). As the body produces heat, it is also losing heat.

Heat produced – heat lost = body temperature

For the body temperature to be maintained, there must be a balance between heat loss and heat production. With aging, the normal temperature range gradually narrows because the mechanisms that control thermoregulation start to deteriorate. Table 10–1 lists factors that affect body temperature.

Body Temperature Measurement Sites

The oral cavity (under the tongue) is the most common site for measuring body temperature. Caution should be taken to prevent inaccurate readings if hot or cold foods have been ingested or if the client has been smoking. Alternative sites such as the ear (tympanic membrane) or axilla (armpit) should be used when the client's safety is a consideration. For example, unconscious clients, infants, small children, or cognitively challenged clients may have difficulty with the oral thermometer under the tongue or may bite the thermometer and break it.

Thermometers

There are four types of thermometers available for measuring body temperature (Table 10–2 and Figures 10–1 to 10–3). Disposable plastic sheaths can be used over the probe end of the thermometers as a protective barrier for infection control. The electronic and the mercury-in-glass thermometers are commonly used at home and in professional practice. The mercury-in-glass thermometer should be handled carefully to avoid breakage and inadvertent spillage of the contents. If a mercury-in-glass thermometer is broken, it should be cleaned up immediately to prevent mercury contamination or poisoning (see Steps to Take in the Event of a Mercury Spill).

Mercury clean-up kits can be purchased from dental supply companies. The electronic (digital) thermometer consists of a probe attached to a digital readout (Figure 10–2). Tympanic membrane (ear) thermometers

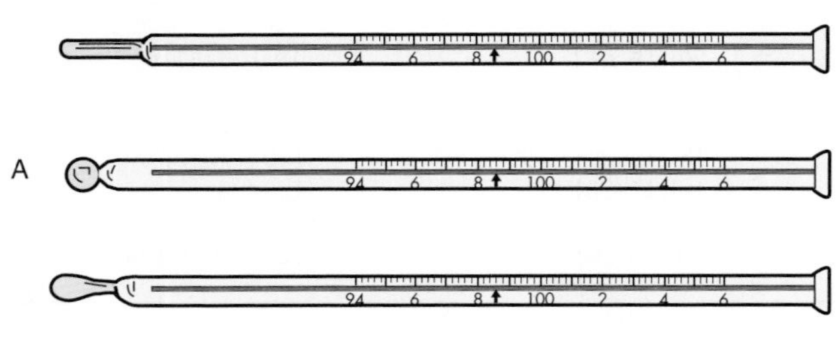

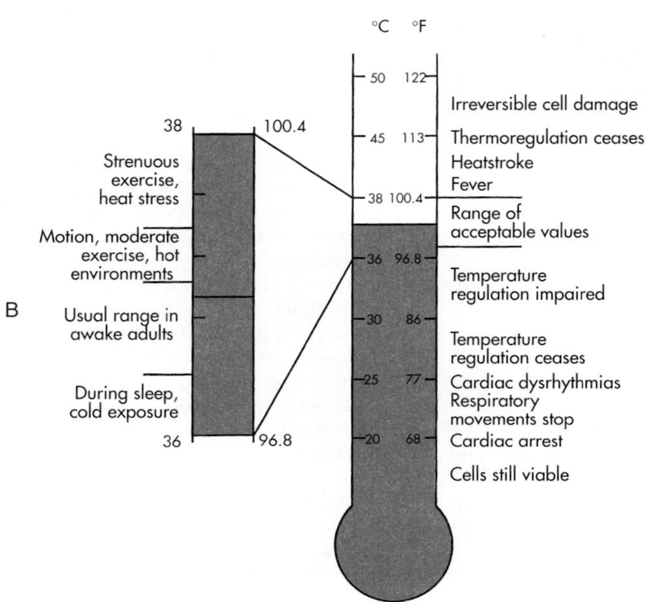

FIGURE 10–1 ✦ **A,** Types of mercury-in-glass thermometers. **B,** Ranges of normal temperature values and physiological consequences of abnormal body temperature. *(From Potter PA, Perry AG:* Fundamentals of nursing, *ed 5, St Louis, 2001, Mosby.)*

Steps to Take in the Event of a Mercury Spill

1. Do NOT touch spilled mercury droplets. If skin contact has occurred, immediately flush area with water for 15 minutes.
2. If possible, remove client from contaminated environment.
3. Change any clothing or linens contaminated with mercury. Wash hands thoroughly after changing. Wash clothing before reuse.
4. Notify the environmental services department or obtain a mercury spill kit.
5. Follow procedures for mercury removal as directed by Material Safety Data Sheet (MSDS). Spills are removed using special absorbent materials, filtered-vacuum equipment, and protective clothing.
6. Reduce concentration of mercury vapors with exhaust ventilation.
7. Complete *incident report* as directed by institution procedure (see Chapter 6, Figure 6–30).

From Potter PA, Perry AG: *Fundamentals of nursing,* ed 5, St Louis, 2001, Mosby.

TABLE 10–2 TYPES OF THERMOMETERS FOR MEASURING BODY TEMPERATURE

Name	Types Available	Disadvantages	Advantages
Mercury-in-glass thermometer	Oral (elongated tip) Stubby (used for any site) Rectal (pear-shaped tip)	Longer reading time (must control environmental factors such as recent intake of hot or cold fluid, smoking) Caution needed to avoid breakage	Low price Availability Reliability Accuracy
Electronic thermometer	Oral Rectal Axillary	Potential for inaccuracies due to shorter reading time (must control environmental factors such as recent intake of hot or cold fluid, smoking)	Short reading time Decreased client discomfort Efficient for healthcare professional Easy to read
Disposable thermometer	Oral	Cost	Short reading time Disposable Good for maintaining infection control
Tympanic membrane thermometer	Ear	Not as accurate as other methods in detecting fever in children under 6 years of age	Less invasive Short reading time

(Figure 10–3) are easy to use, are less invasive, and can achieve a reading within 2 to 5 seconds; however, its use is not recommended for children under 6 years of age. Oral and axillary disposable, single-use thermometers can indicate a client's temperature within 70 seconds. Disposable thermometers are used mostly for oral temperature screening. See Procedures 10–1 and 10–2 for taking basal body temperature orally using two different types of thermometers. Temperature is recorded in degrees Fahrenheit.

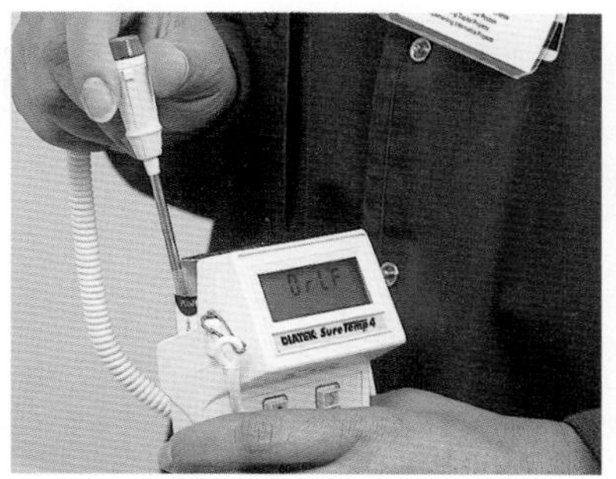

FIGURE 10–2 ✦ Electronic thermometer. *(From Potter PA, Perry AG:* Fundamentals of nursing, *ed 5, St Louis, 2001, Mosby.)*

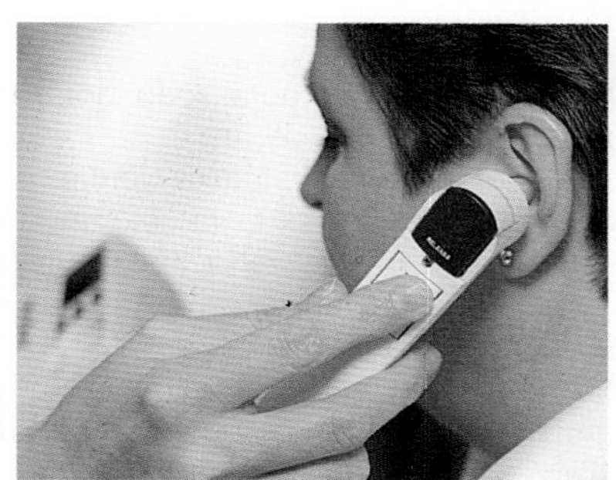

FIGURE 10–3 ✦ Tympanic membrane thermometer. *(From Potter PA, Perry AG:* Fundamentals of nursing, *ed 5, St Louis, 2001, Mosby.)*

Procedure 10–1 TAKING AN ORAL TEMPERATURE MEASUREMENT WITH A MERCURY-IN-GLASS THERMOMETER

EQUIPMENT

Mercury-in-glass thermometer, disposable sheath
Personal protective equipment for the clinician, accurate timepiece

STEPS	RATIONALE
1. Wash hands with antimicrobial soap; don barriers.	Reduces chances of transmitting infectious microorganisms
2. Explain the procedure to the client.	To inform the client of the hygienist's intent
3. Ask the client if hot or cold substances were recently ingested.	This can alter the client's true temperature
4. Hold the end of the thermometer opposite the mercury end with your fingertips.	This prevents contamination of the bulb to be inserted into the client's mouth
5. Before inserting the thermometer into the client's oral cavity, read the mercury level.	Mercury is to be below 35.5°C (96°F); thermometer reading must be below the client's actual temperature before use
6. If the mercury is above the desired level, shake the thermometer so that the mercury moves toward the bulb. Grasp the tip of the thermometer securely and stand away from any solid objects. Sharply flick the wrist downward as though you were cracking a whip. Continue until the reading is at the appropriate level.	Brisk shaking lowers the mercury level in the glass tube; standing in an open spot prevents breakage of the thermometer
7. Place disposable cover or sheath on thermometer.	This prevents cross-contamination
8. Ask client to open his or her mouth and gently place the thermometer under the tongue lateral to the lower jaw.	Heat from lingual arteries under the tongue produces the temperature readings
9. Ask client to hold the thermometer with the lips closed. Warn client to avoid biting down on the thermometer.	The lips hold the thermometer in the proper position during recording to prevent breakage of the thermometer
10. Leave the thermometer in place for 3 full minutes or as directed by the manufacturer.	The thermometer should remain in place for a minimum of 3 minutes and no longer than 6 minutes
11. Carefully remove the thermometer.	
12. Remove and discard the disposable cover.	The cover should be removed to allow maximum visibility and should be discarded in the appropriate manner to prevent cross-contamination
13. Read thermometer as it is held in a horizontal position.	To obtain an accurate reading
14. Wash the thermometer in soap and water. Disinfect the thermometer.	Prevents cross-contamination in the event that the disposable cover breaks or tears
15. Store the thermometer in its proper container.	Proper storage prevents breakage and contamination
16. Record client's temperature, the date, and the time of day on the chart.	Vital signs should be recorded immediately, before they are forgotten
17. Inform dentist of readings above 38°C (99.6°F).	A client experiencing fluctuations in temperature should be referred to his or her physician for immediate consultation

Adapted from Potter PA, Perry AG: *Fundamentals of nursing,* ed 5, St Louis, Mosby, 2001.

Procedure 10–2 TAKING AN ORAL TEMPERATURE MEASUREMENT WITH AN ELECTRONIC THERMOMETER

EQUIPMENT

Electronic thermometer, disposable sheath
Personal protective equipment for the clinician

STEPS	RATIONALE
1. Wash hands with antimicrobial soap; don barriers.	Reduces chances of transmitting infectious microorganisms
2. Explain procedure to the client.	Inform client of the hygienist's intent
3. Ask client if hot or cold substances were recently ingested.	May alter the client's true temperature
4. Remove thermometer pack from charging unit, check to make sure the oral probe is attached to the unit.	To prepare the unit
5. Insert the oral probe into the plastic, disposable cover until it locks into place.	Prevents cross-contamination
6. Ask the client to open his or her mouth and gently place the probe under the tongue, posterior and lateral to the lower jaw.	Body heat from the lingual arteries under the tongue produces the temperature readings; more-accurate readings are obtained with electronic oral thermometers if placed in the posterior area
7. Ask the client to hold the probe with the lips closed.	The lips hold the probe in the proper position
8. An audible tone will signal that the temperature has been taken and will be displayed.	
9. Remove the probe and discard the disposable cover by pushing the ejection button.	Prevents cross-contamination
10. Place probe back into original storage well in the unit.	Prevents damage to probe and clears digital readout
11. Return the thermometer to the charger.	Keeps unit charged and ready for use
12. Record the client's temperature, the date, and the time of day on the chart.	Vital signs should be recorded immediately before they are forgotten
13. Inform the dentist of readings above 38°C (99.6°F).	A client experiencing fluctuations in temperature should be referred to his or her physician for immediate consultation

Adapted from Potter PA, Perry AG: *Fundamentals of nursing*, ed 5, St Louis, 2001, Mosby.

Decision Making Based on Observed Temperature

Usually, a high temperature is an indication that the body is fighting an infection. If the client's temperature exceeds 99.6 degrees Fahrenheit, the client should be evaluated for causative factors (Table 10–1); the client may need to be rescheduled for another oral care appointment, and a physician referral may be indicated. A low temperature can occur with hypothyroidism, some viral infections, chronic debilitation, and excess alcohol intake.

TABLE 10–3 ACCEPTABLE RANGES OF PULSE DATA

Age	Pulse Rate (Beats Per Minute)
Infants	120–160
Toddlers	90–140
Preschoolers	80–110
School-agers	75–100
Adolescents	60–90
Adults	60–100

Modified from Potter PA, Perry AG: *Fundamentals of nursing*, ed 5, St Louis, Mosby, 2001, p. 697.

PULSE

The *pulse* is the intermittent beat of the heart that is felt through the walls of an artery, an indicator of the integrity of the cardiovascular system. *Tachycardia* is an abnormally elevated heart rate, above 100 beats per minute in adults. However, it is a normal response to stress or physical exercise. *Bradycardia* is an abnormally slow heart rate, below 60 beats per minute in adults (Table 10–3). Athletes may be bradycardic at rest due to physical conditioning. Table 10–4 describes factors that influence pulse rate.

Pulse Measurement Sites

The most common site for assessing the pulse is the thumb side of the inner wrist *(radial pulse)* (Figure 10–4, Procedure 10–3). The fingertips of the first two fingers are used to feel for the pulse (a throbbing sensation). *Never use the thumb to feel for the pulse, since it has a pulse of its own that can be mistaken for the client's.* If the radial pulse cannot be felt, the carotid pulse, located on the side of the neck, is an alternative. The pulse is recorded in beats per minute (BPM).

Decision Making Based on Observed Pulse Rate

If the client's heart rate falls under 60 BPM or rises above 110 BPM, the client should be evaluated for causative factors or conditions. If no cause can be determined, a

TABLE 10–4 FACTORS INFLUENCING PULSE RATES

Factor	Increased Pulse Rate	Decreased Pulse Rate
Exercise	Short-term exercise	A conditioned athlete who participates in long-term exercise will have a lower heart rate at rest
Temperature	Fever and heat	Hypothermia
Emotions	Acute pain and anxiety increase sympathetic stimulation, affecting heart rate.	Unrelieved severe pain increases parasympathetic stimulation, affecting heart rate; relaxation
Drugs	Positive chronotropic drugs such as epinephrine	Negative chronotropic drugs such as digitalis
Hemorrhage	Loss of blood increases sympathetic stimulation	
Postural changes	Standing or sitting	Lying down
Pulmonary conditions	Diseases causing poor oxygenation	

From Potter PA, Perry AG: *Fundamentals of nursing*, ed 5, St Louis, 2001, Mosby.

Procedure 10–3 MEASURING THE RADIAL PULSE

EQUIPMENT

Wristwatch with a second hand

STEPS	RATIONALE
1. Use a wristwatch with a second hand.	Allows the clinician to make an accurate assessment
2. Wash hands with antimicrobial soap.	Reduces the chances of transmitting infectious microorganisms
3. Explain the purpose and method of procedure to the client.	Relieves the client's anxiety and facilitates cooperation during the procedure
4. Have the client assume a sitting position, bend the client's elbow 90 degrees, and support the client's lower arm on the armrest of the chair. Extend the wrist with the palm down.	Proper positioning exposes the radial artery for palpation
5. Place the first two fingers of your hand along the radial artery and lightly compress them against it (Figure 10–4).	The fingertips are most sensitive to vibration
6. Obliterate the pulse initially, and then relax pressure so that the pulse is easily palpable.	The pulse is more accurately assessed with moderate finger pressure; too much pressure occludes the pulse, and too little prevents the examiner from feeling the pulse with regularity
7. When the pulse can be felt regularly, use the watch's second hand and begin to count the rate, starting with 0 and then 1, and so on.	The rate is determined accurately only after the examiner is certain that the pulse can be palpated. Timing should begin with 0. The count of 1 is the first beat felt after timing begins
8. If the pulse is regular, count for 30 seconds and multiply the total by 2.	A regular rate is accurately assessed in 15 seconds
9. If the pulse is irregular, count for a full minute.	The longer time ensures an accurate count
10. Assist the client to a comfortable position.	
11. Record heart rate (BPM), rhythm of the heart (regular or irregular), the quality of the pulse (thready, weak, bounding), and the date in the chart. Pulse rates outside the normal range should be evaluated by the client's physician.	Vital signs should be recorded immediately on the client's record

Adapted from Potter PA, Perry AG: *Fundamentals of nursing*, ed 5, St Louis, 2001, Mosby.

medical consultation should be obtained from the client's physician.

If the client is experiencing five or more *premature ventricular contractions (PVCs)* per minute, a medical consultation should be considered. A PVC is a break, or skip, in the normal rhythm, and the dental hygienist will detect an interruption in successive pulse waves.

A medical consultation is recommended for a client who presents with alternating strong and weak heartbeats, which may indicate ventricular failure, high blood pressure, or coronary heart disease.

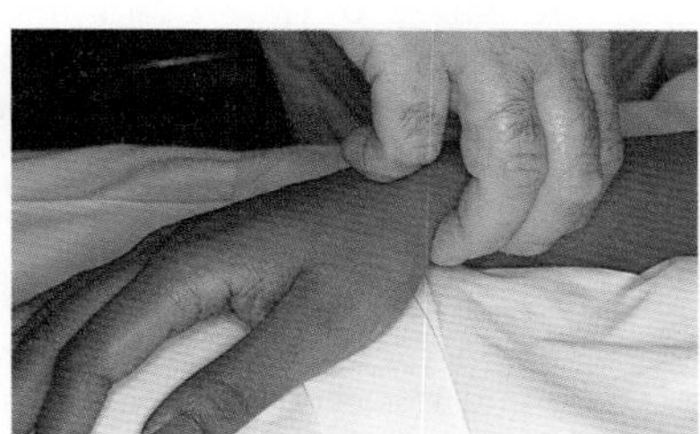

FIGURE 10–4 ✦ Position of the fingers in measuring the radial pulse. *(From Potter PA, Perry AG:* Fundamentals of nursing, *ed 5, St Louis, 2001, Mosby.)*

A full, bounding pulse may indicate high blood pressure. A weak, thready pulse usually is found in persons with hypotension and is a sign of shock.

RESPIRATION

Respiration rate is assessed by counting the rise and fall (inspiration and expiration) of the client's chest, and is recorded as respirations per minute or RPM. The dental hygienist makes this assessment without the client's awareness to prevent the client from changing breathing patterns.

Respiration Measurement Site

The respiration rate may be measured before or after taking the client's pulse rate. The dental hygienist's hand remains on the client's radial pulse while the hygienist *inconspicuously* counts the respiratory rate.

Normal adult range for respiration rate is 12 to 20 RPM. Children have a more rapid respiratory rate (20 to 30 RPM for a 6-year-old child) than that of adults. Young children also tend to have a less regular breathing cycle. Advancing age produces an increase in the respiration rate. Steps for measuring respirations are shown in Procedure 10–4.

Decision Making Based on Observed Respiration

If an abnormal respiratory rate is detected, the dental hygienist refers the client to the physician of record for a medical consultation and evaluation. Table 10–4 presents acceptable range of respiratory rates by age.

BLOOD PRESSURE

Blood pressure, the force exerted by the blood against the arterial walls when the heart contracts, is an important indicator of current cardiovascular function. Blood pressure also indicates the risk of future cardiovascular morbidity and mortality. Chronic hypertension causes thickening and loss of elasticity in the arterial walls, which can lead to serious disorders such as heart failure, stroke, and kidney failure. There are no adverse effects from low blood pressure *(hypotension)* unless the client is in a state of shock or is affected by a disorder or condition that may lower the blood pressure. In fact, the lower the blood pressure, the better the long-term prognosis for cardiovascular health. An acute change in blood pressure can indicate an emergency situation such as shock or rapid hemorrhaging.

Blood pressure is measured in millimeters of mercury (mm Hg). The two measurements taken for blood pressure are the systolic blood pressure and the diastolic blood pressure:

- ✦ *Systolic blood pressure* measures the maximum pressure occurring in the blood vessels during cardiac ventricular contraction (systole) and is the number on the sphygmomanometer when the first sound is heard.
- ✦ *Diastolic blood pressure* measures the minimum pressure occurring against the arterial walls as a result of cardiac ventricular relaxation (diastole) and is the number on the sphygmomanometer when the last sound is heard.

When documenting blood pressure, the dental hygienist records the date and arm used. Blood pressure is recorded as a fraction. The optimal systolic and dia-

Procedure 10–4 MEASURING RESPIRATIONS

EQUIPMENT

Wristwatch with second hand

STEPS	**RATIONALE**
1. Use a wristwatch with a second hand.	Allows the dental hygienist to make an accurate assessment
2. Place your hand along the client's radial artery and inconspicuously observe the client's chest.	Allows the dental hygienist to make the assessment without the client's awareness of the process
3. Observe the rise and fall of the client's chest. Count complete respiratory cycles (one inspiration and one expiration).	The respiratory rate is equivalent to the number of respirations per minute; young infants and children breathe in an irregular rhythm
4. For an adult, count the number of respirations in 30 seconds and multiply that number by two. For a young child, count respirations for a full minute.	
5. If an adult has respirations with an irregular rhythm, or if respirations are abnormally slow or fast (<12 or >20 breaths/minute), count for a full minute.	Accurate interpretation requires assessment for at least a minute
6. While counting, note whether depth is shallow, normal, or deep and whether rhythm is normal or one of the altered patterns.	The character of ventilatory movements may reveal specific alterations or disease states
7. Record the date and the client's respirations per minute (RPM) in the chart; respiration rate that is outside of the normal range should be evaluated by the physician.	Vital signs should be recorded immediately

Adapted from Potter PA, Perry AG: *Fundamentals of nursing*, ed 5, St Louis, 2001, Mosby.

stolic measurements for adults 18 years and older is 120/80 mm Hg. The top number of a given blood pressure is the systolic measurement, and the bottom number is the diastolic measurement (d = down). A client has high blood pressure (hypertension) if the systolic blood pressure is 140 mm Hg or greater and the diastolic blood pressure is 90 mm Hg or greater. Table 10–5 presents average optimal blood pressure for different ages, and Table 10–6 classifies blood pressure for adults ages 18 and older. Table 10–7 describes factors that influence blood pressure.

Decision Making Based on Observed Blood Pressure

A medical consultation is indicated for persons with abnormal blood pressure (Table 10–8). Blood Pressure Guidelines Used in the Dental Hygiene Process of Care provides guidance regarding the ranges of blood pressure and their relationship to the ASA classification and dental hygiene care.

Blood Pressure Equipment and Measurement

SPHYGMOMANOMETER. Commonly referred to as a *blood pressure cuff,* the *sphygmomanometer* consists of a pressure-measuring device called a *manometer* and an inflatable cuff that wraps around the arm or leg (Table 10–9).

The *mercury manometer* (Figure 10–5) is an upright tube containing mercury. The column of mercury is moved upward by the pressure created by the inflation of the bladder. The height of the mercury column is marked by millimeter calibration. When the cuff is deflated, the mercury must be at zero. Although mercury manometers are more accurate than aneroid manometers, the potential for breakage and spilling of mercury is a disadvantage. Mercury is a health hazard if not properly contained.

TABLE 10–5 AVERAGE OPTIMAL BLOOD PRESSURE BY AGE

Age	Blood Pressure (mm Hg)
Newborn 3000 g (6.6 lb)	75/40 (mean)
1 month	85/54
1 year	95/65
6 years	105/65
10–13 years	110/65
14–17	120/75
Middle adult	120/80
Older adult	140/90

From Potter PA, Perry AG: *Fundamentals of nursing,* ed 5, St Louis, 2001, Mosby.

TABLE 10–6 CLASSIFICATION OF BLOOD PRESSURE FOR ADULTS AGES 18 AND OLDER

Category	Systolic (mm Hg)		Diastolic (mm Hg)
Optimal	<120		<80
Normal	<130		<85
High normal	130–139		85–89
Hypertension			
Stage 1 (mild)	140–159	or	90–99
Stage 2 (moderate)	160–179	or	100–109
Stage 3 (severe)	≥180	or	≥110

From Potter PA, Perry AG: *Fundamentals of nursing,* ed 5, St Louis, 2001, Mosby.

TABLE 10–7 FACTORS INFLUENCING BLOOD PRESSURE

Factors	Effects
Age	Blood pressure rises with age. Newborns have the lowest mean systolic blood pressure (75 mm Hg), which peaks at puberty and then declines slightly. As people age, elasticity in the arteries declines, producing an increase in blood pressure. Hypertension is common in the elderly (≥60 years).
Race	Prevalence of hypertension in African and Hispanic Americans is considerably higher than in the white population, and hypertension tends to appear earlier in life in these groups.
Weight	Blood pressure tends to be elevated in overweight and obese persons. Oversized blood pressure cuffs are necessary for accurate readings.
Gender	Hormonal variation causes females to have lower blood pressure after puberty than males. Preeclampsia is abnormal hypertension experienced by some women during pregnancy. Postmenopausal women experience higher blood pressure than before.
Emotional stress	Stress stimulates the sympathetic nervous system, which in turn increases cardiac output and vasoconstriction. The outcome is elevated blood pressure.
Pain	Pain decreases blood pressure, and if severe, can cause shock.
Oral contraceptives	These can increase blood pressure; however, the change is usually within normal limits.
Medications	Medications vary in their ability to increase and decrease blood pressure. Medications must be reviewed at each appointment to determine effects on blood pressure.
Diurnal variation	Blood pressure varies with metabolic rate. Pressure is lowest in the morning, then rises and peaks in the late afternoon or early evening.
Chronic disease	Diseases that affect cardiac output, blood volume, blood viscosity, or arterial elasticity will increase blood pressure.
Tobacco, alcohol, and caffeine use	Chronic, heavy intake of nicotine, alcohol, and and/or caffeine elevates blood pressure.

TABLE 10–8

CLASSIFICATION OF ADULT BLOOD PRESSURE AND DENTAL TREATMENT MODIFICATIONS

Category	Systolic Pressure (mm Hg)	Diastolic Pressure (mm Hg)	Dental/Dental Hygiene Treatment
Normal	<130	<85	No modification of care
High normal	130–139	85–89	No modification of care
Hypertension			
Stage I	140–159	90–99	No modification of care; medical referral; inform client
Stage II	160–179	100–109	Selective dental care*; medical referral
Stage III	180–209	110–119	Emergent nonstressful procedures†; immediate medical referral/consultation
Stage IV	≥210	≥120	Emergent nonstressful procedures†; immediate medical referral/consultation

* Selective dental care may include, but is not limited to, oral prophylaxis, nonsurgical periodontal therapy, restorative procedures, and nonsurgical endodontics.
† Emergent nonstressful procedures may include, but are not limited to, dental procedures that may help alleviate pain, infections, or masticatory dysfunction. These procedures should have limited physiologic effects. An example of an emergent nonstressful procedure might be a simple incision and drainage of an intraoral fluctuant abscess. The medical benefits achieved by performing emergent nonstressful procedures in state III and IV hypertensive persons should outweigh the risk of complications secondary to the client's hypertensive state.
From Muzyka BC, Glick M: The hypertensive dental patient, *Journal of the American Dental Association* 128(8):1109, 1997.)

BLOOD PRESSURE GUIDELINES USED IN THE DENTAL HYGIENE PROCESS OF CARE

Blood Pressure (mm Hg)	ASA Physical Status Classification*	Dental and Dental Hygiene Therapy Considerations and Interventions Recommended
<140 systolic and <90 diastolic	I	No unusual precautions related to client management based on blood pressure readings Recheck in 6 months
140–159 systolic and/or 90–94 diastolic	II	No unusual precautions related to client management based on blood pressure readings needed unless blood pressure remains above normal after three consecutive appointments Recheck blood pressure prior to dental or dental hygiene therapy for three consecutive appointments; if all exceed these guidelines, seek medical consultation Stress-reduction protocol if indicated, such as administration of nitrous oxide–oxygen analgesia, should be considered
160–199 systolic and/or 95–114 diastolic	III	Recheck blood pressure in 5 minutes; if still elevated, seek medical consultation prior to dental or dental hygiene therapy No unusual precautions related to client management based on blood pressure readings after medical approval is obtained Stress reduction protocol if indicated, such as administration of nitrous oxide–oxygen analgesia
>200 systolic and/or >115 diastolic	IV	Recheck blood pressure in 5 minutes; immediate medical consultation if still elevated Dental or dental hygiene therapy, routine, or emergency treatment may be performed if nitrous oxide–oxygen analgesia lowers the blood pressure below >200 systolic or >115 diastolic If blood pressure is not reduced using nitrous oxide–oxygen analgesia, only (noninvasive) emergency therapy with drugs (analgesics, antibiotics) is allowable to treat pain and infection Refer to hospital if immediate dental therapy is indicated

Adapted from Malamed SF: *Medical emergencies in the dental office*, ed 5, St Louis, 2000, Mosby.
* See Chapter 9 for an explanation of ASA Physical Status Classification.

Portable and lightweight, the *aneroid sphygmomanometer* has a glass-enclosed circular gauge containing a needle that registers millimeter calibrations. Aneroid manometers require periodic biomedical calibration to assure their accuracy. The aneroid model has metal parts that expand and contract due to temperature changes and therefore are less reliable than the mercury type.

The *electronic manometer* determines blood pressure automatically (Figure 10–6).

A baseline blood pressure should be obtained using a mercury manometer before applying automatic devices. Comparison assists in evaluation of a client's blood pressure status and allows proper programming of the device. Electronic devices are easy to use, but are more susceptible to error. Error is due to the fact that electronic devices are sensitive to outside interference such as client movement or noise. Such factors interfere with the sensor signal of the manometer.

TABLE 10–9 MAIN TYPES OF MANOMETERS USED IN BLOOD PRESSURE MEASUREMENT

Name	Advantages	Disadvantages
Mercury sphygmomanometer (Figure 10–5)	Most accurate	Bulky Possible mercury spillage
Aneroid sphygmomanometer (Figure 10–5)	Lightweight Portable Compact	Needs to be recalibrated to mercury manometer
Electronic sphygmomanometer (Figure 10–6)	Easy to use Stethoscope not required	Needs to be recalibrated to mercury manometer Sensitive to outside interference Susceptible to error

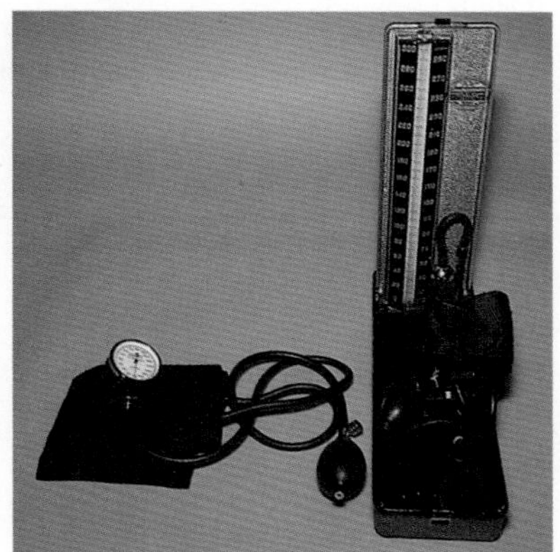

FIGURE 10–5 ✦ Portable sphygmomanometers. Mercury manometer *(right)*. Aneroid manometer *(left)*. *(From Potter PA, Perry AG:* Fundamentals of nursing, *ed 5, St Louis, 2001, Mosby.)*

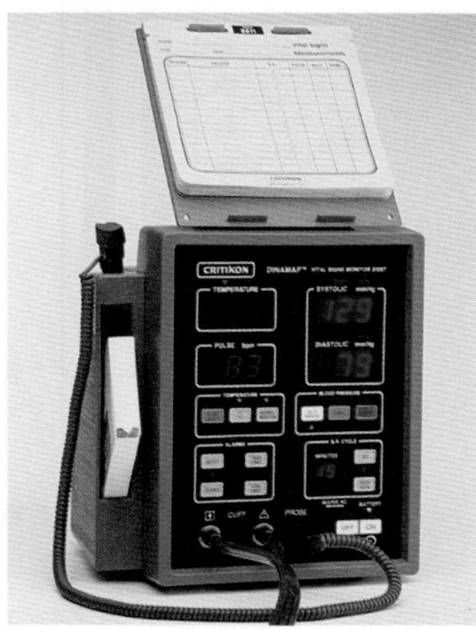

FIGURE 10–6 ✦ Automatic blood pressure monitor. Dinap Vital Signs monitor is a trademark of Critikon, Inc. *(Courtesy Critikon, Inc., Tampa, Fla.) (From Potter PA, Perry AG:* Fundamentals of nursing, *ed 5, St Louis, 2001, Mosby.)*

Parts of a manometer are similar regardless of the type. The parts include an occlusive cloth cuff that encloses an inflatable rubber bladder and a pressure bulb with a release valve that inflates the bladder. Large adult cuffs and thigh cuffs also are available.

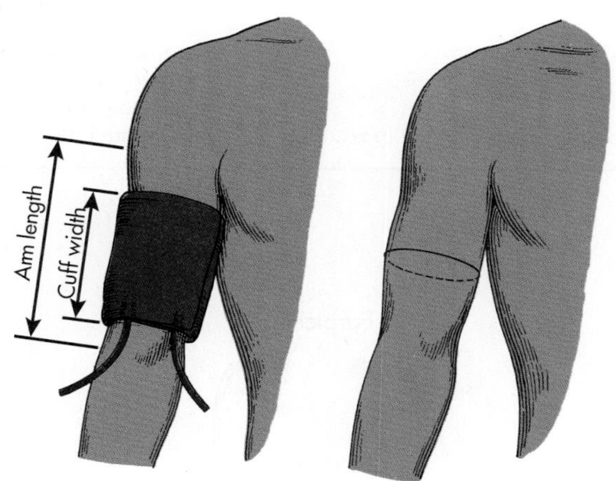

FIGURE 10–7 ✦ Guidelines for proper blood pressure cuff size. Cuff width = 20% more than upper arm diameter or 40% of circumference and two thirds of arm length. *(From Potter PA, Perry AG:* Fundamentals of nursing, *ed 5, St Louis, 2001, Mosby.)*

Proper cuff size of the sphygmomanometer is necessary for an accurate blood pressure reading. The size selected is proportional to the circumference of the midpoint of the upper arm being assessed (Figure 10–7). In an adult, the bladder within the cuff should encircle at least two thirds of the arm and an entire arm of a child.

False high readings can occur if the cuff is too narrow; false low readings can occur if the cuff is too wide. Moderately obese individuals require use of a large adult cuff. Morbidly obese individuals (arm circumference >41 cm) require use of a thigh cuff (18 cm wide). Although cuffs may be labeled newborn, infant, child, small adult, and large adult, the practitioner should not rely on client age as the basis of cuff selection (Table 10–10).

STETHOSCOPE. The *stethoscope,* an instrument used to amplify sound, consists of two earpieces, plastic or rubber tubing, and a chestpiece. The chestpiece has two sides, the bell and the diaphragm (Figure 10–8).

Either end of the chestpiece can be used; however, the bell end is recommended because it transmits low-pitched

TABLE 10–10 COMMON MISTAKES IN BLOOD PRESSURE ASSESSMENT

Effect	Error
False high reading	Bladder or cuff too narrow Cuff wrapped too loosely or unevenly Deflating cuff too slowly (false high diastolic reading) Arm below heart level Arm not supported Inflating too slowly or deflating too quickly (false high diastolic reading) Stethoscope that fits poorly or impairment of examiner's hearing causing sounds to be muffled (false low systolic reading) Cold hands of examiner; cold equipment
False low reading	Bladder or cuff too wide Deflating cuff too quickly (false low systolic reading) Arm above heart level Stethoscope that fits poorly or impairment of examiner's hearing causing sounds to be muffled (false low systolic reading) Repeating assessments too quickly (false low systolic reading)
Inaccurate interpretation of readings	Inaccurate inflation level

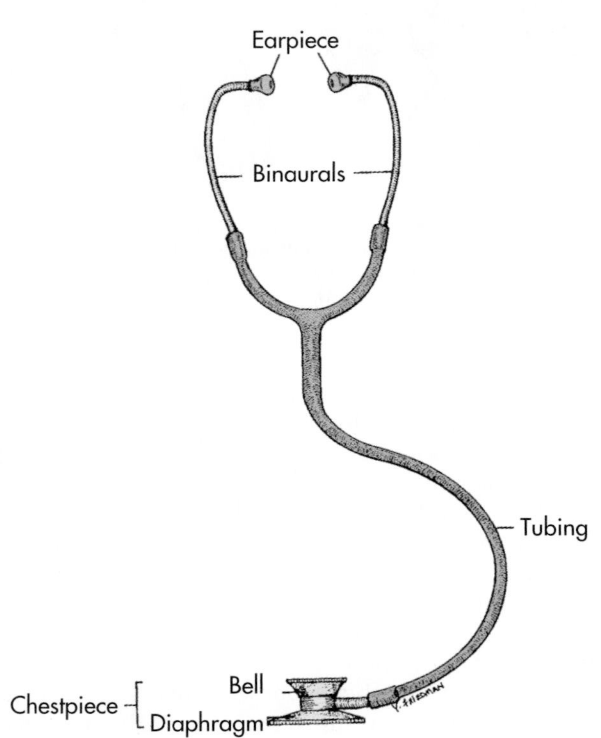

FIGURE 10–8 ✦ Parts of a stethoscope. *(From Potter PA, Perry AG:* Fundamentals of nursing, *ed 5, St Louis, 2001, Mosby.)*

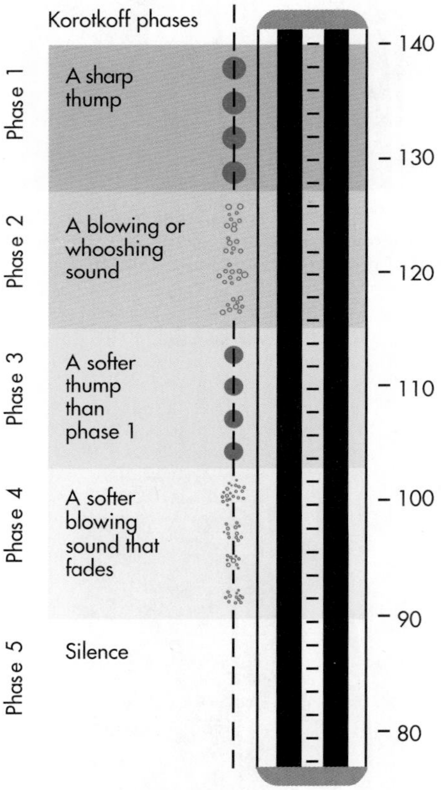

FIGURE 10–9 ✦ Korotkoff phases. *(From Potter PA, Perry AG:* Fundamentals of nursing, *ed 5, St Louis, 2001, Mosby.)*

sounds if held lightly against the skin. Hearing the pulse is difficult if the bell-shaped end is pressed too tightly against the skin.

When the bladder within the occluding cuff is deflated, the blood begins to flow intermittently through the brachial artery, producing rhythmic, knocking sounds. These sounds are referred to as *Korotkoff sounds*. As the cuff is deflated further, the Korotkoff sounds become less audible, and the pulse eventually disappears. There are five Korotkoff sounds that are described in phases (Figure 10–9).

An *auscultatory gap* is often present in hypertensive clients. This gap appears between the first and second systolic sounds. Therefore, it is important that the dental hygienist assess the point at which the pulse is obliterated while increasing the pressure in the bladder prior to taking the blood pressure by auscultation. Moreover, the clinician should increase the bladder pressure 30 mm Hg higher than the point at which the pulse is obliterated when measuring blood pressure (Procedure 10–5). Once taken, blood pressure should be documented in writing and dated in the client's chart (e.g., "7/13/03—Blood pressure in right arm, 160/9 mm Hg with auscultatory gap between 160 and 120").

Procedure 10–5 ASSESSING BLOOD PRESSURE BY AUSCULTATION

EQUIPMENT

Blood pressure cuff or sphygmomanometer
Stethoscope

STEPS	RATIONALE
1. Determine the proper cuff size. Inspect the parts of the release valve and the pressure bulb. The valve should be clean and freely movable in either direction.	The proper cuff size is necessary so that the correct amount of pressure is applied over the artery. Cuffs that are too small for a client's arm produce artificially high blood pressure readings; cuffs that are too large produce artificially low readings. If the valve sticks or becomes too tightly closed, the deflation of the pressure cuff will be hard to regulate.
2. Wash hands with antimicrobial soap.	Washing reduces the chances of transmitting infectious microorganisms.
3. Explain the purpose of the procedure.	Explanations reassure the client and increase the likelihood of compliance in the event of an abnormal reading.
4. Assist the client to a comfortable sitting position, with arm slightly flexed, forearm supported, and palm turned up.	This position facilitates cuff application. Having the arm above heart level would produce a falsely low reading.
5. Expose the upper arm fully.	Exposing the upper arm ensures proper cuff application.
6. Palpate the brachial artery. Position the cuff approximately 1 inch above the brachial artery.	Proper positioning of the cuff facilitates an accurate reading.
7. Center the arrows marked on the cuff over the brachial artery.	Inflating the bladder directly over the brachial artery ensures that proper pressure is applied during inflation.
8. Be sure the cuff is fully deflated. Wrap the cuff evenly and snugly around the upper arm.	This ensures that proper pressure will be applied over the artery.
9. Be sure the manometer is positioned for easy reading.	Eye-level placement ensures accurate reading of the mercury level.
10. If the client's normal systolic pressure is not known, palpate the radial artery and inflate the cuff to a pressure 30 mm Hg above the point at which radial pulsation disappears. Deflate the cuff and wait 30 seconds.	This determines the maximal inflation point and prevents auscultatory gap. The 30-second delay prevents venous congestion and falsely high readings.
11. Place the stethoscope earpieces in the ears and be sure sounds are clear, not muffled.	Each earpiece should follow the angle of the examiner's ear canal to facilitate hearing.
12. Place the diaphragm (or the bell) of the stethoscope over the brachial artery.	Proper stethoscope placement ensures optimal sound reception. The American Heart Association recommends use of the bell for hearing low-pitched Korotkoff sounds clearly.
13. Close the valve of the pressure bulb clockwise until tight.	Tightening the valve prevents air leaks during inflation.
14. Inflate the cuff to 30 mm Hg above the client's normal systolic level.	Proper cuff inflation ensures accurate pressure measurement.
15. Slowly release the valve, allowing the mercury (or the needle of the aneroid gauge) to fall at a rate of 2 to 3 mm Hg per second.	Too rapid or slow a decline in the mercury level may lead to an inaccurate reading.
16. Note the point on the manometer at which the first two consecutive beats are heard.	The first Korotkoff sound indicates the systolic pressure. Blood pressure levels should be recorded in even numbers.
17. Continue cuff deflation, noting the point on the manometer at which the sound disappears (phase V).	Note: The American Heart Association recommends recording the fifth Korotkoff sound as the diastolic pressure in adults and children.
18. Deflate the cuff rapidly. To determine an average blood pressure and to ensure a correct reading, wait 30 seconds and then repeat the procedure for the same arm.	Continuous cuff inflation causes arterial occlusion, resulting in numbness and tingling in the arm. The delay prevents venous congestion and falsely high readings and provides an accurate assessment of the client's blood pressure. Blood pressure reading is repeated on the same arm because there may be as much as 10 mm Hg difference in readings between arms.

Continued on following page

Procedure 10-5 ASSESSING BLOOD PRESSURE BY AUSCULTATION—CONT'D

STEPS	RATIONALE
19. Remove the cuff from the client's arm. Assist the client to a comfortable position and cover upper arm.	Maintains client's comfort.
20. Fold the cuff and store it properly in a cool, dry place.	Proper maintenance of supplies contributes to instrument accuracy. Sunlight and heat may compromise rubber tubing.
21. Record in the client's chart the systolic over the diastolic blood pressure reading in mm Hg, the date, cuff size if it was an atypical size, and arm used for measurement (use guidelines in Normal Values for Vital Signs in Children and Adults on p. 177 to determine need for a physician referral).	Vital signs should be recorded immediately.

Adapted from Potter PA, Perry AG: *Fundamentals of nursing,* ed 5, St Louis, 2001, Mosby.

CLIENT EDUCATION ISSUES

- ✦ Educate client when abnormal vital signs are present and to initiate the proper physician referrals, when appropriate.
- ✦ Encourage compliance with recommended physician referrals and prescriptive medications to control abnormal vital signs.
- ✦ Explain risk factors for abnormal vital signs. Clients with high blood pressure may have no overt symptoms, yet the condition increases their risk of cardiac arrest and stroke.

LEGAL, ETHICAL, AND SAFETY ISSUES

- ✦ Always record the client's vital signs on the treatment record and refer to the client's baseline readings for comparison.
- ✦ Refer clients to their physicians for medical consultation when vital signs exceed normal ranges. Include copies of the referral letter in the client's chart for access and confirmation.
- ✦ Disinfect earpiece of stethoscope before and after use to avoid disease transmission.
- ✦ Never provide dental hygiene care for a client with an ASA IV classification.
- ✦ Vital signs must be measured and recorded during a medical emergency.
- ✦ Clients in hypertension-prone groups should have their blood pressure measured at each dental/dental hygiene appointment.

KEY CONCEPTS

- ✦ Abnormal vital signs can be due to client conditions, equipment failure, or operator error. The dental hygienist must take the vital signs accurately and control factors that contribute to errors.
- ✦ Most dental care environments take blood pressure, pulse, and respiration for baseline measurements as a comparison for subsequent appointments.
- ✦ Temperature is usually not regularly taken; however, the dental hygienist should take the temperature if the client has signs or symptoms of a fever.
- ✦ Pulse rate is recorded in BPM. The radial or carotid artery is often measured for the pulse using the first two fingers of the clinician's hand.
- ✦ The normal pulse rate for an adult at rest can range from 60 to 100 BPM. Children usually have a more rapid pulse rate than adults.
- ✦ If the client is experiencing five or more premature ventricular contractions (PVCs) per minute, a medical consultation should be considered.
- ✦ Respiration rate is determined by observing the rise and fall of the client's chest and is recorded as RPM.
- ✦ Normal adult range for respiration rate is 12 to 20 RPM. Children have a more rapid respiratory rate (20 to 30 RPM for a 6-year-old child) than adults.
- ✦ Two measurements taken for blood pressure are the systolic blood pressure and the diastolic blood pressure.
- ✦ Optimal systolic and diastolic measurements for adults 18 years and older are less than or equal to 120/80 mm Hg.
- ✦ Rhythmic, knocking sounds heard on the stethoscope when measuring blood pressure are referred to as Korotkoff sounds.

Critical Thinking Exercises

1. The client, a 30-year-old medical resident who works at a hospital in the emergency room, has a history of missing several dental appointments, numerous cancellations, and rescheduled appointments. She is 10 minutes late for her appointment and on arrival is still dressed in scrubs and looks weary. On inquiry, she states that she has had about 20 hours of sleep in the last week because of her residency assignment. Her health and pharmacologic history reveals migraine headaches, depression, mitral valve prolapse, and petit mal and grand mal epilepsy. She is currently taking a nonsteroidal antiinflammatory agent for her migraines when needed, a tricyclic antidepressant for depression, and Depakote (an anticonvulsant) medication for her epilepsy. She is taking her antidepressant and anticonvulsant on a regular basis and states that she has taken the medications the day of the appointment. She must also take amoxicillin for her mitral valve prolapse and reports an allergy to aspirin products, which has been confirmed by her physician. Her vital signs are pulse 70 BPM, respirations 16 breaths/minute, and blood pressure 120/90 mm Hg.
   - **A.** Prior to initiating dental hygiene care, what should the dental hygienist do?
   - **B.** The dental hygienist administers 2% lidocaine with 1:100,000 epinephrine for the PSA injection, giving a total of 3/4 of the total cartridge with no complications. Proper local anesthetic technique was given to the client, including aspiration that was negative. The client unexpectedly has a petit mal seizure. What is the most likely cause of the seizure?
   - **C.** After the seizure, the client admits that she forgot to take her prophylactic amoxicillin premedication for her mitral valve prolapse. The dental hygienist reschedules the client for treatment, and no treatment other than the local anesthesia administration was given. What recommendation concerning the premedication is indicated prior to dismissing the client?
   - **D.** The client calls the next day and reports difficulty with mouth opening and soreness of her jaw. What is the most likely cause of the problem?
2. The dental hygienist takes the client's blood pressure and obtains a reading of 125/90 mm Hg. The dental hygienist waits and measures the blood pressure again in 5 minutes and the blood pressure is 110/70 mm Hg. What circumstances could have caused the differences observed in the two readings? Discuss how the problem could be prevented in the future.
3. The dental hygienist takes the client's pulse several times and measures more than five preventricular contractions per minute. The finding is discussed with the client and the client is resistant to seeing his or her physician concerning the problem. Role play with a partner to demonstrate how to effectively manage the situation.

For References, Suggested Readings, and Related Websites, visit

http://evolve.elsevier.com/Darby/hygiene/

CHAPTER 11

Pharmacologic History

OBJECTIVES

Mastery of the content of this chapter will enable the reader to:

- Identify fundamental questions to gather a comprehensive pharmacologic history
- Identify resources to obtain current drug information and indications for drug use
- Differentiate between drug side effects, drug toxicity, and drug hypersensitivity
- Describe common side effects caused by medications
- Describe drug interactions significant to dental hygiene practice
- Explain how normal aging and youth alter drug pharmacokinetics
- Describe strategies to improve client compliance with medication use
- Discuss dental hygiene interventions to manage the oral side effects of medications
- Reduce risk of medical emergencies associated with drug use

KEY TERMS

Adverse drug effects
Cross-sensitivity
Dose schedule
Drug hypersensitivity
Drug idiosyncrasy
Drug interactions
Herbal medicine
Neutraceuticals
Over-the-counter drugs (OTC)
Pharmacokinetics
Pharmacologic history
Side effects
Teratogenicity/teratogenic effect
Tolerance
Toxicity reactions

Assessment includes taking a comprehensive *pharmacologic history* that provides information regarding past and present medications taken and offers clues about the client's health status and health behaviors. Often, a client does not consider a systemic health condition or information about medications to be within the scope of dental hygiene care, and will simply not report it on a health questionnaire. Omission of information about a medical condition or medications may be intentional if the client knows that divulging the information may require that the course of treatment be altered or that additional medical testing or treatment will be required. This situation is encountered with clients who do not wish to confirm the presence of a heart murmur by undergoing an echocardiogram, or those who dislike having to take prophylactic antibiotic premedication. Information also may be omitted when the client fears discrimination due to a violation of confidentiality. Sensitive issues such as taking medications for HIV, sexually transmitted diseases, or mental illness are managed to ensure client privacy and respect. Conversely, a conscientious client may forget to report medications simply because the client does not view these drugs as "medications." This often is the case with oral contraceptives, antacids, vitamin supplements, herbal supplements, and aspirin. Because many medications interact with drugs used in dentistry, or produce side effects, drugs have the potential to compromise client safety and function. The pharmacologic history enables the dental hygienist to assess risks associated with clients taking medications.

COMPREHENSIVE PHARMACOLOGIC HISTORY

Medication List

The first step of the pharmacologic history is compiling a list of all medications that the client is currently taking, including both prescription and nonprescription herbs and OTC (*over-the-counter*) drugs, with the name of the medication, the *dose schedule* (frequency of taking the medication), and any special instructions for use. Clients are asked about their own perceptions regarding their medications, and a physician consultation may be necessary to verify this information. Assistance may also be obtained from the clients' pharmacist or caregiver.

This list is helpful for assessing the client's attitude toward health and wellness. For example, clients using OTC vitamins and nutritional supplements, or "all natural" products known as *neutraceuticals,* may be more interested in nutritional counseling, or seek alternative medicine services. At times, unhealthy behaviors and attitudes may be determined by a client's misuse of drugs, such as abusing OTC stimulants for weight loss or illegal drugs and alcohol for recreational use.

Some people take drugs without understanding why they have been prescribed or knowing the expected outcome of medication therapy. Clients should be encouraged to keep written records of their medications, including dose schedules and the name of the prescribing physician, on their person at all times. This written record is helpful to all health professionals treating the client, and may be especially useful during an emergency situation. The dental hygienist helps the client develop this record as a health promotion activity, and updates it at each appointment. Chairside Drug References contains current drug information.

Chairside Drug References

American Dental Association: *ADA guide to dental therapeutics,* ed 2, Chicago, 2001, ADA.

Gage TW, Pickett FA: *Mosby's dental drug reference,* ed 6, St Louis, 2003, Mosby.

Haveles EB: *Pharmacology for dental hygiene practice,* ed 2, Albany, NY, 2003, Delmar.

PDR for herbal medicines, ed 2, Montvale, NJ, 2000, Medical Economics.

Requa-Clark B: *Applied pharmacology for the dental hygienist,* ed 4, St Louis, 2000, Mosby.

Wynn RL, Meiller TF, Crossley HL: *Drug information handbook in dentistry,* ed 8, Hudson, Ohio, 2002, Lexi-Comp.

Eight Fundamental Assessment Questions

QUESTION 1: WHY IS THE CLIENT TAKING MEDICATION? The dental hygienist assesses why the client is taking medication. Generally, medications are taken:

- *To treat an acute systemic condition:* Medications taken for acute conditions are generally recommended or prescribed for a defined time frame, usually of short duration, to manage the symptoms of the condition or to eliminate an infection (e.g., cough and cold preparations, antibiotics, antifungals, antidiarrheals, and pain relievers). The assumption is that when the medication is gone, so too will be the cause of the symptoms/problem in question.
- *To treat a chronic systemic condition:* Medications may be taken for longer duration or for extended periods throughout the lifetime (e.g., hypoglycemics, allergy drugs, and antihypertensives).
- *To prevent a condition from occurring:* Medications may be indicated for the prevention of a disease or condition (e.g., oral contraceptives to prevent pregnancy and daily aspirin to prevent stroke).
- *To prevent a recurrence of an existing condition:* Medications may be used preventively to ward off the recurrence of a chronic problem (e.g., inhaled steroids for asthma and anticonvulsants to prevent seizures).
- *To satisfy a habit, with no clinical indication or need:* Illegal street drugs have no clinical indication to justify usage. Alcohol consumption, caffeine, and nicotine may also be included in this category. Other drugs, such as daily aspirin and vitamin supplements, may be taken habitually without any documented clinical need, or because of a perceived health benefit, which may or may not exist. Table 11–1 lists common drug classes with indications for their use.

QUESTION 2: ARE SYMPTOMS REPORTED DURING THE CLIENT'S HEALTH HISTORY INTERVIEW CAUSED BY A MEDICAL CONDITION OR ARE THEY DRUG SIDE EFFECTS? Answering this question is a difficult challenge; therefore, attention must be paid to findings from the health history interview. The dental hygienist attempts to match the physical findings/symptoms reported by the client with existing medical/dental conditions. Drugs from the medication list should be suitable for the medical and dental conditions for which the client is being treated. Sometimes a doctor will prescribe an off-label use of a medication. When symptoms do not correlate with known conditions, the dental hygienist must then discern whether the client's medications may be contributing to the problem or if there may be an undiagnosed condition, either of which could explain the findings.

The following questions facilitate problem solving:

- Does the client have a known systemic condition?
- What are the symptoms reported by the client?
- Do these symptoms correlate with the client's known systemic condition?

TABLE 11-1 COMMON DRUG CLASSES ASSOCIATED WITH INDICATIONS FOR DRUG USE

Indications for Drug Use	OTC Drugs	Prescription Drugs
Management of an acute condition	Cold/sinus drugs Aspirin Acetaminophen NSAIDS Antiseptics Antifungals Laxatives Allergy drugs Cough preparations Antidiarrheals Antibacterials Antacids	Antibiotics Antifungals Pain medications Steroids
Management of a chronic condition	NSAIDS	Antihypertensives Antiarrhythmics Antidepressants Insulin Steroids NSAIDS Antianginals Inhalers (asthma) Diuretics Hormones Pain medications Oral hypoglycemics
Prevention of a potential condition	Aspirin Vitamins	Anticoagulants Antibiotics Antiepileptics Oral contraceptives
Prevention of recurrence of a condition	Allergy drugs	Gastric ulcer medications Antiepileptics Antianginals Anticoagulants Allergy drugs
Taken habitually—no clinical indication	NSAIDS Alcohol Vitamins	Illegal drugs Steroids Pain medications NSAIDS

NSAIDS, Nonsteroidal antiinflammatory drugs.
From Spolarich AE, Gurenlian JR: Deductive reasoning with pharmacology: a prescription for quality patient care, *Compendium in Continuing Education in Oral Hygiene* 1(4):5, 1994.

- Do the symptoms reported indicate the presence of an undiagnosed condition?
- What are the indications for the drugs being taken?
- Could the drug(s) be causing or contributing to the symptoms in question?

QUESTION 3: WHAT ARE THE ADVERSE EFFECTS OF THIS DRUG? All drugs have the potential to cause harm. When a drug is selected for use, the potential harm must be carefully weighed against its benefits. Drugs are extensively tested and regulated by the U.S. Federal Drug Administration (FDA) to ensure safety and efficacy. The FDA requires the reporting of all known adverse effects, which can be found in drug reference guides and accessed from the FDA Web sites (see Chairside Drug References and Web Site Information and Resources at http://evolve.elsevier.com/Darby/hygiene/).

Adverse drug effects, undesirable outcomes from drug therapy, include *side effects, toxicity reactions,* and *drug hypersensitivity.* When a drug is administered, the drug produces an exaggerated effect on its primary target tissue, so that when the correct therapeutic dose is given, the client experiences an extension of the desired drug effect. For example, a client with elevated blood glucose takes an oral hypoglycemic agent to adjust his blood glucose level within the normal range. However, the client experiences hypoglycemia, or a blood glucose level that is below normal. In this example, the drug produced the desired effect of lowering blood glucose; however, the level became too low, reflecting an extension of the therapeutic effect.

Conversely, when a drug is administered, it also produces an effect on nontarget tissue, where the effects produced by the drug differ from the desired therapeutic effects. For example, a client takes an ACE inhibitor to treat her hypertension, and although it lowers her blood pressure, she experiences a persistent dry cough. All drugs produce side effects, but most are tolerable and disappear when the drug is discontinued (see Common Side Effects of Medications).

Drug *toxicity* refers to toxin-induced cell damage and cell death from a medication. Usually, a drug does not produce damage directly to the cell itself. Rather, the damage is due to an active metabolite formed during metabolic breakdown by the liver or kidneys. Metabolites cause biochemical damage to cellular components, resulting in altered metabolism of the affected cell, cell mutation, or cell death. Unlike side effects, toxicity reactions cannot be tolerated, and cause permanent tissue damage on either the microscopic or macroscopic level. These are especially dangerous if major organ systems are involved. Drugs that produce these types of reactions may be labeled as hepatotoxic (causing liver damage), nephrotoxic (causing kidney damage), neurotoxic (causing nerve damage), or cardiotoxic (causing heart damage).

Drug hypersensitivity occurs when either the drug or its metabolites act as immunogens, triggering the immune response. Repeated exposure to the same drug produces this allergic response. Signs of a true allergic reaction include skin rash, itching, hives, bronchospasm, and rhinitis. Life-threatening allergic reactions include anaphylaxis, hemolysis, and bone marrow suppression. Allergic reactions are managed with epinephrine, corticosteroids, antihistamines, and assistance from emergency support personnel. The most dangerous aspect of allergic reactions is that they are not predictable and are not dose related. Clients with a history of allergy to a drug in any given class will be allergic to all of the drugs in the same class. In addition, some drugs, such as the penicillins and the cephalosporins, show *cross-sensitivity* to other drug groups with similar chemical structures. The dental hygienist must recognize the warning signs of an allergic reaction, so that appropriate treatment interventions can be administered promptly.

Common Side Effects of Medications

Hyperexcitability
Dizziness
Central nervous system effects
Changes in bleeding time
Hypertension
Weight changes
Edema
Photosensitivity
Blurred vision
Skin changes
Insomnia
Drowsiness
GI disturbances (nausea, vomiting, diarrhea)
Hypotension/fainting
Respiratory difficulties
Sweating
Appetite changes
Sexual dysfunction
Opportunistic infections (yeasts, fungal)
Loss of hair
Cardiac arrhythmias

From Spolarich A: Understanding pharmacology: Adverse drug effects, *Access* 9(10):29, 1995.

Other adverse drug effects include negative effects on fetal development, or *teratogenicity*. Many drugs cross the placenta and are secreted in breast milk; therefore, drugs are not tested on pregnant and lactating women. The FDA labels each drug with a pregnancy risk factor (A, B, C, D, X), which corresponds to one of five categories indicating the potential of a systemically absorbed drug to cause birth defects (see Chapter 46, Table 46–3). FDA pregnancy categories are published in all major drug reference texts.

Occasionally, a client experiences a side effect that is completely unexpected or different from any known published side effects. This unique response to a drug is called a *drug idiosyncrasy*. Clients may also report drug *tolerance*, which manifests as the need to take larger doses of the drug to produce the same response. This is one mechanism that can lead to drug addiction.

To answer Question #3, the dental hygienist assesses the following:

- ✦ What are the known published side effects of the drug(s)?
- ✦ Could the symptoms reported by the client be side effects of the drug(s)?
- ✦ Are reported symptoms indicative of a drug allergy?

QUESTION 4: ARE THERE POTENTIAL DRUG INTERACTIONS? Adverse drug effects can also be caused by *drug interactions*, the negative effects that can occur when two drugs are taken simultaneously. Drug interactions range in severity from mild alterations in drug action to life-threatening conditions in the client (e.g., alterations in drug efficacy, toxicity reactions, or other dangerous reactions such as hypertensive crisis, extended bleeding time, or respiratory depression).

Adverse drug interactions are prevented by knowing drug relationships. Dental professionals keep apprised of drug interactions by routinely reviewing lists of known interactions in standard drug reference texts and scientific publications. Drug interactions arise from a variety of mechanisms, and result in either a decreased or increased effect of one or more drugs. The greater the

SCENARIO 1

ASSESSMENT OF THE CLIENT'S PHARMACOLOGIC HISTORY

At his routine appointment, a 46-year-old Caucasian male reports that for the past two weeks he has been experiencing headaches on a daily basis, and occasional stomach pain that has progressively gotten more frequent and intense. He is scheduled to see his physician at the end of the month for a follow-up on the new hay fever medication that was prescribed two weeks ago. The health history review reveals arthritis of the knees, seasonal allergies, and hospitalization six months ago for surgery to reset a broken wrist. The client is taking ibuprofen PRN for arthritis pain and loratadine daily for allergy symptoms.

On further questioning, the hygienist finds that the client is taking 600 mg of ibuprofen qid, and has been taking loratadine, 10 mg/day as prescribed, for two weeks. The high doses of ibuprofen suggest that his arthritis pain is not well controlled. The client states that he always takes the same amount of ibuprofen, regardless of his pain level, "whether I need it or not, because that seems to keep the pain under control." He saw his physician two weeks ago to get a prescription-strength allergy medication because "the over-the-counter stuff just wasn't working anymore."

Case Analysis: The client has two known systemic conditions: arthritis and seasonal allergies. He reports two symptoms that require assessment: daily headaches and stomach pain of increasing frequency and intensity. When attempting to match the known conditions with the symptoms reported, a possible correlation can be found between the headaches and a sinus-related condition (seasonal allergies). No correlation can be made between stomach pain and arthritis or allergies. Several possible undiagnosed conditions may account for the client's daily headaches, including tooth clenching or grinding, a sinus infection, or hypertension; and a GI disorder, stomach virus, or stomach ulcer could explain his stomach pain.

The indications for the drugs taken by the client match his known conditions: ibuprofen for arthritis pain and loratadine for seasonal allergies. Medications may be contributing to the client's symptoms in question. First, chronic use of ibuprofen causes GI ulceration and bleeding, known side effects for NSAIDS. In this case, the client is taking three times the OTC dose for ibuprofen, four times per day, which is most likely contributing to his stomach pain. Second, headaches are a known side effect of loratadine, and the client has only experienced headaches for the past two weeks, which correlates with the time he has been taking this medication. The client is referred to his physician for further evaluation of his arthritis pain, a potential stomach ulcer, and his headaches, as these may be medication-related problems.

TABLE 11–2 COMMON DRUG INTERACTIONS SIGNIFICANT IN ORAL CARE

Drug	+	Drug	=	Adverse Effect
Oral contraceptives	+	Antibiotics	=	Reduced efficacy of oral contraceptives
Tetracyclines	+	Antacids	=	Reduced serum concentration and efficacy of tetracycline
	+	Penicillin	=	Impaired efficacy of penicillin
Erythromycin	+	Penicillin	=	Impaired efficacy of penicillin
	+	Theophylline (bronchodilator)	=	Nausea, vomiting, seizures
	+	Carbamazepine (Tegretol)	=	Carbamazepine toxicity: nausea, drowsiness, headache, dizziness, blurred vision
	+	Triazolam (Halcion)	=	Triazolam toxicity: psychomotor impairment and memory dysfunction
Ibuprofen	+	Oral anticoagulants	=	Increased bleeding
	+	Lithium	=	Lithium toxicity: nausea, vomiting, slurred speech, mental confusion
Aspirin	+	Oral anticoagulants	=	Increased bleeding
	+	Probenecid (Benemid)	=	Aspirin inhibits uricosuric action of probenecid
Epinephrine	+	Tricyclic antidepressants (Elavil)	=	Hypertension
	+	Monoamine oxidase inhibitors (Nardil, Parnate)	=	Hypertension
Narcotic analgesics	+	Cimetidine (Tagamet)	=	Increased adverse effects of narcotics (increased CNS effects)
Benzodiazepines (Valium)	+	Alcohol	=	Dangerous inebriation, ataxia, and respiratory depression

From Wynn RL et al: *Drug information handbook for dentistry*, ed 8, Hudson, Ohio, 2002, Lexi-Comp.

number of medications taken, the greater the likelihood of experiencing an interaction (Table 11–2.) To assess whether the client is experiencing a drug interaction, the dental hygienist consults a drug reference text and assesses:

- ✦ Are there any known drug interactions for this medication?
- ✦ Could the client's symptoms be indicative of a drug interaction?

QUESTION 5: DO THESE FINDINGS SUGGEST A PROBLEM WITH DRUG DOSAGE? Standard drug dosing schedules may be too strong for children and elderly clients, and may need to be altered to prevent adverse drug effects. The need to reduce drug dosages in these populations is directly related to drug *pharmacokinetics*. Children demonstrate an increased skin and mucous membrane permeability; therefore, they absorb medications much more readily and more quickly than their adult counterparts. In general, dosing schedules for children are half of the standard adult dose.

In the elderly, normal physiologic changes of aging dictate the need for a reduction in dosing. Increased stomach acidity alters drug absorption into circulation. Normally, the liver converts lipid-soluble drugs to water-soluble metabolites, thus inactivating the drug and allowing for filtration and elimination by the kidney. Both liver and kidney function decline with age; therefore, more drug stays active after passing through the liver, and the portion of the drug that remains lipid soluble is scavenged by the kidneys and either put back in circulation or stored in body fat. Production of plasma proteins, the binding sites for drugs in circulation, also declines with age. The portion of the drug that is unbound in the circulation is the active drug. The amount of active drug in circulation increases when the client takes multiple medications, all of which are competing for fewer binding sites. These physiologic changes manifest as an increased drug effect in the client, and contribute to unwanted adverse drug effects such as sedation, confusion, and extensions of desired therapeutic effects. As with children, doses for the elderly may need to be reduced to half of the standard adult dosing schedules. To assess the potential for complications caused by drug dosage, the dental hygienist considers:

- ✦ Have the client's age and weight been taken into account when determining drug dosage?
- ✦ Could the symptoms be attributed to altered drug pharmacokinetics due to normal physiologic changes of aging?

QUESTION 6: HOW IS THIS CLIENT MANAGING MEDICATIONS? Most clients take multiple medications and are treated by multiple healthcare providers. The lack of communication among these providers, all of whom may be prescribing medications, results in an increased risk for adverse drug reactions. The dental hygienist, as client advocate, encourages client compliance and assesses risks associated with medication use.

The client's ability to manage medications is confounded by a number of variables. First, the client may be self-medicating with either OTC or prescription medications, or both. Clients are usually unaware of potential adverse drug effects that can occur as a result of mixing medications, altering recommended dosing schedules, or mixing medications with supplements, alcohol, or certain foods. Second, clients may not read the warning labels on the medication packaging, or may not understand what they are reading. This is especially true when labels warn against using certain classes of drugs, or warn against using the medication because of a preexisting condition. The client may not be aware that he or she has a preexisting condition, such as enlarged prostate, hypertension, or thyroid disease. Others simply choose to ignore the warnings, and take the medication anyway. The small typeface on many labels poses yet another challenge for the visually impaired.

Failure to comply with medication use, intentional or unintentional, must be discerned by the dental hygienist. The dental hygienist never assumes that the client intuitively understands the prescribed regimen or reads the instructions from the pharmacy. Whenever a drug is dispensed or prescribed from the dental office, the dental hygienist provides detailed instructions. Even clients who are normally compliant are given instructions and an opportunity to ask questions to reinforce adherence to the prescribed regimen.

Familiarity with a routine can breed laziness in compliance. Just as clients learn proper dosing schedules, they can also learn to give the "right answer" to inquiries about taking their medications. In these instances, the dental hygienist must rely on the client's physical presentation as well as personal intuition to discern whether the client is truly following instructions. How well a client complies with medication use can reflect the client's willingness to comply with other professional recommendations, including self-care instructions and referrals.

Dental hygienists also facilitate information transfer between the client and other healthcare professionals. A call to the client's physician can clarify discrepancies in the client's understanding of her medications, and confirm that it is safe to provide treatment. Conversations between the dental hygienist and other practitioners should be documented in the services rendered portion of the client record. When assessing client compliance with medications, the dental hygienist focuses on:

- ✦ How many medications is the client taking?
- ✦ When was the client last seen by a physician? By the physician who prescribed the medication?
- ✦ What is the prescribed regimen for the medications?
- ✦ How many providers are prescribing medications for the client?
- ✦ How long is the client to remain on this medication?
- ✦ Does the client understand why the medication was prescribed?
- ✦ Have client instructions been provided for taking the medications? If so, by whom?
- ✦ Does the client understand the instructions for using the medications?

SCENARIO 2

ASSESSMENT OF THE CLIENT'S PHARMACOLOGIC HISTORY

The client is a 36-year-old African American female with a periodontal abscess associated with a 6 mm pocket on the mesiobuccal surface of tooth number 30. After thorough periodontal debridement under local anesthesia and irrigation with 0.12% chlorhexidine, the client is given oral hygiene instructions for keeping the site clean. The client also is instructed to take ibuprofen 200 mg for pain as necessary, and given prescriptions for penicillin 500 mg qid for 10 days and 0.12% chlorhexidine for rinsing bid. The client is scheduled to return in 10 days for evaluation.

When the client returns, the site is still inflamed and exudate is draining from the periodontal pocket. Upon questioning, the client states, "my gum looked so sore that I was afraid to touch it, but the medicine made it feel better after about three days, so I didn't think that I needed it anymore. Besides, it was giving me an upset stomach, so I figured that it was all right to stop taking it. The mouthwash left an aftertaste, which didn't help my upset stomach, so I rinsed my mouth out with water, but it made it taste even worse. I used it though, every day." Furthermore, the client took the ibuprofen twice on the day of the procedure only, then stopped, as she reported no additional pain.

Case Analysis: Assessment of the client's compliance suggests that she did not understand the need for the antibiotic or what to expect while taking this medication. The client should have been informed about: a) GI upset that commonly occurs with antibiotic use, and how to manage this side effect; b) the importance of taking the antibiotic until it was gone to ensure that the infection was treated completely and to reduce the risk of bacterial resistance. Also, this client demonstrated willingness to comply with the mouthrinse, but should have been informed about taste alteration as a side effect. By rinsing with water after using the 0.12% chlorhexidine mouthwash, the client was rinsing away the flavoring agent, and ended up tasting more of the medication that remained. Chlorhexidine will not resolve the remaining infection deep within the pocket. With the incomplete course of antibiotic therapy, the infection persists, and now requires re-treatment.

- ✦ Is the client self-medicating? Undermedicating or overmedicating?
- ✦ How many refills are there for the medication?
- ✦ Has the medication expired?

QUESTION 7: WILL ANY ORAL SIDE EFFECTS OF THIS MEDICATION REQUIRE INTERVENTION? Management of oral side effects is an ongoing challenge (see Common Oral Side Effects of Medications). Oral side effects cause client discomfort and interfere with the ability to chew, swallow, and digest food. Some oral side effects place the client at risk for oral trauma, and others lead to infection, pain, and possible tooth loss. Dental hygienists need to recognize these oral conditions in a timely manner and recommend appropriate treatment interventions. Professional intervention is often necessary to improve client comfort and function.

Common Oral Side Effects of Medications

Xerostomia
Dental caries
Change in taste
Difficulty with mastication
Difficulty wearing appliances
Oral ulcerations
Atrophic mucosa
Hairy tongue
Infection
Mucositis/stomatitis
Burning mouth/tongue
Difficulty with speech
Difficulty with swallowing
Increased periodontal disease progression
Opportunistic infections (candidiasis)
Bleeding
Gingival enlargement

From Spolarich A: Understanding pharmacology: Adverse drug effects, *Access* 9(10):29, 1995.

Classes of Drugs that Cause Xerostomia

Anorexiants
Antiacne drugs
Antianxiety agents
Anticholinergics
Anticonvulsants
Antidepressants
Antidiarrheals
Antihistamines
Antihypertensives
Antiinflammatory analgesics
Antinauseants
Antiparkinsonian agents
Antipsychotics
Antispasmodics
Bronchodilators
Decongestants
Diuretics
Muscle relaxants
Narcotic analgesics
Sedatives

Over 500 medications cause xerostomia, making it the most commonly reported oral side effect (see Classes of Drugs that Cause Xerostomia). Drug-induced xerostomia is a combination of reduced salivary flow rate and a change in both the nature and quality of the residual saliva. Residual saliva is more mucinous and viscous, facilitating food and plaque adherence to tooth surfaces, appliances, dentures, and oral tissues. The client will retain more food in the buccal vestibule after eating, due to the loss of natural salivary cleansing. The pH of the mouth becomes more acidic which, combined with plaque biofilm and food accumulation, places the client at increased risk for dental caries. Xerostomia-induced dental caries are evident along the gingival margin on exposed buccal and lingual root surfaces, at and underneath crown margins, and in root furcations. Caries can lead to extensive tooth destruction and possible tooth loss, which is particularly significant for teeth that serve as anchors to dental prostheses. Increased plaque acidity also contributes to dentinal hypersensitivity. Clients with xerostomia should be placed on supplemental daily fluoride therapy to reduce caries and dentinal hypersensitivity risks (see Chapters 26 and 33). Symptomatic relief of dry mouth and dry throat may be obtained through the use of artificial salivary substitutes or by taking pilocarpine, a drug that stimulates serous salivary flow (see Chapter 43, Table 43–2 and Recommendations for Clients with Xerostomia).

Under normal conditions, saliva maintains the balance of the oral ecosystem with immunologic and antibacterial processes that regulate the population of oral flora. When the ecosystem becomes unbalanced, the proportions of pathogenic and opportunistic organisms increase. Thus, the client is at greater risk for oral infections, including gingivitis, periodontitis, and both viral and fungal infections. Xerostomic clients greatly benefit from the use of daily antimicrobial therapy at home. Chlorhexidine and essential oil mouthrinses have demonstrated efficacy against periodontal pathogens and fungal organisms (see Chapter 24). Fungal infections are associated with use of antibiotics, immunosuppression, and underlying systemic diseases such as diabetes mellitus. Prescription antifungal therapy (e.g., Nystatin) is indicated, and often repeated, in xerostomic clients with recurrent fungal infections. Fungal infections may manifest as white plaques overlying red oral mucosa, burning mouth syndrome, symptomatic geographic tongue, and angular cheilitis (see Chapters 46 and 49).

Salivary mucins lubricate the oral mucous membranes, protect against ulceration and penetration of toxins, and assist with wound healing and repair. Xerostomic clients present with friable mucous membranes, which are highly susceptible to trauma from toothbrushing, mastication, and rubbing against appliances and dentures. Essential oil mouthrinse has been shown to reduce the incidence and severity of aphthous ulcerations when used preventively on a daily basis. There are numerous OTC products available for topical pain control associated with aphthous ulcerations and oral mucositis; most contain benzocaine to improve comfort. Prescription lidocaine in the form of a rinse may also be used for pain relief (see Chapter 43 for the treatment of oral mucositis).

Salivary mucins also play a role in initiating the breakdown of food in preparation for swallowing and digestion. Often, xerostomic clients will experience gastrointestinal disorders related to their inability to adequately digest food. These problems are further compounded in clients taking medications that cause taste alteration as a side effect. These adverse effects may lead clients to make poor food choices and stop eating due to discomfort, disinterest, or chewing difficulties. Clients may experience weight loss, which alters the fit and comfort of dentures and appliances, leading to a cycle that requires intervention. Weight loss and poor nutritional status are of great concern in those with serious medical conditions or those undergoing cancer therapy (see Chapter 43).

Phenytoin (seizure medication), cyclosporine (organ transplant antirejection drug), and some calcium channel blockers (antihypertensives) all cause drug-influenced gingival enlargement as a side effect. Black, hairy tongue is typically associated with antibiotics. Other medication-induced oral side effects include glossitis, erythema multiforme, and lichen planus. The dental hygienist should consult a drug reference guide to verify the potential for a drug to produce these adverse effects. For a list of strategies to manage oral side effects associated with medication use, see Dental Hygiene Interventions to Manage the Oral Side Effects of Medications. To determine the need for intervention, the dental hygienist considers:

- Is the client having difficulty speaking, chewing, swallowing, wearing dental appliances?
- Is the client taking medications that could be contributing to these problems?
- Has the client reported changes in weight that could be attributed to a change in nutritional status?
- Are oral assessment findings consistent with known side effects of the drugs that the client is taking?

QUESTION 8: GIVEN THE PHARMACOLOGIC HISTORY AND OTHER ASSESSMENT DATA, WHAT ARE THE RISKS OF TREATING THIS CLIENT? Assessing the risk of proceeding with treatment is the final and most important determination made. Treatment risks associated with medication use vary in nature and severity and are not always obvious. To assess risk, the following questions must be considered:

- If treatment is initiated, will the client be placed in a situation that is potentially dangerous or life threatening?
- Will the planned treatment temporarily or permanently compromise the client's health or ability to function?
- Will the treatment compromise the client's safety or comfort?
- Will the treatment compromise the provider's safety or comfort?

The dental hygienist assesses whether the client's ability to function has been affected by medications. Medications can alter function temporarily, such as antihistamines that cause drowsiness, or permanently, such as insulin that improves metabolic function in a diabetic. Drug side effects are often responsible for causing temporary alterations in cognitive or behavioral functions. Dizziness, drowsiness, and confusion are all cognitive alterations caused by central nervous system side effects that place the client at risk for falling and injury. Slowed reaction time is an alteration in behavior caused by central nervous system side effects that compromise driving ability. Inappropriate behaviors and poor judgment are associated with excessive alcohol intake and use of illegal substances. Temporary effects such as nausea from antibiotics or drug-induced xerostomia generally affect client comfort more than safety, and can be eliminated by discontinuing the medication. When a temporary effect compromises client safety, such as inadequate insulin with resultant hyperglycemia, treatment should be delayed until the client is stable.

If the client will be taking a medication for extended periods of time, delaying treatment is not always an alternative, and the hygienist must be prepared to respond appropriately should an emergency intervention be required. For example, a client on long-term antidepressant therapy is more susceptible to orthostatic hypotension, and hence falling, when arising from the dental chair. In this case, the antidepressant cannot be

Dental Hygiene Interventions to Manage the Oral Side Effects of Medications

Fluoride Therapy
Prescription dentifrices, gels, and rinses (dental caries, dentinal hypersensitivity)
Custom trays (dental caries)
Professional in-office application of topical fluorides
OTC dentinal hypersensitivity protection dentifrices
Professional in-office treatment for dentinal hypersensitivity

Salivary Replacement Therapy
Artificial saliva
Water, ice

Salivary Stimulation
Pilocarpine (Salagen) (prescribed by dentist)
Sugarless candy/lozenges
Sugarless gum
Powered toothbrush

Daily Antimicrobial Therapy
0.12% chlorhexidine mouthrinse
Essential oil mouthrinse
Biotene alcohol-free mouthwash

Antifungal Therapy
Prescription drugs: topical ointments, liquids, and troches; systemic medications
Daily antimicrobial therapy with 0.12% chlorhexidine or essential oil mouthrinse

Antiviral Therapy
Prescription topical ointments, systemic medications
OTC topical ointments for pain control

Topical Pain Control for Ulcerations/Mucositis
OTC benzocaine ointments
OTC liquid Benadryl
Prescription lidocaine rinse
Prescription amlexanox (Aphthasol) ointment (aphthous ulcerations)

Oral Hygiene Devices
Powered toothbrush and flosser
Oral irrigator
Interdental cleaning aids

eliminated; however, by knowing which medications the client is taking, the hygienist anticipates the possibility of a fall, and manages the situation by allowing the client to remain in an upright position for several minutes before rising. Determining the risk of falling (risk assessment) allows the hygienist to minimize the risk for injury (risk prevention). In this situation, treatment does not need to be delayed; rather, the medication-related temporary effect is managed as a part of the care plan. Other temporary effects that alter dental hygiene care include vomiting from drug ingestion (fluorides), swallowing difficulty from spray-type topical anesthetics, and trauma, pain, and difficulty speaking from local anesthesia.

Life-threatening risks are associated with conditions for which the client is taking medication or with side effects. Clients who are immunocompromised from cancer chemotherapy, organ transplant antirejection therapy, or AIDS are at greater risk for developing infections from poor oral hygiene or invasive dental hygiene procedures. Good oral self-care practices, preprocedural antimicrobial rinsing, and prophylactic antibiotic premedication are strategies to minimize the risk for infection. Antibiotic therapy associated with professional care is determined by the dentist on a case-by-case basis (see Chapter 9).

Risk for hypertensive crisis and stroke is associated with the use of vasoconstrictors, and the dental hygienist must verify the compatibility of administering epinephrine with all medications taken by the client before giving an injection. Use of cocaine sensitizes clients to norepinephrine, posing an even greater risk for hypertensive crisis, heart attack, and stroke in the oral care environment. Myocardial infarction, stroke, and anaphylaxis from an unexpected allergic reaction are perhaps the most dangerous risks. Insulin shock, aspiration, and seizures are mostly preventable with proper client assessment and use of safety precautions.

The dental hygienist is exposed to personal health risks when treating clients with medications. Pregnant practitioners should never be in the presence of nitrous oxide, a drug that causes spontaneous abortion as a *teratogenic effect* (capable of producing genetic mutations). Inhalation risks are associated with general anesthetics and nitrous-oxide and oxygen systems with inadequate scavenging systems. Topically applied agents have the potential to come in contact with the skin, mucous membranes, and eyes, requiring the use of personal protective equipment. The hygienist must also assess the treatment environment for potential hazards to protect both hygienist and client in case a client falls or has a seizure.

All dental hygienists must be currently certified in CPR and managing medical emergencies in the dental office. The dental hygienist can be especially helpful in establishing a safety plan that includes monitoring oxygen tanks to ensure that adequate levels are always available, the expiration dates on emergency medications, and the use of medications dispensed from the office (see Chapter 7).

Dental hygienists should utilize laboratory test results, medical records, and information obtained from the dentist, physician, and pharmacist to assist with clinical decision making. Maintaining a client's systemic health always takes priority over dental hygiene care needs, and treatment should never be initiated when there is concern about the client's safety. Both the client and the dental hygienist must know about any medication risks associated with treatment, and they should be thoroughly explained and documented in the treatment record.

Client Education Issues

- ✦ Inform clients about why medications are being prescribed.
- ✦ Describe what the client should expect while taking the medications.
- ✦ Explain in simple terms what the medication will do, its potential side effects, and proper dosing schedule.
- ✦ Explain the difference between side effects and drug allergies.
- ✦ Describe the signs of an allergic reaction (itching, hives, shortness of breath, or respiratory distress).
- ✦ Explain what to do in case of an allergic reaction
- ✦ Identify known drug interactions ("Do not take drug X when taking drug Y").
- ✦ Give any special instructions relevant to the medication (avoid sun exposure, take the medication until it is gone, etc.).
- ✦ Suggest ways to minimize side effects (drink a full glass of water, eat before taking the medication, etc.).
- ✦ Emphasize that no herbal medication should be taken without a physician's approval.

Legal, Ethical, and Safety Issues

- ✦ Ensure that all instructions and answers to client questions are accurate and complete. Ask for assistance if it is necessary to answer questions completely.
- ✦ Check clients' previous history for known allergies or previous reactions to ensure compatibility.
- ✦ Give written instructions the client can refer to at home.
- ✦ Document in the treatment record what the client was told
- ✦ Caution clients about the dangers of drug interactions and overmedication possible with over-the-counter and herbal medications.

Key Concepts

- The pharmacologic history provides clues regarding a client's general health status and health behaviors, and protects the client's health and safety.
- Using a logical, systematic approach to history taking helps the dental hygienist formulate questions and evaluate client responses to safely provide care.
- Interpreting data obtained from the eight fundamental questions of the pharmacologic history enables the dental hygienist to assess the risks of treating clients taking medications.
- All drugs have the potential to cause adverse effects.
- Drug interactions range in severity from mild alterations in drug action to life-threatening conditions in the client.
- Standard drug dosing schedules are too strong for children and the elderly, and need to be altered to prevent adverse effects.
- The dental hygienist is a client advocate who facilitates client compliance and education on medication use.
- Clients may fail to comply with medication use for several reasons including multiple providers prescribing multiple medications, self-medication, and failure to comply accurately with the prescribed dosing regimens.
- Oral side effects of medications cause client discomfort; interfere with the ability to chew, swallow, and digest food; and increase risk for infection and tooth loss.

Critical Thinking Exercises

1. To learn about new medications and known oral side effects, use the computer to access the many drug databases that are available via the Internet. Present to colleagues those sites that appear to be most valuable and why.
2. Document recommendations made to clients experiencing oral side effects, and monitor clinical outcomes across time. Interview clients about the efficacy of the products/procedures recommended, personal likes and dislikes about the products/procedures, and factors that influenced their compliance.

For References, Suggested Readings, and Related Websites, visit
http://evolve.elsevier.com/Darby/hygiene/

CHAPTER 12

Extraoral and Intraoral Clinical Assessment

OBJECTIVES

Mastery of the content in this chapter will enable the reader to:

- ✦ Recognize the normal anatomy of the head and neck area
- ✦ Recognize and describe common signs of oral disease and deviations from normal
- ✦ Follow proper methods and sequence in performing extraoral and intraoral assessments
- ✦ Describe and document significant findings in the client's record using precise descriptive terms
- ✦ Apply appropriate follow-up and referral protocol when abnormal or atypical tissue changes warrant further medical or dental evaluation
- ✦ Explain self-examination techniques for the oral cavity to the client
- ✦ Discuss the procedures for using an OralCDx brush biopsy and other techniques for early detection of oral cancer

KEY TERMS

Anterior
Anterior faucial pillar
Atrophy
Auscultation
Bidigital palpation
Bilateral
Bilateral palpation
Bimanual palpation
Biopsy
Buccal mucosa
Bulla
Circular compression
Circumvallate papillae
Coalescing
Consistency
Contralateral
Cratered
Crust
Differential diagnosis
Digital palpation
Disposable chemiluminescent light
Distribution
Emptiability
Erythroplakia
Excisional biopsy
Filiform papillae
Fixation
Fluctuance
Foliate papillae
Foramen cecum
Fungiform papillae
Generalized
Incisional biopsy
Incisive papilla
Induration
Inferior
Ipsilateral
Labial frenum
Labial mucosa
Lateral
Leukoplakia
Localized
Lymphadenopathy
Macule
Mandibular torus
Manual palpation
Maxillary tuberosity
Medial
Median palatine raphae
Nodule
Observation
Olfaction
Oral cytology
OralCDx brush biopsy
Palatal torus
Palatine rugae
Palatine tonsils
Palpation
Papillary
Papule
Parotid papilla
Pedunculated
Plaque
Plica fimbriata
Posterior
Posterior tonsillar pillar
Pustule
Retromolar pad
Sensitivity of a test
Separate
Sessile
Sign
Specificity of a test
Sublingual caruncle
Superficial
Superior
Symptom
Texture
Toluidine blue staining
Ulceration
Unilateral
Uvula
Verrucous
Vesicle
Wheal

Careful overall observation of the client and a thorough assessment of the areas in and around the oral cavity are essential to planning and providing optimum client care. The oral tissues are sensitive indicators of general health. Changes in these structures may be the first indication of subclinical disease processes in other parts of the body. For example, some systemic diseases that first manifest themselves in the oral cavity include diabetes, human immunodeficiency virus (HIV) infection, nutritional deficiencies, and leukemia. A variety of skin and oral mucosal lesions observed may or may not be symptomatic.

It has been estimated that 5% to 10% of dental patients have some unusual or atypical finding in the oral cavity.[1] Although the majority of these findings are benign, some may be serious and even fatal. It is the responsibility of the dental hygienist to recognize oral tissue changes from their normal state and to refer clients with changes to the dentist for further evaluation. Taking appropriate action following the recognition of an abnormal extraoral or intraoral condition is imperative for promoting optimal client wellness, low morbidity, and, in the case of cancer, possibly preventing premature death. To meet this challenge, the dental hygienist must be thoroughly familiar with normal and atypical anatomy of the head and neck to recognize abnormal changes.

This chapter focuses on the clinical assessment of extraoral and intraoral structures other than those related to tooth structure, oral hygiene, and the periodontium. (They are covered in detail in Chapters 13, 14, and 15, respectively.) For in-depth treatment of intraoral radiographs, an essential adjunct to extraoral and intraoral clinical assessments, the reader is referred to an oral radiology text.[2]

CLINICAL ASSESSMENT

The skills of *observation, palpation, auscultation,* and *olfaction* are basic to client assessment. These skills and examples of their application are described in Table 12–1. Types of palpation techniques used are described in Table 12–2. Basic anatomical terms of orientation regularly used in describing head and neck anatomy are defined in Basic Anatomical Terminology.

Before performing extraoral and intraoral assessments, the dental hygienist reviews clients' health, personal and social histories, examines their radiographs, and explains the procedure to them. Establishing an assessment sequence and following it systematically

Basic Anatomic Terminology

Anterior: The front of an area in relationship to the entire body
Posterior: The back of an area in relationship to the entire body
Superior: An area that faces toward the head and away from the feet
Inferior: An area that faces away from the head and toward the feet
Medial: Structures toward the midline of the body
Lateral: Structures away from the midline of the body
Ipsilateral: Structures on the same side of the body
Contralateral: Structures on the opposite side of the body
Superficial: Structures located toward the surface of the body
Deep: Structures located inward, away from the body surface

TABLE 12–1 SKILLS USED IN CONDUCTING THE EXTRAORAL AND INTRAORAL ASSESSMENT

Skill	Definition	Examples of Application
Observation	The act of viewing and watching the client to collect data to detect variations from normal and potential disease states	Noting client movement; body structure and symmetry; skin and mucous membrane color, texture, consistency, contour, and form; and client knowledge, attitude, and behavior.
Palpation	The act of using the sense of touch to collect client data to detect variations from normal and potential disease states	Noting tenderness, texture, masses, variations in structure, and temperature
Auscultation	The act of listening to and detecting body sounds to determine variations from normal	Noting sounds made by the temporomandibular joint, e.g., clicking; hoarseness and general quality of speech, which may be indicative of problems with the vocal cords; problems with breathing, which may indicate a respiratory or emotional condition; clicking of dentures indicating a poor fit
Olfaction	The act of sensing body odors to detect variations from normal and potential disease states	Noting alcohol breath caused by alcohol abuse; smoker's breath from cigarette use; halitosis associated with dental caries and periodontitis; necrotizing periodontal disease; sweet fruity ketosis associated with diabetic acidosis

TABLE 12–2 PALPATION METHODS FOR ASSESSING THE ORAL CAVITY

Type	Definition	Technique	Example
Digital palpation	Using index finger to move or press against tissue		Use to palpate the lingual border of the mandible
Bidigital palpation	Using finger and thumb of same hand to move or compress tissue using a rolling motion		Use to palpate the lips, labial and buccal mucosa, and tongue
Manual palpation	Using all fingers of one hand to simultaneously move or compress tissues		Use to palpate the thyroid gland or lymph nodes
Bimanual palpation	Using index finger of one hand and fingers and thumb of other hand simultaneously to move or compress tissue, holding the fingers closely together to avoid missing areas		Use to palpate floor of the mouth, submandibular and sublingual glands, and associated nodes
Bilateral palpation	Using a finger or fingers of both hands simultaneously to move or press tissues on opposite sides of the head/body		Use to palpate lymph nodes of the head and neck
Circular compression	Moving the finger tips in a deliberate, rotating fashion over tissues to be examined, exerting pressure		Use to palpate suspected lesion for more information

during client assessment reduces the possibility of overlooking any area to be examined. A suggested sequence for a thorough extraoral and intraoral assessment is outlined and illustrated in Procedures 12–1 and 12–2 later in the chapter.

EXTRAORAL CLINICAL ASSESSMENT

An extraoral assessment includes an overall appraisal of the client's general characteristics and a thorough evaluation of the client's head, face, and neck areas, especially the skin and associated lymph nodes.

Overall Appraisal

Initially, the client is observed during reception and seating to note any physical characteristics and abnormalities that may require special modification of dental hygiene care or the need for medical and/or dental consultation. This general appraisal includes the level of function of hands, arms, and legs; speech; and personal hygiene. For example, the level of function of the hands and arms may indicate the need to modify oral hygiene instruction. The level of function of the arms and legs may indicate the need for an alteration in seating position or affect the client's ability to easily attend subsequent appointments. The quality of speech may be indicative of problems such as damaged vocal cords or history of stroke. Personal hygiene may give an indication of the care given to the oral cavity.

Specific Appraisal of the Head, Face, and Neck Areas

The client should be seated in an upright position for the extraoral assessment of the head and neck area. Good lighting and exposure of the area being assessed

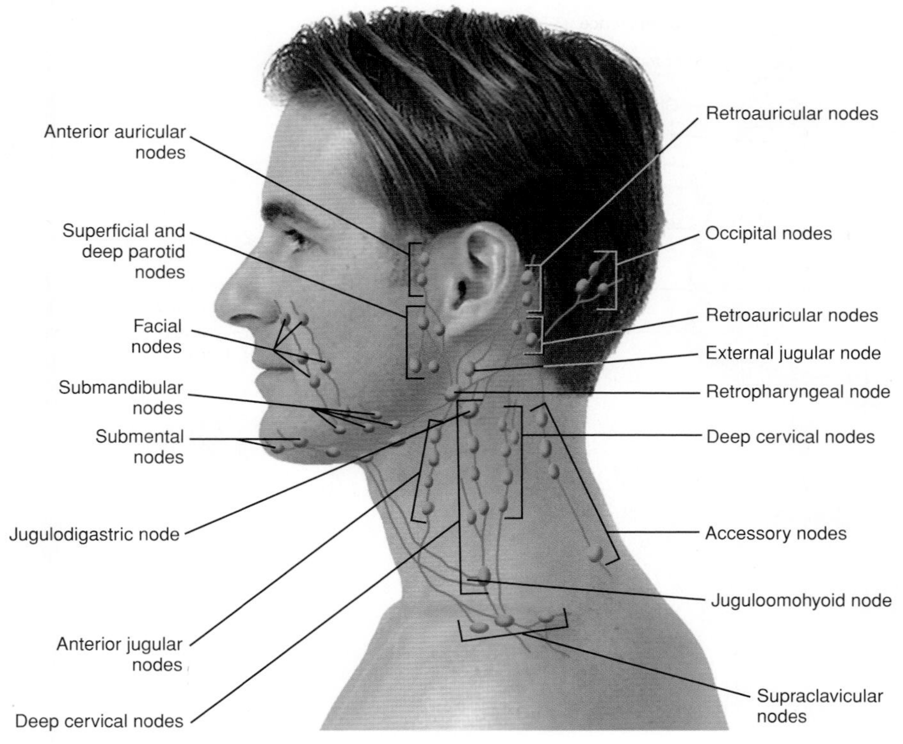

FIGURE 12–1 ✦ Lymphatic drainage system of the head and neck. *(Modified from Seidel HM et al. In Potter PA, Perry AG:* Fundamentals of Nursing, *ed 5, St Louis, 2001, Mosby.)*

are essential (e.g., collar and tie loosened, glasses removed). Before asking the client to open his or her mouth, an overall evaluation is performed of the client's head, neck, eyes, face, lips, and surrounding skin. Normally, the head, face, and neck should have symmetry and the skin should be continuous, firm, and pigmented in relation to the normal variations associated with race and ethnicity. If lesions are initially observed, clients should be asked how long they have had the lesions, if the lesions have changed, and whether they are painful. In addition, lymph nodes, salivary glands, and the temporomandibular joints (TMJ) should be *palpated* (examined by touch). These structures are described in depth in the following sections. Suspected abnormalities require consultation with the dentist.

Lymph Nodes

Lymph nodes are bean-shaped bodies grouped in clusters along the connecting lymphatic vessels, positioned to filter toxic products from the lymph to prevent their entry into the blood (Figure 12–1). In healthy clients, nodes are usually small, soft, and mobile in the surrounding tissue and cannot be visualized or palpated. The nodes can be superficial in position with the superficial veins, or deep in the tissue with the deep blood vessels. All the nodes of the head and neck drain either the right or left tissues in the area, depending on their location (except for the midline submental nodes, which drain the tissues in the region bilaterally).

Palpable lymph nodes are those that have undergone *lymphadenopathy,* or enlargement of the lymph nodes resulting from an increase in size and change in consistency of the lymphoid tissue. This change in node consistency can range from firm to hard. Lymph nodes can also become attached or fixed to the surrounding tissues as the disease process progresses. They can also feel tender to the client when palpated due to the pressure on the area nerves from the node enlargement.

The nodes that are palpable may pinpoint where a disease process, such as infection or cancer, is active. The assessment of lymph node involvement may also help determine if the disease process has become widespread. Some 30% of clients with oral cancer will present with palpably enlarged nodes, and, of those who do not, a further 25% will develop nodal metastases within two years (see Chapter 43). Documentation of history concerning palpable nodes will assist in the diagnosis, treatment, and outcome of any disease process that may be present in the client. It is important to understand the relationship between the lymph node location and its drainage patterns. It is also important to keep in mind that the nodes of the head and neck drain not only intraoral structures such as the teeth, but also the eyes, ears, nasal cavity, and deeper areas of the pharynx.

Head and Neck Regions

The extraoral clinical assessment of the client's head and neck area begins with visually dividing the head and neck into the following regions[3] and then palpating each region in order from superior to inferior, including both sides of the body (Figure 12–2).

PARIETAL AND OCCIPITAL REGIONS. These regions are covered by the scalp overlying the cranium. The occipital

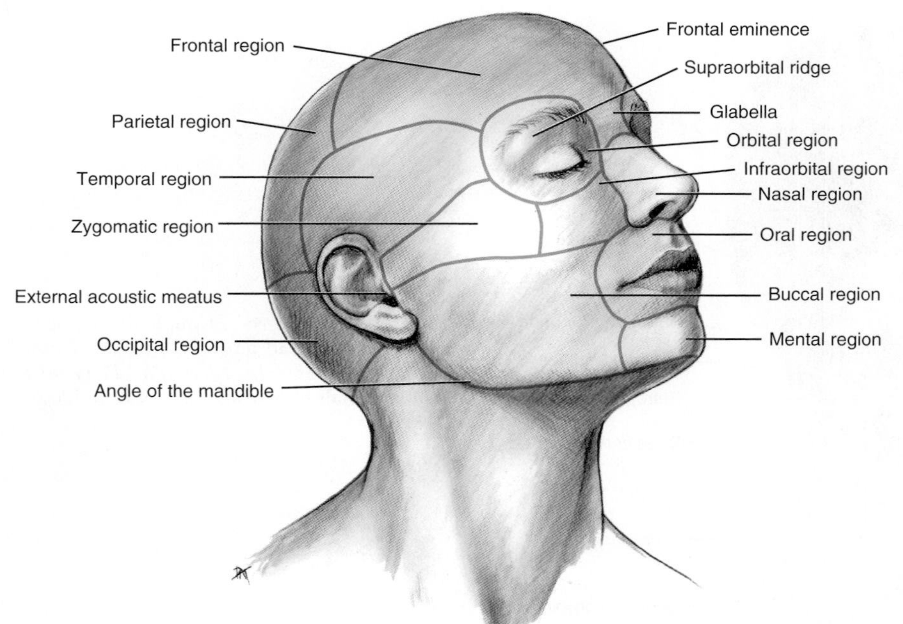

FIGURE 12–2 ✦ Regions of the head for extraoral examination. *(From Fehrenbach MJ, Herring SW:* Illustrated anatomy of the head and neck, *Philadelphia, 1996, WB Saunders.)*

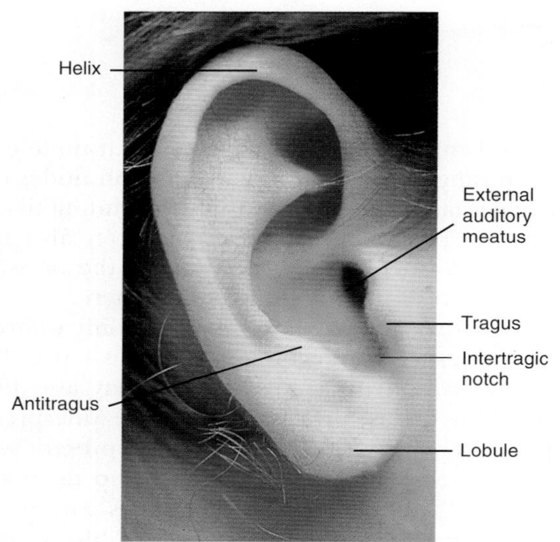

FIGURE 12–3 ✦ Anatomic structures of the auricle of the external ear. *(Modified from Seidel HM et al. In Potter PA, Perry AG:* Fundamentals of nursing, *ed 5, St Louis, 2001, Mosby.)*

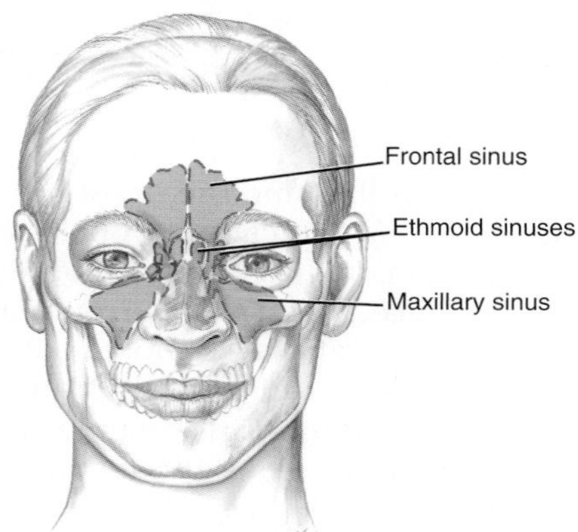

FIGURE 12–4 ✦ Anterior view of the skull and the paranasal sinuses. *(From Fehrenbach MJ, Herring SW:* Illustrated anatomy of the head and neck, ed 2, *Philadelphia, 2002, WB Saunders.)*

nodes are located bilaterally on the posterior base of the head in the occipital region and drain this portion of the scalp (Figure 12–1). The occipital nodes empty into the inferior deep cervical nodes of the neck.

TEMPORAL REGION. Within this region is the external ear (Figure 12–3), which is composed of an auricle (overflap of the ear for collecting sound waves) and the external acoustic meatus (the tube through which sound waves are transmitted to the middle ear within the skull). The superior and posterior free margin of the auricle is the helix, which ends inferiorly at the ear lobe. The part of the auricle anterior to the external acoustic meatus is a smaller flap of tissue called the tragus. The other flap of tissue opposite the tragus is the antitragus. The auricular nodes are located anterior and posterior (retro) to the external acoustic meatus of the ear (Figure 12–1). These nodes drain the external ear, the lacrimal (tear) gland above the eye, and adjacent regions of the scalp and face, and empty into the superior deep cervical nodes.

FRONTAL REGION. This region includes the forehead and the area above the eyes. The paired frontal sinuses are located in the frontal bone just superior to the nasal cavity and each communicates with and drains into the nasal cavity (Figure 12–4).

ORBITAL AND NASAL REGIONS. In the orbital region, the eyeball and all its supporting structures are contained in the bony socket called the orbit. The conjunctiva is the delicate and thin membrane lining the inside of the eyelids and the front of the eyeball. The outer corner where the

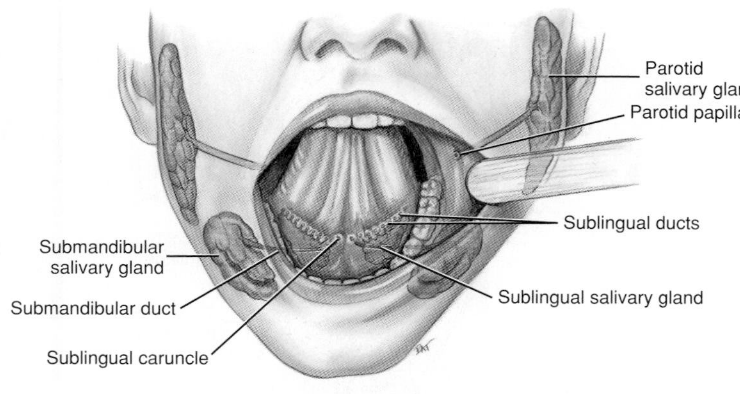

FIGURE 12–5 ✦ The salivary glands and associated structures. *(From Fehrenbach MJ, Herring SW:* Illustrated anatomy of the head and neck, ed 2, *Philadelphia, 2002, WB Saunders.)*

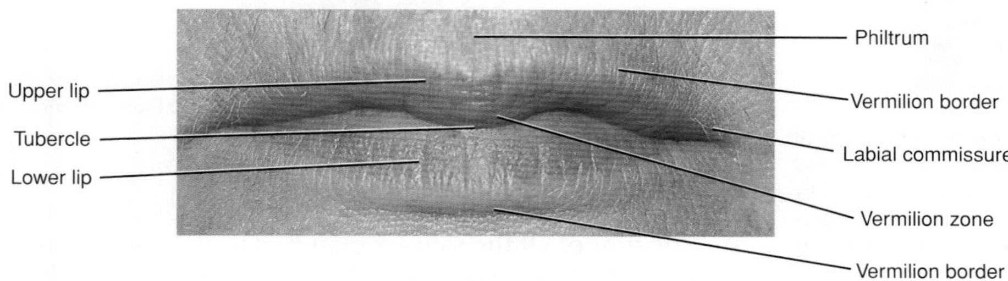

FIGURE 12–6 ✦ Frontal view of the lips. *(From Fehrenbach MJ, Herring SW:* Illustrated anatomy of the head and neck, ed 2, *Philadelphia, 2002, WB Saunders.)*

upper and lower eyelids meet is called the outer canthus. The inner angle of the eye is called the inner canthus (Figure 12–4). The main feature of the nasal region is the external nose. The tip is flexible when palpated.

INFRAORBITAL AND ZYGOMATIC REGIONS. These regions are all located on the face. The infraorbital region is located inferior to the orbital region and lateral to the nasal region. Farther laterally is the zygomatic region, which overlies the cheek bone, the zygomatic arch (Figure 12–2). The zygomatic arch extends from just below the lateral margin of the eye toward the upper part of the ear.

Facial lymph nodes are positioned along the length of the facial vein and are typically small and variable in number (Figure 12–1). Each facial node group drains the skin and mucous membranes where they are located and finally drains into the submandibular nodes. The paired maxillary sinuses are each located in the body of the maxilla, just posterior to the maxillary canine and premolars (Figure 12–4) and drain into the nasal cavity. Inferior to the zygomatic arch, and just anterior to the ear, is the TMJ. This is where the upper skull forms a joint with the lower jaw: the two temporal bones and the two condyles of the mandible. The movements of the joint can be felt when one opens and closes the mouth or moves the lower jaw to the right or left, and forward. The TMJ should be palpated and the movement of the mandible observed as clients open and close their mouths.

BUCCAL REGION. The buccal region forms the side of the face and is a broad area of the face between the nose, mouth, and ear (Figure 12–2). Most of the upper cheek is fleshy, mainly formed by a mass of fat and muscles. One of these is the strong masseter muscle, which is felt when clients clench their teeth together. The sharp angle of the lower jaw inferior to the earlobe is the angle of the mandible. (The anatomy of the mandible is illustrated in Chapter 34). Also within this region is the parotid salivary gland, which occupies the area behind the mandibular ramus, anterior and inferior to the ear (Figure 12–5). The parotid gland is the largest salivary gland.

ORAL AND MENTAL REGIONS. The oral region contains the lips and oral cavity. The lips are outlined from the surrounding skin by a transition zone, the vermilion border (Figure 12–6). Each lip's vermilion zone has a darker appearance than the surrounding skin. On the midline of the upper lip, extending downward from the nasal septum, is a vertical groove called the philtrum, which terminates in a thicker area or tubercle. The upper and lower lips meet at each corner of the mouth, or the labial commissure. The chin is the major feature of the mental region.

ANTERIOR AND POSTERIOR CERVICAL REGIONS. The large strap muscle, the sternocleidomastoid muscle (SCM), divides each side of the neck diagonally into two triangular regions (Figure 12–7). The SCM muscle originates from the clavicle and sternum and passes posteriorly and superiorly to insert on the temporal bone, just posterior and inferior to the ear. When the client's head is tilted to the side, the SCM is more prominent.

The anterior region of the neck corresponds to the two anterior cervical triangles, which are separated by the midline. The lateral region of the neck posterior to each SCM muscle forms the posterior cervical triangles

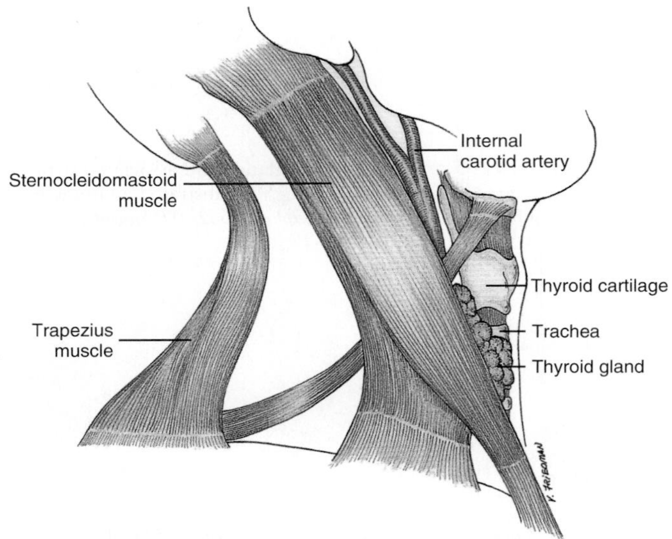

FIGURE 12–7 ✦ Major neck structures. Note the anterior cervical triangle formed by the sternocleidomastoid muscle, lower jaw, and anterior border of neck; and the posterior cervical triangle, created by the sternocleidomastoid muscle, trapezius muscle, and lower neck posteriority. *(From Potter PA, Perry AG:* Fundamentals of nursing, *ed 5, St Louis, 2001, Mosby.)*

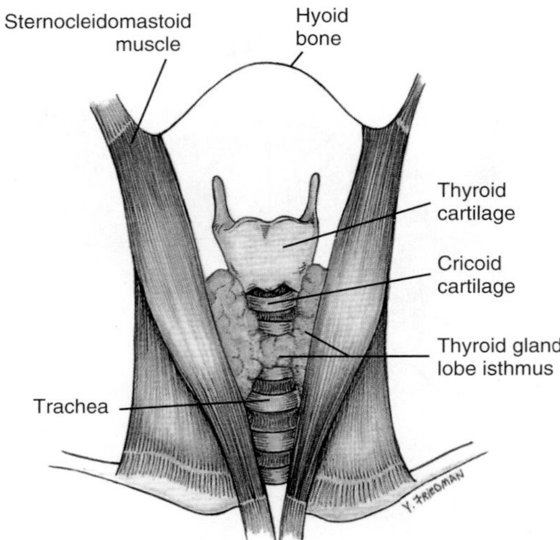

FIGURE 12–8 ✦ Anterior view of the thyroid cartilage, thyroid gland, and associated structures. *(From Potter PA, Perry AG:* Fundamentals of nursing, *ed 5, St Louis, 2001, Mosby.)*

(Figure 12–7). There are many superficial cervical nodes, such as the external jugular nodes, in this region, located on each side of the neck and superficial to the SCM (Figure 12–1). The deep cervical nodes are located along the length of the neck on each side of the neck, deep to the SCM (Figure 12–1). These nodes drain the nasal cavity, posterior portion of the hard palate, soft palate, base of the tongue, maxillary third molars, esophagus, trachea, and thyroid gland. In addition to the deep cervical nodes, there are also nodes in the most inferior portion of the neck. For example, the supraclavicular nodes are located along the clavicle and drain the anterior cervical triangles (Figure 12–1).

SUBMANDIBULAR AND SUBMENTAL TRIANGLE REGIONS. The anterior cervical triangle of the neck can be further subdivided into smaller triangular regions by portions of neck muscles and the mandible. The submandibular region is the superior portion of the anterior cervical triangle on each side of the neck. Both submandibular salivary glands are located in this region posterior to the sublingual gland. The submandibular gland is the second-largest salivary gland (Figure 12–5).

The submandibular nodes are located at the inferior border of the ramus of the mandible, just superficial to the submandibular gland (Figure 12–1). They drain the cheeks, upper lip, body of the tongue, anterior portion of the hard palate, sublingual and submandibular salivary glands, and all the teeth and associated tissues, except the mandibular incisors and maxillary third molars. The submandibular nodes empty into the superior deep cervical nodes.

Near the midline of the anterior cervical triangle is the submental region where both the sublingual salivary glands are located (Figure 12–5). The sublingual gland is the smallest of all the salivary glands. The sublingual and submental nodes are located below the chin in this region (Figure 12–1). These nodes drain both sides of the chin, lower lip, floor of the mouth, tip of the tongue, and the mandibular incisors and the associated tissues, and then empty into the submandibular nodes or directly into the deep cervical nodes.

ANTERIOR MIDLINE CERVICAL REGION. Figure 12–8 shows the thyroid gland located in the anterior midline cervical region. The hyoid bone, which has many muscles attached to it and which controls the position of the base of the tongue, is suspended in the neck. The hyoid bone can be effectively palpated below and medial to the angles of the mandible. When palpating the neck, do not confuse the hyoid bone with the inferiorly placed thyroid cartilage, which is also found in the anterior midline. The thyroid cartilage is the prominence of the "voice box" or larynx. The anterior portion of this skeletal landmark is visible as the "Adam's apple," especially in adult males. The vocal cords or ligaments of the larynx are attached to the posterior surface of the thyroid cartilage. The thyroid gland is located inferior to the thyroid cartilage, at the junction of the larynx and the trachea.

Procedure 12–1 details the steps and rationale for examining recommended structures, and lists examples of normal, atypical, and abnormal findings that may be observed during an extraoral assessment.

INTRAORAL CLINICAL ASSESSMENT

The intraoral clinical assessment includes appraisal of the oral cavity and associated structures (e.g., the palate, pharynx, tongue, floor of the mouth, teeth, and periodontium). The client should be seated in a supine position. After making an initial general inspection

Text continued on page 212

Procedure 12–1 CONDUCTING EXTRAORAL ASSESSMENTS

EQUIPMENT

Hand mirror, periodontal probe or small metric ruler, paper towel, glass of water, personal protective equipment

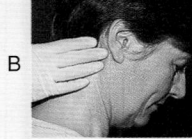

EXTRAORAL REGIONS	STEPS	RATIONALE	NORMAL FINDINGS	ATYPICAL FINDINGS	ABNORMAL FINDINGS
Overall evaluation of the head, face, and neck, including the skin (Figure 12–9). 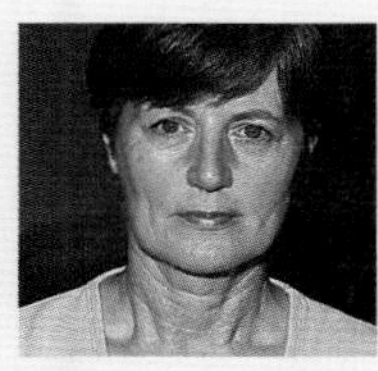 **FIGURE 12–9** ✦	With client sitting upright and relaxed, visually observe symmetry and coloration. Ask client to remove glasses. Ask client about history of lesion if it presents during general evaluation.	Allows the clinician to check for signs of nutritional deficiency and signs of systemic disease, possible asymmetry from neoplasm or abnormal growth and development.	Face and head should be symmetric; skin should be continuous, firm, and pigmented in relation to the normal variations associated with race and ethnicity.	Moles, freckles, scars, or tattoos.	Needle marks due to drug use, trauma due to domestic abuse.
Parietal and occipital regions, including scalp, hair, and occipital nodes (Figure12–10). 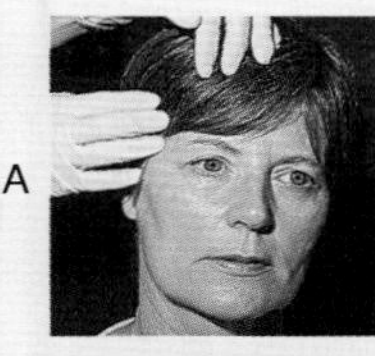 **FIGURE 12–10** ✦ **A,** Parietal and occipital regions including scalp, hair, and occipital nodes. **B,** Palpating the occipital lymph nodes by bending the client's head forward.	Visually inspect the entire scalp by moving the hair, especially around the hairline, starting from around one ear and proceeding to the other ear. Standing behind the client, have the client lean his or her head forward for bilateral palpation of occipital nodes located at base of the head.	Allows the clinician to inspect the scalp where many lesions may be hidden by hair, and inspect the occipital nodes to check for tender, enlarged nodes or masses indicating local or systemic involvement. These nodes drain the area and may indicate disease state in that area.	Scalp should be firm and continuous and without any changes noted, and the hair should be free of debris. Nodes should not be clinically palpable or visible.	Debris found on the scalp and in the hair. Palpable nontender node may be the result of scar tissue from a past chronic infection.	Lesions on the scalp that are hidden by the hair, such as skin cancer; tender, soft, enlarged, and freely movable nodes suggesting acute infection; hard, nontender, and fixed nodes suggesting a chronic infection, malignancy, or trauma due to domestic abuse.
Temporal region, including anterior and posterior auricular nodes and ears (Figure 12–11). 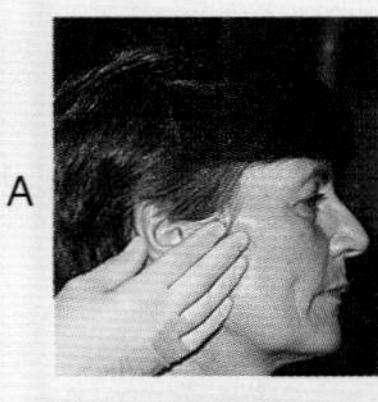 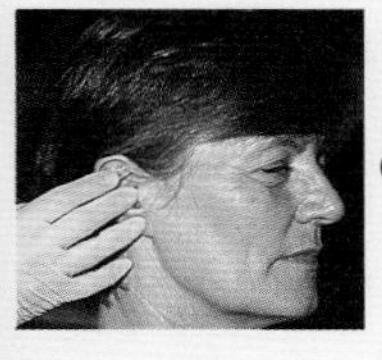 **FIGURE 12–11** ✦	Standing near the client on each side, visually inspect and use bilateral palpation of the auricular nodes and scalp and face around each ear. Visually inspect the ear.	Allows the clinician to check for tender, enlarged nodes or masses indicating local or systemic involvement. These nodes drain the areas around the ear and may indicate a disease state in that area. Also allows for inspection of the ear itself to check for infection or skin cancer.	Skin should be firm and continuous, without any changes noted in the surface. Nodes should not be clinically palpable or visible. Ears should not have discharge or inner canal redness.	Discharge from the ears or redness on the inner canal.	Tender, soft, enlarged, and freely movable nodes; hard, nontender, and fixed nodes.

Continued on following page

Procedure 12–1 CONDUCTING EXTRAORAL ASSESSMENTS—CONT'D

EXTRAORAL REGIONS	STEPS	RATIONALE	NORMAL FINDINGS	ATYPICAL FINDINGS	ABNORMAL FINDINGS
Frontal region, including forehead and frontal sinuses (Figure 12–12) 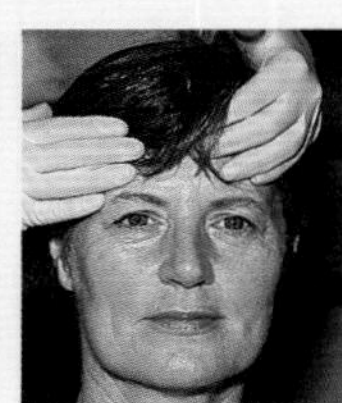 FIGURE 12–12 ✦	Visually inspect and use bilateral palpation of the forehead, including the frontal sinuses.	Allows the clinician to check for any changes in the frontal bone and sinuses by checking for masses, tenderness, and increased skin temperature.	Area should be firm and smooth, without tenderness or increased temperature.	Frontal sinusitis.	Skin cancer.
Orbital region, including the eyes (Figure 12–13) FIGURE 12–13 ✦	Visually inspect the eyes and their movement and response.	Allows the clinician to check for any changes in the cranial nerves that serve the eyes, which may first exhibit as changes in the eye's movement, constriction of the pupil, or changes in the visual acuity or field.	Eyes should be clear and exhibit normal responses to light stimulus by the pupil. Client is able to open and close eyes.	Eyes may show tearing and redness from emotional distress or respiratory condition. Client may wear eyeglasses or contacts.	Yellowish or bluish coloration of sclera showing jaundice or trauma to the eye area; iris cloudy due to eye disease or pinpoint due to drug intake; yellowish discharge from eye showing infection; excessive tearing and redness from drug or alcohol intake; trauma due to domestic abuse; an inability to close eye on affected side with facial paralysis.
Nasal region, including the nose (Figure 12–14) 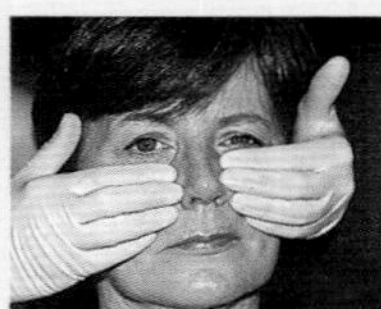 FIGURE 12–14 ✦	Visually inspect and use bilateral palpation for the nasal region, starting at the root of the nose and proceeding to its tip.	Allows the clinician to assess for symmetry of the nose and for any signs of respiratory conditions.	Nose should be symmetric and show no signs of discharge, redness, or ulceration of the surrounding skin.	Nasal discharge may be present and the surrounding skin may show some redness due to respiratory conditions such as allergies or colds; loss of symmetry may be due to deviated septum or broken nose.	Inflammation, infection, necrosis of tissues, and possible nasal septum perforation due to repeated cocaine snorting, possibly forming a saddlenose deformity; skin cancer; trauma due to domestic abuse.

Procedure 12–1 CONDUCTING EXTRAORAL ASSESSMENTS—CONT'D

EXTRAORAL REGIONS	STEPS	RATIONALE	NORMAL FINDINGS	ATYPICAL FINDINGS	ABNORMAL FINDINGS
Infraorbital and zygomatic regions, including the muscles of facial expression, facial nodes, maxillary bone and sinuses, and TMJ (Figure 12–15)	Visually inspect the infraorbital and zygomatic regions, noting the use of the muscles of facial expression. Visually inspect and use bilateral palpation of the facial nodes by moving from the infraorbital region to the labial commissure and then to the surface of the mandible. Visually inspect and use bilateral palpation of the maxillary sinuses. Gently place a finger into the outer portion of the external acoustic meatus. To assess the TMJ and its associated muscles, use bilateral palpation and ask client to open and close mouth several times. Then ask client to move the opened jaw left, then right, and then forward. Ask clients if they experienced any pain or tenderness. Note any sounds made by the joint.	Checks for a lack of expression, which may indicate a change in the cranial nerve that serves the facial muscles. Checks the maxillary sinus for tenderness and increased skin temperature. Allows the clinician to assess for TMD (temporo-mandibular disorders).	Client should have all modes of facial expression. Joint movement should be smooth, continuous, and silent; both sides of the joint should function similarly; both joint and associated musculature should be free of pain.	Maxillary sinusitis; noise or deviation of lower jaw upon opening.	Facial paralysis due to Bell's palsy or stroke; TMD, with limitations of movement and discomfort during appointment; subluxation or pain on TMJ movement.
Buccal region, including the masseter muscle, mandible, and parotid salivary gland (Figure 12–16)	Standing near the client on each side, visually inspect and use bilateral palpation of the masseter muscle and parotid gland by starting in front of each ear and moving to the cheek area and down to the angle of the mandible. Place the fingers of each hand over the masseter muscle and ask client to clench the teeth together several times.	Allows the clinician to check for tender, enlarged nodes or masses indicating local or systemic infection. These nodes drain the area of the cheek and may indicate a disease state in that area. Also allows the clinician to check the masseter muscle for development and that the parotid gland is free of tenderness and enlargement.	Area should be firm and smooth, without tenderness or increased size or firmness.	Overdeveloped masseter muscle in a person with parafunctional habits.	Tenderness and pain in the masseter muscle related to TMD; tender, soft, enlarged, and freely movable nodes; hard, nontender, and fixed nodes; constant pain in gland indicating possible malignancy: skin cancer; extraoral lesion from oral infection.

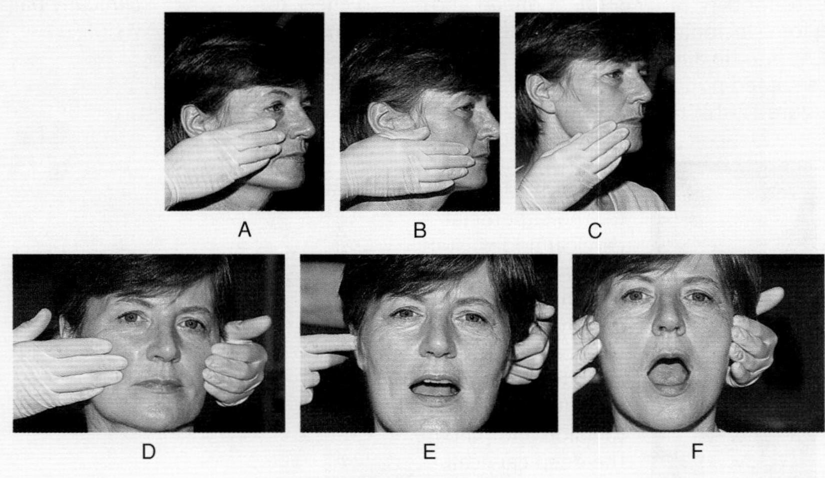

FIGURE 12–15 ✦

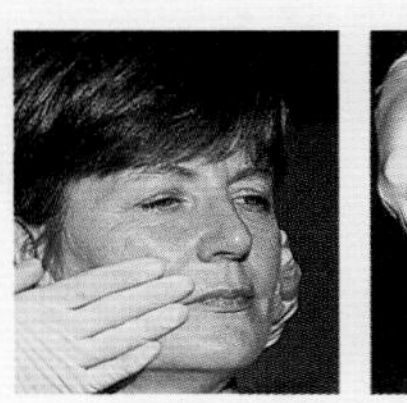

FIGURE 12–16 ✦

Continued on following page

Procedure 12–1 CONDUCTING EXTRAORAL ASSESSMENTS—CONT'D

EXTRAORAL REGIONS	STEPS	RATIONALE	NORMAL FINDINGS	ATYPICAL FINDINGS	ABNORMAL FINDINGS
Oral and mental region, including the chin (Figure 12–17) 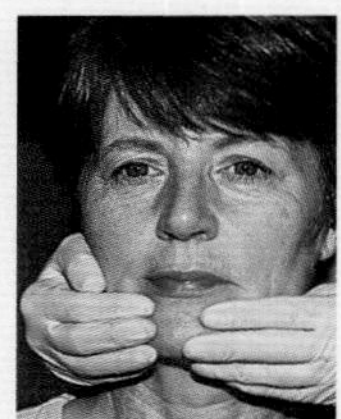 FIGURE 12–17 ✦	Standing near the client on each side, use bilateral palpation and visual inspection of the chin.	Allows the clinician to detect enlargement or masses, as well as any abnormal growth of soft tissue or bone, surface lesions, and tenderness.	Area should be firm and smooth, without tenderness.	May have dimple or slight cleft in central area of chin.	Trauma due to domestic abuse or other scars due to accidents; extraoral lesion from oral infection.
Anterior and posterior cervical regions, including SCM muscle and associated nodes (Figure 12–18) A 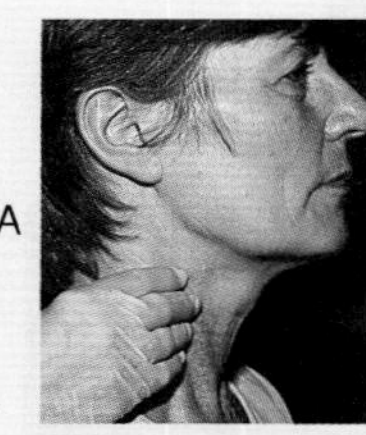 B 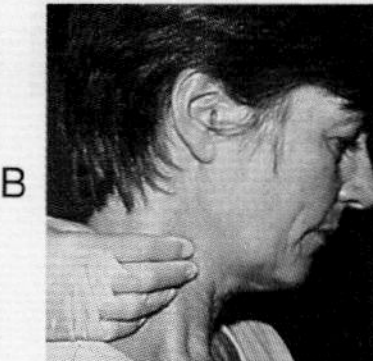 C 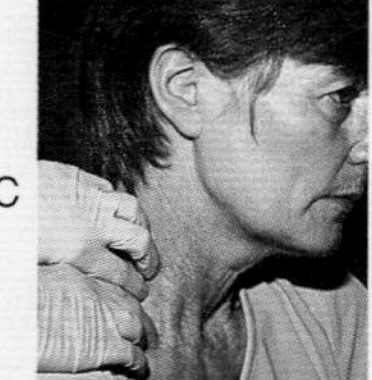 D 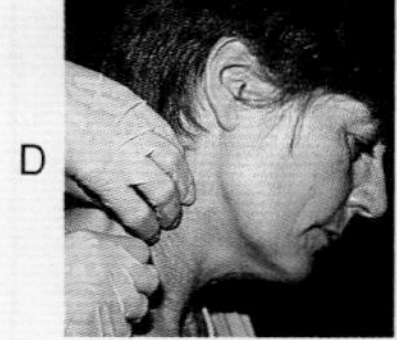 FIGURE 12–18 ✦	Have client look straight ahead and then turn head to the side to make the SCM more prominent. Using manual palpation with two hands on each side of the neck for the superficial cervical nodes, start below the ear and continue the whole length of the SCM surface to the clavicles. Then have the client tilt head to the side and palpate the deep cervical nodes on the underside of the anterior and posterior aspects of the SCM. For those nodes in the most inferior portion of the neck in the area of clavicles, have the client raise shoulders up and forward and then use manual palpation using one hand on each side.	Allows the clinician to check for enlarged nodes or masses indicating local or systemic disease.	Nodes should not be clinically palpable or visible.	Palpable, nontender node may be the result of scar tissue from a past chronic infection. The jugulodigastric (tonsillar node) becomes palpable when the palatine tonsils and/or pharynx are inflamed.	Tender, soft, enlarged, and freely movable nodes; hard, nontender, and fixed nodes suggesting a chronic infection or even malignancy, especially if the client has breast cancer (due to the connection to the axillary nodes).

Procedure 12–1 CONDUCTING EXTRAORAL ASSESSMENTS—CONT'D

EXTRAORAL REGIONS	STEPS	RATIONALE	NORMAL FINDINGS	ATYPICAL FINDINGS	ABNORMAL FINDINGS
Submandibular and submental triangle regions, including submandibular and sublingual salivary glands and associated nodes (Figure 12–19) A 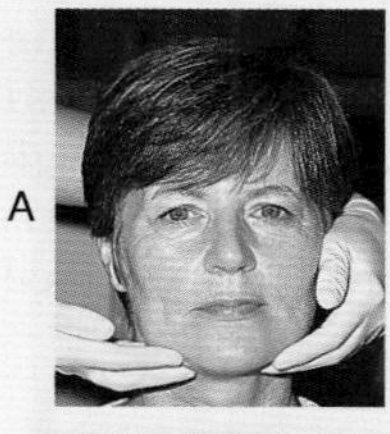 B 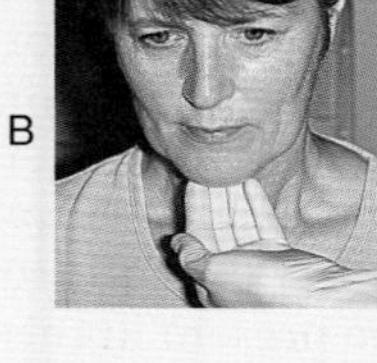	Standing slightly behind the client on each side, have client lower chin for manual palpation of the submental and submandibular triangular region with its nodes and submandibular gland. Push the tissue in the area from the client's one side over to the opposite side, rolling it over the angle of the mandible. The opposite side is examined in the same way. **FIGURE 12–19** ✦	Allows the clinician to assess the submental, sublingual, and submandibular glands, associated lymph nodes, and mandible.	Mandible should be symmetric, with continuous borders. Nodes should not be clinically palpable or visible.	Palpable, nontender node may be the result of scar tissue from a past chronic infection.	Sialolithiasis and blocked duct; excessive salivary flow or xerostomia; tender, soft, enlarged, and freely movable nodes; hard, nontender, and fixed nodes; extraoral lesion from oral infection.
Anterior midline cervical region, including hyoid bone, thyroid gland, and cartilage (Figure 12–20) A 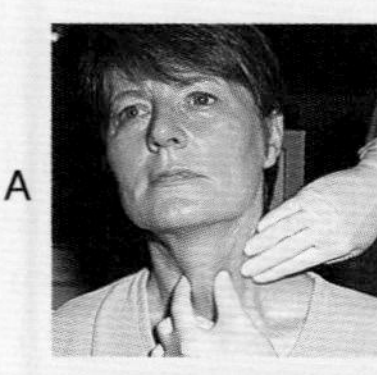 B 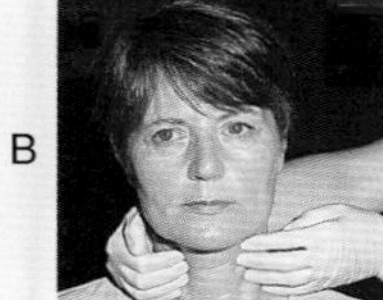 **FIGURE 12–20** ✦	To palpate the thyroid gland, stand to the side of the client. Instruct the client to bend the neck forward and laterally toward the side being examined. Using manual palpation, place one hand on one side of the trachea, then with the other hand gently displace the thyroid tissue to that side of the neck and manually palpate the gland. Then compare the two lobes of the thyroid using bimanual or manual palpation and visual inspection. Ask the client to swallow to check for mobility of the gland by visually inspecting it while it moves superiorly. Client may need a glass of water in order to swallow.	This neck position relaxes the muscles and allows the clinician to check the thyroid for masses. Enlargement or immobility may be a manifestation of thyroid disease.	Thyroid gland should not be clinically visible; gland should rise up and down during swallowing; larynx should be freely movable when palpated and deliberately moved.	Prominent "Adam's apple" or thyroid cartilage.	Enlargement of gland; hard tissue masses; evidence of thyroid surgery; lack of movement during swallowing.

Steps from Fehrenbach MJ, Herring SW: *Illustrated anatomy of the head and neck*, ed 2, Philadelphia, 2002, WB Saunders. Photos courtesy Dr. M. Walsh, University of California – San Francisco.

intraorally with a mouth mirror, the intraoral clinical assessment of a client begins with the systematic assessment of the following smaller regions using visualization and palpation.

Oral Cavity

The oral cavity is the inside of the mouth. The anatomic landmarks in the oral cavity, as shown in Figure 12–21, can be used as a general point of reference during an intraoral examination.

The oral cavity is lined by nonkeratinized oral mucosa (Figure 12–22). The inner portions of the lips are thick *labial mucosa* that are glistening pink or pigmented with melanin. The labial mucosa are continuous with the equally pink and thick *buccal mucosa* that lines the inner cheek. The buccal mucosa covers a dense pad of inner tissue, the buccal fat pad. On the inner portion of the buccal mucosa, just opposite the maxillary second molar, is a small elevation of tissue called the *parotid papilla,* which contains the opening of the parotid gland (Stensen's duct) (Figures 12–5 and 12–21).

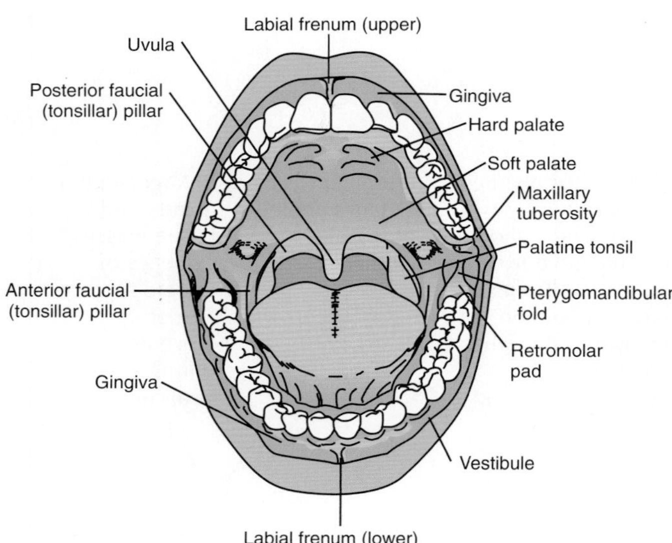

FIGURE 12–21 ✦ Anatomic landmarks in the oral cavity. *(Modified from Massler M, Schour I:* Atlas of the mouth, *ed 2, Chicago, 1958, American Dental Association.)*

The upper and lower spaces between the cheeks, lips, and gums are the maxillary and mandibular vestibules. Deep within each vestibule, the pink and thick labial or buccal mucosa meet the redder and thinner alveolar mucosa at the mucobuccal fold (Figure 12–21). The *labial frenum* is a fold of tissue located at the midline between the labial mucosa and the alveolar mucosa on each jaw. Teeth of the oral cavity are located within the upper and lower jaws of the oral cavity. Just distal to the last tooth of the maxilla is a rounded elevation, the *maxillary tuberosity.* Just distal to the last tooth of the mandible is a dense pad of tissue, the *retromolar pad* (Figure 12–21).

Surrounding the teeth are the attached gingiva, composed of a firm pink keratinized mucosa that tightly adheres to the bone around the roots of the teeth, the alveolar ridges. The line of demarcation between the firmer and pinker attached gingiva and the movable and redder alveolar mucosa is the scallop-shaped mucogingival junction. The gingiva between the teeth, the interdental papilla, is an extension of attached gingiva (see Chapter 15).

Palate and Pharynx

The roof of the mouth has two parts: the firmer anterior portion is the hard palate, and the looser posterior portion is the soft palate (Figures 12–21 and 12–23). A midline ridge of tissue on the hard palate is the *median palatine raphe.* Bony projections known as *palatal torus* are atypical but normal structures that may be present in this area (Figure 12–24). A small bulge of tissue at the most anterior portion, lingual to the anterior teeth, is the *incisive papilla,* and directly posterior to this papilla are *palatine rugae,* which are firm, irregular ridges of tissue.

Palatine foveae, small depressions from the opening of excretory ducts of minor salivary glands, are found at the junction of the hard and soft palates. A midline muscular structure, the *uvula,* hangs from the posterior margin of the soft palate. The pterygomandibular fold is a fold of tissue that extends from the junction of hard and soft palates down to the mandible, just behind the retromolar pad. It stretches when the client opens his or her mouth wider, separating the buccal mucosa from the pharynx (Figure 12–21).

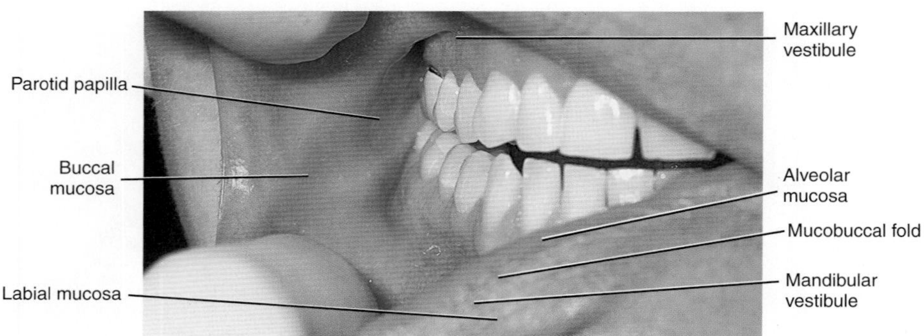

FIGURE 12–22 ✦ View of the buccal and labial mucosa of the oral cavity with landmarks noted. *(From Fehrenbach MJ, Herring SW:* Illustrated anatomy of the head and neck, ed 2, *Philadelphia, 2002, WB Saunders.)*

The oral cavity also provides the entrance into the pharynx, which is a muscular tube that serves both the respiratory and digestive systems. Portions of the nasopharynx and oropharynx are observable; the laryngopharynx is more inferior and is not observable. The portion of the pharynx that is superior to the level of the soft palate is the nasopharynx, which is continuous with the nasal cavity. The portion of the pharynx that is between the soft palate and the opening of the larynx is the oropharynx. The opening from the oral cavity into the oropharynx is the fauces. The fauces are formed laterally by folds of tissue called the *anterior and posterior faucial (tonsillar) pillars*. The *palatine tonsils* are masses of lymphoid tissue located between these pillars (Figure 12–21). Tonsils, like lymph nodes, contain lymphocytes that remove toxic products. Lymphadenopathy can also occur in the tonsils, causing tissue enlargement.

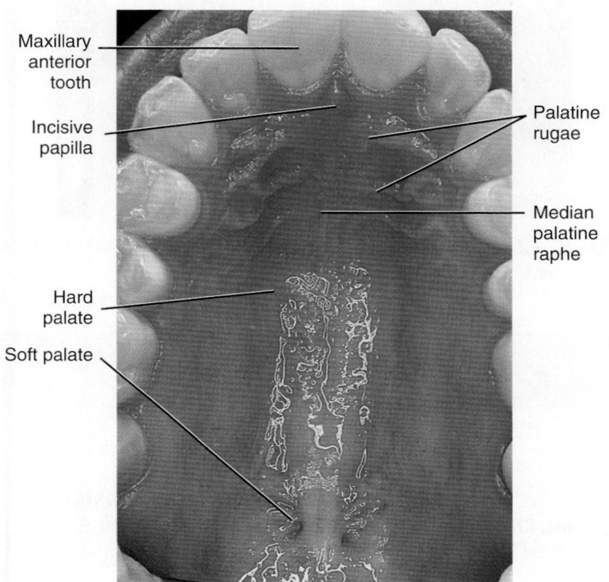

FIGURE 12–23 ✦ View of the palate with its landmarks noted. *(From Fehrenbach MJ, Herring SW:* Illustrated anatomy of the head and neck, ed 2, *Philadelphia, 2002, WB Saunders.)*

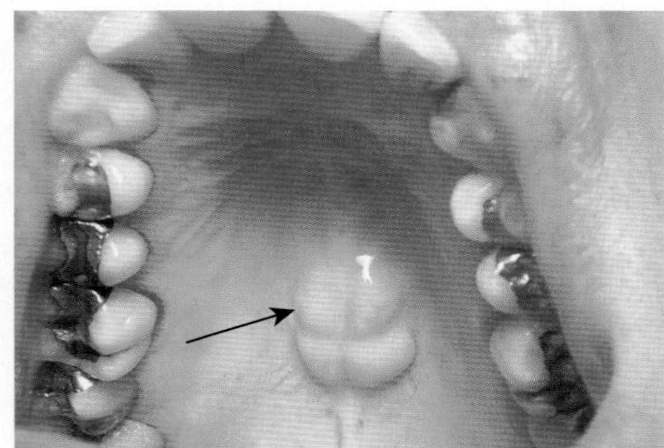

FIGURE 12–24 ✦ Palatal torus. *(Courtesy Dr. M. Walsh, University of California – San Francisco.)*

Tongue

The tongue is an important potential lesion site and must be examined carefully. The posterior one-third of the tongue is its base, which attaches to the floor of the mouth. The base of the tongue does not lie within the oral cavity, but within the oral part of the pharynx. The anterior two-thirds of the tongue is termed the body and it lies within the oral cavity. The top or dorsal surface of the tongue has a midline depression called the median lingual sulcus. The dorsal surface also has small elevated structures of specialized mucosa called lingual papillae that serve in taste sensation. The slender, threadlike, whitish *filiform papillae* give the dorsal surface its velvety texture. The less numerous red, mushroom-shaped dots are the *fungiform papillae.* Figure 12–25 shows the normal anatomy of the dorsal surface of the tongue. Because of these lingual papillae, the dorsal surface of the tongue should not be exceptionally smooth.

Farther posteriorly on the dorsal surface of the tongue and more difficult to visualize clinically is a V-shaped groove, the sulcus terminalis (Figure 12–25). The sulcus terminalis separates the base from the body of the tongue; where it points backward toward the throat is a small pit-like depression called the *foramen cecum.* The *circumvallate papillae* (10 to 14 in number) line up along the anterior side of the sulcus terminalis on the body of the tongue. These large, mushroom-shaped lingual papillae also have taste buds. Farther posteriorly on the dorsal surface of the tongue base is an irregular mass of tonsillar tissue, the lingual tonsil, which is more difficult to see clinically. The side or lateral surface of the tongue is noted for its vertical ridges, the *foliate papillae* (Figure 12–25).

Figure 12–26 identifies the normal anatomy of the ventral surface (under surface) of the tongue and other associated structures. The ventral surface is noted for its visible large blood vessels and the deep lingual veins that run close to the surface. Lateral to each deep lingual vein is the *plica fimbriata,* a feathery fold of tissue.

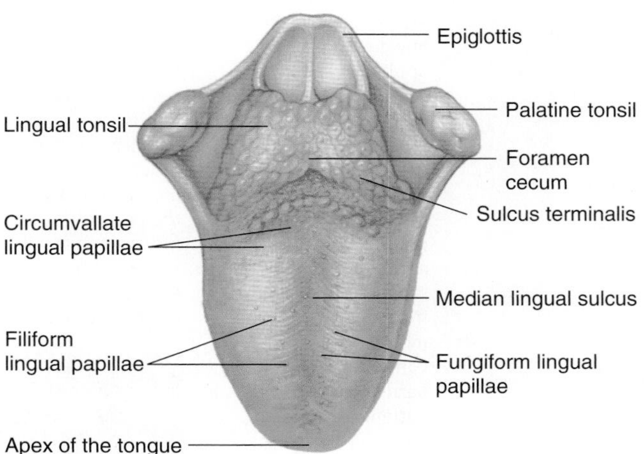

FIGURE 12–25 ✦ Normal anatomy of the dorsal surface of the tongue and relationship of papillae. *(From Fehrenbach MJ, Herring SW:* Illustrated anatomy of the head and neck, ed 2, *Philadelphia, 2002, WB Saunders.)*

Floor of the Mouth

This area is inferior to the ventral surface of the tongue (Figure 12–26). The lingual frenum is a midline fold of tissue between the ventral surface of the tongue and the floor of the mouth. There is also a ridge of tissue on each side of the floor of the mouth, the sublingual folds, that together form a V-shaped configuration from the lingual frenum to the base of the tongue. The sublingual folds contain duct openings from the sublingual salivary gland. The small papilla or *sublingual caruncle* at the anterior end of each sublingual fold contains the submandibular and sublingual duct openings (Wharton's and Bartholin's, respectively) from both the submandibular and sublingual salivary glands. Bony projections known as *mandibular tori* are atypical but normal structures that may be found on the lingual surface of the mandible in the premolar area (Figure 12–27).

Procedure 12–2 details the steps and rationale for examining recommended structures, and lists examples of normal, atypical, and abnormal findings that may be observed during an intraoral assessment. Following this portion of the intraoral assessment, the dental hygienist initiates specific tooth, oral hygiene, and periodontal assessments (see Chapters 13, 14 and 15).

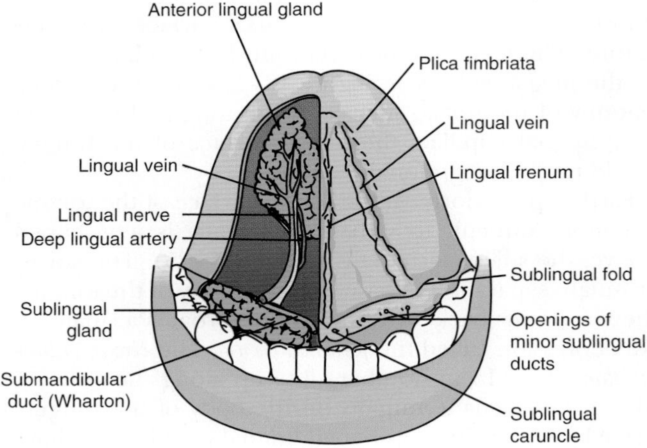

FIGURE 12–26 ✦ Normal anatomy of the ventral surface of the tongue and associated structures. *(From Massler M, Schour I:* Atlas of the mouth, *ed 2, Chicago, 1958, American Dental Association.)*

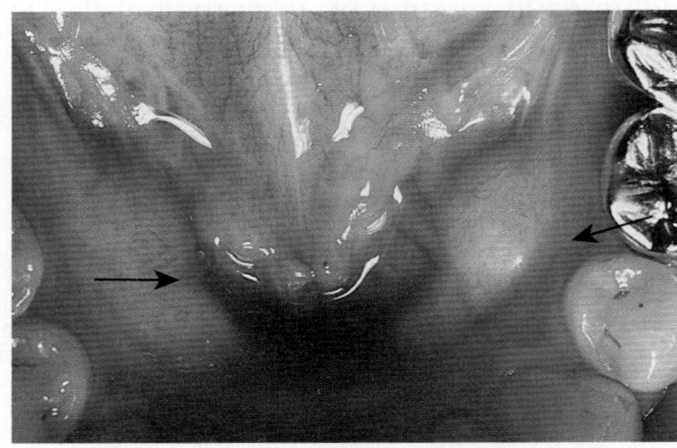

FIGURE 12–27 ✦ Mandibular torus. *(Courtesy Dr. M. Walsh, University of California – San Francisco.)*

Procedure 12–2 CONDUCTING INTRAORAL ASSESSMENTS

EQUIPMENT

Mouth mirror, explorer, periodontal probe, hand mirror, 2 × 2 gauze, paper towel, glass of water, personal protective equipment

INTRAORAL REGIONS	STEPS	RATIONALE	NORMAL FINDINGS	ATYPICAL FINDINGS	ABNORMAL FINDINGS
Lips (Figure 12–28)	Seat the client in a supine position and sit alongside. Remove any dentures or appliances and place in cup of water or mouthrinse. Ask client if he or she is experiencing any areas of discomfort in the mouth. Provide preprocedural antimicrobial mouthrinse. Visually inspect the lips, including the commissures. Ask patient to close. Ask patient to smile.	Allows the clinician to observe the lips and vermilion border and surrounding skin, and the relationship between lips and teeth. Rinsing with an antimicrobial mouthrinse decreases oral microbes prior to the procedure. A functioning facial nerve can be evaluated with symmetric smile.	Lips should be continuous in color, firm in texture, free of lesions, semimoist, with an apparent border between the lips and the skin of the face. Commissures should be continuous and intact. Patient should be able to make lips meet.	Lip dryness, cracks and irritation; angular cheilitis (inflammation and fissuring of the corners of the mouth); herpetic lesions (vesicles that rupture and form crusting of the surface).	Signs of skin and lip cancer; lichen planus (flat, slightly elevated lesions with striae that may have ulcerations); candidiasis (white, loose, curdlike accumulations in the mucosa that can be detached, leaving a red, bleeding surface); sagging lips on affected side with facial paralysis.

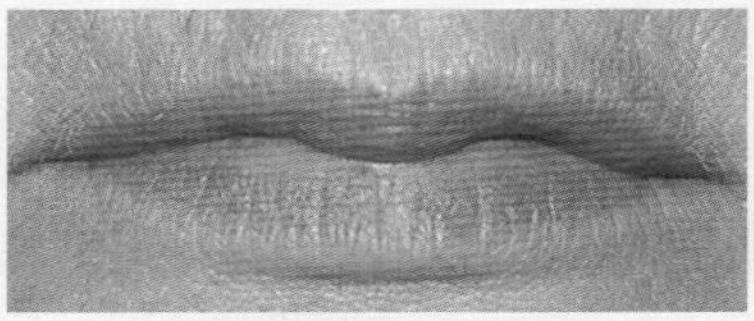

FIGURE 12–28 ✦

Procedure 12–2 CONDUCTING INTRAORAL ASSESSMENTS—CONT'D

INTRAORAL REGIONS	STEPS	RATIONALE	NORMAL FINDINGS	ATYPICAL FINDINGS	ABNORMAL FINDINGS
Oral cavity, including buccal and labial mucosa, parotid glands and ducts, alveolar ridges and attached gingiva (Figure 12–29)	Bidigitally palpate the lower lip systematically from one corner of the mouth to the other, checking the labial frenum. Use same technique for the uper lip. Have the client open his or her mouth slightly and gently pull the lower lip away from the teeth to observe the labial mucosa. Then gently pull the buccal mucosa slightly away from the teeth to palpate bidigitally, using circular compression. Dry the area and observe the flow of saliva from each duct. Retract mucosa enough to visually inspect the vestibular area. Palpate and visually examine the alveolar ridges and attached gingiva. Palpate the maxillary tuberosity and the retromolar area using digital compression.	This step allows the clinician to further assess lips, as well as the oral mucosa for changes in color, form, texture, signs of nutritional deficiency, or fungal infection, and check the labial frena for tightness, tissue tags, or scarring. Allows assessment for enlargements or masses within the gland or duct. This step also allows the clinician to observe swelling, lesions, and color changes of the attached gingiva; and gross signs of periodontal disease or caries.	Oral mucosa should be a continuous pinkish-red color, or pigmented in relation to the normal coloration of the client's skin, firm in texture, free of lesions, and moist. Parotid papilla and duct should be visible and same color and firmness as surrounding mucosa and able to produce saliva. Labial and buccal mucosa will have a pebbly consistency and rough surface texture when palpated due to minor salivary glands. The texture (surface) of the gingiva is generally stippled, and stippling is usually present in varying degrees on facial surfaces of the attached gingiva. A stippled surface is often described as "orange peel" in appearance. The consistency of the gingiva upon palpation should be firm and the attached part tightly anchored to the teeth and underlying alveolar bone.	Mouth breathing; traumatic lesions; abrasions; signs of spit tobacco use; tight labial frena attachment; cheek or inner lip lip biting or chewing; Fordyce's spots (ectopic sebaceous glands); amalgam tattoo; linea alba (white line on buccal mucosa at line of occlusion due to hyperkeratosis); hyperpigmentation; exostosis (benign bony projection from the surface of bone) or mandibular torus; scarring from third molar extractions; impacted third molars.	Signs of oral cancer, lichen planus, or candidiasis; excessive salivary flow or xerostomia (dry mouth); abscesses, fistulas, swellings of the alveolar ridges; alcohol and smoker's breath; halitosis associated with dental caries, periodontitis, necrotizing periodontal diseases; sweet, fruity ketosis associated with diabetic acidosis; trauma associated with domestic abuse

A
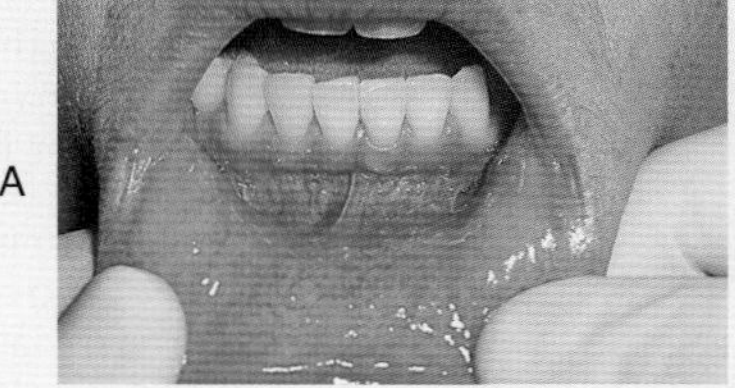

B
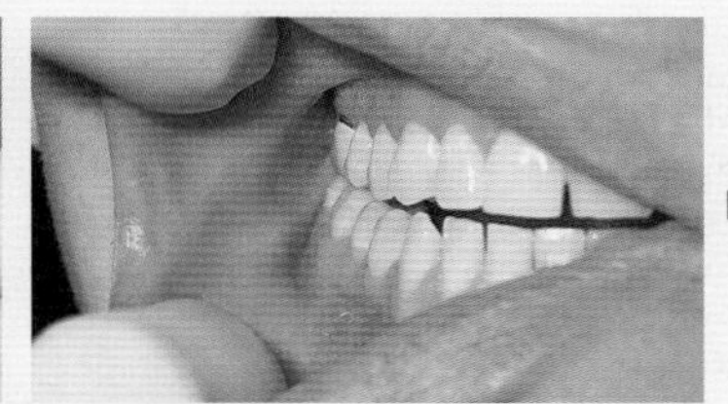

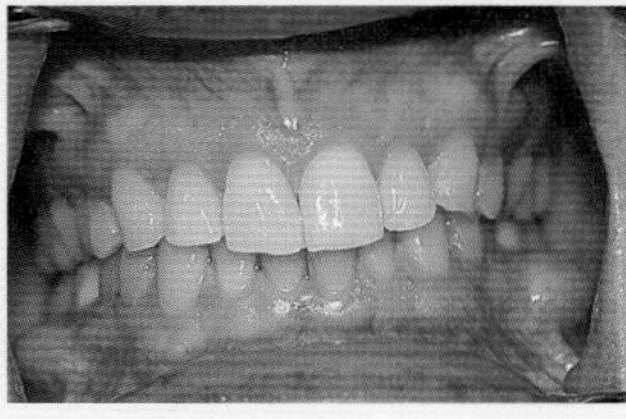
C

FIGURE 12–29 ✦ **A,** View of labial mucosa, labial frenum, mucogingival line, and attached gingiva. **B,** View of the buccal mucosa, parotid papilla, maxillary vestibule, mandibular vestibule, and alveolar mucosa. **C,** Frontal view of periodontium.

Continued on following page

Procedure 12–2 CONDUCTING INTRAORAL ASSESSMENTS—CONT'D

INTRAORAL REGIONS	STEPS	RATIONALE	NORMAL FINDINGS	ATYPICAL FINDINGS	ABNORMAL FINDINGS
Palate and pharynx, including the hard and soft palate, tonsillar pillars, uvula, portions of the oropharynx and nasopharynx (Figure 12–30)	Have client tilt head back slightly. Use mouth mirror to intensify light source and view the palatal and pharyngeal regions. Extend the tongue and observe the soft palate. Gently place the mouth mirror (mirror side down) on the middle of the tongue and ask the client to say "ah." As this is done, visually observe the uvula and the visible portions of the pharynx. Compress hard and soft palate with first or second finger of one hand. Avoid circular compression on the soft palate to prevent initiating the gag reflex.	Allows the clinician to check palatal and pharyngeal tissues for changes in color, form, and texture. 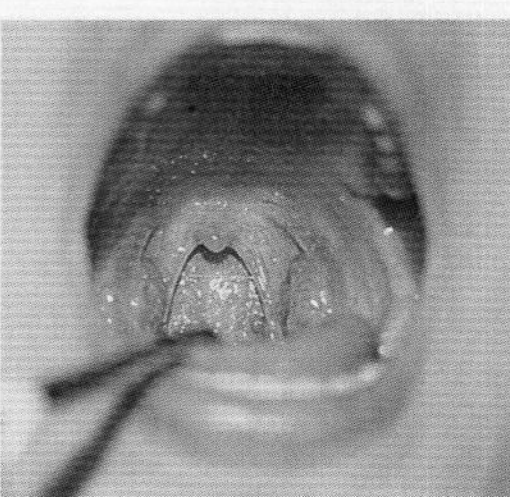 FIGURE 12–30 ✦	Palatal and pharyngeal tissues should be pink in color or pigmented in relation to the normal coloration of the client's skin (with a yellowish hue in the soft palate area), well-hydrated, and devoid of lesions.	Petechiae (pin-point hemorrhagic spots); palatal torus; food burns; nicotine stomatitis (white palatal tissue due to hyperkeratosis or red palatal tissue due to inflamed salivary glands from smoking); bifid (cleft) uvula; prominent tonsillar tissues in children; sore throat.	Denture stomatitis; oral cancer; tonsillitis; trauma due to child abuse. With certain nerve disorders, soft palate will sag on affected side and uvula will be pulled to unaffected side.
Tongue, including all surfaces and swallowing pattern (Figure 12–31) 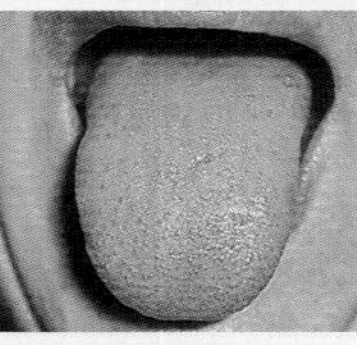 A 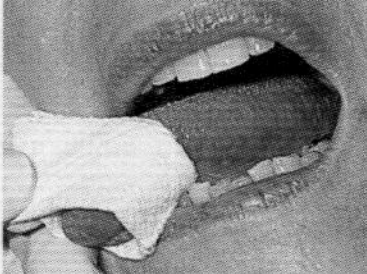 B 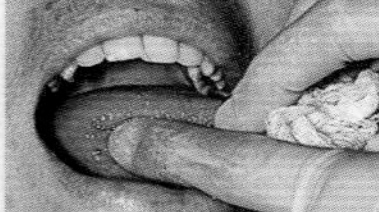 C FIGURE 12–31 ✦	To assess the dorsal and lateral surfaces of the tongue, ask the client to extend the tongue. Wrap a gauze square around the anterior one-third of the tongue to obtain a firm grasp. Digitally palpate the dorsal surface of the tongue. (If the client is forced to extend the tongue too far the gag reflex is triggered.) Turn the tongue slightly on its side to inspect its base and lateral borders. Bidigitally palpate the lateral surfaces of the tongue. To assess the ventral surface, have the client lift the tongue to inspect and digitally palpate the surface. Release the tongue. While holding lips apart, ask client to swallow, and observe swallowing pattern. Client may need glass of water in order to swallow.	Allows the clinician to assess the tongue, especially its base and lateral borders, for abnormal color, swellings, masses, or lesions. Allows for the labial frena to be checked for tightness, tissue tags, or scarring. Allows the clinician to check lingual papilla, foramen cecum, and lingual tonsils; allows evaluation of swallowing pattern.	Bilateral symmetry, extremely vascular, reddish-pink in color all over and moist; may be pigmented in relation to the normal coloration of the skin. Full range of movement, with no excessive movement during swallowing.	Fissured tongue (tongue with clefts or narrow slits in the dorsal surface) or geographic tongue (tongue with areas void or denuded of papillae that appear over time to migrate due to ongoing degeneration and regeneration of lingual papillae); central papillary atrophy (smooth elevation without papillae on the posterior one-third of dorsum of tongue); lingual varicosities; coated or stained tongue; macroglossia (enlarged tongue); tongue thrusting behavior during swallowing; lateral surface may be scalloped from being pressed into the embrasures.	Hairy leukoplakia; tenderness, color changes on tongue; ankyloglossia (short lingual frenum causing limited movement of the tongue); any enlargement, induration, or signs of oral cancer; extreme loss of papilla on tongue related to nutritional disorders; trauma due to child abuse; dysphagia (difficulty swallowing) with certain nerve disorders or oral/pharyngeal cancers.

Procedure 12–2 CONDUCTING INTRAORAL ASSESSMENTS—CONT'D

INTRAORAL REGIONS	STEPS	RATIONALE	NORMAL FINDINGS	ATYPICAL FINDINGS	ABNORMAL FINDINGS
Floor of the mouth, including the submandibular and sublingual salivary glands and ducts (Figure 12–32) 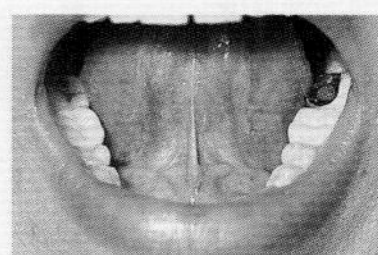 A 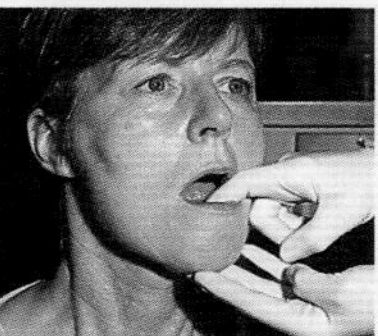 B **FIGURE 12–32** ✦	Use the mouth mirror to facilitate lighting and direct observation. While the client lifts the tongue to the roof of the mouth, observe the mucosa of the floor of the mouth. Check the lingual frenum. Wipe the sublingual caruncle with gauze and observe the saliva flow from the duct. Bimanually palpate the sublingual area by placing the right index finger intraorally and the fingertips of the left hand extraorally under the chin to feel the tissue between the two hands. Use bidigital palpation for the sublingual gland on the floor of the mouth, behind each mandibular canine, by placing the index finger of one hand intraorally and one extraorally with the gland compressed between.	Allows the clinician to detect enlargement or masses, and to note any abnormal growth of soft tissue, gland, or bone, surface lesions, and tenderness.	Bilateral symmetry, extremely vascular, reddish-pink in color, and moist. Sublingual caruncle should be visible and same color and firmness as surrounding mucosa and able to produce saliva.	Tight lingual frenum attachment; mandibular torus/tori.	Sialolithiasis (stones) and blocked duct; ranula; excessive salivary flow or xerostomia; tenderness, color changes; ankyloglossia; any enlargement, induration, or oral cancer.

Steps from Fehrenbach MJ, Herring SW: *Illustrated anatomy of the head and neck*, ed 2, Philadelphia, 2002, WB Saunders. Photos courtesy Dr. M. Walsh, University of California – San Francisco.

DESCRIBING AND DOCUMENTING SIGNIFICANT FINDINGS

Following the observation of atypical or abnormal findings, the dental hygienist describes and documents them accurately in the client record. Precise descriptive terms enable the dental hygienist to communicate with the dentist and other healthcare professionals to facilitate an accurate dental diagnosis. Table 12–3 provides the terminology used to describe lesions.

A sample form used for collecting data during an extraoral and intraoral assessment is shown in Figure 12–33. Figure 12–34 has sample descriptions of lesions for entry into a client record. Specific descriptive items that need to be included in the client record when describing a lesion are discussed in the following sections.

Location and Distribution

When documenting the location of a lesion, it is important to be as accurate as possible so that follow-up examination may be made correctly even if the lesion has healed and no longer remains. The location also is important because some lesions characteristically occur in specific areas or tissues and this information can help the dentist formulate a differential dental diagnosis. For example, hairy leukoplakia occurs usually on the lateral borders of the tongue in HIV-positive clients. When describing the location of an oral lesion, the dental hygienist should identify the nearest anatomic landmark (e.g., upper lip, labial mucosa, tongue, and specific teeth) and note the lesion's anatomic relationship to the structure (e.g., anterior/posterior, lateral/medial, or inferior/superior).

The lesion's location must also specify whether it is located on the right side or on the left side for *unilateral* lesions; for *bilateral* lesions, specify that the lesion is located on both sides of the face/neck/oral cavity. Some lesions may be located in the midline. Generally, bilateral structures are normal anatomic structures but a unilateral structure may indicate a pathologic lesion.

In addition to location, *distribution* of the lesion needs to be described. The distribution of a lesion is either single or multiple in number. For example, a mucocele (an elevated lesion due to accumulation of saliva from a blocked duct) is a single lesion, whereas herpes simplex virus manifesting on the gingiva often presents as multiple lesions.

Multiple lesions may be described as being either separate or coalescing. Multiple lesions that are discrete and do not run together are *separate,* whereas lesions with margins that merge are *coalescing.* In addition, multiple lesions may be localized or generalized. *Localized* refers to lesions that are limited to a single area, whereas *generalized* describes lesions involving more than one area

TABLE 12–3

CATEGORIES OF ORAL LESIONS

Lesion	Term	Size (cm)	Description	Example
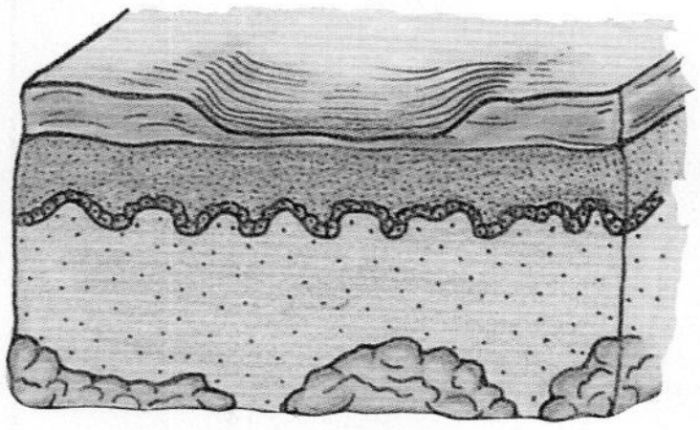	Atrophy	Varies	Thinning of tissue layers with loss of normal skin furrow, with shiny and translucent appearance	Oral mucosa with certain dermatologic disorders
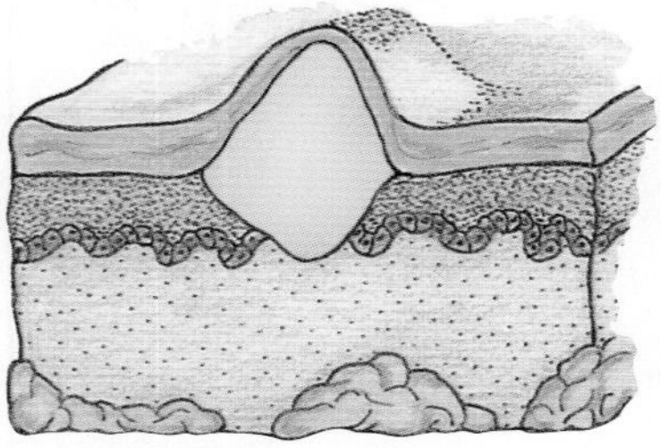	Bulla	> 0.5	Circumscribed lesion containing clear, watery fluid or blood	Large blister in pemphigus or pemphigoid
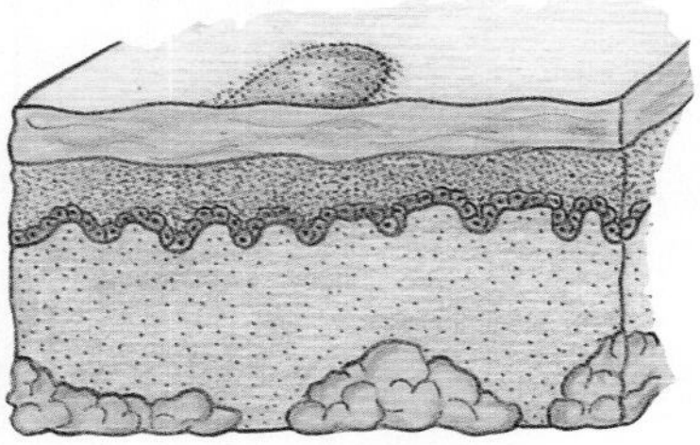	Macule	< 1	Flat, nonpalpable	Freckle, petechiae
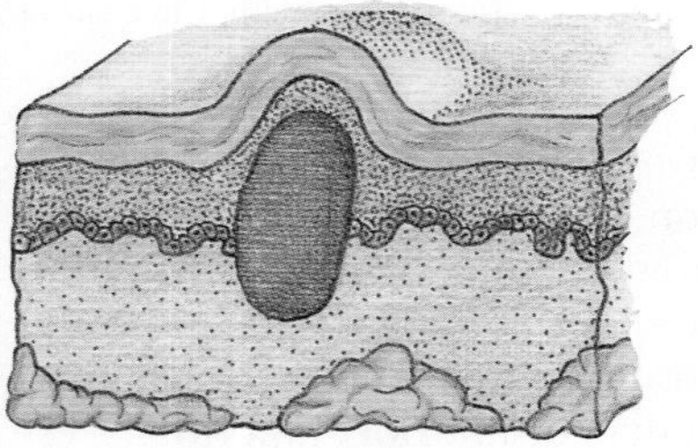	Nodule	0.5-2	Elevated solid mass, deeper and firmer than papule	Wart
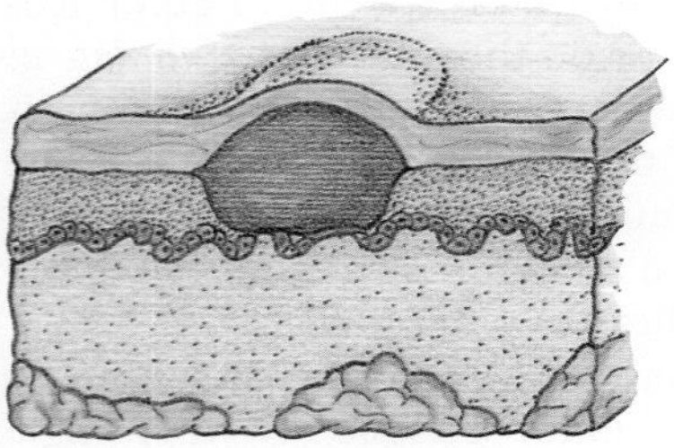	Papule	< 0.5	Palpable, circumscribed, solid elevation	Elevated freckle
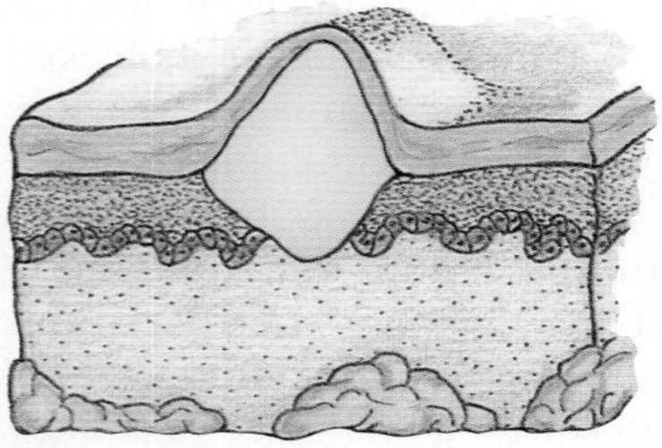	Pustule	Varies	Similar to vesicle; lesion filled with pus	Acne pimple

TABLE 12–3 CATEGORIES OF ORAL LESIONS—CONT'D

Lesion	Term	Size (cm)	Description	Example
	Plaque	> 0.5	Discrete, slightly elevated area of altered texture or coloration	Candidiasis
	Ulcer	Varies	Deep loss of epithelial layer; may extend to connective tissue layers	Recurrent aphthous ulcer
	Vesicle	< 0.5	Circumscribed elevation filled with serous fluid	Herpes labialis blister
	Wheal	Varies	Elevated area of superficial localized edema; irregularly shaped	Hive

Modified from Potter PA, Perry AG: *Fundamentals of nursing*, ed 3, St Louis, 2001, Mosby.

and may indicate a systemic disease of a dermatologic nature (e.g., lichen planus).

Size and Shape

The size of a lesion is determined by using a periodontal probe to measure its length, width, and height. The size of oral lesions varies, but generally a lesion is not apparent to the client when it is smaller than 1 to 2 cm. In addition, the height of a lesion, whether it is raised *(papule)* or flat *(macule),* and the contour of its borders relate to its shape. The borders of the lesion need to be documented as being either well defined or poorly defined. Generally, benign lesions have well-defined borders and are round or ovoid in shape. In contrast, malignancies have poorly defined borders and thus an irregular shape due to the infiltration process of malignancies and inflammation and fibrosis of surrounding tissues.

Color

Any unusual color changes in oral tissues may signal an abnormal condition. Lesion colors observed normally are red and white. Other less common colors may include blue, purple, yellow, black, or gray. Lesions can even exhibit the same color as the adjacent tissue. Lesions of a red color may be the result of thinning of the surface epithelium, increased vascularity, or dissolution of connective tissue. White lesions may be the result of hyperkeratosis of the surface epithelium, decreased vascularity of the connective tissue, or an increased amount of collagen tissue or fibrosis.

Brownish, bluish, or black lesions indicate that there is a deposit of melanin, blood, or heavy metal in the tissues, such as amalgam particles (an amalgam tattoo). In addition, fluid-filled lesions or lesions with extra or large blood vessels can appear bluish. Yellow lesions usually

ORAL/FACIAL SOFT TISSUE EXAMINATION RECORD

PATIENT'S NAME: ______________________

PATIENT'S I.D. #: ______________________

N = Normal   O = Other
use "Notes" section

Date:	____		____		____		____	
EXTRAORAL	**N**	**O**	**N**	**O**	**N**	**O**	**N**	**O**
Skin –Face	☐	☐	☐	☐	☐	☐	☐	☐
–Neck	☐	☐	☐	☐	☐	☐	☐	☐
* Vermilion Borders	☐	☐	☐	☐	☐	☐	☐	☐
Parotid Glands	☐	☐	☐	☐	☐	☐	☐	☐
Lymph Nodes	☐	☐	☐	☐	☐	☐	☐	☐
Anterior Cervical	☐	☐	☐	☐	☐	☐	☐	☐
Posterior Cervical	☐	☐	☐	☐	☐	☐	☐	☐
Submental	☐	☐	☐	☐	☐	☐	☐	☐
Submandibular	☐	☐	☐	☐	☐	☐	☐	☐
Supraclavicular	☐	☐	☐	☐	☐	☐	☐	☐
INTRAORAL								
Labial Mucosa	☐	☐	☐	☐	☐	☐	☐	☐
Labial Vestibules	☐	☐	☐	☐	☐	☐	☐	☐
Anterior Gingivae	☐	☐	☐	☐	☐	☐	☐	☐
Buccal Vestibules	☐	☐	☐	☐	☐	☐	☐	☐
Buccal Gingivae	☐	☐	☐	☐	☐	☐	☐	☐
Tongue–Dorsal	☐	☐	☐	☐	☐	☐	☐	☐
* –Ventral	☐	☐	☐	☐	☐	☐	☐	☐
* –Lateral	☐	☐	☐	☐	☐	☐	☐	☐
* Lingual Tonsils	☐	☐	☐	☐	☐	☐	☐	☐
* Floor of Mouth	☐	☐	☐	☐	☐	☐	☐	☐
Lingual Gingivae	☐	☐	☐	☐	☐	☐	☐	☐
* Tonsillar Pillars	☐	☐	☐	☐	☐	☐	☐	☐
* Pharyngeal Wall	☐	☐	☐	☐	☐	☐	☐	☐
* Soft Palate	☐	☐	☐	☐	☐	☐	☐	☐
Uvula	☐	☐	☐	☐	☐	☐	☐	☐
Hard Palate	☐	☐	☐	☐	☐	☐	☐	☐
Palatal Gingivae	☐	☐	☐	☐	☐	☐	☐	☐
Submandibular Glands	☐	☐	☐	☐	☐	☐	☐	☐

* *High risk sites for squamous carcinoma*

RIGHT LEFT

NOTES

RECOMMENDATIONS:

1. Establish an examination sequence and follow it routinely.
2. Tell the patient you are performing a complete Soft Tissue Examination.
3. Examine ALL areas each time.
4. Use visual inspection AND palpation.
5. Record ALL findings—Normal or Abnormal.
6. Remove dental appliances before the examination.
7. Suggested descriptive terms: hard, soft, well-circumscribed, ill-defined, indurated, sessile, pedunculated, hemorrhagic, ulcerated, edematous, normal in color, red, white, speckled, color other than normal.

FOLLOW-UP TAKEN

Biopsy ______________________

Results ______________________

Referral to Dr. ______________________

Other ______________________

This chart is a general guideline. Neither the American Cancer Society nor the California Dental Association assume liability for individual evaluation or recommendations.

American Cancer Society® CALIFORNIA Developed by the Dental Education Subcommittee American Cancer Society, California Division, Inc.

FIGURE 12–33 ✦ Extraoral and intraoral assessment form. *(Courtesy American Cancer Society.)*

Example No. 1:

Chart Entry:
Positive finding on intraoral examination: lower right labial mucosa, single white sessile nodule 2 x 3 x 2 mm with a slightly rough surface; nonmobile on palpation. Client is asymptomatic with no associated lymphadenopathy. Client has been informed and will return for follow-up visit in 2 weeks—possible biopsy or referral to oral surgeon if the lesion changes in nature or does not resolve.

Date the entry; have the entry initialed by DDS and RDH.

Example No. 2:

Chart entry:
Positive finding on extraoral examination: upper left vermilion border, multiple coalescing vesicles 5 x 3 x 7 mm in total area; slightly red in color with a crust. Lesions have been known to the client for 5 days and began with associated tingling and itching in the area prior to appearance of the lesions. Client reports a history of similar "cold sores" in the area.

Date the entry; have the entry initialed by DDS and RDH.

FIGURE 12–34 ✦ Sample descriptions of lesions for entry into the client's dental record

contin sebaceous glands or adipose tissue. Sometimes these color modifications can occur simultaneously in the same lesion area and the dental hygienist must note this. Also it should be noted if the lesion is hemorrhaging (bleeding) spontaneously or easily with touch.

Texture

The *texture* of a lesion refers to the surface appearance, which is taken into account when establishing a list of possible differential dental diagnoses. (A *differential diagnosis* is the identification of one of several diseases or conditions as the one responsible for producing symptoms reported and signs observed.) Terminology used to describe the surface texture of a lesion is described in Table 12–4. Most normal oral mucosae are smooth in texture on the surface, except in the areas of the palatal rugae and stippling of the attached gingiva. Lesions of surface epithelial tissues frequently have a rough surface, whereas those of deeper tissues may have a smooth surface.

Attachment and Depth

If a lesion has a broad base of attachment as wide as the lesion itself, its attachment is described as *sessile*. In contrast, *pedunculated* lesions have a narrow pedicle, or stalk-like base of attachment (Figure 12–35). Superficial or deep depth is determined by checking with palpation.

Consistency

Consistency refers to the degree of firmness or density of the tissue. Palpation is required to categorize the consistency of a lesion. This categorization can be accomplished by palpating the lesion and then comparing its felt degree of softness, hardness, or firmness to normal tissues of the body. The terminology used to indicate the consistency of a lesion and normal tissue comparisons is described in Table 12–5.

TABLE 12–4 TERMINOLOGY USED TO DESCRIBE SURFACE TEXTURE OF A LESION

Term	Description
Cratered	Centrally depressed like a bowl or saucer
Crust	Hard outer layer or covering composed of dried serum, pus, blood, or a combination
Indurated	Hardness primarily as a result of an increase in the number of epithelial cells
Papillary	Rough surface resembling small nodulations or elevated projections
Pseudomembrane	Loose membranous layer of exudate containing organisms formed during an inflammatory reaction of the surface tissue
Smooth	Deep lesions that push up and stretch surface tissue
Verrucous	Rough, wart-like surface with multiple irregular folds

Modified from Wilkins EM: *The clinical practice of the dental hygienist,* Philadelphia, 1989, Lea & Febiger.

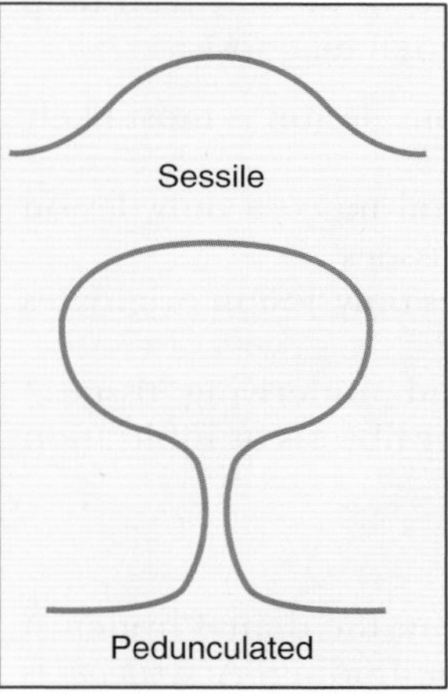

FIGURE 12–35 ✦ Types of base or attachment of a lesion.

All soft lesions over 1 cm in diameter should also be tested for *fluctuance* by placing the fingers of one hand on one side of the lesion and gently pressing on the lesion with the fingers of the other hand. If the fingers can detect a wave or force passing through the lesion, the lesion is said to be fluctuant. The lesion should also be checked for *emptiability,* which is the temporary loss of fluctuance due to brief removal of the fluid of the lesion into the surrounding tissues.

Mobility

It is important to note if a lesion is free or fixed in relationship to the neighboring tissues. This is done by fixing the lesion with the fingers of one hand, while moving the oral mucosa or skin over the lesion with the other hand to see if it is fixed to its overlying tissues. Then an attempt is made to move the lesion independently from its underlying structures/tissues; this will demonstrate if the lesion is freely movable in all directions. Note that certain areas of the oral mucosa do not normally allow movement of the oral mucosa separate from the deeper structures such as

TABLE 12–5 TERMINOLOGY TO INDICATE CONSISTENCY OF A LESION

Term	Description	Normal Tissue Comparison
Soft	Lesion or tissue composed chiefly of cells without much intervening fibrous connective tissue	Adipose tissue, loose connective tissue or glandular tissue
Firm	Lesion or tissue that is harder than the adjacent softer mucosa, indicating a high content of fibrous connective tissue	Cartilage
Hard	Lesion or tissue that contains bone or other calcified material	Bone or enamel

Modified from Wilkins EM: *The clinical practice of the dental hygienist*, Philadelphia, 1989, Lea & Febiger.

the attached gingiva, median palatine raphe, or hard palate.

Generally, the following aspects of mobility can help the dentist make a differential dental diagnosis:

- If freely movable in all directions, lesion is most likely benign and/or encapsulated
- If fixed to overlying skin or oral mucosa only, lesion originates from the overlying tissues
- If fixed to underlying structures only, lesion originates from the underlying tissues
- If fixed to both overlying and underlying tissues/ structures, lesion involves either fibrosis or infiltration of a malignancy

Symptomatology

By directing questions to the client, the dental hygienist can elicit symptoms related to the finding. A *symptom* is a subjective condition reported by the individual. In contrast, a *sign* is an objective condition that can be directly observed. Specifically, the dental hygienist needs to determine and then document in the client record the following information related to symptoms:

- Whether the lesion is known or unknown to the client
- If the lesion is known to the client, how long it has been present, and if there have been any changes in its size and appearance
- Whether the client has related neurologic symptoms: pain, tingling, burning, or numbness; generally, painful lesions are due to inflammation
- Laboratory findings related to radiographs, blood tests, ultrasound readings, histologic evaluation, and any test performed by the client's physician must be documented in the client record.

ORAL CANCER

One of the most serious conditions that can occur in the oral cavity is oral cancer. Oral cancer is a devastating disease when detected in its later stages. Late-stage treatment usually involves major facial surgery, radiation, and chemotherapy, with only half of such patients surviving past five years.[4] Annually, oral cancer in the United States kills more people than cervical cancer and costs society more than $3.7 billion in treatment.[5]

Squamous cell carcinoma (cancer) makes up 90% of all malignant neoplasms of the oral cavity.[5] There is a higher risk of malignant transformation in red and ulcerated areas than in white patches, although the latter can also be malignant. Squamous cell cancer is associated with certain risk factors such as tobacco use, alcohol abuse, human papillomavirus, and, for extraoral lesions, excessive sun exposure.

Although cancer may arise at any site in the oral cavity, the most common sites in order are:

- Lateral border of the tongue
- Soft palate complex (posterior soft palate, uvula, and faucial arches)
- Floor of the mouth
- Lower lip

A cancerous lesion does not show healing and resolution within a two-week window of time, as most traumatic or infective lesions do, and does not respond to treatment. Instead, the cancerous lesions show changes in color, shape, and size over time. Table 12–6 presents terminology used to describe common signs of oral cancer. (For information on dental hygiene care for persons with cancer, see Chapter 43.)

Client Self-examination

The client–dental hygienist interaction is an opportunity to instruct clients in simple self-examination techniques, empowering them with the skills to note any changes in their own extraoral or intraoral conditions. (See http://evolve.elsevier.com/Darby/hygiene/ for oral cancer self-examination procedures.)

The Need for Early Detection

Approximately 30,000 new cases of oral cancer are diagnosed each year, a figure that represents about 3% of all cancers in the United States.[5] Oral cancer is more common than cancers of the brain, liver, bone, stomach, cervix, and ovaries. Oral cancer is more common than leukemia. Approximately 8000 deaths from oral cancer occur in the United States each year.[5] The mortality rate from oral cancer has changed little over the last 40 years and approximately 50% of those who develop oral cancer die from the disease within 5 years. This high mortality rate is due to late detection of the disease. Over 50% of oral cancers are in advanced stages when diagnosed and show evidence of invasion and metastasis.[6,7] This late diagnosis of the disease is tragic because the cure rate is over 90% when oral cancer is detected early (when the lesion is <2 cm).

Public awareness of oral cancer as compared with other cancers is low and this contributes to delays in diagnosis. Also, many early oral cancers appear clinically benign, and it is not possible to determine with certainty which are malignant without performing a biopsy. Since scalpel biopsy often seems extreme for what appears to

TABLE 12–6 TERMINOLOGY FOR COMMON SIGNS OF CANCER

Term	Definition
Chronicity	Failure to heal
Erythroplakia	Used to identify a red patch that is smooth, granular, and velvety and that cannot be diagnosed as any other disease
Fixation	Nonmobile lesion occurring as a result of abnormally dividing cells invading to deeper areas and into muscle and bone
Induration	Hardness primarily as a result of an increase in number of epithelial cells from an inflammatory infiltrate
Leukoplakia	Used to identify a white, plaque-like lesion that cannot be wiped off and cannot be diagnosed as any other disease
Lymphadenopathy	Disease process affecting the lymph nodes resulting in hardening and enlargement of the nodes
Ulceration	Loss of skin surface resulting from destruction of epithelial integrity owing to discrepancy in cell maturation, loss of intercellular attachments, and disruption of the basement membrane

be an innocuous lesion, many early oral cancers remain undiagnosed and progress to a more advanced stage.

Because many clients are seen more regularly for preventive periodontal care than for medical visits in the United States, dental hygienists have a unique opportunity during client assessment to detect oral cancer while it is still asymptomatic, innocuous, and unsuspected. Several techniques have been suggested for early evaluation of lesions to determine whether they show cellular changes that may be cancerous and hence need a scalpel biopsy. These methods include oral cytology, toluidine blue staining,[8] disposable light for identification of abnormal oral tissue, and OralCDx brush biopsy.[9] These methods are intended as adjuncts to and not a substitute for scalpel biopsy.

To understand and compare the relative value of these techniques, it is important to understand the structure of oral epithelial tissue. Oral epithelium consists of three layers: the basal cell layer, the intermediate layer, and the surface layer. Normally, cell division occurs in the basal cell layer. Cells then move through the intermediate layer to the surface where they are exfoliated naturally. An important feature of a method for early detection of oral cancer and precancerous lesions is that it evaluates cells from all layers of the epithelium.

Oral Cytology

In the *oral cytology* method, also known as exfoliative cytology, the oral practitioner collects cells by scraping the surface of a lesion with a cotton swab (Figure 12–36), spreads them on a slide, fixes and stains the specimen on the slide, and sends the slide to a competent pathologist for evaluation. The chief disadvantage of this method is that it is only likely to harvest superficial cells, which may have little diagnostic value. Therefore, oral cytology in practice has a minor role in the detection of precancerous and cancerous lesions.[10]

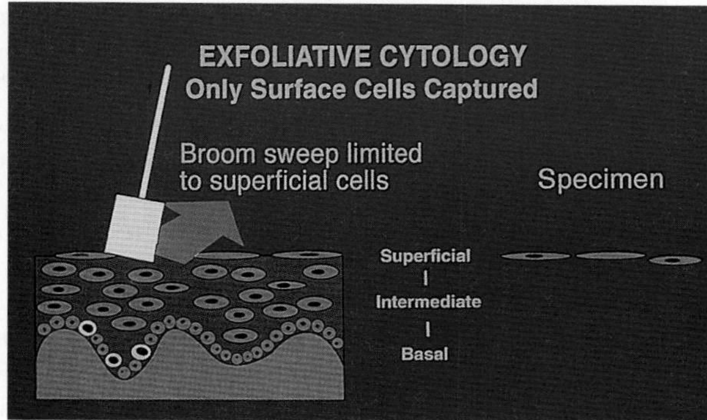

FIGURE 12–36 ✦ Oral cytology. *(Courtesy CDx Laboratories, Inc., Suffern, NY.)*

Toluidine Blue

Toluidine blue is a metachromatic dye (stains certain tissue a different color) that stains cells differentially depending on their nuclear configuration and other cellular characteristics. Because toluidine blue is regarded as a nuclear stain, selective dye uptake by dysplastic (abnormal) and malignant cells, which contain quantitatively more nucleic acids than normal tissue, is the premise for its use to confirm clinical impressions of abnormal cellular changes.[8] A drawback to using toluidine blue on the surface of a lesion to detect dysplasia is that inflammatory cells, often present on the surface of lesions, also take up the stain and make interpretation of the test difficult. Toluidine blue often is used, however, during biopsy to define margins of the lesions and secondary lesions.

Disposable Light for Identification of Abnormal Oral Tissue

Used in conjunction with a conventional visual oral mucosal examination, a new disposable light test improves identification, evaluation, and monitoring of oral mucosal abnormalities in those at increased risk for cancer. The test kit includes a hand-held disposable chemiluminescent light and flavored 1% acetic mouth rinse that work together to help detect abnormalities in the oral cavity that might not be visible to the unaided eye. It is a painless, noninvasive procedure that can be performed in less than 2 minutes. The rinse helps to disrupt the glycoprotein barrier of mucosal surfaces, improving visualization of abnormal tissue. Normal epithelium will absorb the device's illumination and appear dark, while abnormal epithelium will reflect it and appear bright white. As a cell becomes more dysplastic, the nucleus becomes larger compared with the rest of the cell. The enlarged nucleus reflects light and appears bright white, focusing the health professional's attention on lesions that might not be seen otherwise and that may, upon biopsy, reveal cancer and precancerous cells.

OralCDx Brush Biopsy

OralCDx (CDx Laboratories, Inc., Suffern, NY; 800-560-4467) has developed a lesion evaluation technique that uses a specially designed brush to remove cells from lesions that might not otherwise be subjected to biopsy due to their benign appearance. The supplied brush in the *OralCDx brush biopsy* captures a specimen of all three layers of epithelium to help the oral practitioner determine if a lesion is in fact benign or if it should be submitted for scalpel biopsy and histology (Figure 12–37).[10] The brush containing the cells is then spread on a slide that is sent to CDx laboratories for computer-assisted analysis and confirmation by a pathologist.

OralCDx brush biopsy has received the Seal of Acceptance by the American Dental Association. Dental hygienists are specifically permitted to perform the brush biopsy procedure in certain states, including Nevada, Utah, Maryland, Louisiana, New Mexico, and Oregon. The technique for performing an OralCDx brush biopsy is described in Procedure 12–3. All of the materials required are provided in an OralCDx test kit, supplied to practitioners free of charge (Figure 12–38). The kit consists of:

- ✦ A coded test requisition form on which a client's demographic information is recorded as well as all relevant clinical information (e.g., a detailed description of the lesion and the area from which the brush biopsy was taken)
- ✦ A precoded glass slide that matches the code on the requisition form
- ✦ Fixative
- ✦ A sterile oral brush instrument
- ✦ A plastic protective container for the slide
- ✦ A prestamped and addressed mailing carton in which to send the slide to the laboratory

All specimens are examined at OralScan Laboratories in Suffern, NY. Slides are scanned by the OralCDx computer system, which is programmed to search for any of the variations of cell morphology and keratinization that are seen in dysplasia or carcinoma of oral epithelium. Any abnormal cells identified by the computer system are noted, and a pathologist then reviews these computer-selected abnormal cells to determine whether there is evidence of dysplasia or carcinoma.

Specimens are classified into the following categories:

- ✦ **Negative:** No epithelial abnormality detected
- ✦ **Atypical:** Epithelial changes of uncertain diagnostic significance
- ✦ **Positive:** Definitive evidence of epithelial dysplasia or carcinoma
- ✦ **Inadequate:** The specimen did not show evidence of cells from all layers of the epithelium

When the pathologist judges the biopsy to show cells suspicious for precancer or cancer, representative cells are displayed on the computer and the images are printed onto the report form, which is provided to the dentist performing the oral brush biopsy. A scalpel biopsy is recommended for any lesions with an "atypical" or "positive" report.[10]

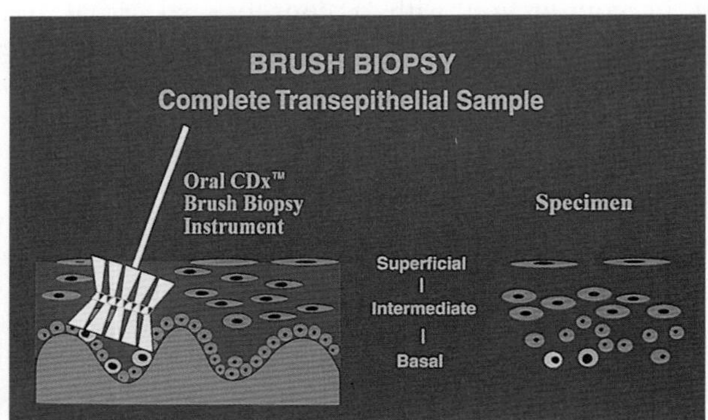

FIGURE 12–37 ✦ OralCDx brush biopsy. *(Courtesy CDx Laboratories, Inc.)*

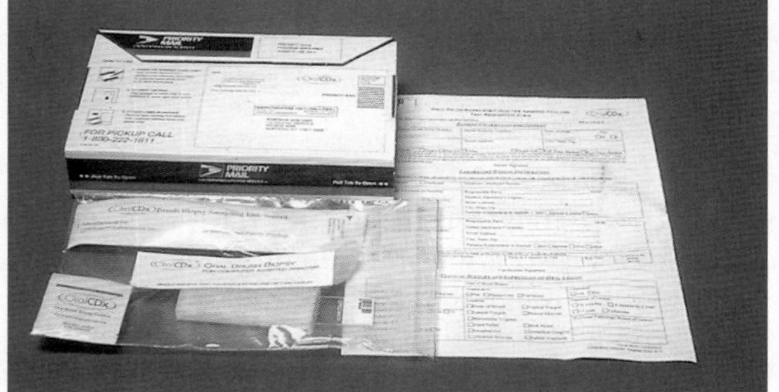

FIGURE 12–38 ✦ OralCDx test kit. *(Courtesy CDx Laboratories, Inc.)*

SPECIFICITY AND SENSITIVITY. *Sensitivity of a test* is the probability that an abnormality will be correctly reported as positive. The results of a multicenter study on the effectiveness of the OralCDx technique reported that its measured sensitivity was 100%.[9] The calculated biostatistical sensitivity (i.e., that which would apply to the general population) is at least 96%. This means that if 100 lesions were known to be positive, OralCDx would be expected to properly report at least 96 of them as "positive," yielding at most a 4% false negative rate.

The *specificity of a test* is the probability that a normal specimen will be correctly reported as "negative." The specificity of the OralCDx positive result was reported to be 100%.[8] The calculated biostatistical specificity of the OralCDx positive result is at least 97%. This means that if 100 lesions were known to be negative, OralDCx would be expected to properly report at least 97 of them as negative, yielding at most a 3% false positive rate. For comparison, the sensitivity and specificity of mammography for women ages 40 and higher is 75% and 90%, respectively. Thus, the OralCDx brush biopsy determines the significance of an oral lesion definitively and detects innocuous-appearing oral cancers at early curable stages with great accuracy. A lesion that is present for two weeks or more without a satisfactory explanation should be tested by brush biopsy to determine if a scalpel biopsy is needed. If used widely by dentists and dental hygienists, many precancerous and oral cancer lesions could be detected much earlier, leading to significant improvements in the mortality rates for oral cancer.[10]

Scalpel Biopsy

Biopsy with a scalpel or "punch" biopsy instrument is the traditional method of diagnosing a cancer. The decision to perform a biopsy, after any unusual oral lesion is identified, is made by the dentist. *Biopsy* is the surgical removal of a section of tissue or other material from the living body for the purpose of diagnosis, to estimate prognosis, and to monitor the cause of disease when the tissue

Procedure 12–3 CONDUCTING AN ORALCDX BRUSH BIOPSY

EQUIPMENT

OralCDx test kit with instructions, return mailing box, barcoded specimen slide and holder, sterile brush instrument, fixative packet; personal protective equipment

STEPS	RATIONALE
1. Put on personal protective equipment before handling brush instrument and slide.	Prevents contamination of the slide and maintains infection control protocol
2. Remove brush from kit (Figure 12-39). Slightly moisten the brush with the client's saliva if the lesion is dry. Neither local nor topical anesthetic is required and should not be used because it may distort the sample.	Prevents the cells from drying and becoming distorted

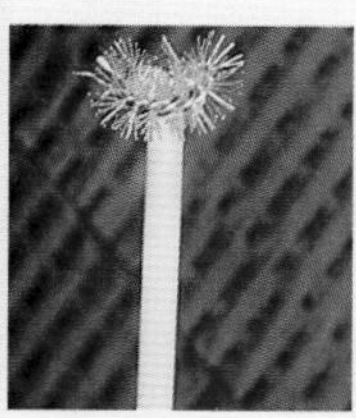

FIGURE 12–39 ✦ OralCDx brush. *(Courtesy CDx Laboratories, Inc.)*

STEPS	RATIONALE
3. Press the brush firmly against the lesion and rotate 5 to 10 times (depending on the thickness of the lesion) until pink tissue or pinpoint microbleeding is observed (Figure 12-40).	Allows a full transepithelial collection of sample cells from the lesion

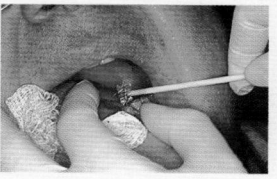

FIGURE 12–40 ✦ Pressing the brush firmly against the lesion. *(Courtesy CDx Laboratories, Inc.)*

STEPS	RATIONALE
4. Spread the cellular sample from the brush onto the slide by rotating and dragging the brush lengthwise (Figure 12-41).	Ensures that the greatest possible amount of material is transferred from the brush to the slide

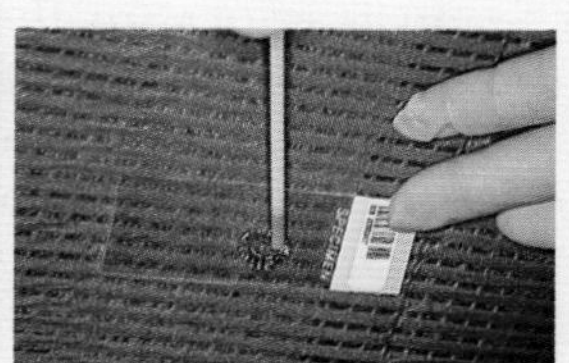

FIGURE 12–41 ✦ Spreading cellular sample on OralCDx slide. *(Courtesy CDx Laboratories, Inc.)*

STEPS	RATIONALE
5. Immediately fix the cells by squeezing the entire contents of one fixative package onto the slide, flooding the slide. Set the slide aside to dry for 15 minutes and then place in slide holder.	Ensures that the cells do not dry out and become distorted
6. Complete the test requisition form and send the specimen to the laboratory in the box provided.	Allows for completion of information such as the dentist's name and address, client's name and address, and a complete clinical description of the lesion necessary for documentation
7. Document procedure in the client record and note on calendar when the pathology report is due back.	Done for legal purposes and to facilitate continuity of care and ensure that the report is not overlooked or ignored
8. Read the pathology report from the laboratory and make sure that findings are shared with the client.	Ensures that client is informed and that appropriate follow-up care is obtained
9. Guide the client to receive the appropriate follow-up care, as recommended by the dentist.	Increases the likelihood that client will adhere to recommendations

later undergoes microscopic assessment.[8] *Excisional biopsy* indicates that the entire lesion is removed for assessment. *Incisional biopsy* indicates that only a representative section is taken.

After the specimen is obtained and properly packaged for transport to a laboratory, it is analyzed by a pathologist. A report of the findings is then issued by the pathologist, who assesses the histologic appearance of the suspected lesion in conjunction with the clinical diagnosis. This report is then sent to the dentist to determine any further action. The report should be discussed with the client and placed, as well as noted, in the client record.

CLIENT EDUCATION ISSUES

- Discuss the importance of annual oral assessment for early detection and diagnosis of oral diseases.
- Instruct the client in simple self-examination techniques for early detection of oral cancer.
- Discuss the elimination of high-risk behaviors that predispose to oral cancer, such as tobacco use, alcohol abuse, and sun exposure.

LEGAL, ETHICAL, AND SAFETY ISSUES

- Dental hygienists have the responsibility to refer all clients with head and neck or oral lesions to the dentist for dental diagnosis.
- Dental hygienists need to perform extraoral and intraoral assessment following the proper standards for infection control.
- On identification of a lesion, the client must be informed of its existence. The clinician should use appropriate verbal skills, and pertinent information must be provided in writing if the client is referred to a specialist for further treatment. The dental hygienist collaborates with the dentist, who determines the course of action to take to protect the client's well-being.
- Biopsy is the only method of definitively diagnosing a cancer.
- All services rendered, including radiographic imaging, must be documented in ink and the entry dated in the client's record. Documentation should include information on the number and type of radiographs exposed and the diagnostic information obtained from them. This information will ensure integrity of the client's record for both the client's health and the legal protection of the practitioner.
- It is the legal responsibility of the dental hygienist to practice within the scope of practice authorized by state law concerning performance of a brush biopsy.

KEY CONCEPTS

- Careful overall observation of the client and a thorough assessment of the areas in and around the oral cavity are essential to planning and providing optimum client care.
- The oral tissues are sensitive indicators of general health. Changes in these structures may be the first indication of subclinical disease processes in other parts of the body.
- It is the responsibility of the dental hygienist to recognize oral tissue changes from normal and to refer clients with such changes to the dentist for further evaluation.
- The dental hygienist must establish an assessment sequence and follow it systematically during client assessment, incorporating the skills of direct observation, palpation, auscultation, and olfaction.
- During the assessment, a dental hygienist needs to examine clients carefully for any palpable lymph nodes and document if any are present. The lymph nodes that are palpable may pinpoint where a disease process is active and will assist in the diagnosis, treatment, and outcome of the disease.
- Following the observation of atypical or abnormal findings, the dental hygienist must describe and document them accurately in the client record. The ability to describe an oral lesion is critical to the assessment process because precise descriptive terms enable the dental hygienist to communicate with the dentist and other referring healthcare professionals to identify the lesion and facilitate its accurate dental diagnosis.
- Because many clients are seen more regularly for preventive periodontal care than for medical visits, dental hygienists have a unique opportunity during client assessment to detect oral cancer while it is still asymptomatic, innocuous, and unsuspected.
- Oral cytology in practice has a minor role in the detection of precancerous and cancerous lesions because this method captures only surface cells as a specimen, which may have little diagnostic value.
- OralCDx captures a specimen of all three layers of epithelium to help the oral practitioner determine if a lesion is in fact benign or if it should be submitted for scalpel biopsy and histology.
- The OralCDx brush biopsy allows a dentist to evaluate lesions that might not otherwise be submitted for scalpel biopsy due to their benign appearance.

Critical Thinking Exercises

1. Structure Identification Exercise: Head and Neck Regions
   Directions: When examining a peer, check off the structures identified in an extraoral examination of a head and neck. Describe and list atypical and abnormal findings. Report any abnormal findings to your supervising instructor.

	Identified	Atypical Findings	Abnormal Findings
Regions of the Head **Parietal, Occipital, and Temporal Regions**			
Scalp and Hair			
Occipital Lymph Nodes Location			
Ears			
Auricular Lymph Nodes Location			
Frontal, Orbital, and Nasal Regions			
Forehead			
Eyes			
Frontal Sinuses			
Nose			
Infraorbital, Zygomatic, and Buccal Regions			
Zygomatic Arches			
Facial Lymph Nodes Location			
Maxillary Sinuses and Maxillary Bone			
Facial Expression and Masseter Muscles			
Temporomandibular Joints and Parotid Salivary Glands			
Mandible			
Oral and Mental Regions			
Chin			
Regions of the Neck **Anterior and Posterior Cervical Regions**			
Sternocleidomastoid Muscles			
External and Anterior Jugular Lymph Nodes Location			
Superior and Inferior Deep Cervical Lymph Nodes Location			
Accessory and Supraclavicular Lymph Nodes Location			
Submandibular and Submental Triangle Regions			
Submandibular Salivary Glands			
Submandibular Lymph Nodes Location			
Sublingual Salivary Glands			
Submental Lymph Nodes Location			
Anterior Midline Cervical Region			
Hyoid Bone			
Thyroid Cartilage and Gland			

Continued on following page

Critical Thinking Exercises—cont'd

2. Structure Identification Exercise: Oral Cavity and Associated Regions
Directions: When examining a peer, check off the items noted in an intraoral examination of an oral cavity and associated regions. Note any atypical findings and report any abnormal findings to your supervising instructor.

	Identified	Atypical Findings	Abnormal Findings
Oral Cavity			
Lips, labial mucosa, and vestibules			
Buccal mucosa and buccal fat pads			
Parotid papillae, parotid salivary glands and ducts			
Alveolar mucosa and labial frena			
Mucogingival junction			
Maxillary bone, teeth, gingiva, and tuberosity			
Mandibular bone, teeth, gingiva, and retromolar pad			
Palate and Pharynx			
Hard palate, median palatine raphe, and incisive papilla			
Soft palate and uvula			
Tonsillar pillars and palatine tonsils			
Tongue			
Sulcus terminalis, lingual papillae, and foramen cecum			
Lingual tonsil			
Ventral surface, lingual veins, and plica fimbriatae			
Floor of the Mouth			
Lingual frenum			
Sublingual folds and caruncles			
Sublingual salivary glands and ducts			
Submandibular salivary glands and ducts			

For References, Suggested Readings, and Related Websites, visit
http://evolve.elsevier.com/Darby/hygiene/

CHAPTER 13

Assessment of the Dentition

OBJECTIVES

Mastery of the content in this chapter will enable the reader to:

- Discuss the purposes, characteristics, and procedures of dental charting
- Describe the classification of quadrants and sextants in dental charting
- Describe the classification of permanent and primary teeth
- Explain the major tooth numbering systems
- Describe Black's classification of types of dental caries and restorations
- Describe common tooth anomalies and tooth damage that may be observed during tooth assessment
- Chart a dentition accurately
- Describe normal occlusion in the permanent and primary dentitions
- Describe centric occlusion and its relationship to movement of the mandible
- Describe Angle's classification of malocclusion
- Describe parafunctional habits and their relationship to occlusion

KEY TERMS

Abfraction
Abrasion
Acquired tooth damage
Acute caries
Amelogenesis imperfecta
Anodontia
Apical third
Arrested caries
Attrition
Bruxism
Buccal
Centric occlusion
Centric relation
Centric stops
Cervical third
Chronic caries
Class I malocclusion
Class II malocclusion
Class III malocclusion
Clenching
Complex caries
Compound caries
Dens evaginatus
Dens in dente
Dental caries
Dental charting
Dentin dysplasia
Dentinogenesis imperfecta
Developmental anomalies
Dilaceration
Distal
Early childhood caries
Enamel dysplasia
Enamel hypocalcification
Enamel hypoplasia
Enamel pearl
End-to-end bite
Erosion
Facial
Gemination
Hidden caries
Hyperdontia
Hypodontia
Incisal
International Numbering System
Intrinsic staining
Lingual
Macrodontia
Malocclusion
Mesial
Mesial step
Microdontia
Midline
Occlusal
Occlusion
Overbite
Overjet
Pit and fissure caries
Quadrant
Rampant caries
Recurrent caries
Root caries
Sextant
Simple caries
Smooth surface caries
Straight (flush) terminal plane
Talon cusp
Taurodontism
Thumb or finger sucking
Universal Numbering System

Tooth assessment is used to determine whether the client's need for a biologically sound and functional dentition is met and is related to the client's human needs for freedom from pain and for wholesome facial image. Tooth assessment and its documentation initially occur during the assessment phase of the dental hygiene process, and are updated regularly during the implementation and evaluation phases of dental hygiene care.

DOCUMENTATION

Documentation of tooth assessments on a client's dentition chart serves the following purposes:

- *Care Planning:* Provides the visual description of the client's current dental status. After collection of tooth assessment and other data, the clinician is able to formulate an accurate and comprehensive care plan.
- *Communication:* Accurate documentation of findings enhances communication with the client, and about the client to other members of the oral healthcare team. It also assists communication with third-party payers, such as insurance companies and health maintenance organizations.
- *Legal Documentation:* The client's record is a legal document and admissible evidence in a court of law. Comprehensive charting of tooth assessment findings documents the level of care provided.
- *Forensic Uses:* During forensic investigations, the record of the client's dentition is often the only means of identifying a deceased person; therefore, accuracy and completeness of these records are essential.
- *Financial Audits:* The client's dentition chart assists in the verification of oral healthcare provided and may be the key record in a financial audit.[1]
- *Quality Assurance Audits:* The client chart contains a detailed chronologic history of the client's clinical examination findings, dental diagnosis, and treatment.[2] Therefore, the dental chart contains a vital record for assessing the quality of treatment.[1]

TYPES OF CHARTS FOR DOCUMENTATION

Dental charting is the graphic representation of the condition of the client's teeth observed on a specific date. The data recorded are based on clinical and radiographic assessments and the client's report of symptoms. The exact location and condition of all teeth and restorations, including normal and abnormal findings, are documented carefully on a detailed dentition chart as a permanent part of the client's record.

An ideal chart for documentation should be comprehensive, and should contain sufficient space for initial recording of data as well as for successive findings. However, the format should be uncomplicated so that all oral health professionals can interpret it with ease. The chart should be accessible for reference during all appointments, thus facilitating continuity, sequencing, and ongoing documentation of care.[1]

The most commonly used charts for recording dental conditions present anatomic or geometric representations of the teeth (Figure 13–1). In anatomical diagrams, the illustrations resemble actual teeth. The anatomy of the crown and root(s) of each tooth is usually provided with *facial* views (tooth surfaces toward the face), *occlusal* views (biting or chewing surfaces), and *lingual* views (surfaces toward the tongue). In a geometrical diagram, each tooth is represented by a circle that is divided into five parts to represent each tooth surface (Figure 13–2). In all charting designs, the teeth are arranged as though one is looking in the mouth of the client. Thus, the right side of the mouth is on the left side of the chart and the left side of the mouth is on the right side of the chart.

Quadrant and Sextant Classification

To facilitate communication about specific areas of the dentition and individual teeth, the dentition is divided into quadrants and sextants, and each tooth is divided into specific surfaces and zones.

QUADRANTS. If one were to draw an imaginary line dividing the client's face into two equal halves longitudinally, then the maxillary and mandibular arches of the mouth would be divided into two mirror images or halves. This imaginary longitudinal line that bisects the client's face is referred to as the *midline.* If one were to draw horizontally a second imaginary line that divided the maxillary arch from the mandibular arch, the combination of the imaginary horizontal and vertical midlines would divide the client's mouth into four equal sections termed *quadrants (Q)* (Figure 13–3). Each quadrant of the mouth contains either five or eight teeth, depending on whether the client has primary or permanent dentition. Quadrants of the permanent dentition are numbered 1 through 4, and those of the primary dentition 5 through 8. The maxillary right is referred to as quadrant 1 in the permanent dentition or quadrant 5 in the primary dentition. Continuing in a clockwise pattern around the dentition, the maxillary left is designated as quadrant 2 (permanent) or quadrant 6 (primary). The mandibular left is referred to as quadrant 3 (permanent) or quadrant 7 (primary), and the mandibular right is designated as quadrant 4 (permanent) or quadrant 8 (primary).

SEXTANTS. Another means of dividing the primary and permanent dentition into sections is created by drawing additional imaginary lines to create divisions between the anterior and the posterior teeth. Dividing the dentition in this manner creates six areas called *sextants (S).* Each anterior sextant contains incisors and canines, and premolars or molars are found in the posterior sextants.

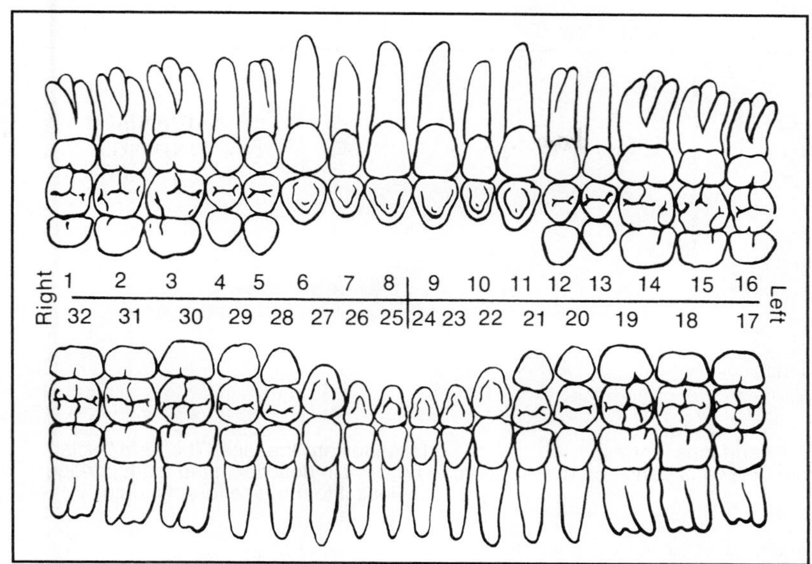

FIGURE 13–1 ✦ Example of an anatomic chart. *(Courtesy Colwell Systems, a division of Patterson Supply, Inc.)*

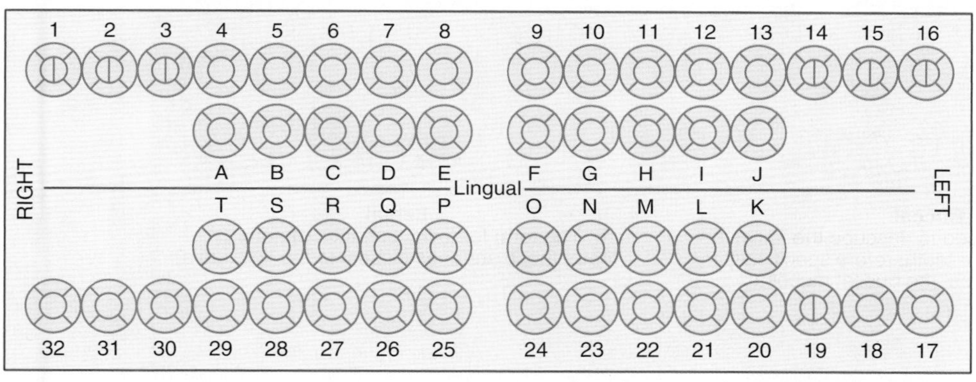

FIGURE 13–2 ✦ Example of a geometric diagram. *(Courtesy Colwell Systems, a division of Patterson Supply, Inc.)*

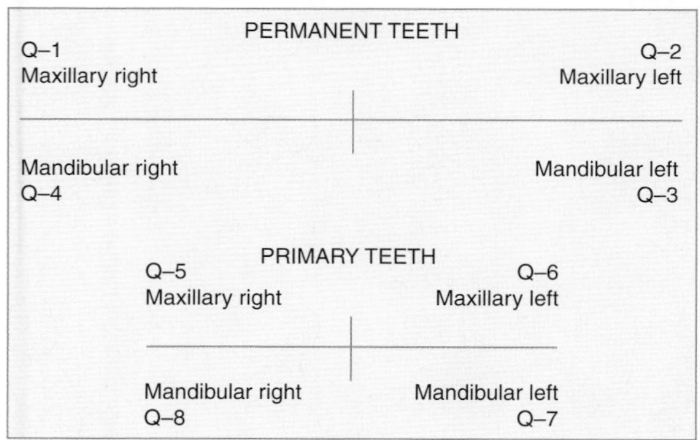

FIGURE 13–3 ✦ Numbering of quadrants (Q) in the permanent and primary dentitions.

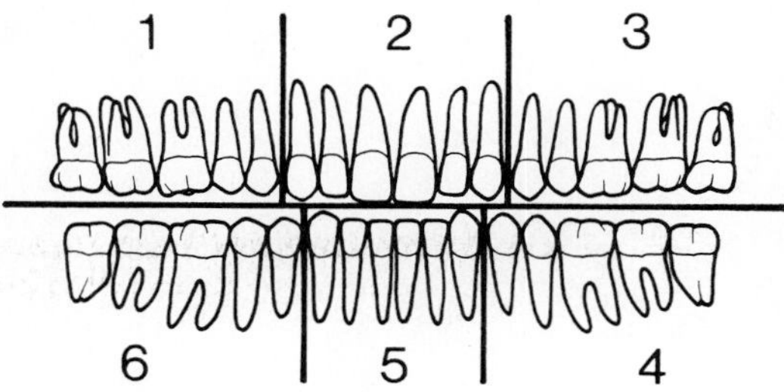

FIGURE 13–4 ✦ Sextant classification in the permanent dentition.

Like quadrants, sextants are numbered clockwise beginning at the client's maxillary right (Figure 13–4).

Tooth Surfaces and Zones

The differentiation of tooth surfaces and zones provides a means of pinpointing specific areas of the tooth for accurate assessment, charting, treatment, and evaluation. There are six tooth surfaces (Figure 13–5):

Occlusal (O)
Incisal (I)
Mesial (M)
Distal (D)
Facial (F) (includes buccal & labial)
Lingual (L) (includes palatal)

TOOTH ZONES. Teeth also are divided into zones of imaginary thirds (Figure 13–6). The root of the tooth is

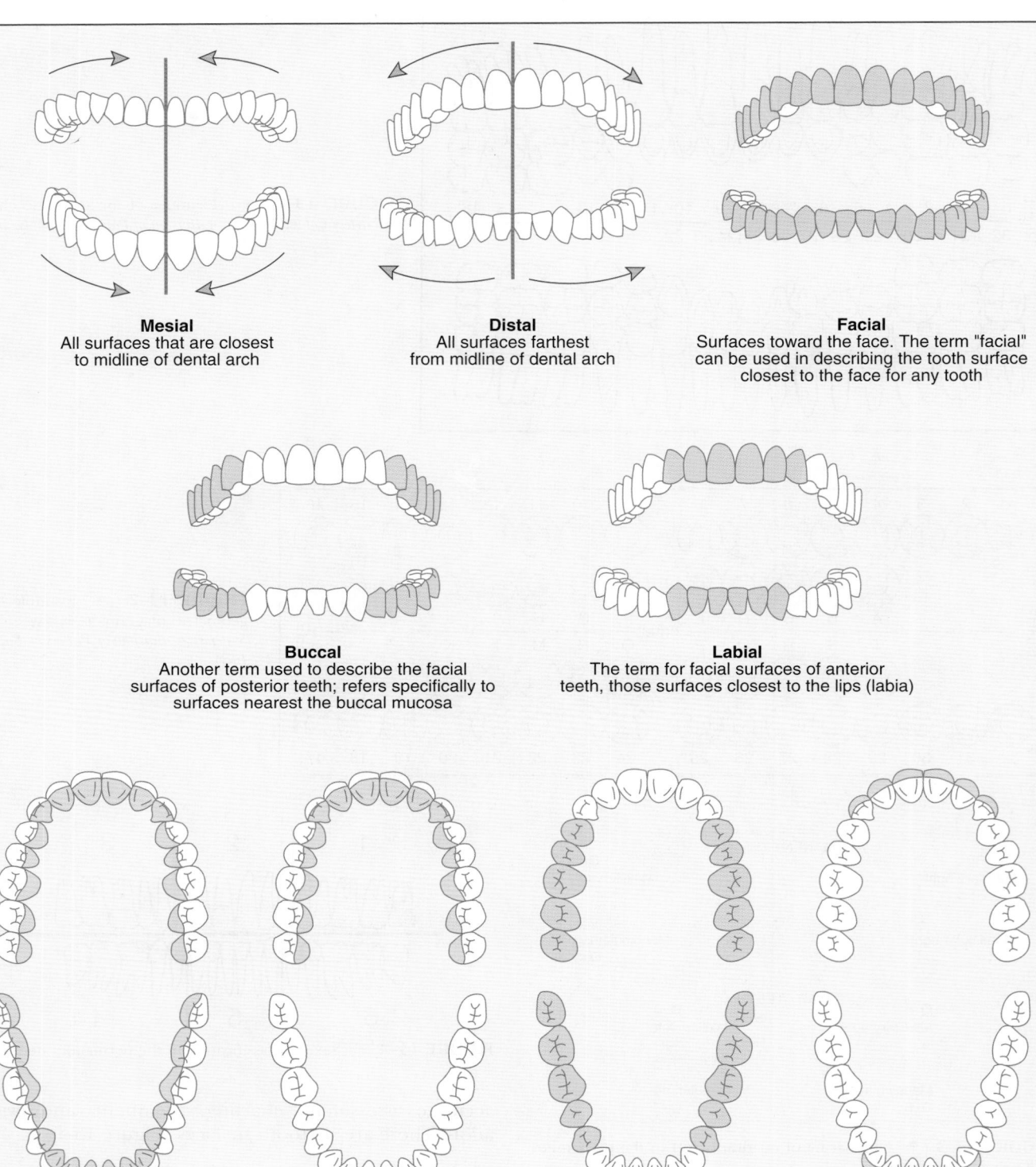

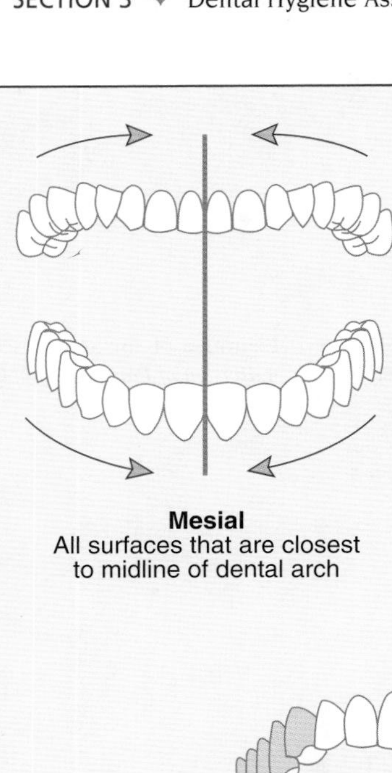

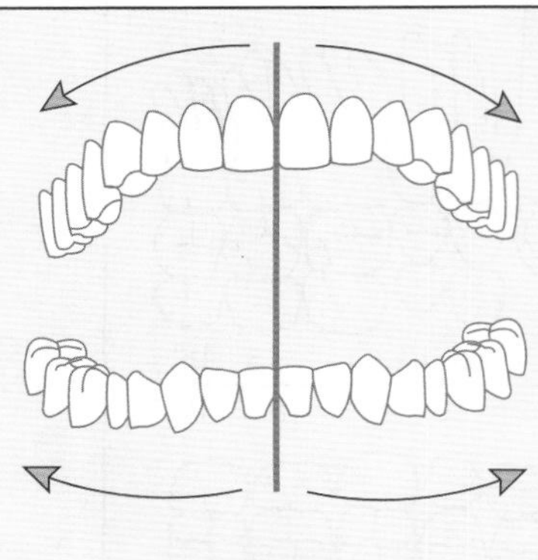

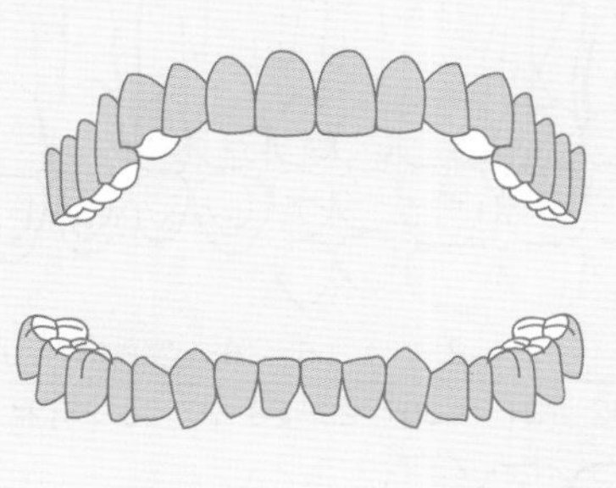

Facial
Surfaces toward the face. The term "facial" can be used in describing the tooth surface closest to the face for any tooth

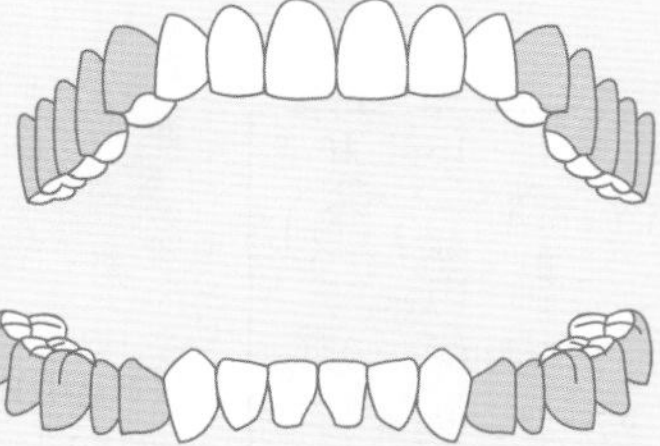

Buccal
Another term used to describe the facial surfaces of posterior teeth; refers specifically to surfaces nearest the buccal mucosa

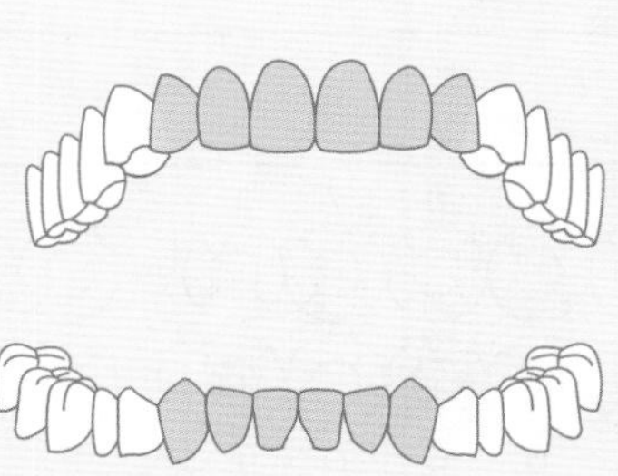

Labial
The term for facial surfaces of anterior teeth, those surfaces closest to the lips (labia)

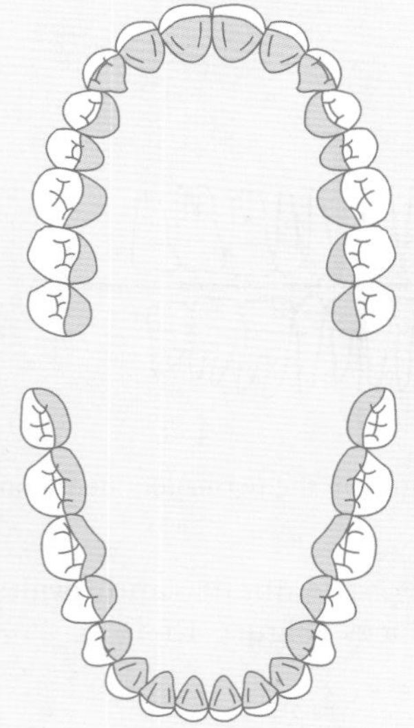

Lingual
Surface of the maxillary and mandibular teeth nearest the tongue. This term may be applied to both maxillary and mandibular teeth

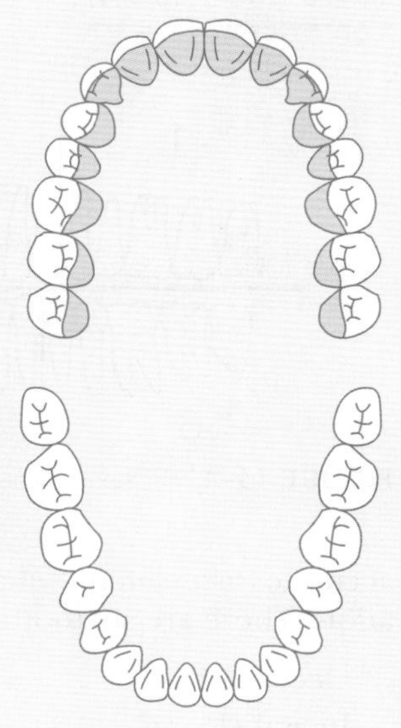

Palatal
Another name for the lingual surface of the maxillary teeth—indicates the surface nearest the palate. The term "lingual" is more frequently used than "palatal"

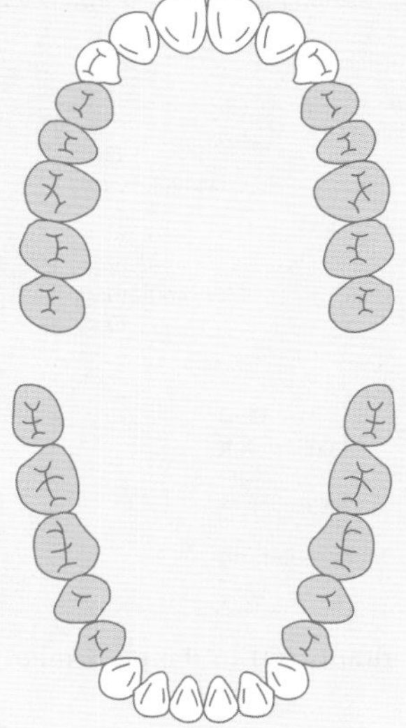

Occlusal
This term indicates the contacting, or biting, surfaces of all posterior teeth

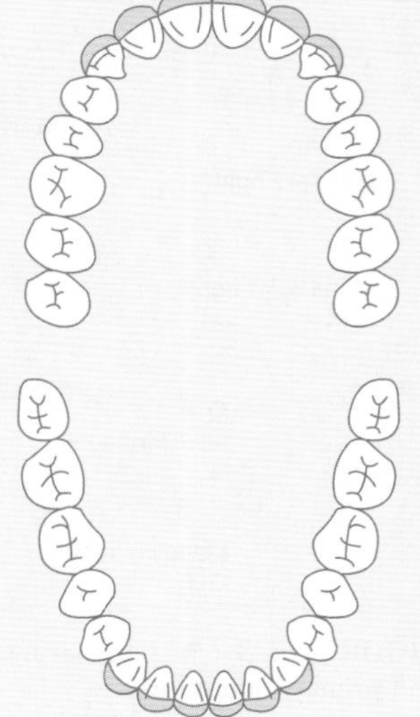

Incisal (or Incisal Edge)
The edge of all anterior teeth. The incisal edge is not considered a full surface

FIGURE 13–5 ✦ Classification of tooth surfaces. *(Adapted from Wootton D:* The art of dental scaling, *Burlington, Vt, 1991, University of Vermont.)*

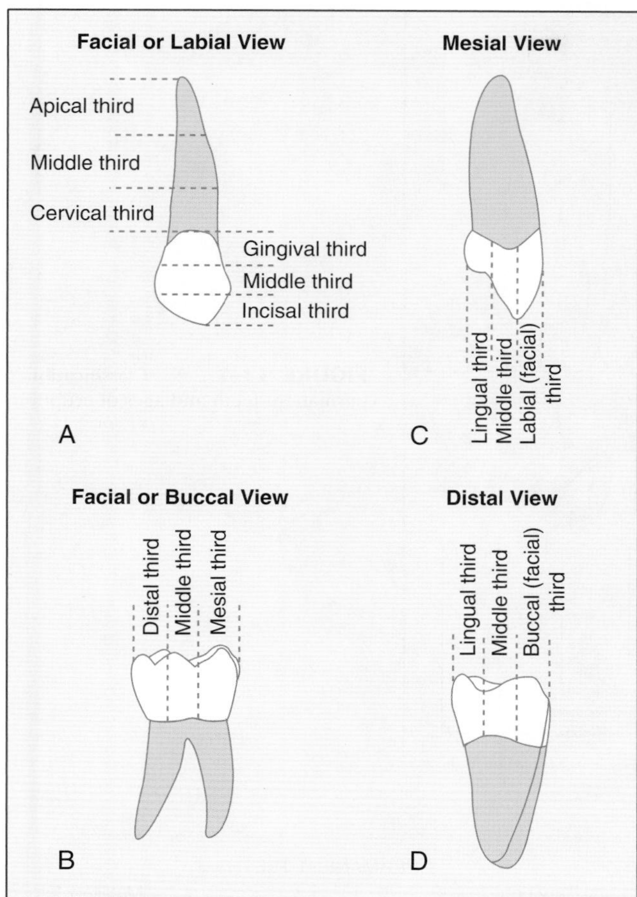

FIGURE 13–6 ✦ Diagram of a maxillary canine and a mandibular first molar showing how the parts of a tooth may be divided.

divided into thirds: the *apical third* (the area involving the tip or apex of the root), the *middle third,* and the *cervical third* (the area closest to the "neck" of the crown of the tooth). The crown of the tooth can be divided into the following three directions:

- *Cervico-occlusal Division:* Dividing the crown of the tooth horizontally, from cervical to occlusal areas, creates thirds called occlusal (for posterior teeth, or incisal for anterior teeth), middle, and gingival thirds (Figure 13–6, *A*).
- *Mesiodistal Division:* Dividing the crown vertically on the facial or lingual surface, from mesial to distal, creates the mesial, middle, and distal thirds (Figure 13–6, *B*)
- *Faciolingual (or Buccolingual) Division:* Dividing the crown vertically on the mesial or distal view creates thirds called facial (in lieu of labial for anterior teeth or buccal for posterior teeth), middle, and lingual (Figure 13–6, *C* and *D*).

Classification of Types of Teeth

In their lifetime, humans have two sets of natural teeth, commonly referred to as the primary and the permanent dentitions. The primary dentition is made up of 20 teeth, 5 in each quadrant: 2 incisors, 1 canine, and 2 molars.

The full permanent, or secondary, dentition contains 32 teeth, 8 in each quadrant: 2 incisors, 1 canine, 2 premolars, and 3 molars. The functions of the individual tooth types are similar in the primary and the permanent dentition. The classification of primary and permanent teeth along with age of eruption are provided in Figures 13–7 and 13–8.

TOOTH NUMBERING SYSTEMS

Tooth numbering systems were developed to simplify the task of identifying individual teeth without using their full name designations. Such systems are essential for charting and recording procedures. The two most commonly used are the Universal Numbering System and the International Numbering System.

Universal Numbering System

The *Universal Numbering System,* officially adopted by the American Dental Association, is widely used. This system provides a standard sequential numbering system for all permanent teeth. The permanent teeth are numbered 1 through 32, starting with the maxillary right permanent third molar designated as tooth number 1, and following around the maxillary arch to the left maxillary third molar, designated tooth number 16. The left mandibular third molar is designated as tooth number 17, and numbering follows clockwise around the mandibular arch to the right mandibular third molar, designated tooth number 32 (Figure 13–9). The primary dentition is identified in the same order; however, alphabetical letters, capitals A to T, identify the individual teeth. Letter "A" designates the maxillary right second molar, and following clockwise around the maxillary and mandibular arches the mandibular right second molar is designated by the letter "T" (Figure 13–9).

International Numbering System (Federation Dentaire International)

The *International Numbering System* uses a two-digit system to identify each tooth. The first digit indicates the quadrant in which the tooth is located, and the second digit identifies the specific tooth. For quadrant designations, numbers 1 to 4 are used to specify permanent quadrants, and numbers 5 to 8 to designate primary quadrants. The second digit identifies the specific tooth in the quadrant: the numbers 1 through 8 are used for permanent teeth, and the numbers 1 through 5 for primary teeth. In each dentition, tooth number 1 is the central incisor. In primary dentition, tooth number 5 is the second primary molar, and in secondary dentition tooth number 8 is the third permanent molar (Figure 13–10). The pronunciation of the International system is emphasized by the hyphenated notation; for example, "1-6" is pronounced "one six," rather than "sixteen."

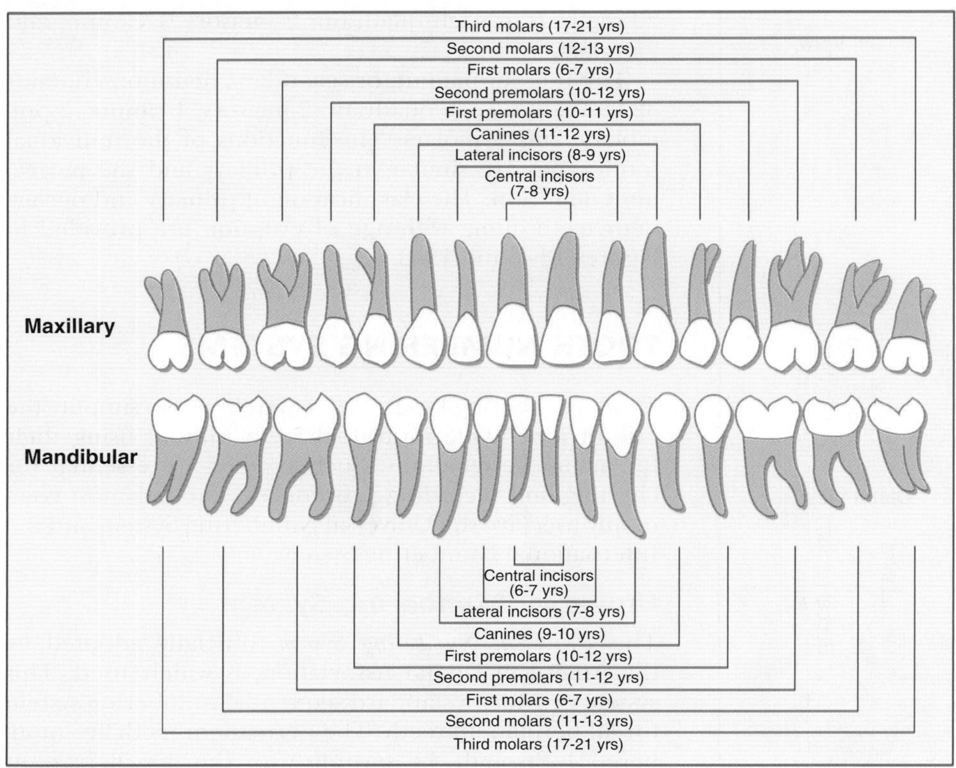

FIGURE 13–7 ✦ Classification of permanent teeth and ages of eruption.

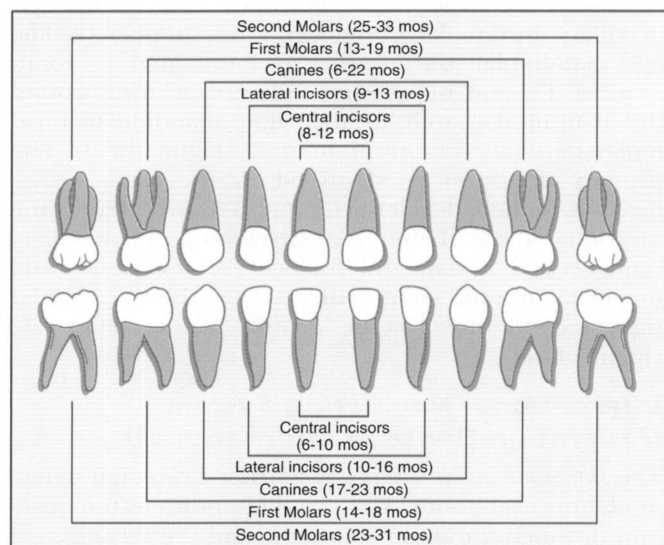

FIGURE 13–8 ✦ Classification of primary teeth and ages of eruption.

PERMANENT TEETH

Maxillary right															Maxillary left
1	2	3	4	5	6	7	8	9	10	11	12	13	14	15	16
32	31	30	29	28	27	26	25	24	23	22	21	20	19	18	17
Mandibular right															Mandibular left

PRIMARY TEETH

Maxillary right					Maxillary left				
A	B	C	D	E	F	G	H	I	J
T	S	R	Q	P	O	N	M	L	K
Mandibular right					Mandibular left				

FIGURE 13–9 ✦ Universal Numbering System adopted by the American Dental Association.

CLINICAL ASSESSMENT

Tooth assessment includes both radiographic and clinical evaluations. Direct clinical examination can be done well only if the teeth are clean and dry and illuminated with good light. When plaque biofilm and saliva coat the teeth, defects and signs of disease may go undetected. The dental examination should proceed systematically, beginning, for instance, with the most distal tooth in the maxillary right quadrant. The examination continues around the arch, through the last tooth in the maxillary left quadrant. Then the mandible is examined in reverse order, beginning with the most distal tooth in the mandibular left quadrant and ending with the last tooth in the mandibular right quadrant. Cotton roll isolation can be helpful in maintaining a dry environment, and air-drying of the teeth is essential for the individual examination of each tooth.

An explorer is commonly used to check grooves and pits in enamel, discolored root surfaces along the gingival margin, and suspicious margins of restorations. Light pressure should be applied with the explorer, using a proper fulcrum to control it. Care should be exercised to avoid exploring known sensitive areas. Clinicians have been advised to use "sharp eyes and blunt explorers."[3]

PERMANENT DENTITION	
Q-1 1-8 1-7 1-6 1-5 1-4 1-3 1-2 1-1	Q-2 2-1 2-2 2-3 2-4 2-5 2-6 2-7 2-8
Q-4 4-8 4-7 4-6 4-5 4-4 4-3 4-2 4-1	Q-3 3-1 3-2 3-3 3-4 3-5 3-6 3-7 3-8

PRIMARY DENTITION	
Q-5 5-5 5-4 5-3 5-2 5-1	Q-6 6-1 6-2 6-3 6-4 6-5
Q-8 8-5 8-4 8-3 8-2 8-1	Q-7 7-1 7-2 7-3 7-4 7-5

FIGURE 13–10 ✦ The International Numbering System.

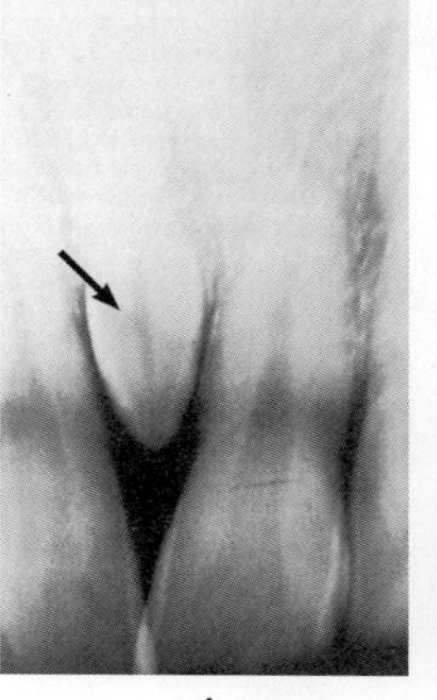

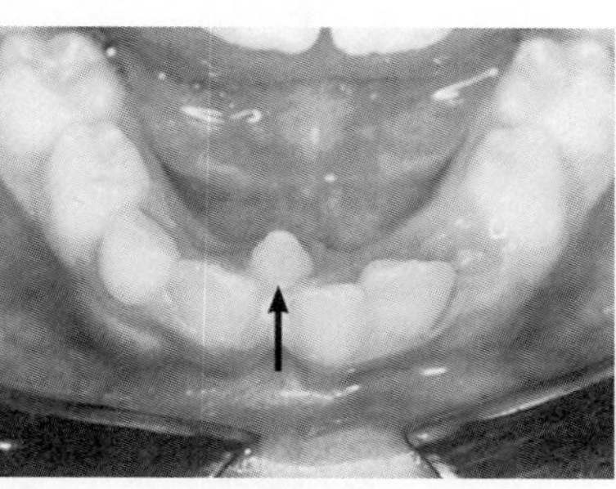

A B

FIGURE 13–11 ✦ Mesiodens *(arrow)*. **A,** Radiographic appearance. **B,** Clinical appearance. *(From Regezi JA, Sciubba JJ:* Oral pathology: Clinical-pathologic correlations, *ed 3, Philadelphia, 1999, WB Saunders.)*

The clinical examination is used to assess developmental anomalies and signs of acquired tooth damage and defective restorations. These conditions are described in the following sections.

DEVELOPMENTAL ANOMALIES AND ACQUIRED TOOTH DAMAGE

The goal of tooth assessment for the dental hygienist is to recognize signs of developmental anomalies and acquired tooth damage and call them to the attention of the dentist, thus optimizing client care.

Developmental Anomalies

Developmental anomalies may arise from a disruption in the stages of tooth development (odontogenesis), causing one or more of the tissues of the tooth bud to be disrupted. These disturbances may be the result of local, systemic, or hereditary factors. The extent of the manifestation of the disturbance is dependent on the stage of dental development at which the disruption occurs and the duration and nature of the assault.

Dental anomalies include anomalies of the number of teeth and anomalies of dental tissues. The following discussion briefly describes the more frequently noted dental anomalies. (Tooth anomalies with variation in root form are presented in Chapter 21.)

ANOMALIES OF NUMBER OF TEETH. *Hyperdontia* is the presence of extra teeth beyond the normal complement. Hyperdontia is commonly referred to as "supernumerary" or "supplemental" teeth. Supernumerary teeth are extra teeth of abnormal shape, whereas supplemental teeth are extra teeth of normal shape. When an extra tooth occurs in the midline between the maxillary anterior incisors, it is referred to as a mesiodens (Figure 13–11). These supernumerary teeth are usually misshapen, small, and peglike. A natal tooth is a supernumerary tooth that erupts prior to birth, and a neonatal tooth is a supernumerary tooth that erupts shortly after birth.[4]

Hypodontia is the absence of one or more teeth and also may be called *anodontia.* The failure of all teeth to develop is termed complete anodontia, and the absence of one or several teeth is called partial anodontia. Anodontia is usually associated with defects of ectodermal structures, such as are found with the disorder ectodermal dysplasia.

Although complete anodontia is extremely rare, partial anodontia is more common. The teeth most frequently observed as congenitally missing are third molars, followed sequentially by maxillary lateral incisors and mandibular premolars. The teeth least frequently absent are first permanent molars.

ANOMALIES OF THE DENTAL TISSUES. Anomalies of the teeth can be subdivided into several categories: those affecting the total tooth and those affecting the individual dental tissues, including enamel, dentin, cementum, and pulp.

Anomalies of the Whole Tooth. Macrodontia refers to larger than normal teeth. These teeth may be larger in width, length, or height.[4] *Microdontia* is a developmental anomaly in which the teeth are smaller than normal. This condition may affect one tooth, several teeth, or all teeth within the dentition. Many supernumerary teeth are small and can be classified as microdonts (Figure 13–12).

In *gemination,* a large tooth results from the splitting of a single tooth germ that attempts to form two teeth (Figure 13–13). This twinning usually results in a partially or completely divided crown attached to a single root with one canal.[4]

Dens in dente is defined as a tooth within a tooth (Figure 13–14). It is caused by invagination of the enamel organ during development and is most frequently observed on the lingual aspect of the maxillary lateral incisors. A deep crevice usually runs between the oral and the inner surface of the tooth where the anomaly is found.[4] This crevice increases the likelihood of early dental caries; consequently, a preventive restoration may be considered to prevent internal decay.

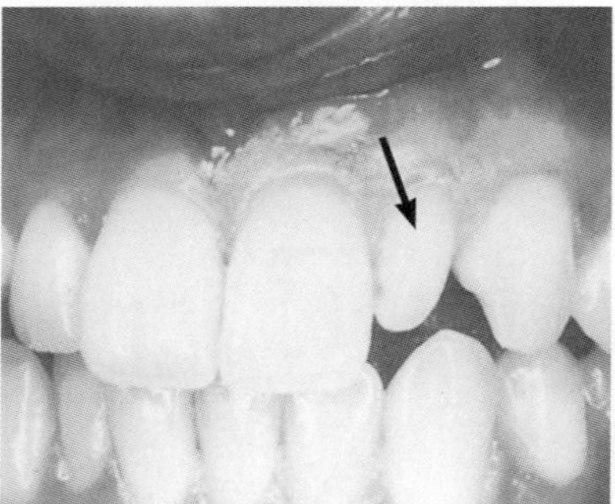

FIGURE 13–12 ✦ Microdontia *(arrow). (Courtesy Dr. George Blozis.)*

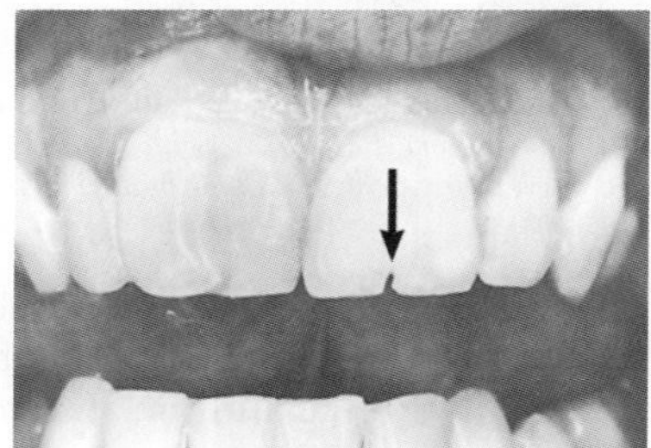

FIGURE 13–13 ✦ Gemination *(arrow). (Courtesy Dr. George Blozis.)*

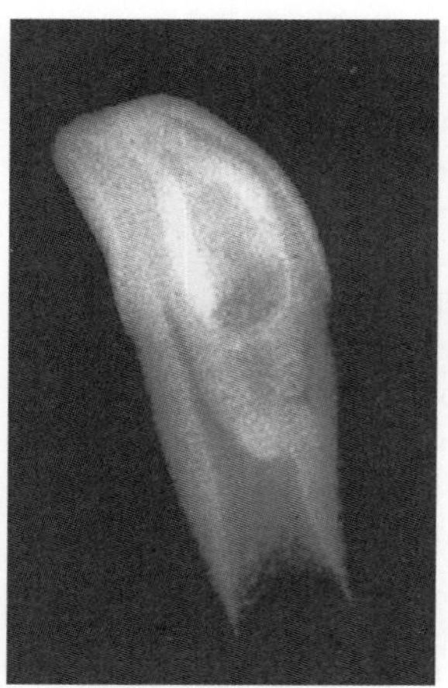

FIGURE 13–14 ✦ Dens in dente. *(Courtesy Oral Pathology, University of Alberta, Canada.)*

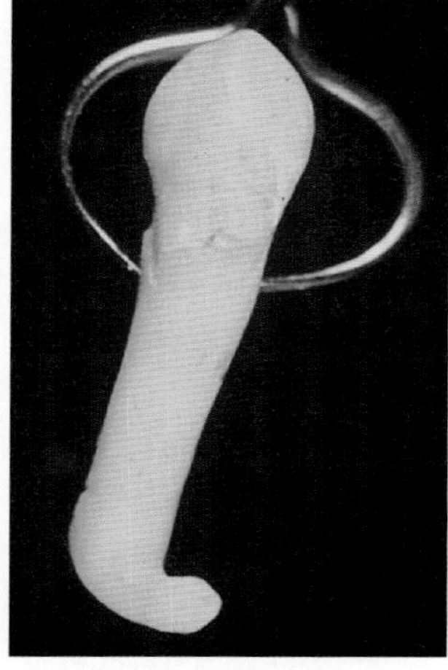

FIGURE 13–15 ✦ Dilaceration. *(Courtesy Oral Pathology, University of Alberta, Canada.)*

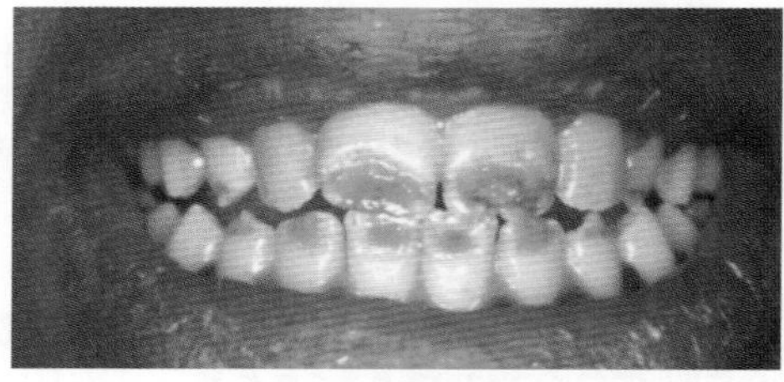

FIGURE 13–16 ✦ Enamel hypoplasia. *(From Ibsen OAC, Phelan JA:* Oral pathology for the dental hygienist, *ed 3, Philadelphia, 2000, WB Saunders.)*

Dilaceration is the severe distortion of a crown or root caused by trauma during tooth formation. It is usually manifested as a severely angulated root (Figure 13–15). Extraction of a tooth with a dilacerated root often creates a treatment problem for the dentist because of the root angulation.[5]

Intrinsic staining of dental tissues may occur when the antibiotic tetracycline is administered during tooth formation. The tetracycline is deposited in the forming enamel and dentin, resulting in permanent staining ranging from mild yellow to yellowish-brown or gray coloration.

Anomalies of Enamel Formation. An insult to ameloblasts during tooth formation may result in abnormal enamel development, referred to generally as *enamel dysplasia.* Enamel dysplasia encompasses two types of abnormal enamel development: enamel hypoplasia and enamel hypocalcification.

Enamel hypoplasia is the result of a disturbance of the ameloblasts during matrix formation that produces a pitted or rough, striated enamel surface (Figure 13–16). *Enamel hypocalcification* is a defect occurring in the enamel as the result of a disturbance during mineralization. The clinical appearance of enamel hypocalcification is that of white spotting of the enamel surface; however, the enamel surface is generally smooth in texture.

Many factors—local (e.g., trauma), systemic (e.g., diseases, nutritional deficiencies, excess systemic fluoride), hereditary, and idiopathic (unknown)—may cause anomalies of enamel formation. When excessive amounts of systemic fluoride are responsible for enamel hypoplasia or enamel hypocalcification, this condition is classified as *dental fluorosis.* This condition may range from mild fluorosis, associated with white flecking, to severe situations in which the teeth are deeply pitted or brown stained. Clients who live in a rural setting may be candidates for fluoride supplements; however, prior to initiating a supplement program it is important to determine the concentration of fluoride in the drinking water through analysis of water samples. Water samples can be analyzed by local health departments.

Congenital syphilis is another, now rare, cause of enamel hypoplasia, and several hypoplastic characteristics are often associated with this condition. "Hutchinson's inci-

A

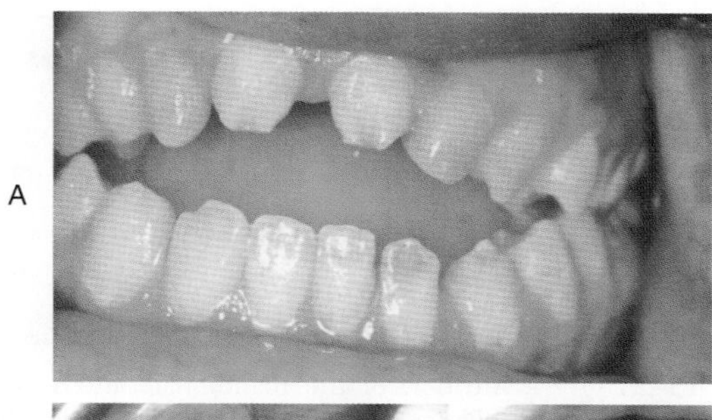

B

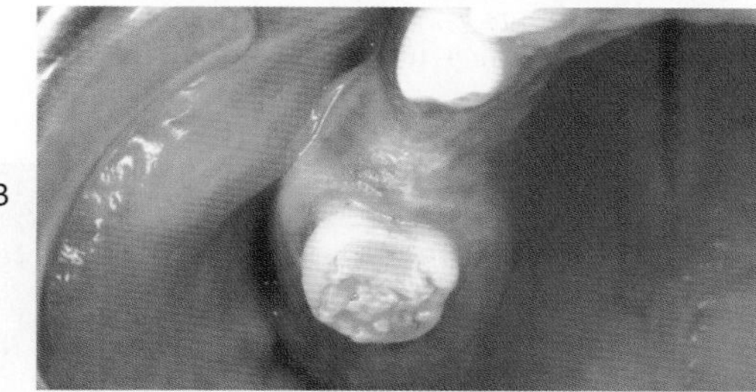

FIGURE 13–17 ✦ Syphilitic enamel hypoplasia. **A,** Hutchinson's incisors. **B,** Mulberry molars. *(Courtesy Dr. George Blozis. From Ibsen OAC, Phelan JA:* Oral pathology for the dental hygienist, *ed 3, Philadelphia, 2000, WB Saunders.)*

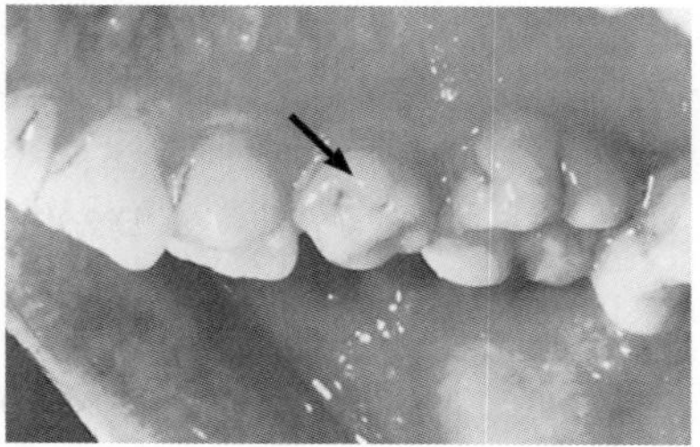

FIGURE 13–18 ✦ Den evaginatus *(arrow). (Courtesy Dr. Margot Van Dis.)*

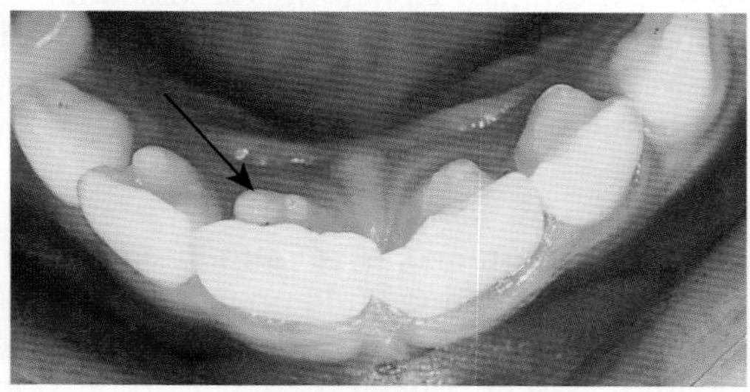

FIGURE 13–19 ✦ Talon cusp *(arrow). (Courtesy Dr. Geoffrey Sperber, University of Alberta, Canada.)*

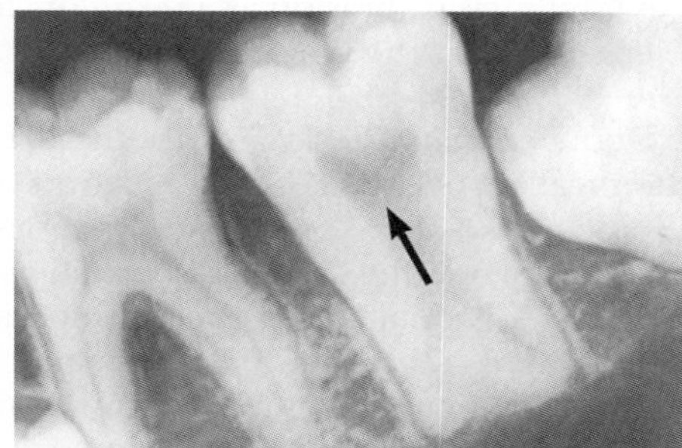

FIGURE 13–20 ✦ Taurodontism *(arrow). (Courtesy Dr. George Blozis.)*

sors" is the term used to denote the notched or screwdriver appearance of syphilitic incisor teeth (Figure 13–17, *A*). When the lateral incisors display a conical shape, they are often referred to as peg-laterals. It is important to note that not all peg-laterals occur as the result of syphilis. A peg-lateral is, in essence, a microdont and can stem from a variety of other causes. The term "mulberry molars" is used to describe the mottled mulberry-shaped molars also associated with congenital syphilis[4] (Figure 13–17, *B*).

Amelogenesis imperfecta is a form of enamel dysplasia resulting from hereditary factors. Many patterns of inheritance are associated with this disorder, such as autosomal dominant, recessive, or X-linked. Amelogenesis imperfecta is the partial or total malformation of enamel. The dentin and pulp of these teeth develop normally, but the enamel is easily chipped or worn away.

Several anomalies involving enamel are not classified as enamel dysplasia, two of which are *enamel pearls* (see Chapter 21) and dens evaginatus. *Dens evaginatus,* also referred to as *tuberculated cusp,* is a small mass of enamel or accessory cusp projecting on the occlusal surface of molars and premolars (Figure 13–18). It is believed to form from an outpouching of the enamel epithelium during the early stages of odontogenesis. The mass of tissue contains normal pulp and is subject to occlusal wear, risking exposure of the evaginated pulp chamber.[5]

Talon cusp is an extra well-delineated cusp found on the lingual surfaces of maxillary and mandibular anterior teeth. It was thought that this cusp resembled an eagle's talon and therefore was named accordingly[5] (Figure 13–19). The talon cusp has well-developed enamel and dentin but varying levels of pulp tissue.[6]

Anomalies of Dentin Formation. Dentinogenesis imperfecta is the irregular formation or absence of dentinal development. Dentinogenesis imperfecta is associated with a dominant inherited disorder characterized by faulty formation of connective tissues. The dentin displays a softer than normal consistency as a result of increased water and organic content. Enamel formation occurs normally. The enamel easily breaks away from the dentin, however, and the teeth are prone to rapid wear[5] and dentinal hypersensitivity. Dental treatment usually includes placement of crowns to preserve existing crown structure.

Dentin dysplasia is a mesenchymal dysplasia and differs from dentinogenesis imperfecta in that the enamel does not readily chip away. The teeth exhibit normal color and little evidence of attrition. However, teeth with dentin dysplasia show retarded root formation and a lack of supporting bone. The lack of periodontal support may have serious periodontal implications; therefore, referral to a periodontist is recommended.

Anomalies of Pulp Formation. Taurodontism, meaning bull-like teeth, is an inherited phenomenon and thus is genetically determined (Figure 13–20). The crowns of these teeth develop normally; however, the pulp chambers are much enlarged at the expense of the dentinal walls.[4]

Acquired Tooth Damage*

Acquired tooth damage can be caused by any process that results in a loss of the integrity of the tooth surface. Dental caries is a bacteria-caused form of tooth damage. The other common forms of tooth damage (attrition, abrasion, erosion, and fracture) are the result of mechanical or chemical assault to the tooth structure.

ATTRITION. Dental *attrition* is the tooth-to-tooth wear of the dentition. All teeth wear from opposing tooth contact. Excessive wear is pathologic and may be caused by bruxism, grinding, or clenching, discussed later in this chapter (Figure 13–21). The restoration of teeth presenting excessive attrition may include the complete tooth coverage offered by a crown.

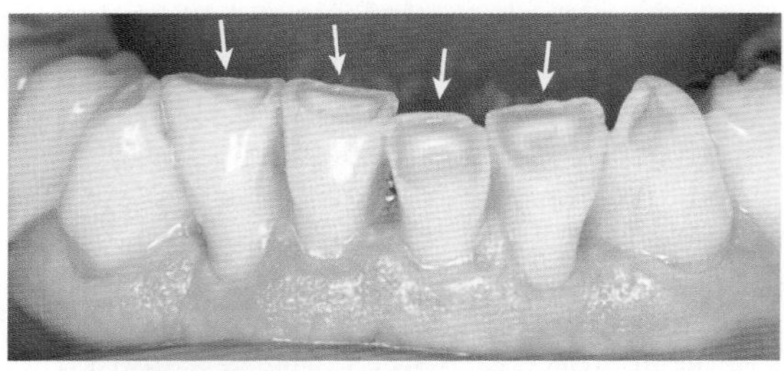

FIGURE 13–21 ✦ Attrition of the mandibular anterior teeth *(arrows). (From Ibsen OAC, Phelan JA:* Oral pathology for the dental hygienist, *ed 3, Philadelphia, 2000, WB Saunders.)*

ABRASION. Dental *abrasion,* pathologic tooth wear due to a foreign substance, is commonly seen as a result of traumatic toothbrushing and appears as notches worn into the teeth near the gumline (Figure 13–22). Occlusal abrasion often is seen on teeth that oppose porcelain crowns. Very coarse diets, uncleaned foods, and dusty environments also can contribute to the loss of occlusal enamel. It is not uncommon for pipe smokers and seamstresses to exhibit incisal abrasion as a result of clenching foreign objects between the anterior teeth.

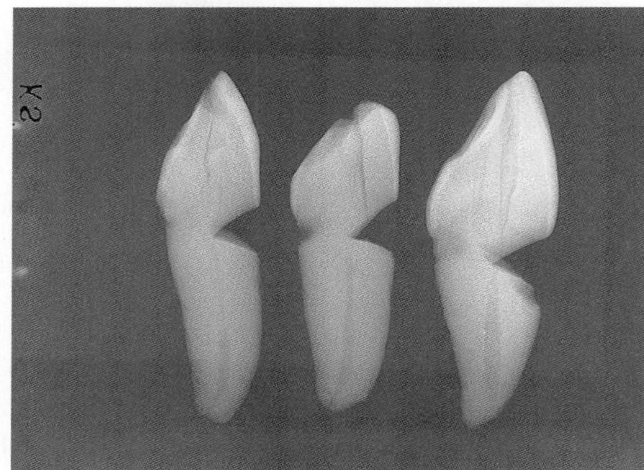

FIGURE 13–22 ✦ Abrasion. *(Courtesy Dr. Geoffrey Sperber, University of Alberta, Canada.)*

EROSION. Dental *erosion,* the loss of tooth surface as a result of chemical agents, has recently received considerable attention because of the prevalence of anorexia and bulimia.[7] Excessive vomiting can be associated with these disorders as the individual strives for the ultimate thinness. The repeated regurgitation of stomach acids through the oral cavity results in the dissolution of the dental tissues on the lingual and incisal/occlusal surfaces of the maxillary teeth. Tooth erosion also results from habits such as sucking on lemons or holding mouth fresheners, cough drops, or candies in the mucobuccal fold. The erosive action of these chemicals causes local destruction of tooth enamel (Figure 13–23).

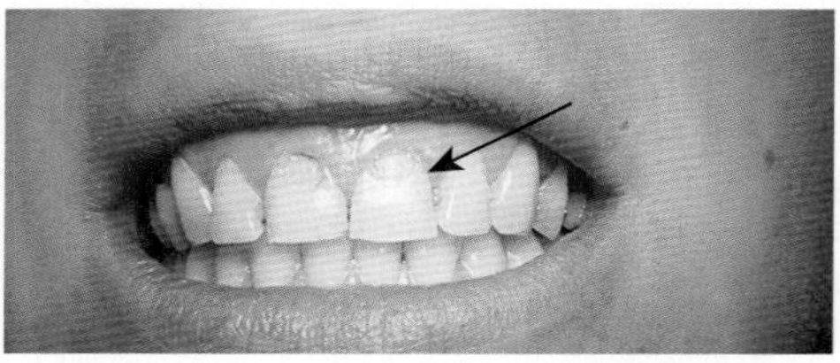

FIGURE 13–23 ✦ Erosion from sucking on lemons *(arrow). (Courtesy Dr. M. Walsh, University of California – San Francisco.)*

ABFRACTION. *Abfraction* is believed to be a cervical stress lesion that is manifested as a V- or wedge-shaped defect at the cementoenamel junction (CEJ). It is believed that abfraction defects are due to "eccentrically applied"[8] occlusal forces, which causes tooth flexure and resulting cervical wear. This concept is currently only a proposed hypothesis[9] and further research is needed to provide greater understanding.

TOOTH FRACTURE. Tooth fractures may range from small chips of the enamel to breaks that penetrate deeply into the tooth (Figure 13–24). Minor enamel fractures often require nothing more than polishing of the rough surfaces. More severe fractures require various levels of restoration. Some fractured teeth may not be restorable and, as a result, require removal.

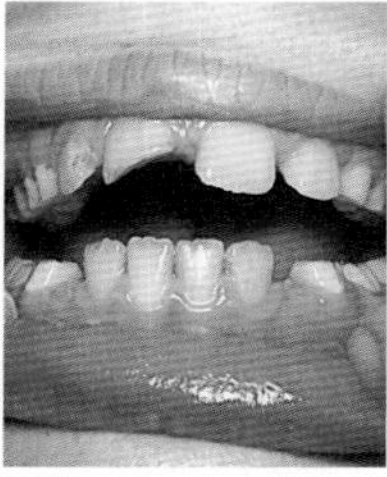

FIGURE 13–24 ✦ Tooth fracture. *(Courtesy Dr. M. Walsh, University of California – San Francisco.)*

DENTAL CARIES. *Dental caries* is an infectious and transmissible bacteria-caused disease characterized by the acid dissolution of enamel and the eventual breakdown of the more organic, inner dental tissues.[10] *Mutans streptococcus* is the microorganism identified as the primary causative agent in this process, which leads to cavitation and possible tooth loss. Through a complex process, a sticky dextran matrix is produced and colonized by these acidogenic bacteria. This inhabited mucogelatinous

---

* Portions of this section were contributed by Cheryl Cameron, RDH, PhD, and Glen E. Gordon, DDS, University of Washington–Seattle.

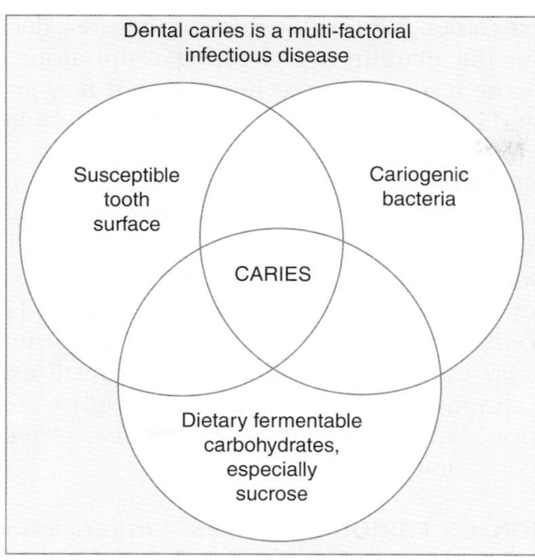

FIGURE 13–25 ✦ Primary factors of dental caries.

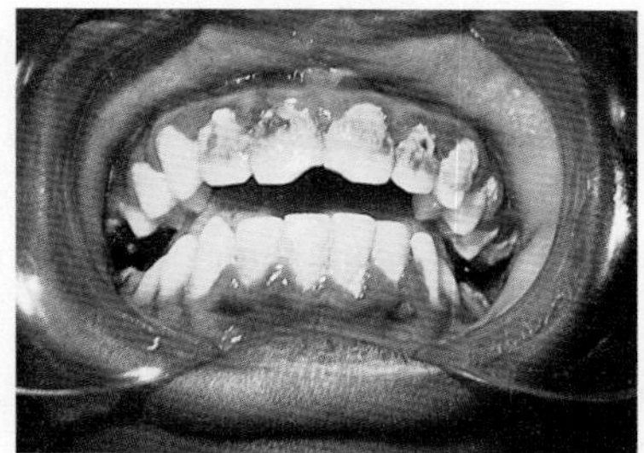

FIGURE 13–26 ✦ Rampant caries. *(Courtesy Dr. M. Walsh, University of California – San Francisco.)*

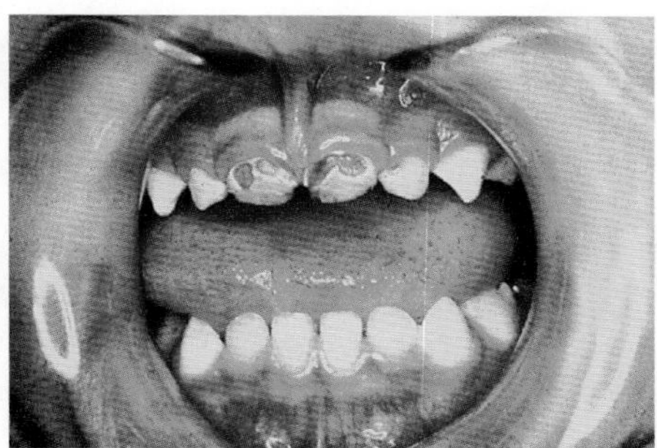

FIGURE 13–27 ✦ Early childhood caries. *(Courtesy Dr. S. El Badrawy, University of Alberta, Canada.)*

coating, called plaque biofilm, is harbored in the recesses in and around the dentition. It is nourished by elements within the diet. Refined sugars (sucrose in particular) are efficiently assimilated by the bacteria and result in the production of acid and a rapid drop in pH. The release of acid over an extended period of time demineralizes the tooth structure adjacent to the plaque biofilm and eventually results in cavitation (Figure 13–25). Within this cavitation the demineralization continues, promoted by episodes of acid release as the bacteria act on new substrate. Tooth cavitation is best referred to as a *carious lesion.* However, it is more commonly called a cavity, and the affected tooth is said to be carious or decayed.

Types of Dental Caries. The classification of dental caries is intended to describe the rate, direction, and/or type of disease progression. The terms of classification include acute, or rampant, caries; chronic caries; arrested caries; recurrent caries; and backward caries. These terms permit the oral healthcare practitioner to communicate the urgency with which restorative therapy should be delivered. As these terms are not specific regarding tooth and surface, they must be combined with other cavity classification terminology to permit location-specific communication.

Acute, or Rampant, Caries. *Acute,* or *rampant, caries* describes a rapidly progressive decay process that requires urgent intervention. The lesions are usually numerous and may be large. The decayed dentin is very soft and moist and is often light in color (Figure 13–26). Rampant caries is often associated with the effects of early childhood caries (nursing bottle caries) in infants.

Early Childhood Caries (ECC). *Early childhood caries* is a relatively new term that is defined as the occurrence of any dental caries in the first three years of a child's life. The most common condition associated with ECC is nursing bottle caries resulting from prolonged use of the baby bottle while sleeping. This condition has been referred to in several other ways, including nursing caries, nursing bottle syndrome, and baby bottle caries. This type of ECC appears rapidly, commonly affecting maxillary anterior teeth, particularly the facial surfaces that are generally considered to be at lower risk for decay (Figure 13–27). Lesions may first appear as a cervical band of demineralization, rapidly progressing to overt caries. Mandibular teeth are often not affected, probably because the child's tongue covers these teeth during the caries challenge.[11]

The evidence clearly shows that high levels of *mutans streptococci* transmitted from the mother are associated with ECC. These elevated bacteria levels combined with frequent carbohydrate intake produce high acid levels over long exposure periods. To provide early intervention strategies the dental hygienist should identify the risk factors (see Risk Factors for the Development of Early Childhood Caries) for ECC as early as possible.[8] For early identification of risk factors, Milgram and Weinstein (1999) have suggested several questions to ask parents (see Early Childhood Caries: Questions for Parents).[9]

Chronic Caries. *Chronic caries* describes a slowly progressive decay process that requires routine intervention. The carious dentin is firm and often brown to black. In large, open cavities the decayed dentin can be scooped out in large segments and has the consistency of firm leather (Figure 13–28).

Arrested Caries. Dental decay is not a continuous demineralization process. Evidence supports a continuous demineralization–remineralization process that can be tipped out of balance by changes in diet and oral envi-

Risk Factors for the Development of Early Childhood Caries

Sleeping with a bottle (containing anything other than water)
Snacking three or more times per day
Visible plaque biofilm on maxillary incisors
Parents/caregivers do not brush child's teeth
Siblings/parents have caries
Child drinks low-fluoride water and does not receive fluoride supplements
Little or no fluoride in diet

Adapted from Milgrom P, Weinstein P: *Early childhood caries: A team approach to prevention and treatment,* Seattle, 1999, University of Washington, Continuing Dental Education.

Early Childhood Caries: Questions for Parents

Do the parents clean the child's teeth regularly?
Do other family members have active dental caries?
Does the child drink water containing less than the optimal fluoride content or not receive fluoride supplements?
Does the child sleep with a bottle containing anything other than water?
Does the child eat more than three cariogenic snacks in a day?
Does the child drink bottled water or bottled fruit juice?

Adapted from Milgrom P, Weinstein P: *Early childhood caries: A team approach to prevention and treatment,* Seattle, 1999, University of Washington, Continuing Dental Education.

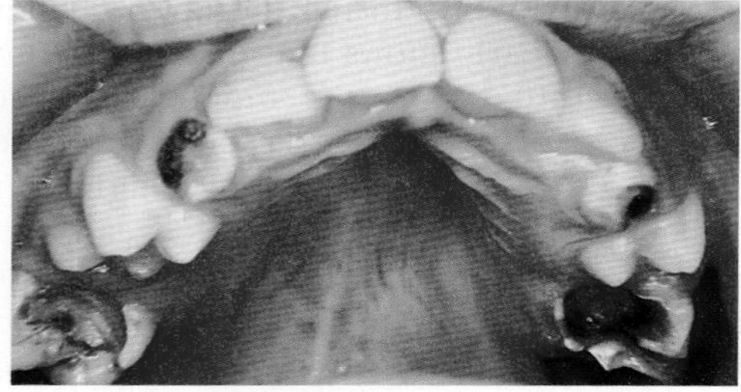

FIGURE 13–28 ✦ Chronic caries.

ronment. Because saliva provides the constituents that enable enamel to remineralize after an acid attack, a reduction in salivary flow or salivary buffering capacity may cause rapid demineralization. Conversely, demineralized lesions may recalcify as a result of an improved oral environment, especially in the presence of frequent use of .05% sodium fluoride mouthrinses. *Arrested caries* describes such a demineralization–remineralization process. Arrested lesions may be noticed because of their light or brown color, but they feel firm and glass-like when explored.

Recurrent Caries. *Recurrent caries* describes new decay that occurs at the margin(s) of existing restorations. These lesions pose a special threat because they may go undetected and invade the tissue beneath the restoration.

Hidden or Backward Caries. *Hidden caries* describes the lateral spread of decay at the dentinoenamel junction. This undermining process frequently results in a carious lesion with a small opening at the surface and extensive breakdown and cavitation within the tooth. The significance of this progression of caries relates primarily to cavity preparation and treatment. On clinical examination, a carious lesion may appear to require a simple restoration, but during dental treatment may require a complex restoration.

LOCATION OF CARIOUS LESIONS. Carious lesions are often referred to by their specific location on a tooth. This mechanism of description may be best suited for describing the dental problem to the client. The description of the location may include anatomic representations such as pit and fissure caries, smooth surface caries, and root caries. Another method of describing the location of a carious lesion is to identify the specific surface(s) on a tooth with a lesion. It is not uncommon for noncarious tooth surfaces to become involved in the restoration process because of the need for access or cavity design. For example, a tooth with a carious lesion on the distal surface may require the involvement of the occlusal surface or a disto-occlusal cavity preparation for restoration. Thus, another form of classification is by the number or identification of involved surfaces rather than carious surfaces.

Pit and Fissure Caries. *Pit and fissure caries* is most frequently found in the grooves and crevices of the occlusal surfaces of premolars and molars (Figure 13–29). It is also found in the lingual pits of maxillary incisors, facial pits of mandibular molars, and lingual grooves of maxillary molars. Pits and fissures are particularly susceptible to a carious attack because of the protected bacterial niche provided by the inadequately coalesced developmental lobes of enamel.

Smooth Surface Caries. *Smooth surface caries* is found on the facial, lingual, mesial, and distal surfaces of the dentition. The proximal smooth surfaces are the most susceptible to dental caries because of the shelter they provide for the bacterial plaque colonies. The gingival one-third of the facial and lingual surfaces also are more susceptible to caries because of the increased difficulty associated with cleaning this less-bulbous portion of the crown.

Root Caries. *Root caries* is found on the root surfaces of teeth. Root caries is most frequently found in the elderly population, in whom root exposure is common because of gingival recession. Root caries presents a unique set of considerations for restorative therapy because of the location of the lesions, the difficulty of adequate plaque

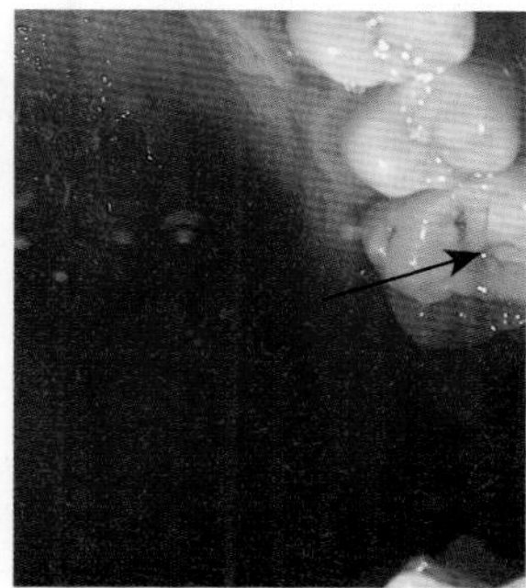

FIGURE 13–29 ✦ Pit and fissure caries.

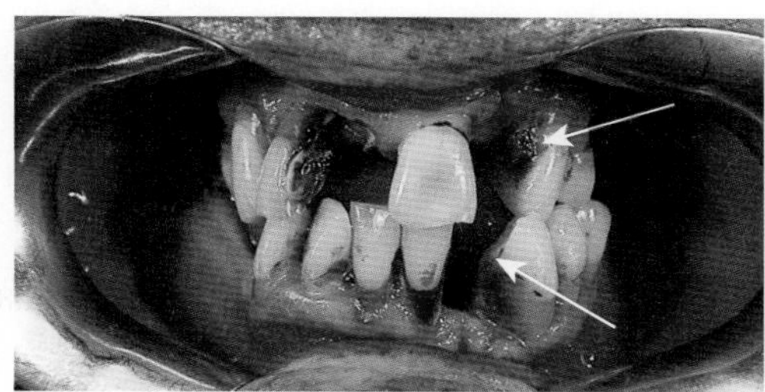

FIGURE 13–30 ✦ Root caries found on the root surfaces of teeth *(arrow)*.

control, and the chemical composition of the root surface.[12] As the lesion progresses, it may encircle the tooth at the gumline, making it very difficult to isolate and restore (Figure 13–30).

CLASSIFICATION OF DENTAL CARIES AND RESTORATIONS

Dental caries and dental restorations are commonly classified either by Black's classification or by the complexity classification system.

Black's Classification of Dental Caries and Restorations

The most commonly used system to describe the types and locations of both dental caries and restorations was established by G. V. Black in the early 1900s. This descriptive system consists of six classifications shown in Table 13–1.

Classification by Complexity

This system of classification identifies dental caries and restorations by the names of the surfaces they involve. *Simple caries* or restorations are those involving only one tooth surface. Those that involve two surfaces are classified as *compound caries* or restorations, and *complex caries* or restorations involve more than two surfaces. The usual practice is to refer to the caries or restoration using the abbreviation of the surfaces affected, such as O for occlusal, DO for disto-occlusal and MOD for mesio-occlusodistal. When doing so, the letters are pronounced separately, such as a D-O caries or an M-O-D restoration.

Table 13–2 outlines examples of simple, compound, and complex designations for dental caries or restorations named with nomenclature as described in the following section.

Nomenclature

In describing a cavity or a restoration, specific nomenclature is used that involves the combination of anatomic terms. Basic rules for nomenclature used to describe a cavity or restoration are as follows:

Rule #1: The terms mesial and distal precede all other terms, with mesial taking precedence (e.g., mesial occlusal distal).

Rule #2: The terms labial, buccal, facial, and lingual follow mesial and distal in that order and precede incisal and occlusal (e.g., mesial buccal occlusal).

Rule #3: The terms incisal (for anterior teeth) and occlusal (for posterior teeth) occur last in any combination, except when they connect two surfaces not connected (e.g., mesial occlusal distal).

Rule #4: In two-term combinations, the final letters "al" are dropped from the first term and replaced by "o" (e.g., mesiolingual).

Rule #5: In three-term combinations, the final letters "al" are dropped from each of the first two terms and replaced by "o" (e.g., mesiolabioincisal).

Rule #6: Whenever dropping of an "al" results in a double "o," a hyphen is added, separating them (e.g., disto-occlusodistal).

Rule #7: In three-term combinations where two nonconnected surfaces are connected by a third surface, the mesial or distal surface is first, followed by facial, lingual, incisal, or occlusal, then the remaining surface (e.g., disto-occlusobuccal).

Rule #8: In three-term combinations where all surfaces are connected, rules 1 through 3 apply.

ASSESSMENT OF SIGNS OF CARIES AND OTHER ACQUIRED TOOTH DAMAGE*

Tooth assessment includes both radiographic and direct (clinical) evaluations. Bite-wing radiographs (radiographs that include images of the crown and some of the roots of several teeth in both arches) are standard diagnostic tools for posterior teeth. Periapical radiographs (radiographs that include the tips of roots of teeth in a single arch) may be used for anterior teeth if they are determined to be necessary during the clinical examination. In addition, periapical radiographs are required of any tooth where the health of the pulp and the tip of the root are in question. A radiolucent (black) area at the tip

* Portions of this section were contributed by Cheryl Cameron, RDH, PhD, and Glen E. Gordon, DDS, University of Washington – Seattle.

TABLE 13–1

BLACK'S CLASSIFICATION OF DENTAL CARIES AND RESTORATIONS

Classification	Description
Class I 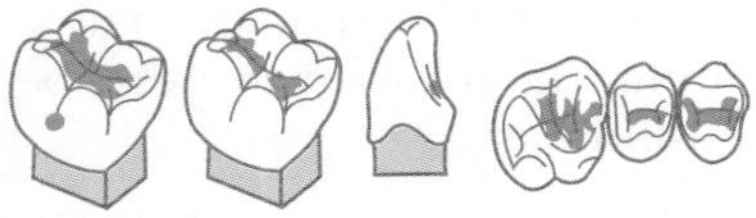	Caries/restoration in the pits and fissures on the occlusal surfaces of molars and premolars, facial (buccal) or lingual pits of molars, and lingual pits of maxillary incisors
Class II 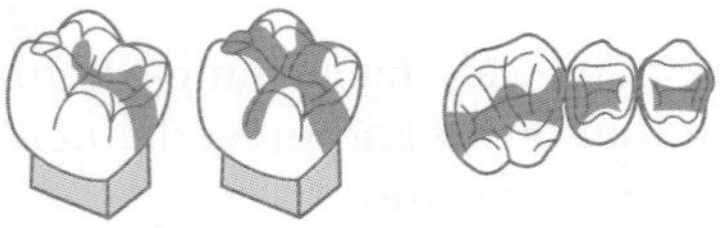	Caries/restoration on the proximal (mesial or distal) surfaces of the premolars and molars involving two or more surfaces
Class III 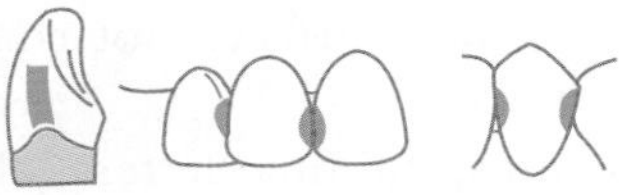	Caries/restoration on the proximal (mesial or distal) surfaces of incisors and canines
Class IV 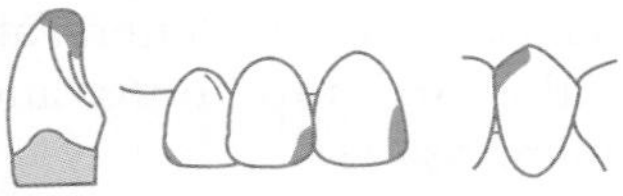	Caries/restoration on the proximal (mesial or distal) surfaces of incisors and canines and also involving the incisal angle
Class V 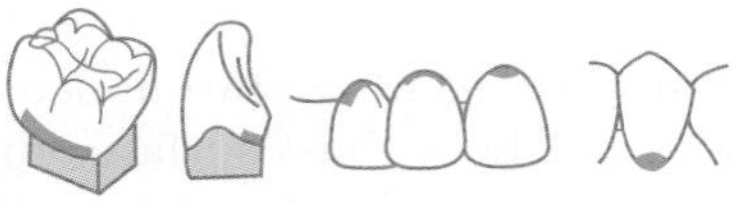	Caries restoration on the gingival third of the facial or lingual surfaces of any tooth
Class IV 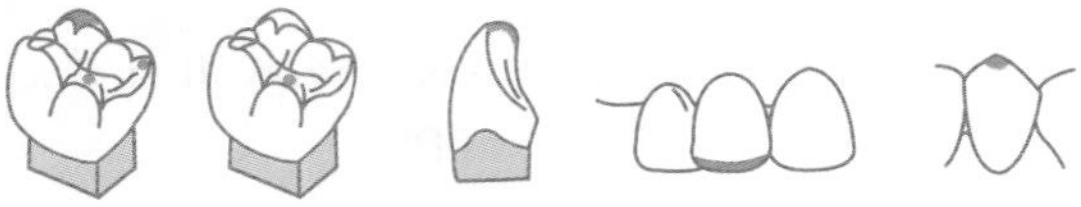	Caries restoration on the incisal edge of anterior teeth or the cusp tips of posterior teeth

Adapted from Robinson D, Bird D: *Torres and Erlich: Essentials of dental assisting,* ed 6, Philadelphia, 1999, WB Saunders. Figures redrawn from Northern Alberta Institute of Technology, Resource No 1399, 1999.

TABLE 13–2

SIMPLE, COMPOUND, AND COMPLEX DESIGNATIONS FOR DENTAL CARIES AND RESTORATIONS

Simple	Abbreviation	Compound	Abbreviation	Complex	Abbreviation
Buccal	B	Mesio-occlusal	MO	Mesioincisodistal	MID
Facial	F	Disto-occlusal	DO	Mesiolinguodistal	MLD
Gingival	G	Occlusobuccal	OB	Mesio-occlusobuccal	MOB
Incisal	I	Distolingual	DL	Mesio-occlusodistal	MOD
Lingual	Li	Disto-occlusal	DO	Mesio-occlusodistobuccolingual	MODBL
Labial	La				
Occlusal	O				

of the root of a tooth may indicate the presence of a periapical abscess and the need for immediate referral to the dentist for treatment.

The bite-wing radiograph, however, produces the best image of the tooth crowns, the main area of concern for tooth restoration. Carious lesions appear as radiolucent (black) images on radiographs because dental caries causes localized demineralization and loss of tooth tissue. In the early stages of decay, classic patterns of the carious process may be seen on radiographs, because the destruction proceeds in line with enamel rods and along dentinal tubules. Depending on their density, restorative materials produce relatively radiopaque (white) images. Due to the contrast between the oral tissues and the restorative materials, radiographs readily illustrate the fit and contours of restorations (Figure 13–31). For example, all suspected overhanging margins of fillings can be verified by radiographs.

As discussed earlier, an explorer is commonly used to check grooves and pits in enamel, discolored root surfaces along the gingival margin, and suspicious margins of restorations. Light pressure should be applied with the explorer, using a proper fulcrum. Care should be exercised to avoid exploring known sensitive areas. It is proposed that exploring may cause early carious lesions to become cavitated due to the rupturing by the explorer of remineralizing enamel crystals. Also, the explorer may transfer cariogenic microorganisms from tooth to tooth.[13]

Currently several other methods for caries detection are being evaluated, including fiberoptic transillumination (Foti) and laser fluorescence (LF). Laser fluorescence utilizes an argon laser beam to illuminate the tooth surface and provides good visibility of early enamel changes. These or other technologies may soon replace the use of an explorer.

Color is not a foolproof sign of caries, since carious dentin can range in color from nearly white to shades of black. If a dark area on a tooth is hard, regardless of the color, it is rarely an active carious lesion. The caries process often undermines otherwise intact enamel (hidden caries), producing a "pearly" appearance. In this case, color may be an indicator of the extent of the carious lesion. Marginal ridges, especially in anterior teeth, should be examined under a well-directed light. The careful use of a nonmagnifying, front-surface mirror for transillumination may show signs of undermining decay, which can then be substantiated by the dentist's exploring the lesion.

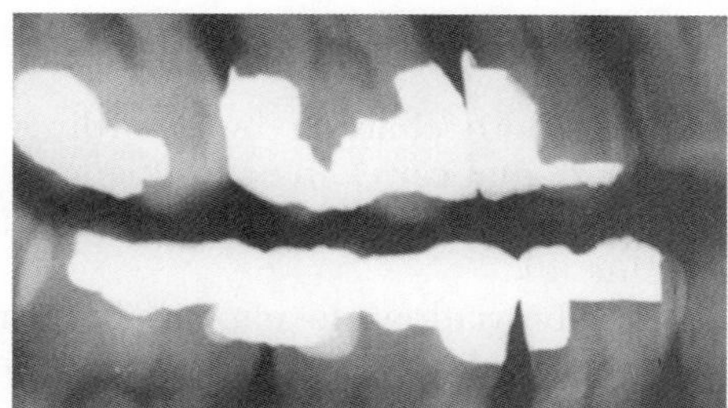

FIGURE 13–31 ✦ Radiograph showing restorations.

ASSESSMENT OF CLIENT SYMPTOMS

Client reports of pain elicited by sugar intake, sensitivity to cold stimuli, and objectionable taste are frequently due to advanced carious lesions or leaking/defective restorations. Tooth abrasions and erosions may be sensitive to toothbrushing, acidic foods, and cold stimuli. Fractures of teeth may elicit sharp pain during chewing and contact with cold foods.

When pain is reported, questioning the client is an important way to gain information about location, duration, postural changes, and qualities of the pain.[14] Questioning should begin with a general question like "Tell me about your pain," followed by more specific questions that focus on provoking factors, attenuating factors, frequency, and intensity (see Questions to Determine Quality of Pain). These questions can be followed by further exploration in which the client is asked to expand on previous responses.

These symptoms are essential to the dental diagnosis and should be communicated to the dentist immediately. Factors indicating the need for immediate referral to a dentist for an endodontic diagnosis[14] are listed in Factors Related to a Dental Diagnosis of a Periapical (Endodontic) Abscess.

Questions to Determine Quality of Pain

General: "Tell me about your pain."
Provoking factors: "Does heat (cold, biting, or chewing) initiate the pain?" (Ask each separately to avoid confusing the client.)
Attenuating factors: "Does anything relieve the pain?"
Intensity: "When you have pain, is it mild, moderate, or severe?"
Location: "Please point to the tooth/area that hurts."
Duration: "Does heat (or cold) cause pain?" "How long does the pain last?"
Postural: "Do you have any pain when you lie down? Bend over?"
Quality: "What is the nature of the pain? Sharp? Dull? Stabbing? Throbbing?"

Factors Related to Dental Diagnosis of a Periapical (Endodontic) Abscess

Sharp, severe, intermittent pain that may be hard to localize
Clinical and/or radiographic evidence of tooth damage such as caries, tooth fracture, or defective restorations
Observation of soft tissue redness or swelling and presence of a fistula (sinus tract drainage)
A rounded radiolucency at the apex of the tooth
Pulpal vitality test results.
Facial asymmetry due to swelling
Skin lesions (occasionally facial lesions may be traced to a tooth source (i.e., sinus tract drainage)

Procedure 13–1 USE OF AN ELECTRIC PULP TESTER TO DETERMINE PULP VITALITY

EQUIPMENT

2 × 2 gauze, saliva ejector, cotton rolls, toothpaste, electric pulp tester

STEPS	RATIONALE
1. Review health history.	Use of the electric pulp tester is contraindicated for a client with a pacemaker or any electronic life-support device because it can interfere with the device's function and cause a serious health threat.
2. Assemble equipment.	Manufacturers' instructions must be followed. When the tester rheostat is separate from the applicator tip, an assistant is needed.
3. Explain briefly to the client the purpose of the test and what is to be done.	This familiarizes the client with the procedure. For some pulp testers, the client lightly holds the handle with the gloved clinician to complete the circuit.
4. Dry the teeth to be tested and isolate them with cotton rolls and insert saliva ejector.	Drying the teeth prevents the current from passing to the gingiva.
5. Moisten the end of the tip of the tester with a small amount of toothpaste or another electrolyte with the same consistency.	Toothpaste acts as a conductor, and its consistency allows it to remain in place.
6. Instruct client to raise a hand or make a sound when he or she feels a sensation.	This promotes effective communication to enhance testing effectiveness.
7. Apply tester tip, without pressure but with definite contact, first to at least one tooth other than the one in question, preferably to an adjacent tooth or the same tooth on the opposite side of the arch.	This determines a normal response for the client and familiarizes the client with the procedure.
8. Apply tip on sound tooth structure on the middle third of the crown of a single-rooted tooth and the middle third of each cusp of a multirooted tooth.	These locations allow the tester to detect the presence of vital pulp tissue.
9. Avoid contact with gingival or other soft tissue.	A low-resistant circuit can be formed to by-pass the tooth.
10. Avoid contact with metallic restorations. Insert a nonconductive plastic matrix strip to separate two metallic restorations.	The metal forms a more rapid conductor than does tooth structure. When approximal restorations are in contact, the circuit can be transmitted to the adjacent tooth and prevent a reading from being obtained from the tooth in question.
11. Start with the rheostat at zero and advance slowly but steadily, stopping only momentarily after each number.	This allows time for client to discriminate response to a specific reading of current flow.
12. Test each tooth at least twice. Avarage the readings.	Responses may vary with each test.
13. Record in client's chart the pulp tester used and the lowest number (average) at which a minimal stimulus induced a response for all teeth tested.	The same pulp tester should be used for a specific client at continuing comparative tests to obtain consistent readings. This also provides a legal record.

Although thermal testing using hot or cold appliances is used to detect vital pulp tissue, electrical pulp testers are considered more reliable. Electrical pulp testing is based on electrical stimulation to create pain to which one can react (Procedure 13–1). Electrical pulp testing may not always be accurate because pulp vitality depends on blood supply, not nerves (see Factors that Affect Client Response to Pulp Testing).

CHARTING TOOTH ASSESSMENT DATA

The tooth assessment charting procedure is conducted at the client's assessment appointment and updated at each reappointment. Although no set sequences are required for charting, a fixed routine avoids omitting important information (Table 13–3). The systematic approach advocated is as follows:

1. Chart all missing or unerupted teeth first, to prevent the wrongful identification of existing teeth.
2. Note the presence of partial and/or complete dentures.
3. Chart in blue ink existing amalgam or tooth-colored restorations.
4. Chart in blue ink gold restorations, crowns, and bridges.
5. Complete the tooth charting by recording signs of early or overt dental caries in red ink and other miscellaneous chartable items (e.g., hypoplasia, appliances) in blue ink.
6. The use of abbreviations to explain the symbols is optional for recording on the chart (Table 13–2). Figure 13–32 illustrates an example of a completed

Factors that Affect Client Response to Pulp Testing

Necrotic pulp: A necrotic pulp gives no response.
Pulpal inflammation: An inflamed pulp responds at varying degrees from no response to a full normal response depending on degree of inflammation.
Blockage of nerve transmission: Anesthetics or injury to nerve blocks nerve trasmission.
Metal restorations: Metal restorations or bridgework adjacent to tooth being tested can form a circuit that bypasses the tooth in question.
Pain perception: Client's reaction to pain depends on such things as pain threshold, premedication, the size of the pulp, and the thickness of dentin, especially secondary dentin.

chart along with a descriptive key of the charted symbols.

7. Periodontal charting of gingival and mucogingival lines, probing depth, attachment loss, recession, furcation involvement, mucogingival problems, abnormal frenum attachments, and mobility of teeth is described in Chapter 15.
8. Protocol for updating the chart should be established in each oral healthcare setting to avoid a cluttered and unreadable chart.

OCCLUSION

Thorough assessment of the dentition includes classifying occlusion and documenting any malrelationships of teeth present. *Occlusion* is defined as the contact relationship between maxillary and mandibular teeth when the jaws are in a fully closed position, as well as the relationship between the teeth in the same arch. As the primary teeth erupt in the child, occlusion develops and is influenced by the development of facial muscles and neuromuscular patterns. Occlusion of the erupting permanent teeth is dependent on that of the primary teeth as they are being shed.[15]

Centric Occlusion

An ideal occlusion, with 138 occlusal contacts when the 32 permanent teeth are in closure, rarely, if ever, exists. Consequently, centric occlusion serves as the standard point of reference for describing a normal occlusion. *Centric occlusion* is the voluntary, habitual position of the teeth that allows maximum contact when the teeth are closed. When the teeth of a normal occlusion are in centric position, each tooth of one arch is in occlusion with two teeth in the opposite arch, except for the mandibular central incisors and the maxillary third molars. This positioning of the teeth serves to equalize the forces of occlusion. Because of this arrangement, the alignment of the opposing jaw is not immediately disturbed if a tooth is lost. However, if restorative treatment is not performed for a long period, the neighboring teeth begin to drift mesially in an effort to fill the space. The teeth become tilted and supereruption of the tooth opposite the space in the opposing arch occurs. Thus, the loss of one tooth can change the occlusion of the entire dentition.

When teeth do not occlude (come together) properly, unnatural stress is placed on them and their periodontal tissues, so that they may be unable to perform their functions. This occlusal disharmony may lead to pain and/or occlusal trauma. Although occlusal trauma does not directly cause periodontal disease, it may be an adverse factor in an already diseased periodontium. An important role of the dental hygienist is to explain to clients the importance of tooth replacement to prevent occlusal disharmonies. To prevent occlusal disharmony, all clients should have an occlusal evaluation by the dentist before and after completion of their dental treatment.[15]

OVERJET. When teeth normally come together in centric occlusion, the maxillary dentition overhangs the mandibular dentition facially, a position called *overjet* (Figure 13–33). This normal horizontal overlap is important because it keeps the soft tissue out of the way of the mandible during mastication.

Overjet is measured when the client's teeth are closed in centric occlusion and the tip of the periodontal probe is placed at a right angle to the labial surface of the mandibular incisor at the base of the incisal edge of the maxillary incisor. The measurement is taken from the labial surface of the mandibular incisor to the lingual surface of the maxillary incisor. The labiolingual width of the maxillary incisor is not included in the recorded measurement. The dental hygienist is then able to measure and record the overlap in millimeters.

OVERBITE. In centric occlusion, the maxillary incisors overlap the mandibular incisors, a position called *overbite.* This vertical overlap allows maximum contact between the posterior teeth during mastication. Overbite is classified as normal, moderate, or severe based on the depth of the overlap. Overbite is considered normal if the maxillary incisors overlap within the incisal third of the mandibular incisors. Moderate overbite occurs when the maxillary incisors overlap into the middle third of the mandibular incisors, and severe overlap when the incisal edges of the maxillary teeth reach to the gingival third of the mandibular incisors (Figure 13–34).

Overbite is measured when the client's maxillary and mandibular teeth are closed in centric occlusion. The tip of the periodontal probe is placed at the incisal edge of the maxillary incisor at right angles to the mandibular incisor. As the client slightly opens his or her mouth, the probe then is placed vertically against the mandibular

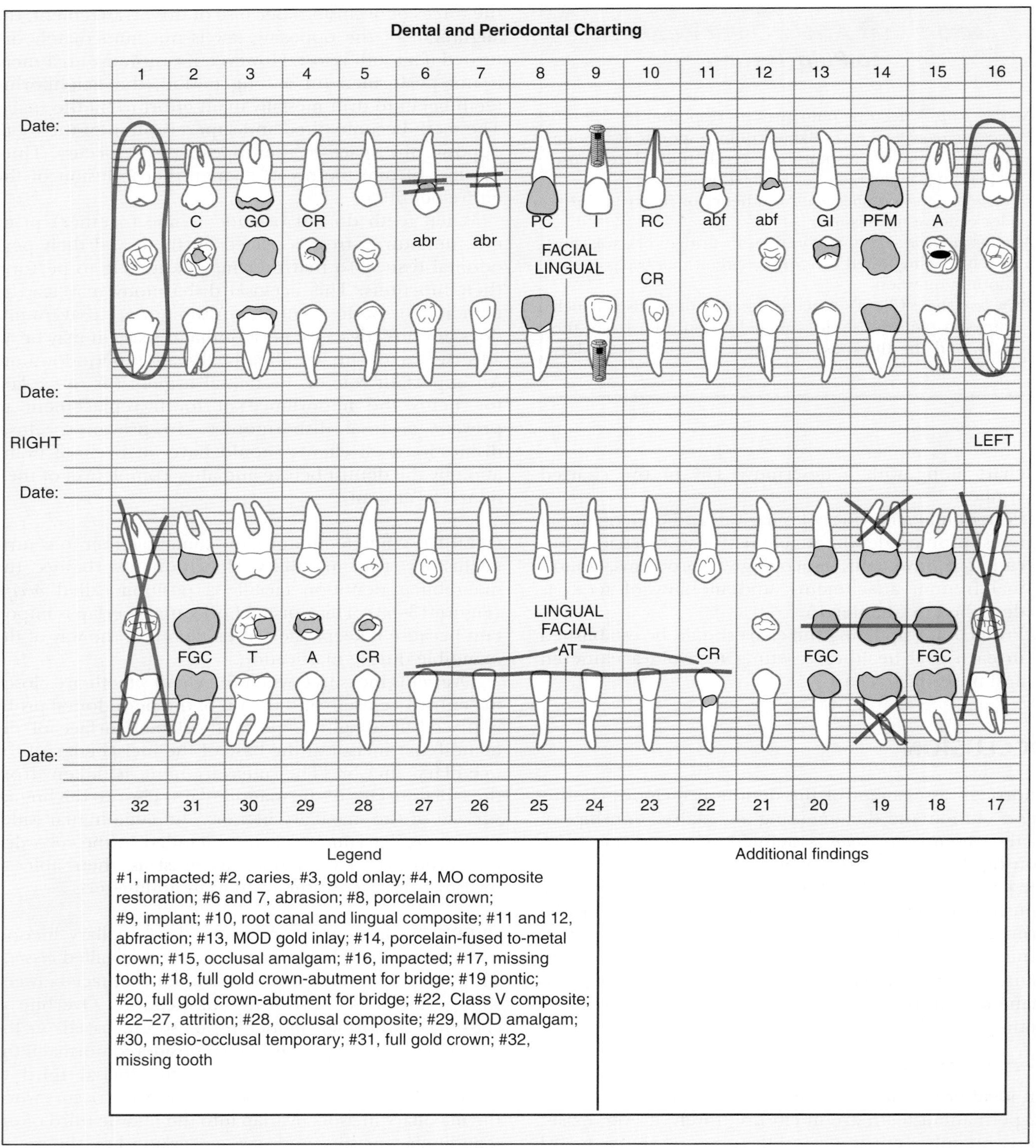

FIGURE 13–32 ✦ Charting symbols. *(Adapted from Nelson DM:* Review of dental hygiene, *Philadelphia, 2000, WB Saunders.)*

incisor to measure the distance to the incisal edge of the mandibular incisor. It is customary to measure the overbite in millimeters and to include a classification of normal, moderate, or severe with the recorded measurement. These variations should be documented in writing on the client's chart.[15]

Centric Relation

Centric relation is the endpoint of closure of the mandible. Ideally, the mandible is in centric relation when the dentition is in centric occlusion. Usually the teeth slide about 1 mm when clients shift their occlusion from centric relation to centric occlusion.[15]

Text continued on page 251

TABLE 13–3 CHARTING SYMBOLS FOR TOOTH ASSESSMENT

Chartable Item	Description	Charting Procedure	Charting Symbol	Abbreviations
Missing teeth	Teeth that are not present because of extraction or are congenitally missing	Place vertical line or X through facial, occlusal, and lingual surfaces Chart in blue ink	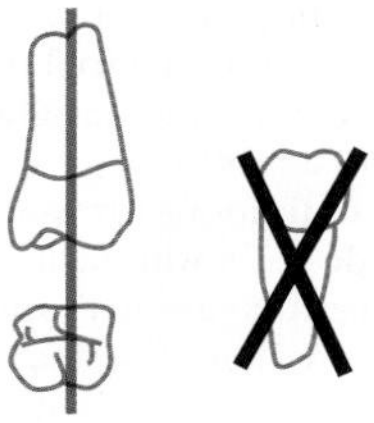	M
Unerupted teeth	Teeth that have not yet erupted or are impacted	Circle facial, occlusal, and lingual surfaces of tooth Chart in red ink	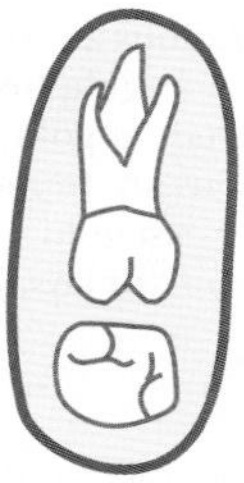	U
Teeth to be extracted	Teeth to be extracted because of pathologic or orthodontic reasons	Draw a red diagonal line through the tooth, or an alternative method is to draw two red parallel lines through the tooth	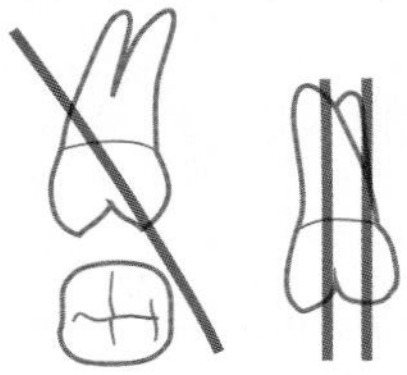	Ex
Amalgam restorations	Alloy of silver and mercury; silver or dark gray in color; widely used as a restorative material	Chart surfaces where the restorations appear Outline and shade in blue the shape of restoration For precise notation, Black's classification can be used	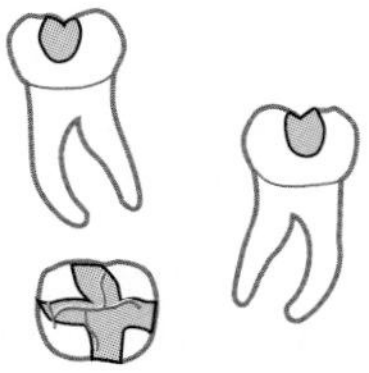	A
Tooth-colored restorations	Composite resin is a tooth-colored restorative material. Usually placed in anterior teeth for restoring facial and/or proximal surfaces where aesthetics are a major concern, but found in posterior areas for the same reason	Outline exact size and shape of restoration Shade with blue ink Chart surfaces involved Can be further identified using Black's classification	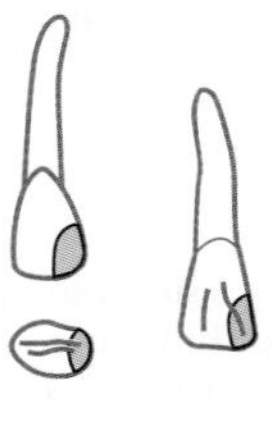	R = resin CR = composite resin
Temporary restorations	Temporary filling cements (i.e., a zinc oxide–eugenol cement) may be placed as an interim measure for a displaced restoration or between phases of treatment while observing pulpal reaction. Distinguishable by its creamy yellow color	Chart temporary restorations the same as amalgam or tooth-colored restorations in blue ink, but distinguish from amalgams with the abbreviation	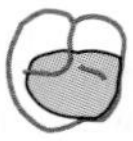	Temp T

Table continued on following page

TABLE 13–3 CHARTING SYMBOLS FOR TOOTH ASSESSMENT—CONT'D

Chartable Item	Description	Charting Procedure	Charting Symbol	Abbreviations
Veneer	An aesthetic veneer or layer of tooth-colored material that is used to cover the unsightly area of a tooth Typical indications for veneers include teeth with facial surfaces that are malformed, discolored, or abraded. Technique for replacing labial surface is used.	Outline and shade in surface of tooth where veneer is found Chart in blue ink	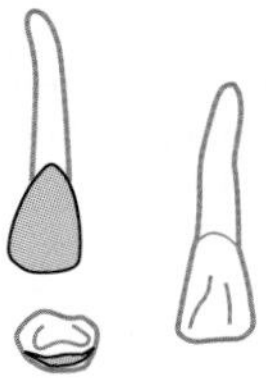	Ven
Gold restorations	Gold restorations are noted by the yellow gold luster. Several types of gold restorations are found, including cast gold restorations (onlays, inlays, crowns)	See below		
Full gold crown	A cast yellow-gold crown covering the entire surface and all of the crown surfaces	Outline and fill in with diagonal lines covering all surfaces of the crown Chart in blue ink	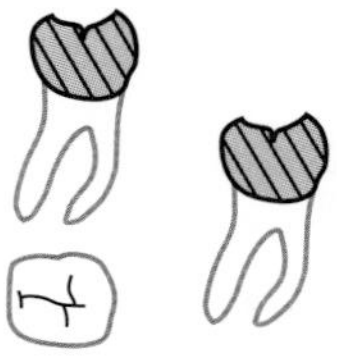	FGC
¾ gold crown	Covers less than ¾ of tooth surfaces	Outline and fill in with diagonal lines placed on all surfaces or portion of surfaces covered by crown Chart in blue ink	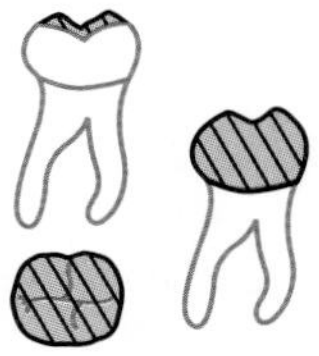	¾ GC
Ceramic-metal crowns	White-gold alloy crown with bonded acrylic or porcelain facing. Provides a tooth-colored appearance.	Chart similarly to gold crowns Abbreviation can be used to distinguish it from full gold or ¾ gold crowns Chart in blue ink	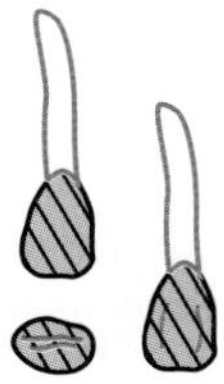	GCPF = gold crown, porcelain face GCAF = gold crown, acrylic face
Gold inlay	A cast gold restoration that is placed within the prepared tooth cavity and does not cover the cusps	Outline the shape of the restoration on the surfaces where it appears Chart in blue ink	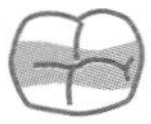	GI
Gold onlay	A cast gold restoration with the cusp tips covered in gold for added strength	Outline and color the shape of the restoration on the surfaces where it appears Chart in blue ink	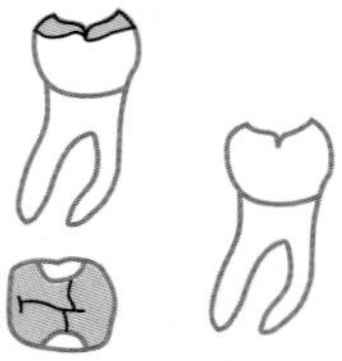	GO

TABLE 13–3 CHARTING SYMBOLS FOR TOOTH ASSESSMENT—CONT'D

Chartable Item	Description	Charting Procedure	Charting Symbol	Abbreviations
Fixed bridges	A bridge unit serves to restore a functional unit by replacing one or more missing teeth. A fixed bridge consists of abutment and pontic teeth splinted together	Outline abutment and pontic teeth in blue ink and fill in with diagonal lines on occlusal, facial, and lingual surfaces Chart the pontic teeth as extracted. The type of crowns may be identified with abbreviations (e.g., FGC, GCPF) Place two horizontal lines between the occlusal surfaces of the teeth to represent the splinted unit		Each tooth may be labeled with the appropriate abbreviations FGC, GCPF, and ¾ GC
Dental implants	A stable functional replacement for one or more missing teeth that consists of an osseointegrated anchor, an abutment, and a prosthetic tooth or appliance	Place a dental implant stamp over the teeth involved. If no stamp is available, make a written comment under the teeth involved		IMPL
Dental caries (see pp. **239-243** for further discussion)	Technically known as carious lesions, commonly referred to as cavities	Outline the carious area(s) in red on the surfaces where the caries appear. Suspect carious surfaces can be labeled for observation On completion of the restorations, fill in the red areas with blue ink		C
Recurrent decay	Recurring caries around the margin of an existing restoration	Outline the area of recurrent decay in red		RD
Defective restorations	Defective restoration may be the result of, for example, marginal ditching, voids, fracture lines, or improper anatomical contours	Chart the defective restoration similarly to recurrent decay Outline the restoration in red and label it with an abbreviation Differentiate between recurrent decay and defective restoration with suitable abbreviation		DR
Appliances Partial or complete dentures	Removable dentures for partial or full replacement of the dentition	Chart the missing teeth with vertical lines or Xs through all surfaces. Join vertical lines or Xs with a horizontal line at the root apex and label appropriately to indicate upper or lower and partial or complete denture.	PUD PUD CLD	PUD = partial upper denture PLD = partial lower denture CUD = complete upper denture CLD = complete lower denture

Table continued on following page

TABLE 13–3 CHARTING SYMBOLS FOR TOOTH ASSESSMENT—CONT'D

Chartable Item	Description	Charting Procedure	Charting Symbol	Abbreviations
Orthodontic/temporomandibular (TMJ) appliance	Placed for the shifting or stabilization of teeth (i.e., bands, night guards, retainers, space maintainers)	These appliances need not be charted on the tooth surfaces but should be identified as present in the record section of the chart		
Overhanging restorations	Projections of restorative material that extend beyond the curvature of the tooth	Chart with triangular symbols in the interproximal area Chart in blue ink	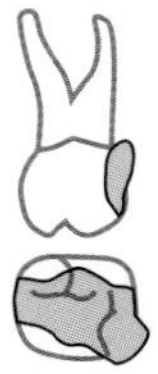	OH
Dental sealants	A plastic resin coating placed on occlusal surface to seal pits and fissures against caries	Encircle and place abbreviation inside the circle Chart on occlusal surface in yellow or green pencil	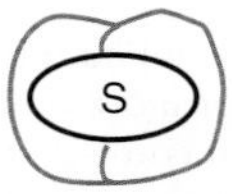 S	S
Root tip	A remaining root tip, likely from surgical extraction of tooth	Chart tooth as missing and place abbreviation symbol near root apex Chart in blue ink	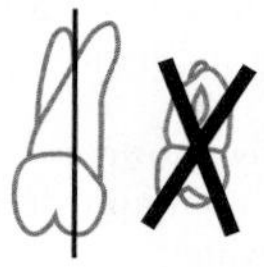	RT
Root canal	Removal of pulp tissue and replacement with endodontic filling material	Place vertical line through pulpal area of root Label with abbreviation Chart in blue ink	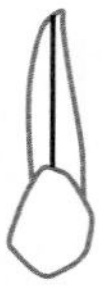	RC
Acquired Dental Defects (see pp. **238-241** for further discussion)				
Decalcification or hypocalcification	Appears chalky white in color, possibly an incipient carious lesion. Usually softer than adjacent enamel	Outline the area and label with abbreviation Chart in blue ink	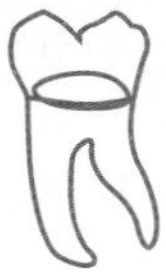	Decal
Enamel hypoplasia or enamel hypocalcification	Enamel defect resulting from a variety of systemic or traumatic influences. The surface is pitted and rough with enamel hypoplasia, and white flecking appears with enamel hypocalcification	Chart using wavy lines to denote the irregularity of enamel with symbol Indicate with abbreviation	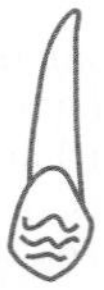	Hypoplas
Erosion	Chemical wear from acidic substances	Shade area in blue and place symbol	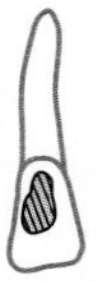	Ero
Attrition	Mechanical wear from the forces of mastication of the incisal or occlusal surfaces	Place a horizontal line over the affected surfaces Chart in blue ink	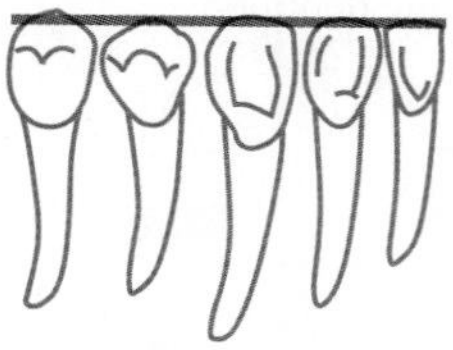	Att

TABLE 13–3 CHARTING SYMBOLS FOR TOOTH ASSESSMENT—CONT'D

Chartable Item	Description	Charting Procedure	Charting Symbol	Abbreviations
Abrasion	Mechanical wear caused by improper toothbrushing or other habits (i.e., chewing on pencils, pipe smoking)	Chart two horizontal lines in blue ink		Abr
Dental Anomalies (see pp. **235-238** for further discussion)				
Supernumerary teeth	Extra teeth	Draw additional tooth in location found Chart in blue ink Label with abbreviation		Su
Other Dental Anomalies	Other anatomic variations, such as dens in dente, should be clearly indicated in the record section of the dental chart			

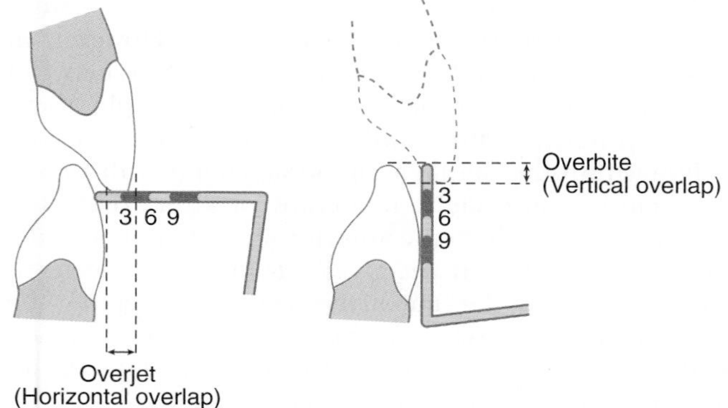

FIGURE 13–33 ✦ Comparison between overjet, the horizontal overlap between the two arches, and overbite, the vertical overlap between the two arches. *(From Bath-Balogh M, Fehrenbach M:* Illustrated dental embryology, histology and anatomy, *ed 1, Philadelphia, 1997, WB Saunders, 1997).*

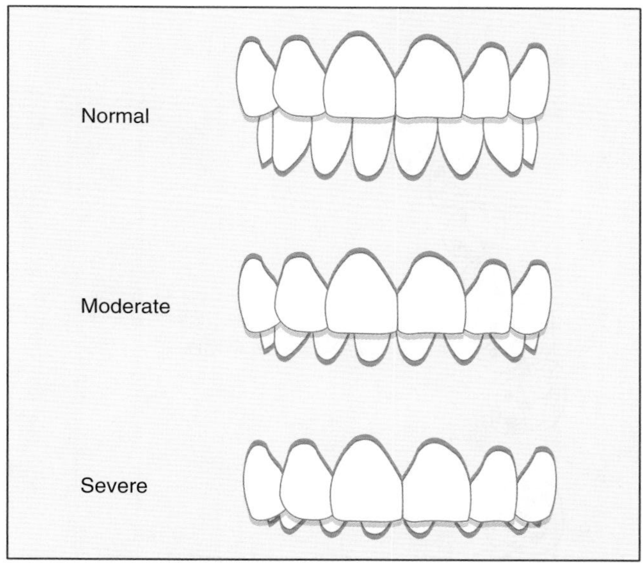

FIGURE 13–34 ✦ Classification of overbite.

Centric Stops

When the maxillary and mandibular teeth are locked in centric occlusion they should be touching each other maximally. These points of touching are called *centric stops.* The ideal centric stops are the height of cusp contour, marginal ridges, and central fossae (Figure 13–35). With attrition, the cusps become closer to the central fossae, increasing the risk of losing a definite locking of the teeth together in centric occlusion. The height of the lower one-third of the face (the vertical dimension) is determined by centric stops and the height of the alveolar bone. Attrition and bone loss cause loss of vertical dimension, which affects physical appearance and proper functioning of the teeth and jaws.[15]

Contact Areas

In the ideal dental arch, there are contact areas where the teeth touch their same arch neighbor on their proximal surfaces. These contact areas protect the interdental gingiva and stabilize each tooth in the dental arch. When there is no contact area between teeth, these *open contacts* trap food, resulting in gingival inflammation, and do not contribute to tooth stability. Suspected open proximal contacts should be visually corroborated by viewing through the contact against a white background, such as the rubber glove surface. If light passes through the contact, it is judged to be open. The use of floss only in assessing the status of an open contact may result in an inaccurate diagnosis. A slightly open contact may resist the passing of dental floss and yet result in food impaction and gingival inflammation. Open contacts need to be called to the attention of the dentist for evaluation and treatment.[15]

Normal Occlusion

In the late 1800s, Dr. Edward H. Angle established a system of classification of occlusion. Angle's method of classification was based on the principle that the maxillary first molars are the keys to occlusion. Because of their stability within the dental arch, the permanent first molars and later the canines were added as the indicator teeth to assess the relationship between the maxilla and the mandible. In a normal molar relationship, the mesiobuccal cusp of the maxillary permanent first molar occludes with the buccal groove of the mandibular permanent first molar. In a normal canine relationship, the maxillary permanent canine occludes with the distal half of the mandibular permanent canine and the mesial half of the mandibular first premolar.

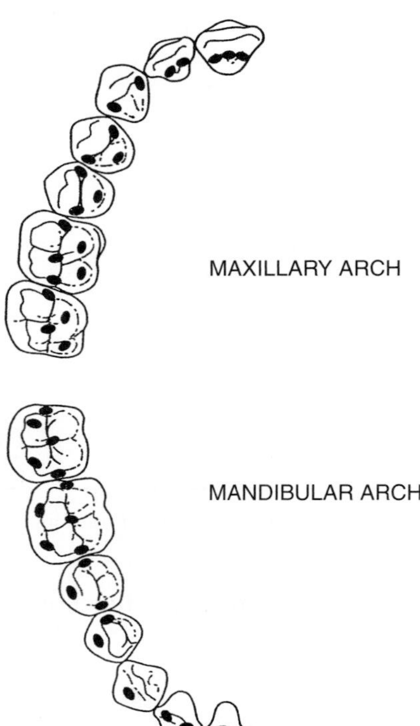

FIGURE 13–35 ✦ The ideal centric stops between the two arches are highlighted. *(From Bath-Balogh M, Fehrenbach M:* Illustrated dental embryology, histology and anatomy, *ed 1, Philadelphia, 1997, WB Saunders, 1997).*

MALOCCLUSION

Malocclusion results when there is a lack of overall ideal form in the dentition while in centric occlusion. In addition, excessive overjet and/or overbite are classified as malocclusion.

Malocclusion may have a negative effect on the client's personal appearance and may make it more difficult for the client to perform effective oral hygiene. Because plaque biofilm causes periodontal disease, individuals with malocclusion are at increased risk for periodontal disease. Malocclusion also may affect bodily function because of temporomandibular joint pain and inadequate nutrition associated with malocclusion. As part of the dental hygiene assessment, occlusion is classified on both the right and left sides of the dentition.[15] Malocclusion and temporomandibular joint dysfunctions, such as pain or popping on opening and closing the mandible, are referred to the dentist for further evaluation and referral (see Chapter 51 for detailed discussion of malocclusion and orthodontic treatment).

In Angle's system there are three types of malocclusion in the permanent dentition: Class I, Class II, and Class III. Class II malocclusion is subclassified into divisions 1 and 2 (Figure 13–36).

Class I Malocclusion

In *Class I malocclusion* the molar and canine relationships are similar to those in normal occlusion. However, in Class I malocclusion there are mal-relationships between individual teeth or groups of teeth. For example, there may be problems with crowding where the teeth are out of line within the dental arch. Some clients with Class I malocclusion have slight, moderate, or severe overbites, or an *open bite* in which the anterior teeth do not occlude. Some clients have an *end-to-end bite* in which the teeth occlude without the maxillary teeth overlapping the mandibular teeth, or a *crossbite* in which the maxillary teeth are positioned lingually to mandibular teeth, an abnormal buccolingual tooth position (Table 13–4). The facial profile associated with Class I malocclusion is classified as straight or orthognathic[15] (Figure 13–36).

Class II Malocclusion

Class II and III malocclusions are referred to as skeletal malocclusions because of the differences in size or the abnormal relationship between the maxilla and the mandible. *Class II malocclusion,* also referred to as distal occlusion, is characterized by the buccal groove of the mandibular first permanent molar being distal to the mesiobuccal cusp of the maxillary first permanent molar by at least the width of a premolar. The canine relationship is such that the distal surface of the mandibular permanent canine is distal to the mesial surface of the maxillary permanent canine by at least the width of a premolar. If the distance is less than the width of a premolar, it is classified as having a "tendency toward Class II." An individual with a Class II malocclusion usually has

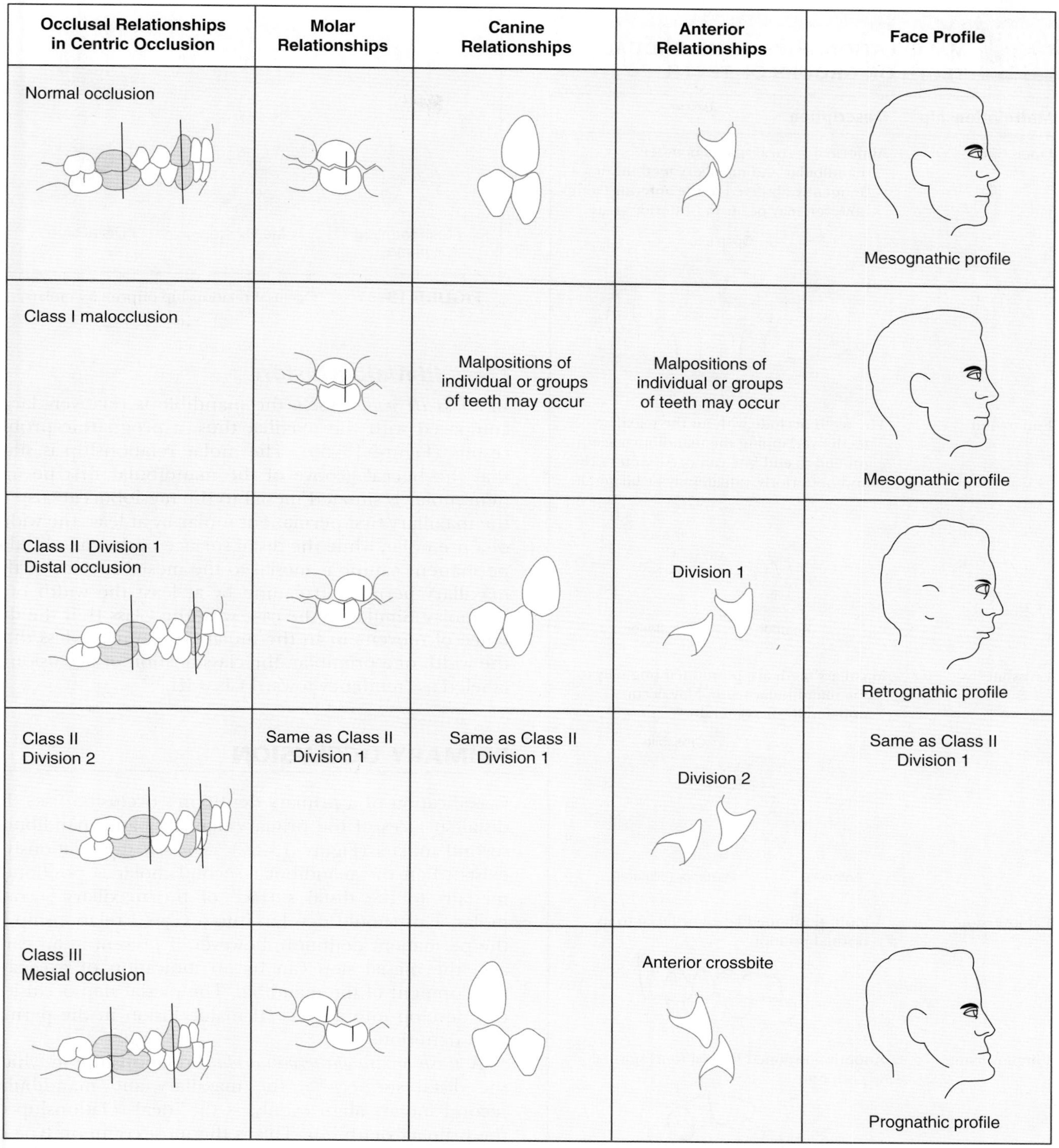

Occlusal Relationships in Centric Occlusion	Molar Relationships	Canine Relationships	Anterior Relationships	Face Profile
Normal occlusion				Mesognathic profile
Class I malocclusion		Malpositions of individual or groups of teeth may occur	Malpositions of individual or groups of teeth may occur	Mesognathic profile
Class II Division 1 Distal occlusion			Division 1	Retrognathic profile
Class II Division 2	Same as Class II Division 1	Same as Class II Division 1	Division 2	Same as Class II Division 1
Class III Mesial occlusion			Anterior crossbite	Prognathic profile

Figure 13–36 ✦ Classification of malocclusion. *(Adapted and redrawn from Woelfel JB:* Dental anatomy: Its relevance to dentistry, *ed 5, Philadelphia, 1997, Lippincott Williams & Wilkins.)*

a retrognathic facial profile, that is, a small, receded chin due to the apparently small mandible in relationship to the maxilla.

Two subdivisions of the Class II malocclusion are used to indicate the relationship of the anterior teeth. In Class II division 1, the maxillary incisors protrude facially from the mandibular incisors. As a result the mandibular incisors over-erupt, causing a severe overbite. Often the palate is deep and narrow and the facial profile includes a protruding upper lip. In class II division 2, one or more of the maxillary central incisors are lingually inclined or retruded (Figure 13–36). The maxillary lateral incisors

TABLE 13–4 MALRELATIONSHIPS OF INDIVIDUAL TEETH OR GROUPS OF TEETH

Malrelationship	Description
Open bite	Abnormal vertical spaces between mandibular and maxillary teeth most frequently observed in the anterior teeth; however, may occur in posterior areas Open bite
End-to-end	The teeth occlude without the maxillary teeth overlapping the mandibular teeth. An end-to-end bite can occur anteriorly and posteriorly, unilaterally or bilaterally Anterior Posterior
Crossbite	Maxillary teeth are positioned lingually to the mandibular teeth. May occur unilaterally or bilaterally Crossbite Anterior Posterior (bilateral)
Labioversion	A tooth positioned labial or facial to its normal position
Linguoversion	A tooth positioned lingual to its normal position

First three figures from Bath-Balogh M, Fehrenbach MJ: *Illustrated dental embryology, histology and anatomy,* Philadelphia, 1997 WB Saunders.

may overlap the central incisors. Overbite is severe, but the palate is wide in comparison to division 1.[15]

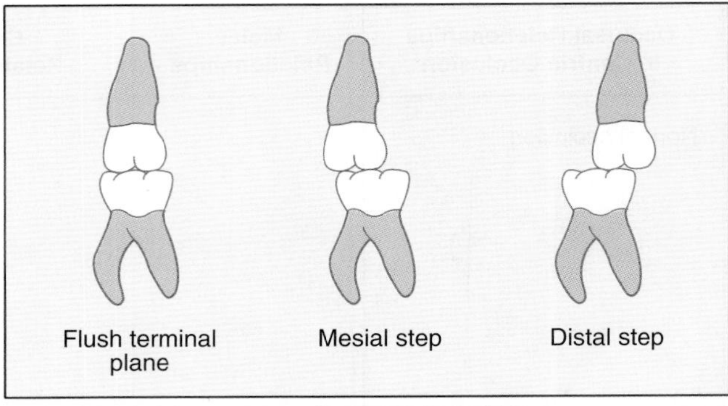

FIGURE 13–37 ✦ Occlusal relationship of primary molars.

Class III Malocclusion

In *Class III malocclusion* the mandible is relatively large compared with the maxilla; thus, a prognathic profile results (Figure 13–36). The molar relationship is such that the buccal groove of the mandibular first permanent molar is situated mesial to the mesiobuccal cusp of the maxillary first permanent molar by at least the width of a premolar, while the distal surface of the mandibular permanent canine is mesial to the mesial surface of the maxillary permanent canine by at least the width of a premolar. Similar to the case with the Class II, if the distance of movement in the molars or canine is less than the width of a premolar, the classification of occlusion is labeled as "tendency toward Class III."[15]

PRIMARY OCCLUSION

Classification of a primary dentition's occlusion uses the distal surfaces of the primary maxillary and mandibular second molars (Figure 13–37). A *mesial step* relationship exists when the mandibular second molar is positioned mesially to the distal surface of the maxillary second molar. This should develop into a Class I relationship in the permanent dentition; however, if present at an early age, the mesial step can be an indication of excessive development of the mandible. The mesial step occlusion can develop into a Class III malocclusion in the permanent dentition.

A *flush or straight terminal plane* relationship, in which the distal surfaces of the maxillary and mandibular second molars align evenly, is the ideal relationship of the primary dentition. This is the most common type of primary occlusion occurring in the majority of children and can guide the permanent molars into a Class I occlusion or Class II malocclusion, depending on the conditions existing elsewhere in the primary dentition.

If spacing between the primary mandibular first molar and canine exists (primate space) in the primary dentition, the first permanent molar, when it erupts at age six, will move the primary molars mesially to close the primate space distal to the primary canines. This movement converts the straight terminal plane relationship to a mesial step and allows the permanent molars to erupt into a Class I relationship.

If the child has no primate spaces in the primary dentition and a straight terminal plane relationship of the primary molars, the permanent molars will initially erupt in an end-to-end relationship. The development of a Class I occlusion in the permanent dentition, however, is still possible. At approximately 11 years of age, the primary mandibular second molars are exfoliated, leaving a space called the leeway space. The permanent mandibular first molars migrate mesially into this leeway space provided by the mesiodistal dimensions of the primary second molars and the permanent second premolar teeth. Given adequate space, this movement will convert the straight terminal plane to a mesial step and provide for a Class I relationship of the permanent first molars.

A *distal step* relationship of the primary second molars is the least frequent occlusal relationship of the primary teeth and exists when the mandibular second molar is distal to the distal surface of the maxillary second molar. The distal step relationship may be a sign of a deficiency in the development of the mandible and will probably develop into a Class II relationship in the permanent dentition. Deficiency in mandibular development may be apparent in a child as young as three years of age. At best, a distal step will lead to an end-to-end molar relationship in the permanent dentition.

Parafunctional Habits

Parafunctional habits are movements of the mandible that are not associated with eating, speech, or respiration. These habits include clenching of the teeth, bruxing (grinding) of the teeth, and thumb/finger(s) sucking. These parafunctional habits often occur subconsciously during sleep or while concentrating deeply on something.

Clenching occurs when the teeth occlude for a long time while in centric position without giving the mandible a rest. Persons who clench their teeth may have enlarged masseter muscles and may consider it normal to feel tension in the facial and masticatory muscles. Directed relaxing of these muscles may help in some cases. Clenching may be due to stress or the way individuals process neurologic impulses.[15]

Bruxism is the forceful grinding of the teeth together, often making an audible noise. Attrition of the incisal or occlusal surfaces of the teeth, especially of the canine cusp tips, results from bruxism. Persons who clench or grind their teeth should be referred to a dentist for a "night guard," which can be worn during waking hours and/or when sleeping. A night guard is an oral appliance that covers the dentition. It protects the teeth from further attrition and helps to spread the occlusal force generated by the habit throughout the dentition.

Thumb or finger sucking usually occurs in children and can cause extreme overjet of the maxillary incisors, irreversibly stretched lips, a deep palate, and a callused thumb or finger (see Chapter 51, for suggested interventions to break the thumb/finger sucking habit).[15]

Client Education Issues

- ✦ Identify developmental anomalies and provide clients with care strategies to prevent disease onset in these areas.
- ✦ Inform clients of the areas of acquired tooth damage and provide individual caries preventive strategies to address needs.
- ✦ Provide clients with an interpretation of the charted findings.
- ✦ Inform pregnant women and mothers about intrinsic staining of their child's teeth caused by tetracycline consumption during pregnancy and early childhood.
- ✦ Inform clients about the many factors—local (e.g., trauma), systemic (e.g., diseases, nutritional deficiencies, excess systemic fluoride), hereditary, and idiopathic (unknown)—that may cause anomalies of enamel formation.
- ✦ Educate clients about the urgency with which restorative therapy should be obtained.
- ✦ Educate the client about the importance of tooth replacement to prevent occlusal disharmonies.
- ✦ Educate about the importance of addressing attrition and bone loss to prevent loss of vertical dimension, which affects physical appearance and proper functioning of the teeth and jaws.
- ✦ Educate about the need to treat open contacts because they trap food, resulting in gingival inflammation, and do not contribute to tooth stability.
- ✦ Inform clients about strategies to control parafunctional habits and their importance.

Legal, Ethical, and Safety Issues

- The ADHA code of ethics states that clients must be kept informed of their treatment progress and health status.
- It is essential to keep accurate records of care and maintain confidentiality of this information.
- Clients must be informed about their treatment alternatives to meet their oral health needs.
- The client's record is a legal document and is admissible evidence in a court of law.
- Comprehensive charting of tooth assessment findings documents the level of care provided and is an essential tool for quality assessment.
- During forensic investigations, the record of the client's dentition is often the only means of identifying a deceased person; therefore, accuracy and completeness of these records are essential.

Key Concepts

- Documentation of tooth assessments is important for care planning, communication, legal documentation, and quality assurance.
- Dental charting is the graphic representation of the condition of the client's teeth observed on a specific date. The data recorded are based on clinical and radiographic assessment and the client's report of symptoms.
- Quadrants are the graphic divisions of the client's mouth into four equal sections.
- Imaginary lines between anterior and posterior regions divide the mouth into six sextants.
- The Universal Numbering System sequentially numbers permanent teeth 1 through 32; primary teeth are alphabetically labeled A through T.
- Using quadrant and tooth designations, the International Numbering System provides a two-digit system to identify teeth.
- An ideal chart for tooth assessment contains sufficient space for initial recording of data and for successive findings.
- The dental chart should be a part of the permanent client record and be accessible for reference during all appointments, thus facilitating continuity, sequencing, and ongoing documentation of care.[1]
- The clinical examination is used to assess developmental anomalies and signs of acquired tooth damage and defective restorations.
- Dental caries and dental restorations are commonly classified either by Black's classification or by the complexity classification system.
- There are basic rules for nomenclature used to describe a cavity or a dental restoration.
- Direct examination can be done well only if the teeth are clean and dry and illuminated with good light. Care should be exercised to avoid exploring known sensitive areas.
- The goal of tooth assessment for the dental hygienist is to recognize signs of developmental anomalies and acquired tooth damage and call them to the attention of the dentist, thus optimizing client care.
- Teeth with signs of disease and client reports of dental pain should be communicated to the dentist immediately.
- The dental hygienist most often uses percussion, a cold stick, or an electric pulp tester to test for pulp vitality. These tests, along with a well-organized and thorough clinical assessment of signs, symptoms, and radiographs, provide additional information to assist the dentist in making an endodontic diagnosis.
- Thorough assessment of the dentition includes classifying occlusion and documenting any malrelationships of teeth present.
- Occlusion of the erupting permanent teeth is dependent on that of the primary teeth as they are being shed.
- Contact areas protect the interdental gingiva and stabilize each tooth in the dental arch. Open contacts need to be called to the attention of the dentist for evaluation and treatment.
- Malocclusion results when there is lack of overall ideal form in the dentition while in centric occlusion.
- Malocclusion may have a negative effect on clients' personal appearance and may make it more difficult for them to perform effective oral hygiene. Because plaque biofilm causes periodontal disease, individuals with malocclusion are at increased risk for periodontal disease.
- Parafunctional habits are movements of the mandible that are not associated with eating, speech, or respiration (i.e., clenching, bruxing [grinding], and thumb sucking).

Critical Thinking Exercises

Marie Smith, a 49-year-old female, reports her last dental examination was 18 months ago. Her health history reveals that she is currently being treated for depression and is taking an antidepressant medication. Her chief concerns are the recent sensitivity of several teeth and an uncomfortable dry mouth that she experiences most of the time. Gingivitis and moderate generalized plaque biofilm are present, with heavy accumulations in posterior lingual areas. Upon assessment of Marie's teeth, the dental hygienist observes the following:

Porcelain crowns on teeth #7 and #10

Teeth #8 and #9 have veneers

Full gold crowns are on teeth #18 and #31

Amalgam restorations are found on #2 MOD, #3 O, #4 DO, #19 MO, #28 MOD, #29 DO

Composite restorations are on #6 MO, #21 F, #22 F, #25 F, #26 F

Teeth #1, #14, #16, #17, and #32 have been extracted

A porcelain fused to metal bridge is found on teeth #13 through #15

Tooth #15 has a root canal

Teeth #3 MO, #5 D, #11 F, and #30 MOD have signs of carious lesions

Attrition is noted on teeth #12 through #16 and on #22 through #27

Record your tooth assessment findings on a dental chart for documentation in Marie's permanent record. Propose preventive strategies needed to control the occurrence of future caries. Propose other interventions to address other tooth damage noted.

For References, Suggested Readings, and Related Websites, visit

http://evolve.elsevier.com/Darby/hygiene/

CHAPTER 14

Oral Hygiene Assessment: Soft Deposits, Plaque Biofilm, Calculus, and Stain

OBJECTIVES

Mastery of the content in this chapter will enable the reader to:

- Define microbial plaque as a biofilm
- Describe the process of plaque biofilm accumulation and maturation
- Describe clinical assessment methods to quantify bacterial plaque biofilm, calculus, and stain
- Describe at least three indices for measuring bacterial plaque clinically
- Discuss how oral hygiene assessment is used for client education and motivation

KEY TERMS

Acquired pellicle
Bacterial plaque (microbial plaque, dental plaque biofilm, bacterial plaque biofilm, plaque, plaque biofilm)
Biofilm
Dental calculus
Dental index
Chromogenic bacteria
Extrinsic stain
Food debris
Intrinsic stain
Materia alba
Oral contributing factors
Oral hygiene assessments
Oral hygiene indices
Plaque disclosing solution
Slime matrix or layer
Soft deposit
Subgingival calculus
Supragingival calculus
Tooth stain

ORAL HYGIENE ASSESSMENT

Before the dental hygienist can influence a client's oral health behavior, it is necessary to assess and document the current state of his or her oral hygiene. *Oral hygiene assessment* is the process of determining the client's:

Amount of hard and soft tooth deposits

Awareness of his or her oral hygiene status and motivation related to oral self-care

Home care regimen

It includes the assessment of *soft deposits* such as food debris, materia alba, and bacterial plaque biofilm; hard deposits composed of stain and calculus; and the significance of such deposits.

Assessment Tools

Basic oral hygiene assessment tools include:

Light: Helps to visualize all areas of the mouth

Compressed air: Aids in the detection of both supragingival and subgingival soft and hard deposits

Mouth mirror: Permits visualization of entire oral cavity, in addition to readily accessible areas

Periodontal explorer: Allows access to deep pockets; ODU 11/12 or 3-A is preferred for accurate assessment of subgingival calculus and optimal tactile sensitivity

Gauze: To maintain a clean instrument tip, rather than moving soft deposits around the mouth

Plaque disclosing solutions (*disclosants*): Allow visualization of supragingival plaque throughout the mouth and determination of effectiveness of oral self-care

Concepts for Oral Hygiene Assessment

Oral hygiene assessment includes observation and measurement of the hard and soft deposits on the teeth according to their:

Location
Degree (amount)
Extent

Assessment also involves evaluating the client's knowledge, skill, and motivation related to oral self-care. Table 14–1 describes the soft and hard deposits that accumulate on the teeth. Of these deposits, *bacterial plaque* is a risk factor for dental caries and periodontal diseases. Stain and calculus assist in the retention of bacterial plaque on teeth and supporting structures, and have important aesthetic implications. The location, amount, and extent of plaque, stain, and calculus, and to a lesser degree, food debris and materia alba, are important variables to measure and record during baseline assessment and at continued-care intervals. These findings must also be understood by clients to encourage self-care and oral disease prevention.

Recognition of bacterial plaque as a biofilm and as a major risk factor for dental caries and periodontal disease is key to effective care planning, client education, and client motivation. Oral hygiene assessments allow the dental hygienist to determine unmet human needs (e.g., responsibility for oral health, conceptualization and understanding), communicate these unmet needs to clients, and instruct them in effective self-care techniques. By understanding the level of bacterial load present in the oral cavity, interventions can be aimed at reducing plaque biofilm and achieving optimal oral health. Quality of the plaque and the client's host response to that bacterial challenge guide both clinician and client. For example, a client with a high plaque score in the lingual region of the mouth, with none on the facial tooth surfaces and healthy gingival tissue, clearly requires instructions tailored to accessing the lingual areas, while reinforcing current good techniques for the facial aspect. A client with a small amount of plaque accumulation, but with severe gingival bleeding, requires a different approach to care.

About 50% to 90% of the population exhibits some type of periodontal disease, and there is a corresponding deficit in personal responsibility for oral health.[1,2] These findings underscore the importance of effective oral hygiene assessment and the corresponding client education that assessment results facilitate. Individualized oral hygiene instruction is important in motivating a client; no one wants the "brush and floss lecture" that comes in a "one size fits all" format. When clients recognize their individual needs, they are more receptive to professional recommendations and are more likely to implement lifestyle changes.

TOOTH DEPOSITS

Bacterial Plaque Biofilm[1–5]

Bacterial plaque (also known as microbial plaque, dental plaque biofilm, bacterial plaque biofilm), a host-associated *biofilm,* is a dense, nonmineralized, highly organized mass of bacterial colonies in a gel-like intermicrobial, enclosed matrix, or slime layer[1] (Figure 14–1). The slime matrix or layer may protect the bacteria from the defensive cells

TABLE 14–1 HARD AND SOFT ACQUIRED DEPOSITS

Term	Classification	Definition
Acquired pellicle and exogenous dental cuticle	Acellular, nonmineralized layer	An unstructured, homogenous film adhering to tooth surfaces, firm surfaces in the oral cavity, and old calculus. May be stained by tar products and tannin.
Bacterial plaque biofilm	Cellular, nonmineralized layer	A dense, transparent, nonmineralized, highly organized mass of bacterial colonies in a gel-like intermicrobial, enclosed matrix; a host-associated biofilm.
Materia alba	Cellular, nonmineralized layer	Loose deposit of microorganisms, desquamated epithelial cells, and broken down food debris; white to yellowish-white in color; has cottage cheese–like appearance. Can be displaced with rinsing and water irrigation.
Food debris	Cellular, nonmineralized layer	Unstructured particles that remain in the mouth after eating and are removed with irrigation unless impacted between the teeth.
Extrinsic stain	Cellular, may be mineralized or nonmineralized	Discolorations that accumulate on the external surface of the tooth via pellicle, plaque biofilm, or calculus and can be removed by toothbrushing, scaling, and/or polishing.
Supragingival calculus	Cellular, mineralized layer	Mineralized bacterial plaque permeated with moderately hard calcium phosphate crystals; superficially covered with bacterial plaque biofilm; usually white or yellowish-white in color but may be stained darker.
Subgingival calculus	Cellular, mineralized layer	Mineralized bacterial plaque; adheres to tooth structure in gingival sulcus; organic matrix of bacteria permeated with hard calcium phosphate crystals. May be stained dark green to greenish-black; superficially covered with bacterial plaque biofilm.

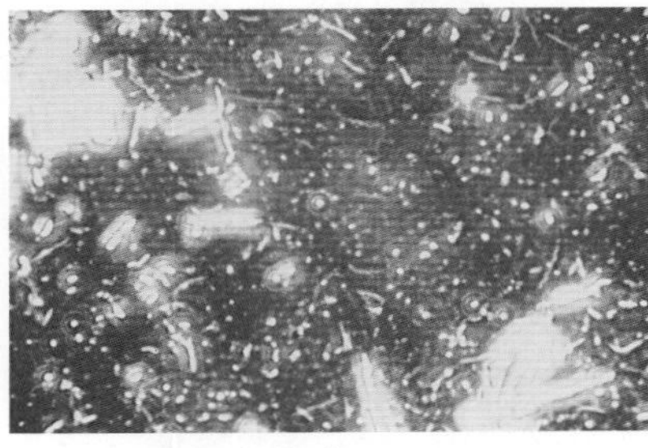

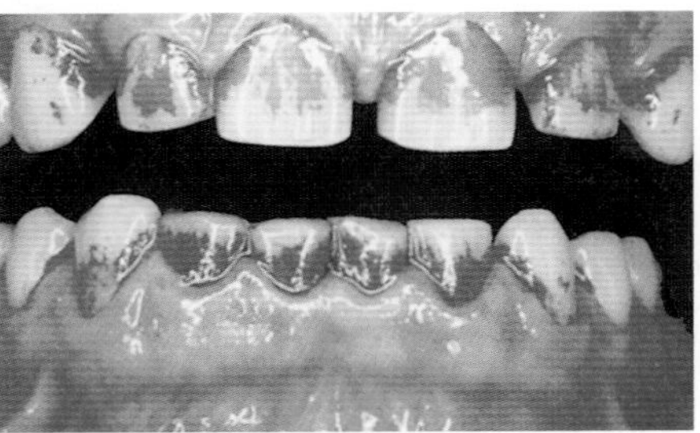

FIGURE 14–1 ✦ Microbial plaque. **A,** Plaque stained and viewed with microscopy. Note cocci, rods, and filamentous forms. **B,** Disclosed supragingival plaque covering one-half to two-thirds of the clinical crown. *(From Newman MG, Takei HH, Carranza FA:* Clinical periodontology, *ed 9, Philadelphia, 2002, WB Saunders. Courtesy Dr. S. Socransky, Boston, Mass).*

(neutrophils, macrophages, and lymphocytes) in the host's immune system as well as from antimicrobial and antibiotic agents. Bacteria within the biofilm adhere to each other and to other surfaces. There are also some loosely attached and unattached bacteria at the surface of the plaque biofilm. The clinical significance of the biofilm is that it creates its own renewing source of lipopolysaccharide for the long-term survival of microorganisms. The biofilm lends other protective properties to the associated bacteria, including resistance to antibacterial agents such as chlorhexidine, systemic antibiotics, and host defense mechanisms such as leukocytes. Biofilm-enclosed bacteria benefit by the concentration and retention of metabolites that are produced by the bacteria, which enhances interactions between the species of bacterium. In addition to the protective nature of the biofilm, there is also the influence of fluid dynamics to consider. The structure of the plaque biofilm includes channels that use the motion of saliva within the oral cavity to extend bacterial colonization, as well as receive nutrients and transport bacterial wastes. Due to these protective and self-sustaining properties of the biofilm, associated bacteria are more likely to survive within the mouth.[1,3] Recognition of the self-sustaining nature of the biofilm community helps explain why periodontal disease has been difficult to control and why periodontal pathogens are resistant to antimicrobial agents, antibiotic therapies, and host-defense mechanisms.[4,5]

In healthy mouths bacterial plaque is mainly supragingival and confined to enamel surfaces. The bacteria associated with healthy dental plaque are primarily aerobic Gram-positive rods and cocci; very few motile species, are present. The bacterial species associated with periodontal health include *Streptococcus mitis, Actinomyces* species and *Streptococcus oralis (sanguis II).* As plaque matures, the bacterial population changes; this change in bacterial species brings signs of disease in the oral tissues. In dental plaque–induced gingival disease, there is an increase in both the quantity and quality of plaque. Bacterial species associated with dental plaque–induced gingival disease include Gram-negative spirochetes and motile rods such as *Fusobacterium nucleatum,* species of *Prevotella* and *Treponema,* and *Campylobacter rectus.* In advancing periodontal disease, plaque is characterized by a zone of Gram-positive organisms attached to the tooth surface, and a loosely adherent zone of Gram-negative species adjacent to the pocket wall. The bacteria associated with advancing periodontal disease are predominantly anaerobic and include *Porphyromonas gingivalis, Prevotella intermedia, Bacteroides forsythus,* and *Peptostreptococcus micros.*

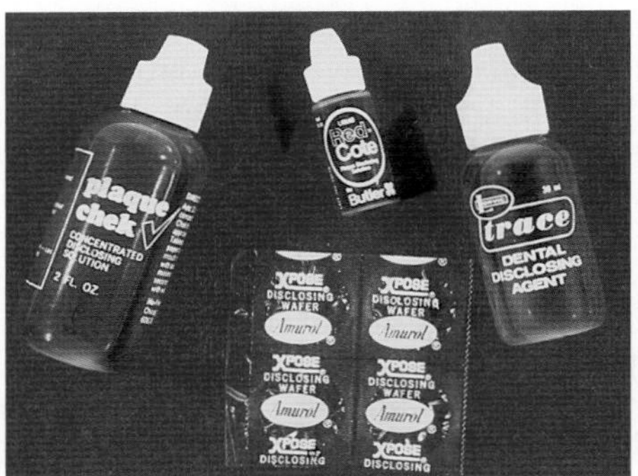

FIGURE 14–2 ✦ Examples of plaque disclosants.

Clinically, plaque presents as a transparent film that accumulates every 12 to 24 hours. Because it is transparent, plaque can be difficult to visualize. Plaque can be detected in several ways. It can be discriminated by direct vision, particularly if there are thick deposits of plaque; the dental hygienist and client may see yellowish, fur-like deposits. Plaque can also acquire stains, allowing for direct visualization. Some people can feel plaque and describe it as a fuzzy coating on their teeth and dental appliances. Most commonly, however, plaque is detected with an explorer or plaque disclosing solution. An explorer can be passed over the tooth surface near the gingival margin to collect plaque, making it easier to see.

For greatest ease in assessment, a *plaque disclosing solution* that stains the invisible plaque can reveal the extent and location of the accumulation (Figure 14–1, *B*). *Disclosants* come in liquid form that may be swabbed onto the tooth surfaces, and tablet form that must be chewed and swished over the teeth and gingiva (Figure 14–2). Both types temporarily stain the plaque with a safe, temporary dye. Staining the plaque for visibility in a client's mouth is a powerful teaching aid for in-office and at-home use.

The first assessment of plaque is its *location.* Plaque can be found both supragingivally, coronal to the gingival margin on the clinical crown of the tooth, and subgingivally, apical to the margin of the gingiva.

Supragingival locations include the occlusal surfaces (most common in areas without opposing teeth), buccal or lingual fissures and pits, interproximal tooth surfaces, and free gingival margin. Subgingival plaque accumulates in the sulcus, or periodontal pocket on all four aspects of the tooth (buccal, lingual, mesial, and distal interproximal spaces).

In assessing plaque, it is important to consider the client's *oral contributing factors,* the presence of which influence the growth and retention of plaque biofilm. These predisposing factors include missing teeth, malocclusions, a short lingual frenum, mouth breathing, orthodontic bands, faulty restorations, calculus, and stain. Oral contributing factors can be physiologic in nature, such as a tight lingual frenum, which interferes with the natural oral cleansing action of the tongue, or restorative, such as faulty restorations with open or overhanging margins or poorly contoured surfaces that readily harbor plaque. Missing teeth contribute to plaque retention and inhibit the ability of the client to self-clean occlusal surfaces via mastication. Malocclusions can result in crowding and tipping of teeth, which can make plaque removal difficult, or lead to traumatic occlusion, resulting in widened PDL spaces that lend themselves to greater plaque accumulation.

Mouth breathing, with its drying effects on the oral tissues, favors the growth of plaque biofilm in the absence of the natural bactericidal action of the saliva. Calculus is a common predisposing factor, as its rough surface allows bacteria to readily attach. Likewise, stain can also provide a rough surface for bacteria to colonize. All of these factors influence the retention of bacterial plaque and can contribute significantly to poor plaque control for the client.

The plaque biofilm is influenced by host mediating factors. In health, there is a balance point between the plaque and the host where no irreparable damage occurs. If the biofilm bacteria cause tissue destruction that exceeds the reparative ability of the host, disease occurs. The oral hygiene assessment includes an evaluation of possible oral contributory factors and the host response to the plaque.

Three Stages of Bacterial Plaque Biofilm Formation

Plaque formation occurs in three distinct stages: pellicle formation, bacterial colonization, and plaque maturation (Figures 14–3 and 14–4). Within these three stages, several important changes are taking place within the overall plaque biofilm.

PELLICLE FORMATION.[4,5] The first stage is the attachment of the *acquired pellicle,* a tenacious, acellular protein film composed of glycoproteins found within saliva. Although pellicle performs a protective function, acting as a barrier to acids, it also serves as the initial site of attachment for free-swimming bacteria and begins the first stage of biofilm development. Immediately following cleansing of tooth surfaces, the pellicle begins to re-form on exposed oral surfaces.

BACTERIAL COLONIZATION.[4,5] Early plaque, one to two days old, consists primarily of aerobic, Gram-positive cocci such as *Streptococcus mutans* and *Streptococcus sanguis.*

On days two through four, filamentous forms grow on the surface of the coccal colonies and begin to infiltrate the colonies, replacing the cocci. The second stage consists of bacterial colonization that occurs in stratified layers against the tooth surface. Initial formation is within distinct colonies that form from the indigenous oral microflora, but as the growth process continues an intermicrobial matrix, the protective slime layer, is formed, connecting the bacterial colonies. The matrix is composed of saliva and polysaccharides produced by the bacteria in response to dietary sucrose. The polysaccharides are sticky, and thus further facilitate plaque adhesion; a client may experience this phenomenon as the "furry" or "filmy" feeling sometimes detected on the teeth; that furry feeling is the polysaccharides produced in response to the ingestion of fermentable carbohydrates. In addition to providing a method of adherence for the bacterial colonies, these polysaccharides are a reserve food source for the bacteria and contribute to the other protective functions of the biofilm. Due primarily to the methods of bacterial adhesion, plaque is not removed by oral irrigation; removal of the plaque biofilm requires mechanical action, such as toothbrushing and interdental cleaning with floss, brush, or wooden wedge.

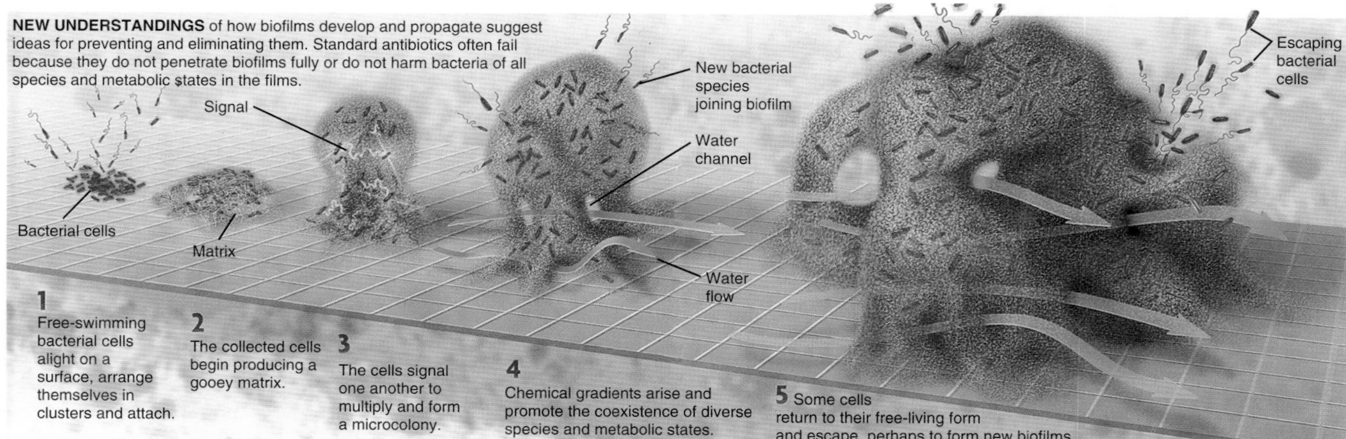

NEW UNDERSTANDINGS of how biofilms develop and propagate suggest ideas for preventing and eliminating them. Standard antibiotics often fail because they do not penetrate biofilms fully or do not harm bacteria of all species and metabolic states in the films.
Signal
New bacterial species joining biofilm
Water channel
Escaping bacterial cells
Bacterial cells
Matrix
Water flow
1 Free-swimming bacterial cells alight on a surface, arrange themselves in clusters and attach.
2 The collected cells begin producing a gooey matrix.
3 The cells signal one another to multiply and form a microcolony.
4 Chemical gradients arise and promote the coexistence of diverse species and metabolic states.
5 Some cells return to their free-living form and escape, perhaps to form new biofilms.

FIGURE 14–3 ✦ How biofilms form. *(Illustration by Keith Kasnot. Licensed for use, Philips Oral Healthcare Inc.)*

By days four through seven, filamentous forms increase and rods and fusobacteria appear. Vibrios and spirochetes appear during days seven through fourteen; overall, the load of Gram-negative anaerobic species increases, and white blood cells are found within the plaque. Clinically, signs of inflammation begin to be observed.

PLAQUE MATURATION.[4,5] During the third stage of plaque formation, the plaque ages and undergoes a distinct change in population. By days 14 through 24, gingivitis is generally clinically evident, and the plaque is composed of densely packed vibrios, spirochetes, and filamentous bacteria. As the biofilm colony matures, it blooms into a mushroom shape attached by a narrow base and incorporates channels that capitalize on the fluid movement present in the oral cavity. These fluid channels distribute nutrients, remove wastes, and allow for free-swimming bacteria to leave and begin new biofilm colonies. It is easy to appreciate the importance of thorough and consistent mechanical plaque disruption and removal to inhibit the destructive processes of plaque maturation. The longer the plaque biofilm remains undisturbed, the greater its pathogenic potential for the host (Figure 14–4).

Tooth Stain

Tooth stain is a discolored spot or area on a tooth contrasting with the rest of the tooth color (Figure 14–5). Stains are divided into two different types: intrinsic stains and extrinsic stains.

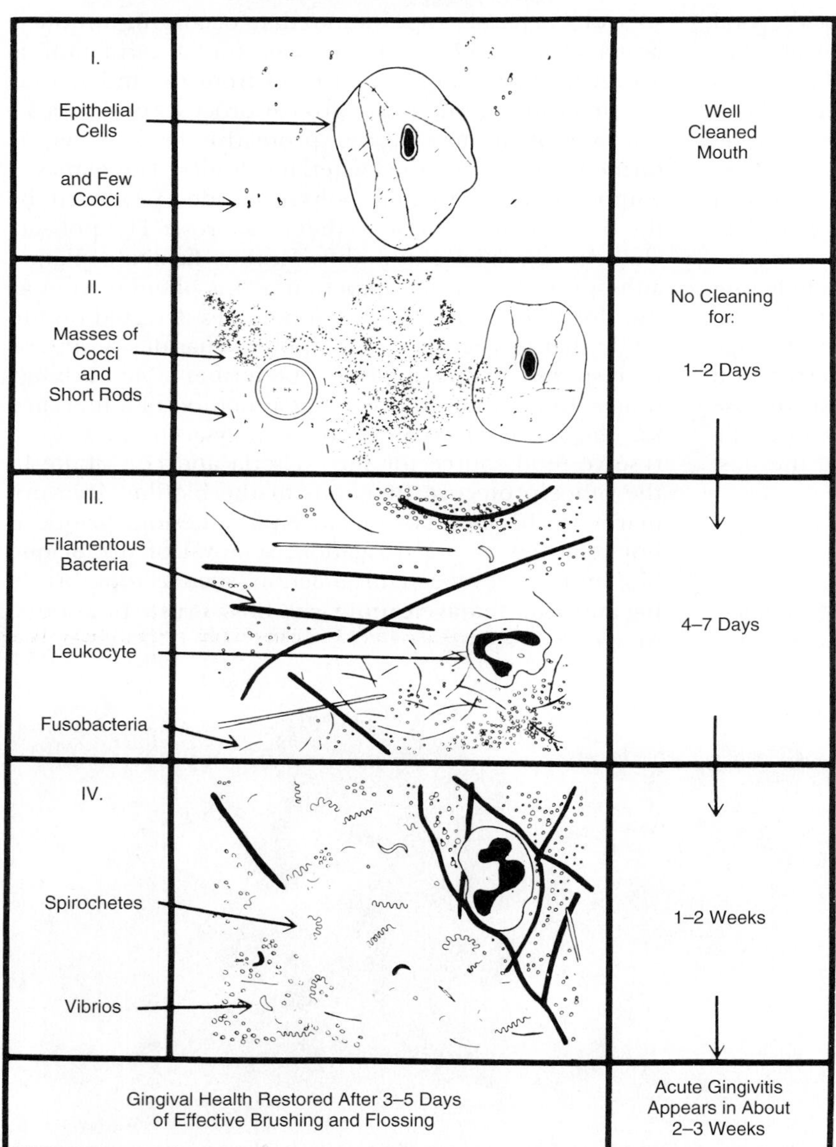

FIGURE 14–4 ✦ Plaque microorganisms. On the right are the time intervals from 1 day to 3 weeks. On the left are the changes in the plaque content that take place as plaque ages. As the numbers of microorganisms increase, the numbers of defense cells (leukocytes) also increase. *(From Crawford JJ. In Barton RE, Matteson SR, Richardson RE, eds:* The dental assistant, *ed 6, Philadelphia, 1988, Lea & Febiger.)*

Intrinsic stains are incorporated within the tooth structure itself and cannot be removed by scaling or polishing. Such stains are the result of alterations during the development of the tooth (embryonic to 6 years of age), associated with antibiotic use, fever, trauma, infection, and exposure to high amounts of systemic fluoride. Examples of intrinsic stains include dental fluorosis (a mottled, opaque or brownish discoloration caused by ingesting excessive amounts of systemic fluoride during enamel formation) and tetracycline stain (a yellow, brown, gray or orange discoloration within the substance of the tooth from ingestion of the antibiotic when the tooth is developing) (Figure 14–5, *A* and *B*).

Extrinsic stains are located on the surface of the tooth; the majority of these stains may be removed by coronal polishing or scaling. These stains develop due to the presence of certain bacteria or the use of staining substances such as tobacco, wine, tea, coffee, soda, and drugs. Again, the method of attachment of dental stain is the acquired pellicle: without pellicle, stains cannot adhere to the smooth enamel surfaces.

Tooth stains occur in various colors. The source can often be identified by the color of the stain and client self-reported information about lifestyle behavior and dietary and oral habits. Identification of the stain assists the dental hygienist in developing a specific self-care plan that facilitates a more aesthetic appearance for clients. The client can often reduce stain formation with improved oral hygiene practices and appropriate over-the-counter product selection (e.g., whitening toothpaste). Table 14–2 describes common dental stains. Professional techniques

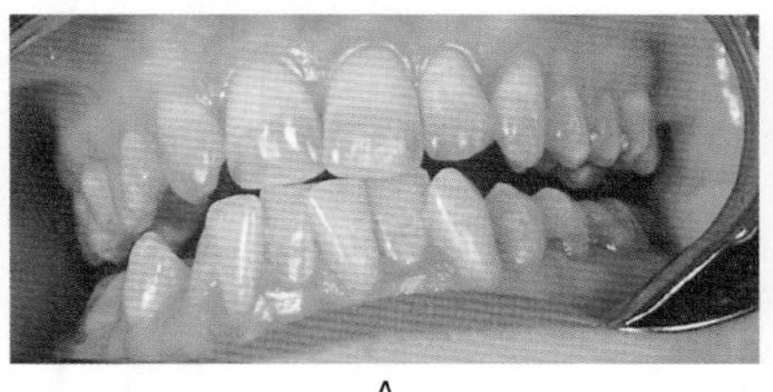
A

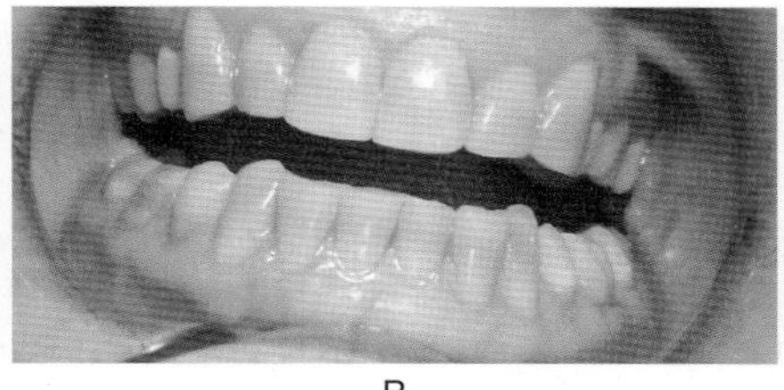
B

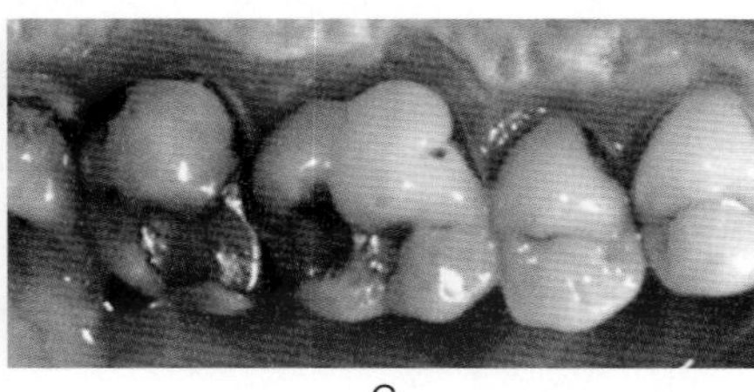
C

FIGURE 14–5 ✦ Intrinsic and extrinsic tooth stains. **A,** Dental fluorosis. **B,** Tetracycline stain. **C,** Green stain. *(A and B from Ibsen OAC, Phelan JA:* Oral pathology for the dental hygienist, *ed 3, Philadelphia, WB Saunders. C from Newman MG, Takei HH, Carranza FA:* Clinical periodontology, *ed 9, Philadelphia, 2002, WB Saunders)*

TABLE 14–2 TYPES OF TOOTH STAINS

Type	Source	Clinical Approach
Extrinsic Stain		
Green	Chromogenic bacteria from poor oral hygiene; most often seen in children with enamel irregularities	Should not be scaled because of underlying demineralized enamel. Have client remove during toothbrush instruction or lightly polish; may use hydrogen peroxide to help with bleaching and removal.
Black-line stain	Iron in saliva; often seen in females with good oral hygiene	Firmly scale because of calculus-like nature and selective polish for complete removal.
Orange	Chromogenic bacteria from poor oral hygiene	Lightly scale and then polish selectively.
Brown stains		
Tobacco	Tars from smoking and chewing and dipping spitting tobacco	Lightly scale and then polish selectively.
Food	Food and beverage pigment	Lightly scale and then polish selectively.
Drug	Chlorhexidine, stannous fluoride, extended antibiotic use	Scale and then polish selectively.
Yellow	Bacterial plaque biofilm	Have client remove during toothbrush instruction and reinforcement.
Intrinsic Stain		
Dental fluorosis (white-spotted to brown-pitted enamel)	Excessive fluoride ingestion during enamel development	Cannot be removed by scaling or selective polishing.
Hypocalcification (white spots on enamel)	High fever during enamel formation; endocrine and other metabolic causes	Cannot be removed by scaling or selective polishing.
Decalcification (white to brown enamel, may be smooth or rough)	Acid erosion of enamel caused by bacterial plaque biofilm	Cannot be removed by scaling or polishing. Recommend daily 0.05% sodium fluoride rinses for remineralization.
Tetracycline (grayish brown discoloration)	Ingestion of tetracycline during tooth development	Cannot be removed by scaling or selective polishing.

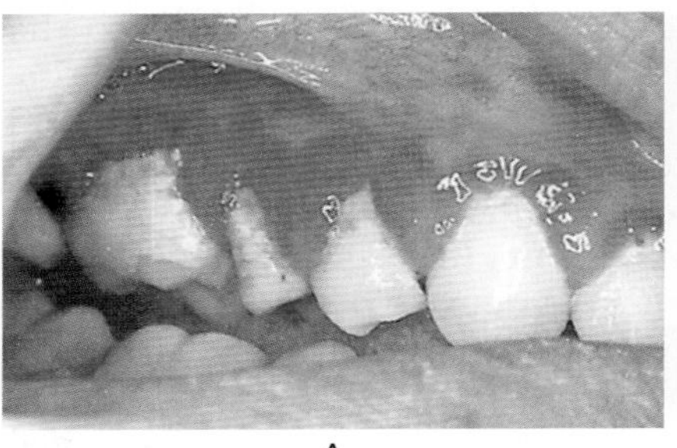
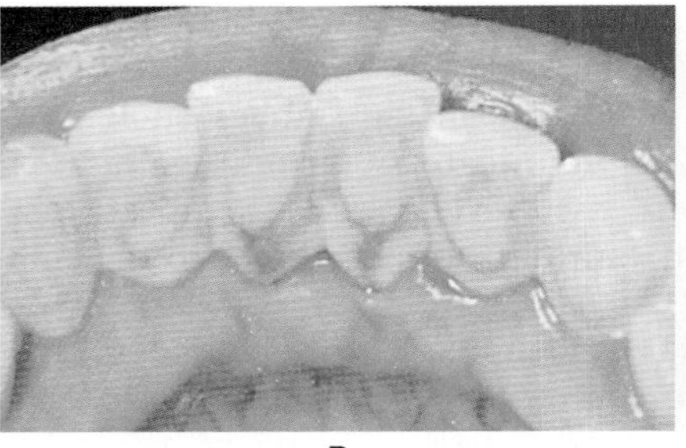
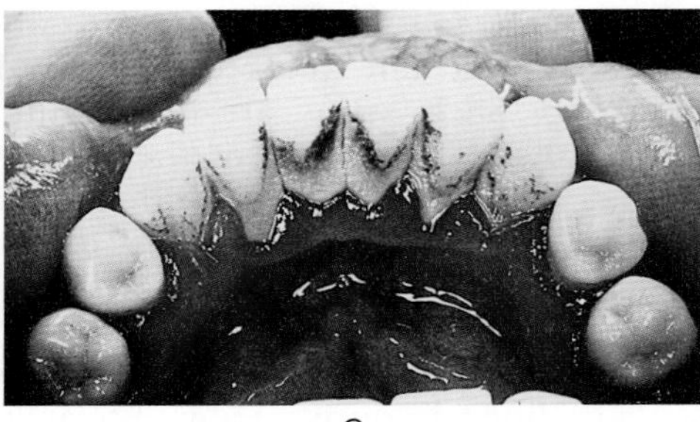

A B C

FIGURE 14–6 ✦ Dental calculus. **A,** Heavy calculus on molar and premolars in area opposite Stenson's duct. Note severe gingival inflammation and edema. **B,** Calculus and stain on the lingual surface in relation to orifice of the submaxillary and sublingual salivary glands. **C,** Calculus superimposed with tobacco stains. *(B from Newman MG, Takei HH, Carranza FA:* Clinical periodontology, *ed 9, Philadelphia, 2002, WB Saunders.)*

for removing and managing tooth stains are found in Chapter 22.

Of the stains found on the dentition, two are attributed to color-producing bacteria called *chromogenic bacteria.*

Green stain is due to poor oral hygiene, and occurs near the cervical region of the teeth. This type of staining can easily become incorporated within decalcified enamel, and should not be scaled to avoid the risk of removing demineralized tooth surface. Due to the likelihood of decalcification, green stain is an indication for fluoride therapy. The organisms responsible for green stain are thought to be *Penicillium* and *Aspergillus* (Figure 14–5, *C*).

Orange stain is less common than other types of stains, and is also associated with poor oral hygiene. This stain is most likely to occur on anterior teeth, and is believed to be due to the presence of *Serratia marcescens* and *Flavobacterium lutescens.*

These chromogenic stains usually can be removed. If the area under the stain is decalcified, scaling is contraindicated. Chromogenic stain can usually be removed safely with 3% hydrogen to loosen and bleach the stain, followed by selective polishing.

Other dental stains include brown stain, yellow stain, and black stain. Brown stains can have multiple causes. Tobacco use causes dark brown, tenacious stains that can become intrinsic and do not necessarily correlate with the amount of tobacco used. Food stains may also be tan to brown and result from the ingestion of foods with tannins, such as wine, sodas, coffee, tea, and certain fruits. Agents such as 0.12% chlorhexidine mouthrinse and stannous fluoride dentifrice may also impart a brown stain if used daily over two to three months. These stains may be somewhat difficult to remove and often require scaling in addition to selective polishing. Yellow stain is most commonly associated with heavy plaque accumulation, and can often be removed by the client with improved toothbrushing techniques. Black stain, or black-line stain, can occur in clients with meticulous oral hygiene. These stains are found on the tooth surface near the gingival margin and are associated with iron in the saliva. Middle-aged females with good oral hygiene are the most likely population to have black-line stain.

Dental Calculus

Dental calculus, commonly referred to as tartar, is plaque that has been mineralized by calcium and phosphate salts within the saliva. Although calculus itself is not the causative factor in periodontal infection, it plays a role in the attachment and retention of plaque bacteria. Like plaque, calculus is classified by its location (either supragingival or subgingival), degree, and extent.

Supragingival calculus, calculus above the gingival margin, is most commonly located adjacent to salivary ducts such as the sublingual and parotid salivary glands, resulting in deposits on the lower anterior lingual surfaces and maxillary posterior facial surfaces of teeth (Figure 14–6, *A* and *B*). However, supragingival calculus can be found in any area of the mouth where there is poor oral hygiene. Supragingival calculus can be identified using direct visualization and compressed air. Generally the deposits are yellowish-white, but may take on surface stains and appear dark (Figure 14–6, *C*). Drying the teeth with compressed air allows for a more complete assessment of the amount of the deposit; as the calculus is dried, it takes on a chalky white appearance, making it easier to visualize.

Subgingival calculus is mineralized plaque formed below the gingival margin, often on the root surface. Unlike supragingival calculus, subgingival calculus is more likely to have a dark color due to the absorption of blood products from the gingival sulcus or periodontal pocket. These deposits may be tenacious, and occasionally may be seen by deflecting the gingival margin with compressed air. The most accurate method of subgingival calculus detection is via subgingival exploration using a periodontal explorer.

Subgingival calculus may take many forms, including granular deposits, veneers, or thin sheets; spurs that have dimension from the root surface; or rings that extend around several surfaces of the tooth. It is this change in surface texture and dimension that the dental hygienist explores when assessing for subgingival calculus. Some deposits are mineralized to the extent that they become visible on radiographs (Figure 14–7; see Chapter 15). The greatest area of occurrence is in the interproximal spaces, because these areas are the most difficult for a client to clean effectively.

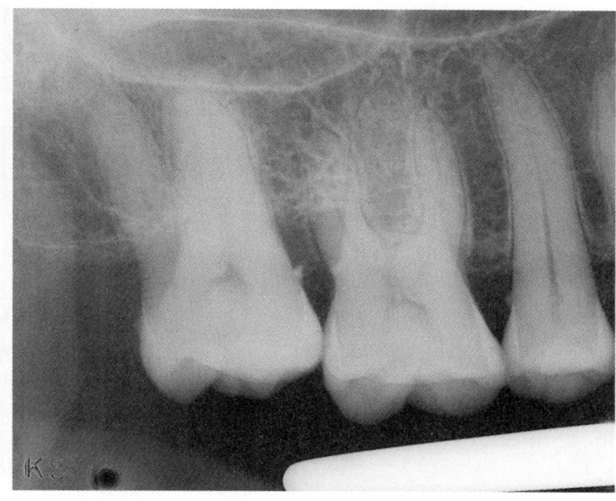

FIGURE 14–7 ✦ Radiograph of teeth with subgingival calculus deposits on mesial surface of maxillary second molar.

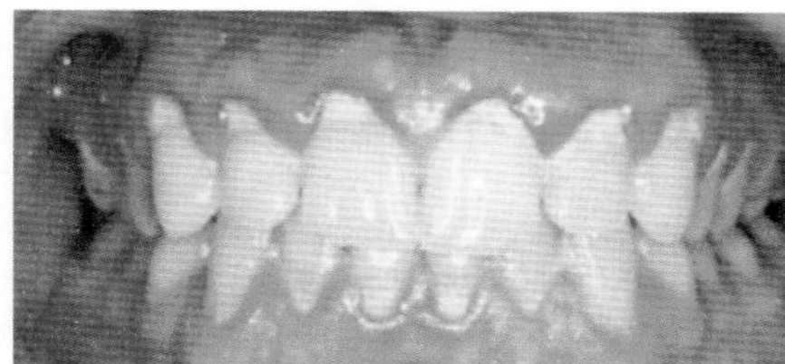

FIGURE 14–8 ✦ Materia alba generalized throughout the mouth, with heaviest accumulation near the gingiva. Note the plaque-induced gingivitis present. *(From Newman MG, Takei HH, Carranza FA:* Clinical periodontology, *ed 9, Philadelphia, 2002, WB Saunders.)*

Materia Alba and Food Debris

Other soft deposits that may be found on the teeth are materia alba and food debris. *Materia alba* is a loosely attached collection of oral debris and bacteria that is seen as a whitish mass on the teeth or overlying plaque (Figure 14–8). *Food debris* is composed of remnants of food retained after a meal. Rinsing and the self-cleansing action of the tongue and saliva can remove both materia alba and food debris. The primary problem with these deposits is that they can impede the dental hygienist's ability to accurately assess the level of plaque and calculus if they are present in great amounts. However, their presence may indicate poor oral hygiene skill, poor manual dexterity, or low motivation level of the client when routinely found upon examination.

SKILL, MOTIVATION, AND COMPLIANCE[4,5]

The dental hygienist assesses the client's ability to manage personal oral care. A client may be capable of performing the necessary mechanical interventions, but have little desire to do so, or the client may be highly motivated, but have physical limitations that render home care difficult. Some clients may be totally dependent on a caregiver for daily oral care. The dental hygienist assesses the factors that limit the client's ability to perform daily self-care to make appropriate recommendations that meet individual needs. Assessment can occur through questioning the client (or caregiver) about oral care practices, direct observation of the techniques used by the client (or caregiver), and measurement of the client's oral hygiene status and dental history (Procedure 14–1) (see Chapter 9). Once an accurate assessment is made, the dental hygienist educates and motivates the client (or caregiver) in small steps aimed at long-term changes that will lead to optimal oral health.

Discussing the characteristics of the oral deposits found in the mouth as part of dental hygiene care can serve as a useful motivator for clients having difficulty adhering to a daily program that targets the disruption of the biofilm community. For example, client knowledge of the biofilm provides a rationale for frequent subgingival root debridement by the dental hygienist, since biofilm in deep periodontal pockets cannot be reached by brushes, interdental cleaners, and mouthrinses. Moreover, clients can be taught that if left undisturbed, the plaque biofilm acts as a higher level organism capable of coordinating efforts, communication among its members, and defense of its bacterial colony. Teaching the client about the resistant nature of the biofilm and the importance of mechanically disrupting and removing biofilm via effective daily oral hygiene measures remains the most effective means for its control (see Chapters 18 and 19).[4,5]

ORAL HYGIENE INDICES

To objectively monitor the oral hygiene of an individual or group, dental indices are used as measures of oral status at baseline and over time (see Chapter 15 for periodontal indices and Chapter 50 for indices used with dental implant clients). A *dental index* is a data collection tool that allows the practitioner (or researcher) to convert specific clinical observations into numerical values that can be summarized, analyzed, and interpreted. *Oral hygiene indices* that measure levels of oral hygiene are used to:

- Establish a baseline and monitor, over time, an individual's oral self-care progress and motivate the client to achieve higher levels of oral wellness
- Survey the oral hygiene status within a population, as is done in epidemiologic research
- Establish a baseline and monitor, over time, the oral health status of a target population in order to evaluate the effectiveness of a community-based program or intervention
- Evaluate an intervention, drug, or device, as is done in a clinical trial

It is important to use an index that meets set criteria for validity, reliability, and usability (see Criteria for Determining an Effective Dental Index).

Procedure 14–1 ORAL DEPOSIT ASSESSMENT

EQUIPMENT

Mouth mirror, periodontal explorer, gauze, plaque disclosing solution, cotton tip applicators, compressed air, intraoral light source, client hand mirror, oral hygiene assessment form, personal protective equipment

STEPS	RATIONALE
1. Place client in supine position and position light source to illuminate client's mouth.	Allows visualization of both arches.
2. Using compressed air, dry the supragingival tooth surfaces a sextant at a time; using mouth mirror and direct and indirect vision, examine for supragingival calculus deposit.	Makes the deposits more visible; deposits will appear chalky against the tooth surface. Drying a sextant at a time is comfortable for the client and manageable for the clinician. Using both direct and indirect vision allows the clinician to maintain proper ergonomic positioning.
3. Identify tooth surfaces with supragingival calculus and surfaces with stain and record these areas on assessment form.	Allows for assessment of change over time and illustrates areas requiring additional oral hygiene.
4. Apply plaque disclosing solution with cotton tip applicator, rinse, and dry with compressed air.	Makes the supragingival plaque easy to identify for both the clinician and the client; rinsing removes the excess solution and drying improves visibility.
5. Examine tooth surfaces with mouth mirror for areas stained with plaque; during this examination, have client watch with a hand mirror.	Engages client in the assessment and begins the education process.
6. Record plaque-covered tooth areas on assessment form using red ink.	Allows for the assessment of change over time and illustrates areas requiring additional oral hygiene. Recording in red ink will correlate with the red disclosing solution to assist clients in making the connection between what they see in their mouths and on the forms.
7. Using the periodontal explorer and mouth mirror, explore subgingival tooth surfaces for calculus deposits.	A periodontal explorer will access the root surfaces and transmit information due to the finer gauge of the tip, allowing the clinician to discriminate root deposits.
8. Record subgingival calculus deposits on assessment form.	Assists the clinician in removing the deposits during instrumentation.
9. Communicate findings to client.	Client must be informed to participate in decision making regarding oral health.
10. Record service in "services rendered" section of client record (e.g., "Computed a plaque-free score of 75%".)	Allows for ongoing quality care and prevents risk of malpractice.

Criteria for Determining an Effective Dental Index

An effective dental index:

- Is simple to use
- Is painless to the client
- Takes a minimal amount of time to execute
- Is cost-effective in terms of time, money, and armamentarium
- Has clear criteria for standardization and reproducibility
- Uses numerical values on a smooth, graduated scale
- Is statistically valid and reliable

Indices Used for Assessing Deposits in Client Care

Use of a standardized method of assessment can be valuable for motivating a client. The ability to show improvement is a powerful motivator and a method of positive reinforcement that can help a client remain compliant. An index can also illustrate repeated neglect of a specific area of the mouth and thus assist a client in making necessary alterations to a self-care regimen. For maximum effectiveness, an index performed with an individual should evaluate the entire dentition rather than specific teeth, as is often done when working with a group in a clinical trial. Even indices that were originally designed to measure a sample of teeth in a research subject's mouth can be used to measure all teeth present in a client.

A simple plaque index is O'Leary's Plaque Control Record, illustrated in Figure 14–9 and described in Table 14–3. This record provides a simple method of recording plaque on the mesial, distal, facial, and lingual surfaces at the gingival margin. Plaque observed is recorded by striking a dash through the appropriate surface or surfaces. After all teeth are examined and scored for plaque, the index is computed by dividing the number of plaque-containing surfaces by the total number of available surfaces. The resulting score is the percentage of tooth surfaces in the mouth with plaque. Use of the form over time allows clients to visualize and monitor their own plaque control progress and therefore facilitates client motivation and behavior change. This index can also be used to quantify stain in the same manner. Commonly used oral hygiene indices are in Table 14–3.

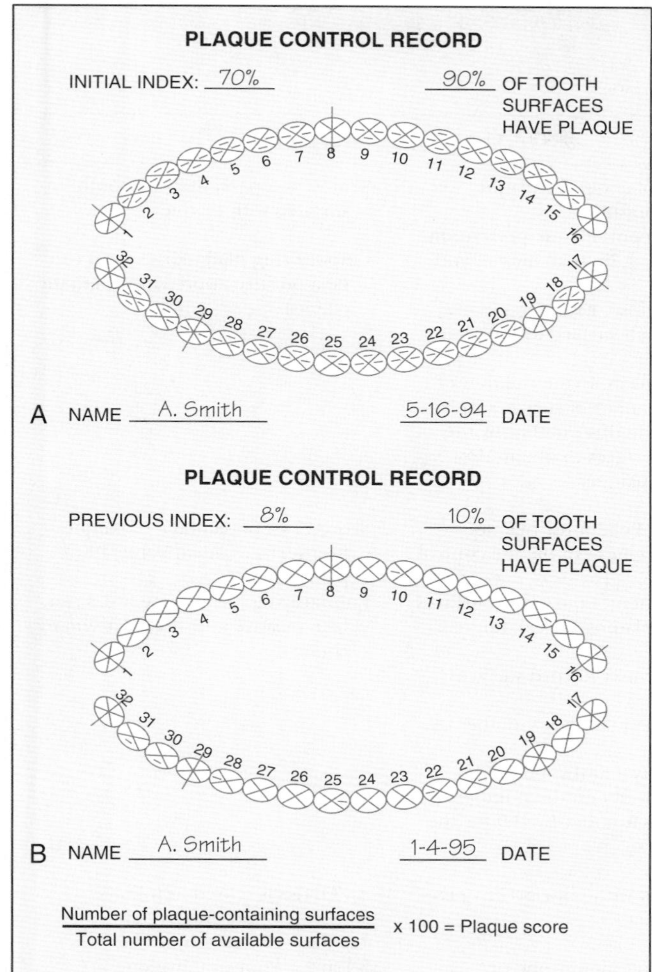

FIGURE 14–9 ✦ Plaque control record form. **A,** 70% of tooth surfaces have plaque at initial appointment. **B,** 8% of tooth surfaces have plaque at a follow-up visit. *(Redrawn from O'Leary TJ, Drake RB, Naylor JE: The plaque control record,* Journal of Periodontology *48:38, 1972.)*

Simple Scoring System for Oral Hygiene

0 = No plaque present
1 = Light plaque (at gingival margin)
2 = Moderate plaque (covering half the tooth surface)
3 = Heavy plaque (up to the incisal/occlusal edges)

Courtesy S. Kramer and P. Rhodes.

RECORD-KEEPING AND DOCUMENTATION

Maintaining a record of a client's oral hygiene status is part of the dental hygiene assessment phase of care. Such records provide baseline reference for subsequent visits and a basis for making professional care or product recommendations. Clinician awareness of oral hygiene products used and previous instruction given to the client provides continuity of care and assures that educational interventions are appropriate.

One simple method for documenting oral hygiene status is the Kramer-Rhodes Periodontal Maintenance Record (Figure 14–10). On the Kramer-Rhodes Periodontal Maintenance Form, client plaque scores, self-care routine, demonstrated oral hygiene techniques, and products dispensed can be recorded. The mouth is divided into upper and lower arches with corresponding scoring boxes for the upper right (UR), upper anterior (UA), upper left (UL), lower right (LR), lower anterior (LA), and lower left (LL) sextants of the dentition. With the aid of a disclosing agent, the hygienist scores plaque for facial, interproximal, and lingual surfaces of all teeth on a scale of 0 to 3 as described in the Simple Scoring System for Oral Hygiene chart (see Simple Scoring System for Oral Hygiene). The dental hygienist then determines the mean plaque scores for buccal (bucc), interproximal (ip), and lingual (ling) surfaces in each sextant and records each in the corresponding box. The scores in the boxes are totaled and the sum for the entire dentition is recorded in the largest square. A score of 10 or less is an indication of client success with bacterial plaque control.[6] Host response to the oral deposits present must be considered in the interpretation of any plaque score.

Documenting the client's plaque index score at each appointment serves to monitor plaque accumulation over time and motivate clients to initiate or continue positive self-care behavior. Also, the hygienist is provided with information about the efficacy of client oral hygiene efforts in each sextant of the mouth. This information is used to:

- ✦ Refine oral hygiene techniques
- ✦ Recommend appropriate oral hygiene devices
- ✦ Demonstrate the relationship between bacterial plaque biofilm and clinical parameters of oral disease

Comparing plaque scores at subsequent appointments facilitates evaluation of client skill development and acceptance of oral hygiene recommendations. This documentation allows the clinician to reinforce instructions and encourages effective use of techniques and products. Clients expect a continuing conversation about their success with recommended oral care products and devices, and a form that documents this information supports such interaction (see Chapters 18 and 19).

At the top of the Kramer-Rhodes Periodontal Maintenance Form is an area in which to enter the date and fee. The term "DDS" is circled and initialed when the dentist examines the client after the dental hygienist has completed the assessment and care. At the bottom of the Kramer-Rhodes form shown in Figure 14–10, the dental hygienist circles the specific dental hygiene care provided (scaling/root planing [RP], selective polishing [polish], and/or topical fluoride application [F]) and initials the form. Quadrants receiving quadrant root planing (QRP) on that date are identified by circling UR, UL, LR, or LL, on the QRP line, allowing records to reflect when treatment concentration is rotated by quadrant or arch from one appointment to the next.

TABLE 14–3 ORAL HYGIENE INDICES

Index/Purpose	Procedure for Use	Interpretation
Plaque Control Record (O'Leary, Drake and Naylor, 1972). Purpose: to record the presence of plaque on all individual tooth surfaces so that the client may monitor progress over time	Best suited for use with an individual client for plaque visualization and oral hygiene motivation. All teeth are included in the assessment. Plaque present on 4 tooth surfaces is recorded: buccal, lingual, mesial, and distal. Apply plaque disclosing agent and rinse. Examine gingival margin for plaque, and record each surface with plaque with a slash (Figure 14–9). Multiply the number of teeth present by 4 (the number of surfaces examined), count the number of surfaces with plaque, and multiply by 100. Divide this number by the total number of available tooth surfaces to obtain the percentage of tooth surface with plaque.	Scored as a percentage of tooth surfaces with plaque. Emphasizing plaque-free areas can be a positive approach with many clients.
Plaque-Free Score (Grant, Stern, and Everett, 1979) Purpose: to measure the location, number, and percentage of plaque-free surfaces in the entire mouth.	Best suited for use with an individual client for plaque visualization and positive reinforcement of plaque control behaviors. All teeth are included in the assessment. Four tooth surfaces are evaluated for the absence of plaque: buccal, lingual, mesial, and distal. Apply plaque disclosing agent and rinse. Record surfaces with plaque. Add the total number of teeth present, and the number of surfaces with plaque. Multiply the total number of teeth by 4 and subtract the number of surfaces with plaque to obtain the number of plaque-free surfaces. Multiply this number by 100 for the percentage of plaque-free surfaces.	Scored as a percentage of plaque-free surfaces, ideal being 100% plaque free. Emphasizing plaque-free areas can be a positive approach with many clients.
Simplified Oral Hygiene Index (OHI-S) (Greene and Vermillion, 1964) Purpose: to measure the presence of debris and calculus on select teeth as an indication of cleansing efficiency	Useful for either an individual client with poor oral hygiene or for a population-based assessment. Divide the dentition into sextants. Using the side of the tip of the periodontal probe or explorer estimate oral debris and supragingival and subgingival calculus on the facial and lingual surfaces of the teeth. Select one tooth from each sextant with the greatest amount of debris or calculus and score the facial and lingual surfaces using the following criteria: Oral Debris Index (DI) 0 = No debris or stain present 1 = Soft debris covering not more than one-third of the tooth surface being examined, or the presence of extrinsic stains without debris, regardless of surface area covered 2 = Soft debris covering more than one-third but not more than two-thirds of the exposed tooth surface 3 = Soft debris covering more than two-thirds of the exposed tooth surface Calculus Index (CI) 0 = No calculus present 1 = Supragingival calculus covering not more than one-third of the exposed tooth surface being examined 2 = Supragingival calculus covering more than one-third but not more than two-thirds of the exposed tooth surface, or the presence of individual flecks of subgingival calculus around the cervical portion of the tooth 3 = Supragingival calculus covering more than two-thirds of the exposed tooth surface, or a continuous heavy band of subgingival calculus around the cervical portion of the tooth Separately determine the DI and CI by totaling the scores and dividing the total by the number of sextants. Add the DI and CI to determine the OHI–S.	An OHI-S is scored as follows: 0.0–1.2 = Good oral hygiene 1.3–3.0 = Fair oral hygiene 3.1–6.0 = Poor oral hygiene Individually, the DI-S and CI-S are scored as follows: 0.0 to 0.6 = Good oral hygiene 0.7 to 1.8 = Fair oral hygiene 1.9 to 3.0 = Poor oral hygiene

TABLE 14–3 ORAL HYGIENE INDICES—CONT'D

Index/Purpose	Procedure for Use	Interpretation
Plaque Index (PI) (Silness and Loe, 1967) Purpose: to assess the thickness of plaque at the gingival area and general plaque accumulation	Useful for either an individual client who has significant plaque accumulation or a population-based assessment. Four gingival scoring units (mesial, distal, buccal, and lingual) are examined on the following teeth: numbers 3, 9, 12, 19, 25, and 28. A mouth mirror, dental explorer, and air are used to score the above tooth surfaces for plaque using the following criteria: 0 = No plaque 1 = A film of plaque adhering to the free gingival margin and adjacent area of the tooth. The plaque may be recognized only after application of disclosing agent or by running the explorer across the tooth surface 2 = Moderate accumulation of soft deposits within the gingival pocket that can be seen with the naked eye or on the tooth and gingival margin 3 = Abundance of soft matter within the gingival crevice and/or the tooth and gingival margin For individual clients, the PI is obtained by totaling the 4 plaque scores per examined tooth and dividing by 4. *A PI score within a group is obtained by adding PI scores per tooth and dividing by number of teeth examined. A PI may be obtained for a segment or group of teeth.*	A PI is scored as follows: 0.0 = Excellent oral hygiene 0.1 to 0.9 = Good oral hygiene 1.0 to 1.9 = Fair oral hygiene 2.0 to 3.0 = Poor oral hygiene
Patient Hygiene Performance (PHP) (Podshadely and Haley, 1968) Purpose: to assess the extent of plaque and debris over a tooth surface as an indication of oral cleanliness	Most useful with individual clients who have significant plaque accumulation. Apply disclosing solution to the following teeth: numbers 3, 8, 14, 19, 24, and 30. Divide each tooth into 5 areas: 3 longitudinal thirds, distal, middle, and mesial; the middle third is subdivided horizontally into incisal, middle, and gingival thirds. Individual client score is obtained by totaling 5 subdivision scores per tooth surface and dividing by the number of tooth surfaces examined.	The PHP is scored as follows: 0.0 = Excellent 1.7 = Good 1.8 to 3.4 = Fair 3.5 to 5.0 = Poor
Plaque Index (PI) (Ramfjord, 1967) Purpose: to measure the presence of plaque on all tooth surfaces as an indication of oral cleanliness	Useful for either an individual client who has significant plaque accumulation or a population-based assessment. Four gingival scoring units, mesial, distal, buccal, and lingual, are examined on the following teeth: numbers 3, 9, 12, 19, 25, and 28. Apply a plaque disclosing solution and rinse. Score the plaque present as follows: 0 = No plaque 1 = Plaque present on some but not all interproximal, facial, and lingual surfaces 2 = Plaque present on all interproximal, facial, and lingual surfaces, but covers less than one-half of these surfaces 3 = Plaque extending over all interproximal, facial, and lingual surfaces, covering more than one-half of these surfaces. Add the plaque scores for each tooth and divide by the number of teeth examined.	A PI is scored as a numerical expression ranging from 0 to 3: 0 = Excellent; no plaque 3 = Poor; abundant plaque
Calculus Index (CI) (Ramfjord, 1967) Purpose: to assess the presence and extent of both supragingival and subgingival calculus	Useful for either an individual client who has significant calculus accumulation or a population-based assessment. An explorer or probe may be used to locate subgingival calculus and determine its extent. For teeth numbers 3, 9, 12, 19, 25, and 28, four surfaces (facial, lingual, mesial, and distal) are scored using the following criteria: 0 = No calculus 1 = Supragingival calculus extending only slightly below the free gingival margin (not more than 1 mm) 2 = Moderate amount of supragingival and subgingival calculus, or subgingival calculus only 3 = Abundance of supragingival and subgingival calculus Add scores for each surface and divide by the number of surfaces (4) for tooth score. Add the scores for the individual teeth and divide by the number of teeth to determine the calculus score for an individual.	A CI is scored as a numerical expression ranging from 0 to 3: 0 = Excellent; no calculus 3 = Poor; abundant calculus

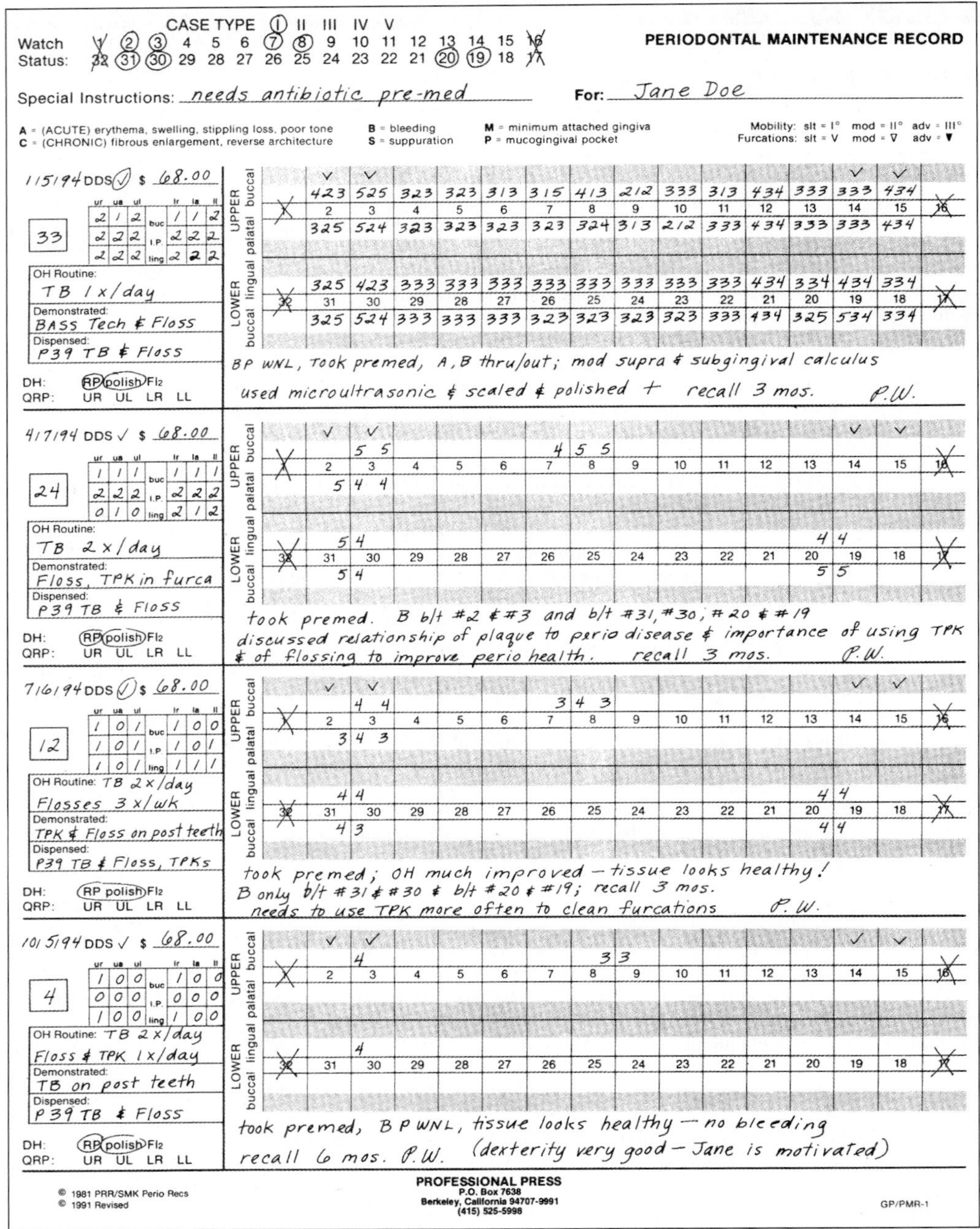

CASE TYPE ① II III IV V

Watch 1 ② ③ 4 5 6 ⑦ ⑧ 9 10 11 12 13 14 15 16

Status: 32 ㉛ ㉚ 29 28 27 26 25 24 23 22 21 ⑳ ⑲ 18 17

PERIODONTAL MAINTENANCE RECORD

Special Instructions: *needs antibiotic pre-med* For: *Jane Doe*

A = (ACUTE) erythema, swelling, stippling loss, poor tone
C = (CHRONIC) fibrous enlargement, reverse architecture
B = bleeding
S = suppuration
M = minimum attached gingiva
P = mucogingival pocket
Mobility: slt = I° mod = II° adv = III°
Furcations: slt = V mod = ∇ adv = ▼

Visit 1/15/94 DDS ✓ $ 68.00 — Score: 33

Index (ur ua ul / lr la ll): buc 2 1 2 / 1 1 2; I.P. 2 2 2 / 2 2 2; ling 2 2 2 / 2 2 2

OH Routine: TB 1x/day
Demonstrated: BASS Tech & Floss
Dispensed: P39 TB & Floss
DH: RP polish Fl2
QRP: UR UL LR LL

	1	2	3	4	5	6	7	8	9	10	11	12	13	14	15	16
Upper buccal	X	423	525	323	323	313	315	413	212	333	313	434	333	333	434	X
Upper palatal		325	524	323	323	323	323	324	313	212	333	434	333	333	434	

	32	31	30	29	28	27	26	25	24	23	22	21	20	19	18	17
Lower lingual	X	325	423	333	333	333	333	333	333	333	333	434	334	434	334	X
Lower buccal		325	524	333	333	333	323	323	323	323	333	434	325	534	334	

BP WNL, Took premed, A, B thru/out; mod supra & subgingival calculus used microultrasonic & scaled & polished + recall 3 mos. P.W.

Visit 4/7/94 DDS ✓ $ 68.00 — Score: 24

Index: buc 1 1 1 / 1 1 1; I.P. 2 2 2 / 2 2 2; ling 0 1 0 / 2 1 2

OH Routine: TB 2x/day
Demonstrated: Floss, TPK in furca
Dispensed: P39 TB & Floss
DH: RP polish Fl2
QRP: UR UL LR LL

Upper buccal: #3 5 5; #7–8 4 5 5. Upper palatal: #2–3 5 4 4.
Lower lingual: #31–30 5 4; #20–19 4 4. Lower buccal: #31–30 5 4; #20–19 5 5.

took premed. B b/t #2 & #3 and b/t #31, #30; #20 & #19 discussed relationship of plaque to perio disease & importance of using TPK & of flossing to improve perio health. recall 3 mos. P.W.

Visit 7/6/94 DDS ✓ $ 68.00 — Score: 12

Index: buc 1 0 1 / 1 0 0; I.P. 1 0 1 / 1 0 1; ling 1 0 1 / 1 1 1

OH Routine: TB 2x/day, Flosses 3x/wk
Demonstrated: TPK & Floss on post teeth
Dispensed: P39 TB & Floss, TPKs
DH: RP polish Fl2
QRP: UR UL LR LL

Upper buccal: #3 4 4; #7–8 3 4 3. Upper palatal: #2–3 3 4 3.
Lower lingual: #31–30 4 4; #20–19 4 4. Lower buccal: #31–30 4 3; #20–19 4 4.

took premed; OH much improved — tissue looks healthy! B only b/t #31 & #30 & b/t #20 & #19; recall 3 mos. needs to use TPK more often to clean furcations P.W.

Visit 10/5/94 DDS ✓ $ 68.00 — Score: 4

Index: buc 1 0 0 / 1 0 0; I.P. 0 0 0 / 0 0 0; ling 1 0 0 / 1 0 0

OH Routine: TB 2x/day, Floss & TPK 1x/day
Demonstrated: TB on post teeth
Dispensed: P39 TB & Floss
DH: RP polish Fl2
QRP: UR UL LR LL

Upper buccal: #3 4; #8 3 3. Lower lingual: #30 4.

took premed, BP WNL, tissue looks healthy — no bleeding recall 6 mos. P.W. (dexterity very good — Jane is motivated)

PROFESSIONAL PRESS, P.O. Box 7638, Berkeley, California 94707-9991, (415) 525-5998
© 1981 PRR/SMK Perio Recs © 1991 Revised GP/PMR-1

FIGURE 14–10 ✦ Kramer-Rhodes periodontal data collection form for comparisons at successive visits. *(Courtesy S. Kramer and P. Rhodes.)*

Client Education Issues

- ✦ Explain the role of bacterial plaque biofilm and host response in the development of gingival inflammation and periodontal disease.
- ✦ Explain bacterial plaque as a complex biofilm community that is self-sufficient, secure, and self-sustaining, rather than as a mere accumulation of bacteria.
- ✦ Use of disclosing agents and bleeding points identifies areas of the mouth that need improved self-care.
- ✦ Discuss how and where calculus is formed and methods of calculus management.
- ✦ Explain the causative factors in oral deposit accumulation.
- ✦ Explain the relationship between oral hygiene index scores and the client's current oral health status.

Legal, Ethical, and Safety Issues

- Prophylactic antibiotic premedication is indicated for clients at risk for infective endocarditis during subgingival exploration.
- Dental hygienists have a responsibility to document oral hygiene assessment data over time and clients' compliance with oral hygiene recommendations in the treatment record.
- Documenting lack of compliance is a risk management strategy and can be used, if necessary, to establish contributory negligence on the part of the client.

Key Concepts

- Oral hygiene assessment gives the clinician an accurate understanding of the client's oral hygiene status. Host response to the oral deposits present must be considered in the interpretation of oral hygiene assessment data.
- Oral hygiene assessments are teaching tools to motivate the client to achieve or maintain oral health.
- Assessment of soft and hard deposits, their origin and location, is essential for oral hygiene care planning.
- Many factors contribute to the retention of bacterial plaque biofilm, including stain, calculus, local predisposing factors, and oral contributing factors.
- The clinical significance of the plaque biofilm is that it creates its own renewing source of lipopolysaccharide for the long-term survival of microorganisms. Biofilm also lends other protective properties to the associated bacteria, such as resistance to antibacterial and antibiotic agents such as chlorhexidine and systemic amoxicillin, respectively.
- Mechanical removal is the most effective method to control plaque biofilm.
- Without disrupting and removing the plaque biofilm daily and frequent supportive periodontal therapy (see Chapter 23), antimicrobial and antibiotic therapies are unlikely to penetrate the resistant biofilm community.
- Although calculus and stain are not in themselves causative agents in gingival inflammation, they contribute significantly by providing bacterial plaque biofilm an environment for attachment.
- Tracking plaque indices over time gives an objective measure of a client's personal progress with self-care techniques.

Critical Thinking Exercises

1. While working with a client you notice a decrease in the amount of plaque on the posterior lingual surfaces of the mandibular teeth from the last time a plaque index was performed. By reviewing the chart, you note that at the last dental hygiene care visit, particular attention was paid to these areas during oral hygiene instruction. What is the best means of conveying this information to your client to maximize positive reinforcement?
2. Upon examination you note a moderate amount of brown stain on a client's teeth and the client indicates to you that he is troubled by the appearance of his teeth. What is the most effective way of exploring the nature of the stains and assisting the client in maintaining a more aesthetic appearance between dental hygiene care visits?
3. Select an appropriate oral hygiene assessment index for a client and provide the rationale for its selection. Use a client you are currently treating.
4. For images and information about biofilms, visit the Center for Biofilm Engineering at Montana State University at *www.erc.montana.edu*, the American Society for Microbiology at *http://dev.asmusa.org/edusrc/biofilms/*, and the MicrobeLibrary at *www.microbelibrary.org* (search for "biofilm").

For References, Suggested Readings, and Related Websites, visit
http://evolve.elsevier.com/Darby/hygiene/

CHAPTER 15

Periodontal and Risk Assessment

OBJECTIVES

Mastery of the content in this chapter will enable the reader to:

- Describe healthy periodontium by clinical signs, histologic characteristics, and radiographic findings.
- Identify and assess risk factors that affect onset, progression, and severity of periodontal disease, and health maintenance.
- Identify four objective parameters of the periodontal assessment.
- Evaluate radiographs for signs of periodontal disease.
- Explain the importance and limitations of radiographs and digital radiographs in periodontal assessment.
- Distinguish between gingivitis and periodontitis.
- Identify four types of plaque-induced gingival diseases.
- Identify the eight categories of periodontitis.
- Identify three methods of microbiologic identification of periodontitis.
- Differentiate between pocket depth and clinical attachment levels.
- Assess client need for specific periodontal treatment modalities.
- Use a standard notation system for periodontal recordkeeping.
- Describe at least two indices for measuring periodontal disease.

KEY TERMS

Alveolar mucosa
Attached gingiva
Basement lamina
Bone loss (horizontal and vertical)
Cementum
Clinical attachment level (CAL)
Cytokines
Digital radiography
Digital subtraction
Disease activity
Disease severity
Epithelial attachment
Erythema
Exudate
Fremitus
Frenectomy
Genetic testing
Gingival crevicular fluid (GCF)
Gingival margin
Gingival recession
Gingival sulcus
Gingivitis
Hemidesmosomes
Iatrogenic factors
Inadequately attached gingiva (IAG)
Infrabony pocket
Interdental papilla
Junctional epithelium (JE)
Microbiologic testing
Mucogingival conditions
Mucogingival junction
Non–plaque-induced gingivitis
Occlusal traumatism/occlusal trauma
Periodontal ligament (PDL)
Periodontal pocket
Periodontal Screening and Recording (PSR)
Periodontal Susceptibility Test (PST)
Periodontitis
Periodontium
Plaque-induced gingivitis
Prostaglandin E2 (PGE2)
Pseudo-pocket
Relative attachment level
Risk factors
Sulcular epithelium
Suppuration
Suprabony pocket
Tumor necrosis factor alpha (TNF)
Triangulation

RISK ASSESSMENT DEFINED[1–3]

Risk factors influence one's susceptibility to periodontitis. Assessment and analysis of risk factors provide information about a client's periodontal disease susceptibility beyond traditional clinical assessment parameters. *Although pathogenic bacteria are necessary for disease initiation, they are not sufficient to cause periodontal destruction.* Many host, environmental, and systemic risk factors modify the body's response to bacterial pathogens in plaque, resulting in great variability in individual susceptibility to periodontal disease. Hence the number and type of client risk factors present modulate the onset, degree, and severity of periodontal disease (Figure 15–1). Risk factor assessment is important because conditions associated with increased risk may affect treatment, client management, and outcomes. Risk factor assessment is based on information obtained through client interviews; the comprehensive health, dental, and pharmacologic history; and the clinical and radiographic examination.

RISK FACTORS

Risk factors are attributes or exposures that significantly increase the risk for onset and or progression of a specific disease and affect treatment outcomes. Risk factors are categorized as:

- *Modifiable*, those that can be changed
- *Nonmodifiable*, those that cannot be changed

MODIFIABLE RISK FACTORS
Smoking
Diabetes
Specific bacterial pathogens
Poor oral hygiene
Osteoporosis
HIV/AIDS
Stress
Bleeding on probing
Medications
Local factors
NON-MODIFIABLE RISK FACTORS
History of periodontitis
Age
Gender
Race
Genetic disorders
Genetic marker

FIGURE 15–1 ✦ Risk factors for periodontal disease.

Modifiable (Mutable) Risk Factors[1–3]

SMOKING.[4-6] Cigarette smoking is one of the most important risk factors for periodontal disease. Studies reveal that smokers have greater loss of attachment, bone loss, periodontal pocket depths, dental calculus formation, and tooth loss than nonsmokers. Both surgical and nonsurgical interventions are less effective in those who smoke, and disease recurrence is more common compared to nonsmokers. The effects of smoking on the periodontium are evidenced at an early age, usually beginning at age 20 to 30. Not only is the onset of disease earlier in smokers, but the disease progresses more rapidly. The association between level of disease and the amount of plaque is minimal. Greater pocket depths are found in the anterior areas and maxillary lingual sites; recession is commonly found in these areas as well because of concentrated exposures of heat and toxins from tobacco smoke.

The negative effects of smoking on the periodontium are linked with an altered host response and direct local damage to periodontal tissues. Gingiva in smokers is thickened and fibrotic with minimal redness. Smoking masks gingival inflammation by reducing gingival blood flow caused by constriction of blood vessels of the gingiva. Local damage may also be related to direct thermal damage. Immunosuppressive effects result from decreased salivary antibodies and impaired neutrophil functioning.

Length of time used and amount of smoking exposures are important assessment factors. A positive linear relationship exists between an increased amount of smoking and an increased loss of attachment (dose-response effect). For example, heavy smokers are 5 to 7 times more likely to develop severe periodontitis when compared to individuals who have never smoked. Attachment loss is greater in heavy smokers when compared to individuals who are light smokers. Smoking cessation seems to have positive effects on the gingiva, and normal anatomy and contour have been reported in individuals after one year of tobacco cessation. Dental hygienists incorporate smoking cessation strategies into care plans as appropriate (see Chapter 29 on tobacco cessation).

DIABETES MELLITUS.[7,8] Diabetes is a strong risk factor for periodontal disease. In both type 1 and type 2 diabetics, greater prevalence of periodontal disease is observed. Individuals with diabetes are up to 3 times more likely to have attachment loss and bone loss than are nondiabetics. For diabetics older than age 40, severity of periodontal disease increases with years of disease duration. Risk for edentulousness is 15 times greater in the diabetic population than the nondiabetic.

Prevalence of periodontal disease increases significantly when the diabetic's blood glucose is poorly controlled or uncontrolled. Persons who maintain good control have less attachment and bone loss than those with poor control, and they respond well to therapy. A diabetic's increased susceptibility to periodontal infections has been linked to immune dysfunction and impaired polymorphonuclear leukocyte functioning.

A two-way relationship exists between periodontal disease and diabetes. Periodontal disease appears to complicate diabetes by making control of blood glucose levels more difficult. Diabetic clients who have a compromised immune system are predisposed to bacterial infection associated with periodontal disease. Conversely, periodontal disease influences the course of diabetes; once successfully treated for periodontal disease, the diabetic's need for insulin can be reduced. Thus control of periodontal infections is critical for maintaining long-term control of diabetes.

SPECIFIC BACTERIAL PATHOGENS. Specific anaerobic, Gram-negative bacteria must be present in the gingival fluid for periodontal disease to occur. Strong evidence links *Actinobacillus actinomycetemcomitans, Porphyromonas gingivalis,* and *Bacteroides forsythus* with periodontal disease. Bacteria associated with moderate evidence for etiology are listed in Table 15–1. These periodontopathic bacteria, also known as *putative bacteria,* can cause direct tissue damage resulting from the production of bacterial enzymes and toxins and play a major role in the immunopathologic processes that destroy periodontal tissues. Presence of one or more of the bacteria in plaque biofilm does not predict that periodontal disease will occur. Other host and environmental factors must be involved.

POOR ORAL HYGIENE. Lack of oral hygiene has a strong association with periodontitis among all age groups. Poor oral hygiene increases the risk for periodontal breakdown. In contrast, excellent oral hygiene greatly reduces the risk for severe periodontitis. Daily plaque control in conjunction with regular professional care prevents attachment loss in most individuals. Studies reveal that a lack of supragingival plaque control following professional treatment minimizes effective results and interferes with resolution of inflammation and periodontal disease control.

OSTEOPOROSIS.[9,10] Evidence indicates an association between alveolar bone loss and osteoporosis. Increased alveolar bone resorption, attachment loss, tooth loss, and edentulousness have been found in women with osteoporosis when compared to women without this condition. Estrogen deficiency also has been linked to decreases in alveolar bone density. For osteoporotic women who smoke, the risk for tooth loss is extremely high. Estrogen replacement therapy (ERT) may be beneficial in preventing tooth loss in women with osteoporosis and lower gingival inflammation and frequency of attachment loss (see Chapter 46, section on osteoporosis).

TABLE 15–1 BACTERIAL ETIOLOGY OF PERIODONTAL DISEASE

Strong Evidence	Moderate Evidence
Actinobacillus actinomycetemcomitans	*Campylobacter rectus*
Porphyromonas gingivalis	*Eubacterium nodatum*
Bacteroides forsythus	*Fusobacterium nucleatum*
	Prevotella intermedia
	Peptostreptococcus micros
	Streptococcus intermedius-complex
	Treponema denticola

American Academy of Periodontology: Consensus report: Periodontal diseases—Pathogenesis and microbial factors, *Annals of Periodontology* 1:928, 1996.

HIV/AIDS.[11] Human immunodeficiency virus (HIV) and acquired immunodeficiency syndrome (AIDS) are suspected risk indicators for periodontal disease. Individuals infected with HIV may exhibit linear gingival erythema (LGE) characterized by acute gingival inflammation around the gingival margin that affects all teeth. There is a disproportionate amount of plaque present compared to the degree of inflammation. About 3% to 17% of persons with HIV disease have necrotizing ulcerative periodontitis (NUP), which results in severe, rapidly progressive periodontal destruction (see Chapter 44, The Individual with HIV Infection).

STRESS.[12] Psychological stress is associated with depression of the immune system, and studies reveal a link between stress, poor coping skills, and periodontal attachment loss. Evidence also suggests that financial stress in individuals with poor coping skills is a risk indicator for more severe periodontal disease in adults. Individuals with adequate coping behaviors have less periodontal tissue destruction even with high financial stress than those individuals with inadequate coping skills. Research is ongoing to determine the link between psychological stress and periodontal disease.

BLEEDING ON PROBING.[13,14] As a predictor of periodontal breakdown, bleeding on probing has minimal value. Numerous studies reveal that bleeding is not a predictor of future attachment loss; however, treated clients with a high number of bleeding sites at maintenance visits have an increased risk for continued periodontal destruction. Repeated absence of bleeding on probing, especially on two or more occasions, generally indicates good periodontal health. Cessation of bleeding correlates with reduced gingival inflammation, repair of gingival connective tissue, and pocket reduction.

MEDICATIONS. Another important aspect of risk assessment is evaluation of client medications (see Chapter 11, Pharmacologic History). Although some medications, such as tetracycline and nonsteroidal anti-inflammatory drugs (NSAIDS), have a beneficial effect on the periodontium, others have a negative impact. Xerostomia is associated with more than 400 medications, including diuretics, antihistamines, antipsychotics, antihypertensives, and analgesics. Decreased salivary flow facilitates plaque accumulation, especially at the cervical one-third of the tooth, and diminishes resolution of gingival inflammation. The dental hygienist assists clients with xerostomia by recommending salivary substitutes as well as alcohol-free mouthrinses, frequent continued-care visits, and excellent self-care behaviors.

Several categories of drugs cause drug-influenced gingival enlargement. Calcium channel blockers such as nifedipine, immunosuppressive drugs such as cyclosporin, and antiseizure drugs such as phenytoin have all been implicated. Sex hormones such as estrogen and progesterone also have been reported to cause gingival enlargement. Gingival enlargement associated with these types of drugs and hormones is co-dependent on bacterial plaque and generally can be minimized with good plaque control.

LOCAL CONTRIBUTING FACTORS. As a part of periodontal risk assessment, the dental hygienist identifies local contributing factors that may augment periodontal disease progression. *Iatrogenic factors* (caused by the practitioner) can contribute to the initiation and progression of periodontal disease. Overhanging restorations, subgingival margin placement of crowns and restorations, orthodontic appliances, and removable partial dentures are examples of iatrogenic factors that may contribute to disease progression. Other local factors include malpositioned teeth, improper tooth contacts, size and shape of the root, calculus, minimal amount of attached gingiva, and traumatic factors such as toothbrush abrasion. Many local contributing factors make plaque removal difficult; the dental hygienist should work with the dentist to modify these factors.

Nonmodifiable (Nonmutable) Risk Factors[1–3]

HISTORY OF PERIODONTITIS. The presence and severity of existing periodontitis are strongly linked with future periodontal breakdown. Persons who have experienced previous episodes of periodontal disease are at a greater risk for future attachment loss than individuals who have not had periodontitis. Because individuals who have existing periodontitis are at great risk for continued periodontal destruction, frequent continued-care appointments are especially important to assist with maintenance of attachment levels.

AGE. Aging is a nonmodifiable risk factor associated with enhanced susceptibility to periodontal disease. Aging has been associated with increased attachment loss and bone and tooth loss. Increased prevalence and severity of periodontal disease in the aging population do not result from specific changes associated with aging, as was once thought. The cumulative effects of periodontal breakdown over a lifetime are the cause of the increased periodontal disease seen with advanced aging.

GENDER AND RACE. Other background characteristics that increase the risk for periodontal disease are race and gender. Studies report more bone loss, attachment loss, and tooth loss in males than females even when oral hygiene, age, and socioeconomic status were considered. African-Americans have greater susceptibility to both aggressive and chronic periodontitis. Some studies of race suggest that socioeconomic class may be more of a factor than race in itself. Research is needed to determine the degree to which periodontal disease susceptibility is a function of race and gender.

GENETIC DISORDERS. Several genetic and inherited disorders are nonmodifiable risk factors linked with depressed immune system and increased periodontal disease susceptibility. Phagocyte dysfunction, cyclic neutropenia, Papillon-Lefevre syndrome, Down syndrome, and Chediak-Higashi syndrome are highly associated with early-onset types of periodontal disease. (See a current pathology textbook for specific information on these diseases.)

GENETIC MARKER.[15] An advance in risk factor assessment was the discovery of a genetic marker highly associated with severe periodontal disease. This discovery resulted in the development of a genetic susceptibility test for periodontal disease. The *Periodontal Susceptibility Test* (PST) is a saliva-based genetic test that identifies a specific interleukin-1 (IL-1) gene type that is associated with increased susceptibility to chronic periodontal disease. Studies indicate that approximately 30% of the population test positive for this IL-1 gene type. IL-1 is a key regulator in the inflammatory process and, in high concentrations, causes tissue destruction. The overproduction of IL-1 helps explain the more generalized and severe periodontal disease seen in genotype-positive clients. The PST involves the collection of saliva from a client by a DNA filter paper. The saliva-soaked filter paper is sent to a DNA laboratory for analysis. Results are returned to the ordering dentist, and only one test is ever needed.

Clients who may benefit from PST include:

- Persons who continue to experience destruction of the periodontium with no clear etiology
- Maintenance clients with continuing signs of disease
- Biologic family members of individuals who test positive
- New clients in a periodontal practice as a part of the initial examination
- Clients who are noncompliant and resistant to accepting recommended therapies and treatment

The PST can identify potential high-risk clients and therefore the need for more aggressive treatment and perhaps improved client compliance. Importantly, the PST is not a diagnostic test but a prognostic test (e.g., some clients will test positive for the genotype and never develop severe periodontal disease, and some clients who test negative will develop severe periodontal disease). Although *genetic testing* provides important information concerning the risk for periodontal disease, the multifactorial nature of this disease must also be considered when assessing risk for periodontal disease.

CLINICAL APPLICATION OF RISK ASSESSMENT

Using a risk assessment screening form assists in identifying risk factors, determining which are modifiable versus nonmodifiable, and determining appropriate treatment interventions (Figure 15–2). Information to complete the risk assessment screening form is obtained through the comprehensive health and dental history and client interview. The more risk factors that a client has increases susceptibility for periodontal breakdown; however, even one risk factor may substantially increase the client's degree of risk. The most significant risk factors are:

- Smoking
- Diabetes
- Poor oral hygiene
- Genotype-positive status

In fact, heavy smokers (10 or more cigarettes per day), combined with a genotype-positive status, are at the greatest risk for periodontal disease breakdown. Persons with these two risk factors are more than 7 times more likely to lose teeth than those without these risk factors. After periodontal and risk assessment, suggestions for eliminating or modifying risk factors that can be altered are addressed. For example, the dental hygienist could consult a client's physician to determine if medications not associated with gingival enlargement can be substituted for those that do. Clients who smoke can be referred to tobacco cessation programs; clients experiencing high levels of psychosocial stress could be provided with stress management strategies; and clients with osteoporosis could consult with their physician about the use of ERT.

If risk factors are identified in a client without periodontal disease, the client is educated about his or her increased susceptibility and encouraged to improve self-care, maintain frequent maintenance care, cease smoking, and reduce other risk factors as appropriate. Clients with periodontitis and risk factors are treated aggressively (e.g., scheduled for 2- to 3-month maintenance care visits; referred for periodontal surgery earlier; and encouraged to follow a rigorous self-care program, including local antimicrobial therapy, oral irrigation, systemic antibiotics, local controlled drug delivery, or subantimicrobial doses of doxycycline to control collagenase activity). Eliminating as many risk factors as possible is vital to long-term periodontal health.

Periodontal Disease Links to Systemic Conditions[16–19]

Systemic conditions increase a client's susceptibility to periodontitis, and periodontal disease may increase a client's susceptibility to certain systemic conditions. Periodontitis may be a risk factor for cardiovascular disease, preterm low-birthweight deliveries, and respiratory disease.

CARDIOVASCULAR DISEASE[20] (see Chapter 40). Individuals with periodontitis have a higher incidence of coronary heart disease, resulting in a greater occurrence of strokes and heart attacks, than individuals with similar characteristics (i.e., age, gender) but being free of periodontitis. Individuals with severe periodontal disease have 3 times the risk of stroke and 3.6 times the risk for coronary heart disease when compared to individuals without periodontitis. In fact, clients with periodontal infection have a 1.5 to 2 times greater risk of incurring fatal cardiovascular disease than clients without periodontal disease.

Several explanations for this association may be related to the development of atheromas, fatty deposits that form along the walls of blood vessels. Studies link coronary heart disease and periodontal infection through immunologic factors, bacteremias, and inflammatory mediators. In periodontal disease, the high level of Gram-negative anaerobic bacteria present in the oral cavity easily spreads into the bloodstream. Oral bacteria can enter the bloodstream, attach to fatty plaques in the coronary arteries, and contribute to clot formation and heart attacks. Inflammation caused by periodontal disease increases arterial plaque buildup (atheroma formation), which contributes to arterial swelling. Periodontal disease can also exacerbate existing cardiovascular conditions.

PRETERM LOW BIRTHWEIGHT[21-23] (see Chapter 46). *Preterm birth* (PTB) is defined as a pregnancy of less than 37 weeks, and *low birthweight* (LBW) is less than 5.5 pounds (2400 grams). PTB and LBW remain the two most significant predictors of infant health and survival. Multiple risk factors such as smoking, alcohol use, drug use, and infections contribute to preterm low birthweight (PLBW).

A link has been established between PLBW babies and periodontal disease. Mothers of PLBW infants having otherwise low risk factors for PLBW had significantly more periodontal attachment loss than mothers who have normal-weight babies at birth. Women who have LBW infants because of preterm labor or premature rupture of membranes tend to have more severe periodontal disease than mothers with normal-birthweight infants. Women with severe periodontal disease have 7 times the risk for PLBW deliveries than individuals with minimal or no periodontal disease. The exact cause of this association may be related to the release of certain biochemical mediators associated with periodontitis, such as *prostaglandin E2* (PGE2), which may create hormonal and cytokine abnormalities that precipitate early uterine contractions and labor. *Cytokines*—soluble proteins released by living cells to regulate bodily functions—remodel tissue that occurs with infection, wound healing, and inflammation. During pregnancy, hormones and cytokines help regulate the onset of labor, uterine contractions, and delivery. Cytokines include mediators of inflammation and growth factors. Also, lipid mediators of inflammation such as PGE2 play a vital role in inflammation and bone loss.

How periodontal disease influences PTB and LBW is explained in the relationship between Gram-negative bacteria and cytokine levels. Gram-negative anaerobic bacteria found in periodontitis or bacterial byproducts

NAME: ______________________ AGE: ______________________ DATE __________

INITIAL PERIODONTAL ASSESSMENT

NON-MODIFIABLE RISK FACTORS

Race	______________									
Gender	Female	☐	Male	☐						
Periodontitis case type	Type 1	☐	Type 2	☐	Type 3	☐	Type 4	☐	Type 5	☐
Family history of early tooth loss	No	☐	Yes	☐						
Genetic disorders	No	☐	Yes	☐	______________					
PST marker test	Negative	☐	Positive	☐						

MODIFIABLE RISK FACTORS **MODIFIERS**

Self care behaviors	Good	☐	Fair	☐	Poor	☐	
Bleeding on probing	No	☐	Yes	☐			% of sites
Diabetes	No	☐	Yes	☐			Controlled
Osteoporosis	No	☐	Yes	☐			ERT
Stress	No	☐	Yes	☐			
HIV Disease	No	☐	Yes	☐			
Medication linked to:							
Gingival overgrowth	No	☐	Yes	☐			
Smoking	No	☐	Yes	☐			Amount/Day
Local risk factors	______________						

TOTAL ______________________________

FIGURE 15–2 ✦ Client risk assessment.

and/or cytokines, which are produced by the infected periodontium and found in the systemic circulation, can target the placenta. More likely, bloodborne bacteria and/or bacterial products, especially lipopolysaccharide, target the placenta to mediate local prostaglandin (a lipid mediator of inflammation) and *tumor necrosis factor alpha (TNF)* synthesis (a cytokine mediator of inflammation). Amniotic fluid levels of PGE2 rise throughout pregnancy, and when a critical threshold occurs, labor, cervical dilation, and delivery are induced.

RESPIRATORY DISEASE[24] (see Chapter 42). Individuals with periodontal disease may be at an increased risk of respiratory infection, especially hospitalized intensive care, acute care, and nursing home residents. The exact role of oral bacteria in the pathogenesis of respiratory infection seems to be linked to the teeth serving as a reservoir for respiratory pathogen colonization and subsequent nosocomial pneumonia. Inflammatory mediators such as cytokines released from periodontal pathogens may alter respiratory epithelium, resulting in increased susceptibility to respiratory infection. In addition, periodontal pathogens can be aspirated into the lungs, causing aspiration pneumonia.

Pneumonias, chronic bronchitis, emphysema, and chronic obstructive pulmonary disease may be adversely influenced by oral conditions. Bacterial respiratory infections may be caused by inhaling fine droplets from the oral cavity and throat into the lungs. These droplets contain bacteria that multiply within the respiratory tract and cause infections or aggravate existing lung conditions.

Periodontal Assessment Instruments[25–27]

(See Chapter 20, section on assessment and treatment instruments)

Basic tools to assess clinical parameters include a good source of light, compressed air to dry the tissues, a mouth mirror, an explorer, a periodontal probe, and a current set of radiographs.

Many kinds of periodontal probes are available. All are calibrated in millimeters for use in assessing the health of the periodontium. Figure 15–3 shows the Marquis probe with colored bands to indicate different measurement levels of 3, 6, 9, and 12 mm, and the Williams probe, which is calibrated with 4- and 6-mm calibrations missing to facilitate reading the probe. When a probe is inserted into the space between the tooth and the gingiva, the calibrations show the depth of the space in millimeters (Figure 15–4). Probing depths are used to monitor periodontal health and disease.

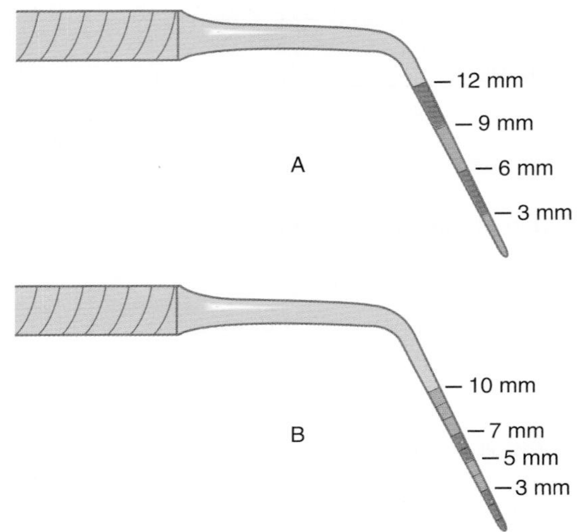

FIGURE 15–3 ✦ **A,** Marquis probe calibrated with color bands to indicate 3-, 6-, 9-, and 12-mm levels of penetration. **B,** Williams probe calibrated in 3-, 5-, 7-, and 10-mm increments.

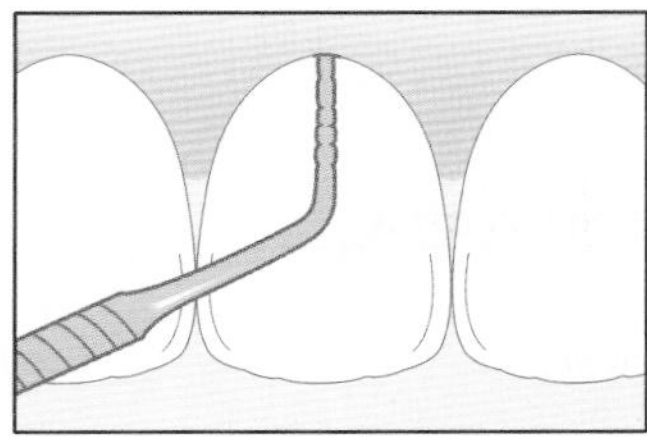

FIGURE 15–4 ✦ Williams probe inserted into a gingival sulcus. Calibrations show a depth of 4 mm. (Probe readings are rounded up to the next highest mm. Here, the 3-mm mark is covered up, so the measurement is read "4 mm.")

Periodontal Screening and Recording (PSR)[25–27]

PSR is a rapid and effective method to screen clients for the presence of periodontal disease. This screening tool, developed by the American Dental Association (ADA) and the American Academy of Periodontology, requires a specially designed probe that has a 0.5-mm ball tip and is color coded from 3.5 to 5.5 mm. The client's mouth is divided into six sextants, and each tooth is probed by walking the probe around the entire sulcus. At a minimum, six areas of the tooth are examined: mesiofacial, midfacial, distofacial, and the corresponding palatal/lingual areas. Only the highest score is recorded for each sextant according to the codes found in Figure 15–5. Clients found to be at high risk receive comprehensive periodontal examinations. All clients should receive a comprehensive periodontal examination annually.

Healthy Periodontium[25–27]

Healthy *periodontium* consists of four physical units: gingiva, periodontal ligament, alveolar process (supporting bone), and cementum.

GINGIVA. Gingiva is masticatory oral mucosa that surrounds the teeth. It covers the alveolar process and the cementoenamel junction (CEJ) of the tooth. Histologically, the gingiva has a protective layer of stratified squamous epithelium, covering a dense, fibrous connective tissue. Gingiva is divided into the free or marginal gingiva, the attached gingiva, and the interdental gingiva or interdental papilla (Figure 15–6).

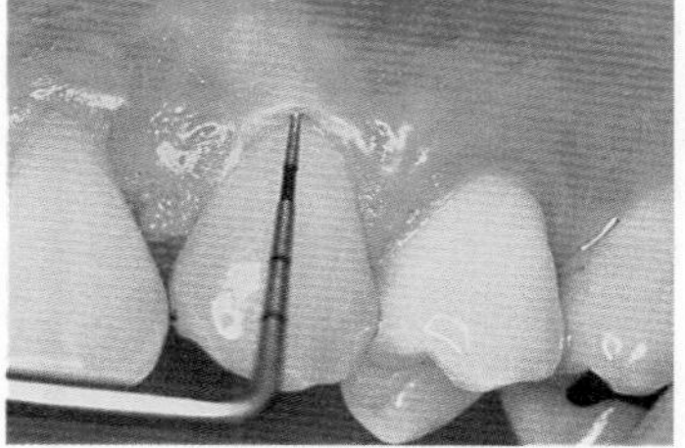
CODE 0

CODE 0

Colored area of probe remains completely visible in the deepest probing depth in the sextant.

- ✦ No calculus, bleeding, or defective margins detected
- ✦ Gingival tissues are healthy

Treatment recommendations:
Appropriate preventive care

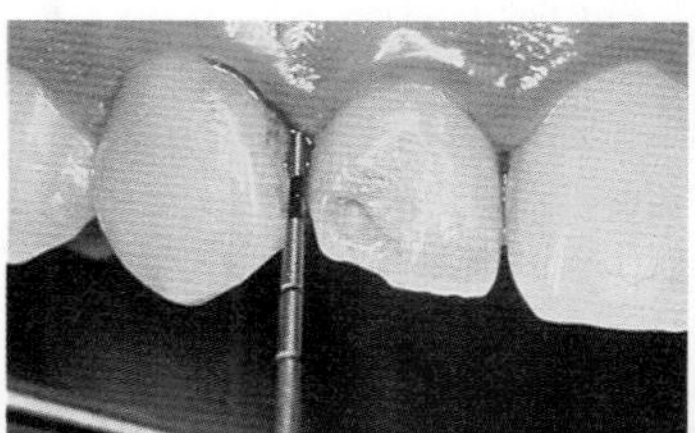
CODE 1

CODE 1

Colored area of probe remains completely visible in the deepest probing depth in the sextant.

- ✦ No calculus or defective margins detected
- ✦ There *is* bleeding on probing

Treatment recommendations:
Oral self-care instructions
Appropriate therapy, including:

- ✦ Subgingival plaque removal

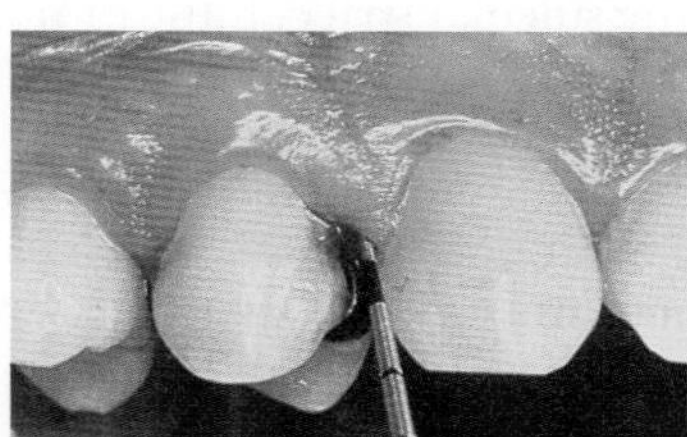
CODE 2

CODE 2

Colored area of probe remains completely visible in the deepest probing depth in the sextant.

- ✦ Supra- or subgingival calculus detected, and/or
- ✦ Defective margins detected

Treatment recommendations:
Self-care instructions
Appropriate therapy, including:

- ✦ Subgingival plaque removal
- ✦ Removal of calculus
- ✦ Correction of overhanging and defective margins of restorations

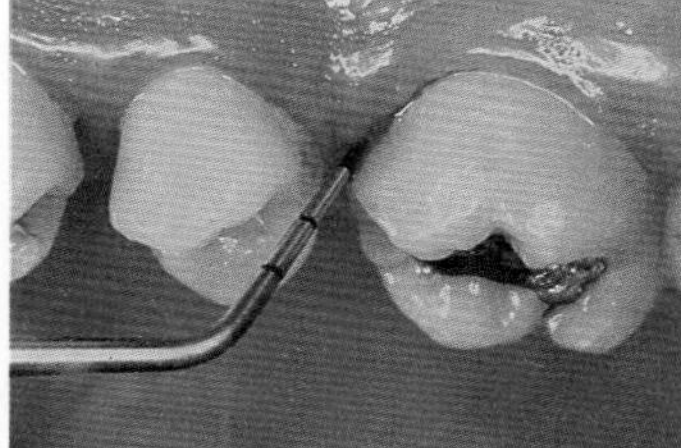
CODE 3

CODE 3

Colored area of probe remains partly visible in the deepest probing depth in the sextant.

Treatment recommendations:
Comprehensive periodontal assessment and charting of the affected sextant are necessary to determine an appropriate treatment plan.
Examination and documentation should include:

- ✦ Identification of probing depths
- ✦ Mobility
- ✦ Gingival recession
- ✦ Mucogingival problems
- ✦ Furcation invasions
- ✦ Radiographs

NOTE: if two or more sextants score CODE 3, a comprehensive periodontal assessment and evaluation are indicated.

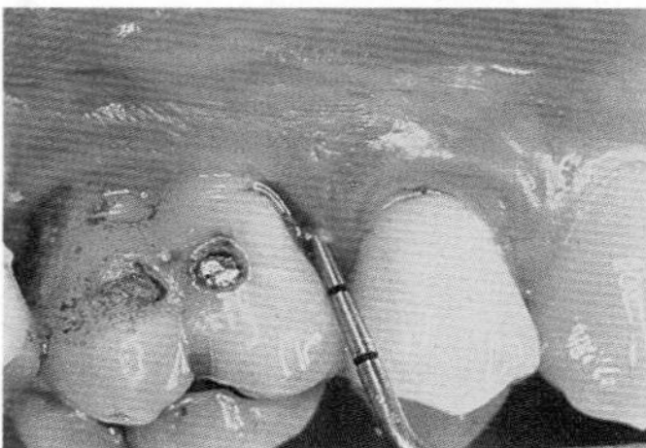
CODE 4

CODE 4

Colored area of probe completely disappears (probing depth greater than 5.5 mm).

Treatment recommendations:
Comprehensive full-mouth periodontal assessment and evaluation are necessary to determine an appropriate treatment plan.

CODE*

The symbol * should be added to sextant score whenever findings indicate clinical abnormalities such as:

- ✦ Furcation invasion
- ✦ Mobility
- ✦ Mucogingival problems
- ✦ Recession extending to the colored area of the probe (3.5 mm or greater)

NOTE: Comprehensive full-mouth examination and charting are necessary to determine an appropriate treatment plan.

FIGURE 15–5 ✦ Periodontal screening and recording. *(From the American Dental Association.)*

Gingival tissue closest to the crown is the marginal gingiva. Free gingiva is not directly attached to the alveolar bone. In healthy adult dentitions, the free gingiva is located on the tooth enamel 0.5 to 2 mm coronal to the CEJ and fits tightly around each tooth. The edge of the free gingiva nearest to the incisal or occlusal area of the tooth is the *gingival margin* or the crest of the gingiva. The gingival margin marks the opening of the gingival sulcus (Figure 15–7).

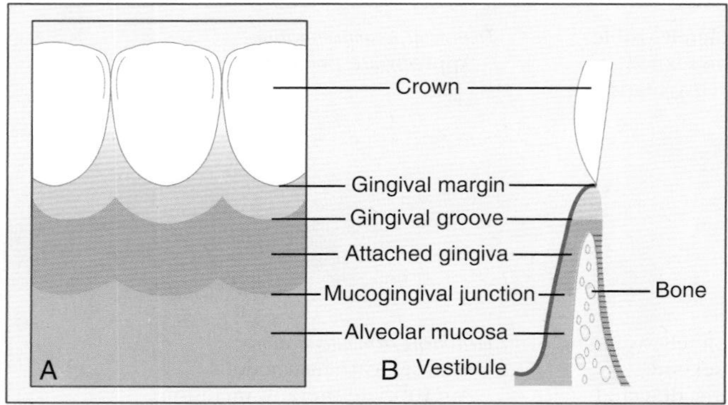

FIGURE 15–6 ✦ Anatomic relationship of normal gingiva. **A,** Facial view. **B,** Cross-section.

Gingival Sulcus. The space between the marginal gingiva and the tooth is the *gingival sulcus* or gingival crevice. A healthy gingival sulcus generally measures 0.5 to 3 mm from the gingival margin to the base of the sulcus. Boundaries of the gingival sulcus are the sulcular epithelium and the tooth. *Sulcular epithelium* is the nonkeratinized continuation of the keratinized epithelium covering the marginal gingiva. Sulcular epithelium is clinically significant in that it is a semipermeable membrane, which in the presence of plaque biofilm may allow bacterial endotoxins to penetrate into the underlying tissue.

Junctional Epithelium (JE). Inside the gingival sulcus, the sulcular epithelium attaches to the tooth at the coronal portion of the JE. The *JE* is a cufflike band of squamous epithelium that completely encircles the tooth. The apex, or base of the sulcus, is formed by the JE (Figure 15–7). Histologically, the JE is 15 to 20 cells thick where it joins sulcular epithelium and tapers down to 1 or 2 cells thick at the apical end. The *epithelial attachment* is the innermost part of the JE attached to the tooth by hemidesmosomes and the basement lamina. A *hemidesmosome* is half of a dense plate near the cell surface that forms a site of attachment between the JE and the surface of the tooth. *Basement lamina* is a thin layer of delicate, noncellular material underlying the epithelium, with the principal component being collagen.

Gingival Crevicular Fluid (GCF). *GCF,* sometimes called sulcular fluid, is a serumlike fluid secreted from the underlying connective tissue into the sulcular space. Little or no fluid is found in the healthy gingival sulcus, but gingival crevicular fluid has been found to flow after one day without bacterial plaque control and to increase with the presence of gingival inflammation. The GCF, which is part of the body's defense mechanism, is able to transport antibodies and certain systemically administered drugs.

Attached Gingiva. Free gingiva connects with the alveolar gingiva at the gingival groove. The *attached* or *alveolar gingiva* is continuous with the free gingiva and is covered

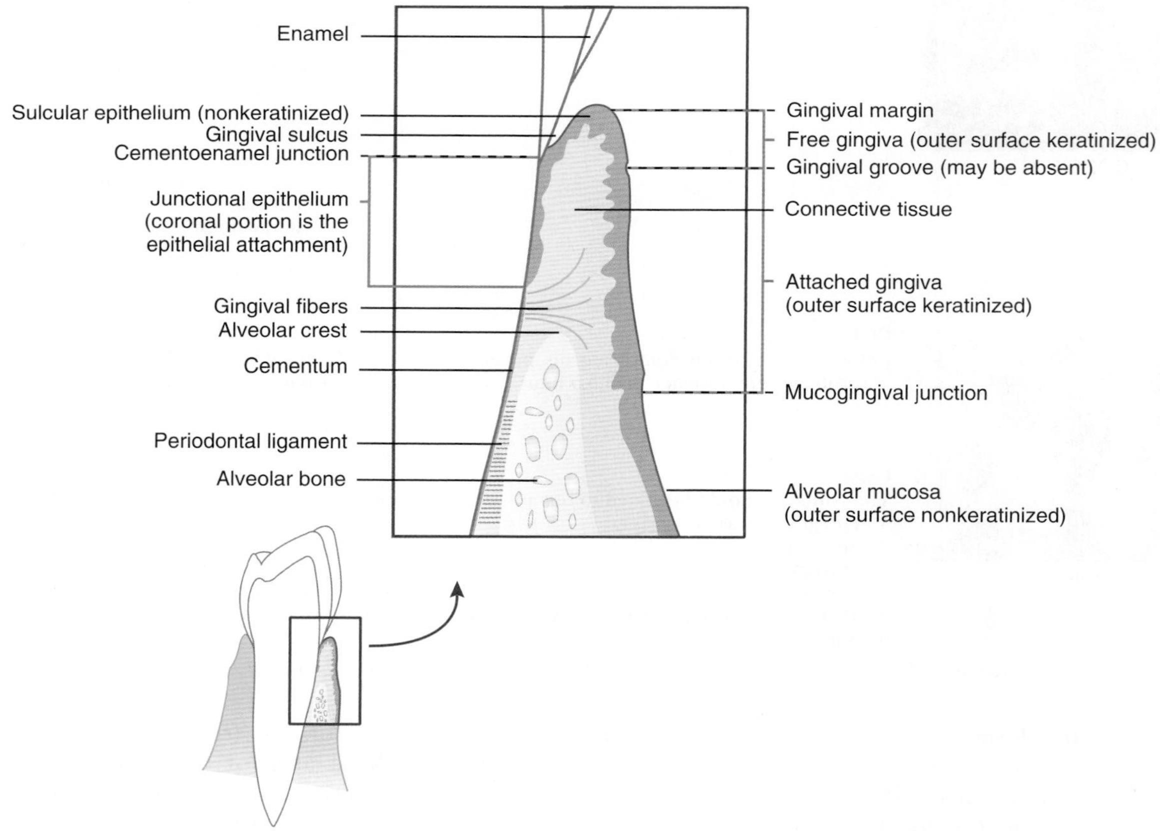

FIGURE 15–7 ✦ Gingiva and other periodontal tissues in cross-section.

with stratified squamous epithelium. The free marginal gingiva joins to the attached gingiva at the gingival groove. This shallow groove is clinically visible in less than half of the population. Alveolar gingiva covers the crestal portion of the alveolar bone and the roof of the mouth. It is firmly attached to the alveolar bone, unlike the marginal gingiva, which has no attachment fibers. Mandibular facial and lingual attached gingiva and the maxillary facial attached gingiva are demarcated from the alveolar mucosa by the *mucogingival junction* (MGJ); the width of alveolar gingiva varies throughout the mouth (from 1 to 9 mm). The facial aspect of the maxillary anterior teeth has the widest alveolar gingiva. In general, at least 1 mm of alveolar gingiva is sufficient for gingival health.[1] This 1-mm minimum width measurement has significance for planning educational and clinical interventions for persons with periodontal disease.

Gingival Papilla. An interdental or gingival papilla is located in the interdental space between two adjacent teeth (Figure 15–7). The tip and lateral borders of the *interdental papilla* are continuous with the marginal gingiva, and the center is composed of alveolar gingiva. The shape of the interdental papilla varies with the space or distance between two adjacent teeth. Given a wide space, the papilla is flat or saddle-shaped. If the interdental space is narrow, the papilla is pointed or pyramidal. When two teeth are in contact, the facial and lingual aspects of the papilla are connected by the col, a nonkeratinized area of interdental gingiva. Because the col is not keratinized, it is highly susceptible to disease. Most periodontal infections begin in the col area (Figure 15–8).

Alveolar Mucosa. Alveolar mucosa is movable tissue, loosely attached to underlying alveolar bone. Its surface appears smooth and shiny and is composed of thin, nonkeratinized epithelium. The alveolar mucosa is separated from the alveolar gingiva at the mucogingival junction. The alveolar mucosa blends into the palatal gingiva in the maxilla so that no MGJ is distinguishable there. Alveolar mucosa is a darker shade of red than gingiva because of its richer blood supply.

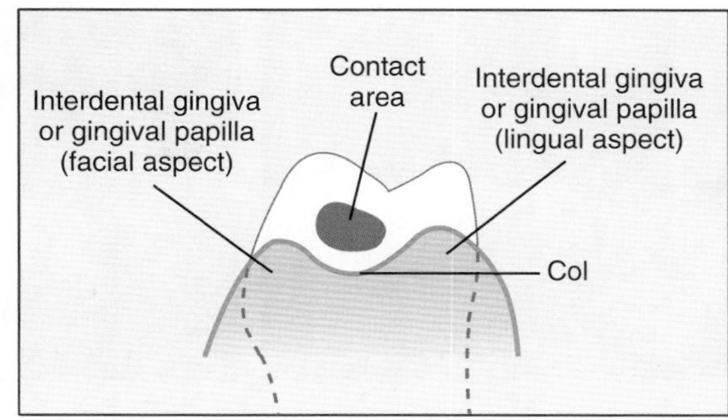

FIGURE 15–8 ✦ The col.

APPEARANCE OF GINGIVA. Clinically, gingiva has distinctive *color, consistency, surface texture, contour,* and *size* in health and disease (Table 15–2).

Healthy Gingiva. Gingival color varies according to the degree of vascularity, the amount of melanin pigmentation present, the degree of epithelial keratinization present, and the thickness of the epithelium. Pigment-containing cells in the basal layer of epithelium are commonly present in persons of dark complexion (Figure 15–9, *A* and *B*). Therefore, some individuals normally have brown melanin pigmentation distributed throughout the gingiva. The healthy attached gingiva is resilient and firm. It is tightly bound to the underlying bone by gingival fibers running between connective tissue and the alveolar periosteum.

TABLE 15–2 CLINICAL GINGIVAL CHARACTERISTICS IN HEALTH AND DISEASE

Characteristic	Health	Disease
Color	Uniformly pale pink with or without generalized dark brown pigmentation	Bright red Dark red, blue-red Pink if fibrotic
Consistency	Firm, resilient	Soft, spongy, dents easily when pressed with probe Bleeds readily to probing
Surface texture	Free gingiva—smooth Attached—stippled	Loss of stippling, shiny Fibrotic with stippling Nodular Hyperkeratotic
Contour	Gingival margin is 1-2 mm above CEJ in fully erupted teeth. Marginal gingiva is knife-edge, flat; follows a curved line around the tooth and fits snugly around the tooth Papilla is pointed and pyramidal; fills interproximal spaces	Irregular margins from edema, fibrosis, clefting, and/or festooning. May be rounded, rolled, or bulbous; therefore more coronal to CEJ. May show recession so that the anatomic root is exposed. Bulbous, flattened, blunted, cratered
Size	Free marginal gingiva is near CEJ and adheres closely to the tooth	Enlarged from excess fluid in tissues or fibrotic from the formation of excess collagen fibers. Free marginal gingiva may be highly retractable with air.
Probing depth	0-4 mm; no apical migration of JE	More than 4 mm with or without apical migration of JE

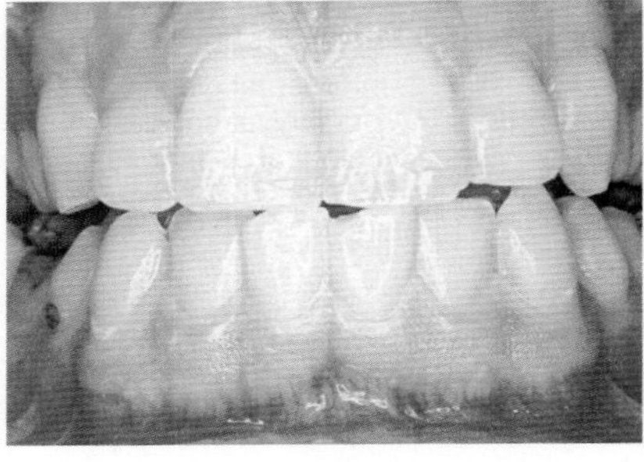
A

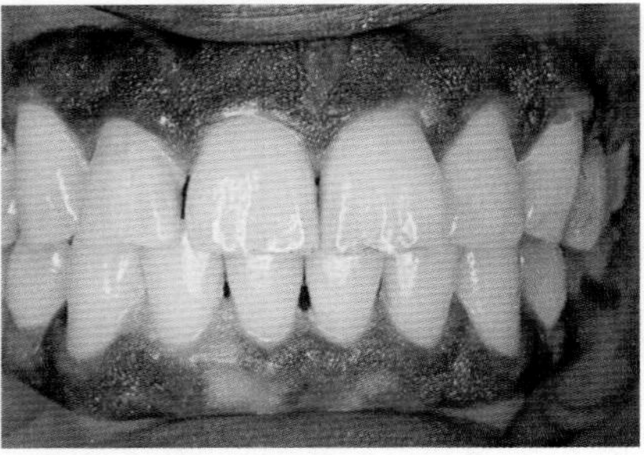
B

FIGURE 15–9 ✦ **A,** Clinically normal gingiva in light-skinned individuals. **B,** Clinically normal pigmented gingiva in dark-skinned individuals. *(From Glickman I, Smulow JB:* Periodontal disease: Clinical, radiographic, and histopathologic features, *Philadelphia, 1974, WB Saunders.)*

The healthy gingiva, when visually examined, air-dried, and probed, does not bleed or exude fluids. The healthy attached gingiva usually has an overall stippled texture. The presence of stippling varies with individuals and areas of the mouth. The gingival margin in health is located 1 to 2 mm above the CEJ. The gingival contour in health follows the contour of the teeth. In addition, the contour, size, and shape of the gingiva depend on location, tooth size, and tooth alignment (Figure 15–10). Healthy gingiva does not feel hypersensitive to air or touch.

CEMENTUM. *Cementum,* a mineralized bonelike substance that covers the roots of teeth, provides attachment and anchorage for the periodontal fibers. Cementum is usually a very thin cellular layer, not as hard as dentin, and it lacks blood vessels and nerves. In health the cementum is not exposed to the oral environment but is protected by the periodontal ligament.

PERIODONTAL LIGAMENT. The *periodontal ligament (PDL)* is the fibrous connective tissue that surrounds and attaches the tooth roots to the alveolar bone. The width of the PDL, seen in radiographs only as a black (radiolucent) space, depends on age, stage of eruption, function of the tooth, and angle of the film. Collagen fibers of the ligament are inserted into the cementum, and they prevent tooth mobility by anchoring the tooth into its alveolar socket. The PDL is connected to cementum and bone by collagen fibers called Sharpey's fibers. Functions of the ligament also include formation and maintenance of fibrous and calcified tissue, nutritional metabolite transport, and the sensory functions of pain and displacement sensitivity.

ALVEOLAR BONE. The alveolar bone is composed of compact or cortical bone and of spongy bone that is marked by trabecular spaces seen on radiographs. The compact bone is the outside wall of the alveolar bone, where the PDL fibers are anchored and the rich vascular supply penetrates. Spongy bone is the interior of the alveolar bone. It can increase and decrease in response to physical pressure, function, and bacterial infection and inflammation. The alveolar crest—the portion of the alveolar bone located between the teeth—varies in size and shape, depending on tooth position.

Diseased Periodontium[25–27]

The histopathology of periodontal disease is explained in four stages (Table 15–3). Three of the stages describe a sequence of events resulting in gingivitis, and the last stage describes events resulting in periodontitis. The progression of periodontitis involves the destruction of connective tissue attachment at the most apical portion of a periodontal pocket. Associated with this attachment loss is the apical downgrowth of the subgingival flora, apical migration of the JE, and resorption of alveolar bone. Table 15–4 compares the clinical characteristics of gingivitis and periodontitis.

GINGIVITIS.[28] Understanding the characteristics of the healthy periodontium provides a foundation on which to recognize signs of disease and to make evidence-based decisions regarding dental hygiene care. The term *periodontal disease* includes both gingivitis and periodontitis. *Gingivitis* means inflammation of the gingival tissue. In gingivitis, the marginal gingiva shows signs of inflammation, but there is no apical migration of the JE beyond the CEJ or bone loss (Figure 15–10).

Although most forms of gingivitis are plaque-induced, host and systemic factors modify the clinical characteristics of the disease and have resulted in two classifications of gingival diseases: plaque-induced gingival diseases and non–plaque-induced gingival lesions (Figure 15–11, *A*).

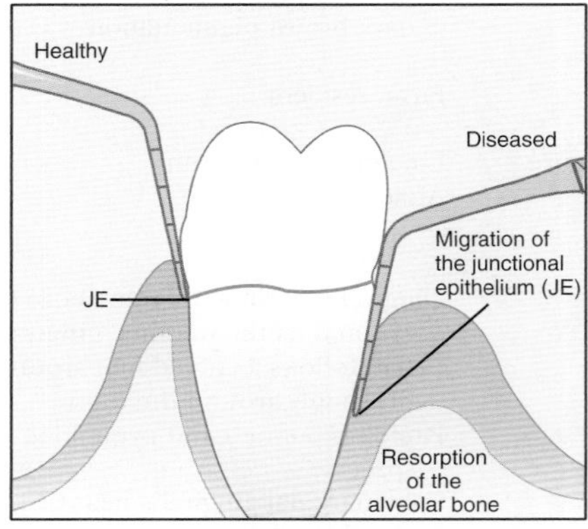

FIGURE 15–10 ✦ Some clinical parameters in health and in periodontitis.

TABLE 15–3 HISTOPATHOLOGY OF PERIODONTAL DISEASE: PAGE AND SHROEDER MODEL OF INFLAMMATION

Stage	Histopathology	Time	Clinical Signs
Initial lesion	Vasoconstriction followed by migration and infiltration of PMNs into junctional epithelium and gingival sulcus Alteration of most coronal part of junctional epithelium Increase in gingival crevicular fluid flow Loss of perivascular collagen	2 to 4 days of plaque accumulation	None Subclinical infection
Early lesion	Accentuation of initial lesion features Chronic inflammatory cells such as lymphocytes accumulate in the connective tissue Junctional and oral epithelium form rete pegs 70% loss of collagen fibers	4 to 7 days of plaque accumulation	Acute signs of inflammation Redness Edema Loss of tissue tone Bleeding on provocation
Established lesion	Persistence of acute inflammation manifestations Plasma cells predominate in the connective tissue Increased collagen loss with loss of connective tissue fiber support Junctional and oral epithelium continue to proliferate with areas of ulceration; epithelium is more permeable Junctional epithelium moves apically with early pocket formation; no bone loss	2 weeks or more	Chronic signs of inflammation Continuation of changes from early lesion; may become more severe Chronic changes such as fibrosis occur over time
Advanced lesion	Continuation of features in established lesion Pocket epithelium extends deep into connective tissue Extensive destruction of collagen and gingival fibers Extension of irritants into alveolar bone and PDL resulting in bone loss Formation of periodontal pockets Conversion of bone marrow distant from the lesion into fibrous connective tissue Periods of quiescence and exacerbation	Varies, may never progress to this stage; depends on host response	Signs of periodontitis Attachment loss Crestal bone resorption Periodontal pockets

TABLE 15–4 CLINICAL CHARACTERISTICS IN GINGIVITIS AND PERIODONTITIS

Characteristic	Gingivitis	Periodontitis
Gingival inflammation	Acute or chronic	Acute or chronic
Position of junctional epithelium	At the CEJ	Below the CEJ (attachment loss)
Position of gingival margin	Greater than 1-2 mm above the CEJ (gingival pocket)	Variable
Bleeding on probing	Present	May be present
Exudate	May be present	May be present
Furcation involvement	Absent	May be present
Tooth mobility	Absent	May be present
Bone loss	Absent	May be present

Dental *plaque-induced gingivitis* has been divided into four main types of gingival diseases:

✦ Plaque-induced gingivitis resulting from dental plaque being the *only* etiologic agent (most common type)

The other types are plaque-induced but modified by host and systemic factors:

✦ Gingival diseases modified by systemic factors (i.e., endocrine disorders and blood diseases)
✦ Gingival diseases modified by medications (i.e., anticonvulsive drugs)
✦ Gingival diseases modified by malnutrition (ascorbic acid deficiency) (Figure 15–12)

Non–plaque-induced gingivitis includes a wide variety of disorders that affect the gingiva:

✦ Gingival diseases of viral, bacterial, fungal and genetic origin
✦ Gingival manifestations of systemic conditions, such as allergic reactions, traumatic lesions, and mucocutaneous disorders

I. Gingival Diseases
- A. Dental plaque-induced gingival diseases*
  - 1. Gingivitis associated with dental plaque only
    - a. without other local contributing factors
    - b. with local contributing factors (See VIII A)
  - 2. Gingival diseases modified by systemic factors
    - a. associated with the endocrine system
      - 1) puberty-associated gingivitis
      - 2) menstrual cycle-associated gingivitis
      - 3) pregnancy-associated
        - a) gingivitis
        - b) pyogenic granuloma
      - 4) diabetes mellitus-associated gingivitis
    - b. associated with blood dyscrasias
      - 1) leukemia-associated gingivitis
      - 2) other
  - 3. Gingival diseases modified by medications
    - a. drug-influenced gingival diseases
      - 1) drug-influenced gingival enlargements
      - 2) drug-influenced gingivitis
        - a) oral contraceptive-associated gingivitis
        - b) other
  - 4. Gingival diseases modified by malnutrition
    - a. ascorbic acid-deficiency gingivitis
    - b. other
- B. Non-plaque-induced gingival lesions
  - 1. Gingival diseases of specific bacterial origin
    - a. *Neisseria gonorrhoeae*-associated lesions
    - b. *Treponema pallidum*-associated lesions
    - c. streptococcal species-associated lesions
    - d. other
  - 2. Gingival diseases of viral origin
    - a. herpesvirus infections
      - 1) primary herpetic gingivostomatitis
      - 2) recurrent oral herpes
      - 3) varicella-zoster infections
    - b. other
  - 3. Gingival diseases of fungal origin
    - a. *Candida* species infections
      - 1) generalized gingival candidosis
    - b. linear gingival erythema
    - c. histoplasmosis
    - d. other
  - 4. Gingival lesions of genetic origin
    - a. hereditary gingival fibromatosis
    - b. other
  - 5. Gingival manifestations of systemic conditions
    - a. mucocutaneous disorders
      - 1) lichen planus
      - 2) pemphigoid
      - 3) pemphigus vulgaris
      - 4) erythema multiforme
      - 5) lupus erythematosus
      - 6) drug-induced
      - 7) other
    - b. allergic reactions
      - 1) dental restorative materials
        - a) mercury
        - b) nickel
        - c) acrylic
        - d) other
      - 2) reactions attributable to
        - a) toothpastes/dentifrices
        - b) mouthrinses/mouthwashes
        - c) chewing gum additives
        - d) foods and additives
      - 3) other
  - 6. Traumatic lesions (factitious, iatrogenic, accidental)
    - a. chemical injury
    - b. physical injury
    - c. thermal injury
  - 7. Foreign body reactions
  - 8. Not otherwise specified (NOS)

* Can occur on a periodontium with no attachment loss or on a periodontium with attachment loss that is not progressing.

FIGURE 15–11 ✦ Classification of periodontal diseases and conditions. **A,** Gingival diseases.

PERIODONTITIS.[29] *Periodontitis* means inflammation of the supporting tissues of the teeth. In periodontitis there is apical migration of the JE with associated loss of attachment and alveolar bone. Periodontitis, therefore, is the extension of the inflammatory process into the connective tissue and alveolar bone that supports the teeth. To classify periodontal disease, the practitioner decides if gingival disease or periodontitis is present. The American Academy of Periodontology has classified periodontitis into seven categories (Figure 15–11, *B*).

Describing the extent (localized or generalized) and severity of sites affected can further identify types of disease:

- ✦ If less than 30% of sites in the mouth are affected, the disease is considered *localized.*
- ✦ If more than 30% of sites in the mouth are affected, the disease is considered *generalized.*

Disease severity is determined by the amount of clinical attachment loss (Figure 15–13):

- ✦ Slight or early
- ✦ Moderate
- ✦ Severe or advanced

In general, chronic periodontitis is most prevalent in adults, with those affected averaging about 0.25 mm attachment loss per year. It thus progresses much more slowly than the aggressive forms of periodontitis; however, progression rates vary widely. Periodontitis is cyclic in nature, with extended periods of quiescence or inactivity followed by short periods of exacerbation or activity. Connective tissue attachment loss during the active stage can vary from minor changes to extensive tissue loss. All forms of periodontal disease, however, appear to be related to specific Gram-negative anaerobic bacteria found in the subgingival flora. *The mere presence*

II. Chronic Periodontitis†
 A. Localized
 B. Generalized
III. Aggressive Periodontitis†
 A. Localized
 B. Generalized
IV. Periodontitis as a Manifestation of Systemic Diseases
 A. Associated with hematologic disorders
  1. Acquired neutropenia
  2. Leukemias
  3. Other
 B. Associated with genetic disorders
  1. Familial and cyclic neutropenia
  2. Down syndrome
  3. Leukocyte adhesion deficiency syndromes
  4. Papillon-Lefevre syndrome
  5. Chediak-Higashi syndrome
  6. Histiocytosis syndromes
  7. Glycogen storage disease
  8. Infantile genetic agranulocytosis
  9. Cohen syndrome
  10. Ehlers-Danlos syndrome (Types IV and VIII)
  11. Hypophosphatasia
  12. Other
 C. Not otherwise specified (NOS)
V. Necrotizing Periodontal Diseases
 A. Necrotizing ulcerative gingivitis (NUG)
 B. Necrotizing ulcerative periodontitis (NUP)
VI. Abscesses of the Periodontium
 A. Gingival abscess
 B. Periodontal abscess
 C. Pericoronal abscess
VII. Periodontitis Associated With Endodontic Lesions
 A. Combined periodontic-endodontic lesions
VIII. Developmental or Acquired Deformities and Conditions
 A. Localized tooth-related factors that modify or predispose to plaque-induced gingival diseases/periodontitis
  1. Tooth anatomic factors
  2. Dental restorations/appliances
  3. Root fractures
  4. Cervical root resorption and cemental tears
 B. Mucogingival deformities and conditions around teeth
  1. Gingival/soft tissue recession
   a. facial or lingual surfaces
   b. interproximal (papillary)
  2. Lack of keratinized gingiva
  3. Decreased vestibular depth
  4. Aberrant frenum/muscle position
  5. Gingival excess
   a. pseudopocket
   b. inconsistent gingival margin
   c. excessive gingival display
   d. gingival enlargement (See I.A.3. and I.B.4.)
  6. Abnormal color
 C. Mucogingival deformities and conditions on edentulous ridges
  1. Vertical and/or horizontal ridge deficiency
  2. Lack of gingiva/keratinized tissue
  3. Gingival/soft tissue enlargement
  4. Aberrant frenum/muscle position
  5. Decreased vestibular depth
  6. Abnormal color
 D. Occlusal trauma
  1. Primary occlusal trauma
  2. Secondary occlusal trauma

† Can be further classified on the basis of extent and severity.

FIGURE 15–11 ✦ *Cont'd* **B,** Periodontitis. *(From Armitage G:* Annals of Periodontology *4(1):2, 1999.)*

of these bacteria is not sufficient for periodontitis to occur because bacterial virulence and susceptibility of the host are critical contributing factors.

Immunopathology[16,19,26]

Two distinct etiologic components are responsible for periodontal destruction:

- ✦ Gram-negative periodontal pathogens located next to the periodontium
- ✦ Host-mediated response to the periodontal pathogens

With adequate removal of bacterial plaque and an intact immune system, pathogen growth is held in check through neutrophil chemotaxis and phagocytosis. When bacterial plaque is not adequately removed, it accumulates at the gingival margin. This plaque accumulation over several days results in bacterial byproducts and toxins such as lipopolysaccharides (LPSs) being released, penetrating into the JE, and gaining access to connective tissue and blood vessels. An imbalance in the host defense system that may be a result of bacterial virulence, altered host defense, or other periodontal risk factors weakens the body's ability to fight the pathogens and results in an overproduction of inflammatory mediators. *Instead of being protective, the overproduction of these inflammatory mediators results in destruction of the periodontal tissues.*

The body responds to the bacteria and their byproducts by triggering the immune system and sending in B- and T-lymphocytes, macrophages, and plasma cells (Figure 15–14). LPS interacts with monocytes and macrophages to produce cytokines (inflammatory mediators) such as interleukin-1 (IL-1), PGE2, TNF, and matrix metalloproteinases (MMPs). IL-1 stimulates the synthesis of MMPs and PGE2. TNF, PGE2, and IL-1 have been shown to mediate or enhance bone resorption thus promoting periodontal destruction. An overproduction of MMPs resulting from the host's inflammatory reaction results in destruction of collagen in the connective tissue of the periodontium. Degradation of collagenous connective tissue and bone resorption results in the clinical manifestations of periodontal disease. *Thus the host's own immunoinflammatory response is responsible for the tissue destruction associated with periodontal disease.*

I. Dental Plaque-induced Gingivitis

Dental Plaque-induced Gingivitis [19]	Inflammation of the gingiva with plaque present at the gingival margin. Characterized by absence of attachment loss, clinical redness, bleeding upon provocation, changes in contour, color and consistency. No radiographic evidence of crestal bone loss. Local contributing factors may enhance susceptibility.

II. Plaque-induced Gingival Diseases Modified by Systemic Factors

Endogenous Sex Steroid Hormone Gingival Disease	Includes puberty associated-gingivitis, pregnancy-associated gingivitis and menstrual cycle gingivitis; characterized by an exaggerated response to plaque, reflected by intense inflammation, redness, edema, and enlargement with absence of bone and attachment loss; in pregnancy may progress to a pyogenic granuloma (pregnancy tumor)
Diabetes Mellitus-Associated Gingivitis	Found in children with poorly controlled type 1 diabetes mellitus. Characteristics similar to plaque-induced gingivitis but severity is related to control of blood glucose levels rather than plaque control
Hematologic (Leukemic) Gingival Diseases	Swollen, glazed and spongy gingival tissues which are red to deep purple in color; enlargement is first observed in the interdental papilla; plaque may exacerbate condition but is not necessary for it to occur
Drug-influenced Gingival Enlargement	Occurs as a result of the use of phenytoin, cyclosporin, and calcium channel blockers such as nifedipine and verapamil. Onset is usually within 3 months of drug use and is more common in younger age groups. Characterized by an exaagerated response to plaque resulting in gingival overgrowth (most commonly occurring in the anterior area and beginning in the inderdental papilla.); found in gingiva with or without bone loss but is not associated with loss of attachment
Gingival Diseases Associated with Nutrition	Associated with a severe vitamin C deficiency and scurvy. Gingiva appears red, bulbous, spongy, and hemorrhagic.

FIGURE 15–12 ✦ Characteristics of plaque-induced gingival diseases. *(Based on American Academy of Periodontology Proceedings of the World Workshop in Clinical Periodontics, July 15-17, 1996, Lansdowne, Va; American Academy of Periodontology Classification of Periodontal Diseases and Conditions.)*

SIGNS OF GINGIVAL DISEASE[30,31]

Clinical Signs of Inflammation (Gingivitis) (Figure 15–15). Inflammation begins in the epithelium of the col and of the marginal gingiva as a result of bacterial invasion or endotoxin irritation. Bacterial endotoxins and enzymes released from Gram-negative bacteria cause a breakdown of epithelial intercellular substances that produce ulceration of the sulcular epithelium. This ulceration permits enzymes and toxins to penetrate further into the underlying connective tissue. Inflammation in the connective tissue results in dilation and increased permeability of capillaries, resulting in redness of tissue, edema, bleeding, and an exudate. Thus four characteristic signs of gingival or periodontal inflammation are:

- ✦ Changes in color
- ✦ Bleeding on probing
- ✦ Swelling or edema
- ✦ Presence of exudate from the gingival sulcus

Oral tissue is assessed for these signs after it has been dried with compressed air.

Color Change. During assessment, the first characteristic to note is the color of the gingival tissue. *Erythema* (reddened gingiva) is common in the process of inflammation. Reddened gingiva indicates an increase in the vascular supply as a result of the body's effort to defend itself against bacterial plaque or foreign objects (e.g., a popcorn shell). Bright red color indicates acute gingival inflammation. Blue or purple color indicates venous congestion (cyanosis) in the connective tissue as a result of chronic inflammation.

It is important to monitor and record the slightest change of color in the gingiva, as well as changes in its contour, consistency, and texture. Documentation should note the location, distribution, severity, and quality of such changes. Table 15–5 summarizes this terminology and provides examples. Clients should be informed of clinical findings and taught to monitor their own gingival health. Using the hand mirror, the dental hygienist should point out gingival color to the client and compare an inflamed gingival area of the client's mouth to one that is healthy. This instruction assists the client in conceptualizing and understanding periodontal health.

Bleeding on Probing (BOP). Use of a periodontal probe to measure the depth of a healthy sulcus (one with an intact layer of sulcular epithelium) does not produce bleeding. Therefore, BOP is one of the earliest clinical signs of the presence of inflammation:

I. Chronic Periodontitis [9]

Onset at any age but is most prevalent in adults. Characterized by inflammation of the supporting structures of the teeth, loss of clinical attachment due to destruction of the periodontal ligament and loss of adjacent bone. Prevalence and severity increases with age. The following levels of chronic periodontal classifications have been identified:

- **Slight or Early Periodontitis**: Progression of gingival inflammation into the alveolar bone crest and early bone loss resulting in slight attachment loss of 1 to 2 mm with periodontal probing depths of 3 to 4 mm
- **Moderate Periodontitis**: A more advanced state of the previous condition, with increased destruction of periodontal structures, clinical attachment loss up to 4 mm, moderate-to-deep pockets (5-7 mm), moderate bone loss, tooth mobility and furcation involvement not exceeding Class I in molars
- **Severe or Advanced Periodontitis**: Further progression of periodontitis with severe destruction of the periodontal structures, clinical attachment loss over 5 mm, increased bone loss, increased pocket depth (usually 7 mm or greater), increased tooth mobility and furcation involvement greater than class I in molars

II. Aggressive Periodontitis [26]

Occurs prior to age 35 and is associated with rapid rate of progression of tissue destruction; host defense defects and composition of subgingival flora. The following subclassifications have been identified:

- **Prepubertal Periodontitis**: onset occurs between eruption of the primary teeth and puberty; occurs in localized forms usually not associated with a systemic disease and generalized forms usually accompanied by alteration of neutrophil functioning; clinically manifests as attachment loss around primary and or permanent teeth
- **Juvenile Periodontitis**: localized and generalized forms. Generalized form (GJP) occurs late in the teenage years with a variable microbial etiology that may include *Actinobacillus actinomycetemcomitans* (Aa), *Porphyromonas gingivalis* (Pg) and affects most teeth;

Localized form is associated with less acute clinical signs of inflammation than would be expected based on the severity of destruction. The localized form (LJP) is associated with bone and attachment loss confined mostly to permanent first molars and/or incisors. Age of onset is at or around puberty; associated with *Actinobacillus actinomycetemcomitans* (Aa) and neutrophil dysfunction.

III. Necrotizing Periodontal Diseases [20]

- **Necrotizing Ulcerative Gingivitis (NUG)**- A gingival infection of complex etiology (e.g., plaque, temporary depression of PMN functioning, stress, poor diet) characterized by sudden onset of pain, necrosis of the tips of the gingival papillae (punched out appearance) and bleeding. Secondary features include fetid breath and a pseudomembrane covering. Fusiform bacteria, *Prevetella intermedia* and spirochetes have been associated with gingiva lesions
- **Necrotizing Ulcerative Periodontitis (NUP)**
  Characterized by necrosis of gingival tissues, periodontal ligament and alveolor bone. Associated with immune disorders such as HIV infection and individuals on immunosuppressive therapies; characteristics include severe and rapid periodontal destruction. Extensive necrosis of the soft tissue occurs simultaneously with alveolar bone loss resulting in a lack of deep pocket formation

FIGURE 15–13 ✦ Characteristics of periodontitis.

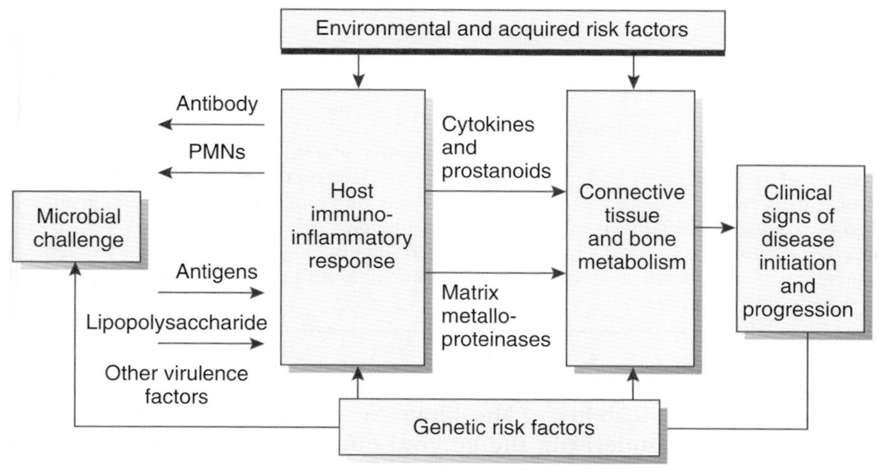

FIGURE 15–14 ✦ Current model of periodontitis. *(From Armitage G:* Supplement to Compendium of Continuing Education in Dentistry *19(1):9, 1999).*

✦ BOP predicts attachment loss only 30% of the time. Furthermore, fibrotic tissue that results from chronic inflammation may bleed very little or not at all.

✦ BOP always signals the presence of inflammation and has value in identifying clients at risk for periodontal disease progression.

✦ Gingival bleeding occurring at several sequential continued-care visits is associated with an increased risk for loss of attachment.

✦ The absence of bleeding is associated with a lack of disease progression; however, the mere presence of bleeding does not predict periodontal breakdown.

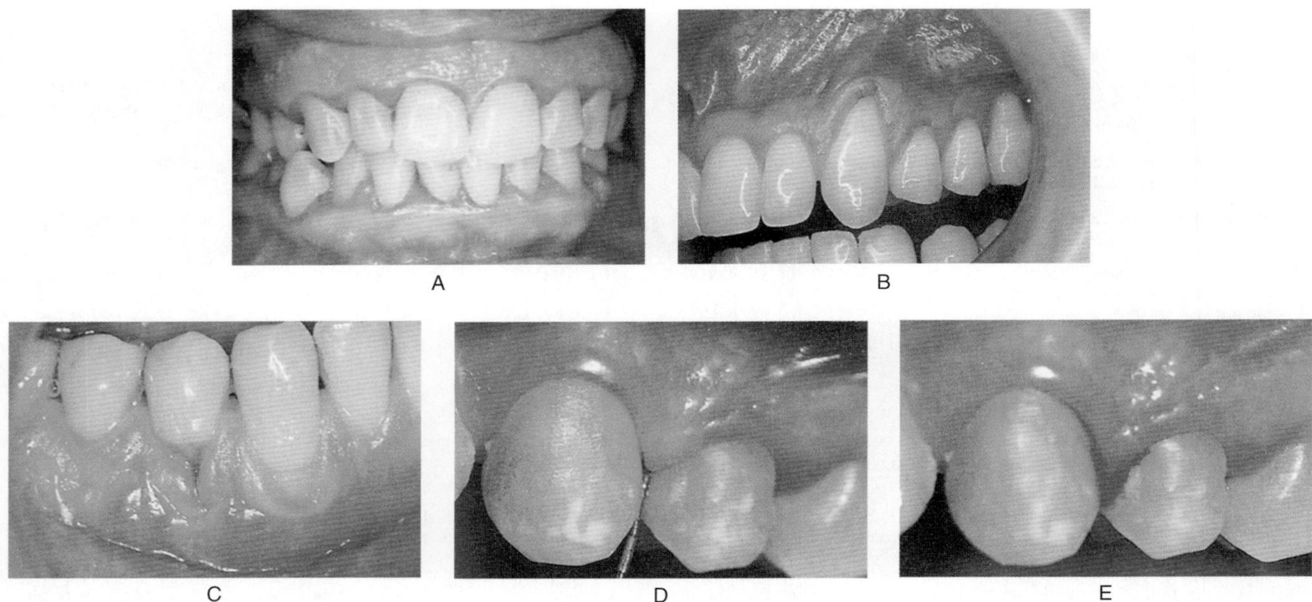

FIGURE 15–15 ✦ **A,** Edema associated with papillary gingivitis. **B,** Lifesaver-like enlargement of the gingival margin characteristic of McCall's festoons and severe gingival recession on maxillary canine. **C,** Different degrees of recession. Recession is slight in teeth numbers 26 and 29 and significant in 27 and 28. Note irregular contours of the gingiva in 28 denoting a gingival cleft and inadequately attached gingiva on 27 and 28. **D,** Insertion of a probe into the gingival sulcus. Note the lack of stippling, the slightly rolled gingival margins, and the dark red color. **E,** Bleeding appears about 30 seconds after probing area in slide D. *(B from Newman MG, Takei HH, Carranza FA:* Carranza's clinical periodontology, *ed 9, Philadelphia, 2002, WB Saunders; E from Carranza FA, Newman MG:* Clinical periodontology, *ed 8, Philadelphia, 1996, WB Saunders.)*

TABLE 15–5 TERMINOLOGY USED TO DESCRIBE OBSERVATIONS ASSOCIATED WITH CLINICAL ASSESSMENT OF GINGIVA

Characteristic	Terminology	Description	Example
Gingival color	Location: Distribution: Severity: Quality:	Generalized or localized Diffuse, marginal, or papillary Slight, moderate, severe Red, bright red, pink, cyanotic	Localized slight marginal redness linguals of numbers 18, 19, 30, 31; all other areas coral pink, uniform in color
Gingival contour	Location: Distribution: Severity: Quality:	Generalized or localized Diffuse, marginal, or papillary Slight, moderate, severe Bulbous, flattened, punched-out, cratered	Localized moderately cratered papilla numbers 6-11, 22-27; all other areas within normal limits
Consistency of gingiva	Location: Distribution: Severity: Quality:	Generalized or localized Diffuse, marginal, or papillary Slight, moderate, severe Firm (fibrotic), spongy (edematous)	Generalized moderate marginal sponginess more severe on facial numbers 8, 9; all other areas coral pink with moderate, generalized melanin pigmentation
Surface texture of gingiva	Location: Distribution: Quality:	Generalized or localized Diffuse, marginal, or papillary Smooth, shiny, eroded, stippling	Localized smooth gingiva on facial numbers 7, 8; all other areas with generalized stippling

BOP is recorded in the client record and monitored. The dental hygienist explains to the client that BOP is caused by soft tissue inflammation and is a significant sign of gingival infection. Moreover, the hygienist points out that bleeding, or its absence, upon brushing or interdental cleaning gives the individual a self-test for monitoring gingival health status at home.

Swelling or Edema. Microorganisms in plaque produce harmful toxins and enzymes that result in increased permeability of the blood vessels in the connective tissue underlying the gingival epithelium. This increased permeability of blood vessels allows lymphocytes, plasma cells, and extracellular fluid to accumulate in gingival connective tissue. This accumulation results in enlarged, edematous tissue. When there is no apical migration of the JE, the sulcus becomes deepened from this edematous enlargement of the gingival tissue, producing a gingival pocket. This gingival pocket is also called an artificially deepened sulcus or a *pseudo-pocket* because the

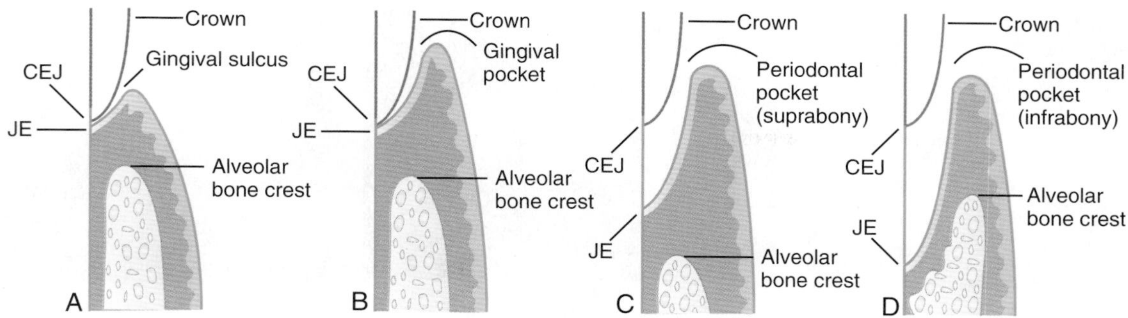

FIGURE 15–16 ✦ **A,** Comparison of the relationship of the junctional epithelium (JE) to the cementoenamel junction (CEJ) and alveolar bone in health. **B,** Gingival pocket. **C,** Suprabony periodontal pocket (periodontitis), JE above alveolar bone crest. **D,** Infrabony periodontal pocket (periodontitis), JE below alveolar bone crest.

marginal gingiva has moved coronally, not apically (Figure 15–16). Deeper periodontal structures are not involved, and there is no migration of the JE.

A gingival pocket can be reversed to a healthy gingival sulcus by the client's daily plaque control regimen supplemented by professional mechanical oral hygiene care. When bacterial plaque is controlled and calculus is removed, the inflammation subsides and the gingival enlargement decreases, with a resultant decrease in the depth of the gingival pocket.

Changes in Texture and Contour. Swelling or edema produces texture and contour changes in the gingiva (Figure 15–15). In gingivitis, the texture of the gingiva becomes shiny and smooth as a result of loss of stippling and edema. Contour changes occur as a result of gingival enlargement, such that the position of the gingiva is high on the enamel, partly or nearly covering the anatomic crown. The marginal gingiva becomes rounded or rolled, rather than knife-edged or slightly rounded, and closely adapted to the tooth. In chronic inflammation the gingival surface may even become nodular or fibrotic (Figure 15–17).

Interdental Papillae Changes. While examining the color, texture, size, and shape of the gingiva, the clinician gives careful attention to the gingival papilla. When the col area is inflamed, degeneration of the epithelial and connective tissue layer can result in a blunted papilla, a split interdental papilla, or a cratered papilla (Figure 15–18). Such degradation usually indicates a loss of the alveolar bone. Self-induced trauma from improper use of dental floss may cause laceration of the gingival papillae.

Exudate. GCF rarely is found in healthy gingiva but significantly increases in the presence of inflammation. GCF is measured by isolating a site, drying it with air, and inserting a small paper strip into the pocket or sulcus for 3 to 5 seconds. Electronic devices can measure the GCF volume of the paper strip.

GCF is called *suppuration* when it is a clear serous liquid and *purulent exudate* when it contains living and dead polymorphonuclear neutrophilic leukocytes (PMNs), bacteria, necrotic tissue, and enzymes. When purulent exudate is present in the pocket, pus can be noticed during probing and expressed by applying pressure to the base of a pocket with one's finger and moving it coronally. Although purulent exudate is a dramatic sign of inflammation, it does not indicate the severity of inflammation or pocket depth. Some shallow and some deep pockets have pus formation, and some do not. *The presence of pus is, however, a good indicator of active periodontal destruction. Suppuration correlates with specific attachment loss only 2% to 30% of the time, so it is not a reliable indicator of active periodontal destruction.* Suppuration is not always clinically evident. When suppuration or purulent exudate is observed, it is recorded for each area found.

Documentation of the Clinical Gingival Assessment. When assessing the gingiva, changes in gingival color, consistency, surface texture, contour, and size are described with regard to:

- ✦ *Location* (generalized throughout or localized to a specific area)
- ✦ *Distribution* (diffuse, marginal, or papillary)
- ✦ *Severity* (slight, moderate, severe)
- ✦ *Quality*

Table 15–2 compares gingival characteristics associated with health and disease. The term *healthy periodontium* is appropriate for sites that are disease-free but have extensive attachment loss and recession resulting from previous episodes of periodontitis. For example, sites that have been successfully treated fall into this category. When successfully treated periodontitis sites become inflamed at the gingival margin, this condition is termed *plaque-induced gingivitis on a reduced periodontium.*

SIGNS OF DISEASE PROGRESSION (PERIODONTITIS)[30,31]

Periodontal Pocket. Probing depth is the distance from the gingival margin to the base of the sulcus or pocket, as measured by the periodontal probe (Figure 15–19). Unlike a gingival or pseudo-pocket, a *periodontal pocket* is a pathologically deepened sulcus caused by bacterial infection. When the coronal end of the JE (the surface that forms the actual sulcus/pocket bottom) comes in contact with bacterial plaque, it detaches from the tooth. At the same time, the apical end of the JE migrates apically,

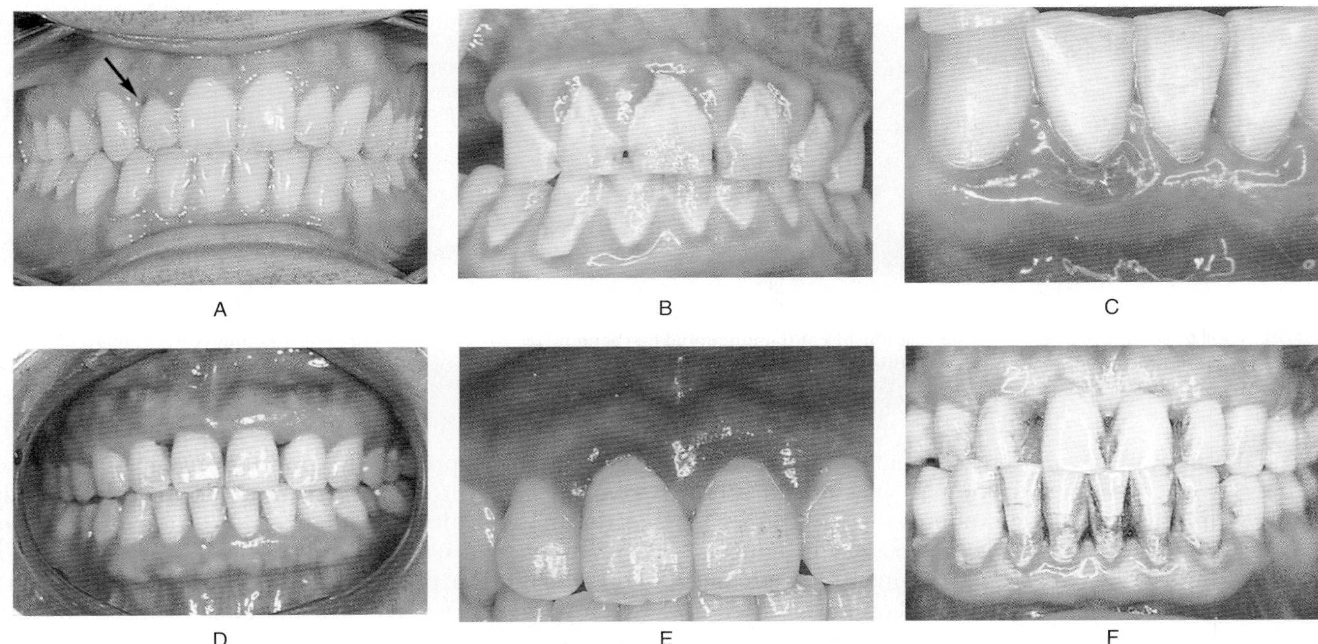

FIGURE 15–17 ✦ **A,** Slight plaque-induced gingivitis. Note that gingival margins and interdental papillae have lost their sharpness and now have puffy, rolled borders. **B,** Edematous gingiva. Note loss of stippling; increase in size of gingiva; abundant plaque, calculus, and material alba; and change in color and consistency. Note red, shiny, smooth gingiva. **C,** Close-up view of edematous gingiva. Note the red, shiny, smooth gingiva. **D,** Fibrotic gingiva. Pockets of moderate depth are present, but the gingiva retains its stippling in some areas. **E,** Severe generalized gingival inflammation and gingival enlargement. **F,** Fibrotic gingiva. Note color and consistency of gingiva, calculus, tobacco stain, plaque, gingival recession, blunted papilla, open contacts. *(From Carranza FA, Newman MG:* Clinical periodontology, *ed 8, Philadelphia, 1996, WB Saunders.)*

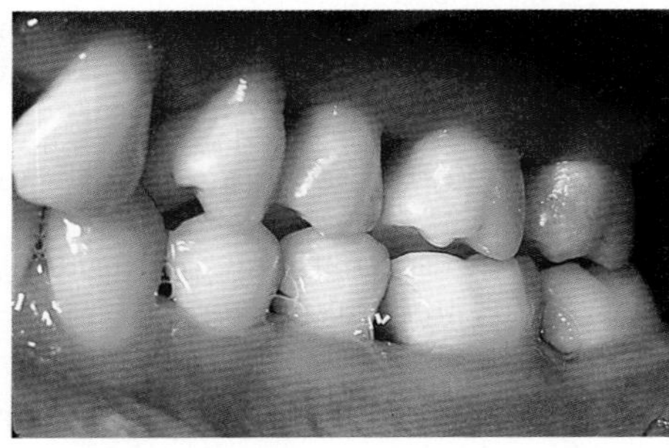

FIGURE 15–18 ✦ Cratered and missing interdental papilla.

thus deepening the sulcus into a periodontal pocket. As inflammation causes apical migration of the JE, it also causes gradual alveolar bone resorption, which reduces the level of bone support for the tooth (Figure 15–10).

Periodontal pockets are classified as follows (Figure 15–16):

- *Suprabony periodontal pocket* when the JE has migrated below the CEJ but remains above the crest of the alveolar bone. Suprabony pockets are most commonly associated with horizontal bone loss.
- *Infrabony periodontal pocket* when the JE has migrated below the crest of the alveolar bone. Infrabony pockets are associated with vertical bone loss.

Periodontal pockets may be present in the absence of clinical signs of gingival inflammation. Therefore, *clinical probing is the only accurate way to assess the gingiva for the presence of periodontal pockets.* Because periodontal pockets can develop at any point around a tooth, the probe must be inserted around the entire circumference of the tooth. The deepest reading at each of the six tooth surfaces is the one that should be recorded on the client's periodontal charting form (Figure 15–20). The probe is moved or *walked* along the pocket bottom and angled to keep the tip in contact with the tooth (Figure 15–21). If calculus is encountered, the probe is teased over the calculus, or the calculus should be removed to allow insertion of the probe to the bottom of the pocket (Figure 15–22).

The interproximal area is the most difficult area for the client to clean and, therefore, is where periodontal pockets tend to form. To probe the interproximal area just apical to the contact, place the probe up against the interdental contact and tilt the probe mesially or distally as appropriate to keep the tip touching the tooth (Figure 15–23). Failure to tilt the probe enough to keep its tip in contact with the tooth surface is a common error and causes inaccurate interproximal probing depth readings (Figure 15–24). The interproximal tooth surfaces should be probed from both the facial and lingual sides of each tooth so that all of the epithelial attachment of the JE is explored (Figure 15–25; see Procedure 20–2 in Chapter 20).

Gingival Recession. *Gingival recession* is a reduction of the height of the marginal gingiva to a location apical to the CEJ (Figure 15–15, *A*). It has importance in the periodontal assessment because it signifies attachment loss and can

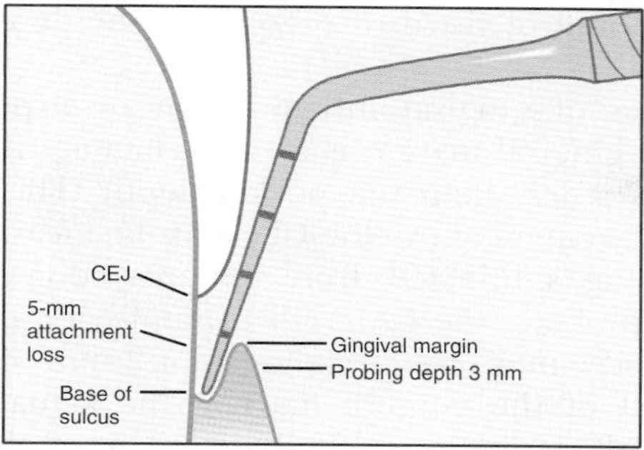

FIGURE 15–19 ✦ Probing depth and attachment loss measurement on same tooth using the Williams probe.

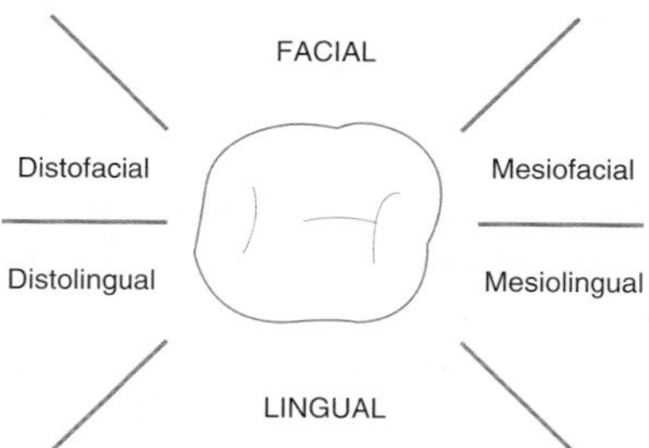

FIGURE 15–20 ✦ Occlusal view of the six surfaces measured in periodontal probing.

produce significant discomfort for the client. Causes of gingival recession are numerous. Chronic exposure to bacterial plaque, toothbrush abrasion, orthodontia, floss cuts, occlusal trauma, abfraction root instrumentation, and tooth polishing with an abrasive prophylaxis paste or air polisher have all been known to result in migration of the JE and cause recession. Once the root surface is exposed to the oral environment by gingival recession, the connective tissue rarely reattaches because collagen breaks down when exposed to the oral environment, and cementoblasts grow only on root surface adjacent to the PDL. Areas of recession may be sensitive because the exposed cementum may be lost, exposing dentin. As a result, exposed nerve endings in the dentin may be stimulated mechanically (e.g., by toothbrushing), chemically (e.g., by acidic foods or bacterial plaque), or thermally (e.g., by cold air or food at extreme temperature), producing sensitive teeth (see Chapter 33 on Dentinal Hypersensitivity).

Noting areas of dentinal hypersensitivity on the client record provides information for planning care because clients with hypersensitivity may require more time and possibly a local anesthetic agent and/or nitrous oxide–oxygen analgesia for effective tooth instrumentation (see Chapter 34, Local Anesthesia, and Chapter 35, Nitrous Oxide–Oxygen Analgesia).

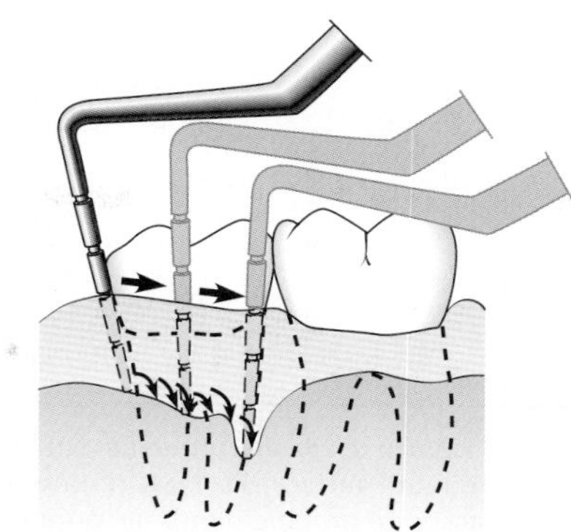

FIGURE 15–21 ✦ Facial view showing how the probe is moved around the tooth in short steps, reestablishing contact with the pocket bottom at each step. *(From Newman MG, Takei HH, Carranza FA:* Carranza's clinical periodontology, *ed 9, Philadelphia, 2002, WB Saunders.)*

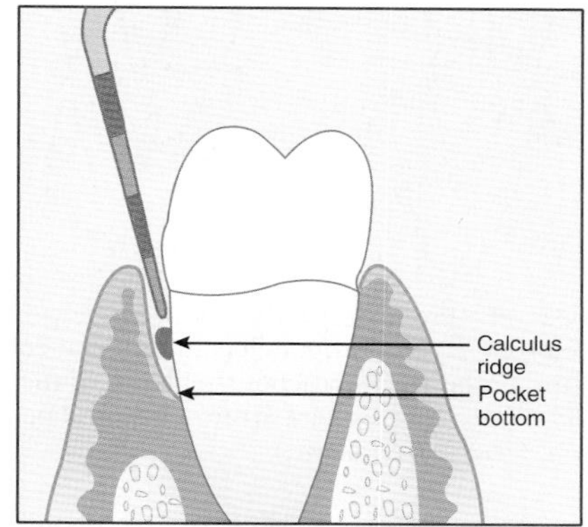

FIGURE 15–22 ✦ Probe blocked by calculus. *(Courtesy Praxis Publishing. From Instructional Design, Department of Periodontology, UCSF School of Dentistry, 1978.)*

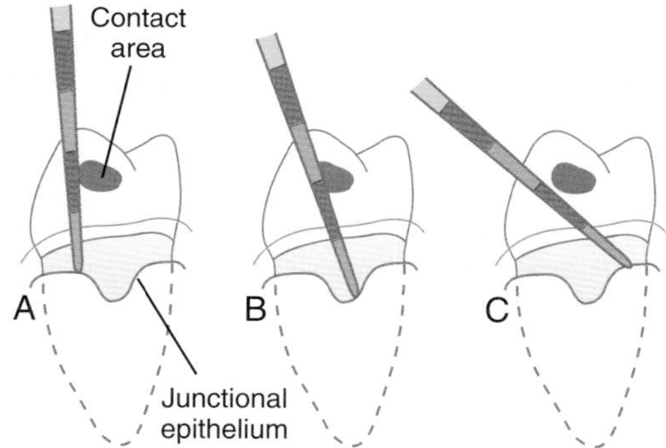

FIGURE 15–23 ✦ **A,** Incorrect technique for probing the interproximal area. **B,** Correct technique. **C,** Incorrect technique. *(Redrawn from Perry D, Beemsterboer P, Carranza FA:* Techniques and theory of periodontal instrumentation, *Philadelphia, 1990, WB Saunders.)*

Clinical Attachment Level (CAL) (Figure 15–26). *CAL* is the position of the attached periodontal tissues at the base of the pocket. It is determined by comparing the distance from the CEJ to the base of the sulcus or pocket. The location of the gingival margin is important in determining the CAL, which includes both periodontal pocket depth and recession measurements. When the gingival margin coincides with the CEJ, the CAL and the pocket depth are equal. When the gingival margin is apical to the CEJ, the CAL is greater than the pocket depth and equal

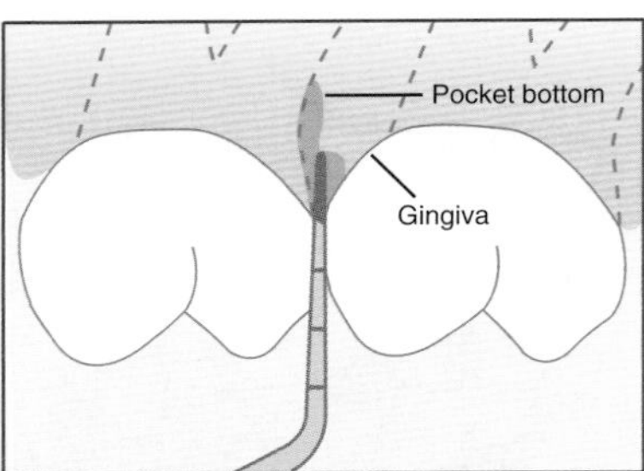

FIGURE 15–24 ✦ Failure to tilt the probe far enough to keep its end in contact with the tooth surface. Probe is resting on the pocket wall, resulting in an inaccurate probing depth measurement.

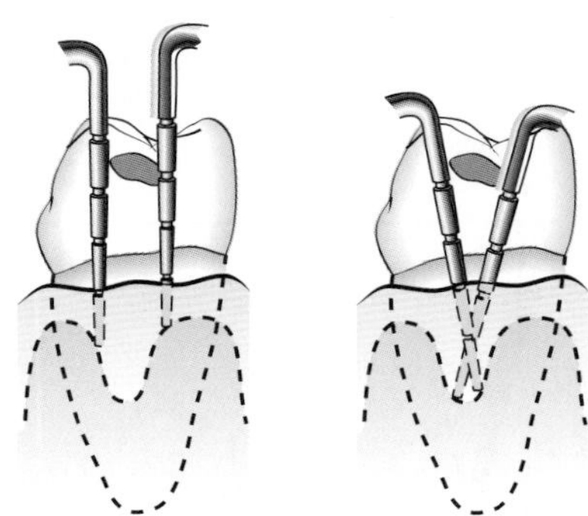

FIGURE 15–25 ✦ Proximal view of tooth being probed. Vertical insertion of the probe (*left*) may not detect interdental craters; oblique positioning of the probe (*right*) reaches the depth of the crater. *(From Newman MG, Takei HH, Carranza FA:* Carranza's clinical periodontology, *ed 9, Philadelphia, 2002, WB Saunders.)*

to the amount of visual recession plus the depth of the pocket.

In cases of gingival inflammation or hypertrophy, when the gingival margin is on the enamel, the attachment loss is less than the pocket depth. The gingival margin placement above the CEJ must be measured and this reading subtracted from the periodontal probe reading to obtain the CAL. For example, if a client has generalized 6-mm probe readings but 2 mm of coronal movement of the gingival margin, the actual CAL is 4 mm. If this 2 mm is not subtracted from the probe reading, a realistic assessment of the CAL cannot be obtained. In this situation, a client with only 4 mm of attachment loss might be misclassified as a higher periodontal class than what is actually apparent. If a client has generalized 3 mm of recession and 3-mm pocket readings, the recession and the pocket reading must be added together to obtain the actual CAL of 6 mm. If they were not added together, the client might be classified as having slight periodontal disease when 6 mm CAL would indicate severe disease.

Attachment loss over time (*disease activity*), not periodontal pocket readings, indicates actual progression of periodontal disease and is considered its defining feature. Consequently, regular documentation of attachment loss in the client record is important to track periodontal disease activity.

Relative Attachment Level (RAL). *RAL* is the measurement from a fixed reference point on a tooth (CEJ) or a stent

Clinical attachment levels

A
Inflamed gingival margin

Gingival margin
3 mm above CEJ

Pocket reading
6 mm

GM subtracted from pocket reading
(6 – 3 = 3 mm clinical attachment level)

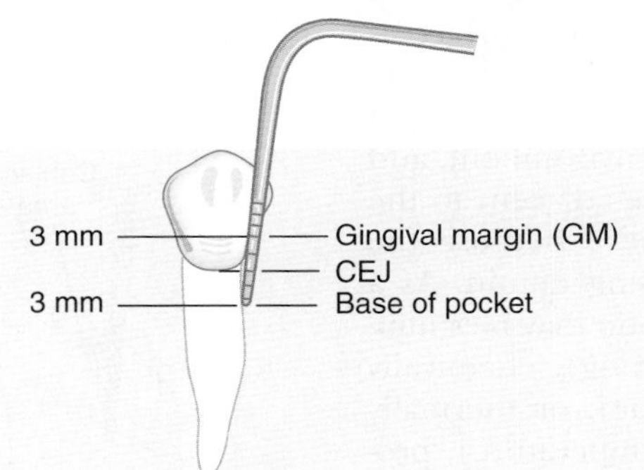

B
Gingival recession

Gingival margin
3 mm below CEJ

Pocket reading
3 mm

GM from CEJ added to pocket reading
(3 + 3 = 6 mm clinical attachment level)

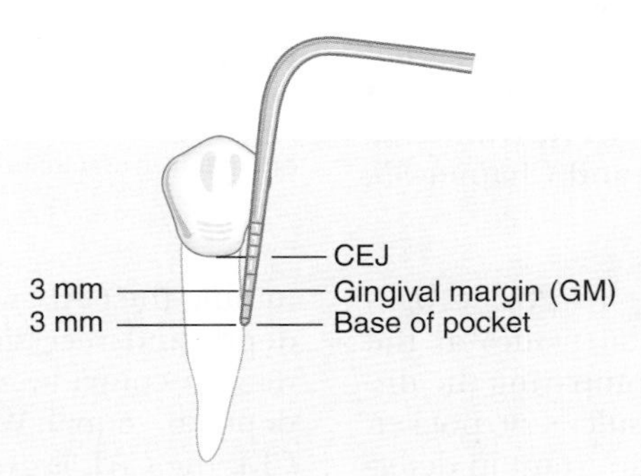

FIGURE 15–26 ✦ Measuring clinical attachment levels. **A,** Gingival margin 3 mm above CEJ. **B,** Gingival margin 3 mm below CEJ (gingival recession).

to the JE. Such measurements are taken using a periodontal probe, and they are a record of past disease activity.

Furcation Involvement (Figures 15–27 and 15–28). Furcation involvement (or loss of attachment between the roots of posterior teeth), is identified, classified, and monitored (Table 15–6). The client is informed about areas of furcation involvement and taught home care techniques to manage these areas. The Nabers furcation probe is often used to detect and measure furcation involvement. Radiographs confirm but do not always reveal this condition. A separate notation indicating the use of the Nabers probe must be made or a serious misunderstanding may result, especially if the furcation reading is mixed up with mobility readings (see Chapter 20, Figure 20–25).

Tooth Mobility. Tooth mobility is the degree to which a tooth is able to move in a horizontal or apical direction. Although caused by the loss of PDL and bone support in periodontitis, tooth mobility varies during the day according to diet and stress. Children, young adults, and some women exhibit more movement than other groups. Tooth mobility, which is not a cause of periodontal disease, may contribute to it. Thus it is assessed along with attachment levels. To test for mobility, the practitioner places an instrument handle on the lingual surface of the tooth and gently pushes on the facial surface with another instrument (e.g., a periodontal probe or mouth mirror). The feeling of movement is most acute at the contact points between two teeth. The classification of mobility should be recorded directly on the dental chart to allow comparative readings at successive appointments (Table 15–7).

Fremitus. *Fremitus* is the vibration or movement of the teeth when in contacting positions. The vibrations result from the client's own occlusal forces. To assess fremitus, the clinician places his or her index finger along the facial aspects of the cervical one-third of each maxillary tooth, and the client is asked to tap the teeth together. The teeth that are displaced are then identified (Table 15–8).

TABLE 15–6 CLASSIFICATION OF FURCATIONS

Class	Description
Class I	Beginning involvement. Concavity of furcation can be detected with an explorer or probe, but it cannot be entered. Cannot be detected radiographically.
Class II	The clinician can enter the furcation from one aspect with a probe or explorer but cannot penetrate through to the opposite side.
Class III	Through-and-through involvement, but the furcation is still covered by soft tissue. A definite radiolucency in the furcation area on a radiograph is visible.
Class IV	A through-and-through furcation involvement that is not covered by soft tissue. Clinically it is open and exposed.

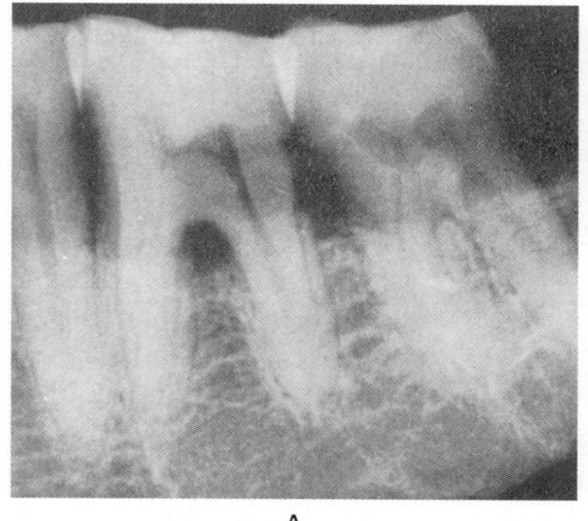

A

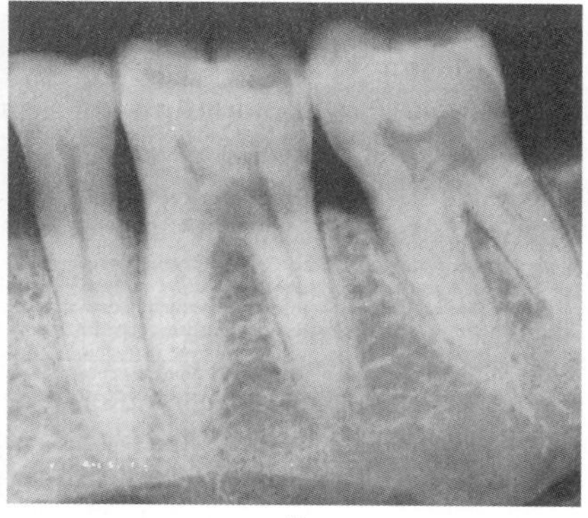

B

FIGURE 15–27 ✦ Furcation involvement. **A,** Triangular radiolucency in bifurcation area of mandibular first molar indicates furcation involvement. **B,** Same area, different angulation. The triangular radiolucency in the bifurcation of the first molar is obliterated, and involvement of the second bifurcation is apparent. *(From Carranza F: Glickman's clinical periodontology, ed 7, Philadelphia, 1990, WB Saunders.)*

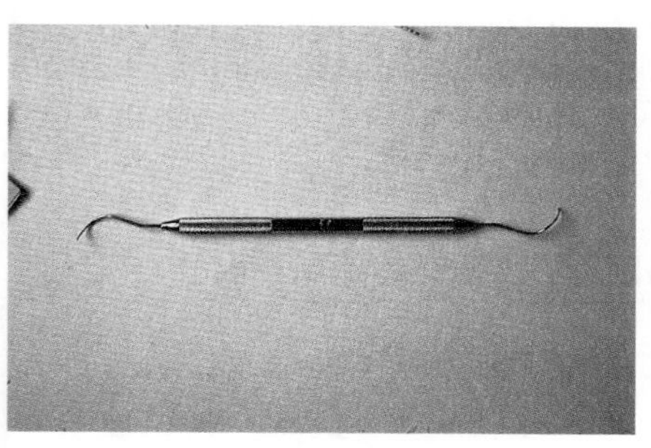

A

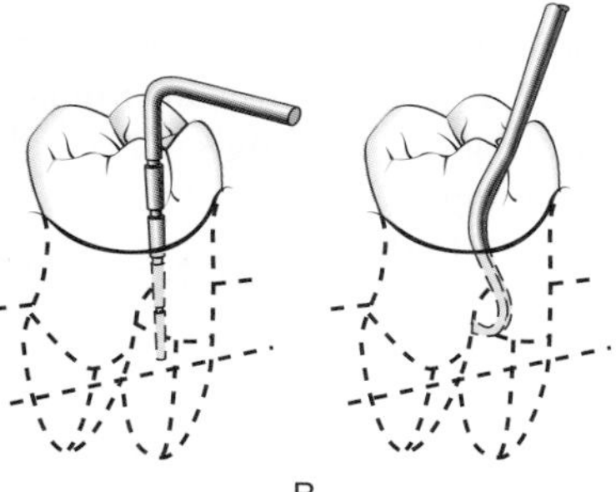

B

FIGURE 15–28 ✦ **A,** Nabers probe. **B,** Exploring with a periodontal probe (*left*) may not detect furcation involvement. Specially designed instruments (Nabers probe) (*right*) can enter furcation area. *(From Newman MG, Takei HH, Carranza FA:* Carranza's clinical periodontology, *ed 9, Philadelphia, 2002, WB Saunders.)*

Occlusal Traumatism. *Occlusal traumatism* is a degenerative, noninflammatory periodontal condition resulting in the destruction of the periodontium because the supporting structures of the teeth cannot withstand the heavy forces. Excessive occlusal force may be from bruxism, clenching, malocclusion, or iatrogenic factors such as a poorly made dental restoration or appliance.

Because clinical signs and symptoms associated with occlusal traumatism often indicate other conditions, use of pulp vitality testing and evaluation of parafunctional habits is indicated.

Occlusal trauma causing destruction of the supporting structures may be primary or secondary:

- *Primary occlusal traumatism* is caused by excessive occlusal forces acting on an otherwise normal periodontium.
- *Secondary occlusal traumatism* is caused by excessive occlusal forces acting on an already diseased periodontium.

Occlusal trauma exacerbates periodontal disease because the supporting structures are already weakened or damaged. Elimination of the etiologic factors of gingivitis and periodontitis comes first, with occlusal therapy a secondary intervention by the dentist.

Mucogingival Conditions (Figure 15–29). Deviations from the normal anatomic relationship between the gingival margin and the MGJ are termed *mucogingival conditions.*[1] Recession, absence or reduction of attached gingiva, and probing depths that reach and extend beyond the MGJ resulting in no attached gingiva are common mucogingival conditions. When pockets extend up to or beyond this point, the area must be monitored closely for the potential of tooth loss because of reduced periodontium and vascular supply to this defect. Conscientious home care and precise root planing are indicated. In the absence of pocket formation, gingival grafts may be performed by the dentist to cover root surfaces with a transplanted piece of gingival tissue from a donor site, such as the palate. In many cases, however, the condition can be maintained nonsurgically. *Frenectomy* is a surgical technique to correct a high frenum attachment associated with pocket formation and mucogingival problems. It is usually performed in conjunction with pocket elimination methods.

Inadequately Attached Gingiva (IAG). Areas with a limited zone of attached gingiva are noted, shown to the client, and explained during the periodontal assessment. To measure the amount of attached gingiva, the clinician uses a periodontal probe to measure the total width of the gingiva from the free gingival margin to the mucogingival junction. Next the periodontal pocket depth is obtained and subtracted from the total width of the gingiva (Figure 15–30). *IAG* is defined as less than 1 mm of keratinized attached gingiva. Areas with IAG are often sensitive, can be difficult to maintain, and can develop into a mucogingival problem because the thin zone of attachment usually reflects a reduced blood supply and a potential for quick loss of supporting bone and connective tissue. Recession and high frena or muscle attachments may add to the reduction of alveolar mucosa. These chronic conditions must be recorded and monitored. Although good oral hygiene can maintain periodontal health with almost no alveolar gingiva, high frenum attachments or the use of the tooth as a crown and bridge abutment may indicate surgical intervention to widen the zone of attached gingiva (Procedure 15–1).

TABLE 15–7 CLASSIFICATION OF MOBILITY

Class	Description
Class I	Tooth can be moved up to 1 mm in any direction.
Class II	Tooth can be moved more than 1 mm in any direction but is not depressible in the socket.
Class III	Tooth can be moved in a buccolingual direction and is depressible in the socket.

TABLE 15–8 CLASSIFICATION OF FREMITUS

Class	Description
Class I	Mild vibration or movement detected
Class II	Easily palpable vibration but no visible movement
Class III	Movement that is clearly visible

Signs of Occlusal Trauma

Clinical Signs

Tooth pain or discomfort on chewing or percussion
Tooth migration
Wear facets exceeding expected levels for the client's age and diet
Fremitus
Chipped enamel
Tooth mobility
Root fracture

Radiographic Signs

Widening of the periodontal ligament space
Loss of lamina dura
Radiolucencies at tooth apices in a vital tooth
Root resorption

RADIOGRAPHIC ASSESSMENT[32–35]

Clinical Use of Radiographs

Periodontal assessment includes diagnostic radiographs. Good-quality radiographs are indispensable in assessing

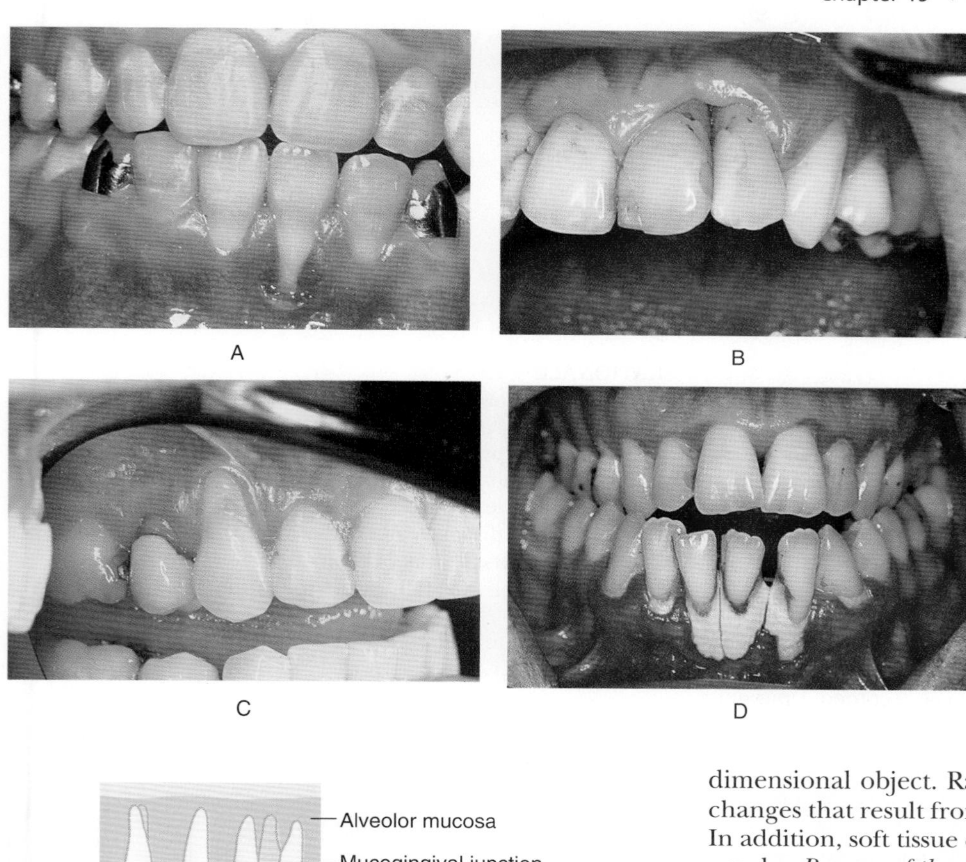

FIGURE 15–29 ✦ Mucogingival defects. **A,** Irregular gingival contours and recession with severe gingival inflammation. **B,** Gingival recession and chronic inflammation with fibrotic tissue. Bottom of the pocket is beyond mucogingival junction. **C,** Recession on maxillary canine with presence of shallow pocket and absence of attached gingiva. **D,** Advanced gingival recession and inflammation caused by heavy plaque and calculus accumulation. *(Courtesy Dr. Kenneth Marinak, Adjunct Clinical Instructor, School of Dental Hygiene, Old Dominion University, Norfolk, Virginia.)*

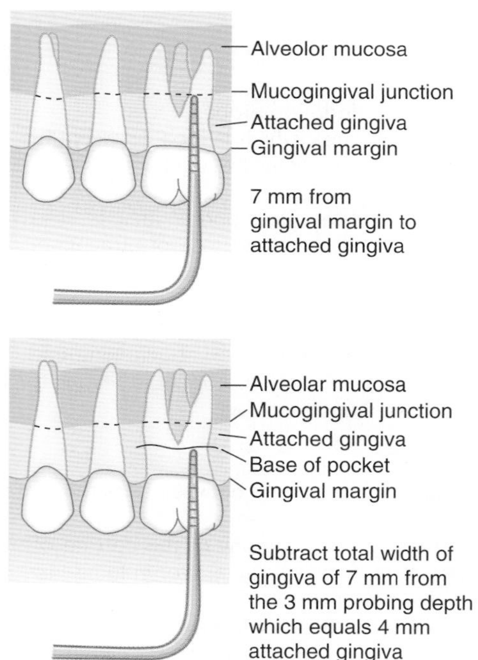

FIGURE 15–30 ✦ Measuring attached gingiva.

the amount of alveolar bone present as well as the pattern, location, and extent of alveolar bone loss. Radiographs are also helpful in identifying local etiologic factors involved in periodontal disease, such as calculus and overhanging restorations (Figure 15–31), as well as dental caries. Not all periodontal defects are visualized on radiographs, however, because the image produced is a two-dimensional representation of a three-dimensional object. Radiographs indicate alveolar bone changes that result from past disease activity, not current. In addition, soft tissue changes are not reflected on radiographs. *Because of these limitations, radiographs must always be used in conjunction with a thorough clinical assessment.*

Before any radiographic examination, a clinical examination and risk assessment of the client are conducted. Care is taken to consider health and dental history, clinical assessment data, safety concerns, and radiographic history when exposing clients to radiation.

Selection criteria have been established for client radiographic exposures (Table 15–9). In general, for new clients who present with generalized signs or history of periodontal disease, a complete intraoral radiographic survey is recommended. When disease is localized, selected periapical or bitewing films should be exposed. Dental office radiographic exposure policies that fail to recognize the individual's risk for oral diseases, but rather require annual or biannual radiographs for everyone, border on malpractice.

Selecting Types and Techniques

Periapical and/or vertical bitewing radiographs should be used to evaluate periodontal disease. Vertical bitewing radiographs are recommended over horizontal bitewings because moderate to severe bone loss cannot be adequately imaged on a horizontal bitewing film. When the long dimension of the film packet is positioned vertically instead of horizontally, the area of bone on the radiograph increases by more than 1 cm (Figure 15–32).

Panoramic projections are not recommended for evaluating periodontal disease. Magnification encountered with this type of image minimizes its usefulness in

Procedure 15–1 PERIODONTAL CHARTING AND ASSESSMENT

EQUIPMENT

Personal protective equipment
Periodontal probe
Nabers probe or other furcation probe
Mouth mirror
Dental light
Red and blue pencils
Compressed air

STEPS	RATIONALE
1. Use direct and indirect lighting, mouth mirror, and compressed air to determine findings (Table 15–2).	For visualizing even minor changes in color, consistency, surface texture, contour, size of the gingiva; for reading the periodontal probe.
2. Use proper client and operator body mechanics.	Improves visualization and comfort, and prevents recurrent trauma injuries.
3. Question client about existing conditions.	Many systemic diseases are linked with periodontal diseases; determines risk status of client.
4. Hold probe with modified pen grasp and establish appropriate fulcrum.	Provides control and stability of the instrument.
5. Gingival recession: Use periodontal probe to determine location of the gingival margin in relation to the CEJ. Recession of 1 mm or greater is to be recorded. Draw gingival margin in blue on chart (Figure 15–26).	Necessary to later determine clinical attachment levels.
6. Frenal involvement: Determine abnormal muscle pull on the gingiva and/or short frenum by drawing a right angle in blue pencil, with the apex occlusally oriented in the area of involvement.	Muscle pull may contribute to recession and inadequate attached gingiva. These areas are at risk of disease progression.
7. Measure periodontal pockets with periodontal probe:	
a. Insert tip to JE and maintain tip against tooth structure.	Ensures accurate periodontal probe depths.
b. Angle the probe slightly on proximal surfaces to reach directly apical to the contact point (Figures 15–22 and 15–23).	Ensures that the col area, which is highly susceptible to periodontal disease, is measured correctly.
c. "Walk" tip along JE in 1-mm increments (Figure 15–20).	Ensures that the entire sulcus/pocket area is assessed and that periodontal pockets and loss of attachment are not overlooked.
d. Recognize when deposits obstruct probe measurement readings and manipulate probe around calculus deposits (Figure 15–21).	Calculus can stop the probe prematurely, underestimating the depth of the periodontal pocket, rendering an inaccurate assessment of probe depths and attachment levels.
8. Record proximal, facial, and lingual readings in excess of 3 mm (+ or – 1 mm) where there is no recession. Where recession is present, record all measurements to reflect CAL.	Ensures that CAL around each tooth that is beyond the normal limit is identified and recorded.
a. Record measurements in blue pencil and circle bleeding points in red.	Allows clinician to differentiate between sites that are healthy and those with active disease.
9. Draw clinical attachment level in red throughout complete dentition.	Displays location and topography of the bottom of the periodontal pockets. Serves as an aid for guiding instrumentation and client instructions.
10. Furcation involvement: Use a Nabers probe to determine which classification of involvement is present (Table 15–6, Figure 15–28).	Avoids overlooking a furcation. Serves as an aid for guiding instrumentation and client instructions.
11. Mobility: Use handles of two instruments to rock the tooth and classify the amount of movement obtained (Table 15–7).	Important for determining long-term prognosis of tooth.
12. Evaluate drifting, extrusion, and malalignment.	Movement of teeth is often associated with periodontitis and mobility.
13. Evaluate areas of food impaction.	Serves as a guide to contributory factors and client instructions.
14. Evaluate open contacts with dental floss.	Serves to identify areas at risk of periodontal disease.
15. Assess fremitus, occlusal disharmonies, and wear facets (Table 15–8).	Helps clinician identify occlusal trauma that may be contributing to the periodontal disease.

Procedure 15–1 PERIODONTAL CHARTING AND ASSESSMENT—CONT'D

STEPS	RATIONALE
16. Gingival examination (on periodontal chart):	Assures evaluation in terms of color, contour, consistency, and surface texture.
a. Record the gingival disease entity, severity, and location (Table 15–5).	
b. Use correct dental terminology when describing severity (slight, moderate, or severe) and location (localized or generalized) (Table 15–5).	Ensures that gingival condition is accurately described and documented.
17. Amount of attached gingiva: Determined by subtracting the depth of the pocket from the distance from the gingival margin to the mucogingival line (Figure 15–30). The difference will be the amount of attached gingiva.	Areas of inadequately attached gingiva must be identified and treated, or else disease progression is likely.
a. Less than 2 mm should be noted as IAG (inadequately attached gingiva).	
b. Less than 1 mm should be noted as NAG (no attached gingiva) in the apical area of the facial aspect of the tooth in red pencil.	
18. Periodontal examination (on periodontal chart):	
a. Record severity of periodontitis (slight, moderate, or advanced). Necessary for planning appropriate professional therapy, self-care interventions, and referral to a periodontist.	Necessary for planning therapy, self-care interventions, and referral to a periodontist.
b. Record location of periodontitis (generalized or localized).	
19. Record disease (gingivitis and/or periodontitis) location and severity under periodontal assessment.	Necessary for planning professional therapy, self-care interventions, and referral to a periodontist.
20. Assign the appropriate periodontal classification number according to the AAP and record (Table 15–11).	Necessary for filing dental insurance forms (see Chapter 23, section on insurance codes).
21. Use appropriate charting symbols (Figure 15–39).	Ensures accurate documentation that can be interpreted over time and by other professionals.
22. Correlate radiographic and clinical readings (Table 15–10).	Assists in diagnosis and documentation of disease.
23. Use appropriate infection control protocols.	Protects clinician, client, and others from disease transmission.
24. Record service in client chart under "services rendered" (e.g., 9/19/03: periodontal and risk assessment complete. Communicated signs of periodontitis to client. Recommended referral to periodontist.)	Provides legal evidence that the standard of care was provided and that client was informed of findings.

(Adapted from the process evaluation form used at the School of Dental Hygiene, Old Dominion University, Norfolk, Virginia.)

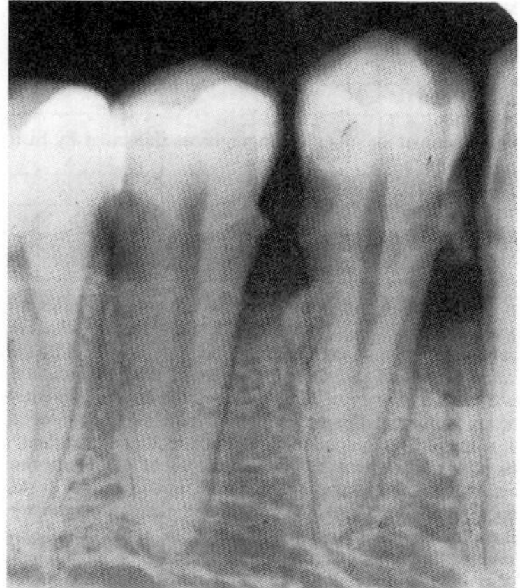

FIGURE 15–31 ✦ Radiograph showing bone destruction and dental caries in the mandibular premolar area. Note heavy calculus and thickening on the lamina dura. *(From Carranza F:* Glickman's clinical periodontology, *ed 7, Philadelphia, 1990, WB Saunders.)*

accurately detecting bone changes. The paralleling technique is recommended for periodontal disease assessment over the bisecting angle technique. The paralleling technique produces standardized films that are more anatomically correct, and the height of the crestal bone appears more accurate. The bisecting angle technique can create a foreshortened image, resulting in a film that may show more or less bone than is actually present.

Radiographic Interpretation

Radiographically determining changes in the alveolar bone associated with periodontal disease is based on the appearance of the crestal lamina dura (Figure 15–33). In health, the crestal lamina dura appears radiographically as a continuous, radiopaque line running parallel to an imaginary line drawn between the CEJs of adjacent teeth. In health, the difference between the normal crest of the alveolar bone and the CEJ can range from 0.4 to 2.9 mm. In general, however, a distance greater than 2 mm from

TABLE 15–9 CLIENT SELECTION CRITERIA FOR PRESCRIBING DENTAL RADIOGRAPHS

CHILDREN			
Primary Dentition (before eruption of first permanent tooth)	**Transitional Dentition** (after eruption of first permanent tooth)	**Adolescents** (all permanent teeth present except third molars)	**Adults**
I. Radiographic examination of new client without previous radiographs*			
Posterior bitewing examination if proximal surfaces of primary teeth cannot be visualized and probed and if child can be expected to cooperate for exposure	Full-mouth examination and posterior bitewings or panoramic examination with posterior bitewings†	Full-mouth examination with posterior bitewings	Full-mouth examination and posterior bitewings‡
II. Radiographic examination of recall client			
A. Caries or other high-risk factors§			
Posterior bitewing examinations at 6-month intervals or until no caries are evident		Posterior bitewing examination at 6- to 12-month intervals or until no caries are evident	Posterior bitewing examination at 12- to 18-month intervals
B. No caries and no other high-risk factors			
Posterior bitewing examination if proximal surfaces of primary teeth can be visualized and probed and if child can be expected to cooperate for exposure; posterior bitewing examination repeated every 12 to 24 months	Posterior bitewing examination every 12 to 24 months	Posterior bitewing examination every 18 to 36 months	Posterior bitewing examination every 24 to 36 months
C. Periodontal diseases or history of periodontal treatment			
Selected periapical or bitewing should be made for those areas where periodontal diseases (except gingivitis) can be demonstrated clinically			
D. To assess growth and development			
	Full-mouth or panoramic examination	Periapical or panoramic radiographs to view third molars	
E. With signs or conditions other than caries or periodontal disease*			
Radiographs as indicated by history, signs, or symptoms			

These guidelines are to be used by the dentist only after a review of the health history and a clinical examination are completed. The recommendations used in the chart are subject to clinical judgment and may not apply to every client, given individual susceptibility, healthcare practice, and experience.

* Clinical situations for which radiographs may be indicated include previous pulpal therapy; deep carious lesions; large or deep restorations; history of pain; evidence of swelling; positive neurologic findings in face and jaws; trauma to teeth, jaws, or lips; mobility of teeth; unexplained bleeding; unexplained sensitivity of teeth; evaluation of sinus condition; unusual spacing or migration of teeth; unusual tooth structure, calcification, or color; evaluation of growth abnormalities or eruption; altered occlusal relationships; aid in diagnosis of systemic disease; familial history of dental anomalies; postoperative evaluation for diagnostic purposes; missing teeth because of unknown history of unexplained absence; localization of foreign bodies within jaws; or evaluation of temporomandibular joint.

† Clinical evidence of periodontal disease (except gingivitis) indicates periapical and bitewing views rather than panoramic.

‡ Full-mouth examination with bitewings is preferred, but panoramics and bitewings may be substituted in the clinical absence of periodontal diseases (except gingivitis).

§ High-risk group includes clients demonstrating any of the following: high level of caries experience, history of recurrent caries, existing poor-quality restorations.

From U.S. Food and Drug Administration: The selection of clients for x-ray examinations: Dental radiographic exposures, HHS Pub No 88-3273, Washington, DC, 1987, US Government Printing Office.

CEJ to bone is considered evidence of disease. An early radiographic change associated with periodontal disease is a fuzziness or break in the continuity of the lamina dura at the mesial or distal aspect of the interdental area. This change results from a loss of crestal density. As the inflammation spreads, a wedge-shaped widening of the PDL occurs, manifesting as a radiolucent area between the tooth and the crestal bone, known as *triangulation*. The V of the wedge of the triangle points apically. As the inflammation spreads deeper into the connective tissue, bone degenerates with a subsequent reduction in bone height.

The pattern of bone loss is described as either horizontal or vertical. The CEJ of adjacent teeth can be used to determine bone loss. If teeth are erupted at varying levels or if they are tilted, the lamina dura crest will be slanted to match the variation in crown level. The normal slanting may be confused with bone loss (Figure 15–34).

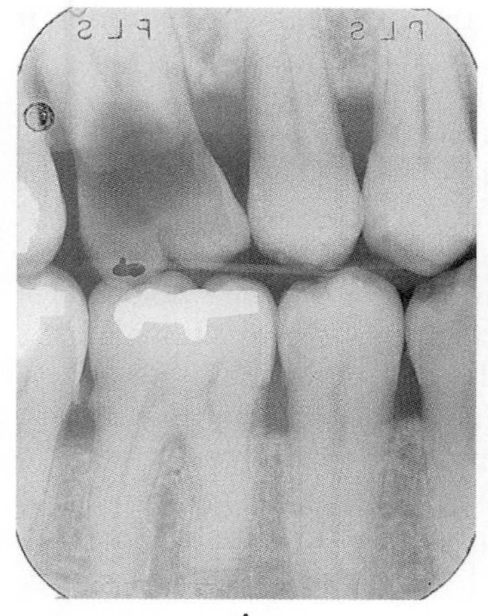
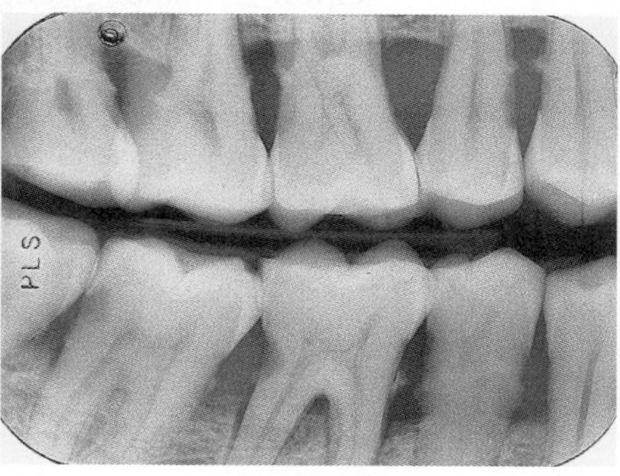

A B

FIGURE 15–32 ✦ **A,** Vertical bitewing radiograph. **B,** Horizontal bitewing radiograph.

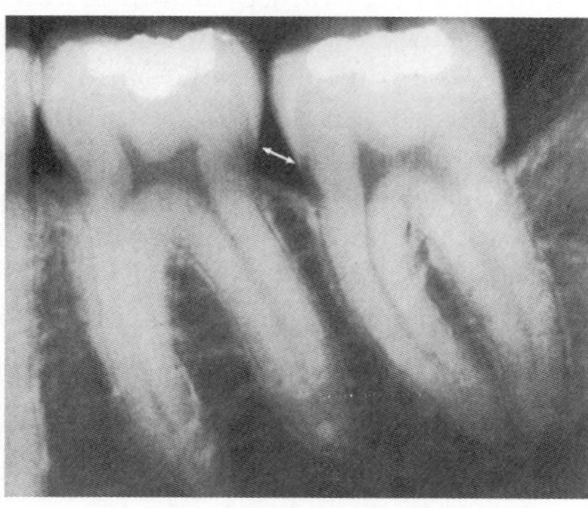

FIGURE 15–33 ✦ Crest of interdental septum normally parallel to a line drawn between the cementoenamel junction of the adjacent teeth (*arrow*). Note the radiopaque lamina dura around the roots and interdental septa. *(From Carranza FA, Newman MG:* Clinical periodontology, *ed 8, Philadelphia, 1996, WB Saunders.)*

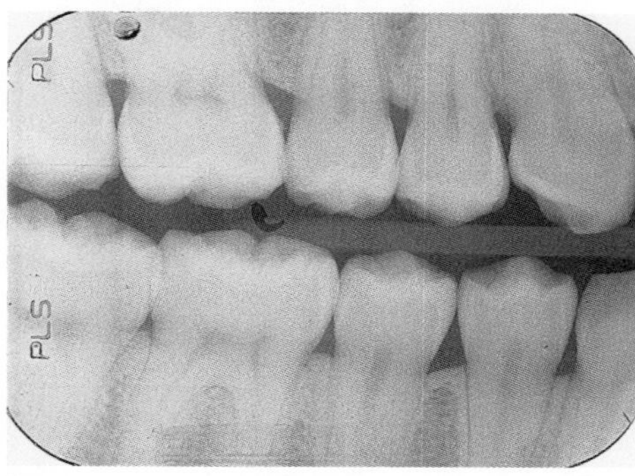

FIGURE 15–34 ✦ Normal bone slanting on teeth numbers 2, 3, 4, and 5; often confused with bone loss.

✦ If the bone loss is parallel to the CEJ of adjacent teeth, *horizontal bone loss* is present (Figure 15–35, *A*).
✦ When the bone height is oriented diagonally to the CEJ of adjacent teeth, *vertical bone loss* is present (Figure 15–35, *B*).

Bone loss typically does not occur uniformly throughout the mouth; loss in one area may be more severe than in another. The distribution of bone loss is described as *localized* or *generalized.* With localized destruction, bone loss occurs in a few areas; in generalized destruction, bone loss is distributed throughout the mouth.

The severity of bone loss is described as *mild, moderate,* or *severe.* The severity is assessed as a percentage loss of the normal amount of bone. To obtain the percentage loss, the radiograph and probe are used to measure the total root length (from the CEJ to the root apex). Next, the distance from the CEJ to the alveolar crest is determined. The percentage of bone loss is a ratio of these two measurements (the distance from the CEJ to alveolar crest divided by total root length). For example, a 6-mm distance from the CEJ to the crest of the bone with a 15-mm root length would equal a 25% loss of bone (6 mm divided by 15 mm). Table 15–10 correlates percentage of bone loss to the severity of periodontal disease.

Furcation Involvement (Figure 15–28)

Radiographs may be used to detect alteration in the furcations of multirooted teeth. When the bone in the furcation area is destroyed, it will appear as a radiolucency in the furcal area. Importantly, lack of radiolucency in the furcation does not mean that the disease has not spread to the area. Clinical examinations must always be implemented to ensure a true representation of furcation involvement. Exposing radiographs at differing angles may also assist in radiographically detecting furcation involvement.

Limitations of Radiographs

A major limitation of radiographs is that they reveal less severe bone loss than what is actually present. Early bone changes are not visible radiographically. Typically 30% of the bone mineral must be destroyed before it can be seen on a radiograph. *Clinically, radiographs confirm oral findings.* For example, if the dental hygienist obtains probing depth readings of 2 to 3 mm but observes bone loss on

A

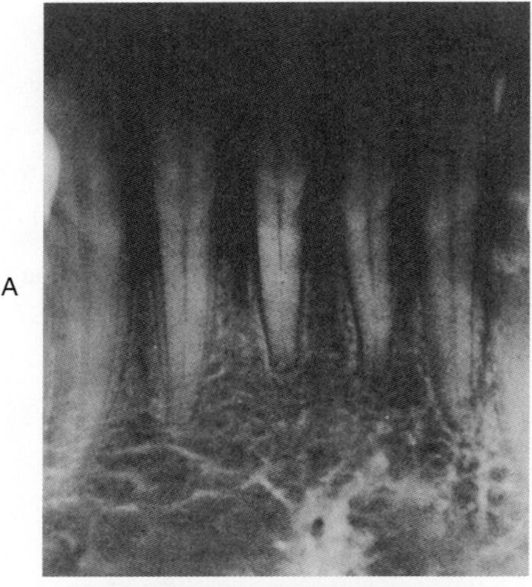

B

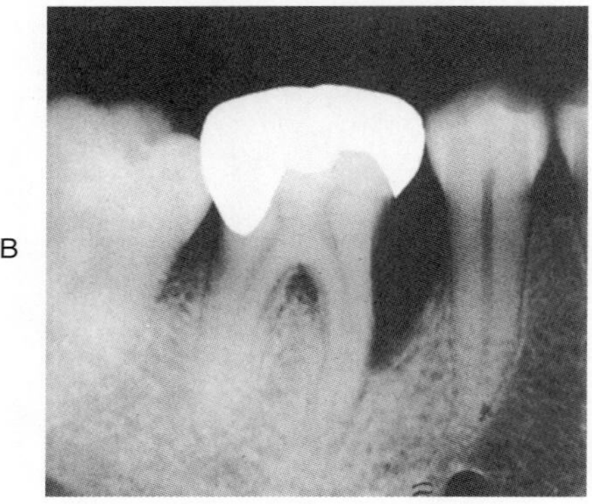

FIGURE 15–35 ✦ **A,** Horizontal bone loss around mandibular anterior teeth. Note thickening of periodontal ligament space and lamina dura. **B,** Vertical bone loss on the mesial surface of the first molar. Note also the furcation involvement. *(From Carranza FA, Newman MG:* Clinical periodontology, *ed 8, Philadelphia, 1996, WB Saunders.)*

TABLE 15–10 RELATIONSHIP BETWEEN PERIODONTAL DISEASE SEVERITY AND RADIOGRAPHIC FINDINGS

Disease	Radiographic Evidence
Gingivitis	No bone loss
Slight periodontitis	Less than 30% bone loss
Moderate periodontitis	30 to 50% bone loss
Severe periodontitis	More than 50% bone loss

the radiograph, probing depth measurements should be rechecked. In this case the radiographs provide a check of clinical findings for periodontal probing.

Radiographs provide a serial record of the client's periodontal status, affording a basis for comparison with new findings. Radiographs show the history of disease progression, allowing the dental hygienist to follow bone levels over time. As a part of periodontal risk assessment, absence of bone loss is associated with a lower risk of future periodontal destruction; however, the presence of bone loss on a radiograph does not indicate that the client will experience continued destruction; rather it indicates an increased risk of future bone loss.

Standardized radiographs of like projections are most helpful in making longitudinal comparisons and providing objective documentation of clinical findings. For example, periapical projections of posterior teeth should not be compared with subsequent bitewing radiographs because an accurate comparison of the bone level cannot be made with two different projection angles. Periodontal probing depths and other clinical findings are subjective assessments, but radiographs present objective data that two or more clinicians can observe at the same time.

Limitations of radiographs in periodontal assessment are as follows:

- Projection factors such as cone-to-film distance, angulation, technique, and film positioning can distort or obscure radiographic images. For example, healthy alveolar bone is evenly located 1 mm apical to the tooth's CEJ, and the alveolar crest should parallel an imaginary line drawn from the CEJ of one tooth to the CEJ of the adjacent tooth. In the radiographic view, this bone position may be distorted by x-ray angulation, suggesting vertical bone loss.
- Exposure errors such as cone cuts and imbalance of kilovolt peak (kVp) and milliamperage (mA) disguise anatomy and pathosis. Proper exposure of the complete dental and bitewing series utilizes the widest range of contrast (grays) so that minute changes in bone density and mineralized calculus are visualized. Increased kVp and lower mA produce this broad contrast range and reduce exposure time for the client, but this combination also lengthens processing time. Shortened processing time decreases contrast and reduces diagnostic information for the clinician.
- Facial and lingual supporting bone are not visualized because they are obscured by the radiodense tooth structure. Therefore, facial and lingual bone loss cannot be detected from radiographs.
- Early interdental bone loss is not detectable on radiographs because horizontal alveolar bone loss may not be seen until 30% of the original bone height and density is lost. By the time one sees it radiographically, the bone loss is so far advanced that it is easily detected clinically by probing.
- Bony interdental craters, resulting from vertical bone loss, are not well imaged because facial and lingual ridges of the teeth may be superimposed, and because the dense facial and lingual walls of bone obscure the crater. Interdental craters, therefore, are detected only with the periodontal probe.
- Radiographs do not show soft tissues or connective tissue attachment and consequently cannot show soft tissue changes. Pockets cannot be measured from radiographs except by using radiopaque markers, such as a periodontal probe or silver point placed at the depth of the sulcus before exposure.

- Although such radiographic images as a "moth-eaten" alveolar crest, a discontinuous lamina dura, increased trabeculation, and a thickened PDL space are suggestive of periodontal abnormality, they are not indicators of periodontitis.
- Normal anatomy can be mistaken for abnormalities on radiographs. Darkened or radiolucent areas, such as the mental and incisive foramina located in apical regions, may masquerade as lesions.
- Although all teeth are radiographically examined for the presence of calculus, films are not the best indicators of calculus. Only highly mineralized deposits may be seen as radiopacities on the radiograph.

In general, however, the radiographic examination is helpful in observing many conditions related to overall periodontal status.

Digital Radiography[35]

Digital radiography uses intraoral sensors and a radiation source to display radiographic images on a computer monitor following client exposure (Figure 15–36). A sensor, which is available in a variety of sizes, is positioned in the client's mouth in place of dental film (Figure 15–37). This method of producing radiographic images requires no chemicals for developing, thus eliminating processing supplies and equipment. Trips to the darkroom to develop and retrieve films are eliminated. Treatment is not interrupted for development of digital radiographic images as with the use of conventional radiographs. Rather, with digital radiography, images are displayed on a computer monitor within seconds of a client's exposure. A major advantage of digital radiography is reduced client exposure to ionizing radiation by 60% to 80% when compared to E-speed film.

A direct digital imaging system requires a radiation source, typically a conventional dental x-ray unit with the timer modified, an intraoral sensor, and a computer monitor. The sensor is covered with a protective barrier before intraoral placement. Sensor-holding devices similar to traditional film-holding devices used for the paralleling technique are recommended. Figure 15–38 displays a full-mouth series of radiographs on a computer monitor.

Digital imaging has 256 colors of gray compared to the 16 to 25 shades of gray found with conventional dental x-ray film. Thus diagnosis can be improved with enhanced image contrast. When used as a part of the periodontal assessment, diagnostic decision making is improved by the excellent images of the lamina dura, bone trabeculation, calculus, furcation involvement, and bone levels that are produced with minimal distortion.

Digital subtraction, another aspect of digital imaging, can improve diagnostic information by comparing a previously stored image with a current image. Subtraction radiography eliminates distracting background information. Radiographs, taken at different times throughout the course of disease or treatment, can be compared by subtracting one image from another. The similar areas of the two films will cancel each other out, leaving a neutral gray appearance, whereas changes will be highlighted. Areas of bone loss will appear darker gray, and areas of bone gain will be isolated as lighter gray.

By removing all structures that do not exhibit change between radiographic examinations, differences can be easily identified. Using digital radiography during periodontal assessment provides excellent opportunities for

Periodontal Conditions Observed on Radiographs

Normal anatomy and the tooth crown-to-root ratio
Confirmation of clinical findings and topography of root surfaces
Status of the lamina dura
Remaining bone height
Changes of PDL space
Local irritants such as calculus and overhanging restorations
Pattern or extent of the disease
Possible furcation involvement
Disease progression or remission by serial radiography

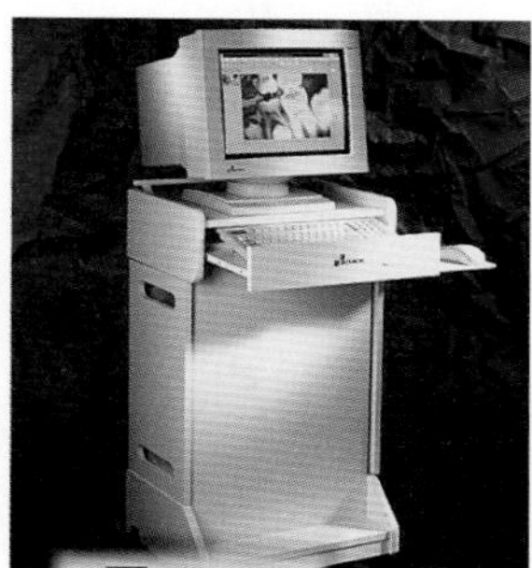

FIGURE 15–36 ✦ Digital dental radiography system. *(Courtesy Schick Technologies.)*

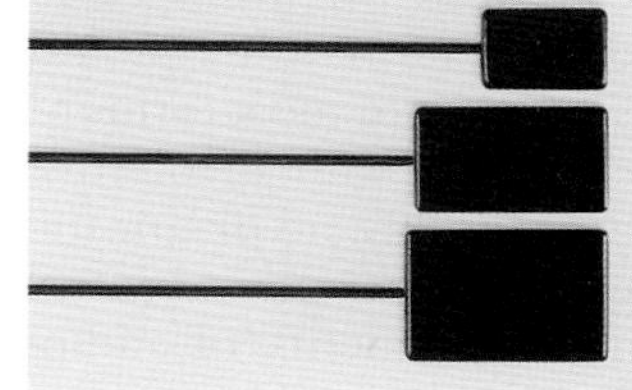

FIGURE 15–37 ✦ Three sizes of sensors for adult and primary dentitions. *(Courtesy Schick Technologies.)*

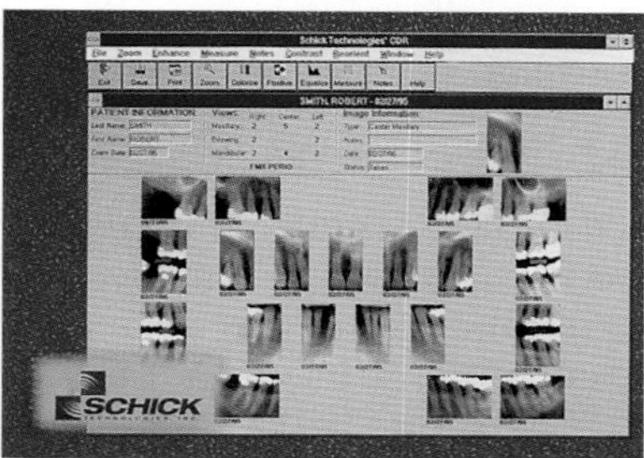

FIGURE 15–38 ✦ Full-mouth series of radiographs displayed in computer monitor using digital technology. *(Courtesy Schick Technologies.)*

immediate client discussion, education, and consultation because of the almost-instantaneous images that result. Images can be manipulated to change and improve the contrast and enlarged or zoomed for enhanced viewing. This manipulation of the image affords opportunities to focus on particular client conditions and improve client education, interaction, understanding, and compliance.

Importantly, digital radiography systems can be integrated with dental office software. Clinicians can electronically archive the dental images and transmit them via modem to insurance companies and specialists. Network-configured workstations allow radiographic images to be accessed by clinicians at any time from a variety of locations.

The disadvantages of digital radiography include initial startup costs, which can exceed $10,000; the bulky sensor, which may result in more client discomfort than with dental x-ray film; and the inability to heat-sterilize the sensor. Controversy surrounds the image quality and image manipulation, which may present legal concerns in lawsuits.

ASSESSMENT OF PERIODONTAL DISEASE ACTIVITY[25–27]

Periodontal disease progression is the pathologic process in which connective tissue attachment at the most apical portion of a periodontal pocket is destroyed. Related to this attachment loss is the apical migration of the JE and resorption of alveolar bone. Progression of most forms of periodontitis appears to be associated with qualitative changes in the subgingival flora. Currently, no diagnostic tests can identify progressing or active periodontitis lesions other than longitudinal assessments of radiographs and probing attachment levels. Many tests designed for this purpose will be marketed in the future, however. Before purchasing these tests, only valid data from well-controlled studies justify their use.

Measure of Attachment Loss[36]

An increase in the distance measured from the CEJ to the base of the sulcus or pocket currently is the best measure for disease progression. Flaws in this measure are related to the fact that the probe's penetration can vary with its thickness, the insertion force, and the degree of inflammation in the tissues. In addition, it is difficult to position the periodontal probe in exactly the same position from one appointment to another. These limitations are minimized by using standardized equipment and techniques.

Clinical Signs of Inflammation

Redness, swelling, bleeding on probing, and suppuration have relatively good diagnostic value. Two long-term studies found that sites without BOP were almost certain not to show further loss of attachment. Of sites that did bleed on probing at four consecutive visits, 30% lost 2 mm or more of probing attachment. Whereas BOP may have some clinical value as an indicator of increased risk of progression, the continuous absence of BOP is a reliable indicator that periodontal health will be maintained.

MICROBIOLOGIC ASSESSMENT OF SUBGINGIVAL PLAQUE[37]

Several bacteria have been suggested as possible periodontopathogens (Table 15–1). Which of these organisms, singly or in groups, is responsible for the progression of periodontitis is not known. Nevertheless, sufficient research exists to implicate these microorganisms as potential periodontopathogens, so that methods have been devised to detect their presence in subgingival flora as a measure of disease activity. Such testing is limited, however, because the tests do not project progression of disease or identify specific types of periodontal diseases. Therefore, microbial testing in clients with chronic periodontitis is not recommended. Microbiologic assessments may prove useful in high-risk clients when there is the suspected presence of unusual microorganisms and in aggressive forms of periodontal disease when treatment interventions may include antibiotics. But even with a complete understanding of the specific microbes responsible for the disease, the treatment for it changes very little. Methods of microbiologic assessment include:

- ✦ Microbiologic cultural analysis
- ✦ Immunologic methods
- ✦ DNA probes
- ✦ Bacterial enzymatic activity test

Microbiologic Cultural Analysis

A sample of subgingival plaque is collected and cultured in the laboratory to determine the presence of specific microorganisms—marker bacteria—associated with the progression of periodontitis (e.g., *Actinobacillus actinomycetemcomitans* and *Porphyromonas*). The advantage of *microbiologic testing* is its ability to determine antibiotic susceptibility and resistance; however, this method is time-consuming, costly, and relies on living bacterial samples that must be specially handled to survive transport to the laboratory. Consequently this test is not readily used in private practice settings.

Immunologic Methods

Antibodies specific for particular bacterial species are applied to plaque samples, and antibody–antigen reactions are detected by a variety of methods, such as direct and indirect immunofluorescence, rapid enzyme immunoassay, and latex agglutination tests. Although direct and indirect immunofluorescence is valuable as a research tool, it requires considerable expertise and expense to perform in evaluating plaque samples.

DNA Probes

Fragments of bacterial DNA are used in hybridization reactions to "probe" for complementary DNA in subgingival plaque samples. In-office tests are available, but these tests cannot be used to determine antibiotic sensitivity. Only organisms for which tests are sensitive can be identified.

Bacterial Enzymatic Activity Test

Chemicals that indicate the presence of enzymes produced by periodontopathogens are applied to plaque samples. These tests identify the presence of a group of pathogenic bacteria by detecting tissue-destructive enzymes. Such tests may have value in detecting relative levels of certain periodontopathogens; however, their use in practice is limited because they do not identify specific bacterial species and are unable to determine antimicrobial susceptibility.

PERIODONTAL INDICES

There are many ways of quantifying periodontal health. If the dental hygienist is to survey the prevalence of periodontal disease in a particular population (epidemiologic research), it is important to use indices employed by other researchers so that the results can be compared. If the intent is to assess a single individual's periodontal status for the purpose of developing a dental hygiene care plan, however, it is important to select a method that is simple, cost-effective, and easily understood (see Chapter 14, Criteria for Determining an Effective Dental Index).

Indices Used in Client Care

Indices are used to motivate clients to improve their self-care behaviors and to provide an easily understood numerical score for comparison between visits. Once scores are calculated over time, clients can identify changes and improvements in their periodontal health. The Gingival Index (GI) and the Plaque Index (PlI) are easy to use in clinical practice (Table 15–11 and Chapter 14, Table 14–3).

A limitation of indices is that each index usually measures only one variable, and thus the GI (Silness and Loe) provides information about the presence and severity of gingival inflammation in a population at a given time, but it provides no information about the cause of the inflammation. In contrast, the PlI (Podshadley) does provide information on the location and thickness of plaque (the cause of the inflammation), but does not provide information about inflammation (Table 14–3). Moreover, indices that measure the same variable often do not have the same focus. For example, the thickness of plaque is important in the Silness and Loe GI, but not in the Turesky modification of the Quigley-Hein Index (Table 15–11). Note that few teeth are evaluated during use of an index, perhaps missing a problem area in a client's mouth.

Indices Used in Research

Periodontal indices are used in epidemiology to quantify the prevalence and incidence of disease and oral debris in specific populations.

- *Prevalence* refers to the number of cases existing at a specific point in time per specified number of persons. For example, the statement "52% of 1328 college baseball athletes reported using dental floss daily" is a statement of floss use prevalence.
- *Incidence* refers to the number of new cases or diseases per specified number of persons occurring in a specified period of time, typically one year. For example, the statement "40,000 new cases of periodontitis were diagnosed in the United States from 1992 to 1993" is a statement of incidence.
- *Severity* refers to how much destruction is present at one time. For instance, 5 mm of CAL is a standard often used to indicate the need for periodontal treatment.

Periodontal and oral hygiene indices are also used in research to serve as outcome measures when testing the efficacy of approaches to care, such as when an antimicrobial toothpaste is tested to determine its effectiveness in preventing periodontal disease.

Popular periodontal indices used in research are listed in Table 15–11. Usually a subset of teeth described by Ramfjord is used in evaluating groups of people. Based on large-scale studies, Ramfjord determined that measurement of six teeth (numbers 3, 9, 12, 19, 25, 28) was representative of those for the entire dentition. These six teeth are called the Ramfjord teeth and have been applied to the use of many indices.[27] When data are collected on a few representative teeth, the index is called "simplified." Methods of substitution are always calibrated in the simplified index. In some studies missing teeth are not counted, and in others the clinician is required to substitute missing teeth with the next most distal tooth. Other indices require substitution by going mesially or across the arch to the contralateral tooth. More than one index is often needed.

It is essential to calibrate examiners before using any oral index for research purposes. With regard to measuring probing depths, examiners are considered calibrated if each one's measurements are within 1 mm, plus or minus, of the others. Some plaque indices require that disclosing solutions be applied and rinsed away after application, whereas others require no rinsing or the use of no disclosant. Whether in research or practice, the dental hygienist should standardize all aspects of data gathering to increase the likelihood of comparable results.

Procedures for use may vary with different indices (Table 15–11). The Community Periodontal Index of Treatment Needs (CPITN) is of special interest because it provides information on periodontal status as well as treatment needs. A special periodontal probe with color-coded gradations, designed for this index, has a 0.5-mm ball tip to prevent severing of JE and to allow some tactile sensation as the clinician probes the tooth surface in the pocket. Shallow pockets, represented by reporting a sulcus less than a color-coded gradation from 3.5 to 5.5 mm, indicate that no special treatment is needed. Deeper pockets measuring within the color gradation require therapeutic scaling. The deepest pockets, where the color-coded gradation cannot be seen (more than

TABLE 15–11 PERIODONTAL INDICES

Index/Purpose	Procedure for Use	Rating Score/Interpretation
Community Periodontal Index of Treatment Needs (CPITN) (Ainamo, 1982) To assess priorities for periodontal treatment of an individual or a group	For adults (20 years and older), divide the dentition into sextants. Evaluate all teeth except third molars. For children and adolescents (7-19 years of age), divide dentition into sextants but evaluate only first molars in posterior; right central incisor in maxilla; and left central incisor in mandibular anterior. Use WHO periodontal probe (CPITN-E probe) marked at 3.5-, 2.0-, 3.0-, and 3.0-mm intervals from the tip with color coding between 3.5 and 5.5 mm and a ball 0.5 mm in diameter at the working tip. Criteria used: Code 0 = Healthy periodontal tissues Code 1 = Bleeding after gentle probing Code 2 = Supragingival or subgingival calculus or defective margin of filling or crown Code 3 = 4- or 5-mm pocket Code 4 = 6-mm or deeper pathologic pocket Mark one score to represent each sextant. Record only highest code that corresponds with most severe condition. Clients are classified (0, I, II, III) into treatment needs according to the highest coded score recorded during the examination.	Calculations of the number and percentage of individuals with the following can be made: a. No sextant scoring each code b. 1 to 2 sextants scoring code 1, 2, 3, or 4 c. 3 to 4 sextants scoring code 1, 2, 3, or 4 d. 5 to 6 sextants scoring code 1, 2, 3, or 4 0 = No need for treatment (code 0) I = Oral hygiene instruction (code 1) II = Oral hygiene instruction plus scaling and root planing, including elimination of plaque retentive margins of fillings and crowns (codes 2 and 3) III = I + II + complex periodontal therapy that may include surgical intervention and/or deep scaling and root planing with local anesthesia (code 4)
Gingival Index (GI) (Loe and Silness, 1963) To assess gingival inflammation based on color, consistency, and bleeding on probing; based on the assumption that a slight color change is indicative of gingival inflammation	A score of 0 to 3 is assigned to mesial, distal, buccal, and lingual surfaces of teeth numbers 3, 9, 12, 19, 25, and 28. A blunt instrument, such as a periodontal probe, is used to assess bleeding potential based on the following criteria: 0 = Normal gingiva 1 = Mild inflammation: slight change in color, slight edema. No bleeding on probing 2 = Moderate inflammation: redness, edema, and glazing. Bleeding on probing 3 = Severe inflammation: marked redness and edema. Ulceration. Tendency to spontaneous bleeding Totaling scores around each tooth yields GI score for area; divide by 4, score for tooth is determined. Totaling all scores and dividing by number of teeth examined provides GI score per person. Can be used on selected or all erupted teeth.	0.0 = No gingivitis (excellent) 0.1 to 1.0 = Mild gingivitis (good) 1.1 to 2.0 = Moderate gingivitis (fair) 2.1 to 3.0 = Severe gingivitis (poor)
Periodontal Index (PI) (Russell, 1967) To measure the overall periodontal condition from health, gingival inflammation, to advanced destruction of the periodontium	Score for each individual is obtained by arriving at a score for mesial, distal, facial, and lingual surfaces of all teeth in the mouth, adding the scores, and dividing by the total number of teeth. Criteria used: 0 = Negative: neither overt inflammation in the investing tissues nor loss of function due to destruction of supporting tissues 1 = Mild gingivitis: an overt area of inflammation in the free gingiva, but this area does not circumscribe the tooth 2 = Gingivitis: inflammation completely circumscribes tooth, but there is no apparent break in epithelial attachment 4 = Not used in the field study 6 = Gingivitis with pocket formation: epithelial attachment has been broken and there is a pocket (not merely a deepened gingival crevice caused by swelling in the free gingivae). No interference with normal masticatory function; tooth is firm in its socket and has not drifted 8 = Advanced destruction with loss of masticatory function: tooth may be loose; may have drifted; may sound dull on percussion with a metallic instrument; may be depressible in its socket	0.0 to 0.2 = Clinically normal 0.3 to 0.9 = Gingivitis 0.7 to 1.9 = Incipient destructive disease 1.5 to 5.0 = Established destructive disease 3.8 to 8.0 = Terminal states of disease

TABLE 15–11 PERIODONTAL INDICES—CONT'D

Index/Purpose	Procedure for Use	Rating Score/Interpretation
Periodontal Disease Index (PDI) (Ramfjord, 1967) To measure the extent of periodontal disease (i.e., assesses gingivitis, gingival sulcus depth, calculus, plaque, occlusal and incisal attrition mobility, and lack of contact)	Six teeth are examined: numbers 3, 9, 12, 19, 25, and 28. Criteria used: 0 = Absence of inflammation 1 = Mild to moderate inflammatory gingival changes not extending all around tooth 2 = Mild to moderately severe gingivitis extending all around tooth 3 = Severe gingivitis, characterized by marked redness, tendency to bleed, and ulceration 4 = Gingival crevice in any of 4 measured areas (mesial, distal, buccal, lingual), extending apically to CEJ but not more than 3 mm 5 = Gingival crevice in any of 4 measured areas extending apically to CEJ (3-6 mm) 6 = Gingival crevice in any of four measured areas extending apically more than 6 mm from CEJ PDI score is obtained by totaling scores of the teeth and dividing by number of teeth examined	Group score of 3.5 = Severe gingivitis for epidemiologic purposes. Care must be taken when interpreting the PDI on an individual basis.
Sulcus Bleeding Index (SBI) (Muhlemann and Son, 1971) To assess clinical signs of inflammation; based on the assumption that bleeding on probing is the first clinical sign of inflammation	Four gingival units are scored on each tooth: the marginal gingiva, labial and lingual (M units), and the papillary gingiva, mesial and distal (P units). Probe each of the four areas. Hold probe parallel with long axis of the tooth for M units and direct probe toward the col area for P units. Wait 30 seconds after probing and score using the following criteria: 0 = Healthy appearance of P and M, no bleeding on sulcus probing 1 = Apparently healthy P and M showing no change in color and no swelling, but bleeding from sulcus on probing 2 = Bleeding on probing *and* change of color caused by inflammation. No swelling or macroscopic edema 3 = Bleeding on probing *and* change in color and slight edematous swelling 4 = Bleeding on probing *and* change in color *and* obvious swelling; or bleeding on probing and obvious swelling 5 = Bleeding on probing and spontaneous bleeding *and* change in color, marked swelling with or without ulceration Scores for the four units are totaled and divided by 4. By totaling scores for individual teeth and dividing by the number of teeth, the SBI is determined.	Scores may range from 0 to 5: 0 = Health 5 = Severe gingival inflammation
Eastman Interdental Bleeding Index (Caton and Polson, 1985) To assess interdental gingival bleeding and enable the clinician and client to monitor interproximal gingival health	All interdental gingival areas are examined 0 = Absence of bleeding when a triangular toothpick is horizontally depressed 2 mm interproximally four times, and checked 15 seconds later 1 = Bleeding after above procedure	Yields a score that reflects the percentage of bleeding sites. The higher the percentage of bleeding sites, the more generalized the interdental bleeding.

5.5 mm), require complex treatment, described as scaling and root planing under local anesthesia, with or without surgical exposure for access.

Sextants of the mouth or the full mouth can be assessed by the CPITN, but in epidemiologic studies only 10 teeth are examined. Only the worst score per sextant is recorded. This approach may underestimate the number of deep pockets in older adult populations that generally have many areas of attachment loss and overestimate shallow pockets in younger age groups that have many healthy sulci. Other periodontal indices are shown in Table 15–11; oral hygiene indices can be found in Chapter 14, Table 14–3.

DOCUMENTATION AND RECORDKEEPING (see Chapter 54)

The dental hygienist evaluates information collected throughout the assessment phase of care and records all pertinent findings at each appointment. Such records allow the hygienist to monitor the effects of the client's personal oral hygiene efforts, the progress of healing after professional care, and the status of periodontal health. Data collected on periodontal and oral hygiene status facilitate assessment of several client human needs: skin and mucous membrane integrity of the head and neck, a biologically sound and functional dentition, responsibility for oral health, and conceptualization and understanding.

Recordkeeping includes efficient recording of and access to important information. The format should be brief, complete, comprehensible, and permanent. Legal and insurance regulations require thorough documentation of the client's periodontal and general health status at each visit. Documentation protocols should be based on current information related to plaque accumulation and to the following anatomic changes: inflammation, attachment levels (probing depth and gingival recession), furcation involvement, tooth mobility, the width of alveolar gingiva, mucogingival problems, and bone loss determined from radiographs. Records must demonstrate the dental hygienist's awareness of the client's periodontal and general health status to legal authorities, as well as to the client.

The record must provide a form for documentation of the baseline or initial data collected about the client. This form should be carefully organized before the client is seen, so that all required data are included and there is one standard location for the information. A well-organized record form eliminates having to search for more details or for critical information, thus signaling inadequate recordkeeping to the client or to the health-care professionals with whom the dental hygienist collaborates. At subsequent client visits, changes in the baseline conditions are further documented, and these data are compared with baseline information. Diligent recordkeeping is the key to tracking frequency of care, disease episodes, client response, and the success rate of interventions. Trend analysis is based on comparing findings with the baseline data and is as critical to the practitioner as it is to the researcher.

Noting conditions beyond normal limits, or variations from previous conditions, allows for analysis of trends. Longitudinal evaluation is critical for providing optimal care and for meeting third-party requirements for periodontal data on client needs and treatment outcomes. Moreover, objective notations of client perceptions, needs, and desires alert other personnel of special considerations and facilitate oral health education and continuity of care.

Documentation

Periodontal status is monitored from appointment to appointment. Findings of inflammation, recession, pocket probe readings, aberrant tissue forms, bleeding, suppuration, minimum attached gingiva, tooth mobility, and furcation involvement are recorded. Initially, complete six-point probing measurements are recorded for each tooth; however, only changes can be recorded at subsequent visits. The practitioner is able to identify an improvement or disease progression by comparing assessment parameters and charting data from visit to visit. Comparison of notations facilitates diagnosis, care planning, and monitoring by the oral care team.

The documentation form should list factors that may negatively affect the outcome of care. For example, the dental hygienist notes when gingival inflammation, disease progression, and healing may be affected by risk factors. Client noncompliance, tardiness, cancellations, and missed appointments also are recorded to demonstrate that the client may be responsible for a less than satisfactory result (contributory negligence).

Recordkeeping Formats

Recorded findings provide a graphic display of the client's periodontal health status. Figure 15–39 is an example of a chart showing gingival margin and probing measurements. Recession is visualized by the gingival margin. Other codes, such as for mobility, are added to the form, using the criteria described in the Classification of Mobility chart (Table 15–7), and bleeding is specified by circling probe readings in red.

DECISION-MAKING MATRIX

Figure 15–40 illustrates a decision-making matrix used in providing dental hygiene care. Decisions are the result of objective clinical and radiographic information collected and recorded during the assessment phase of dental hygiene care, the current research evidence base, and collaboration with the dentist and the client. Objective assessment data can be further evaluated in follow-up assessments.

The health, dental, pharmacologic, and personal history information influence choice of treatment modalities. For example, the host defense mechanisms and presence of systemic disease may compromise care results, as can nutritional status, substance use, medications, oral habits, and emotional factors. Client motivation and degree of assumption of responsibility also affect self-care instruction and therapeutic outcomes. Such factors are considered in the decision-making process.

Dental factors such as occlusal trauma and oral appliances also influence the outcome of care (e.g., occlusal trauma may exacerbate periodontal disease). Orthodontic treatment often entails trauma to gingival tissue and compromises oral hygiene. In addition, each situation needs to be assessed to identify the client's per-

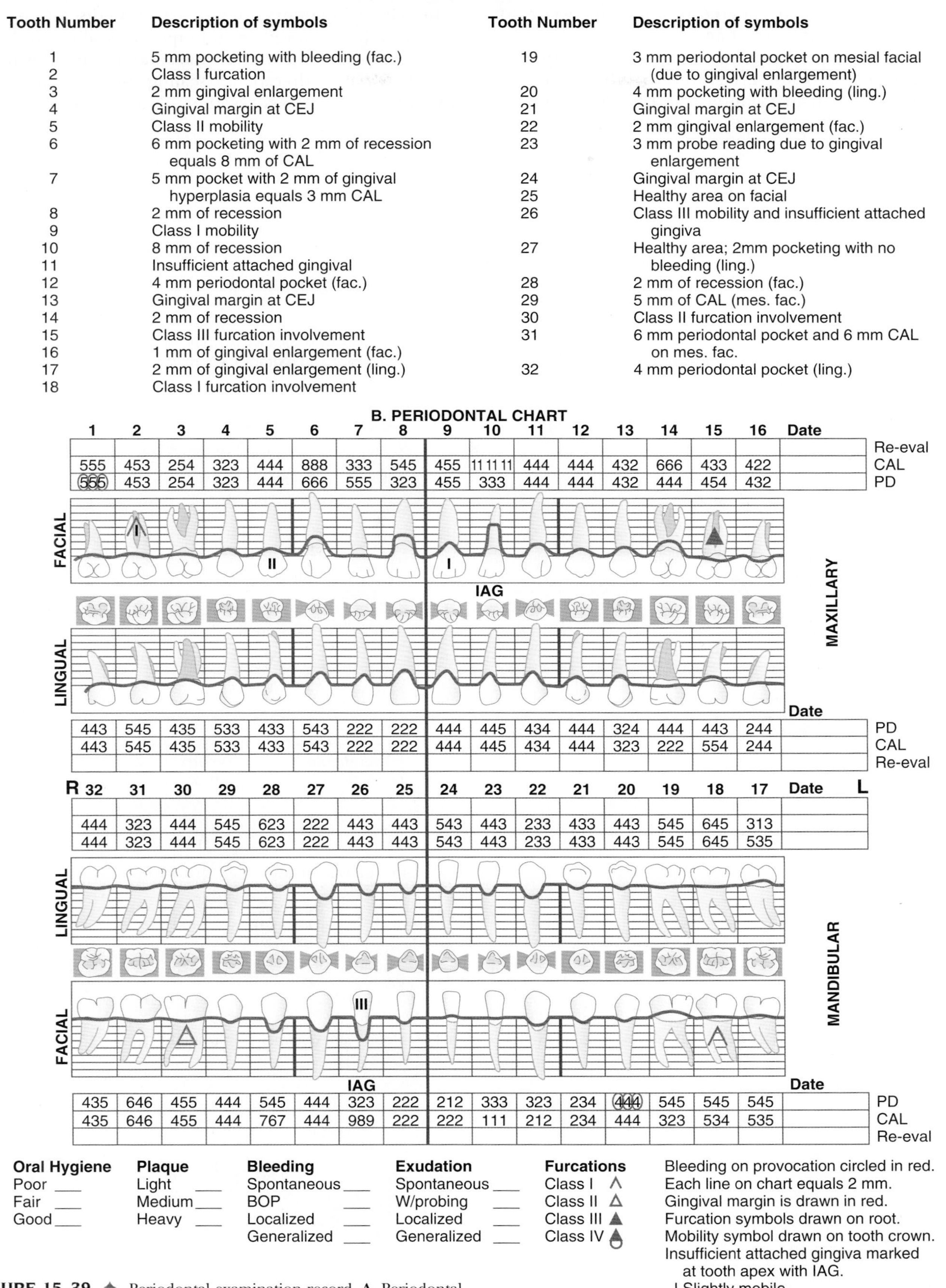

A. PERIODONTAL CHARTING CODE

Tooth Number	Description of symbols	Tooth Number	Description of symbols
1	5 mm pocketing with bleeding (fac.)	19	3 mm periodontal pocket on mesial facial (due to gingival enlargement)
2	Class I furcation	20	4 mm pocketing with bleeding (ling.)
3	2 mm gingival enlargement	21	Gingival margin at CEJ
4	Gingival margin at CEJ	22	2 mm gingival enlargement (fac.)
5	Class II mobility	23	3 mm probe reading due to gingival enlargement
6	6 mm pocketing with 2 mm of recession equals 8 mm of CAL	24	Gingival margin at CEJ
7	5 mm pocket with 2 mm of gingival hyperplasia equals 3 mm CAL	25	Healthy area on facial
8	2 mm of recession	26	Class III mobility and insufficient attached gingiva
9	Class I mobility	27	Healthy area; 2mm pocketing with no bleeding (ling.)
10	8 mm of recession	28	2 mm of recession (fac.)
11	Insufficient attached gingival	29	5 mm of CAL (mes. fac.)
12	4 mm periodontal pocket (fac.)	30	Class II furcation involvement
13	Gingival margin at CEJ	31	6 mm periodontal pocket and 6 mm CAL on mes. fac.
14	2 mm of recession	32	4 mm periodontal pocket (ling.)
15	Class III furcation involvement		
16	1 mm of gingival enlargement (fac.)		
17	2 mm of gingival enlargement (ling.)		
18	Class I furcation involvement		

B. PERIODONTAL CHART

	1	2	3	4	5	6	7	8	9	10	11	12	13	14	15	16	Date
Re-eval																	
CAL	555	453	254	323	444	888	333	545	455	11 11 11	444	444	432	666	433	422	
PD	555	453	254	323	444	666	555	323	455	333	444	444	432	444	454	432	

	1	2	3	4	5	6	7	8	9	10	11	12	13	14	15	16	Date
PD	443	545	435	533	433	543	222	222	444	445	434	444	324	444	443	244	
CAL	443	545	435	533	433	543	222	222	444	445	434	444	323	222	554	244	
Re-eval																	

R	32	31	30	29	28	27	26	25	24	23	22	21	20	19	18	17	Date L
	444	323	444	545	623	222	443	443	543	443	233	433	443	545	645	313	
	444	323	444	545	623	222	443	443	543	443	233	433	443	545	645	535	

	32	31	30	29	28	27	26	25	24	23	22	21	20	19	18	17	Date
PD	435	646	455	444	545	444	323	222	212	333	323	234	444	545	545	545	
CAL	435	646	455	444	767	444	989	222	222	111	212	234	444	323	534	535	
Re-eval																	

Oral Hygiene	Plaque	Bleeding	Exudation	Furcations
Poor ___	Light ___	Spontaneous ___	Spontaneous ___	Class I ∧
Fair ___	Medium ___	BOP ___	W/probing ___	Class II △
Good ___	Heavy ___	Localized ___	Localized ___	Class III ▲
		Generalized ___	Generalized ___	Class IV

Bleeding on provocation circled in red.
Each line on chart equals 2 mm.
Gingival margin is drawn in red.
Furcation symbols drawn on root.
Mobility symbol drawn on tooth crown.
Insufficient attached gingiva marked at tooth apex with IAG.
I Slightly mobile
II Greater than 1 mm
III Tooth can move in all directions

FIGURE 15–39 ✦ Periodontal examination record. **A,** Periodontal charting code. **B,** Periodontal chart. *(Courtesy School of Dental Hygiene, Old Dominion University, Norfolk, Virginia.)*

ception of his or her needs, the level of dexterity in plaque control, and the degree of anatomic access for professional and self-maintenance.

The levels of nonsurgical periodontal therapy that the dental hygienist provides are shown in Table 15–12 and explained in detail in Chapter 23. The data collected during the periodontal assessment determine the appropriate level of care to be recommended to the client. If eliminating inflammation and arresting disease progression can be achieved by therapeutic scaling and root planing, then no further periodontal treatment is necessary. If, however, therapeutic scaling and root planing fail to achieve these objectives, then periodontal surgery may be necessary.

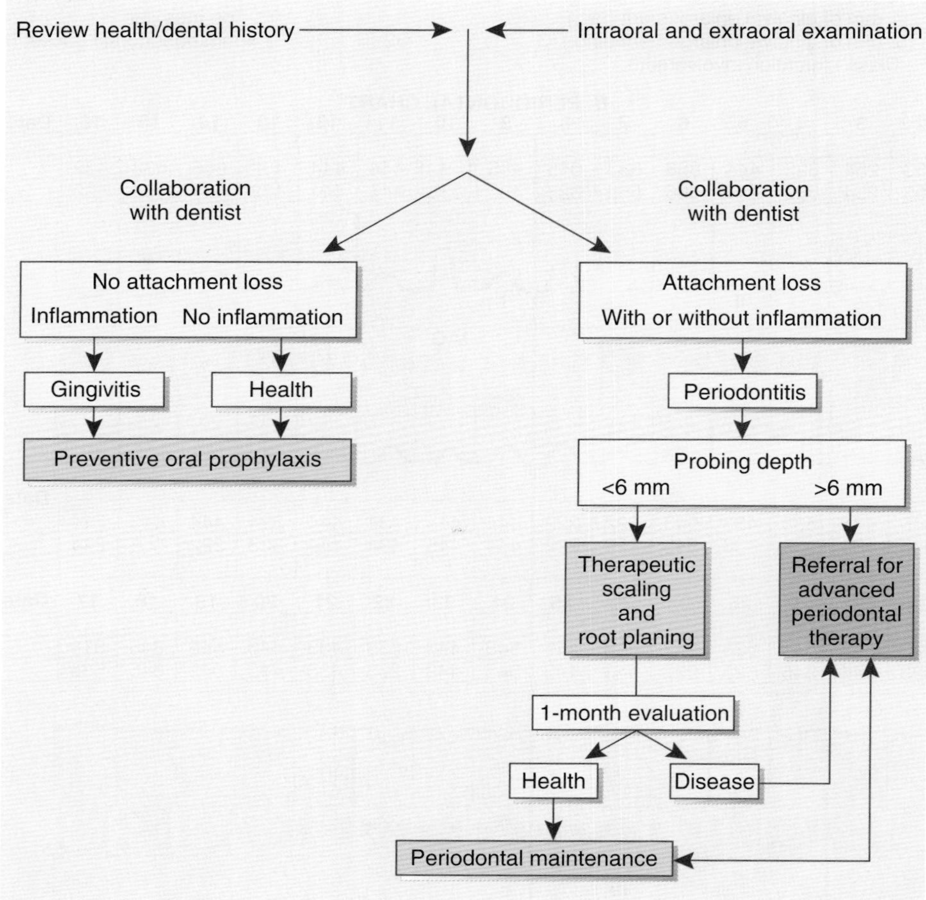

FIGURE 15–40 ✦ Decision tree for periodontal assessment and treatment of the adult.

TABLE 15–12 PROFESSIONAL MECHANICAL DENTAL HYGIENE CARE MODALITIES

	Preventive Oral Prophylaxis	Therapeutic Scaling and Root Planing	Professional Periodontal Maintenance Care
Objective	To prevent/control gingivitis	To treat periodontitis; to achieve connective tissue reattachment	To maintain attachment level and periodontal health in individuals who have been treated for periodontitis
Continued care interval	3 to 6 months or as needed	1 month evaluation; repeat as needed	3 to 4 months or as needed
Dental hygiene action*	Scaling to remove calculus, extrinsic stain, and bacterial plaque to promote a healthy oral environment	Scaling and root planing to eliminate microorganisms, endotoxins, and calculus to reduce inflammation, promote connective tissue regeneration, and make root surface biologically acceptable to gingival tissues	Closely monitors periodontal status, scaling, and root planing to prevent return of pathogenic subgingival microflora
Required time	Usually one appointment	Several appointments (up to 8 hours) with use of a local anesthetic	One appointment

* Includes assessment of oral health behaviors and client education.

Client Education Issues

- ✦ Importance of a comprehensive periodontal examination and risk factor assessment.
- ✦ Clinical appearance of healthy gingiva, periodontal pocket readings, bleeding on probing and other signs of disease prepares clients to participate knowledgeably in care and is fundamental for teaching self-examination techniques.
- ✦ Development of client's ability to self-monitor clinical signs of oral disease.
- ✦ Relationship of periodontal health to overall health, especially with regard to cardiovascular diseases, diabetes, pregnancy, and respiratory disease. *Risk estimates are useful when explaining the relationship between periodontal disease and systemic disease to clients.*
- ✦ Explanation of periodontal risk factors to enhance client understanding of personal degree of risk for periodontal disease or disease progression.
- ✦ Importance of self-care interventions and regular professional care to maintain periodontal health.

Legal, Ethical, and Safety Issues

- ✦ Comprehensive periodontal assessment is a critical component of dental hygiene assessment and risk management.
- ✦ Documentation of all clinical and radiographic oral findings related to health, at both the initial visit and all subsequent continued-care visits, is vital to evidenced-based decision making, care planning, referral, and evaluation of clinical outcomes.
- ✦ Periodontal assessment findings need to be communicated to clients so they have an understanding of their current periodontal disease status and potential risk for future periodontal disease, based on their degree of risk
- ✦ Information from the periodontal assessment provides the basis for client informed consent.

KEY CONCEPTS

- Individual susceptibility to periodontal disease varies widely.
- Periodontal risk factors modulate periodontal disease susceptibility and influence the onset, progression, and severity of periodontal disease.
- The most significant periodontal risk factors are smoking, poor oral hygiene, genotype-positive status, and diabetes mellitus.
- Systemic conditions can increase a client's susceptibility to periodontitis, and periodontitis may increase a client's susceptibility to certain systemic conditions such as cardiovascular disease, respiratory disease, and diabetes mellitus.
- The origin of periodontal disease is strongly linked to three periodontal pathogens: *Actinobacillus actinomycetemcomitans, Porphyromonas gingivalis, and Bacteroides forsythus.*
- Clinical signs of inflammation, clinical attachment levels, probing depths, and radiographs are the primary indicators for assessing periodontal health and determining diagnosis and treatment.
- Gingivitis is inflammation of the gingiva with no loss of clinical attachment.
- Gingival color, contour, consistency, and texture vary in health and disease.
- Although most forms of gingivitis are plaque-induced, host and systemic factors modify the clinical characteristics of the disease. Hence the two classifications of gingival diseases: dental plaque-induced gingival diseases and non–plaque-induced gingival lesions.
- Periodontitis is inflammation of the supporting structures of the teeth and gingiva with resulting loss of clinical attachment and alveolar bone.
- The host immunoinflammatory response is responsible for tissue destruction in periodontal disease.
- Absence of bleeding on probing is a sign of periodontal health.
- Gingival bleeding occurring at several sequential continued-care visits is associated with an increased risk for periodontal destruction.
- Radiographs reveal the amount of alveolar bone present and the pattern, extent, and loss of bone.
- Because of the limitations of radiographs, they must always be used in conjunction with a thorough clinical assessment.
- Vertical bitewing radiographs are recommended over horizontal bitewings for evaluation of periodontitis.
- Attachment loss over time, not periodontal pocket depths, indicates periodontal disease progression.
- Periodontitis is cyclic in nature, with extended periods of quiescence (inactivity) followed by short periods of exacerbation (disease activity).
- Microbiologic assessment of subgingival plaque has minimal value in clinical practice settings.
- Documentation of periodontal assessment findings at every visit is essential for accurate diagnosis, periodontal disease management, and risk management.

Critical Thinking Exercises

SYNOPSIS OF CLIENT HISTORY	
Age: 62 years **Gender:** Female **Height:** 5' 6" **Weight:** 180 lb **Race:** Pacific Islander	**VITAL SIGNS** **Blood Pressure:** 130/80 mm Hg **Pulse Rate:** 80 bpm **Respiration Rate:** 15 rpm
1. **Under care of a physician:** Yes / No **Conditions:** Coronary heart disease 2. **Hospitalized within the last 5 years:** Yes / No **Reason:** Back surgery 3 years ago 3. **Has or had the following conditions:** high blood pressure, basal cell carcinoma on face 4. **Current medications:** Cardizem, Advil 5. **Smokes or uses tobacco products:** Yes / No	**Health History:** Last medical exam was three weeks ago when the client had an evaluation for her angina history. Client reports an allergy to tetracycline. **Dental History:** Last dental visit was two years ago when a prophylaxis was completed. Client remembers being told she had periodontal disease. She brushes with a hard-bristled toothbrush and uses fluoride toothpaste. She just started flossing daily. **Social History:** Client lives with her husband and works as a receptionist at a senior center. Client complains about being on a limited income and is concerned about how she can afford dental treatment. She reports smoking more than one pack of cigarettes per day. **Chief Complaint:** "My mouth is sore when I brush. I don't like the stains on my teeth and my gums bleed a lot when I brush."

Supplemental Examination Findings. Client reports she had a full-mouth series of radiographs exposed two years ago. Clinical examination reveals severely inflamed gingiva in the maxillary anterior area and a whitish coat to the gingival margin in the posterior areas with moderate enlargement. Heavy subgingival calculus is found throughout the mouth.

Periodontal assessment reveals generalized 5-mm pocket depths in all posterior areas, 6-mm pocket depths in the maxillary lingual area, and 4-mm pocket depths in all other areas; 3-mm recession on teeth numbers 7, 27, and 28. Use the case information to answer the following questions:

1. List at least four periodontal risk factors for this client. Identify which risk factors are modifiable and those that are nonmodifiable.
2. Explain why this client has a whitish coating on the marginal gingiva in the posterior areas.
3. What would be the best type of radiographs to expose on this client?
4. Based on the periodontal assessment findings, what would be the attachment level on teeth numbers 28 and 29?
5. How would you classify this client's periodontal disease: slight, moderate, or severe?
6. What is the most likely explanation for the increased pocket depths found in the maxillary lingual area?
7. Explain to this client the link between periodontitis and coronary heart disease. Role play this dialogue with one of your peers.
8. Explain to your client the role of the host response in the tissue destruction observed in periodontal disease. Role play this dialogue with one of your peers.
9. How would you determine if this client had mucogingival involvement in any areas?

For References, Suggested Readings, and Related Websites, visit
http://evolve.elsevier.com/Darby/hygiene/

SECTION 4

Dental Hygiene Diagnosis, Care Plan, and Evaluation

CHAPTER 16

DENTAL HYGIENE DIAGNOSIS

OBJECTIVES

Mastery of the content in this chapter will enable the reader to:

- Explain the dental hygiene diagnostic process.
- Differentiate between a dental hygiene diagnosis and a dental diagnosis.
- Cite advantages of using the dental hygiene diagnosis.
- Write dental hygiene diagnostic statements.
- Identify interventions that support various dental hygiene diagnoses.
- Apply human need theory to diagnostic decision making.

KEY TERMS

At-risk problem
Diagnosis
Defining characteristics (signs and symptoms)
Dental diagnoses
Dental hygiene diagnosis
Dental hygiene diagnostic classification
Diagnostic process
Oral health condition
Unmet human needs (human need deficits)

DIAGNOSIS DEFINED

A *diagnosis* is an analysis of the cause and nature of a problem, condition, or situation.[1] The diagnostic process is generic but can be applied to specific disciplines. A diagnosis becomes discipline-specific when it is applied to the practice of that discipline. The dental hygienist diagnoses client conditions within the scope of dental hygiene to prevent oral disease, minimize the risk of oral disease, and promote wellness.

Miller introduced the concept of the dental hygiene diagnosis to describe the expression of dental hygiene judgment and decision making.[2] The dental hygiene profession has accepted diagnosis as part of the dental hygienist's role. The American Dental Education Association's *Competencies for Entry into Dental Hygiene,* the American Dental Hygienists' Association's *Code of Ethics,* and the Commission on Dental Accreditation's *Standards for Dental Hygiene Education Programs* all address the dental hygiene diagnosis.[3-5]

DENTAL HYGIENE DIAGNOSIS

A *dental hygiene diagnosis* is a clinical decision made by a dental hygienist that identifies an actual or potential human need deficit that the dental hygienist is educated and licensed to treat, and/or to refer for care. A dental hygiene diagnosis:

- Focuses on client conditions, behaviors, or risk factors related to oral health and disease.
- Derives from client data collected during assessment.
- Requires interventions within the scope of dental hygiene practice.
- Is necessary for planning and implementing effective dental hygiene care and evaluating its outcomes.

Therefore, after completing the assessment phase of the dental hygiene process, the diagnostic process begins (Figure 16–1). Making a dental hygiene diagnosis includes identifying:

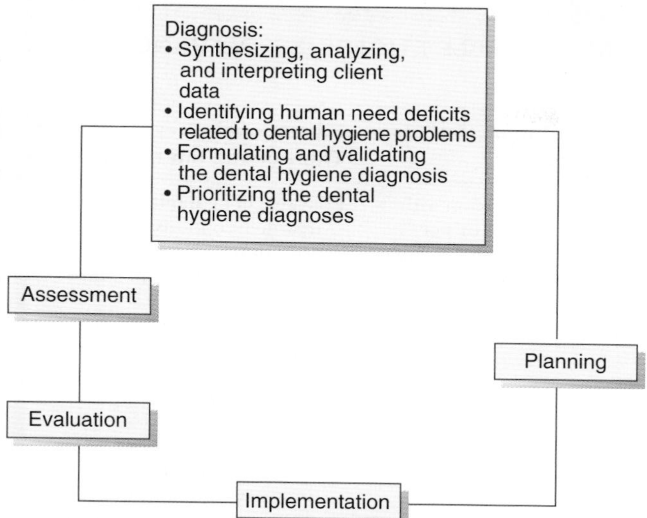

FIGURE 16–1 ✦ The concept of diagnosis within the dental hygiene process. The term *dental hygiene diagnosis* is used to describe actual or potential oral health problems that can be prevented or resolved by dental hygiene interventions.

- ✦ Unmet human needs that can be met through dental hygiene care
- ✦ Factors contributing to or causing the unmet human needs (etiologies and risk factors)
- ✦ Evidence to support the dental hygiene diagnosis (signs and symptoms)

In making a dental hygiene diagnosis, the dental hygienist works within the scope of dental hygiene practice. Hence the dental hygiene diagnostic process requires a concrete understanding of the scope of dental hygiene and collaboration between the dental hygienist and dentist.[6]

Historically, dental hygienists were cautioned to not diagnose, but to identify dental problems and then communicate their observations using phrases such as:

Mr. Jones has *suspicious* areas on teeth numbers 14, 19, and 32.

Ms. Smith has *signs* of gingival and periodontal disease around teeth numbers 22 to 26.

There *appears* to be a radiolucent area at the apex of tooth number 8.

Such observations are neither dental nor dental hygiene diagnoses and create confusion for the client. If state law permits preliminary diagnostic services provided by the dental hygienist, the dental hygienist could say:

Mr. Jones, my preliminary diagnosis suggests dental caries on several of your teeth; the final dental diagnosis must be made by the dentist.

Ms. Smith, the periodontal probing depths of 5 to 7 mm, mobility of 2, and bleeding around the lower front suggest moderate periodontitis; however, the final diagnosis must be confirmed by the dentist.

TABLE 16–1 DENTAL HYGIENE DIAGNOSIS VERSUS DENTAL DIAGNOSIS

Dental Hygiene Diagnosis	Dental Diagnosis
Identifies an unmet human need (human need deficit)	Identifies a specific oral disease
Identifies conditions or problems (unmet human needs) within the scope of dental hygiene practice	Identifies conditions or problems for which the dentist directs the primary treatment
Often deals with the client's perceptions, beliefs, attitudes, and motivations regarding his or her own oral status	Often deals with the actual pathophysiologic changes
May change as the client's responses and behaviors change	Remains the same for as long as the disease is present

Mrs. Carson, your son has a radiolucent area on the root tip of his top front tooth suggesting a pathologic condition; however, a dental diagnosis must be made by the dentist.

When a dental hygienist identifies oral disease, such as gingivitis or early periodontitis, this is called a *preliminary diagnosis,* which must be referred to a dentist for a definitive diagnosis and treatment or for possible delegation by the dentist back to the dental hygienist for nonsurgical periodontal care. When the client manifests signs and symptoms of oral conditions that require treatment by a dentist, a dental referral is indicated for quality client care and for the legal protection of the dentist, dental hygienist, and client.

Dental Hygiene Diagnosis Versus Dental Diagnosis

Legal, professional, and social responsibilities require clear distinctions between a dental hygiene and a dental diagnosis. Diagnostic decision making and therapeutic care fall within precise legal and professional boundaries. *Dental diagnoses* identify diseases or conditions for which the dentist directs or provides the primary treatment; dental hygiene diagnoses identify *unmet human needs* (also known as *human need deficits*) that can be met by dental hygienists within the scope of dental hygiene practice. Both types of diagnoses serve different purposes as related to the professional's scope of practice (Table 16–1).

Dental Hygiene Diagnostic Classifications[7] (Table 16–2)

Diagnosis is a critical thinking and decision-making process by which clinical data about the client are analyzed and assigned a diagnostic label. Therefore, making diagnoses requires a classification system for naming the diagnosis. Currently, a classification of eight possible diagnoses creates a standardized language for identifying client oral health conditions amenable to dental hygiene

TABLE 16–2 DENTAL HYGIENE DIAGNOSES: THEIR DEFINITIONS, POSSIBLE ETIOLOGIES, DEFINING CHARACTERISTICS, AND INTERVENTIONS

Dental Hygiene Diagnosis	Causes/Etiologies	Signs and Symptoms (Defining Characteristics)	Educational, Preventive, and Therapeutic Interventions
Wholesome Facial Image: The need to feel satisfied with one's own oral-facial features and breath.	Acquisition of oral prosthesis Visible dental disease or disorder Halitosis Malocclusion Acquisition of orthodontic appliances	Client reports dissatisfaction with the appearance of his or her teeth, gingiva, facial profile, or breath.	Educate client about dental treatment options such as orthodontics or dental implants to eliminate body image stressors. Refer client to a general dentist, periodontist, prosthodontist, or orthodontist for care beyond the scope of dental hygiene practice. Encourage client to seek other support systems to deal positively with body image stressors, such as individual counseling and group therapy.
Protection from Health Risks: The need to avoid medical contraindications to dental hygiene care, and includes the need to be protected from health risks related to dental hygiene care	Participation in sports Improper use of oral healthcare product Educational or knowledge deficit Paresthesia, anesthesia Oral habit Potential for infection Potential for oral injury Concern about infection control, radiation safety, fluoride safety, previous negative experience Risky lifestyle behaviors	Evidence on health history for immediate referral to, or consultation with, a physician regarding uncontrolled diseases (e.g., signs of cardiac problem, signs of uncontrolled diabetes, or abnormal vital signs) Evidence of need for antibiotic premedication because of heart murmurs, heart valve replacement, joint replacement, or organ transplant Evidence that client is at risk for oral injury (e.g., plays a contact sport without an athletic mouth protector or has impaired eyesight, tremor, or limited dexterity) Evidence that client is at risk for oral or systemic disease Evidence that client is in a life-threatening situation	Assess client need for precautions during care. Work to prevent emergencies from occurring. Discuss dental hygiene care plan with the client. Address safety factors with the client. Use current standards for infection control, radiation safety, and fluoride therapy.
Biologically Sound and Functional Dentition: The need to have intact teeth and restorations that defend against harmful microbes, provide adequate function, and reflect appropriate nutrition and diet	Nutrition and diet Mutable and nonmutable risk factors Educational deficit Inadequate self-monitoring Lack of regular dental care	Teeth with signs of disease Missing teeth Defective restorations Teeth with abrasion or erosion Teeth with signs of trauma Ill-fitting prosthetic appliances Chewing difficulty	Teach clients strategies for maintaining healthy teeth, including nutritional strategies. Advocate for a healthy dentition. Refer to a general dentist when dental caries or dental dysfunction is evident.
Skin and Mucous Membrane Integrity of Head and Neck: The need to have an intact and functioning covering of the person's head and neck area, including the oral mucous membranes and periodontium, which defend against harmful microbes, resist injurious substances and trauma, and reflect adequate nutrition	Inadequate oral health behaviors Inadequate nutrition Mutable and nonmutable risk factors Use of tobacco Inadequate control of a systemic disease (e.g., diabetes, HIV) Lack of regular dental care	Presence of extra/intraoral lesions, tenderness, or swelling; gingival inflammation Bleeding on probing; probing depths or attachment loss greater than 4 mm; mucogingival problems Presence of xerostomia, with accompanying oral mucous membranes that are not uniform in color Oral manifestations of nutritional deficiencies	Perform periodontal debridement, chemotherapy to control plaque biofilm and gingivitis. Refer client to a specialist (e.g., periodontist, nutritionist). Provide dietary assessment and counseling for oral disease. Discuss link between periodontal health status and systemic health.

TABLE 16–2 DENTAL HYGIENE DIAGNOSES: THEIR DEFINITIONS, POSSIBLE ETIOLOGIES, DEFINING CHARACTERISTICS, AND INTERVENTIONS—CONT'D

Dental Hygiene Diagnosis	Causes/Etiologies	Signs and Symptoms (Defining Characteristics)	Educational, Preventive, and Therapeutic Interventions
Freedom from Head and Neck Pain: The need to be exempt from physical discomfort in the head and neck area.	TMJ discomfort Oral surgery, dental procedure, dental hygiene procedure Untreated dental disease Inadequate access to care/ lack of regular dental care	Extra/intraoral pain or sensitivity before commencing dental hygiene care Tenderness on palpation during the extra/intraoral examination Discomfort during dental hygiene care	Refer client to the dentist for immediate care/pain relief. Initiate pain control strategies that will ensure the client's comfort (e.g., reassurance, utilization of desensitizing agents, skillful instrumentation techniques). Administer topical and local anesthetic agents, or nitrous oxide–oxygen analgesia.
Freedom from Anxiety and Stress: The need to feel safe and to be free from fear and emotional discomfort in the oral healthcare environment	Past negative dental experience Fear of the unknown Lack of financial resources	Client fear Client has concern about confidentiality, cost of care, disease transmission, fluoride toxicity, mercury toxicity, radiation exposure, or dental hygiene care planned.	Provide reassurance. Use desensitizing agents. Perform instrumentation techniques with care and gentleness. Use a topical anesthetic agent, local anesthesia and/or nitrous oxide–oxygen analgesia.
Responsibility for Oral Health: The need for accountability for one's oral health as a result of interaction between one's motivation, physical capability, and environment.	Nonadherence/ noncompliance Uses oral care aids or products inappropriately Need for parental supervision of oral hygiene Partial self-care deficit Total self-care deficit Skill deficit Impaired physical, mental ability Inadequate oral health behaviors Lack of financial resources	Client presents with inadequate plaque control. Inadequate parental (guardian) supervision of child's daily oral hygiene regimen Inadequate self-monitoring of oral health status No dental examination within the last two years	Teach specific self-care behaviors to maintain oral and systemic health. Evaluate the client's oral health behaviors for effectiveness. Appeal to the client's sense of self-care. Encourage the client's active participation in formulating goals for dental hygiene care. Facilitate choices and decision making by the client.
Conceptualization and Understanding: The need to grasp ideas and abstractions in order to make sound decisions about one's oral health	Educational deficit Knowledge deficit Lack of exposure to information	Client has questions, misconceptions, or lack of knowledge about oral diseases. Client does not understand the rationale for daily self-care (e.g., bacterial plaque and host factors and their relationship to oral disease or the importance of daily plaque removal). Client does not understand the link between some systemic diseases and oral disease. Client has misinterpreted information.	Explain the rationale for the prevention and control of oral disease as a method to reduce the risk of some systemic diseases. Teach the client about the disease process and how it can be interrupted by appropriate, daily self-care. Measure the client's oral health knowledge and teach new concepts accordingly. Promote self-evaluation of the oral cavity and head and neck by the client as a way of maintaining health and client participation in health care.

From Darby ML, Walsh MM: Application of the human needs conceptual model to dental hygiene practice, *Journal of Dental Hygiene* 74(3):230, 2000.

care. The *dental hygiene diagnostic classification* uses descriptors that focus on the client's human needs, thus emphasizing the client as an integrated human being rather than as a disease entity. The diagnostic classification allows dental hygienists to focus on client needs and to communicate this information to the client and other health professionals.

DENTAL HYGIENE DIAGNOSTIC PROCESS

The *diagnostic process*, a problem-solving approach to clinical decision making, guides the intellectual activity of the dental hygienist (Figure 16–2). The dental hygiene diagnostic process uses as a foundation eight human

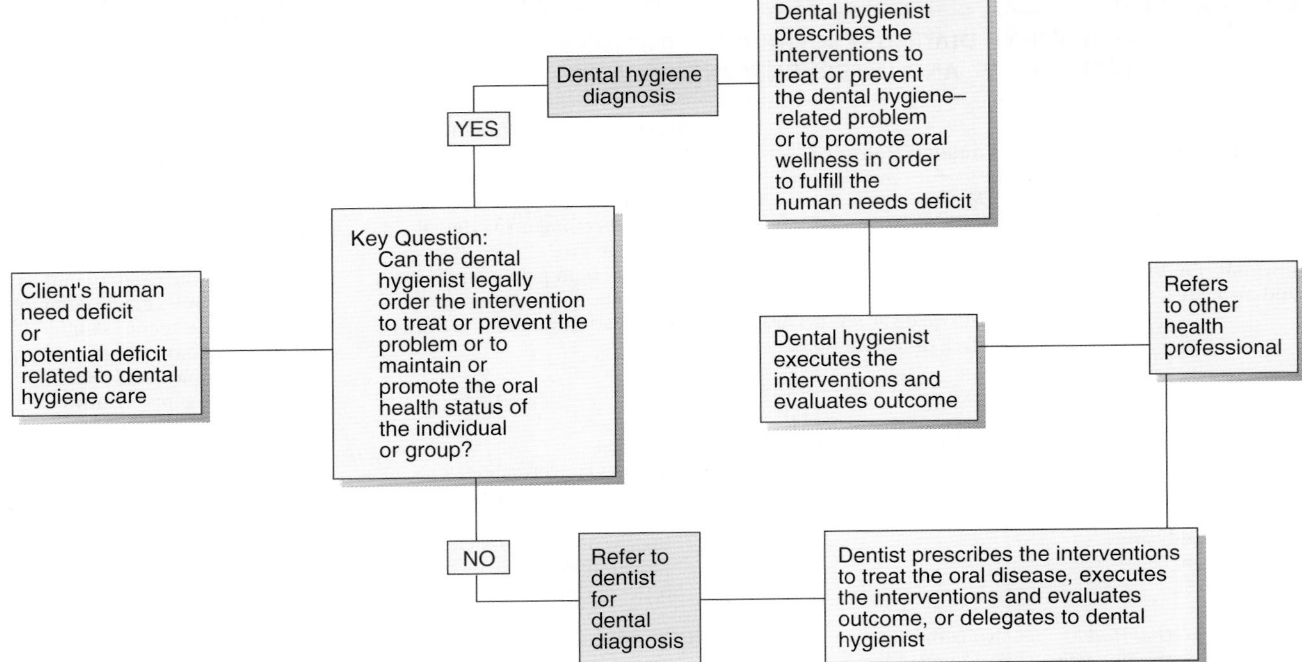

FIGURE 16–2 ✦ Flowchart of the dental hygiene diagnostic process.

needs related to dental hygiene care (Table 16–2). Dental hygiene diagnoses focus professional care and allow dental hygienists to assess and manage client conditions within their scope of practice. After diagnosis, goals are developed in conjunction with the client. Client goals—the desired outcome of care—clarify what the client needs to do to promote, maintain, or achieve oral health and wellness. Planning care and evaluation of clinical outcomes are guided by the dental hygiene diagnosis (see Chapter 17).

Synthesis, Analysis, and Interpretation of Assessment Data

Dental hygienists begin data synthesis, analysis, and interpretation during assessment. Figure 16–3 provides a tool that can be used to assess the client's unmet human needs. The dental hygienist looks for significant clusters of data that signal the presence of an actual or potential unmet human need, formulates a diagnosis, and develops a care plan (see Chapter 17).

Using Standards to Validate Diagnoses

To arrive at a valid dental hygiene diagnosis, the dental hygienist can compare observed data (objective and subjective) with an accepted standard. Appropriate standards include normative values for the client's age, race, and oral disease status. For example, a child's gingival architecture may be normal given the child's developmental level, but abnormal at another age. Similarly, a blood pressure of 130/90 mm Hg might be within the expected range for an individual with hypertension under the control of a physician but abnormal for a person not under a physician's care. The following may be used to recognize significant data:

- ✦ Changes in a client's usual oral or systemic health patterns that are unexplained by expected norms for growth, development, and maturation
- ✦ Oral and systemic health status that deviates from normal limits
- ✦ Behavior or condition indicating a developmental lag or risk to health or personal safety

Recognizing Patterns

Dental hygiene diagnoses should always be based on a cluster of significant information rather than on a single sign or symptom. The danger of arriving at a dental hygiene diagnosis from a single factor is evident from this example: The dental hygienist diagnosed an Eastern Indian woman as having an unmet human need for a wholesome facial image, related to a lack of dental care as evidenced by malpositioned teeth and a prognathic profile, but may have misinterpreted the observed data. The dental hygienist erroneously identified the cause as lack of dental care when really it is rooted in the belief system of the client's culture that accepts malocclusion as being within the range of normal. The woman has had regular dental care throughout her life. Gathering complete data to support a recognizable pattern prevents the dental hygienist from formulating an erroneous diagnosis.

Identifying Unmet Human Needs

The next step in the diagnostic process is to determine the client's unmet human needs. The dental hygienist

ASSESSMENT (circle signs and symptoms present)	
1) WHOLESOME FACIAL IMAGE *expresses dissatisfaction with appearance –teeth –gingiva –facial profile –breath –other ______	5) FREEDOM FROM HEAD AND NECK PAIN *extra-/intraoral pain or sensitivity •other ______
2) FREEDOM FROM ANXIETY/STRESS *reports or displays: –anxiety about proximity of clinician, confidentiality, or previous dental experience –oral habits –substance abuse *concern about: –infection control, fluoride therapy, fluoridation, mercury toxicity	6) BIOLOGICALLY SOUND & FUNCTIONAL DENTITION *reports difficulty in chewing *presents with: –defective restorations –ill-fitting dentures, appliances –teeth with signs of disease –abrasion erosion –missing teeth –rampant caries –other ______
3) SKIN & MUCOUS MEMBRANE INTEGRITY OF HEAD AND NECK –extra-/intraoral lesion –pockets >4 mm –swelling –attachment loss > 1 mm –gingival inflammation –xerostomia –bleeding on probing –other ______	7) RESPONSIBILITY FOR ORAL HEALTH *plaque & calculus present *inadequate parental supervision of oral health care *no dental exam within the last 2 years *other ______
4) PROTECTION FROM HEALTH RISKS *BP outside of normal limits *need for prophylactic antibiotics *potential for injury *risk factors *other ______	8) CONCEPTUALIZATION & UNDERSTANDING *has questions about DH care and/or oral disease *other ______

DENTAL HYGIENE DIAGNOSIS (List the human need not met, then be specific about the etiology and signs & symptoms evidencing a deficit)

(Unmet Human Need) DUE TO (Etiology) EVIDENCED BY (Signs & Symptoms)

CLIENT GOALS	INTERVENTIONS (Target etiologies)	EVALUATION (goal met, partially met, or unmet)

Appointment Schedule: ______

Continued-care recommendations:

FIGURE 16–3 ✦ Human Needs Assessment Form. *(Darby ML, Walsh MM:* Journal of Dental Hygiene *74(3):230, 2000.)*

distinguishes between oral health conditions that only a dentist is qualified to treat (dental diagnosis), therefore requiring a dental referral, and oral health conditions that require dental hygiene care (dental hygiene diagnosis). Critical thinking determines whether the identified condition requires a dental diagnosis, a dental hygiene diagnosis, or a medical diagnosis.

The client also may present information during the assessment indicating that he or she is at risk for developing an unmet human need (i.e., an *at-risk problem*). For example, the dental hygienist records that a client has signs of possible uncontrolled diabetes mellitus, but the results were not confirmed at the last medical examination. The dental hygienist then predicts the problems this client is likely to experience as a result, such as a diabetic emergency, longer healing period than normal, and a risk for infection. These potential problems are related to the unmet human needs for protection from health risks and for skin and mucous membrane integrity.

Dental hygiene diagnoses have implications for planning interventions. For example, interventions may include collaboration with and referral to the dentist and physician of record, analysis of the client's diet and nutrition, review of the client's medication schedule, reduction in length of appointment, prophylactic antibiotic premedication, use of antibacterial agents, and establishment of a personal oral self-care program.

Identifying Strengths

At times, a client may present with no unmet human needs. These individuals may not know how to build on this strength for greater levels of oral wellness. This situation is an opportunity for the dental hygienist to discuss observed strengths with the client and to reinforce oral health promotion interventions to maintain and augment wellness. Strengths may include good general health status, not smoking, valuing health, regular professional healthcare, and good self-care behaviors.

FORMULATING AND VALIDATING DENTAL HYGIENE DIAGNOSES

Writing Dental Hygiene Diagnostic Statements

After interpreting and analyzing the client's data, the dental hygienist reaches one of four basic conclusions, all of which require different actions. These conclusions and actions are shown in Table 16–3.

If the action requires a diagnosis, the dental hygienist formulates, validates, and prioritizes dental hygiene diagnoses before care. Formulation of the dental hygiene diagnosis is based on the identification of the client's human needs as supported by the assessment data. Because most people are motivated to satisfy their human needs, the dental hygienist is able to engage the client as an active participant in care to facilitate human need fulfillment. More than one unmet human need may be found, and multiple dental hygiene diagnoses may be identified.

Three components comprise a diagnostic statement (Figure 16–4):

- ✦ The *oral health condition* or potential (at-risk) health problem amenable to dental hygiene intervention
- ✦ The probable cause, etiologic factor(s), or risk factors and risk indicators
- ✦ The defining characteristics (signs and symptoms)

A diagnostic statement links the client's problem and etiology, guides the selection of interventions, and facilitates the definition of expected outcomes to evaluate the efficacy of care (see Chapter 17 for a discussion of expected outcomes).

Table 16–4 presents examples of dental hygiene diagnostic statements. Eight diagnostic categories presented in Table 16–2 delineate possible dental hygiene diagnoses. In this approach to diagnosing, the organizing principle guiding the diagnosis is human needs theory. The diagnostic categories enable the dental hygienist to summarize the data collected during client assessment. More important, the diagnostic statement provides a focus so that the traditional shotgun approach characteristic of routine dental hygiene care (a 45-minute appointment for an oral prophylaxis, bitewing radiographs, fluoride application, and 6-month continued care) is no longer an appropriate standard.

Each diagnosis has a cluster of defining characteristics that must be observed in the client during the assessment. The *defining characteristics* are the signs and symptoms that must be evident for the diagnostic label to be used correctly (Table 16–2). The *signs and symptoms* are predictors for judging the presence of an unmet human need related to an oral health condition or a potential

TABLE 16–3 POSSIBLE CONCLUSIONS AND ACTIONS TAKEN BY THE DENTAL HYGIENIST AFTER ANALYZING CLIENT ASSESSMENT DATA

Conclusion	Dental Hygiene Actions
No unmet human needs related to dental hygiene care	Initiate oral health promotion strategies to achieve higher levels of oral and systemic wellness. Reinforce client's oral health beliefs and behaviors.
Possible unmet human needs related to an oral health problem	Collect more assessment data to validate suspected problem that may require a dental hygiene diagnosis, a dental diagnosis, or a medical diagnosis.
Actual or potential unmet human needs related to dental hygiene care (dental hygiene diagnosis)	Plan, implement, and evaluate dental hygiene care.
Actual or potential unmet human needs requiring a diagnosis by another healthcare professional	Consult with and refer to appropriate healthcare professional and work collaboratively to solve the problem.

problem. The client's signs and symptoms enable the dental hygienist to focus on the true problem and to eliminate others. (This process is referred to as the *differential diagnosis*).

Sometimes the client may not have a problem yet, but presents with risk factors and risk indicators suggesting that he or she is at risk for a problem. At-risk problems are conditions that should also be diagnosed so that actions can be taken to prevent the problem from developing further. If the client is at risk for an oral health problem, there may not be signs and symptoms because the problem has not yet occurred; rather, it is still preventable.

A diagnosis should be accompanied by noting the following:

✦ Factors that led to the condition or at-risk problem (cause or etiology)

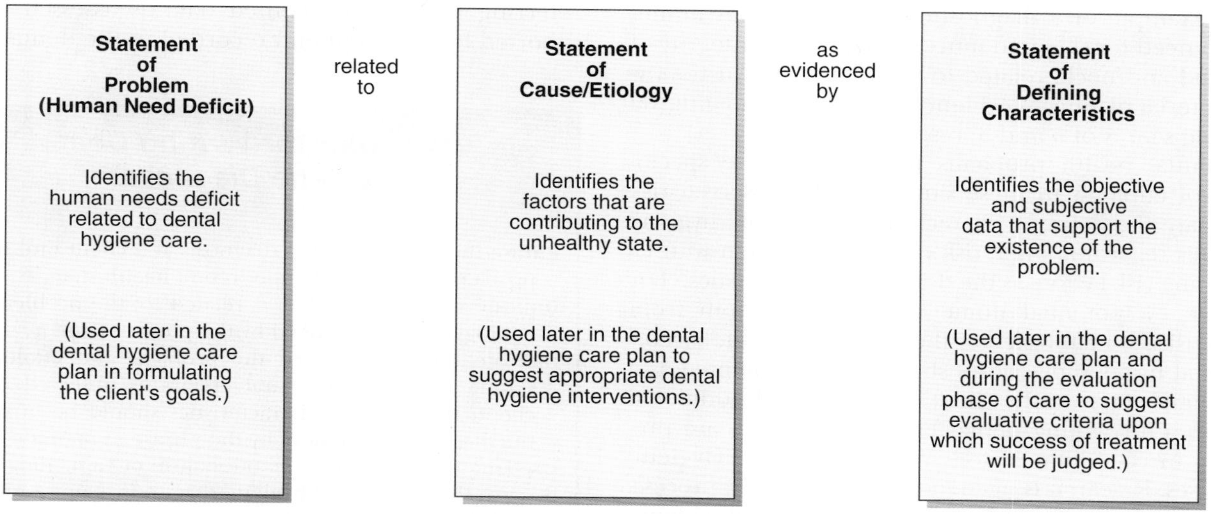

Statement of Problem (Human Need Deficit)	related to	**Statement of Cause/Etiology**	as evidenced by	**Statement of Defining Characteristics**
Identifies the human needs deficit related to dental hygiene care.		Identifies the factors that are contributing to the unhealthy state.		Identifies the objective and subjective data that support the existence of the problem.
(Used later in the dental hygiene care plan in formulating the client's goals.)		(Used later in the dental hygiene care plan to suggest appropriate dental hygiene interventions.)		(Used later in the dental hygiene care plan and during the evaluation phase of care to suggest evaluative criteria upon which success of treatment will be judged.)

FIGURE 16–4 ✦ Three parts of a dental hygiene diagnostic statement. *(Darby ML, Walsh MM:* Journal of Dental Hygiene *74(3):230, 2000.)*

TABLE 16–4 FORMULATION OF DENTAL HYGIENE DIAGNOSTIC STATEMENTS

Dental Hygiene Diagnosis	Causes/Etiologies	Signs and Symptoms
Definitions		
Client's unmet human needs related to dental hygiene care for which the dental hygienist is educated and licensed to treat	Factors causing or maintaining the unhealthy oral state or response, or factors putting the client at risk of a health problem	Subjective and objective data collected in the dental hygiene assessment that supports the existence of a problem or potential problem
Examples		
Skin and mucous membrane integrity of the head and neck	Related to mutable and nonmutable risk factors (e.g., diabetes, smoking, and plaque biofilm accumulation)	As manifested by moderate gingival bleeding, periodontal probing depths of 5-7 mm
Responsibility for oral health	Related to impaired physical ability	As manifested by arthritis in the hands and shoulders
Protection from health risks (potential for oral infection)	Related to the presence of risk factors or risk indicators	*Note:* Potential problems may not have signs or symptoms in the diagnostic statement because the problem has not yet manifested.
Protection from health risks (potential for oral injury)	Related to participation in contact sports Client does not wear a mouth protector	*Note:* Potential problems may not have signs or symptoms in the diagnostic statement because the problem has not yet manifested.
Responsibility for oral health	Related to inadequate parental supervision of daily oral hygiene	As manifested by gingival bleeding, signs of active caries, and parent indicating that "John brushes his own teeth."
Wholesome facial image	Related to a Class II, Division I malocclusion	As manifested by client's consistent derogatory remarks about her teeth

- Objective signs observed by the dental hygienist and the subjective symptoms reported by the client (defining characteristics as evidence of the problem)

Thus a dental hygiene diagnosis is written as a three-part diagnostic statement:

- The unmet need (human need deficit)
- The etiology (*related to* or *due to*)
- The defining characteristics (signs and symptoms, *as evidenced by*)

An example of a diagnostic statement is "an unmet human need for skin and mucous membrane integrity of the head and neck, related to skill deficiency in removing bacterial plaque, as evidenced by plaque and gingival bleeding scores of 5 and 3, respectively."

Potential health problems may not require specification of etiology. In these situations, the observed risk factors are the defining characteristics. A dental hygiene diagnosis regarding an at-risk problem is written with its presenting risk factors as the defining characteristics.[8] For example, "a potential unmet need for freedom from health risks, as manifested by the use of chewing tobacco."

Dental hygiene diagnoses should be documented as a permanent entry on the client's record. Some additional guidelines for writing dental hygiene diagnoses are presented in Guidelines for Writing Dental Hygiene Diagnoses. Research is needed on the diagnostic process, the validation of dental hygiene diagnoses, and the identification of interventions that work for each diagnosis.

Errors in Writing a Dental Hygiene Diagnostic Statement

The most frequent errors found in dental hygiene diagnostic statements include the presence of emotional terms, a dental diagnosis, a medical diagnosis, etiology presented as the diagnosis, or signs and symptoms presented as the diagnosis rather than in terms of the client's unmet needs. These common errors are listed in Table 16–5, with guidelines on how these errors can be corrected. The dental hygienist must also avoid personal beliefs and values in the diagnostic statement by always referring to the documented data as assessed and/or reported by the client and recorded in the dental chart.

Guidelines for Writing Dental Hygiene Diagnoses

Phrase the dental hygiene diagnosis as a client oral health problem, risk, or alteration in oral health state.

Indicate what the problem is related to; the problem and etiology should be linked by the phrase *related to.*

Indicate the evidence for the problem and etiology by stating the defining characteristics as observed in the client; the defining characteristics should be linked to the diagnostic statement by the phrase *as indicated by.*

Use language that avoids emotionalism or value judgment.

Be sure that the dental hygiene diagnosis is not a medical or dental diagnosis.

TABLE 16–5 COMMON ERRORS IN WRITING DENTAL HYGIENE DIAGNOSES

Type of Error	Poor Dental Hygiene Diagnosis	Correction Required	Corrected Dental Hygiene Diagnosis
Emotionalism expressed in the diagnosis	Poor self-care related to laziness	Eliminate words that express emotionalism.	Unmet need for responsibility for oral health related to lack of adherence to self-care regimen, as evidenced by heavy plaque accumulation and client's self report.
Dental diagnosis instead of a dental hygiene diagnosis	Moderate, localized aggressive periodontitis	Avoid using dental diagnostic terms.	Unmet need in skin and mucous membrane integrity due to heavy plaque and cigarette smoking, as indicated by continued loss of clinical attachment since the last 3-month continued-care appointment. Refer to dentist for dental diagnosis.
Citing etiology as the diagnosis	Deficit related to nonadherence	Use human need framework.	Unmet need for responsibility for oral health related to a lack of manual dexterity and self-care deficit, as evidenced by a Plaque Index score of 3 and an inability to grasp a toothbrush.
Identifying signs and symptoms as the client problem	Generalized gingival bleeding and attachment levels of 5-8 mm	Use signs and symptoms to define and validate the actual problem.	Unmet need for skin and mucous membrane integrity related to inadequate oral health behaviors and smoking, as manifested by moderate gingival bleeding, clinical attachment loss of 5 to 8 mm, and signs of nicotine stomatitis.
Writing the diagnosis in terms of what the dental hygienist will do	Needs education on the disease process	Write the diagnosis in terms of the client rather than what the dental hygienist needs to do.	Unmet need in conceptualization and understanding related to a lack of knowledge about disease process, as evidenced by client's misconceptions about the causes of tooth decay.

Nothing should be recorded that insinuates negligence on the treatment rendered by another practitioner. For example, "an unmet need for a biologically sound dentition, due to poor dentistry, as manifested by overhanging restorations." Table 16–6 provides examples of conditions that are *not* dental hygiene diagnoses.

Validation of the Dental Hygiene Diagnosis

Once the diagnosis is formulated, it must be validated. An affirmative response to each of the statements in Figure 16–5 validates the dental hygiene diagnosis[9] (see Chapter 17). The format in Figure 16–6 can be used to practice the process of diagnostic decision making. The dental hygienist can begin by reviewing the following three scenarios that exemplify the dental hygiene diagnostic process applied clinically.

OUTCOMES OF DENTAL HYGIENE DIAGNOSES

Collaboration and independent decision making are important dimensions of professionalism. Dental hygiene diagnoses require critical thinking and facilitate the development of autonomy and accountability by focusing on the phenomena that are within the scope of dental hygiene practice and by providing a language for communication of the scope. *Autonomy* is the "right to self-determination and governance without external control in which its membership defines and delineates the services that constitute practice."[10] *Accountability* is the "responsibility incurred by individuals and members to

1. The database is complete, accurate, and based on a concept of dental hygiene. Yes ___ No ___
2. Data reflect the existence of a pattern. Yes ___ No ___
3. Both subjective and objective data support the existence of the human need deficit identified in the dental hygiene diagnosis. Yes ___ No ___
4. The dental hygiene diagnosis is based on scientific knowledge and evidence. Yes ___ No ___
5. The dental hygiene diagnosis can be prevented, controlled, or resolved by dental hygiene interventions. Yes ___ No ___
6. Given the same data, other qualified practitioners would formulate the same dental hygiene diagnosis. Yes ___ No ___

FIGURE 16–5 ✦ "Yes" answers to all of these statements validate the dental hygiene diagnosis.

TABLE 16–6 WHAT A DENTAL HYGIENE DIAGNOSIS IS NOT

It Is Not ...	Examples	Rationale
A dental diagnosis	Myofascial pain disorder Class III malocclusion Advanced chronic periodontal disease Oral carcinoma Early childhood caries Prepubertal periodontitis	Although there is dental hygiene care associated with dental diagnoses, the disease or disorder is not primarily amenable to dental hygiene intervention. Dental hygiene's concern is for the person and the oral health behaviors in which they engage.
A dental pathology	Leukoplakia Aphthous ulcer Oral cancer	Dental hygienists need to understand the pathology underlying disease states to plan appropriate dental hygiene care; however, the focus is on the person's response and not the pathology. The person's response to the pathology and its prevention is the domain of dental hygiene.
A diagnostic test, treatment, or appliance	Pulp tester Antibiotic therapy Antimicrobial therapy Oral prosthetic appliances	Dental hygiene's concern is the individual's oral health behavior and response to the diagnostic test, treatment, or equipment. If assessment data or data gathered throughout care reveal an unmet need, this becomes the dental hygiene diagnosis.
A goal of the hygienist or a dental hygiene intervention	To develop the client's responsibility to control oral disease by referring him or her to the dentist and by providing education.	The dental hygiene diagnosis should be written from the client's perspective, not the dental hygienist's perspective. Example: Unmet need for responsibility for oral health, related to lack of financial resources, as evidenced by no professional care for 5 years and no dental insurance.
A single sign or symptom	Microbial plaque on lingual surfaces of all teeth	A dental hygiene diagnosis is not developed until a pattern or cluster of significant cues is identified. The clustering of signs and symptoms leads to the dental hygiene diagnosis but it is not the diagnosis. In this situation, no dental hygiene diagnosis is indicated until more data are collected, synthesized, analyzed, and interpreted.
An unvalidated dental hygiene diagnosis	Previous example leads dental hygienist to the dental hygiene diagnosis: Unmet need in conceptualization and understanding.	Unvalidated, this premature dental hygiene diagnosis may not focus on the client's true problem. More defining characteristics (signs and symptoms) need to be identified before the dental hygiene diagnosis can be validated.

Dental Hygiene Diagnosis	Due To	Evidenced By	Goal/Behavior

FIGURE 16–6 ✦ Worksheet for making a dental hygiene diagnosis.

SCENARIO 1

YOUNG WOMAN WHO RECENTLY OBTAINED ORTHODONTIC APPLIANCES

Brenda Smith, age 16, Asian American, and a junior in high school, received full orthodontic appliances 1 month ago. Although she wanted the orthodontic appliances to correct the severe crowding of her anterior teeth, she now is experiencing an adjustment problem. She decided to visit her dental office of record for a 3-month checkup. She was treated last for gingivitis before placement of the orthodontic appliances. Upon assessment, the dental hygienist found loss of weight, slight plaque-induced gingivitis, and fair bacterial plaque control. All other findings were within normal limits.

Ms. Smith verbalized that not very many 16-year-olds at her school wear braces, that she couldn't wait to get them off, and that she can't stand to look at herself in the mirror. One of her high school friends said that she looked weird. She obviously is experiencing high anxiety since the orthodontic appliances were placed. She said that she has a difficult time eating because food sticks to the appliances, and she feels embarrassed if the appliances are retaining food. She no longer likes to eat with her friends in the school cafeteria or when she is out on weekends.

Dental Hygiene Diagnosis (Unmet Need)	Due to or Related to (Causes/Etiologies)	As Evidenced by (Signs and Symptoms)	Client Goal (Expected Outcomes)
Wholesome facial image	Acquisition of orthodontic appliances	Unwillingness to smile Constant negative referral to the appliances and the way she looks Anxiety about wearing the appliances	Verbalizes acceptance of appliance after 2 months
Freedom from stress and anxiety	Inability to eat Acquisition of orthodontic appliances	Loss of weight Anxiety about wearing the orthodontic appliances	Verbalizes acceptance of appliance after 1 month Reports stabilized weight after 2 months

DENTAL HYGIENE INTERVENTIONS

1. Assess Ms. Smith's perception of her oral condition and appearance before wearing orthodontic appliances.
2. Listen to client's comments.
3. Compliment client on appearance.
4. Assist Ms. Smith in visualizing her altered facial image and the temporary status of the orthodontic appliances. Emphasize that the altered facial image is a normal part of wearing orthodontic appliances.
5. Assist Ms. Smith in concentrating on the positive aspects of her oral health (e.g., no decay, no periodontal disease).
6. Actively reinforce accomplishments such as bacterial plaque control, no gingival bleeding.
7. Encourage Ms. Smith to talk with others who wear orthodontic appliances in order to share concerns and feelings.
8. Conduct nutritional counseling with Ms. Smith to identify nutritional foods that can be eaten with orthodontic appliances.
9. Describe the dietary needs of adolescents.
   - Explain using basic food pyramid.
   - Review a basic food plan.
10. Instruct Ms. Smith in how to record a food diary.
11. After about 1 week, review food diary and lead Ms. Smith to identify areas of concern that might be contributing to undernutrition.
    - Discuss alternative food choices (e.g., foods that are less retentive).
    - Explain how good nutrition will enable her to cope better with the appliances.
12. Review oral hygiene care for orthodontic appliances, with specific emphasis on what can be done to keep appliances looking clean while away from home.
13. Continually monitor her anxiety level, emotional status, and attitude toward orthodontic appliances.
14. After 1 month, evaluate client's eating habits, body weight, and anxiety level.
15. After 2 months, evaluate client's eating habits, body weight, and anxiety level.

be morally obligated and answerable to a higher authority for services rendered."[10] The dental hygiene diagnosis, by identifying the client's unmet human needs that can be fulfilled through dental hygiene care, clarifies the role of the dental hygienist and allows for a defined scope, domain, and focus of dental hygiene practice. "Diagnosis by dental hygienists is not, and should not be, an attempt to move into the domain of the dentist; it is a vehicle for distinguishing roles professionally and legally."[2]

Dental hygiene diagnosis facilitates the delivery of quality dental hygiene care and quality management, and it provides a mechanism for establishing dental hygiene fees. Because dental hygiene diagnoses are based on a diagnostic classification system, communication and collaboration among oral health professionals are facilitated, as is the application of computerized information systems for operation and research. For example, the future use of dental hygiene diagnoses appears promising for the development of a computerized system of diagnosis and care planning, with expansion to a system of cost accounting for dental hygiene. Diagnosis fosters clinical practice that is focused and capable of outcomes evaluation, which has implications for education, research, regulatory mechanisms, direct access to care, and direct reimbursement.

SCENARIO 2

CHILD WITH AGGRESSIVE PERIODONTITIS

Devan Prince, age 12, female, and African American, is a new client in the dental practice and has been scheduled for dental hygiene care. Devan is in the seventh grade and is one of the star players on the girls' soccer team. She is with her mother Margaret (age 32) and her sister Bridget (age 10). After completing health and dental histories, the dental hygienist initiates the assessment phase of the dental hygiene process of care, including a baseline assessment of human needs related to dental hygiene care, a complete tooth and periodontal assessment, and dental hygiene education and skill level assessment. Significant findings include 6-mm probing depths around tooth numbers 19 and 30 and 4- to 5-mm loss of clinical attachment around tooth numbers 22 to 27. Oral hygiene was generally poor, and tooth mobility of periodontally involved teeth ranged from 2 to 3. Client has a knowledge deficit regarding bacterial plaque, periodontal disease process, and status of the oral cavity.

Dental Hygiene Diagnosis (Unmet Need)	Due to or Related to (Causes/Etiologies)	As Evidenced by (Signs and Symptoms)	Client Goal (Expected Outcomes)
Freedom from health risks	Participation in contact sport and does not use a mouth protector	*Note:* Potential problems may not have defining characteristics in the diagnostic statement (no defining characteristics necessary because client is at risk for a problem; problem has not yet occurred)	Verbalizes belief in the value of a mouth protector Reports wearing mouth protector at all soccer games and practice sessions by next appointment Parent verbalizes emergency care for an avulsed tooth
Skin and mucous membrane integrity of the head and neck.	Presence of bacterial plaque Nonmutable risk factors for juvenile periodontitis	4- to 5-mm clinical attachment loss, poor oral hygiene, tooth mobility of 2 and 3	Decrease bacterial plaque score from 3 to 0 within 1 month Referral to periodontist
Conceptualization and understanding	Knowledge deficit about the periodontal disease process, bacterial plaque, and state of oral cavity	Misconceptions about what is an unhealthy mouth	Identify unhealthy and healthy signs in her mouth by end of this appointment Explains periodontal disease process by 1 month

DENTAL HYGIENE INTERVENTIONS

1. Assess client's present level of knowledge about mouth protectors.
2. Teach client about the value of wearing a mouth protector during contact sports.
3. Teach parent and client emergency care for an avulsed tooth.
4. Construct a mouth protector and discuss use and care with the client; fit mouth protector.
5. After 1 week, evaluate fit and client response to the mouth protector.
6. Teach both child and parent about the periodontal disease process.
   - Explain the disease process of aggressive periodontitis.
   - Use signs and symptoms of health and disease found in the client's own mouth as a teaching aid.
7. Work collaboratively with the dentist and periodontist to carry out successful root planing and antimicrobial therapy. Support therapeutic recommendations of the periodontist.
8. Teach child and parent about bacterial plaque and other mutable and nonmutable risk factors.
9. Teach child and parent appropriate self-care (e.g., toothbrushing and interdental cleaning).
10. Evaluate knowledge and skill acquisition after 1 month.
11. Modify plan as needed.
12. Refer back to dentist or periodontist.

SCENARIO 3

YOUNG CHILD WITH EARLY CHILDHOOD CARIES

Blake Olds, age 4 and Caucasian, was brought to the dental hygiene clinic by his mother Caren, age 28. Caren is unemployed and on public assistance; therefore, finances are always a major concern. Blake has been in pain associated with his teeth. His mother reported that "he has been crying on and off for about four days, saying that his mouth hurt." She indicates that she tries to appease his discomfort with sweets to eat. The dental hygienist conducted a complete health, dental, and cultural history and initiated the assessment phase of the dental hygiene process. Because of the immediacy of the need for relieving the child's pain, she collaborated with the attending dentist, who extracted J, K, and L at that visit and who prescribed an antibiotic to control the infection. After the oral surgery, the client was given postoperative instructions, dismissed, and the dental hygienist analyzed the findings. Blake's significant findings included early childhood caries and periapical abscesses on J, K, and L, with caries also on teeth A, B, E, F, I, M, O, P, S, and T. Because of extraction and interproximal caries, the maintenance of space for the permanent teeth is a major concern. Although there were no significant periodontal probe depths, there is green and orange extrinsic stain, heavy materia alba, and bacterial plaque throughout the mouth.

Dental Hygiene Diagnosis (Unmet Need)	Due to or Related to (Causes/Etiologies)	As Evidenced by (Signs and Symptoms)	Client Goal (Expected Outcomes)
Freedom from head and neck pain	Untreated caries	Client's expression of pain, mother's report of pain, and signs of severe caries	Parent complies with referral to dentist for emergency care.
Biologically sound and functional dentition	Risk factors for dental disease	Signs of early childhood caries	Parent complies with referral to dentist for care.
	Lack of dental care/ financial resources	Signs of periapical abscesses on radiographs	Parent lists two dental care resources (e.g., the government-funded Children's Health Insurance Program, local public health dental clinic)
	Cariogenic diet	Space loss that could create a future malocclusion	Parent explains nutritional and chemotherapeutic strategies to control tooth decay. Parent identifies cariogenic foods to avoid and healthful foods to substitute.
Responsibility for oral health	Lack of parental supervision of daily plaque control	Heavy materia alba and bacterial plaque Green/orange extrinsic stain present	Decrease Plaque Index score by 2 within 1 month. Mother reports that client cleans oral cavity once a day by himself by next appointment.
	Skill deficit of parent and client	Lack of a systematic and efficient method of toothbrushing	Mother reports cleaning client's oral cavity once a day by end of next appointment. Mother demonstrates effective mouth cleaning technique on Blake by end of appointment.
Conceptualization and understanding	Knowledge deficit of parent about the caries process	Misconceptions about the causes of tooth decay	Parent explains the disease process and etiology; client explains disease process in age-appropriate terms by next appointment.
		Does not understand oral disease can be prevented in a cost-effective manner	Parent verbalizes the value of preventing further tooth loss by next appointment.

DENTAL HYGIENE INTERVENTIONS

1. Assess oral hygiene knowledge, attitude, and skill level of the client and the parent.
2. Instruct client and parent on basic oral hygiene:
   - Knowledge of etiology
   - Use of a toothbrush and positioning of client
   - Frequency of toothbrushing
3. Conduct nutritional analysis and counseling for caries control with the parent.
4. Discuss value of daily fluoride treatment until caries are controlled.
5. Discuss reasons for restoring the primary teeth:
   - Maintenance of space
   - Prevention of malocclusion and costly orthodontics
6. Compliment client on the good job he is doing.
7. Refer parent to community facility where oral healthcare can be obtained on a sliding-scale payment basis.
8. Complete scaling, selective polishing, and fluoride therapy; obtain prescription for daily fluoride therapy.
9. One month after, evaluate effectiveness of interventions.
10. Modify as necessary; maintain collaboration with treating dentist.

Client Education Issues

- Explain the dental hygiene diagnosis to the client so that the client understands the condition or problem and how it can best be resolved.
- Explain how the goals established will, if achieved, meet the client's need.

Legal, Ethical, and Safety Issues

- Dental hygiene diagnoses should reflect the scope of dental hygiene practice and never the scope of the dentist's practice. Avoid terminology in the diagnostic statement that implies blame or malpractice, which could lead to litigation.
- When the client manifests signs and symptoms of oral conditions that require dental treatment by a dentist, a dental referral is indicated for quality care and legal protection.
- Dental hygiene diagnoses must be validated to ensure that the focus of care is accurate.
- Dental hygiene diagnostic statements should be recorded in the client record and used to develop client goals and throughout the dental hygiene process of care.

Key Concepts

- A dental hygiene diagnosis states the client's actual or potential (at-risk) problem related to oral health and disease.
- Diagnosis is a decision-making process that requires critical thinking and professional judgment.
- Current standards (e.g., ADEA *Competencies for Entry into Dental Hygiene* and the ADHA *Code of Ethics*) expect dental hygienists to make dental hygiene diagnoses.
- The diagnostic process includes analysis of assessment data; identification of the client's problem, health risks, and strengths; and formulation of the diagnostic statements.
- Dental hygiene diagnoses improve communication among the dental hygienist, the client, and other health professionals.
- The *related to* part of the diagnostic statement provides the dental hygienist with direction regarding selecting interventions.
- The *as evidenced by* part of the diagnostic statement provides the dental hygienist with defining characteristics to evaluate the outcome of care.
- The client goal reflects the desired outcome of care.
- The dental hygiene diagnostic statement allows the dental hygienist to focus care on the client problems and individualize care.
- Each dental hygiene diagnostic statement should be clear, client centered, based on reliable assessment data, and reflect only one problem.
- Eight dental hygiene diagnoses are based on human needs related to oral health and disease.
- The development of dental hygiene diagnoses is an ongoing project that requires research.

Critical Thinking Exercises

1. Select one new client that you are scheduled to treat. Using all of the subjective and objective information from assessment, including data collected on the form displayed in Figure 16–3, prepare at least one diagnostic statement. What client goals could be established? What dental hygiene interventions will you use to achieve the client goals? Use the information in Table 16–1 to help you identify possible etiologies and defining characteristics. The previous scenarios can serve as examples.
2. How would you validate this diagnostic statement?
3. What interventions can be used to elevate a client to higher levels of wellness?

For References, Suggested Readings, and Related Websites, visit
http://evolve.elsevier.com/Darby/hygiene/

CHAPTER 17

DENTAL HYGIENE CARE PLAN

OBJECTIVES

Mastery of the content in this chapter will enable the reader to:

- Identify purposes of the dental hygiene care plan and the client's role in its development.
- Identify phrases used to increase client participation in care planning.
- Write client-centered goals that contain a subject, verb, criterion for measurement, and time dimension.
- Apply concepts of informed consent and informed refusal to care planning.
- Develop a care plan derived from a dental hygiene diagnosis.
- Collaborate with other healthcare professionals during care planning.
- Integrate the dental hygiene care plan with the appointment plan.
- Define evaluation according to its purpose, relationship to other steps in the dental hygiene process, and legal rationale.
- Evaluate achievement of client goals as established in the plan of care.
- Discuss the dental hygiene prognosis and its impact on continued dental hygiene care.

KEY TERMS

Affective goals
Client-centered goals
Cognitive goals
Collaboration
Continued care
Dental hygiene care plan
Dental hygiene intervention
Evaluation
Express consent
Implied consent
Informed consent and refusal
Oral health status
Planning
Psychomotor goals
Reevaluation
Supervised neglect

PLANNING

Planning is that phase of the dental hygiene process in which priorities are set, client goals are established, and interventions and outcome measures are determined (Figure 17–1). Its purpose is to develop the plan of care that will target the resolution of an oral health problem amenable to dental hygiene care, the prevention of a problem, or the promotion of oral health. Therefore, the phrase *care plan,* rather than treatment plan, is consciously used to denote the broad range of preventive, educational, therapeutic, and support services within the scope of dental hygiene practice. Given the human need for responsibility for oral health, the dental hygienist actively involves clients, according to their ability and motivation, in the process and obtains the informed consent of the client (or client's guardian) before initiation of care. The tangible outcome of the planning phase is the dental hygiene care plan.

To formulate a care plan, the dental hygienist must:

- Possess a sound background in dental hygiene theory.
- Be thoroughly familiar with the parameters or standards of dental hygiene care.
- Possess the ability to collect, analyze, and interpret client data.
- Develop dental hygiene diagnoses.
- Formulate client goals.
- Select supportive dental hygiene interventions.

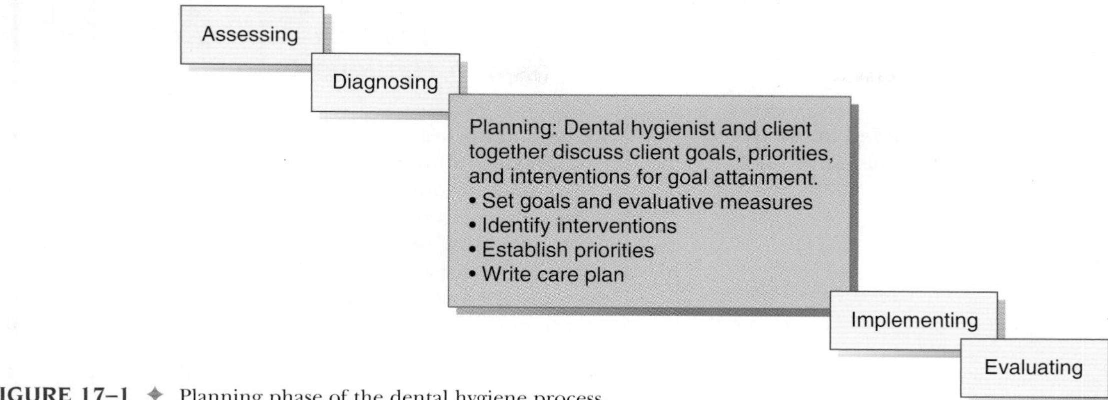

FIGURE 17–1 ✦ Planning phase of the dental hygiene process.

- ✦ Synthesize this aforementioned information into a written plan.
- ✦ Communicate oral health needs to clients effectively.
- ✦ View the dental hygiene care plan within the context of the total treatment plan developed by the dentist.

Overall Dental Treatment Plan

The general dentist, or dental specialist, develops a total dental treatment plan for the client. This usually includes the dental diagnosis; the essential services that need to be carried out by the dentist, dental hygienist, and client to eliminate or control disease; and the prognosis. The total dental treatment plan is shown in Table 17–1. The dental hygiene care plan supports the overall dental treatment plan. This requires communication and collaboration between the dental hygienist, the dentist, and the client.

Dental Hygiene Care Plan[1,2]

The *dental hygiene care plan* is the written blueprint that directs the dental hygienist and client as they work together to meet the client's oral health goals. Primarily, the plan increases the likelihood that the oral healthcare team will work collaboratively to deliver client-focused, goal-oriented, individualized care to clients. The plan facilitates the monitoring of client progress, ensures continuity of care, serves as a vehicle for communication among healthcare professionals, and increases the likelihood of quality care.

The dental hygiene care plan is prepared on the day that the dental hygienist completes the assessment and diagnosis phases of the dental hygiene process and in conjunction with the overall dental treatment plan prepared by the dentist. The plan specifies the dental hygiene diagnoses, client goals, dental hygiene interventions, and evaluative strategies to measure the proposed and expected outcomes. For efficiency, the plan may use standardized abbreviations and key phrases as specified in the policy manual of the healthcare institution with which the dental hygienist is affiliated.

Once written and shared with the client, the care plan becomes a legal contract between the dental hygienist and the client. When one begins to write the dental hygiene care plan, each assessment finding is scrutinized to determine its relationship to a human need deficit. Human need deficits and related assessment findings become the dental hygiene diagnoses in the care plan. Once the diagnosis is made, client-centered goals are established by the dental hygienist in conjunction with the client. From the established client goals, interventions and expected outcomes can be drafted. With client input, priorities for each goal are established, and then appointment planning can begin.

Once priorities are established, the dental hygienist estimates the time necessary to complete each intervention. The speed and experience of the dental hygienist and the oral condition and host response of the client affect the ultimate time required.

The dental hygienist assesses the comprehensiveness of the care plan by answering the following questions:

1. Does the care plan address the client's unmet human needs related to oral health that are amenable to or affect the outcomes of dental hygiene care?
2. Has the cultural diversity of the client been considered?
3. What might the client's response to the care plan be? For example, will the client express interest, commitment, worry, fear, discontent, or lack of enthusiasm?
4. How can the dental hygienist best present the care plan to elicit client cooperation?

Rationale for Developing a Formal Dental Hygiene Care Plan

Individualize dental hygiene care.
Focus care on priorities.
Facilitate communication and collaboration among healthcare professionals.
Establish client-centered goals.
Provide a foundation on which evaluation of dental hygiene interventions can be based.
Evaluate the client's response to dental hygiene care (outcomes).
Promote professional dental hygiene practice.

TABLE 17–1 COMPONENTS OF THE OVERALL DENTAL CARE PLAN

Components	Included in the Dental Hygiene Care Plan
Preliminary Phase: Emergency Care	
Relief of pain	
Laboratory tests for suspected pathology	
Removal of hopeless teeth	
Temporary replacement to restore function	
Emergency needs (e.g., treatment of periodontal or periapical abscess)	
Phase I: Etiotropic Therapy	
Client education/self-care instruction	*
Diet assessment	*
Tobacco cessation	*
Fluoride therapy	*
Placement of pit and fissure sealants	*
Debridement (scaling/root planing)	*
Hard tissue desensitization	*
Correction of restorative and prosthetic irritational factors, excavation of caries	
Antimicrobial therapy (local or systemic)	*
Occlusal therapy, minor orthodontics	
Selective polishing	*
PHASE I: EVALUATION OF RESPONSE TO ETIOTROPIC THERAPY	
Reassessment of gingival and periodontal health, hard and soft deposits, host response	*
Renew and reinforce self-care	*
Phase II: Surgical Phase	
Periodontal surgery	
Implant surgery	
Endodontic therapy	
Phase III: Restorative Therapy	
Restorative care/final management of dental caries	
Fixed/removable prosthetics	
Reevaluation of periodontal status and host response	
Phase IV: Maintenance Therapy	
Frequency of continued care	*
Supportive preventive and periodontal maintenance therapy	*
Self-care education	*
Evaluation of continued-care interval	*

Adapted from Fermin A, Carranza FA, Takei HH: The treatment plan. In Newman MG, Takei HH, Carranza FA, eds: *Clinical periodontology,* ed 9, Philadelphia, 2001, WB Saunders; and Lautar CJ, Pimlott JFL: Periodontal diagnosis and care planning. In Hodges KO, ed: *Concepts in nonsurgical periodontal therapy,* Albany, NY, 1998, Delmar.

5. How can client involvement be maximized in the care plan?
6. What alternative plans should be offered to the client?
7. What is the dental hygienist's response if the client refuses care?

LINK BETWEEN DIAGNOSIS AND CARE PLAN. Basing care plans on dental hygiene diagnoses, rather than on oral symptoms alone, ensures that care will be comprehensive, individualized, and focused on the needs of the client. A complete dental hygiene diagnosis includes a statement of the problem (deficit), cause of the problem (etiology), and its signs and symptoms. Therefore, it directs the dental hygienist's attention to the causes of the signs and symptoms and, hence, to what interventions can be used to control or eliminate them and their causes, as opposed to providing the same routine care to all. Because signs and symptoms related to dental hygiene problems may have numerous etiologies, interventions must be carefully selected to ensure that the fundamental cause is being addressed in dental hygiene care.

For example, a dental hygiene diagnosis of an unmet human need in the area of wholesome facial image may result from any of the following:

- ✦ Client dissatisfaction with the color of his teeth
- ✦ Client embarrassment because of a disfiguring malocclusion
- ✦ A middle-aged man's loss of self-esteem associated with mobile teeth and halitosis from chronic periodontal disease
- ✦ A resident of a nursing home who has misplaced her dentures and who no longer wants to interact with friends and family

These problems require the establishment of unique client goals and varying dental hygiene interventions to resolve them. Figure 17–2 uses the aforementioned examples as the basis for establishing goals and planning dental hygiene interventions that focus on the unique needs of the client who is dissatisfied with the color of his teeth.

Many suggestions for dental hygiene care plans appear in the dental hygiene literature. Each dental hygiene care

Characteristics of a Well-Written Dental Hygiene Care Plan

Reflects purposes of dental hygiene to (1) develop and maintain the individual's capacity to perform behaviors essential to oral health and the mastery of self-care and the environment; (2) prevent oral disease whenever possible using primary, secondary, and tertiary preventive interventions; and (3) promote oral wellness.
Is consistent with the needs of the client.
Identifies the dental hygiene diagnoses, related client goals, and dental hygiene interventions.
Is compatible with the dental treatment plan prepared by the dentist.
Identifies the dental hygienist's responsibilities, if any, for fulfilling components of the dental treatment plan.
Is based on current standards of evidence-based dental hygiene care.
Meets the psychosociocultural and physical needs of the client.
Reflects the dental hygienist's role as clinician, educator/health promoter, manager, researcher, change agent, and client advocate.
Establishes priorities of care.

<table>
<tr><td colspan="3">Client Profile: Personal, dental, medical, and pharmacologic history reveals no significant findings. Assessment reveals slight supragingival calculus, soft deposits, and extrinsic stain. The client verbalized "I wish that my teeth were a whiter color," and "My teeth seem to be darkening with age."</td></tr>
<tr><td colspan="3">Dental Hygiene Diagnosis
Human need for wholesome facial image due to client's dissatisfaction with the color of his teeth as evidenced by the client asking if there is anything that can be done to make his teeth whiter.</td></tr>
<tr><td>Client Goals:</td><td>Intervention:</td><td>Evaluative Statement:</td></tr>
<tr><td>♦ Client will seek cosmetic bleaching consultation with dentist by 6/28.</td><td>♦ Refer client to dentist for cosmetic bleaching consultation.</td><td>♦ Goal unmet. Client did not seek cosmetic bleach consult with dentist.</td></tr>
<tr><td>♦ Client will use tooth whitening dentifrice by 6/14.</td><td>♦ Educate client about tooth whitening dentifrice with fluoride and whitening strips available over-the-counter
♦ Educate client about the normal color of teeth.
♦ Remove all extrinsic stains and deposits from the client's teeth.</td><td>♦ Goal met. Client reports using a tooth whitening dentifrice and is satisfied with the results.</td></tr>
</table>

FIGURE 17–2 ✦ Example of a dental hygiene diagnosis, goals, interventions and evaluative statements for a client who wants whiter teeth.

facility may have its own format. The care plan format should provide the dental hygienist with an opportunity to document assessment findings, dental hygiene diagnoses, client-centered goals, dental hygiene interventions, evaluative outcomes anticipated from care, and the expected date of goal attainment. Although formats may differ, the critical point is that these factors are documented in the client's permanent record and are followed rigorously to ensure quality dental hygiene care. See Figure 17–3, a proposed dental hygiene care plan for unmet human needs form.

ESTABLISHING PRIORITIES.[1,2] To establish priorities in care, the dental hygienist considers the dental and dental hygiene diagnoses and, in collaboration with the dentist, determines their urgency.

Priorities can be based on the degree to which the dental hygiene diagnosis:

- ✦ Threatens the client's well-being (it is important to distinguish deficits that pose the greatest threat to the client's comfort, health, and safety from those that are non–life-threatening and/or not related to a current oral disease)
- ✦ Can be addressed simultaneously with other diagnoses
- ✦ Is viewed as a priority by the client (client's primary concern)

Once these criteria are applied to the dental hygiene diagnoses, the dental hygienist ranks the human need deficits in the priority that they will be addressed. Other than meeting the client's human need for safety, which in some instances constitutes emergency care, most dentists and dental hygienists would probably identify the client's ability to assume responsibility for oral health as a top priority.

The establishment of priorities is always influenced by factors such as:

- ✦ Attitudes of the client
- ✦ Philosophy of the healthcare provider
- ✦ Goals of the collaborating dentist
- ✦ Health status of the client
- ✦ Whether the client is experiencing any discomfort

After the list of dental hygiene diagnoses is prioritized, goal setting begins.

GOAL SETTING.[1,2] *Client-centered goals* are the desired end result that the client is to achieve through specific dental hygiene interventions. Goals may be cognitive, psychomotor, affective, or health status–oriented in nature. *Cognitive goals* target increases in the client's knowledge. *Psychomotor goals* reflect the client's skill development and skill mastery. The dental hygienist must recognize that knowledge and skill development alone may not correlate with client compliance. The client must internalize the desire to make modifications in behavior. Therefore, *affective goals* address the desired changes in client values, beliefs, and attitudes. Health status goals target the signs and symptoms of oral disease and reflect the desired health outcome achievable through dental hygiene interventions.

All client-centered goals must be directly related to the dental hygiene diagnosis. The direct link between the dental hygiene diagnosis and the client-centered goal is the reported signs and symptoms of the client. Thus intervention strategies that focus on client-centered goals will satisfy specific client needs rather than being task oriented. To measure achievement of client-centered goals, the clinician must evaluate whether the goals have been achieved in terms of changes in the signs and symptoms reported in the original diagnosis.

Writing Client-Centered Goals. Adopting a format for each client-centered goal simplifies the act of goal writing (see Guidelines for Writing Client-Centered Goals). Each client-centered goal should have a subject, a verb, a criterion for measurement, and a time dimension. The subject is the client (or client's caregiver); the verb is the action desired of the client; the criterion is the observable behavior or tangible outcome expected; and the time dimension denotes when the subject is to have achieved the goal. At least one goal and one intervention should be established for each dental hygiene diagnosis (Table 17–2).

Client Involvement. Too often, individuals receiving care are referred to as the "Class II cavity preparation in

ASSESSMENT (circle signs & symptoms present)	
1) **WHOLESOME FACIAL IMAGE:** * expresses dissatisfaction with appearance - teeth - gingiva - facial profile - breath - other ________	5) **FREEDOM FROM HEAD AND NECK PAIN** * extra-/intraoral pain or sensitivity * other ________
2) **FREEDOM FROM ANXIETY AND STRESS:** * reports or displays: - anxiety about proximity of clinician, confidentiality or previous dental experience - oral habits - substance abuse * concern about: - infection control, F_2 therapy, fluoridation, mercury toxicity	6) **BIOLOGICALLY SOUND AND FUNCTIONAL DENTITION** * reports difficulty in chewing * presents with: - defective restorations - ill fitting dentures, appliances - teeth with signs of disease - abrasion erosion - missing teeth - rampant caries - other ________
3) **SKIN & MUCOUS MEMBRANE INTEGRITY OF HEAD AND NECK** - extra-/intraoral lesion - pockets > 4 mm - swelling - attachment loss > 1 mm - gingival inflammation - xerostomia - BOP - other ________	7) **RESPONSIBILITY FOR ORAL HEALTH** * plaque & calculus present * inadequate parental supervision of oral healthcare * no dental exam within the last 2 years * other ________
4) **PROTECTION FROM HEALTH RISKS** - BP outside of normal limits - need for prophylactic antibiotics - potential for injury - other ________	8) **CONCEPTUALIZATION AND UNDERSTANDING** * has questions about DH care and/or oral disease * other ________

DENTAL HYGIENE DIAGNOSIS (List the human need not met; then be specific about the etiology and about signs & symptoms evidencing a deficit)

(Unmet Human Need) due to (Etiology) as evidenced by (Signs & Symptoms)

CLIENT GOALS	**INTERVENTIONS** (target etiologies)	**EVALUATION** (goal met, partially met, or unmet)

APPOINTMENT SCHEDULE:

CONTINUED-CARE RECOMMENDATION:

FIGURE 17–3 ✦ Proposed dental hygiene care plan for unmet human needs form.

TABLE 17–2 EXAMPLES OF CLIENT-CENTERED GOALS AS RELATED TO THE DENTAL HYGIENE DIAGNOSIS

Dental Hygiene Diagnosis	Goals
Unmet human need for protection from health risk *due to* organic heart murmur, *as evidenced by* self-report on health history.	Client will report taking prescribed antibiotic premedication 1 hour before dental hygiene care.
Unmet human need in wholesome facial image *due to* abuse of smokeless tobacco, *as evidenced by* client dissatisfaction with stained teeth.	Client will successfully complete a formal program for smokeless tobacco cessation, by 12/30.
Unmet human need for skin and mucous membrane integrity of the head and neck *due to* subgingival plaque accumulation in 4-mm pockets, *as evidenced by* gingival bleeding.	Client will exhibit a gingival bleeding score of no more than 2, by 6/15

treatment room 2" or "the perio case at 4 p.m." These apparently harmless phrases communicate insensitivity to the individual, who is the focus of dental hygiene care. The oral healthcare professional who views the person as the focus of attention is more likely to establish a collaborative, co-therapeutic relationship with the client. This philosophy of care sets the stage for active client participation in identifying needs, priorities, goals, and interventions. Clients who are encouraged to participate in the process of care are more likely to communicate their wants, needs, and expectations than to relinquish decision making about their oral care to the dentist or dental hygienist. Individuals are more likely to express commitment to a care plan if they shared in the development of goals, priorities, interventions, and even appointment planning. Furthermore, when persons are a part of the planning process and have a key role in the overall success of the plan, compliance is augmented. Phrases that can be used by the dental hygienist to maximize the client's involvement in the care planning are

Guidelines for Writing Client-Centered Goals

Prepare each goal, or set of goals, from only one dental hygiene diagnosis.
Make sure that goals, if met, will resolve the problem reflected in the dental hygiene diagnosis.
Collaborate with the dentist to ensure that the dental hygiene and dental care plans are mutually supportive.
Involve the client in goal setting.
Make sure the client values the goals set.
Write goals that are observable and measurable.
Include a target time when a goal will be met by the client.
Use active verbs to denote critical client behavior expected in the goal, such as the following:

affirm	detect	plan
attend	discuss	purchase
choose	eliminate	remove
communicate	exhibit	replace
complete	explain	report
decrease	finish	stop
define	guide	use
demonstrate	increase	verbalize
describe	perform	

Common Phrases Used by the Dental Hygienist to Maximize Client Involvement

Here is a hand mirror. Let's examine your mouth together.
What was your primary reason for seeking dental hygiene care?
Is this set of priorities acceptable to you?
Is this care plan acceptable to you?
What would you like to achieve as a result of dental hygiene care?
How will you feel if this goal is attained?
Are you satisfied with the plan of care we just discussed?
How important is your oral health?
Where would you like me (the dental hygienist) to start first?
When and where is it easiest for you to clean your mouth (or your dependent's mouth)?
Can you think of a better way that we can accomplish this goal?
Let's compare how your gingiva looks today with how it looked two weeks ago.
What are you willing to do to keep your mouth healthy?

listed in Common Phrases Used by the Dental Hygienist to Maximize Client Involvement.

There are times when specific goals are valued more highly by the dental hygienist than by the client. When this occurs, the dental hygienist should provide an explanation for this professional judgment, with a clear message that the client's wants and needs are equally important to the overall care plan. Although these points are important for obtaining client commitment and compliance with the final dental hygiene care plan, dental hygienists must also keep in mind that respecting the client's role as a co-therapist and as a partner in decision making is an effective risk management strategy for avoiding malpractice.

At times the client may disagree with the dental hygienist's recommended care plan. The client may not want certain procedures or may choose to delay care despite the dental hygienist's careful explanations and rationales. Such disagreements between dental hygienist and client may manifest themselves in the client's following actions:

- Refusal of fluoride therapy, radiographs, or antimicrobial agents
- Noncompliance with referral to a dental specialist or physician
- Nonadherence to a specific oral self-care technique
- Decision to terminate care before goal attainment
- Refusal to give up a behavior that increases the risk of periodontal disease progression, such as use of tobacco

Although disappointing, such client responses must be analyzed to determine how or why the client arrived at that decision. In such situations, further discussion with and education of the client are warranted. If the client continues to refuse professional advice, this occurrence is documented in the client's permanent record. Documenting informed refusal is a risk management strategy for the potential threat of malpractice (see section on informed refusal and Chapter 54). In some situations, the client may request care that, in the opinion of the dentist or dental hygienist, is unwarranted, inappropriate, or dangerous. If the dental hygienist is faced with this dilemma, she or he should refuse to provide the care and encourage the client to seek a second professional opinion.[3]

SELECTING DENTAL HYGIENE INTERVENTIONS.[1,2] *Dental hygiene interventions,* like client goals, are derived from the dental hygiene diagnosis and address the factors contributing to the diagnosis. If dental hygiene care is to be effective, the dental hygienist must select evidence-based interventions that specifically address the factors contributing to the client's unmet human need related to dental hygiene care. Various factors may contribute to a client's unmet need for a biologically sound and functional dentition (e.g., lack of knowledge about dental caries prevention strategies, high intake of fermentable carbohydrates, skill deficit in self-care, low value on oral health, low self-esteem, and inadequate financial resources or culture as a barrier to professional care, just to mention a few). Thus not every client with a high caries risk is cared for in the same way. Professional dental hygiene care involves the careful tailoring of interventions to meet the unique needs of the client, as directed by the dental hygiene diagnosis.

Interventions are the evidence-based strategies that resolve a client's unmet human need. These strategies or services are the steps that guide the clinician and client in achieving the proposed client-centered goals and desired health outcomes.

APPOINTMENT PLANNING

Planning Appointment Time

Once the dental hygiene interventions have been decided, they must be operationalized at planned appointments. The appointment schedule becomes a guide for implementing the proposed interventions and specifies the following:

- Number of visits
- Time needed for each visit
- Interventions to be implemented at each visit

The number of visits and sequencing of interventions into planned appointments will vary among clinicians and clients. Consider the following when planning appointments:

- Time needed for each intervention (e.g., self-care education, pain management)
- The logic of grouping interrelated procedures
- Status and severity of unmet human need
- Client's tolerance for long sessions
- Client's scheduling requirements (e.g., early morning only, time limitations)

When unmet client needs and proposed care plan goals are easily attainable, the related intervention may be implemented in one visit. Multiple appointments are indicated to successfully manage dental hygiene care when diagnoses, client goals, and interventions are complex.

Consideration must be given to scheduling time for client education. Too often self-care instruction is squeezed in at the end of an appointment as time permits. Effectively addressing the client's cognitive, psychomotor, and affective needs influences the outcome of care and the client's long-term responsibility for self-management. Sequencing small increments of client education into each visit may successfully shape the client's self-care responsibilities. For example, multiple appointment care plans may spread client education over several visits, including time to review and reinforce self-care education at each visit. Consider the following client education issues when planning appointments:

- Include self-care education in each visit.
- Link self-care instruction with related dental hygiene interventions.
- Manage client variables such as dexterity, technical skill, knowledge, disabilities, and personal preference.
- Actively involve the client during self-care instruction (e.g., have client demonstrate technique intraorally, clarify questions).
- Pace and monitor self-care instruction to encourage client success (e.g., small steps, review, remediate, reinforce).
- Include parent or caregiver when instructing a young child or a mentally or physically impaired client.
- Assess the client's ability to access recommended oral health aid regarding cost and availability.
- Educate the client to accept responsibility for health maintenance.

Informed Consent

Most consumers no longer view healthcare professionals as infallible. Clients expect to participate in their care and know that they have a right to accept or refuse care. For the client to participate in care, the care plan must be presented to the client. Failure to present the care plan to the client can result in services performed without the client's knowledge or permission. This scenario can result in a violation of tort law known as *technical assault* (see Chapter 54).

Informed consent means that the client must be knowledgeable about what the healthcare provider plans to do and must give permission for the plans to be carried out. To achieve informed consent, the client must have enough information to make a rational choice. The client must receive, in understandable language, the following information:

- Nature of the condition
- Proposed care plan
- Risks involved (if any)
- Potential for failure
- Expected outcomes if the problem goes untreated
- Alternative procedures that might be used

In addition to the requirements of informed consent, the client giving consent must:

- Be legally competent.
- Be informed.
- Give consent to a specific treatment.
- Give consent to a procedure that is legal.
- Give consent under truthful conditions (e.g., the consent cannot be obtained through fraud, deceit, misrepresentation, or trickery).

Although informed consent is given when a client voluntarily comes to the oral care setting and sits in the dental chair, *implied consent* applies only to the assessment, diagnosis, and planning components of the dental hygiene process of care. The dental hygienist cannot assume that the client consents to any further care (see Chapter 54). The dental hygienist must obtain the client's *express consent,* orally or in writing, for specific procedures to be performed.

Informed Refusal[3]

Given all information necessary for a client to make an informed decision, the possibility exists that a client may decline all or part of the proposed care plan. Some reasons for declining care include the following:

- Cost
- Fear
- Lack of understanding
- Low value placed on dental care
- Lack of dental insurance coverage

When a client refuses care, the clinician should listen and evaluate the client's reasons for refusing care. At this time, the clinician may choose to reopen the discussion of treatment needs and include the following:

- Acknowledgment of the client's concerns
- Further clarification of the proposed plan
- Consequences of declining care

If the client continues to decline the recommended care, the client must sign an informed refusal document. Informed refusal implies that the client has made an educated decision to decline care based on knowledge of the following:

- His or her personal health needs
- Treatment recommendations and procedures
- Prognosis of care
- Consequences without care

An alternative treatment option may be considered with the client when appropriate. A copy of the refusal form can be given to the client and a copy kept in the client's record. An informed refusal form should include the following:

- A brief explanation of proposed treatment recommendations
- Specific treatment procedures being declined
- The risks or consequences to the client's health without treatment
- Date
- Signature of the client, dentist, and a witness

CARE PLAN EVALUATION[1,2]

Goal of Evaluation

Evaluation in the dental hygiene process ensures quality dental hygiene care that facilitates the client's human need fulfillment related to oral health and wellness. Evaluation is a critical component to the successful outcome of dental hygiene care. Specifically, evaluation allows the clinician to measure the short-term achievements of client-centered goals as well as to anticipate the client's long-term prognosis in maintaining the goals achieved.

Evaluation includes monitoring or reassessing the client's self-care, changes in self-care behaviors, and/or parameters of oral health and disease at continued care. Although evaluation is indicated as the fifth phase of the dental hygiene process, an evaluation strategy is determined in conjunction with the planning phase and is evident during the implementation of care (Figure 17–4).

Evaluation is ongoing during the implementation of dental hygiene interventions to monitor the client's progress toward achieving proposed goals. A dental hygienist may perform an intervention competently, but if the action does not help the client achieve the desired goal, the action is ineffective and a new intervention must be implemented. The evaluation of dental hygiene interventions directed at the achievement of client goals occurs periodically so that the dental hygienist can decide to:

- Modify the plan because the client is having difficulty in achieving the goal.
- Continue the plan because the client needs more time to achieve the goal.
- Terminate the plan of care because the client has achieved the goals.

At each appointment, the dental hygienist and client measure the client's progress toward achieving the desired goals. Failure to evaluate the client can lead to what has been referred to as supervised neglect. *Supervised neglect* occurs when the client continues to require further dental hygiene care to achieve higher levels of oral wellness or to prevent or control oral disease progression, yet the client has been erroneously discharged from care thinking that a healthy state was achieved. Supervised neglect can occur in practices that have a one-approach-fits-all philosophy (e.g., "Just do what you can in the time allotted," or "Do your best given the schedule," or "Everyone in this office gets a prophy and four bitewings" or "Everyone gets a professional topical fluoride treatment").

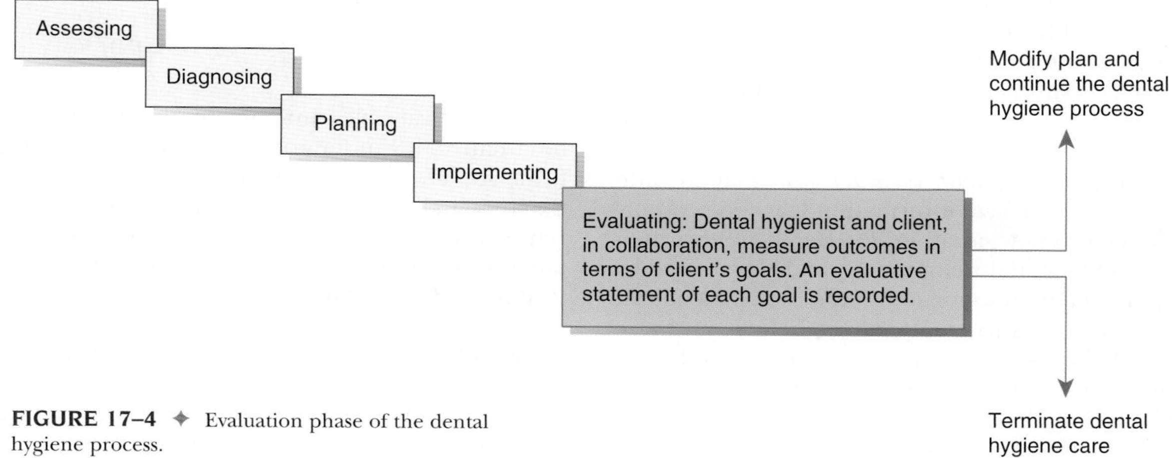

FIGURE 17–4 ✦ Evaluation phase of the dental hygiene process.

In situations such as these, emphasis is on the mechanics of doing, with too little regard for the needs of the person, risk factors, and the influences of care on the client's health status. Evaluation is always needed to determine whether the client's treatment goals have been attained, reactivating the cycle of the dental hygiene process of care. Evaluation does not meet every person's need, but it provides the assurance that unmet needs will not be overlooked or neglected.

Evaluation of Client-Centered Goals

The evaluation process determines the quality of dental hygiene care by judging whether goals are met, partially met, or unmet. As indicated in the previous guidelines, client goals must be observable, measurable, and reflect a time dimension for evaluation. Examples of criteria reflected in well-written client goals are as follows:

- ✦ Client achieves a score of 1 on the Patient Hygiene Performance (PHP) index after using the new toothbrushing and flossing technique (3/28).
- ✦ Parent observes no more than three areas of gingival bleeding after flossing the child's teeth (4/16).
- ✦ Probing attachment levels remain the same or are reduced by 1 mm (5/10).
- ✦ Parent of client reports cleaning the child's teeth once each day (6/15).
- ✦ Client reports using gingival bleeding as an indicator of active oral infection for 1 month (7/8).

Observable, measurable goals allow for concrete evidence that will be used to determine if a client's goal was successfully met, partially met, or not met. Therefore, each goal must correspondingly have an expected outcome that is achievable by self-care and professional intervention. In addition, clients need time to absorb information, integrate new knowledge, practice new skills, experience physical and attitudinal changes related to oral health and wellness, and assess the importance of these changes to their lifestyle. Time must be provided to the client to process information and to make lifestyle modifications. Therefore, a timeframe is established and incorporated into the client goal for determining whether the specified change in the client has been observed. Client goals evaluated too early restrict the dental hygienist's (and the client's) ability to determine the impact of the care provided. Failure to evaluate client goals leaves the dental hygienist unaware of the client's health status and whether the care made any difference.

Methods used to evaluate *cognitive goals* may include having the client verbalize information learned or apply the knowledge in a new situation. *Psychomotor goals,* which reflect the client's skill development, can be evaluated by observing the client demonstrate the newly acquired skill. Desired changes in client values, beliefs, and attitudes are *affective goals.* Affective goals can be evaluated by observing the client's verbal and nonverbal behavior. Desired changes in the client's *oral health status*(signs and symptoms) reflect tangible outcomes and are the most definitive way of evaluating the effectiveness of dental hygiene care. For example, a client may intellectually grasp the importance of daily bacterial plaque control in a Class III furcation (cognitive) but still need instruction from the dental hygienist in using an interdental brush and antimicrobial agent to control disease in the area (psychomotor). Both cognitive and psychomotor goals would need to be established in the dental hygiene care plan of this client; however, the final measure of success would be the health of the tissue surrounding the Class III furcation (oral health status).

During the evaluation phase, the dental hygienist measures the degree to which the client goal has been achieved (Figure 17–5). The dental hygienist makes one of the following decisions:

- ✦ Goal met
- ✦ Goal partially met
- ✦ Goal not met

An evaluative statement is written into the client's permanent record, signed, and dated by the dental hygienist. The evaluative statement contains the dental hygienist's decision on how well the goal was achieved and concrete evidence that supports the decision. Samples of evaluative statements as they relate to the dental hygiene diagnosis and client goal are displayed in Table 17–3.

When client goals are met, the client is placed on a continued-care schedule appropriate to maintain optimum oral health. If a client goal was partially met or not met, the dental hygienist reassesses the client, discusses the findings with the dentist, and perhaps modifies the dental hygiene diagnosis and care plan. Hence the cyclical nature of the process of care is again in motion. Without an evaluative statement, the value of dental hygiene care is too easily overlooked.

From a legal perspective, failure to evaluate the status of the client after care may be grounds for negligence or malpractice charges because the client's oral health knowledge, behaviors, status, or values may still be contributing to an oral health deficit. When a dental hygienist evaluates the *outcome* of dental hygiene care and records that outcome in the permanent record, it is an indication of willingness to assume responsibility for the quality of care provided.

Factors Influencing Client Goal Attainment

Numerous variables interact in the healthcare setting to enhance or hinder goal attainment. The astute dental hygienist identifies both positive and negative factors that affect client goal attainment. Positive factors can be reinforced and negative factors can be resolved to facilitate the achievement of the desired oral health outcome.

Positive factors might include:

- ✦ Client's interest in oral health, motivation, or sense of inquiry
- ✦ A family environment that values personal and profession oral healthcare and oral wellness

TABLE 17–3 SAMPLE OF EVALUATIVE STATEMENTS AS RELATED TO THE DENTAL HYGIENE DIAGNOSIS AND CLIENT-CENTERED GOAL STATEMENTS

Dental Hygiene Diagnosis	Goal Statement	Evaluative Statement
Human need for responsibility for oral health *due to* impaired physical ability, *as evidenced by* a plaque free index score of 30%.	Client will use a manual toothbrush modified with an enlarged, elongated handle at least one time each day by 11/1. Client will increase plaque free index score by 11/1.	11/1 *Goal met.* Client reported using modified toothbrush twice daily and plaque free index has increased to 80%.
Human need for wholesome facial image *due to* wearing a denture and halitosis, *as evidenced by* client's concern with appearance of dentures and self-report of bad breath.	Client will meet at least two other individuals who successfully wear dentures by 12/1. Client will clean dentures, tongue, and oral cavity with appropriate brushes and dentifrice by 11/25.	12/5 *Goal partially met.* Client met one person who successfully wears dentures and verbalized that the dentures looked natural. 11/25 *Goal met.* Client reported cleaning mouth twice daily as directed and that spouse no longer complained about her bad breath.
Human need for conceptualization and understanding *due to* a knowledge deficit about the periodontal disease process, *as evidenced by* bleeding on probing and attachment loss.	Client will verbalize the periodontal disease process and identify plaque as a prime etiologic agent by 9/20.	9/20 *Goal met.* Client can describe the role of bacterial plaque and the periodontal disease process.
Human need for biologically sound dentition *due to* infrequent dental visits, *as evidenced by* signs of four carious lesions.	Client will follow up on a referral made to the dentist of record and have the four carious lesions diagnosed and restored by 8/1.	8/15 *Goal not met.* Client canceled dental appointment.
Human need for skin and mucous membrane integrity of the head and neck *due to* inadequate self-care, *as evidenced by* gingival bleeding and inflammation.	Client will decrease bleeding and inflammation by 5/8.	5/10 *Goal met.* Client no longer shows clinical signs of gingival bleeding and inflammation.

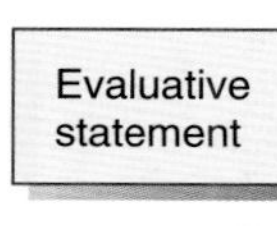

FIGURE 17–5 ✦ Components of an evaluative statement.

✦ A dental hygienist who keeps abreast of current knowledge in the discipline
✦ A work environment that values quality healthcare and offers incentives for dental hygiene care that meets or exceeds national standards

Table 17–4 presents common negative variables that can detract from quality dental hygiene care. Possible dental hygiene responses are presented to initiate thinking about overcoming variables that impede client goal attainment.

Modifying or Terminating the Care Plan

When the evaluation reveals that the client has made little progress toward goal attainment, the dental hygienist again initiates the dental hygiene process of care with the assessment (reassessment). New assessment data may be collected; dental hygiene diagnoses may be altered; goals may need modification; client's attitudes, beliefs, and practices must be considered; and interventions must be changed. On reassessment, the dental hygienist may find some common problems in how the dental hygiene process was used.

Some common problems may include:

✦ Improperly developed client goals; goals that, if achieved, do not guarantee a resolution of the problem
✦ Unrealistic goals for the client to achieve; unmeasurable goals
✦ Care plan that does not specifically address the client's goals and unique socioethnocultural characteristics; plan contains only general information
✦ Care plan that has not been updated
✦ Failure to evaluate
✦ Inadequate documentation

Once the dental hygienist understands why the client has failed to achieve goals, the evaluative statement can be used to redirect the care plan.

When all of the client goals have been achieved and no new problems have been identified, the dental hygienist and client have achieved the ultimate purpose of dental hygiene care, placing the responsibility for oral health maintenance under the full control of the individual. Throughout dental hygiene care, the client has been educated to assume control over his or her own oral health. Written and verbal instructions should be given to the client to take home, and signs and symptoms of any possible future problems should be fully understood.

TABLE 17–4 CLIENT, DENTAL HYGIENIST, AND ENVIRONMENTAL FACTORS THAT MAY DETRACT FROM QUALITY DENTAL HYGIENE

Variables/Factors	Possible Dental Hygiene Response
Client Variables	
Client who refuses to cooperate with therapeutic regimen.	Determine underlying reason for the observed behavior; consider possible socioethnocultural factors. Counsel and educate appropriately.
Client who rarely communicates needs.	Encourage client to communicate by asking questions. Be nondirective in the educational approach. Consider need to involve primary caregiver, family, or interpreter in communication process.
Dental Hygiene Variables	
Dental hygienist who gives 200% of self when others do not.	Learn to leave work on time, avoid assuming work of others, leave work-related concerns at the workplace. Work to resolve work-related problems positively; seek strategies that improve motivation and morale of colleagues and self. Learn to view problems as challenges rather than insurmountable obstacles. Develop a realistic sense of what can be accomplished in the given amount of time. When resources do not permit quality care and strategies do not result in positive change, explore other employment options.
Dental hygienist is bored.	Seek avenues within the employment setting for growth and development; participate in staff development and continuing education programs; identify a project and become involved in it; initiate strategies that result in positive change. Evaluate long-term career goals; seek advanced degrees. Participate in professional associations. Search for new position.
Dental hygienist is under stress from outside concerns (e.g., illness or death of significant others; marriage, childbirth, divorce, separation; conflict with roles as professional, parent, spouse; significant life changes).	Evaluate whether this is the exception or the rule, and assess whether performance at work is less than optimal. May need to reduce work hours rather than "cheat" clients. Seek counseling.
Environmental Variables	
Inadequate supplies and equipment	Identify and document problems with supplies and equipment. Talk with co-workers about their experiences. Identify specific supply and equipment needs and discuss with employer.
Inadequate time allotted to provide quality care	Identify and record the type of dental hygiene care required. Relate client needs and outcomes to the level of care provided. Demonstrate and document how more time can make a difference in client outcomes. Discuss with employer.
Inadequate respect, recognition, and reward from employer	Identify and document incidents when respect, recognition, or reward were withheld. Talk with employer about the specific incidents. Give employer suggestions on how situation can be improved. Search for new position. Initiate cultural diversity training in the workplace.

Adapted from Taylor C, Lillis C, LeMone P: *Fundamentals of nursing*, ed 3, Philadelphia, 1997, Lippincott.

Dental Hygiene Prognosis and Continued Care

Termination of the care plan initiates a new phase of dental hygiene care: periodic *reevaluation* and *continued care*. At the final appointment, the dental hygienist recommends a continuing care plan that will support the client's efforts to maintain the level of oral health achieved during active therapy. This recommendation for re-care is determined by the dental hygiene prognosis of continued oral health.

The dental hygiene prognosis reflects an overall appraisal of the expected outcome evaluative statements and is contingent on the client's continued compliance with self-care as well as the level of optimum oral health achieved. A favorable prognosis occurs when the risk for a new disease or recurrence of the previous conditions is low. A prognosis is guarded when the risk for a new disease or recurrence of the previous condition is high.

Client-centered goals may be successfully achieved during active therapy; however, the prognosis may be guarded because of risk factors such as cigarette smoking or poorly controlled diabetes mellitus. The client and dental hygienist would select a frequent continued-care interval to monitor oral health. The frequency of periodic continued-care appointments ranges from 2 to 12 months, with 3 and 6 months being the most common. The continued-care plan must periodically be reviewed and adjusted to meet client needs. See the following case scenarios and sample care plans.

SCENARIO 1

CLIENT WITH PLAQUE-INDUCED GINGIVITIS AND SAMPLE DENTAL HYGIENE CARE PLAN

Susie S., a healthy 19-year-old single female who does not have dental insurance, is a second-year student and resident at the local university. Her last preventive dental appointment was two years ago and included a prophylaxis and four bitewing radiographs. She brushes twice daily with a fluoride toothpaste and flosses occasionally. Her chief complaint is brown stain on her teeth.

The clinical examination reveals soft tissues within normal limits, Class I occlusion with a slight anterior overbite, and crowding in mandibular anteriors. Evaluation of her gingiva indicates localized slight papillary erythema and edema in sextant 5. Sulcus depths are within 3 mm, no attachment loss, and slight bleeding on probing in sextant 5. Plaque free index is 85%. Dental examination indicates 30 teeth present, including partially erupted third molars (17/32), extrinsic brown stain from coffee, and slight lingual and proximal calculus in sextant 5. No restorations are present; however, her molars have pit and fissure sealants. Bitewing radiographs reveal Class II carious lesions mesial of #2 and #15, incipient carious lesions mesial of #19 and #30. Further questions reveal that Susie drinks three to four cups of coffee a day with two teaspoons of sugar.

Dental Hygiene Client Goals	Interventions	Evaluation
Dental Hygiene Diagnosis *Unmet human need* for skin and mucous membrane integrity of head and neck *due to* anterior malocclusion, plaque retention in sextant 5, *as evidenced by* localized papillary erythema/edema, bleeding on probing, plaque free score of 85%.		
The client will: Demonstrate proper flossing technique by end of appointment. Eliminate bleeding and inflammation of sextant 5 by next continued-care visit.	Instruct client on relationship between bacterial plaque and gingival health. Review client's flossing skills. Provide periodontal debridement.	Goal met, client's flossing technique modified. Goal met, no evidence of bleeding/inflammation.
Dental Hygiene Diagnosis *Unmet human need* for biologically sound and functional dentition *due to* frequent coffee and sucrose intake, *as evidenced by* smooth surface carious lesions and extrinsic stain.		
The client will: Decrease the frequency of sucrose and coffee intake by choosing an alternative beverage with a noncariogenic sweetener, by next continued-care visit. Use daily sodium fluoride rinse to decrease risk for future smooth-surface carious lesions, by next continued-care visit. Have current carious lesions restored, by next continued-care visit.	Instruct client on impact of bacterial plaque and frequent sucrose exposure to the caries process. Instruct client on role of fluoride in prevention of caries risk. Perform selective polishing to remove extrinsic stain. Refer to dentist of record for restorative treatment. Recommend use of powered toothbrush and an ADA-approved whitening toothpaste to control stain.	Goal met, carious lesions restored and no evidence of new lesions. Goal met, client reports using daily fluoride rinse and noncariogenic sweetener.

APPOINTMENT SCHEDULE

Appointment 1 (50 minutes)	CDT-4 Procedure Code
Comprehensive oral assessment: initial personal, dental, medical, pharmacologic history, measure vital signs, head and neck exam, dental/periodontal chart	D0150
Bitewing radiographs: four films	D0274
Inform client of diagnosis and recommended care plan, including clinical findings, and obtain informed consent (or informed refusal)	
Oral self-care instruction: flossing	D1330
Client education: bacterial plaque/gingival health and caries process. Benefits of daily fluoride to prevent smooth surface caries. Benefits of a powered toothbrush and whitening toothpaste.	
Adult prophylaxis: full-mouth debridement, selective coronal polishing with mild abrasive	D1110
Continued-care interval: 6 months	

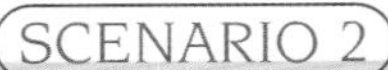

CLIENT WITH PLAQUE-INDUCED GINGIVITIS MODIFIED BY SYSTEMIC FACTORS (PREGNANCY-ASSOCIATED GINGIVITIS) AND SAMPLE DENTAL HYGIENE CARE PLAN

Renee B. is a 29-year-old female, married with a five-year-old child. Renee, who is eight months pregnant and in good health, is taking Pepcid at bedtime for heartburn. She reports that her pregnancy is becoming uncomfortable.

Last oral prophylaxis was six months ago and included oral hygiene instruction. Full-mouth radiographs were taken one year ago. She brushes one time a day and flosses sometimes. Her chief complaint is that "gums are bleeding when she brushes and bad taste in her mouth."

Clinical examination reveals soft tissues within normal limits, Class I occlusion. Gingival and periodontal assessment indicates generalized moderate marginal erythema and edema, moderately bulbous papilla and enlarged marginal gingiva, spontaneous heavy bleeding on probing, probing depths of 4-5 mm with no attachment loss evident. Plaque free index is 75.8%. Supragingival calculus is present lingual of the mandibular anterior teeth and facial of the maxillary molars. Generalized subgingival calculus is noted. Dental examination indicates 28 teeth present, third molars were previously extracted, and multiple Class I and II amalgam restorations are present.

Dental Hygiene Client Goals	Interventions	Evaluation
Dental Hygiene Diagnosis *Unmet human need* for conceptualization and understanding *due to* client's lack of knowledge and understanding of bacterial plaque, *as evidenced* by the client's bleeding gums when brushing.		
The client will: Explain the composition of bacterial plaque and impact on gingival tissue and halitosis by 4/16. Verbalize how pregnancy can enhance gingivitis in the presence of bacterial plaque by 4/16.	Instruct client on composition of bacterial plaque and impact on gingival tissues and halitosis. Instruct client on how pregnancy can enhance the incidence of gingivitis.	Goal met, client verbalized role of bacterial plaque and effects on oral health. Goal met, client explained pregnancy-associated gingivitis.
Dental Hygiene Diagnosis *Unmet human need* for wholesome facial image *due to* plaque retention and pregnancy hormones, *as evidenced by* plaque free index of 75.8%, gingivitis, and client's concern about bad taste in her mouth and bad breath.		
The client will: Recognize the importance of efficient daily plaque control for oral health by 4/26. Increase plaque free index score to 90% by 4/16.	Assist the client in identifying plaque-retentive sites with bleeding points and disclosing agent.	Goal met, client reports daily flossing and extended brushing time. Goal met, client increased plaque free index score to 95%.
Dental Hygiene Diagnosis *Unmet human need* for skin and mucous membrane integrity of the head and neck *due to* plaque retention, infrequent flossing, hormonal changes associated with pregnancy, *as evidenced by* gingival erythema and edema, spontaneous bleeding.		
The client will: Decrease bleeding by 80% by 4/26. Decrease probing depths by 1 mm by 4/26.	Instruct client on modified Bass toothbrushing. Utilizing sulcus toothbrush for the disruption of subgingival plaque. Instruct client on flossing to disrupt proximal bacterial plaque. Full-mouth periodontal debridement: one visit for quadrants 1 and 4; second visit for quadrants 2 and 3 Selective polishing	Goal partially met, bleeding points decreased by 70%. Goal met, decreased probing depths by 1 mm.
Dental Hygiene Diagnosis *Unmet human need* for protection from health risk *due to* risk of orthostatic hypotension, *as evidenced by* client report that her pregnancy is becoming uncomfortable in the eighth month.		
The client will: Identify comfortable chair position at each dental hygiene appointment to prevent orthostatic hypotension.	Position client in semi-upright position (45-degree angle) to alleviate fetal pressure on vena cava.	Goal met, client was asymptomatic of orthostatic hypotension during appointment.

SCENARIO 2

CONT'D

APPOINTMENT SCHEDULE

Appointment 1 (1 Hour)	CDT-4 Procedure Code
Periodic oral assessment: update personal, social, dental, medical, pharmacologic history; measure vital signs; head and neck examination; dental/periodontal assessment	D0120
Inform client of diagnosis and recommended care plan, including clinical findings, and obtain informed consent	
Oral self-care instruction: modified Bass	D1330
Client education: bacterial plaque/gingivitis/halitosis/hormone-influenced gingivitis	
Nonsurgical periodontal debridement of quadrants 1 and 4	D4341
Appointment 2 (1 Hour)	**CDT-4 Procedure Code**
Update health history/measure blood pressure	
Assess tissue response to self-care and periodontal debridement of quadrants 1 and 4	
Self-care instruction: review toothbrushing if needed and instruct on flossing	D1330
Nonsurgical periodontal debridement of quadrants 2 and 3	D4341
Appointment 3 (1 Hour)	**CDT-4 Procedure Code**
Update health history/measure blood pressure	
Assess all quadrants for tissue response to home care and periodontal debridement (gingival color, contour, consistency, bleeding/probe/PFI)	
Reinforce oral self-care instruction	D1330
Dispense literature on preventive oral health for infants and early childhood caries	
Adult prophylaxis to remove residual calculus (if any), and extrinsic stain with mild abrasive	D1110
Continued-care interval: 4 months	

SCENARIO 3

CLIENT WITH CHRONIC PERIODONTITIS AND SAMPLE DENTAL HYGIENE CARE PLAN FOR PHASE I: THERAPY

Mark B. is a 43-year-old single male, residing in a rural community. He is unemployed, receiving public assistance for basic needs, and does odd jobs to supplement his income. He has no dental insurance. Mark reports being in good health except for being hospitalized seven years ago for an ulcer, no recurrence. No medications were reported. Smokes a half-pack of cigarettes per day.

Last dental appointment was five months ago for extraction of an abscessed molar tooth. He reports brushing twice daily with a soft toothbrush and fluoride toothpaste. He wants to keep his remaining teeth. Chief complaint is "I have pain in my upper left back teeth."

Clinical examination reveals soft tissues within normal limits. Gingiva exhibits generalized moderate marginal erythema, generalized slight edematous papilla with localized moderate edematous papilla in sextant 5. Facial gingiva of #14 is enlarged, smooth, and shiny. Spontaneous bleeding on probing. Generalized recession of 2 mm. Probing depths within 3 to 4 mm, with attachment loss of 6 mm on facial of #14 and exudate present. Generalized moderate interproximal calculus and localized supragingival calculus lingual of sextant 5. Plaque free index is 71%. Extrinsic brown stain evident in sextant 5. Dental examination notes several missing teeth (teeth present include 2, 4, 5, 9-12, 14, 15, 21-28, 31, 32), Class I and II amalgam restorations. Full-mouth radiographs with vertical bitewings show generalized slight horizontal bone loss with localized moderate horizontal bone loss on #14, which is slightly supererupted due to lack of opposing tooth. Radiographs confirm Class II furcation facial #14 with evidence of a periodontal abscess.

Continued on following page

SCENARIO 3

CONT'D

Dental Hygiene Client Goals	Interventions	Evaluation
Dental Hygiene Diagnosis *Unmet human need* for freedom from anxiety and stress *due to* infection around tooth 14, *as evidenced by* exudate on palpation and client report of pain in upper left quadrant.		
The client will: Comply with initial palliative (emergency) treatment and recommended therapeutic care of periodontitis by 2/24.	Local chemotherapeutic subgingival oral irrigation Local ultrasonic debridement Instruct client on use of periodontal aid (toothpick in holder); disrupt bacterial plaque on tooth 14.	Goal met, client reported pain has subsided. Goal met, client returned for dental hygiene therapeutic care.
Dental Hygiene Diagnosis *Unmet human need* for conceptualization and understanding *due to* client's lack of knowledge of the periodontal disease process and the increased risk of smoking on disease progression, *as evidenced by* the signs and symptoms of periodontal disease and history of smoking.		
The client will: Explain the relationship of bacterial plaque and the periodontal disease by 2/10. Explain the impact smoking has on periodontal disease progression by 2/24.	Educate client on relationship between bacterial plaque and periodontal disease process. Educate client on the impact of smoking on periodontal disease progression, the immune system, and healing. Introduce client to smoking cessation literature and indicate willingness to help.	Goal met, client verbalized the periodontal disease process. Goal met, client reported enrolling in a smoking cessation program at local community center.
Dental Hygiene Diagnosis *Unmet human need* for wholesome facial image *due to* multiple missing teeth, financial insecurity, *as evidenced by* client's desire to maintain teeth that he has.		
The client will: Complete several therapeutic appointments for care of generalized moderate gingivitis and stabilize the progression of periodontal disease by 3/24. Adhere to a more frequent preventive care schedule to maintain oral health by 3/24. Investigate options for replacement of missing teeth by 4/15.	Refer client to local dental school for affordable dental hygiene care. Educate client on importance of a regular continued-care schedule to monitor oral health. Referral to dentist of record for consultation for future replacement of missing teeth.	Goal met, client completed all scheduled appointments. Goal partially met, client scheduled 3-month continued-care visit at final dental hygiene care appointment. Goal met, client scheduled consultation appointment with dentist.
Dental Hygiene Diagnosis *Unmet human need* for skin and mucous membrane integrity of the head and neck *due to* supragingival and subgingival plaque removal. Class II furcation on tooth 14, *as evidenced by* bleeding on probing, plaque free index score of 71%, gingival bleeding, edematous gingiva, exudate.		
The client will: Maintain periodontal tissues in a health state with no future destruction by 3/24.	Instruct client on modified Bass toothbrushing technique utilizing a sulcus toothbrush for the disruption of bacterial plaque. Instruct client on flossing to disrupt interproximal bacterial plaque. Full-mouth nonsurgical periodontal debridement Selective polishing Instruct the client on PerioAid for furcation.	Goal partially met, client decreased bleeding on probing by 50%. Goal met, client maintaining clinical attachment levels. Goal met, client increased plaque free index score to 50%. Goal met, client decreased pocket depths by 1 mm.

SCENARIO 3

CONT'D

APPOINTMENT SCHEDULE

Appointment 1 (1 hour) (2/10)	CDT-4 Procedure Code
Comprehensive oral assessment: initial personal, medical, dental, pharmacologic history, measure vital signs, head and neck examination, dental/periodontal assessment, plaque free index	D0150
Full-mouth series radiographs and four vertical bitewings	D0210
Inform client of diagnosis and recommended care plan, including clinical findings, and obtain informed consent (or informed refusal)	
Client education on bacterial plaque and periodontal disease process, instruction on PerioAid	D1330
Ultrasonic periodontal debridement of tooth 14	D9110
Chemotherapeutic subgingival oral irrigation of tooth 14	D9999
Postoperative instructions	

Appointment 2 (1 hour) (2/24)	CDT-4 Procedure Code
Update health history/measure blood pressure	
Assess tissue response around tooth 14; document findings	
Self-care instruction: modified Bass	D1330
Client education on smoking as a risk factor for periodontal disease, disease severity, disease progression, and healing	
Local anesthesia if needed quadrant 2 and 3	D9215
Nonsurgical periodontal debridement with ultrasonic and hand instruments as needed quadrants 2 and 3	D4341
Postoperative instructions	

Appointment 3 (1 Hour) (3/10)	CDT-4 Procedure Code
Update health history	
Assess quadrants 2 and 3 for tissue response to home care and periodontal debridement (gingival color, contour, consistency, pocket depths, bleeding, PFI); document findings	
Self-care instruction: flossing	D1330
Local anesthesia: quadrants 1 and 4 if needed	D9215
Nonsurgical periodontal debridement with ultrasonic and hand instruments as needed quadrants 1 and 4	D4341
Postoperative instructions	

Appointment 4 (1 hour) (3/24)	CDT-4 Procedure Code
Update health history	
Assess all quadrants for tissue response to home care and periodontal debridement (gingival color, contour, consistency, pocket depths, bleeding, PFI); document findings	
Adult prophylaxis to remove residual calculus (if any), and selective polish with mild abrasive	D1110
Refer to dentist of record for reevaluation and consultation for missing teeth replacement	
Continued-care interval: 3 months	

SCENARIO 4

DENTAL HYGIENE CARE PLAN FOR ORAL HEALTH MAINTENANCE (SUPPORTIVE PERIODONTAL THERAPY)

Pauline D. is a 70-year-old female and a widow of 10 years who lives a productive, independent lifestyle. Her health history indicates high blood pressure and an organic heart murmur. She has slight hearing loss and wears a hearing aid in one ear. Pauline took prophylactic antibiotic premedication as prescribed one hour before her scheduled preventive appointment.

Last continued-care appointment was three months ago. She was instructed on the use of an interdental brush for plaque removal in open embrasure areas. Bitewing radiographs were taken six months ago, indicating no evidence of dental caries. Pauline brushes two times a day. She inconsistently uses the interdental brush because she finds the aid difficult to work with.

Clinical examination indicates soft tissue findings within normal limits, generalized fibrotic gingival tissue in the posterior, with slight marginal erythema and edema in sextant 5. Generalized slight marginal recession, probing depths of 3 to 4 mm, and attachment loss of 3 to 5 mm. Slight bleeding on probing. Plaque free index improved to 86.3%. Supragingival calculus is present on the lingual and interproximal of sextant 5.

Dental examination indicates two five-unit fixed bridges from teeth numbers 2 to 6 replacing 3 to 5 and from 11 to 15 replacing 13 and 14. Teeth numbers 18, 19, 21, 29, 30, and 31 have gold crowns. All third molars have been extracted. The remaining posterior teeth have Class II amalgam restorations.

Dental Hygiene Client Goals	Interventions	Evaluation
Dental Hygiene Diagnosis *Unmet human need* for skin and mucous membrane integrity of head and neck *due to* inadequate plaque control by the client, *as evidenced by* localized slight bleeding on probing, localized slight gingival inflammation, and recurrence of supragingival calculus within 3 months.		
The client will: Eliminate bleeding and inflammation in sextant 5, by next 3-month continued-care visit.	Periodontal debridement Selective polishing Reinforce daily self-care and need for frequent professional maintenance care	Goal partially met, no evidence of bleeding on probing, erythema and edema sextant 5. Slight bleeding on probing is evident in sextant 6.
Dental Hygiene Diagnosis *Unmet human need* for responsibility for oral health *due to* infrequent plaque control of proximal surfaces, *as evidenced by* supragingival calculus sextant 5 and client admits to finding interdental cleaner difficult to manage.		
The client will: Demonstrate use of rotary-powered toothbrush to remove bacterial plaque by next 3-month continued-care visit.	Instruct client on use of rotary-powered toothbrush for facial, lingual, and interproximal surfaces. Reteach use of interdental brush.	Goal met, client increased plaque free index to 93% and eliminated supragingival calculus.

APPOINTMENT SCHEDULE

Appointment 1 (50 minutes)	CDT-4 Procedure Code
Periodic oral assessment: update personal, social, medical, dental, pharmacologic history; measure blood pressure; update head and neck examination and dental/periodontal assessment; confirm prophylactic antibiotic premedication	D0120
Document findings	
Inform client of diagnosis and recommended care plan, including clinical findings, and obtain informed consent	
Self-care instruction: rotary-powered toothbrush; review use of interdental brush	D1330
Periodontal maintenance care: debridement and selective polishing	D4910
Continued-care interval: 3 months	

Client Education Issues

- Explain to the client the importance of developing a plan of care.
- Explain how the dental hygiene care plan is integrated with the overall dental care plan.
- Explain how the needs and values of the client are incorporated into the care plan (e.g., client's chief complaint, client-centered goals).
- Be sure the client has participated in the development of client-centered goals and is committed to the goals.
- Explain to the client how the goals will be used and how clinical outcomes of care will be related to the original goals.
- Reinforce that the dental hygienist and client are working in partnership, as co-therapists, to achieve the client-centered goals.

Legal, Ethical, and Safety Issues

- Inherent in the process of care is the legal and ethical responsibility of healthcare providers to:

  Complete a comprehensive assessment of client unmet need.

  Formulate a diagnosis and care plan based on that assessment.

  Communicate the recommended care plan to the client.

  Secure informed consent before implementing the care plan.

  Implement the care plan.

  Evaluate the outcome of care.

  Recommend a continued-care schedule.
- Keep adequate client records that are legible, dated, and signed with the title of the individual making the entry.
- Document clinical and radiographic findings as evidence that the diagnosis and care plan are based on client needs.
- Provide evidence of medical consultation, when needed, and written response, addressing information requested.
- Provide evidence of informed consent before implementation of care, signed and dated.
- Provide evidence of informed refusal when client refuses care or recommendations.
- Document self-care education, status of client compliance, failed or canceled appointments, postoperative instructions, modifications made in care plan and supportive facts, referrals, and continued-care schedule.
- Never release client record without written authorization from the client.

Key Concepts

- A dental hygiene care plan is an evidence-based, client-centered written proposal to meet the unmet human needs of a client that are related to oral health.
- The care plan reflects the dental hygiene diagnosis, client-centered goals, dental hygiene interventions, detailed appointment schedule, and proposed expected outcomes.
- A well-formulated and executed care plan will assure a positive outcome in the dental hygiene care process.
- Evaluation is a critical component of the dental hygiene process to document dental hygiene success in achieving a desired outcome in the client's oral health status.
- The dental hygiene care plan is a management strategy to minimize the risk of litigation.
- Without evaluation, a dental hygienist's contribution to the oral health of the client becomes invisible and undervalued.

Critical Thinking Exercises

1. Critique several client records for completeness of documentation. Discuss the strengths and limitations of the entries. Use the results for quality improvement.
2. Review various samples of dental hygiene care plans and discuss the strengths and limitations of each document.
3. Role-play a clinician-client interaction about the assessment findings, client needs, and goal development. Include the clinician's presentation of the care plan to the client for informed consent.
4. Given dental hygiene diagnoses for unmet human needs, formulate related client-centered goals and dental hygiene intervention.
5. Write dental hygiene diagnoses, client-centered goals, and appointment schedule for the following two scenarios:

SCENARIO 5

Kelly T., a 28-year-old single female and assistant manager of a local retail shop, reports a history of seasonal allergies and mitrovalve prolapse that requires antibiotic premedication for dental care. Her last preventive dental appointment was six months ago, and her most recent bitewing radiographs were one year ago. She brushes two times a day with fluoride toothpaste and flosses three to four times per week. Her chief complaint is a periodic dull ache in the lower right posterior region.

The clinical examination reveals soft tissue within normal limits, Class II malocclusion with a moderate anterior overbite, and slightly rotated mandibular central incisors. Dental examination indicates 32 teeth are present, including partially erupted third molars, and no evidence of calculus, stain, or carious lesions. She has three Class I amalgam restorations. The gingival assessment reveals localized slight marginal erythema and edema #32 and sextant 5, sulcus depths within 3 mm, no attachment loss, and localized slight bleeding on probing #32 and sextant 5. Plaque free index is 93%.

SCENARIO 6

James W., a 50-year-old male, is a long-haul truck driver who is taking hydrochlorothiazide for hypertension, drinks two to three cups of coffee per day, and smokes one pack of cigarettes per day. His last dental appointment was one month ago for extraction of tooth number 2 that was periodontally involved and before that 10 years had passed. He brushes once daily with fluoride toothpaste. His chief complaint is discomfort in the upper left molar region, and he does not want to lose additional teeth.

Clinical examination reveals nicotine stomatitis, Class II occlusion with a moderate overbite, and a coated tongue. Dental examination indicates that all third molars are missing, as well as the maxillary right second molar, generalized moderate brown stain, slight subgingival calculus, localized moderate supragingival calculus sextant 5, and Class I and II amalgam restorations.

Gingival and periodontal assessment findings reveal generalized moderate marginal erythema and edema, generalized slight recession, localized moderate recession facial of sextants 3 and 4, bleeding on probing, pocket depths of 3 to 5 mm, with attachment loss at 4 to 5 mm, Class II and III furcations, and Class I mobility on tooth numbers 14 and 15. Full-mouth periapical and vertical bitewing radiographs show evidence of a recurrent carious lesion on tooth 30 and root caries on the distal of tooth 14, generalized moderate horizontal bone loss in molar regions, and localized vertical bone loss on the distal of tooth 14.

For References, Suggested Readings, and Related Websites, visit
http://evolve.elsevier.com/Darby/hygiene/

SECTION 5

Implementation

CHAPTER 18

Mechanical Plaque Control: Toothbrushes and Toothbrushing

OBJECTIVES

Mastery of the content in this chapter will enable the reader to:

- List the characteristics of an acceptable manual toothbrush.
- Describe the advantages of various power toothbrushes and indications for their use.
- Explain the technique, advantages, and disadvantages of each of the following toothbrushing methods: Bass, Stillman's, and Charter's.
- Describe the methods for evaluation of toothbrushing effectiveness.
- Discuss legal and ethical considerations related to the client in an effective plaque control program for personal oral hygiene care education.

KEY TERMS

Biofilm
Brushing plane
Manual toothbrush
Multitufted toothbrush
Plaque control
Power toothbrush
Self-care
Tufted toothbrush

Plaque control refers to the daily removal of plaque *biofilm* from the teeth and adjacent oral tissues. Mechanical removal of plaque biofilm, through the use of toothbrushes and other oral physiotherapy aids, is the most widely accepted mechanism for plaque control. These cleansing devices are indispensable because there are, to date, no chemotherapeutic agents that totally prevent the formation of plaque biofilm in the oral cavity. This chapter focuses on toothbrushes and toothbrushing as important elements of a comprehensive plaque control regimen. Effective Toothbrush Characteristics lists characteristics of an effective toothbrush identified by the American Dental Association (ADA).[1,2]

Effective Toothbrush Characteristics

Size, shape, and texture conforms to individual user's needs
Effectively and easily used
Inexpensive and durable
Functional in terms of flexibility, softness, and diameter of filaments, and strength, rigidity, and weight of handle
End-rounded nylon filaments
Designed for cleanliness, aeration, and efficiency

MANUAL TOOTHBRUSHES

The manual toothbrush is the most commonly used device for removing plaque biofilm from the facial, lingual, and occlusal surfaces. The Chinese are given credit for developing the first bristle toothbrush, which was introduced into the Western world in the sixteenth century.[3] Since that time, many improvements have been made and many varieties of toothbrushes have been developed. Currently, no evidence suggests that one type of manual toothbrush is superior in reducing plaque and gingivitis as long as individuals are properly motivated and instructed.

Parts of the Toothbrush

Manual toothbrushes have several parts (Figure 18–1). The *head,* or working end, contains the tufts of bristles or filaments. The head of an adult toothbrush should be approximately 1 to 1 1/4 inches (25.4 to 31.8 mm) long and 5/16 to 3/8 inches (7.9 to 9.5 mm) wide. The size of the head should be selected based on the size of the client's mouth. It should be large enough to remove plaque efficiently, yet small enough to facilitate access to all areas of the mouth.

There are various toothbrush sizes on the market. Smaller sizes are available for children. The *handle* is the portion of the toothbrush that is grasped by the hand during use. Some handles are aligned in a straight plane with the head of the toothbrush, although many designs have modified the handle. Handles may be angled like a dental mirror, curved, or offset. Consumers can select the handle shape of their preference, with only a few considerations. The toothbrush handle should be easy to grasp, free from sharp projections, durable, and lightweight, regardless of its design. The *shank* of the toothbrush is the segment that connects the head and the handle. It is frequently constricted so that it is narrower than the rest (Figure 18–1).

The head of the toothbrush contains tufts made of nylon filaments (Figure 18–2) or natural bristles made of boar's hair (Figure 18–3). *Tufted toothbrushes* are five or nine tufts long and two or three tufts across; *multitufted toothbrushes* have 10 or 12 tufts in three or four rows (Figures 18–4 and 18–5). Multitufted filaments or bristles are in closer proximity, allowing the user to generate greater force while brushing and, thus, to achieve better cleansing action. The multitufted design also allows for improved delivery of dentifrice to the tooth surfaces. The filaments or bristles take long to dry between uses, so many professionals recommend that their clients rotate use of more than one toothbrush per day. Toothbrush filaments or bristles should be allowed to air dry between uses. One advantage of synthetic nylon filaments is that they dry faster than natural filaments.

The *brushing plane* is the surface of the brush used for cleaning the teeth and tissues (Figure 18–1). In some toothbrushes, it is flat with all filaments or bristles of the same length. Other manual toothbrushes have uneven planes (Figure 18–6).[3] Little evidence exists to document that any of these designs is superior in reducing plaque and gingivitis to a clinically significant level. Some studies have shown plaque removal advantages of bristles specifically designed to adapt to areas of the mouth that are difficult to access during toothbrushing. Further evidence is needed for any manual toothbrush design to claim superiority in reducing gingivitis. The ADA's Council on Scientific Affairs states that the proper type of toothbrush depends largely on the toothbrushing method employed, the positioning of the teeth, and the manipulative skills of the user. The brush must, however, conform to individual requirements in size, shape, and texture, and be easily and efficiently manipulated, readily cleaned and aerated, impervious to moisture, durable, and inexpensive.[2]

It is clear, however, that nylon filaments are superior to natural bristles. Nylon filaments flex up to 10 times more before breaking; rinse clean and dry more readily; do not split or abrade; and are more resistant to accumulation of

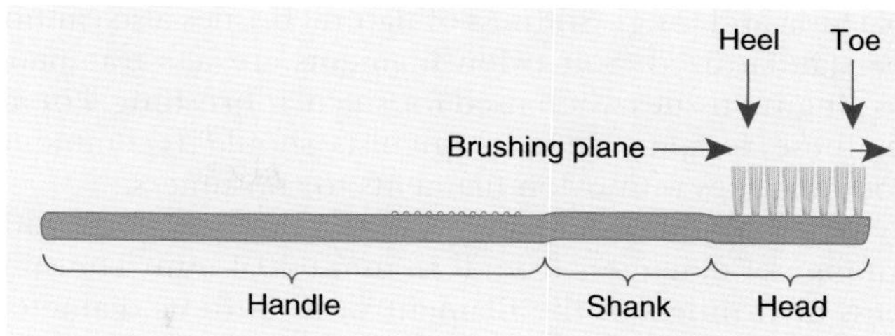

FIGURE 18–1 ✦ Parts of a manual toothbrush.

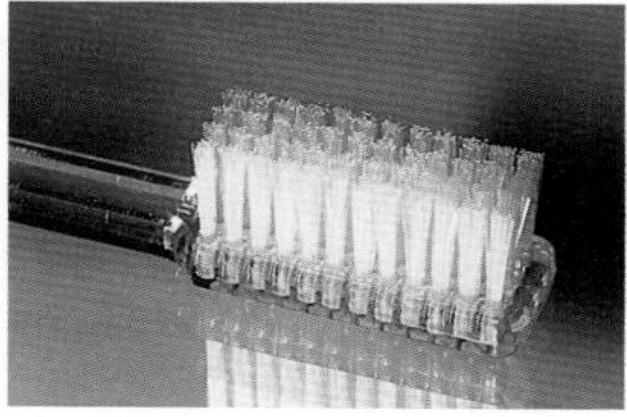

FIGURE 18–2 ✦ Toothbrush with tufts of nylon filaments. *(Courtesy Dr. M. Walsh, University of California–San Francisco.)*

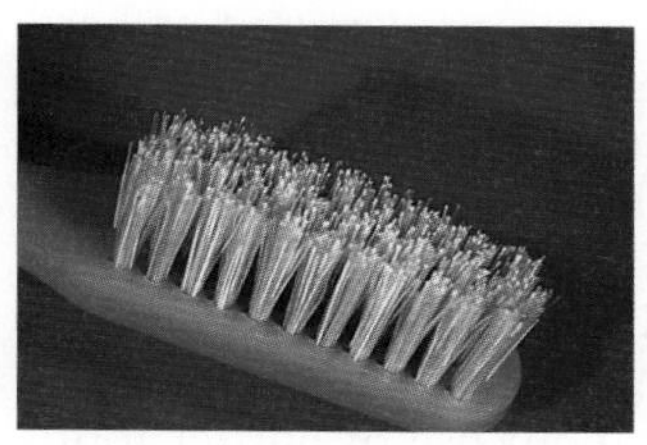

FIGURE 18–3 ✦ Toothbrush with tufts of natural bristles made of hog or boar hair. *(Courtesy Dr. M. Walsh, University of California–San Francisco.)*

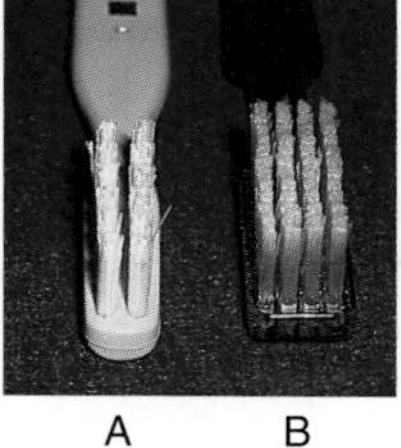

FIGURE 18–4 ✦ Tufts. **A,** Tufted toothbrush head, two tufts wide. **B,** Multitufted toothbrush head, four tufts wide. *(Courtesy Dr. M. Walsh, University of California–San Francisco.)*

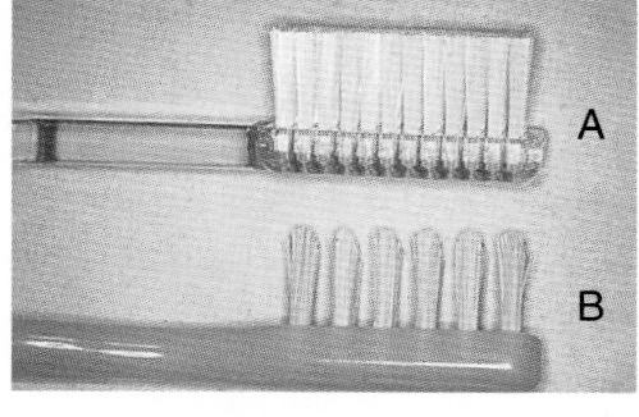

FIGURE 18–5 ✦ **A,** Multitufted toothbrush, 12 tufts long. **B,** Tufted toothbrush, six tufts long.

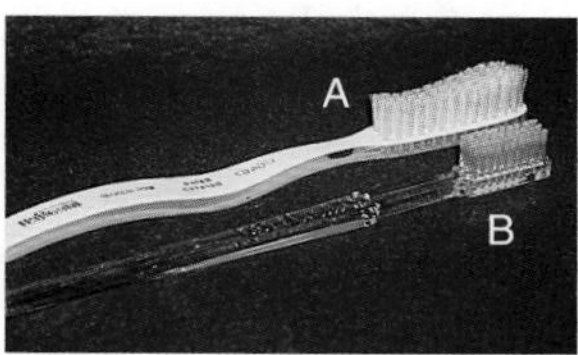

FIGURE 18–6 ✦ Brushing plane. **A,** Toothbrush head with uneven brushing plane. **B,** Toothbrush head with flat brushing plane. *(Courtesy Dr. M. Walsh, University of California–San Francisco.)*

bacteria and fungi. Stiffness of natural bristles also cannot be standardized. Soft nylon filaments are less traumatic to gingival tissues when used for sulcular brushing. For all of these reasons, dental hygienists should recommend toothbrushes with nylon filaments to consumers.

Nylon toothbrush filaments have a uniform shape with a range of diameters from 0.15 mm to 0.4 mm. The stiffness or firmness of the filament varies with its diameter. Filament hardness is primarily related to its diameter and length. Traditionally, most filaments were 10 to 12 mm long. Today, many manufacturers vary the length of the filaments mounted in a single head. A shorter filament will have increased stiffness over a longer one. As a result, a manufacturer might vary the diameter of individual filaments to compensate for variations in length. Toothbrushes are marketed for consumers as extra soft, soft, medium, and hard. Generally, with filaments of standard, traditional length, those from 0.007 to 0.009 mm are considered soft, 0.010 to 0.012 mm are considered medium, and 0.013 to 0.015 mm are classified as hard. Soft filaments are recommended for sulcular cleaning and have been shown to be more flexible and to clean proximal surfaces more effectively than medium or hard filaments.[4]

Some people prefer medium-hard brushes because they feel that their teeth are cleaner after brushing with a stiffer brush. The concern about use of harder toothbrush filaments or bristles relates primarily to the potential for hard and soft tissue abrasion. Soft filaments are universally considered preferable for sulcular brushing.[5,6]

The end of the toothbrush filament can be cut bluntly or rounded. Originally, all brush ends were cut; however, end-rounding has become increasingly more common in manufacturing processes to reduce gingival abrasion (Figure 18–7).

Several other factors, besides quality of bristle end-rounding, may affect toothbrushing-induced trauma. Hardness of the bristle, worn bristles, pressure applied by the client during brushing, improper brushing techniques, and abrasiveness of dentifrices used can all influence the degree of trauma. Detrimental effects of toothbrushing are discussed in more detail later in this chapter.

It is generally recommended that toothbrushes be replaced before the first sign of the bristles becoming worn, splayed, or frayed. The average life of a toothbrush has been estimated to be 2 to 3 months. As toothbrushes deteriorate, plaque removal becomes less effective.[4,7]

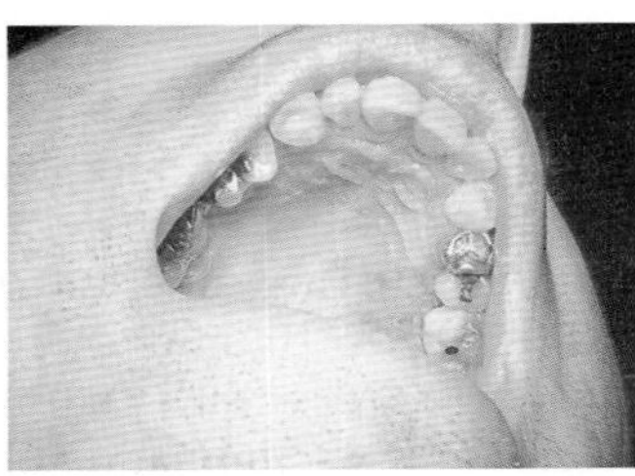

FIGURE 18–7 ✦ Toothbrush abrasions of gingival and palatal tissue. *(Courtesy Dr. M. Walsh, University of California–San Francisco.)*

Studies of dentists' and dental hygienists' attitudes toward toothbrush replacement indicate that practitioners recommend that their clients replace their toothbrushes usually at 2 to 3 months when filaments are bent or splayed.[8,9] Another consideration affecting frequency of toothbrush replacement relates to toothbrush contamination. Some authors recommend that individuals change toothbrushes as often as every 2 weeks to 1 month because toothbrushes are a source of pathogens, especially after an oral or systemic infection.[10] It is unknown whether these organisms have any relevance to oral disease in clients who use toothbrushes harboring pathogens. Clients can be instructed to soak their toothbrushes in a solution of 1% sodium hypochlorite or household bleach and water (1:10) or in 0.12% chlorhexidine gluconate to control toothbrush contamination and cross infection.[11]

Dental hygiene clinicians, as educators and consumer advocates, are influential in helping consumers select toothbrushes. For most clients, a soft multitufted toothbrush with soft, end-rounded nylon filaments; a small enough head to adapt to all areas of the mouth; and a wide and long handle designed to secure a good grasp is desirable. If a client perceives some benefit from a specific design feature and no detrimental effects are noted, the dental hygienist should not change the type of toothbrush.

POWER TOOTHBRUSHES

The first toothbrush powered by electricity was developed by Bermann and Woog in Switzerland and was introduced in the United States in 1960 as the "Broxodent."[12] In 1961, a cordless rechargeable model was introduced by General Electric.[13] These early power toothbrushes consisted of an electric motor encased in plastic and detachable toothbrushes. They used a battery or an alternating current to operate (Figure 18–8). Studies of these early electric toothbrushes showed that there was no difference in plaque removal when compared with a manual toothbrush; however, when assessing effects on controlling gingivitis, results were mixed.[14]

Since the 1980s, tremendous advances have been made in the technology of electrically powered tooth-

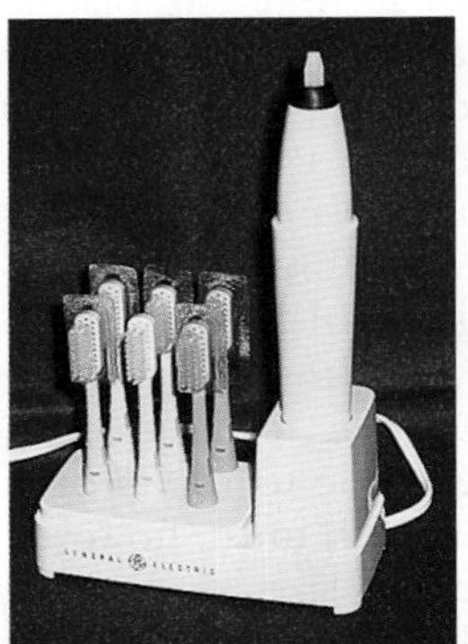

FIGURE 18–8 ✦ Early electric toothbrush.

brushes, now called *power toothbrushes*. Instruments produced include the Braun Oral-B Ultra Plaque Remover, the Braun Oral-B 3D, the Interplak, the Rota-dent, and the Sonicare. Although these brands have different mechanisms of action, studies report they are safe when applied to hard and soft tissues in the mouth.[14] Studies also indicate that these modern power toothbrushes are more effective than manual toothbrushes in removing plaque and reducing gingivitis.[15-31] Indications for Use of a Power Toothbrush lists clients who may benefit from the use of a modern power toothbrush.[15,16]

Evidence also shows a high rate of acceptance and compliance with use of power toothbrushes.[32] Perhaps client preference is the most compelling reason for recommending them. Moreover, some of the power toothbrushes enhance client motivation and compliance by using timing devices set at 2 minutes. Because most individuals brush their teeth for about 45 to 60 seconds, power toothbrushes with timers provide a means for clients to accurately assess time spent brushing. Modern power toothbrushes also have been shown to use significantly less brushing force (80–190 g/f) than manual toothbrushes (over 250 g/f).[16,17] Caregivers often prefer using a power toothbrush without dentifrice for bedridden or comatose clients, or for people who cannot control swallowing reflexes. Foam brushes often are used by caregivers; however, data do not support efficacy in maintaining gingival health.[33] The most widely studied brands of modern power toothbrushes are discussed in the following sections.

Indications for Use of a Power Toothbrush

- Individuals with fixed orthodontic appliances
- Children and adolescents with decalcification
- Adults requiring periodontal maintenance
- Individuals with periodontal disease (gingivitis or periodontitis)
- Individuals with poor oral hygiene
- Adults with extensive prosthodontics or endosseous implants
- Older adults
- Individuals with dexterity problems
- Individuals with gingival recession or toothbrush abrasion

Braun Oral-B Power Toothbrushes

The Braun Oral-B Ultra/D9 has a small, round toothbrush head. The head contains 26 tufts that move in a 60-degree, counter-rotational motion 7600 times per minute (Figure 18–9).[14] This power toothbrush has an oscillating/rotating action and has been found to be more effective than a manual toothbrush in reducing plaque and gingivitis.[34,35] In addition, it has been found to be safe for children[36] and for clients after periodontal treatment.[34]

The Braun Oral-B 3D/D15 and 3D Excel/D17 have a three-dimensional oscillating/rotating/pulsating action. The high-frequency pulsating action is in the direction of the long axis of the filaments (Figure 18–10).[14] When compared to the Braun Oral B Ultra/D9, the Braun Oral-B 3D models have a deeper penetration of occlusal and interproximal surfaces resulting in improved plaque biofilm removal.[37] When compared to the manual toothbrush, the Braun Oral-B 3D models demonstrated greater reduction in plaque biofilm and gingivitis.[31,38]

The oscillating/rotating brush (Braun Oral-B Ultra/D9) and the oscillating/rotating/pulsating toothbrushes (Braun Oral-B 3D/D15 and 3D Excel/D17) have round heads with a cup-shaped bristle design. Most models have a two-minute timer and a slower speed for areas of recession or cosmetic dental restorations. The 3D Excel also includes an interproximal brush attachment. The difference between the earlier models (D7, D9) and the 3D models is faster oscillation and the addition of pulsating as well as oscillating/rotating movement.

Interplak

The Interplak, a counter-rotational brush, has 10 tufts of two different lengths. Each tuft independently rotates 1.5 turns in one direction and then reverses 1.5 turns in the opposite direction at a rate of 4200 rotations per minute (Figure 18–11).[14] A full-size head or a compact head is available, as well as a power flosser, tongue cleaner, and

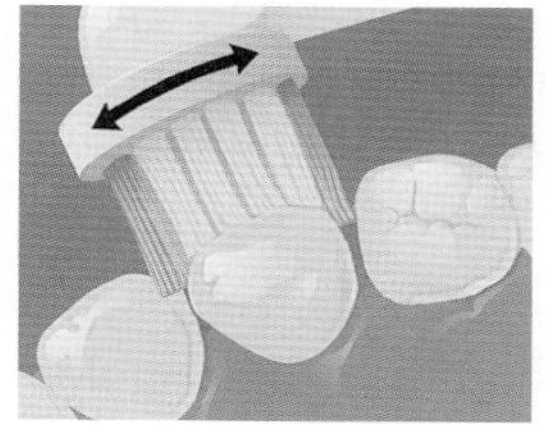

FIGURE 18–9 ✦ Braun Oral-B Ultra Plaque Remover toothbrush head action. *(From Barnes CM:* Oral Hygiene *7(2):8, 2000.)*

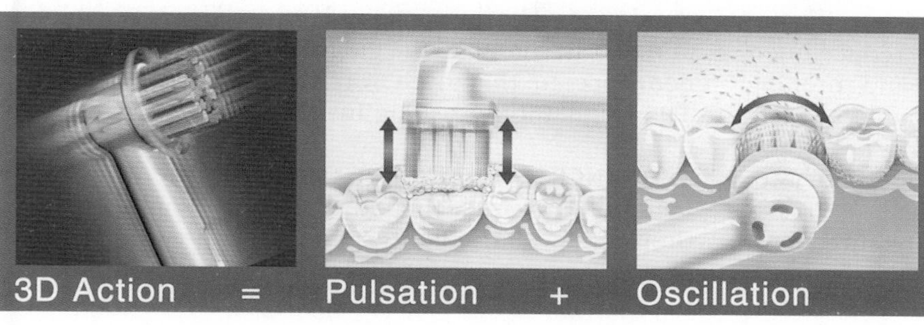

FIGURE 18–10 ✦ Braun Oral-B 3D toothbrush head action. *(From Barnes CM:* Oral Hygiene *7(2):8, 2000.)*

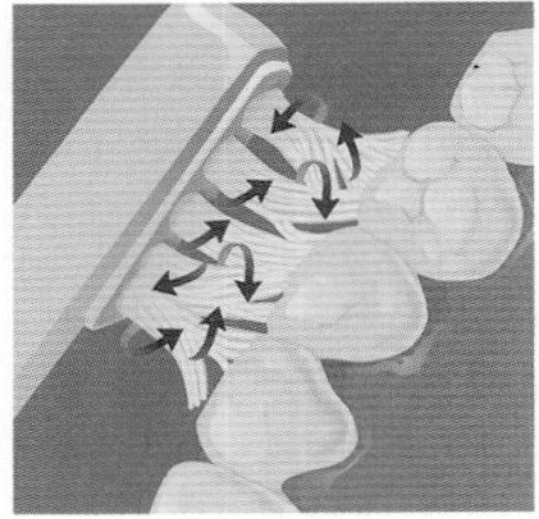

FIGURE 18–11 ✦ Interplak toothbrush head action. *(From Barnes CM: Oral Hygiene 7(2):8, 2000.)*

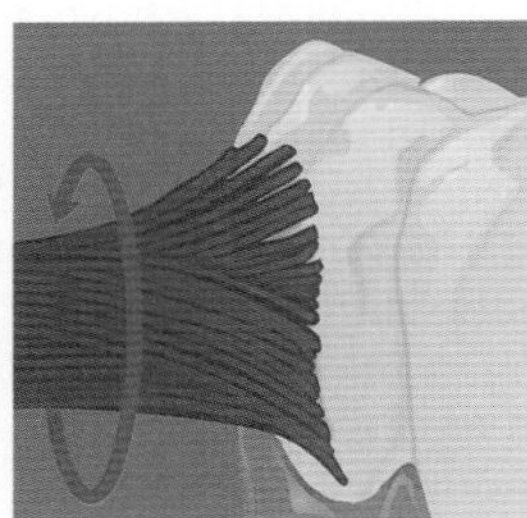

FIGURE 18–12 ✦ Rota-dent toothbrush head action. *(From Barnes CM: Oral Hygiene 7(2):8, 2000.)*

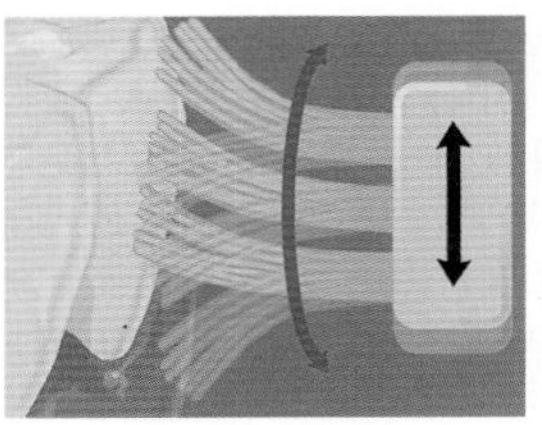

FIGURE 18–13 ✦ Sonicare toothbrush head action. *(From Barnes CM: Oral Hygiene 7(2):8, 2000.)*

interproximal brush attachments. Some models have a 2-minute timer to encourage longer brushing. Originally the Interplak required use of its own dentifrice; however, it has been redesigned to function well with regular dentifrice. The Interplak has been reported to be more effective than a manual toothbrush in reducing plaque and gingivitis in orthodontic and dental implant patients.[20,39-41]

Rota-dent

The Rota-dent, a rotary electric brush, has movement resembling a professional dental rotary instrument. It has three interchangeable hollow-cup tips: a hollow-cup that is similar in shape to a professional prophylaxis cup; a single tuft of bristles similar to a professional prophylaxis brush; and an elongated brush tip that rotates (Figure 18–12).[14] The Rota-dent must be purchased from a dental professional because instruction is needed for proper use and safety. Studies have shown the Rota-dent to be more effective than manual brushing for reducing plaque, gingival inflammation, and bleeding.[42,43] Moreover, it has been shown to be safe and effective for use by clients undergoing orthodontic and periodontal maintenance treatment.[29,40]

Sonicare

The Sonicare is an electronic toothbrush that employs low-frequency acoustic energy to alter bacterial adherence and increase filament movement.[14] The Sonicare Elite vibrates at 31,000 brush strokes per minute (Figure 18–13) and has been shown to significantly reduce interproximal plaque, bleeding on probing, and probing depths.[39] In addition, it has been demonstrated to be safe and effective among orthodontic patients[29,39,44] and among residents in long-term care facilities who were unable to brush their own teeth.[45]

All clinical studies use the manufacturers' directions, which instruct users to apply light pressure to the tooth for plaque removal. One six-year study on dental implants showed safety and effectiveness in removing plaque and reducing gingival bleeding significantly better than a manual brush after 6 months of use.[46] See Table 18–1 for a summary of recommendations for toothbrushes.

TABLE 18–1 SUMMARY OF RECOMMENDATIONS FOR TOOTHBRUSHES

Type of Toothbrush	Recommendation
Manual Toothbrushes	
Nylon filament	Highly recommended Soft-bristled toothbrushes are safe and effective in removing bacterial plaque and controlling gingivitis.
Natural filaments	Not recommended Natural bristles are stiff and dry slowly, causing safety concerns.
Foam brushes	Not recommended Data do not support efficacy in maintaining gingival health.
Power Toothbrushes	
Oscillating/rotating, rotary, counter-rotational, and electronic designs	Highly recommended Long-term studies show safety and effectiveness, as well as benefits for plaque, gingivitis, and bleeding reduction; orthodontic clients; periodontal maintenance; dental implants; special needs; noncompliant individuals; stain removal.

TOOTHBRUSHING

Toothbrush Instruction

Both manual toothbrushes and power toothbrushes have greater benefit when dental professionals provide advice and instruction in methods for using these devices.[47-50] Many different methods of toothbrushing have been developed. The best methods dislodge plaque biofilm and debris, stimulate the gingiva, and deliver fluoridated dentifrice to the tooth surface. (See Components of Thorough Toothbrushing Instruction.)

SEQUENCE. Regardless of the specific toothbrushing method employed, the client must be taught to brush thoroughly. Many clients spend too little time brushing or they brush haphazardly. Dental hygiene practitioners need to stress the importance of thorough plaque

Components of Thorough Toothbrushing Instruction

Toothbrush selection and replacement
Sequence of toothbrushing
Duration of toothbrushing
Frequency of toothbrushing
Toothbrushing method(s)
Evaluation of toothbrushing effectiveness
Detrimental effects of improper toothbrushing (safety evaluation)
Tongue brushing (or scraping)

biofilm removal when teaching others about proper toothbrushing. Clients should be encouraged to develop a standardized sequence of toothbrushing. For example, the hygienist may suggest that the client begin brushing on the facial surface of the most posterior tooth in the maxillary right arch. The brushing sequence may follow around the arch from the right molar region, to the right premolars, to the anteriors, to the left premolars, and finally to the left molar regions.

The client then begins on the maxillary lingual surfaces of the left posterior segment, brushing each surface until reaching the right posteriors. The same sequence is then repeated on the mandible. After brushing all maxillary and mandibular facial and lingual surfaces, the occlusal surfaces in each quadrant are brushed. There are many possibilities for sequencing, but the individual should be encouraged to select a logical sequence and to use it consistently to avoid omission of any area. Also, each brush placement must overlap the previous one for thorough coverage.

DURATION. Duration of toothbrushing also should be stressed during toothbrushing instruction. It has been shown that the average brushing time varies from approximately 45 to 60 seconds. Dental professionals frequently recommend that clients brush their teeth for 3 minutes; however, it has been shown that thorough manual toothbrushing actually requires 5 minutes to consistently yield adequate reductions in plaque biofilm.[51] Even with 5 minutes of toothbrushing, interproximal cleansing aids are needed to achieve effective plaque control. Research also has shown that 2 minutes of power toothbrushing can be as effective as 6 minutes of manual toothbrushing.

Different teaching strategies can be used with clients to increase their brushing time. The client can be instructed to count 10 brushing strokes in each area before proceeding to the next area of the mouth. Another strategy involves timing manual toothbrushing with an egg timer or a clock. People using power toothbrushes with 2-minute timers can brush 30 seconds in each quadrant.

FREQUENCY. In addition to thoroughness of toothbrushing, frequency must be considered. There is no standard recommendation for how many times per day all clients should brush because of variable plaque biofilm–retention factors, variations in client dexterity, and various plaque biofilm–formation rates. It could be hypothesized that, for the average person, thoroughly cleaning the teeth once every 24 hours should prevent gingival disease because plaque biofilm is colonized in that amount of time. Unfortunately, most people cannot attain the goal of 100% plaque removal in a single oral hygiene session. Therefore, it is generally recommended that clients brush *at least* twice daily in order to control plaque biofilm and halitosis. Brushing before bedtime and after a period of sleep should be encouraged, and thus clinicians often suggest cleaning the teeth in the morning and at night. The frequency of toothbrushing should be increased in people with more rapid plaque biofilm and calculus formation, for people with oral habits such as smoking, and for those with systemic diseases compromising the immune system.

Several toothbrushing methods vary in their efficiency in controlling plaque biofilm (Table 18–2). Dental hygienists can teach their clients the toothbrushing methods suited to their oral health needs. Over time, at continued-care or maintenance appointments, reinforcement of instruction and observation of the client's technique are the most effective means of improving plaque biofilm removal techniques.

Toothbrushing Methods

BASS METHOD. The *Bass*, or sulcular, *toothbrushing method* is universally accepted as the most effective; therefore, it is the most commonly recommended. This technique is designed to clean the cervical one-third of the crown of the tooth as well as the area beneath the gingival margin. It has been demonstrated to be more effective than other methods in cleaning the gingival zones of the teeth.[52] Thus, it can be recommended for clients who are periodontally healthy, for clients with periodontal disease, or for periodontal maintenance clients.

The toothbrush can be grasped with a palm grasp or a pen grasp. The toothbrush bristles are directed apically and angled 45 degrees to the long axis of the teeth (Figure 18–14). Gentle force is then applied to insert the bristles into the gingival sulcus and interproximal embrasures until the gingiva blanches. The stroke is activated with a gentle but firm vibratory motion. This vibratory motion consists of short back-and-forth strokes. Approximately 10 gentle strokes should be completed without removing the bristle ends from the sulcus before proceeding to the next area. The brush head is moved to the next tooth or group of teeth by overlapping with the completed area. It must be repositioned at the proper 45-degree angle, with the bristles directed apically into the sulcus.

On the facial and lingual surfaces of the posterior teeth, the toothbrush head is positioned parallel with the arch. The rows of bristles closest to the tooth surface are angled into the sulcus. On the anterior teeth, the

TABLE 18–2 **TOOTHBRUSHING METHODS AND INDICATIONS FOR USE**

Method	Technique	Indications
Bass (sulcular)	Bristles are directed apically at a 45-degree angle to the long axis of the tooth. Gentle force is applied to insert bristles into sulcus. Use gentle but firm vibratory strokes without removing bristle ends from sulcus.	Sulcular cleansing Periodontal health Periodontal disease Periodontal maintenance
Stillman's	Bristles are directed apically and angled similar to Bass. Bristles are placed partly on cervical portion of teeth and partly on adjacent gingiva. Short back-and-forth strokes are employed, and the brush head is moved occlusally with light pressure.	Progressive gingival recession Gingival stimulation
Charter's	Bristles are directed toward the crown of the tooth. Bristles are placed at the gingival margin and angled 45 degrees to the long axis of the tooth. Short back-and-forth strokes are used for activation.	Orthodontics Temporary cleaning of surgical wounds Fixed prosthetic appliances Gingival stimulation
Modified Bass, Stillman's, and Charter's	Add a roll stroke. Roll tufts occlusally after cervical area is cleaned by prescribed method.	Cleaning of entire facial and lingual surfaces
Horizontal scrub	Bristles are activated in a gentle, horizontal scrubbing motion.	Not recommended because transition to another technique may be difficult
Fone's (circular)	Bristles are activated in a circular motion.	Young children with primary teeth; otherwise not recommended
Leonard	Vertical strokes are used with teeth in an edge-to-edge position.	Not recommended
Roll stroke	Bristles are pointed apically and rolled occlusally.	Used in conjunction with Bass, Stillman's, or Charter's

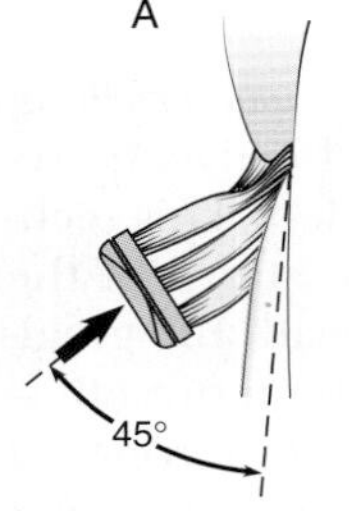

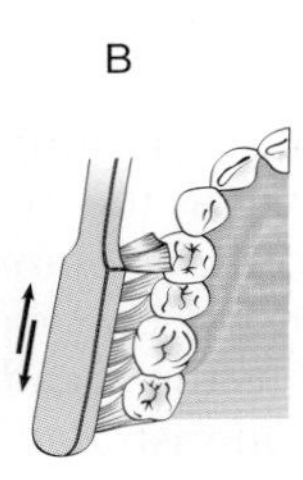

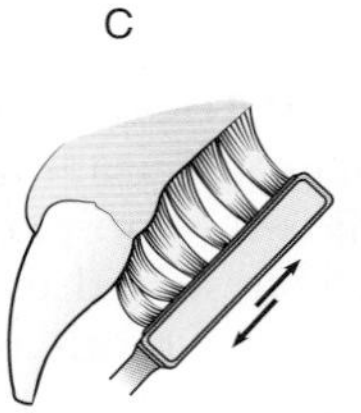

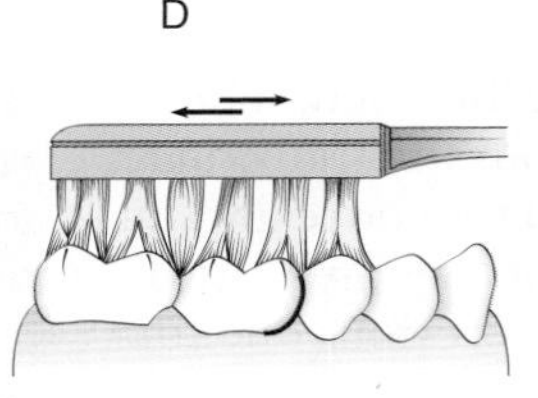

FIGURE 18–14 ✦ The Bass toothbrushing method. **A,** Intrasulcular position. **B,** Correct position on facial surface of posterior teeth. **C,** Correct position of lingual surfaces of anterior teeth. **D,** Correct position on occlusal surfaces. *(From Newman MG, Carranza FA, Takei H:* Carranza's clinical periodontology, *ed 9, Philadelphia, 2001, WB Saunders.)*

toothbrush head can also be placed parallel to the arch (or horizontally) when brushing the labial surfaces, but it should be placed parallel with the long axis of the teeth (or vertically) when brushing the lingual surfaces (Figure 18–14). Thus on the lingual surfaces of the anterior teeth, the heel of the toothbrush is used and the vibratory motion is changed to a short up-and-down stroke. After brushing all facial and lingual surfaces in a sequence, the occlusal surfaces should be cleaned. The bristles are pressed firmly into the occlusal surface so that the ends can penetrate into the pits and fissures and a back-and-forth brushing stroke is activated. The brush is advanced section by section until all occlusal surfaces have been cleaned.

Use of a soft, nylon-bristled brush is indicated when the Bass method is employed.[53] Otherwise, the potential for gingival trauma exists. Dental hygiene clinicians should also be aware of common technique problems encountered by individuals who have been taught to use the Bass technique. Some clients exert too much pressure or use too long a stroke, when attempting the vibratory motion. These errors can result in tissue laceration or gingival sensitivity. Obtaining the proper angle of the bristles is also difficult to achieve, and the toothbrush bristles may not be angled into the sulcus. This error results in inefficient strokes, and plaque biofilm is allowed to remain at the gingival margin.

Sometimes clients place the bristles on the attached gingiva rather than at the gingival margin, thereby neglecting the tooth surface and traumatizing the attached gingiva. The lingual surfaces of the anterior teeth can be problematic for the client because of the need to position the brush vertically in those areas. If the arm is not raised high enough to direct the bristles toward the gingival margin, only the incisal one-third of these surfaces is cleaned. It is critical for the dental hygienist to observe and evaluate each client's toothbrushing skills so that problems or errors can be corrected. Oral hygiene skill assessment must be repeated periodically to help clients achieve optimal efficiency while toothbrushing.

STILLMAN'S METHOD. *Stillman's toothbrushing method* was developed originally to provide gingival stimulation.[54] The toothbrush is positioned and angled (toward the apex of the tooth) similarly to the Bass method, but the bristles are placed partly on the cervical portion of the tooth and partly on the adjacent gingiva (Figure 18–15). The strokes are activated in a short back-and-forth motion, while the brush head is moved simultaneously in an occlusal direction. Approximately 5 to 10 strokes are completed in each region, and the brush is moved to the next area. This process is repeated in a sequence until all regions are thoroughly cleaned. Once again, brush placement is vertical on the anterior lingual surfaces, and the heel of the brush is used. The occlusal surfaces are brushed with the bristles perpendicular to the occlusal plane.

In Stillman's method, the toothbrush bristle ends are not directed into the sulcus; therefore, this method can be recommended for clients with progressing gingival recession. It is considered less traumatic to the gingival tissue than scrub or sulcular brushing. An extra-soft brush and light pressure should be recommended in these cases. The added advantage of gingival stimulation has been questioned because, although it has been found to increase circulation and keratinization, no definite clinical benefits have been demonstrated.

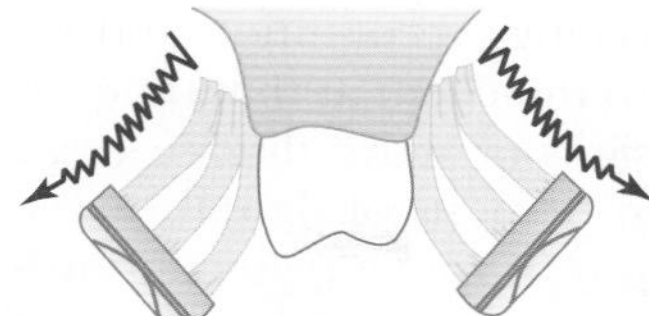

FIGURE 18–15 ✦ Stillman's toothbrushing technique—position and placement of bristles. *(From Newman MG, Carranza FA, Takei H:* Carranza's clinical periodontology, *ed 9, Philadelphia, 2001, WB Saunders.)*

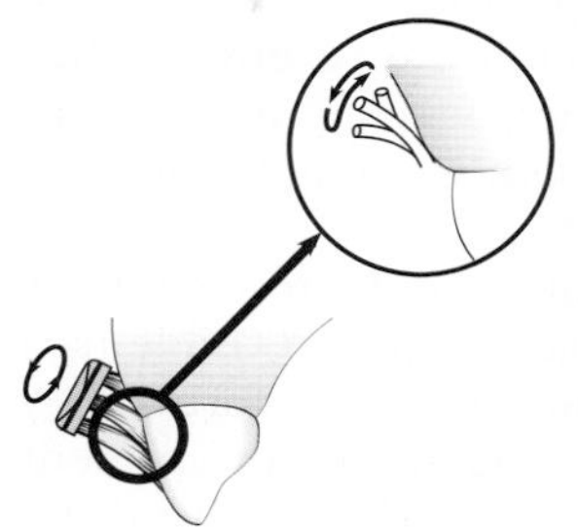

FIGURE 18–16 ✦ Charter's toothbrushing method—position and placement of bristles. *(From Newman MG, Carranza FA, Takei H:* Carranza's clinical periodontology, *ed 9, Philadelphia, 2001, WB Saunders.)*

CHARTER'S METHOD. *Charter's method* was originally developed to increase cleansing effectiveness and gingival stimulation in the interproximal areas.[55] It is now known that interproximal surfaces are not cleaned adequately by any toothbrushing method, but Charter's technique has its advantages. In this technique, the bristles are pointed toward the crown of the tooth rather than apically (Figure 18–16). Like the Bass and Stillman methods, the toothbrush is positioned horizontally and parallel with the arch in all areas except the lingual area of the anterior teeth and the occlusal surfaces. The bristles are placed at the gingival margin and directed toward the occlusal surface at a 45-degree angle to the long axis of the tooth. A short back-and-forth motion is used for activation.

The process is repeated in a sequence around the mouth until all areas are cleaned. Charter's method can be recommended for orthodontic clients or for clients with fixed prosthetic appliances to clean the area between the appliance and the gingival margin. It also is useful for clients immediately after periodontal surgery during healing of surgical wounds.

MODIFIED BASS, MODIFIED STILLMAN'S, AND MODIFIED CHARTER'S METHODS. The Bass, Stillman's, and Charter's methods of toothbrushing were designed to concentrate on the cervical portion of the teeth and the adjacent gingival tissues. Each of these methods can be modified to add a roll stroke. The toothbrush bristles are rolled occlusally to clean the entire facial and lingual surfaces after the cervical area is cleaned. Clinicians need to stress the importance of thoroughly completing the original stroke before rolling the toothbrush bristles occlusally. If the client rolls too prematurely, the vibratory or back-and-forth strokes are ineffective for plaque biofilm removal at the concave gingival third of the tooth.

HORIZONTAL SCRUB. The horizontal scrub technique is probably the most commonly used toothbrushing method. It is considered detrimental because the unlimited scrubbing motion exerts pressure on the facial tooth prominence, resulting in gingival recession and gingival and tooth abrasion.

CIRCULAR METHOD. The circular method may be recommended as an easy-to-learn first technique for young children. With the teeth closed, the upper and lower facial surfaces of the teeth are brushed simultaneously with large, circular strokes. For lingual surfaces, small, circular strokes are used on each arch separately.

Evaluation of Toothbrushing

Before presentation of oral hygiene instruction, the clinician begins by questioning the client about the type of toothbrush used, frequency of toothbrushing, duration of toothbrushing, and toothbrush replacement practices. Next, the client is asked to demonstrate the toothbrushing method routinely used at home. Observation of the client's technique and skill is important in determining the need for modification and reinforcement. The information gained through the client interview and the observation of toothbrushing then is correlated with gingival conditions found during the periodontal assessment and with presence of plaque biofilm and calculus.

If the client is using an acceptable toothbrushing technique, the teeth are relatively plaque-free, the gingival tissues are healthy with no bleeding, and no detrimental effects are noted, there is no need to modify the current methods used by the client. Positive recognition and reinforcement should be given to the client at that time. In contrast, clients who exhibit signs of active disease (e.g., signs of gingival inflammation or signs of dental caries, plaque biofilm deposits, or signs of trauma) need toothbrushing instruction to assist them with improving their oral health. Instruction and practice are indicated at that time, as well as at subsequent appointments, to evaluate client progress. Positive approaches are received better than negative feedback, fear tactics, or scolding. A discussion of methods used to assess toothbrushing follows.

DISCLOSING AGENTS. Disclosing agents are materials used to make the presence of plaque biofilm visible (see Chapter 14). Available in liquid or tablet form, they contain an ingredient that stains plaque biofilm present on the teeth so that it can be seen. Erythrosin dye is the most commonly employed agent; it stains plaque biofilm red. Fluorescein is a dye that can be applied to the teeth without obvious staining. A special ultraviolet light is used to make this agent visible to the client and clinician. Two-tone disclosing agents that stain thicker plaque biofilm blue and thinner plaque red are also available. Disclosing agents ideally should provide a distinct staining of deposits that does not rinse off immediately, should have a pleasant taste, and should be nonirritating to the oral soft tissues.

Because staining of the oral soft tissue inhibits the clinician's assessment of signs of disease, disclosing agents should not be applied to the teeth until after completing the oral and periodontal assessment and after findings are shown to the client. Theory regarding plaque biofilm and gingival inflammation also should be presented before disclosing deposits, so that the client understands the correlation between oral hygiene and gingival inflammation. After performing the gingival assessment and providing the client with needed theoretical background about the composition and effects of plaque biofilm, a non–petroleum-based jelly can be applied to the lips or to cosmetic dental restorations to prevent them from staining. Petroleum-based jellies are not recommended because they can break down latex and contribute to weakening the protective barrier of the clinician's gloves.

The technique for disclosing depends on the type of product used. Solutions can be applied as a concentrate with a cotton swab or diluted with water in a cup for the client to use as an oral rinse. Tablets are chewed and swished around in the mouth by the client. Excess disclosing agent is expectorated or suction and evacuation devices are used to remove it from the mouth after staining. Clean tooth surfaces do not absorb the dye unless roughness is present (e.g., decalcification, hypocalcification, restorations, cementum). Pellicle, plaque biofilm, debris, and calculus absorb the disclosing agent. This discriminate staining characteristic makes the disclosing agent an excellent oral hygiene aid because the client is able to use it at home for self-evaluation and motivation. Being able to see the plaque biofilm deposits helps individuals improve the effectiveness of their self-care.

After application of the disclosing agent, the client is given a hand mirror to observe the location of stained deposits. The dental hygienist assists the client in identifying deposits and correlates findings with signs of gingival inflammation identified before staining. Toothbrushing techniques are then modified to improve efficacy in areas of concern. Instruction and demonstration by the clinician are followed by observation of the client's technique during practice. Each area of concern should be practiced because the client may have difficulty adapting the toothbrushing method in a particular region.

GINGIVAL EVALUATION. The color, size, shape, and consistency of the gingiva are examined for signs of inflammation. Periodontal probing also is completed to detect bleeding on probing and pocket formation. These findings are then reviewed with the client and correlated with the presence of plaque biofilm. The client also should be commended for areas of improvement. Quadrants that have been treated with nonsurgical periodontal therapy can be compared and contrasted with untreated quadrants. Gingival or bleeding indices also can be used to calculate a numerical score for the client (see Chapter 15).

DETRIMENTAL EFFECTS OF IMPROPER TOOTHBRUSHING. In addition to toothbrushing effectiveness, damage resulting from toothbrushing needs to be evaluated. The client may be removing plaque biofilm deposits but also causing trauma from improper toothbrushing, horizontal scrubbing, excessive pressure, use of medium to hard bristles or worn bristles, use of an abrasive dentifrice, and/or adaptation difficulties around prominent root surfaces. Changes can be detected anywhere in the mouth, although they are most often seen on the facial tooth surfaces. Canines are particularly susceptible because of their position in the mouth and the prominence of their roots. Location of trauma is often inversely related to left- or right-handedness.

Initially, toothbrush trauma results in gingival abrasion, which can appear as redness, scuffing, brushing, or punctate lesions (Figure 18–7). Long-term detrimental effects include gingival recession, gingival clefts, or festooning of the gingiva (Figure 18–17). In addition, tooth abrasion, the wearing away of the tooth surface, usually cementum and dentin, in the cervical areas, can be caused by toothbrush trauma. Tooth abrasion can result in cervical notches apical to the cementoenamel junction and dentinal hypersensitivity.

If detrimental effects from toothbrushing are noted, the dental hygienist should question the client in an attempt to discover the causative factors. Observation of the client's toothbrushing is also indicated, and corrective measures are then discussed and correlated with the clinical findings indicating toothbrush trauma (Figure 18–18). When changing toothbrushing method, it is often helpful

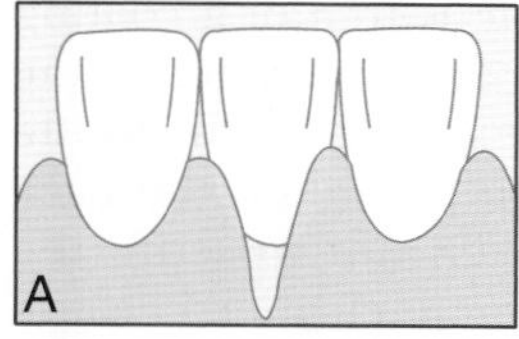

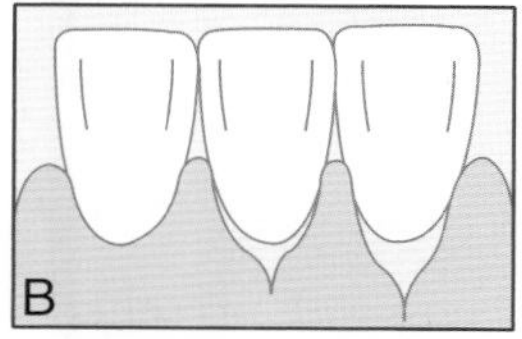

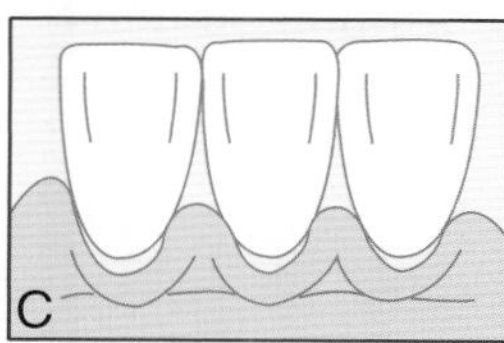

FIGURE 18–17 ✦ **A,** Gingival recession. **B,** Gingival clefting. **C,** Gingival festooning.

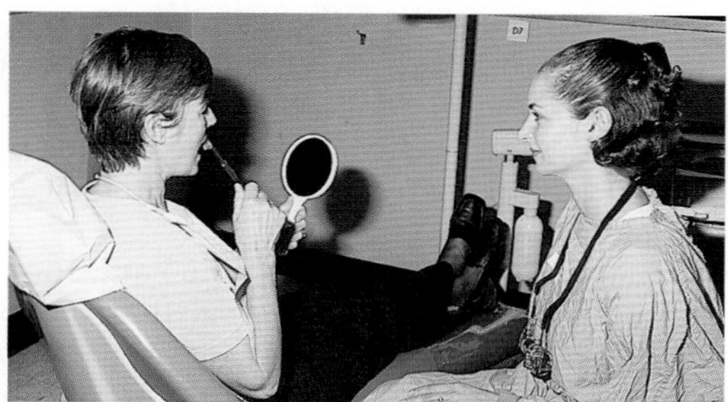

FIGURE 18–18 ✦ Observing toothbrushing technique. *(Courtesy Dr. M. Walsh, University of California–San Franscisco.)*

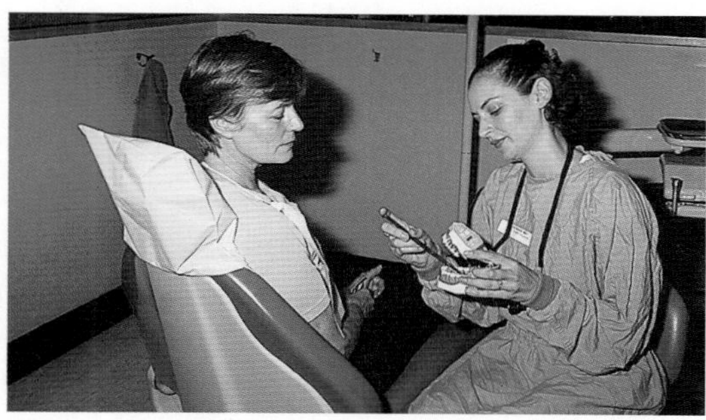

FIGURE 18–19 ✦ Demonstrating corrective measures on a typodont. *(Courtesy Dr. M. Walsh, University of California–San Franscisco.)*

to demonstrate the new technique on a typodont model before demonstrating the technique in the client's mouth (Figure 18–19); however, the client's performance of the new technique must also be observed in the client's own mouth and feedback provided to ensure that the proper skill level is obtained. Recommendations to Correct Toothbrush Trauma lists strategies to correct trauma caused by improper toothbrushing.

Also, because power toothbrushes exert less toothbrushing force than manual toothbrushes and their handles generally are larger in diameter, allowing a fingertip grip, they can be recommended to people who are overzealous manual toothbrush users.

Recommendations to Correct Toothbrush Trauma

- Use soft toothbrush with end-rounded bristles.
- Replace worn toothbrush.
- Use a less abrasive toothpaste.
- Modify toothbrushing technique.
- Use a fingertip grip rather than a palm grip on the toothbrush.
- To decrease brushing force and detrimental effects of "scrubbing" or overzealous toothbrushing, use a power toothbrush.

Long-term Evaluation

Long-term evaluation of the effectiveness of oral hygiene practices is based on the client's periodontal health status, rather than on the presence of plaque biofilm deposits. Plaque biofilm may be present because the person was unable to brush before the dental hygiene appointment. Absence of plaque may be the result of thorough brushing immediately before the appointment rather than daily plaque removal. Evaluation of the gingival tissues for signs of inflammation yields more valid findings. Comparisons of previous and current probing depths and periodontal attachment levels at a 4- to 6-week interval and a 3-month interval after active treatment also provide valuable information regarding long-term effectiveness.

Special Toothbrushing Considerations

At times, clients avoid toothbrushing because it is uncomfortable for them. This avoidance syndrome usually compounds problems because of the effects of accumulated plaque biofilm. Special toothbrushing instructions are needed for individuals who may want to avoid toothbrushing. Clients who are in pain have a basic need to free themselves from pain. For example, persons with necrotizing ulcerative gingivitis or acute injuries to the soft tissue may be sensitive to toothbrushing. Recommending supragingival brushing and an extra-soft brush and explaining the importance of oral cleanliness helps these clients. Clients who are undergoing periodontal or oral surgeries need similar instructions. Some people also want to avoid toothbrushing around new dental appliances. Teaching them specific methods for toothbrushing (e.g., Charter's) and interdental care in the healing or recently restored areas is important for maintenance of oral health.

Tongue Brushing

To cleanse the mouth thoroughly, tongue brushing or cleaning should be incorporated with toothbrushing. The dorsum of the tongue is a primary source of oral microorganisms. Tongue cleaning can reduce the number of these organisms, improve the client's taste perception, and contribute to overall cleanliness. Tongue cleaning also is essential to treating bad breath. The reduction in anaerobic bacteria that produce volatile sulfur compounds has been shown to reduce oral malodor.

After extending the tongue, the toothbrush head is placed horizontally across the tongue and the bristles are directed posteriorly. The bristles are then drawn forward with light pressure to cleanse the tongue. This brushing motion is repeated until the tongue is free of a coating or debris. Tongue cleaners also are available. Some people prefer these devices because the size of the toothbrush head produces gagging when placed on the back of the tongue. Care should be taken not to scrub the tongue with the toothbrush or tongue cleaner because damage to the tongue can result.

Client Education Issues

- Inform about appropriate toothbrushes and toothbrushing methods to meet the client's needs
- Explain effects of tongue brushing
- Correlate toothbrushing effectiveness with presence of gingival inflammation, toothbrushing trauma, and disclosed plaque

Legal, Ethical, and Safety Issues

- According to the *Principles of Ethics* of the American Dental Hygienists' Association, it is the dental hygiene practitioner's ethical responsibility to "provide oral health care using the highest level of professional knowledge, judgment and ability" and to "use every opportunity to increase public understanding of oral health practices."
- The dental hygienist has an ethical obligation to make a lifelong commitment to reviewing scientific literature related to preventive interventions and applying the knowledge gained to client care.
- Dental hygiene care requires allocation of time for instruction, repetition, reinforcement, and continual assessment of each client's oral health practices.
- The legal standard of care requires that dental hygienists educate clients about oral self-care.
- Care plans should include evaluation of the presence and distribution of bacterial plaque and calculus, plans for educating the client in daily personal oral hygiene, consideration of adjunctive chemotherapeutic agents, assessment of the client's bacterial plaque control effectiveness, and reinstruction where needed.
- Upon completion of dental hygiene care, the legal records of the client should reveal that the client has been counseled on why and how to perform an effective daily personal oral hygiene program. Monitoring the client's progress also should be recorded.
- Malpractice cases for failure to recognize and treat periodontal disease can be related to failure to teach adequate plaque control measures to clients.

Key Concepts

- The manual toothbrush is the most commonly used device for removing bacterial plaque from the facial, lingual, and occlusal surfaces.
- A soft, multitufted toothbrush with soft, end-rounded nylon filaments; a small enough head to adapt to all areas of the mouth; and a wide and long handle designed to secure a good grasp is desirable.
- Nylon filaments are superior to natural bristles.
- Hardness of the bristle, worn bristles, pressure applied by the client during brushing, improper brushing techniques, and abrasiveness of dentifrices used can all influence degree of trauma.
- Both manual toothbrushes and power toothbrushes have greater benefit when dental professionals provide advice and instruction in methods for using these devices.
- The average life of a toothbrush is approximately 2 to 3 months.
- Studies indicate that modern power toothbrushes improve plaque removal, gingival inflammation, and gingival bleeding when compared with manual toothbrushing.
- Thorough toothbrush instruction addresses issues related to toothbrush selection and replacement; sequence, duration, frequency, and method of toothbrushing; evaluation of toothbrushing effectiveness; and tongue brushing.
- A standardized sequence of toothbrushing is important to avoid omission of any area.
- Each brush placement must overlap the previous one for thorough coverage.
- The Bass method of toothbrushing is the most effective method for cleaning the gingival areas of the teeth.
- Use of a soft, nylon-bristled brush is indicated when the Bass method is employed.

KEY CONCEPTS—CONT'D

- Stillman's method can be recommended for clients with progressing recession.
- The horizontal scrub technique is detrimental and causes gingival recession and gingival and tooth abrasion.
- The circular method is an easy-to-learn first technique for young children.
- Disclosing agents are materials used to make the presence of plaque visible. Being able to see plaque deposits helps individuals improve the effectiveness of their home care.
- Because staining of the oral soft tissue inhibits the clinician's assessment of signs of disease, disclosing agents should not be applied to the teeth until after completing the oral and periodontal assessment, and findings are shown to the client.
- Evaluation of the effectiveness of toothbrushing includes observation of the client's toothbrushing, a gingival evaluation for signs of inflammation and detrimental effects of improper toothbrushing, and using disclosing agents. Corrective measures are related to clinical findings.
- To cleanse the mouth thoroughly, tongue brushing or cleaning should be incorporated with toothbrushing.

CRITICAL THINKING EXERCISES

Mrs. Truman is a 65-year-old female being seen by the dental hygienist. Upon disclosing her teeth, she has heavy plaque throughout, with generalized gingival inflammation and bleeding on probing. During the dental hygienist's conversation with Mrs. Truman, the client says "You know my arthritis has been bothering me in my hands, and I find it difficult to brush my teeth sometimes." What type of toothbrush and toothbrushing method would you recommend for Mrs. Truman and why?

For References, Suggested Readings, and Related Websites, visit
http://evolve.elsevier.com/Darby/hygiene/

CHAPTER 19

Mechanical Plaque Control: Interdental Care and Supplemental Aids

OBJECTIVES

Mastery of the content in this chapter will enable the reader to:

- ✦ Discuss the appropriate use and indications for interdental and supplemental plaque control devices.
- ✦ Discuss ethical, legal, and safety considerations related to the client in an effective plaque control program for personal oral hygiene care.

KEY TERMS

Clasp brush
Dental floss
Dental tape
Denture brush
Embrasure spaces
End-tuft brush
Floss holder
Floss threader
Foam sticks/foam brushes
Gauze strip
Interdental swab tip
Interdental tip stimulators
Interproximal/interdental
Interproximal brushes
Knitting yarn
Pipe cleaner
Single-tuft/uni-tuft brush
Sonic action/motion
Supplemental aids
Tongue cleaners
Toothpick
Toothpick holder
Tooth towelettes
Tufted dental floss
Wedge stimulators

The most common method of mechanical plaque control is toothbrushing. Toothbrushing, however, does not reach the proximal surfaces of teeth or the area immediately under the contact point of adjacent teeth (*embrasure spaces*). These areas are known as the *interproximal* or *interdental* area.[1] Because plaque biofilm in the interdental area is not accessible to toothbrushing, a means for plaque biofilm removal in this area is necessary for complete preventive care.

Removal of plaque biofilm from the interdental area is important for the following reasons:

- ✦ To prevent periodontal diseases, most of which commonly begin in the interdental col area, a depressed concave area of gingival tissue under the contact area of two teeth. The col area connects the lingual and facial papillae, and because of its saddle-like shape, it harbors plaque biofilm. The epithelium covering the col area is thin and less resistant to disease. When inflammation is present in the gingival papilla, the papilla is enlarged and the col becomes deeper (see Chapter 15). The interdental col area is inaccessible to toothbrushing.
- ✦ To prevent proximal dental caries in combination with fluoride therapy.
- ✦ To prevent oral malodor (halitosis) caused by interdentally trapped plaque biofilm.

Toothbrushing is an automatic habit for most clients, but interdental cleaning is not. Therefore, it is recommended that interdental cleaning be implemented before toothbrushing. A newly developing habit, such as flossing, should be implemented before the established habit of toothbrushing to avoid skipping the new habit.[1] Also, as the mouth begins to feel clean after toothbrushing, it is easier for clients to establish a false sense of thorough plaque biofilm removal and skip interdental cleaning.

In addition to interdental plaque control devices, supplemental plaque control aids target the tongue, gingival margins, buccal mucosa, and removable and fixed appliances. When circumstances prevent proper toothbrushing and interdental care (e.g., immune disorders or hospitalization), alternative *supplemental aids* other than toothbrushes and interdental devices are necessary for thorough cleaning.

SELECTION OF INTERDENTAL AND SUPPLEMENTAL AIDS

A wide variety of interdental and supplemental plaque control aids are available. In general, when the interdental gingiva fills the embrasure spaces, plaque biofilm removal from proximal tooth surfaces and shallow pockets is best accomplished with dental floss or tape, provided the client has the dexterity to use them. When the interdental gingiva is reduced or missing, however, the embrasures are open and other methods of interdental cleaning are needed (Figure 19–1). The dental hygienist needs to evaluate information gained during the assessment phase of care to select the most appropriate interdental and supplemental aids for the client. To accomplish this, it is important to keep in mind the following client conditions and risk factors:

- ✦ Contour and consistency of the gingival tissues
- ✦ Probing depths
- ✦ Gingival attachment levels
- ✦ Size of the interproximal embrasures
- ✦ Tooth position and alignment
- ✦ Condition and types of restorative work present
- ✦ Susceptibility of the client to disease (risk assessment)
- ✦ Level of dexterity and ability to use an aid
- ✦ Client motivation
- ✦ Cost, safety, and effectiveness of the recommended aids
- ✦ Client preference

Once an assessment is made, the dental hygienist reviews the planned care and goals for the client to determine which oral hygiene aid will most effectively clean the interdental areas. The simplest, least time-consuming procedures that will effectively control bacterial plaque biofilm and maintain oral health should be recommended. Also, if one device works, the dental hygienist should choose it over two devices that would accomplish the same goal. Studies demonstrate that both client acceptance and effectiveness of oral hygiene recommendations improve when the number of aids is limited.

If the client's current oral hygiene regimen is effective in maintaining oral health, the dental hygienist should reinforce it rather than change it. Even the ideal interdental aid is not effective if the client does not use it. Thus, if a client prefers a specific interdental strategy, the clinician can evaluate its use, modify the technique to maximize effectiveness, and discuss potential detrimental effects that can result from incorrect use. These factors are considered when selecting the most appropriate interdental aid for a particular client. Table 19–1 summarizes a variety of mechanical oral hygiene interdental devices available.

TYPES OF INTERDENTAL AIDS

Dental Floss and Tape

Dental floss is the most frequently recommended aid for cleaning proximal tooth surfaces with normal gingival contour and embrasure spaces. Figure 19–2 provides an illustration of the various embrasure types and their recommended interdental care. Dental floss should be recommended only for individuals with type I embrasures. There is consensus that floss is more effective when interdental spaces are covered by the papillae;

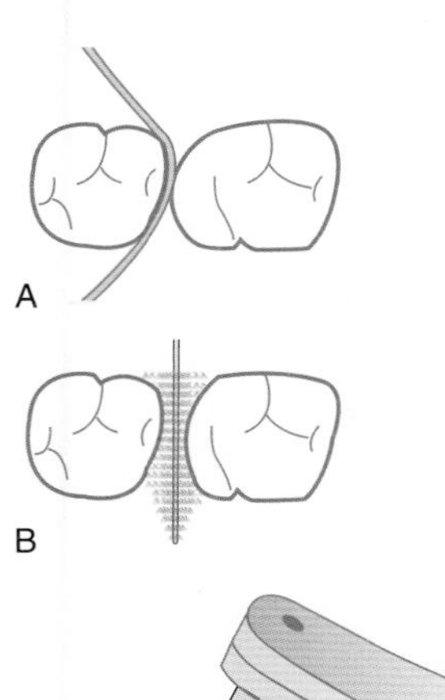

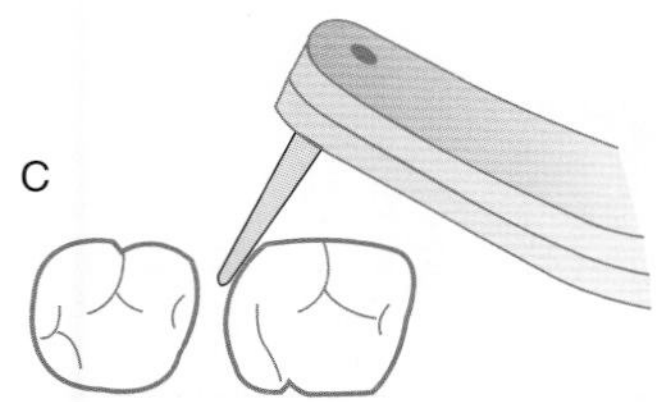

FIGURE 19–1 ✦ Use of interdental plaque control devices. **A,** Dental floss. **B,** Interdental brush. **C,** Toothpick in holder.

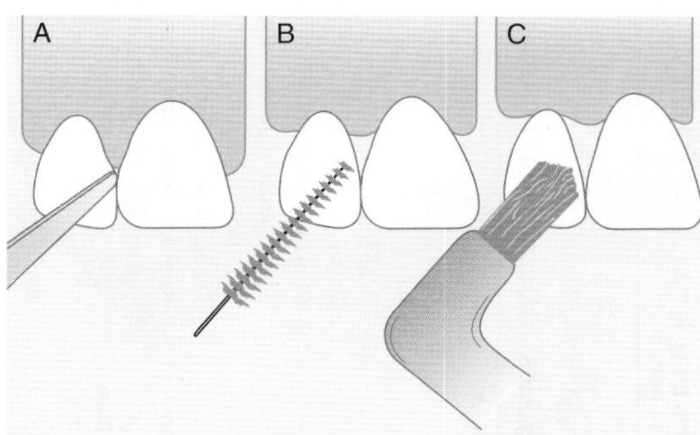

FIGURE 19–2 ✦ Interproximal embrasure types and corresponding interdental cleansers. **A,** Type I—no gingival recession: dental floss. **B,** Type II—moderate papillary recession: interdental brush. **C,** Type III—complete loss of papillae: uni-tufted brush. *(From Carranza FA, Newman MG:* Clinical periodontology, *ed 8, Philadelphia, 1996, WB Saunders.)*

TABLE 19–1 INTERDENTAL MECHANICAL ORAL PHYSIOTHERAPY (OPT) AIDS

Interdental Mechanical Oral Physiotherapy Aids	Description/Types	Indications	Contraindications/ Limitations	Common Problems that may be Experienced During Use/Misuse
Floss	Unwaxed vs. waxed Dental tape PTFE Braided G-floss Plain vs. flavored Therapeutic agents added (fluoride, baking soda, calculus inhibitors)	Type I embrasures Floss reaches 2 to 3.5 mm subgingivally Braided and G-floss are used with implants	Type II and III embrasures	Floss cuts Floss clefts Circulation to fingers cut off from wrapping too tight; wear finger cots or gloves to reduce this problem Inability to reach posterior teeth for some clients
Tufted dental floss (also known as variable diameter floss, Super Floss, Nu Floss)	Regular floss, yarn, floss threader combination	Type II and III embrasures Mesial and distal of abutment teeth Under pontics of fixed partial dentures Under orthodontic appliances (e.g., wires)	Type I embrasures	Trauma from forcing threader into tissues Yarn portion may catch on appliances and become stuck if appliances are rough If yarn portion becomes stuck to appliance, client may damage appliance trying to remove floss
Floss holder	Flossing aid Handle with two prongs in Y shape or C shape	Type I embrasures Clients with use of one hand Clients lacking manual dexterity Clients with large hands Clients with strong gag reflex Caregivers	Type II and III embrasures	Unable to maintain tension of floss Need to unwrap and rewrap floss to move to new area of floss after each tooth Need to set fulcrum to avoid floss cuts
Floss threader	Flossing aid Clear plastic with closed eye Tinted plastic with open eye Soft plastic loop Flexible wire Twisted wire	Type I embrasures Insert floss under tight contacts Floss between and under abutment teeth and pontics of fixed prosthesis Floss under orthodontic appliances (e.g., wires, lingual bar) Floss under bars for implants	Type II and III embrasures	Trauma from forcing threader into tissues
Toothpick	Round Triangular	Type II and III embrasures from facial aspect only Trace gingival margin Accessible furcations Small root concavities	Type I embrasures Healthy tissue Toothpick does not clean area of tooth contact	Wearing down of papilla and marginal tissues from incorrect usage Splaying of wood ends may cause tissue trauma/cuts or abrasions Enamel abrasion from incorrect use Can force bacteria or debris into gingival attachment if used improperly = risk of abscess formation
Toothpick holder (also known as periodontal aid)	Round vs. triangular toothpick Metal vs. plastic handle	Type II and III embrasures from facial or lingual aspect Trace gingival margin at 45-degree angle to tooth surface Accessible furcations Concave surfaces in interproximal areas Fixed prosthetic and orthodontic appliances Maxillofacial surgery client wired shut Sulcular cleansing in areas of shallow pocketing Application of fluoride, antimicrobial, or desensitizing agents	Type I embrasures Healthy tissue	Wearing down of papilla and tissues from incorrect use Splaying of wood ends may cause tissue trauma/cuts or abrasions Possible damage of epithelial attachment if used incorrectly subgingivally

Wedge stimulator (also known as wood interdental cleaner, balsa wood wedge, Stimudent)	Wood wedge Plastic wedge	Type II and III embrasures from facial aspect only Trace gingival margin for supragingival plaque removal (maintains a plaque-free region for 2 to 3 mm subgingivally) Accessible furcations Application of fluoride, antimicrobial, or desensitizing agents	Type I embrasures Healthy tissue Stimulator does not clean area of tooth contact Periodontal pockets (not effective in removing debris or decreasing inflammation in apical regions)	Wearing down of papilla and marginal tissues from incorrect use Splaying of wood ends may cause tissue trauma/cuts or abrasions Enamel abrasion from incorrect use Can force bacteria or debris into gingival attachment if used improperly = risk of abscess formation
Interproximal brush (also known as interdental brush, proxa brush, proxi brush)	Bristle inserts: tapered (conical) or straight Variety of sizes With or without handles	Type II and III embrasures Diastemas Exposed root furcations Orthodontic and fixed appliances Maxillofacial surgery client wired shut (appliances) Difficult access areas Application of fluoride, antimicrobial, or desensitizing agents		Trauma to tooth surface or gingiva from sharp wire center of some
Interdental swab tip	E-Z Floss Handle with swab tip (cotton strands tightly held together on a twisted stainless steel wire)	Type II and III embrasures Root concavities Furcations Orthodontic appliances Fixed dental appliances Application of fluoride, antimicrobial, or desensitizing agents	Type I embrasures	Some have metal wire in center, which can cause trauma to tissue if used improperly
Knitting yarn	Flossing adjunct May need to use with floss threader	Type II and III embrasures Isolated teeth Diastemas Abutments of partials Under sanitary pontics Distal of most posterior teeth in mouth	Type I embrasures	Yarn may catch on appliances and become stuck if appliances are rough If yarn becomes stuck to appliance, patient may damage appliance trying to remove it
Gauze strip	2 × 2 gauze 4 × 4 gauze (cut)	Type III embrasure Diastemas Teeth adjacent to edentulous areas	Type I and II embrasures	Gauze may catch on rough surfaces or appliances and become stuck If gauze becomes stuck to appliance, client may damage appliance trying to remove it
Pipe cleaner	Same as pipe cleaners used for arts and crafts	Type III embrasure Exposed root furcations Malpositioned or separated teeth (areas of bone loss and severe loss of tissue)	Type I and II embrasures	Trauma to tooth surface or gingiva from sharp wire center of pipe cleaner

however, as recession becomes more pronounced, floss becomes progressively less effective.[1] Dental floss is recommended for adults because it is more effective than toothbrushing alone in controlling gingivitis and periodontitis; however, its value in preventing gingivitis in children is questionable.[2] The main reason for flossing in children is to habituate the behavior into adulthood.

Most types of dental floss are made of nylon and some are impregnated with flavorings, fluoride, baking soda, or calculus-inhibiting agents. The following general types of dental floss are available commercially:

- Unwaxed
- Waxed, including dental tape
- Polytetrafluoroethylene (PTFE)
- Braided
- G-floss and tapered G-floss
- Tufted (variable diameter)

UNWAXED VERSUS WAXED FLOSS. Studies have shown no difference in the effectiveness of unwaxed versus waxed dental floss.[3,4] *Unwaxed dental floss* is generally recommended for clients with normal tooth contacts because it slides through the contact area easily. It is the thinnest type of floss available, yet when it separates during use, it covers a larger surface area of the tooth than waxed floss.

Waxed dental floss is recommended for clients with tight proximal tooth contacts, moderate to heavy calculus deposits before scaling and root planing, or defective and overhanging restorations. In these clients, unwaxed floss may shred or tear more easily, resulting in frustration and discomfort. Waxed floss is preferred by some clients because of its ability to slide through tight contacts and resist fraying. Concern that waxed floss may be inappropriate to use because it leaves a waxy film on tooth surfaces has been dispelled. Wax residue is not left on teeth coated by saliva.[4] *Dental tape* or ribbon is a waxed floss product that is wider and flatter than conventional dental floss. The flat-sided surface of dental tape is preferred by some, particularly when the surface area to be flossed is large.

POLYTETRAFLUOROETHYLENE (PTFE) FLOSS. PTFE floss (e.g., Glide) is another type of floss that slides through contacts easily. Coated with a type of Teflon material that is resistant to fraying, its uses are similar to waxed dental floss.

BRAIDED NYLON FLOSS, G-FLOSS, AND TAPERED G-FLOSS. These types of floss are intended for cleaning dental implants. Braided floss (e.g., Postcare) is sold on a spool or as a precut piece with a stiff nylon end for threading. The braided nylon resembles a cord, can be washed after use, and is reused after drying. G-floss has a mesh or gauze appearance and is meant for one-time use. More information on both types of floss can be located in Chapter 50 on osseointegrated dental implants.

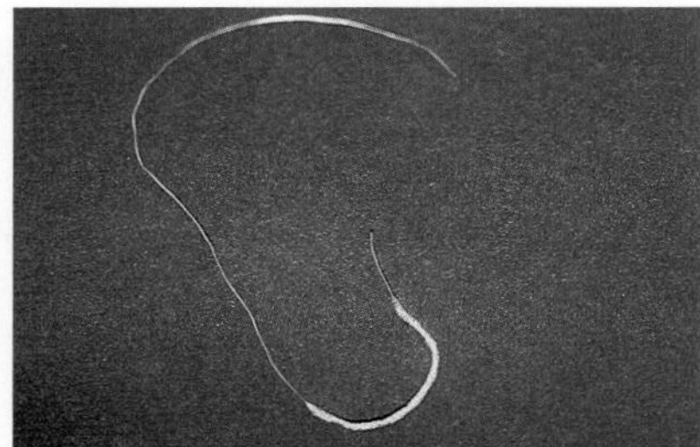

FIGURE 19–3 ✦ Tufted dental floss.

TUFTED FLOSS. Tufted floss (e.g., Super Floss), or variable-diameter dental floss, has been found to be equally as effective as waxed or unwaxed dental floss for removing plaque biofilm. Some evidence, however, suggests that it may be more effective.[5] *Tufted dental floss* is designed to have three continuous segments: a length of waxed or unwaxed dental floss; a shorter segment of cylindrical, nylon meshwork; and a relatively rigid nylon needle capable of being threaded beneath the contact or under fixed bridges (Figure 19–3). The segment of dental floss is used in areas of normal gingival contour, and the other segments are used as indicated in Table 19–1.

Flossing Methods

The two primary methods of dental flossing are the spool method and the loop method. Procedure 19–1 reviews the spool method of flossing, a method used by many teens and adults.

The spool method of flossing requires manual dexterity. Children or those who have less manipulative ability with their hands may prefer to use the loop method of flossing instead of the spool method. The loop method of flossing is described in Procedure 19–2. In either method, when the tooth surface is clean, the person can hear a squeaky-clean sound during flossing. The squeaky-clean sound is more definitive when unwaxed floss is used as compared with waxed or PTFE floss.

Evaluation of Flossing

Evaluation of flossing is similar to the evaluation of toothbrushing. The clinician observes the client's flossing technique for effectiveness and safety and suggests modifications or alternate interdental aids as necessary. Disclosing solution and the presence of plaque biofilm, gingival bleeding, and periodontal indices are parameters used to assess the effectiveness of removal of plaque biofilm in terms of clinical outcomes. Oral signs of gingival trauma (e.g., floss cuts, gingival clefts, gingival abrasion) are used for the safety evaluation (Figure 19–8). Causes of trauma include using too long a piece of floss between fingers when inserting between teeth, snapping the floss in between the contact area, failing to wrap the floss around the tooth before activating it, and failing to use a finger rest to prevent undue pressure and to provide control. Frequent reinstruction and reinforcement are necessary because flossing is a difficult psychomotor skill to master.

Procedure 19–1 SPOOL FLOSSING METHOD: ADULTS

STEPS / **RATIONALE**

1. Break off a piece of floss from the spool 12 to 18 inches long (Figure 19–4, *A*).

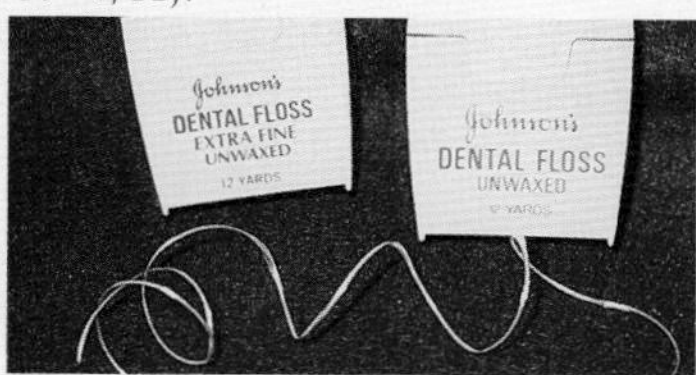

FIGURE 19–4, *A*

Rationale: As a rule of thumb, the appropriate length of floss should be as long as your forearm. This length ensures enough floss to cover the entire mouth, advancing to a new area after completing each interproximal space.

2. Wrap floss around middle fingers; wrap floss around right middle finger 2 to 3 times; wrap remaining floss around left middle finger (or vice versa)(Figure 19–4, *B*).

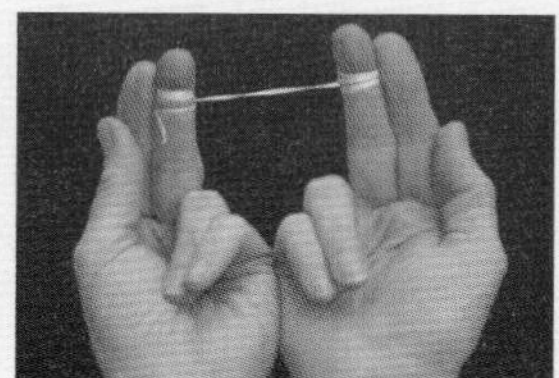

FIGURE 19–4, *B*

Rationale: Wrapping dental floss around the middle fingers allows for increased control since the index fingers and thumbs are then free to control the floss. Be careful to wrap the floss somewhat loosely to avoid cutting off circulation to the middle fingers.

3. For maxillary insertion, grasp floss firmly with thumb and index finger of each hand using ½ inch of floss between fingertips (Figure 19–5, *A*).
   For mandibular insertion, direct the floss down with the index fingers (Figure 19–5, *B*).

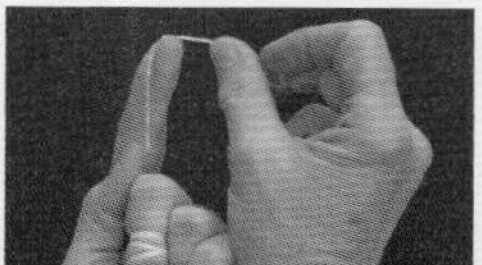

FIGURE 19–5, *A*

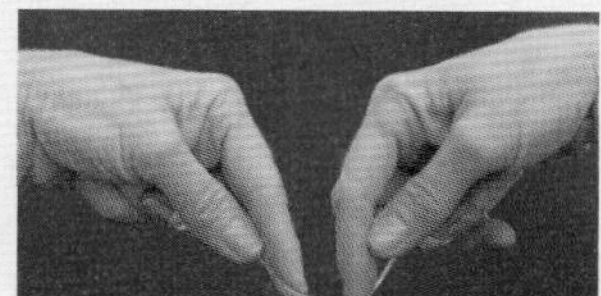

FIGURE 19–5, *B*

Rationale: Grasping the floss with two fingers on both hands improves control. Using only ½ inch of floss between fingers reduces the chance of floss cuts on facial or lingual surfaces adjacent to or across papillae (Figure 19–8).

4. Select area to begin flossing and establish a pattern to progress throughout the mouth.

Rationale: Establishing a pattern for completing flossing avoids missing areas of the mouth. Many people like to start at the midline and progress posteriorly in one quadrant and then the other in the same arch, then switch arches and progress in a similar manner. Others like to start with #1 and continue in order to #32. Each patient should establish a pattern that is comfortable for him or her.

5. Set a fulcrum on the cheek or in the mouth.

Rationale: Setting a fulcrum increases stability and reduces the chance of popping through a contact area, possibly causing a floss cut or cleft.

6. Use gentle seesaw motion to pass through contact area.

Rationale: This motion reduces the chance of popping through a contact, possibly causing a floss cut.

7. Pass floss below gingival margin.

Rationale: Floss will reach 2 to 3 mm subgingivally when placed below the gingival margin.

8. Wrap tightly in **C** shape around tooth (Figure 19–5, *C*).

Rationale: Wrapping the floss in a **C** shape and keeping it tight to the tooth prevents floss cuts and increases the surface area covered by the floss, thereby disrupting more plaque biofilm.

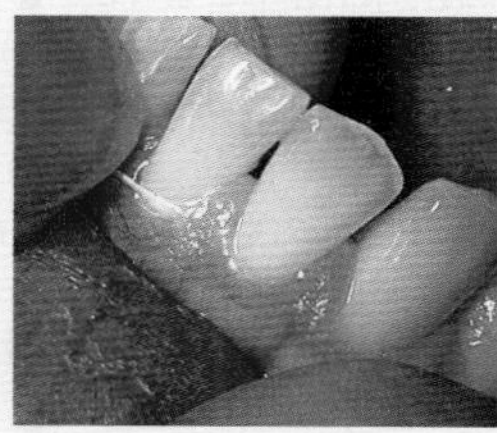

FIGURE 19–5, *C* ✦

Continued on following page

Procedure 19–1 SPOOL FLOSSING METHOD: ADULTS—CONT'D

STEPS	RATIONALE
9. Move floss up and down on mesial of tooth 3 to 4 strokes, then move above papilla (just below contact); wrap in C shape on distal of adjacent tooth, moving floss up and down 3 to 4 strokes.	An up-and-down motion interproximally covers the entire length of the interproximal area, rather than a single area accomplished by a shoeshine motion. Moving the floss above the papilla before wrapping the C shape on the opposite surface avoids a floss cut in the papilla.

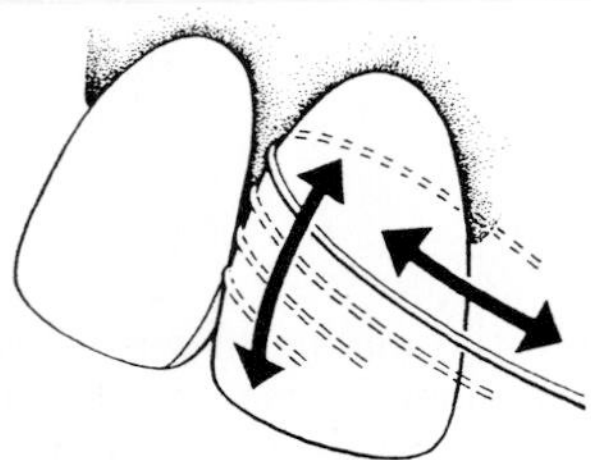

FIGURE 19–6 ✦ Floss wrapped around dental surface. *(From Hoag PM, Pawlak EA:* Essentials of periodontics, *ed 4, St Louis, 1990, Mosby.)*

STEPS	RATIONALE
10. Use a seesaw motion to remove floss through contact.	A seesaw motion back out of the contact allows for more gentle removal of the floss.
11. Advance floss to new area by unwrapping floss from left-hand middle finger and wrapping onto right-hand middle finger (or vice versa; see step 2).	Floss is advanced to a new area after each interproximal space to avoid spreading bacteria from sulcus to sulcus. This is an attempt to contain diseased bacteria to localized sites.
12. Repeat steps 5 to 11 until all teeth have been completed, continuing to grasp the floss with the thumb and index fingers.	The entire mouth should be flossed, including the distal of the most posterior tooth in each quadrant.
13. Dispose of floss in waste receptacle.	Floss is meant for one-time use.

Procedure 19–2 LOOP FLOSSING METHOD: CHILDREN AND CLIENTS WITH LIMITED MANUAL DEXTERITY

STEPS	RATIONALE
1. Break off a piece of floss from the spool 8 to 10 inches long.	Less floss is needed to loop than to wrap around the middle fingers. A midsize piece of floss is still needed, however, to advance the floss to new areas in the mouth.
2. Tie the two ends together in a knot. (Figure 19–7).	Tying the two ends together puts the floss into a complete circle. With this method the floss does not need to be wrapped around the middle finger of each hand, which often causes the blood flow to be reduced in the fingers. A loop is also easier to control.

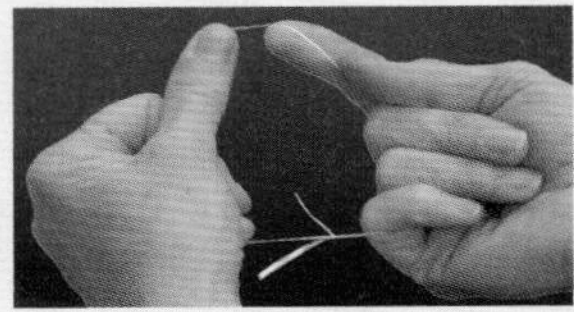

STEPS	RATIONALE
3–10. Follow steps listed for spool flossing method.	Steps 3 to 10 use the same techniques for both methods of flossing.
11. Advance floss to new area by sliding floss away from the knot.	Floss is advanced to a new area after each interproximal space to avoid spreading bacteria from sulcus to sulcus. This is an attempt to contain diseased bacteria to localized sites.
12. Repeat steps 5 to 11 until all teeth have been completed, continuing to grasp the floss with the thumb and index fingers.	The entire mouth should be flossed, including the distal of the most terminal teeth in each quadrant.
13. Dispose of floss in waste receptacle.	Floss is meant for one-time use.

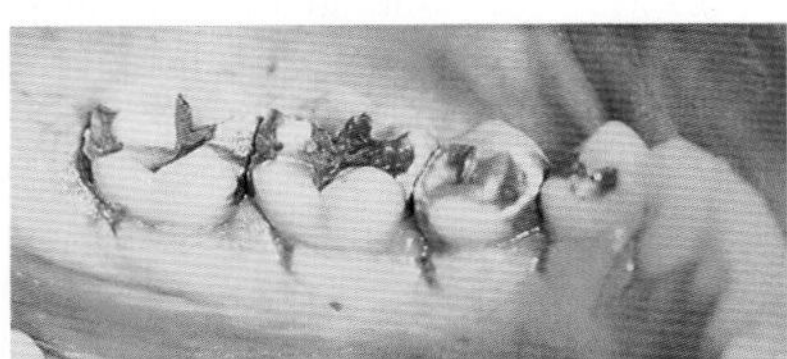

FIGURE 19–8 ✦ Floss cuts. *(Courtesy Dr. M. Walsh, University of California–San Francisco.)*

Gingival bleeding during flossing can be a result of trauma or an indication of inflammation. When clients with gingival inflammation initiate flossing, the gingiva bleeds as a result of the ulcerations in the sulcular lining that occur during the active disease process. Clients must be aware that bleeding is not a sign that flossing should be avoided, but rather an indicator of active disease that needs to be controlled by more frequent flossing. In most cases, bleeding from gingival inflammation sub-

Procedure 19–3 USE OF A FLOSS HOLDER

STEPS	RATIONALE
1. Tightly string floss on holder following the manufacturer's recommendations (Figure 19-9). 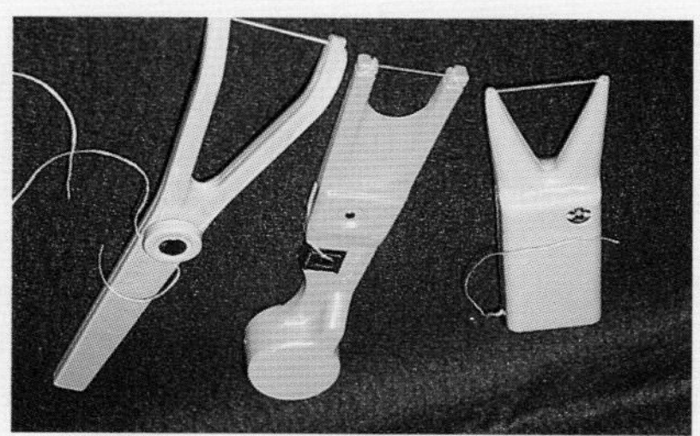 FIGURE 19–9	Each manufacturer will specify the directions for winding the floss on the floss holder in the directions for use. The floss must be taut in order to seesaw the floss through the contact area. If it is not tight, it will fall off the holder and must be restrung.
2. Follow steps 4 to 10 for the spool method of flossing.	The method for flossing with a floss holder does not differ from the spool method of flossing other than the fact that only one hand is needed.
3. To direct floss in a **C** shape toward mesial and distal in step 8, use push or pull motion with floss holder (Figure 19–10). 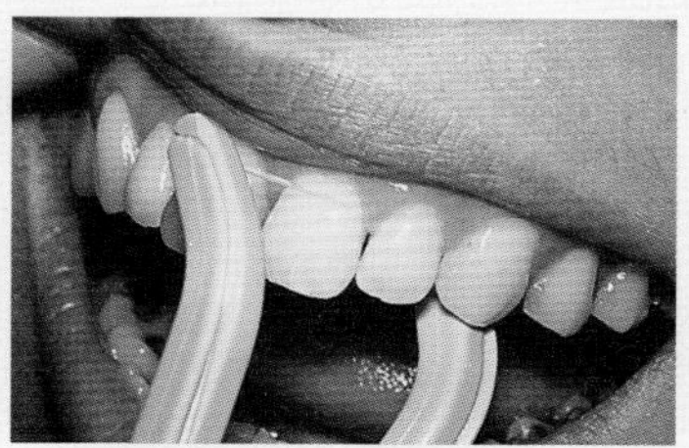 FIGURE 19–10	The floss should still adapt to the tooth in a **C** shape. In the spool method, the index fingers and thumb adapt the floss to the teeth. With a floss holder a push or pull motion adapts the floss to the tooth.
4. To move to a new area of floss (step 11 of the spool method), the holder must be unwrapped, floss advanced, and holder rewrapped.	The only way to advance floss to a new area with most floss holders is to unwrap the holder and rewrap it, ensuring that a clean area of floss is placed between the prongs. In some holders, a dial can be turned in a clockwise motion to advance the floss.
5. Continue until all teeth are completed.	The entire mouth should be flossed, including the distal of the most terminal teeth in each quadrant.
6. Dispose of floss in waste receptacle.	Floss is meant for one-time use.
7. Wash off floss holder with warm water and soap, dry, and store in clean, dry area until next use.	The floss holder may be reused and is normally made of plastic, a material that is durable, lightweight, and able to be cleaned. As the holder shows signs of wear or becomes difficult to clean, it should be replaced. Another recommendation is to replace the holder every 3 months, just as you would a toothbrush.

sides with the regular removal of bacterial plaque biofilm and supportive periodontal therapy.

Irregular flossing also might be a concern for some medically compromised persons. During vigorous flossing, bacteremia may result. The occurrence of bleeding and resultant bacteremia increases when gingival inflammation is present. People with congenital heart disease, rheumatic heart disease, heart or vascular prostheses, joint replacements, immunosuppression associated with cancer therapy, or other conditions that require antibiotic premedication before dental hygiene care should be cautioned about the potential hazards of occasional (rather than routine) flossing.[6] Regular flossing eliminates gingival inflammation and thus presents no problem for clients with these medical conditions.

Flossing Devices

FLOSS HOLDER. Another method of flossing, considered easier for some clients, involves the use of a *floss holder* (Figure 19–9). Floss holders are described in Table 19–1 and their method of use in Procedure 19–3. Research reveals that reductions in bacterial plaque biofilm and gingivitis are equivalent with either the use of hand flossing or floss holders.[7,8]

FLOSS THREADER. Another device designed to assist clients with flossing is the *floss threader* (Figure 19–11). As described in Table 19–1, a floss threader assists in introducing floss into an area such as between an abutment tooth used for support of a fixed bridge and a pontic, the artificial tooth that replaces a missing natural tooth (see Chapter 49). Procedure 19–4 reviews the use of a floss threader.

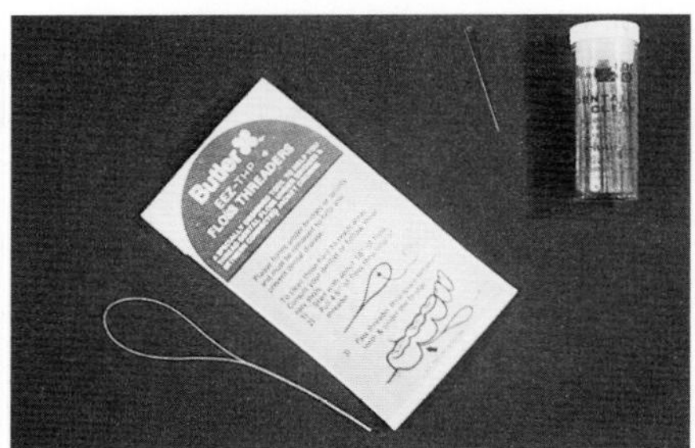

FIGURE 19–11 ✦ Examples of floss threaders.

Wooden Toothpicks and Toothpick Holders

Many people prefer to use *toothpicks* for control of interdental plaque biofilm, particularly on concave proximal surfaces and exposed furcation areas. Studies have shown that the toothpick is as effective as dental floss in reducing interproximal plaque biofilm and gingival bleeding.[1,2] To use toothpicks, however, there must be sufficient interdental space available (see Table 19–1 for indications). Toothpicks are often too long and have the potential to damage tissue while working lingually. To

Procedure 19–4 USE OF A FLOSS THREADER

STEPS	RATIONALE
1. Determine the need to use a floss threader and appropriate areas for use.	See a list of indications for use in Table 19–1.
2. Break off a piece of floss from the spool 4 to 6 inches long.	A smaller piece of floss can be used since only one to two areas are normally flossed using a floss threader.
3. Thread floss through eye of floss threader, overlapping floss 1 to 2 inches.	Threading the floss threader is similar to threading a needle. Once it is threaded, the floss is pulled through so that 1 to 2 inches overlap (double-stranded). Overlapping the floss prevents unthreading of the floss once resistance is met; however, if the entire piece of floss is left double stranded, it is more difficult to remove the floss threader in step 6.
4. Grasp threader with thumb and index finger of one hand.	A stable grasp prevents dropping the threader.
5. Insert tip of threader from the facial surface through an open interproximal area or area between a pontic and an abutment tooth (Figure 19–12). 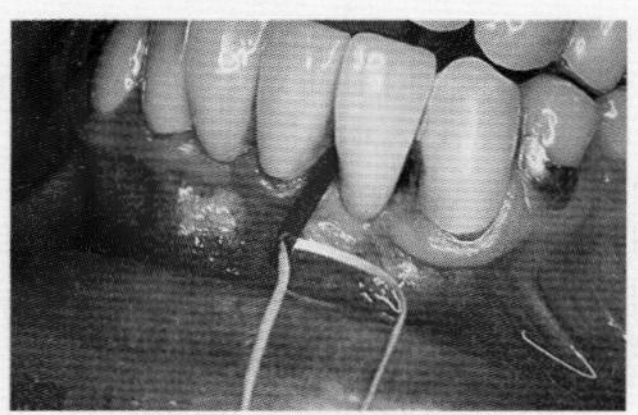 **FIGURE 19–12**	Inserting the threader from the facial allows better visualization of insertion and less chance of tissue trauma at the insertion point.
6. Pull floss threader toward lingual until threader has passed completely through the interproximal space or under a pontic (only floss is now in the space) (Figure 19–13, *A*). 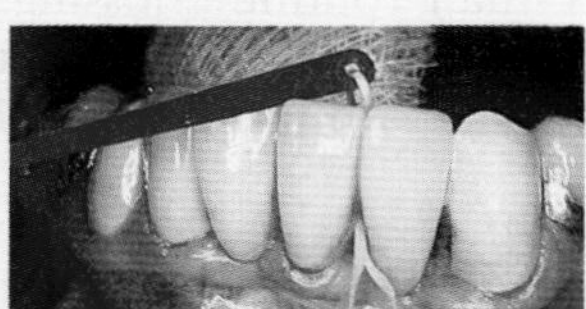 **FIGURE 19–13, A**	To floss correctly, the floss needs to wrap around the mesial or distal side of the tooth. Therefore, the floss must pass all the way from facial to lingual for maximum coverage of surface area.
7. Slide the floss threader off the floss and remove from mouth.	Taking the floss threader off the floss and removing it from the mouth prevents loss of the threader or swallowing the threader.

Procedure 19–4 USE OF A FLOSS THREADER—CONT'D

STEPS	RATIONALE
8. Move floss back and forth several times under the pontic. Then follow steps 8 and 9 of the spool method of flossing (Figure 19–13, *B*).	Once the floss is inserted into the space, the flossing method is the same. Sliding floss back and forth under the pontic removes plaque and food debris from the gingival surface of the pontic.
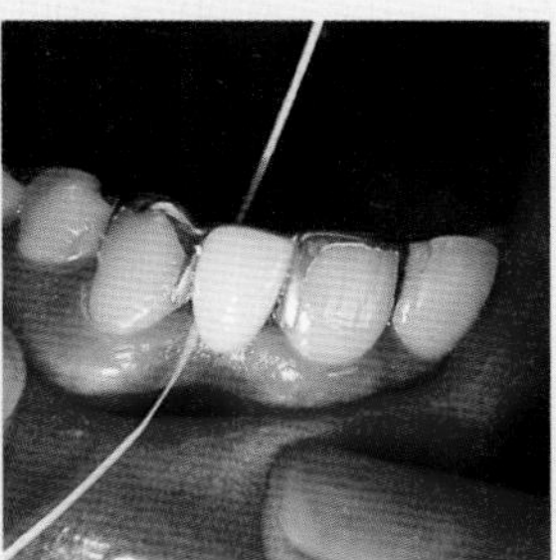 **FIGURE 19–13, B**	
9. Remove floss by letting go with hand that is on the lingual and pulling floss toward the facial.	Since the contact area was blocked (requiring use of a floss threader), the floss will not be able to be removed by see-sawing it through the contact area. Instead, letting go with the hand that is on the lingual side allows for removal from the facial.
10. Dispose of floss and threader in waste receptacle.	Floss and a floss threader are meant for one-time use. Some patients will reuse the floss threader for the sake of cost containment. If the threader is reusable, it should be cleaned with soap and warm water, dried, and stored in a clean, dry place. If the threader becomes bent, splayed, or unusable, it should be replaced.

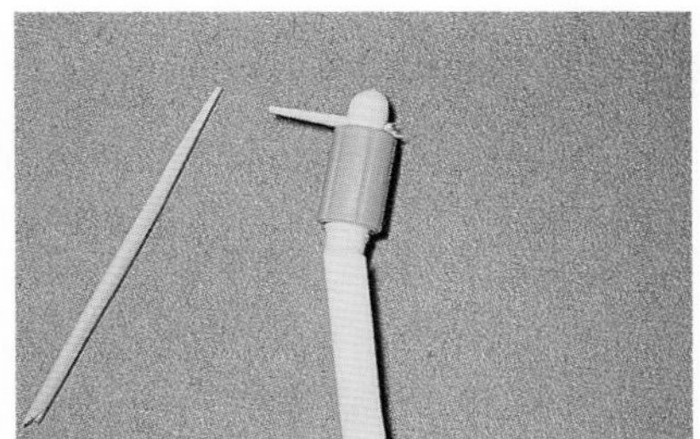

FIGURE 19–14 ✦ Example of a toothpick holder.

prevent damage, use of a *toothpick holder* (e.g., Perio Aid) is recommended for cleaning lingual surfaces. Toothpick holders (Figure 19–14) may be used from the facial or lingual aspect and adapt better interproximally and posteriorly when compared with toothpicks alone.

The main concern regarding use of a toothpick or toothpick holder is avoidance of gingival damage. Clients should be taught the proper use of the toothpick to effectively remove plaque biofilm without causing damage to the gingiva, especially the epithelial attachment (Procedures 19–5 and 19–6 and Figures 19–15 to 19–17.)

Toothpicks and *wedge stimulators* have also been shown to be excellent tools for introducing fluoride and chlorhexidine into proximal areas.[9,10] When chemotherapeutic agents are introduced into proximal areas, the rate of demineralization leading to caries is reduced. In this case, there is an improvement in plaque reduction because of mechanical plaque removal and the chemotherapeutic agents.

Wedge Stimulators—Wood or Plastic

Wedge stimulators are wooden (e.g., Stim-u-dent) or plastic (e.g., Rota-point) oral hygiene devices designed for interdental cleansing and stimulation (Figure 19–18). The indications and contraindications for use are similar to those for toothpicks, as noted in Table 19–1. Wedge stimulators are recommended for use only from the facial aspect, where the proximal surfaces are exposed to avoid traumatizing gingival tissue. The use of wedge stimulators is reviewed in Procedure 19–6. The key difference between the use of toothpicks and wedge stimulators relates to the triangular design of the wedge. Wedges are inserted interdentally, with the base of the triangle resting on the gingival side, the tip pointing occlusally or incisally, and the sides of the triangle against the adjacent tooth surfaces (Figure 19–19). Placing the base of the triangle against the tissue prevents damage, such as gingival cuts and clefts, to the interdental papilla and gingival margins. Triangular wedges have been found to be superior in plaque biofilm removal when compared with round or rectangular wedges or toothpicks.[1] The triangular wedge fits the interdental area more snugly, covering a larger surface area, thereby allowing for the removal of more plaque biofilm.

Procedure 19–5 USE OF A TOOTHPICK IN A TOOTHPICK HOLDER

STEPS	RATIONALE
	See a list of indications for use in Table 19–1.
1. Insert a round tapered toothpick into the end of an angled plastic holder. Twist toothpick securely into holder and break off longer end of toothpick (Figure 19–15). 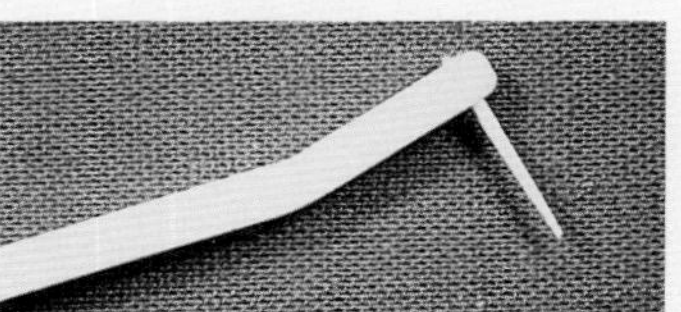 FIGURE 19–15	Once the toothpick is inserted into the holder, it is tightened in place to avoid loosening the toothpick. Breaking off the longer end prevents the toothpick from damaging tissue in the lips or cheek during use and allows for better access to posterior areas.
2. Moisten the end of the toothpick with saliva.	Moistening the toothpick with saliva softens the wood to prevent tissue trauma and reduce splintering.
3. Place the toothpick tip at the gingival margin with the tip pointing at a 90-degree angle to the long axis of the tooth. Trace the gingival margin around the tooth (Figure 19–16, *A*). 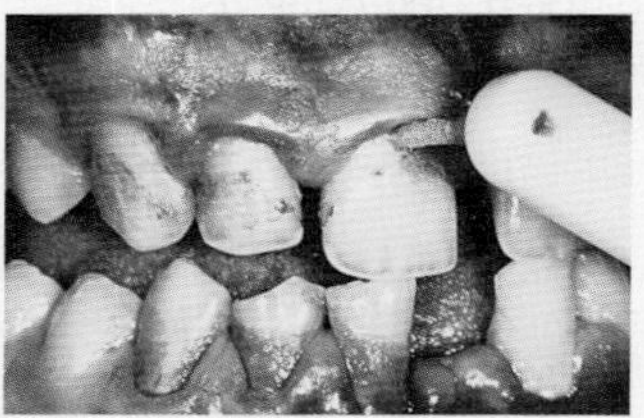 FIGURE 19–16, *A*	Tracing the gingival margin with the toothpick creates mechanical friction to disturb and remove plaque biofilm.
4. Some clients may be dexterous enough to point the tip at less than a 45-degree angle into the sulcus or pocket and trace around the tooth surfaces and root concavities. The tip should maintain contact with the tooth at all times. Insertion should stop once the toothpick meets a slight resistance in the space without the teeth being forced apart interproximally or the tissue being impinged. Keeping the tip on the tooth, use a gentle up-and-down motion to clean concave proximal surfaces (Figure 19–16, *B*). 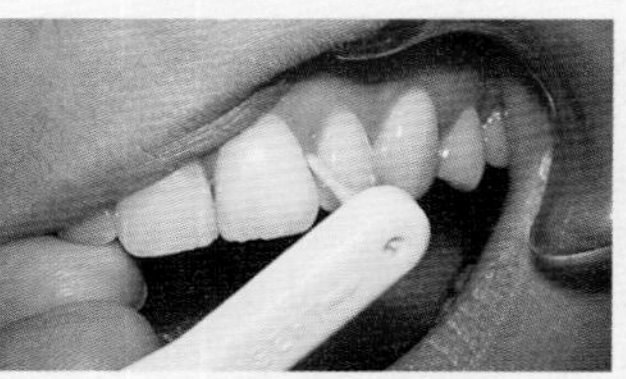 FIGURE 19–16, *B*	Applying the toothpick in this manner disturbs and removes plaque biofilm just below the gingival margin and from root concavities. This step is not recommended for clients with limited dexterity. Tissue damage could result if the toothpick is pointed directly into the epithelial attachment, making the pocket deeper. Inserting the toothpick interproximally should only be done until the space between the teeth is filled. If the teeth are forced apart or tissue impinged, permanent damage could result; teeth may be abraded or tissue worn away.
5. For exposed furcation areas, trace the furcation and use in-and-out motion to clean the furcation. The tip should maintain contact with the tooth at all times (Figure 19–17). 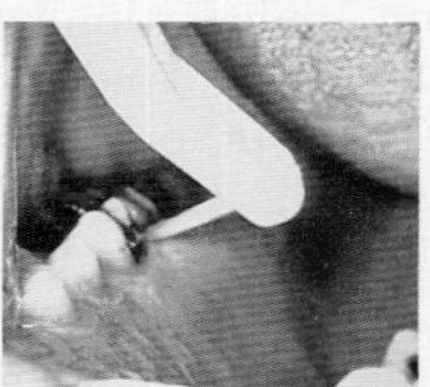 FIGURE 19–17	Keeping the tip in contact with the tooth avoids tissue trauma.
6. If debris accumulates on toothpick, rinse under running water.	Loose debris should be rinsed away and not introduced into a new interproximal area or sulcus.
7. Once all areas of the mouth are completed, dispose of toothpick in waste receptacle.	Toothpicks made of wood will absorb blood, saliva, and bacteria and should be thrown away after one use.
8. Holder may be washed with soap and warm water and stored in a clean, dry place for reuse.	If the wedge is plastic, it can be reused if washed with soap and warm water and then stored in a clean, dry place.

Procedure 19–6 USE OF A WEDGE STIMULATOR

STEPS	RATIONALE
1. Determine the need to use a wedge stimulator and appropriate areas for use.	See a list of indications for use in Table 19–1.
2. If wedge is made of wood, moisten the end of the wedge or toothpick with saliva. Establish a rest by placing the hand on the cheek or chin, or by placing a finger on the gingiva convenient to the place were the tip will be applied.	Moistening the wooden wedge with saliva softens the wood to prevent tissue trauma and reduce splintering. Establishing a rest will help prevent inserting the wedge/ toothpick with too much pressure.
3. Place wedge against the proximal surface of a tooth with the base of the wedge triangle toward gingival border and the tip pointing occlusally or incisally at approximately a 45-degree angle (Figure 19–19).	The base of the triangular wedge is flat instead of pointed, which reduces the possibility of damaging interdental tissue. Pointing the wedge or toothpick occlusally reduces the chance of flattening or wearing away papillae or damaging the gingival border.
4. Use an in-and-out motion interproximally from the facial only. Apply a burnishing stroke with moderate pressure first to the proximal surface of one tooth and then to the other, about 4 strokes each. Stop once wedge meets a slight resistance in the space without the teeth being forced apart or tissue being impinged.	Inserting the wedge interproximally should only be done until the space between the teeth is filled. If the teeth are forced apart or tissue impinged, permanent damage could result; teeth may be abraded or tissue worn away.
5. Trace margin of tissue to remove marginal debris, again with tip pointing occlusally (away from tissue).	Pointing the tip occlusally avoids tissue trauma.
6. If debris accumulates on wedge, rinse under running water.	Loose debris should be rinsed away and not introduced into a new interproximal area or sulcus.
7. Once all areas of mouth are completed, dispose of wedge in waste receptacle.	Wedges made of wood will absorb blood, saliva, and bacteria and should be thrown away after one use. If the wedge is plastic, it can be reused if washed with soap and warm water, then stored in a clean, dry place.

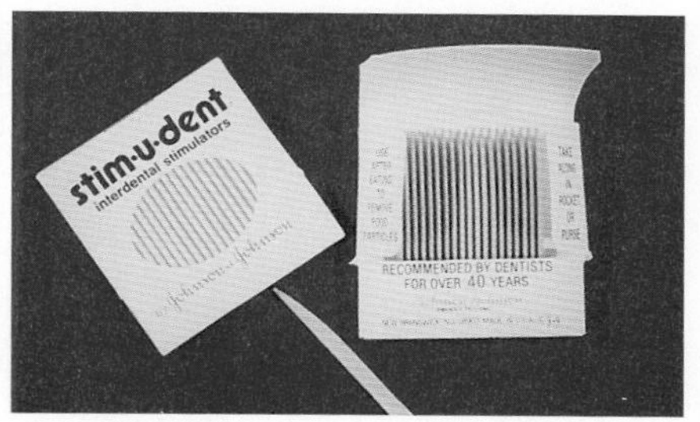

FIGURE 19–18 ✦ Examples of Balsa wood wedge.

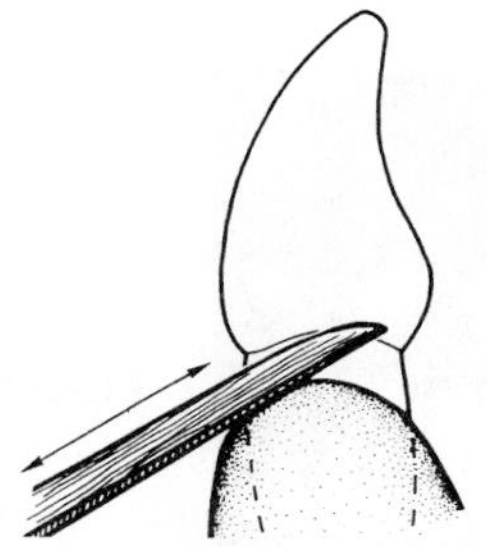

FIGURE 19–19 ✦ Proper placement of the Balsa wood edge against the proximal surface of a tooth. *(From Hoag PM, Pawlak EA:* Essentials of periodontics, *ed 4, St. Louis, 1990, Mosby.)*

Interdental Brushes and Swab Tips

Interdental brushes are available in various sizes and shapes. The most common brushes are conical or tapered (like an evergreen tree) and designed to be inserted into a plastic, reusable handle that is angled to facilitate interproximal adaptation (Figure 19–20). Studies have shown that interproximal brushes are equal to or more effective than floss for plaque biofilm removal and for reducing gingival inflammation in type II embrasures, type III embrasures, and exposed furcation areas.[1,2,11] Further indications for use are discussed in Table 19–1. The brush design selected is related to the size of the gingival embrasure or furcation to be cleaned. The interdental brush should be slightly larger than the embrasure space so that it can effectively clean the designated area. Use of the interdental brush is reviewed in Procedure 19–7 and Figure 19–21.

Interdental swab tips (Table 19–1) also are available in various sizes for plaque biofilm removal in areas similar to interdental brushes. Most are made of a cotton material that absorbs liquid chemotherapeutic agents, such as antimicrobials or desensitizing agents, for transport and target delivery to tooth surfaces. The swab tips are meant for one-time use; the handles may be washed with warm, soapy water and reused.

Knitting Yarn, Gauze Strips, and Pipe Cleaners

Knitting yarn (Figure 19–22) or *gauze strips* (Figure 19–23) can be used to clean proximal tooth surfaces adjacent to wide embrasure spaces, isolated teeth, or distal surfaces of most posterior teeth (Table 19–1). Yarn is used similarly to dental floss, whereas gauze strips are normally wrapped around the tooth in a C shape and used in a shoeshine motion to rub back and forth on the tooth. *Pipe cleaners* also can be used for type II embrasures or exposed furcation areas (Figure 19–24 and Table 19–1). They are used in an in-and-out motion similar to the motion used by wood stimulators and interdental brushes. All three of these items—yarn, gauze, and pipe cleaners—are inexpensive and accessible to most people.

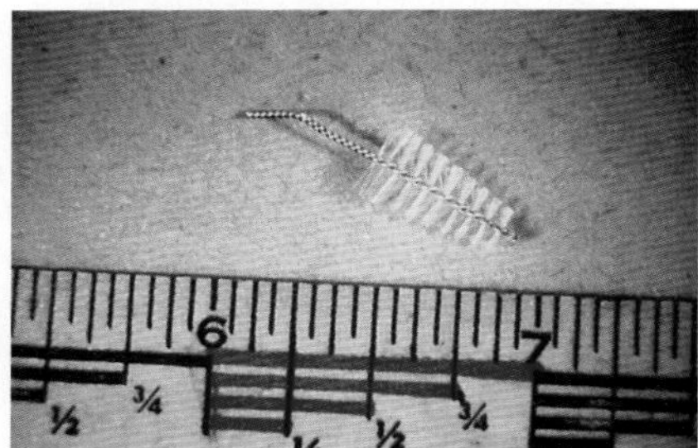

FIGURE 19–20 ✦ Example of an interdental brush.

SUPPLEMENTAL MECHANICAL ORAL PHYSIOTHERAPY AIDS

Table 19–2 summarizes various supplemental mechanical interdental aids for at-home use. As noted in the table, there are indications and contraindications for these aids as well as possible problems encountered during use or misuse.

Interdental Tip Stimulator

Massaging the gingiva with a toothbrush or an interdental oral physiotherapy device can lead to improved circulation, increased keratinization, and epithelial thickening. Whether these gingival changes provide any clinical benefits is questionable. Improved gingival health resulting from oral hygiene practices is more directly related to plaque biofilm removal than to gingival stimulation.

Procedure 19–7 USE OF AN INTERDENTAL BRUSH

STEPS	RATIONALE
1. Determine the need to use an interdental brush and appropriate areas for use.	See a list of indications for use in Table 19–1.
2. Moisten the bristles of the brush with saliva.	Moistening the bristles allows for a softer insertion of the brush.
3. Insert bristles into embrasure at a 90-degree angle to tooth surface (long axis of the tooth) (Figure 19–21).	Inserting the bristles at a 90-degree angle prevents trauma to the sulcus or interdental papilla, yet provides maximum coverage of surface area.

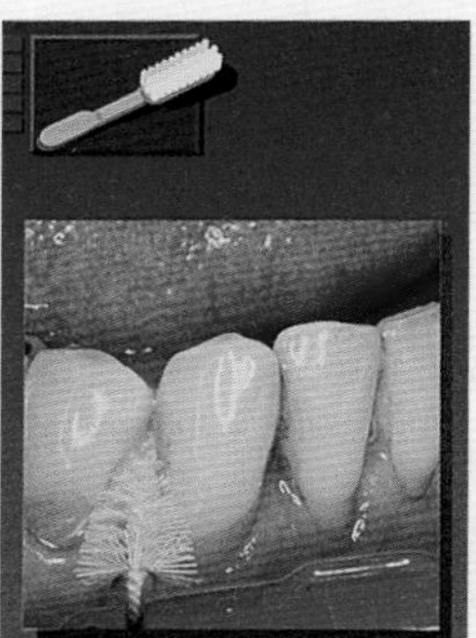

FIGURE 19–21

STEPS	RATIONALE
4. Move brush using in-and-out motion from facial and/or lingual surfaces of appropriate areas.	Because of the handle design, the interdental brush may be used from either the facial or lingual aspects. Most handles are double-ended, with one end angled for the facial surfaces and the opposite end angled for the distal surfaces.
5. Rinse bristles under running water as necessary to remove debris.	Debris that accumulates on the bristles should be rinsed off to avoid contaminating other areas that require use of the brush.
6. Upon completion of use, rinse entire handle and bristles with soap and warm water.	The interdental brush is designed to be reused, just as a toothbrush is reused.
7. Store in a clean, dry place.	Storage is similar to that of a toothbrush. The interdental brush should be kept clean and dry to prevent bacterial growth.
8. Replace bristles as they become worn or splayed, after an illness, or every 3 months. Replace handle after an illness or every 3 months.	Bristles and handle should be replaced as needed to ensure cleanliness and to prevent the spread of harmful bacteria.

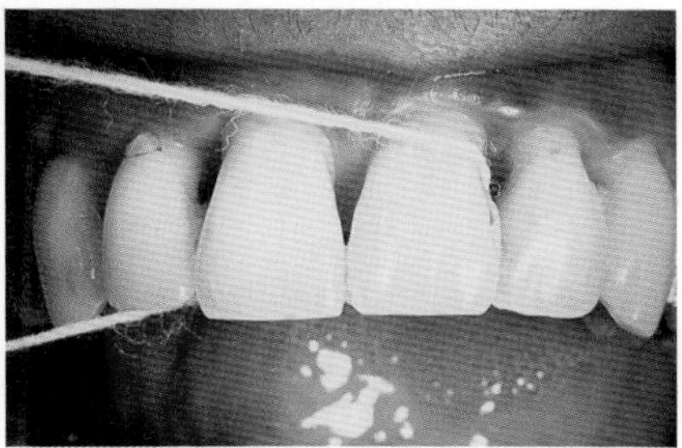

FIGURE 19–22 ✦ Use of knitting yarn to clean large embrasures.

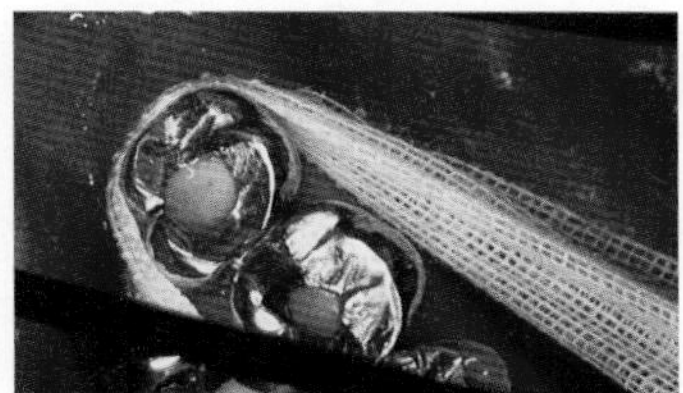

FIGURE 19–23 ✦ Use of gauze strip to clean distal of most posterior tooth.

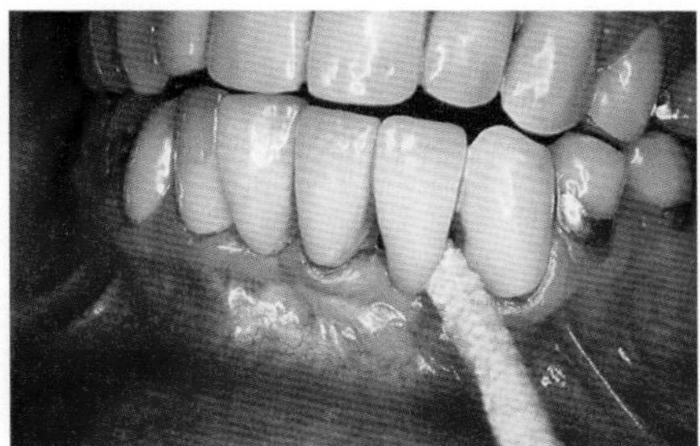

FIGURE 19–24 ✦ Use of pipe cleaner to clean large embrasure.

The *interdental tip stimulator*, or rubber tip stimulator, attached to the end of a toothbrush or to a plastic handle (Figure 19–25), has been suggested for use to remove plaque biofilm by rubbing the exposed tooth surfaces, to stimulate the gingiva, and to recontour gingival papillae following periodontal therapy (Table 19–2). With regard to plaque biofilm removal, the literature provides conflicting findings, with some studies indicating that the rubber tip is effective in removing plaque biofilm and others showing that it does not remove plaque biofilm effectively.[2] A rubber tip stimulator can cause injury to the gingiva if used improperly (Procedure 19–8 and Figure 19–26). In general, gingival stimulation receives a low priority in a disease control program. Its value in oral health promotion is in need of research.

End-Tuft, Single/Uni-Tuft Brushes

End-tufted or *single/uni-tufted toothbrushes,* indicated for type III embrasures, difficult to reach areas, or around fixed dental appliances (Table 19–2), are designed with a smaller brush head that has a small group of tufts

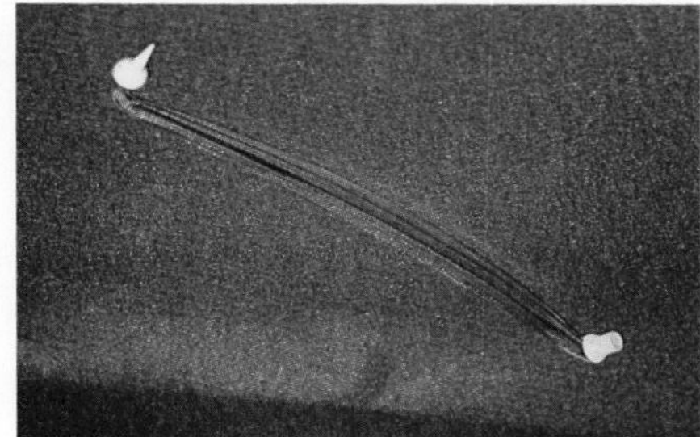

FIGURE 19–25 ✦ Example of a rubber tip stimulator.

(end-tufted) or a single tuft (single- or uni-tufted) (Figure 19–27). The bristles are directed into the area to be cleaned and activated with a rotating motion, similar to the vibratory motion of Bass toothbrushing. End-tuft brushes have been shown to be effective adjuncts to toothbrushing in controlling gingivitis in adults.[2]

Tongue Cleaners

Tongue cleaners or scrapers have not played a role in the reduction of plaque biofilm or gingivitis intraorally.[2] Instead, the primary indication for tongue cleaners is to remove debris and bacteria from the tongue's dorsal surface that play a role in halitosis. Tongue cleaning has been shown to remove the coating responsible for up to 85% of cases of oral malodor.[12] Brushing the tongue with a toothbrush can also clean the tongue, but some believe that the soft filaments that are so beneficial for the gingiva are not stiff enough to remove debris on the tongue, especially when debris is moderate to heavy. For clients with a gag reflex, tongue cleaners have been shown to be effective in cleaning the posterior third of the tongue without instigating a gag reflex. Tongue cleaners come in many shapes, styles, and colors, from a simple plastic strip to a variety of handled devices. Procedure 19–9 outlines use of a tongue cleaner.

Tooth Towelettes

Tooth towelettes are being marketed as a method of plaque biofilm removal when toothbrushing is not possible. The towelettes are gauze squares usually treated with some form of mouthwash that will also help freshen breath. The gauze square is held between the thumb and index finger and wiped on the tooth surface, moving from the cervical margin to the incisal or occlusal edge. Both facial and lingual surfaces are cleaned at the same time. Use of towelettes should be limited and is not meant to replace a daily toothbrushing regimen.

Foam Sticks or Brushes

Foam sticks, also called *foam brushes,* are sponge-tipped applicators on handles, most often associated with oral hygiene care in hospitals, especially for clients undergoing chemotherapy. Toothbrushes can be too rough on friable or ulcerated tissue and in cases of oral mucositis noted in clients undergoing chemotherapy and radia-

TABLE 19–2 SUPPLEMENTAL MECHANICAL ORAL PHYSIOTHERAPY (OPT) AIDS

Supplemental Mechanical Oral Physiotherapy Aids	Description/Types	Indications	Contraindications/ Limitations	Common Problems that May Be Experienced During Use/Misuse
Rubber tip stimulator (interdental tip)	End of toothbrush handle Separate handle	Type II and III embrasures Margins of tissue following periodontal surgery Exposed furcations	Type I embrasures and healthy tissues	Tissue trauma (wearing away of papilla and tissues, especially when used aggressively with increased pressure)
End-tuft brush Single-tuft brush (also known as uni-tuft brush)	Flat or tapered end Straight or angled handle	Type III embrasures Fixed dental prosthesis (e.g., orthodontic appliances, implants, pontics, maxillofacial surgery client wired shut) Difficult-to-reach areas (e.g., lingual of mandible, molars, abutment teeth, distal of terminal teeth, crowded teeth, third molars)	Type I and II embrasures	Tissue trauma Similar to problems associated with improper toothbrushing methods
Tongue cleaner (also known as tongue scraper)	Flat vs. ridged Plastic strip or with handle	Dorsal surface of tongue to remove coating and reduce halitosis		If clients press too hard, they could traumatize papillae
Tooth towelettes	Gauze treated with mouthwash Tooth Towels	Remove plaque from teeth and freshen breath in absence of a toothbrush	Should not totally replace toothbrushing	May be difficult to remove all plaque from teeth; educate clients about limited use
Foam sticks or foam brushes	Sponge-tipped applicators with handles (e.g., Toothette, Poliswab, Ora-Swab)	Cleanse teeth and mucous membranes when WBC drops below 2000/mm Apply fluoride, chemotherapeutic agents, desensitizing agents, xerostomia relief agents	Should not totally replace toothbrushing	May abrade friable tissue Sponge may become worn out during use (may fall off handle and risk chance of client aspiration) If handle is made of cardboard, don't saturate with fluids
Picks of various designs and names	Orapik, Dental Pik	Type II and III embrasures Remove plaque, food, and soft calculus	Type I embrasures and healthy tissues; great care is necessary to avoid trauma; clients with limited dexterity should not use in Type I embrasures	Improper use may cause damage to tissue and papillae
Bridge and clasp brush	Cylindrical brush on one end with tuft on opposite end for difficult-to-reach areas	Metal clasp of removable partial dentures		Use with nonabrasive denture paste to avoid scratching
Denture brush	Flat, trim, firm nylon design, stiffer than manual toothbrushes Some have double-end, flat side for tooth side of denture, pointed bristle end for tissue side	Tooth and tissue sides of dentures		Use with nonabrasive denture paste to avoid scratching

Procedure 19–8 USE OF A RUBBER TIP STIMULATOR

STEPS	RATIONALE
1. Determine the need to use a rubber tip stimulator and appropriate areas for use.	See a list of indications for use in Table 19–2.
2. Place side of rubber tip interdentally and slightly pointing coronally (45-degree angle) (Figure 19–26).	Using the side of the rubber tip allows for more surface area to be covered and less chance for tissue trauma to occur. Pointing the tip coronally also decreases the risk of tissue trauma.

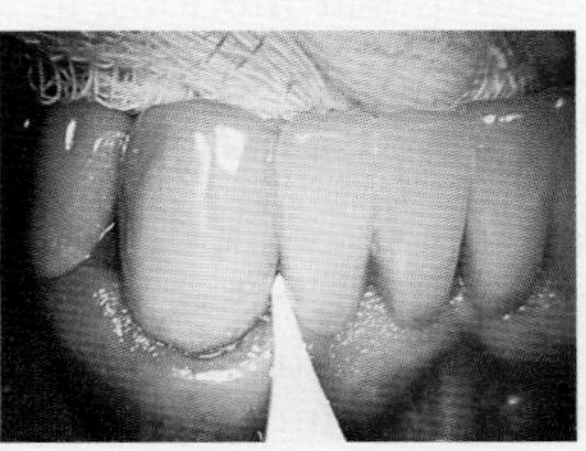

FIGURE 19–26 ✦ Proper placement of a rubber tip stimulator.

STEPS	RATIONALE
3. Move in and out with a slow stroke, rubbing the tip against the teeth and under the contact area.	Movement in and out of the proximal space removes plaque and massages the interdental tissue. The tip should not be forced into the space, however, to avoid trauma.
4. Remove from the interproximal space and trace the gingival margin with the tip positioned just below the margin following the contour of the gingiva.	When the margins are traced, the marginal tissue is stimulated.
5. Once all appropriate areas are completed, rinse stimulator with soap and warm water, then store in a clean, dry place.	The stimulator is meant to be reused after cleaning. Storage is similar to that of a toothbrush.
6. Replace rubber tip as it becomes worn, cracked, or splayed.	The handle may still be kept and reused, but a worn rubber tip should be replaced to improve efficacy and reduce the possibility of tissue trauma.

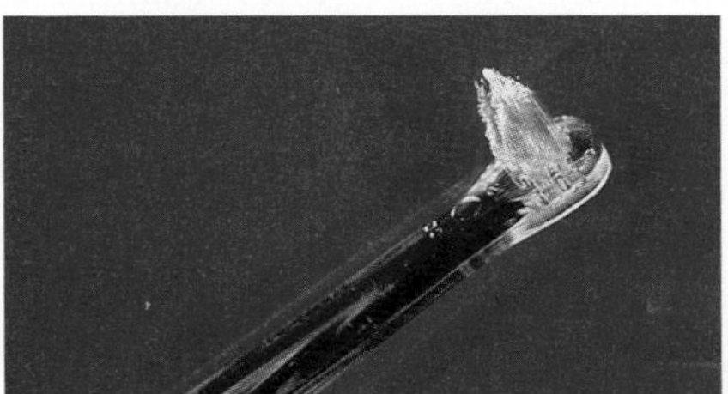

FIGURE 19–27 ✦ End-tuft brush.

Procedure 19–9 USE OF A TONGUE CLEANER

STEPS	RATIONALE
1. Determine the need to use a tongue cleaner.	See a list of indications for use in Table 19–2.
2. Hold the handle of the tongue cleaner, or if it is a strip tongue cleaner, wrap in a U shape by holding both ends of the cleaner.	The grasp on the tongue cleaner should be stable, with light pressure.
3. Start at the posterior part of the tongue and drag the tongue cleaner to the tip of the tongue. If a gag reflex ensues, drag from the lateral border of the tongue to the opposite lateral border.	Drag the tongue cleaner with a light stroke to avoid tissue trauma, especially trauma to the papillae.
4. Rinse tongue scraper with water.	Rinse the tongue cleaner to remove bacteria and debris.
5. Repeat step 3 until tongue cleaner is clean upon removal, being sure to cover all aspects of the tongue, overlapping strokes.	Overlapping strokes on the surface of the tongue will avoid missing any area.
6. Rinse tongue cleaner with soap and warm water to clean. Store in a clean, dry place.	Tongue cleaners are reusable, but should be replaced after 3 months or if they cannot be cleaned adequately.

tion therapy. Foam sticks are used as a more gentle form of oral self-care for a limited duration. Although use of the foam stick often occurs in place of a toothbrush, it was not developed to replace a toothbrush.[2,13] In one study, foam tips helped to remove enough plaque biofilm and debris from the mouth to prevent plaque biofilm formation below 2 mm at the cervical margin of the tooth.[13] In most studies, however, the primary use of the foam stick is to apply chemotherapeutic agents such as fluoride, chlorhexidine, desensitizing agents, and agents to relieve xerostomia. When used in combination with chlorhexidine, the foam brush is more effective in reducing plaque biofilm and gingivitis.[14]

Clasp Brush and Denture Brush

Specialty toothbrushes such as the *clasp brush* and *denture brush* have been designed with firm nylon filaments to clean dentures and the clasps of partial dentures (Table 19–2 and Figures 19–28 and 19–29). Because these prostheses are removable and cleaned outside of the mouth, the firmer filaments cannot cause destruction of gingival tissues (see Chapter 49).

AUTOMATED INTERDENTAL AND SUPPLEMENTAL MECHANICAL DEVICES

In the past several years, automated interdental devices have been increasingly introduced to consumers. Table 19–3 summarizes some of the more recognizable automated aids developed for interdental and supplemental use. The most commonly automated interdental aids are flossing devices, interproximal brushes, and tongue cleaners. Many of these products are continuing to undergo testing, and long-term studies are not always available.

The most common theme shared by automated aids is *sonic action* or *motion*. Sonic motion involves the use of waves or vibrations to assist in the removal of plaque biofilm and debris from the oral cavity. Most of the devices use other electromechanical motions that accomplish mechanical plaque biofilm removal (including rotary, counter-rotational, or elliptical motion) in addition to the sonic action.

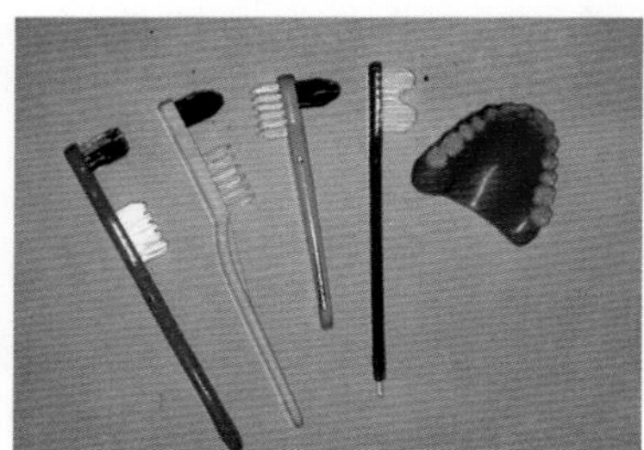

FIGURE 19–28 ✦ Examples of denture brushes.

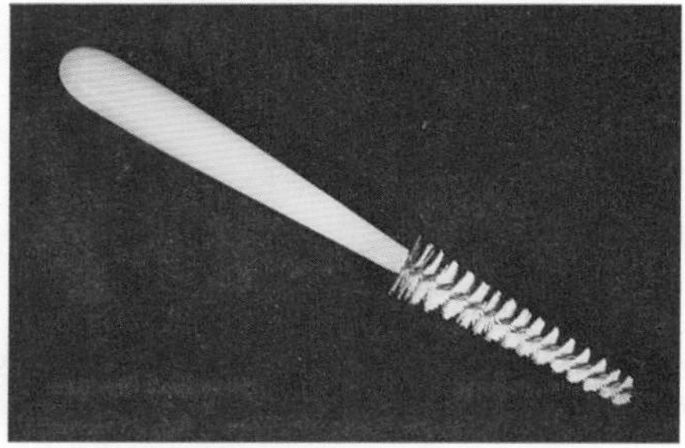

FIGURE 19–29 ✦ Example of a denture clasp brush.

Flossing Devices

The automated flossing devices are similar to floss holders in design and use; the electromechanical devices, some with a sonic motion added, further disrupt plaque biofilm and facilitate the placement of floss interproximally. As with the floss holder, these devices may help clients with poor dexterity, and the novelty may increase the client's motivation to floss.

Interproximal Brushes

Several automated interproximal brushes have been developed with the intent of being an alternative to dental flossing. Included in Table 19–3 are the Braun Oral-B Interclean (ID2); Interplak Interproximal Brush Attachment; Sonex International Corporation SoniPick; and the WaterPik Technologies, Inc. WaterPik Flosser. Automated interproximal brushes were developed for the proximal spaces and not to clean the contact area or interproximal area. Early study results suggest that the various automatic flossing devices are safe and just as effective as manual flossing.[15-18]

Tongue Cleaners

Automated tongue cleaners have been developed to remove plaque and debris from the surface of the tongue and to keep breath fresh. Automation provides a means for additional action that may help clients with dexterity difficulties. Two automated tongue cleaners currently marketed are the Interplak Power Tongue Cleaner Attachment and the Oralgiene Automated Tongue Cleaner. Currently there are no studies on automated tongue cleaners.

MANUFACTURERS OF INTERDENTAL AND SUPPLEMENTAL MECHANICAL ORAL HYGIENE

Questions often arise from clients regarding the newest and most effective products on the market. Although dental hygienists try to keep abreast of most new products and developments, this task can be challenging because numerous interdental and supplemental mechanical plaque control devices exist, and they change regularly. As a starting point, Table 19–4 lists some of the more commonly recognized manufacturers and contact information for the companies, the names of the products produced, and the names of the oral physiotherapy categories in which the aids fit.

TABLE 19–3 AUTOMATED INTERDENTAL AND SUPPLEMENTAL MECHANICAL ORAL PHYSIOTHERAPY (OPT) AIDS

Automated Interdental Mechanical Oral Physiotherapy Aids	Description/Types	Indications	Contraindications/ Limitations	Common Problems that May Be Experienced During Use/Misuse
American Dentronics Incorporated Cybersonic Sonic Flossing Attachment	Attaches to Cybersonic toothbrush handle Works similar to a tuning fork with up and down cleaning strokes at the rate of 31,000 per minute	Type I embrasures	Type II and III embrasures	Limited studies at this time Activation only occurs as pressure of the floss is applied against the tooth via a push or pull stroke; client may not think it is working if not using gentle pressure to activate motion
American Dentronics Incorporated Cybersonic Sonic Tongue Cleaning Attachment	Attaches to Cybersonic toothbrush handle	Removes plaque and food debris from tongue surface Keeps breath fresh and clean	Limited studies at this time	Limited studies at this time
Braun Oral-B INTERCLEAN Interdental Plaque Remover	Thin, flexible, mint-flavored cleaning filament (replaceable) that extends in to the interdental space on activation Alternative to dental floss	Interproximal cleaning to reduce plaque, bleeding, and gingival inflammation Patients with poor manual dexterity	None known at this time; no significant soft or hard tissue damage in studies conducted	Extends straight interdentally; unable to wrap in C shape around tooth
Conair Corporation Interplak Power Flosser Attachment	Attaches to Interplak toothbrush handle Moves in side-to-side orbital motion Use with any type of floss	Type I embrasures	Type II and III embrasures	Limited studies at this time
Conair Corporation Interplak Interproximal Brush Attachment	Attaches to Interplak toothbrush handle Microfine filaments	Ideal for cleaning around braces, crowns, bridgework, and periodontal pockets	Limited studies at this time	Limited studies at this time
Conair Corporation Interplak Power Tongue Cleaner Attachment	Attaches to Interplak toothbrush handle	Removes plaque and food debris from tongue surface Keeps breath fresh and clean	Limited studies at this time	Limited studies at this time
Dentist Preferred, Inc. PowerProxi Plus Sonic Interdental Plaque Removal System	System includes stand, power handle, 2 interdental attachments, 2 conventional toothbrush attachments, 24 coated wire interdental brushes (extra fine conical and tapered), 2 AA batteries, and oral hygiene instruction pamphlet	Cleans plaque missed by brushing and flossing Freshens breath Ideal for crowns, bridges, implants, periodontal pockets, and orthodontic brackets	Consider flossing areas that are too tight for interdental brushes; don't force brush between teeth Direct supervision is necessary with children or those who are mentally or physically challenged	Wear of interproximal tips is expected to occur, so replace as necessary No other known problems
NeoSonics FlossPlus Easy Flosser	SONIC Flossing Wand (designed in shape similar to floss holder; sonic action glides floss between teeth and provides soft massaging action)	Type I embrasures Removes plaque and food particles interproximally	Limited use with Type II and III embrasures	As floss shows wear, need to unwind, advance, and rewind floss on holder Need to rinse floss between areas or rewrap Need to maintain tension of floss
Oralgiene Automated Tongue Cleaner		Removes plaque and food debris from tongue surface Keeps breath fresh and clean	Limited studies at this time	Limited studies at this time
ProDentec Rotadent Electric Toothbrush	Pointed bristles	Type I, II, or III embrasures Margins of tissue Entire tooth surface Accessible furcations Orthodontic appliances Maxillofacial surgery clients wired shut		Toothbrush may cause tickling sensation; repeated use decreases sensation Use of a fulcrum is required for increased stability during use
Sonex International Corporation SoniPick	Sonic interdental plaque remover—sonic-frequency plaque remover Alternative to dental floss	Implants Braces Bridges Gingival pockets	Limited studies at this time	Limited studies at this time
WaterPik Technologies, Inc. WaterPik Flosser (models FL-110 and FL-310)	Electromechanical flossing device with a single nylon filament that reaches in between teeth and oscillates at 10,000 strokes per minute Alternative to dental floss	Control of plaque, bleeding, and gingivitis Normal interdental spaces Braces Crowns Bridges	None known at this time; no significant soft or hard tissue damage in studies conducted	Extends straight interdentally; unable to wrap in C shape around tooth

TABLE 19–4 MANUFACTURERS OF INTERDENTAL AND SUPPLEMENTAL MECHANICAL ORAL PHYSIOTHERAPY (OPT) AIDS (INCLUDING AUTOMATED AIDS)

Company Name, Address, Phone Number, and Internet Address	Product Name	Type of OPT Aid
AIT Dental 8920 Wilshire Blvd., Suite 305 Beverly Hills, CA 90211 www.aitdental.com	Proxi-Tip with standard handle or pocket traveler (3 tips: Proxi-Tip, Proxi-Pik, Perio-Brush) Proxi-Floss	Interproximal brush/stimulator, toothpick, interdental brush Floss threader and floss
Alwin 27104 Patriot Dr. Salisbury, MD 21801 1-800-749-4553	Pickleen 2—tongue cleaner and dental massager/stimulator	Tongue cleaner
American Dentronics, Inc. 503 Vista Bella, Suite 2 Oceanside, CA 92057-7006 1-800-770-7525 email: csonic@earthlink.net	Cybersonic System Sonic Toothbrush Sonic Flossing Attachment Sonic Ortho Brush Attachment Sonic Tongue Cleaning Attachment	Toothbrush Floss holder Orthodontic brush Tongue cleaner
Boji Distributors P.O. Box 15074 San Diego, CA 92115	FLOSSPAN	Floss holder
Breathaid LLC 1015 Fair Street Camden, SC 29020 1-888-2REFRESH www.breathaid.com	Breathaid (formerly known as NuBreath)	Tongue cleaner
Sunstar Butler Company 4635 W. Foster Ave. Chicago, IL 60630 312-777-4000 www.jbutler.com	EEZ-Lok Proxabrush handle (single- or double-ended plastic handle or single-ended aluminum handle) Butler G-U-M Proxabrush brushes (ultrafine cylindrical, ultrafine tapered, cylindrical, tapered, large cylindrical) Butler Trav-Ler (cylindrical, tapered)	Interdental brush handles and replacement brushes
	Butler Stimulator (gold with replacement tips)	Rubber tip stimulator
	End Tuft Brush (flat or tapered trim)	End-tuft brush
	Butler G-U-M EEZ-Thru Floss ButlerWeave Dental Floss (waxed, mint waxed, unwaxed) Butler G-U-M Fine Floss (waxed, mint waxed, unwaxed)	Dental floss
	Butler G-U-M Dental Tape (mint waxed, unwaxed)	Dental tape
	G-U-M EEZ-Thru Floss Threader	Floss threader
	Flossmate Handle (blue or red) Flossbrush Flosser (all-in-one floss and flosser; lightly waxed, lightly waxed mint)	Floss holder
	Soft-Pick Interdental Cleaner	Plastic wedge stimulator
	POSTCARE (regular or thin)	Braided floss for implants
	Bridge and Clasp Brush (blue or red)	Partials clasp brush
	Denture Brush (blue or red)	Denture brush
Calba Corporation P.O. Box 4125 Grand Central Station New York, NY 10163-4125 1-800-601-6647 www.allny.com/flossawl	FlossAwl	Floss holder
Colgate Oral Pharmaceuticals 1 Colgate Way Canton, MA 02021 1-800-225-3756 www.colgate.com	Colgate Precision Floss Colgate Dental Floss Colgate Total Dental Floss (regular waxed and mint waxed)	Dental floss
	Colgate Precision Tape	Dental tape
Conair Corporation One Cummings Point Rd. Stamford, CT 06904 1-800-633-6363 www.interplak.com	Interplak Power Flosser Attachment Interplak Power Tongue Cleaner Attachment Interplak Power Interproximal Brush Attachment Toothtowels	Floss holder Tongue cleaner Interproximal brush Tooth towels
Crescent Dental Manufacturing Co. 7750 W. 47th St. Lyons, IL 60534 708-447-8050	Perio Holders Spiral Brushes (soft or medium) Stimulator tips Soft Rubber Massage Cups	Interdental handle Interdental brush Rubber tip stimulator

TABLE 19–4 MANUFACTURERS OF INTERDENTAL AND SUPPLEMENTAL MECHANICAL ORAL PHYSIOTHERAPY (OPT) AIDS (INCLUDING AUTOMATED AIDS)—CONT'D

Company Name, Address, Phone Number, and Internet Address	Product Name	Type of OPT Aid
Curaprox 1605 South Farwell St. Eau Claire, WI 54701 1-877-387-2779 www.curaprox.com	Curaprox UHS Curaprox CPS Curaprox TP930 Brushpic Curaprox TP919 MicroSticks Curaprox CS001 Single Tuft Toothbrush—CS Sulcular	Universal holder system Interproximal brushes Interdental brush and ultrafine toothpick Wooden stimulators Single-tuft brush
Custom Medical Arts 13882 N. Kendall Dr. Miami, FL 33186 1-800-682-5840	Breathtique	Tongue cleaner
Deep Trading Corporation P.O. Box 273653 Tampa, FL 33688 1-813-931-0390	OOLITT Low Ripple Edge (normal use) OOLITT High Ripple Edge (thicker coating on tongue) OOLITT Comfort EZE (children) OOLITT One-Hand Use (reduced-dexterity patients)	Tongue cleaner
Dental Concepts, Inc. 9 North Goodwin Ave. Elmsford, NY 10523 1-914-592-1860	Orapik	Pick (supplemental aid to remove plaque and food particles)
Denteco, Inc. Internet Sales 74 Highland St. Worcester, MA 01609 1-888-640-3344 www.denteco.com	Denteco Tongue Cleaner (red, blue, teal, white, hot pink)	Tongue cleaner
Denticator 13705 Shoreline Court E. Earth City, MO 63045 1-800-227-3321 www.denticator.com	Handle with Cup Handle with Flat Brush Handle with Gum Massager Handle with Spirex Brush (tapered, extra long, narrow) Travel Spirex Brush (tapered, narrow) Handle with Gum Massager and Brush Handle with Gum Massager and Mirror Pick-A-Dent Tip-A-Dent	Supplemental aid End-tuft brush Rubber tip stimulator Interdental brush Rubber tip and interdental brush Rubber tip and mirror Plastic wedge stimulator Rubber tip
Dentist Preferred, Inc. 113 Floral Vale Blvd., Suite 10 Yardley, PA 19067 1-800-997-7694 fax: 215-504-9366	PowerProxi Plus Sonic Interdental Plaque Removal System Tongue Cleaner	Sonic toothbrush and interdental brushes Tongue cleaner
Discus Dental 8550 Higuera St. Culver City, CA 90232 1-800-422-9448 www.discusdental.com	BreathRx Gentle Tongue Scraper	Tongue cleaner
DreamCastle, Inc. www.dreamcastle.com/tungs	Dr. Tung's Tongue Cleaner	Tongue cleaner
E-Z Floss Co. P.O. Box 954 Palm Springs, CA 92262	E-Z Floss E-Z Handle Interproximal and Subgingival Cleaning Device—Inter–proximal Brush and Swab Tip	Floss holder Interdental handle Interdental brush and swab tip
Floss Aid Corporation P.O. Box 624 Santa Clara, CA 95052	FLOSSAID Holder BRIDGEAID Threader	Floss holder Floss threader
Flossrite Corporation 6932 Gettysburg Pike Fort Wayne, IN 46804 1-800-648-1453	Dr. Flosser	Floss holder

Table continued on following page

TABLE 19–4 MANUFACTURERS OF INTERDENTAL AND SUPPLEMENTAL MECHANICAL ORAL PHYSIOTHERAPY (OPT) AIDS (INCLUDING AUTOMATED AIDS)—CONT'D

Company Name, Address, Phone Number, and Internet Address	Product Name	Type of OPT Aid
Halbrand, Inc. Willoughby, OH 44094 1-800-321-3654	PoliSwab	Foam stick
Health-Tech, Inc. 15 Jackson Rd. Totowa, NJ 07512 973-785-8121	Sweet Breath Interdental Stimulators	Interdental brush
Hydro Floss Technologies, Inc. P.O. Box 159 Round Rock, TX 78680 1-800-338-8411	Hydro Floss	Oral irrigator
International Dental Design Specialists, Inc. 629 9th St. Imperial Beach, CA 91932 1-888-437-3749 www.breathsofresh.com/front.html	Breath-So-Fresh Tongue Cleaner	Tongue cleaner
Johnson & Johnson Professional Dental Care 199 Grandview Rd. Skillman, NJ 08558 908-874-2682	Reach Stim-U-Dent (mint flavored)	Wedge stimulator
	Reach Floss (regular, unwaxed, waxed, mint waxed cinnamon, fluoride mint waxed)	Dental floss
	Reach Floss Easy Slide Ultra Shred-Resistant Dental Floss waxed (mint waxed)	
	Reach Gentle Gum Care Dental Floss (mint, baking soda, mint fluoride, mint waxed, tartar control)	
	Reach Woven Floss (mint, mint tartar control, mint with fluoride)	
	Floss for Kids (grape)	
	Reach Floss DENTOTAPE (waxed, mint waxed)	Dental tape
	Wild Flossers Dental Floss Holder (single use)	Floss holder
NeoSonics Corporation P.O. Box 4053 Joliet, IL 60435 Attn: Customer Service Department 1-815-740-0001 or 1-800-99-FLOSS	FlossPlus Easy Flosser SONIC Flossing Wand (shape is similar to floss holder)	Automated flosser
Oral-B Laboratories 600 Clipper Dr. Belmont, CA 94002 1-800-44ORALB www.oralb.com	Stimulator	Rubber tip stimulator
	End-Tufted Brush—Tapered	End-tuft brush
	End-Tufted Brush—Flat	
	Interdental Brush—Handle	Interdental brush
	Interdental Brush—Bristles (extra fine brush refills [tapered, cylindrical], soft foam refills)	
	Interdental Brush—Compact (tapered, cylindrical)	
	Dental Floss Cirée (waxed, unwaxed, mint waxed)	Dental floss
	ULTRA FLOSS (mint, regular)	
	SATINfloss Dental Floss (mint, regular)	
	SATINtape	Dental floss
	Super Floss (mint, regular)	Super floss
	Braun Oral-B INTERCLEAN Interdental Plaque Remover	Automated interdental plaque remover
Oralgiene USA, Inc. 5811 Uplander Way Culver City, CA 90230 1-800-933-6725 or 8460 Higuera St. Culver City, CA 90232	Oralgiene Tongue Cleaners (white, blue, purple, green)	Tongue cleaner
	Oralgiene Automated Tongue Cleaner	
Oral Health Products, Inc. P.O. Box 470623 Tulsa, OK 74147 1-800-331-4645	POH Floss	Dental floss

TABLE 19–4 MANUFACTURERS OF INTERDENTAL AND SUPPLEMENTAL MECHANICAL ORAL PHYSIOTHERAPY (OPT) AIDS (INCLUDING AUTOMATED AIDS)—CONT'D

Company Name, Address, Phone Number, and Internet Address	Product Name	Type of OPT Aid
OraLine 823 NYS Rt. 13 Cortland, NY 13045 1-800-566-8772	Interdental Wooden Picks Dental Floss (waxed, unwaxed, mint flavored, smooth wax) Bubble Gum Flavor Dental Floss Waxed Dental Tape Interdental Bushes (cone, micro)	Wedge stimulators Dental floss Dental tape Interdental brushes
OraSweet Corporation P.O. Box 900340 Palmdale, CA 93590-0340 1-805-945-2255 or 1832 West Avenue K, Suite 6 Lancaster, CA 93534-5936 1-661-945-2255 or 1-800-549-1556 www.cleanbreath.com	OraSweet Tongue cleaner (crystal clear, aqua green, pink)	Tongue cleaner
PHB, Inc. N48862 US Hwy. 53 Osseo, WI 54758-9116 1-800-553-1440 (order line) 1-715-597-3935 www.phbinc.com	Peri-O-Floss PHB Floss (flat waxed) PHB Flosser and Refill EZeee Floss (toothbrush and floss handle) Interproximal Brushes (3 sizes) Denture Brush (large and small) PHB Tongue Scraper	Super floss Dental floss Floss holder Interdental brushes Denture brushes Tongue cleaner
Polteco, Inc. 23595 Cabot Blvd., Suite 110 Hayward, CA 94545 Mailing address: P.O. Box 2055 Burlingame, CA 94011 1-800-830-4849	Poly-Floss Ultra Thin Tape (waxed) Textured Dental Tape (waxed)	Dental floss Dental tape
Preventive Dentistry Products, Inc. P.O. Box 754 Corona del Mar, CA 92625	EZ Denta Flosser	Floss holder
Pro-Dentec P.O. Box 4129 Batesville, AR 72503 1-800-752-2565 www.prodentec.com	Rota-Points RotaDent	Wedge stimulator Electric toothbrush
Sakool Co. P.O. Box 5439 Dearborn, MI 48128-5439 1-888-551-1986 www.sakool.com	Sakool Tongue Cleaners (Scrapers) (scented [cinnamon, spearmint] or unscented [white, blue, pink])	Tongue cleaner
sb products, inc. 1872 S. Tamiami Trail, Suite D Venice, FL 34293	ToothTowels	Tooth towelettes
ShowerFloss, Inc. P.O. Box 4055 Niagara Falls, NY 14304 1-800-959-3567	ShowerFloss (hooks to shower head)	Oral irrigation
SONEX International Corporation 2022 Route 22 P.O. Box 533 Brewster, NY 10509-0533 1-800-633-7858	SoniPick	Sonic interdental plaque remover, sonic-frequency plaque remover

Table continued on following page

TABLE 19–4 MANUFACTURERS OF INTERDENTAL AND SUPPLEMENTAL MECHANICAL ORAL PHYSIOTHERAPY (OPT) AIDS (INCLUDING AUTOMATED AIDS)—CONT'D

Company Name, Address, Phone Number, and Internet Address	Product Name	Type of OPT Aid
Sulcabrush, Inc. 4600 Witmer Industrial Estates, Unit #2 Niagara Falls, NY 14305 1-800-387-8777 www.sulcabrush.com	Sulcabrush Sulcabrush Replacement Tips	Single-tuft brush
The Tongue Cleaner Co. P.O. Box 1070 Capitola, CA 95010 1-831-662-9500 http://tonguecleaner.com/	The Tongue Cleaner (white with blue print, green with gold print, purple with gold print, blue with gold print)	Tongue cleaner
Thornton International, Inc. Home Dental Care Division P.O. Box 52 Rowayton, CT 06853 1-800-445-3567	Thornton's 3-in-1 Floss Thornton's Perio Floss	All-purpose super floss Special-purpose super floss (bridges, implants, braces, perio home care) (thicker than 3-in-1 floss)
Tongue Sweeper, Inc. 3054 West Tuscarawas St. Canton, OH 44708 1-800-589-3043 www.tonguesweeper.com	Tongue Sweeper	Tongue cleaner
U.S. Dentek Corporation 1-800-433-6835 www.usdentek.com	Gingibrush Super Pik Dental Pik with Mirror Dental Pik Sensitive with Mirror Flossers (regular, mint) Breath Remedy Tongue Scraper	Gumline and interdental brush Wedge stimulator Plaque and soft tartar remover Travel flosser and wedge stimulator Tongue cleaner
Venk Enterprises, Inc. 6 Castle Creek Place Shawnee, OK 74801	Lila Tongue Cleaners	Tongue cleaner
Waterpik Technologies 1730 East Prospect Rd. Fort Collins, CO 80553-0001 1-800-525-2020 www.waterpik.com	Waterpik Flosser (model FL-110 [replaceable battery] and model FL-310 [rechargeable battery])	Automated flossing device
W.L. Gore & Associates 100 Airport Rd. Blvd. P.O. Box 1010 Elkton, MD 21922-1010 1-800-645-4337 or 1500 N. Fourth St. Flagstaff, AZ 86003 www.gore.com/glidefloss	Glide Floss Floss Travel Package Floss Trial Package Floss Single-Use Sachet Floss Dispenser Glide Tape Tape Trial Package Tape Dispenser	Dental floss Dental tape

Client Education Issues

- ✦ Explain the importance of interdental cleaning to the prevention and control of periodontal disease.
- ✦ Demonstrate proper use of interdental cleaning aids as dictated by the needs of the client.
- ✦ Explain that breath freshness may be improved by using a tongue cleaner.
- ✦ Explain that dexterity and visual acuity problems may be solved with automated or adaptive aids (see Chapter 36).
- ✦ Explain that supplemental oral physiotherapy aids become increasingly necessary as embrasure spaces progress from type I to type II or III.
- ✦ Explain that as probe readings become deeper and loss of attachment increases, floss may no longer be effective; other oral physiotherapy aids are required.
- ✦ Explain that adequate plaque control at home must be maintained to prevent caries and periodontal disease and to maintain health.
- ✦ Explain that clients must understand their own interdental anatomy and how specific interdental cleaning devices can be used to control plaque biofilm in hard-to-reach areas.
- ✦ Question clients to determine which interdental aids are currently used and the reason(s) other aids are not. If they simply do not like or value the procedure, find out why and perhaps recommend an alternative interdental aid.
- ✦ Instruct clients based on their unique human needs to promote client acceptance.

Legal, Ethical, and Safety Issues

- ✦ The legal standard of care requires that dental hygienists educate clients about oral self-care. Upon completion of dental hygiene care, the legal records of the client should reveal that the client has been counseled on why and how to perform an effective daily personal oral hygiene program.
- ✦ Monitoring the clients' progress should be recorded.
- ✦ Malpractice cases for failure to recognize and treat periodontal disease can be related to failure to teach adequate plaque control measures to clients, especially since proximal areas are a focal site for infection.
- ✦ Many oral physiotherapy aids can cause damage in the oral cavity if used incorrectly.
- ✦ Properly educating the client regarding use of the various oral physiotherapy aids will help prevent misuse and increase safety.

Key Concepts

- ✦ Interdental cleaning is essential in the prevention of periodontal disease and dental caries. Poor interdental cleaning has been linked to cardiovascular disease and premature, low-birthweight infants.
- ✦ Risk assessment is an important part of determining which oral physiotherapy aids to recommend.
- ✦ Thoroughness of plaque removal rather than frequency appears to be more important in preventing gingivitis. Use of oral physiotherapy aids helps improve thoroughness and may often be used in combination to reach maximum benefits.
- ✦ Although additional aids are best when used in combination, oral physiotherapy aids should be kept to a minimum and related to the dexterity and preferences of the client. Clients must be involved in the selection of supplemental aids.

Critical Thinking Exercises

1. Scenario: As a result of a recent automobile accident, one of your teenage clients suffered a broken jaw. To allow healing, her mouth is wired shut, keeping her from moving her jaw. She is seeking advice on how to care for her oral cavity. Several wires are present, and staples appear at the cervical margins of all teeth. She also has several intraoral cuts and abrasions, making any form of cleaning somewhat painful. Discuss possible oral physiotherapy aids that could be used and make recommendations for home care.
2. With samples of floss provided in class by your instructor, identify each as unwaxed or waxed dental floss, dental tape, PTFE floss, braided floss, G-floss, or Super Floss.

Continued on following page

Critical Thinking Exercises—cont'd

3. Demonstrate proper flossing techniques for spool and loop methods on a typodont. Once mastered on a typodont, demonstrate flossing in your own mouth and then on a partner while using proper infection control.
4. Identify and demonstrate proper use of a floss holder and floss threader on a typodont.
5. With a partner, role-play flossing instructions as if providing home care instructions to a client.
6. Identify the name of various aids provided in class by your instructor. Also describe various areas in which each aid may be used in the mouth.
7. On a periodontal typodont, demonstrate use of the various oral physiotherapy aids.
8. With a partner, role-play instructions on how to use the supplemental aids as if providing home care instructions to a client.
9. Give each student in the class one oral physiotherapy aid to research. Students should deliver oral reports to the class, including key points to teach the client.

For References, Suggested Readings, and Related Websites, visit
http://evolve.elsevier.com/Darby/hygiene/

CHAPTER 20

INSTRUMENTS AND INSTRUMENTATION THEORY

OBJECTIVES

Mastery of the content in this chapter will enable the reader to:

- Describe assessment and treatment instruments for periodontal instrumentation
- Discuss variations in instrument shank length, curvature, flexibility, and blade-to-shank angulation
- Discuss proper instrument blade adaptation and angulation
- Customize fulcrum placement for a tooth surface
- Describe dental perioscopy during periodontal hand instrumentation
- Describe protective scaling strategies and reinforcement scaling
- List some intraoral and extraoral fulcrums for periodontal instrumentation

KEY TERMS

Adaptation
Angle (shank)
Angulation
Area-specific curets
Assessment instruments
Chisel scaler
Dental perioscopy
Exploratory stroke
Explorer
Extended-shank curets
File scaler
Fulcrum (intraoral, extraoral, same arch, cross arch, opposite arch)
Handle
Hoe scaler
Insertion
Lateral pressure
Mini-bladed curets
Modified pen grasp
Mouth mirror
Palm-thumb grasp
Pen grasp
Periodontal probe
Reinforcement scaling
Reinsertion
Root planing stroke
Scaling stroke
Sickle scaler
Strength (shank)
Stroke direction
Stroke length shank
Tactile sensitivity
Treatment instruments
Universal curet
Working end

BASIC INSTRUMENT DESIGN

Assessment and Treatment Instruments

Instruments used in caring for clients with healthy or diseased periodontium may be divided into two categories:

- *Assessment instruments* provide the operator with periodontal assessment information.
- *Treatment instruments* are used to perform periodontal scaling and root planing (Tables 20–1 and 20–2).

Examples of assessment and treatment instruments are shown in Figure 20–1. All of these instruments consist of three functional parts:

- Handle
- Shank
- Working end

Variations in these functional parts determine the purpose, effectiveness, efficiency, and comfort of use for the operator. A good assessment or treatment instrument supports all of these functions.

TABLE 20–1 ASSESSMENT INSTRUMENTS

Assessment Instruments	Basic Use	Assessment Instruments	Basic Use
Mouth mirror	Indirect vision, indirect illumination, transillumination, and retraction of buccal mucosa and tongue; for use throughout appointment.	Nabers probe	A furcation classification instrument to be used during assessment and again during the evaluation phase of the process of care.
Periodontal probe	Measurement of probing depth, clinical attachment level, relative attachment level, amount of attached gingiva, gingival recession, furcation invasion, bacterial plaque biofilm, gingival inflammation, assessment of bleeding points, and pathological lesions. Used during assessment and again during the evaluation phase of the process of care.	Explorer	Detection of calculus, irregular cementum, junctional epithelium, dental caries, irregular root anatomy, margins or restorations, external resorption and osseous exposures. For use during assessment, implementation, and evaluation phases of the process of care.

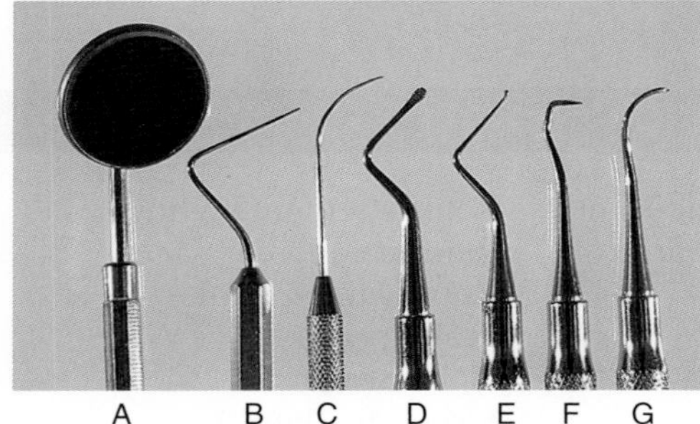

FIGURE 20–1 ✦ Assessment instruments: mirror *(A)*, periodontal probe *(B)*, explorer *(C)*. Working instruments: file *(D)*, hoe *(E)*, sickle *(F)*, curet *(G)*.

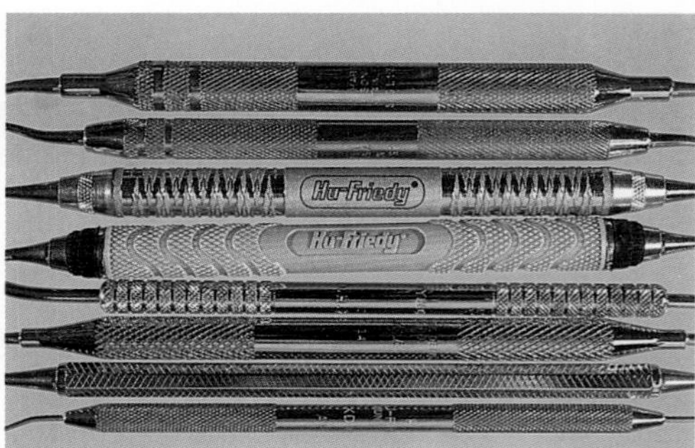

FIGURE 20–2 ✦ Instrument handle variations in size, shape, and pattern.

Parts and Characteristics of Dental Instruments

HANDLE. When selecting an instrument, handle specifications primarily benefit operator comfort. Nevertheless, handles *should not* be considered less important than any other part of the instrument. In response to a heightened concern for operator comfort and to lessen the effect of repetitive strain injuries, instrument manufacturers offer a variety of handle options relating to size and weight. The larger-diameter grips are more comfortable than the smaller handles, but because of the extra circumference, posterior access may be more difficult, especially if the client has limited mouth-opening ability. Slender handles can lead to cramping of the hands after prolonged use.

Handle shape or circumference may be round or hexagonal. Both are quite comfortable when a suitable surface pattern is used. The depth of the pattern cut into the handle can determine the practitioner's comfort level. Some patterns are cut so deeply that they feel as if they are biting into the skin when pressure is placed on the instrument.

Handle weight is the final consideration in handle selection. There are solid-handled and hollow-handled instruments. Most clinicians find that hollow handles are lighter and less strenuous to use and improve tactile sensitivity more than solid-handled instruments (Figure 20–2).

SHANK. The *shank* of an instrument connects the *working end* to the handle, and is the major factor determining the use of each particular instrument. Differences among instruments in shank design relate to the following:

- ✦ Length of shank
- ✦ Angle of shank
- ✦ Strength of shank

TABLE 20–2 TREATMENT INSTRUMENTS

Treatment Instruments	Basic Use	Treatment Instruments	Basic Use
Universal curet	Depending on design, may be used in all areas of the mouth for supragingival and subgingival scaling and root planing. Used during the implementation phase of the dental hygiene process for periodontal scaling and root planing.	Hoe	Used for supragingival and subgingival calculus removal where tissue is retractable, and during initial scaling; *should not* be used for root planing.
Gracey curets	Area-specific curets that, depending on design, may be used in various areas of the mouth for supragingival and subgingival scaling, root planing, and bacterial plaque biofilm removal. Used for periodontal scaling and root planing.	Plastic and graphite instruments	Used for assessment as well as calculus and bacterial plaque biofilm removal around titanium dental implant abutment cylinders; gold instruments are also used.
Sickle	Principally a supragingival calculus removal instrument. Used for gross calculus removal. This instrument is *not* used for root planing.	Ultrasonic and sonic scaling devices (see Figures 23–9 and 23–17)	Used for supragingival and subgingival calculus removal, bacterial plaque biofilm recommended for titanium dental implant abutment cylinders, unless working end is a specially designed rubber-coated tip (see Table 23–10 and Figures 50–59 and 50–60).
File	Used for supragingival and subgingival calculus removal where tissue is retractable. For use during initial scaling; *should not* be used for root planing.	Slow-speed handpiece (see Figure 22–1)	Used for bacterial plaque biofilm and extrinsic stain removal after scaling and root planing are complete. Recommended for use with a fine abrasive agent for polishing titanium dental implant abutment cylinders. The prophylaxis angle, rubber cup, point or brush, and polishing agent are part of the armamentarium.
		Air polishing/ airbrasion system (see Figure 22–21)	Used for bacterial plaque biofilm and stain removal after scaling and root planing are complete. Contraindicated for use around titanium dental implant abutment cylinders.

Length of Shank. Instrument shank length ranges from short to long (Figure 20–3). An instrument with a long shank is preferred for instrumenting anterior or posterior teeth with deep periodontal pocket depths or recession, or when the operator needs to fulcrum a great distance from the area being instrumented. An instrument with a short shank is best suited for instrumenting anterior teeth, when fulcruming close to the area being instrumented, and when there are shallow pocket depths.

Angle of Shank. Most periodontal instruments have shanks that are curved or bent in at least one and usually two places (Figure 20–4). The degree and angle of this curvature also determine the area(s) in which the instrument is effective:

- The smaller the angle and fewer the number of bends in an instrument's shank, the more suitable the instrument is for use on anterior teeth.
- The more acute the angle and greater the number of bends, the more suitable the instrument is for use on posterior teeth.

The fulcrum plays a major role in directing the use of the instrument, despite the angle of the shank. Although

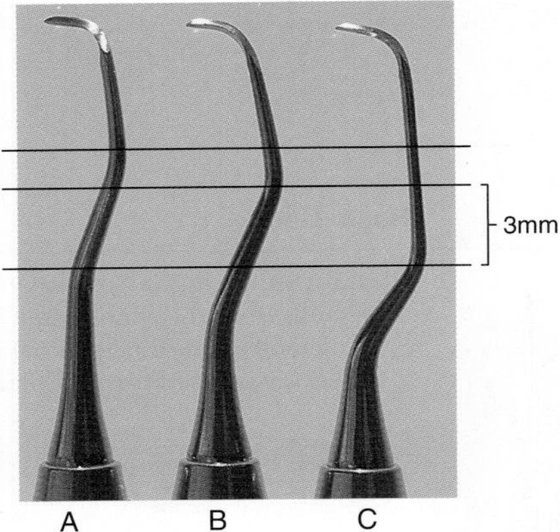

FIGURE 20–3 ✦ Comparison of instrument shank lengths. **A,** Gracey 1/2. **B,** Gracey 5/6. **C,** Gracey After-Five series 5/6.

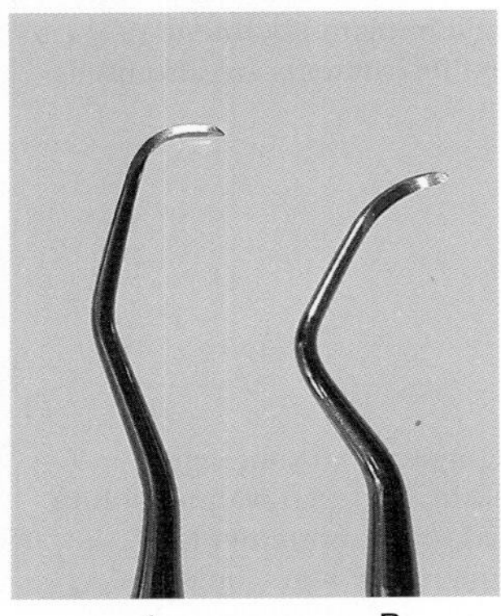

FIGURE 20–4 ✦ Comparison of shank angles or curvatures. **A,** Gracey curet 5/6. **B,** Universal curet.

generally the straighter-shanked instruments are used in anterior areas and the more curved-shanked instruments are used in posterior areas, this does not always have to be the case. For example, clinicians who use a variety of fulcrums ranging from intraoral to extraoral to allow the working end access to deep periodontal areas find that shank angle does not limit the usefulness of the instrument. In other words, fulcrum versatility allows greater flexibility in use of instruments in nontraditional areas. Thus, in some cases straighter-shanked instruments may be used for scaling of posterior teeth and considerably more curved instruments may be used in anterior areas.

The portion of the shank from the last bend or curve to the working end is termed the *terminal shank.* Its position as it relates to the working end is important in determining the correct positioning of the angulation of the curet blade and usually is kept parallel to the long axis of the tooth.

Shank Strength. All shanks taper in diameter from the handle as they approach the working end. *Shank strength,* categorized as extra rigid, rigid, moderately flexible, or flexible, is a function of the thickness and type of metal used:

- Extra-rigid shanks are designed for removing very tenacious calculus. A step down are rigid shanks, also designed for heavy, tenacious calculus. Both are ideal when additional strength is needed and the clinician does not want dissipation of pressure against the tooth surface felt with more flexible shanks. Tactile sensitivity detecting changes in tooth surface smoothness is not compromised using extra rigid and rigid shank curets. Sickles, files, and rigid Gracey curets are examples of instruments with rigid shanks.
- Moderately flexible shanks, found in most universal curets, are ideal for removal of moderate to light calculus providing adequate resistance against this type of tooth deposit.
- Flexible shanks are used to detect and remove light subgingival calculus deposits or plaque biofilm. They are characteristic of area-specific curets and explorers, and their flexibility provides the best tactile sensation but least strength as compared to other shank strengths.

Some manufacturers designate the flexibility of their instruments' shanks. There are definite benefits in using instruments with less-flexible shanks. When scaling teeth with heavy calculus, much less operator effort is needed if the instrument does not bend or flex away from the tooth when pressure is exerted. The practitioner must work harder to direct equivalent lateral pressure against the tooth when the instrument shank flexes. In addition, if the instrument shank is long or if fulcruming away from the working area is required, shank flexibility results in further dissipation of pressure exerted by the operator. Consequently, in these cases use of an instrument with a strong shank is important.

In scaling teeth of individuals with light calculus or in fulcruming close to the working area there are also savings in operator effort, although this is less noticeable when using an instrument with a strong shank. However, if the operator's saved effort is multiplied by 8 to 10 clients treated per day, the savings become more meaningful.

Nevertheless, arguments against rigid-shanked instruments claim a decreased tactile sensitivity compared to flexible-shanked instruments. Many clinicians find the rigid shanks comfortable with all types of clients. Others find that flexible shanks are better to use when scaling. The decision to select a rigid-shanked or flexible-shanked instrument is largely a matter of habit and the type of instrument one is accustomed to using. However, it is prudent to learn to use instruments with rigid shanks. The savings in operator effort and possible avoidance of operator injury such as tendonitis of the wrist are most likely to be felt when scaling and root planing teeth with rigid-shanked instruments (see Chapter 8, section on hand, wrist, and finger injuries).

WORKING END. The *working end* (terminal end) of the instrument attached to the shank determines the general purpose of the instrument. This is probably the most important detail in instrument selection. There are slight differences between manufacturers as to shape, length, width, bend or curvature, and metallurgy of the working ends of identically named and numbered instruments. These small details are important considerations when selecting instruments.

The working end of an instrument is designed for a specific task. For example, if an instrument is needed for assessing the distance between the marginal gingiva and the base of the periodontal pocket, the dental hygienist selects an instrument that has a working end calibrated to measure distance (e.g., the periodontal probe). The general shape and length of the probe's working end are fairly consistent among all manufacturers. However, there are differences in the working ends of periodontal probes with respect to their thickness, intervals of millimeter markings, and the presence or absence of color-coded probe markings for easier reading.

The design of the working ends among scaling instruments varies considerably. Therefore, when deciding on which instrument to use for scaling, the criteria for instrument selection are more complex. The decision is based on experience with using different scaling and root planing instruments, periodontal probing depths present, the gingival tissue tone, and the quantity and type of calculus to be scaled. If there is heavy subgingival calculus, one type of treatment instrument option is the curet. Within this category of treatment instrument, there is a range in variation among manufacturers of the same instrument (e.g., differences in blade size, length, shape, and metallurgy). Curet selection should be based on the amount and tenacity of calculus, pocket depth, alignment of teeth, root proximity, use of intraoral or extraoral fulcrums, and tissue tone. For example, a wide, heavy blade is needed for removal of heavy subgingival calculus; a long blade is necessary for removal of deep subgingival and interproximal calculus. The curvature of the blade is important for specific area(s) being scaled.

Curets are further subdivided based on blade metal.

- ✦ Stainless steel instruments maintain adequate sharpness for scaling and root planing and do not rust or discolor when sterilized with saturated steam or with formalin-alcohol vapor.
- ✦ Carbon steel blades tend to feel sharper clinically and hold their sharpened edges longer after prolonged use than do stainless steel blades.[1,2] However, carbon steel is more brittle and breaks more easily than does stainless steel. Carbon steel instruments also may corrode or rust when sterilized. Carbon steel has a tendency to oxidize (rust) after saturated steam sterilization,[3] or when moisture content of a formalin-alcohol vapor sterilizer reaches 15% or greater. Because of this tendency for oxidation of the carbon steel metal, commercially available corrosion inhibitors are recommended for use with the autoclave to reduce oxidation. Manufacturer instructions concerning dilution of ultrasonic cleaners and chemical disinfection solutions and length of time instruments should remain in solution must be carefully monitored. Dry heat sterilization, however, does not present a problem for carbon steel instruments.

The final selection of a treatment instrument for scaling purposes usually involves personal preference relative to which instrument works best with a given instrumentation technique (grasp, fulcrum, wrist, and finger action), scaling and root planing objectives, and desired efficiency in terms of time management. If, for example, a practitioner's scaling technique involves using extraoral fulcrums, area-specific curets are ideal instruments to use. If the client presents with no significant periodontal disease, universal curets may accomplish the scaling with more efficiency in terms of time management than area-specific curets that require different instruments for different areas of the tooth.

Depending on the manufacturer, the working end of an instrument may be:

- ✦ Double-ended, with exact, mirror images on the opposite ends. This is necessary because the same curvature of blade does not adapt to each side of the same tooth. For example, the distal surface from the facial aspect of the tooth requires the mirror image of the same instrument to scale the distal surface from the lingual aspect.
- ✦ Single-ended, with only one end having a working blade, requiring the practitioner to have twice as many instruments. Single-ended instruments are inefficient because of the necessity of picking up and replacing instruments to and from the work area every time the dental hygienist chooses to work from the opposite aspect of the same tooth. Instrument cleaning, packaging, sterilization, and storage efforts also are doubled.

Some assessment instruments do not have mirror-image working ends, such as the periodontal probe and the straight explorer. Such instruments may be manufactured so that one end is a periodontal probe and the other is an explorer. They are double-ended but have two different instruments on the same handle (Figure 20–5).

Balanced Instruments. See Chapter 8, Figure 8–11 and section on balanced instruments.

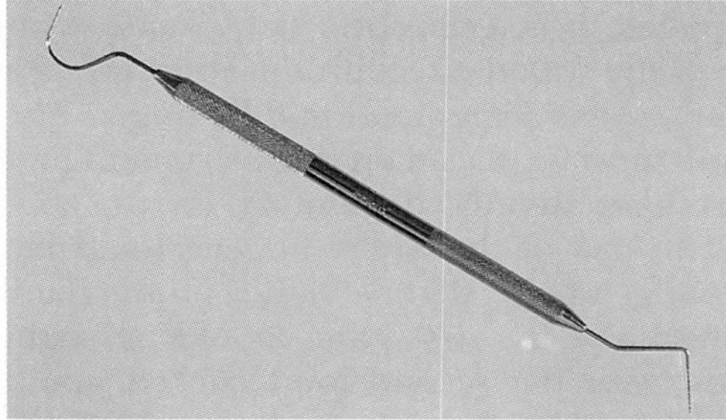

FIGURE 20–5 ✦ Double-ended instrument with a periodontal probe on one end and an explorer on the opposite end.

FUNDAMENTALS OF INSTRUMENTATION

Operator and Client Positions[4]

Operator and client positioning facilitate proper instrumentation technique. In operator positioning, the dental hygienist attempts to achieve a state of musculoskeletal balance that protects the body from strain and cumulative injury (see Chapter 8, section on positioning factors).

Instrument Blade Selection

After the appropriate instrument has been selected, the hygienist determines the correct working end of the instrument to use for the tooth surface to be scaled. For some instruments, such as the periodontal probe and the #3-A EXD explorer, the working end is universal (i.e., used on all surfaces). However, the practitioner may find some instruments that work well on all mesial and distal surfaces but only on the anterior teeth, for example, the straight sickle scaler. The majority of treatment instruments are site-specific, with a definite side of the blade that should be used against the tooth.

After establishing a comfortable operator position and selecting the appropriate instrument and working end, the dental hygienist begins scaling and/or root planing. For discussion purposes, this procedure is broken down into its component parts of grasp, fulcrum, insertion, adaptation, angulation, lateral pressure, stroke direction, stroke length, and reinforcement.

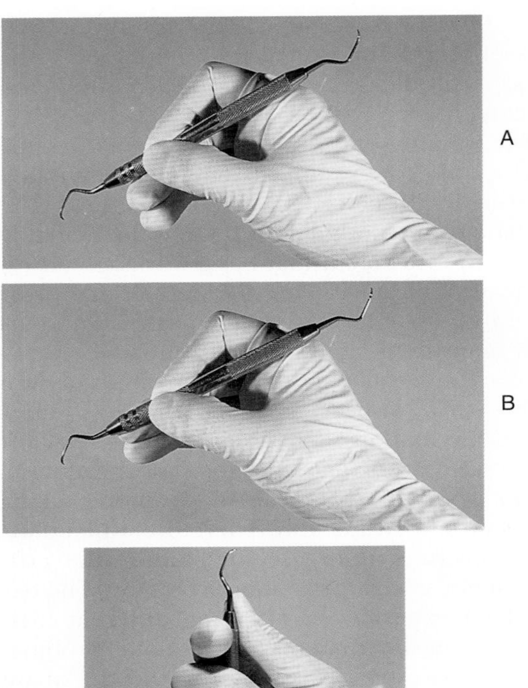

FIGURE 20–6 ✦ Comparison of instrument grasps. **A,** Pen grasp. **B,** Modified pen grasp. **C,** Palm grasp.

Grasp

Table 8-4 in Chapter 8 categorizes grasp by instrument selection. The *pen grasp* (Figure 20–6, *A*) is used when the exacting or directive type of pressure in scaling and root planing is not required. The thumb and index finger pads are well situated on the instrument handle, but the middle finger slips down and the instrument rests on the side of the finger near the first knuckle. The pen grasp may be used when light, easy probing or exploring into nonperiodontally involved areas is performed. Much heavier pressure also may be used with this grasp on the mouth mirror for retraction of the buccal mucosa, tongue, or other soft tissues.

The *modified pen grasp* (Figure 20–6, *B*) is the standard grasp used for periodontal instrumentation. When correctly applied, it is a sensitive, stable, and strong grasp because of the tripod effect produced by the position of the thumb, index finger, and middle finger. The pad of the thumb must be placed on the instrument handle and the joint bent slightly, depending on the area being scaled. The pad of the index finger should be on the instrument at a point slightly higher on the handle than the thumb, and the first joint should be slightly bent downward with the second joint cocked upward. The side of the middle finger near the nailbed should be placed opposing the thumb and further down the instrument on the shank toward the working end. The middle finger may remain straight when using extended fulcrums (e.g., cross arch, opposite arch, and extraoral fulcrums), or it may be angled on the first and second knuckles similar to the position of the index finger but less pronounced, especially when working with fulcrums in close proximity to the area being scaled.

Once instrumentation is initiated, the modified pen grasp must be continually reestablished on the instrument handle to accommodate the minute rolling of the instrument into and around depressions of tooth structure. Otherwise, the instrument can roll and slip out of the grasp, or the thumb and fingers can end up in an undesirable position on the instrument handle, which may not allow for optimal pressure to be placed against the instrument for adequate assessment or instrumentation.

The thumb, index, and middle fingers also are flexed to allow the instrument to be manipulated in various directions around the tooth surface and to allow equal pressure to be applied against root structure during the course of the stroke. Although historically dental hygienists were taught to avoid digital movement during instrumentation, it now appears that such digital movement, when combined with the movement of the wrist, facilitates accurate, even scaling and root planing strokes in deep periodontal pockets during nonsurgical periodontal therapy. Moreover, the most protective situation for the dental hygienist when scaling in deep pockets occurs when both finger movement and wrist (or arm) movement can be used, minimizing stress to one particular area such as the hand or wrist. The degree to which finger flexing is required for successful instrumentation (versus wrist movement and even arm movement) varies according to the fulcrum used, the area being scaled, the instrument used, and the depth of the periodontal pocket. In certain areas, either finger flexing or wrist movement is used.

The *palm–thumb grasp* (Figure 20–6, *C*) is achieved with all four fingers wrapped tightly around the handle and the thumb placed on the shank in a direction pointing toward the tip of the instrument. This is a very awkward, uncontrolled grasp because the thumb provides the only source of pressure and the opposing fingers clumsily wrap around the handle and do not provide a means of turning the instrument or modifying the effect of the thumb. The palm–thumb grasp provides little in the way of tactile sensitivity during scaling procedures and is not recommended for periodontal instrumentation either supragingivally or subgingivally. Because the palm–thumb grasp is a very stable grasp that does not allow the instrument to move on its own, it is ideal for use during instrument sharpening.

Fulcrum

The action of applying lateral pressure against the tooth surface with a sharp blade or pointed instrument necessitates a stable fulcrum. The *fulcrum* is the source of stability or leverage on which the finger rests and against which it pushes to hold the instrument with control during stroke activation. When there is no fulcrum, the instrument uncontrollably slips off of the tooth surface when even a slight amount of lateral pressure is exerted. There are two basic fulcrums: intraoral and extraoral.

INTRAORAL FULCRUM. The *intraoral fulcrum,* established inside the mouth against a tooth surface, is used for scaling in shallow pockets. The pad of the ring finger usually is positioned on the occlusal, incisal, or facial surface of a tooth close to the one being instrumented. The middle finger should remain in contact with the ring finger even when it is bent during finger flexing or when making digital movements. If the middle finger splits away from the ring finger, control and strength diminish from the stroke. With the added support of the middle finger, a built-up stable fulcrum is accomplished.

Depending on the area to be scaled, the angle of access, and the pocket depth, intraoral fulcrums may be positioned on the following:

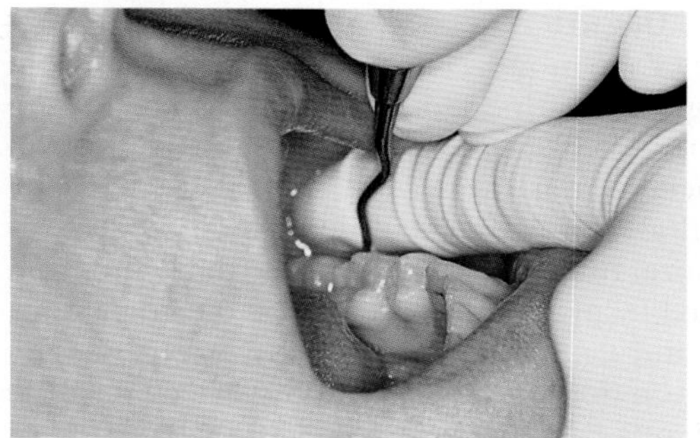
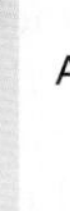
A

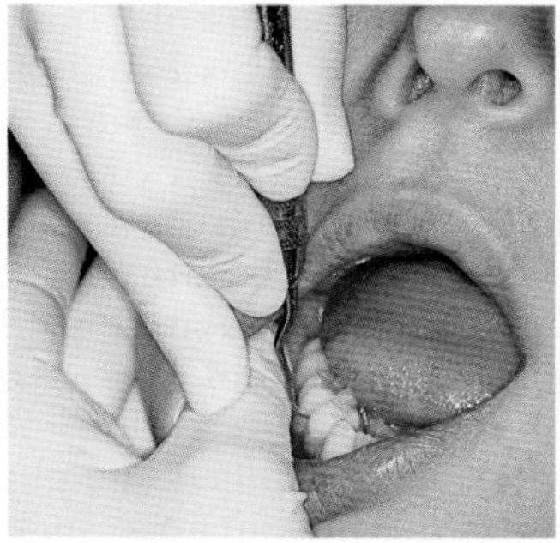
B

FIGURE 20–7 ✦ Intraoral fulcrums. **A,** Fulcrum on operator's index finger. **B,** Fulcrum on operator's thumb.

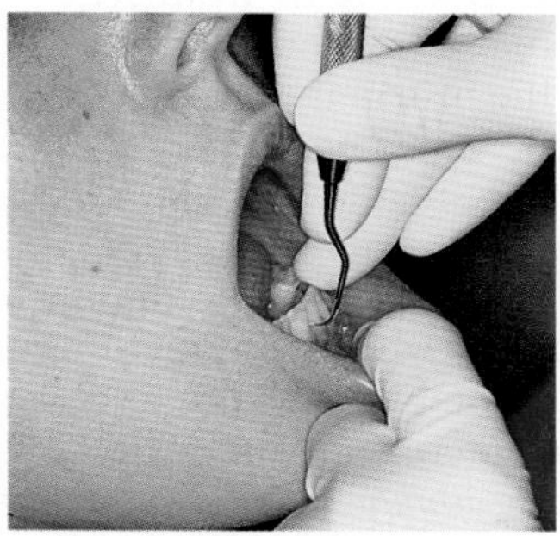

FIGURE 20–8 ✦ Same arch fulcrum positioned near area being scaled.

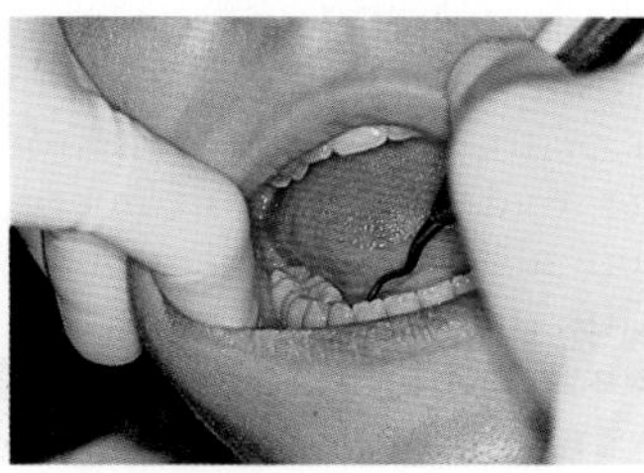

FIGURE 20–9 ✦ Cross arch fulcrum is positioned on the same arch but across from area being scaled; fulcrum on opposite quadrant.

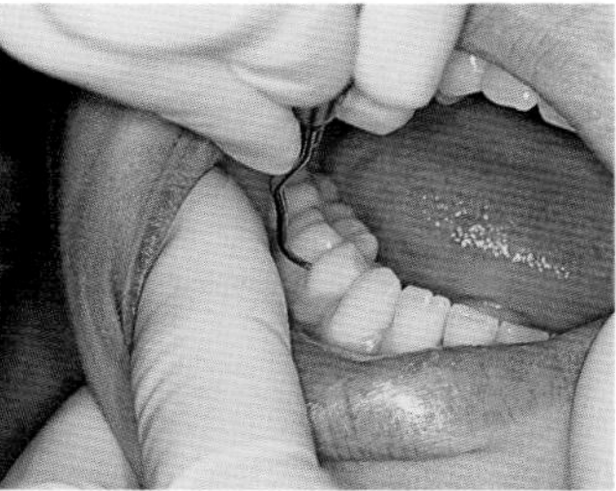

FIGURE 20–10 ✦ Opposite arch fulcrum from the arch being scaled.

- ✦ The operator's own finger (e.g., fulcrum on index or thumb) that is located within the oral cavity (Figure 20–7, *A* and *B*)
- ✦ A tooth surface on the same arch near to the area being scaled (*same arch fulcrum*) (Figure 20–8)
- ✦ A tooth surface on the same arch but across from the area being scaled (i.e., on the opposite quadrant or cross arch), creating a *cross arch fulcrum* (Figure 20–9)
- ✦ A tooth surface on the opposing arch from the arch being scaled (*opposite arch fulcrum*) (Figure 20–10)

EXTRAORAL FULCRUM. The *extraoral fulcrum,* established outside of the mouth, is used predominantly when instrumenting teeth with deep periodontal pockets. The extraoral fulcrum is placed against the client's jaw or on a broad surface such as the side of the face. The extraoral fulcrum does not use a small finger point source as does the intraoral fulcrum. Rather, the extraoral fulcrum is accomplished by placing the broad side of the palm or back of the hand against the chin or outer cheek. The extraoral fulcrum does not use light pressure against the skin of the client's face. Rather, the palm or backside of the hand rests with moderate pressure against the bony structures of the face and/or mandible. This extraoral fulcrum has been described as a palm-up, palm-down, knuckle-rest, and chin-cup position.[5,6] The extraoral fulcrum provides an excellent means of control and stability for access into periodontally involved areas that may be cumbersome or physiologically strenuous for the dental hygienist to instrument using intraoral fulcrums. Often, the extraoral fulcrum allows a direct "line of draw" in which the instrument may be pulled straight down, as opposed to twisting with the wrist in areas such as the maxillary posterior regions.

Criticism of extraoral techniques stems from fear of loss of fulcrum stability when fulcruming farther from the working area, when grasping the instrument farther from the working end, and/or when stabilizing the instrument against a slightly mobile surface such as the skin rather than on a solid tooth. In reality, fulcruming away from the immediate working area does not necessarily diminish the stability of the fulcrum. Rather, when instrumenting a tooth surface in a deep periodontal pocket, the leverage and lateral pressure may be increased and extended throughout the length of a long *working stroke* (scaling or root planing stroke). The loss of control from extending the grasp away from the working end of the instrument can be easily overcome by using reinforcement from the nonworking index finger or thumb to the shank or handle close to the working end of the instrument. Finally, the extraoral fulcrum allows the operator to change the action of pulling the stroke from the wrist to the lower arm, upper arm, and shoulder. Using instrumentation techniques such as these may protect the operator from future injury and stress to the nerves, tendons, and ligaments of the wrist and elbow.

Insertion

Insertion is the act of placing an assessment or treatment instrument into subgingival areas. The purpose of insertion may be to measure the sulcus or pocket depth, to explore the subgingival areas, or to scale and/or root plane subgingival areas. Whatever the purpose is, the procedure must be as nontraumatic and accurate as possible. As with all sharp-pointed instruments, extreme care must be taken when the point is inserted directly toward the junctional epithelium. Too much pressure and lack of proper grasp, fulcrum, and contact points with the instrument as it glides subgingivally may cause perforation through the attachment apparatus.

Straight instruments such as the periodontal probe are easily manipulated as long as the side of the tip and the rest of the working end stays in contact with the root when inserting the tip. A delicate touch using fairly light pressure is required when probing or initially exploring subgingivally. With such exploratory strokes, the junctional epithelium offers a moderate amount of resistance, feels slightly elastic to the touch, and gives with a slight amount of pressure from the instrument. Pressure on the instrument may be increased after the topography of the pocket is understood, to interpret cemental irregularities, calculus, and restorative margins. When inserting a curved explorer, the tip should be pointed apically and the side of the tip should be in contact with the tooth surface being explored. Care must be taken to avoid tissue distention with the rounded bend and to avoid directing the point right at the root surface. Inaccurate deposit assessment and possible scratching of the root surface result if the pointed tip is directed into the root surface. The only time this is done intentionally is when the dental hygienist suspects root caries or furcation involvement. When evaluating dental caries, probing pressure, as opposed to forceful penetrations, is used against suspected carious areas to avoid worsening the breakdown of the lesion. (See Chapter 12, section on dental caries detection.)

Careful insertion of a bladed treatment instrument into subgingival areas involves closing the angle of the cutting edge of the blade relative to the tooth surface to avoid tissue trauma with the opposite side of the blade and to reach the base of the pocket on the downstroke of insertion. With the curet, the closed blade angulation is from 0 to 10 degrees. With sickle scalers (sharp-pointed back and triangular design), the angulation of insertion is slightly more than 10 degrees, but much less than the more open "working" angulation (the angle of the cutting edge of the blade against the tooth that produces a grip or bite to the tooth surface).

Reinsertion is the act of returning the instrument down into the subgingival areas after an assessment or working stroke has been accomplished. The reinsertion stroke angulation is slightly closed compared to that of a working stroke. The working end of the instrument should remain in contact with the tooth until instrumentation is complete. A common error with the reinsertion stroke is lifting the instrument from the tooth surface during the act of reinsertion. The dental hygienist should use the same guidelines of following tooth structure down on reinsertion as in the initial insertion to avoid tissue trauma and to accurately replace the blade for continuous, overlapping strokes.

Adaptation

With regard to pointed assessment instruments, instrument *adaptation* refers to the alignment or placement of the side of the first few millimeters of the periodontal probe or straight explorer against the tooth. Adaptation is important with assessment instruments because it provides the clinician with an accurate measurement or with information about the smoothness of the tooth surface. If the instrument is not well aligned against the tooth surface, it will be off the tooth and into soft tissue. This leads to client discomfort as well as to misinterpretations regarding probing depths and the presence of calculus deposits or cemental irregularities. Only in instances in which a tooth surface is being assessed for dental caries is the point or tip of such an instrument used directly against the tooth.

Assessment instruments such as the periodontal probe and the explorer are always thin, pointed instruments by design to reach deep, sometimes tight subgingival pockets, and to facilitate tactile sensitivity. Because they have to reach under tight tooth contacts to detect calculus and into minute pits and fissures to detect dental caries, explorers have fine, delicate working ends. As indicated earlier, the point or tip of an explorer may be used for caries detection. However, the side of the tip should always be in contact with the tooth structure to avoid tissue trauma when assessing the presence of cemental irregularities and acquired deposits. The remainder of the explorer's working end should be as closely adapted to the subgingival tooth surface as possible to avoid excessive distention of tissues, excessive pressure against the instrument from the pocket wall, and the possible use of the point instead of the side of the tip of the instrument. There is only one working end on the straight periodontal probe and explorer. Although the correct working end is automatically determined, proper adaptation to the tooth surface must be maintained.

With a bent explorer such as the double-ended pigtail explorer, there is a correct and incorrect working end for different tooth surfaces. The first 2 to 3 mm of the side of the toe (or side of the tip of the instrument) must adapt to an area between the base of the pocket and the contact of the next tooth. The rest of the working end should not excessively distend the sulcular tissues.

With treatment instruments used for scaling and root planing, adaptation is the close relationship of the working blade to the tooth surface. When the working blade is well adapted to the tooth surface, it instruments more root surface than does a poorly adapted blade and causes less damage to the root surface and/or soft tissues. If only the toe or tip is in contact with the tooth, there is a chance that the tooth surface may become gouged or over-instrumented. If the middle or upper third of the blade is in contact with tooth surface and the lower third is off the tooth, the toe is in an open position and may cause tissue trauma to sulcular epithelium (Figure 20–11, *A* and *B*). The adaptation position most effective and causing the least amount of hard or soft tissue damage occurs when the lower third of the working blade remains in contact with the tooth surface during scaling and root planing procedures (Figure 20–11, *C*).

For treatment instruments that have sharp, pointed tips, such as sickle scalers, the dental hygienist uses adaptation guidelines similar to those presented for assessment instruments. If the instrument is a simple straight sickle scaler, for example, there is only one end to use. Proper adaptation with the side of the toe to avoid tissue trauma is as important with the sickle scaler as it is with the periodontal probe and the explorer.

If the sickle scaler has a bent shank and is double-ended, one bladed side is preferable for each tooth surface. The correct end produces the closest adaptation of the blade to the tooth surface and maintains a shank position parallel to the plane of the tooth surface being scaled. The *angulation* (relationship of the cutting edge to the tooth surface) should be between 45 and 90 degrees to the tooth surface (Figure 20–12).

Adaptation of the curet follows many of the same principles previously discussed. In general, the lower third of the blade is the most desirable portion of the curet blade to contact the tooth surface. However, when broad, flat areas of tooth surface are scaled, the middle third of the blade can be used in addition to the lower third. Most

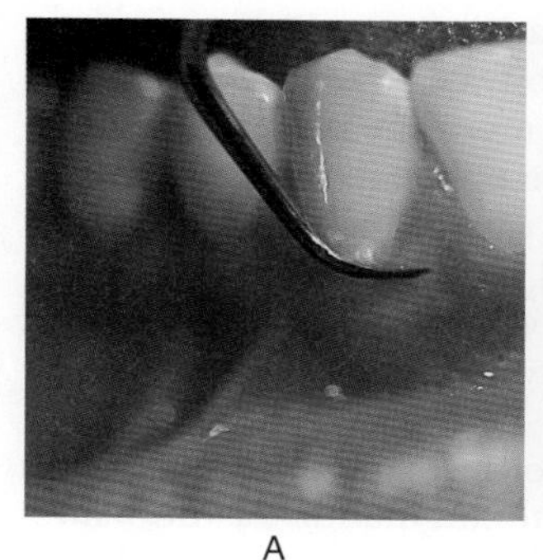
A

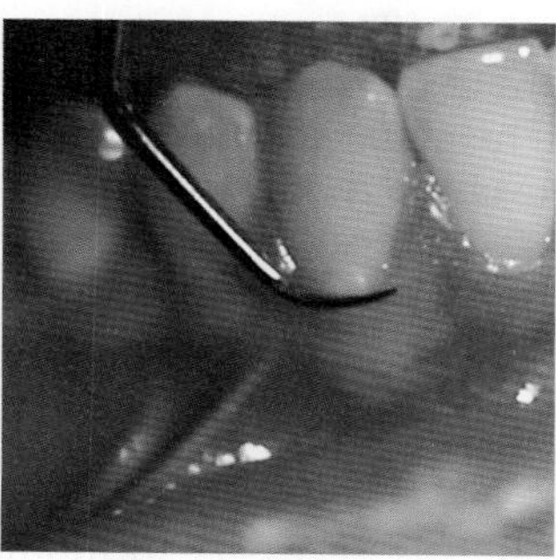
B

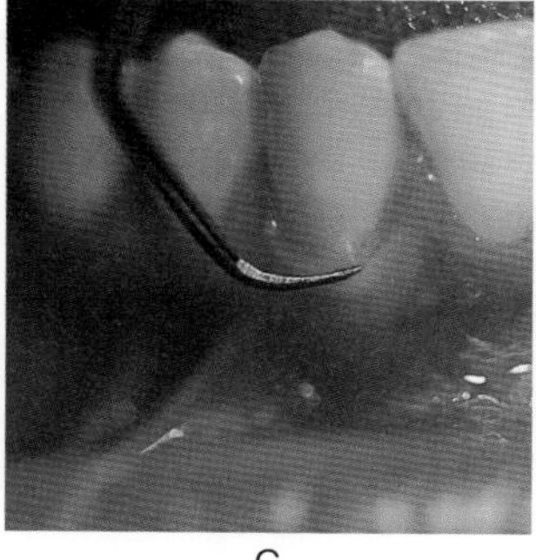
C

FIGURE 20–11 ✦ Comparison of various adaptations of bladed instrument. **A,** Upper third of blade. **B,** Middle third of blade. **C,** Lower third of blade.

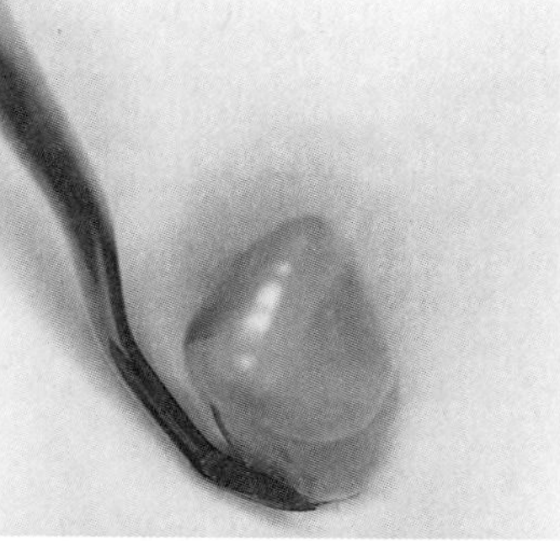

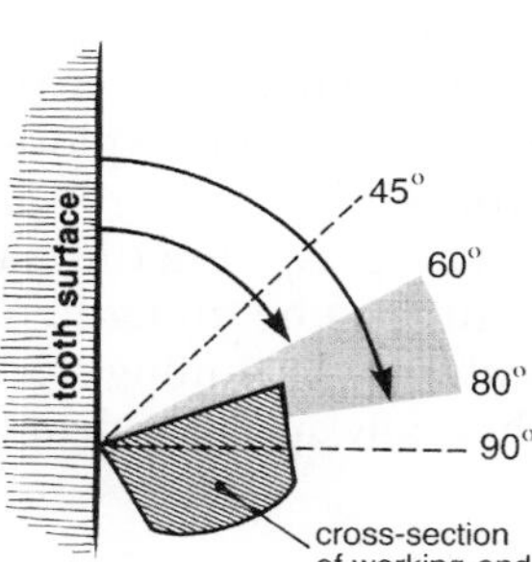

FIGURE 20–12 ✦ The correct working angulation of the blade to the tooth should be between 45 and 90 degrees; 60 to 80 degrees is ideal for debridements.

instrumentation difficulties lie in conforming instruments to the varying convexities and concavities found on tooth structures (see Chapter 21). Especially when instrumenting periodontitis-affected teeth, proper adaptation of the curet blade is a continuing process because of root morphology. Instrumentation is further complicated when there is close root proximity on multiple-rooted teeth or from adjacent teeth. Tooth alignment also complicates procedures, particularly for the novice. In situations such as these, the most successful adaptation is use of the lower third of the blade.

Angulation

Angulation of a bladed instrument refers to the relationship of the cutting edge to the tooth surface (Figure 20–12). Specifically, this is the measurement from the face of the blade to the tooth surface being scaled.

An angulation of between 45 and 90 degrees is ideal for removing calculus and planing roots. This standard allows a range of 45 degrees in which to modify the angulation. The closer the angulation is to 45 degrees, the more the instrument cuts or bites into the tooth surface. The closer to 90 degrees, the more the instrument slides over the tooth surface. A more open angulation (close to 90 degrees) is recommended when a smoothing, shaving root planing stroke is desired. A closer angulation (near 45 degrees) is recommended when there is heavy deposit to remove and it is necessary to grab the root surface effectively.

Just as in performing proper instrument adaptation, it often is necessary to modulate angulation of the blade. An example of such a situation is when there is heavy calculus only at the base of a 6-mm pocket with smooth cementum directly above. Angulation of the blade is closer and the pressure applied is heavier at the base of the pocket to remove the calculus. The angulation is more open and the pressure applied is lighter toward the mouth of the pocket for root planing. The procedure is followed by several more strokes at less than 90 degrees for root planing from the junctional epithelium to the cementoenamel junction.

Lateral Pressure

Lateral pressure is the pressure of the tip and anterior third of the working end of the instrument against the tooth. This pressure may range from very light to firm, depending on the nature of the roughness of the tooth surface. Therefore, it is necessary to use gradations of pressure during exploratory, scaling, and root planing strokes.

The grasp, fulcrum, and basic control of the instrument must be strengthened as pressure is increased. This is why the beginning student may experience difficulty in physically applying firm lateral pressure.

Strokes

EXPLORATORY STROKE. The *exploratory stroke* is used for detection and usually is performed with an explorer or periodontal probe. The curet also may perform an exploratory function to assess the tooth surface during actual scaling or root planing. An exploratory stroke may use light to firm lateral pressure. Light lateral pressure during exploration is recommended for detecting light spicules of subgingival calculus. In this case, heavier lateral pressure is insensitive for fine-deposit exploration. Situations that require the use of moderate to firm pressure during exploration include the detection of flat, burnished calculus or distinguishing restorative margins from tooth anatomy.

SCALING STROKE. The *scaling stroke* is used for removing calculus from supragingival and subgingival areas. The curet is the instrument of choice for definitive scaling and root planing. As in the exploratory stroke, the lateral pressure used with the scaling stroke ranges from light to firm. The difference, however, is that the magnitude of what is considered firm is far greater during scaling than during exploring. During scaling, the action of the instrument may quickly change from a scaling stroke to an exploratory stroke. This change in lateral pressure is done specifically to break off calculus but not to over-instrument a clean area above or below that calculus. It is performed also to assess areas previously scaled without having to stop and pick up an explorer. It is very efficient to be able to work in this manner, and to reserve the actual exploration procedure with an explorer until major areas have been scaled.

The practitioner uses assessment data on pocket depth, clinical attachment, tissue color, tissue consistency, tissue surface texture, tissue size, bleeding, and bone loss to determine the degree of periodontal involvement and the probable amount of lateral pressure needed for calculus detection and scaling. Generally, the more periodontally involved the client's teeth, the more suspicious the dental hygienist should be of local contributing factors such as subgingival calculus. If the calculus occurs in the form of ledges, any amount of pressure is likely to detect it. If, however, the calculus formation is flat and smooth, medium or even firm exploratory strokes may be necessary to detect the deposit.

The density of the calculus may be determined by radiographs and most accurately by "hardness" felt with the explorer. Dense calculus appears more radiopaque than lighter, easier-to-remove calculus. Dense calculus feels hard, like tooth structure, as opposed to the porous feel of lighter calculus. In situations in which there is dense calculus and naturally grainy or rough root surfaces, the calculus is likely to be embedded into the root surface. Calculus deposits that are both dense and tenacious make scaling more difficult than with light calculus deposits.

The older and more dense the calculus, usually the more tenacious it is. The practitioner should increase the lateral pressure of the scaling stroke as the tenacity and density of the calculus increases. Too little lateral pressure on instrumentation may cause burnishing of tenacious calculus on cementum. To avoid indiscriminately applying too much lateral pressure on instrumentation, causing unnecessary gouging and over-instrumentation of root surfaces, the dental hygienist should evaluate the changes occurring on the root surface during instrumentation with the curet using exploratory strokes or by using a dental explorer. Lighter lateral pressure during scaling strokes is indicated for light and easy-to-remove calculus.

ROOT PLANING STROKE. The *root planing stroke* is used for shaving embedded calculus from cemental surfaces and smoothing roots. The rationale for root planing lies in the fact that clean, smooth roots are more biologically acceptable for connective tissue reattachment than are rough roots, accounting for a reduction of periodontopathic bacteria.[7–9] In addition, the client's ability to maintain soft tissue health is improved because bacterial plaque biofilm control is easier when the roots are smooth.

Root planing requires extremely good control and dedication to smoothing subgingival surfaces evenly from the junctional epithelium to the cementoenamel junction. Knowledge of root morphology, a sense of the dimensions of this subgingival space, and the area the curet has covered are important to successful root planing. The root planing stroke is a longer stroke than the scaling stroke and may begin with firm lateral pressure if there is significant root roughness to smooth. The change to lighter lateral pressure should occur rather quickly as the curet moves to even out the surface of the cementum.

The thickness of cementum varies but is thinnest at the cervical third of the tooth (0.02 to 0.05 mm). In scaling and root planing tooth structure with such a thin covering of cementum it is easy to visualize how removal of cementum often occurs during indiscriminate root planing, leading to exposure of dentin and dentinal hypersensitivity (see Chapter 33). To avoid hypersensitive reactions, the dental hygienist explores the area carefully and discriminately uses lateral pressure during scaling and root planing with the purpose of removing only subgingival calculus and altered cementum, smoothing the root surface, and removing as little healthy cementum as possible to achieve good results. (See Chapter 23, section on clinical and therapeutic end points.)

Stroke Direction

For accurate identification and removal of deposits, a combination of three basic *stroke directions* is used with assessment and treatment instruments:

- ✦ Vertical stroke direction is parallel to the long axis of the tooth.
- ✦ Horizontal stroke direction is perpendicular to the long axis of the tooth.
- ✦ Oblique stroke direction is diagonal across the long axis of the tooth.

Using combinations of different stroke directions is referred to as a "basketweave of strokes" (Figure 20–13). Varying stroke direction allows a greater possibility that a piece of burnished or smooth calculus may be detected because the instrument may catch one side of the calculus when all other sides may be smooth. Both the explorer and the probe are activated beginning with a gentle insertion or downward stroke into the pocket. This exploratory stroke is used as part of the detection process as long as the side of the tip is well adapted to the tooth surface.

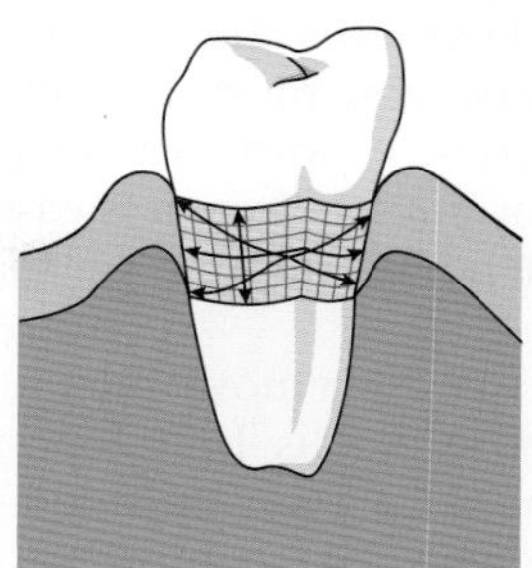

FIGURE 20–13 ✦ This diagram illustrates vertical, horizontal, and oblique stroke directions. *(Redrawn from Pattison A, Pattison G:* Periodontal instrumentation, *ed 2, Norwalk, Conn, 1992, Appleton & Lange.)*

The working stroke of the curet, sickle, file, and hoe is performed with a pull stroke. The direction of the pull stroke may be vertical, horizontal, or oblique, and it is not directed toward the junctional epithelium. The push or insertion stroke with working pressure is not recommended with treatment instruments because it could potentially violate the integrity of the client's intact junctional epithelium by forcing dental calculus and bacterial plaque biofilm through the membrane, potentially causing periodontal abscess formation.

Once an efficient stroke direction has been established, it is best to keep moving forward in the direction of the toe of the instrument. Short, overlapping strokes for calculus removal and longer, overlapping strokes for root planing maximize root coverage.

Stroke Length

The *stroke length* is limited by the tissue tone, the morphology of the tooth structure, and the client's periodontal probing depth measurements. Loose and inflamed tissue accommodates the movement of long, sweeping, overlapping strokes. However, if the tissue is healthy or fibrotic in tone and positioned tightly against the tooth, short, overlapping, well-adapted strokes are indicated to prevent trauma to the tissue.

Short, overlapping strokes and a firmly planted fulcrum provide for good operator-controlled strokes. When managing the curvatures common to most root surfaces, shorter strokes do not pass over deposits in root depressions as easily as longer strokes and therefore are more reliable. On relatively flat areas such as the palatal roots of maxillary molars, however, one may use long stroke lengths and still maintain a controlled, effective movement.

Deep periodontal pockets allow for greater flexibility in stroke length than do shallow pockets because of greater root surface area from clinical attachment. Where there is recession there also may be significant root surface. Therefore, with greater pocket depth or more exposed root surface area, it is easier to vary stroke length than where pocket depth is very shallow with little recession.

The scaling stroke to remove calculus is a short pull stroke. The short stroke is best for calculus removal because the increased pressure needed to remove a calculus deposit reduces stroke control. A short stroke facilitates a controlled stroke. For root planing, the stroke length should be increased and the pressure lightened once the calculus has been removed.

Reinforcement

Reinforcement scaling is the use of the nondominant hand to support the instrument or the working hand, providing additional lateral pressure during instrumentation procedures. In general, the index finger and thumb of the nondominant hand do the work of reinforcing. Either finger or both may be applied to the instrument or to the operator's working hand, usually near the thumb or the muscle area near the thumb (thenar muscle; see Chapter 8). Reinforcements are used only with treatment instruments such as curets. They are not necessary with assessment instruments because control and lateral pressure are not difficult with these instruments. Reinforcements provide additional support and lateral pressure in deep periodontal pockets, particularly when using extended fulcrums (cross arch, opposite arch, and extraoral) placed away from the immediate area being scaled. Several reinforcements make scaling easier and more controlled and accurate; each is discussed later in this chapter.

Customizing Instrumentation for Periodontitis-Affected Teeth

When instrumenting periodontally involved teeth, the method of scaling and root planing varies because of individual facial anatomy, alignment of teeth, and extent of periodontitis. Some individuals have large dental arches, and others have very small ones; some present with nearly perfect tooth alignment, and others have severely crowded teeth; some clients have limited ability to open their mouths for access into posterior regions. Clients may have normal, healthy periodontium or moderate to severe periodontal problems even within the same arch. Each of these general variations requires customization of basic instrumentation technique to treat a particular individual successfully. The procedure for customizing instrumentation in periodontitis-affected areas allows the clinician to reach almost any area of the mouth, to reach both sulcus areas and deep periodontal pockets, and to manage difficult root anatomy with the control and strength needed for effective care (see Guidelines for Customizing Instrumentation).

Customizing instrumentation successfully depends on finding the correct fulcrum. To accomplish this, the dental hygienist:

- ✦ Uses a sitting or standing position and moves in different positions around the client
- ✦ Fulcrums intraorally near the tooth being scaled, cross arch, opposite arch, or on the index finger or thumb of the nondominant hand, or finds a comfortable position using extraoral fulcrums
- ✦ Uses reinforcement techniques during scaling procedures

If the shape of the tooth surface changes to the degree that one fulcrum position no longer works, the process must be repeated from that point and the fulcrum altered to accommodate the change. With experience, the entire process becomes second nature and adjustments may be made within seconds. Because treatment is customized, the working environment is safer, less stressed, and more effective in meeting client needs.

Traditional instrumentation is based on setting the fulcrum first. Establishing the fulcrum first does not allow for variations in probing depths or alterations in root anatomy, which affect the amount and direction of lateral pressure that can be applied to the root surface. For instance, as probing depth increases on the distal aspect of a mandibular molar from 3 mm to 10 mm, the dental hygienist may find a change in the plane of the root surface from a vertical to a slightly more oblique or horizontal inclination. In subgingival instrumentation of periodontitis-affected teeth, such slight changes in the plane of a tooth surface alter stroke effectiveness. By setting the fulcrum first and not readjusting the fulcrum as the instrument maneuvers into pocket depth, the practitioner is limited in producing effective lateral pressure.

INSTRUMENT SHARPENING

Rationale

The major objective of *instrument sharpening* is to restore blade sharpness while preserving the original contours and angles of the instrument. The basic clinical outcome of using sharp versus dull instruments is delineated in Table 20–3. By using sharp instruments, the practitioner improves the comfort level of the client and decreases operator fatigue by working to remove dental deposits effectively. Moreover, sharp instruments are easier to control than dull instruments because they do not slip as easily over tooth surfaces.

To maintain effectiveness and quality of client care, at the first sign of instrument dullness, the dental hygienist should sharpen the instrument. Methods for sharpening individual instruments are discussed under each instrument subheading.

Sharpening Stones

Natural and synthetic sharpening stones for sharpening dental instruments are composed of abrasive crystals that are harder than the metal of the instrument (Figure 20–14).

Guidelines for Customizing Instrumentation

Grasp the instrument with a modified pen grasp.
Remember that this is the best grasp when applying a treatment instrument against a tooth surface.

Find the general operator position for the area to be scaled.
Refer to the general operator positions in Chapter 8, Table 8–7 and Figure 8–8.

Find the general fulcrum position for the area to be scaled.
This may be intraoral (same quadrant, cross arch, or opposite arch) or extraoral.

Close angulation and insert the instrument to reach the base of the sulcus or pocket.
This is to avoid trauma and, most important, to reach the bottom of the pocket.

Adapt the instrument to the tooth surface.
Initially adapt at least the first 2 to 3 mm of the blade to the tooth surface.

Angulate the instrument to the tooth surface.
Adjust the angulation of the blade between 45 and 90 degrees for scaling and root planing. The dental hygienist should feel the instrument bite the tooth surface.

Stabilize or firm up the grasp on the instrument handle.
During the manipulations that occur while adapting and angulating the instrument to the tooth surface, the grasp may have changed. Because the handle is positioned for the tooth surface, it changes the angulation if the handle is moved back to the original grasp; therefore, the position of the grasp must be adjusted to the new position of the instrument handle.

Establish a firm fulcrum.
The hand may now be in a slightly different position than it was when the general fulcrum position was found. Within the space of this newfound position that the grasp has moved into, a stable fulcrum position may be established. This fulcrum may be moved to the opposite arch or to an extraoral position if the fulcrum close to the area being scaled does not allow correct adaptation and angulation.

Establish a stable and comfortable operator position to facilitate unit movement.
The practitioner moves to a body position that keeps the hand, arm, and possibly the shoulder in line with the direction of the stroke and allows them to move as one unit. This helps distribute the workload and mitigates the stress on the hands and wrist. The body position may range from 8:00 to 4:00 for both the right-handed and left-handed clinician, depending on the area to be scaled.

Apply reinforcement with the nondominant hand as needed.
The further the fulcrum is from the area being scaled, the more useful reinforcement with the nondominant hand becomes. The reinforcement hand can provide stabilization, additional pressure, additional pulling strength, support for the client in opening the mouth, and retraction of lips and buccal mucosa.

Initiate the working stroke.
This action should be the final step of the sequence after all previous actions have been satisfied.

TABLE 20–3 CLINICAL OUTCOMES USING SHARP VERSUS DULL INSTRUMENTS

Outcome	Sharp Instrument	Dull Instrument
Tactile sensitivity	Increased	Decreased
Client safety and comfort	Increased	Decreased
Working efficiency	Increased	Decreased
Control	Increased	Decreased
Lateral pressure	Decreased	Increased
Probability of burnished calculus	Decreased	Increased

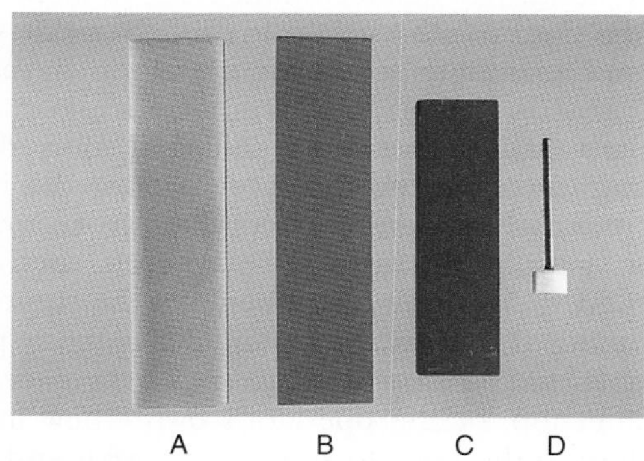

FIGURE 20–14 ✦ Sharpening stones. **A,** Arkansas stone. **B,** India stone. **C,** Ceramic stone. **D,** Mounted composition stone.

NATURAL STONES. The Arkansas stone is an example of a natural stone with a fine texture that is manufactured in a variety of shapes for sharpening instruments. Conical and cylindrical Arkansas stones are available for sharpening the face of curets, a practice that tends to weaken the blade. The India stone also is a natural stone that comes in a medium texture. Natural stones such as the Arkansas and India are usually lubricated with clear, fine oil to facilitate the movement across the stone, reduce friction, and reduce the problem of metallic particles embedding into the surface of the stone. Stones should be washed and/or ultrasonically cleaned before sterilization to remove excess oil. Steam, chemical vapor, or dry heat may be used to sterilize these stones.

SYNTHETIC STONES. These include composition and ceramic stones. The composition stone is a mounted rotary stone and the ceramic stone is manufactured as a hand-held rectangular stone. The rotary stone may be adapted to the face as well as the edge of the curet. The rectangular stone is used only against the side of the curet or scaler. Both of these stones are of medium coarseness and are lubricated with water.

Sharpening stone selection is determined by the amount of sharpening required to reestablish a cutting edge. Fine stones such as the Arkansas or medium-textured India stones are preferable for the novice or for sharpening during client treatment when little sharpening is required for reestablishment of a cutting edge. Coarsely surfaced stones remove metal at a faster rate than do finely surfaced stones, and should be used on instruments requiring significant recontouring. Less pressure, fewer strokes, and greater accuracy are needed with coarsely textured stones. Rotary-mounted stones such as the composition stone are considerably more abrasive than coarse hand-held stones because the stone is mounted on a metal mandrel and used in a motor-driven handpiece. For this reason, the mounted rotary stone should be used only when major recontouring of dental instruments is required. Lack of good control, friction, and rapid wearing of the instrument are disadvantages of the rotary-mounted stone.

Instrument Sharpening Technique

To begin sharpening procedures, select the proper sterilized, lubricated stone for the amount of sharpening to be done. The technique for using hand-held sharpening stones requires either moving the instrument over the stone, or moving the stone over the instrument. In either method, the movement is initiated by the operator's dominant hand. The first technique is recommended for sharpening flat surfaces such as the hoe or sickle scaler. The second technique is recommended for sharpening curets.

To guard against accidental clinician injury during sharpening when moving the stone against the instrument, care must be observed in length of stroke, grasp of stone, and grasp of instrument. Short, even, continuous strokes tend to keep the instrument on the stone. The hand holding the instrument should assume a palm–thumb grasp and be supported against a firm object such as a cabinet top, or the operator's own elbow may be pulled close to the body to support the wrist and hand holding the instrument. The fingers holding the stone should not be wrapped around the stone on the long side exposed to the cutting surface, but positioned behind the cutting surface or at the short ends of the stone (Figure 20–15).

Prior to initiating the sharpening stroke, proper angulation of the stone to the surface of the instrument is assumed and continuous sharpening motions at this constant angle are made across the length of the cutting edge. (Correct angulation of stone to cutting surface will be discussed under each individual instrument.) The amount of pressure applied should be determined by the amount of recontouring necessary to produce a sharp blade. Greater pressure exerted against the blade with the stone removes more metal. Prudent advice for instrument conservation is to limit sharpening procedures to what is necessary. The last sharpening stroke(s) should be away from the face of the instrument in a downward motion to remove small metal particles or flash that adhere to the edges of the instrument. The practitioner should wipe the blade with a 2″ × 2″ gauze square to aid in removing oil and metal shavings floating on the surface of the instrument.

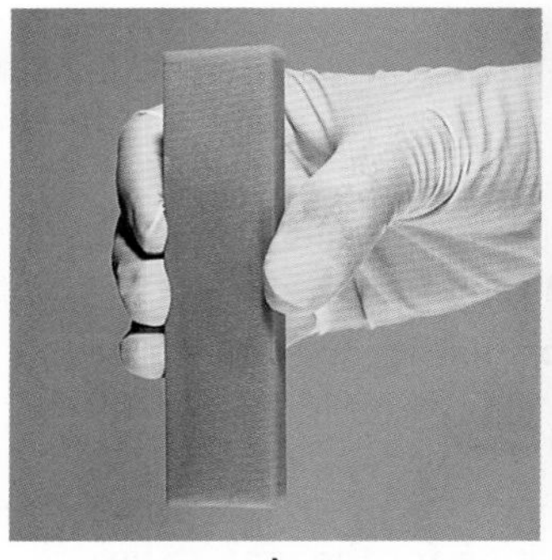
A

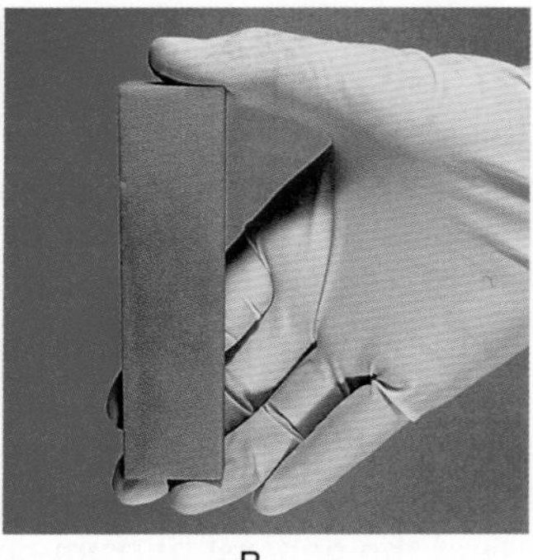
B

FIGURE 20–15 ✦ **A,** Incorrect finger position on stone; fingertips are exposed to possible injury if stone slips. **B,** Correct finger position on stone.

Testing for Instrument Sharpness

Testing for sharpness is done by visual inspection or by comparing the sharpness before and after the procedure using a plastic testing stick. When using visual inspection, it is important to have a strong light such as the dental light for viewing. With this test the sharp instrument does not reflect light at the junction between the face and the lateral side of the instrument. In contrast, the dull instrument is beveled on the cutting edge and reflects light back to the observer. The tactile test requires the use of a hard plastic stick that engages the blade of the instrument at the proper working angulation. It is important when using this method to test the instrument fully across the length of the blade and to resharpen any area that allows the instrument to slip over the stick.

When testing for sharpness, the dental hygienist examines the shape of the sharpened blade. To protect the client against unnecessary instrument breakage, all instruments that have lost their original strength or are too fine to remove heavy deposits or reach deep pockets should no longer be used in such areas. Instruments that have been sharpened down and are of moderate or fine dimensions may be used for the healthier individual with little calculus formation and shallower probing depths. The instrument is retipped or discarded when it is no longer functional or is of danger to the client from possible breakage.

Managing Instrument Tip Breakage

When an instrument breaks subgingivally, only the tip breaks off, leaving it for the dental hygienist to locate. To

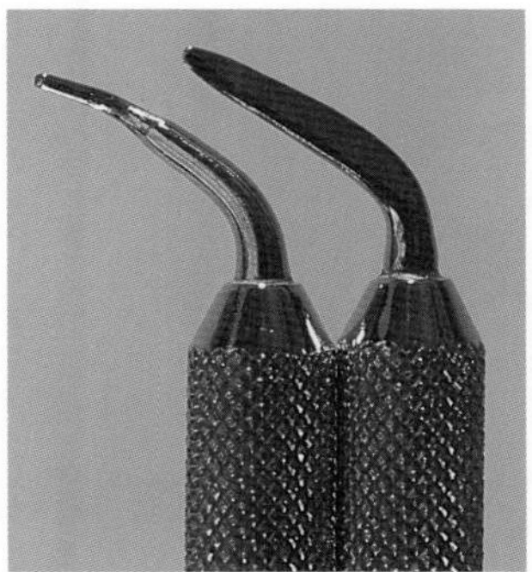

FIGURE 20–16 ✦ Magnetic broken tip retrievers (Schwartz Periotrievers).

retrieve the small metal fragment, the dental hygienist stops instrumentation as soon as the instrument tip has broken and informs the client. Slow-speed or high-speed aspiration (suction) should be discontinued and the client should use a cup to expectorate into (in case the tip is floating in saliva) until the tip is found. Techniques for locating the broken piece include the following:

- ✦ Reinstrumentation with another instrument
- ✦ Use of magnetic-tip Periotrievers shaped like thick explorers or probes (Figure 20–16)
- ✦ Open-flap periodontal surgery

Radiographic examination is helpful during these exploration techniques for more accurate identification of the metal tip. It should be noted that even new instruments, especially curets, break if they are lodged in a tight area such as under a contact and are twisted or pulled in a direction in which the toe may not be released. If the broken tip cannot be clinically located or if it is not visible on a radiograph of the area, the dental hygienist should suspect that the tip may be outside of the sulcus. A complete visual inspection of the oral cavity is begun. Gauze squares are used to wipe out the vestibular areas and areas under the client's tongue. They then are carefully inspected for the broken tip. In the event that the tip cannot be located, a chest radiograph is indicated to rule out the possibility that the client has aspirated it.

INSTRUMENT TYPES

Mouth Mirror

The dental *mouth mirror* is used during all phases of the dental hygiene process for the following (Table 20–4):

- ✦ Indirect vision
- ✦ Indirect illumination
- ✦ Transillumination
- ✦ Retraction of tissues and tongue

Moistening the face of the mouth mirror by gently rubbing it against the buccal mucosa or dipping it in a commercial mouthwash prevents the mirror from fogging up.

The traditional mouth mirror has a handle and mirror, each with a threaded design or cone–socket attachment. The handle and mirror components are separated, washed, and autoclaved after each appointment. Unlike the mirror heads, which eventually become clouded or scratched, handles rarely need to be replaced. Wrapping the mirror heads with 2″ × 2″ gauze squares when packaged with other instruments or separating them during sterilization minimizes scratching.

Mirror heads come in a variety of sizes from 5/8- to 2-inch diameters. Mirror size selection is made by the size of the client's mouth, the operator's ability to place the mirror and instrument within a confined space, and the operator's comfort in holding and using a certain size mirror head. There are also three types of mirror faces (Table 20–5):

- ✦ Front surface
- ✦ Concave surface
- ✦ Flat surface

TABLE 20–4 FUNCTIONS OF THE DENTAL MOUTH MIRROR

Function	Reason for Use
Indirect vision	The most difficult function to master. Reflection in mirror provides indirect vision of area. Use when it is difficult to view the tooth or area directly, e.g., distal surfaces of last molars or when a direct vision requires a strenuous operator position.
Indirect illumination	Use to catch light and direct increased illumination to intraoral areas. When mirror is being used in this capacity, it cannot be used for indirect vision at the same time. Therefore, operator and client position must be adjusted for direct-vision scaling.
Transillumination	Use to reflect light back onto anterior tooth surfaces, which are thin enough to allow light to pass through. Essentially a shadowing technique for visualization of teeth. Areas of various density or darkness such as dental caries and calculus will contrast and be readily visible.
Retraction	A pulling away of soft tissue for illumination, visualization, and protection of client's tissue. Use with the face of the mirror toward the buccal mucosa, lips, or tongue to retract tissues for light to illuminate the working area and/or protect the soft tissues during instrumentation. The face of the mirror should be turned toward the working area to provide indirect vision while at the same time retracting soft tissue.

The mouth mirror generally is held with a modified pen grasp; however, other grasps also may be used. The pads of the thumb, index, and middle fingers all rest on the shank and handle of the instrument with the modified pen grasp. Because of its stability, the modified

TABLE 20–5 TYPES OF MOUTH MIRROR SURFACES

Type	Advantages and Disadvantages
Front surface	Mirror surface is on the front of the glass, therefore, the image produced is the mirror image of the area reflected. Most commonly used because there is no distortion or magnification of the image.
Concave surface	Causes magnification of the image. Because each movement visualized with this mirror is magnified, the operator needs to relate the scale of movement and the image differently from the way it actually appears. More difficult to use than the front-surface mirror. Does not allow the operator to see as wide a range as the front surface and causes distortion, even dizziness, for some clinicians. Not recommended unless eye strain or vision is a significant problem.
Flat surface	The image appears doubled or shadowed. Not recommended for periodontal procedures.

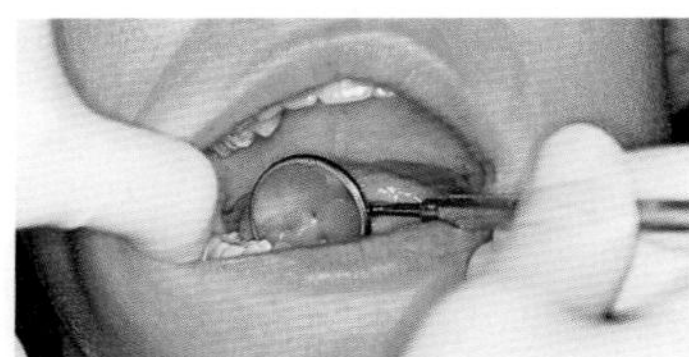

FIGURE 20–17 ✦ The modified pen grasp is used for stability when there is resistance (e.g., the tongue) against the mirror head.

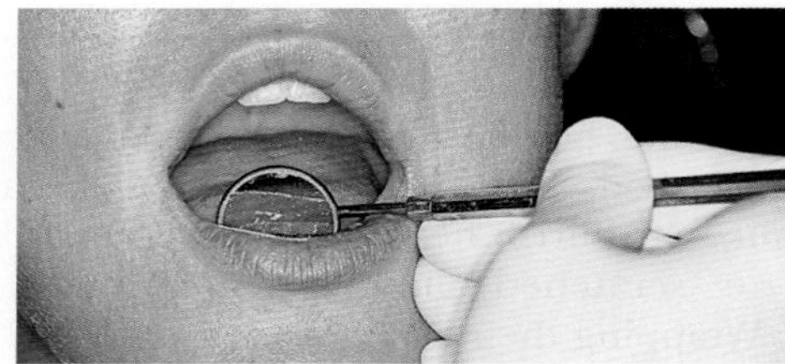

FIGURE 20–18 ✦ The modified pen grasp is used for indirect vision and illumination with mirror.

pen grasp should be used when there is resistance to the mirror head, such as during the retraction of buccal mucosa or the tongue (Figure 20–17).

When there is no resistance and when indirect vision, indirect illumination, and/or transillumination are the goals, the standard pen grasp is adequate and perhaps desirable. The standard pen grasp yields a very loose grasp that generally allows easy, fluid movement of the mirror head around the mouth. This range of movement is beneficial when examining or comparing large oral areas.

For indirect vision or illumination and reinforcement of a curet with the nondominant hand, the mirror is held between the middle and ring fingers. This position allows little manipulation of the mirror; however, in areas where reinforcements with indirect vision are needed, positioning changes of the mouth mirror are minimal (Figures 20–18 and 20–19).

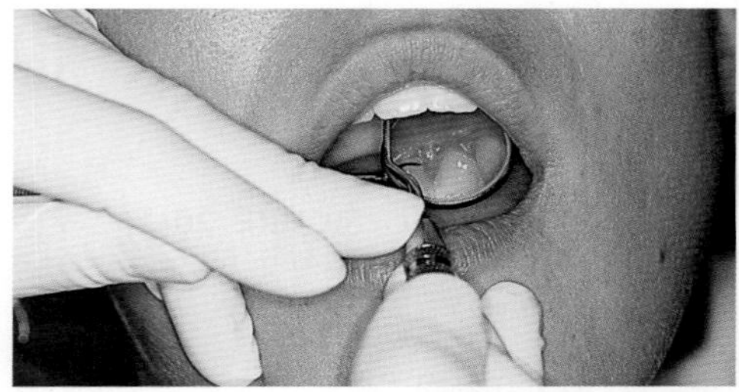

FIGURE 20–19 ✦ Use of the mirror hand for mirror placement and reinforcement of scaling instrument.

Because the mouth mirror is the instrument used for retraction, care is taken to avoid tissue trauma with the handle or shank of the instrument, particularly at the corners of the mouth. This injury may be as slight as soreness or as serious as initiation of herpetic lesions on the client's lips and commissures. Trauma can be avoided by maintaining less pressure on stretched lips. In addition, the mouth mirror should never be allowed to rest on sublingual tissue because doing so causes discomfort to the client (Figure 20–20, *A* to *C*).

Periodontal Probe

DESIGN AND USE (Table 20–6). The *periodontal probe* (see also Chapter 15, section on periodontal probes), a slender, tapered, blunt instrument with millimeter markings, is used to determine the following:

- ✦ Probing depth
- ✦ Clinical attachment level
- ✦ Relative attachment level
- ✦ Amount of attached gingiva
- ✦ Gingival recession
- ✦ Furcation invasion
- ✦ Bleeding on probing
- ✦ Size of atypical or pathologic lesions
- ✦ Distance between teeth

Variations in millimeter markings and other design differences are found among manufacturers. For example, the Marquis probe is marked at the 3-, 6-, 9-, and 12-mm intervals; the Williams probe is marked at the 1-, 2-, 3-, 5-, 7-, 8-, 9- and 10-mm intervals. Differences in markings, color-coding, shapes, and an automated probe are shown in Figure 20–21. Personal operator preference determines selection of interval and color-coded markings of the periodontal probe. In the case of failing dental implants, which require the use of plastic probes (Figure 20–22), safety against further injury and scratching of the titanium implants determines instrument selection (see Chapter 50 on individuals with osseointegrated dental implants.)

When the probe design is flat and too thick or wide, it is difficult to manipulate the instrument into and around narrow, tight areas for accurate measurement. Conversely, if the probe is too fine and sharp, there is

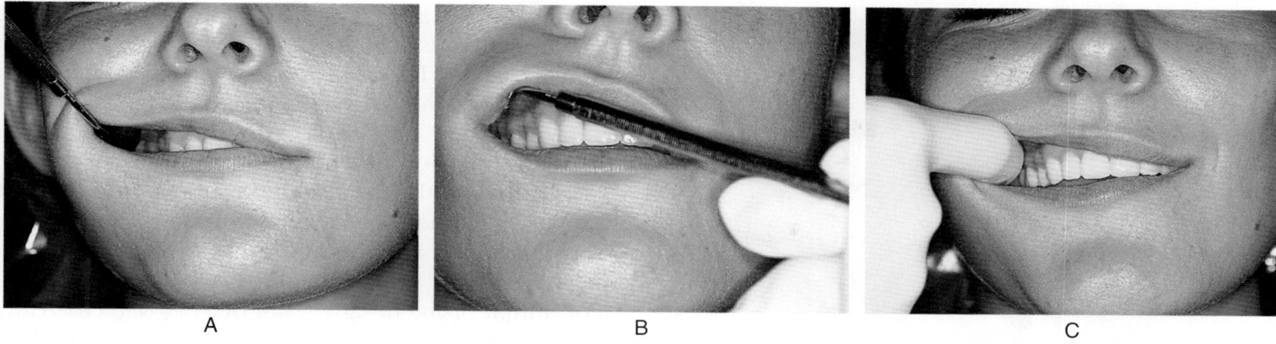

FIGURE 20–20 ✦ **A,** Mouth mirror is traumatic to corners of the mouth. **B,** Mouth mirror is positioned with less trauma to the corner of the mouth. **C,** Index finger is used in place of the mouth mirror for retraction.

TABLE 20–6 PERIODONTAL PROBE: USE, TECHNIQUE, AND SIGNIFICANCE OF RESULTS (See Chapter 15)

Measurement	Technique and Significance of Results
Probing depth	Measures probing depth from marginal gingiva to junctional epithelium. Six measurements are taken around each tooth (distofacial, facial, mesiofacial, distolingual, lingual, and mesiolingual). The deepest measurements are recorded for each surface. Within any sextant, it is easier to record all facial surfaces, then all lingual surfaces. Probing depth is an important indicator of past disease activity (Procedure 20-2).
Clinical attachment level	The clinical attachment level is the measurement from the cementoenamel junction to the junctional epithelium. The technique is similar to probing depth, except that the depth is measured from the junctional epithelium to a fixed reference point. When measuring from a fixed reference point, a clearer picture of bone loss can be determined, especially when there is recession and minimal probing depths.
Relative attachment level	The relative attachment level is the measurement from a fixed reference point on the tooth or a stent to the junctional epithelium. The technique is similar to assessing probing depth and offers a record of past disease activity.
Amount of attached gingiva	Attached gingiva is the keratinized stratified squamous epithelium firmly attached to the cementum and alveolar bone. Adequate attached gingiva is an important safeguard against future mucogingival defects and recession when there is bone loss.
Gingival recession	Gingival recession is the measurement from the gingival margin to the cementoenamel junction. This measurement is another indicator of apical migration of the attachment apparatus.
Furcation invasion	Furcation invasion is classified (see Chapter 15). The No. 2 Nabers probe is a specialized probe used for furcation detection and classification. Detection of furcation invasion is critical to the therapy and long-term prognosis of the tooth and adjacent bone.
Bleeding on probing	Observation of bleeding on light probing should be noted because it is a primary clinical indicator of gingival inflammation.
Pathological lesions	An important aspect of assessment is an accurate description of the size and shape of the lesion. The periodontal probe is used for measurement of pathologic lesions.
Distance between teeth	The periodontal probe may be used to measure the distance between teeth (diastema), overjet, and migration of teeth with severe periodontal disease.

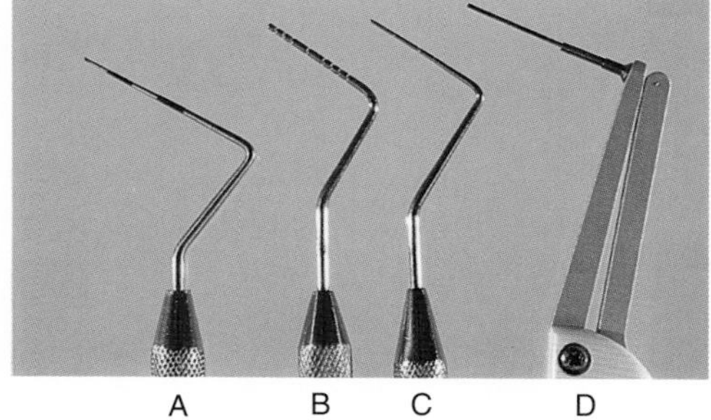

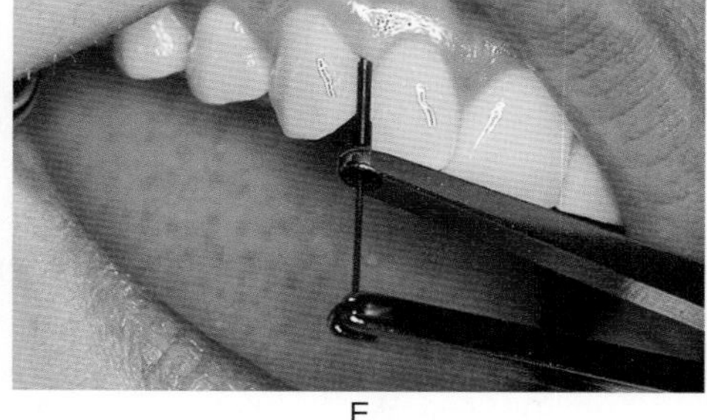

FIGURE 20–21 ✦ Examples of periodontal probes. Note the differences in markings. **A,** Marquis color-coded probe with markings at intervals of 3, 6, 9, and 12 mm. **B,** Williams probe with marking at intervals of 1, 2, 3, 5, 7, 8, 9, and 10 mm. **C,** Michigan "O" probe with markings at intervals of 3, 6, and 8 mm. **D,** Florida Probe Computerized Periodontal Probing and Patient-Education System. **E,** Florida Probe positioned in periodontal pocket. *(Courtesy Florida Probe Corporation.)*

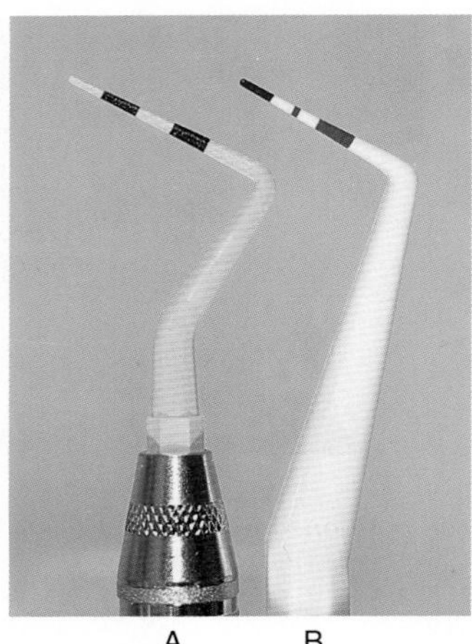

FIGURE 20–22 ✦ Examples of plastic perio probes. **A,** The Hu-Friedy black and yellow color-coded replaceable plastic periodontal probe tip. **B,** The Premier Dental Products Co. reusable plastic periodontal probe.

danger of trauma and perforation through the nonkeratinizing junctional epithelium, resulting in inaccurate readings. If too fine a probe is selected, client comfort and safety become important factors to consider. Thin instruments are also subject to bending and damage during sterilization procedures.

Variations of the periodontal probe, criteria for selection, design, and procedures are found in Table 20–7 and Procedures 20–1 and 20–2. A variation in shank design of the periodontal probe is shown in Figure 20–23. This periodontal probe design (Hu-Friedy Novatech) features a right-angle tip that is color-coded. It offers ease of access in posterior distal surfaces.

Probing inaccuracy is related to probe design, pressure applied, contour of the tooth, contour of the periodontal defect, degree of inflammation, and accompanying loss of collagen fibers. Probing depth usually correlates with attachment loss, but it is always an objective measure of the distance between the base of the pocket and the crest

TABLE 20–7 PERIODONTAL PROBE DESIGN AND SELECTION

Common Design Specifications of All Periodontal Probes

This slender, often tapered assessment instrument is used to measure sulcus and periodontal pocket depth, clinical attachment levels, and amount of attached gingiva.

Calibrated markings are engraved or color-coded onto the angulated tip design.

Tips are blunted or rounded.

Cross-sectional view is rounded, oval, or rectangular.

Probe Examples	Rationale for Use	
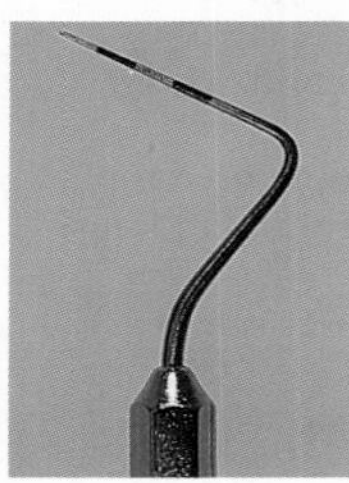	***Marquis color-coded probe***	
	Shank	Thin, round, and tapered.
	Measurement	Alternately color-coded at 3, 6, 9 and 12 mm.
	Tip design	Thin tip.
	Advantages	Color-coding every 3 mm makes it easy to read. Thin shank allows access into tight fibrotic sulci.
	Disadvantages	Markings must be estimated between color bands. Thin tip may penetrate junctional epithelium if too much pressure is applied.
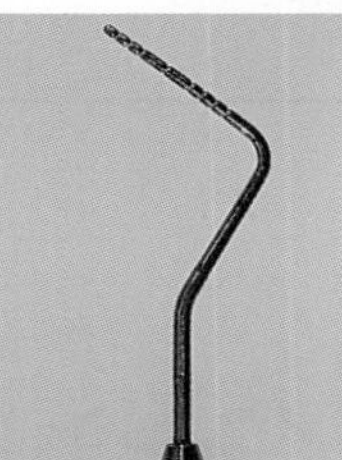	***Williams probe***	
	Shank	Round and tapered.
	Measurement	1, 2, 3, 5, 7, 8, 9, 10 mm.
	Tip design	Thin to thick, depending on manufacturer.
	Advantages	Spaces between 3 to 5 and 5 to 7 minimize confusion.
	Disadvantages	Markings are difficult to read.
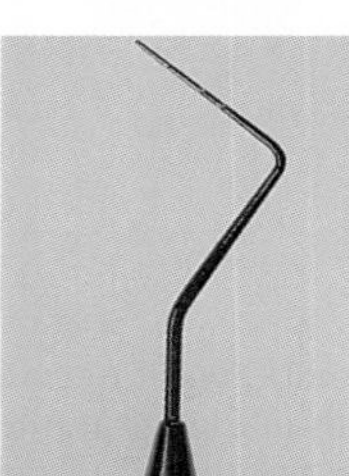	***Michigan "O" probe***	
	Shank	Thin, round, and tapered.
	Measurement	3, 6, 8 mm.
	Tip design	Thin tip.
	Advantages	Thin shank allows access into tight fibrotic sulci.
	Disadvantages	Markings end at 8 mm.

TABLE 20–7

PERIODONTAL PROBE DESIGN AND SELECTION—CONT'D

Probe Examples	Rationale For Use	
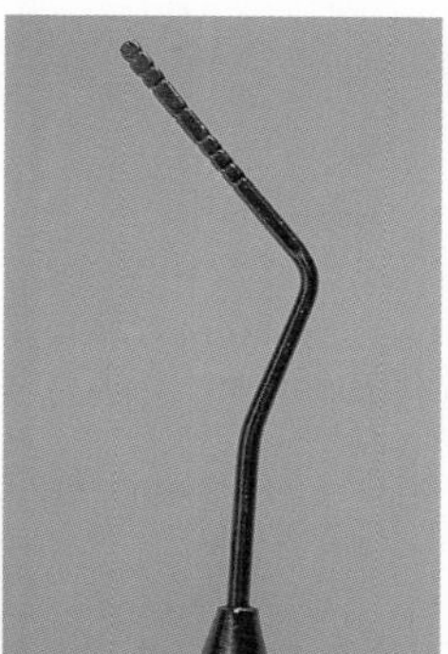	***Goldman Fox probe***	
	Shank	Flat.
	Measurement	1, 2, 3, 5, 7, 8, 9, 10 mm.
	Tip design	Blunt or wide.
	Advantages	No mark at 4 and 6 mm.
	Disadvantages	Flat shank does not allow easy access into tight fibrotic pockets.
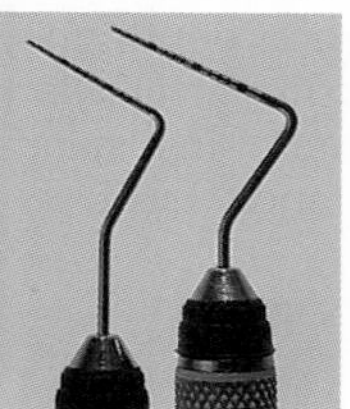	***UNC-12 probe and UNC-15 probe (University of North Carolina)***	
	Shank	Thin, round, and tapered.
	Measurement	UNC-12: 1, 2, 3, 4, 5, 6, 7, 8, 9, 10, 11, 12 mm. UNC-15: 1, 2, 3, 4, 5, 6, 7, 8, 9, 10, 11, 12, 13, 14, 15 mm.
	Tip design	Thin tip.
	Advantages	UNC-12 color coded at 4 and 9 mm. UNC-15 color coded at 4, 9, and 14 mm. Thin shank allows access into tight fibrotic sulci.
	Disadvantages	UNC-12 is used for maintenance and UNC-15 for clients with significant attachment loss.
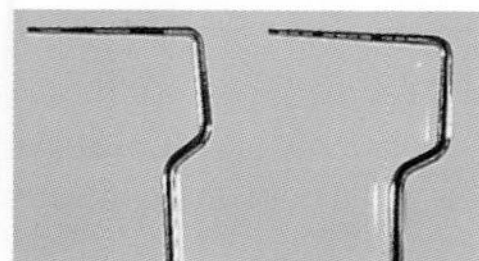	***Novatech probe***	
	Shank	Upward and right-angled bend.
	Measurement	Available in a variety of designs.
	Tip design	Available in a variety of designs.
	Advantages	Easier access in posterior distal areas.
	Disadvantages	May feel bulky due to angulation.
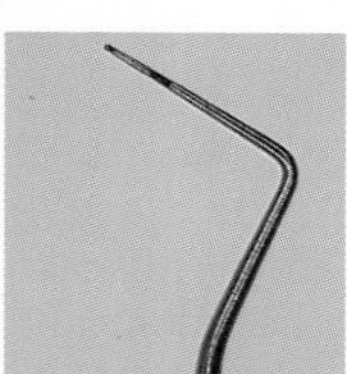	***PSR screening probe (World Health Organization probe)***	
	Shank	Thin, round, and tapered.
	Measurement	0.5, 3.5, 5.5, 8.5, 11.5 mm.
	Tip design	Thin tip with ball tip.
	Advantages	Ball tip (.5 mm) for client comfort. Color-coded at 3.5 mm. Easy-to-read markings. Thin shank allows access into tight fibrotic sulci.
	Disadvantages	Markings at 0.5 mm.
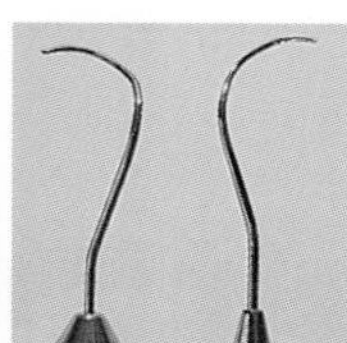	***Naber's furcation probe***	
	Shank	Round, tapered, and curved.
	Measurement	Available with or without measurement markings.
	Tip design	Blunted tip.
	Advantages	Ideal for detection of mesial and distal furcations in maxillary molars. Measurement markings are helpful.
	Disadvantages	May feel bulky when clinician is accustomed to using a periodontal explorer for furcation detection.
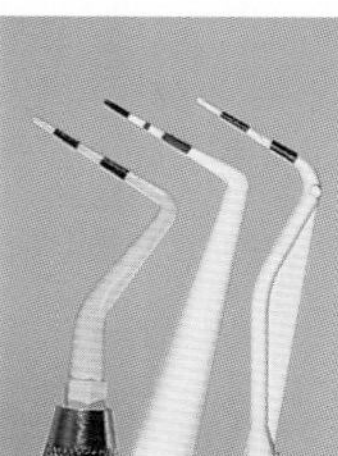	***Plastic probe (for dental implants)***	
	Shank	Thin, round, and tapered.
	Measurement	Color coded and variable measurements depending on manufacturer.
	Tip design	Thin tip or ball tip.
	Advantages	Ball tip for client comfort and less chance of penetration. Color-coded, easy to read markings. Thin shank allows access into tight fibrotic sulci Sterilizable for reuse. Will not scratch implants.
	Disadvantages	When markings wear away, entire probe or probe tip unscrewed and disposed of.

Procedure 20–1 BASIC POSITIONING FOR ASSESSMENT AND TREATMENT

EQUIPMENT
Ergonomically designed dental chair and operator chair
Personal protective equipment
Protective eyewear for client
Assessment and treatment instruments (as needed)
Air/water syringe and evacuation equipment

STEPS	RATIONALE
CLIENT POSITIONING	
1a. Mandibular occlusal plane positioned parallel to floor.	Maximizes accuracy of observation and measurement.
1b. Maxillary occlusal plane positioned nearly perpendicular to floor.	Optimal accessibility for assessment and instrumentation.
1c. Client's head turned for maximum direct vision of instrumentation when possible.	Enhanced client comfort.
OPERATOR POSITIONING	
2a. Right-handed operator: 8 to 10 o'clock for shallow or healthy client. The 10 to 4 o'clock positions are recommended for instrumentation of mandibular posterior teeth with moderate to severe periodontal pocket depth and sides of anterior teeth facing away from the operator. These positions usually require the use of extraoral fulcrums. The operator is often in a standing position.	Accessibility to all surfaces is generally optimal from a comfortable, seated operator position next to the client. Moderate to advanced mandibular posterior depth may require an extended operator position using a maxillary reach-down extraoral fulcrum with the operator in a standing position for optimal instrument adaptation and insertion to the base of the pocket. Extended operator positioning usually allows direct vision and better control of the instrument.
2b. Left-handed operator: 2 to 4 o'clock for shallow or healthy client. The 8 to 2 o'clock positions are recommended for instrumentation of mandibular posterior teeth with moderate to severe periodontal pocket depth and sides of anterior teeth facing away from the operator. These positions usually require the use of extraoral fulcrums. The operator is often in a standing position	Accessibility to all surfaces is generally optimal from a comfortable, seated operator position next to the client. Moderate to advanced mandibular posterior depth may require an extended operator position using a maxillary reach-down extraoral fulcrum with the operator in a standing position for optimal instrument adaptation and insertion to the base of the pocket. Extended operator positioning usually allows direct vision and better control of the instrument.
LIGHT/AIR/WATER AND EVACUATION	
3. Central beam illuminates working area.	Aids in comfortable instrument insertion, reducing client anxiety and stress.
4. Maintain good, unobstructed lighting; use water/air syringe and saliva evacuation when necessary: Depending on the procedure, evacuation may include the use of a saliva ejector or high-volume evacuation by a dental assistant.	Allows operator to visualize instrument-to-tooth relationships, aiding in complete tooth surface assessment and instrumentation; improves efficiency and quality of care.

Procedure 20–2 USE OF THE PERIODONTAL PROBE

EQUIPMENT
Periodontal probe
Mouth mirror

STEPS	RATIONALE
1. Begin with Basic Positioning in Procedure 20–1.	Allows for ergonomic practice and the prevention of repetitive stress injuries.
GRASP	
2. Use a light, modified pen grasp.	Allows clinician to carefully insert and walk tip of instrument along junctional epithelium with minimal client discomfort. Increases maneuverability of the instrument around the tooth.

Procedure 20–2 USE OF THE PERIODONTAL PROBE—CONT'D

STEPS	RATIONALE
FULCRUM AND FULCRUM PRESSURE	
3. Use relatively light fulcrum pressure.	Allows movement with good adaptation of the tip and first few millimeters of probe to base of deep periodontal pockets.
Flexible fulcrum placement: Intraoral near the tooth being probed; Cross arch; Opposite arch; Extraoral	Allows probe to be positioned with the working end parallel to long axis of tooth. Fulcrum position may be raised, lowered, tilted, and/or rotated in response to surface being measured. Since probing is an assessment function, fulcrum pressure on the tooth or extraorally is light compared to a calculus removal or debridement stroke.
INSERTION AND ADAPTATION	
4a. *All periodontal probes*: Insert with the lower 1–3 mm of the probe adapted against the tooth structure until the junctional epithelium is found. Insertion is parallel to the long axis of the tooth.	Avoids injury and penetration of junctional epithelium, leading to client comfort and accurate readings. Parallel insertion to base of pocket leads to accurate pocket depth measurement.
4b. When the probe reaches the contact area, slant tip to the area directly under the contact (col) and with the shank touching the contact, record measurement.	
4c. Carefully negotiate tip of probe around ledges of calculus when possible.	
4d. If significant ledges of calculus prevent insertion or comfortable adaptation, remove calculus first and then take readings for baseline assessment.	Ledges of calculus oftentimes interfere with the periodontal probe reaching base of the pocket.
5a. *Naber's furcation probe*: Using radiographs, previously recorded probe depths, and knowledge of root anatomy as a guide, wrap and insert the furcation probe into the furcation; note extent of penetration and classification of involvement.	Provides information to accurately diagnose furcation involvement as treatment options, planning, and prognosis depend on assessment accuracy. Because the furcation is a concavity of the tooth, the curved furcation probe is ideal in identifying mesial and distal furcations of maxillary molars.
5b. *Plastic probe*: Insert plastic probe adapted to the implant surface until resistance is met with very light pressure.	Prevents scratching of metal surfaces. Avoid trauma and distention of soft tissue around implants.
ACTIVATION AND DIRECTION OF STROKE	
6a. Move probe in small increments along the base of the sulcus/pocket. Under gentle pressure, the junctional epithelium feels soft and resilient.	Careful and accurate activation of periodontal probe is important because this procedure is usually done without the benefit of local anesthesia.
6b. Move distally in small increments until the center (no contact) or col area (under contact) of the tooth is reached. One side of the probe must be touching tooth surface.	Avoids penetrating tissue or measuring too shallowly.
6c. Note deepest reading on the distal surface.	Deepest readings offer the most accurate picture of periodontal status.
6d. Lift probe and reinsert at the distal line angle; walk forward until the mesial col area is reached. The probe is straightened until the upper portion touches the contact.	Assures that complete pocket area is assessed.
6e. Continue throughout the mouth buccally and lingually.	Assures that complete pocket area is assessed.
RECORDING PROBE READINGS	
7a. Record deepest buccal and lingual readings from the distal, buccal/lingual, and mesial surfaces. Six readings are recorded per tooth.	Deepest readings offer the most accurate picture of periodontal status. Assists dentist in formulating the dental diagnosis and care plan.
7b. Stop to record in the periodontal assessment section of the client record after several surfaces are complete.	Enhances efficiency when clinician can remember probe readings for several teeth and chart them all at once or when a dental assistant can be used to record. Participation of a dental assistant can improve infection control and more easily avoid the contamination of charts.

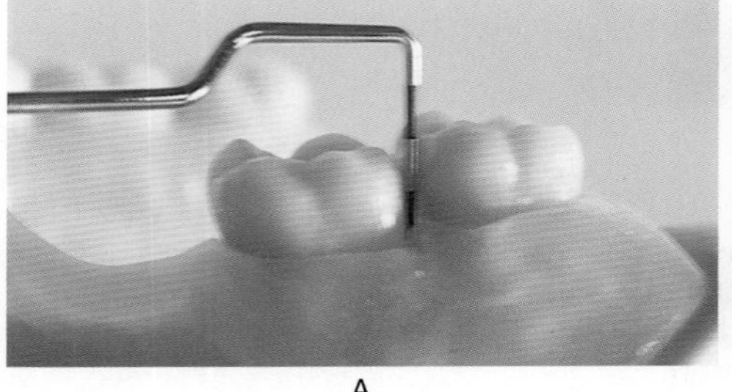

A

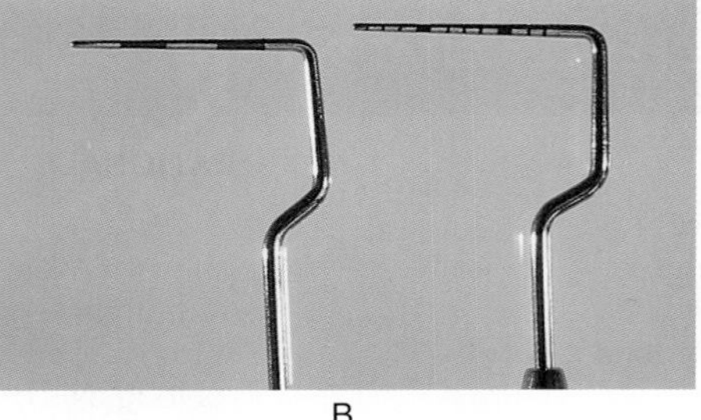

B

FIGURE 20–23 ✦ **A,** The Hu-Friedy Novatech periodontal probe with its upward bend is designed for access in posterior areas. **B,** The type of probe tip may differ, as illustrated in this photograph.

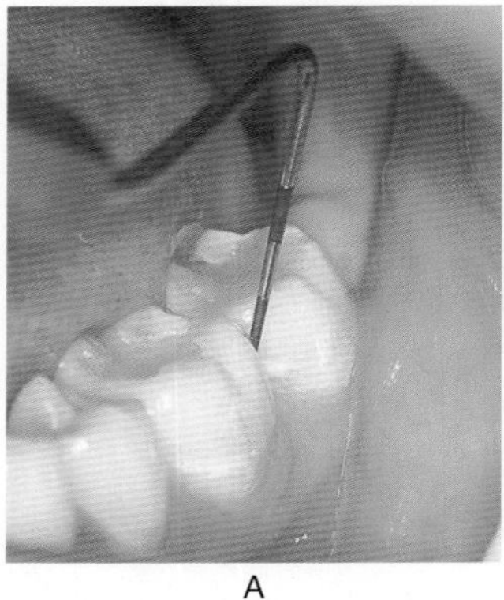

A

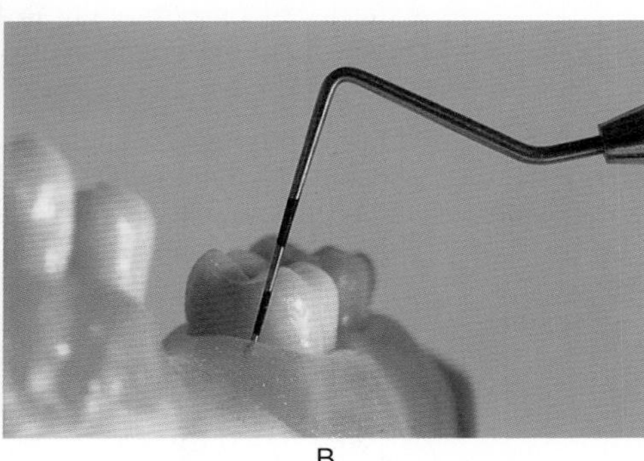

B

FIGURE 20–24 ✦ For proximal readings, the periodontal probe is slightly angled under the col and positioned vertically to touch the contact area between the adjacent teeth.

of the gingiva regardless of the degree of attachment loss (recession). Readings may change over time due to changes in the position of the gingival margin.[10]

When probing the full mouth, the practitioner begins the probing sequence from the distal surface. The periodontal probe is held with a pen grasp or a modified pen grasp because control and sensitivity may be accomplished with either grasp. The dental hygienist selects any intraoral or extraoral fulcrum that allows access into the area being assessed. The instrument is advanced by moving up and down and forward in 1- to 2-mm increments, gently inserting to the junctional epithelium on each downstroke. The least amount of trauma to the client occurs when the side of the probe maintains contact with the tooth during stroke activation. When using a flat-shaped periodontal probe, it is important for the operator to keep the flat side of the instrument against the tooth. For accuracy of interproximal readings, the probe should be slightly angled to examine the site under the col area and at the same time positioned vertically to touch the contact between the adjacent teeth (Figure 20–24).

Measurement of the probing depth is made by reading the marking on the probe where the gingival margin lies or by adding the increments above the gingival margin and subtracting from the total number of markings on the probe. For information on the measurement of probing depth, clinical attachment, relative attachment, adequacy of attached gingiva, and gingival recession, see Chapter 15 and Table 20–6.

Computerized periodontal probes are also available, for example, the Florida Probe (Figure 20–21, *D* and *E*). The tip of the probe is inserted into the sulcus or pocket and, with the use of a foot pedal, the system automatically records pocket depth, attachment loss, bleeding, mobility, and other clinical parameters. Once data are collected, a graphic chart can be printed and used as part of the dental record and for client education. The computerized probe is designed to apply 15 grams of pressure each time it is used. This design feature increases consistency in the probing technique over time and between practitioners. Some computerized probes are accurate to 0.2 mm, which is far better than the accuracy of a traditional marked probe.

The #2 Nabers probe is a specialized probe used for the detection and classification of furcations. Because classification of furcation involvement is based on the degree of penetration of a probe between the roots of multirooted teeth, the Nabers probe, with its curved shank and blunted tip, is well suited for subgingival insertion and furcation classification. The color-coded Nabers probe allows the clinician to more accurately classify furcations (Figure 20–25).

The blunted tip of the periodontal probe makes it ideal to determine (but not measure) bleeding tendencies on probing. If gentle probing elicits bleeding, this observation should be noted on the client's record as a clinical indication of inflammation. Gingival bleeding is associated with significant increases in spirochetes, motile bacterial forms, and increased flow of gingival crevicular fluid.[11–17] Evidence of bleeding has been shown to have only a 30% predictive value in determining future clinical attachment loss. Cessation of bleeding has been related to a significant reduction in gingival inflammation and is used to monitor the effects of periodontal treatment.[10,18,19]

By compressing the side of the probe tip against the attached gingiva, the dental hygienist evaluates tissue

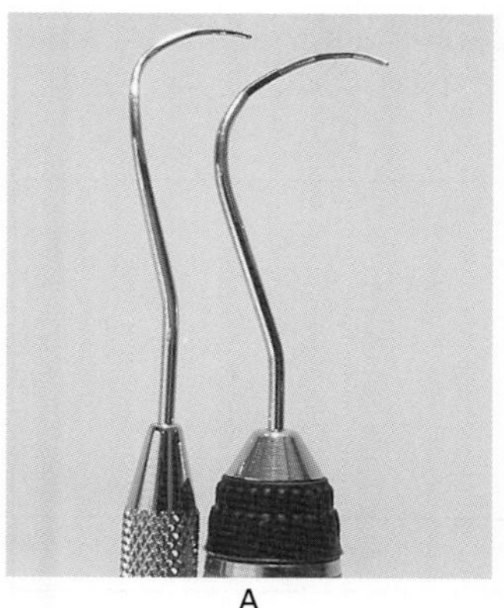
A

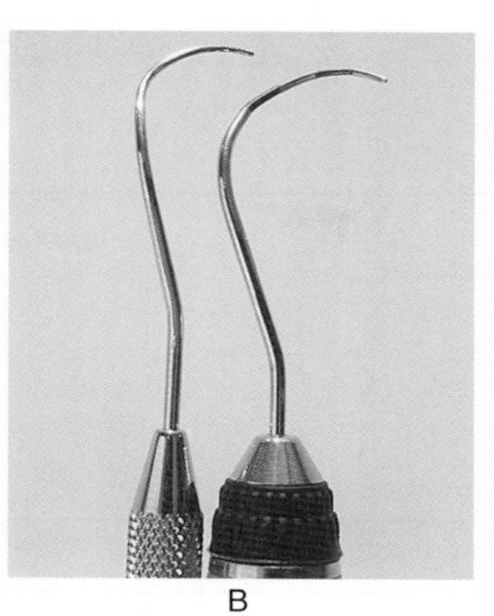
B

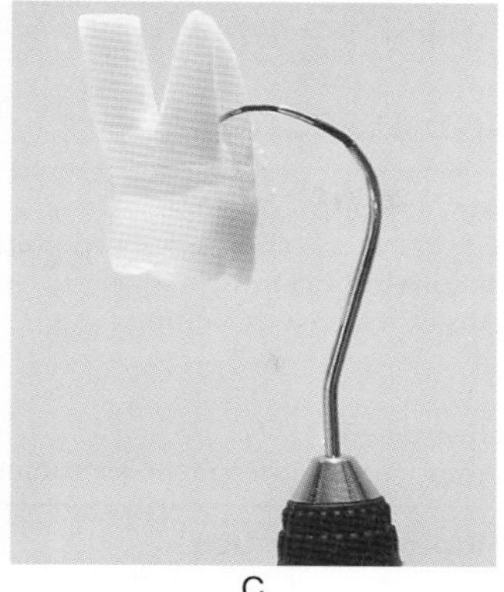
C

FIGURE 20–25 ✦ **A,** Nabers probe is plain or color-coded *(B)* and is used for furcation classification *(C)*.

tone without producing trauma. More information may be obtained from a standard dental index such as the Silness and Löe Plaque Index, which uses the periodontal probe in the assessment (see Chapter 14, Table 14–3). Some practitioners use the periodontal probe to identify subgingival calculus; however, most find the dental explorer more reliable for deposit assessment because of its curvature and fine tip.

Measurement of suspected pathologic lesions is important for complete documentation, in addition to a diagram of the shape and verbal description of intraoral and extraoral lesions, whether or not the lesions are biopsied. The periodontal probe is used to measure the dimensions of small lesions, and the side and tip of the instrument are used to palpate, lift, or rub over the lesion to examine other characteristics that may be helpful to the dentist making a differential diagnosis. If not excisionally biopsied, the lesion should be monitored by evaluating the size (with a periodontal probe), shape, and visual description on subsequent appointments (see Chapter 12 on extraoral and intraoral clinical assessment).

The periodontal probe also is used to measure the distance between teeth (diastema) and the amount of overjet a person may exhibit. In individuals with severe periodontal disease, tooth migration is an indicator of further loss of support structures, and the stability or degree of movement over time may be monitored with the periodontal probe.

Explorer

DESIGN AND USE. Clinicians use many diagnostic indicators such as tissue response, bleeding, and radiographic surveys to determine the presence of subgingival deposits. However, tissue response to calculus varies by individual, and radiographs are two-dimensional, making it difficult to visualize flat, burnished calculus deposits obscured by restorations or located on facial or lingual surfaces of teeth. The *explorer*, designed for angulation around the tooth, is used to detect and assess the following:

- ✦ Supragingival calculus
- ✦ Subgingival calculus
- ✦ Cemental irregularities
- ✦ Dental caries
- ✦ Decalcification
- ✦ Irregularities in margins of restorations
- ✦ Secondary caries around restorations
- ✦ Morphologic crown and root anomalies
- ✦ External root resorption

The explorer consists of a very fine, wire-like tip with a sharp point that comes in a variety of lengths, diameters, and bends. Shank diameter is narrow for increased tactile sensitivity. The differences in curvature of the shank, length, and diameter make different explorers useful for specific purposes dependent on tissue, calculus, probing depth, tooth alignment, and other details specific to individual clients.

An explorer is selected for the task it is to perform:

- ✦ Heavier, wider, or even medium-diameter explorers are best suited for caries detection or exploration around restorations. Such explorers are sturdy and do not deform or bend as they are manipulated under and around caries and metallic margins. Fine, elongated explorers are more difficult to use for caries detection because of the deflection of the instrument during use.
- ✦ Fine-diameter explorers are best suited for subgingival exploration of root structure and identification of calculus, and allow for tactile sensitivity. Explorers that are too thin flex and catch in tissue or on root structure in fibrotic or tight areas, relaying incorrect messages about subgingival deposits.
- ✦ For deep periodontal pockets, the explorer should be slightly bent and long enough (such as the Hu-Friedy #3-A EXD or the #EXD 11/12AF) to reach to the apical regions (i.e., 12 mm or deeper).
- ✦ For shallow sulcus areas, cementoenamel junctions, and under contact areas, a short explorer (such as a pigtail explorer) is easily adapted because it is short and acutely bent. These short, curved explorers are usually double-ended and area-specific, that is, each end works best on specific surfaces of the tooth.

Comparisons of these and other explorers are seen in Figure 20–26. Criteria for design, selection and procedure for use of the explorer are found in Table 20–8 and Procedures 20–1 and 20–3.

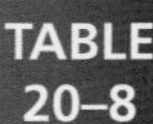

TABLE 20–8

EXPLORER DESIGN AND SELECTION

Common Design Specifications of Explorers

A wirelike, flexible assessment instrument that always ends in a sharp pointed tip.
Cross-sectional view is rounded with variations in thickness.
Variations in regular and extended lengths of selected explorers.
Available as:
Universal single-ended instrument.
Area specific, double-ended and paired instrument.
Double-ended instrument with two different types of assessment instruments on each end.

Instrument Examples	Rationale for Use
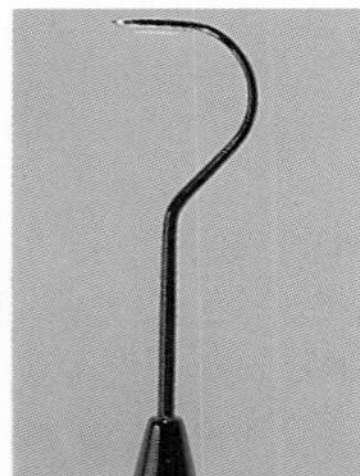	***#23 Shepherd's hook explorer (supragingival exploration)*** Design: A single-ended explorer with a short lower shank and large rounded hook design. Function: Use for supragingival detection of dental caries on all crown surfaces and around restorations. Not recommended for subgingival calculus or caries detection.
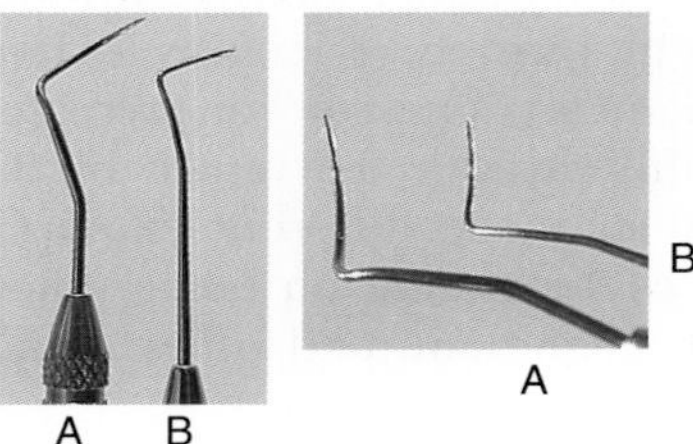	***Pigtail explorer (short and long)*** Design: Double-ended, paired, short, curved explorer. Function: The longer pigtail explorer (A) is designed for improved interproximal access. The shorter version (B) is excellent for supragingival detection of dental caries on all crown surfaces and around restorations, and caries and calculus detection in normal shallow sulci. The pigtail is not recommended for subgingival calculus or caries detection in moderate to deep periodontal pockets.
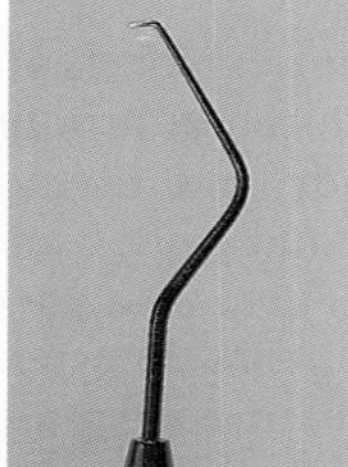	***#17 explorer (limited-use periodontal exploration)*** Design: A single-ended explorer with a 90-degree angled 2-mm fine tip. Function: Use for calculus detection in deep narrow pockets. Best suited for deep, narrow pockets in anterior teeth and facial or lingual surfaces of posterior teeth. Difficult to use around line angles and proximal surfaces of posterior teeth.
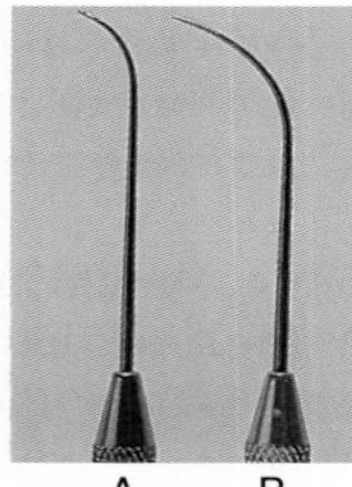	***#3-A explorer (periodontal exploration; regular length and extended length)*** Design: Single-ended, gently curved and tapered explorer. Function: The shorter version (A) is excellent for subgingival calculus detection in normal sulci. The thinner, extended version (B) is excellent for deep periodontal pockets and furcations. Both versions are excellent for caries detection supragingivally and subgingivally.
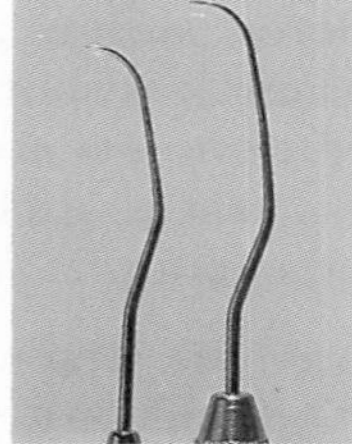	***11/12 explorer (periodontal exploration; regular length and extended length)*** Design: A double-ended, paired explorer. Shank design is similar to the Gracey 11/12 area-specific curet. Function: Used primarily for subgingival calculus detection in deep periodontal pockets. Exceptional tactile sensitivity and adaptation for anterior as well as posterior shallow and deep pocket depths. The regular length (A) limits access in deep distal proximal areas of posterior molars; this is corrected with the extended version (B).

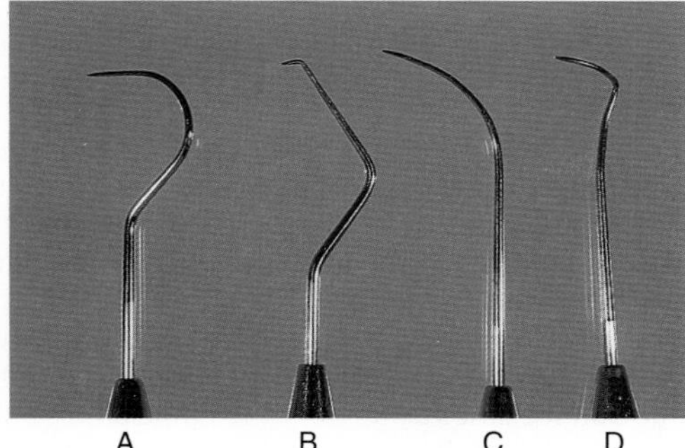

FIGURE 20–26 ✦ **A,** No. 23 Shepherd's hook explorer. **B,** No. 17 Orban explorer. **C,** Hu-Friedy No. 3-A extralong explorer. **D,** Pigtail explorer (double-ended).

Procedure 20–3 USE OF THE PERIODONTAL EXPLORER

EQUIPMENT

Periodontal explorer (3-A explorer or 11/12 explorer)
Mouth mirror

STEPS	RATIONALE
1. Begin with Basic Positioning in Procedure 20–1.	Allows for ergonomic practice and the prevention of repetitive stress injuries.
SELECTING CORRECT WORKING END	
2. The 3-A extended explorer has only one working end. 11/12 extended explorers are paired with two working ends. Use the end whose curvature adapts toward the tooth surface to be explored.	Both the 3-A and 11/12 explorers are curved explorers. When the curve is adapted toward the tooth surface, the tip is also adapted, minimizing tissue discomfort to the client.
GRASP	
3a. Use a light to moderate modified pen grasp.	Enhances tactile, sensitivity allowing operator to feel slight vibrations conducted through shank and handle with pads of tripod of fingers. Increases maneuverability of instrument around tooth and reduces muscle fatigue in operator's hands and fingers.
3b. Grasp pressure is slightly increased when explorer pressure against the tooth must be increased to distinguish between tooth structure, restorative material(s), and/or calculus.	Grasp strength is increased when more pressure is necessary to interpret density and topography of harder structures such as burnished calculus, irregular cementum, or restorative materials.
3c. Move grasp further away from the working end as you go from anterior to posterior teeth. When fulcrum moves cross arch, opposite arch, or extraorally, move grasp away from the working end of the explorer.	Accessibility to posterior pockets improves with extension of fulcrum away from the tooth being explored. This extension requires movement of the grasp away from the working end.
FULCRUM AND FULCRUM PRESSURE	
4. Use relatively light fulcrum pressure. Flexible fulcrum placement: Intraoral near the tooth being explored; Cross arch; Opposite arch; Extraoral	Allows extended movement with good adaptation to base of deep periodontal pockets. Allows movement of the explorer in a variety of directions (vertical, horizontal, oblique). Fulcrum position may be raised, lowered, tilted, and/or rotated in response to the changing topography of a tooth surface. Since exploring is an assessment function, fulcrum pressure on the tooth or extraorally is light compared to a calculus removal or debridement stroke.
INSERTION AND ADAPTATION	
5a. Insertion with the lower 1–3 mm of the explorer adapted or curved toward tooth structure until the junctional epithelium is found.	**3-A and 11/12 Extended Explorers:** Tactile evaluation of irregularities on the root surface and subgingival calculus exploration begins with the insertion of the explorer.
5b. Adapt explorer tip to the root surface.	Reduces the possibility of soft tissue injury.

Continued on following page

Procedure 20-3 USE OF THE PERIODONTAL EXPLORER—CONT'D

5c. In anesthetized clients or after the clinician understands the pocket topography, reinsert tip of the explorer pointed downward like a periodontal probe. The adaptation of the explorer curves toward tooth surface.	Insertion with the tip in a downward direction (first 1–2 mm must be adapted to root) enhances the clinician's ability to reach the base of moderate to deep pocket depth and maneuver around line angles and significant curvatures. **11/12 Extended Explorer:** *Anterior teeth*: The 11/12 explorer is more effective when the clinician uses the opposite end of the instrument to explore the surface sides away from the clinician on anterior teeth. It is easier for the curvature of the instrument to adapt to the root surface. *Posterior teeth*: Using the same end of the 11/12 explorer on the distal, buccal, and mesial surfaces on posterior teeth allows tip to remain in contact with root surface and accessible to base of pocket.
ACTIVATION, DIRECTION OF STROKE, AND EFFICIENCY	
6a. Begin activation with the insertion stroke (vertical direction). Stroke activation is both a push and pull stroke.	Push/downward action is important in identifying roughness that may be detectable only from the upper edge of a piece of calculus. Burnished calculus is usually smoothest at the base and may not easily be detected from the bottom. Therefore, multidirection exploration is important.
6b. Assess root surfaces in multiple directions (vertical, horizontal, oblique): – Use sweeping strokes to initially determine surface irregularities. – Strokes are short and restricted around pieces of calculus or surface irregularities. – Strokes are long and sweeping to evaluate root smoothness. – Use many strokes from many directions when there is need to assess calculus, burnished calculus, root caries, or restorative margins. – Use fewer strokes when the surface is smooth during the final evaluation phase of treatment.	Results in accurate identification of size and location of calculus. Long, sweeping exploratory strokes allow the clinician to evaluate the shape of tooth surface and effectively compare surfaces.
PRESSURE	
7a. Use light pressure when assessing light calculus, little pocket depth, and friable soft tissue.	Easier to feel calculus and irregularities when lightly exploring tooth surface. Easier to feel heavy, tenacious calculus with either light or moderate pressure strokes.
7b. Increase pressure with moderate to heavy calculus to detect burnished calculus and root irregularities.	Moderate pressure strokes allow the clinician to assess the hardness for appropriate treatment planning and instrument selection for removal.
7c. Use light pressure to assess root planing outcomes.	Evaluation of scaling and root planing requires light, long, fluid strokes that do not hang up or inadvertently catch on root anatomy. At this point in treatment, it is important to assess overall smoothness over large areas.

The modified pen grasp is used with the dental explorer. When exploring shallow, light, or obvious calculus, the dental hygienist uses a grasp with light to moderate strength. The grasp should become firmer when more pressure needs to be exerted against the tooth or when the dental hygienist needs to distinguish between tooth structure and burnished calculus.

The most important rule governing fulcrum placement when exploring is that the fulcrum be flexible enough to allow the explorer to move from the cementoenamel junction to the apex of the pocket with correct insertion and adaptation. Almost any scaling fulcrum could be used as an exploring fulcrum; however, the reverse may not always be true because a scaling fulcrum needs more stability. The exploratory fulcrum could be located close to the area being explored, cross arch, or extraoral. As the fulcrum moves further from the area being explored, the clinician's grasp on the instrument handle also moves further away from the working end. This distance does not diminish the hygienist's ability to explore the area, nor does it lessen instrument control. Rather, it enhances access into interproximal regions and deep periodontal pockets.

TACTILE SENSITIVITY. *Tactile sensitivity* is the ability to distinguish relative degrees of roughness and smoothness on the tooth surface. Experience in detecting light calculus when it is almost completely scaled and in feeling heavy calculus when it has been burnished is a prerequisite for developing good tactile sensitivity. The skill may be improved by attention to stroke direction, pressure, type of calculus, and type of root surface being explored.

For calculus detection with an explorer, the practitioner uses a variety of stroke directions (vertical, horizontal, and oblique) to form a basketweave of strokes, as described in a previous section (Figure 20–13). This is particularly helpful when problems of differentiation between calculus and root structure occur. The dental hygienist should practice different strokes when instrumentation has been particularly difficult in a certain area or when it is necessary to be particularly thorough in calculus detection (such as in a very deep pocket or in an area where there is a periodontal abscess).

Tactile sensitivity also is important in distinguishing between the sulcular soft tissue wall, the junctional epithelium, and possible osseous exposures. The explorer tip should not stop on the sulcular wall if the instrument is inserted properly and the tip remains well adapted to the tooth surface to the base of the pocket. If the explorer contacts soft tissue, it bounces and snags along the wall until the instrument is properly adapted. As one follows the root of the tooth down to the base of the pocket, the nonkeratinizing junctional epithelium is the base of the pocket. The junctional epithelium feels different at different states of periodontal health:

- In healthy sulci, the junctional epithelium is firm and elastic in nature.
- In the inflamed state, the junctional epithelium is soft and easily penetrable with a sharp-pointed instrument.
- If osseous exposure occurs because of heavy instrumentation and exceptionally friable soft tissue, the sensation at the base of the pocket is much like that of heavy, porous calculus. To differentiate calculus from an osseous exposure, the dental hygienist attempts to move around and under the area. If it is calculus, the junctional epithelium is felt under the deposit. If the roughness is an osseous exposure, the dental hygienist will find it impossible to move the explorer down and under the area.

The practitioner uses light pressure when faced with light calculus, little pocket depth, and friable tissue. Increased pressure is required when trying to distinguish burnished calculus or when over-instrumentation may have caused irregular changes in root structure. Pressure should be decreased, however, after thorough root planing to get an overview of the final product.

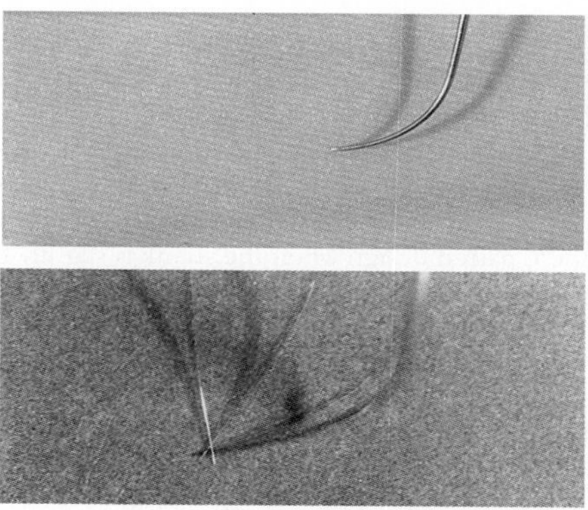

FIGURE 20–27 ✦ The dental explorer is sharpened by lightly dragging and rotating the first 2 to 3 mm along the sharpening stone.

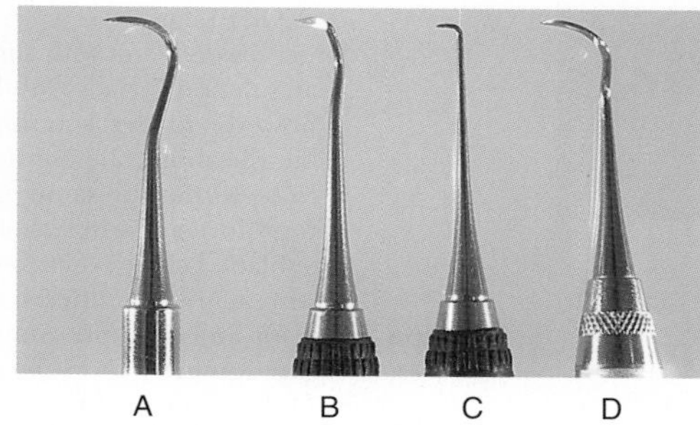

FIGURE 20–28 ✦ Comparison of various sickle scalers. **A,** Curved anterior sickle. **B,** Jacquette (double-ended) sickle. **C,** Morse anterior sickle. **D,** posterior sickle.

SHARPENING TECHNIQUES. Fine explorers become dull through general use and from caries detection in pits and fissures and around restorations. Decreased tactile sensitivity is evident when fine changes in root texture cannot be distinguished or when the explorer glides over the plastic testing stick instead of catching on irregularities. To sharpen the tip of an explorer, the instrument is held with a modified pen grasp, dragged, and rotated along the stone at an angle that keeps the tip and 2 to 3 mm of the terminal end in contact with the stone. Two to three rotations around the tip on the stone sufficiently sharpens the dental explorer (Figure 20–27). Because the periodontal explorer's length is important, an explorer shortened through wear should be replaced.

Sickle Scaler

DESIGN AND USE. The *sickle scaler* is designed with either a straight or bent shank (contra-angle) design (Figure 20–28.) The straight-shanked sickle scalers are anterior scaling instruments and are often single-ended because the same end may be used mesially and distally (Procedures 20–1 and 20–4 and Table 20–9). The bent-shanked sickle scalers may be used for anterior as well as posterior areas of the mouth, and are usually double-ended with one end designed for scaling mesial tooth surfaces and the other end for scaling distal tooth surfaces (Procedures 20–1 and 20–5 and Table 20–10).

TABLE 20–9 ANTERIOR SICKLE SCALER DESIGN AND SELECTION

Common Design Specifications of All Anterior Sickle Scalers
Single-ended straight shank.
Double-ended, paired design when the shank is slightly bent.
Blade, shank, and handle are in the same plane.
Two cutting edges on a straight blade that end in a point *or* two cutting edges on a curved blade that end in a sharp point.
Cross-sectional view is triangular.
Back is a sharp edge of the meeting of the two sides or flattened depending on manufacturer.

Instrument Examples	Rationale for Use	
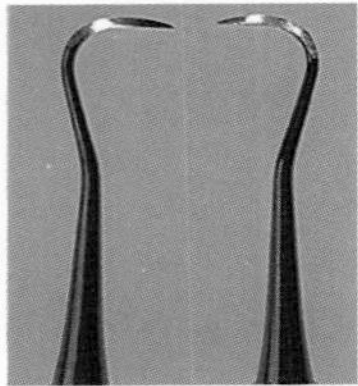	***SH 6/7***	
	Design	Paired, contra-angle, curved sickle design. Short lower shank with slight angulation for accessibility; however, blades, shank, and handle should be considered to be within the same plane, therefore are anterior sickles. The blade is long, relatively thin, with a large rounded back.
	Function	Use for anterior and premolar supragingival and subgingival (1–2 mm) calculus removal. Contra-angle design allows easier access interproximally than a straight shank. With good adaptation, this instrument could be used to remove heavy ledges of calculus on lingual surfaces of posterior teeth in a horizontal direction. Not recommended for subgingival calculus removal 3 mm or deeper or root planing.
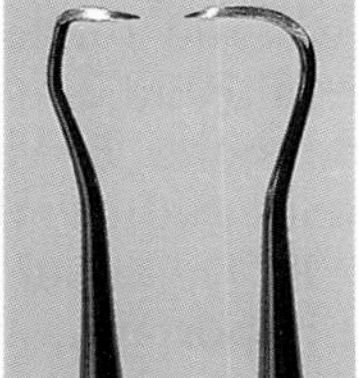	***SH 5/33***	
	Design	Double-ended with a straight sickle on one end and a curved sickle on the other end. Both blades are within the same plane as the shank and handle. Both blades are relatively thin.
	Function	Use both ends for anterior supragingival and subgingival (1–2 mm) calculus removal. Not recommended for subgingival calculus removal 3 mm or deeper or root planing.

TABLE 20–10 POSTERIOR SICKLE SCALER DESIGN AND SELECTION

Common Design Specifications of All Posterior Sickle Scalers
Double-ended, paired design with a bent shank for posterior interproximal access.
Two straight or curved cutting edges that end in a sharp point.
Cross-sectional view is triangular.
Back is a sharp edge of the meeting of the two sides or flattened depending on manufacturer.

Instrument Examples	Rationale for Use	
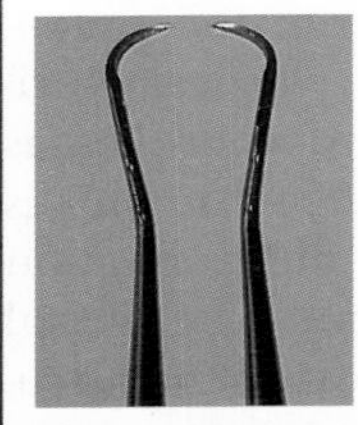	***S204SD***	
	Design	Paired, contra-angle, curved sickle design. Shank is bent in two places. The blade is small, about half the width and length of the anterior SH 6/7 sickle scaler.
	Function	Bent lower shank allows access interproximally in anterior and posterior areas. Short narrow blade allows access subgingivally. Use for supragingival and subgingival calculus removal (where tissue permits).
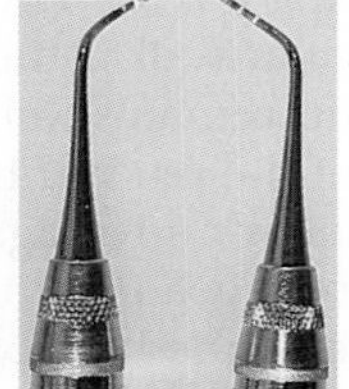	***SJ 34/35***	
	Design	Paired, contra-angle, straight sickle design (Jacquette scaler). Shank is bent in two places. The 34/35 is a miniature sickle scaler.
	Function	Bent lower shank allows access interproximally and subgingivally in anterior and posterior areas. Access may be limited due to size of blade.
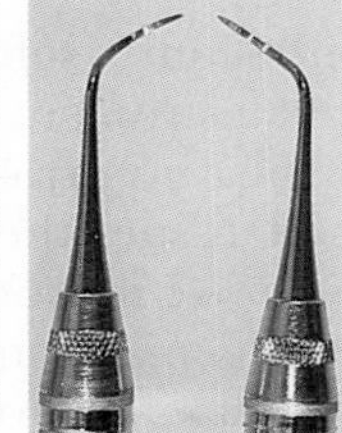	***SCNEVI2***	
	Design	Paired, contra-angle, curved sickle design. Shank is acutely bent. The blade is long and thin.
	Function	Bent lower shank allows ideal access interproximally in anterior and particularly posterior areas. Use for supragingival and subgingival calculus removal (where tissue permits).

The working end of the sickle scaler is a two-sided blade with the face and two sides forming the two cutting edges. The two sides join together in a V shape or are slightly flattened, depending on the manufacturer, to form the back of the instrument. Because the sides form a V shape, this instrument is very sturdy in terms of strength even after it has been sharpened many times. Therefore, it is valuable for removal of heavy calculus. However, the extra width from the face to the back of this working end makes it difficult to close the angulation of most sickles without traumatizing the sulcular epithelium with the V-shaped back during subgingival instrumentation. This problem is accentuated with large sickle scalers.

Procedure 20–4 USE OF THE ANTERIOR SICKLE SCALER

EQUIPMENT
Anterior sickle scaler
Subgingival explorer
Mouth mirror

STEPS	RATIONALE
1. Begin with Basic Positioning in Procedure 20–1.	Allows for ergonomic practice and the prevention of repetitive stress injuries.
SELECTING CORRECT WORKING END	
2a. Select correct adaptation and working end based on the amount of calculus present and tissue tone.	Selection of the correct end reduces possible injury from sharp point and allows better adaptation to tooth surfaces.
2b. Use straight end of the SH 5/33 on anterior interproximal surfaces.	
2c. Use the slight contra-angle design of the SH 6/7 in anterior and premolar areas.	
GRASP	
3. Use a moderate modified pen grasp.	Allows clinician to carefully engage tip of sickle scaler under calculus and remove it with light to firm force, depending on tenacity of calculus.
FULCRUM AND FULCRUM PRESSURE	
4. Use stable, moderate fulcrum pressure during working stroke.	Allows the cutting edge and tip to be well adapted to tooth surface.
Fulcrum placement: Intraoral near the tooth being scaled	Fulcrum position may be raised, lowered, tilted during calculus removal.
Opposite arch	Maximizes stability.
INSERTION AND ADAPTATION	
5a. Engage lower edge of interproximal supragingival ledge of calculus. Engagement may extend, when soft tissue permits, 1–2 mm subgingivally.	Enhances the probability of popping off pieces of calculus rather than relying on multiple shaving motions, which may burnish the calculus.
5b. Adapt cutting edge of sickle to tooth surface.	Proper adaptation of a large-pointed instrument prevents possible injury from slippage. The slightly offset position of the lower shank allows access interproximally and subgingivally. The long blade with large, rounded back does not permit comfortable and atraumatic adaptation and insertion deeper than 1–2 mm.
ACTIVATION, DIRECTION OF STROKE AND PRESSURE	
Supragingival use:	
6a. Engage large pieces of calculus with a vertical to oblique stroke direction.	An oblique stroke directed toward contact area prevents losing control of the instrument beyond the immediate area and injuring the client's soft tissues.
6b. Use a pull stroke with moderate pressure.	Allows clinician to use safest method of calculus removal without injuring soft tissue.
Subgingival use:	
7. Activate with a pull stroke in a vertical direction with moderate pressure.	Because the toe of the sickle scaler is a sharp point, the vertical stroke avoids injury to the soft tissue or cementum.

There are medium posterior sickle scalers with a curved blade contra-angle design, which are very effective for moderate to heavy subgingival calculus removal in anterior and posterior areas. Small straight-shanked sickle scalers such as the Morse scaler (Figure 20–28, *C*) cause even less trauma and may be easier to use for subgingival scaling in tight anterior areas.

The tip of the sickle scaler always ends in a sharp point. This tip is the major difference between a sickle scaler and a curet, especially when comparing the curved blade, contra-angle designed sickle scalers with a curet. The advantage of the sickle scaler is its ability to reach between very tight contacts. The disadvantage is that the sharp tip and straight cutting edge do not adapt well to rounded tooth surfaces; some part of the instrument is always off the tooth. This problem of adaptation and a V-shaped back imposing on the sulcular wall makes the sickle scaler largely a supragingival scaling instrument. Only in situations of moderate to heavy subgingival calculus and very loose tissue may the sickle

Procedure 20–5 USE OF THE POSTERIOR SICKLE SCALER

EQUIPMENT
Posterior sickle scaler
Subgingival explorer
Mouth mirror

STEPS	RATIONALE
1. Begin with Basic Positioning in Procedure 20–1.	Allows for ergonomic practice and the prevention of repetitive stress injuries.
SELECTING CORRECT WORKING END	
2a. Select correct adaptation and working end based on amount of calculus present, tissue tone, and pocket depth.	Selection of the correct end of the sickle scaler reduces possible injury from the sharp point and enhances clinician effectiveness.
2b. Use the SCNEVI2 rather than the S204SD for more periodontally involved clients.	
GRASP	
3. Use a moderate modified pen grasp.	Allows clinician to carefully engage tip of sickle scaler under calculus and remove it with light to firm force, depending on tenacity of calculus.
FULCRUM AND FULCRUM PRESSURE	
4. Use stable, moderate fulcrum pressure during working stroke.	Bends in posterior sickles allow for fulcrum placement away from the area being scaled.
Fulcrum placement:	Allows the cutting edge and tip to be well adapted to tooth surface.
Intraoral near the tooth being scaled Cross arch Opposite arch	Fulcrum position may be raised, lowered, tilted during calculus removal. Maximizes stability.
INSERTION AND ADAPTATION	
5a. Insert to greatest depth tissue allows. Side of tip remains well adapted to root surface.	Proper adaptation and engagement of calculus are critical to safe subgingival instrumentation with a sickle scaler. Avoid possible injury to soft tissue and cementum.
5b. Engage lower edge of supragingival ledge of calculus.	Inserting subgingivally to find the deepest part of the ledge of calculus is a safer stroke than attempting to fracture the calculus simply to stay supragingival.
5c. Tilt tip slightly downward.	Enhances the probability of popping off pieces of calculus rather than relying on multiple shaving motions, which may burnish the calculus.
5d. Engage ledge of subgingival calculus. (Use opposite end for alternate sides of the tooth.)	In loose, deep periodontal pockets, the curved, thin sickle blade inserts subgingivally and the curvature allows proper adaptation to root surfaces.
ACTIVATION, DIRECTION OF STROKE AND PRESSURE	
Supragingival use:	
6a. Engage large pieces of calculus with a vertical to oblique stroke direction.	Allows the clinician to use safest method of calculus removal without injuring soft tissue.
6b. Use pull stroke with moderate pressure, moving across tooth surface until all gross calculus is removed.	Prevents losing control of instrument beyond immediate area and injuring client's soft tissues.
Subgingival use:	
7a. Activate stroke with a pull stroke in a vertical direction using moderate pressure.	Because toe of sickle scaler is a sharp point, the vertical stroke avoids injury to soft tissue or cementum.
7b. Move across subgingival area until all gross calculus is removed.	

scaler be used subgingivally. Because of the need to control adaptation of the toe and cutting edge of this instrument, instrumentation techniques for sickle scalers require a stable modified pen grasp and fulcrum relatively close to the area being scaled. A pull stroke action in a vertical or oblique direction is made against the tooth surface.

SHARPENING TECHNIQUE. The sharpening method for the sickle scaler requires the stone to remain stationary and the instrument to move over the stone. The stone is secured with the nondominant hand, the instrument held with a modified pen grasp, and the lateral surface positioned at an angle of 100 to 110 degrees to the stone. The entire lateral surface on a flat-surfaced sickle scaler lies against the stone. For curved sickle scalers, small portions of the lateral surfaces are sharpened at a time, beginning from the portion nearest the shank. The working hand is stabilized with a fulcrum on the stone, and short, firm strokes are applied for sharpening. Because the sickle scaler has two cutting edges, the instrument is turned over and the procedure is repeated for the other lateral surface of the blade. Occasionally the face of the sickle scaler is sharpened. For this surface, the stone either must be positioned near the edge of the table or held up so that the entire face may be sharpened against the surface of the stone. The practitioner tests for sharpness using the visual or tactile methods described earlier.

Universal Curet

DESIGN AND USE. The *universal curet,* used for supragingival and subgingival scaling and root planing in all areas of the mouth, is designed with paired mirror-image working ends placed on a single-handle instrument. These working ends are identified by the name of the manufacturer, inventor, or school that developed the particular design. On double-ended instruments the name is followed by two numbers, each designating a working end (e.g., Columbia 13/14). Universal curets are available also as single-ended instruments that must be purchased in pairs because both ends are necessary in instrumenting a tooth (Procedures 20–1 and 20–6 and Table 20–11).

The universal curet blade has two lateral surfaces that form two parallel cutting edges on both sides of the flat face (inner surface) of the blade. The two cutting edges form a rounded tip (or toe) at the terminal end of the blade. The lateral surfaces converge to form the rounded back of the blade. This design reduces the chances of subgingival trauma to both sulcular tissues and tooth structure. Both cutting edges of a universal curet blade are parallel and curved upward toward the toe of the blade (Figure 20–29). The curvature of the blades defines the areas in which the instrument is most useful.

The face of the universal curet blade is positioned at a 90-degree angle to the lower shank. There is a bend above the lower shank so that the handle is not parallel with the lower shank (Figure 20–30). Therefore, to close angulation for scaling to an angle between 45 and 90 degrees, the handle and lower shank of the universal curet must be tilted slightly toward the tooth (Figure 20–31).

One double-ended (or a pair of single-ended) universal curets can be used to scale all areas of the dentition of a periodontally healthy mouth. Scaling with a universal curet is more difficult with increased pocket depth. In these cases, combinations of universal curets may be necessary to extend the reach. The Columbia 13/14, for instance, is a short, acutely curved universal curet. This

TABLE 20–11 UNIVERSAL CURET DESIGN AND SELECTION

Common Design Specifications of All Universal Curets

Double-ended, mirror image working ends.
Two curved cutting edges that end in a rounded toe.
Face is at 90 degrees or perpendicular to the lower shank.
Cross-sectional view is semicircular.
Back is round.
Differences in shank length, design, and blade size affect use.
One curet can be used throughout the healthy mouth of a child, adolescent, or adult.

Instrument	Rationale for Use	
Posterior and Anterior Application (A) Columbia 13/14 (B) Barnhardt 5/6 (C) Younger Good 7/8 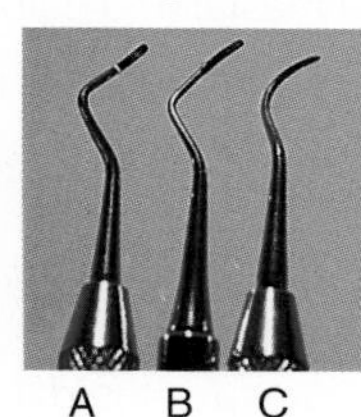 A B C	Design	Short lower shank. Rigid or regular flexibility in shank.
	Function	Scaling and root planing of supragingival and subgingival plaque biofilm and calculus. Use on all anterior tooth surfaces. May be useful in posterior areas of the healthy mouth.
Posterior Application (A) Columbia 4R/4L (B) Columbia 2R/2L (C) Barnhardt 1/2 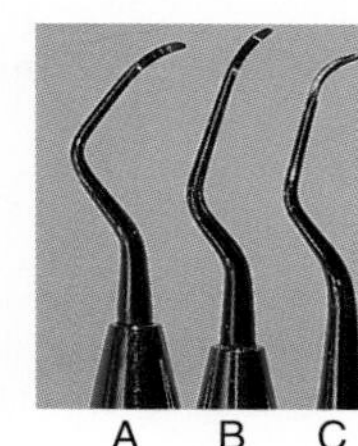 A B C	Design	Long lower shank. Rigid or regular flexibility in shank.
	Function	Scaling and root planing of supragingival and subgingival plaque biofilm and calculus. Use on all posterior tooth surfaces in clients with moderate to deep pocket depth. The more bent the shank, the easier it is to reach interproximally (A and C). The straighter the shank, the easier it is to reach buccally and lingually (B). May be useful on anterior teeth where there are deep pockets and or recession.

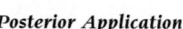

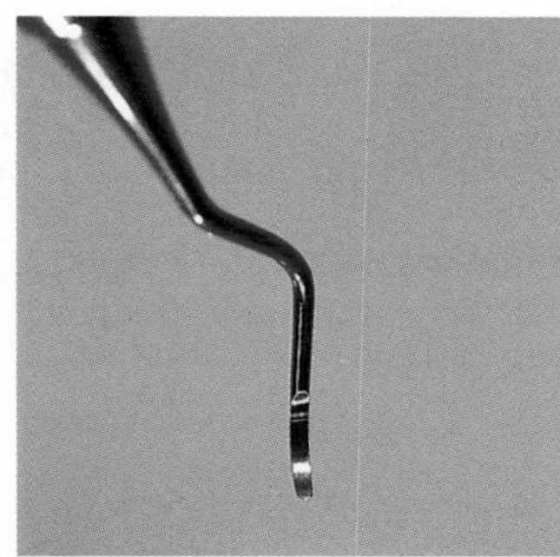

FIGURE 20–29 ✦ Both cutting edges of a universal curet blade are parallel and curved upward toward the toe of the blade.

Procedure 20–6 USE OF THE UNIVERSAL CURET

EQUIPMENT
Universal curet
Subgingival explorer
Mouth mirror

STEPS	RATIONALE
1. Begin with Basic Positioning in Procedure 20–1.	Allows for ergonomic practice and the prevention of repetitive stress injuries.
SELECTING CORRECT WORKING END	
2a. See Table 20–11 to determine anterior versus posterior instrument usage.	
2b. Posterior instrument end selection is simple if the clinician first positions the blade against the buccal surface. Choose the end that offers a more closed adaptation to the tooth. This same end is used on the mesial and distal surface from the buccal aspect.	Correct blade selection avoids excessive hard and soft tissue trauma and allows instrument to reach base of periodontal pocket.
2c. Follow this same rule for the lingual aspect.	
2d. For anterior instrument end selection, select either end of the universal curet.	Blade selection of anterior areas is based on thickness of instrument blade, tightness of tissue, pocket depth, and amount of calculus present.
GRASP	
3a. Use a moderate modified pen grasp. Grasp should be secure but responsive to changes during calculus removal and root topography such as line angles and concavities.	Maximizes tactile sensitivity.
3b. Roll handle of instrument around convexities and into concavities with fluid motion.	A moderate grasp (versus a heavy grasp) responds better to the anatomy of calculus and root structure(s), which is important for skillful scaling and root planing.
FULCRUM AND FULCRUM PRESSURE	
4. Use stable, moderate fulcrum pressure during working stroke. Fulcrum placement: Intraoral near the tooth being scaled Cross arch Opposite arch Extraoral	Allows cutting edge and tip to be well adapted to tooth surface. Maximizes stability. Fulcrum position may be raised, lowered, tilted during calculus removal.
INSERTION, ADAPTATION, AND ANGULATION	
5a. Insert blade in a relatively closed position to base of pocket.	Correct blade selection and subsequent insertion avoid excessive soft tissue trauma.
5b. Adapt blade of instrument to tooth surface using tactile sensations to feel that the first 2–3 mm are positioned against tooth surface.	Correct alignment of shank in posterior areas allows vertical access and instrumentation of deep subgingival depths. Correct blade adaptation of lower 1/3 of blade is critical to efficient scaling and root planing. Incorrect blade adaptation may cause slippage and trauma to the tooth or sulcular soft tissue.
5c. Open angulation to between 45 and 90 degrees.	An opened angulation achieves an effective working stroke that does not burnish calculus.
ACTIVATION, PRESSURE, AND DIRECTION OF STROKE	
6a. Resecure grasp and fulcrum to achieve an effective working stroke activated initially in a pulling, vertical direction.	Increased grasp and fulcrum pressure during the working stroke is needed to increase the force of the blade against calculus.
6b. Modify pressure against tooth by the type, amount, and position of calculus and/or root irregularity.	Generally, light calculus requires light pressure, whereas heavy, tenacious calculus requires increased pressure. Pressure during root planing is modulated by the degree of roughness and the changes that are occurring during instrumentation.
6c. Following a series of vertical strokes, use a variety of stroke directions (oblique, horizontal) to complete calculus removal and root planing.	Stroke variety ensures consistent root coverage.

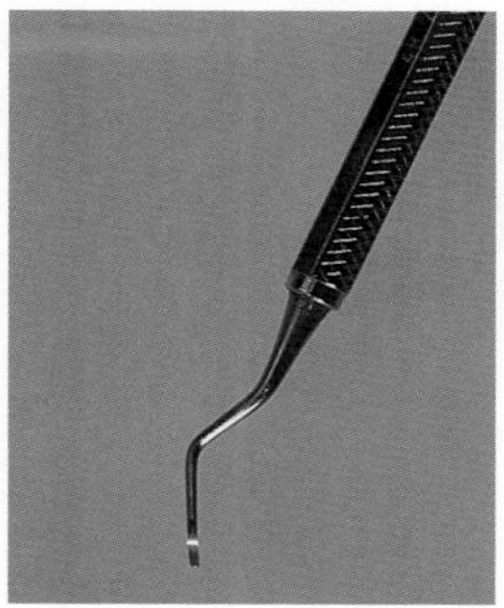

FIGURE 20–30 ✦ The handle of the universal curet is not parallel with the lower shank.

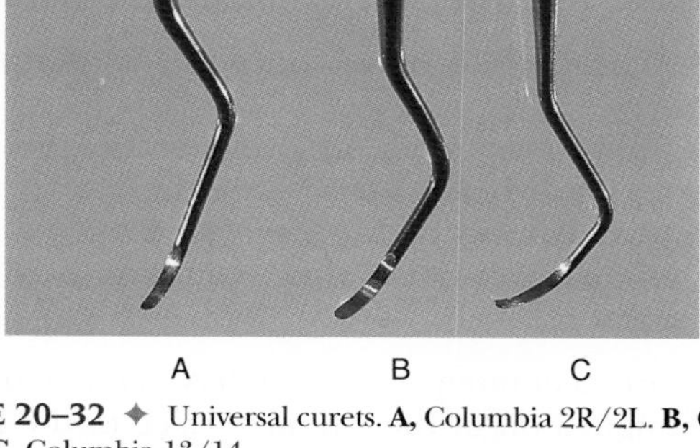

FIGURE 20–32 ✦ Universal curets. **A,** Columbia 2R/2L. **B,** Columbia 4R/4L. **C,** Columbia 13/14.

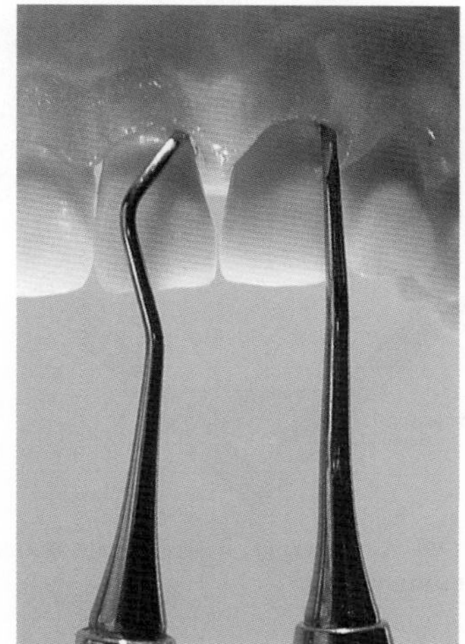

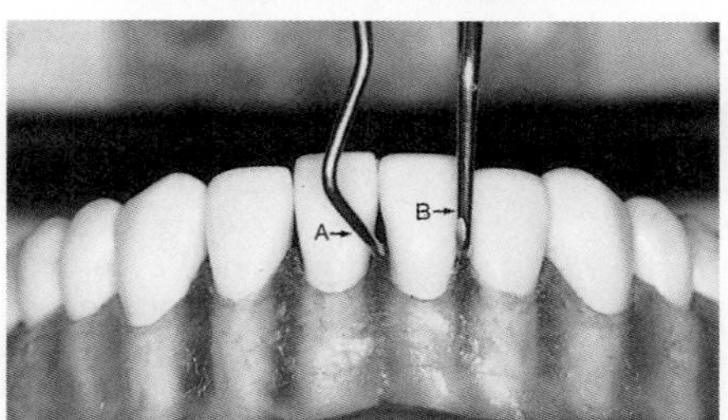

FIGURE 20–31 ✦ To close angulation with the universal curet *(A)*, the handle is tilted toward the tooth surface more than is necessary with the Gracey curet *(B)*. This angulation is due to the differences in the relationships of the faces of the blades and the lower shanks of the two instruments.

instrument works well in anterior areas or in areas with slight to moderate probing depths, and is often paired with the Columbia 4R/4L for use in deeper, more posterior areas. The Columbia 2R/2L is even longer than the Columbia 4R/4L and is ideal in areas of deep facial or lingual pocket depth (Figure 20–32).

BLADE SELECTION FOR POSTERIOR TEETH. Because the ends of a double-ended universal curet or paired universal curets are mirror images, they are used in the same manner but for mirror-image surfaces. This application is especially true in posterior regions. If, for example, one end is used for the distal interproximal surface from the facial surface, then the opposite end is used for the mesial interproximal surface from the lingual aspect. The end that works best for the straight facial aspect is the same end used for the mesial surface. The end that works best for the straight lingual aspect is the same end used again for the mesial aspect from the lingual surface. Therefore, the working ends of the universal curet are not the same for the facial and lingual surfaces in posterior areas.

Blade Selection for Anterior Teeth. In anterior areas, the correct side of the instrument is not so critical. Both cutting edges of the universal curet blade may be used for scaling and root planing in anterior areas. Only the angulation or the degree to which the blade is open is different from one end to the other when the ends of the instrument are exchanged. The cutting edge that offers a more open angulation is better for traction and reduces calculus burnishing. However, the type of tissue is a major consideration in selecting the cutting edge for anterior scaling. If the tissue is tight and fibrotic and the pocket depth very shallow, the dental hygienist should choose the cutting edge that offers a closer blade angulation to the tooth surface. If the tissue is loose, the cutting edge that offers a more open angulation, better traction, and less burnishing action is a better choice because there is less chance of inadvertent soft tissue curettage against the wall of the pocket with the opposite cutting edge.

Curet Selection. Because the curets are critically important instruments in scaling and root planing, the dental hygienist needs to select the best instruments made from many different manufacturers. The universal curets are made in several varieties of metals, each with specific strengths and weaknesses (see the section on the working end in this chapter). The shank strength and thickness of the blade when new are also factors to consider in instrument selection.

The practitioner uses a modified pen grasp and selects an intraoral or extraoral fulcrum based on the techniques used in customizing the stroke to a particular tooth surface. Basically, the more periodontally involved the tooth, the more the dental hygienist will find the need to fulcrum away from the working site. A working stroke is initiated in a vertical, horizontal, or oblique direction.

SHARPENING TECHNIQUES. A curet has lost sharpness if:

- ✦ Tactile sensitivity decreases during light root planing strokes.
- ✦ It does not grasp tooth structure unless the practitioner uses inordinate lateral pressure.
- ✦ Its angulation must be further closed for the instrument to maintain a working relationship with the tooth surface.

The more accurately the curet has been sharpened (i.e., the angulation of the lateral surface to the face of the blade is correct and a definite cutting edge has been established), the longer the curet remains sharp. Thus, accurate sharpening lengthens the time interval between sharpening and thus preserves the metal. Because the cutting edge of the universal curet is two-sided and includes the rounded toe, the method for sharpening this curet includes all of these areas. It is recommended, however, that the toe of the universal curet be preserved as long as possible because the toe itself is not usually used in instrumentation except occasionally under the floor of furcations or under tooth contacts. When the toe is sharpened each time the lateral surfaces are sharpened, there is unnecessary reduction of the length of the blade, eventually making the instrument inaccessible to interproximal areas. Both sides of the blade should be sharpened if dull.

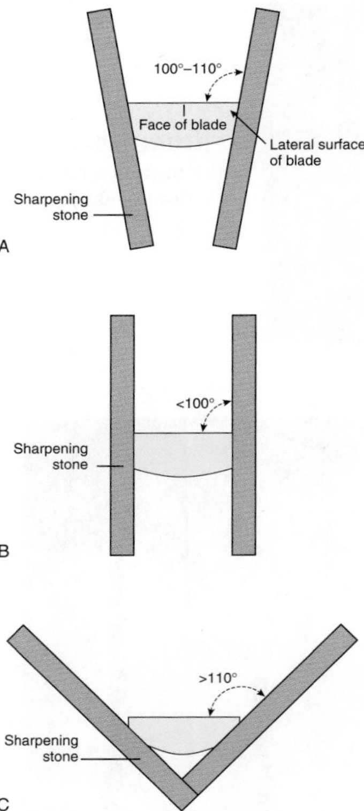

FIGURE 20–33 ✦ **A,** Correct instrument sharpening. **B** and **C,** Common sharpening errors.

Sharpening the Lateral Sides. The universal curet may be sharpened in two ways:

- ✦ Moving the instrument over the stone requires the stone to be placed on a stable surface such as a tabletop, the curet held in a modified pen grasp, angulation of the face to the surface of the stone positioned between 100 and 110 degrees, and the curet blade moved at this angulation from the lower third of the blade to the midline of the toe. Each side of the universal curet blade is sharpened as needed.
- ✦ Moving the stone over the blade requires the stone to be held in the dominant hand and the instrument held with a palm–thumb grasp secured against a firm surface (tabletop) or the elbow drawn close to the body for support. The instrument is held with the face of the blade parallel to the floor and the stone positioned on the lateral surface at a 100- to 110-degree angle. The stone is moved with short, light to firm vertical strokes, depending on the amount of sharpening needed, and is slowly passed across the entire cutting edge at consistent angulation. It is important to maintain consistent angulation for an evenly sharpened blade. To do this, the stone should not be lifted from the blade; both the upward and downward stroke are used for sharpening. Even pressure should be used along the cutting edge to prevent changing the normal shape of a curet blade.

Figure 20–33 illustrates the cross-sectional views of curet blades resulting from common sharpening errors. The most common error is to increase the pressure as the stroke nears the toe, producing a blade with converging lateral sides connected by a point instead of parallel lateral sides connected by a rounded toe (Figure 20–34). The method of moving the stone over the instrument is slightly easier than moving the instrument because as the stone is moved, a light film of lubricant and/or sharpening byproducts (sludge) accumulate on the surface of the face, and angulation of lateral surface to stone is easier to visualize. The last stroke(s) should be in a downward motion toward the back of the instrument to reduce the possibility of a wire edge on the face of the blade. Figure 20–35 compares both methods of sharpening the universal curet.

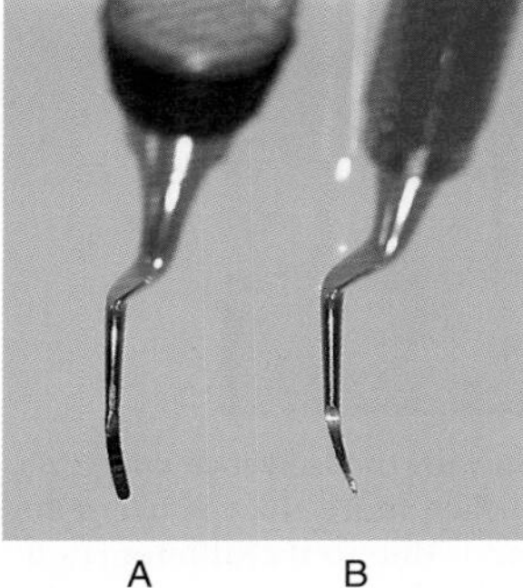

FIGURE 20–34 ✦ **A,** Parallel lateral cutting edge of a Gracey curet 7/8. **B,** Converging lateral cutting edge due to too heavy pressure of the sharpening stone near the toe of the blade of a Gracey curet 7/8.

Sharpening the Face. The face of the curet blade may be sharpened with a cone-shaped sharpening stone, the

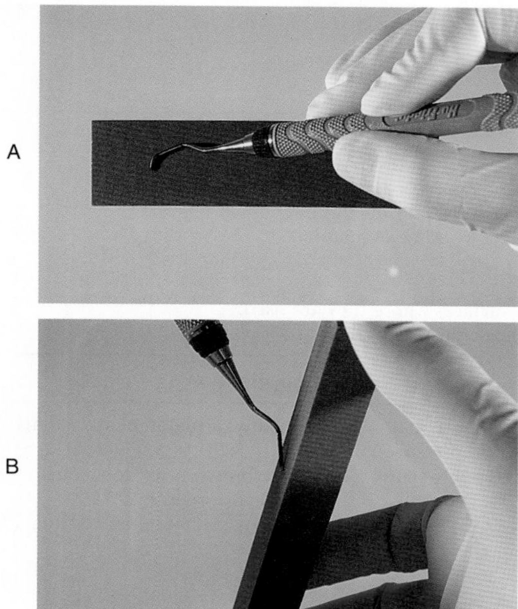

FIGURE 20–35 ✦ **A,** Sharpening by moving instrument over the sharpening stone. **B,** Sharpening by moving sharpening stone over instrument.

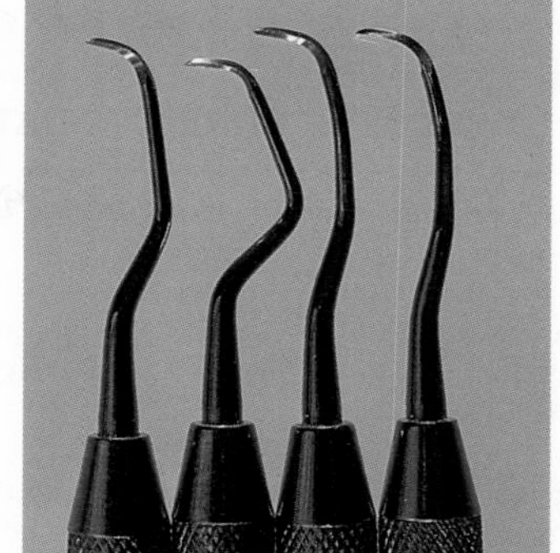

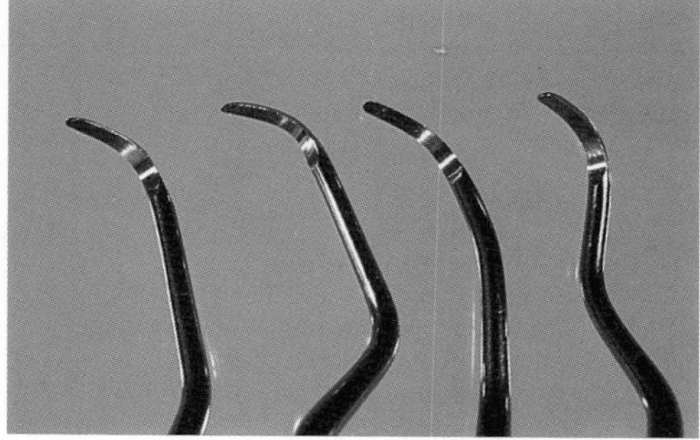

FIGURE 20–36 ✦ Gracey curets 5/6, 7/8, 11/12, and 13/14.

rounded side of a sharpening stone, or a mounted rotary stone. Often these methods produce unreliable results because it is difficult to maintain even pressure across the face. If too much metal is removed (as with the rotary stone) the strength of the blade from face to back is weakened. This dimension from face to back is significant because it is an important factor in providing strength to an instrument that uses a pulling action, as does the curet. When all sharpening has been completed, the instrument is wiped with a 2″ × 2″ gauze square and tested for sharpness.

Area-Specific Curets

DESIGN AND USE. The designation of *area-specific curets* means that each of the instruments in the collection is designed to scale specific areas of the mouth (e.g., anterior versus posterior) and specific tooth surfaces (e.g., mesial versus distal). Gracey curets are particularly effective for instrumenting teeth with slight to severe periodontitis in individuals who require therapeutic scaling and root planing by quadrant or sextant.

Gracey curets consist of nine mirror-image pairs of instruments: the Gracey 1/2, 3/4, 5/6, 7/8, 9/10, 11/12, 13/14, 15/16, and 17/18. Although Gracey curets were designed to be used in designated areas of the mouth (area-specific), it is possible to use Gracey curets in a variety of places. Because of this, dental hygiene educators often provide instruction for full-mouth periodontal instrumentation using a select few of the entire collection. The instruments selected usually represent basic anterior-, posterior-, mesial-, and distal-specific instruments. An example of such a selection is the Gracey 5/6, 7/8, 11/12, and 13/14 (Figure 20–36). Table 20–12 outlines the variations of design in area-specific curets. Table 20–13 summarizes the design of and selection criteria for the use of each of the Gracey area-specific curets. Procedures 20–1 and 20–7 outline the steps for their use.

The basic reason Gracey instruments are ideal for instrumenting periodontitis-affected teeth lies with the relationship of the face of the blade to the lower shank. The Gracey curet is honed so that the face is "offset" or at an angle to the lower shank. (The lower shank is the last bend of the shank closest to the working end.) Whereas the universal curet's face is at 90 degrees, the Gracey curet is at a 60- to 70-degree angle to the lower shank. With this angle of the face to the lower shank, the lower shank is parallel to the tooth surface being scaled when proper angulation of the cutting edge to the tooth surface is achieved. This automatically places the blade against the tooth at a 40-degree angle. Therefore, when using Gracey curets, it is important to observe the relationship of the lower shank to the surface being scaled to help determine if correct angulation is achieved.

Like the universal curet, the Gracey curet has two bladed sides that come together to form a rounded toe. But unlike the universal curet, which has two useful cutting edges because both blades run parallel to each other, the Gracey curet has only one designated cutting edge. The correct cutting edge is determined by examining the curvatures of the blade. The blade of the Gracey curet not only is bent in a curve, but also is bent so that one cutting edge is elongated. This longer curved side of the Gracey curet, as shown in Figure 20–37, is the correct cutting edge. When the lower shank is held perpendicular to the floor with the face of the blade up, this cutting edge is slightly lower than the shorter edge.

TABLE 20–12 AREA-SPECIFIC CURET VARIATIONS

Common Design Specifications of All Area-Specific Curets
Double-ended, mirror-image working ends.
Each blade has two curved cutting edges that end in a rounded toe; however, only one cutting edge per working end is used.
When the lower shank is held vertically, only the lower edge of the blade is identified as the cutting edge.
Face is offset or tilted at approximately 60 to 70 degrees to the lower shank for perfect working angulation.
Cross-sectional view is semicircular.
Back is round.
Shank design varies with each instrument, making them specific to areas and tooth surfaces where they are used.
All Gracey curets may be used for supragingival and subgingival plaque biofilm and calculus removal and root planing.

Variations	Options	Comparisons	Application
Shank strength	Standard	Slight flexion with moderate to heavy instrumentation pressure	Healthy or maintenance clients
	Rigid and extra rigid	Larger, stronger, less-flexible shank	Moderate to heavy tenacious calculus removal
Shank length	Standard	Area specificity allows for deep scaling, root planing, and periodontal debridement	Healthy or maintenance clients
	Examples by manufacturer: After Five (Hu-Friedy) Extended Gracey (Hartzell)	Terminal shank elongated by 3 mm	Deep periodontal pockets
Blade size	Standard	Offset blade relative to the lower shank, curved upward with a curved blade producing an elongated cutting edge	Healthy to periodontally involved clients
	Examples by manufacturer: Mini Five (Hu-Friedy) Mini-Extended Gracey (Hartzell)	Terminal shank elongated by 3 mm and blade length reduced by 1/2 standard blade	Deep, narrow periodontal pockets and furcations

TABLE 20–13 AREA-SPECIFIC CURET DESIGN AND SELECTION

Instrument		Rationale for Use
A B	***Gracey 1/2***	
	Design	Straight shank in the Gracey 1/2 (A) similar to that of a Gracey 5/6 (B), but shorter.
	Function	Maxillary and mandibular anterior incisors and canines. The shorter shank length limits this instrument to shallower depth than the Gracey 5/6.
A B	***Gracey 3/4***	
	Design	Bent shank in the Gracey 3/4 (A) similar to that of a Gracey 7/8 (B), but shorter
	Function	Maxillary and mandibular anterior incisors and canines. The shorter shank length limits this instrument to shallower depth than the Gracey 7/8.
(See comparison above with Gracey 1/2)	***Gracey 5/6***	
	Design	Similar straight shank as that of a Gracey 1/2, but longer.
	Function	Maxillary and mandibular anterior incisors, canines, and premolars.
(See comparison above with Gracey 3/4)	***Gracey 7/8***	
	Design	Similar shank bend as that of a Gracey 3/4, but longer.
	Function	Maxillary and mandibular anterior incisors, canines, premolars, and molars. Limitations on distals of molars.

TABLE 20–13 AREA-SPECIFIC CURET DESIGN AND SELECTION—CONT'D

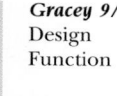

Instrument	Rationale for Use	
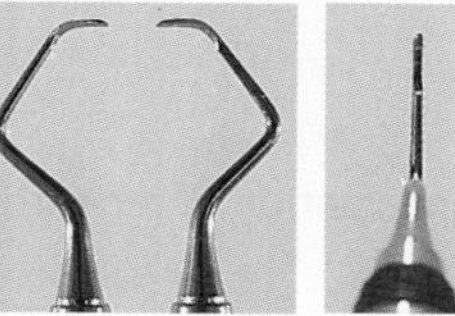 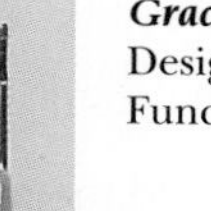	***Gracey 9/10***	
	Design	Shank bend is more pronounced than a Gracey 7/8.
	Function	Maxillary and mandibular molar buccal and lingual surfaces.
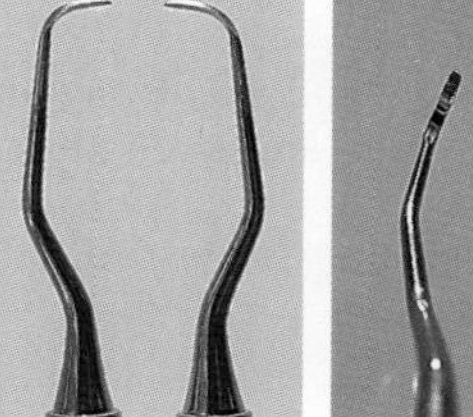	***Gracey 11/12***	
	Design	Shank is slightly angulated at two points for adaptation to mesial surfaces.
	Function	Maxillary and mandibular molar and premolar mesial surfaces.
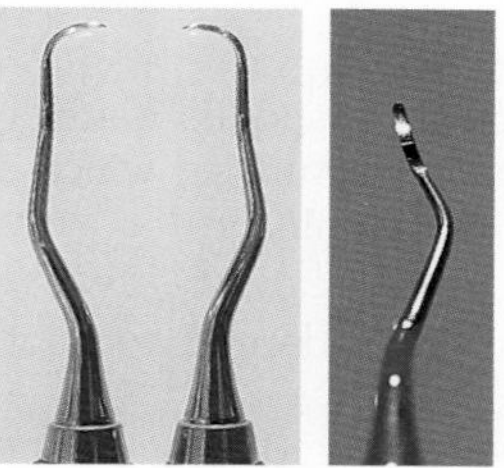	***Gracey 13/14***	
	Design	Shank is angulated for adaptation to distal surfaces.
	Function	Maxillary and mandibular molar and premolar distal surfaces. Using extraoral fulcrums and a variety of operator positions around the client, the clinician also may be able to use the 13/14 in nontraditional areas such as lingual surfaces.
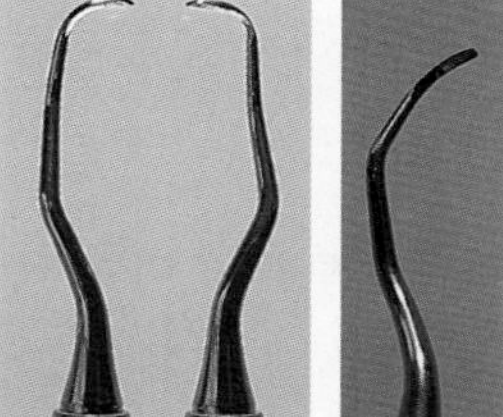	***Gracey 15/16***	
	Design	Same shank angulation as the Gracey 13/14, but nonworking blade is now the cutting edge, thereby positioned to reach mesial posterior surfaces.
	Function	Maxillary and mandibular molar and premolar mesial surfaces.
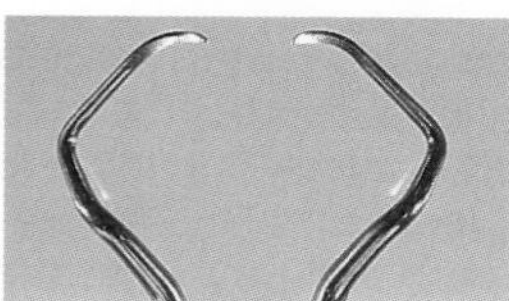 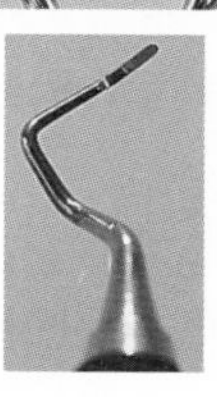 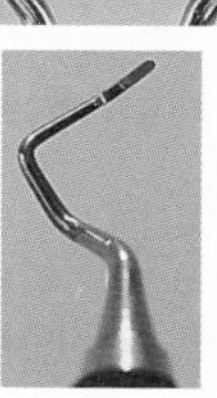	***Gracey 17/18***	
	Design	Accentuated shank angles for access to distal posterior surfaces. Smaller blade and slightly longer terminal shank.
	Function	Maxillary and mandibular molar distal surfaces.

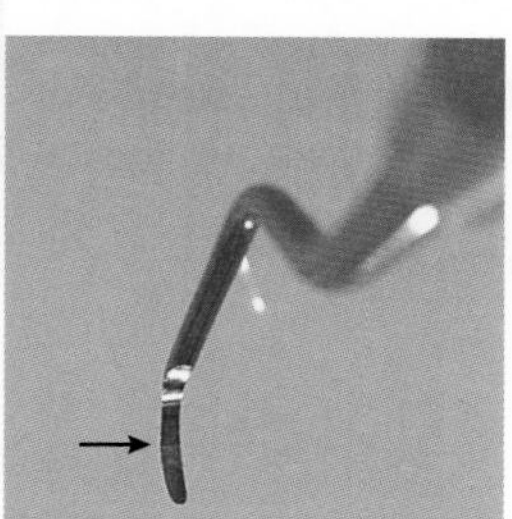

FIGURE 20–37 ✦ The longer curved side of the Gracey curet blade is the cutting edge *(arrow)*.

Together with the basic bend of the blade, this elongation makes Gracey instruments particularly efficient in adapting to root morphology.

Extended-Shank Curets

DESIGN AND USE. In response to the continued challenge of periodontal instrumentation and new knowledge about the value of nonsurgical periodontal therapy, two

Procedure 20–7 USE OF AREA-SPECIFIC CURETS

EQUIPMENT
Area-specific curets, e.g., Gracey curets
Subgingival explorer
Mouth mirror

STEPS	RATIONALE
1. Begin with Basic Positioning in Procedure 20–1.	Allows for ergonomic practice and the prevention of repetitive stress injuries.
SELECTING CORRECT WORKING END	
2. See Table 20–12 for area-specific curet variations. See Table 20–13 for design and selection criteria of area-specific curets.	Area-specific curets are uniquely designed for deep periodontal scaling and root planing. The offset blade, one cutting edge design, and shank angulation require knowledge of specific usage and strengths of each instrument in set. Experienced clinicians traditionally use the Gracey 5/6, 7/8, 11/12, and 13/14 as a basic set.
GRASP	
3a. Use a moderate modified pen grasp. Grasp should be secure but responsive to changes during calculus removal and root topography, such as line angles and concavities.	Maximizes tactile sensitivity.
3b. Grasp allows the handle to roll around convexities and into concavities with fluid motion.	A moderate grasp (versus a heavy grasp) responds better to the anatomy of calculus and root structure(s), which is important for skillful scaling and root planing.
FULCRUM AND FULCRUM PRESSURE	
4. Use stable, moderate fulcrum pressure during working stroke. Fulcrum placement: Intraoral near the tooth being scaled Cross arch Opposite arch Extraoral	Allows cutting edge and tip to be well adapted to tooth surface. Maximizes stability. Fulcrum position may be raised, lowered, tilted during calculus removal.
INSERTION, ADAPTATION, AND ANGULATION	
5a. Select the correct end of curet by positioning the longer, lower cutting edge of blade against tooth. (The correct end positions the face of the blade toward the root surface; with a vertical stroke, the lower shank should be parallel to the long axis of the tooth.)	Correct blade selection, alignment, and subsequent insertion.
5b. Insert blade in a relatively closed position to base of pocket.	Avoids excessive soft tissue trauma and allows vertical access and instrumentation of deep subgingival depths.
5c. Adapt blade of instrument to tooth surface using tactile sensations to feel that the first 2–3 mm are positioned against tooth surface.	Correct blade adaptation of lower 1/3 of blade is critical to efficient scaling and root planing. Incorrect blade adaptation may cause slippage on the tooth and trauma to the tooth or sulcular soft tissue.
5d. Open angulation to between 45 and 90 degrees.	Angulation must be opened to achieve an effective working stroke that does not burnish calculus.
ACTIVATION, PRESSURE, AND DIRECTION OF STROKE	
6a. Resecure grasp and fulcrum to achieve an effective working stroke activated initially in a pulling, vertical direction.	Increased grasp and fulcrum pressure during the working stroke are needed to increase force of the blade against calculus.
6b. Modify pressure against tooth by type, amount, and position of calculus and/or root irregularity.	Generally, light calculus requires light pressure, whereas heavy, tenacious calculus requires increased pressure. Pressure during root planing is modulated by the degree of roughness and the changes that are occurring during instrumentation.
6c. Following a series of vertical strokes, use a variety of stroke directions (oblique, horizontal) to complete calculus removal and root planing.	Stroke variety ensures consistent root coverage.

variations of Gracey curets have been introduced: the Gracey extended series and the mini-extended series. The extended series is a modified set of Gracey curets that are exactly like the traditional Gracey curets except that the lower shank of each instrument is 3 mm longer (Figure 20–38). Extended Gracey curets are particularly useful in areas with significant pocket depth or recession. The Hu-Friedy Mfg. Co., Inc. calls its extended Gracey curet the Hu-Friedy After Five and G. Hartzell & Son uses the name Extended Gracey curet. Some manufacturers offer a blade thinned by 10% for ease in gingival insertion and to reduce tissue distention. Because the shanks are longer than those of the traditional Gracey curets, they often require an extended fulcrum such as an opposite arch, cross arch, or extraoral fulcrum. Reinforcement with the nondominant hand often is helpful for additional control.

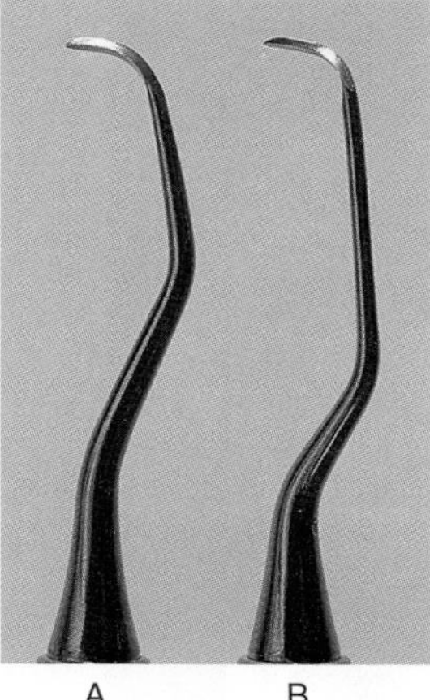

FIGURE 20–38 ✦ **A,** Gracey curet. **B,** Gracey extended series with the elongated shank.

Mini-Bladed Curets

DESIGN AND USE. The second variation of the basic curet is the Gracey mini series of curets, which have a terminal shank that is 3 mm longer than and a working blade that is half the length of the traditional Gracey curet (Figure 20–39). Like the extended-shank curets, each manufacturer labels the mini series differently: the Hu-Friedy Mfg. Co., Inc. calls their mini Gracey curet the Hu-Friedy Mini-Five and G. Hartzell & Son uses the name Mini-extended Gracey curet. The mini-bladed Gracey curet is particularly useful in areas of narrow, deep pocketing in which it is impossible to vertically insert a long, regular blade straight down into the pocket or vertically instrument interradicular root surfaces of furcations. The options for the dental hygienist in these situations are to use a horizontal stroke with the toe directed to the junctional epithelium or to use a shortened instrument such as the mini series with a vertical stroke. This instrument is also used in rounded convexities or concavities found going into and out of root depressions and around line angles.

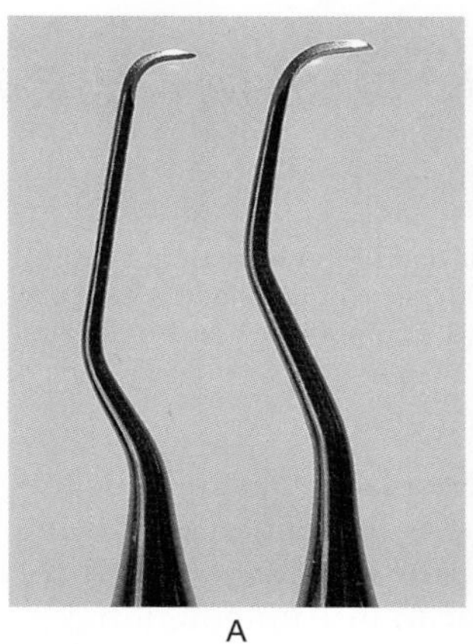

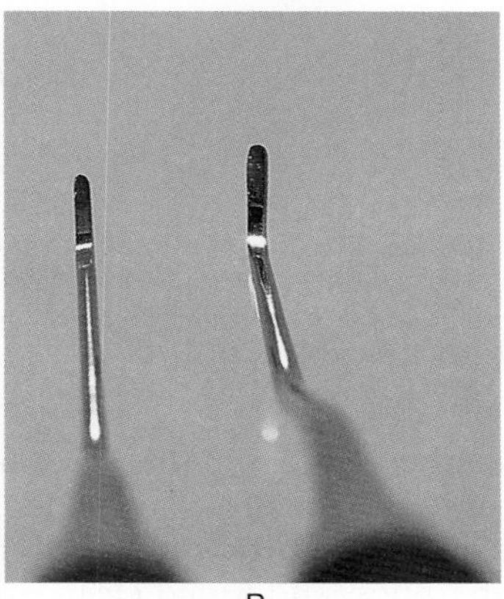

FIGURE 20–39 ✦ **A,** The Mini series with a shorter working blade compared with the traditional Gracey curet *(B)*.

Shank Design and Metallurgy

Certain manufacturers make the Gracey curet with a rigid and even extra-rigid strength shank that does not dissipate the power used in a working stroke. This design differentiates the rigid Gracey from the finishing Gracey curet, which has a more flexible shank. The rigid shank is essential when performing heavy scaling and root planing. It is also quite effective when less lateral pressure is required. The rigid shank does not diminish tactile sensitivity. Rather, it enhances control and reduces energy needed to make any direction of stroke under any degree of pressure.

Because the finishing Gracey has a more flexible shank, it bends under pressure. A significant amount of lateral pressure is lost in the flexion that occurs under firm working strokes. Therefore, this instrument is indicated for times when light scaling and root planing are needed.

The basic modified pen grasp and fulcrum placement techniques used with the universal curet are also used with Gracey curets. Instrumentation in deep periodontal defects or when using elongated, specialized Gracey curets requires the use of extended fulcrums and reinforcement scaling techniques.

Sharpening Technique

The major difference between sharpening the Gracey and the universal curet is that the Gracey curet blade is offset. Both instruments may be sharpened with movement of the instrument or the stone. Grasp positions, angulation of 100 to 110 degrees, and movement across the blade are the same for the Gracey and universal curets. The Gracey curet blade face is offset at 60 to 70 degrees to the shank (as opposed to 90 degrees for the universal curet), which opens the angle of the stone on the Gracey when the lower shank of each is held perpendicular to the floor. When the Gracey curet blade face is held parallel with the floor (like the universal curet), the stone is positioned like the universal curet, but the handle and shank of the Gracey curet are tilted away from the stone and not perpendicular to the floor. Figure 20–40 shows a comparison of stone and handle when the faces of a Gracey and a universal curet are held parallel to the floor. On the Gracey curet, only the lower, longer

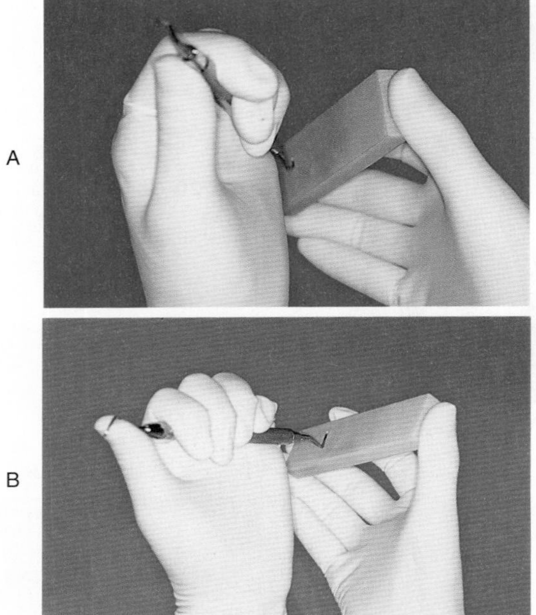

FIGURE 20–40 ✦ Comparison of handle position of a universal curet *(A)* and a Gracey curet *(B)* when the face of the blade is held parallel to the floor for sharpening (from the point of view of the clinician looking down to floor).

cutting edge from the area where blade sharpness begins and occasionally around the toe is sharpened. Following sharpening procedures, the blade should be tested for sharpness and wiped clean prior to instrumentation.

Hoe Scaler

DESIGN AND USE. The *hoe scaler* is used for heavy supragingival calculus removal. Because of design limitations, it is best used in subgingival areas where access is easy, such as facial and lingual surfaces (as opposed to interproximal surfaces), and when tissue tone is loose and edematous. It is not well suited for fine subgingival scaling and root planing.

The hoe scaler may be double-ended or single-ended. The hoe has paired working ends, and a set of four working ends is needed to instrument each tooth surface. Shank length on a hoe may vary from long to short and may also be bowed in a slight or more acute angle (Figure 20–41). These variations in shank length and angle help determine the best areas in which to use the hoe scaler. The longer and more angled the shank is, the better suited the instrument is for posterior areas. The shorter, less acutely angled shank is better suited for anterior areas.

The terminal end of the blade is bent to a 99- to 100-degree angle and the tip is beveled at a 45-degree angle to form a single cutting edge. The upper edge forms the actual cutting edge because the hoe scaler is a pull instrument. The cutting edge is a straight, thick, short blade with two sharp corners on each end. These corners may be rounded with a sharpening stone to prevent grooving or gouging of tooth structure.

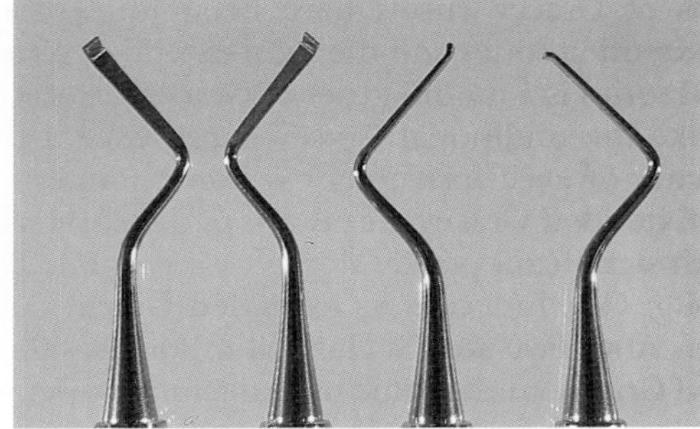

FIGURE 20–41 ✦ Hoe scaler.

When the instrument is inserted subgingivally and the blade is well adapted to the tooth surface, the side of the shank should form a two-point contact with the tooth surface. This improves stability and leverage during instrumentation.

The limitations of the hoe scaler begin with the bow or angle in the shank. This characteristic angle of hoe scalers seriously limits the ability of the dental hygienist to instrument to the base of pocket depth unless the tissue is very loose. The short, straight, bulky blade also poses a problem of adaptation when instrumenting curved root surfaces. Tactile sensitivity also is limited.

The modified pen grasp should be used with the hoe scaler. A fulcrum close to the immediate working area is suggested for maximal control. The cutting edge is positioned under the deposit and a pull stroke in a vertical direction is applied to remove the calculus.

SHARPENING TECHNIQUES. The hoe is sharpened by placing a stationary stone on a tabletop and positioning the entire blade surface on the stone. It is important to maintain the 45-degree bevel. The instrument is held with a modified pen grasp and stabilized with a fulcrum on the stone. Movement of the instrument across the stone is made in short, moderate pull strokes. A push-pull or grinding stroke is not recommended. The corners at each cutting edge are occasionally rounded with light rolling strokes to prevent injury to soft tissue and tooth structure. The hoe is tested for sharpness on a testing stick and wiped of debris prior to instrumentation.

File Scaler

DESIGN AND USE. The *file scaler,* which is similar in design to the hoe scaler, is a pull instrument used supragingivally or subgingivally for crushing or breaking up heavy subgingival calculus. It consists of a series of miniature hoe blades on a pad attached to the shank. Each blade is bent at an angle of between 90 and 105 degrees from the shank. Each blade possesses sharp corners that together pose a hazard to tooth structure if adaptation is not maintained during stroke activation. These corners may be slightly rounded with a sharpening stone before the file is used (Figure 20–42).

Roughening up the surface of tenacious, burnished calculus helps to prepare the surface, making it easier for the curet to latch onto to break the piece away from the

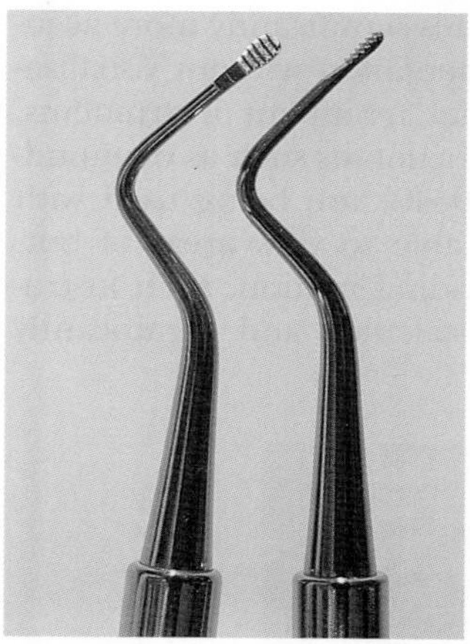

FIGURE 20–42 ✦ File scaler.

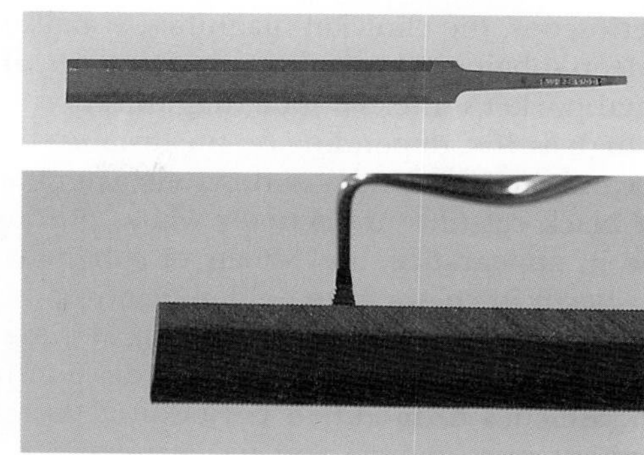

FIGURE 20–43 ✦ A tanged file for sharpening the file.

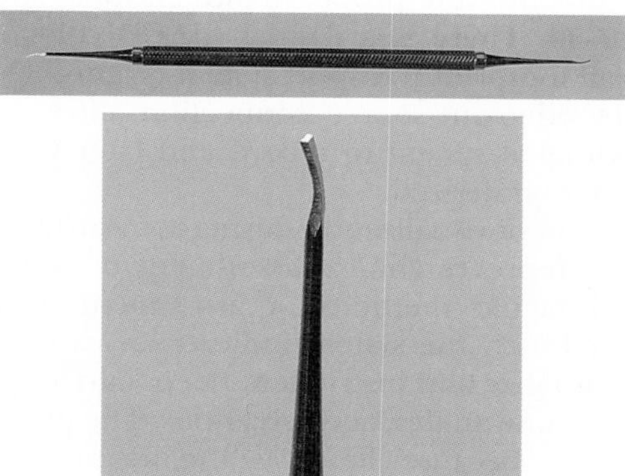

FIGURE 20–44 ✦ Chisel scaler.

tooth. Because this instrument has many of the limitations of the hoe scaler, it should not be used for definitive subgingival scaling and root planing.

The instrument may be double-ended or single-ended. The file has paired ends, and like the hoe, four working ends are needed to instrument each of the four surfaces of a tooth (mesial, distal, facial, and lingual). As with the hoe, the longer, more angled shanks are better suited for posterior areas. The shorter, less angled shanks are better suited for anterior areas. The shank of the file is fairly rigid, which is advantageous when applying pressure against the tooth.

The pad or base of the working end of the file may come in a variety of shapes (round, oval, or rectangular) and in numerous sizes, depending on the manufacturer. It is obvious that the larger the base, the more difficult it becomes in adapting to rounded root surfaces. The size, adaptation, and bend of the shank create problems for working in interproximal areas. Like the hoe, the easiest areas are the facial and lingual surfaces and mesial and distal surfaces where there are no contacts. Loose, edematous tissue is necessary for reaching areas close to the base of the pocket.

The modified pen grasp should be used with the file scaler with a fulcrum close to the immediate working area and the entire series of blades positioned against tooth surface.

SHARPENING TECHNIQUES. The file is a difficult instrument to sharpen because of the miniature size of each blade. Sharpening may be accomplished with a tanged file sharpener positioned against each small, flat-bladed surface (Figure 20–43). To begin the sharpening procedure, the instrument is stabilized on a firm surface (tabletop) and the practitioner stabilizes the working hand near the instrument on the tabletop to perform light, short, push-pull strokes across each blade. Consistently good results are difficult to achieve when sharpening this instrument.

Chisel Scalers

DESIGN AND USE. The *chisel scaler* is a double-ended instrument with either a straight or a curved shank. The blade is continuous with the shank, and the narrow cutting edge is formed with the tip beveled at a 45-degree angle (Figure 20–44). This instrument should be used only on heavy interproximal ledges of calculus, especially on lower anterior teeth. It should not be used for scaling and root planing procedures. The chisel is very limited and is not often used by dental hygienists because of the better versatility and advantages of other scaling instruments.

The chisel scaler is a push instrument. To avoid unnecessary trauma to soft tissues, it should be used only in a horizontal direction. The instrument should be stabilized against a tooth structure and used with a pushing motion to dislodge heavy interproximal, facial, and lingual calculus from mandibular anterior teeth. Because the corners of the chisel are sharp, care should be taken to keep the blade evenly on tooth structures during stroke activation. A modified pen grasp with an intraoral fulcrum close to the working area aids the practitioner in stabilizing this instrument. Sharpening objectives and procedures for the chisel scaler are similar to those for the hoe scaler.

DENTAL PERIOSCOPY

Fiberoptic imaging of the periodontal pocket, called *dental perioscopy*, allows subgingival visualization for diagnosis as well as treatment (DentalView Perioscopy). Using dental perioscopy, the clinician magnifies, visualizes, and accesses deep subgingival calculus, root fractures, and the periodontal pocket's internal wall. Magnification is from 24× to as high as 46×, depending on the distance between the object and the lens. Under endoscopic magnification, ledges of black calculus are actually white, porous, and crystalline in appearance, and sheets of subgingival calculus may occur in colors from golden brown to black.

The system is composed of a disposable sterile sheath that houses a fiberoptic endoscope, provides continuous irrigation, attaches to modified periodontal assessment and treatment instruments, and has a metal soft tissue shield that keeps the soft tissue away from the tube (Figure 20–45). The actual size of the hand-held sheath and instrument with proper hand grasp is shown in Figure 20–46. There is a flat-panel LCD color display, and a small footprint transport system (Figure 20–47). A composite video-out source connection allows users to employ a digital system to record and later view endoscopic images if desired.

This system of visualization during root surface instrumentation improves clinical assessment of results over traditional tactile methods of assessment. Clinicians experienced with the system indicate an extraordinary ability to visualize and instrument deep, narrow pockets, depressions, line angles, and furcations. The process also is educational, because clients see the intricacies of their disease and treatment on the monitor, and judge the effectiveness of oral self-care procedures. Figure 20–48 illustrates a cross-sectional view of the endoscope in place subgingivally.

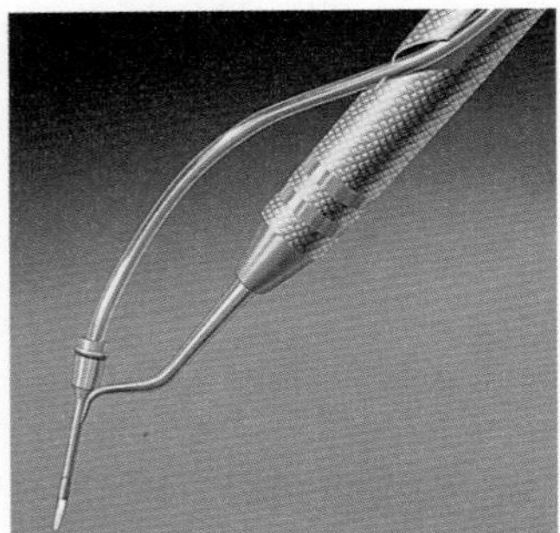

FIGURE 20–45 ✦ The endoscope explorer with sheath and fiberoptic bundle in the "thistle" adapter. *(Courtesy DentalView Inc., Irvine, Calif.)*

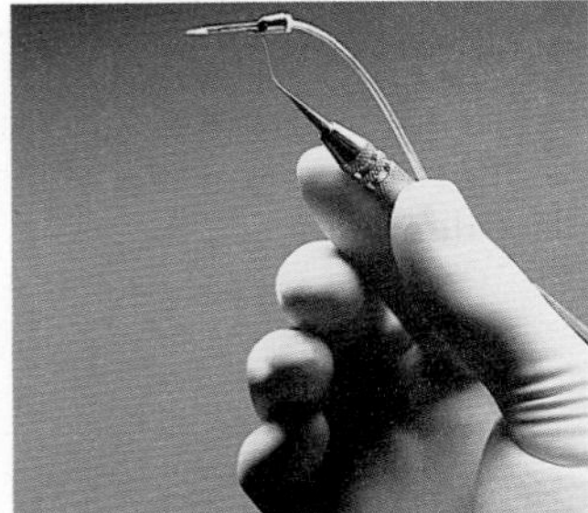

FIGURE 20–46 ✦ Proper grasp for the endoscope explorer. *(Courtesy DentalView Inc., Irvine, Calif.)*

Periodontal instrumentation is significantly more accurate and specific than instrumentation without visualization. In addition to traditional treatment instruments, nontraditional periodontal instruments such as diamond-coated instruments (Figure 20–49) are being used with success when the clinician is able to view areas of burnished calculus. Used in a sanding motion, such instruments remove flat, smooth calculus and significantly

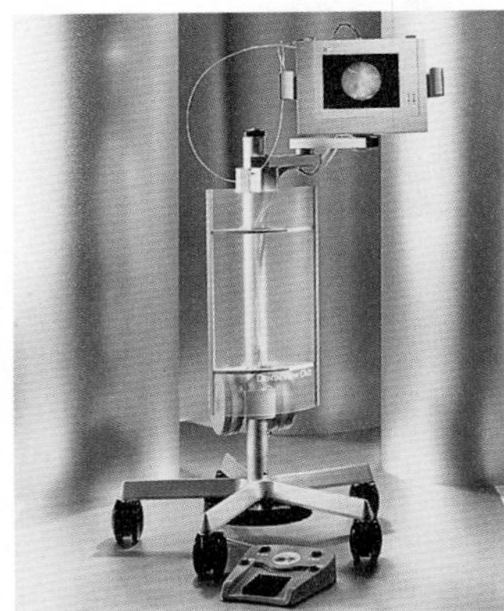

FIGURE 20–47 ✦ The DentalView 2 endoscope with an image of the subgingival sulcus on the monitor screen. *(Courtesy DentalView Inc., Irvine, Calif.)*

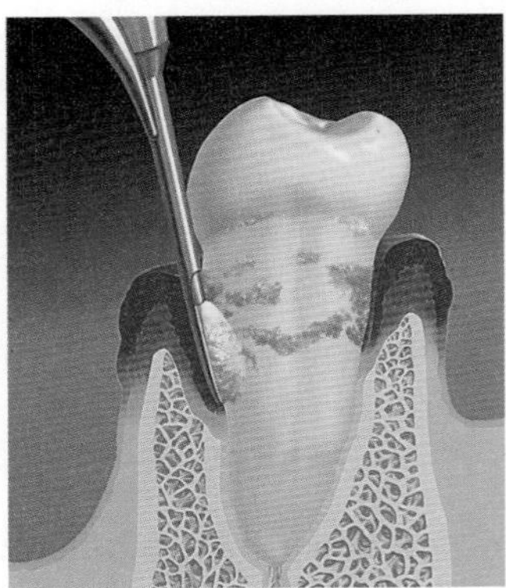

FIGURE 20–48 ✦ Diagrammatic illustration of the endoscope's explorer examining the subgingival root surface and calculus deposits. *(Courtesy DentalView Inc., Irvine, Calif.)*

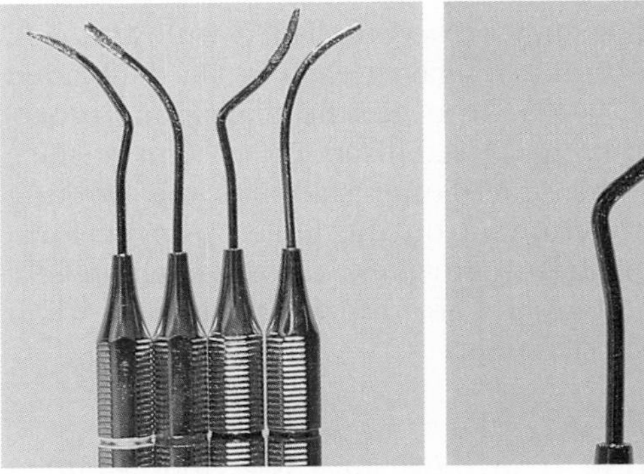

FIGURE 20–49 ✦ Brassler diamond-coated instruments.

reduce root over-instrumentation that might have resulted with curet use. Even with visualization, successful instrumentation is still dependent on the clinician's ability to use a variety of fulcrums, stroke directions, and periodontal instruments.

REPETITIVE STRAIN INJURIES

The dental hygienist uses protective strategies of positioning and instrumentation to prevent or lessen risk of injury (see Chapter 8, section on repetitive strain injuries). The term "protective scaling" (established by Tsutsui) denotes operator and client positioning, fulcrums, and reinforcements that seek to minimize practitioner injury (see Procedure 20–8). Protective techniques of operator and client positioning and instrumentation offer viable solutions to the problems of occupational injury to dental hygienists.

To reduce the possibility of developing repetitive strain injuries, the dental hygienist must look at the ergonomics of the work environment—beginning with basic operator positioning, client positioning, grasp, and fulcrum—and monitor the effects of instrumentation on practitioner hand, wrist, elbow, shoulder, and back movements (Table 20–14 and Figure 8–2). Self-evaluation may be

Procedure 20–8 BASIC OPERATOR POSITIONING STRATEGIES OF PROTECTIVE SCALING

EQUIPMENT

Ergonomically designed dental chair, equipment, and operator chair

STEPS	RATIONALE
1. Position self comfortably in chair with weight distributed evenly on the seat. 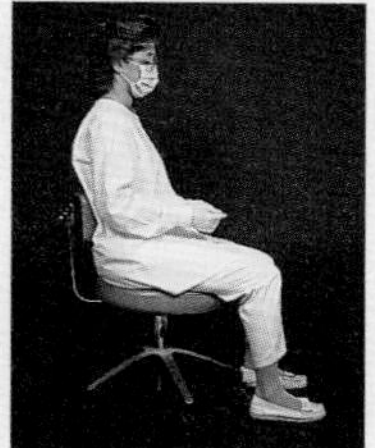	Dental operator chairs are small and tip over or move if operator's weight is not evenly distributed over the seat. Safe, effective periodontal instrumentation requires a balanced body.
2. Lower back should be straight but does not have to be against the back of the seat. At times, when speaking with the client (e.g., reviewing the health history) or if a moment of relaxation is required, the backrest may be used for support.	It is impossible to keep the lower back against the backrest during scaling because it is necessary to lean over the client to distribute body weight over the scaling arm to transfer some of the workload to the upper arm and shoulder. Maintain a straight lower back for much of the time during the appointment. A straight lower back reinforces good postural habits and minimizes possible back injury.
3. Knees should be bent in a sitting position. They should not be crossed or straight.	It is easier to control the movable operator's stool when knees are bent to lessen the chance that the chair will flip out from under the operator. From this position, it is then easier to lean over the client, concentrating more total body effort to control scaling actions. Bent knees are more balanced and allow changes in upper body position at a moment's notice.
4. Legs do not have to be kept together (i.e., they may straddle the chair). Pant dressing is essential. 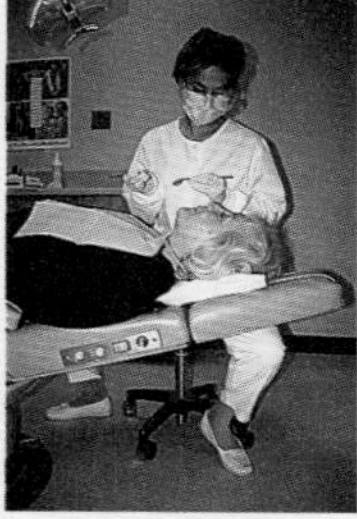	Straddling the client's chair provides better stability when it is necessary to lean over the client.

Continued on following page

Procedure 20–8 BASIC OPERATOR POSITIONING STRATEGIES OF PROTECTIVE SCALING—CONT'D

STEPS	RATIONALE
5. Both feet do not have to be positioned squarely on the floor. Either knee or both knees may be dropped, which changes the foot position to a side or toe placement instead of feet flat on the floor. 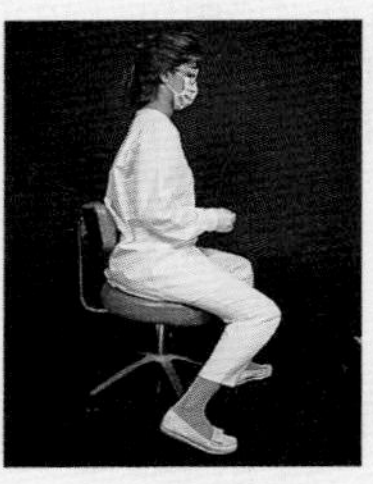	A right-angle knee position limits the ability to position the client's chair in a low supine position. A variety of foot positions allows the clinician to stretch and maintain agility, thereby improving balance throughout the day.
6. The right-handed or left-handed operator may move anywhere from an 8:00 to a 4:00 seated position around the client.	Some areas of the mouth are easier to reach from different angles. Allows clinician to move to positions that are ergonomically sound and safe for both clinician and client.
7. A standing approach is useful in all positions from 8:00 to 4:00. 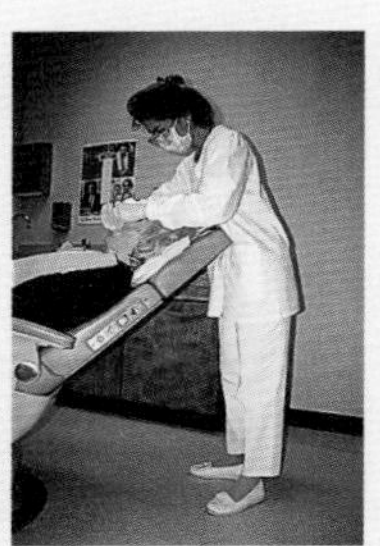	The standing position is easier in some areas of the mouth (e.g., mandibular posterior mesial surfaces) because it allows traction and versatility to move over a client. Clinician may need to perform instrumentation without the risk or need to control a movable stool
8. The standing position is useful when it becomes difficult to see (e.g., in situations where the client is seated slightly upright, the mouth is small, or the client's chair does not drop low enough).	Allows the clinician to reach down and use a pull stroke while keeping the wrist and arm in line with the shoulder.
9. In the standing position, the feet may be positioned squarely on the floor but may lift off onto the ball of the left foot (right-handed clinician) with the right hip leaning against the client's chair. 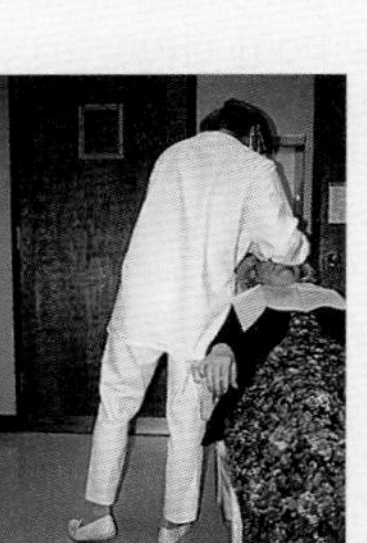	By lifting slightly up on the toes and bracing the lower body against the client's chair, the clinician may lean across the client and work with maximal control.

TABLE 20–14 SELF-EVALUATION OF BASIC OPERATOR TECHNIQUE

Problem	Solution
Did you rely on your legs and feet to stay in your seat at any point during the appointment?	You may have been sitting too close to the edge of seat and even if the chair is designed to prevent tipping, you unnecessarily used your lower body for stability when it may have been more efficient to conserve energy or direct it towards control during scaling.
At the end of the appointment or day of work, straighten your lower back. Does it feel stiff, tight, or sore?	If your back feels tight or achy, you have bent over from the lower back too often for long periods during the day (instead of keeping it straight as often as possible).
Does your right side around the waistline feel sore or stiff?	Indicates a scaling posture that utilizes an excessive leaning position for long periods of time. It would have been better to straddle the chair or stand, lean hip against the chair, and work over the client.
Are your wrist, hand, or fingers and shoulders unusually tired and aching after scaling?	Indicates one or more of the following: Need to change operator from standard 8 to 9 o'clock approach to another angle. Client position too high. Either lower dental chair and/or operator chair or stand during instrumentation. Clinician's body position should have been in better alignment with scaling hand to eliminate exertion at hand and wrist level. Possibility of repetitive strain injury.

done at any time during the instrumentation process. It requires that the practitioner be aware of areas of stress in the working hand, arm, or spine. If it is possible to transfer or equalize the stress of working from the hand and wrist to include the arm or even the shoulder, doing so will minimize occupational injury.

REINFORCEMENT SCALING TECHNIQUES

Reinforcement scaling is used to gain additional stability and control of the instrument when scaling with both the intraoral and extraoral fulcrums.[5] In most cases, reinforcement scaling means that the nondominant hand is used for additional support of the instrument instead of holding the mouth mirror. In some cases (Figure 20–19), it is still possible to hold the mouth mirror and provide reinforcement with the nondominant hand. Reinforcement scaling is protective to the dental hygiene practitioner.

The added support from reinforcement may come from the index finger, thumb, or thenar region (radial palm or fleshy mass on lateral side of palm) of the nondominant hand. The dominant hand must continue to play the major role in adapting and angulating the blade against the tooth surface. It also must exert control over the direction in which the instrument is pulled over the tooth. The benefits of reinforcement include the following:

- ✦ Provides additional lateral pressure in the same direction to which the dominant hand's fingers are directing pressure
- ✦ Guides the instrument in a longer pull stroke when an extended extraoral fulcrum is used

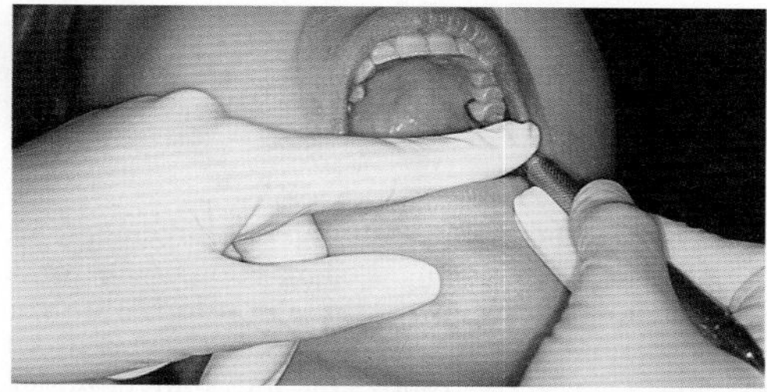

FIGURE 20–50 ✦ Index finger reinforcement. Left maxillary mesial surface from lingual approach. Operator is at the 8:00 to 9:00 position. The Gracey curet 11/12 is being used. Position of the working hand is extraoral fulcrum, palm down. The position of the reinforcement hand shows the index finger on the instrument applying pressure in the same direction of lateral pressure in which the dominant hand is working.

- ✦ Supports the thenar region of the dominant hand, which provides protective qualities during often strenuous and intensive instrumentation processes

The beneficial aspects of reinforcement scaling are found only when the operator uses both intraoral and extraoral fulcrum techniques. Pattison and Pattison have illustrated the index finger and thumb reinforcement on the instrument.[5] Two additional reinforcements are the index finger–thumb reinforcement and thumb-to-thumb (or thenar) reinforcement. The names of the reinforcements tell the operator where the reinforcements originate. The placement of the index finger and thumb may be on or around the instrument between the working end and the dominant hand. The reinforcing thumb also may be positioned against the dominant thumb or thenar region for support and comfort to the operator. Examples of reinforcement scaling in selected areas of the mouth are shown in Figures 20–50 to 20–54.

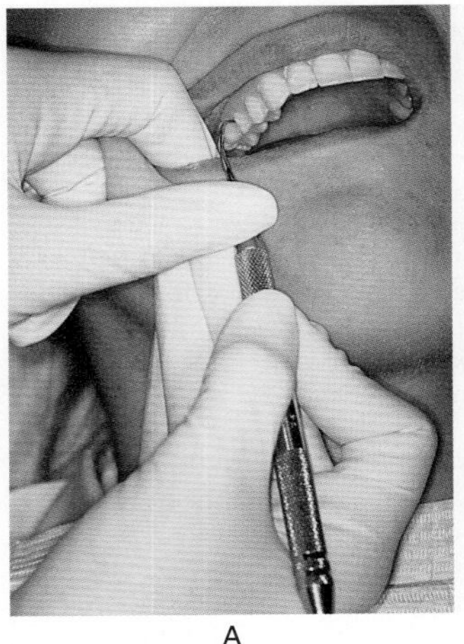

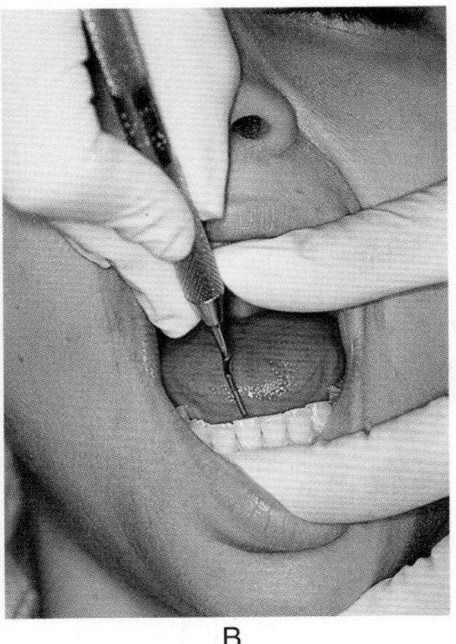

FIGURE 20–51 ✦ Thumb reinforcement. **A,** Right maxillary posterior mesial surface from facial approach. Operator is at the 8:00 to 9:00 position. The Gracey curet 11/12 is being used. Position of the working hand is extraoral fulcrum, palm up. The position of the reinforcement hand shows the index finger retracting buccal mucosa, and the thumb on instrument applying pressure in the same direction of lateral pressure in which the dominant hand is working. **B,** Mandibular anterior lingual interproximal surface. Operator is at the 12:00 position. The Gracey curet 7/8 is being used. Position of the working hand is opposite arch fulcrum. The position of the reinforcement hand shows the index finger retracting the lower lip, and the thumb applying pressure in the same direction of lateral pressure in which the dominant hand is working or supports in upward movement.

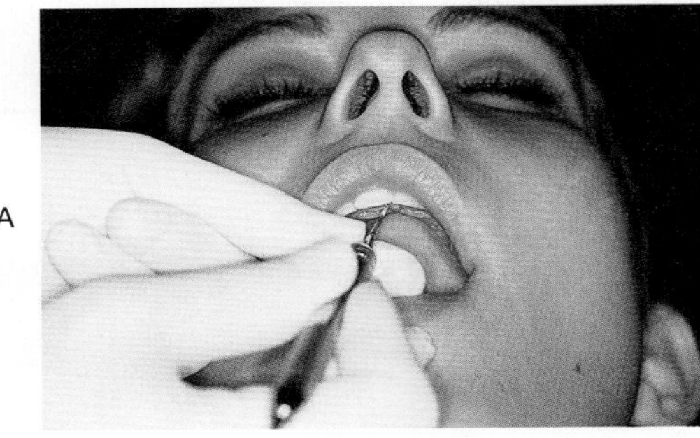

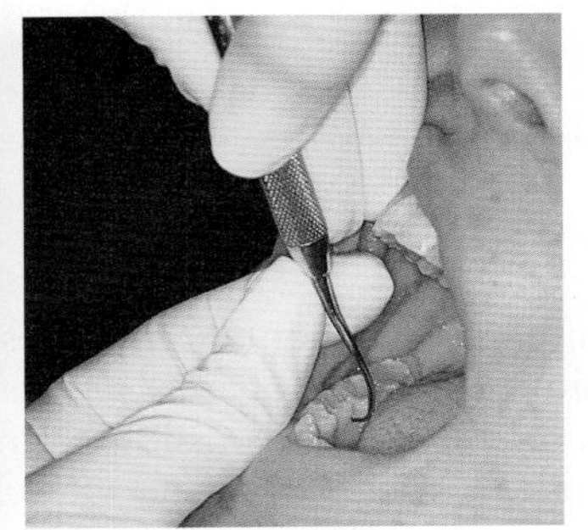

FIGURE 20–52 ✦ Index finger–thumb reinforcement. **A,** Maxillary anterior lingual interproximal surface. Operator is at the 8:00 to 9:00 position. The Gracey curet 5/6 is being used. Position of the working hand is extraoral fulcrum, palm up. The position of the reinforcement hand shows the index finger under instrument, thumb on top of instrument in pinchlike grasp. **B,** Mandibular right posterior mesial surface from lingual approach. Operator is at the 1:00 position. The Gracey curet 11/12 is being used. Position of the working hand is opposite arch fulcrum. The position of the reinforcement hand shows the index finger under the instrument, thumb on top of the instrument in pinchlike grasp.

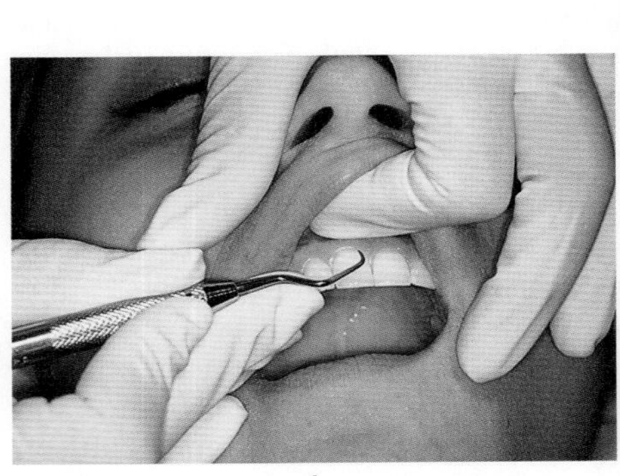

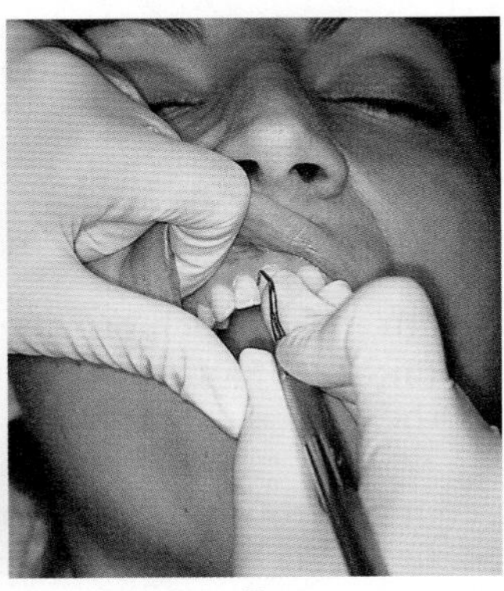

FIGURE 20–53 ✦ Thenar support reinforcement. **A,** Maxillary anterior facial surface from labial approach. Operator is at the 12:00 position. The Gracey curet 7/8 is being used. Position of the working hand is intraoral fulcrum close to working area. Position of the reinforcement hand shows the index finger retracting the lip, and thumb supporting working thumb. **B,** Maxillary anterior interproximal surface from labial approach. Operator is at the 8:00 to 9:00 position. The Gracey curet 7/8 is being used. Position of the working hand is intraoral fulcrum close to the working area. The position of the reinforcement hand shows the index finger retracting the upper lip, and thumb supporting working thumb near thenar area.

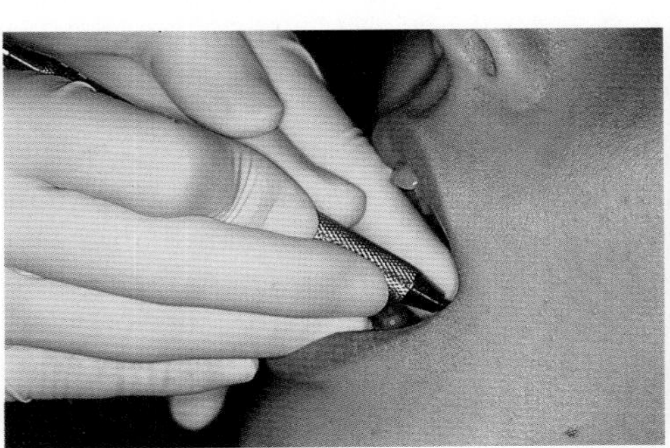

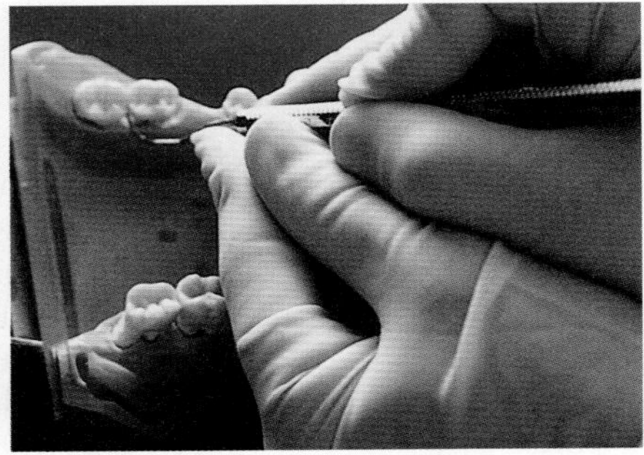

FIGURE 20–54 ✦ Index thenar reinforcement. Mandibular right posterior distal line angle from lingual approach. Operator is at the 8:00 to 9:00 position. The Gracey curet 13/14 is being used. Position of the working hand is fulcrum same quadrant as area being scaled. Position of the reinforcement hand is index finger on instrument, and thumb of reinforcement hand along thumb of working hand.

Client Education Issues

- ✦ Assist clients in visualizing a diseased pocket by using dental perioscopy.
- ✦ Educate clients to visualize health and disease by using a mouth mirror, periodontal probe, and explorer in the client's own mouth while the client observes by looking into a hand mirror.
- ✦ Ensure that clients are aware of the significance of clinical attachment loss and periodontal pocket depths in terms of oral health and disease.

Legal, Ethical, and Safety Issues

- ✦ The dental hygienist uses appropriate instrumentation techniques to safely, efficiently, and effectively treat clients.
- ✦ The dental hygienist manages the work environment to minimize risk of injury to the client, self, and others.
- ✦ The dental hygienist retrieves broken instrument tips and documents such occurrences in the client record. When broken instrument tips cannot be found, a chest x-ray for the client is indicated.

Key Concepts

- ✦ A comfortable, well-designed and functional treatment area is necessary for optimal and safe dental hygiene care.
- ✦ Basic dental hygiene assessment instruments include the mouth mirror, periodontal probe, and explorer.
- ✦ The shape, length, and markings of periodontal probes and explorers vary; selection is dependent on the client's oral disease status and clinician preference.
- ✦ A variety of periodontal hand instruments are available and selection is dependent on function, the client's oral health status, and clinician preference and experience.
- ✦ Variations in periodontal treatment instruments are found in handle size, shape, and pattern.
- ✦ Major classifications in blade design, shape, and size dictate use and effectiveness of periodontal instruments.
- ✦ Small variations in periodontal treatment instruments in shank length, curvature, and flexibility profoundly affect use and effectiveness.
- ✦ A proper grasp and fulcrum placement is essential for safe and effective periodontal instrumentation technique.
- ✦ Excellent periodontal instrumentation technique encompasses a complex set of skills, assessment of relationships, and movements with the goal of performing subgingival scaling and root planing to treat and arrest periodontal disease.
- ✦ Dental perioscopy magnifies the subgingival periodontal pocket for visualizing the area during assessment, instrumentation, and client education.
- ✦ Instrumentation techniques include protective scaling strategies and the application of ergonomic principles as a means of minimizing repetitive strain injuries.

Critical Thinking Exercises

1. Stretch a thick rubber band over a ceramic coffee cup so that it crosses the opening of the cup. Practice using the periodontal probe across the resistance of the rubber band. Do this first with your eyes open, then with your eyes closed.
2. To facilitate the development of tactile sensitivity, take a few monetary coins and practice exploring the relief on the coin with a periodontal explorer designed for calculus detection. Do this first with your eyes open, then with your eyes closed.
3. Apply artificial calculus on models. Practice using a variety of assessment and treatment instruments to simulate the assessment and removal of calculus.

For References, Suggested Readings, and Related Websites, visit

http://evolve.elsevier.com/Darby/hygiene/

Acknowledgments

Instruments generously provided courtesy of Brasseler USA; G. Hartzell & Son; Hu-Friedy Manufacturing Company, Inc.; Florida Probe Corporation; and Premier Dental Products Company.

CHAPTER 21

Root Morphology and Instrumentation Implications

OBJECTIVES

Mastery of the content in this chapter will enable the reader to:

- Identify anatomic landmarks of the roots of permanent teeth
- Discuss significance of root morphology to root surface management
- Compare the contour of the cementoenamel junction on the facial (lingual) and proximal surfaces of anterior and posterior teeth
- Compare the numbers and shapes of the roots of the permanent teeth
- Explain the significance of root concavities and where they are most likely to occur
- Discuss the numbers of roots and furcations of teeth with two and three roots and the challenges this presents to root instrumentation
- Discuss the axial positioning of teeth and its importance in root instrumentation
- Discuss the specific anatomic features of the root(s) of any permanent tooth
- Describe variations in root morphology and their effects on the process of care

KEY TERMS

Accessory roots
Anatomic root
Axial positioning
Cementoenamel junction
Cervical enamel projections
Clinical crown
Concrescence
Dilaceration
Enamel pearls
Furcation
Furcation entrance
Furcation roof
Fused roots
Fusion
Hypercementosis
Interradicular area
Periapex
Periapical foramen
Root apex
Root concavities
Root trunk

ROOT ASSESSMENT

The dental hygienist uses various instruments (i.e., the periodontal probe, Nabers probe, dental perioscope) in assessing the characteristics of the root surface. Radiographs, placed on the viewbox and reviewed prior to and during client care, provide information on root number, root shape, furcation location, bone loss, root alterations, calculus, and defective restorations that may affect instrumentation. Radiographs have limitations because they show only the mesial (M) and distal (D) outlines of a tooth from a facial (F) (lingual [L]) view. The complex root anatomy of maxillary molars (mesiobuccal [MB], distobuccal [DB], L roots) compromises their assessment radiographically.

An anatomically correct model of the dentition with transparent gingiva is helpful for visualizing anatomy of individual roots and their positioning within the alveolar processes. Models and Table 21–1 can be used for review. These aid in the assessment and instrumentation of the roots without displacing the gingiva, injuring the periodontal structures, or damaging the root itself. See Chapter 20 for a review of assessment instruments.

TABLE 21–1 CHARACTERISTICS OF ROOTS

Tooth/teeth	Characteristic
Maxillary Arch	
Central and lateral incisor	One cone-shaped root
	Does not have prominent root concavities; lateral incisor may have a palatoradicular groove
	Prominent CEJ incisal curvature on the proximal surface
	Lingual surface is smaller than facial because of proximal surface convergence
	Cervical cross-section is rounded and triangular in shape; central may have flat mesial outline; lateral is rounder
	Root is one and one third times the length of the crown*
Canine	One long cone-shaped root
	Generally has proximal root concavities; their presence and depth are unpredictable
	Distal crest of curvature in the middle third of the crown may hinder access to the mesial surface of the first premolar
	Cervical cross-section is ovoid in shape
	Root is one and one half times the length of the crown*
First premolar	Two roots (40% have one root)
	Prominent mesial concavity begins on the crown apical to the mesial contact
	Bifurcated in apical third to half
	Elliptical in cervical cross-section; narrow facial and lingual; broad proximally
	Root is one and three fourths times the length of the crown*
Second premolar	One root
	Mesial concavity, but not as pronounced as first premolar
	Elliptical in cross-section; broad proximally
	Root is one and three fourths the length of the crown*
First molar	Three roots: mesiofacial, distofacial, and lingual
	Lingual root is longest, extending beyond lingual surface of crown
	Root concavities may be present on the palatal surface of the lingual root and on the furcal surfaces (furcal concavities)
	MF and DF roots may appear as a "pair," their apices curved toward each other; look like pliers
	Furcations are on the facial, mesial, and distal surfaces and begin gradually before the entrance, which is generally located near the junction of the cervical and middle third of the root; the mesial furcation is located more toward the lingual
	Roots are one and three fourths the length of the crown*
Second molar	Three roots: mesiofacial, distofacial, and lingual
	Roots are closer together and more distally oriented; there is less interradicular area
	Longer root trunk
	Roots are one and three fourths the length of the crown*
Third molar	Varies greatly
	May be three-rooted
	Roots are frequently fused
Mandibular Arch	
Central and lateral incisor	One cone-shaped root
	Proximal root concavities are likely
	Cervical cross-section elliptical in shape; narrow facial and lingual; broad proximally
	Root is one and a half times the length of the crown*
Canine	One cone-shaped root
	Proximal root concavities are present
	In cervical cross-section, oval in shape with small lingual surface
	Occasionally bifurcated into a facial and lingual root in apical third
	Root length is one and a half times the length of the crown*
First premolar†	One cone-shaped root
	In cervical cross-section, may be ovoid or elliptical in shape
	May have a deep proximal root concavity on the distal root surface
	Root is one and two thirds the length of the crown*
Second premolar†	One cone-shaped root
	In cervical cross-section, may be ovoid or elliptical in shape
	Root is one and two thirds the length of the crown*
First molar†	Two roots: mesial and distal; distal is narrower
	Furcations on facial and lingual; concavity before the furcation on F begins just after CEJ
	Short root trunk; larger interradicular area
	Proximal and furcal concavities on mesial root
	Cervical enamel projections (CEPs) may be present
	Roots are one and three fourths the length of the crown*

Table continued on following page

TABLE 21–1 CHARACTERISTICS OF ROOTS—CONT'D

Tooth/teeth	Characteristic
Mandibular Arch—cont'd	
Second molar†	Two roots: mesial and distal Roots are likely to be closer together with a longer root trunk Mesial root concavities are not as prominent CEPs may be present Roots are one and three fourths the length of the crown*
Third molar†	Varies greatly Usually has two roots Roots are short and frequently fused

* Knowing the length of the crown of a tooth is helpful in assessing the length of its root and the amount of attachment. Maxillary central and lateral incisor crowns are the longest in the dentition, being approximately one half inch in length. Anterior crowns are 2 to 3 mm longer than posterior crowns. Roots range from 12 to 17 mm in length; incisor roots are the shortest, and canines are the longest. Proportionally, when comparing the length of roots with their crowns, molars have the longest roots (because of their short crowns), and maxillary incisors have the shortest.

† Crowns of all the mandibular posterior teeth are inclined toward the lingual and may make instrument placement more difficult.

GENERAL MORPHOLOGIC CONSIDERATIONS

Root Terminology

The *anatomic root* of a tooth is that part of the dentin covered by cementum and embedded in the alveolar bone; it begins at the *cementoenamel junction.* The end of the root is called the *apex* and the area surrounding the apex is the *periapex.* At the apex is an opening, the *periapical foramen,* where the blood vessels and nerves enter the pulp (root) canal.

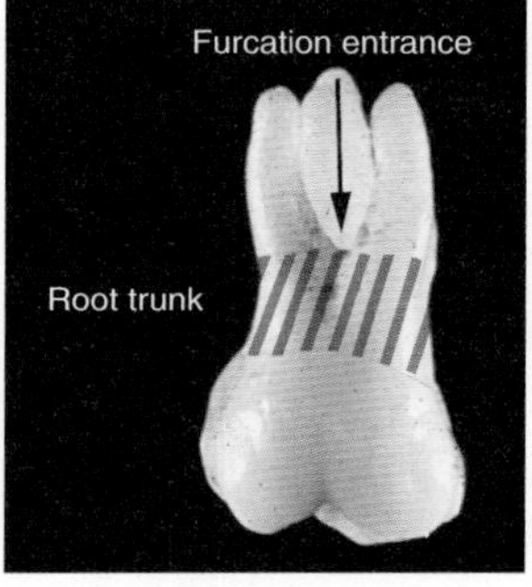

FIGURE 21–1 ✦ Root terminology: root trunk and furcation entrance. *(Courtesy Department of Dental Hygiene, Marquette University.)*

Teeth have one, two, or three roots. Teeth with two or three roots have an unbranched portion called the *root trunk.* The area where the root trunk branches into two roots is the *furcation* or furca. The opening into the furcation is the *furcation entrance* (Figure 21–1). The most coronal portion of the furcation is called the *furcation roof.* Sometimes the furcation roof is more coronal than the furcation entrance. Between the roots of a two- or three-rooted tooth is the interfurcal or *interradicular area.*

When the junctional epithelium has migrated apically and there is attachment loss, portions of the anatomic root are included in the definition of a *clinical crown,* the unattached portion of a tooth. When discussing roots, the concept of thirds is frequently used (i.e., cervical, middle, and apical thirds).

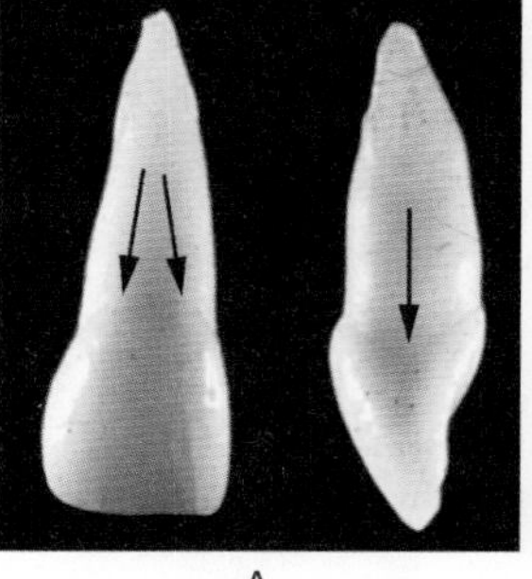

FIGURE 21–2 ✦ Cementoenamel junction contours. **A,** Anterior teeth. **B,** Posterior teeth. *(Courtesy Department of Dental Hygiene, Marquette University.)*

Cementoenamel Junction

The *cementoenamel junction (CEJ)* or cervical line (see Chapter 15) is a structure that the dental hygienist must be able to identify subgingivally with an instrument. A 1993 study of the relationship of the cementum and enamel using scanning electronic microscopy on teeth that had not been exposed to the oral environment showed 76% having an edge-to-edge relationship of the cementum to enamel, and 14% with cementum overlapping the enamel. Ten percent of the teeth, which initially appeared to have a gap between the cementum and enamel, showed a ditch in the cementum with no exposed dentin under high magnification.[1] These findings update the 60% overlap, 30% meets, and 10% gap relationship of cementum to enamel reported in many current texts from a 1917 study.

The curvature of the CEJ differs on anterior and posterior teeth (Figure 21–2). The facial and lingual contours of the CEJ on anterior and premolar teeth are convex. The CEJ curvature on molars is much straighter. Sometimes there is an apical dip, termed a cervical enamel projection (CEP), of the CEJ toward the furcation on molars.

The proximal curvature of the CEJ is much more pronounced on anterior than on posterior teeth. On anterior teeth the curvature is V shaped and prominent on the mesial surfaces of incisors, especially the maxillary central incisor. These areas are particularly difficult to instrument because of limited access and may contribute to incomplete deposit removal.

Root Surface Texture

Surface texture of crowns and roots differs due to the differential degree of mineralization of enamel and cementum (also dentin, which is frequently exposed in root planing) and how it is altered by bacterial plaque biofilm.

The surface texture of enamel (anatomic crown) is analogous to glazed pottery—it is smooth, hard, and glassy when unaltered. The surface texture of cementum (anatomic root) is not as smooth, hard, and glassy, but is more porous. The texture of cementum can be altered by loss of periodontal attachment, plaque by-products, and unintentional injury by the client or clinician. Scaling instruments with pointed tips should not be used on root surfaces. Cementum is intentionally removed in root planing, using ultrasonic instruments and curets to produce a clean, smooth, hard surface conducive to connective tissue reattachment. Sometimes all of the cementum is removed and dentin is exposed. The amount of root planing necessary for promoting periodontal health and tissue reattachment continues to be studied.

Root Shapes

The roots of the permanent teeth vary from one individual to another. The following discussion presents the typical versus normal root morphology, and focuses on the anatomy between the CEJ and mid-root, where most nonsurgical periodontal therapy occurs.

TEETH WITH ONE ROOT. All of the anterior teeth and the maxillary second and mandibular premolars have one root. Characteristics of these teeth include:

- Basically cone shaped with their facial, lingual, and proximal surfaces converging (tapering) apically with different degrees of convergence
- Widest in the cervical third and taper to a small apex
- Show a distal inclination from a facial (lingual) view
- In cervical cross-section (crown cut off the root horizontally at CEJ) are one of these basic shapes (Figure 21–3, *A* and *B*):

  Triangular: Appears to be three-sided with broad (equal) facial, mesial, and distal surfaces and a very narrow lingual surface. The proximal surfaces converge markedly to the lingual (e.g., maxillary central incisors).

  Ovoid: Oval, "egg-shaped," with facial surface broader than lingual and proximal surfaces equal and broader than either facial or lingual (e.g., canines).

  Elliptical: Opposite sides are relatively equal; facial and lingual sides are approximately the same size but smaller than the proximal. Roots are broad FL and narrower MD. The roots of mandibular incisors and maxillary premolars are elliptical in cervical cross-section.

- In mid-root sections shapes of roots are generally the same as in cervical section, though smaller
- Roots that are triangular or ovoid in cross section have smaller lingual than facial surfaces because of proximal surface convergence (taper) toward the lingual
- Cervical cross-section shapes may be altered by the presence of root concavities
- Cervical half of a conical-shaped root has more than 50% of the root surface area because of the convergence of surfaces apically

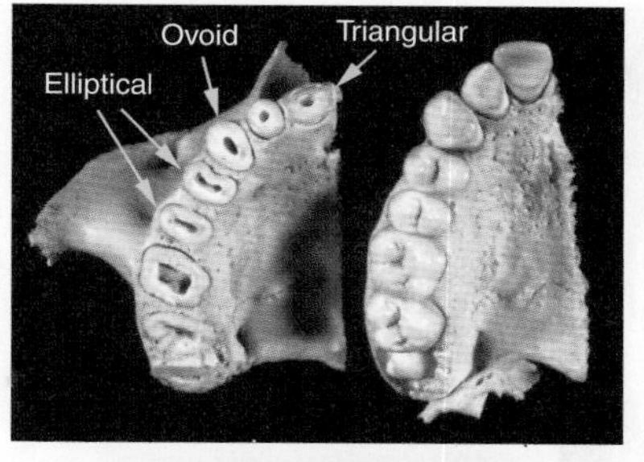

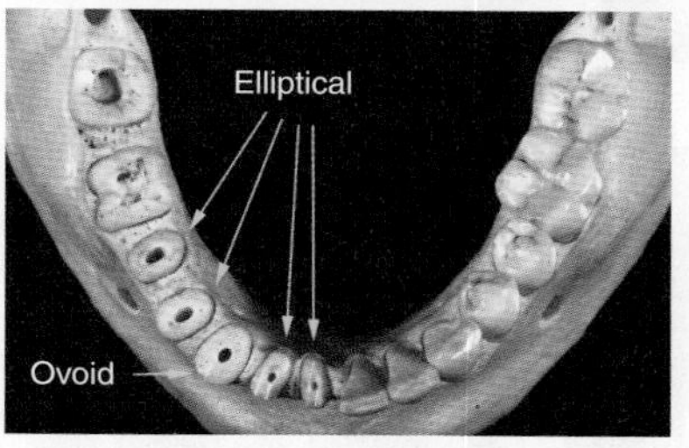

Figure 21–3 ✦ Root shapes in cervical cross-section. **A,** Maxillary teeth: triangular, elliptical, and ovoid. **B,** Mandibular teeth: elliptical and ovoid. *(Courtesy Department of Dental Hygiene, Marquette University.)*

TEETH WITH TWO OR THREE ROOTS. Periodontal assessment and instrumentation on teeth with two or three roots is challenging and time consuming. Posterior teeth are more difficult to reach, and the clinician's competence influences the therapeutic outcome. Characteristics of these teeth are as follows:

- Maxillary first premolars generally have two roots, facial and lingual. Furcations are on the mesial and distal (Figure 21–4).
- Maxillary molars have three roots, mesiobuccal, distobuccal, and lingual. Furcations are on the buccal between the MB and DB root, on the mesial between the MB and lingual root, and on the distal between the DB and lingual root (Figure 21–5).
- Mandibular molars have two roots, mesial and distal. Furcations are on the buccal and lingual surfaces between the mesial and distal roots (Figure 21–6).
- Roots on second molars are more likely to have longer root trunks, be closer together, and have more distal orientation.

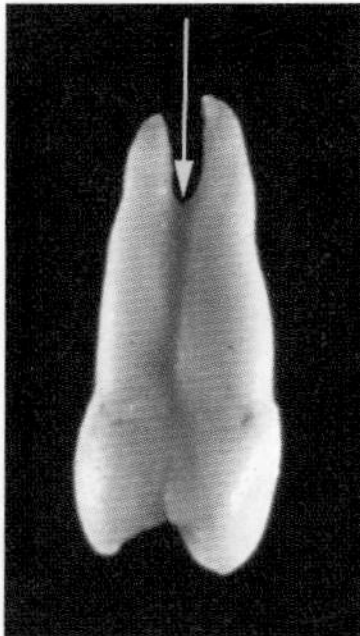

FIGURE 21–4 ✦ Mesial furcation on a maxillary first premolar. *(Courtesy Department of Dental Hygiene, Marquette University.)*

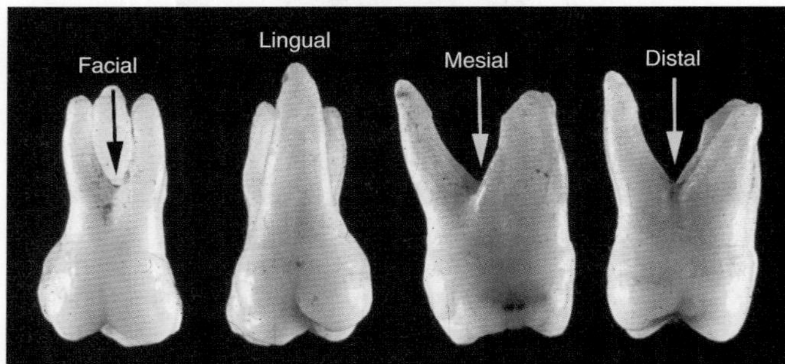

FIGURE 21–5 ✦ Furcations on a maxillary (first) molar. *(Courtesy Department of Dental Hygiene, Marquette University.)*

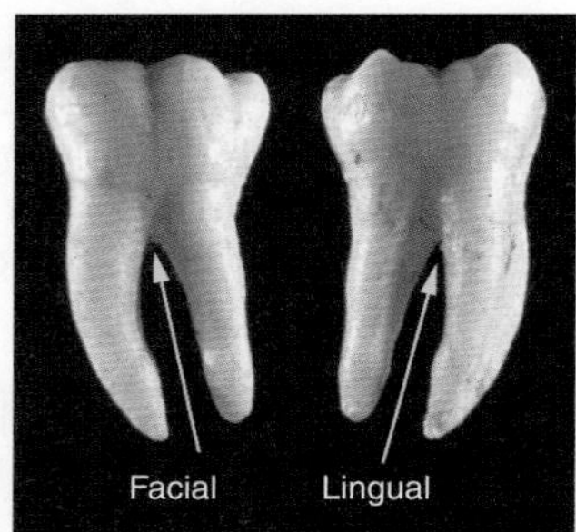

FIGURE 21–6 ✦ Furcations on a mandibular (first) molar. *(Courtesy Department of Dental Hygiene, Marquette University.)*

✦ Therefore, each root of a multirooted tooth needs to be treated individually; a two-rooted tooth is like treating two single-rooted teeth.

Furcations

Furcations generally begin as very narrow openings from a shallow depression on the root trunk. Frequently this opening is too narrow for instruments. The precision thin and furcation inserts for ultrasonic instruments and the mini-bladed curets with smaller and narrower working ends are indispensable to the debridement of the furcation area (see Chapter 23 section on mechanized instruments). A very narrow furcation entrance can be surgically enlarged with burs by a periodontist. Characteristics of furcations are:

✦ The more cervical the furcation, the more stable the tooth because of the divergence (separation) of the roots.

✦ Furcations are generally more cervical on first molars; the root trunk of a first molar is shorter than the root trunk of second or third molars.

✦ Furcations close to the cervical are more likely to become involved with periodontal disease, though access for instrumentation is easier.

✦ Furcation involvement occurs when there is a loss of attachment apical to the furcation

It is important to know the expected location of a furcation in both horizontal ↕ and vertical ↔ directions. In a horizontal direction most furcations are located midway on the root trunk. The mesial furcation of a maxillary first molar is generally located more toward the lingual in a horizontal direction, and therefore instrumentation of the mesial furcation of this tooth is easier from the lingual approach (Figure 21–5).

In a vertical direction, the furcations on a maxillary premolar are in the apical third to half (Figure 21–4). Furcations on a maxillary molar are located near the junction of the cervical and middle thirds of the root (Figure 21–5). Furcations on maxillary second and third molars are more apical. Furcations on a mandibular first molar are apical to the cervical one-fourth of the root, making this the shortest root trunk in the permanent dentition (Figure 21–6). It is also the furcation most likely to experience furcation involvement due to attachment loss to this level and furcation proximity to the CEJ. The furcations on the mandibular second and third molars are more apical than furcations on the first mandibular molar.

R oot Concavities

Root concavities are shallow vertical depressions on the surfaces of the roots. They function to protect the tooth from forces that could rotate it in its alveolus, to provide more root surface area, and to provide direction for periodontal fiber attachment. Root concavities most frequently occur on proximal root surfaces such as *proximal root concavities* (Figure 21–1). The maxillary first molars have a concavity on the palatal surface of their lingual root, called *lingual concavity* (Figure 21–5). Molars may have root concavities on the surface of their root toward the furcation; these are termed *furcal concavities.* A root concavity on the distal surface of the mesial root of the mandibular first molar is a furcal concavity. The presence of root concavities complicates root instrumentation, especially when there are prominent proximal root concavities.

Axial Positioning

For placement of instruments on root surfaces, consider:

✦ Morphology of the individual root
✦ Position of the tooth in the alveolar bone
✦ Encumbrances of the crown
✦ Periodontal status of the client
✦ Size of the arch
✦ Instrument design
✦ Axial positioning

Axial positioning is the relationship of an imaginary vertical line representing the long axis of a tooth in relationship to a horizontal plane. This concept is more easily defined visually than verbally (Figure 21–7). The functions of this positioning are to bring the maxillary and mandibular teeth into an interarch relationship that facilitates incision and mastication and distributes forces throughout the bones of the skull.

Following the vertical lines in Figure 21–7, it is clear that in a faciolingual dimension the roots of all the teeth except the mandibular posteriors have a more lingual inclination than do the crowns. The mandibular posterior crowns are more inclined than the roots that are more facially oriented. Plaque removal in this area is especially difficult for clients.

Again following the vertical lines in Figure 21–7, it is clear that in a mesiodistal dimension the roots of the canines, premolars, and molars have a distal inclination, which is more pronounced posteriorly. The roots of the incisors do not incline distally. See Root Instrumentation Checklist for more information.

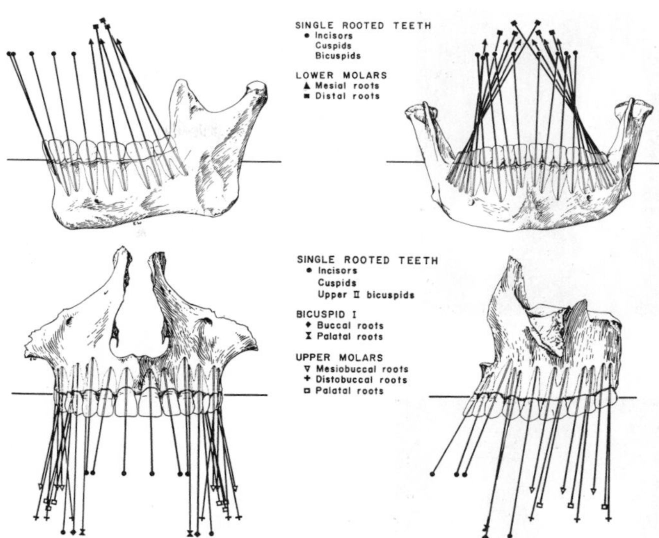

FIGURE 21–7 ✦ Axial positioning of the maxillary and mandibular teeth in an anterior and lateral view. The slant of the roots along their long axis is shown by vertical lines that have been extended to represent the direction of the slant in both faciolingual and mesiodistal directions. *(From Dempster et al:* Journal of the American Dental Association *67:779, 1963.)*

VARIATIONS IN ROOT FORM

Root alterations, anomalies, or abnormalities should be recognized and documented in the dental hygiene care plan. Some variations do not influence periodontal instrumentation but are recorded in the dental chart for subsequent client education.

Fused Roots, Fusion, and Concrescence

Molar roots may be fused together, especially second and third molar roots, and are a result of limited space during tooth development (Figure 21–8). *Fused roots* frequently can be observed on radiographs. Their presence, and the variations that follow, should be noted in the client's record, and instrumentation adapted accordingly.

Teeth may be joined together in an anomaly called *fusion,* in which two tooth buds fuse together during development and form one large tooth with a large crown and a single root that has two pulp canals. This needs to be confirmed by radiographs. *Concrescence* occurs when two teeth become joined by cementum after they have been formed.

Accessory Roots

Accessory roots are extra roots. Sometimes the mandibular permanent canines are bifurcated into facial and lingual roots in the apical third (Figure 21–9). Maxillary first premolars are sometimes seen with three roots—two buccal and one lingual. Buccal roots are very thin, which makes treatment difficult if periodontal disease is present. Third molars sometimes have extra roots. Accessory roots may be assessed via radiographs, recorded on the client's chart, and instrumented if the attachment level is apical to their occurrence.

Root Instrumentation Checklist

Review radiographs	Remove deposits
Probe sulcus depths	Root plane/debride
Identify attachment level	Reassess
Assess root structure	

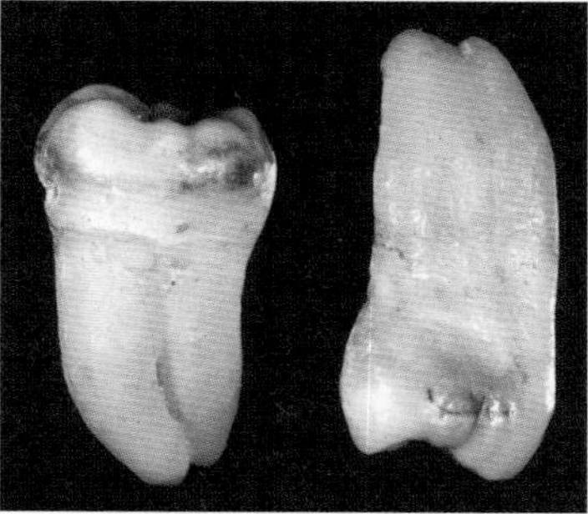

FIGURE 21–8 ✦ Fused roots on a mandibular and maxillary molar. *(Courtesy Department of Dental Hygiene, Marquette University.)*

Hypercementosis

Hypercementosis, the excessive formation of cementum in the apical third to half of the tooth after the tooth has erupted (Figure 21–10), may be caused by trauma, chronic inflammation of the pulp, or metabolic disturbances. It is assessed radiographically and recorded on the client's chart. If areas of hypercementosis are

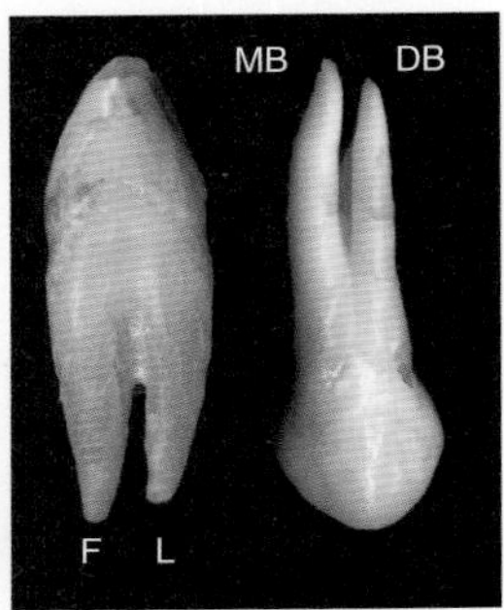

FIGURE 21–9 ✦ Accessory roots on a mandibular canine and maxillary first premolar. *(Courtesy Department of Dental Hygiene, Marquette University.)*

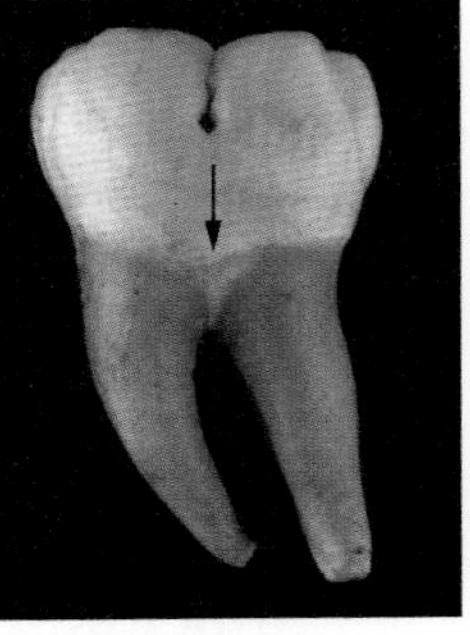

FIGURE 21–11 ✦ Cervical enamel projection on a mandibular first molar. *(Courtesy Department of Dental Hygiene, Marquette University.)*

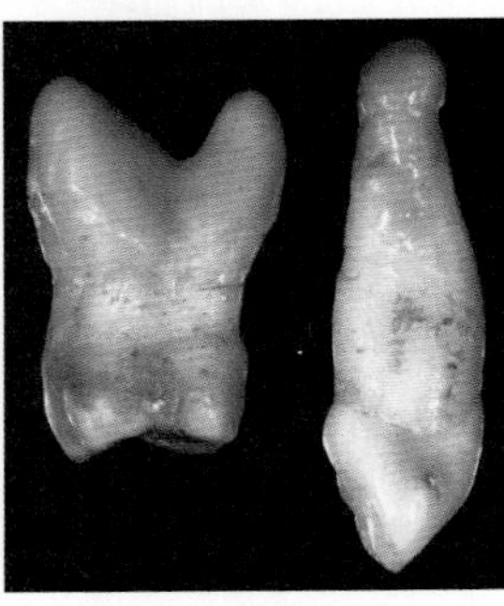

FIGURE 21–10 ✦ Hypercementosis *(Courtesy Department of Dental Hygiene, Marquette University.)*

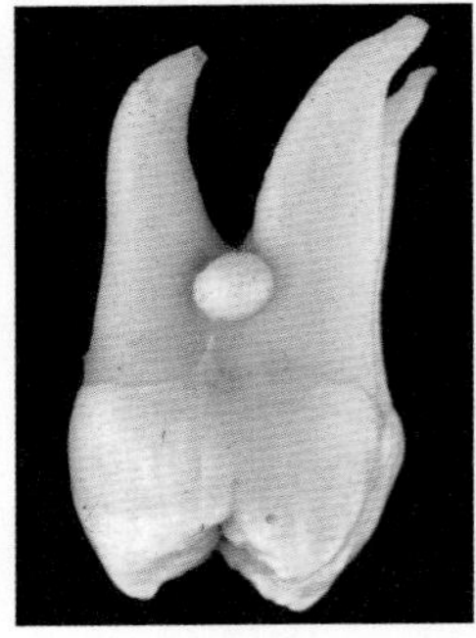

FIGURE 21–12 ✦ Enamel pearls near the furcation of a maxillary molar. *(Courtesy Department of Dental Hygiene, Marquette University.)*

exposed with apical migration of the junctional epithelium, decisions on the extent of root instrumentation will be more difficult.

Cervical Enamel Projections

Cervical enamel projections (CEP) are apical extensions of the CEJ toward the furcation of a molar (Figure 21–11). CEPs are classified by their degree of extension:

- ✦ Grade I CEPs slightly extend toward the furcation and occur frequently.
- ✦ Grade II CEPs approach the area of root separation.
- ✦ Grade III CEPs extend into the furcation.

Periodontal attachment loss is more likely in the CEP area because periodontal fibers do not form the same type of attachment to enamel as does cementum. A CEP can be removed surgically to expose dentin and facilitate reattachment of periodontal fibers.

Enamel Pearls

Enamel pearls, most frequently seen on maxillary molars, are "droplets" of enamel in the furcation area (Figure 21–12). They are thought to be due to a genetic error in the developing root sheath as it reaches the area of furcation. As periodontal fibers will not attach to enamel, they may encourage periodontal disease. Exploration of an enamel pearl can sometimes be puzzling to a dental hygienist if it is not visible on radiographs, because it may feel like subgingival calculus.

Dilaceration

Dilaceration is a sharp bend or curvature in the root surface caused by the displacement of the root during tooth development (Figure 21–13).

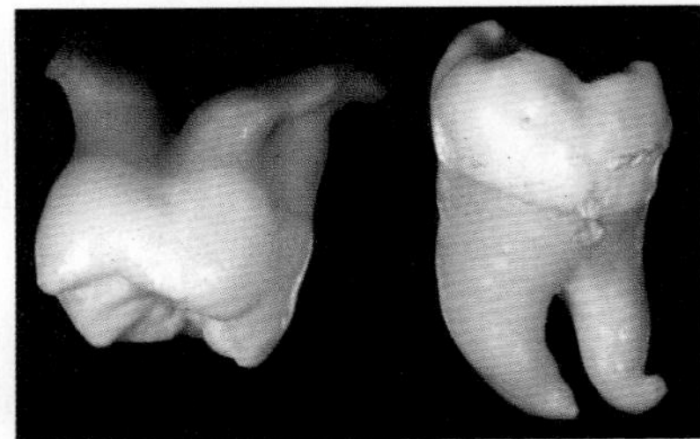

FIGURE 21–13 ✦ Dilaceration. *(Courtesy Department of Dental Hygiene, Marquette University.)*

Client Education Issues

- ✦ Educate clients about root morphology and related periodontal structures as a rationale for recommended self-care.
- ✦ Individualize oral self-care methods and appropriate adjunctive aids as related to each client's root morphology, oral health or oral disease status, level of understanding, and capability.

Legal, Ethical, and Safety Issues

- ✦ Knowledge of root morphology is critical to successful root instrumentation. Only competent dental hygienists should perform root assessment and instrumentation.
- ✦ Root variations that influence professional and self-care should be recorded in the client's chart, discussed with the client, and accounted for in the plan of care.

Key Concepts

- Root assessment, instrumentation, and management require thorough knowledge of root morphology.
- Periodontal assessment includes the identification of root anatomy and root surface characteristics prior to the development of the plan for care.
- Incisors, canines, and all of the premolars except the maxillary first premolars have one root.
- Approximately 60% of maxillary first premolars have two roots.
- Mandibular molars have two roots, one mesial and one distal, with furcations on the facial and lingual surfaces.
- Maxillary molars have three roots—mesiobuccal, distobuccal, and lingual—with furcations on the mesial, facial, and distal surfaces.
- Teeth with more than one root have a root trunk before division into two or three roots.
- The area of division is called the furca; the furcation entrance may be very narrow.
- The CEJ on posterior teeth has much less-pronounced curvatures on all surfaces.
- Cementum is not as hard as enamel and only instruments with a rounded toe should be used on it.
- The number and shape of the roots determine the selection and adaptation of assessment, scaling, and root planing instruments.
- Root surfaces converge (taper) apically; there is more surface area to the root in the cervical than in the apical thirds.
- More of the proximal surface of a single-rooted tooth with broader facial than lingual surfaces can be reached from the lingual because of the proximal convergence toward the lingual.
- The horizontal and vertical location of the furcation determines the selection and placement of instruments.
- Roots may have shallow, longitudinal vertical depressions on their surfaces, which add curvature and dimension to the instrumentation.
- The axial positioning of each individual tooth in its alveolus needs to be considered when placing instruments on the root surface.

Critical Thinking Exercises

1. Root surface characteristic exercise.
Materials: autoclaved extracted tooth with subgingival deposit, curets, dissecting microscope (7×), tray cover, gauze square, gloves, protective eyewear
Exercise:

1. Observe the root of the tooth under the microscope (7×).
2. Select one area of the root surface and remove the deposit with a curet.
3. Observe the root again, noticing the residual deposit microscopically.
4. Root plane the area until it is smooth and hard.
5. Observe the root again.
6. Document the observations.

2. Root anatomy exercise:
Materials: autoclaved extracted maxillary and mandibular first molars, black nail polish, black crayon, 11 to 14 area-specific curets, tray cover, gauze square, gloves, protective eyewear
Preparation: paint the cervical third to half of the root to the distal half of the root surface (simulate deposit, altered cementum); color the mesial half of the root with crayon (simulate subgingival plaque)
Exercise:

1. Identify tooth and hold it in the correct orientation.
2. Select the appropriate curet for an area and remove deposit from root trunk and roots.
3. Observe how each root is approached as if it were a single tooth.
4. Observe how each of the surfaces needs to be approached.
5. Count the number of strokes needed to remove all the deposit.

For References, Suggested Readings, and Related Websites, visit
http://evolve.elsevier.com/Darby/hygiene/

CHAPTER 22

Extrinsic and Intrinsic Stains and their Management

OBJECTIVES

Mastery of the content in this chapter will enable the reader to:

- Identify types and characteristics of tooth stains
- Describe a variety of stain removal and management procedures, including tooth bleaching and alternative restorative procedures, and advantages and disadvantages of each
- Explain the philosophy of selective polishing
- Describe indications, contraindications, and techniques for rubber cup and air polishing
- Describe precautions and preventive measures for clients and clinicians prior to, during, and following rubber cup and air polishing
- Describe the effects of rubber cup and air polishing on teeth, gingiva, restorations, and treatment area environment
- Describe maintenance and sterilization procedures for instruments and materials used in rubber cup and air polishing

KEY TERMS

Air polishing (air-powder polishing)
Enamel pearls
Endogenous stain
Exogenous stain
Extrinsic stain
Home bleaching
In-office bleaching
Intrinsic stain
Laser bleaching
Nonvital tooth bleaching
Rubber cup polishing
Selective polishing
Stain
Tooth bleaching
Vital tooth bleaching

A *stain* is a discolored spot or area on a tooth that contrasts with the rest of the tooth color. Stains may be classified as *extrinsic* (surface stain) or *intrinsic* (stain occurring within the tooth), and *exogenous* (caused by factors external to the tooth) or *endogenous* (caused by factors within the tooth). Extrinsic stains are always exogenous, but intrinsic stains may originate from exogenous or endogenous sources.

EXTRINSIC STAINS

Extrinsic stains can be caused by smoking cigarettes, cigars, or pipes; using spit (smokeless) tobacco or marijuana; rinsing with antimicrobial agents such as chlorhexidine; and brushing with stannous fluoride products. Other common sources of stains include tea, coffee, cola beverages, berries, iron tablets, red wine, and poor oral hygiene. In addition, teeth may become stained from environmental factors such as metallic dust in industrial employment settings. Stain colors may be yellow, brown, gray, green, orange, or black.

Extrinsic stains usually can be removed by a variety of methods, including scaling with hand, sonic, and ultrasonic instruments, and by rubber cup or air polishing. Once removed, extrinsic stains may be prevented by a client's change in self-care practices or intake of stain-producing products.

INTRINSIC STAINS

Intrinsic stains occur for many reasons, and may be hereditary or developmental in nature. Defects in enamel or dentin during tooth development due to high fevers, trauma, excessive intake of fluoride, or tetracycline may result in a mottled or stained appearance to the tooth. The morphology may range from slight pitting to gross defects. Color changes may be slight or severe, including yellow, light to dark brown, gray, and black. Due to the translucent nature of enamel, discolorations may also result from large restorations, pulpal necrosis, and dental caries.

Because intrinsic stains cannot be removed by traditional methods, they may be managed by alternative techniques such as *tooth bleaching* (use of a chemical oxidizing agent, sometimes in combination with heat, to lighten tooth discolorations) or restorative procedures. The severity of the intrinsic tooth staining usually determines which technique is recommended. Recognition of intrinsic staining and referral for appropriate treatment address the client's human need for a wholesome facial image.

SELECTIVE POLISHING PHILOSOPHY

It is important to assess the value of tooth polishing for each client, because research has demonstrated adverse effects of tooth polishing on tooth structures, gingival tissues, restorations, and the treatment room environment.[1-7] *Selective polishing* is the practice of omitting tooth polishing in areas where there is no stain, and when tooth polishing could cause damage. It is based on the concept that not all teeth need to be polished on a routine basis. Enamel is approximately 2.5 millimeters in thickness on the cuspal surfaces, with considerable thinning occurring at the cervical portions of the tooth.[8] Polishing with pumice for 30 seconds removes approximately 4 microns of the fluoride-rich, outer layer of enamel.[1,9] Cumulative effects may be greater over many years of polishing during maintenance visits.

Moreover, because stain and plaque do not prevent fluoride uptake in enamel, topical fluoride applications may be provided without first polishing the teeth.[10,11] In addition, polishing the teeth as part of a routine oral prophylaxis has not been shown to have any therapeutic value in terms of periodontal health.[12]

Although stain itself is not a pathologic concern, it may be a cosmetic concern. The value of stain removal lies in the client's need to have white teeth and a pleasing appearance. Therefore, selective polishing of only tooth surfaces with stain instead of routine polishing of all teeth has been advocated for many years.[13-20] To enable clients to make an informed decision about polishing, they need to be educated on the potential harmful effects of tooth polishing, the lack of therapeutic value, and the purely cosmetic nature of the polishing process.[12,21,22] In addition, clients should be informed about any available alternative methods of stain removal or stain management.

STAIN REMOVAL PROCEDURES

Identification of the type of stain present and the client's oral health behaviors that may contribute to the stain occurs during the oral assessment. With these data, the client and the dental hygienist select an appropriate stain removal or stain management intervention. When extrinsic stain remains following scaling and root planing, the dental hygienist considers the advantages and disadvantages of various stain removal methods and selects the least harmful to remove the stain. More than one method may be indicated for the same client in different areas of the mouth.

Rubber Cup Polishing

Rubber cup polishing is the removal of tooth stains following scaling using a slow-speed handpiece and prophylaxis polishing paste. This procedure is the traditional method used for removal of extrinsic stains from tooth surfaces, is quite effective for stain removal, and generally has good client acceptance. The procedure rapidly removes stain and is a relatively easy procedure to learn and to perform.

ADVERSE EFFECTS ON TEETH. It is well accepted that rubber cup polishing removes tooth structure from the outer layer of enamel. Because the highest content of fluoride is in the outermost layer, performing rubber cup polishing routinely over many maintenance visits could affect clients negatively, especially those who are at an increased risk for dental caries.[1,9] Use of a fluoride-containing prophylaxis paste may replace some of the fluoride lost from abrasive polishing procedures, but a professional topical fluoride is necessary to compensate fully for the lost fluoride.[23] Demineralized tooth surfaces lose three times more surface structure during polishing than does intact enamel.[24] Because newly erupted teeth are not mineralized completely, polishing should be avoided on these teeth.[19]

Dentin and cementum are less resistant to abrasion than are enamel surfaces.[4] Because dentin and cementum are potentially removed during rubber cup polishing, using this procedure on roots also should be avoided. Moreover, tooth sensitivity to rubber cup polishing may occur in cervical areas of enamel due to the thinness of enamel in these areas and the possible exposure of dentin or cementum.[25] Finally, coarse abrasives may actually roughen tooth surfaces, causing increased plaque biofilm accumulation and, if used for stain removal, should be followed with a less abrasive paste to minimize enamel scratches.[26]

ADVERSE EFFECTS ON RESTORATIONS. Rubber cup polishing may damage restorations by making surfaces rough.[5] Gold, amalgam, conventional composites, and microfilled composites exhibit surface roughness following polishing with a prophylaxis paste.[5] If polishing of dental implants is desired, a nonabrasive prophylaxis paste (ImplantCleanic, Premier Dental Products Co., Morristown, PA. 19404-0111) or a mild toothpaste is used.

ADVERSE EFFECTS ON SOFT TISSUES. Irritation of soft tissues can result from rubber cup polishing if the tissues are inflamed, because gritty particles of the polishing paste can become embedded in the gingiva and may delay healing. Trauma to gingiva can also occur with improper technique, especially with the rubber cup used at high speed, with excessive pressure, or kept in one place too long.[2] Pressure should be enough to flatten one edge of the cup so it slips under the gingiva, but not enough so that the entire lip of the cup is flattened. Generation of heat with the handpiece and rubber cup may initiate or promote pulpal necrosis, especially in deciduous teeth with large pulps.[19] Pulpal discomfort may also occur if pressure, speed, and abrasiveness of the polishing paste are sufficient to generate heat.

ADVERSE EFFECTS ON ENVIRONMENT. Bacterial aerosol production during rubber cup polishing may provide a means of disease transmission to dental personnel. Bacteria remain suspended in the air for hours and settle on environmental surfaces. Inhalation of bacterial aerosols generated throughout the polishing procedure could be problematic for those with respiratory problems. The clinician may also be subject to occupational injury from the weight of the handpiece. Most of these problems can be eliminated or minimized by adhering to appropriate protocols for technique and infection control, and by using rubber cup polishing only when it is indicated.

RISK MANAGEMENT STRATEGIES. Due to the adverse effects discussed in the preceding section, contraindications to rubber cup polishing are numerous (see Contraindications to Rubber Polishing). Rubber cup polishing should be limited to stain removal on enamel surfaces only or when the client requests the procedure even after education on its harmful effects. It should be followed by a professional topical fluoride application.

Because rubber cup polishing is a procedure that may cause bleeding, the American Heart Association (AHA) recommends antibiotic premedication to prevent bacterial endocarditis for clients having specific moderate and high-risk medical conditions.[27] The AHA also recommends preprocedural antimicrobial rinses for these at-risk clients to reduce the possibility of developing a bacteremia.[27,28] Chlorhexidine is the antimicrobial of choice and should be rinsed gently in the mouth for 1 to 2 minutes prior to treatment.[29]

All clients, however, should have a preprocedural antimicrobial rinse to decrease the aerosol production.[30] Protective safety glasses for the client are recommended for all intraoral procedures, but especially for those that involve splatter such as that produced during rubber cup polishing. The dental hygienist follows the Centers for Disease Control (CDC) guidelines for infection control[31] and wears gloves, a facemask, a protective gown, and safety glasses or a face shield. Following these guidelines ensures that clients are treated safely during the rubber cup polishing procedure and that they and the clinician have their human need for protection from health risks satisfied.

Contraindications to Rubber Cup Polishing

Absence of extrinsic stain
Newly erupted teeth, especially primary teeth
Decalcification or hypocalcification
Enamel hypoplasia
Areas of recession where cementum or dentin is exposed
Areas of hypersensitivity
Acute gingival or periodontal inflammation
Immediately following deep scaling, root planing, or soft tissue curettage
Xerostomia
Composite restorations and bonding, glass ionomer, porcelain, and gold restorations
Rampant caries
Allergy to ingredients in paste
Radiation to head and neck area, particularly the salivary glands
Respiratory problems, i.e., asthma or emphysema*
Communicable diseases*
High-risk clients needing antibiotic premedication must be premedicated for polishing*

*Precautions needed, but these are not strict contraindications.

ARMAMENTARIUM FOR RUBBER CUP POLISHING. Commercial polishing pastes are available in different grits (i.e., fine, medium, and coarse) and may have different flavoring agents. These pastes may also contain fluoride and replace some of the fluoride lost by the abrasive action of the polishing procedure. These pastes, however, are *not* a substitute for a professionally applied topical fluoride treatment.[23,29] Toothpastes also contain abrasives and may be used for polishing enamel with a toothbrush or a slow-speed handpiece.[26] The least abrasive type of paste necessary for stain removal should be used at a slow speed with moderate pressure.[7]

A prophylaxis angle, attached to a slow-speed, lightweight handpiece, may contain disposable rubber cups or brushes of various types: screw-type, latch-type, or snap-on. The rubber cups may be used on all surfaces, but flat or pointed brushes are designed for stain removal on occlusal surfaces. Disposable prophylaxis angles are also available. (Figure 22–1). All disposable items, such as rubber cups, brushes, saliva ejectors, and plastic prophylaxis angles, are used only once and then discarded. Handpieces and stainless steel prophylaxis angles are cleaned, lubricated, and sterilized according to manufacturers' directions. The materials and procedures for rubber cup polishing are outlined in Procedure 22–1.

Hand Scaling

Hand instruments such as curets and scalers are designed primarily for calculus removal, but can also be used for extrinsic stain removal. When stain adheres to calculus, it may be efficiently removed with the calculus. Because hand instruments are small, they can remove

Text continued on page 447

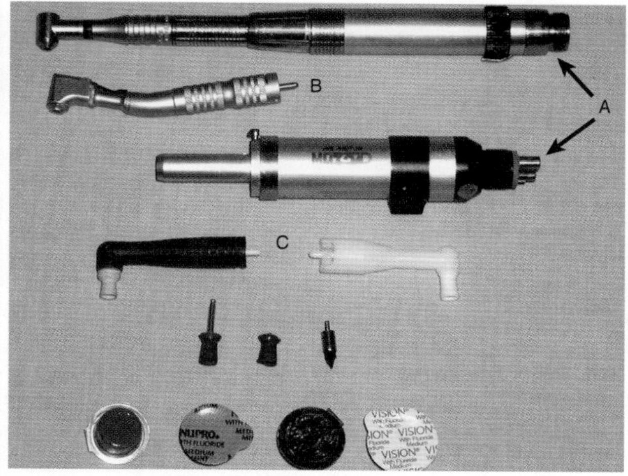

FIGURE 22–1 ✦ Armamentarium for rubber cup polishing. **A,** Slow-speed handpieces. **B,** Latch-type prophylaxis angle. **C,** Disposable prophylaxis angles. **D,** Latch-type rubber cup. **E,** Screw-type rubber cup and tapered brush. **F,** Examples of commercial prophylaxis pastes.

Procedure 22–1 RUBBER CUP POLISHING TECHNIQUE

MATERIALS

Polishing paste and toothpaste
Prophylaxis angle and toothbrush
Dental floss or tape
Floss threader (if needed)
Rubber cups and/or brushes
Slow-speed handpiece
Gauze squares
Mouth mirror, air/water syringe
Disclosing solution
Preprocedural antimicrobial mouthrinse
Saliva ejector or high-volume evacuation (HVE) tip
Safety glasses for client
Personal protective equipment

PREPARATION/POSITIONING	RATIONALE
1. Evaluate client's health history to determine need for antibiotic premedication	Ensures safe treatment
2. Identify tooth surfaces indicated and contraindicated for polishing	Prevents unnecessary removal of tooth structure
3. Educate client about selective polishing procedure	Facilitates client acceptance
4. Select polishing abrasive based on type of stain and oral conditions and assemble basic setup (Figure 22–2)	Prevents unnecessary removal of tooth structure

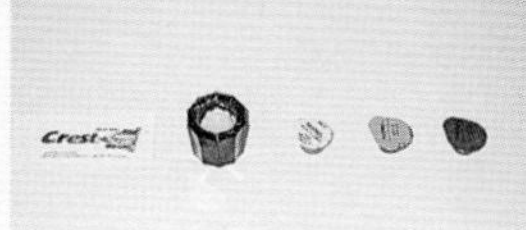

FIGURE 22–2 ✦ Pastes of different grits for polishing.

5. Use appropriate personal protective equipment and provide protective eyewear for client	Prevents cross-contamination and protects client's eyes from splatter
6. Provide a preprocedural antimicrobial rinse for the client to use before polishing	Reduces aerosol microorganisms and minimizes occurrence of bacteremia in at-risk clients
7. Sit in the 8:00 to 9:00 o'clock position • Have the client tilt head up and turn slightly away when polishing maxillary and mandibular right buccal surfaces of posterior teeth, and maxillary and mandibular left lingual surfaces of posterior teeth	Enhances access and visibility and prevents occupational injury

GRASP

8. Use modified pen grasp (Figure 22–3)	Facilitates movement of handpiece

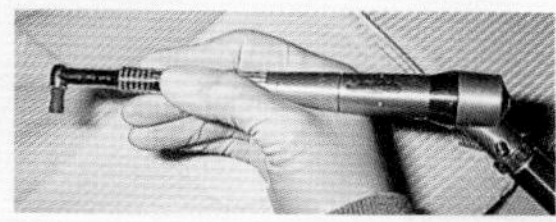

FIGURE 22–3 ✦ Handpiece grasp.

9. Rest handpiece in V of hand	Transfers handpiece weight from fingers to hand to decrease fatigue
10. Have all fingers in contact as a unit	Facilitates wrist–forearm motion

Continued on following page

Procedure 22–1 RUBBER CUP POLISHING TECHNIQUE—CONT'D

PREPARATION/POSITIONING	RATIONALE
FULCRUM	
11. Establish intraoral fulcrum close to working area	Enhances control of handpiece
12. Fulcrum on ring finger	Facilitates pivoting for wrist forearm motion
13. Use moderate fulcrum pressure	Enhances stabilization
ADAPTATION	
14. Angle rubber cup to flare at gingival margin	Enhances stain removal at cervical third of tooth
15. Adapt rubber cup to reach distal, facial/lingual, or mesial surfaces	Ensures access to all surfaces with stain
16. Maintain adaptation of the cup to tooth by rotating handpiece or pivoting on fulcrum, as necessary	Decreases tissue trauma and provides adequate tooth coverage
17. Adapt cup or brush to occlusal surface	Removes stain from pits and grooves
STROKE	
18. Fill cup with paste and evenly apply to surfaces to be polished	Ensures adequate and even distribution of paste
19. Place cup on tooth and activate handpiece by gently stepping on foot pedal. Stroke from the gingival third to the incisal third with just enough pressure to make the cup flare while using wrist forearm motion to polish the teeth	Controls speed of handpiece and prevents or reduces finger fatigue
20. Use intermittent, dabbing, overlapping strokes with moderate pressure and slow speed in a cervical to occlusal/incisal direction. Use overlapping strokes (Figure 22–4)	Dissipates heat, reduces abrasion, ensures complete tooth coverage

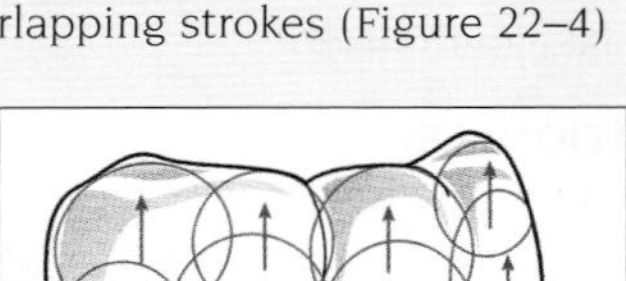

FIGURE 22–4 ✦ Overlapping strokes to ensure complete coverage of the tooth. *(From Robinson DS, Bird DL:* Ehrlich and Torres essentials of dental assisting, *ed 3, Philadelphia, 2001, WB Saunders.)*

PREPARATION/POSITIONING	RATIONALE
21. Remove rubber cup from tooth at completion of stroke and readapt cup for next stroke	Dissipates heat
SEQUENCE	
22. Hold mirror in nondominant hand and use it to retract buccal mucosa. Instruct client to close mouth halfway and to tilt head slightly toward the ceiling. Polish the buccal surfaces of the maxillary right posterior quadrant (Figure 22–5)	Mirror use facilitates access and direct vision of buccal and mesial surfaces and indirect vision of distal surfaces

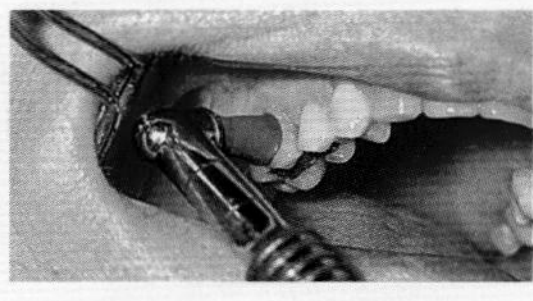

FIGURE 22–5 ✦ Polishing the buccal surfaces of the maxillary right posterior quadrant.

PREPARATION/POSITIONING	RATIONALE
23. Polish the facial surfaces of the maxillary anterior teeth. Palm mirror and retract lip with fingers of non-dominant hand. (Figure 22–6)	Allows for direct vision and keeps mirror accessible

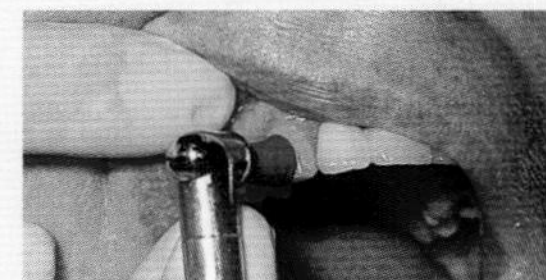

FIGURE 22–6 ✦ Polishing the facial surfaces of the maxillary anterior teeth.

Procedure 22–1 RUBBER CUP POLISHING TECHNIQUE—CONT'D

SEQUENCE	RATIONALE
24. Hold mirror in nondominant hand and use it to retract buccal mucosa. Instruct client to close mouth halfway and to tilt head slightly toward the ceiling. Polish the buccal surfaces of the maxillary left posterior quadrant (Figure 22–7)	Mirror use facilitates access, direct vision of buccal and mesial surfaces, and indirect vision of distal surfaces

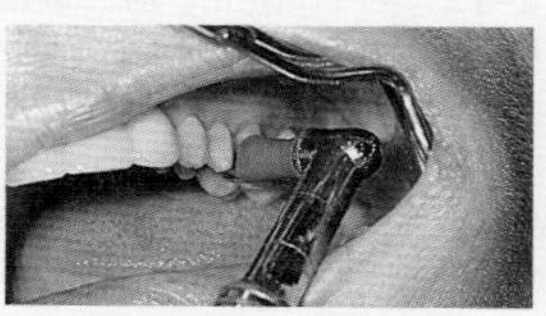

FIGURE 22–7 ✦ Polishing the buccal surfaces of the maxillary left posterior quadrant.

SEQUENCE	RATIONALE
25. Polish the lingual surfaces of the maxillary right posterior quadrant. Use mirror for indirect vision and indirect lighting (Figure 22–8)	Use of indirect vision promotes good posture and visibility of lingual surfaces

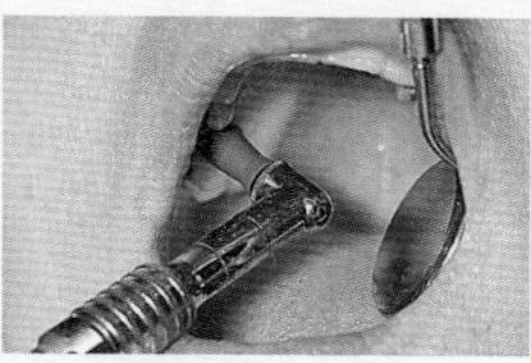

FIGURE 22–8 ✦ Polishing the lingual surfaces of the maxillary right posterior quadrant.

SEQUENCE	RATIONALE
26. Polish the lingual surfaces of the maxillary anterior teeth. Use mirror for indirect vision (Figure 22–9)	Use of indirect vision promotes good posture and visibility of lingual surfaces

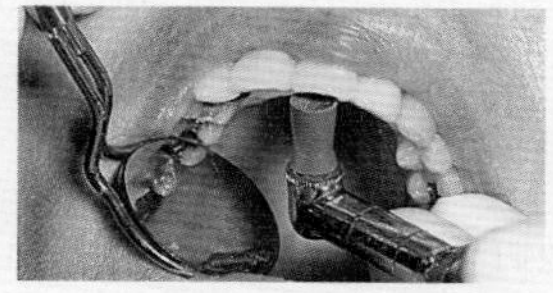

FIGURE 22–9 ✦ Polishing the lingual surfaces of the maxillary anterior teeth.

SEQUENCE	RATIONALE
27. Polish the lingual surfaces of the maxillary left posterior quadrant. Use mirror for indirect vision (Figure 22–10)	Use of indirect vision promotes good posture and good visibility of lingual surfaces

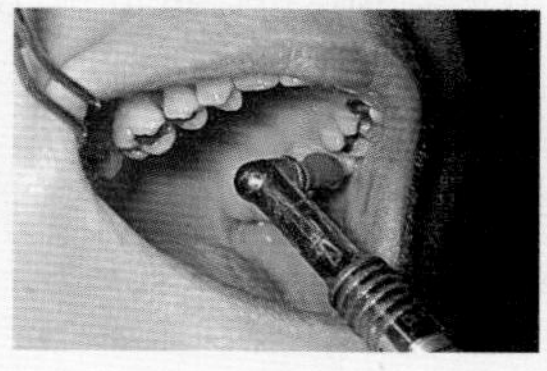

FIGURE 22–10 ✦ Polishing the lingual surfaces of the maxillary left posterior quadrant.

SEQUENCE	RATIONALE
28. Rinse client's teeth	Removes prophylaxis paste from client's mouth
29. Hold mirror in nondominant hand and use it to retract right buccal mucosa. Polish the buccal surfaces of the mandibular right posterior quadrant (Figure 22–11)	Retracting buccal mucosa with mirror facilitates access, direct vision of buccal and mesial tooth surfaces, and indirect vision of distal surfaces

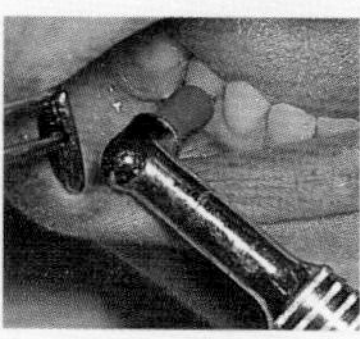

FIGURE 22–11 ✦ Polishing the buccal surfaces of the mandibular right posterior quadrant.

Continued on following page

Procedure 22–1 RUBBER CUP POLISHING TECHNIQUE—CONT'D

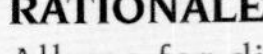

SEQUENCE	RATIONALE
30. Palm mirror and retract lip with fingers of nondominant hand. Polish the facial surfaces of the mandibular anterior teeth (Figure 22–12)	Allows for direct vision and keeps mirror accessible

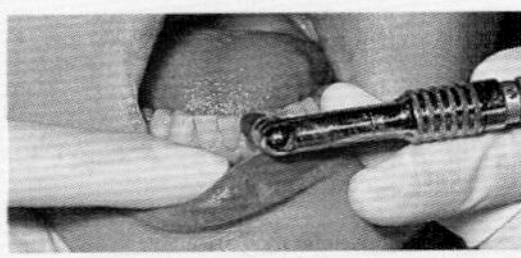

FIGURE 22–12 ✦ Polishing the facial surfaces of the mandibular anterior teeth.

SEQUENCE	RATIONALE
31. Retract buccal mucosa with mirror and polish buccal surfaces of the mandibular left posterior quadrant (Figure 22–13)	Allows for direct vision of buccal and mesial surfaces and indirect vision of distal surfaces

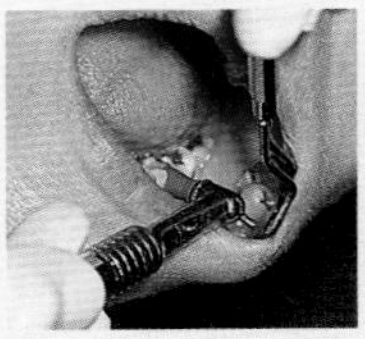

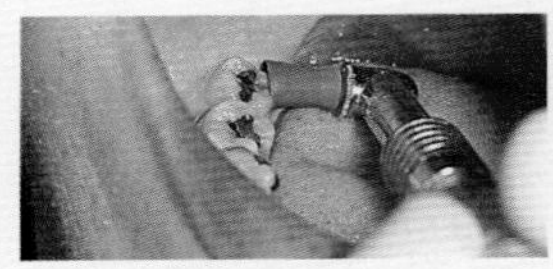

FIGURE 22–13 ✦ Polishing the buccal surfaces of the mandibular left posterior quadrant.

SEQUENCE	RATIONALE
32. Polish lingual surfaces of mandibular right posterior quadrant. Use mirror to retract tongue and for indirect vision and lighting (Figure 22–14)	Retracting the tongue facilitates direct and indirect vision

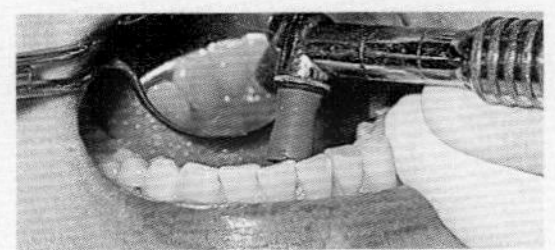

FIGURE 22–14 ✦ Polishing the lingual surfaces of the mandibular right posterior quadrant.

SEQUENCE	RATIONALE
33. Polish lingual surfaces of mandibular anterior teeth (Figure 22–15). Use mirror for indirect vision and indirect lighting. Be careful *not* to rest mirror on sublingual mucosa	Resting the mirror on sublingual mucosa is very uncomfortable for the client

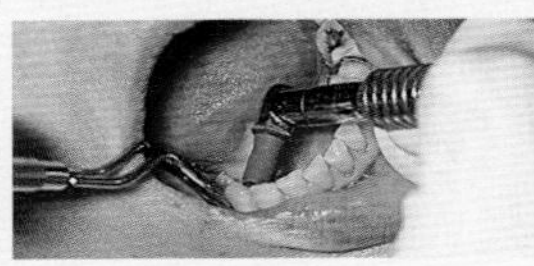

FIGURE 22–15 ✦ Polishing the lingual surfaces of the mandibular anterior teeth.

SEQUENCE	RATIONALE
34. Polish lingual surfaces of mandibular left posterior quadrant (Fig 22–16). Use mirror to retract tongue, and for indirect vision and lighting. Replace rubber cup with flat or pointed brush and remove stain on occlusal surfaces	Use of mirror facilitates access and visibility of lingual surfaces. Brushes adapt to pits and fissures.

FIGURE 22–16 ✦ Polishing the lingual surfaces of the mandibular left posterior quadrant.

SEQUENCE	RATIONALE
35. Rinse client's teeth. Floss client's teeth (Figure 22–17)	Removes prophylaxis paste from client's mouth

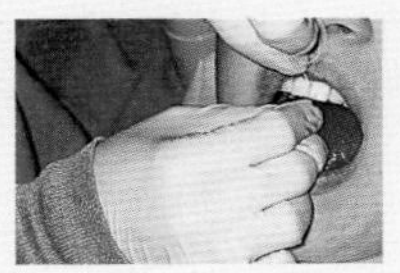

FIGURE 22–17 ✦ Flossing the client's teeth.

SEQUENCE	RATIONALE
36. Apply topical fluoride (Figure 22–18) (See Chapter 26)	Replaces fluoride removed from the outer surfaces of enamel by polishing

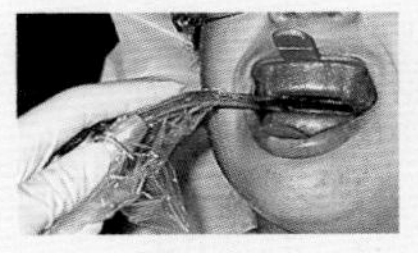

FIGURE 22–18 ✦ Applying topical fluoride.

Photos courtesy Dr. M. Walsh, University of California–San Francisco

stain in areas inaccessible to a rubber cup. In addition, hand instruments are not abrasive to enamel surfaces.

Hand instruments, however, can remove cementum on root surfaces so over-instrumentation should be avoided.[32] When moderate to heavy stain is present on root surfaces, the dental hygienist is faced with the problem of removing the stain with the least alteration of cementum. Because stain removal is only a cosmetic concern, one possible choice is to explain to the client that stain is not associated with oral disease and will not harm the teeth or gingiva if it is not removed. However, this may not be a viable choice to a client because appearance is considered so important in today's society. Some authors recommend removing as much stain as possible during root planing with curets.[19] Others support use of the air polisher over curets on root surfaces.[17,32] The less root structure that is removed, the less likelihood there is of root surface sensitivity occurring after the procedure. At present, any method capable of removing stain from root surfaces might also remove cementum.

Sonic/Ultrasonic Scaling

Ultrasonic and sonic scaling to remove extrinsic stain have the same advantages and disadvantages as when these devices are used for calculus removal. Efficiency and efficacy are the primary benefits for selecting these instruments for stain removal. In addition, a slender tip is able to remove stain on occlusal surfaces and in areas of rotated or overlapped teeth. There is usually good client acceptance, and operator fatigue is minimized significantly when compared to hand instrumentation.

Aerosols are created with sonic/ultrasonic instrumentation and the instrumentation, if used improperly, can generate heat and cause tissue trauma. Aerosols can be minimized with the use of a safety suction, an aerosol reduction device[33] (Figures 22–19 and 22–20, *A* and *B*). When comparing the results of studies on hand instruments to sonic/ultrasonic instruments on root surface roughness, the findings are ambiguous. Rough cementum and lost tooth structure are encountered with both instruments (see Chapter 20 for a complete discussion of sonic/ultrasonic instruments).

Air Polishing

Air polishing (air-powder polishing) is a method of stain removal that uses a specially designed device with a handpiece that delivers a spray of warm water and sodium bicarbonate under pressure. Air polishing was introduced to dentistry in the late 1970s as a device to remove extrinsic stain quickly and easily from tooth surfaces. The air polisher (Figure 22–21) is an efficient and effective method of stain removal.[32,34–37] Air polishing requires less time than traditional polishing methods do and removes stain three times as fast as hand scaling.[32,34] Less operator fatigue is also an important benefit of air polishing.

EFFECTS ON ENAMEL, CEMENTUM, AND DENTIN. Intact enamel surfaces are not damaged when stain removal is accomplished with the air polisher.[36,38–41]

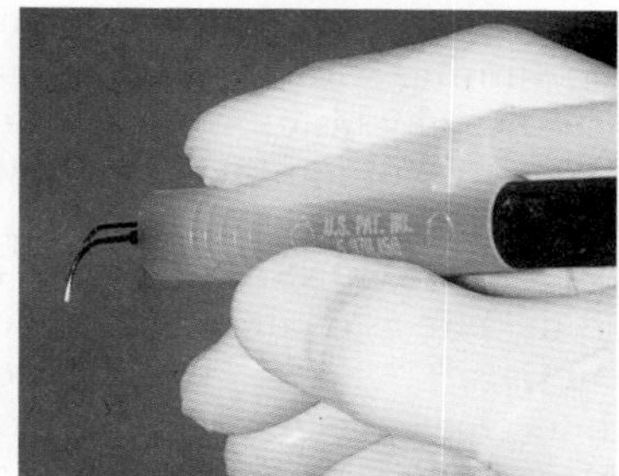

FIGURE 22–19 ✦ Safety Suction *(Courtesy Dental Designs of Dallas, Dallas, Tx.)*

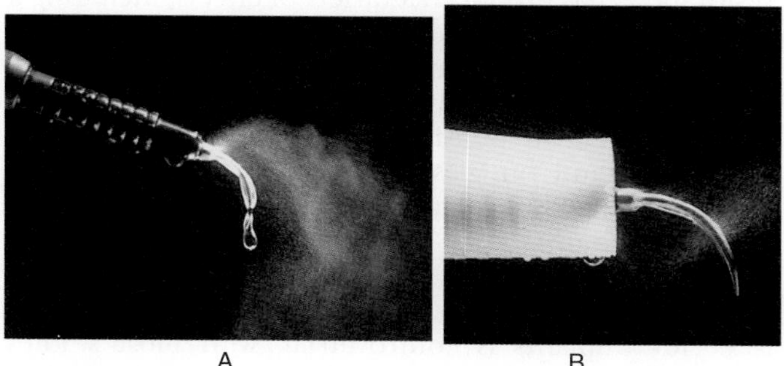

FIGURE 22–20 ✦ **A,** Excessive spray emitted without use of Safety Suction. **B,** Reduced spray with use of Safety Suction. *(Courtesy Dental Designs of Dallas, Tx.)*

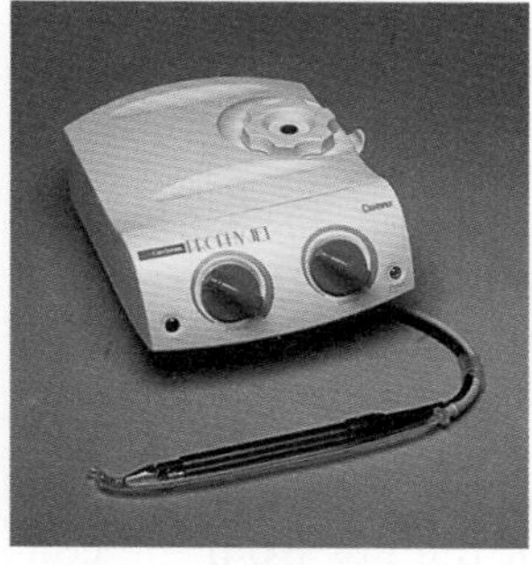

FIGURE 22–21 ✦ Prophy-Jet air polisher with aerosol reduction device attached. *(Courtesy Dentsply Preventive Care Division, York, Pa.)*

However, prolonged use of air polishing on cementum and dentin can remove significant tooth structure and should be avoided.[39] Results are inconsistent on which method is ideal for stain removal on root surfaces. Presently, it appears that air polishing may be the least damaging and most efficient means of removing stain on enamel, but no method is risk-free on cementum.

EFFECTS ON SOFT TISSUES. Gingival bleeding and abrasion are the most common effects of air polishing on soft tissues.[42,43] These results are temporary, healing occurs quickly, and effects are not clinically significant.[37,42,43] In addition, no complications were seen with healing at extraction sites following air polishing of teeth prior to extraction.[44] The tip of the air polisher, however, should be pointed away from the gingiva to avoid tissue trauma.

Clients have noticed a salty taste with air polishing but it was not objectionable.[44] Covering the tongue with a moist gauze square may prevent irritation and an excessively salty taste. Rinsing with water or mouthwash also helps to reduce the salty taste. Another option to mask the salty taste is the use of mint-flavored powder.

EFFECTS ON RESTORATIONS. Numerous investigators have examined the effects of air polishing on a variety of restorative materials.[45–55] Some results have been positive, and others have recommended caution near restorations. Most studies suggest not using air polishing on or near composite restorations to avoid causing surface roughness or pitting.

Air polishing of amalgam alloys and other metal restorations has produced a variety of effects, including a matte finish, surface roughness, morphologic changes, and structural alterations. Studies also report surface roughness, staining, pitting, and loss of marginal integrity when air polishing is used on porcelain and gold alloys and on glass ionomers. Clinicians should avoid extended use of air polishing on all restorative dental materials.

EFFECTS ON IMPLANTS. Research on using the air polisher for implants is controversial, with most studies showing that the air polisher can be effectively used to polish implants.[56–58] Implant surfaces were generally smooth and plaque biofilm formation was also inhibited following air polishing.[57,59–61] One study, however, found slight surface alterations on all types of implants.[60] Therefore, until more definitive research assures safe use of the air polisher on implants, avoidance is recommended on sapphire and pure titanium implants.[60]

SAFETY ISSUES. Safety concerns for the client, the operator, and others in the treatment room appear in the dental literature regarding use of the air polisher.[61–64] Client concerns include systemic problems from absorption of the sodium bicarbonate polishing powder, respiratory difficulties from inhaling aerosols that contain oral microorganisms, stinging of the lips from the concentrated spray, and eye problems from the spray entering the eyes, especially if contact lenses are worn. Some of these problems could be addressed by coating a client's lips with a protective lubricant, using the appropriate technique, removing contact lenses, wearing safety glasses, and placing a protective drape over the client's nose and eyes.

Despite these safety concerns, limited credible information is available on the systemic effects of sodium bicarbonate absorption from air polishing powder. It is important, however, for the body to maintain a very specific balance between acids and bases. Some individuals cannot adjust readily to disturbances to this balance. It is for this reason, due to the potential absorption of sodium bicarbonate by the oral mucosa, that air polisher manufacturers caution against its use with such clients.[65]

Because of the marked rise in aerosols with air polishing, additional health hazards potentially exist for clients or healthcare professionals present in the treatment room during or after a procedure.[62] To decrease any potential risks, oral healthcare personnel can employ several measures, such as adhering to universal precautions in the operatory. This includes wearing a well-fitting mask with recommended Bacterial Filtration Efficiency (BFE) scores of 74 to 98%.[62–64,66,67] Using high-volume evacuation will reduce aerosols better than a saliva ejector will.[64,66] However, if working without an assistant, use of an aerosol reduction device (Jet-Shield, Dentsply Preventive Care Division, York, PA) attached to a saliva ejector can significantly reduce aerosol production[68,69] (Figure 22–22). Rinsing with a preprocedural antimicrobial, such as chlorhexidine, for up to two minutes also reduces production of aerosols.[62,70] To help prevent cross-contamination between clients, disinfection of contaminated surfaces as far away as six feet from the immediate treatment area should be considered.[63] A synopsis of the medical contraindications to air polishing, which are based on a client's health history findings, can be found in Medical Contraindications to Air Polishing.

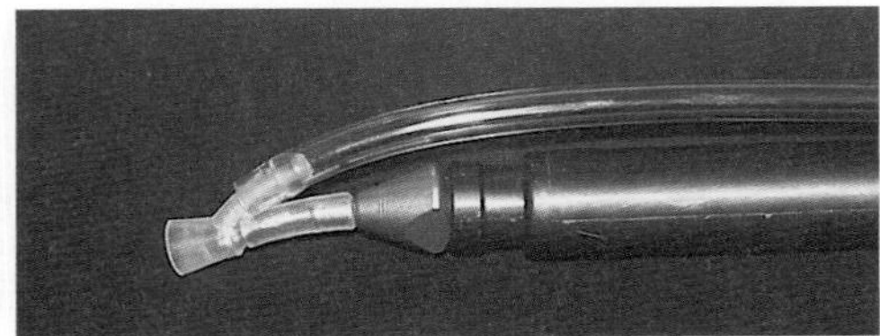

FIGURE 22–22 ✦ Jet-Shield *(Courtesy of Dentsply Preventive Care Division, York, Pa.)*

Medical Contraindications to Air Polishing

Low-sodium diet or history of hypertension
Respiratory illness
Infectious disease
Renal insufficiency
Addison's disease
Cushing's disease
Metabolic alkalosis
Medications such as mineralocorticoid steroids, antidiuretics, or potassium supplements

Dental Contraindications and Precautions Related to Air Polishing contains a listing of other contraindications and precautions that should also be considered when evaluating the appropriateness of air polishing for a particular client.

AIR POLISHING TECHNIQUE. Air polishing should be included in the dental hygiene care plan only after a careful review of the client's medical and dental history and a thorough examination of the oral hard and soft tissues. Indications and contraindications to air polishing are discussed in the preceding section.

Dental Contraindications and Precautions Related to Air Polishing

Composite restorations or bonding
Porcelain restorations, including crowns, veneers, inlays, onlays
Gold (foil or castings) restorations
Amalgam restorations
Glass ionomer restorations
Absence of stain
Exposed cementum or dentin
Areas of hypersensitivity
Immediately following deep scaling, root planing, or soft tissue curettage where acute gingival or periodontal inflammation is present
High-risk clients needing antibiotic premedication must be premedicated for air polishing*
Clients wearing contact lenses should remove them first and wear safety glasses*

*Precautions needed, but these are not strict contraindications

Because air polishing is a procedure that may cause bleeding, the American Heart Association (AHA) recommends antibiotic premedication to prevent bacterial endocarditis for clients having specific moderate and high-risk medical conditions.[27] The AHA and others also recommend a preprocedural antimicrobial rinse for these at-risk clients to reduce the possibility of developing a bacteremia.[27,28] Chlorhexidine is the antimicrobial of choice and should be rinsed gently in the mouth for one to two minutes prior to treatment.[29] All clients, however, should have a preprocedural antimicrobial rinse to decrease the aerosol production.[30,70,71] Removal of contact lenses, lubrication of the lips, and protective safety glasses for the client are recommended. Following these guidelines will ensure that clients are treated safely and comfortably during the air polishing procedure and have their human need for protection from health risks satisfied.

To ensure safety of clinicians, the CDC guidelines for infection control as outlined previously for rubber cup polishing should be followed.[31] The materials and sequence of procedures for air polishing with an aerosol reduction device are outlined in Procedure 22–2, and are based on the manufacturer's guidelines for the Cavitron Prophy-Jet (Dentsply/Preventive Care Division, York, PA). Procedures for air polishing with and without an aerosol reduction device are listed in Procedures 22-2 and 22–3.

All disposable items, such as aerosol reduction devices and saliva ejectors should be used only once and then discarded. Handpieces and stainless steel tips or nozzles should be cleaned and sterilized according to manufacturers' directions. All contaminated surfaces, if not covered with disposable plastic drapes, should be cleaned and disinfected with an approved high-level surface disinfectant. Manufacturers' directions should be followed for maintenance and care of equipment.

STAIN MANAGEMENT PROCEDURES

Clients unsatisfied with the appearance of their teeth have a deficit in their human need for a wholesome facial image. If the deficit results from intrinsic staining or stain that reaccumulates shortly after its removal, the client may benefit from one or more stain management procedures. Stain management includes client education and clinical services such as bleaching or restorative procedures. An attempt to identify the cause of the stain must be made before treatment planning its management. Some stains cannot be modified, and others can be altered only slightly. This determination will ultimately direct the dental hygiene care plan for the client.

Often, the dental hygienist's focus in extrinsic stain management is primarily on self-care plaque removal practices, which may prevent the recurrence of stain. Often, education is the most long-lasting solution for extrinsic stain management and should always be based on the client's health history, oral assessment, and self-care assessment.

Bleaching the teeth, however, is a viable alternative for stain management when tooth stains are intrinsic. Tooth bleaching is primarily a cosmetic procedure. Many techniques, ranging from over-the-counter (OTC) products to sophisticated in-office bleaching systems, are available. *In-office bleaching* is any bleaching procedure performed in the dental office by a dental health professional. All bleaching procedures must be approached with caution. The dental hygienist has a responsibility to understand the processes involved in tooth bleaching, including indications, contraindications, precautions, products, protocols, efficacy, and safety issues. It is also important to ensure that clients understand thoroughly the ramifications of any bleaching treatment prior to its initiation. The dental hygienist's role is summarized in Dental Hygienist's Role in Tooth Bleaching.

Over-the-Counter Products

There are three types of OTC whitening toothpastes. The first type uses an abrasive to remove extrinsic stains and has been available for many years.[72,73] All toothpastes, however, contain some abrasives and are capable of potentially removing stains whether they are labeled "whitening" or not. Toothpastes with a high content of abrasives should not be recommended for daily use. The second type of OTC whitening toothpaste is newer and actually contains a bleaching agent, such as peroxide, but the Council on Scientific Affairs of the ADA does not recommend them for long-term use.[74] The third type of cosmetic toothpaste contains titanium dioxide, covers extrinsic stains like paint covers a wall, and does not change the internal tooth color.[73]

Commercial bleaching kits, containing an oxidizing agent and materials to form a "boil and fit" mouth tray, are also available. An acidic prerinse is available with some kits. Over-the-counter products are a cause for concern in terms of efficacy and safety due to the potential for overuse and abuse by uninformed clients.[75]

Procedure 22–2 AIR POLISHING TECHNIQUE USING AEROSOL REDUCTION DEVICE

MATERIALS

Sodium bicarbonate powder and toothpaste
Air polisher device and toothbrush
Dental floss or tape
Mouth mirror, air/water syringe
Disclosing solution
Lubricant for client's lips
Preprocedural antimicrobial mouthrinse
Saliva ejector
Aerosol reduction device
Safety glasses for client
Personal protective equipment

PREPARATION/POSITIONING	RATIONALE
1. Evaluate client's health history to determine need for antibiotic premedication	Ensures safe treatment
2. Identify tooth surfaces indicated and contraindicated for polishing	Prevents unnecessary removal of tooth structure
3. Educate client about selective polishing procedure	Facilitates patient acceptance of procedure
4. Attach aerosol reduction device to air polisher and saliva ejector	Reduces amount of aerosol released into atmosphere
5. Verify that slurry exits from the cup when held outside the mouth and adjust saliva ejector as necessary	Ensures adequate evacuation
6. Use appropriate personal protective equipment and provide protective eyewear for client.	Reduces aerosol microorganisms and minimizes occurrence of bacteremia in at-risk clients
7. Clinician, client, and equipment must be in appropriate position for each area	Enhances access and visibility and prevents occupational injury
GRASP	
8. Use modified pen grasp	Facilitates movement of handpiece
9. Rest handpiece in V of hand	Transfers handpiece weight from fingers to hand to decrease fatigue
10. Have all fingers in contact as a unit	Facilitates wrist–forearm motion
11. Tuck excess cord around pinkie finger, if desired	Decreases pull from handpiece cord
FULCRUM	
12. Use external soft tissue fulcrums	Facilitates access
ADAPTATION	
13. Apply cup to middle third of tooth with light pressure	Enhances slight flaring of the cup
STROKE	
14. Pivot nozzle inside the cup to incisal, gingival, mesial, or distal surfaces.	Provides adequate coverage of tooth surface
15. Apply 2 seconds of spray for each segment of the tooth, releasing the foot pedal each time.	Removes stain while minimizing spray
16. Readjust cup to maintain flat contact with tooth surface, if spray escapes	Prevents escape of spray
17. Adjust angle by pivoting nozzle inside the aerosol reduction device's cup	Ensures adequate stain removal
OTHER	
18. Brush tooth surfaces without stain with a toothbrush and fluoride toothpaste (or have client do so)	Provides a pleasant aftertaste and ensures adequate plaque removal
19. Rinse with water and floss all teeth	Removes any remaining polishing paste
20. Evaluate effectiveness with disclosing solution, compressed air, and good lighting	Ensures complete stain removal
21. Provide topical fluoride treatment	Replenishes any fluoride lost from outer fluoride-rich surface layer of enamel
22. Dispose of aerosol reduction device's assembly according to federal, state, and local regulations	Ensures compliance with the law
23. Properly disinfect/sterilize all other equipment	Prevents cross-examination between clients
24. Document in ink the completion of this service in the client's record under "Services Rendered" and date the entry. For example, "Removed tobacco stain with air polishing on #'s 6-11L, 22-27L, and client removed plaque biofilm from remaining teeth with a soft toothbrush and fluoride toothpaste. Flossed all teeth. APF topical fluoride treatment—tray method—provided for 4 minutes. Advised client not to eat, drink, or rinse for 30 minutes."	Ensures integrity of the client's record for both the client's health and the legal protection of the practitioner

Modified from Dentsply Preventive Care Division, York, Pa.

Procedure 22–3 AIR POLISHING TECHNIQUE WITHOUT USE OF AN AEROSOL REDUCTION DEVICE

MATERIALS

Sodium bicarbonate powder and toothpaste
Air polisher device and toothbrush
Dental floss or tape
Gauze squares (2 × 2 or 4 × 4)
Mouth mirror, air/water syringe
Disclosing solution
Lubricant for client's lips
Preprocedural antimicrobial mouthrinse
Saliva ejector or high-volume evacuation (HVE) tip
Safety glasses for client
Personal protective equipment

PREPARATION/POSITIONING	RATIONALE
See Procedures 22–2, steps 1 through 7	
GRASP	
See Procedures 22–2, steps 8 through 11	
FULCRUM	
1. Use external soft tissue fulcrums	Facilitates access
ADAPTATION	
2. Hold nozzle tip 3–4 mm from tooth in a slightly apical direction on the incisal to middle third of the tooth	Facilitates complete stain removal
3. Angle nozzles for posterior teeth at 80°, anterior teeth at 60°, occlusals at 90° (Figure 22–23)	Protects gingival tissues

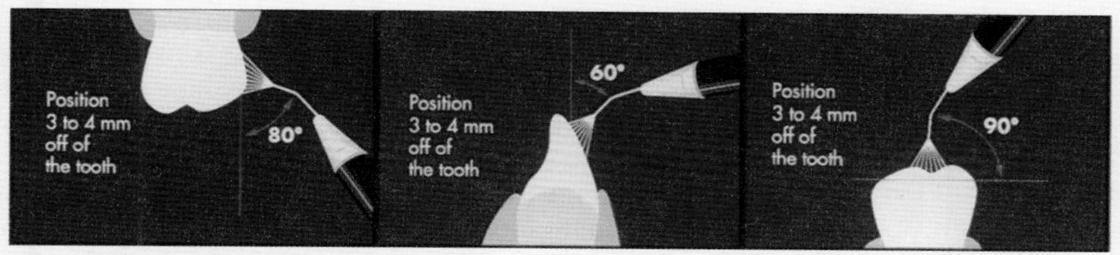

FIGURE 22–23 ✦ Recommended angulations of Prophy-Jet nozzle to tooth surface. *(Modified from DENTSPLY Preventive Care Division, York, Pa.)*

STROKE	
4. Activate foot pedal by pushing halfway down for water and all the way down for combined air, water, and sodium bicarbonate spray	Allows frequent rinsing without removing handpiece from mouth
5. Use constant circular sweeping motions, from proximal to proximal	Facilitates complete stain removal
6. Polish one or two teeth for one to two seconds and rinse	Increases client comfort
7. Use index finger and thumb to hold client's lip or cheek	Facilitates pooling of liquid in the vestibule for easier evacuation and containment of aerosols
OTHER	
8. See Procedure 22–2, steps 21 through 24	
9. Place all disposable supplies in trash container	Prevents cross-contamination between clients
10. See Procedure 22–2, steps 26 and 27	

Modified from Dentsply Preventive Care Division, York, Pa.

Without a comprehensive oral examination to determine the etiology of the stain and the safest, most appropriate method to use in treating the stain, clients may neglect to seek appropriate care for serious oral problems. For example, a dark area on a tooth may be due to a carious lesion or an amalgam restoration visible through the surface enamel. Bleaching would not remedy either situation. In addition, gel may seep out of improperly fitted trays and harm the soft tissues. Lay persons may not know how to deal with side effects that may be encountered. The Council on Scientific Affairs of the ADA does not recommend any over-the-counter products and suggests that clients seek professional care to lighten teeth.[74]

Home Bleaching with Professionally Supplied Products

Home bleaching with a custom-fitted tray and bleaching agent has become very popular (Figure 22–24). This procedure is also called nightguard vital bleaching (NGVB).[73] (See Chapter 30 for fabrication of custom-fitted bleaching trays.) In most cases, an oxidizing agent, usually 10% carbamide peroxide, is placed in a flexible polyvinyl, custom-made tray that the client wears one to two hours a day overnight for a two to six week period. The carbamide peroxide concentration, however, may vary from 10–22% or the bleaching agent may be 3% hydrogen peroxide. In addition to the oxidizing agent,

Dental Hygienist's Role in Tooth Bleaching

Provide client education on the ramifications of any bleaching treatment prior to its initiation.

Determine etiology of the stains, any allergies to ingredients in the bleaching agents, and client expectations.

Assess for any lesions that contraindicate bleaching.

Assess for any signs of caries or defective restorations that need to be addressed prior to initiation of any bleaching procedure.

Assess for any tooth sensitivity, because clients with extreme tooth sensitivity are not good candidates for tooth bleaching.

Evaluate the translucency of the teeth for alternative lightening procedures, because highly translucent teeth may appear more gray than white after bleaching.

Assess the presence and extent of gingival recession that may contraindicate bleaching.

Use radiograph, percussion, thermal, and electrical pulp testing to help determine the vitality and size of the pulp and the most appropriate method to meet a client's needs.

Assess client self-care to gather data on needed educational services.

Assist the client in setting realistic expectations and in making pretreatment and posttreatment comparisons using a shade guide, intraoral photographs, computer imaging, or an intraoral video camera.

Assess the presence of cracks during a fiberoptic examination of the teeth. An intraoral camera also may help to verify and measure enamel cracks. Deep cracks may be a contraindication to tooth bleaching, depending on their direction.

Remove calculus and extrinsic stains prior to any tooth bleaching procedure.

Take impressions and fabricate custom bleaching trays for home use.

If the dental practice act permits, provide in-office bleaching. The exact technique for in-office bleaching is dependent on the specific bleaching system used.

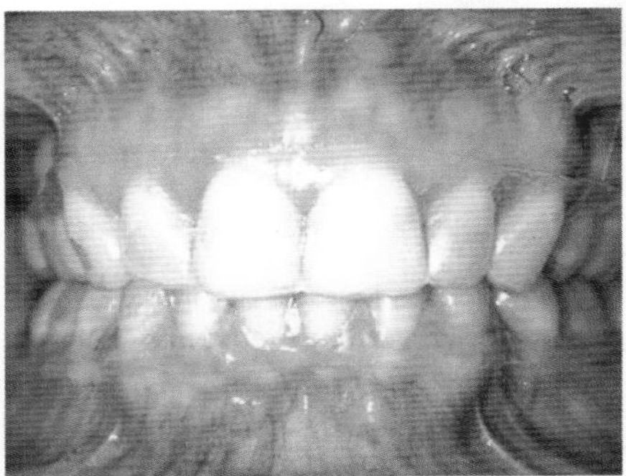

FIGURE 22–24 ✦ Custom-made maxillary and mandibular bleaching trays. *(Courtesy Dr. Brent B. Hutson.)*

an additive called carbopol (carboxypolymethelene polymer) may be added to thicken the gel, improve adherence to the tooth surface, and prolong the release of oxygen.[76] This additive keeps the gel contained within the tray and slows the chemical reaction.

Home bleaching is effective in producing a lightened tooth surface, but clients should be informed that the degree of change, especially with tetracycline-stained teeth, may be unpredictable. Therefore, client expectations must be clarified prior to initiation of any treatment. Stains in the yellow to brown range respond better than stains in the blue to gray range. Teeth with horizontal bands or striations of various colors, such as occurs with tetracycline-stained teeth, may bleach at different rates, making the defects more noticeable. Clients need to understand that although the teeth may look lighter, they may not necessarily be whiter, due to the normal, intrinsic color of the tooth. This type of treatment is temporary and additional treatments may be necessary in one to three years. Clients also need to know that any composite restorations subjected to bleaching will not change color and may need to be replaced because they may no longer match the color of the teeth following the bleaching procedure.[75] Finally, longevity of success will vary from client to client.[74]

Studies report that short-term side effects are usually minimal and disappear on cessation of treatment.[73,75] The most common side effects are mild thermal tooth sensitivity and gingival irritation. Tooth sensitivity is attributed to the easy passage of the hydrogen peroxide through the enamel and dentin to the pulp, resulting in a reversible pulpitis.[75,77] Use of a prescription brush-on fluoride gel or a shortened exposure time may decrease the sensitivity.[75] Clients with recession should not have bleaching because of the possibility of exposed dentin, which provides the hydrogen peroxide a direct route to the pulp. In 10% of the population, there is a gap at the cementoenamel junction between the enamel and the cementum, leaving exposed dentinal tubules that can lead to extreme sensitivity.[78] Gingival irritation may occur if the bleaching tray is overfilled. Use of a syringe dosage system, a highly viscous gel, and a properly fitted tray may prevent any excess from escaping the trays.

Occasionally, sore throats, tooth pain, tingling of tissues, and headaches are reported as side effects of tooth bleaching.[79] Slight morphologic changes in the enamel have also been noted with the vital bleaching gels.[80,81] A recent study, however, showed that 10% carbamide peroxide did not significantly alter enamel microhardness.[82] Localized microstructural and chemical changes were seen, but these were not clinically significant.[82]

Although wide variations in data exist concerning composite restorations, it seems reasonable to suggest that some composites are more susceptible to alterations and that some bleaching agents with higher concentrations are more likely to cause these alterations.[83] These changes,

Contraindications to Tooth Bleaching

Pregnancy*
Breastfeeding*
Allergy to any of the ingredients
Cervical erosion†
Large, defective restorations (should be replaced prior to bleaching)
Gingival, periodontal, or mucosal conditions that could be irritated by use of a bleaching tray or rubber dam
Recession†
Enamel cracks†
Tooth sensitivity†
Caries†

* No research is available on these population groups because they are not generally used as research subjects
† Tooth sensitivity may increase.

Sample ADA-Approved Dentist-Dispensed Home-Use Tooth Bleaching Products*

Colgate Platinum Daytime Professional Tooth Whitening System (Colgate Oral Pharmaceuticals, Canton, MA 02021)
Colgate Platinum Overnight Professional Tooth Whitening System (Colgate Oral Pharmaceuticals, Canton, MA 02021)
Rembrandt Lighten Bleaching Gel (Den-Mat Corporation, Santa Maria, CA 93455)
Nite White Classic Whitening Gel (Discus Dental Inc., Culver City, CA 90232)
Opalescence Whitening Gel (Ultradent Products Inc., South Jordan, UT 84095)
Patterson Brand Tooth Whitening Gel (Patterson Dental Supply, Inc., St. Paul, MN 55120)
Contrast P.M. (Spectrum Dental, Inc., Culver City, CA 90232)

*All products contain 10% carbamide peroxide

however, are unlikely to be clinically significant. Bleaching of teeth containing amalgams is not contraindicated but should be approached with caution because some changes in amalgam have been noted.[84,85] Another possible side effect involves the temporomandibular joint (TMJ).[86] When fabricating the bleaching tray, a thin material should be used to avoid interference with the client's occlusion. No effects on porcelain or ceramic materials have been reported and no long-term systemic effects have been identified. See Contraindications to Tooth Bleaching for a complete list of contraindications.

The ADA's Council of Scientific Affairs has approved several at-home bleaching products based on the manufacturers' submission of safety and efficacy studies (see Sample ADA-Approved Dentist-Dispensed Home-Use Tooth Bleaching Products). At present, the only concentration of carbamide peroxide approved by the Council on Scientific Affairs of the ADA is 10%. In general, the preponderance of research on bleaching techniques supports the safety and efficacy of ADA-approved products when prescribed protocols are followed. Ongoing studies are evaluating higher concentrations of carbamide peroxide and longer wearing times. Due to the rapid changes occurring in this area of dentistry, it is important to remain informed.

In-Office Bleaching

If the bleaching system is considered a topical medication under the dental practice act, then dental hygienists may, in some states, provide in-office bleaching. The dental practice act in each jurisdiction will determine the extent of the dental hygienist's involvement in bleaching or restorative services and should be consulted prior to providing any clinical bleaching service. The exact technique for in-office bleaching is dependent on the specific bleaching system used. The dental hygienist should follow the manufacturers' directions for maximum safety and efficacy. Protection of the client's gingiva, lips, eyes, and clothing is recommended. Several types of in-office or professional bleaching procedures are available. Techniques may differ based on a number of factors, including etiology of the stain, tooth vitality, and the number of teeth (a single tooth, multiple teeth, one arch, or both arches) needing the procedure. In addition, office time involved, client preference and compliance, cost, provider's preference, and the oral assessment are additional factors to consider when selecting the most appropriate procedure. Vital tooth bleaching is bleaching of a tooth with a vital pulp, and nonvital tooth bleaching is bleaching of an endodontically treated tooth.

In-office techniques for bleaching vital teeth can be classified as professional bleaching, power bleaching, conventional or traditional bleaching, laser bleaching, or combination bleaching. Often, the combination of office and home bleaching procedures enhances the desired effect. For a nonvital tooth or teeth, the bleaching procedure is usually intracoronal and may also be combined with one of the procedures indicated for vital teeth.

Each manufacturer of in-office bleaching systems has specific instructions for use of the product. In general, the in-office bleaching procedure for vital teeth involves several steps:

- Placement of a rubber dam or use of a light-cured paint-on dam and protection of the gingival tissues with a petroleum jelly is necessary.
- Teeth may or may not be etched prior to placement of the bleaching agent. A gel or liquid bleaching agent, usually 35% hydrogen peroxide, is then applied to the enamel surface (see ADA-approved In-Office Bleaching Products). If the liquid form is used, gauze squares saturated with the bleaching agent are placed on the facial surfaces. The bleaching agent is allowed to remain on the teeth for 20 to 30 minutes. A heat source, usually a visible light curing lamp or a

laser, is then applied to accelerate the chemical reaction (Figure 22–25).

- ✦ Local anesthetic must never be used during bleaching. Client discomfort must be monitored at all times to avoid tissue burns or excess heat build-up in the pulp. Analgesics may be recommended for the first 24 hours if any tooth sensitivity is noted.
- ✦ At the end of the procedure, all excess bleaching agent should be removed with water before removing the rubber dam.

The in-office bleaching procedure lasts from 30 to 60 minutes and may involve one to three appointments at two- to four-week intervals until teeth sufficiently lighten or no further color change is noted. This time interval between appointments allows the pulp to settle down in case irritation develops from the initial procedure. Clients should be informed that white spots on the tooth might become whiter and result in a splotchy appearance. If tooth-colored restorations need to be done, it is advisable to wait two to three weeks to determine the correct color shade. In addition, resin bonds are significantly reduced after tooth bleaching, so this time interval will help prevent failed restorations due to inadequate bond strength.[80] Side effects may include gingival burns and tooth sensitivity. Although rare, more serious side effects such as acute irreversible pulpitis and pulp necrosis may occur following vital bleaching with 35% hydrogen peroxide. Long-term stability is unknown because there are no controlled clinical studies that follow clients for years after bleaching.

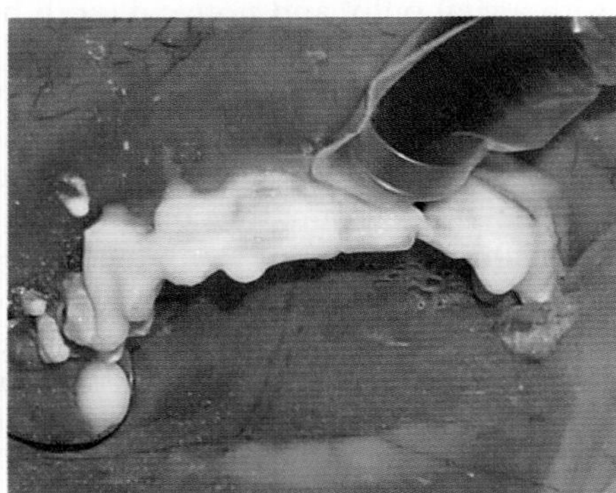

FIGURE 22–25 ✦ In-office bleaching procedure with a rubber dam, bleaching gel, and a resin curing light as the heat source. (*Courtesy Dr. Brent B. Hutson.*)

ADA-Approved In-Office Tooth Bleaching Products*

Starbrite In-Office Bleaching Gel (Spectrum Dental, Inc., Culver City, CA 90232)
Superoxyl (Sultan Chemists, Inc., Englewood, NJ 07631)

* Both products contain 35% hydrogen peroxide.

In addition to a resin curing light, other heat sources are available, such as the use of a specially designed bleaching light to catalyze the oxidizing agent. Many of these lights are currently marketed. The primary advantage of using a specially designed bleaching light is decreased chair time. An average of two 45-minute appointments is adequate to accomplish most bleaching procedures to a client's satisfaction.

Another heat source is the laser. Laser manufacturers claim that laser bleaching is faster, produces fewer side effects, and increases the whitening results. *Laser bleaching,* however, has not been supported by clinical studies to confirm safety and efficacy. Lasers currently are used primarily to accelerate the chemical reaction of the bleaching gel and do not bleach teeth alone (laser-assisted bleaching).[76] However, future research may confirm that lasers are effective for deep stains that conventional bleaching cannot alter. Lasers appear to be more costly and technique sensitive than traditional in-office methods. The ADA Council on Scientific Affairs has not approved the carbon dioxide laser because a number of unanswered questions exist regarding its safety and efficacy.[87] The argon laser is approved for use only as a heat source.[87] Some state dental practice acts specifically state that only licensed dentists may provide laser bleaching.

Clients who desire immediate whitening results may have one preliminary in-office procedure to begin the process, followed by one or two weeks of using home trays to complete the process. Alternatively, instead of the heat-activated in-office procedure, a high concentration of hydrogen peroxide, 30 to 50%, can be placed in the client's custom-fabricated bleaching trays and worn for about 30 minutes without the application of heat. The client is monitored in the office for color change and any discomfort.[88] Following the one-time high-concentration office procedure, the client continues the traditional at-home bleaching process with the lower-concentration bleaching agent. Both of these methods seem to be gaining in popularity.

INTRACORONAL BLEACHING. This method of in-office bleaching is used only for bleaching endodontically treated teeth and is usually performed by endodontists. Nonvital bleaching techniques usually fall into two categories: the thermocatalytic and the walking bleach techniques.[89] With both techniques, the bleaching agent is placed within the tooth. With the first method, the bleaching agent is usually 30% hydrogen peroxide, sodium perborate, or sodium hypochlorite.[73] The agent is placed within the coronal portion of the pulp chamber with a cotton pellet after the cervical portion has been sealed with zinc phosphate or zinc oxide-eugenol cement to prevent penetration of the bleaching agent into the patent dentinal tubules and the possibility of cervical resorption. Heat (heat lamp, heated instrument, electric heating device, or an ultraviolet light) is applied to hasten the reaction.[89]

The *walking bleach* method is so called because a paste of sodium perborate and hydrogen peroxide is placed in the coronal portion of the pulp chamber, the tooth is sealed, and the client is seen again in a week. At that time, the paste may be reapplied if further alteration in color is necessary. Often, only a small amount of color change can be achieved, but it may be sufficient to satisfy the client. This procedure is technique sensitive, and failure to follow exact protocols may result in severe pain during or following the procedure. If the cervical area is not sealed well, a cervical resorptive process may also occur. To enhance the final effect, both nonvital bleaching methods may be combined with the professional or home bleaching methods for vital teeth.[73]

MICROABRASION. Microabrasion is a dental procedure that removes superficial dark stains or "white spot" decalcified areas of enamel. This procedure involves removal of a thin layer of enamel and uses a paste of abrasives and hydrochloric acid on a specially designed prophy angle attachment.[90] Some commercially prepackaged kits are available. Although considered effective, this procedure is technique sensitive, may require multiple applications of the abrasive paste and hydrochloric acid, and removes some tooth structure. Side effects may include burns, sensitivity, pulpal damage, and noticeable removal of the outermost fluoride-rich layer of tooth enamel. It is sometimes difficult for the dentist to determine the exact amount of enamel to remove, and a restorative procedure may be needed if the stain is too deep. Microabrasion is more effective on mild stains than in moderate or severe cases. Long-term studies are not available. Home bleaching may be recommended following microabrasion to enhance the effect.

Restorative Management of Stained Teeth

Deep stains, mottled or pitted teeth, and grayish blue stains may need restorative procedures by the dentist, such as composite bonding, veneers, or full crowns to provide the client with a more aesthetic appearance. All bleaching of teeth that will not be restored should be done prior to the restorative procedures to ensure that crowns, bondings, and veneers will match the new enamel shade. Although not as conservative as bleaching, these procedures may assist the client in achieving a more wholesome facial image. The psychological and emotional benefits could be great. A dentist performs most restorative procedures, but the dental hygienist should be able to explain all procedures to the client.

VENEERS. Veneers are shell-like facings, usually made of composite resin or porcelain, that are bonded onto the facial surfaces of the teeth. Indirect composite veneers are fabricated in a dental laboratory on a stone die made from an impression. A small amount of tooth structure must be removed for this indirect composite restoration.

A direct technique for composite bonding is also available and does not require as much removal of tooth structure. Teeth indicated for composite bonding are isolated, polished with pumice, and acid-etched. A bonding agent and an optional opaquer can be added before the composite is molded onto the facial surface. This procedure can change the appearance and shape of the tooth. After curing, the bonded area must be contoured, finished, and polished. This procedure is done quickly and requires only one visit. It is relatively inexpensive, is good for young teeth with large pulps, and does not remove much tooth structure. However, it can look bulky, and has the potential to chip and stain over time.[72]

A porcelain veneer is ideal for older teeth. Fabrication of a porcelain veneer uses an indirect technique and involves preparation of the tooth by removing a thin layer of enamel, making an impression, and sending the impression to the laboratory for construction of the porcelain veneer. A temporary veneer is made and worn until the second visit. On the second visit, the temporary veneer is removed and the permanent veneer is checked for proper fit. The tooth is then isolated, polished with pumice, etched, rinsed, and dried. A bonding agent and an optional opaquer are applied. The inside of the veneer is conditioned and composite is added to bond the veneer to the tooth. The veneer is placed and excess composite is removed. Porcelain veneers can be bulky if they are not done properly, can stain at the margins, and can chip. Porcelain veneers are expensive but have good aesthetic properties and are more durable than composite veneers.

FULL-COVERAGE CROWNS. Full crowns are used when caries or restorations on the teeth are extensive. In some cases, they may be indicated following endodontic treatment. Good aesthetics can be achieved with crowns, but a large amount of tooth structure must be removed. Crowns should not be recommended just to make the teeth appear whiter. More conservative techniques are available and should be discussed with the client.

Client Education Issues

- ✦ Explain self-care plaque removal to prevent the recurrence of extreme stains.
- ✦ Explain the etiology, types, prevention, and management of extrinsic and intrinsic stains.
- ✦ Explain adverse effects of tooth polishing on tissues, restorative materials, and the environment.
- ✦ Explain the rationale for selective polishing.
- ✦ Explain tooth bleaching and aesthetic restorative procedures for stain management, including safety, efficacy, side effects, advantages, disadvantages, and indications and contraindications.

LEGAL, ETHICAL, AND SAFETY ISSUES

- ✦ All recommended guidelines on the safe use of rubber cup and air polishing must be followed to minimize risk to the client.
- ✦ Clients must be informed of procedures that may be harmful to hard tooth structures, oral soft tissues, and restorations prior to the performance of those procedures.
- ✦ Risk management strategies for treating medically compromised clients must be followed.
- ✦ State statutes regarding the legality of polishing teeth by allied dental personnel must be followed. Delegation of rubber cup polishing procedures to dental assistants in states where assistants are not legally allowed to perform is illegal. An ethical issue presents when delegation to dental assistants is legal, but a lack of background knowledge exists to determine when polishing is contraindicated.
- ✦ The dental hygienist must adhere to state statutes regarding the dental hygienist's role in home or in-office bleaching procedures.
- ✦ Client education about the advantages, disadvantages, risks, and potential adverse effects of treatment is essential for informed consent to all aesthetic procedures.

KEY CONCEPTS

- ✦ Rubber cup polishing, air polishing, and bleaching are selective procedures that should be included in dental hygiene care plans only after a comprehensive oral assessment.
- ✦ Although not a pathologic concern, the presence of stain may be a cosmetic concern.
- ✦ Selective polishing is the practice of omitting tooth polishing in areas where there is no stain to avoid removing some of the fluoride-rich outer layer of enamel and other adverse effects on teeth.
- ✦ Knowledge of the indications, contraindications, and various home and in-office techniques for aesthetic management of extrinsic and intrinsic stains is essential for client education.
- ✦ For all stain removal and stain management procedures, the dental hygienist must use the recommended techniques and products for safe and effective client care.

CRITICAL THINKING EXERCISES

1. In small groups, read and discuss a published paper (see References and Suggested Readings) dealing with selective polishing, air polishing, tooth bleaching, or aesthetic restorative procedures, and then report findings to the entire class.
2. Conduct a mock classroom debate on selective polishing or tooth bleaching. All students should participate, some as part of the debate team, some as literature reviewers, some as witnesses (dentists, dental hygienists, clients, parents, insurance company representatives). Half of the class should advocate for the "pro" position and half for the "con" position.
3. Conduct a survey (electronic or paper and pencil) of practicing dentists, dental hygienists, and clients about preferences for or experiences with selective polishing, air polishing, or bleaching. Discuss the findings during a designated class session.

For References, Suggested Readings, and Related Websites, visit
http://evolve.elsevier.com/Darby/hygiene/

CHAPTER 23

Nonsurgical, Supportive, and Mechanized Periodontal Therapies

OBJECTIVES

Mastery of the content in this chapter will enable the reader to:

- Differentiate between an oral prophylaxis, nonsurgical periodontal therapy, and supportive periodontal therapy
- Integrate nonsurgical periodontal therapy (NSPT) into the dental hygiene process of care
- Discuss advanced manual instrumentation techniques used in nonsurgical periodontal therapy
- Differentiate between ultrasonic (magnetostrictive and piezoelectric) and sonic instrumentation
- Discuss the procedure for instrumentation with mechanized devices using both standard and precision thin designs
- Apply a periodontal pack to a surgical site

KEY TERMS

Active therapy
Active tip area
Acoustic microstreaming
Amplitude
Autotuned unit
Cavitation
Clinical endpoint
Clinical power
Cycle
Defect volume
Deplaquing
Evaluation/Reevaluation
Final diagnosis
Final evaluation
Frequency
Full-mouth disinfection
Initial therapy
In phase
Lavage
Load
Magnetostrictive
Manual-tuned unit
Mechanical action
Mechanical nonsurgical pocket therapy
Mechanized instrumentation
Nonsurgical periodontal therapy (NSPT)
Out of phase
Periodontal debridement
Periodontal diagnosis
Periodontal maintenance procedures (PMP)
Periodontal pack
Pharmacotherapeutic nonsurgical pocket therapy
Piezoelectric
Power
Precision thin designs
Preliminary or presumptive dental diagnosis
Reevaluation
Supportive periodontal therapy (SPT)
Therapeutic endpoint
Tip displacement
Ultrasonic and sonic instruments

BASIC CONCEPTS IN NONSURGICAL PERIODONTAL THERAPY

Purposes

Nonsurgical periodontal therapy (NSPT) encompasses "plaque removal, plaque control, supragingival and subgingival scaling, root planing, and the adjunctive use of chemical agents."[1] Plaque removal alone will not resolve inflammation in all cases. Supragingival plaque biofilm control alone will not control all microorganisms in periodontal pockets. Thus, supragingival and subgingival plaque biofilm control must occur simultaneously in therapy to enhance the outcome of NSPT (plaque biofilm removal and control are discussed in Chapters 18 and 19).

Purposes of nonsurgical periodontal therapy are to:

- ✦ Eliminate or suppress infectious microorganisms
- ✦ Eliminate or control infection to prevent reinfection
- ✦ Establish an environment that helps resolve inflammation
- ✦ Modify host and environmental risk factors
- ✦ Employ antimicrobial agents when indicated

Scaling, instrumentation of the crown and root to remove plaque biofilm, calculus, and stains, is used for the treatment of clients with healthy gingiva or gingivitis. *Oral prophylaxis* combines both supragingival and subgingival scaling with selective polishing. This procedure is preventive in nature and not therapeutic as is NSPT. The dental hygienist performs an oral prophylaxis when periodontal health or gingivitis is diagnosed. *Root planing* is a definitive procedure to remove cementum or surface dentin that is rough, impregnated with calculus, or contaminated with toxins or microorganisms. The objective of therapeutic scaling and root planing is to remove as little root structure as possible while returning adjacent tissues to health.

Periodontal debridement is the "removal of all subgingival plaque and its by-products (as evidenced by clinical signs of inflammation), clinically detectable plaque-retentive factors (calculus and overhangs), and detectable calculus-embedded cementum to finish the root surface during periodontal instrumentation while preserving as much tooth surface as possible."[2] This intervention blends scaling and root planing into one procedure (periodontal debridement), and focuses on all plaque-retentive factors, not just calculus. Because plaque is a necessary factor in gingivitis and periodontitis, the emphasis on subgingival plaque removal is essential. Removal of calculus is secondary and important only because of its plaque-retentive nature.

Periodontal debridement strives to achieve tissue healing with minimal iatrogenic damage (e.g., damage from professional treatment) to the soft tissue and cementum. Periodontal debridement is divided into the following:[3]

- ✦ Coronal debridement
- ✦ Root surface debridement
- ✦ Deplaquing

Deplaquing, the removal or disruption of bacterial plaque biofilm and its toxins subgingivally following the completion of supragingival and subgingival debridement,[2] is performed mechanically using a curet or mechanized instrument at the reevaluation visit and during maintenance therapy. Because of the resistant nature of plaque biofilm, mechanical removal of bacterial plaque is the most effective mechanism of control. In addition to periodontal debridement, chemical agents via mouthrinses, local controlled delivery, or systemic antibiotics are sometimes used to suppress infectious microorganisms (see Chapter 24).

The *therapeutic endpoint* is the restoration of gingival health, reduction in pocket depth, and a gain in or maintenance of a stable clinical attachment level. These parameters can be expected only after a four- to six-week healing interval post-NSPT. This appointment, called periodontal *reevaluation,* is scheduled to reassess the clinical parameters of health after NSPT. Without a reevaluation visit, the therapeutic endpoint of active therapy is never assessed or documented.

Assessment, Diagnosis, and Care Planning

For a discussion on periodontal assessment, see Chapter 15. The *periodontal diagnosis* is determined after analyzing information collected during the assessment phase of therapy. The dental hygienist, and ultimately the dentist, must make an informed decision about the disease classification, extent, and severity. To accomplish this the hygienist considers the following:

- ✦ Presence or absence of inflammation
- ✦ Extent and pattern of clinical attachment loss
- ✦ Rate of disease progression
- ✦ Presence or absence of additional signs such as pain, ulceration, and familial aggregation
- ✦ Amount of plaque biofilm and calculus
- ✦ Client risk factors

To classify periodontal diseases, the practitioner decides if gingival disease or chronic or aggressive periodontitis is present. (See Chapter 15, Table 15–11 for a complete review of the Classifications of Periodontal Diseases and Conditions.)

An individual simultaneously may have areas of health and chronic periodontitis with slight, moderate, and advanced destruction. A system of periodontal classification used by practicing dental professionals for third-party insurance payments is shown in Table 23–1.

Identification of disease includes overall disease severity and disease activity. Disease severity is the measure of the destruction that occurred prior to the assessment. An important determination is whether the periodontitis is a slowly progressing form such as chronic periodontitis, or rapidly progressing, such as aggressive periodontitis. This determination is critical in planning the course of nonsurgical care and predicting the prognosis. The clinician considers multiple factors when classifying disease and it might not be possible to determine all these factors for a new client. For example, rate of disease progression can be determined only after multiple periodontal examinations are performed. Therefore, the initial diagnosis can be altered over time as more data become available. For this reason, the clinical examination results in a *preliminary or presumptive diagnosis* during initial or active therapy. A *final diagnosis* is the result of clinical findings and the response to nonsurgical or surgical care at the reevaluation visit. The diagnosis might change over time as periodontal maintenance occurs at appropriate time intervals (see Chapter 15, Figures 15–11 and 15–13).

More difficult to establish than disease severity, disease activity refers to the bone or attachment loss that

TABLE 23–1 CONSIDERATIONS FOR CLASSIFICATION OF PERIODONTAL DISEASES FOR INSURANCE REPORTING

Classification	Extent	Severity
Chronic periodontitis	Localized: ≤ 30% of sites involved Generalized: > 30% of sites involved	Slight: 1 or 2 mm CAL Moderate: 3 or 4 mm CAL Severe: ≥ 5 mm CAL
Aggressive periodontitis	Localized: ≤ 30% of sites involved Generalized: > 30% of sites involved	Slight: 1 or 2 mm CAL Moderate: 3 or 4 mm CAL Severe: ≥ 5 mm CAL

From American Academy of Periodontology, *Current procedural terminology for periodontics and insurance reporting manual*, ed 8, Chicago, 2002, American Academy of Periodontology and Armitage, GC; Development of a classification system for periodontal disease and conditions, Ann Periodontal, 4 (1), 1999.

is ongoing at the time of the examination. Periodontal disease activity involves periods of quiescence (inactivity) and periods of exacerbation (activity) evident in active disease. Periods of quiescence are characterized by a reduced inflammatory response and little or no loss of bone and connective tissue attachment. Unattached plaque and anaerobic bacteria (Gram-negative, motile) initiate periods of exacerbation that, in conjunction with other risk factors and the host's response, result in loss of bone and connective tissue attachment, creating deeper periodontal pockets.

Periods of exacerbation might last for days, weeks, or months and eventually quiescence may follow. This description of activity and inactivity explains the episodic nature of periodontal diseases. Clinically, disease activity can be measured only retrospectively by comparing the current examination with previous data. Thus, disease activity routinely is assessed at continued-care appointments.

Periodontal diagnosis is different from, yet related to, the dental hygiene diagnosis. NSPT relates to a variety of unmet human needs, but the clinical parameters of periodontal disease focus on the human need of skin and mucous membrane integrity of the head and neck. Bleeding, gingival inflammation, pocket depth, and attachment loss are all deficits related to this need and each requires interventions, such as NSPT.

Sequencing of therapeutic procedures follows a traditional model of periodontal care planning involving four phases of periodontal care (see Table 17–1). Nonsurgical periodontal therapy is part of Phase I therapy and is often referred to as *initial therapy*, initial preparation, or anti-infective therapy. Much of Phase I therapy is the responsibility of the dental hygienist working in concert with the general dentist or periodontist. *Active therapy* is either nonsurgical or surgical care or both, depending on the needs of the client. Active therapy includes Phase I care and can also extend to Phase II care.

After a series of appointments for NSPT and surgery, if indicated, the client is moved from active therapy to maintenance therapy. *Supportive periodontal therapy (SPT)* is Phase IV care that is an extension of periodontal therapy performed at selected intervals to assist the client in maintaining oral health. It continues at client-dependent intervals for the life of the dentition or its implant replacements. SPT might be discontinued and active therapy reinstituted if recurrent disease is detected. Other terms to describe this phase of care include periodontal maintenance therapy, periodontal maintenance, or periodontal recare. The *2002 Code on Dental Procedures and Nomenclature*[4] uses the term *periodontal maintenance procedures* (following active therapy) for clients who have completed periodontal treatment (surgical or nonsurgical).

Care planning approaches to periodontal therapy vary by the following:

- ✦ Classification and diagnosis of periodontitis
- ✦ Severity of periodontitis
- ✦ Systemic health or disease of the client
- ✦ Client's human needs and informed consent
- ✦ Practitioner's philosophy of care

In planning care, interventions are decided on and scheduled. The number, sequence, and length of appointments are determined to best meet the client's human needs. Table 23–2, a synopsis of clinical features and interventions for the most common forms of periodontal disease, is not intended to be all inclusive, but instead outlines treatment options and emphasizes where surgical intervention might be needed.

Chronic Disease States[5–8]

Chronic disease states (see Figure 15–12) of dental plaque–induced gingivitis and periodontitis progress slowly and respond in a relatively predictable manner to NSPT directed at reducing disease-causing bacteria. The main focus of NSPT for chronic disease states is oral self-care education and mechanical removal of plaque biofilm and plaque-retentive factors by both the client and professional. Oral self-care is ultimately the client's responsibility; instrumentation and selective polishing are the professional's responsibility.

Therapy for gingivitis includes oral self-care education, supragingival and subgingival debridement (scaling), and antimicrobial and antiplaque agents. Correction of plaque-retentive factors also is essential,

TABLE 23–2 CLINICAL FEATURES AND INTERVENTIONS FOR COMMON CLASSIFICATIONS OF PERIODONTAL DISEASES (see Chapter 15)

Class	Form	Clinical Features	Interventions
Gingival diseases	Dental plaque induced	Bacterial plaque biofilm present at gingival margin Disease begins at margin Change in gingival color Sulcular temperature change Increased gingival exudate Bleeding upon provocation Absence of attachment loss Absence of bone loss Histologic changes Reversible with plaque removal	Self-care education Client removal of plaque Periodontal debridement/scaling Correction of plaque retentive factors Antimicrobial mouthrinses Irrigation with antimicrobial
Periodontitis	Chronic	Most prevalent in adults, can occur in children and adolescents Amount of destruction is consistent with presence of local factors Subgingival calculus present Variable microbial pattern Slow to moderate rate of progression, maybe periods of rapid progression Further classified based on extent and severity Can be associated with local predisposing factors May be modified by and/or associated with systemic disease Modified by risk factors such as smoking and stress	Elimination, alteration, or control of risk factors Self-care education Periodontal debridement/scaling/root planing Reevaluation for surgery needs
Periodontitis	Aggressive	Clients otherwise clinically healthy Rapid attachment loss and bone destruction Familial aggregation Secondary features (usually present) Amounts of microbial deposits are inconsistent with severity Elevated proportions of *Actinobacillus actinomycetemcomitans* and *Porphyromonas gingivalis* Phagocyte abnormalities Hyper-responsive macrophage phenotype, including elevated levels of PGE 2 and IL-IB Progression of attachment loss and bone loss may be self-arresting	Self-care education Debridement/scaling/root planing Control of risk factors Systemic antibiotics (tetracyclines) Local controlled delivery of antibiotics Microbial diagnostic testing (DNA probe analysis) 0.12% chlorhexidine rinses Surgery Genetic testing Evaluation and counseling of family members

From American Academy of Periodontology: 1999 International Workshops for a Classification of Periodontal Diseases and Conditions, *Annals of Periodontology* 4(1):7, 1999.

including overhanging margins, open margins, overcontoured crowns, narrow embrasure spaces, open contacts, ill-fitting fixed or removable partial dentures, caries, and tooth malposition. Infrequently, surgical correction of gingival deformities that hinder the client's oral self-care is needed to aid control of bacterial plaque. Following Phase I active therapy, the client's condition should be reevaluated to determine future periodontal care.

Therapy for chronic periodontitis with slight to moderate loss of periodontal support includes active therapy and SPT. Systemic diseases and other risk factors must be considered because of the effect on the therapeutic outcome of NSPT. Diabetes mellitus, cardiovascular disease, HIV infection, smoking, substance abuse, and medications must be eliminated, altered, or controlled based on the client's needs assessment. Consultation with the client's physician(s) is appropriate. Oral self-care and periodontal debridement are the main therapeutic foci. Antimicrobial agents or devices might be useful when treating periodontitis with coexisting gingivitis. Implant therapy can be initiated during the initial phase of care or considered as Phase II therapy.

Periodontal surgery might also be indicated for advanced sites; however, most cases of slight and moderate involvement can be treated nonsurgically provided access to subgingival deposits and plaque-retentive factors is achievable. If the results of initial therapy resolve the periodontal infection and conditions, then SPT is scheduled. If results of initial therapy do not resolve the periodontal condition, then surgery is considered.

When advanced chronic periodontitis is present, additional considerations for therapy are necessary and include subgingival microbial samples for analysis, antibiotic sensitivity testing, and extraction of hopeless teeth. In specific cases optimal results may not be attainable because of the client's health, age, uncontrolled systemic condition, and extent of disease; initial therapy might be the endpoint of periodontal care. Periodontal surgery is also a problem-focused surgical therapy aimed at enhancing root debridement and tissue regeneration, and reducing gingival recession for clients who have effective self-care practices. In any form of periodontal disease, client compliance with self-care practices and recommended maintenance intervals is crucial to a successful long-term outcome.

Aggressive Disease States[9] (See Figure 15–12)

Aggressive periodontitis and some uncommon forms of gingivitis will not respond predictably to NSPT. Aggressive periodontitis is seen in clients who otherwise appear healthy, tends to have a familial aggregation, and progresses rapidly. Traditional NSPT is the basic therapeutic modality for aggressive periodontitis; however, quantity of bacterial plaque and calculus deposits is less important than the host response to specific periodontal pathogens present. Initial periodontal therapy alone often is not effective at controlling host response to specific pathogens. Other care planning considerations include the following:

- General medical evaluation to determine if systemic disease is present
- Consultation with physician to coordinate medical care with periodontal care
- Modification of risk factors
- Adjunctive antimicrobial therapy
- Microbiologic identification
- Antibiotic sensitivity testing
- Evaluation and counseling of family members to determine genotype status

Tooth extraction and occlusal therapy might also be part of therapy. The SPT interval should be short (one to three months) to slow rapid disease progression. Clients with aggressive periodontitis are referred to the periodontist more often than those with chronic disease. Diagnosis of aggressive periodontitis might occur after active therapy, reevaluation, and several intervals of SPT; at this point, referral to the periodontist is indicated.

Appointment Planning

One major consideration that affects the appointment plan (see Chapter 17) during NSPT is the use of pain control strategies such as behavior modification, nitrous oxide–oxygen analgesia, or local anesthetic. Need must be established based on assessment data and client-related factors. Pain control modalities might require more appointment time and thus should be included in the care plan. Length of appointment could vary from 40 to 90 minutes depending on client needs (Table 23–3).

Case Presentation and Informed Consent (See Chapter 17)

Objectives of case presentation are to do the following:

- Encourage collaborative treatment between the client and clinician
- Satisfy legal responsibilities

Through case presentation and gaining informed consent, the clinician is able to communicate to the client the following:

- Periodontal assessment findings indicating disease, much like other chronic disease states
- How NSPT differs from the oral prophylaxis
- Extensive nature of periodontal debridement and why the number of appointments and time involved are critical to achieving an optimal outcome

Because reevaluation and SPT are vital to continued success, the purpose and intent for each must be explained to the client.

IMPLEMENTATION OF NSPT

Implementation includes the delivery of preventive and therapeutic procedures identified in the individualized care plan to meet client human needs. Preventive and therapeutic entities of nonsurgical periodontal therapy such as self-care education, manual and mechanized instrumentation, pharmacotherapeutic interventions, pain control strategies, if indicated, and selective polishing are performed. Other supportive interventions in achieving the ultimate goals of NSPT are overhang removal (margination), desensitization, dietary assessment and counseling, dental caries management, and occlusal therapy. Therapeutic procedures include the following:

- *Mechanical nonsurgical pocket therapy:* scaling and root planing (periodontal debridement) using manual and/or mechanized instruments.
- *Pharmacotherapeutic nonsurgical pocket therapy:* use of systemic, topical, and controlled delivery antimicrobial agents to selectively remove or inhibit pathogenic bacteria (also known as antimicrobial therapy or periodontal chemotherapy).

Recently, the concept of full-mouth disinfection has been proposed as a treatment strategy. *Full-mouth disinfection* is the scaling and root planing of all pockets within a 24-hour time period, including the application of 0.12% chlorhexidine to all periodontal pockets followed by daily 0.12% chlorhexidine mouthrinsing for two months.[10] The rationale underlying this concept is that the traditional method of four consecutive appointments for scaling and root planing without proper disinfection might permit reinfection of previously disinfected pockets by bacteria from an untreated region of the mouth.

TABLE 23–3 FACTORS TO CONSIDER WHEN DETERMINING NEED FOR LOCAL ANESTHETIC AGENTS

Factor	Comment
Periodontal Assessment Factors	
Pocket depth greater than 4 mm	Limited accessibility and visibility decrease chance of complete deposit removal; pain control increases client comfort and operator confidence
Tissue tone	Tight or nonelastic tissue may limit access to deep pockets or challenging root anatomy Local anesthetic may be used to increase the turgor of the gingiva if injected into an edematous interdental papilla
Pocket topography	Cratering at epithelial attachment or narrow intrabony pockets; pain control enhances deposit removal
Furcations	Limited accessibility and visibility decrease chance of complete deposit removal; pain control increases client comfort and operator confidence
Root anatomy	Anatomic variations may require pain control for NSPT Limited access Unusual longitudinal depressions Deeper pockets with more complex root anatomy Increases sensitivity Overscaled roots (Coke-bottle appearance) Gingival recession Abrasion
Inflammation	Inflamed tissue likely to be painful Incidental curettage will occur inadvertently in some areas Hemostasis may be a concern
Hemorrhage	Use vasoconstrictor when hemostasis is a concern such as with bleeding upon probing or spontaneous hemorrhage
Client-related Factors	
Pain threshold	If pain threshold is low, administer local anesthetic to control pain and/or reduce anxiety level
Sensitivity	Determine type of sensitivity (pulpal or soft tissue) Determine type of instrumentation (hand vs. mechanized instruments)

From Hodges KO: *Concepts in nonsurgical periodontal therapy,* ed 1, Albany, NY, 1998, Delmar.

Mechanical Nonsurgical Pocket Therapy (Advanced Manual Instrumentation)

"The critical determinant of periodontal therapy is not the choice of treatment modality, but the detailed thoroughness of the root surface debridement and the patient's standard of oral hygiene care."[11] Advanced manual instrumentation is an extension of basic instrumentation. Instrumentation in deep pockets of 6 mm or greater in and adjacent to furcations and where mobility exists, is significantly impaired when providing NSPT; therefore, subsequent periodontal surgery should be considered. Options for treating areas affected by periodontal disease include traditional armamentarium such as files, universal curets, and area-specific curets (see Chapter 20). The clinician selects these instruments based on the following:

- Type of deposit or plaque-retentive factor being removed
- Pocket depth
- Inflammation
- Tissue tone
- Access
- Root morphology
- Pocket topography

A single instrument is not likely to produce the desired clinical and therapeutic endpoints because multiple clinical factors require periodontal debridement with a host of instruments. For example, during initial therapy the clinician might experience generalized heavy and tenacious subgingival deposit requiring removal with files and standard unmodified ultrasonic inserts. Then both universal and area-specific hand instruments are used to debride because the clinician is treating most root surfaces of most teeth. Universal instruments enable the clinician to treat the midline of proximal areas of the tooth and adapt as far subgingivally as is reasonable, depending on the tissue tone and pocket topography. The final periodontal debridement then is accomplished with area-specific instruments with flexible shanks to remove bacterial plaque and calculus deposits and create a relatively smooth root environment.

Options for instrumentation in pockets 5 mm or greater include extended shank curets and mini-bladed curets.[12] Extended shank curets have a terminal shank that is 3 mm longer than the standard area-specific curet to access deep periodontal pockets and improve oral clearance around the crown (Figure 23–1). The blade itself is also thinner to enhance insertion and reduce tissue distention (Figure 23–2).

Mini-bladed curets combine features of the extended shank designs with a 50% reduction in blade length as compared to the extended shank or standard design (Figure 23–1). Mini-bladed curets enhance adaptation on narrow facial and lingual surfaces of anterior teeth (Figure 23–3), in furcations, and on root surfaces in

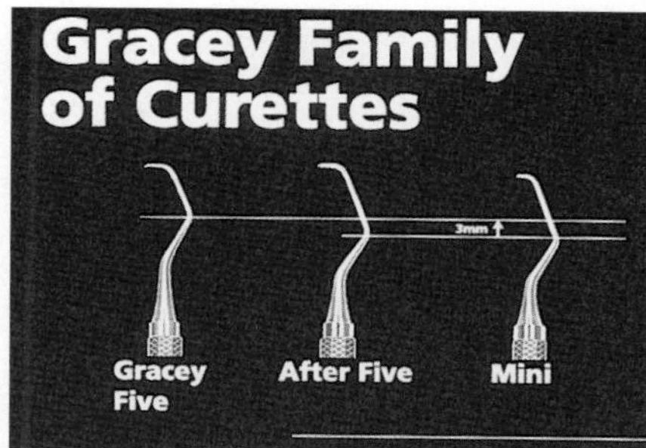

FIGURE 23–1 ✦ Gracey family of curets: Gracey (standard area-specific design), After-Five (extended shank area-specific design), and Mini-Five (mini-bladed area-specific design). *(Courtesy Hu-Friedy Manufacturing Co.)*

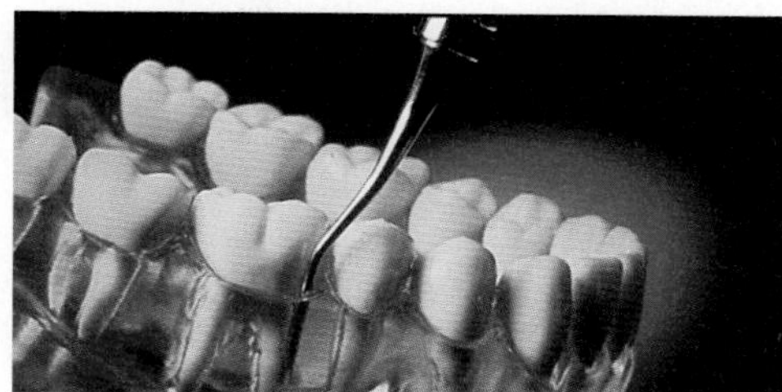

FIGURE 23–2 ✦ After-Five root planing curet. Adapting to the root in a deep periodontal pocket. *(Courtesy Hu-Friedy Manufacturing Co.)*

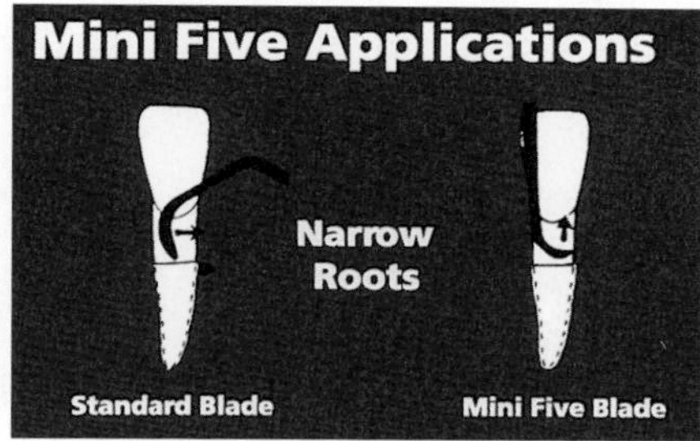

FIGURE 23–3 ✦ Mini Five applications: narrow roots. The short blade of the mini-bladed design permits access to the epithelial attachment on the facial surface without the use of the toe-down approach. *(Courtesy Hu-Friedy Manufacturing Co.)*

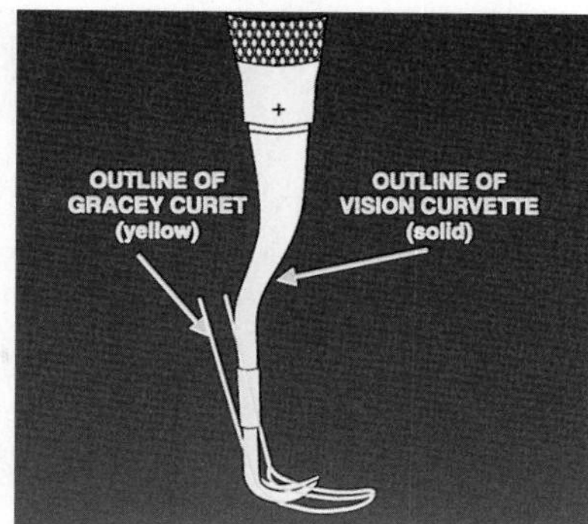

FIGURE 23–4 ✦ Comparison of Vision Curvette with Gracey curet. *(Courtesy Hu-Friedy Manufacturing Co.)*

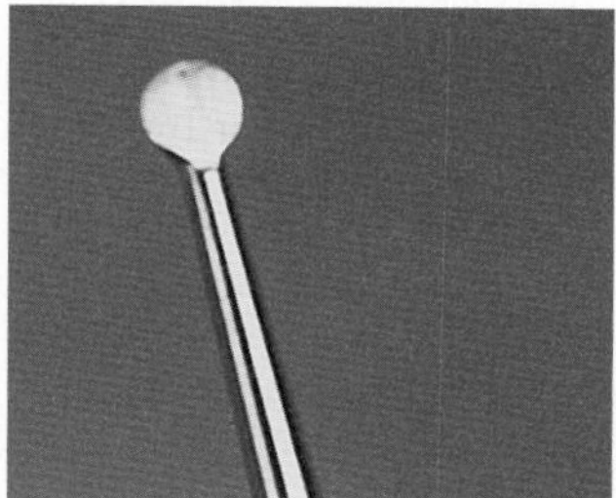

FIGURE 23–5 ✦ Debridement curet. In a close-up view, the instrument blade appears similar to a small spoon excavator. The entire circumference of the blade is a cutting edge. *(Courtesy Hu-Friedy Manufacturing Co.)*

narrow and deep periodontal pockets. A limitation of mini-bladed curets is the extension to the midline of proximal surfaces. Also, because of the small size of the blade, their longevity after sharpening is reduced when compared to other instruments. Both the extended shank and mini-bladed versions are available in any area-specific pattern except the 9/10 and 17/18 (Hu-Friedy Manufacturing Corporation, Chicago, Illinois). The 9/10 and 17/18 designs both have accentuated shank bends and long terminal shanks, enhancing their use in deeper pockets and difficult to reach areas without the extended shank feature (see Procedure 23–1 for use of extended and mini-bladed curets).

Other area-specific instruments include the following:[12]

- *Vision Curvettes* have curved blades and are 50% shorter than the standard design. The shank has a 5 mm and 10 mm mark for a visual cue to pocket depth during instrumentation. Curvature of the blade is what distinguishes this set of instruments from mini-bladed curets (Figure 23–4). Curvettes, designed to enhance adaptation on teeth with deep periodontal pockets, have four configurations:
  - Subzero with a long shank for instrumentation on the facial and lingual surfaces and around line angles on premolars and anterior teeth
  - 1/2 for anterior and premolar surfaces and interproximal areas
  - 11/12 for the mesial proximal surfaces of molars and for furcations
  - 13/14 for the distal proximal surfaces of molars and for furcations
- A disadvantage of Vision Curvettes is the short working end, which limits extension to the midline of proximal surfaces and the upward curvature of the blade, which could cause gouging or striations in the root if not adapted properly.
- *Debridement curets* are designed for gentle removal of residual deposits and for smoothing root surfaces after ultrasonic instrumentation (Figure 23–5). They are ideal for furcations (Figure 23–6), developmental grooves, and line angles. The entire edge of the blade is a cutting edge, which enables the clinician to use a vertical, horizontal, or oblique push or pull stroke (see Chapter 20 on area-specific curets).
- *Furcation curets* are designed for root concavities and for furcation instrumentation. The blade width is less than that of other curets, ranging from 1.3 mm to 0.9 mm.[12]

Procedure 23–1 USE OF EXTENDED SHANK AND MINI-BLADED CURETS

EQUIPMENT

Personal protective equipment
Subgingival periodontal explorer
Set of extended shank area-specific curets (minimum recommendations for a quadrant include an anterior curet such as the Gracey 1/2 and posterior curets 11/12 and 13/14 (or 11/14 and 12/13).
Set of mini-bladed area-specific curets for specific locations.
Pockets greater than 5 mm
2″ × 2″ gauze

STEPS	RATIONALE
1. Refer to periodontal assessment.	Identifies pocket depths greater than 5 mm, gingival contour and tone, pocket topography.
2. Self-assess operator and client positioning.	Ensures positioning for area-specific design and pocket depth or root anatomy.
3. Use modified-pen grasp with thumb and index finger across from one another near the junction of the shank and handle, or further up on the handle, depending on the fulcrum used.	Facilitates tactile sensitivity, adaptation, activation, and comfort for client and operator.
4. Select an appropriate fulcrum such as conventional or opposite arch. Vary fulcrum position when negotiating deep pockets. It is advisable to extend to the depth of the pocket or underneath the calculus, adapt the blade, and then place the fulcrum.	Provides stability for activation. Fulcrums are modified depending on the depth of pocket. Conventional fulcrums are still the most useful and the opposite arch is useful for molars, especially on the maxillary arch.
5. Use dental mirror.	Needed for retraction, indirect vision, reflection, and/or trans-illumination depending on area and surface.
6. Select appropriate working end and blade. Hold instrument so that terminal shank is perpendicular with the floor. Viewing face of the blade from above, the larger, convex curved lower blade is the correct blade, or adapt the cutting edge that tilts away from the terminal shank.	Only one cutting edge is appropriate to use on a specific surface.
7. Insert working end into pocket with blade as closed as possible to reach the epithelial attachment or to extend 1mm below the calculus, whichever is appropriate.	Reaches base of pocket in a nontraumatic manner.
8. Use vertical position of terminal shank as a visual cue to recognize correct working end and blade.	Terminal shank should be parallel with surface being treated.
9. Use handle position as a visual cue to recognize correct working end and blade.	Handle should be as parallel as possible with the long axis of tooth in the buccolingual dimension. Handle should not cross the occlusal plane.
10. Adapt terminal 1 to 2 mm of blade to the root.	Using too much of the blade (more than the terminal one-third) hinders effective channeling, can be uncomfortable for the client, and/or does not provide correct adaptation to convex and concave root surfaces.
11. Acquire correct blade-to-root angle for the procedure (from 45° to 90° depending on mode of attachment of the lighter calculus).	Provides appropriate angle to meet the purpose of the stroke (exploratory, working, or debridement).
12. Activate with appropriate lateral pressure, length of stroke, and direction of stroke.	Lateral pressure and length of the stroke (1 to 3 mm) depend on the purpose of stroke (light calculus deposit removal or debridement). Direction of stroke depends on the purpose. Oblique strokes are necessary on proximal surfaces of molars and premolars to maintain adaptation and achieve oral clearance of handle from opposite arch.
13. Use the rock, roll, and pivot to maintain adaptation.	Facilitates adaptation to the many convex and concave surfaces encountered.
14. View radiographs throughout procedure.	Complements tactile sensitivity.
15. Evaluate instrument sharpness throughout procedure.	Effectiveness depends on a sharp blade.
16. Evaluate root surface with the explorer.	Determines relative smoothness and clinical endpoint.
17. Record in client record the curets used and where, e.g., periodontal debridement of maxillary right quadrant using Gracey 11/12 and 13/14.	Aids in instrument selection at subsequent NSPT and/or SPT appointments; maintains accurate documentation for legal purposes.

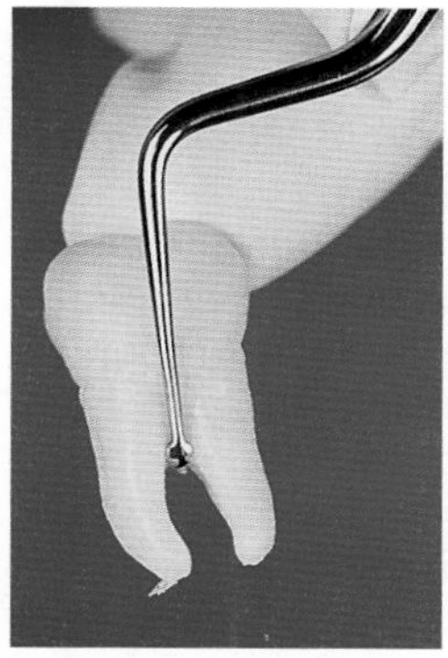

FIGURE 23–6 ✦ Debridement curet (SOH 1/2) in furcation. The small disc-shaped blade curves into the tooth, easily adapting to the furcations. The long terminal shank (15 mm in length) facilitates access to deep and narrow periodontal pockets. *(Courtesy Hu-Friedy Manufacturing Co.)*

SHANK STRENGTH. See Chapter 20 on strength of shanks.

FURCATION INVOLVEMENT. Presence of furcation involvement seriously compromises the prognosis of the tooth; therefore, detection and thorough periodontal debridement are essential at the earliest point in NSPT. When a 4-mm periodontal probe reading is recorded on a multirooted tooth adjacent to a buccal or lingual furcation, a furcation involvement should be suspected. In some cases, especially in mandibular molars where the bifurcation is located only 3 mm from the cervical line, invasion can occur in the early stages of periodontitis with attachment loss of only 2 to 4 mm.

Furcation entrance diameters are relatively small, so access with an explorer, Nabers probe, and especially a curet is challenging. The estimated furcation entrance width of maxillary first molars is from 0.5 mm to 0.75 mm, depending on the surface. The average width of the furcation entrance on a mandibular molar buccal surface is 0.75 mm and the lingual width is 1 mm. The blade face width of curets is from 0.75 mm to 1 mm. Area-specific curets (Gracey's), however, are slightly narrower in blade width than are universal designs. Curets that have been sharpened, creating a thinner blade, are recommended for furcation debridement. When curet blade width is compared to the furcation entrance width, it is easy to see why it is difficult to adequately debride these areas without surgery. The clinician refers to the degree of invasion of the furcation to aid in instrument selection and instrumentation.

Location of the furcation involvement, the relationship of the gingiva and furcation entrance, and pocket depth also are factors to consider when deciding how to instrument the area. When access permits, the best approach is to treat each root as a separate tooth, using a combination of strokes. The distal surface of each root is instrumented, then the buccal/lingual surfaces, and last, the mesial surfaces of each root. The clinician overlaps strokes, especially in the concavity where the roots meet (Figure 23–7). Next, the clinician concentrates on the concavity coronal to the furcation entrance by employing horizontal and oblique strokes with a toe-down approach, if applicable. An area-specific curet designed for mesial surfaces such as the 11/12 Gracey or

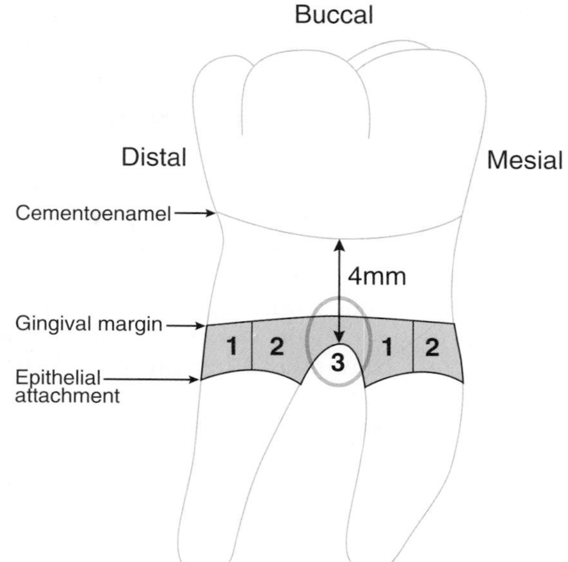

FIGURE 23–7 ✦ Periodontal debridement of a furcation. The distal surface of each root is instrumented *(area 1)*. The buccal, lingual, and mesial surfaces are then treated *(area 2)*. Last, the concavity is debrided *(area 3)*.

one with a straight shank such as the 7/8 Gracey can be used in the concavity.

When the gingiva occludes the furcation, the pocket depth is shallow, or the furcation entrance is barely detectable, the clinician may not be able to treat each root separately. Instead, the area is treated with a combination of strokes, including the toe-down approach. The mini-bladed curet is especially appropriate for these situations.

Maxillary mesial and distal furcations present a unique challenge. Access to the mesial furcation is best from the lingual surface because the furcation is located lingually and not in the midline. An extended shank, area-specific, mesial surface design and a universal design with a long terminal shank might be used in combination to treat this area.

The distal furcation entrance is located near the midline of the proximal surface; therefore, access from the lingual or buccal is equal. Furcation involvement on proximal surfaces of maxillary teeth requires extreme rolling and pivoting to adapt explorers and curets into the defect. Alternative fulcrum placement such as finger-on-finger, opposite arch, and cross-arch placement might be useful to negotiate the furcation (see Chapter 20).

MOBILITY. The clinician's mirror hand is used to stabilize the tooth during instrumentation. Stabilization occurs on the incisal or occlusal edge if mobility is slight, and stability might be needed on the surface opposite or adjacent to the one being treated if significant mobility is present.

If the facial surface of a mobile mandibular anterior tooth is being treated, then the index finger on the mirror hand is placed on the lingual surface near the incisal edge. If the mesial buccal surface of a mobile molar is being treated, the tooth will be stabilized from the lingual.

Mobile teeth interfere with optimal fulcrum placement; therefore, problem solving is indicated. The finger-on-finger rest, in which the fulcrum is established on the index finger or thumb of the nonoperating hand, is especially useful in this situation. Also, periodontal debridement of a tooth adjacent to a mobile tooth is challenging when the mobile tooth would usually be used for the fulcrum placement. Again, alternative fulcrums must be used, such as a conventional fulcrum placed farther away from the tooth being treated, or use of an opposite arch or cross-arch approach (see Chapter 20).

PHARMACOTHERAPEUTIC NONSURGICAL POCKET THERAPY. See Chapter 24.

CLINICAL OUTCOMES OF PERIODONTAL DEBRIDEMENT[11]

Despite incomplete calculus removal, nonsurgical instrumentation arrests periodontitis. After scaling and root planing, most studies have observed a loss of clinical attachment at sites with initially shallow pockets and a gain in attachment level at sites with deeper pockets. Loss in attachment at shallow sites is thought to relate to over-instrumentation and overzealous self-care. Also, the buccolingual gingival thickness (thin gingival walls) experiences more loss, and instrumentation at deeper sites adjacent to shallow sites damages shallow sites.

Shallow sites (1 to 3 mm) had a mean clinical attachment level change of –0.34 mm. Pockets with initial depth of 4 to 6 mm had an attachment level gain of 0.55 mm. Pockets 7 mm or greater had an attachment gain of 1.29 mm. Clinical attachment level gain from mechanical therapy is 2.9 mm and for surgical methods the clinical attachment gain is 4.2 mm. Mean probing depth reduction for 4- to 6-mm sites was 1.29 mm versus 2.16 mm for sites 7 mm or greater. Pocket depth reduction is greater postsurgery than postscaling and root planing; however, over time the differences become insignificant.

These findings highlight the need for clinicians to educate clients about the expected outcome of mechanical therapy during NSPT, the need for continued care at appropriate SPT intervals, and the potential for additional treatment as indicated. Bleeding on probing has been used by clinicians as an indicator of disease activity. Because there is a lack of correlation between bleeding on probing and risk for future clinical attachment loss, it is best to use absence of bleeding as a criterion for stability. Mechanical NSPT predictably reduces the level of inflammation. After scaling and root planing, several outcomes are expected:[11]

- ✦ Percentage of motile microbes and spirochetes, *Porphyromonas gingivalis,* and other Gram-negative anaerobic microbes, are reduced and the percentage of cocci and nonmotile microbes increases.
- ✦ Microbes that repopulate the subgingival environment after therapy have two origins: residual following incomplete instrumentation, or an extension of supragingival plaque.
- ✦ Microbial repopulation of subgingival pockets can be inhibited by effective oral self-care practices. Presence of supragingival bacterial plaque facilitates repopulation of pockets with high percentages of spirochetes and motile rods within four to eight weeks.[11]
- ✦ Predictable elimination of *Actinobacillus actinomycetemcomitans* associated with aggressive disease does not occur.
- ✦ There is minimal or no bone repair after scaling and root planing.

As previously discussed, furcations associated with periodontitis present a particularly challenging environment to accomplish the objectives of mechanical therapy. Research suggests[11] that 19 to 57% of teeth diagnosed with furcation involvement were lost over a 15-year period as compared to 5% to 10% of teeth without furcation involvement that were lost during the same period of time. Typically, problems with mechanical therapy adjacent to furcation involvement include:

- ✦ Identification during the periodontal assessment
- ✦ Furcal anatomy
- ✦ Lack of access
- ✦ Persistence of pathogenic microflora

These same factors affect the clients' ability to perform self-care.

Aggressive instrumentation to remove endotoxin is unwarranted because endotoxin is loosely bound to the root surface.[13] Also, treated root surfaces become recontaminated over short periods of time. Another outcome of mechanical instrumentation to consider is the role root surface roughness plays in microbial recolonization and in achieving the desired clinical endpoint. Both surface free energy and roughness play major roles in the initial adhesion and retention of microbes.[14] These findings are particularly true in regard to supragingival root surfaces; however, they are also important to subgingival root surfaces. Clinicians need to achieve the smoothest root surface possible without resorting to over-instrumentation.

Clinical and Therapeutic Endpoints

The clinical endpoint measures the tooth surface's preparation for healing of adjacent tissues. It is determined immediately after periodontal therapy when the subgingival environment is assessed with an explorer. To assess the clinical endpoint a variety of explorers may be used, accompanied by air and illumination:

- ✦ Curved universal curets (Suter 2R-2L; Hu-Friedy 2, 2H, or 2R/2L)
- ✦ Area-specific designs (Hu-Friedy EXD 11/12 or 11/12 After Five)
- ✦ Pocket feelers (Hu-Friedy 20 F Orban)

Of particular interest to NSPT is the 11/12 extended shank design. It, like the extended shank curets, has a longer terminal shank (3 mm) when compared to the standard design. It is indicated for deep pockets and anterior teeth. A limitation might be midline extension on posterior proximal surfaces due to the short working end (Figure 23–8).

The therapeutic endpoint of therapy determined at the evaluation visit includes the measurement of critical criteria such as probing depth, clinical attachment level, and gingival inflammation accompanied by bleeding. If bleeding and inflammation are present, site-specific therapy is performed including instrumentation, consideration of chemotherapeutic agents, and further client education in self-care practices. Evaluation is the only mechanism for determining if inflammation has been eliminated as evidenced by the absence of bleeding and swelling, and whether the level of attachment is maintained. If the clinical endpoint yields the desired therapeutic endpoint, then the appropriate level of calculus and/or cementum removal and removal of plaque retentive factors has been attained.

The dental hygiene practitioner is constantly evaluating whether the clinical endpoint of instrumentation during NSPT is sufficient. Because removal of subgingival plaque biofilm and its by-products cannot be measured clinically, the topography of the tooth surface is the best criterion to make this decision. The clinical endpoint for the majority of clients is a tooth surface devoid of detectable plaque-retentive factors. If the subgingival area remains rough or irregular, the clinician should attempt to remove the roughness. To decide when instrumentation is complete, the clinician considers factors such as:

- Self-evaluation of proper instrumentation technique
- Progress towards removing the irregularity
- Probable root anatomy in the areas (see Chapter 21)
- Radiographic appearance of the tooth surface
- Extent of gingival inflammation
- Severity of periodontitis
- Generalized characteristics of the client's calculus and other plaque retentive factors.

If the clinician is in doubt about certain areas, these sites should be recorded in the record of services to ensure their evaluation at the next visit during active therapy, or at the reevaluation visit.

When instrumentation technique is sound and further instrumentation is not changing root roughness and irregularity, then the clinician stops instrumentation. The area is then reexamined at the evaluation visit to assess if the clinical endpoint was appropriate. If the area warrants further instrumentation because of persistent inflammation or bleeding, then instrumentation continues. This decision making process and evaluation build the clinician's experience base and expertise in providing NSPT. Also, the clinician must recognize the client's role in the healing process; therefore, home care must be evaluated along with other clinical parameters of health.

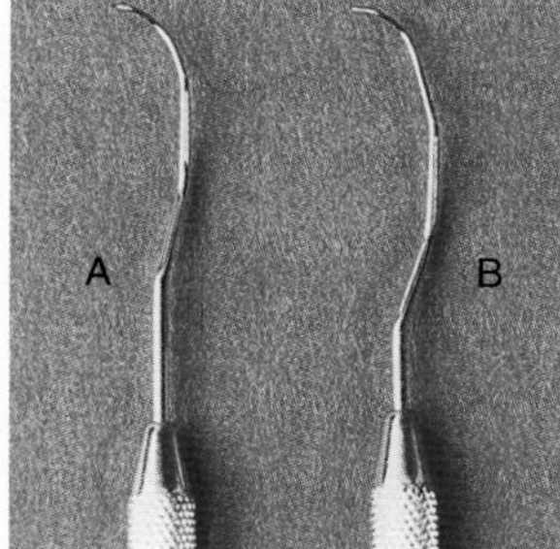

FIGURE 23–8 ✦ 11/12 explorers for use in NSPT. **A,** Standard design. **B,** Extended shank. *(Courtesy Hu-Friedy Manufacturing Co.)*

It is important to note that the basic definition of periodontal debridement includes the removal of all plaque-retentive factors, including removal of detectable calculus, and that the therapeutic endpoint of periodontal debridement is periodontal health. Removal of 100% of the calculus and diseased cementum is not possible or even desirable because of the amount of lost tooth structure and probable dental hypersensitivity. Although meticulous periodontal debridement may remove some cementum, the use of aggressive root planing to intentionally remove cementum is not recommended.

In contrast, periodontal debridement requires complete removal of clinically detectable calculus. Because calculus retains bacterial plaque biofilm, its removal is critical to the success of periodontal therapy. Also, because gingivitis and periodontitis both relate to the systemic health of the client, the immune response, and self-care practices, there will probably never be one easy standard for assessing the clinical endpoint. Sound professional judgment must be practiced to determine endpoints of NSPT. Intentionally leaving detectable calculus, therefore, constitutes unethical or substandard care.

EVALUATION. *Final evaluation* compares the initial assessment data with client data at the completion of care to determine if therapeutic and client goals were met. The clinician should remember, however, that evaluation occurs continually throughout the implementation phase of NSPT. Because of the extent of therapy and the multiple visits involved, the clinician has the opportunity to reexamine areas previously treated to assess gingival healing via color change and shape, deposit removal, the client's oral self-care practices, and/or results from diagnostic testing or medical screening. Generally, the first evaluation of the gingival healing takes place two weeks after completion of periodontal debridement of a sextant, quadrant, or half mouth. This two-week period represents the time required for epithelial adaptation; assessment for plaque-retentive factors also occurs at the next appointment after each segment of periodontal debridement is completed. With additional information, the care plan is revised to include the new information and to assess client needs.

Part of evaluation is the reevaluation visit that occurs four to six weeks after the completion of initial or active therapy. The purpose of reevaluation is to:

- Evaluate the response to initial therapy and recommend additional therapy as needed
- Make a final periodontal diagnosis by modifying the presumptive diagnosis, if indicated

Elements of the reevaluation visit include:

- ✦ Reassessing initial periodontal and risk factor assessment to evaluate host response
- ✦ Reevaluating client's self-care practices
- ✦ Reeducating and motivating client
- ✦ Removing residual deposit or plaque-retentive factors
- ✦ Debriding nonresponsive areas as indicated by bleeding upon probing or gingival inflammation
- ✦ Performing any supportive intervention such as desensitization or antimicrobial therapy
- ✦ Reassessing the maintenance interval and adjusting if indicated

The Reevaluation Appointment Guide depicts a reevaluation sequence that can be used in both the educational and practice settings.

Clients who were initially diagnosed with plaque-induced gingival disease should demonstrate a reduction in gingival inflammation, stability of clinical attachment levels, and a reduction in clinically detectable plaque to a level compatible with gingival health. If resolution of conditions does not occur, the following client factors are reassessed:

- ✦ Self-care practices
- ✦ Periodontal disease risk factors
- ✦ Systemic disease status
- ✦ Residual calculus and bacterial plaque biofilm
- ✦ Plaque-retentive factors
- ✦ Compliance with continued-care interval
- ✦ Disabilities

Reevaluation Appointment Guide

Assessment

Probing measurements (expected healing is 1 to 2 mm if periodontitis is chronic and not aggressive)
BOP (should be absent)
Gingival description (should be healthy)
Soft-tissue assessment information (should be healthy)

Periodontal diagnosis

Reevaluation of the presumptive diagnosis

Care planning: Decision making for the appointment

Localized periodontal debridement
Need for generalized periodontal debridement; reappoint for recare
Incorporate adjunctive care; local controlled delivery of antibiotic, antimicrobial rinses, desensitization therapy, etc.
Referral to periodontist; referral to other specialist
Set SPT or continued-care interval
Reinforce self-care (teach, focus on skill or management deficiencies)

Implementation

Delivery of care as planned
Quality of care

For clients who were initially diagnosed with chronic periodontitis, the expected outcome is a reduction in:

- ✦ Periodontal probing depth (1–2 mm)
- ✦ Inflammation (or its resolution)
- ✦ Bleeding upon probing (or its resolution)

If nonresponse is apparent, evaluation of the site(s) or the case is imperative. Nonresponse does not necessarily imply an aggressive disease state. Retreatment should occur and another SPT visit be arranged at the appropriate interval. For clients with aggressive periodontitis, stability and control of the disease are the objectives of reevaluation. If control is not possible, then slowing the progression of disease is the next alternative. Inclusion of reevaluation in a care plan is dependent on multiple factors that are assessed during initial therapy (see Factors to Consider for Reevaluation).

Each client who has completed initial or active NSPT should be reevaluated to assess if the objectives of NSPT were met. It is critical that individuals with systemic conditions, risk factors, aggressive forms of the disease, pockets of 5 mm or greater, advanced bone loss or attachment loss, furcations, and/or mobility be evaluated. When the reevaluation visit is presented as an essential part of the NSPT care plan, compliance on the part of the client seems to be better. When the clinician believes that reevaluation is an integral part of the care plan, the ability to relate and discuss this need with the client is enhanced. Some practices consider the evaluation visit part of the initial periodontal debridement (scaling and root planing) fee, and other practices consider the reevaluation visit to warrant a separate fee.

Appointment time for evaluation depends on the services included in the care plan; however, the typical appointment in practice is 30 minutes. If the scheduled 30-minute appointment is not ample time, then reappointment for retreatment is indicated. For example, if a client returns with nonresponsive areas adjacent to furcations where 5- to 6-mm pocket depth was recorded, then nonresponse is identified as a new problem.

Explanations are generated focusing on the potential reasons for the lack of healing, which could include

Factors to Consider for Reevaluation

Gingival inflammation
Bleeding on probing
Depth, number, and location of periodontal pockets
Clinical attachment loss
Furcations and mobility
Expected client response to oral self-care recommendations
Presumptive diagnosis
Other complicating factors such as restorative needs or occlusion
Systemic disease and risk factors present
Client goals for NSPT and degree of compliance
Likelihood of disease progression

incomplete periodontal debridement, systemic disease, inadequate self-care, smoking, or use of inappropriate self-care aids. Probably, more than one course of action will be chosen. The clinician could retreat the area with extended shank curets and/or ultrasonic instrumentation, reevaluate the self care aid(s) recommended or used, reeducate, and/or use an antimicrobial agent (professional irrigation coupled with home irrigation, or local delivery) in the area. These additional therapies will precipitate the need for more discussion and client decision making (informed consent).

At the conclusion of the reevaluation visit, the first supportive periodontal therapy (SPT) (also known as continued-care, recare, or recall) visit is established.[15–17] If the objectives of care are reached, then this visit will occur eight to ten weeks from the reevaluation visit. This represents an SPT interval scheduled three or four months after the last appointment for periodontal debridement.

If the objectives of care are not reached, or if multiple risk factors for continuing periodontal destruction exist, then the appointment for maintenance should occur in four weeks, representing a two-month interval from the last appointment when periodontal debridement was performed.

If the objectives of care are not reached and the preliminary diagnosis is mild to moderate periodontitis, then the client is returned to the initial therapy phase of care versus maintenance. Table 23–4 offers suggested SPT intervals.

REFERRAL TO A PERIODONTIST. The decision to care for the client in the general dental practice or to refer to a periodontal practice is based on:

- Type and severity of disease
- Dental hygienist's acquired skill level
- Time allotted to maintain periodontally involved clients.

For example, if the periodontal diagnosis is advanced periodontitis or an aggressive form of the disease, referral to a periodontist is indicated. A client with moderate chronic periodontitis might also be referred to the periodontist if risk factors exist and the extent of disease is close to an advanced disease status. It is then the responsibility of the general practitioner to strive to maintain periodontal health and inform the client when that goal is not being achieved.

Some clients decline referral because of geographic constraints, cost, or because they do not want to go to a new office setting. When this is the case, documentation of the referral to the periodontist, and the client's response, is imperative.

TABLE 23–4 SUGGESTED SUPPORTIVE PERIODONTAL THERAPY INTERVALS

Characteristics	Interval
First-year client; routine therapy and uneventful healing	3 months
First-year client; difficult case with complicated prosthesis, furcation involvement, poor crown-to-root ratios, questionable client cooperation	1 to 2 months
Excellent results well-maintained for 1 year or more	6 months to 1 year
Client displays good oral hygiene, minimal calculus, no occlusal problems, no complicated prostheses, no remaining pockets, and no teeth with less than 50% of alveolar bone remaining	6 months to 1 year
Generally good results maintained reasonably well for 1 year or more, but client displays some of the following: Inconsistent or poor oral hygiene Heavy calculus formation Systemic disease and risk factors that predispose to disease progression Some remaining pockets Occlusal trauma Complicated prostheses Ongoing orthodontic therapy Recurrent dental caries Some teeth with less than 50% of alveolar bone support	3 to 4 months (select interval based on number and severity of negative factors)
Generally poor results following periodontal therapy and/or client displays some of the following: Inconsistent or poor oral hygiene Heavy calculus formation Systemic disease that predisposes to periodontal breakdown Remaining pockets Occlusal trauma Complicated prosthesis Recurrent dental caries Periodontal surgery indicated but not performed for medical, psychological, or financial reasons Many teeth with less than 50% of alveolar bone support Condition too far advanced to be improved by periodontal surgery	1 to 3 months (select interval based on number and severity of negative factors; consider retreating some areas or extracting severely involved teeth)

Modified from Newman MG, Takei HH, Carranza FM: *Clinical periodontology*, ed 9, Philadelphia, 2002, WB Saunders.

Most periodontists will alternate visits for SPT with the general practitioner. Clients with advanced chronic disease or aggressive disease will probably be maintained at the periodontist's office and be referred to the general dentist once every six months or once a year for restorative examination, depending on the client's caries risk.

Surgical Intervention

Some forms of moderate to advanced periodontitis need to be reevaluated often to determine if the goals for periodontal therapy are achieved and maintained. For clients with moderate to advanced disease, therapeutic goals include:

- Resolution of gingival inflammation
- Decrease in periodontal probing depths
- Maintenance or gain in attachment level
- Radiologic resolution of osseous defects
- Occlusal stability
- Plaque reduction to a level acceptable to the client's immune response

Surgery should be considered when nonsurgical therapy is unsuccessful at reaching these goals. A surgical approach, as opposed to NSPT, is considered when:

- Enhanced access for removal of etiologic factors is needed
- Diseased sites with deep periodontal pockets persist
- Regeneration or reconstruction of the periodontal tissues (e.g., osseous defects) is indicated

NSPT INSURANCE ISSUES

Dental benefit plans (dental insurance) influence the NSPT provided. The dental hygienist needs to know:

- Office philosophy about third-party payment
- Common dental terms associated with the insurance (see Common Dental Terms for Insurance Associated with Nonsurgical Periodontal Therapy)
- Periodontal insurance codes (can be obtained from the *Current Dental Terminology*, CDT-4, version 2002, American Dental Association 2002) (Table 23–5)[4]
- Third-party insurance carriers in the geographic area
- Coverage-of-benefits letters of explanation used with clients (if not, letters can be developed)
- Who is responsible for filing insurance claims, explanations to the client, and communication with the insurance company
- How to maximize insurance benefits

The dental hygienist is a source of information about insurance coverage for periodontal services. The dental hygienist may explain the relationship between the office fees and third-party insurance benefits and the responsibility of the client for the NSPT fee charged. Treatment plans should be developed according to professional standards and client needs, not according to the provisions of the client's insurance policy.[18] This philosophy ensures that clients receive care that meets their individual needs.

When diagnosing and classifying periodontal disease for insurance claims, the clinician uses two considerations:

- Host and microbial parameters (e.g., onset, progression, and response to the disease)
- Disease severity (e.g., probing depth, clinical attachment level, and furcation involvement)

The descriptions of disease progression in Table 23–1 are used to convey information about the client's periodontal disease to the insurance company. A specific diagnosis can be used whenever appropriate. The AAP

Common Dental Terms for Insurance Associated with Nonsurgical Periodontal Therapy

Curettage Scraping and cleaning the walls of a cavity or gingival pocket

Debridement Removal of subgingival and/or supragingival plaque and calculus that obstructs the ability to perform an evaluation; removal of contused and devitalized tissue from a wound surface

Dental Prophylaxis Scaling and selective polishing performed to remove coronal plaque, calculus, and stains

Gingiva Soft tissues overlying the crowns of unerupted teeth and encircling the necks of those that have erupted

Gingivitis Inflammation of gingival tissue without loss of connective tissue

Periodontal Pertaining to the supporting and surrounding tissues of the teeth

Periodontal Disease Inflammatory process of gingival tissues and/or periodontal membrane of the teeth, resulting in an abnormally deep gingival sulcus, possibly producing periodontal pockets and loss of support alveolar bone

Periodontal Maintenance Therapy for preserving the state of health of the periodontium

Periodontal Pocket Pathologically deepened gingival sulcus; a feature of periodontal disease

Periodontist Dental specialist whose practice is limited to the treatment of diseases of the supporting and surrounding tissues of the teeth

Periodontitis Inflammation and loss of the connective tissue of the supporting or surrounding structure of teeth with loss of attachment

Plaque Soft sticky substance that accumulates on teeth composed largely of bacteria and bacterial derivatives

Prophylaxis Scaling and polishing procedure performed to remove coronal plaque, calculus, and stains

Root Planing Procedure designed to remove microbial flora, bacterial toxins, calculus, and diseased cementum or dentin on the root surfaces and in the pocket

Scaling Removal of plaque, calculus, and stain from teeth

From *Current Dental Terminology*, CDT-4, Version 2002, Chicago, 2002 American Dental Association.

TABLE 23–5

INSURANCE CODES RELATED TO NONSURGICAL PERIODONTAL THERAPY

Code	Procedure	Description
D0120	Periodic oral evaluation	An evaluation performed on a patient of record to determine any changes in the patient's dental and medical health status since a previous comprehensive or periodic evaluation. This may require interpretation of information acquired through additional diagnostic procedures. Report additional diagnostic procedures separately.
D0140	Limited oral evaluation–problem focused	An evaluation limited to a specific oral health problem. This may require interpretation of information acquired through additional diagnostic procedures. Report additional diagnostic procedures separately. Definitive procedures may be required on the same date as the evaluation. Typically, patients receiving this type of evaluation have been referred for a specific problem and/or present with dental emergencies, trauma, acute infection, etc.
D0150	Comprehensive oral evaluation	Typically used by a general dentist and/or a specialist when evaluating a patient comprehensively. It is a thorough evaluation and recording of the extraoral and intraoral hard and soft tissues. It may require interpretation of information acquired through additional diagnostic procedures. Additional diagnostic procedures should be reported separately. This would include the evaluation and recording of the patient's dental and medical history and a general health assessment. It may typically include the evaluation and recording of dental caries, missing or unerupted teeth, restorations, occlusal relationships, periodontal conditions (including periodontal charting), hard and soft tissue anomalies, oral cancer screening, etc.
D0160	Detailed and extensive oral evaluation: problem focused, by report	A detailed and extensive problem-focused evaluation entails extensive diagnostic and cognitive modalities based on the findings of a comprehensive oral evaluation. Integration of more extensive diagnostic modalities to develop a treatment plan for a specific problem is required. The condition requiring this type of evaluation should be described and documented. Examples of conditions requiring this type of evaluation may include dentofacial anomalies, complicated perioprosthetic conditions, complex temporomandibular dysfunction, facial pain of unknown origin, severe systemic diseases requiring multidisciplinary consultation, etc.
D0210	Intraoral complete series (including bitewings)	
D0270	Bitewing: single film	
D0272	Bitewings: two films	
D0274	Bitewings: four films	
D0277	Vertical bitewings: 7 to 8 films	
D1310	Nutritional counseling for control of dental disease	Counseling on food selection and dietary habits as a part of treatment and control of periodontal disease and caries.
D1320	Tobacco counseling for the control and prevention of oral disease	Tobacco prevention and cessation services reduce client risk of developing tobacco-related oral diseases and conditions and improve prognosis for certain dental therapies.
D1330	Oral hygiene instructions	This may include instructions for home care. Examples include tooth brushing technique, flossing, use of special oral hygiene aids.
D1110	Prophylaxis: adult	A dental prophylaxis performed on transitional or permanent dentition that includes scaling and polishing procedures to remove coronal plaque, calculus, and stains. Some patients may require more than one appointment or one extended appointment to complete a prophylaxis. Document need for additional time or appointments.
D1120	Prophylaxis: child	Refers to a dental prophylaxis performed on primary or transitional dentition only.
D4341	Periodontal scaling and root planing: four or more continuous teeth per quadrant	This procedure involves instrumentation of the crown and root surfaces of the teeth to remove plaque and calculus from these surfaces. It is indicated for patients with periodontal disease and is therapeutic, not prophylactic, in nature. Root planing is the definitive procedure designed for the removal of cementum and dentin that is rough and/or permeated by calculus or contaminated with toxins or microorganisms. Some soft tissue removal occurs. This procedure may be used as a definitive treatment in some stages of periodontal disease and/or as a part of presurgical procedures in others.
D4342	Periodontal scaling and root planing: one to three teeth per quadrant	This procedure involves instrumentation of the crown and root surfaces of the teeth to remove plaque and calculus from these surfaces. It is indicated for patients with periodontal disease and is therapeutic, not prophylactic, in nature. Root planing is the definitive procedure designed for the removal of cementum and dentin that is rough and/or permeated by calculus or contaminated with toxins or microorganisms. Some soft tissue removal occurs. This procedure may be used as a definitive treatment in some stages of periodontal disease and/or as a part of presurgical procedures in others.
D4355	Full mouth debridement to enable comprehensive periodontal evaluation and diagnosis	The removal of subgingival and/or supragingival plaque and calculus. This procedure does not preclude the need for other procedures.

Table continued on following page

TABLE 23–5 INSURANCE CODES RELATED TO NONSURGICAL PERIODONTAL THERAPY—CONT'D

Code	Procedure	Description
D4381	Localized delivery of chemotherapeutic agents via a controlled release vehicle into diseased crevicular tissue, per tooth,	Synthetic fibers or other approved delivery devices containing controlled-release chemotherapeutic agent(s) are inserted into a periodontal pocket. Short-term use of the timed-release therapeutic agent as supplemental or adjunctive therapy provides for reduction of subgingival flora. This procedure does not replace conventional or surgical therapy required for debridement, resective procedures, or regenerative therapy. The use of controlled-release chemotherapeutic agents is an adjunctive procedure for specific sites that are unresponsive to conventional therapy or for cases in which systemic disease or other factors preclude conventional or surgical therapy.
D0415	Bacteriologic studies for determination of pathologic agents	May include, but is not limited to, tests for susceptibility to periodontal disease.
D4220	Gingival curettage, surgical: per quadrant, by report	The surgical procedure of debriding the soft tissue wall of the periodontal pocket by means of a curet. Root instrumentation is routinely accomplished in conjunction with the procedure, which usually is performed under local anesthesia. Gingival curettage is typically indicated in the treatment of periodontally compromised patients, debridement of localized sites of recalcitrant periodontitis, treatment of juvenile periodontitis, treatment of other types of periodontitis, and when esthetics is of concern. Report should include treatment needs and teeth to be treated.
D9910	Application of desensitizing medicament	Includes in-office treatment for root sensitivity. Typically reported on a "per visit" basis for application of topical fluoride. This code is not to be used for bases, liners, or adhesives used under restorations.
D4910	Periodontal maintenance procedures (following active therapy)	This procedure is for patients who have previously been treated for periodontal disease. Typically, maintenance starts after completion of active (surgical or nonsurgical) periodontal therapy and continues at varying intervals, determined by the clinical diagnosis of the dentist, for the life of the dentition. It includes removal of supra- and subgingival microbial flora and calculus, site-specific scaling and root planing where indicated, and/or polishing of the teeth. When new or reccurring periodontal disease appears, additional diagnostic and treatment procedures must be considered.
D9911	Application of desensitizing resin for cervical and/or root surface, per tooth	Typically reported on a "per tooth" basis for application of adhesive resins. This code is not to be used for bases, liners, or adhesives used under restorations.

From *Current Dental Terminology*, CDT-4, Version 2002, Chicago, 2002, American Dental Association.

recognizes that an extensive range of therapies exists for periodontal therapy and that no one treatment is effective for everyone. In fact, one section of the mouth might require one type of therapy while another area requires a different therapy. Therefore, description of disease in one quadrant of the mouth as reported on the insurance claim might differ from that in another area.

It is useful to develop a fee-for-service schedule for dental hygienists that includes:

- ✦ AAP Classifications[18]
- ✦ ADA Procedure Code[4]
- ✦ Description of the service
- ✦ Fee or range of fees charged

This schedule provides standardized fees for service between dental hygienists in the same practice and enhances communication with the office manager. Although there are ADA codes for various supportive services (local anesthetic, root desensitization), not all dental plans provide reimbursements for these services. In fact, there is variation in insurance coverage by different carriers, as well as in different plans from the same carrier in regard to services covered, frequency of payment for services, and maximum fee reimbursed. For example, some insurance plans reimburse for SPT every three months but others do not. A dental office cannot possibly know the reimbursement rates and plans of each carrier and client; therefore, the ultimate responsibility for the fee rests with the client.

SUPPORTIVE PERIODONTAL THERAPY (SPT)[15–17]

SPT is planned following the active phase of periodontal care at appropriately timed intervals based on client needs. SPT is the preferred term for what was formerly referred to as periodontal maintenance or periodontal recall. Although the dentist has ultimate responsibility for SPT, the dental hygienist also has responsibility to provide comprehensive and individually timed SPT for clients who have participated in NSPT. SPT continues for the life of the dentition or its implant replacements and this recommendation must be explained to clients who have NSPT. Clients with gingivitis and periodontitis should understand that they have a chronic disease entity that must be controlled by frequent periodontal care and daily self-care.

Goals of SPT[15,16]

The goals of SPT are to:

- ✦ Prevent or minimize recurrence and progression of periodontal disease in persons who have been treated for gingivitis, periodontitis, and periimplantitis
- ✦ Prevent or reduce incidence of tooth loss
- ✦ Increase probability of locating and treating other diseases or conditions

Intervals for SPT[17]

Clients with gingivitis and without a history of attachment loss maintain their oral health status when SPT is performed every six months. For clients with periodontitis, a three-month interval, or less, is ideal. Part of the rationale for three-month intervals is that after periodontal pathogens are suppressed, they return to pretreatment levels in 9 to 11 weeks; however, this interval varies significantly among clients. Even though three months is the ideal interval, the SPT interval is customized to the client based on self-care compliance, extent of disease, systemic contributions to disease, risk factors, and client consent. Factors that influence client consent to a specific interval are cost, third-party benefits, cooperation, and needs.

Components of Care

Components of SPT should be similar at each SPT visit; however, the extent of these services may vary depending on client compliance, length of time in SPT, and extent of periodontitis. Table 23–6 presents a summary of care for an SPT visit and associated risk factors.

Appointment Time

The appointment time required to provide effective SPT varies according to:

- ✦ Number of teeth
- ✦ Self-care efficacy
- ✦ Cooperation
- ✦ Systemic health
- ✦ Previous frequency of SPT
- ✦ Instrumentation needs
- ✦ History of periodontal disease
- ✦ Practitioner skill

In practice, 60 minutes is probably practical and adequate; however, 45 minutes may suffice in some cases and others may require 90 minutes. It is challenging in the practice sector to establish a reasonable fee, work with the insurance carriers, and explain needs to the client. A number of insurance carriers will not cover the four annual SPT appointments the client needs. In this case, the client's out-of-pocket expense and consequences of inadequate SPT are discussed.

Compliance[19]

Dental and medical literature suggests that the less threatening the problem appears to be to the individual, the less likely they are to comply. Compliance is also reduced if therapy is time consuming and no symptoms are present. Other reasons for noncompliance include self-destructive behavior, fear, economics, health beliefs, stress, and perceived professional indifference. The rate of compliance with toothbrushing is less than 50%; with interdental aids it is even lower. The dropout rate of clients with SPT is 11% to 45% in university-based settings; in private practice settings, complete compliance is seen in 33% of cases or less. Suggestions[19,20] to improve compliance follow:

- ✦ Enhance client education about therapeutic need
- ✦ Keep recommendations simple and oral care devices to a minimum
- ✦ Pay attention to client questions and needs
- ✦ Remind clients of appointments
- ✦ Inform clients in writing about the disease and self-care practices
- ✦ Provide positive reinforcement
- ✦ Target potential noncompliers early
- ✦ Ensure the dentist's involvement

MECHANIZED PERIODONTAL DEBRIDEMENT

Ultrasonic and sonic instrumentation is collectively referred to as power-driven or *mechanized instrumentation.* The original, larger, traditional working end of the power-driven insert is described as conventional or *standard design.* Thinner working ends of inserts for subgingival access are called micro-ultrasonic, periodontal, slim, or *precision thin designs.*

Ultrasonic and sonic instruments have three modes of action:

Mechanical action, or vibration of the tip, results in deposit removal. Mechanized instruments are said to have *clinical power,* referring to the ability to remove calculus deposits under load. Tip action that provides clinical power is dependent on the stroke, frequency, type of tip motion, and angulation of the motion against the tooth surface. *Load* is the resistance on an instrument tip when placed against the calculus deposit or tooth surface.

Cavitation is the action created by the formation and collapse of bubbles in the water by high-frequency sound waves surrounding an ultrasonic tip. Cavitation results in *lavage,* the therapeutic washing of the pockets and root surface to remove endotoxins and loose debris. Irrigation occurs via the water or the antimicrobial used to replace the water.

Acoustic microstreaming occurs because agitation in the fluids surrounding a rapidly vibrating ultrasonic tip has the potential to destroy or disrupt bacteria.

Ultrasonic Instruments

Ultrasonic instruments convert electrical energy into mechanical energy in the range of 18,000 to 50,000 vibrations per second. The term *ultrasonic* describes a nonaudible range of acoustical vibrations that are a unit of

TABLE 23–6 SPT ASSESSMENT CRITERIA, PROCEDURES, AND ASSOCIATED RISK FACTORS

Criteria	Procedure	Risk Factors to Evaluate
Health and pharmacologic history	Review and update for: Need for prophylactic antibiotics Making sure medications have been taken New diseases/medications Need for medical consultation Smoking status	Age of client Smoking status Systemic diseases such as diabetes, CVD, osteoporosis, immunosuppression, etc. Stress Pregnancy
Dental history	Review and determining the chief complaint	Lack of compliance with the SPT continued-care interval
Extraoral and intraoral soft tissue examination	Examine for significant pathology	Dependent on type of pathology
Restorative examination	Evaluate prosthesis (including implants), caries activity and risk, and restorations	Overhangs or ill-fitting restorations Failing implant
Periodontal examination	Examine the following: Gingival conditions for inflammation, position, contour, and mucogingival involvement	Inflammation Progressive recession Minimal or no keratinized gingiva
	Probing depth	1- to 2-mm increase Moderate to deep probe depths
	Attachment loss	Extent and severity of disease; type of disease present; 2-mm loss of attachment in one year
	Radiographs	Changes in bone levels Vertical bone loss Presence of dental caries
	Bleeding on probing	Presence indicates risk
	Furcation involvement	Presence indicates risk; the more advanced the furcation involvement, the more risk
	Mobility	Presence indicates risk; the more advanced the mobility, the more risk
	Suppuration	Presence indicates risk
Deposit accumulation	Evaluate the location and extent of supragingival bacterial plaque	Presence of supragingival bacterial plaque is strongly correlated with gingivitis
	Supra- and subgingival deposits	Type of bacteria present in the subgingival environment (microbiologic monitoring) Lack of compliance with oral self-care Calculus (plaque-retentive factor)
Radiographic assessment	Evaluate the: Risk of advancing disease Clinical findings, especially progressive attachment loss Client radiographic history	Advancing radiographic bone loss

Adapted from Hodges KO: *Concepts in nonsurgical periodontal therapy,* ed 1, Albany, NY, 1998, Delmar.

frequency referred to as cycles per second (CPS) or hertz (Hz). There are two types of ultrasonic units: *magnetostrictive* and *piezoelectric*. Both units have four similar components: the electric generator, the handpiece, the insert, and the foot pedal control (Figure 23–9, *A*). When the ultrasonic unit receives electrical energy and the foot pedal is activated, an electrical current is sent through the generator, or base of the unit, to the handpiece. The handpiece holds the transducer or insert. The transducer converts the electrical energy to mechanical energy, causing the tip to vibrate. The mechanical action of the tip removes calculus, bacterial plaque, and root surface constituents that are directly contacted by the tip.

MANUAL AND AUTOTUNED UNITS. Ultrasonic units are either manual tuned or autotuned. The *manual-tuned unit* permits the clinician to adjust the frequency via the tuning knob (Figure 23–9, *A*). *Frequency* is the number of times per second that the tip moves back and forth in one cycle. A *cycle* is one complete linear or elliptical stroke path of the tip. The frequency is the speed of movement of the tip. The clinician's ability to control the frequency may assist the operator in meeting the instrumentation needs. For example, using a low frequency when attempting to debride light calculus deposits may enhance client comfort. However, frequent readjustments of the tuning knob to ensure optimal efficiency of the unit may increase treatment time. Manual-tuned units are magnetostrictive ultrasonic devices only. An example of this type of unit is the USI series (Ultrasonic Services Incorporated, Houston, Texas).

The *autotuned unit* has a preset frequency within the instrument that automatically tunes the cycles per

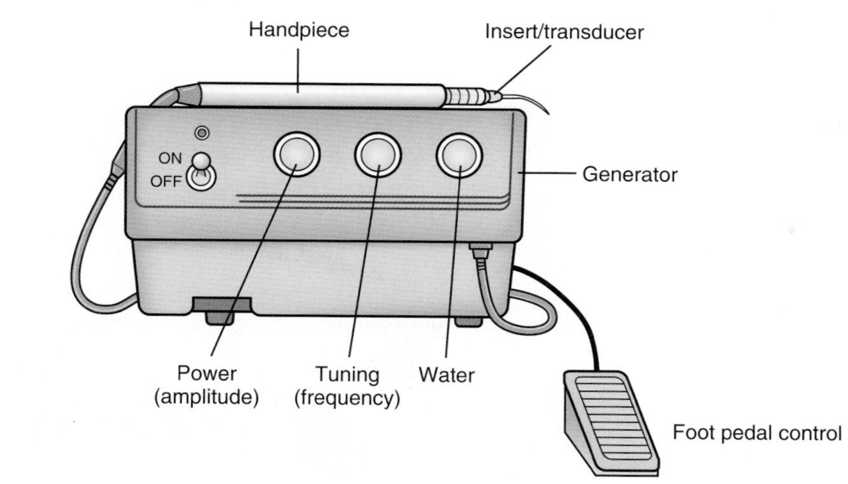

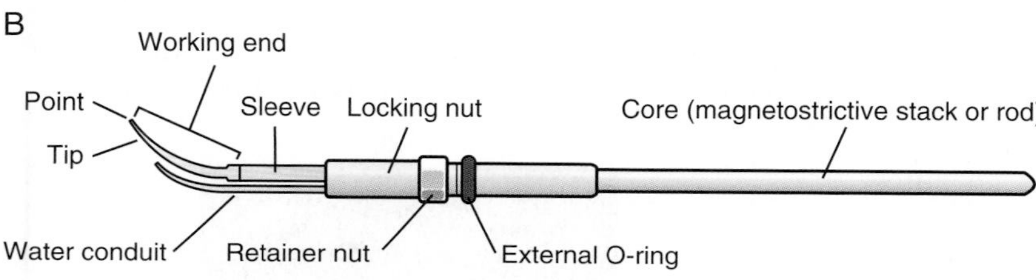

FIGURE 23–9 ✦ Components of an ultrasonic dental unit and insert. *(From Hodges KO: Concepts in nonsurgical periodontal therapy, Albany, NY, 1998, Delmar.)*

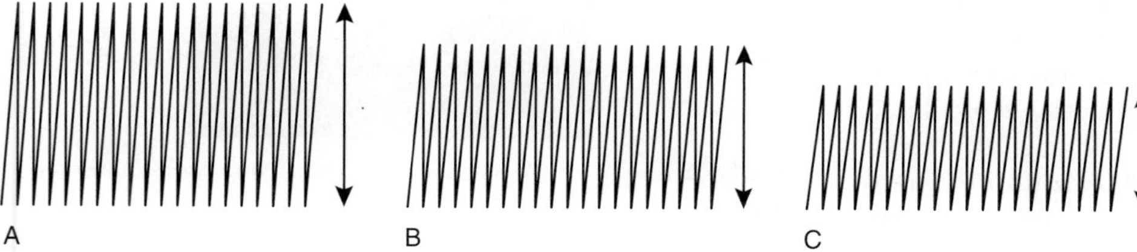

FIGURE 23–10 ✦ Tip displacement or amplitude. *(From Hodges KO: Concepts in nonsurgical periodontal therapy, Albany, NY, 1998, Delmar.)*

second to maximum efficiency for each insert used. Therefore, there is no tuning knob to adjust the speed (frequency) of the tip. The majority of magnetostrictive units and all piezoelectric units are autotuned.

Both manual tuned and autotuned units have power and water control knobs. The *power* is the energy in the handpiece that creates movement of the working end. Increasing the power setting increases the distance the working end moves. This is the length of the stroke (Figure 23–10). *Amplitude* is synonymous with power, and the distance the working end travels in the single vibration is called *tip displacement.* For example, one manufacturer reports that a particular unit has an amplitude from 0.001 to 0.008 of an inch (Ultrasonic Services Incorporated, Houston, Texas). As amplitude increases, the output of power increases, enhancing the efficiency of the action of the tip.

The water control knob adjusts the volume and temperature of the flow from the handpiece. The water flow:

- ✦ Cools the transducer and tip. (Note: Although a piezoelectric transducer can run without water, the tip generates frictional heat that requires water to keep it cool and flush the debris once it is removed. Also, piezoelectric transducers will heat and lose efficiency without water flow. In clinical practice, a piezoelectric unit would never be operated without the addition of water.)
- ✦ Stems bleeding
- ✦ Increases visibility
- ✦ Provides lavage
- ✦ Removes root surface constituents
- ✦ Irrigates sulci and periodontal pockets

Proper water spray is critical to prevent damage to the root surface. The greater the water flow, the lower the water temperature; a decreased water flow creates a higher water temperature. This is why the water temperature should be adjusted if clients experience sensitivity. The water flow is independent from the energy generated from the tip (i.e., increased water flow does not affect the mechanized energy produced). The piezoelectric unit does not require water for cooling of the transducer; however, as mentioned earlier, the water flow provides other advantages and is necessary to cool the tip.

Magnetostrictive Units (Procedure 23–2)

The insert in a magnetostrictive unit is a core attached to the working end (Figure 23–9, *B*). The core is either a stack of metal (permanickel) strips or a ferrite rod, depending on the type of unit. The Cavitron SPS Ultrasonic Scaler (DENTSPLY Professional) and the Cavitron Select SPS Ultrasonic Scaler are examples of magnetostrictive units with a handpiece that houses an insert with metal strips for the core (Figure 23–11, *A* and *B*).

In contrast, the Odontoson-M (Odonto-Wave) is an example of a magnetostrictive unit that uses a ferric rod (Figure 23–12). Some magnetostrictive units are available with an autoclavable handpiece and/or an autoclavable handpiece line.

Inside the handpiece is a copper wire coil that exposes the core to a varying magnetic field when it receives an electrical current. When magnetized, the core contracts; when demagnetized, the core returns to its original size. The alternating electromagnetic field causes the tip of the insert to vibrate in an elliptical or orbital (360°) motion when the transducer is a metal stack. Similarly, when the transducer is a ferrite rod, the tip can also be used on all sides, enhancing its adaptability to tooth surfaces. The *active tip area* is the portion of the working end that performs the instrumentation and it is affected by the frequency. In the 25,000- to 30,000-Hz unit the active tip area is approximately the last 4.3 mm of the working end (Procedure 23–2).

Heat is a by-product of the dimensional change of the transducer and oscillating tip in magnetostrictive units and, thus, water is needed to control the heat to prevent pulp tissue damage. When the water flows to the end of the insert and contacts the moving tip, tiny droplets and a fine spray result. This phenomenon is called atomization because the lavage is reduced to tiny droplets and a fine spray.

INSERT SELECTION.[21] A variety of inserts are available for mechanized instrumentation. When selecting inserts, the dental hygienist considers the following:

- ✦ Designs for periodontal debridement
- ✦ Compatibility with other units in the practice setting
- ✦ Compatibility with the frequency (kHz)
- ✦ Method of fluid delivery

There are two types of magnetostrictive inserts based on the frequency requirements of the unit: either 25 kHz or the newer 30 kHz. The stack of the 30-kHz insert is shorter than the 25-kHz inserts (Figure 23–13). Insert designs are ordered in either type based on the frequency of the equipment being utilized. Most magnetostrictive units accept most manufacturers' 25-kHz or 30-kHz inserts. For example, inserts manufactured by DENTSPLY Professional or Hu-Friedy can be used in Ultrasonic Services Incorporated units. Inserts for the Odontoson–M (Odonto-Wave) unit are not interchangeable with other magnetostrictive units. Some units accept both 25-kHz and 30-kHz size inserts (e.g., Model 2530, Tony Riso Company).

An internal or external fluid hose (conduit) is available in most designs (Figure 23–14). An advantage of the internal hose is that it does not bend like the external tube does. The external hose is available in two types: a tube that is long and not fixed and a shorter external tube that

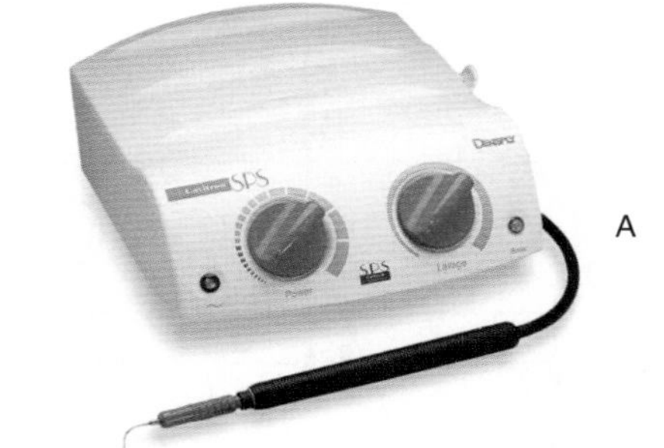

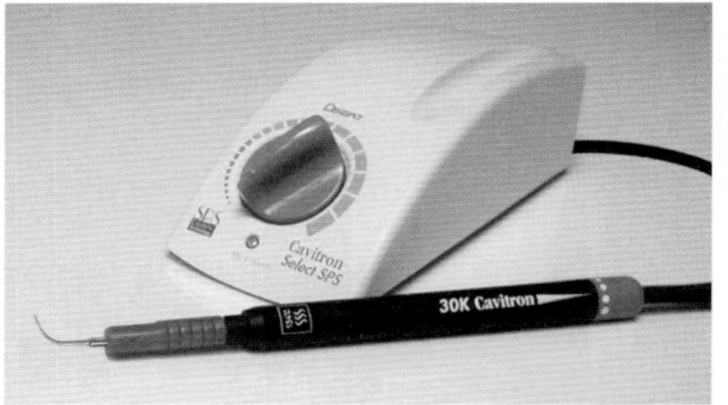

FIGURE 23–11 ✦ Magnetostrictive unit. **A,** Cavitron SPS. **B,** Cavitron Select SPS with 30-kHz insert. *(Courtesy DENTSPLY Preventive Care.)*

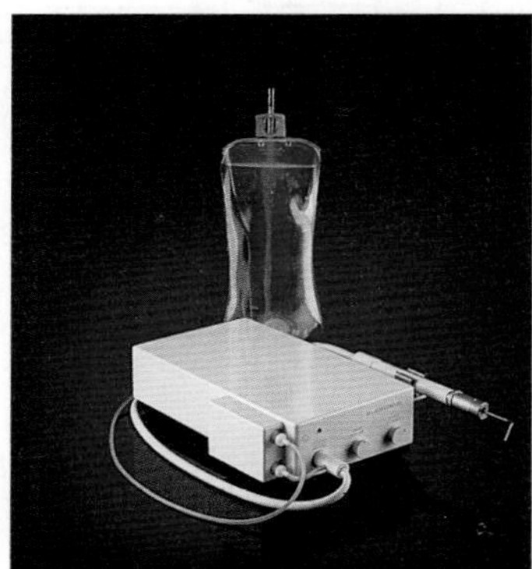

FIGURE 23–12 ✦ Magnetostrictive unit: Odontoson-M. Insert core is a ferrite rod. The Odontson operates at 42,000 Hz and has a small rotational tip movement (0.01–0.02 mm). The tip is equally active on all sides and all the way up the tip. *(Courtesy Odonto-Wave.)*

Procedure 23–2 INSTRUMENTATION WITH THE MAGNETOSTRICTIVE ULTRASONIC UNIT

EQUIPMENT

Personal protective equipment, including face shield
Ultrasonic unit (manual or auto-tuned) tuned appropriately
Inserts (standard and/or precision thin)
Subgingival explorer
Mouth mirror
Files
Curets
High-speed evacuation
Protective eyewear and drape for client

STEPS	RATIONALE
PREPARATION	
1. Connect ultrasonic unit to water source on dental unit and electrical power source.	Provides power source to operate the equipment.
2. Turn ultrasonic unit on and allow water to flow through handpiece for 2–5 minutes (30 seconds between clients).	Allows stagnant water and trapped air to flush through handpiece.
3. Select a straight angled tip and insert into water-filled handpiece of ultrasonic unit.	
4. Holding handpiece over a water receptacle, adjust water and power to desired setting. Tip emits a mist of water without excessive dripping.	The higher the power setting, the more water is needed to keep tip properly cooled.
POSITIONING	
5. Place client in an appropriate supine position: have client tilt head toward right or left depending on area being treated and place suction appropriately. Provide protective eyewear, plastic drape, and paper towels.	Prevents lavage from pooling in client's throat and directs fluid to the suction. Protective barrier protects client's eyes and clothing.
GRASP	
6. Use a pen or modified-pen grasp that is light.	A light feather-like grasp is all that is needed because of the mechanized action.
FULCRUM	
7. Employ a conventional, opposite arch, cross arch, or other fulcrum.	Enhances control and access.
8. Use intraorally for standard designs and extraorally for precision thin designs.	Various fulcrums are needed to perform periodontal debridement with mechanized instrument.
MIRROR USE	
9. Prepare mirror to allow water to pool on its surface.	Enhances care, retraction, and client comfort.
ADAPTATION	
10. Explore or visually locate deposit. Position side of insert tip on deposit (standard) or at epithelial attachment (precision thin).	Using point of working end causes tooth structure damage.
11. Apply insert tip at no more than a 15° angle to tooth surface.	Use of active tip and appropriate surfaces is essential for successful periodontal debridement.
12. Adapt back or lateral surfaces of insert tip parallel to long axis of tooth.	Allows access to larger surface area.
13. Adapt insert tip diagonally (bisecting the long axis) on proximal surface. Back of precision thin insert might be adapted in pocket on proximal surfaces or in furcation invasions.	Allows access to larger surface area.
14. Roll insert within handpiece to adapt to various tooth surfaces. (Hu-Friedy Satin Swivel is designed to facilitate adaptation in an ergonomic manner.)	Facilitates adaptation to variable tooth surfaces.
15. Extend insert tip to midline of proximal surfaces.	Facilitates comprehensive instrumentation.
ACTIVATION	
16. Keep insert in motion at all times.	Prevents unnecessary loss of tooth structure.
17. Use quick, controlled, eraser-like motions with standard inserts. Speed of movement is slower with precision thin inserts, except where smoothing is indicated ("vibrato" stroke).	Speed of movement is adjusted depending on the purpose of the debridement and insert used.

Continued on following page

Procedure 23–2 INSTRUMENTATION WITH THE MAGNETOSTRICTIVE ULTRASONIC UNIT—CONT'D

STEPS	RATIONALE
18. Use overlapping, multidirectional strokes.	Varying stroke direction is essential for complete periodontal debridement.
19. Do not apply excessive lateral pressure.	Prevents unnecessary loss of tooth structure.
20. Stop periodically to allow complete evacuation.	Assists in visibility.
21. Evaluate progress and product with visual examination (light and air) and/or an explorer. Retreat areas with manual or mechanized instruments.	Maximizes efficiency; allows clinician to modify technique as necessary.
DOCUMENTATION	
22. Record services rendered in client record, e.g., oral debridement of mandibular left quadrant using universal tip insert.	Maintains accurate record for legal purposes and monitoring care.
23. Follow current infection control protocol.	Aerosolization of contaminants requires strict infection control.

is fixed. A choice in internal hose design is inserts manufactured with the port close to the insert tip (Focused Spray® Inserts, DENTSPLY Professional). There is no evidence to support use of a particular type of water delivery; therefore, the operator's preference influences this choice. Standard inserts are used for supragingival or subgingival (1 to 3 mm) debridement of the following:

- ✦ Light, moderate, or heavy calculus
- ✦ Bacterial plaque biofilm
- ✦ Extrinsic stain
- ✦ Orthodontic cement

The universal designs (FSI-1000 or FSI-100, DENTSPLY Professional) are standard inserts that can be used supragingivally, primarily for initial debridement of moderate to heavy deposits. Depending on access, gingival contour, and tone, these inserts can also be used subgingivally.

Design affects the efficiency and quality of the periodontal instrumentation. Refer to Table 23–7 for a review of insert tips manufactured by DENTSPLY Professional, Hu-Friedy, and Tony Riso. Other companies make similar inserts (Ultrasonic Services Incorporated).

The clinician must decide on the array of inserts for periodontal instrumentation:

- ✦ A standard insert that has a larger diameter is indicated primarily for removal of moderate to heavy deposits
- ✦ A precision thin insert (Focused Spray Slimline by DENTSPLY Professional or an *After Five Design* by Hu-Friedy) is indicated for light deposits in shallow and deep pockets.

Precision thin inserts are probe-like slim designs indicated for light periodontal debridement. Although they were developed for subgingival use, some supragingival applications occur because they are also used for light deposits and debridement at the gingival margin, or for root surfaces exposed after gingival recession. Precision thin inserts are from 0.3 to 0.6 mm wide, or about 40% narrower in diameter than standard inserts, facilitating subgingival access, client comfort, and tactile sense.

Precision thin inserts are available in three configurations: straight, right, and left. The rationale for using all three designs is to enhance subgingival access and adaptation to root anatomy. The straight design is indicated for periodontal pockets that are 4 mm or less. The right

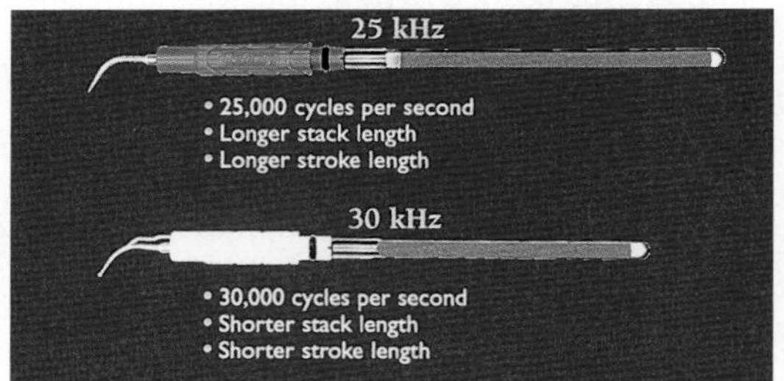

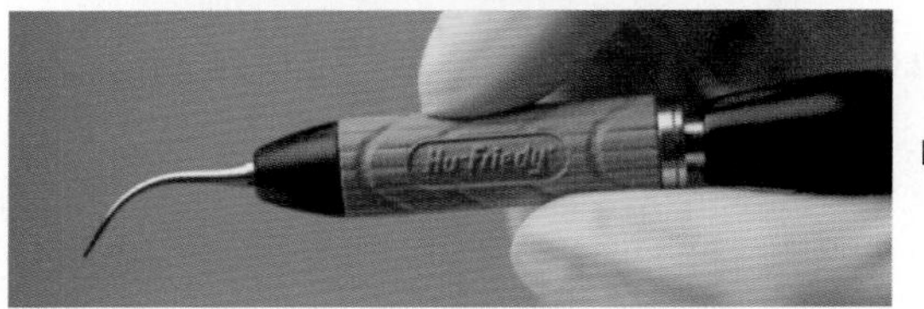

FIGURE 23–13 ✦ **A,** Magnetostrictive inserts: 25 kHz and 30 kHz. **B,** Satin Swivel Ultrasonic inserts with soft silicone grip. Slight swivel increases maneuverability and adaptability. *(Courtesy Hu-Friedy Manufacturing Co.)*

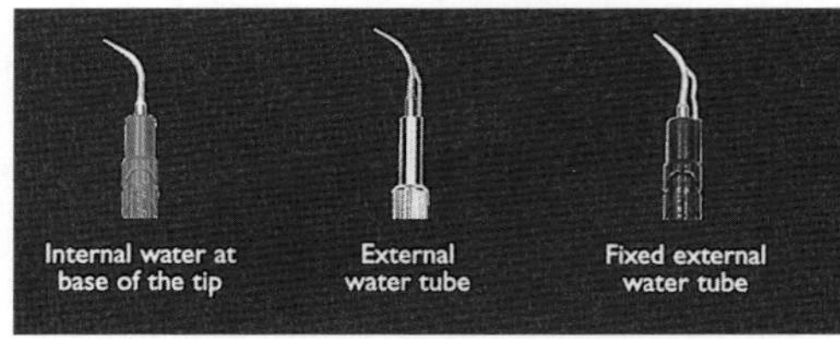

FIGURE 23–14 ✦ Methods of water delivery. *(Courtesy Hu-Friedy Manufacturing Co.)*

TABLE 23–7

SUMMARY OF MECHANIZED INSTRUMENT INSERT DESIGNS

Type of Insert	Design	Power Setting	Indications	Adaptation and Activation
Standard	Chisel type *(Courtesy DENTSPLY International Professional Division.)*	Low to high	Supragingival moderate to heavy calculus interproximally and labial lingual surfaces of anteriors and premolars	Work with tip of insert. Horizontal strokes supragingivally using very light pressure.
Standard	Beavertail *(Courtesy DENTSPLY International Professional Division.)*	Low to high	Supragingival moderate to heavy calculus labial and lingual surfaces of teeth (usually anteriors) Removing stain from all accessible tooth surfaces (recommended for black stain, but *not* light yellow stain.)	Work with end of insert tip; avoid using sides or face of tip. *Stain:* "erasing" motion using very light pressure. *Scaling lingually or buccally:* vertical overlapping strokes using light pressure.
Standard	Fine tipped *(Courtesy DENTSPLY International Professional Division.)*	Low to high	Supragingival calculus and stain from very tight interproximal spaces	Work with tip of insert.
Standard	Universal *(Courtesy DENTSPLY International Professional Division.)*	Low to high	Light, moderate, and heavy calculus removal in all areas (universal)	Work with side of insert tip.
Standard	Universal *(Courtesy DENTSPLY International Professional Division.)*	Low to high	Anterior and posterior subgingival moderate and heavy calculus removal	Use sides of tip for complete deposit removal (cross-hatch). Horizontal or vertical strokes.
Precision thin (straight, left, right designs)	Probe-like *(Courtesy Tony Riso Company.)*	Low to medium	Light subgingival periodontal debridement (calculus and plaque) Shallow and deep pocket depth Concavities and furcations	Adapt sides and back. Horizontal, vertical, and oblique strokes.

Table continued on following page

TABLE 23–7 SUMMARY OF MECHANIZED INSTRUMENT INSERT DESIGNS—CONT'D

Type of Insert	Design	Power Setting	Indications	Adaptation and Activation
Precision thin—cont'd	*(Courtesy DENTSPLY International Professional Division.)*	Low to medium	Light subgingival periodontal debridement (calculus and plaque) Shallow and deep pocket depth Concavities and furcations	Adapt sides and back. Use horizontal, vertical, and oblique strokes. Some furcation insert tips terminate with a small ball at the end (see Figure 23–15).
Ultrasonic rubber tip	Dental implants *(Courtesy Tony Riso Co.)*	Low	Debridement of dental implants	Adapt sides. Use horizontal, oblique, or vertical strokes.
Sonic rubber tip	Dental implants (See Figures 50–59 and 50–60)	N/A	Debridement of dental implants	Adapt sides. Use horizontal, oblique, or vertical strokes.

Note: Manufacturers make a variety of designs.

and left designs are indicated to reach depths greater than 4 mm, concavities, and furcations. Pocket penetration with an unmodified, standard (P-10 DENTSPLY Professional) and precision thin insert (Focused Spray Slimline right and left) was compared. Trends indicate that the precision thin inserts were able to debride the apical plaque border in deep pockets and the standard insert was more effective in shallow pockets.

Another precision thin insert used in NSPT has a 0.8-mm ball end feature (Furcation Designs, Hu-Friedy). The ball end is thought to provide more tip surface area for periodontal debridement of furcations and concavities (Figure 23–15). These inserts are manufactured in right, left, and straight designs.

Researchers[22] found that the mean buccal furcation entrance dimension of first and second molars measured from 0.63 to 1.04 mm. Mandibular molars measured from 0.71 to 0.88 mm. The standard, unmodified P-10 insert (DENTSPLY Professional) measured an average of 0.56 mm in diameter and the width of a new Gracey curet blade measured from 0.76 to 1.00 mm. Therefore, the majority of mean furcation entrance dimensions in second molars were less than the blade width of the Gracey curet. Also, the majority of mean furcation entrance dimensions of first molars were similar to the Gracey curet blade width. For these reasons, the combined use of inserts and curets is required to treat the furcation areas because the curet alone does not provide the clinician with a means to access the furcation under its roof. The dimension of the ball end designed insert should be considered in light of these research findings. Certainly the reduced width of precision thin inserts would enhance the efficiency and effectiveness of NSPT in furcations. Also, the narrow width of the precision thin inserts should be considered when treating deep, narrow pockets in NSPT. The thinner the instrument, the greater chance of negotiating the pocket topography.

INSERT FUNCTION.[21] Inserts for magnetostrictive units deliver energy from all four surfaces: the point, the concave surface, the convex surface, and the sides or lateral surfaces. The point generates the greatest amount of energy and is not used to prevent undue surface alterations to the root and sensitivity. The lateral surfaces generate the least amount of energy. (Refer to Figure 23–16 to evaluate the order of energy generated by these inserts.) The lateral surfaces (sides) and back of the working end are adapted to the tooth.

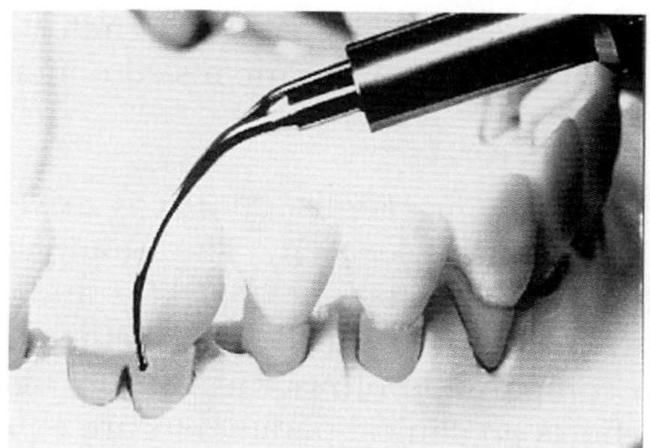

FIGURE 23–15 ✦ Furcation design. *(Courtesy Hu-Friedy Manufacturing Co., Furcation Designs.)*

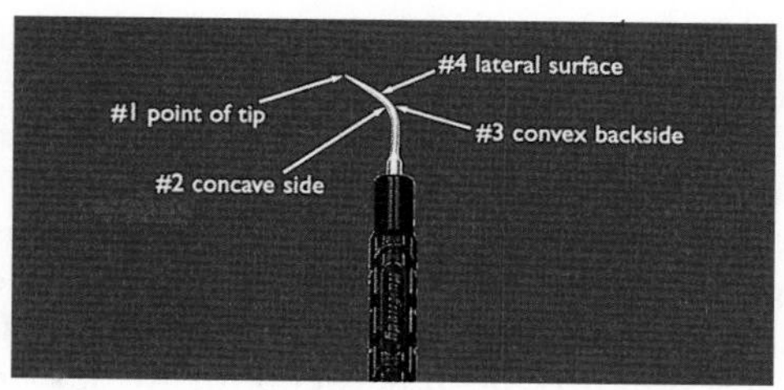

FIGURE 23–16 ✦ Power dispersion of a magnetostrictive insert tip. (1) Point of tip generates the greatest amount of energy. (2) Concave side generates the second greatest amount of energy. (3) Convex backside generates less energy than the point or concave surface. (4) Lateral surface generates the least amount of energy. *(Courtesy Hu-Friedy Manufacturing Co.)*

In addition to the energy generated from the power and frequency settings of a unit, other factors influence the energy emitted from the working end and may compromise client comfort and increase trauma to the tissues:

- Time of exposure: The longer the time spent on the tooth structure, the greater the amount of energy.
- Pressure: Pressure will increase the effects of the tip of the working end. When too much pressure is applied, the tip will stop or dampen and the clinician must reevaluate the pressure used.
- Shape: The sharper the tip of the working end, the greater the amount of energy. Blunt or rounded tip inserts are preferred for light periodontal debridement because less energy output enhances comfort and reduces hard and soft tissue trauma.
- Angle of application: The greater the angle of application of the tip to the tooth, the greater the energy output. Typically, the tooth to tip angle with an insert should be 15 degrees or less.

INSERT CARE AND MAINTENANCE. All inserts must be sterilized according to the manufacturer's instructions, which vary. Prior to autoclaving, most manufacturers recommend that used inserts be rinsed with water and dried. Hu-Friedy inserts can be placed in an ultrasonic cleaning unit for 7–10 minutes, or 15–20 minutes if the insert is in a cassette. For sterilization, inserts should be placed in an all-paper or combination paper and plastic autoclave bag. Use of an all-plastic autoclave bag is not recommended because the bag may build up too much heat during autoclaving and shorten the lifespan of the insert. Inserts should not be placed in disinfectants because the chemicals may disintegrate the plastic grips and alter the metal components, resulting in a shorter insert lifespan. For sterilization, inserts should be placed on top of other instruments in the autoclave or run separately to prevent bending or mishandling.

Magnetostrictive inserts require maintenance of the "O" ring. To aid in inserting the tip into the handpiece, lubricate the ring with water and gently twist the insert into place. These "O" rings can be replaced when worn or cracked to prevent leakage of water at the junction of the handpiece and tip.

Inserts wear out with regular use and with mishandling. Inserts should be examined often to ensure that the metal tips are not bent and that the stacks are not damaged. The length of the insert tip should also be evaluated because wear over time will shorten the tip. Worn insert tips reduce efficiency, resulting in extended instrumentation time, need for increased power settings, and risk of tip fracture. An insert tip worn down 1 mm has lost 25% of its efficiency, and a tip worn down 2 mm has lost 50% of its efficiency.

Replacement of inserts is recommended when 2 mm of the tip is worn away. The "Efficiency Indicator" guide (DENTSPLY Professional) is used to assess tip loss. Some manufacturers will retip inserts, but the stack is still subject to age.

Piezoelectric Units

A piezoelectric unit (Figure 23–17) differs from a magnetostrictive unit in the following ways:

- Transducer material
- Working end pattern
- Activated surfaces of the working end
- Working end and transducer/handpiece design
- Functions of the water source

A piezoelectric unit utilizes a transducer that consists of ceramic crystals. Vibration occurs when alternating electrical currents are applied to the transducer, creating a dimensional change that is transmitted to the tip. The tip moves in a linear pattern and only two sides of the tip are activated and adapted to the tooth surface (Figure 23–18). The lateral surfaces emit the least amount of energy and are adapted to the tooth.

The transducer is contained within the permanently sealed handpiece of the piezoelectric unit. The working end is threaded or screwed into the handpiece with a specialized wrench and is not connected to the transducer as is the insert used with a magnetostrictive unit. Therefore, working ends for piezoelectric units are not transferable to magnetostrictive units nor are they interchangeable among piezoelectric units. Each piezoelectric unit comes with working ends designed for that particular unit. Additional working ends can be purchased. Most manufacturers sell standard and precision thin designs such as the universal, beavertail, and periodontal slim tips. If selecting this type of unit, consider the available designs for NSPT. Some piezoelectric units have removable, autoclavable handpieces.

Although water is not needed to cool the transducer of the piezoelectric unit because it generates less heat than a magnetostrictive unit, water is still required to cool the friction produced between the working end and the tooth (see section on manual and autotuned units). Cavitation is also a by-product of piezoelectric technology. Examples of this type of unit are the Piezon Master 400 (Electro Medical Systems, seen in Figure 23–17) and Amdent US30 (Biotrol International). The active tip area for the 25- to 30-kHz piezoelectric units is from 2.2 to 3.5 mm, depending on the tip design. Frequencies of the units vary from 24,000 to 50,000 kHz. No evidence supports either the piezoelectric or magnetostrictive unit as more efficacious for ultrasonic instrumentation.

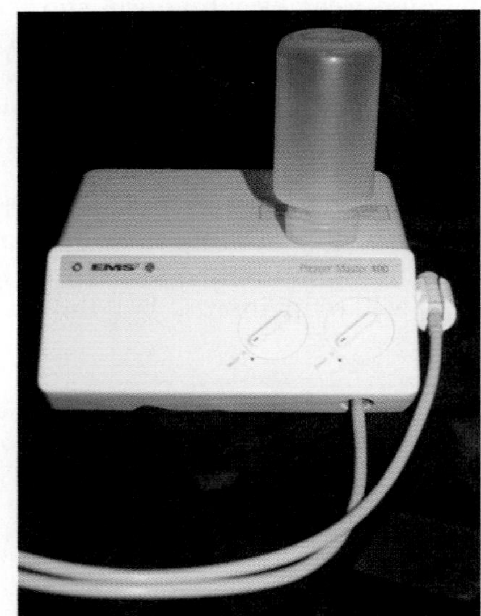

FIGURE 23–17 ✦ The Piezon Master 400 is a piezoelectric unit. *(Courtesy Electro Medical Systems.)*

Sonic Instruments

The sonic instrument (Figure 23–19) is driven by compressed air instead of electricity. The frequency range of sonic instruments is between 3000 kHz and 8000 kHz. This slower vibration results in less-efficient calculus removal as compared to ultrasonic instruments, although results of effects on clinical parameters are equal to ultrasonic and hand instrumentation. The sonic handpiece is connected to the compressed air line and is activated by the dental unit's rheostat. The internal portion of the handpiece is composed of a hollow rod, a rotor, and several rubber "O" rings. The instrument tips screw onto the handpiece and move in an elliptical motion. Water is used in this system to cool the tip and for lavage. The unit itself does not generate heat. Sonic instruments do not offer the array of tip designs that ultrasonic units do, although a rubber-coated sonic tip is available for debridement of implants (Quixonic SofTip Prophy Tips, DENTSPLY Professional; Table 23–7 and Figures 50–59 and 50–60). Refer to Table 23–8 for a summary of the three types of mechanized instruments.

HEALTH-RELATED OUTCOMES OF MECHANIZED INSTRUMENTS

Little difference exists between the clinical response achieved with sonic, ultrasonic, and hand-activated instrumentation:[11,23]

- ✦ A combination of ultrasonic/sonic instrumentation and hand-activated instrumentation provides the best results for NSPT.
- ✦ Interproximal areas, furcations, the cementoenamel junction, and multirooted teeth are most likely to exhibit residual calculus regardless of instrument method.

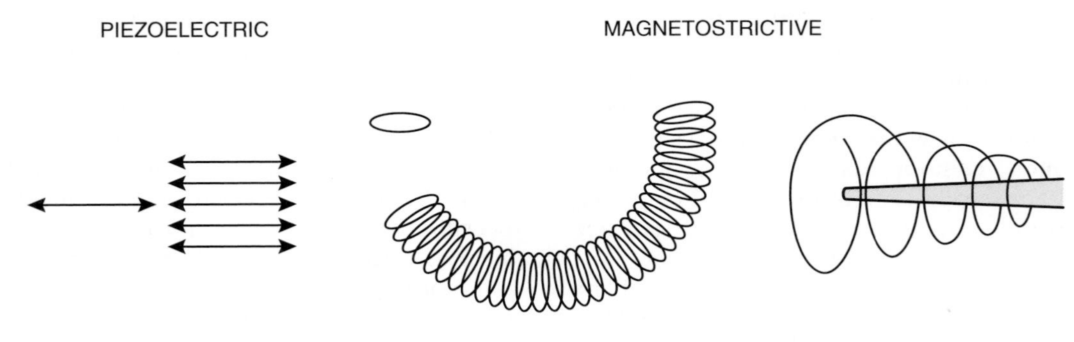

FIGURE 23–18 ✦ Tip motion of the piezoelectric and magnetostrictive units. *(From Hodges KO:* Concepts in nonsurgical periodontal therapy, *Albany, NY, 1998, Delmar.)*

- Bleeding on probing and probing depths are both reduced to equivalent levels when sonic and ultrasonic methods are compared to one another and to hand-activated instrumentation. In some cases, instrumentation takes less time with mechanized instrumentation than with hand instrumentation.
- As probing depth increases, the effectiveness of standard-design power-driven instruments declines due to limitations in design. The exception to this statement, however, is with precision thin insert designs.
- The curet is more efficient than ultrasonic instruments with standard inserts; however, the curet requires more effort, time, and expertise.
- Longitudinal studies measuring clinical attachment level are needed to evaluate clinical parameters after mechanized instrumentation.

Subgingival Microbial Flora[23]

Equal reductions in microbial flora are found with ultrasonic instrumentation and manual curets. Also, reductions of microbial flora appear equivalent when comparing sonic and ultrasonic methods of mechanized instrumentation. Limited studies have determined that spirochetes in particular, as well as Gram-negative microbes, are destroyed at ultrasonic frequencies. Other specific organisms studied include *Porphyromonas gingivalis, Bacteroides forsythus,* and *Actinobacillus actinomycetemcomitans.*

Endotoxin Removal

Ultrasonic instrumentation is effective in removing weakly adherent endotoxin. Endotoxin removal is achieved with less time, effort, and root surface removal because of the powered action versus the manual instrumentation that could ultimately result in over-instrumentation. One study found that about 16 strokes with ultrasonic instruments, rather than intentional cementum removal, resulted in fibroblast reattachment to previously diseased roots.[23]

Acoustic Microstreaming[24]

Acoustic microstreaming is caused by shear force surrounding an oscillation tip. The effects of acoustic microstreaming depend on tip geometry and tip orientation. It is hypothesized that acoustic microstreaming affects the microbial composition of bacterial plaque biofilm because the force generated by the streaming should shear the plaque away from the bacterial colony and tooth. This force accompanies the mechanical and cavitational activity that occurs during ultrasonic

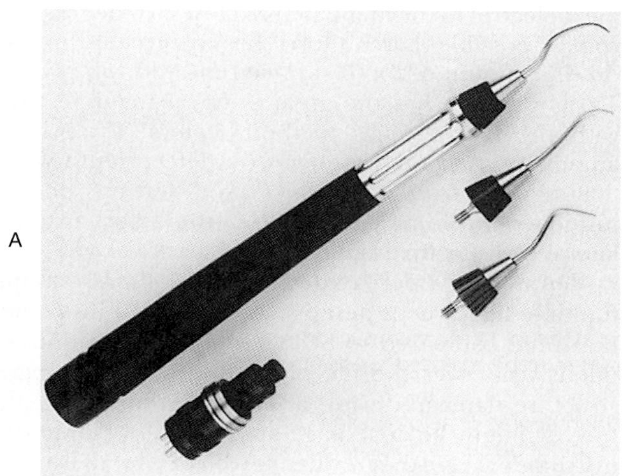

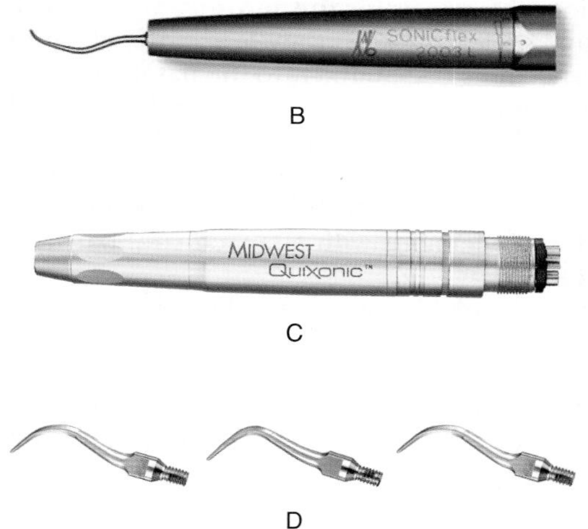

FIGURE 23–19 ✦ **A,** Titan SW sonic instrument and insert tips. **B,** SONICflex. **C,** Quixonic handpiece. **D,** Quixonic Tips. *(B courtesy Tony Riso; C courtesy DENTSPLY.)*

TABLE 23–8 COMPARATIVE SUMMARY OF MECHANIZED INSTRUMENTATION

Type of Unit	Frequency/ Cycles per Second	Type of Transducer	Motion of Insert	Activated Surfaces of Working End	Active Tip Area	Water Used as Coolant
Magnetostrictive ultrasonic	25,000 to 42,000	Stack of metal strips (permanickel) or ferrite rod	Elliptical or orbital	All; back and sides are used most often	4.3 millimeters (ultimately depends on frequency)	Yes for both transducer and tip
Piezoelectric ultrasonic	25,000 to 50,000	Ceramic	Linear	The two sides of the tip	2.3 to 3.5 millimeters	No for transducer Yes for tip
Sonic air-turbine	2,500 to 7,000	None	Elliptical	All		Yes for tip

instrumentation. More evidence is needed to draw conclusions about its therapeutic effect.

Plaque and Calculus Removal

Hand and mechanized instrumentation are equally effective in removing subgingival bacterial plaque and calculus.[23] Also, when hand and mechanized instrumentation have been compared to diamond burrs, diamond-coated ultrasonic tips, plastic-coated tips, and reciprocating systems, plaque and calculus removal has been reported to be equal to removal by manual instrumentation.

Antimicrobial Irrigation

See Chapter 24.

Aerosols and Spatter[25,26,27] (see Chapter 22)

During periodontal debridement a large amount of contaminated aerosols and spatter is produced. Dental aerosols are fine, airborne particles that are liquid, solid, or a combination of both and are 50 μm or less in size. Spatter includes particles greater than 50 μm that travel a considerable distance from the source and splash on environmental surfaces, masks, and the operator's skin and clothes. The sources of the contamination are the client's blood, saliva, and bacteria, and the water spray coolant provides the means for the aerosols. When particles are 50 μm or less in size, they are more likely to remain airborne and to be pulled into the nasal passages, penetrating into the respiratory system. Even large liquid particles eventually evaporate and leave smaller particles called droplet nuclei that carry respiratory bacteria such as *Mycobacterium tuberculosis.* Both large and small particles contain blood elements with attached viral particles such as HIV or HBV.[25]

No evidence is available on the number of potentially pathogenic organisms in the aerosol and spatter produced by mechanized instrumentation. In addition, no epidemiologic studies link dental aerosols to disease transmission; however, the dental hygienist should still be concerned about this potential.

A comparative study revealed that magnetostrictive, piezoelectric, and sonic instruments all produced an equal amount of contamination that contained bacteria as small as 0.65 μm. Despite different volumes of coolant water, there is no difference in the amount of aerosols emitted.[26] However, in another study comparing piezoelectric and magnetostrictive units, the piezoelectric unit produced the greatest amount of contamination because of the linear motion of the tip.[25] A greater production of aerosols and spatter also was observed in some of the precision thin inserts when compared to standard inserts. This finding probably is related to the ultrasonic energy being applied to a thinner piece of metal, causing more movement than the same amount of energy applied to a standard insert tip. More movement enhances greater aerosol production at a given power setting. One recent study evaluated a new focused spray insert design (FSI–10, DENTSPLY Professional, York, Pennsylvania), which produced fewer aerosols and thus less contamination than a traditional insert (Thru Flow Insert [TFI–10], DENTSPLY Professional, York, Pennsylvania).[13] Both inserts produced equal amounts of aerosol contamination.

Root Surface Roughness

Studies have arrived at conflicting conclusions regarding instrumentation and root surface roughness. For example, manual instrumentation produces a smoother surface than ultrasonic instrumentation, manual instrumentation produces a rougher surface than ultrasonic instrumentation, and both methods produce an equally smooth surface.[11] In studies in which ultrasonic instrumentation left a rougher surface than hand instrumentation, roughness was not shown to be significant in terms of gain in clinical attachment.[28,29] Tip angulation, exposure time, lateral pressure, and intensity of settings are all critical factors to consider to avoid over-instrumentation. When root smoothness with sonic and ultrasonic methods were compared with each other, results revealed either equal outcomes or that the ultrasonic method produced smoother surfaces.[23]

Root Substance Removal[30,31]

To prevent root surface damage it is imperative that the piezoelectric tip be angulated as close to 0 degrees to the root as possible. Lateral force has the greatest influence on the amount of tooth surface removed (*defect volume*). Tip angulation has the greatest effect for defect depth with the piezoelectric method. Lateral force and tip angulation had similar effects on defect depth with the magnetostrictive method. Power setting does not influence the volume or depth of the defect as much as lateral force or tip angulation.

Removal of calculus during initial therapy requires multiple instrument designs and increased instrumentation time compared to SPT; however, SPT requires frequent visits over the life of the tooth. Preventing root structure damage during SPT is a consideration; therefore, it might be advantageous to employ power-driven instruments. Further evidence related to these factors will help dental professionals select appropriate interventions for NSPT and SPT based on client need, safety, and effectiveness.

MECHANIZED INSTRUMENTS IN PRACTICE

Advantages (see Advantages and Disadvantages of Mechanized Instruments as Compared to Manual Instruments)

There is increased efficiency of removal for large calculus deposits when compared to hand instrumentation. This advantage must be considered in clinical treatment because moderate to large calculus deposits can be tenacious. Burnished calculus often results if ultrasonic instruments alone are used for tenacious deposit. In this case, the clinical power of the unit is increased and hand-activated instruments, such as the periodontal file, are incorporated into debridement therapy. Overall, the increased efficiency is a benefit for both the operator and client.

Multiple surfaces of the tip can be utilized to remove deposits rather than the single surface cutting edge of a curet. The curet blade must be adapted at a precise tooth-to-blade angle to remove calculus and stain deposits in a channeling fashion. This is one reason why manual debridement (scaling and root planing) is technically demanding.

Tips never need sharpening as hand instruments do, saving time and effort for the operator and client. Also, inserts/working ends are replaced less often than curets.

A larger diameter handpiece is an advantage for the clinician because it does not require much pinching motion to hold it as compared to a smaller diameter manual instrument handle. In addition, lateral pressure is not needed to enhance activation of the working end, therefore, the chance of developing repetitive strain injuries could be reduced (see Chapter 8).

It is possible that less tissue distention occurs with precision thin designs than with manual curets because of the greater width of a new curet blade.

Water is an advantage. Lavage and irrigation might enhance healing and client comfort when compared to manual instrumentation. Enhanced comfort could be due to the warm lavage and/or less lateral pressure needed to remove the deposit. Acoustic microstreaming is another byproduct of the water coolant.

Advantages and Disadvantages of Mechanized Instruments as Compared to Manual Instruments

Advantages

Increased efficiency
Multiple surfaces of tip are capable of removing deposits
No need to sharpen
Less chance for repetitive stress injuries
- Handpiece size
- Reduced lateral pressure

Less tissue distention
Water
- Lavage
- Irrigation
- Acoustic microstreaming

Disadvantages

More precautions and limitations
Client comfort (water spraying)
Aerosol production
Temporary hearing shifts
Noise
Less tactile sensation
Reduced visibility

Disadvantages (see Advantages and Disadvantages of Mechanized Instruments as Compared to Manual Instruments)

Water flow can interfere with client comfort because of unavoidable spray on the cheeks and chin. Aerosol production is a concern, although further evidence is needed to study its effects on the clinician and client. An aerosol reduction device attached to a handpiece reduces aerosol contamination.[27]

Temporary hearing shifts have been observed in clinical experience. Further research is indicated to assess the prevalence of the hearing loss and the long-term effects it has on the individual's health. At times the noise produced may be uncomfortable for the client.

Reduced tactile sensation as compared to curets has been experienced by dental hygienists. Limited tactile sense is developed over time with precision thin designs and an explorer is always employed to determine progress and the clinical endpoint.

Water spray interferes with the operator's visibility of the tooth and gingiva. Continued evacuation is a must, and commercially prepared solutions to prevent mirror fog might be useful. Recommendations to reduce mirror fog are discussed in the instrumentation section.

Indications

With the advent of precision thin designs, the clinician can remove lighter deposits supragingivally and subgingivally without changing inserts/working ends. Subgingival instrumentation for calculus, bacterial plaque (loosely attached and attached), root surface constituents, and periodontal pathogens is accomplished primarily with precision thin designs. Standard inserts, however, probably extend subgingivally about 1 to 3 mm depending on the tissue tone, access to the area, insert selection, and gingival sensitivity of the client. Mechanized instruments can also assist in the removal of excess cement and bonding agents around orthodontic appliances and residual cement after appliance removal. In these cases, manual instrumentation is usually not as effective. Other indications include dental hygiene care for necrotizing periodontal diseases or pericoronitis, or treatment during surgical interventions (removal of residual deposits and granulation tissue).

Precautions

Caution should be exercised when a client reports having a pacemaker. Some pacemakers may be disrupted by external electrical fields. The demand pacemaker is the most common type and the most sensitive to external electromagnetic forces. Older models were unipolar and less insulated, creating more problems from dental equipment. Newer models are bipolar and well insulated, so the small amount of electromagnetic radiation generated by dental equipment does not pose much threat to their function.[32] Consultation with the appropriate physician will provide the needed information on the type of pacemaker involved.

Communicable diseases such as hepatitis, tuberculosis, strep throat, and respiratory infections could all be transmitted via aerosols. Therefore, clients with communicable disease should not receive NSPT until the disease has been treated for a period of time. When it is appropriate for NSPT to take place based on health status, universal precautions are employed to protect the client and clinician (see Chapter 6).

Demineralized tooth structure, exposed dentin associated with sensitivity, restorative materials, and restorations such as veneers, cast crowns, and titanium implants do not prevent the clinician from using mechanized instruments; however, these localized areas and restorations should be avoided. The clinician refers to the periodontal and restorative chartings to make decisions about which surfaces to treat with the mechanized instrument, which will be best treated with manual instrumentation, and which should not be instrumented. Tip placement should occur adjacent to these conditions and not on or within these entities. If restorative material is on the clinical crown and the tip of the mechanized instrument can be placed apical to the restoration, then the insert can be used. Restorative materials can be adversely affected by creating roughness or striations (e.g., on composite restorations, black-colored striations can result because the composite material will abrade the metal tip). Also, undue wear to the working end can occur when it is placed against metal restorations. The tip of the mechanized sonic instrument should be covered with a specially designed plastic sheath to prevent damage to the titanium implant.

Contraindications

Mechanized instrumentation should *not* be used with clients who report:

IMMUNOSUPPRESSION. Immunosuppression from a disease or from chemotherapy, e.g., HIV infection, organ transplants, cancer, systemic lupus erythematosus, Crohn's disease, or corticosteroid therapy, increases the risk of opportunistic infection from breathing contaminated aerosols and from ingesting contaminated dental unit water.

UNCONTROLLED DIABETES. Clients with uncontrolled diabetes should be referred to the physician to achieve control prior to providing NSPT. Most diabetics who receive initial NSPT or SPT will be indicated for mechanized instrumentation (see Chapter 41).

CHRONIC PULMONARY DISEASE. This includes asthma, emphysema, cystic fibrosis, or pneumonia. The risk for infection probably would increase if microorganisms in the bacterial plaque were aspirated into the lungs (see Chapter 42).

CARDIOVASCULAR DISEASE WITH SECONDARY PULMONARY DISEASE. The risk of aspiration of plaque microorganisms into the lungs could adversely affect the cardiovascular system.

DYSPHASIA OR SWALLOWING DIFFICULTY (due to the water flow). Also, muscular dystrophy, multiple sclerosis, paralysis, or a psychological disorder might affect the client's swallowing.

CHILDREN. Use with children is a concern because the vibrations might negatively affect the young growing tissue. Also, primary and newly erupted teeth have large pulp chambers that are more susceptible to heat generated by dental instruments.

A summary of the indications, precautions, and contraindications is found in Indications, Precautions, and Contraindications for Use of Mechanized Instruments. Recommendations for Discussion and Demonstration of Mechanized Instrumentation with a Client is used to guide client discussions.

Unit Tuning

AUTOTUNED UNITS (Magnetostrictive and Piezoelectric). In an autotuned unit, frequency is already preset within the unit; the clinician only controls energy output by adjusting the power knob. The lowest powered setting that is effective should be selected. A low- to medium-powered setting for most procedures and insert/working end designs is usually adequate. A higher-powered setting might be warranted for heavier, tenacious deposits. The water flow must be adjusted with the water knob to achieve a fine mist or spray.

MANUAL-TUNED UNITS. In a manual-tuned unit, the frequency, in addition to power and water, are controlled by the clinician. The option to tune frequency is only available in manual-tuned units. Being able to manually tune the instrument increases the clinician's control over insert performance. First, the power knob is adjusted to the lowest setting, and the frequency knob is adjusted so that no vibration is emitted from the tip. The external water conduit is positioned 1 mm from the back of the tip and not contacting the insert. With the desired insert in place, the handpiece is held in a horizontal position in relation to the floor. The insert tip is pointed upward toward the ceiling, and the water knob is adjusted until an arch of water from 1 to 1 ½ inches occurs over the tip. This arch of water assures adequate water flow. With the tip pointed downward toward the floor, the frequency knob is adjusted so that a light aerosol of water is emitted.

The terms *in phase* and *out of phase* are used to describe the frequency adjustment of an insert. In phase means that the insert is adjusted to resonance frequency for maximum energy output. This level of tuning puts the insert at peak efficiency suitable for light to heavy deposit removal. Usually, the in phase adjustment is used with traditional inserts and a fine mist of water. Out of phase means that the insert is

Indications, Precautions, and Contraindications for Use of Mechanized Instruments

Indications
Supragingival debridement of calculus and stain
Subgingival debridement of calculus, bacterial plaque biofilm, root surface constituents, and periodontal pathogens
Removal of orthodontic cement
Gingival and periodontal conditions/diseases
Surgical interventions
Margination (reduces amalgam overhangs)

Precautions
Some pacemakers
Communicable diseases: hepatitis, tuberculosis (active stages)
Demineralized tooth surface
Exposed dentin (especially associated with sensitivity)
Restorative materials (porcelain, amalgam, gold, composite)
Titanium implant abutments unless using Quixonic SofTip Prophy tips or ITStip

Contraindications
Immunosuppression from disease or chemotherapy
Uncontrolled diabetes
Chronic pulmonary disease: asthma, emphysema, cystic fibrosis, or pneumonias
Cardiovascular disease with secondary pulmonary disease
Swallowing difficulty (dysphagia)
Children

Recommendations for Discussion and Demonstration of Mechanized Instrumentation with a Client

Operation. Discuss how instrument operates by electrical energy that is converted to mechanical energy or through the air-driven handpiece, depending on the unit.

Water Use. Discuss why water is needed. Cavitation, lavage, and acoustic microstreaming are addressed in lay terms.

Water Evacuation. Discuss how water will be evacuated using either high-volume or low-volume suction. A demonstration is effective.

Feel of Instrumentation. Discuss what instrument will feel like. Clients need to know they should not experience discomfort.

Discomfort. Discuss what to do if the instrumentation is uncomfortable. Explain that the water, the tip, and heat are all factors that can create a problem with the client's comfort level. If any of these factors are present, advise the client to raise a hand so that proper adjustments can be made. Assure the client that, in most cases, adjustment can occur to achieve comfort.

Sound. Demonstrate what instrument will sound like (high-pitched noise). Any extended noise exposure can produce temporary hearing shifts. If sound is too bothersome, direct the client to let you know. If a hearing aid is worn, it should be turned off.

Adjunct Instrumentation. Discuss use of manual instrumentation. The client is informed that mechanized instrumentation alone will not accomplish the clinical and therapeutic goals of instrumentation, and that manual instrumentation will also be incorporated to complete the therapy.

Informed Consent. All questions should be answered to the client's satisfaction. A two-way discussion occurs to gain informed consent for the procedure.

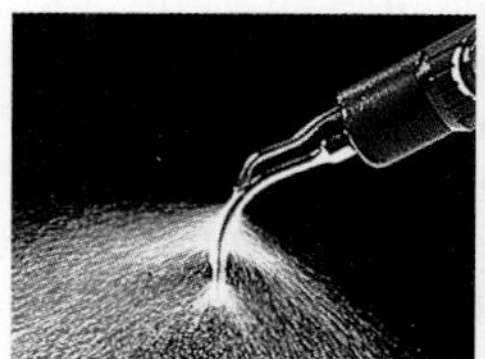
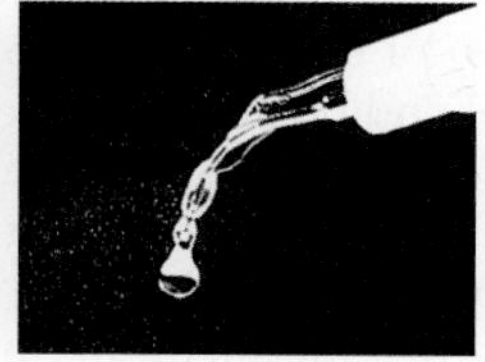

FIGURE 23–20 ✦ Tuning options. "In Phase" *(left)*. "Out of Phase" *(right)*. *(Courtesy Hu-Friedy Manufacturing Co.)*

detuned from resonance frequency. The out of phase adjustment is usually used with precision thin inserts and a fine mist with a water drip (Figure 23–20). Out of phase is thought to enhance client comfort and results in less vibration for deplaquing procedures.

SONIC UNIT. Tuning of a sonic unit is different because air pressure is the mode of operation. The handpiece is connected to the handpiece tubing. The air pressure is adjusted to 40 to 50 pounds per square inch (psi). With the water switch on, the unit is operated at about 45 psi and the dental unit water supply value is slowly opened. Handpiece lubricant is used prior to autoclaving.

INSTRUMENTATION TECHNIQUE FOR MECHANIZED INSTRUMENTS

Positioning

The client is placed in a normal supine position appropriate for the maxillary or mandibular arch. For example, if instrumenting the mandibular right lingual, have the client turn to the right. The water will pool in the right posterior corner of the oral cavity, where suction can remove it efficiently and the potential for gagging is reduced. The client turns to the right to treat the right side of the mouth and the left for treatment on the left side.

Suction and Retraction

High-volume suction that requires the assistance from another individual is recommended. High-volume suction reduces the aerosols created and diminishes the pathogens and dislodged deposits from being aspirated into the client's pulmonary system. The aerosols emitted into the air also will be reduced for the benefit of all persons involved in the procedure and any others in close proximity.

If assistance is not possible, suction occurs via slow-speed saliva ejectors. Slow-speed suction can be monitored by the clinician and controlled by the client. Slow-speed suction is with either a straight saliva ejector or a curved circular ejector (Hygoformic, Pulp Dent). With the straight device, the client participates by holding and placing the ejector intraorally as needed. If using the curved circular ejector, the suction hose is extended behind the dental chair to place the ejector in the mouth. The weight of the hose stabilizes the ejector. This ejector is used to retract the buccal mucosa when placed between the buccal plane of the teeth and the cheek mucosa. The circular end is twisted to adapt to the contour of the cheek and to expose the holes where the water exits to the suction hose. Retracting the client's lips helps control the water. In the anterior regions the lips can form a cuplike space between the facial surfaces and mucosa of the lips. For posterior regions, the lips can be retracted away from the teeth to form a space or "cup" for the water.

Grasp

A light grasp, similar to that used with exploration, is mandatory because it increases tactile sensitivity and reduces the likelihood of excessive lateral pressure. The light grasp is all that is necessary because the activation of the tip removes the calculus deposit. The handpiece is grasped when necessary to facilitate instrumentation. At times, the grasp will occur next to the junction of the handpiece and insert, or the grasp might be placed further up the handpiece to enhance access.

The cord to the handpiece should be straight and not twisted to prevent undue stress on the operator's shoulder, arm, and hand. The cord can be draped over the clinician's shoulder, over the light handle, or held between the ring finger and the little finger. When the clinician is adapting the tip to the tooth and rolling the handpiece within the grasp, strain is also placed on the arm of the clinician. The insert itself should, therefore, be rotated (using the nondominant hand) within the handpiece of the magnetostrictive unit to prevent some of this strain. Rotation of the insert within the handpiece occurs when the operator is attempting to achieve adaptation of the tip between the distal and buccal/lingual surfaces, as well as between the buccal/lingual surfaces and the mesial surfaces. If the handpiece alone is rotated, the cord could get twisted, causing ergonomic problems. (Table 23–7). Ergonomics can be enhanced by using a handpiece that is capable of rotating to eliminate twisting of the cord, reduce cable drag, and minimize stress on internal tubings. The Satin Swivel by Hu-Friedy and the Cavitron Steri-Mate handpiece with swivel by DENTSPLY Professional have been designed to address this adjustment and ergonomic issue.

Fulcrum

An intraoral fulcrum is used most of the time with standard inserts, whereas an extraoral fulcrum is acceptable and recommended with precision thin designs. The fulcrum is placed extraorally because only an extremely light stroke is needed to debride. The extraoral fulcrum seems to enhance the tactile sensitivity the clinician develops with experience. The dental hygienist does not need a firm fulcrum on the tooth surface as with manual instrumentation because strength to exert lateral pressure is not indicated for power-driven instrumentation. The fulcrum placement is either conventional, opposite arch, or cross arch, depending on the surface being treated. The grasp relates to the fulcrum placement just as with manual instrumentation. In other words, a cross-arch fulcrum requires the clinician to place the grasp further back on the handpiece.

Dental Mirror Use

The mirror is still used, but visibility is impaired. Operators tend to use direct vision as much as possible while striving to attain correct client and operator positioning.

Adaptation

Key factors for adapting the working end are:

- ✦ Use the correct part of the active tip
- ✦ Cover all tooth surfaces where periodontal debridement is indicated

For supragingival debridement the clinician focuses on the visible deposit or stain (Figure 23–21). For general periodontal debridement, the easiest way to adapt any universal insert/working end to the tooth surface is to think of the application in relation to a universal curet. In other words, the tip is directed toward the distal surface when the clinician is inserting the tip at the distal line angle (Figure 23–22). The clinician then activates the tip towards the distal surface while adapting the side (lateral surface) of the tip. To keep the tip adapted, the clinician will roll and pivot while advancing the tip to extend to the midline of the distal proximal surface.

Next, the clinician will reinsert, adapting the tip parallel to the long axis at the distal line angle, will advance across the buccal or lingual surface, and will roll and pivot (or turn the insert in the handpiece) at the mesial line angle to keep the side of the tip adapted to the tooth surface (Figure 23–23, *A* and *B*). The clinician ensures that the tip reaches the midline of the mesial proximal surface. The tip is applied somewhat perpendicularly or diagonally to the long axis of proximal surfaces (Figure 23–23, *C*). Another approach to the buccal or lingual of a sextant or quadrant is to complete the distal of each tooth first, then to approach the buccal/lingual surfaces, then the mesial surfaces one by one. This method involves less rolling and pivoting and allows the clinician to move the insert in the handpiece less often.

With magnetostrictive units the inserts also can be used on the back (convex) surface. Adapting the back to the enamel and cementum is indicated for loss of attachment, periodontal pockets, concavities, and furcations

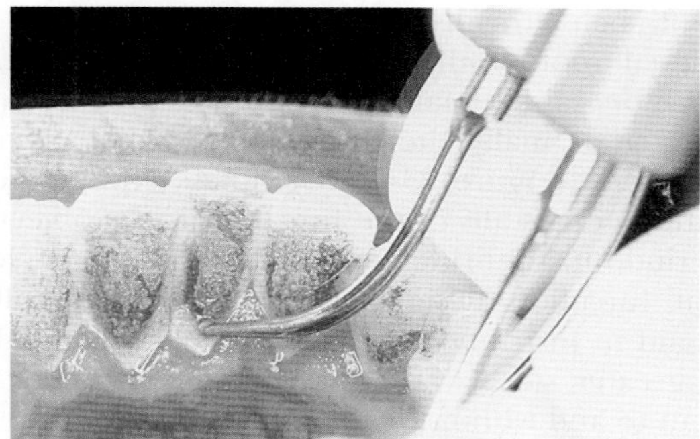

FIGURE 23–21 ✦ Insert adapted for supragingival debridement. *(Courtesy Hu-Friedy Manufacturing Co.)*

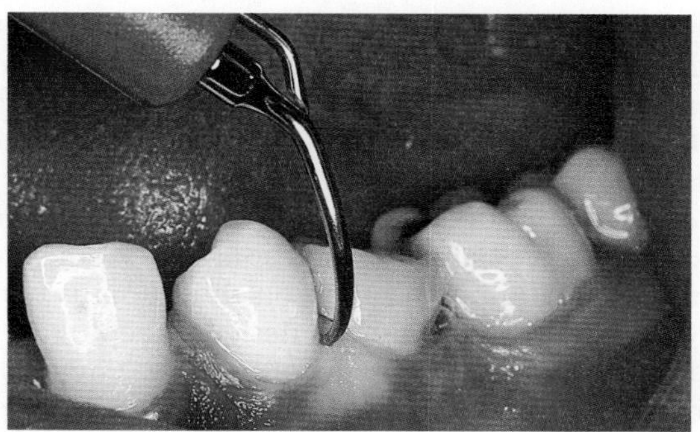

FIGURE 23–22 ✦ Precision thin insert adapted to distal surface covered with dental calculus. *(Courtesy Hu-Friedy Manufacturing Co.)*

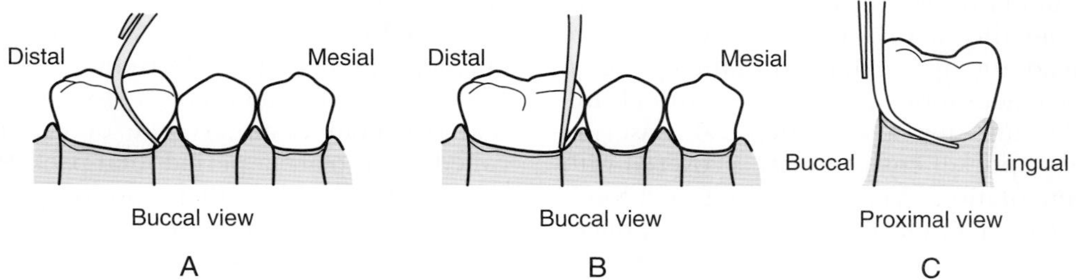

FIGURE 23–23 ✦ Right precision thin insert used to debride the buccal surfaces. **A,** Select insert based on its curvature toward the mesial surface. Adapt tip below contact area. **B,** Roll tip onto the proximal surface. Keep tip against tooth. **C,** Extend tip toward the lingual surface to negotiate the CEJ and proximal surfaces. *(From Hodges KO:* Concepts in nonsurgical periodontal therapy, *Albany, NY, 1998, Delmar.)*

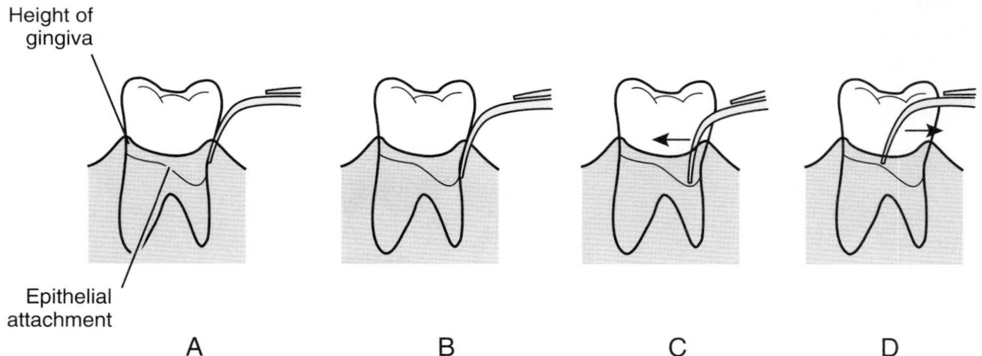

FIGURE 23–24 ✦ Pocket negotiation. **A,** Enter pocket using the back surface. Keep tip in contact with root and parallel to the long axis of the root. **B,** Negotiate tip to the apical extent of the pocket using minute overlapping strokes. NOTE: Weight of the instrument and the oscillations generated by the tip will guide the tip subgingivally. **C,** To move the tip along the epithelial attachment, use the back of the tip and a push-like stroke to avoid trauma and client discomfort. **D,** Avoid using a pull stroke with front or concave surface when tip is against the epithelial attachment. Place current periodontal charting and radiographs within view for reference during instrumentation. *(From Hodges KO:* Concepts in nonsurgical periodontal therapy, *Albany, NY, 1998, Delmar.)*

(Figure 23–24). At all times the tip to tooth angle is 15 degrees or less. The point of the insert is never placed on the tooth surface because it could cause iatrogenic damage to the enamel or cementum. With the use of the standard size inserts, extension to the epithelial attachment is not an objective.

Activation

Activation of the tip is initiated by wrist movement or rocking from the fulcrum as with hand instrumentation. The tip must be moving at all times to prevent iatrogenic damage (clinician-caused damage) to the root or crown of the tooth, excessive heat, or a "shock" effect felt by the client. Strokes will be overlapping and multidirectional. Oblique and vertical strokes are used primarily; however, horizontal and combination strokes on a surface also are employed. Movement in different directions helps break up heavy calculus deposits and aids in treating all root surfaces in periodontal pockets.

Different designs of standard inserts require different instrumentation. (See Table 23–7 to review the designs, indications, and applications.) For example, a standard periodontal probe-like design insert is used at the margin of the gingiva. The insert is inserted like a periodontal probe on top of the calculus deposit and the deposit is removed from the top towards the epithelial attachment. A cross-hatching pattern is used after the deposit is fractured. Extension subgingivally depends on tissue tone, access, and the tenaciousness of the deposit.

Instrumentation with precision thin designs parallels instrumentation with standard designs, keeping in mind the differences in the purpose of therapy. The right and left insert are used successfully in the posterior regions and adapted like a universal curet, as previously described. The straight design is used in deep periodontal pockets and furcations and adapts well in anterior regions of the mouth. Activation of the tips is essentially the same as for standard designs; however, the clinician will not work from the margin towards the epithelial attachment. Instead, the tip is extended to the epithelial attachment prior to activation, and then activation is initiated. The strokes are slow and methodical, ensuring that the subgingival pocket environment is covered with the power instrumentation. When smoothing of a tooth surface is indicated, a faster motion can be applied, sometimes termed a "vibrato" stroke. Manual instrumentation is always considered as an adjunct to power-driven instrumentation, and an explorer is always used to evaluate the clinical endpoint.

Instrumentation of furcations is achieved with multiple precision thin designs. They are adapted using the sides or back into the concavities adjacent to the furcation and on the mesial and distal surfaces of the furcation itself. The tooth can be divided into two teeth, with one tooth being the distal root and the other tooth being the mesial root. Both distal surfaces are treated first, then the buccal/lingual surfaces of the roots are instrumented, and finally the mesial surfaces of each root are debrided (Figure 23–7). Complete coverage of the roof and lateral walls of the furcation is the objective of the periodontal debridement therapy. The right, left, or straight furcation designs with the 0.8-mm ball end might aid in instrumenting the furcation. The ball end offers greater surface area to adapt to the concavities adjacent to and within the exposed furcation.

PERIODONTAL SURGERY

A discussion of periodontal surgical options for clients who need more than NSPT is beyond the scope of this chapter. The reader is referred to any major dental textbook on periodontal therapy. However, after a client has had periodontal surgery, the dental hygienist may be called on to place a periodontal pack. A *periodontal pack* is a puttylike bandage that is positioned over the surgical site to protect the area for about one week. To prepare the pack material (Coe-Pak), equal parts of the two pastes are squeezed onto a paper mixing pad. The two pastes are mixed thoroughly for about two to three minutes. Most clinicians use a wooden tongue depressor for mixing because the material is very tacky and difficult to clean up. When the tackiness is gone, the material is rolled into two cylinders for placement on the facial and lingual surfaces of the surgical site. See Figure 23–25 for a diagram of the pack placement procedure.

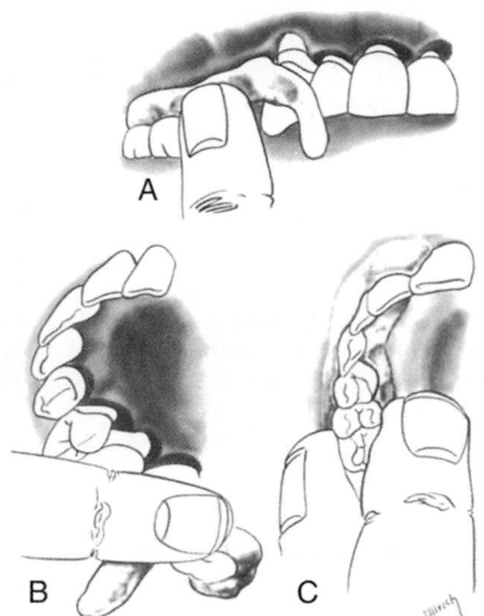

FIGURE 23–25 ✦ Inserting the periodontal pack. **A,** Strip of pack is hooked around the last molar and pressed into place anteriorly. **B,** The lingual pack is joined to the facial strip at the distal surface of the last molar and fitted into place anteriorly. **C,** Gentle pressure with fingers or with the heel of a curet on the facial and lingual interproximal surfaces joins the pack interproximally. *(From Newman MG, Takei HH, Carranza FA:* Clinical periodontology, *ed 9, Philadelphia, 2002, WB Saunders.)*

Client Education Issues

- Gingivitis is reversible but periodontitis is not; periodontitis is a chronic disease.
- Oral prophylaxis is not indicated for treatment of periodontitis.
- Evaluation is an integral aspect of NSPT, especially in reference to the initial therapy phase of care.
- Prevention and successful treatment of periodontal diseases depend on the co-therapy approach in which the client performs adequate self-care and complies with the continued-care interval.
- Self-care, alone, will not maintain or prevent further recurrence of periodontitis.
- The care plan for NSPT and SPT is dependent on the client's systemic and oral conditions, and not on the client's third-party payment plan benefits.
- SPT at the recommended interval is needed long-term to control progression of periodontitis.
- Risk factors are associated with the development and progression of periodontitis and they should be eliminated, reduced, or controlled depending on the nature of the risk factor itself (see Chapter 15).
- A combination of manual and mechanized instrumentation is recommended to obtain optimal results from periodontal debridement.

Legal, Ethical, and Safety Issues

- The client needs to be informed of the NSPT and SPT care plan, including the mode of periodontal debridement, and be involved in the decision-making process.
- The client must receive information to make an informed decision about the care plan.
- Referral to a medical professional or other dental professional (periodontist) when indicated is essential. Referral might be because of the clinician's lack of skill/knowledge to treat, advancing conditions of disease despite therapy, or an aggressive form of periodontal disease. Clinician needs to acquire informed consent if professional consultation related to a medical condition or periodontal disease arises.
- Failure to assess the periodontium adequately is malpractice.
- Negligence may include the dental hygienist's failure to protect a client from harm when the client has a systemic disease; and failure to record information about the assessment, care plan, informed consent, and interventions related to care. Negligence might occur if NSPT or SPT is needed by a client, but the dental hygienist provides an oral prophylaxis instead.
- The hygienist uses evidence-based decision making to select appropriate interventions for care. The dental hygienist must remain current with information about NSPT, SPT, and mechanized instrumentation by reading research reports and attending continuing education.
- Risks associated with care increase with NSPT that involves subgingival periodontal debridement (root planing) and local anesthetic over multiple appointments. Clients need to be informed of the consequences of local anesthetic (i.e., hematoma or paresthesia) and the consequences of periodontal debridement (i.e., bleeding, periodontal abscess, dentinal hypersensitivity).

Key Concepts

- A disease-free periodontium includes the absence of inflammation and the maintenance of periodontal attachment over time.
- Gingivitis is the presence of inflammation without clinical attachment loss and is treated by oral prophylaxis (scaling and selective polishing).
- Periodontitis is present when there is loss of clinical attachment and supporting bone. It is treated with nonsurgical periodontal therapy and/or surgery.
- NSPT includes plaque removal, plaque control, supragingival and subgingival scaling, root planing, and the use of chemotherapeutic agents.
- Periodontal debridement is the removal of subgingival plaque and its by-products, clinically detectable plaque-retentive factors, and detectable calculus-embedded cementum, sufficient to allow healing of adjacent periodontal tissues.
- Therapeutic endpoint is defined as the restoration of gingival health, reduction in pocket depth, and a gain in or stable clinical attachment level.
- Periodontal infection influences overall health and the course of systemic conditions such as cardiovascular disease, diabetes mellitus, respiratory disease, and preterm low birth weight.
- Periodontal assessment is the foundation for providing successful periodontal care including NSPT, SPT, and referrals to the periodontist for surgery.

Continued on following page

KEY CONCEPTS—CONT'D

- NSPT is Phase I periodontal therapy often referred to as initial therapy and is the responsibility of the dental hygienist working in concert with the general dentist or periodontist.
- Chronic disease states of gingivitis and periodontitis progress slowly and can respond to NSPT in a predictable manner; however, aggressive disease states progress rapidly and do not respond in a predictable manner.
- Periodontal diagnosis is determined from analyzing information during the assessment phase of therapy and includes health, dental, and pharmacologic history data and disease classification, extent, and severity.
- Mechanical pocket therapy is periodontal debridement using manual and/or mechanized instrumentation. Both methods are efficacious.
- Evaluation occurs throughout NSPT because gingival inflammation is reassessed two weeks after periodontal debridement of an area, reassessment for plaque-retentive factors occurs at each subsequent appointment, and reevaluation of the full mouth occurs four to six weeks after initial therapy.
- SPT follows the active phase of therapy, is appropriately timed based on client need, and continues for the life of the dentition or implant replacements.
- SPT prevents or minimizes the recurrence and progression of periodontal disease, prevents or reduces tooth loss, and increases the chances of locating and treating other diseases/conditions.
- Clients with gingivitis maintain their oral health when SPT is performed every six months. Clients with periodontitis require a three-month interval.
- Three modes of mechanized periodontal debridement are magnetostrictive ultrasonic, piezoelectric ultrasonic, and sonic instrumentation.
- Manual-tuned ultrasonic units allow the clinician to adjust the frequency but autotuned units do not. Both types require the clinician to control power and water.
- Two types of working end designs for mechanized instrumentation are standard for supragingival debridement and 1–3 mm of subgingival debridement. Precision thin designs are primarily for subgingival debridement.
- A combination of ultrasonic/sonic instrumentation and manual instrumentation provides the best results for NSPT.

CRITICAL THINKING EXERCISES

1. You are caring for a new client who has not received dental hygiene care for three years due to "financial constraints"; however, prior to this, she had received annual oral prophylaxes. She does not have dental insurance. Dental hygiene assessment findings reveal periodontal pockets ranging from 4 to 6 mm, radiographic early bone loss, bleeding upon probing, and generalized light to moderate deposits. Develop a dialogue explaining the need for NSPT versus oral prophylaxis, the number and length of appointments estimated, the type of interventions recommended, the need for evaluation, the need for supportive periodontal therapy, potential cost, and relationship of insurance coverage. Include what the client needs to know to make an informed decision (informed consent) about NSPT.
2. Compare and contrast the three different types of mechanized instrumentation. Compare the efficacy and efficiency of mechanized instrumentation with manual instrumentation based on evidence in the literature.
3. Identify one of your most challenging periodontally involved clients. Using the Insurance Procedure Codes in Table 23–1, identify all of the services you have provided that may be billed to the insurance company.
4. Obtain and complete the self-study CD-ROM from DENTSPLY Professional, Clinical Education Department, titled *Your Clinical Edge: Ultrasonics and Airpolishing.*

Special thanks to Cynthia Fong, RDH, MS for her expertise in reviewing the mechanized instruments section.

For References, Suggested Readings, and Related Websites, visit
http://evolve.elsevier.com/Darby/hygiene/

CHAPTER 24

PERIODONTAL CHEMOTHERAPY

OBJECTIVES

Mastery of the content in this chapter will enable the reader to:

- Discuss indications for chemotherapeutic intervention as an adjunct to mechanical plaque biofilm control, nonsurgical periodontal therapy, the treatment of gingivitis and periodontitis, and maintenance of periodontal health
- Relate FDA and ADA guidelines for acceptance of chemotherapeutic agents/devices for the control of plaque, gingivitis, and/or periodontitis to the evaluation of related professional literature
- Discuss legal and ethical considerations when involving a client in an effective personal oral hygiene care program

KEY TERMS

ADA Seal of Acceptance
Antimicrobial agents
Biodegradable
Bioresorbable
Chemotherapeutic agent
Chlorhexidine
Controlled drug delivery
Dentifrice (cosmetic and therapeutic)
Doxycycline hyclate
Intracrevicular delivery device
Local drug delivery
Monotherapies
Mouthrinse (cosmetic and therapeutic)
Oral irrigation
Oxidizing agent
Oxygenating agent
Phenolic compounds
Prebrushing mouthrinse
Quaternary ammonium compounds
Sanguinarine
Stannous fluoride
Subantimicrobial dose
Substantivity
Sustained drug delivery
Systemic administration

BACTERIAL PLAQUE AND HOST RESPONSE

Initiation and progression of oral diseases are related to the interaction of host, agent, and environmental factors (see Chapters 15 and 26). Prevention and control of inflammatory periodontal diseases depend, in part, on the control of bacterial plaque biofilm (the agent) because it is a primary risk factor for these diseases. Thus, prevention of bacterial colonization or disruption of plaque via pharmacologic antimicrobial agents is the basis of local drug delivery regimens.

Because total elimination of bacterial plaque biofilm is unrealistic, a more reasonable approach is to prevent disease by methods that can reduce bacterial plaque below the individual's threshold for disease.[1] Interactions between the host and the oral microorganisms are dynamic. In health, there is a balance between the two. If the balance shifts in favor of the microflora, disease results. Diet, stress, systemic disease, genetics, inadequate professional oral care, and environmental risk factors can affect the balance. The disease threshold undergoes changes, and the host is unable to defend itself against the microbial challenge. Thus, continual monitoring of plaque control and revision of methods, when necessary, are fundamental components of a supportive periodontal therapy program.

Another approach to controlling bacterial plaque is to alter its composition. Chemical plaque control is directed toward this goal. Presently, no singular device or agent can prevent plaque formation or render plaque nonpathologic. As a result, regular, efficient mechanical plaque removal is requisite to disease prevention and control. Increasing host resistance may also be an important component of the formula for maintaining a favorable balance between the oral microflora and the host.

Although bacterial plaque biofilm is a major risk factor in periodontal diseases, a susceptible host and the absence of beneficial species together determine the initiation and progression of periodontal diseases. When there is a balance between the host and its parasites, health results. Local or systemic factors that decrease host resistance can alter the balance. Host immunologic response is important to any infection. In periodontal disease, host response can provide protection against infectious agents by modulating the effects of microorganisms, but it also can contribute to tissue destruction and disease pathogenesis through cytotoxic, anaphylactic, or cell-mediated reactions. An impaired immunologic response (e.g., when antibody levels are not adequate in response to certain pathogens) can intensify disease severity.

PRODUCT SELECTION AND EVALUATION

Food and Drug Administration (FDA)

The FDA ensures the safety and efficacy of medical and dental drugs and devices through federally mandated review and approval. Periodontal products reviewed by the FDA include hand-activated and ultrasonic instruments, prescription drugs, controlled-release devices, bone-filling materials, guided tissue regeneration membranes, endosseous dental implants, growth factors, and diagnostic test kits. Evaluation of dental drug products is carried out by the Center for Drug Evaluation and Research. Dental devices are evaluated by the Center for Devices and Radiologic Health, with input from the Dental Products Panel. Products consisting of a combination of any two of the following three categories—drug, device, or biologic—are assigned a primary Center jurisdiction in consultation with other related Centers.[2]

Approval of prescriptive chemotherapeutic agents or products for treatment of gingival and/or periodontal diseases requires submission of clinical data to support therapeutic claims. Studies required for FDA approval are conducted in three phases with periodic consultation and review by the agency (Table 24–1). Approval to begin phases I and II testing is dependent on supportive animal pharmacologic and toxicologic data. Study design characteristics for phase III clinical trials in support of FDA submissions for marketing approval follow:

- Welfare of study participants is assured by adequate safeguards and adherence to institutional review and informed consent guidelines. Adverse events must be well documented.
- Two multicenter, parallel group or crossover clinical trials using the same protocol representative of the indications for use are required.
- The study population consists of adequate numbers and represents typical product users.
- Trained and experienced independent investigators are required.
- Both participants and examiners must be unaware of treatment assignment (double blind).
- The experimental product must be compared with appropriate positive and negative controls.
- Well-defined, appropriate outcome variables to measure responses of study participants to the effects of the product are required.
- Protocol must be strictly adhered to and any modifications or deviations must be well documented.
- Methods of statistical analysis must be described and documented, and account for missing data, participant follow-up, subgroup analysis, and predictors of response.

Efficacy results from FDA-mandated clinical trials are often published in scientific dental journals. Clinicians

TABLE 24–1 TYPES OF STUDIES REQUIRED FOR A NEW DRUG APPLICATION

Phase	Study Type	Primary Purpose
Preclinical	Animal pharmacologic and toxicology	Safety, tolerability
I	Clinical pharmacology studies (10–70 volunteers)	Safety; tolerability; occasionally effectiveness; pharmacokinetics
II	Controlled studies with 50–500 subjects with the disease or condition	Safety and effectiveness; dose ranging; pharmacokinetics-pharmacodynamics
III	Expanded studies for approval (2000 or more additional subjects) monitored for adverse effects and information to be used for setting dose requirements and labeling	Safety and effectiveness
IV	Postmarketing studies; new indications	Safety and effectiveness

can apply the FDA study design characteristics to evaluate related literature with particular interest in determining the value of results for individual patients. Practitioners should be aware that the lag time for professional publications can prolong their review of study outcomes well after release to the public through lay press and commercial marketing. This presents a particularly sensitive dilemma when a client inquires about a new product that the hygienist is either unaware of or has not had the opportunity to critically evaluate.

American Dental Association (ADA) Council on Scientific Affairs

The ADA Council on Scientific Affairs assists professionals in selection and use of therapeutic agents by evaluating new products for safety and effectiveness. Its purview includes the following:

- Dental therapeutic agents that are offered to the public or the profession
- Adjuncts to dental therapeutic agents
- Dental cosmetic agents that are offered to the public or the profession

Evaluation of dental materials and devices is carried out by the ADA Council on Dental Materials, Instruments, and Equipment. When dental materials and devices claim therapeutic value, they are evaluated cooperatively by both Councils.

Commercial products are examined by the ADA Council on Scientific Affairs at the request of the manufacturer or distributor, or at the initiation of the Council. Generally, the manufacturer submits research to substantiate the effectiveness of the product. Products that do not claim therapeutic value (e.g., cosmetic mouthwashes, denture cleansers, etc.) are not considered by the Council. Decisions of the Council are based on available scientific data. Product approval is granted for a three-year period and is renewable. After consideration of a product, the Council classifies it as "accepted," "provisionally accepted," or "unacceptable."

Accepted products have adequate evidence of safety and effectiveness and may use the *ADA Seal of Acceptance* or an authorized statement provided by the Council (Figure 24–1).

Provisionally accepted products have reasonable evidence of usefulness and safety but lack sufficient documentation for acceptance. Further investigation is indicated.

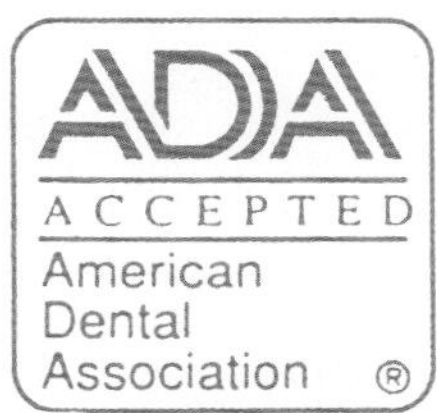

FIGURE 24–1 ✦ American Dental Association seal of acceptance.

Unaccepted products have no substantial evidence of usefulness or have questionable safety. Clinical products that carry these seals have been evaluated by the ADA Council on Scientific Affairs or the Council on Dental Materials, Instruments, and Equipment and have been found safe and effective for specific purposes. The Council on Scientific Affairs periodically prepares and publishes guidelines for acceptance of certain types of products. Guidelines for acceptance of chemotherapeutic products for the control of supragingival bacterial plaque and gingivitis must be followed in research.[3] Guidelines require the following:

- Characteristics of the study population represent typical product users.
- Active product should be used in a normal regimen and compared with a placebo control or, where applicable, an active control.
- Crossover or parallel study designs are acceptable and should be a minimum of six months in duration.
- Two studies should be conducted by independent investigators.
- Additional guidelines regarding microbial sampling and evaluation periods are in the guidelines.
- A product may not receive the ADA Seal of Acceptance if:
  - It does not fall within the purview of the Council on Scientific Affairs.
  - There is insufficient scientific evidence of its safety or effectiveness.
  - It has not been submitted for consideration.[4]

CHEMICAL PLAQUE CONTROL

Although mechanical removal of bacterial plaque biofilm remains the most widely accepted mechanism for plaque control (see Chapters 18 and 19), the bacterial etiology of periodontal diseases justifies supportive use of antimicrobial agents. The application of *antimicrobial agents* to reduce and control microorganisms and hence periodontal diseases is referred to as *local drug delivery*. It includes the transport of antimicrobial agents to the oral cavity using dentifrices, mouthrinses, irrigation devices, systemic administration, and sustained-release or controlled-release devices. Success of local drug delivery systems to treat periodontal infections depends on:

- Delivering the antimicrobial agents to the site of action
- Maintaining a bacteriostatic or bactericidal concentration
- Maintaining the agent at the diseased site for a sufficient duration of time[4]

Numerous local drug delivery systems and antimicrobial agents have been tested both as *monotherapies* (standalone therapies) and as adjuncts to professional debridement, but only a select few have confirmed efficacy for the treatment of gingivitis or periodontitis.[5]

Dentifrices

Dentifrices, sold as toothpastes, gels, or tooth powders, can be cosmetic or therapeutic. *Cosmetic dentifrices* assist in cleaning and polishing the teeth; *therapeutic dentifrices* also contain an active ingredient to reduce dental disease. For example, fluoride dentifrices reduce the occurrence of dental caries, and desensitizing toothpastes reduce dentinal hypersensitivity. Several antimicrobial toothpastes have been marketed to reduce bacterial plaque and gingivitis. The ADA does not consider acceptance for ordinary cleansing dentifrices, but it does consider dentifrices that are marketed for therapeutic, whitening, or prophylactic effects.[3,5]

The dental hygienist makes recommendations to clients regarding dentifrices. Regular use of a fluoride dentifrice is important for clients of all ages. It has been shown to reduce the incidence of dental caries. Sodium fluoride, sodium monofluorophosphate, and stannous fluoride are considered safe and effective agents for use in dentifrices. Safe products proven to have an anticariogenic effect earn the ADA Seal of Acceptance.

Research is ongoing to evaluate the effectiveness of dentifrices containing various antimicrobial agents in reducing bacterial plaque biofilm and gingivitis. Some active ingredients currently under study include sanguinaria, zinc citrate, triclosan, and copper citrate. Although many antimicrobial agents have been investigated, their incorporation into dentifrices presents problems of compatibility with other dentifrice components. For example, chlorhexidine, the most widely accepted antiplaque agent, may be inactivated by agents such as sodium lauryl sulfate and fluoride found in dentifrice. Because the most commonly used oral hygiene device is a toothbrush, it is logical to consider dentifrice as a delivery system for antimicrobials. The American Academy of Periodontology's (AAP) Research, Science and Therapy Committee outlined problems associated with this delivery system.[6] Their primary concern is that a manual toothbrush reaches an average of less than 1 mm subgingivally, and only occasionally 2 to 3 mm. Antimicrobial agents delivered by a toothbrush fail to reach the deeper subgingival sites associated with periodontitis. Presently, only one dentifrice has received the ADA Seal of Acceptance for antiplaque and gingivitis effectiveness (see Triclosan).

Mouthrinses

Like dentifrices, *mouthrinses* can be cosmetic, therapeutic, or both. Mouthrinses are a popular and simple delivery system, and thus present a logical mode for delivery of chemotherapeutic agents. They also provide a mechanism for rinsing oral debris and bacterial deposits dislodged during mechanical oral hygiene practices. Cosmetic benefits include a reduction in number of oral microorganisms, short-term halitosis control, and a pleasant taste and oral sensation. Mouthrinses that claim no therapeutic value are not included in the ADA Seal of Acceptance program.

Commercial mouthrinses generally contain an active ingredient to reduce the number of oral microorganisms, a flavoring agent, an astringent, ethyl alcohol, and water. The active ingredient, such as chlorhexidine, sanguinarine, phenolic compounds (thymol, eucalyptol, menthol, hexylresorcinols), and quaternary ammonium compounds (cetylpyridinium chloride), may or may not have therapeutic qualities. Astringent (e.g., citric acid, zinc chloride) provides an invigorating sensation in the mouth, and the flavoring agent provides the pleasant taste. Ethyl alcohol acts as a solvent and a taste enhancer. Many products contain 11% to 27% alcohol, although a few products are alcohol-free (Table 24–2). Consumers should be advised to read labels on commercial products to determine alcohol content. Alcohol-containing mouthrinses can be dangerous if ingested by small children, resulting in intoxication, illness, or fatalities, depending on dosage and body weight. The American Academy of Pediatrics recommends that alcohol content be limited to less than 5%, that package volume be minimal to prevent lethal dosages, and that safety caps be employed.[7] Adult clients who object to alcohol, recovering alcoholics or substance abusers, clients taking medications that react adversely with alcohol (e.g., Antabuse, metronidazole), or clients with xerostomia should be

TABLE 24–2 EXAMPLES OF MOUTHRINSES: pH, SUBSTANTIVITY, ALCOHOL, AND SODIUM CONTENT

Product	pH	Substantivity	Alcohol Content (%)	Sodium Content (mg/L)	Sodium Retention (mg/15 mL)
Cepacol	6.0	LOW	14.0	144	1.9
Regular Listerine	5.0	LOW	26.9	*	*
Peridex/ Periogard	5.5	HIGH	11.6	*	*
Plax	*	LOW	7.0	5320	28.3
Scope	5.5	LOW	18.0	*	*
Viadent	4.5 (paste 5.2)	MODERATE	11.5	144	0.7

* Data not available.
Data adapted from Ciancio SG: Pharmacology of oral antimicrobials. In Academy of Periodontology: *Perspectives on oral antimicrobial therapeutics,* Littleton, Mass, 1987, PSG; Wagner MJ et al: Sodium retention in mouthwashes, *Journal of Clinical Preventive Dentistry* 11:21, 1989.

informed of alcohol content in commercial mouthrinses and guided to select alcohol-free mouthrinses.

Dental hygiene clinicians also need to consider the pH of the mouthrinse when making recommendations to clients (Table 24–2). A pH below 5 may demineralize exposed cementum. Clients with gingival recession, post-periodontal surgical cases, and those in periodontal maintenance therapy may benefit from a less acidic mouthrinse.

Some mouthrinses also contain sodium, which can result in sodium intake during rinsing.[8] Table 24–2 provides information on sodium content in various products. People on sodium-restricted diets (those with hypertension, congestive heart disease, fluid retention disorders, etc.) should be aware that some brands of mouthwash may be a significant source of sodium.

Some clients prepare their own mouthwashes at home. Ingredients frequently used include sodium chloride (salt), sodium bicarbonate (baking soda), and hydrogen peroxide. When clients prefer a homemade mouthrinse, the hygienist can recommend approximately 1/2 teaspoon of salt or baking soda per 8 ounces of water for a safe preparation. Hydrogen peroxide is diluted with water in equal parts and used two times a day to avoid the development of black hairy tongue.

Extensive short-term and long-term studies evaluating the use of baking soda and peroxide as adjuncts to home care have demonstrated no added value over mechanical oral hygiene alone. Further, chronic use of hydrogen peroxide may have numerous adverse effects (see the AAP position paper on baking soda and hydrogen peroxide use).[9] The routine unsupervised use of medicated mouthwashes is not recommended.

Therapeutic mouthwashes are available over-the-counter and by prescription for control of dental caries, bacterial plaque, and gingivitis. Several products have received the ADA Seal of Acceptance. Mouthrinses that have a beneficial effect on supragingival plaque and gingivitis are discussed within the section on chemotherapeutic agents. Fluoride-containing mouthrinses are discussed in Chapter 26. Mouthwashes do not have a therapeutic effect on subgingival periodontopathic microorganisms because they do not significantly penetrate subgingivally[10] (Table 24–3). Thus, there is currently no mouthrinse accepted by the ADA Council on Scientific Affairs for use in treatment of periodontitis.

Therapeutic mouthrinses for the control of bacterial plaque are recommended for use prior to and during professional oral care. Pretreatment rinsing can reduce the number of microorganisms in the oral cavity and thereby reduce the aerosol contamination occurring during professional care. Clients also appreciate the provision of a pleasant-tasting rinse after completion of professional care.

CHEMOTHERAPEUTIC AGENTS FOR CONTROL OF BACTERIAL PLAQUE AND GINGIVITIS

No linear relationship exists between quantity of bacterial plaque and extent of periodontal disease. Rather, the relationship between the presence of plaque biofilm and the threshold for disease is most likely dependent on the specific bacterial composition of plaque and systemic and environmental factors. A supplemental method for plaque control is to alter the bacterial composition of plaque biofilm in such a way that health cannot convert to disease. Use of antimicrobial agents as adjuncts to mechanical oral hygiene is promising for the prevention and control of periodontal diseases.[1] Figure 24–2 shows a variety of chemotherapeutic products available.

Published studies describe the value of antimicrobial agents such as chlorhexidine, stannous fluoride, essential oils, sanguinarine, cetylpyridinium chloride, and peroxides. Practitioners must be able to evaluate professional literature to determine which findings are valid. The ADA publishes guidelines for acceptance of chemotherapeutic products for the control of bacterial plaque and gingivitis.[3] Any product claiming therapeutic effect that has not been accepted by the ADA Council on Scientific Affairs either has not been submitted for consideration or has been found to be lacking in scientific evidence of therapeutic effectiveness, safety, or both.[1]

Consumers should be advised to look for the ADA Seal of Acceptance when purchasing products containing chemotherapeutic agents for the control of bacterial plaque and gingivitis. Use of chemotherapeutic agents

TABLE 24–3 COMPARISON OF LOCAL DRUG DELIVERY SYSTEMS

Delivery Systems	Site of Action	Adequate Concentration	Adequate Duration
Mouthrinse	Poor	Good	Poor
Subgingival irrigation	Good	Good	Poor
Systemic administration	Good	Fair	Fair
Sustained delivery	Good	Good	Good

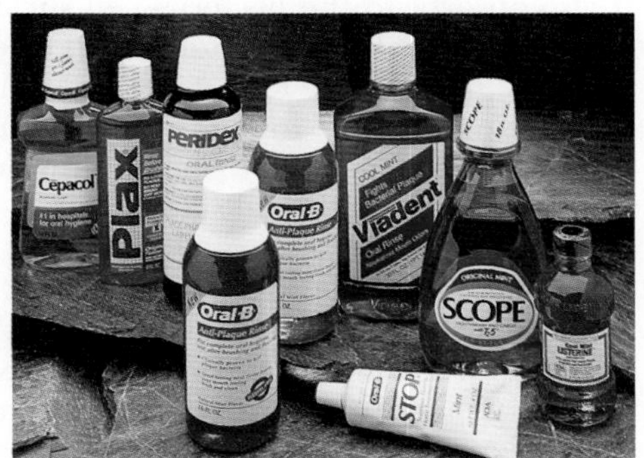

FIGURE 24–2 ✦ Various chemotherapeutic products available to consumers. *(Courtesy Oral-B Laboratories.)*

for the control of periodontitis is discussed later in the section on Controlled-Release Devices.

Evaluating Chemotherapeutic Agents for Control of Plaque and Gingivitis

ADA guidelines for acceptance of chemotherapeutic agents for the control of bacterial plaque and gingivitis specify criteria used by the Council on Scientific Affairs to evaluate product research. The guidelines do not pertain to evaluating agents for the management of periodontitis or other periodontal diseases.

A term that dental hygienists should understand when evaluating chemotherapeutic agents is *substantivity*. Substantivity is the ability of an active agent to be retained in the oral cavity and to continue to be released over an extended period of time without losing its potency. Oral antimicrobial rinses are divided into first-generation agents and second-generation agents. First-generation agents, such as essential oils, sanguinarine, cetylpyridinium chloride, and peroxides, have been available for some time as over-the-counter antibacterial rinses. They are antibacterial, but they have less substantivity than second-generation agents. Therefore, first-generation agents need to be used more frequently to obtain results.

Second-generation agents have antibacterial activity plus proven substantivity. Common second-generation agents include chlorhexidine (with high substantivity) and stannous fluoride (with moderate substantivity). Both of these agents require prescriptions for client use. All of the other agents currently available have lower substantivity and are available over-the-counter.

Chemotherapeutic Agents

CHLORHEXIDINE. *Chlorhexidine* is a bisbiguanide, first synthesized and used as a disinfectant for skin and mucous membranes. Currently, chlorhexidine is the most effective antiplaque and antigingivitis agent approved for clinical use. It has been shown to reduce plaque by 55% and gingivitis by 45%.[6,10] Mouthrinses containing 0.12% chlorhexidine (Peridex and Periogard) are ADA accepted and are available on a prescription basis for treatment of gingivitis; as shown in Table 24–2, the product has 11.6% alcohol and a pH of 5.5.[6,10] The mode of action of chlorhexidine is to bind to hydroxyapatite and glycoprotein to prevent pellicle formation. It also absorbs to the bacterial cell surface and may interfere with cell attachment. Chlorhexidine remains available in an active form for 8 to 12 hours in the mouth. Staining of teeth, tongue, and tooth colored restorations; a bitter taste; soft tissue ulcerations; and transient loss of taste are reported side effects.

Administration and Use. Chlorhexidine rinses are recommended for clients who have problems with plaque control; clients with plaque-induced gingivitis, extensive fixed prostheses, splinting, orthodontics, implants, or overdentures; clients undergoing nonsurgical periodontal therapy and clients in the immediate postperiodontal surgery period during the healing phase; and clients with impaired manual dexterity. Although chlorhexidine is not effective in improving periodontal parameters such as pocket depth and clinical attachment, it may enhance nonsurgical outcomes by controlling plaque and reducing the gingivitis superimposed on periodontal diseases.

It is recommended that the client rinse for 60 seconds with 1/2 ounce of chlorhexidine after brushing and flossing twice a day. Clients should be advised to allow at least 30 minutes between rinsing and toothbrushing because of interaction (and possible inactivation) between sodium lauryl sulfate, a common foaming ingredient in dentifrices, and chlorhexidine. Because chlorhexidine may temporarily affect the sensation of taste, it should be used after meals to minimize taste alteration and maximize compliance. Clients should not rinse with water immediately after it is used. Rinsing removes the flavor-masking agents from the oral cavity, making the medicinal taste worse. Practitioners should be cautious about recommending a chlorhexidine mouthrinse for clients with anterior facial restorations with rough or pitted areas because it may stain them permanently. It also is not recommended for children or recovering alcoholics because of its high alcohol content.

STANNOUS FLUORIDE. *Stannous fluoride* (SnF_2) has more antiplaque properties than sodium fluoride (NaF). Interestingly, it is the stannous ion, not the fluoride, that produces the antimicrobial effect. Tin from the stannous ion enters the cell, impairs the metabolism, and affects the growth and adherence properties of bacteria. Studies have demonstrated that 0.4% stannous fluoride gel reduces dental plaque, and some have also indicated a decrease in gingivitis and dentinal hypersensitivity.[11,12] Two large six-month clinical trials evaluated the potential benefits of a stabilized stannous fluoride dentifrice formulation. In both studies, gingival inflammation was reduced by approximately 20%. Surprisingly, corresponding decreases in plaque scores were not observed in either study.[13,14] Reductions in gingival inflammation may be due to the agent's ability to improve gingival health by reducing plaque virulence rather than by reducing plaque volume.[15] Additionally, the increased deposition of pellicle protein layer may affect the clinical assessment of plaque coverage.[16]

Extended use of a stannous fluoride dentifrice results in significantly more extrinsic tooth staining than with a sodium fluoride control dentifrice. Increased tooth staining and weak antiplaque activity significantly limit the potential application of stabilized stannous fluoride formulations. Several 0.4% stannous fluoride gels are also commercially available for caries prevention (e.g., Stop and Gel Kam). ADA acceptance on these products is for anticaries activity and safety; they have not been accepted for reductions in plaque and gingivitis.

Administration and Use. Clients should be instructed to brush with the prescribed gel or dentifrice twice daily. Recommendation for client use of a stannous fluoride product may be warranted for individuals who cannot utilize chlorhexidine, such as teens and recovering alcoholics. It may also be the product of choice for individuals with dentinal hypersensitivity.

PHENOLIC COMPOUNDS (ESSENTIAL OILS). Triclosan and a combination of essential oils are two distinct types of *phenolic compounds* with antimicrobial properties. Triclosan is a noncationic, chlorinated phenol first used as a disinfectant in hand and body soaps and underarm deodorants. The commercially available toothpaste formulation (Total) delivers 0.3% triclosan via a 2.0% copolymer of polyvinyl ether that increases triclosan substantivity, and 0.243% sodium fluoride in a silica base. Triclosan and copolymer dentifrice reduces plaque by 12% to 59% and gingivitis by 20% to 30%.[17–20] Anticaries efficacy of this triclosan/copolymer system is comparable to that achieved by a conventional fluoride dentifrice.[21,22] The dual mechanism of triclosan combines bactericidal activity with bacterial enzyme inhibition. No tooth staining or increased calculus formation can be expected.

Essential oil mouthrinses (Listerine) are a mixture of three phenolic-derived essential oils— thymol, menthol, and eucalyptol—combined with methylsalicylate. The original Listerine formula contains 26.9% alcohol (Table 24–2). Listerine has received the ADA Seal of Acceptance as an effective agent for reduction of bacterial plaque and gingivitis. Mechanism of action appears to be related to alteration of the bacterial cell wall. This product has low substantivity and is safe when used as directed. Adverse effects reported have been a burning sensation, bitter taste, and a possible staining of teeth. Twice daily usage without concern for dentifrice interactions favors compliance. Long-term studies evaluating the clinical effects of Listerine mouthrinse indicate that bacterial plaque can be reduced by 25% to 28% and gingivitis can be reduced by an average of 30% compared to baseline levels.[23,24] Listerine dentifrice is also available over-the-counter but does not demonstrate antiplaque or antigingivitis properties.

Administration and Use. Essential oil rinses and toothpaste with triclosan are recommended for clients who have problems with plaque control; clients with extensive fixed prostheses, splinting, orthodontics, implants, or overdentures; and clients with impaired manual dexterity. Although essential oils are not effective in reducing periodontal parameters such as pocket depth and clinical attachment, they may enhance nonsurgical outcomes by controlling plaque and reducing the gingivitis superimposed on periodontitis.

It is recommended that the client rinse for 30 seconds with 1/2 ounce of Listerine after brushing and flossing twice a day. Due to the relatively high alcohol content, it should not be recommended for persons with xerostomia, children, recovering alcoholics, or persons on medications that interact with alcohol. All clients should be informed of the potential drying effects that may accompany use of a high-alcohol mouthrinse.

SANGUINARINE. *Sanguinarine,* a benzophenathridine alkaloid, is an alcohol extract from the root of the plant *Sanguinaria canadensis.* This antiplaque substance is currently available in over-the-counter mouthrinse and dentifrice products (Viadent) (Table 24–2). The activity of sanguinarine is attributed to its ability to interfere with bacterial glycolysis and bind to plaque to prevent adherence of microorganisms. Sanguinarine is retained for about two to four hours in the mouth. Sanguinarine is less effective than chlorhexidine, and no side effects are observed.[24] Short-term clinical studies employing various experimental conditions suggest that sanguinarine reduces bacterial plaque and gingivitis somewhat; however, a consistent degree of efficacy has not been documented. Effectiveness is enhanced when both the mouthrinse and the dentifrice are used.[25–27] Due to inconsistent efficacy, professional recommendations of *Sanguinaria* products for the reduction of plaque and gingivitis as part of a self-care program are not warranted.

QUATERNARY AMMONIUM COMPOUNDS. *Quaternary ammonium compounds* have been evaluated in a number of short-term studies relative to their effect on plaque and gingivitis. In these studies, an average plaque reduction of 35% less than baseline scores has been reported with mixed effect on gingival health.[10] Cepacol and Scope are two well-known representatives of this group with concentrations of 0.05% and 0.045% cetylpyridinium chloride (CPC), respectively. Mechanism of action is related to increased bacterial cell wall permeability that favors lysis, decreased cell metabolism, and a decreased ability for bacteria to attach to tooth surfaces. These agents are categorized as cationic, which favors their attraction to tooth surfaces and bacterial plaque. They alter surface tension and have a low substantivity and a high safety factor.[16] Given their inconsistent efficacy, professional recommendations of products containing quaternary ammonium compounds for the reduction of plaque and gingivitis as part of a self-care program are not warranted.

PREBRUSHING MOUTHRINSES. Plax is a *prebrushing mouthrinse* containing sodium benzoate, other nontoxic surfactants (Table 24–2), and 7.5% alcohol. Short-term studies have shown some reductions in bacterial plaque; however, some investigations not supported by the manufacturer have shown no effect on plaque reduction when compared to a placebo.[1] Reductions in gingivitis have not been documented. Proof of clinical efficacy of this product awaits long-term studies that include comparisons with normal toothbrushing and measures of periodontal disease. Safety is not a concern. Sodium content contraindicates use for clients on sodium-restricted diets (Table 24–2). Evidence does not support its use in any self-care program.

OXYGENATING AGENTS. Several products containing *oxygenating agents* are available on the market (e.g., Amosan, Gly-Oxide). The American Academy of Periodontology[13] has published a review of oxygenating agents. Long-term studies have shown no beneficial effects on reductions in bacterial plaque and gingivitis when compared to controls. Safety is an issue with hydrogen peroxide. Chronic use of hydrogen peroxide causes serious side effects including carcinogenesis, tissue damage, hyperkeratosis, oral ulcerations, hyperplasia, and black hairy tongue syndrome.[9] Short-term use of oxygenating oral rinses is intended for oral wound cleansing. A soothing effect has been reported. Evidence does not support their use in any self-care program.

OXIDIZING AGENTS. Chlorine dioxide, an *oxidizing agent,* is available in mouthrinse and toothpaste formulations (e.g., Oxyfresh, Clo-Syst II, Enfresh). The proposed mechanism of action is neutralization of volatile sulfur compounds that contribute to bad breath. Product claims are primarily cosmetic (i.e., the elimination of bad breath). To date, there is no evidence to support the use of these products for the reduction of plaque and gingivitis. Evidence does not support their therapeutic use as part of any self-care program.

CHEMOTHERAPY AND SELF-APPLIED ORAL IRRIGATION*

The purpose of self-applied irrigation is to nonspecifically reduce the bacteria and their by-products that lead to the initiation or progression of periodontal diseases. Powered irrigation devices (e.g, Waterpik Oral Cleaning System) designed to deliver a *pulsating* stream of fluid with controlled variable pressure have been shown to be the most effective.[28]

Irrigation can reduce gingivitis, bleeding, pocket depth, and pathogenic microorganisms.[28] Studies have shown that daily water irrigation can modulate chemical mediators that promote or enhance the disease process. Reductions in proinflammatory mediators, interleukin-1 (IL-1) and prostaglandin E2 (PGE2), concurrent with an increase in the antiinflammatory mediator IL-10 have been shown.[29,30] These improvements to the inflammatory response may potentially extend to systemic health as documented by a study on persons with diabetes, in which systemic measures of inflammatory mediators and reactive oxygen species were better reduced by the addition of oral irrigation to the self-care routine.[30]

The penetration of an irrigant is dependent on tip design and pocket depth. Standard jet tips placed at the gingival margin can penetrate 44% to 71% of the pocket depth.[31] Specialized tips (e.g., Pik Pocket subgingival irrigation tip) designed to be placed below the gingival margin can penetrate up to 90% of a 6-mm pocket and 64% if the pocket is 7 mm or greater.[32] Use of a cannula, or needlelike tip, can provide 70% to 80% penetration to the depth of a 4- to 6-mm pocket. However it is highly dependent on the client's dexterity.

Powered oral irrigation devices are an ideal delivery method for antimicrobial agents or water because mouth rinsing has a limited ability to penetrate subgingivally.[32] Comparisons between antimicrobial rinsing and water irrigation have shown equivalent reductions in gingivitis. The use of water reduces the cost and side effects that may influence compliance. In addition, some agents can be diluted and are still effective when delivered with an oral irrigator.

Most periodontal maintenance clients will benefit from the addition of oral irrigation to their self-care routines. Conclusions about self-applied irrigation are as follows:

- Water irrigation has a positive effect on some clinical and microbial parameters. The addition of a chemical agent may further improve the outcomes.
- Irrigation can modulate the host response by the reduction of key proinflammatory mediators.
- Irrigaion is a preventive and therapeutic self-care procedure. It is not intended to treat active periodontitis.
- Not all irrigators are equivalent regarding pulsation and pressure.

Each product should be evaluated individually on its body of evidence. Irrigation-induced bacteremia is a concern for persons susceptible to infective endocarditis. The prevalence of bacteremia following irrigation ranges from 7% to 50%.[33,34] This range of occurrence is not greater than that associated with bacteremia observed following toothbrushing and flossing. As a precautionary measure, the use of irrigation in persons susceptible to infective endocarditis is contraindicated during periods of active treatment of gingivitis or periodontitis.

*Self-Applied Oral Irrigation Technique**

After turning on the unit, the client should:

- Adjust the pressure setting. Begin on lowest setting and increase as comfort permits or as instructed by the dental hygienist.
- Place the jet tip at the gingival margin at a 90-degree angle to the long axis of the tooth. If using a subgingival tip, place the tip at or below the gingival margin according to manufacturer's instructions at a 45-degree angle to the tooth (Figure 24–3).
- Move the tip around the mouth in sequence until all areas needing irrigation are treated.
- Be sure to read all manufacturer's instructions before using.

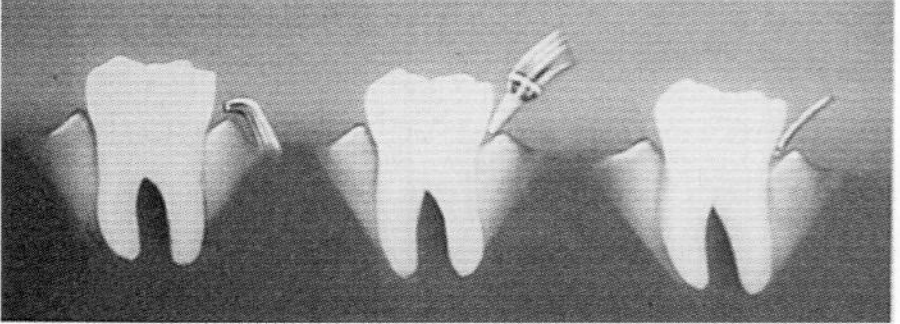

FIGURE 24–3 ✦ Oral irrigation tips and placement. *(Courtesy Waterpik Technologies.)*

* Section contributed by Deborah Lyle, RDH, MS, Manager of Professional Marketing and Education, Waterpik Technologies.

With proper instruction, oral irrigation can be successfully accomplished by most clients. Oral irrigation as an addition to regular oral hygiene has been clinically proven to benefit clients with gingivitis, orthodontic and prosthodontic appliances, implants, and diabetes and for those on periodontal maintenance. Evidence supports the inclusion of oral irrigation in self-care programs.

Professionally Applied Subgingival Irrigation

Subgingival irrigation with antimicrobials such as chlorhexidine, tetracycline, stannous fluoride, oxygenating agents, and others is another therapeutic application. Devices have been developed for in-office use by professionals as well as for home use by clients. When performed professionally by the hygienist, subgingival irrigation takes valuable chair time, is performed only infrequently, and has produced questionable results. Although professionally applied irrigants may reach the base of the periodontal pocket they cannot be retained for sufficient duration, due in part to rapid gingival crevicular fluid (GCF) clearance rates. Professional subgingival irrigation performed in conjunction with root planing has no demonstrated advantage over root planing alone.[35–37]

CHEMOTHERAPEUTIC AGENTS FOR CONTROL OF PERIODONTITIS

Evaluating Chemotherapeutic Agents to Control Periodontitis

Thus far the use of locally delivered antimicrobial agents has focused on control of plaque and gingivitis. Use of dentrifices, mouthrinses, and irrigation for the treatment of periodontitis is impaired by the inability of these delivery systems to reach the base of periodontal pockets and/or maintain agents for sufficient duration at requisite concentrations.[38] GCF is replaced about every 90 seconds, thus rapidly reducing the concentration of any antimicrobial agent placed subgingivally. Commonly used local delivery systems for improving periodontal health are compared in Table 24–3.

Chemotherapeutic Agents: Antibiotics

As clinical attachment loss develops and progresses, traditional therapies such as toothbrushing, flossing, mouthrinsing, irrigation and even professional mechanical debridement lose effectiveness, making the adjunctive use of antimicrobial agents in periodontal pockets desirable. The only clinically efficacious means of administering antimicrobial agents for the treatment of periodontal disease(s) are systemic administration and controlled-release devices.

SYSTEMIC ADMINISTRATION. *Systemic administration* of antibiotics is successful for treatment of periodontitis because doxycycline, penicillins, metronidazole, and clindamycin used singularly or in combination are all effective against anaerobic periodontal pathogens. Efficacy of systemic administration of antibiotic as an adjunct to scaling and root planing is presented in Table 24–4.[39–41] Systemic administration provides a successful means of delivering antibiotics to periodontal pockets, but it is also associated with many contraindications, precautions, and side effects. Systemic administration provides an adequate means to maintain sufficient duration in the pocket

TABLE 24–4 REDUCTION IN PROBING DEPTH (PD) AND GAIN OF CLINICAL ATTACHMENT (CAL) AFTER THERAPY WITH VARIOUS TREATMENT METHODS (RESULTS IN MM)

Reference	PD Reduction (CAL) Initial PD 4–6 mm	PD Reduction (CAL) Initial PD ≥7 mm
Root Planing Studies		
Ramford et al, 1987	1.08 (–0.32)	2.92 (0.69)
Hill et al, 1981	1.16 (–0.10)	2.76 (0.47)
Hammerle et al, 1991	1.03 (0.69)	2.28 (1.52)
Pihlstrom et al, 1981	0.71 (0.41)	1.21 (1.07)
Root Planing Plus Systemic Antibiotics		
Loesche et al, 1992	1.72 (0.79)	2.83 (1.69)
Loesche et al, 1991	0.75 (0.40)	1.91 (0.86)
Magnusson et al, 1989	2.50 (2.0)	
Root Planing Plus Local Drug Delivery		
Newman et al, 1994 (tetracycline fibers)	1.81 (1.56)	
Drisko et al, 1995 (tetracycline fibers)	1.0 (1.1)	2.1 (1.2)
Jeffcoat et al, 1998 (chlorhexidine chip)	0.95 (0.75)	
Soskolne et al, 1997 (chlorhexidine chip)	1.16	1.77
Williams et al, 2001 (minocycline microspheres)	1.31	1.99

Modified from Greenstein G, Polson A: The role of local drug delivery in the management of periodontal diseases: A comprehensive review, *Journal of Periodontology* 69:507, 1998.

only if the client takes and finishes the prescription as directed. This is a major concern, because most clients fail to follow prescriptions. Furthermore, the routine use of antibiotics to treat periodontal diseases is not recommended due to universal concerns regarding the development of antibiotic-resistant organisms. The AAP recommends the use of systemic antibiotics be reserved for clients exhibiting continued loss of attachment after diligent mechanical therapy and clients with forms of the disease recognized for increased risk for periodontal breakdown such as aggressive periodontitis. Persons with acute or severe periodontal infections (e.g., periodontal abscess, necrotizing periodontal diseases) may also benefit from systemic antibiotic therapy.[42]

CONTROLLED-RELEASE DEVICE ADMINISTRATION. *Intracrevicular delivery devices* consist of a drug reservoir that controls the rate of drug release. Such devices provide a means of administering antimicrobial agents directly into the periodontal pocket without the side effects associated with systemic drug administration. In contrast to systemic drug administration, intracrevicular delivery results in GCF levels 1000 times the concentration of antibiotic at the diseased site, but only one-hundredth of the systemic dose in the rest of the body.[43] *Controlled drug delivery* refers to those intracrevicular devices that provide drug delivery for longer than one day.[44,45] *Sustained-release devices* consist of formulations designed to provide drug delivery for less than 24 hours.

Characteristics of the delivery vehicle such as *biodegradability* and *bioresorbtion* may impact the efficacy, cost-effectiveness, and ease of product use. Delivery systems with regulatory approval or pending approval by the FDA or the regulatory bodies of the European Union include tetracycline fibers, chlorhexidine chips, doxycycline hyclate gel, minocycline microspheres, metronidazole gel, and minocycline gel. The American Academy of Periodontology recommends the use of these products as adjuncts to mechanical therapy in localized persistent pockets of depths greater than or equal to 5 mm that do not respond to conventional therapy.[46] Contraindications and precautions for all commercially available controlled-release devices are presented in Table 24–5.

Tetracycline Fiber. The first controlled-release device approved for use in the United States for the treatment of periodontal disease was tetracycline fiber (Actisite). The delivery system consists of a flexible 23 cm long by 0.5 mm diameter ethylene vinyl acetate fiber vehicle containing 12.7 mg of tetracycline (Figure 24–4).

Clinical Efficacy. Pharmacokinetic studies report controlled drug delivery of 1590 μg/ml of tetracycline for up to 14 days.[47] Intercrevicular concentrations far exceeded those achieved by systemic tetracycline administration and exceeded the minimum inhibitory concentration of tetracycline. Although tetracycline fibers demonstrated clinical efficacy both as an adjunct and alternative to scaling and root planing therapy, placement was an arduous task, and retention and removal of the fiber were required.[48–50] Tetracycline fibers are no longer

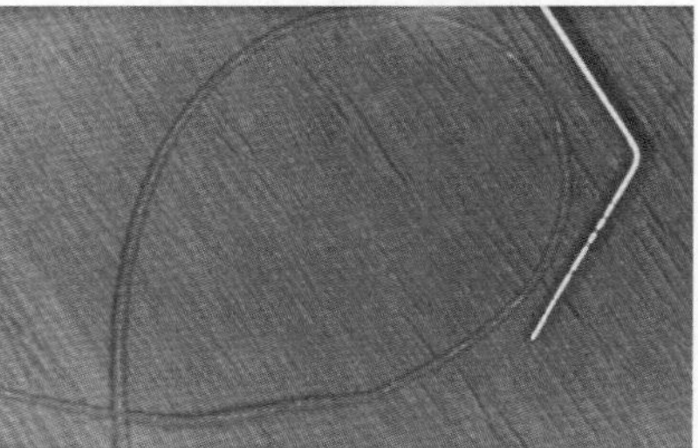

FIGURE 24–4 ✦ Comparing the dimensions of the tetracycline fiber to a periodontal probe.

TABLE 24–5 CONTRAINDICATIONS AND PRECAUTIONS FOR CONTROLLED-RELEASE DEVICES AVAILABLE IN THE UNITED STATES

Contraindications	Precautions*	Product
Allergy to chlorhexidine		PerioChip
Allergy to tetracyclines		Atridox, Arestin, Actisite
	Pregnancy/Nursing	PerioChip (Category C), Atridox (Category D), Arestin (Category D), Actisite (Category D)
	Pediatrics	None have been tested for use in children
	Overgrowth of nonsusceptible organisms	Atridox, Arestin, Actisite
	Oral candidiasis	Atridox, Arestin, Actisite
	Photosensitivity	Atridox, Actisite
	Use during tooth development	Atridox, Arestin, Actisite
	May decrease effectiveness of birth control pills	Atridox, Actisite

* The term *precautions* generally means that the product has not been tested with populations that present with these conditions; therefore, very little is known about the effects of the product on these individuals. In clinical decision making, precautions are typically treated as contraindications.

being manufactured or used in the United States; they are used in other countries.

Administration and Use. See Procedure 24–1 and Figure 24–5.

Contraindications and Precautions. The only absolute contraindication to the placement of tetracycline fiber is allergy to tetracycline.

Chlorhexidine Chip. The chlorhexidine chip (PerioChip), 0.35 mm thick and 4 × 5 mm in dimension, combines a biodegradable hydrolyzed gelatin chip delivery system with 2.5 mg chlorhexidine (Figure 24–7). The biodegradable chip releases and maintains an average GCF concentration of 125 μg/ml chlorhexidine over a 7- to 10-day period. In vitro testing reveals that this concentration inhibits 99% of subgingival bacteria.[51] Suppression of

Procedure 24–1 PLACEMENT OF TETRACYCLINE FIBER CONTROLLED-RELEASE DEVICE

EQUIPMENT

Mouth mirror, periodontal probe, cotton pliers, cord packing instrument, scaler(s), scissors

STEP	RATIONALE
1. Determine need for controlled-release tetracycline therapy. Tetracycline fiber is indicated for reduction of pocket depth in sites ≥ 5 mm not responding to mechanical therapy alone in persons with chronic periodontitis.	Prevents indiscriminate use of an antibiotic and development of antibiotic-resistant microorganisms.
2. Evaluate contraindications and precautions to treatment.	Ensures quality of care and manages legal risks.
3. Explain risks/benefits and alternative to treatment. Obtain informed consent.	Encourages active decision making by the client and manages legal risks.
4. Remove fiber from foil package prior to use. Precut fiber into 3- to 5-inch segments if desired.	Facilitates organization and placement.
5. Insert fiber subgingivally into pocket using a cord packing instrument. Fill entire pocket by overlapping (layering) fiber over itself.	Fiber must be present in the pocket to produce therapeutic effect.

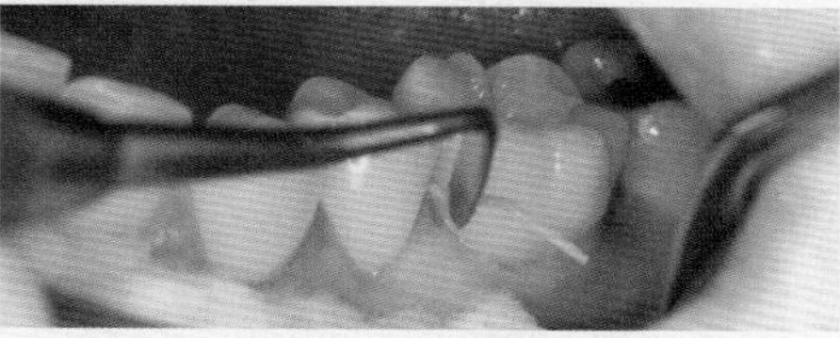

FIGURE 24–5 ✦ Subgingival placement of tetracycline fiber.

STEP	RATIONALE
6. Secure fiber in pocket with cyanoacrylate tissue adhesive. Replace any fiber lost before day 7.	Provides fiber retention. Fiber replacement ensures a therapeutic effect.

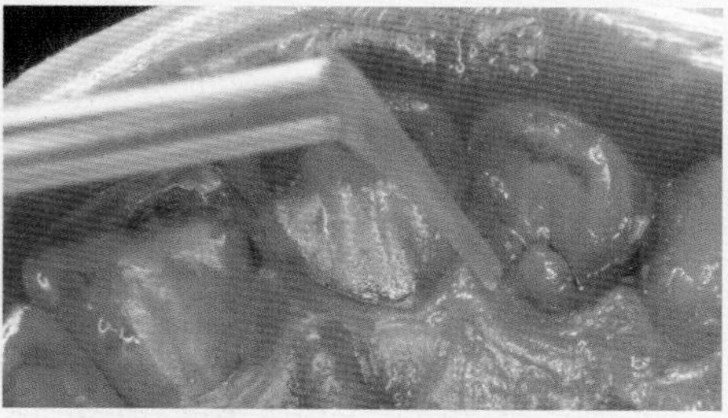

FIGURE 24–6 ✦ Application of cyanoacrylate adhesive to retain tetracycline fiber in periodontal pocket.

STEP	RATIONALE
7. Instruct client not to brush or floss area for 10 days.	Brushing or flossing may prematurely dislodge the fiber.
8. Remove fiber after 10 days with cotton pliers.	Fiber is not bioresorbable. Time required for a therapeutic effect.
9. Schedule reevaluation and/or reapplication. Can coincide with 3-month maintenance visits.	Host response to therapy must be observed and documented.
10. Document in client's record under service rendered and date the entry. For example, "Tetracycline fiber placed in the sites not responding to mechanical debridement alone for the reduction of pocket depths: #2M, #3D, #30 M,D, #31D. Cyanoacrylate adhesive placed for retention at each site. Client instructed not to brush or floss the area for 10 days and to report any loss of fiber before day 7 to the office."	Ensures integrity of client's record for both client's health and legal protection of practitioner.

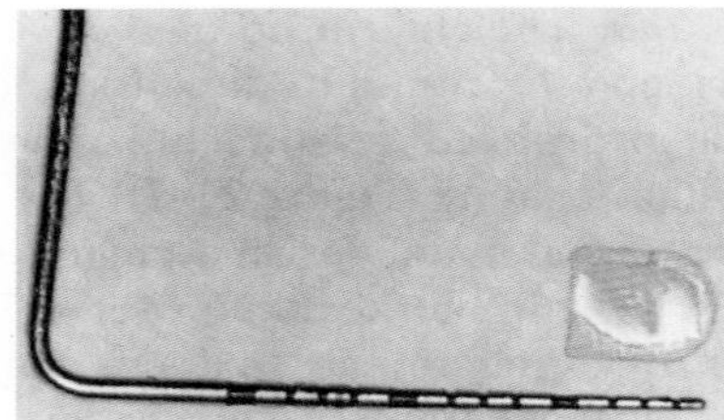

FIGURE 24–7 ✦ Comparing the dimensions of the chlorhexidine chip to a periodontal probe.

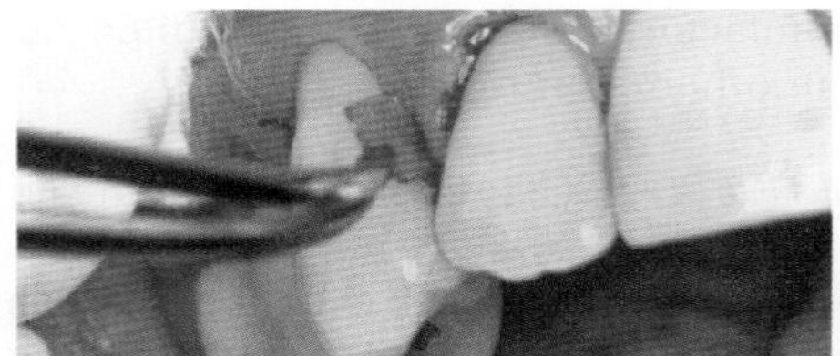

FIGURE 24–8 ✦ Subgingival application of chlorhexidine chip.

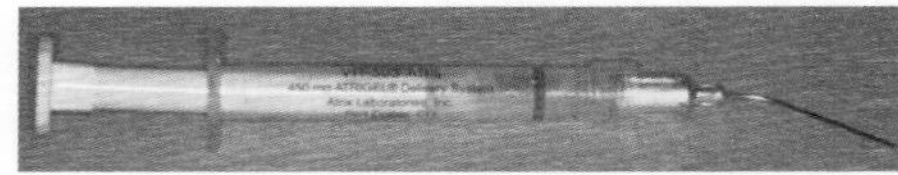

FIGURE 24–9 ✦ Doxycycline gel controlled release product.

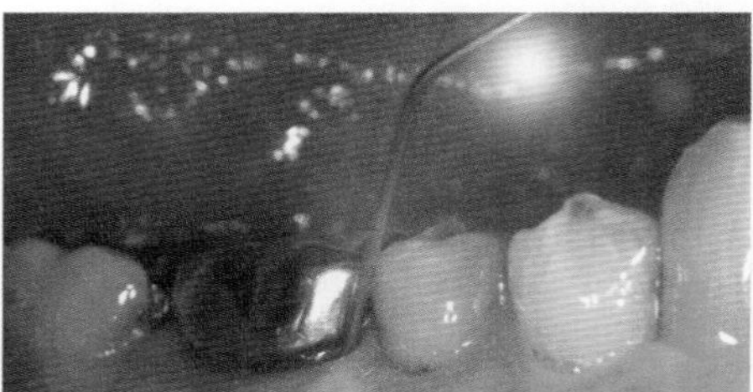

FIGURE 24–10 ✦ Subgingival application of doxycycline gel.

subgingival bacterial flora is evident up to 11 weeks following administration. [52]

Clinical Efficacy. Trials on chlorhexidine chip as an adjunct to scaling and root planing found improved pocket depths compared to scaling and root planing alone (Table 24–4).[53,54] The scaling and root planing plus chlorhexidine chip group showed statistically significant reductions in probing depths at six and nine months compared to both the scaling and root planing plus placebo and scaling and root planing alone. Mean pocket depth reduction at nine months in the scaling and root planing with chlorhexidine chip group was 0.95 mm compared to 0.69 mm in the scaling and root planing with placebo and 0.65 mm in the scaling and root planing alone group. Additionally, the proportion of patients exhibiting a pocket depth reduction greater than or equal to 2 mm was significantly greater in subjects receiving combined scaling and root planing plus chlorhexidine chip therapy.

As determined by digital subtraction radiology, the percentage of sites exhibiting alveolar bone loss in one or more sites was 15% in sites receiving scaling and root planing alone compared to 11% in sites receiving scaling and root planing plus placebo chip therapy. Comparatively, when chlorhexidine chip therapy was used as an adjunct to scaling and root planing, no sites exhibited bone loss.[55] These data suggest that scaling and root planing combined with chlorhexidine chip use at three-month intervals may be an effective therapy for maintaining alveolar bone.

Administration and Use. The amber-colored chip is rounded at one end to facilitate placement into the pocket. Each chip is packaged in an individual foil bubble pack and must be refrigerated upon delivery. Placement of the chlorhexidine chip is presented in Procedure 24–2 and Figure 24–8. Non-serrated pliers are recommended to prevent sticking. Once exposed to GCF, the chip is self-retentive and resorbs over a 7- to 10-day period, eliminating need for removal. Recent reformulation of the product no longer requires that the chip be refrigerated or chilled for successful manipulation or placement. Chips should not be cut; however, if the pocket dimensions prohibit placement of a whole chip, all cut portions should be used in the designated site. Further, it may be helpful in some sites to roll the chip into a cylindrical shape resembling a cigar prior to placement. No retention stent is necessary. One chip per pocket site is used. If a pocket ≥ 5 mm is present on the mesial-buccal and distal-buccal, only one chip is necessary in this site. Manufacturers' directions indicate maximum dosage of eight chips per visit. Patients should be instructed not to floss at the chip placement site for ten days. Reevaluation is crucial and can be conveniently scheduled to coincide with the next supportive periodontal therapy visit because retrieval of the delivery vehicle is unnecessary.

Contraindications and Precautions. The only absolute contraindication to the placement of chlorhexidine chips is the rare allergy to chlorhexidine.

Doxycycline Gel. Doxycycline gel consists of 10% doxycycline hyclate in a flowable polymer delivery system that solidifies on contact with moisture to provide controlled release of doxycycline for seven to ten days (Atridox) (Figures 24–9 and 24–10). Doxycycline hyclate reaches GCF concentrations of over 1200 mg/ml, and is released at the minimum inhibitory concentration (MIC) for most periodontal pathogens for seven to eight days.[56]

Clinical Efficacy. When doxycycline gel was compared to scaling and root planing, a vehicle control, and oral hygiene only, doxycycline gel reduced probing pocket depth, increased clinical attachment levels, and reduced bleeding on probing similar in magnitude to the improvement achieved by scaling and root planing.[57] Both doxycycline gel and scaling and root planing groups

Procedure 24–2 PLACEMENT OF CHLORHEXIDINE CHIP CONTROLLED-RELEASE DEVICE

EQUIPMENT

Mouth mirror, periodontal probe, cotton pliers, scaler(s)

STEP	RATIONALE
1. Determine need for controlled-release chlorhexidine therapy. Chlorhexidine chip is indicated for the reduction of pocket depth in sites ≥ 5 mm not responding to mechanical therapy alone in persons with chronic periodontitis.	Prevents indiscriminate use of a chemotherapeutic agent.
2. Evaluate contraindications and precautions to treatment.	Ensures quality of care and manages legal risks.
3. Explain the risks/benefits and alternative to treatment. Obtain informed consent.	Encourages active decision making by the client and manages legal risks.
4. Remove required number of chips from package prior to application.	Product no longer requires storage in refrigerator or refrigeration prior to placement.
5. Grasp flat end with cotton pliers and insert subgingivally.	Rounded end is for subgingival anatomy.
6. Use cotton pliers or an instrument of choice to advance chip into pocket.	Chip is bioresorbable and self-retentive in pocket.
7. Instruct client not to floss area for 10 days.	Flossing may prematurely dislodge the chip. Time required for the therapeutic effect.
8. Schedule reevaluation and/or reapplication. Reevaluation can coincide with 3-month maintenance visits.	Host response to therapy must be observed and documented. Maximum benefit is attained after 3 consecutive administrations at 3-month Intervals over a 9-month period.
9. Document in client's record under service rendered and date the entry. For example, "Chlorhexidine chip placed in sites not responding to mechanical debridement alone for the reduction of pocket depths: #2M, #3D, #30 M,D, #31D. Client instructed not to brush or floss the area for 10 days and to report any loss of chip to the office."	Ensures integrity of client's record for both the client's health and legal protection of practitioner.

reported a maximum mean gain in clinical attachment level (CAL) of 0.8 mm and 1.3 mm for PPD reduction. About 29% to 31% of subjects in the doxycycline gel group and 31% to 34% of the scaling and root planing group had attachment level gains of ≥ 2 mm at nine months. Periodontal probing depths were reduced similarly, with 31% to 41% of sites reduced by ≥ 2 mm for the doxycycline gel groups and 31% to 43% in the scaling and root planing groups. However, concluding that doxycycline gel improved and maintained periodontal health at a level comparable to scaling and root planing should be made with caution because all subjects had previously received scaling and root planing and were currently undergoing periodontal maintenance care. The decision to use an intracrevicular delivery device as a monotherapy, in the absence of mechanical debridement during any phase of periodontal therapy, remains controversial.

Smokers. Tangible benefits of doxycycline gel therapy extend beyond the local antimicrobial effects in the periodontal pocket. Evidence confirms the adverse effects of smoking on periodontal therapies such as scaling and root planing, flap surgery, guided tissue regeneration, mucogingival surgery, and dental implants. So compelling are the deleterious effects of smoking on periodontal healing that many clinicians forego surgery, placing many smokers in compromised maintenance therapy with few options. Contrary to other periodontal outcomes, research found that although former and current smokers receiving scaling and root planing experienced predictably less-favorable pocket depth reductions and attachment gains, those treated with doxycycline hyclate therapy exhibited pocket depth reductions and gains in clinical attachment equivalent to nonsmokers.[58]

Administration and Use. The flowable delivery vehicle allows the drug to reach and conform to the unique topography of each pocket upon application. Gel solidifies to a wax-like consistency on contact with moisture, such as GCF or blood, assuring its retention in the pocket. Doxycycline gel polymer is both biodegradable and bioresorbable, thus its removal is not necessary.

Application of doxycycline gel requires notable preparation before use. If desired, product can be prepared in advance and stored at room temperature for up to three days. Steps for placement of doxycycline gel are presented in Procedure 24–3. Problems associated with sticking are typically most pronounced during the first couple of applications and generally improve with experience. The setting reaction is triggered by contact of the gel with moisture. The tip of the cannula may become obstructed with solidified material, but the remainder of the gel in the syringe is still flowable, allowing the clinician time to wipe the cannula clean and move gradually to the next site/tooth. The product should remain in the pocket for seven days; however, loss as early as three days after placement shows no diminished effectiveness.

Procedure 24–3 PLACEMENT OF DOXYCYCLINE GEL CONTROLLED-RELEASE DEVICE

EQUIPMENT

Mouth mirror, periodontal probe, scaler(s) or cord packer instrument, lubricant

STEP	RATIONALE
1. Determine the need for controlled-release doxycycline therapy. Indicated for the reduction of pocket depth and gains in clinical attachment in sites ≥ 5 mm not responding to mechanical therapy alone in persons with chronic periodontitis.	Prevents indiscriminate use of an antibiotic and development of antibiotic-resistant microorganisms.
2. Evaluate contraindications and precautions to treatment.	Ensures quality of care and manages legal risks.
3. Explain risks/benefits and alternative to treatment. Obtain informed consent.	Encourages active decision making by the client and manages legal risks.
4. Remove required number of packages from refrigerator 15 minutes prior to use. Each package contains enough material to treat 3–4 teeth.	Product requires storage in refrigeration at 36–46° F.
5. To mix, couple syringe A with syringe B by removing and discarding the white syringe caps. Lock open ends of both syringes together by twisting together until they lock.	Ensures a sealed container for the mix.
6. Mix by holding the coupled syringes together horizontally in both hands. Inject liquid contents of syringe A (purple stripe) into syringe B (yellow powder) and then push the contents back into syringe A again. This constitutes one mixing cycle and should be repeated for one and a half to two minutes for 100 cycles. Finish with contents in syringe A by holding the coupled syringes vertically with syringe A at the bottom. Pull back on syringe A plunger and allow gel to flow down barrel.	Ensures adequate mixing of ingredients.
7. Uncouple syringes and attach enclosed cannula to syringe A by twisting in place. Cannula can be bent at desired angle to resemble a periodontal probe. Product is now ready to use. If product is mixed in advance, refresh mixture with 10 mixing cycles before uncoupling the syringes.	Product can be prepared in advance and stored at room temperature for up to three days.
8. Insert tip of cannula near base of pocket; express gel into pocket while slowly withdrawing tip coronally until material can be seen at gingival margin. Gel will begin setting reaction immediately upon contact with pocket. Separate tip from newly placed material by using a twisting motion or cut material by pushing cannula tip against tooth surface.	Increases likelihood of 100% coverage.
9. Wipe excess material protruding from pocket with a wet cotton swab or pack into pocket and interproximal embrasures with back surface of a curet or cord packer instruments. Use water or lubricant to prevent sticking.	Removal of excess material increases longevity of the material within the pocket.
10. Secure gel in pocket by applying cyanoacrylate tissue adhesive or noneugenol type periodontal dressing.	Provides retention. Gel must be present in the pocket to produce therapeutic effect.
11. Remove retention after 10 days of therapy with cotton pliers.	Removal increases client comfort. Gel is bioresorbable.
12. Instruct client not to brush or floss area for 10 days	Brushing or flossing may prematurely dislodge retention and/or the gel.
13. Schedule reevaluation and/or reapplication. Reevaluation can coincide with 3-month maintenance visits.	Host response to therapy must be observed and documented.
14. Document in client record under service rendered and date the entry. For example, "Doxycycline gel placed in sites not responding to mechanical debridement alone for the reduction of pocket depths: #2M, #3D, #30 M, D, #31D. Cyanoacrylate adhesive placed for retention at each site. Client instructed not to brush or floss the area for 10 days and to report any loss of gel to the office."	Ensures integrity of client's record for both quality care and legal protection of practitioner.

Contraindication and Precautions. The only absolute contraindication to the administration of doxycycline gel is known sensitivity to tetracyclines. Clinicians should be aware that despite the local administration of doxycycline, the product label carries the same precautions for systemic tetracycline use. Precautions are presented in Table 24–5. The product insert lists all contraindications and precautions for the product and should be thoroughly read to assure the standard of care.

Minocycline Microspheres. The minocycline microsphere (Arestin) is a bioresorbable, controlled-delivery device containing 1 mg minocycline in a poly(glycolide-co-dilactide) (PGLA) polymer. The microsphere powder is packaged in a unit dose dispenser, which is inserted into a dispenser handle for subgingival administration (Figure 24–11). The microsphere polymer vehicle is self-retentive in the pocket.

Minocycline concentrations in GCF following application yield a pattern ranging from 66,000 mg/ml at one hour to 340 μg/ml at 14 days.[59] When multiple sites are treated simultaneously with minocycline microspheres, serum levels of minocycline remain below levels expected from a comparable oral dose.[60] High salivary levels of minocycline were maintained after 14 days. Suppression of putative pathogens was maintained for one month following minocycline PTS alone or in combination with scaling and root planing.[61,62]

Clinical Efficacy. Clinical trials found that treatment of all periodontal pockets ≥ 5 mm with minocycline microspheres as an adjunct to scaling and root planing improved pocket depths compared to scaling and root planing alone.[63] At three and six months, minocycline microspheres or the vehicle control were reapplied according to group assignment. After one month of treatment, the scaling and root planing plus minocycline microspheres group showed statistically significant reductions in probing depths, maintained for nine months, compared to both scaling and root planing plus placebo and scaling and root planing alone. Mean pocket depth reduction at nine months in the scaling and root planing plus minocycline microspheres group was 1.32 mm, compared to 1.0 mm in the scaling and root planing plus placebo and 1.08 mm in the scaling and root planing alone group. The greatest pocket depth reductions were achieved in sites with advanced disease (pocket depths ≥ 7 mm). The mean proportion of sites per patients exhibiting a pocket depth reduction greater than or equal to 2 mm were 40.52, 28.98, and 32.87 in the minocycline microspheres, scaling and root planing plus vehicle and scaling and root planing alone groups, respectively.

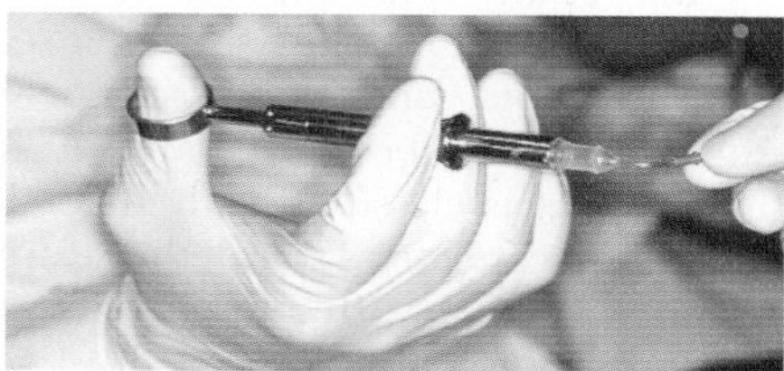

FIGURE 24–11 ✦ Minocycline microspheres delivery system.

Smokers and Persons with Cardiovascular Disease (CVD). Smoking is a significant risk factor for periodontal disease. The relationship between chronic periodontal infections and CVD focuses attention on the systemic impact of periodontal diseases. Although nonsmokers showed greater improvement than smokers did, smokers in the minocycline microspheres group showed significantly greater pocket depth reductions than smokers in the scaling and root planing group.[63] The enhanced treatment result attained by adjunctive minocycline microspheres therapy may be attributed to the anticollagenase properties of minocycline. The minocycline microspheres treatment effect was also proportionally better than scaling and root planing of molars in older persons, and in a small sample of patients with cardiovascular disease.

Administration and Use. The dry powder is packaged in single-unit dose cartridges via an anesthetic syringelike handle. The tip of the disposable cartridge is inserted subgingivally, to the base of the pocket. The powder is expelled from the cartridge by pressing the thumb ring while gradually withdrawing the tip from the pocket. Steps for placement of minocycline microspheres are presented in Procedure 24–4. The handle mechanism is sterilized between patients. No adhesive or dressing is required.

Contraindication and Precautions. The only absolute contraindication to the administration of minocycline microspheres is known sensitivity to minocycline or tetracyclines. Additionally, clinicians should be aware that despite the local administration of minocycline, the product label carries many of the same precautions for systemic minocycline use. Table 24–5 provides a comprehensive review of the contraindications and precautions associated with controlled-release devices. The product insert lists all contraindications and precautions for the product and should be thoroughly read to assure the standard of care.

Metronidazole Gel. Metronidazole gel (Elyzol) is a bioresorbable drug delivery system consisting of 25% metronidazole benzoate in a glycerol and sesame oil mixture. A single subgingival dose applied subgingivally via cannula and syringe reaches peak concentration in gingival crevicular fluid of 480 μg/ml four hours following administration. Concentrations exceeding 1 μg/ml, the MIC for anaerobic pathogens susceptible to metronidazole, are maintained for 36 hours.[64] The microbial effects of this drug delivery system on reducing anaerobic bacteria in vitro are only marginal.[65,66] This poor microbial effect may be due in part to a low proportion of metronidazole-susceptible bacteria in the study sample and/or to the presence of bacterial biofilm.[67]

Clinical Efficacy. As a monotherapy, multiple applications of metronidazole gel resulted in improved clinical outcomes

Procedure 24–4 PLACEMENT OF MINOCYCLINE MICROSPHERES CONTROLLED- RELEASE DEVICE

EQUIPMENT
Mouth mirror, periodontal probe, scaler(s)

STEP	RATIONALE
1. Determine need for controlled-release minocycline microspheres therapy. Indicated for the reduction of pocket depth in sites ≥ 5 mm not responding to mechanical therapy alone in persons with chronic periodontitis.	Prevents indiscriminate use of an antibiotic and development of antibiotic-resistant microorganisms.
2. Evaluate contraindications and precautions to treatment.	Ensures quality of care and manages legal risks.
3. Explain risks/benefits and alternative to treatment. Obtain informed consent	Encourages active decision making by the client and manages legal risks.
4. Remove number of product cartridges need for treatment.	Product does not require refrigeration; store at 68–77° F. Avoid excessive heat.
5. Insert cartridge into sterile cartridge handle to administer product.	Minimizes risk of cross-contamination.
6. Insert tip of cartridge subgingivally to base of pocket; press thumb ring to express powder while gradually withdrawing tip from base of pocket.	Product must be in pocket to produce therapeutic effect.
7. No dressing or adhesive is required.	Product is bioresorbable and self-retentive in pocket.
8. Instruct client not to floss area for 10 days.	Flossing may prematurely dislodge product.
9. Schedule reevaluation and/or reapplication. Reevaluation can coincide with 3-month maintenance visits.	Maximum benefit is attained after 3 consecutive administrations at 3-month intervals over a 9-month period.
10. Document in client record under service rendered and date the entry. For example, "Minocycline microspheres placed in sites not responding to mechanical debridement alone for the reduction of pocket depths: #2M, #3D, #30 M,D, #31D. Client instructed not to brush or floss the area for 10 days."	Ensures integrity of client's record for both quality care and legal protection of practitioner.

similar to those achieved by scaling and root planing alone.[67] Sufficiently large controlled clinical trials have not been conducted to determine the clinical efficacy of metronidazole gel when used as an adjunct to scaling and root planing. This product is currently marketed in Europe and is not commercially available in the United States.

Contraindication and Precautions. Allergy to metronidazole is an absolute contraindication to the use of metronidazole gel. Clients should be advised that any antibiotic use may result in an increase in photosensitivity, an increase in vaginal candidiasis, impaired adsorption of some nutrients, and depressed prothrombin activity, and may render oral contraceptives less effective. Similarly, the product is classified with systemic tetracyclines as pregnancy category D and therefore is NOT warranted during pregnancy. In addition, its use in children and for periodontal abscesses has not been tested. The product insert lists all contraindications and precautions for the product and should be thoroughly read to ensure the standard of care.

Minocycline Ointment. Minocylcine ointment is a drug delivery product marketed in Europe but not commercially available in the United States. This drug delivery system consists of 2% minocycline HCl in a hydroxyethylcellulose matrix. The pharmacokinetics of this delivery system are unknown.

Clinical Efficacy. Clinical efficacy of minocycline ointment is difficult to determine due to limited investigations utilizing sufficiently large samples and observation periods. Minocycline ointment in conjunction with scaling and root planing was not significantly better than scaling and root planing alone.[68] Researchers reported improvement in pocket depth ≥ 7 mm with four adjunctive administrations of minocycline ointment at weekly intervals compared with scaling and root planing plus a vehicle control.[69] Need for multiple applications of minocycline impairs clinical efficiency. Given a lack of data, it remains unclear if minocycline ointment provides a clinical benefit when used as an adjunct to scaling and root planing.

Contraindication and Precautions. The only absolute contraindication to the administration of minocycline ointment is known sensitivity to minocycline or tetracyclines. Clients should be advised that any tetracycline-derived antibiotic use may result in an increase in photosensitivity, an increase in vaginal candidiasis, impaired adsorption of some nutrients, and depressed prothrombin activity, and may render oral contraceptives less effective. Similarly, the product is classified with systemic tetracyclines as pregnancy category D and therefore is NOT warranted during pregnancy. In addition, its use in children and for periodontal abscesses has not been tested. The product insert lists contraindications and precautions for the product and should be thoroughly read to assure the standard of care.

COMPARING CONTROLLED-RELEASE DEVICES

Despite the availability of FDA-approved clinical efficacy data for each controlled-delivery system, inherent study design differences make comparison of clinical efficacy and decisions regarding product selection difficult. The FDA allows controlled-release devices to be tested under protocols for use as either alternatives or adjuncts to treatment. Clinicians may notice differences pertaining to the labeled indications for each product. Products tested as an adjunct to nonsurgical periodontal therapy are required by the FDA to evaluate the reduction in pocket depth as the primary study outcome. The FDA does not allow an adjunct product to make claims regarding clinical attachment gain regardless of the outcome. Conversely, products tested as an alternative therapy may make claims regarding gains in clinical attachment. Although the labeled indications for products tested as alternative treatment may appear to have added benefits of clinical attachment gains, comparative adjunctive treatments may have achieved similar gains in attachment level but the FDA has restricted their labeling. To date, evidence fails to support superiority of one delivery system over another. Product selection should be based on client health history, pertinent precautions, number of sites requiring treatment, ease of use, and degree of client-required compliance.

Postoperative Considerations for Controlled-Release Drug Delivery

Client perceptions and tolerance during product placement are similar to those experienced during a thorough periodontal probing, and placement typically does not require use of a local anesthetic agent. Clients may experience a mildly bitter taste immediately following application, which soon subsides. Clients should be instructed not to floss and/or brush treated areas for one week. During this time an antimicrobial oral rinse such as chlorhexidine can be prescribed. Additionally, retention and avoidance of premature loss of material may be improved if the client avoids hard and sticky foods during this same period. For this reason, it is recommended that the product be used to treat one side of the mouth at a time, leaving one side for normal function. Reevaluation should be scheduled at an interval consistent with scaling and root planing or supportive periodontal therapy (three- to four-month interval).

MODULATING HOST RESPONSE

Periodontal disease initiation and progression are determined by a complex interaction between a susceptible host, the presence of periodontal pathogens, and the absence of beneficial species. For decades, therapeutic interventions and strategies for disease prevention have focused exclusively on controlling the bacterial etiology by mechanical or chemical means. Modifying personal periodontal risk factors (i.e., smoking cessation) provided the only means of addressing the susceptible host aspect of the disease equation.

Historically, the host immunologic response was regarded as protective. Current research has shown that although bacteria and their by-products initiate the inflammatory process, endogenous enzymes are actually responsible for the destruction of periodontal tissues.[70] Specifically, the manufacture and secretion of matrix metalloproteinases (MMPs) degrade certain proteins, most notably collagen. Therefore, researchers are investigating the modulating host response as an approach to treatment.

Subantimicrobial Doxycycline Hyclate

Certain classes of drugs commonly used to treat other conditions such as nonsteroidal anti-inflammatory drugs (NSAIDs) modify host responses. In addition to NSAIDs, subantimicrobial systemic doses of doxycycline have been found to inhibit collagenase, which breaks down collagen in the periodontal disease process. The FDA approved Periostat, a 20-mg doxycycline hyclate capsule, a collagenase inhibitor, as a systemic adjunct to scaling and root planing for the treatment of chronic periodontal disease.

CLINICAL EFFICACY. The efficacy of *subantimicrobial dose* doxycycline therapy as an adjunct to scaling and root planing was investigated in a multicenter clinical trial with 190 patients with adult periodontitis. Scaling and root planing combined with nine-month subantimicrobial doxycycline dosage resulted in greater pocket depth reductions and gains in clinical attachment level compared with scaling and root planing plus placebo treatment.[71] No detrimental shifts in the normal periodontal flora or doxycycline resistance were observed during the study. Duration of clinical improvements attained by subantimicrobial doxycycline therapy following cessation of dosing is not known. Preliminary results suggest that subantimicrobial doxycycline may be a beneficial adjunct to scaling and root planing.

ADMINISTRATION AND USE. Subantimicrobial doxycycline therapy is taken by mouth via a 20-mg capsule twice daily. Clients should be instructed not to double up when a dose is missed in order to maintain subantimicrobial dosing. Based on the observation that most of the clinical benefits occurred by the three-month evaluation period, Periostat is used for three months and then clinical response reevaluated.[72]

CONTRAINDICATIONS AND PRECAUTIONS. The only absolute contraindication to administration of subantimicrobial doxycycline hyclate is known sensitivity to tetracyclines. Clients should be advised that use may result in an increase in photosensitivity, an increase in vaginal candidiasis, impaired adsorption of some nutrients, depressed prothrombin activity, and oral contraceptive ineffectiveness. The product is classified as pregnancy category D and therefore is NOT warranted during pregnancy. The product insert lists contraindications and precautions for the product and should be thoroughly read to assure the standard of care.

Other Host-Modulating Therapies

See Table 23–6.

TABLE 24–6 SUPPORTIVE PERIODONTAL THERAPY: SELF-CARE AND PROFESSIONAL-CARE STRATEGIES FOR MAINTAINING PERIODONTAL HEALTH

Objectives	Self Care	Professional Care
Reducing bacterial load	Compliance with selfcare: Meticulous oral hygiene Regular dental care	Risk assessment Frequent SPT Local chemotherapy Controlled drug delivery (chlorhexidine chip, doxycycline hyclate gel, tetracycline fibers, monocycline hyclate microspheres Systemic antibiotic therapy (tetracyclines, penicillins)
Reducing host modulators	Compliance with: Smoking cessation Prescribed host-modulating drugs	Smoking cessation Host-modulating drugs: Subantimicrobial doses of doxycycline hyclate Nonsteroidal antiinflammatory drugs* (flurbiprofen, naproxen, meclofenamate, ketorolac) Bisphosphonates* (risedronate, alendronate)

* Under investigation.
From Darby ML: Can we successfully maintain risk patients? *International Journal of Dental Hygiene* 1(1): 9-15, 2003.

CLIENT EDUCATION ISSUES

- ✦ Explain that control of bacterial plaque, gingivitis, and periodontitis should be made by personal and professional mechanical disease control methods. When these attempts are unsuccessful, or when problems are anticipated, chemical agents can be introduced and used until health is attained.
- ✦ Discuss that reevaluation of clinical parameters is indicated after a 3- to 12-week period. If clinical outcomes are improved, chemotherapeutic therapy should be discontinued until it is needed again.
- ✦ Note that products with effective chemotherapeutic agents are costly. If mechanical plaque control adequately removes soft deposits, the expense cannot be justified.
- ✦ Discuss possible side effects of antimicrobial agents.

LEGAL, ETHICAL, AND SAFETY ISSUES

- ✦ The American Academy of Periodontology outlines standards of care in a series of *2000 Parameters of Care Documents*.[73] These should be used to guide periodontal therapy.
- ✦ Care plans should include evaluation of the presence and distribution of bacterial plaque and calculus, plans for educating the client in daily personal oral hygiene, consideration of adjunctive chemotherapeutic agents, assessment of the client's bacterial plaque control effectiveness, and reinstruction when needed.
- ✦ Upon completion of dental hygiene assessment, the legal records of the client should reveal that the client has been informed of the current disease status and counseled on why and how to perform an effective personal oral hygiene program. Monitoring the client's progress also should be recorded.
- ✦ Carefully review the health and dental history to be sure that clients selected for antimicrobial therapy have no potential allergies or drug interactions with the agent being recommended. Instruct clients to keep antimicrobial agents out of the reach of children.
- ✦ Oral administration of subantimicrobial doses of doxycycline, the topical use of metronidazole gel, and the topical use of minocycline ointment are contraindicated for pregnant women.
- ✦ Malpractice cases for failure to recognize and treat periodontal disease can be related to failure to teach adequate plaque control measures to clients or failure to document contributory negligence.

Key Concepts

- ✦ Although bacterial plaque biofilm is believed to be a primary etiologic agent in inflammatory periodontal diseases, it is now known that a susceptible host and the absence of beneficial species together determine the initiation and progression of periodontal diseases.
- ✦ Although mechanical removal of bacterial plaque biofilm through the use of toothbrushes and other oral physiotherapy aids remains the most widely accepted mechanism for disease control, the bacterial etiology of periodontal diseases justifies the supportive use of antimicrobial agents.
- ✦ Success of local drug delivery systems in treating periodontal infections is dependent on their ability to deliver the antimicrobial agents to the site of action at a bacteriostatic or bactericidal concentration and maintain the agent for a sufficient duration of time.
- ✦ Dentifrices and mouthrinses do not have a therapeutic effect on subgingival periodontopathic microorganisms because they do not significantly penetrate subgingivally and do not have the necessary level of substantivity.
- ✦ Substantivity is the ability of an active agent to be retained in the oral cavity and to continue to be released over an extended period of time without losing its potency.
- ✦ Supragingival irrigation, as an adjunct to conventional oral hygiene, may be of value in the treatment of gingivitis and for periodontal maintenance care.
- ✦ Professional in-office subgingival irrigation performed in conjunction with root planing has no demonstrated advantage over root planing alone.
- ✦ Intracrevicular delivery devices consist of a drug reservoir that controls the rate of drug release directly into the periodontal pocket without the side effects associated with the systemic drug administration.
- ✦ Controlled drug delivery is an effective adjunct to scaling and root planing in pocket depths ≥ 5 mm not responding to mechanical therapy alone.
- ✦ Antimicrobial agents with high alcohol content are contraindicated for children, persons with a history of alcohol abuse, or persons taking medications that interact negatively with alcohol.

Critical Thinking Exercises

Mr. Thomas is a 59-year-old university professor. He is in generally good health with no known allergies to medications and has been in supportive periodontal maintenance for six years. His prognosis is compromised by his tobacco use (1 1/2 packs of cigarettes a day) and somewhat irregular compliance with prescribed maintenance intervals. Upon reexamination the dental hygienist documents localized pocket depths ≥ 5 mm unresponsive to mechanical periodontal debridement alone. Mr. Thomas is unwilling to consider surgical treatment options. In consultation with the dentist, the dental hygienist offers Mr. Thomas the option of adjunctive controlled-release therapy.

Use this case to answer the following questions:

1. Select the controlled-delivery system and drug combination best suited for this client. Give the rationale for your selection.
2. Are other chemotherapeutic agents indicated? If so, which one(s)?
3. What clinical outcomes can be achieved from the use of controlled drug delivery? What reevaluation interval should be recommended and why?
4. What homecare instruction should be given to Mr. Thomas, based on the controlled-delivery system used?
5. What is the average cost of this therapy? Would it be covered under most dental insurance programs? Does it have an insurance code? (See Chapter 23.)
6. Visit www.perio.org. Explore the site. Click on "Resources and Products." Then click on "Position Papers, Statements, and Parameters." Report on those that apply to dental hygiene practice. Explain how these resources can contribute to evidence-based decision making in practice.
7. Visit www.ada.org. Find information on the site about the role and publications of the ADA Council on Scientific Affairs. Explain how this resource can contribute to evidence-based decision making in practice.

For References, Suggested Readings, and Related Website, visit
http://evolve.elsevier.com/Darby/hygiene/

CHAPTER 25

Acute Gingival and Periodontal Conditions, Lesions of Endodontic Origin, and Avulsed Teeth

OBJECTIVES

Mastery of the content in this chapter will enable the reader to:

- Explain etiology, oral signs and symptoms, and treatment of clients with periodontal abscesses, gingival abscesses, and lesions of endodontic origin
- Explain etiology, oral signs and symptoms, and treatment of acute herpetic gingivostomatitis, pericoronitis, necrotizing ulcerative gingivitis, and necrotizing ulcerative periodontitis
- Practice the collaborative role of the dental hygienist in caring for clients with common periodontal and dental emergencies
- Educate clients about the need for immediate treatment of common periodontal and dental emergencies and expected outcome of emergency care
- Follow standard emergency protocol for an avulsed tooth

KEY TERMS

Acute herpetic gingivostomatitis
Acute periapical abscess
Acute periodontal abscess
Avulsed tooth
Chronic periapical abscess
Chronic periodontal abscess
Combination periodontal and periapical abscess
Dentoalveolar abscess
Endodontic abscess
Fistula
Gingival abscess
Herpes simplex labialis (HSL)
Herpes simplex virus 1 (HSV-1)
Herpes simplex virus 2 (HSV-2)
Herpetic whitlow
Lesion of endodontic origin (LEO)
Necrotizing ulcerative gingivitis (NUG)
Necrotizing ulcerative periodontal diseases
Necrotizing ulcerative periodontitis (NUP)
Operculum
Periapical abscess
Periapical pathosis (PAP)
Pericoronitis (acute, subacute, chronic)
Periodontal abscess
Pseudomembrane
Sinus tract
Trench mouth

The dental hygienist is frequently in a position to identify urgent periodontal conditions in need of treatment. A major part of care provided in these situations is to recognize the disease process. In some situations, the dental hygienist will provide therapeutic or palliative care; in other cases, the responsibility lies solely with referral for care. Postponement of appropriate care can result in prolonged pain, further periodontal tissue destruction, and tooth loss (see Chapter 7 for other dental and medical emergencies).

PERIODONTAL ABSCESS

Periodontal abscess is a general term used to describe an odontogenic infection from various possible sources, including periodontal infections, pulpal infections, and trauma. Prevalence of periodontal abscess is relatively high, and is often the reason a person seeks dental care. Periodontal abscess has been reported as the diagnosis for 6% to14% of all dental emergencies in the United Kingdom and the United States, and is the third most common dental emergency situation behind acute pulpal infections (14% to 25%) and pericoronitis (10% to 11%).[1]

Types of Periodontal Abscesses

Periodontal abscesses can be classified in many ways. Type of periodontal abscess is distinguished by location, either periodontal or gingival:

- A *gingival abscess* is a periodontal abscess that occurs in the gingiva. It occurs in otherwise healthy gingiva and is often found in the absence of periodontal infections of the teeth.
- A *periodontal abscess* is a deeper infection associated with periodontal pockets, furcations, and bone loss. This type of periodontal abscess is also described by the course of the disease (i.e., chronic or acute).
- The *acute periodontal abscess* is a lesion with expressed periodontal breakdown, occurring over a limited period of time, and with easily detectable clinical symptoms.[1] It is characterized by pain, swelling, and other symptoms that lead the client to seek urgent care.
- The *chronic periodontal abscess* is a long-standing infection that often displays a *sinus tract.* This opening permits drainage of the infection and a diminution of acute symptoms such as pain and swelling, thus making the abscess chronic in nature. The sinus tract, an abnormal channel that connects the abscess to another space or the surface, is called a *fistula.*[2]

Periodontal abscesses also have been classified by number as single abscesses and multiple periodontal abscesses:

- Single abscesses are caused by local factors that lead to acute or chronic symptoms.
- Multiple abscesses have been related to factors such as medically compromised systemic health, uncontrolled diabetes mellitus, and systemic antibiotic therapy for nonoral health-related situations.[1]

The importance of recognizing and treating clients with periodontal abscesses cannot be overemphasized. Data show that most abscessed teeth, particularly those receiving regular periodontal maintenance, benefit from treatment and can be preserved. An interesting retrospective study of tooth loss due to periodontal abscess demonstrated that 55% of teeth with periodontal abscess were maintained for an average of 12.5 years, with the range of 5 to 29 years.[3] The importance of recognizing the disease process and encouraging clients to follow through with treatment is significant to one major goal of dental hygiene practice, preserving oral health.

Microbiology of Periodontal Abscess

All periodontal abscesses share a characteristically complex pathogenic microflora similar to that associated with periodontal diseases. In these pathogenic microflora, the preponderance of bacteria changes from approximately 75% Gram-positive facultative rods and cocci associated with gingival health to one harboring approximately 74% Gram-negative rods.[4] These are complex mixed infections that vary from person to person and from one site of infection in the mouth to another within the same person. Those microbial species most associated with abscesses are listed in Microbial Species Most Associated with Periodontal Abscess.

Characteristics and Treatment of Periodontal Abscesses

ACUTE PERIODONTAL ABSCESS. The acute periodontal abscess is a localized accumulation of pus in the gingival wall of a periodontal pocket. It usually occurs on the lateral aspect of the tooth and appears edematous, red, and shiny. It may have a domelike appearance or come to a distinct point.[5] Figure 25–1 presents an example of an acute periodontal abscess with these characteristics. Acute abscesses are frequently associated with preexisting periodontal disease. The anatomic features of periodontal pockets—pocket depth, furcation involvement, and tortuous pocket anatomy—may predispose the client to occlusion of the pocket orifice. This permits an exacerbation of infection in the pocket wall and pus formation. Pus can often be expressed from the pocket with gentle finger pressure.

Abscess formation also can occur when a foreign body becomes lodged in the pocket.[2,6] An exacerbated inflammatory reaction then occurs. If the pocket continues to drain through the orifice, it can stabilize and become a chronic infection that drains pus to relieve pressure in the tissues. Conversion to the chronic state

Microbial Species Most Associated with Periodontal Abscess

Porphyromonas gingivalis
Prevotella intermedia
Bacteroides forsythus
Fusobacterium nucleatum
Actinobacillus actinomycetemcomitans
Capnocytophaga ochraceus
Eikenella corrodens
Campylobacter recta
Selenomonas species
Treponema denticola

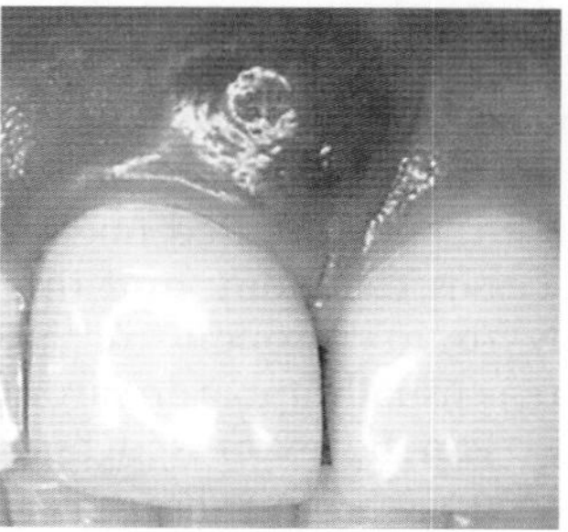

FIGURE 25–1 ✦ Acute periodontal abscess. This abscess is associated with tooth #8, and shows obvious signs of redness and swelling. *(Courtesy Philip R. Melnick, DMD.)*

rarely occurs when foreign objects such as peanut skins and popcorn hulls are embedded in the pocket, provoking the acute response.

Incomplete scaling and root planing that leaves residual calculus at the base of treated pockets has been suggested as a cause of periodontal abscesses.[2] It is postulated that the pocket orifice tightens from improved gingival health, leaving the calculus and associated plaque to infect the deeper pocket tissues. This is a commonly held belief, but few data support it. In an analysis of 29 persons seeking treatment at a postgraduate periodontics clinic and diagnosed with periodontal abscess, 18 of the persons (62%) presented with untreated periodontal disease, 7 (24%) were on periodontal maintenance, and only 4 (14%) reported a history of recent scaling and root planing. Of these 29 persons, 27 were diagnosed with moderate to severe periodontal disease; the other 2 had early periodontitis. The mean probing depths of these abscesses were quite deep, 7.3 mm, ranging from 3 to 13 mm, and were mostly associated with molar teeth.[4]

Given the number of abscesses treated, one would expect to see a much larger proportion of clients returning shortly after scaling and root planing appointments if incomplete treatment were a major cause of acute exacerbation. In another study, four types of periodontal treatment were compared and abscess rate was noted. Quadrants treated with supragingival scaling alone developed abscesses to a far greater extent than those treated with subgingival scaling and root planing or those treated with periodontal surgery.[7] These data suggest that abscess formation is more associated with deep pockets and untreated disease than with recent scaling and root planing treatment. It is also known that residual calculus and plaque biofilm is often left in pockets after even the most thorough scaling and root planing, especially in deep pockets.[8] This information highlights three points:

- ✦ It is extremely difficult to remove all calculus from periodontal pockets.
- ✦ The clinician should scale and root plane as completely as possible with the intention of removing all subgingival deposits.
- ✦ Supragingival scaling alone is totally inadequate in periodontal treatment and may predispose periodontal clients to acute abscess formation.

Signs and Symptoms. Acute periodontal abscess may be associated with any tooth in the mouth; abscesses appear as shiny, red, raised, and rounded masses on the gingiva or mucosa. Abscesses can point and drain through the tissue or simply drain through the pocket opening. Purulent exudate is usually apparent around the opening of the abscess or can be expressed by finger pressure. Signs and Symptoms of Acute Periodontal Abscess lists the signs of acute periodontal abscesses.

The client also may report that the tooth "feels high," because it may become slightly extruded due to swelling.[6]

Signs and Symptoms of Acute Periodontal Abscess[6]

Throbbing and radiating pain
Localized swelling of the gingiva
Deep-red to bluish color of the affected tissue
Sensitivity of the tooth and gingiva to palpation
Tooth mobility
Cervical lymphadenopathy
Systemic symptoms of fever and malaise

Radiographs may be helpful in locating a preexisting area of bone loss and can suggest the origin of the abscess. However, the infection moves through the tissue in the direction of least resistance, so the external features may appear at some distance from the affected tooth.[5]

Treatment. Treatment consists mainly of drainage and appropriate use of antimicrobial agents. The acute phase of the disease must be managed to alleviate pain and prevent spread of infection. The abscess must be drained, either through the pocket opening or through an incision. Drainage through the pocket opening is less invasive and is commonly performed by the dental hygienist. The tooth or teeth in the affected area are anesthetized and scaled. Postoperative instructions call for rest, fluid intake, and warm saltwater rinses to help reduce swelling. The client should be scheduled to return in 24 to 48 hours for reevaluation of the area and planning for required follow–up treatment (e.g., periodontal surgery to eliminate the problem area).[2,9]

The dentist often delegates initial treatment of the acute abscess that does not require surgical intervention to the dental hygienist. However, sometimes treatment requires an incision and reflection of the tissue (surgical flap procedure) to provide access to perform the debridement. If the client is febrile or if lymphadenopathy is present, the dentist may prescribe therapy using penicillin or other antibiotics. An example of debridement therapy for acute periodontal abscess is presented in Figure 25–2.

Repair potential for acute periodontal abscesses is excellent. After treatment, the appearance of the gingiva returns to normal within six to eight weeks. Repair of bone defects requires approximately nine months. Bone is lost rapidly during the acute phase, but with immediate recognition of the problem and proper treatment, the lost tissue can be largely regained.[6] The positive nature of clinical results from healing further emphasizes the importance of recognition and treatment of acute abscesses by the dental hygienist.

CHRONIC PERIODONTAL ABSCESS. Chronic periodontal abscess resembles acute periodontal abscess in that there is an overgrowth of pathogenic organisms in a periodontal pocket that drains inflammatory exudate. Chronic abscesses have communication to the oral cavity, either

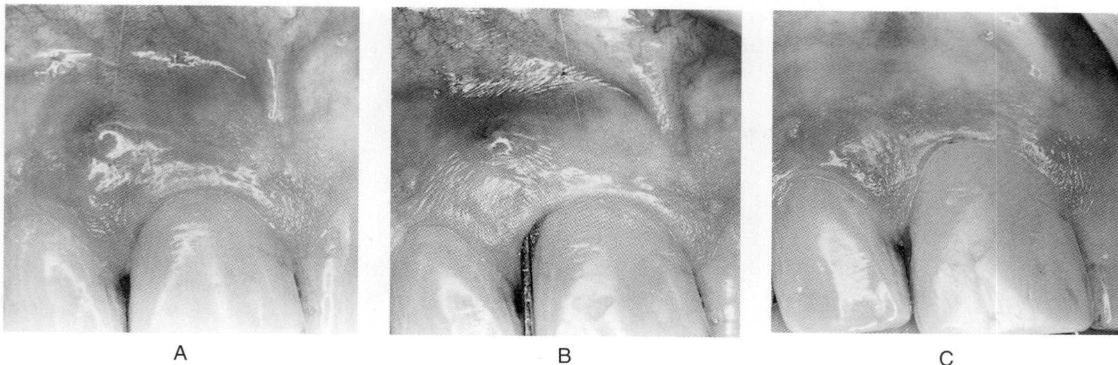

FIGURE 25–2 ✦ Treatment of acute periodontal abscess. Acute abscesses can often be successfully treated without surgical intervention. **A,** Abscess associated with tooth #9, showing swelling and a nondraining fistula. Clinically, the tissue appears very red. **B,** Probe in place to show 9-mm depth of pocket before scaling, root planing, and curettage. **C,** Healing after one month shows normal tissue architecture and little recession. A 7-mm periodontal pocket is still present, but surgical reduction would result in nonaesthetic recession. This situation can continue indefinitely with good home care and frequent periodontal maintenance. *(Courtesy Philip R. Melnick, DMD.)*

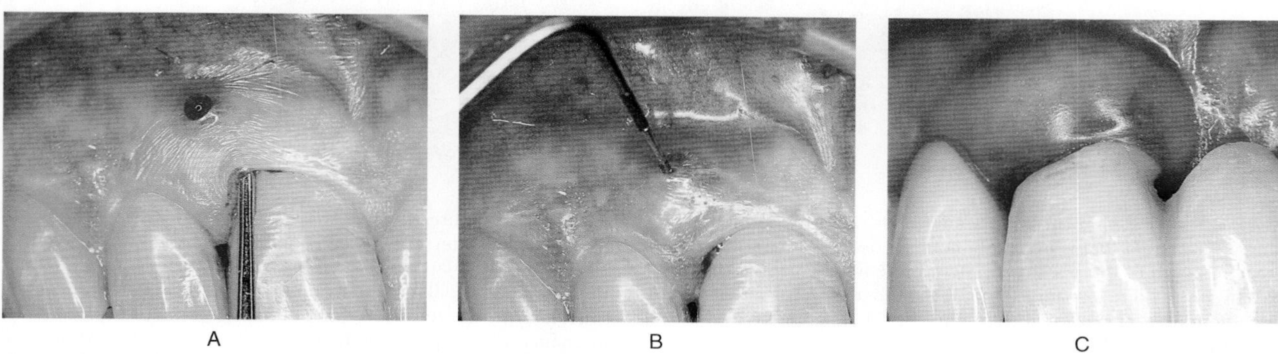

FIGURE 25–3 ✦ Chronic periodontal abscess. **A,** Draining through a sinus tract. **B,** Probe inserted to show communication to periodontal pocket. **C,** Draining through the periodontal pocket. *(Courtesy Philip R. Melnick, DMD.)*

through the opening of the pocket or through a sinus tract that permits regular drainage. The chronic periodontal abscess is usually painless or causes dull, intermittent pain; however, the client may recount previous episodes of painful acute infection.[5] Figure 25–3 provides examples of draining chronic periodontal abscesses.

Signs and Symptoms. The signs and symptoms of the chronic periodontal abscess are similar to those of acute periodontal abscesses; however, the level of pain can be the distinguishing feature. See Signs and Symptoms of Chronic Periodontal Abscess.

The dental hygienist must assess exudate associated with the periodontium as indicative of possible chronic abscess to ensure that appropriate dental referral and treatment are provided.

Treatment. Treatment of chronic periodontal abscess is similar to treatment of acute periodontal abscess. Scaling, usually requiring local anesthesia in the abscess area, must be performed. The client should return within 24 to 48 hours for further diagnosis. The dentist must determine the need for more periodontal treatment to reduce pocket depth and address other periodontal defects. This additional treatment usually includes pocket reduction periodontal surgery but may also include tooth extraction and more frequent periodontal maintenance visits.[9]

Some chronic periodontal abscesses are better treated initially by gaining surgical access. Figure 25–4 shows the surgical treatment sequence for a chronic periodontal abscess.

The dental hygienist plays a major role in educating the client about the chronic nature of this condition. The client must be informed of the likelihood of increased bone loss and future acute episodes if no further treatment is performed, and the need for frequent maintenance care including scaling, root planing, and daily

Signs and Symptoms of Chronic Periodontal Abscess

- Inflammatory exudate seeping into the oral cavity without inducement or when digital pressure is applied to the pocket or sinus tract
- Reddened and swollen gingival tissue in the area
- Varying degrees of pain (a chronic draining abscess is rarely painful)

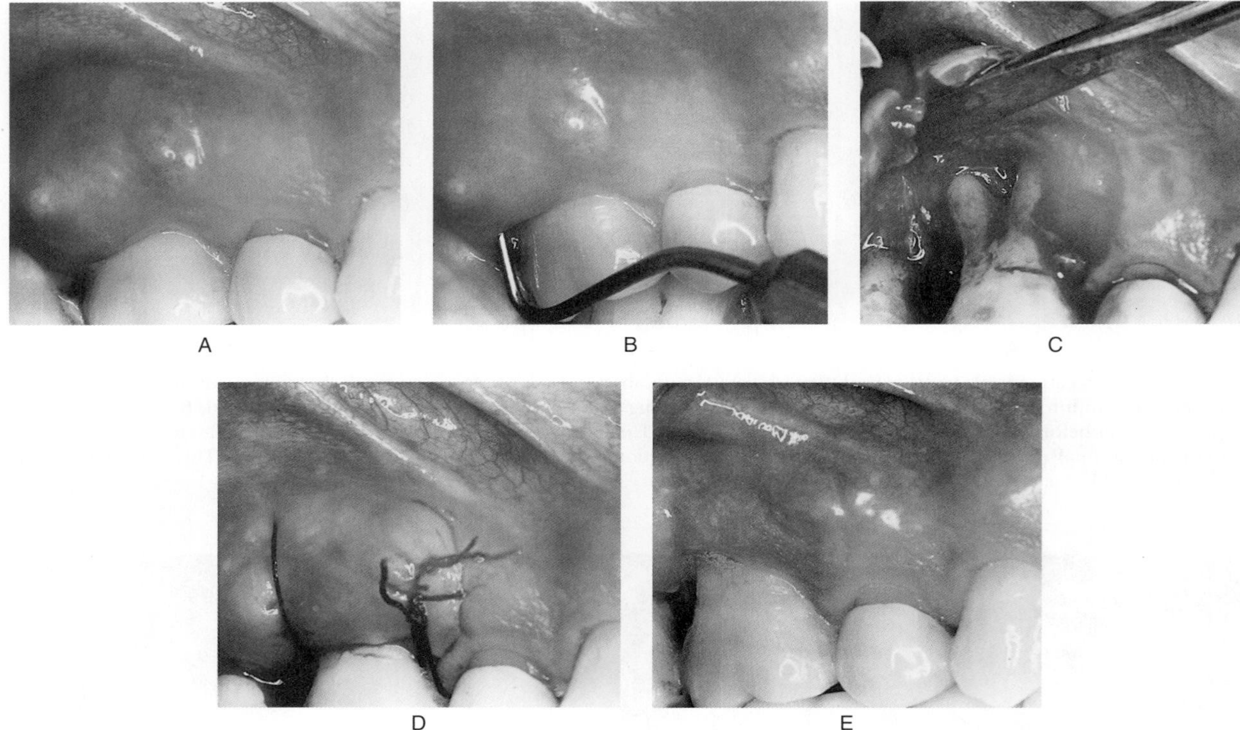

FIGURE 25–4 ✦ Surgical treatment of a chronic periodontal abscess associated with a furcation. **A,** Abscess associated with tooth #3 exhibits swelling and a fistula that is not draining. The tissue is very reddened and the patient has intermittent severe pain. **B,** Periodontal probe inserted to show the depth of the pocket and determine its association with the buccal furcation. **C,** Flap reflected to permit access for debridement. Note the extent of the bone loss and depth of the furcation involvement. **D,** After debridement, the flap is sutured in place. **E,** Healing after one month shows tissue returned to normal color and consistency, and no evidence of the fistula. Note the recession that occurred following surgical treatment. This client must keep the teeth clean and return for frequent periodontal maintenance visits to preserve the tooth. *(Courtesy Philip R. Melnick, DMD.)*

Signs and Symptoms of Gingival Abscess

Reddened tissue
Swelling (pus-filled lesion)
Pain

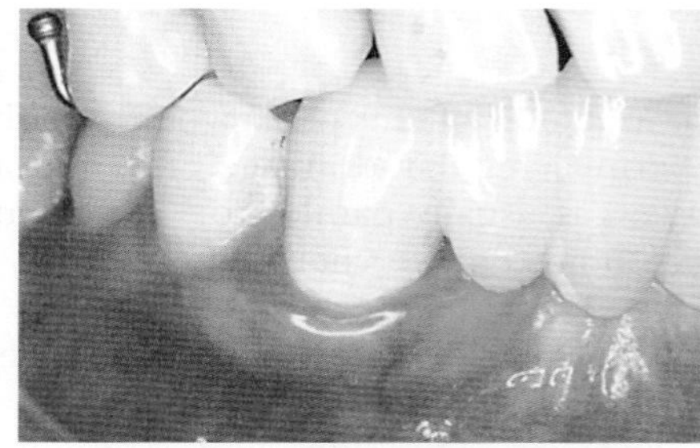

FIGURE 25–5 ✦ Gingival abscess. The gingival abscess is associated with the marginal gingiva and is often the result of inclusion of a foreign body. Note the swelling and color change of the marginal gingiva. *(Courtesy Philip R. Melnick, DMD.)*

control of bacterial plaque biofilm. Often, discussing the risk of rapid bone loss during acute episodes of abscess helps the client value the need to seek further care and better preserve the teeth.

GINGIVAL ABSCESS. The gingival abscess usually occurs in previously disease-free areas and can often be related to forceful inclusion of some foreign body into the area.[2,5] Most frequently, gingival abscesses are found on the marginal gingiva and are not associated with pathology of the deeper tissues.[6]

Signs and Symptoms. The gingival abscess can be observed on the marginal gingiva. The signs and symptoms are listed in Signs and Symptoms of Gingival Abscess.

A pus-filled lesion that is not associated with the sulcular epithelium is often clearly seen. Figure 25–5 shows a gingival abscess in the otherwise healthy periodontium of a teenager.

Treatment. The gingival abscess must be drained and the foreign object removed by the dentist or periodontist. The acute lesion is incised and irrigated with saline solution. Sutures are not usually required. Warm saltwater rinses are recommended for postoperative therapy at home. The client must return for postoperative observation in about 24 hours, at which time the swelling should be greatly reduced and the acute tenderness subsided.[9]

LESIONS OF ENDODONTIC ORIGIN (LEO)

Types of LEOs

The *lesion of endodontic origin,* the most common dental emergency,[1] is also referred to as a *dentoalveolar, apical, periapical,* or *endodontic abscess.* The LEO can result from a variety of noxious stimuli that cause inflammation, death, and dystrophy of pulpal tissues of the teeth.[10] It is sometimes difficult to distinguish a LEO from an acute periodontal abscess because facial pain and tenderness to the tooth are similar. The endodontic abscess commonly results from infection of the pulpal tissues from caries, traumatic fracture of the tooth, or the trauma of a dental procedure. Pulpal infection can be spread laterally to a tooth from an adjacent infected tooth or infected periodontium, through the lateral canals.[9]

Microbiology of LEO

Most commonly, the LEO is caused by microorganisms spreading into the pulp through the dentinal tubules from a carious lesion. Dissemination of the microorganisms and their toxic by-products through the enamel to the dentinal tubules can be very rapid. Although microorganisms are the most common cause of pulpal disease, bacterial toxins also can initiate pulpal disease by penetrating through tubules with pores small enough to block bacteria. The toxins affect the odontoblastic cells, and then penetrate into the pulp, initiating an inflammatory response. The bacterial cells also move toward the pulp by demineralizing the hard tooth structure with acids that they produce along the way. The microorganisms colonize in the pulp and produce a variety of toxins that result in pulp cell death. Bacteria and their metabolic products exit the apical foramen and can cause a localized formation of granulation tissue containing lymphocytes, plasma cells, mast cells, and other elements of the immune response. If the irritation continues, the granulation tissue gradually replaces the normal bone and periosteum at the apex of the tooth and gives rise to the common radiographic appearance of the LEO, a defined radiolucency at the apex of the affected tooth, called a *periapical pathosis (PAP).*[11]

Characteristics and Treatment of LEOs

PERIAPICAL ABSCESSES. There are both acute and chronic periapical abscesses. The *acute periapical abscess* occurs when bacteria or toxins rapidly enter the periradicular tissues, usually from the tooth pulp chamber. The confined abscess can cause severe pain. The pain may subside as the infection spreads toward a surface or space to provide relief to the tissues. Clients typically experience pain and swelling, and may have systemic symptoms of infection, including osteitis (inflammation of the bone) or cellulitis (inflammation of cellular tissue, usually occurring in the loose tissues beneath the skin, in the mucous membranes, or around muscle bundles or around organs, which can be life-threatening. The *chronic periapical abscess* is associated with a more gradual introduction of irritants from the root canal to the periradicular tissues. The inflammatory response is intense, but the client gets relief from an either constantly or intermittently draining sinus tract. These usually drain into the mouth through a fistula in the bone or through the periodontal ligament, but they can also drain through the skin of the face. If the sinus tract is through the periodontal ligament and is left untreated, it will become a true periodontal pocket.[11]

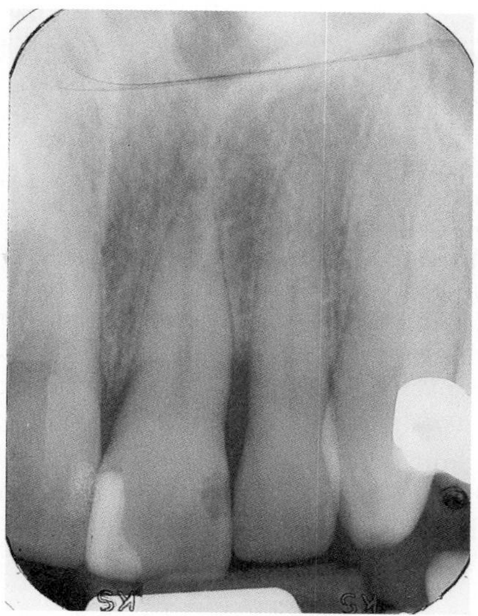

FIGURE 25–6 ✦ Lesion of endodontic origin. The radiographic appearance of an endodontic abscess associated with tooth #9 shows the classic appearance of radiolucency at the apex. Note that the periodontal ligament does not appear to be intact around the apex of the tooth. *(Courtesy Edward J. Taggart, DDS, MS.)*

Signs and Symptoms. The LEO is most identifiable on radiographs as a rounded radiolucency at the apex of the tooth. Figure 25–6 shows the typical appearance. However, early in the abscess formation the radiographic changes are often not obvious. If the LEO drains through a sinus duct in the cortical bone or through the periodontal ligament, it is likely to be much less identifiable on radiographs. LEOs that drain through the periodontal ligament can resemble acute periodontal abscesses because their symptoms are very similar, both exhibiting reddened tissue, swelling, and a sinus tract opening. It is often difficult to determine if the fistula opens into the periodontal pocket or goes to the apex of the tooth (see Signs and Symptoms of the LEO).

In assessing an abscess to determine its origin, it is helpful to know that 85% of tooth pain is pulpal and 15% is periodontal. In addition, many teeth with lesions of endodontic origin are nonvital, which is a good distinguishing clue. However, some populations of clients likely to be treated by the dental hygienist, such as those treated in the periodontal practice, are much more likely to have periodontal abscesses than pulpal ones. Pain may be the distinguishing feature in differentiating between

Signs and Symptoms of the LEO

Sharp pain, likely to be intermittent
Sinus tract often present
Swelling of tissues in a localized area
Redness of tissues in a localized area
History of restoration, trauma, or other source of infection to the tooth
Rounded radiolucency at apex of tooth (appears later in disease process)

periapical and periodontal abscesses. Periapical pain is characterized as sharp, severe, intermittent, and hard to localize. In contrast, periodontal pain tends to be constant, less severe, and localized.[6]

Treatment. Treatment of apical abscesses requires either endodontic treatment to remove the pulp of the tooth and replace it with inert material, or extraction of the tooth. Untreated endodontic abscesses can lead to severe cases of brain abscess[12] or fasciitis of the neck or chest wall that can be life-threatening.[11] The dental hygienist has a responsibility to inform clients with untreated LEOs of the risk of delaying treatment. Clients who do not suffer from acute symptoms due to draining of the abscess are likely to have the need for conceptualizing and understanding the disease process in order to pursue care and avoid further tissue destruction and ill effects from the infection.

COMBINATION ABSCESSES. The periodontium is a continuous unit. Pathology at the apex of the tooth from infection of the root canal system can extend to the marginal tissues, and infection originating in the periodontal tissues can progress to the pulp through openings at the apex or through lateral canals. A true combined lesion is present when both of these infectious processes are present. Whatever the route or source of the infection, when both the periodontal and pulpal tissues are involved and the disease has abscess formation, the abscess is considered *a combination periapical and periodontal abscess.*[13]

Signs and Symptoms. Combination abscesses present with some combination of the signs and symptoms described separately for periapical and periodontal abscesses. They are sometimes difficult to diagnose, and can result in extensive damage to the surrounding periodontium because the intermittent nature of symptoms often causes clients to delay seeking treatment. The dentist diagnoses combination abscesses when symptoms of both pulpal and periodontal infection are identified. Figure 25–7 illustrates a combination abscess.

Treatment. Combination abscesses require treatment of both sources of infection. Both periodontal and endodontic therapy are indicated to preserve the tooth.

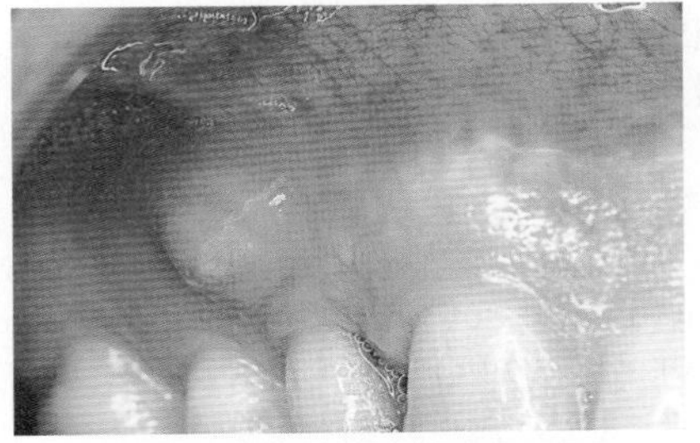

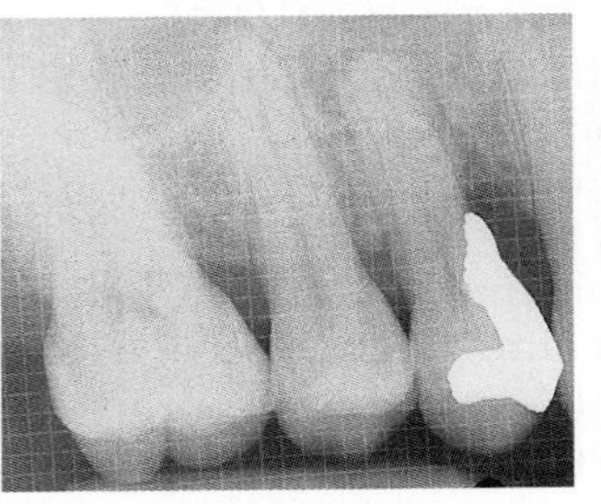

FIGURE 25–7 ✦ Combined periapical and periodontal abscess. The combined abscess is associated with tooth #5. It could have occurred from the spread of pathologic microorganisms from the deep pockets to the tooth pulp, the caries process, or trauma from placement of the very deep restoration. **A**, The sinus tract (fistula) emerges into the oral cavity. **B**, Radiolucency at the apex and significant bone loss appear on the radiograph. *(Courtesy Philip R. Melnick, DMD.)*

In some cases the periodontal tissue destruction is so severe that the tooth must be extracted even though endodontic therapy could be successfully performed.

HERPETIC INFECTIONS

Acute Herpetic Gingivostomatitis

Acute herpetic gingivostomatitis represents the oral manifestations of primary infection with the herpes virus, *herpes simplex virus 1 (HSV-1).* Almost everyone has experienced herpes virus because it is known that up to 90% of the population have antibodies to HSV-1. The virus is spread by physical contact, but there is no documentation that it can be spread through the airborne droplet route, contaminated water, or contact with inanimate objects. Most people encounter the virus and never show signs or symptoms of primary infection.[14]

Historically, primary herpetic gingivostomatitis has been seen predominantly in infants and children. However, in recent decades the disease has been found in young adults in their twenties and thirties. Primary herpetic gingivostomatitis in teenagers and adults is most likely HSV-1, but may be the initial manifestation of *herpes simplex virus 2 (HSV-2),* the form of the virus transmitted sexually, possibly explaining the increase in incidence in those age groups. The clinical manifestations of the infection, whether from HSV-1 or HSV-2, are indistinguishable.[14] Most clients presenting with primary herpetic infections never experience the secondary or recurrent forms. It is estimated that 20% to 40% of the infected population experience recurrent expressions of the virus as herpes labialis, commonly called cold sores

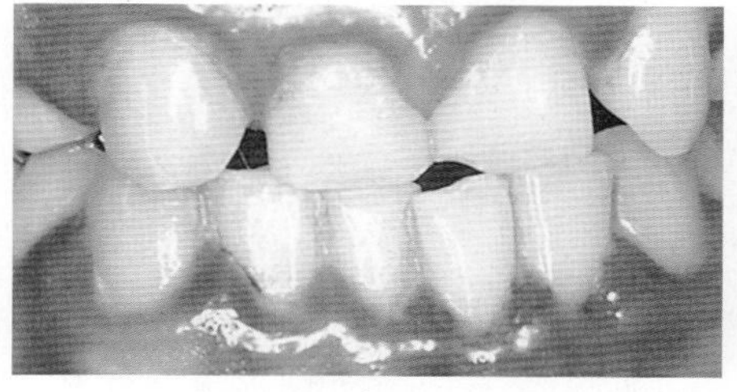
A

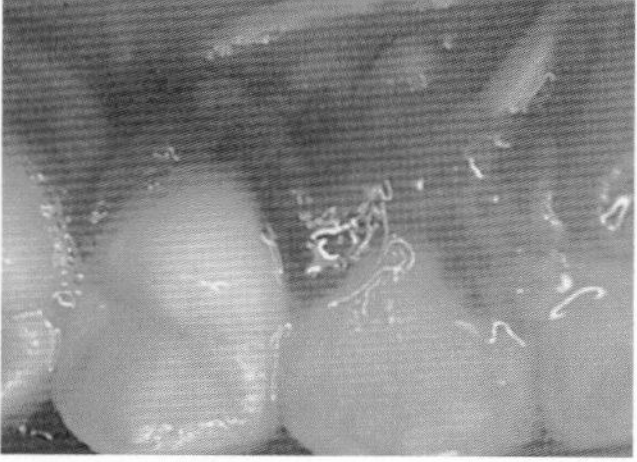
B

FIGURE 25–8 ✦ Primary herpetic gingivostomatitis. This oral infection of the mouth is characterized by bright red gingiva, vesicles, and pain. **A,** Facial gingiva showing swelling and color change. **B,** Lingual view of premolar and anterior teeth showing coalesced vesicles. *(Courtesy Philip R. Melnick, DMD.)*

Signs and Symptoms of Acute Herpetic Gingivostomatitis

Ulcers with the characteristic appearance of red halos of tissue immediately surrounding them (extraorally, on skin, vermilion border of lip; intraorally, on any mucosal surface)
Generally reddened tissues
Pain
Fever
Malaise
Headache
Cervical lymphadenopathy

or fever blisters.[14] The painful herpetic ulcers in the mouth associated with primary infection often cause reduction in food and fluid intake, creating a human need for the understanding of health risks that accompany this disease. Nutritional deficits can be critical in children and infants. Serious dehydration is not uncommon and can lead to hospitalization for infants.

SIGNS AND SYMPTOMS. Acute herpetic gingivostomatitis is recognized by a set of characteristic systemic and intraoral signs and symptoms (see Signs and Symptoms of Acute Herpetic Gingivostomatitis). The vesicular eruptions may occur on the skin, vermilion border, or oral mucous membranes. Intraorally, they may appear on any mucosal or gingival surface, the hard palate, and alveolar mucosa or any other area of oral soft tissue.[14] The discrete grayish vesicles rupture and coalesce within 24 hours to form ulcers. The ulcers have a red, elevated, "halo-like" margin with a depressed yellow or gray central area. They are teeming with shedding viruses. Figure 25–8 exemplifies the intraoral appearance of primary herpetic infection in a teenager. The disease is commonly associated with systemic symptoms including fever, malaise, headache, and cervical lymphadenopathy.[15]

Recognition of primary herpetic gingivostomatitis is based on knowledge of the appearance of the ulcers and assessment of systemic manifestations. Diagnostic tests, such as culturing for herpes virus by the client's physician, can be conducted for confirmation of the presence of the virus but are not routine. In addition, this is a highly infectious disease; therefore, the dental hygienist and client, and the client's parents in the case of children, must work together to prevent transmission of the virus to family members and other members of the oral healthcare team. Figure 25–9 shows a more unusual presentation of primary herpetic infection on the skin of the face.

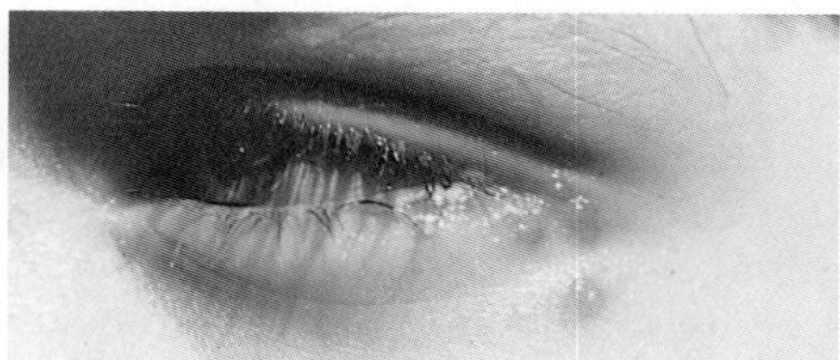

FIGURE 25–9 ✦ Primary herpetic infection on facial skin near eye. This eight-year-old child had to remain out of school for three weeks until the infection ran its course to prevent spread to others.

TREATMENT. Treatment of gingival inflammation and any other elective dental care should be postponed until the primary herpetic gingivostomatitis has run its course. The client is assessed by the dentist to obtain a definitive dental diagnosis. Management of acute herpetic gingivostomatitis is entirely supportive because of the infectious nature of the disease and the fact that it runs its course in seven to ten days. The client should be instructed to rest, take fluids, and make every effort to eat a nutritious diet. The client should also try to clean the teeth at home with an extra-soft toothbrush if it can be tolerated.[14,15]

Professional care should not be performed because of the risk of transmission of the virus to other head and neck areas of the client, or to the dental hygienist and other workers. Even if the hygienist was previously exposed to herpes virus or has had an episode of initial infection with or without recurrent lesions, the dental hygienist can still be inoculated with the virus by an inadvertent finger puncture with an HSV-contaminated instrument. This could result in the development of *herpetic whitlow* (Figure 25–10). Herpetic whitlow is a recurrent herpetic lesion of the finger that can be extremely painful and debilitating. The whitlow can last many weeks longer than the usual two-week course of herpes virus in the oral tissue.[14]

The dental hygienist should educate the client about consuming adequate fluids and soft, nutrient-dense foods; performing oral hygiene as much as possible at home; and using over-the-counter topical anesthetics and

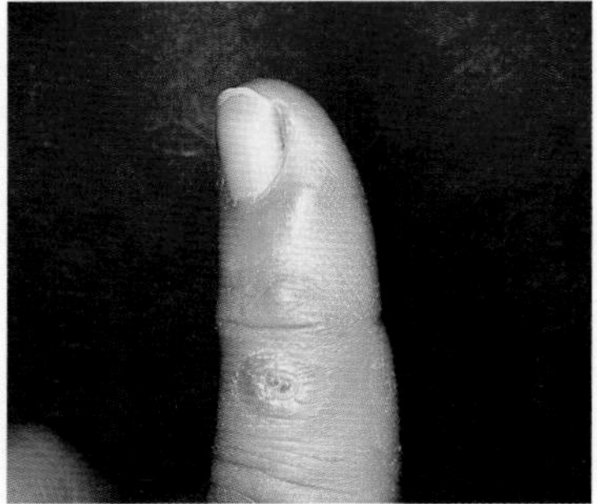

FIGURE 25–10 ✦ Herpetic whitlow.

systemic nonsteroidal antiinflamatory agents to minimize discomfort. The client can swab topical anesthetics onto the lesions for controlled local delivery. Topical anesthetics should be used cautiously with children so as not to anesthetize the throat, which can be frightening to them.

Recurrent Herpetic Infection

Clients often present at dental hygiene appointments when they have recurrent herpetic lesions. These are quite common, as previously mentioned, and do not interfere with activities of daily living, so clients are frequently unaware of the nature of the event. The typical recurrent lesion is on the lip, and is referred to as *herpes simplex labialis (HSL)*. Common names such as fever blister and cold sore reflect the public understanding of what precipitates these recurrences. Unfortunately, they are extremely innocuous names for lesions with serious potential effects for the dental hygienist.

SIGNS AND SYMPTOMS. Clients often have prodromal symptoms of burning, tingling, or pain in the site where the lesion recurs (see Signs and Symptoms of Recurrent Herpetic Infection). Within hours of the prodromal symptoms, vesicles appear, which become ulcerated and coalesce into a large ulcer or ulcers. The lesions heal without scarring in about 14 days, and can recur as often as once per month.[14] Typically, lesions will recur in the same place on the vermilion border and skin around the face. Figure 25–11 is an example of a recurrent herpetic lesion.

TREATMENT. Recurrent lesions shed vast amounts of herpes virus. For this reason, the dental hygienist must not treat the client while the lesions are present. Sometimes this can be very disconcerting because it may require reappointing a client who has waited months for an appointment. However, the dental hygienist is placed at great risk of inoculation, just as with primary herpetic infections. Not only are herpetic whitlow lesions a possibility, but the virus is also shed in the saliva, meaning that spatter during treatment can be hazardous. Figure 25–12 is an example of a recurrent herpetic infection of the cornea acquired from splatter.

Treatment of the herpetic lesion is entirely supportive. There are some antiviral agents available by prescription (e.g., acyclovir) that the client may benefit from using.

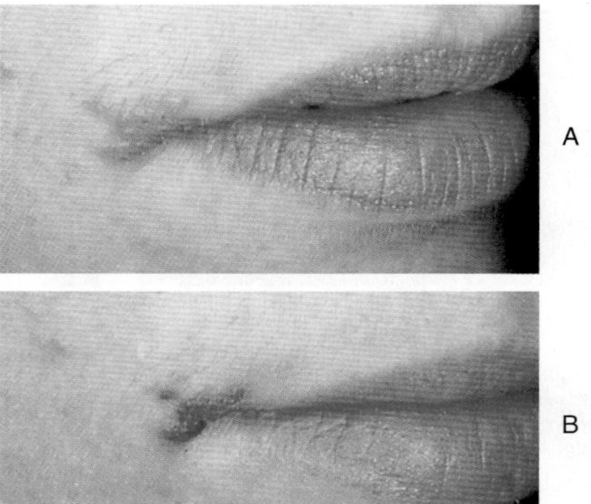

FIGURE 25–11 ✦ Recurrent herpetic infection on the lip—"cold sore." Clients frequently do not recognize these lesions as recurrent herpetic infections that are highly contagious. **A,** Herpes labialis 12 hours after onset. **B,** Herpes labialis 48 hours after onset. *(From Ibsen OAC, Phelan JA:* Oral pathology for the dental hygienist, *ed 3, Philadelphia, 2000, WB Saunders.)*

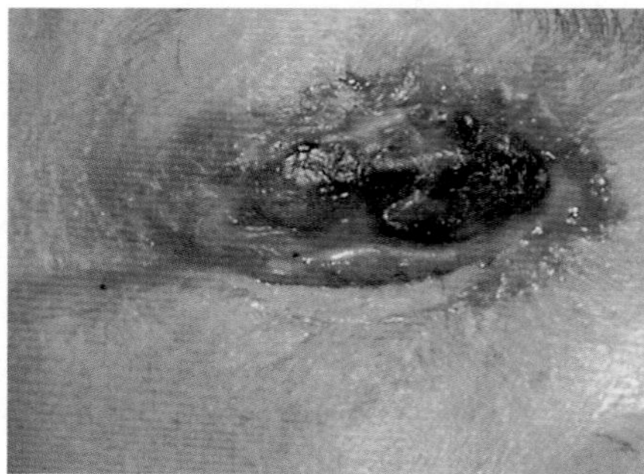

FIGURE 25–12 ✦ Recurrent herpetic infection of the cornea. Without protective eyewear and universal precautions, calculus and other contaminants can enter the eye of the dental hygienist or client and infect the cornea with herpes virus. Recurrences are extremely painful and last months. Partial loss of sight and disability can occur. *(Courtesy Dr. Sidney Eisig; from Ibsen OAC, Phalen JA:* Oral pathology for the dental hygienist, *ed 3, Philadelphia, 2000, WB Saunders.)*

Signs and Symptoms of Recurrent Herpetic Infection

Prodromal symptoms of burning or tingling at the site
Ulcer on the lip and/or perioral skin
Pain
Vesicles early in the course of the infection
Crusting of the ulcer surface as it heals

These agents can reduce the extent and duration of the recurrence. The dental hygienist should inform the client of this possibility and refer the client to the physician or dentist for further information.

It is extremely important for the client to be educated about these lesions and the client's responsibility for preventing the spread of infection. Clients who have

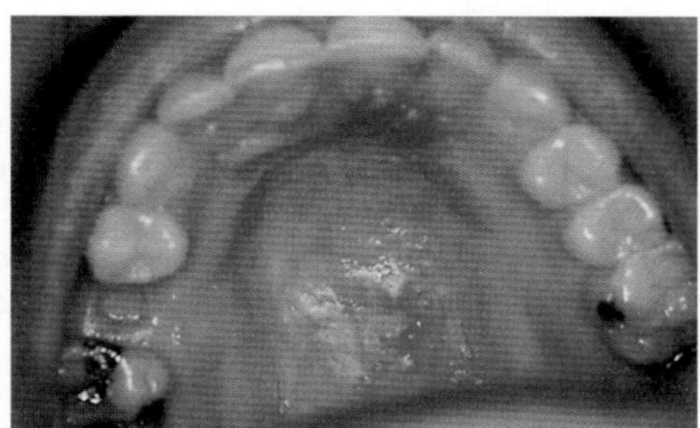

FIGURE 25–13 ✦ Recurrent herpetic infection of the palate. *(From Ibsen OAC, Phalen JA: Oral pathology for the dental hygienist, ed 3, Philadelphia, 2000, WB Saunders.)*

common recurrences are often aware of the prodromal symptoms and should be informed to call and reschedule dental appointments until the disease runs its course.

Recurrent herpetic lesions can occur intraorally and usually appear on the soft palate.[14] These lesions sometimes erupt after therapeutic scaling and root planing when repeated palatal injections have been given to the client to achieve anesthesia. The client will either call or return for a subsequent appointment and the typical oral ulcers will be evident in the area where the injections were given. Figure 25–13 is an example of recurrent palatal herpes subsequent to periodontal therapy in the maxillary quadrant. This situation requires the same management as other herpetic episodes. The client should not be treated until the lesions have healed, and the client must be educated about the situation.

Recurrent intraoral herpetic lesions can almost always be easily distinguished from the more commonly occurring aphthous ulcers. Reviewing the client history for recent trauma or illness may be helpful, but either lesion can result. The more distinguishing characteristic is that recurrent herpetic lesions almost always occur on the gingiva or hard palate, and aphthous ulcers almost always appear on the movable mucosa.

PERICORONITIS

Pericoronitis is soft tissue inflammation associated with a partially erupted tooth. It may be acute, subacute, or chronic in nature.[5] The most commonly affected tooth is the mandibular third molar, but maxillary third molars and other teeth that are the most distal in the arch have been associated with the disease. The flap of tissue that either completely or partly covers the associated tooth is called an operculum. The space between the flap of tissue and the tooth is an ideal location for food debris to collect and bacteria to grow. As bacteria increasingly infect the area, the tissue responds by becoming extremely inflamed and painful.[16] There is constant inflammation in the area, so it is always considered subacute or chronically infected even if the acute symptoms are not present.[15]

Acute pericoronitis involves an extremely high degree of inflammation in the local area. As inflammation increases, the tissue swells and can interfere with the complete closing of the jaws. This can lead to added trauma, increased inflammation, and severe pain. The tissue becomes quite red, suppuration is evident, and the pain can radiate to the throat and ear.

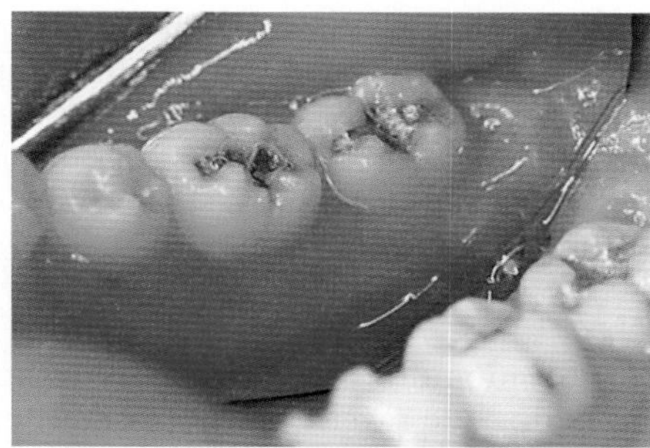

FIGURE 25–14 ✦ Pericoronitis. This condition is most commonly found in the third molar region and can be extremely painful. Note the swelling of the soft tissue distal to the second molar. Clnically, the tissue is intensely red. *(Courtesy Edward J. Taggart, DDS, MS.)*

Signs and Symptoms of Acute Pericoronitis

Extreme pain
Swelling of the operculum and gingiva associated with the most distal tooth in the arch
Redness
Purulent exudate
Foul taste
Swelling of the cheek
Cervical lymphadenopathy
History of recurrence

This disease is a common problem associated with young adults and has been considered to be a serious problem for military personnel, most of whom are in the 17- to 26-year-old group. In fact, 20% of dental emergencies reported by the military in World War II and 16% of those from the Vietnam conflict were acute pericoronitis.[17] Figure 25–14 is an example of acute pericoronitis.

Signs and Symptoms

Oral areas that have an operculum are predisposed to pericoronitis and typically exhibit chronic signs of the disease, increased redness, and some exudate (see Signs and Symptoms of Acute Pericoronitis).

The tissue may be so swollen that it interferes with mastication, and is easily traumatized during eating. The infection can extend very deeply into the tissues and cause peritonsillar abscess formation, cellulitis, and Ludwig's angina.[15] These are rare sequelae, but emphasize the importance of recognition and treatment of the lesions.

A review of military studies documents the extent of symptoms associated with pericoronitis. In a military study of 359 recruits, pain, swelling, and redness were present in every instance. Purulent exudate was reported in half the cases, few cases bled on palpation, and none of that population presented with a fever. In addition, two-thirds of 25 cases in the naval population reported previous episodes of pericoronitis, suggesting that pericoronitis is often a recurrent problem.[17]

Treatment

A number of considerations are involved in treating pericoronitis, including the severity of the case, whether it is a recurrence, and possible systemic complications. The dentist may ask the dental hygienist to participate in the care of the client with pericoronitis, which requires multiple visits.

Initial dental management is aimed at treating symptoms, with the goal of making the client more comfortable. The infected area is debrided, usually by gentle flushing with warm water or dilute hydrogen peroxide delivered in a disposable irrigating syringe with a blunt needle. Topical anesthetic should be applied first. Much manipulation of the tissue may not be possible, but the tissue should be lifted away from the tooth to permit as much debridement as is tolerable at the first treatment appointment.[15] After this initial debridement, the client should be instructed to rest at home, use warm saltwater rinses, and drink fluids to avoid dehydration. The dentist may prescribe antibiotics if the client is febrile or if there is cervical lymphadenopathy. The client should be asked to return the next day. At the second visit, the area should be irrigated again and instrumented if possible, and more thorough home care should be initiated. A marked improvement is usually observed at the second appointment.

After the acute condition has resolved, the client should be assessed by the dentist to determine further treatment. Dental treatment might include extraction of the offending third molar or operculum removal to produce a more normal gingival contour if the tooth is to be retained.[15]

The presence of any operculum should be assessed and viewed with suspicion. There is almost always some amount of inflammation present, and the potential for acute exacerbation is likely. The dental hygienist should inform the client of the potential of the condition to permit the client to conceptualize and understand the situation and take responsibility for his or her oral health.

NECROTIZING ULCERATIVE PERIODONTAL DISEASES

Necrotizing ulcerative periodontal diseases are clinically recognizable diseases distinct from chronic periodontitis. Until 1999,[18] the condition was most commonly called acute necrotizing ulcerative gingivitis (ANUG), or just *necrotizing ulcerative gingivitis (NUG)*. However, the disease is often associated with attachment loss, making the term *gingivitis* inaccurate, so the disease is now referred to as *necrotizing ulcerative periodontitis (NUP)*. It is not certain whether or not the conditions with attachment loss are separate diseases from those confined to the gingiva, so the consensus is to use the more general disease name of necrotizing periodontal diseases.

Necrotizing ulcerative periodontal diseases are opportunistic infections of the gingiva that are associated with lifestyle risk factors such as stress and tobacco use, and also systemic conditions such as blood dyscrasias, acquired immunodeficiency syndrome (AIDS), and Down syndrome.[19]

The disease was first described by Vincent in the late nineteenth century, and was so common among troops fighting in trenches in Europe during World War I that the name *trench mouth* was adopted. It was primarily seen in young adult individuals and was thought to be communicable.[20] The disease is transmissible, able to be maintained through successive passages via a susceptible host, but is not communicable, infectious or spread through direct contact. Necrotizing ulcerative periodontal diseases are recognized to be recurrent diseases with complex bacteriology consisting of a large proportion of spirochetes and Gram-negative organisms. These organisms invade the tissue, causing the characteristic appearance of the disease.[19]

Signs and Symptoms

Necrotizing ulcerative periodontal diseases have specific clinical characteristics that distinguish them from other forms of acute oral infections. The clinical appearance of the disease is one of cratered or "punched-out" papillae, very reddened gingivae, and pain. There is often a collection of debris, dead cells, and bacteria on the gingival surface that appears gray and is referred to as the *pseudomembrane*. The gingival lesions may be localized to specific areas or generalized throughout the mouth, and they progressively destroy the gingiva and underlying periodontal structures. Clients frequently exhibit an extremely offensive and fetid breath odor that can be smelled anywhere in the room occupied by the client. They may also complain of a thick or pasty texture to the saliva. In addition, the acute lesions can be extensive, covering parts of the face, as seen in Third World countries when associated with malnutrition. Figure 25–15 shows the clinical oral features of NUP.

The three most reliable criteria for recognizing the disease are:[21]

- ✦ Acute necrosis and ulceration of the interproximal papillae
- ✦ Pain
- ✦ Bleeding

Other symptoms have been recognized as strongly associated with the disease (see Signs and Symptoms of Necrotizing Ulcerative Periodontitis).

Stress is often related to both initial occurrence and recurrence of this disease. The role of psychological factors involved with stress is not well understood, but it has been postulated that changes in the immune system occurring at stressful times predispose certain individuals to an exuberant bacterial response, resulting in necrotizing ulcerative disease.[19]

Treatment

The course of a single episode of NUP is usually short but painful. Clients come to the oral care setting most often because of pain. Because of the cyclic and recurring nature of the disease, treatment focuses on microbial control through mechanical debridement by both client and clinician. It also requires consultation with the client's physician because of possible predisposing systemic factors such as HIV infection.[15] Treatment should progress daily during the acute phase of the disease because the pain often inhibits thorough cleaning by the client or the dental hygienist at one time. Treatment includes periodontal debridement with ultrasonic scalers, plaque biofilm control, and 0.12% chlorhexidine rinses twice daily. The dentist may prescribe a systemic antibiotic if fever and lymphadenopathy are present. The recommended treatment sequence is described in Table 25–1.

Given the signs and symptoms, most clients with necrotizing periodontal diseases have unmet human needs in the areas of freedom from head and neck pain, skin and mucous membrane integrity of the head and neck, and conceptualization and understanding. Client health and oral health and well-being are the keys to successful treatment of these diseases. The client must be

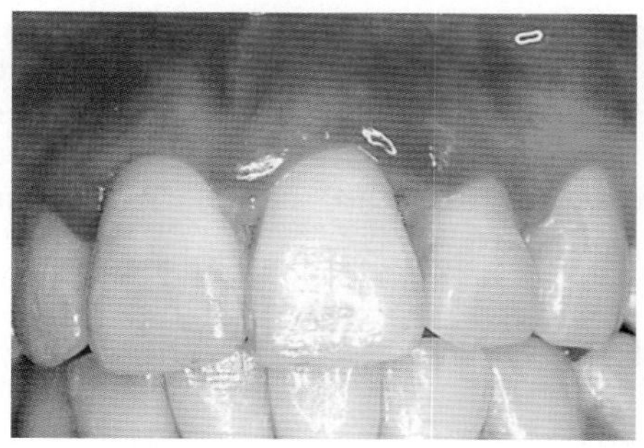

FIGURE 25–15 ✦ Necrotizing ulcerative periodontitis. The classic intraoral signs of this disease, redness, cratered papillae, and pseudomembrane, appear throughout the anterior area. *(Courtesy Philip R. Melnick, DMD.)*

Signs and Symptoms of Necrotizing Ulcerative Periodontitis

Necrosis of interproximal papillae of the gingiva
Bleeding
Pain
Fetid odor
Pseudomembrane over gingiva
Cervical lymphadenopathy
Fever

TABLE 25–1 TREATMENT REGIMEN FOR NECROTIZING ULCERATIVE PERIODONTITIS

Day 1	First visit: Oral therapy	Scale and debride as much as possible Mechanized(ultrasonic) instruments may be more easily tolerated than hand scalers Use topical anesthetic as needed Provide plaque control instruction Frequent rinsing with a mixture of warm water and 3% hydrogen peroxide is soothing and oxygenates the pseudomembranous plaque Twice-daily rinses with 0.12% chlorhexidine are recommended
Day 1	Systemic therapy	Review health history for underlying conditions and consult with physician as needed The use of antibiotics such as penicillin, erythromycin, or metronidazole is indicated if the client has fever and cervical lymphadenopathy
Day 2	Second visit	Pain should be reduced considerably Continue to remove calculus to the limit of the client's tolerance Oral hygiene instructions should be reinforced The home rinsing regimen should be continued
Days 4 to 7	Third visit	Therapeutic scaling and root planing should be completed, taking as many appointments as necessary Oral hygiene must be reinforced Hydrogen peroxide rinses can be discontinued Continue on 0.12% chlorhexidine mouthrinse twice daily for two to three weeks
Month 1	Reevaluation for continued care	Reinforce oral hygiene Scale and root plane if necessary Meticulous and regular debridement by the client and the dental hygienist to control bacterial pathogenicity is required Cratering frequently occurs and can result in significant gingival defects that should be evaluated by the dentist for possible surgical correction
Month 3	Supportive periodontal therapy (maintenance)	Regular professional mechanical dental hygiene care should be encouraged to minimize the risk of recurrence Continued-care interval should be 2 to 4 months

knowledgeable about the roles of stress, bacteria, and nutrition in the disease process and encouraged to take control over his or her oral health and lifestyle behaviors. Suggestions to identify stress management techniques and improve nutrition are necessary components of dental hygiene care.

AVULSED TOOTH

Prevalence

The *avulsed tooth* is one that is separated from the alveolar bone by trauma.[22] Avulsed teeth, though not strictly periodontal emergencies, are traumatized teeth that can be replanted successfully if managed properly. The dental hygienist may have the opportunity to help a parent of a small child or a student or adult participating in athletic activities to preserve an avulsed tooth through quick action.

Avulsion is the most common dental injury to children younger than 15 years of age, as reported in the consumer product–related injury survey of U.S. hospitals from 1979 to 1987.[23] The situation occurs in as many as 1 in every 200 American children, approximately 2 million occurrences per year.[24] To meet the client's need for a biologically sound and functional dentition, it is incumbent on the dental hygienist to respond to this dental emergency. Lost time and improper handling of the avulsed tooth can substantially reduce long-term success of replantation. Moreover, the dental hygienist should inform parents, teachers, and coaches about the procedure so increased awareness can improve the opportunity for successful tooth replantation when injuries causing avulsed teeth occur.

In addition, during the assessment phase of dental hygiene care, clients who play contact sports should be identified as having a potential unmet need for a biologically sound and functional dentition. The appropriate intervention would be education of the client and parent, and construction of a mouth protector to prevent tooth avulsion and other oral injuries. The procedure for constructing a custom-made athletic mouth protector is described in Chapter 30, Procedure Table 30–7. Athletic mouth protectors are highly recommended to prevent tooth avulsion.

Treatment

The dental hygienist might be present at a sporting event or other venue when a tooth is traumatically avulsed, or have a child who experiences a traumatically avulsed tooth. The avulsed tooth is quickly separated from the alveolus from a fall or a strike of some kind. Typically, a layer of periodontal ligament cells remains on the cemental surface of the avulsed tooth and on the bone in the socket, because of the very fast occurrence of the trauma. Successful treatment of avulsed teeth by replantation is dependent on rejoining intact periodontal ligament cells covering the cementum of the tooth to those remaining in the socket.

The object of this emergency treatment is to promote healing of the periodontal ligament once the tooth is replanted in the socket. To maximize the chances of healing, the tooth must be handled only by the crown to prevent damage to the remaining periodontal ligament cells. It is essential that the avulsed tooth not dry out and that it not be debrided in any way. As little as one hour of dry storage prior to replantation negatively affects the success rate of the procedure.[25]

The ideal place to store and transport the avulsed tooth is in the socket, if it can be gently placed and held there while the client is taken to an oral healthcare setting or a hospital emergency room. The socket provides the most nutritious environment for the cells of the periodontal ligament, thereby increasing their survival rate. If it is not possible to replace the tooth temporarily in the socket because of other injuries associated with the trauma, or emotional upset, physiologic saline is a safe alternative. Unfortunately, it may not be handy. Milk is also a good medium because it has physiologic osmolality and relatively few bacteria. Saliva has more bacteria than milk, but is a good way to keep the tooth moist. However, the client may be too upset or too young to hold the tooth in the mouth. Warm saltwater can prevent dehydration but cannot keep the cells alive long. Air-drying or wrapping the tooth in gauze or other materials, even for a short time, is contraindicated because that will kill the periodontal ligament cells.[24] Alternatives may have to be thought through quickly, and a decision made during a stressful situation to avoid dehydration and death of cells. The options for storage and transportation of the avulsed tooth are highlighted in Table 25–2.

At the emergency treatment facility the tooth should be removed from its transport medium, gently rinsed if necessary, replanted in the socket after the blood clot is removed, and splinted into place. A five- to seven-day course of systemic antibiotics typically used for dental infections should be prescribed. Endodontic procedures need to be performed at a later time, usually about two weeks after replantation, to avoid inflammatory root resorption.[26,27] The protocol to manage the avulsed tooth is presented in Procedure 25–1. A comparative summary of the conditions presented in this chapter can be found in Table 25–3.

TABLE 25–2 STORAGE OF AVULSED TEETH DURING TRANSPORTATION FOR TREATMENT

Choice	Transportation Medium
First	Replace in socket
Second	Store in physiologic saline
Third	Store in cold, fresh milk
Fourth	Place in the individual's mouth, under the tongue or in the cheek
Fifth	Store in warm saltwater
Sixth	Store in tap water

TABLE 25–3 SUMMARY COMPARISON OF ACUTE GINGIVAL AND PERIODONTAL CONDITIONS, LESIONS OF ENDODONTIC ORIGIN, AND AVULSED TEETH

Etiology	Risk Factors	Signs and Symptoms	Prevention and Management
Acute Periodontal Abscess			
Periodontal pathogens	Deep pockets Untreated periodontal disease	Swelling Redness Pain Exudate Sinus tract may occur	Education about the disease Scaling and root planing Referral for further treatment
Chronic Periodontal Abscess			
Periodontal pathogens	Deep pockets Untreated periodontal disease	Sinus tract Exudate Pain Swelling Redness Acute episodes	Education about the disease Scaling and root planing Referral for further treatment
Gingival Abscess			
Foreign object	Unknown	Swelling Redness Pain Exudate	Educate to prevent recurrences Refer for incision and drainage of abscess
Lesion of Endodontic Origin (LEO)			
Caries Periodontal disease Tooth fracture Traumatic dental procedures	Dental caries Periodontal disease Traumatic injury	Pain Swelling Sinus tract	Education to reduce likelihood of recurrences Refer for definitive endodontic treatment
Combined Periapical and Periodontal Abscess			
Caries Periodontal disease Tooth fracture Traumatic dental procedures	Dental caries Periodontal disease	Pain Swelling Bone loss	Education to reduce likelihood of recurrences Refer for definitive endodontic and periodontal treatment
Acute Herpetic Gingivostomatitis			
Herpes simplex virus	Age	Ulcers with halos Pain Systemic symptoms	Reappoint for dental procedures Education to prevent transmission to others Supportive care until the virus has run its course
Recurrent Herpetic Lesions			
Herpes simplex virus	History of recurrences Change in immune status	Ulcer on lip or perioral tissues	Reappoint for dental procedures Supportive treatment Inform about antiviral drugs Refer to physician
Acute Pericoronitis			
Bacterial plaque	Partially erupted molars Operculum	Pain Swelling Redness Foul odor	Education to pursue treatment and prevent recurrences Debride and irrigate area
Necrotizing Ulcerative Periodontitis			
Pathogenic bacteria	Systemic disease Stress Smoking	Pain Bleeding Fetid odor Redness Pseudomembrane Cratered papillae	Education to prevent recurrences Debridement over multiple appointments Definitive scaling as soon as possible Consultation with physician
Avulsed Tooth			
Trauma	Contact sports Accidents	Traumatic separation from alveolus	Preserve tooth in an appropriate transport medium Transport immediately to treatment facility for replantation of tooth Refer for endodontic treatment

Procedure 25–1 EMERGENCY MANAGEMENT OF THE AVULSED TOOTH

EQUIPMENT
Clean cup or other container
Transport medium

STEP	RATIONALE
1. Calm the individual or parent.	Quick action is necessary to increase the chance of successful replantation; emotional upset can cause delays.
2. Locate tooth.	Often the child or parent will not know that the tooth can be replanted.
3. Handle only by the crown and do not dry the tooth; do not debride the tooth.	Successful tooth replantation can occur only if periodontal ligament cells are alive and intact on the tooth surface.
4. Place in transport medium (Table 25–2).	Options for keeping the surface cells viable must be thought through quickly. A child may be too young to retain the tooth either in the socket or in the mouth
5. Contact dentist, dental office, or other emergency facility, such as a dental clinic or hospital emergency room.	Client or parent may be too upset to know where to call. Facilitate timely response to this emergency.
6. Arrange for transportation to treatment facility immediately.	If not personally taking the client to the treatment facility, make sure the parent or other driver knows where to go.
7. Record services rendered in dental chart.	Provides continuity of care and manages legal risks.

Client Education Issues

- ✦ Educate clients about disease transmission and lifestyle influences, particularly related to the herpes virus and necrotizing ulcerative periodontal diseases.
- ✦ Educate clients with painful oral infections to consume adequate fluids and nutrient-dense foods, perform oral hygiene, and use over-the-counter topical anesthetics to control discomfort.
- ✦ Review methods to prevent transmission of an active herpetic infection.
- ✦ Teach clients with a history of recurrent herpetic infection to cancel dental appointments when an active oral lesion is present.
- ✦ Review methods and treatment to prevent the recurrence of pericoronitis and necrotizing periodontal diseases.
- ✦ Teach parents, teachers, and coaches about avulsed teeth and their management to improve the probability for successful tooth replantation.
- ✦ Teach clients at risk of tooth avulsion about the need for a mouth protector.

Legal, Ethical, and Safety Issues

- ✦ Dental hygienists have a legal responsibility to recognize and refer emergency conditions and to treat those conditions within the scope of dental hygiene practice.
- ✦ Dental hygienists have an ethical responsibility to educate clients about the significance of their diseases and the potential for recurrence and infection of others.
- ✦ Dental hygienists have a responsibility to educate and refer clients in cases of dental trauma, and to prevent oral injuries when possible.
- ✦ Dental hygienists must consider personal safety from infectious diseases when treating clients with acute infectious conditions such as primary herpetic gingivostomatitis or herpes labialis.

Key Concepts

- Periodontal abscess is a treatable and often preventable disease process.
- LEO is a serious infection that requires consultation and referral for immediate treatment. Left untreated, LEO could develop into a brain abscess or fasciitis of the neck or chest wall, which can be life-threatening.
- Periodontal abscesses have a pathogenic microflora similar to that associated with periodontal diseases.
- Incomplete subgingival scaling and root planing has been suggested as a cause of periodontal abscesses; however, there are few data to support this assumption.
- Abscesses can point and drain through the tissue or simply drain through the periodontal pocket opening.
- Infection moves through tissue along the pathway of least resistance; therefore, clinical features of the infection may appear at a distance from the affected tooth.
- Primary and recurrent herpetic infections are serious but self-limiting conditions that require postponement of elective dental hygiene and dental treatment. Dental hygiene care should not be performed on a client with a herpetic infection because of the risk of transmission of the virus to the dental hygienist and other workers.
- Pericoronitis, at any stage, is a serious infection that requires referral and definitive treatment.
- Pain may be the key feature distinguishing between periapical and periodontal abscesses. Periapical pain is sharp, severe, intermittent, and hard to localize; periodontal pain is constant, less severe, and localized.
- Necrotizing ulcerative periodontal diseases are complex processes that benefit from the dental hygiene process of care.
- Mouth protectors and their fabrication are significant to comprehensive dental hygiene care.
- Avulsion is the most common dental injury to children younger than 15 years. The dental hygienist has a role in the management of avulsed teeth as possibly the most knowledgeable person at the scene of the traumatic injury.
- The ideal place to store and transport an avulsed tooth is in the victim's tooth socket; if this is not possible, physiologic saline is one alternative.

Critical Thinking Exercises

1. A 30-year-old client who has not been treated for several years arrives for a dental hygiene appointment. The client wants to have his "teeth cleaned today" but informs you about some pain and sensitivity in the lower right quadrant, and a tooth that feels "high" in that same area. The pain is intermittent but "very bothersome." After taking the medical and pharmacologic histories, you determine that he is in good general health with no systemic illnesses; he is taking no medications. Your intraoral findings indicate that the client has redness and swelling on the buccal surface of tooth #30. The gingival architecture appears normal, and there is no sinus tract, but pus can be elicited from the site by gentle finger pressure.

   A. What condition *most likely* is causing the client's symptoms?
   B. What is the *most likely* treatment for the condition?
   C. What dental hygiene diagnosis should be addressed first for this client?

2. A 20-year-old client comes to the dental office complaining of severe pain in the mouth. You determine that the client has no systemic illnesses and examine the oral tissues. The oral findings are extreme redness and swollen gingiva throughout the mouth and small, grayish ulcers on the gingiva and mucosa in several areas.

   A. What condition *most likely* is causing the client's symptoms?
   B. What is the *most likely* treatment for the condition?
   C. What dental hygiene diagnosis should be addressed first for this client?

3. The client comes to the dental office without an appointment, complaining of exquisite pain in the jaw. In fact, the client can hardly open her mouth. Based on a review of her medical and pharmacologic histories, the client is in good general health and takes no medications. Intraoral findings reveal extremely reddened and swollen gingiva on the mandibular right posterior area. The client complains of a bad taste in her mouth and says that the condition "comes and goes," but that this is the worst pain she has experienced. The client has many large amalgam restorations and appears to have a partially submerged molar in the quadrant.

   A. What is the *most likely* emergency condition?
   B. How should the dental hygiene component of the overall dental treatment begin?
   C. What dental hygiene diagnosis should be addressed first for this client?

Continued on following page

Critical Thinking Exercises—cont'd

4. A 45-year-old client arrives at the dental office without an appointment and complaining of severe pain. You seat the client, determine that she is in good general health, has no systemic illnesses, and is taking no medications. Intraoral examination reveals a large, pointed fistula associated on the buccal surface of tooth #3, about one-third of the way toward the apex of the tooth. The client has been treated for periodontal disease in the past, including some areas of periodontal surgery, and has many teeth restored with amalgam and composite restorations. There is a large MOD amalgam with a lingual extension on tooth #3. The radiograph you just took shows no obvious apical pathology.
   - **A.** What condition is *most likely* causing the client's symptoms?
   - **B.** What should the dental hygiene component of overall dental treatment that day include?
   - **C.** What dental hygiene diagnosis should be addressed first for this client?
5. A client arrives for his four-month continued-care appointment. He is very excited to be leaving tomorrow for a six-month stay in Europe and is anxious to have his dental hygiene maintenance care before he leaves. You notice a crusted lesion on his lower lip that is 6 mm round with some vesicles on the edge. He relates to you that he has never had such a sore before, that it was hurting a few days ago but is fine now. He requests that you cover the lesion with petroleum jelly so it will not crack while you are treating him.
   - **A.** What is the *most likely* condition present on the client's lip?
   - **B.** What is the dental hygiene care protocol for the client?
   - **C.** What dental hygiene diagnosis should be addressed first for this client?

For References, Suggested Readings, and Related Website, visit
http://evolve.elsevier.com/Darby/hygiene/

CHAPTER 26

FLUORIDES AND CHLORHEXIDINE

OBJECTIVES

Mastery of the content in this chapter will enable the reader to:

- Describe the multifactorial, infectious nature of dental caries
- Explain the process of demineralization and remineralization that occurs in the oral environment
- Distinguish between systemic and topical fluorides in dental caries prevention and management
- Evaluate clients' risk for dental caries based on objective and subjective evidence gathered
- Design a caries management plan based on client needs and the fluoride products available
- Administer a professional fluoride treatment (foam or gel) utilizing the tray technique
- Administer a professional fluoride varnish treatment utilizing the paint-on technique
- Differentiate between acute and chronic fluoride toxicity based on causes and management
- Discuss chlorhexidine delivery systems for dental caries management

KEY TERMS

Acidogenic plaque biofilm
Acute fluoride toxicity
Caries management
Caries risk assessment
Cariogenic plaque biofilm
Certainly lethal dose (CLD)
Chlorhexidine
Chronic fluoride toxicity
Critical pH
Demineralization
Dental caries
Dental caries process
Dental fluorosis
Dentifrices
Early childhood caries (ECC)
Fluorapatite crystals
Fluoridated community
Fluoride
Fluoride varnish
Nonfluoridated community
Professionally applied fluoride
Remineralization
Safely tolerated dose (STD)
Self-applied fluoride
Stephan's Curve
Systemic fluoride
Topical fluoride

REVIEW OF DENTAL CARIES PROCESS

A Continuing Health Issue

"[D]espite the major decline in dental caries prevalence that has occurred in many countries, dental decay remains the single most common disease of childhood that is not self-limiting or amenable to a course of antibiotics."[1] Dental caries is the most common dental disease afflicting children and adults in the United States, and it remains a significant worldwide disease.[2]

Bacterial-based Disease

Dental caries are caused by *mutans streptococci* (a group that includes the *Streptococcus mutans* and *Streptococcus sobrinus* species) and lactobacilli that live in the plaque biofilm that attach to teeth. These bacteria metabolize dietary fermentable carbohydrates (sugars and cooked starch) to produce acids. These acids diffuse into the tooth to dissolve the calcium and phosphate minerals (carbonated hydroxyapatite), a process called *demineralization*.[2a,2b] If the acid attacks are infrequent and of short duration, saliva can help repair the damage by neutralizing the acid and replacing minerals and fluoride lost from the tooth. This process is called *remineralization*. If, however, the flow of saliva is low, the bacterial level is high, and the frequency of client snacking is high, the tooth mineral lost by acid attacks is too great for repair by remineralization. This situation leads to the start of dental caries.

Dental caries involves an interaction among pathologic factors and protective factors. *Pathologic factors* include acidogenic (acid producing) bacteria (*mutans streptococci* and lactobacilli), low saliva flow due to salivary gland dysfunction or the use of many medications, and many fermentable carbohydrates in the diet. Protective factors include calcium, phosphate, proteins, and fluoride in the saliva; normal salivary flow; and antibacterial agents if needed (Figure 26-1).[2a–2c]

DEMINERALIZATION. *Demineralization* is the first stage of dental caries. When teeth have bacterial plaque biofilm adhering to them, acidogenic bacteria in the biofilm metabolize fermentable carbohydrates (sucrose, glucose, starches, etc.) and produce acids. These acids can then dissolve the calcium phosphate mineral of the enamel and dentin. The acids diffuse through the plaque biofilm, dissociate to produce hydrogen ions, move to the enamel surface, and dissolve the tooth mineral. Demineralization results in the greatest loss of calcium and phosphate minerals in the *subsurface zone* of the enamel and the formation of a white spot lesion. The enamel surface of the white spot typically remains intact, but the demineralized area appears white due to the loss of mineral in the subsurface zone of the enamel. By comparison, the enamel surrounding the white spot appears sound and translucent.[4]

The resulting acid environment created when plaque bacteria act on fermentable carbohydrates results in a substantial change in the plaque pH. At rest, the pH of plaque is typically neutral. When fermentable carbohydrates are ingested, the plaque pH drops rapidly to create an acid environment conducive to demineralization. Demineralization occurs when the pH drops to 5.5; this is the *critical pH*.

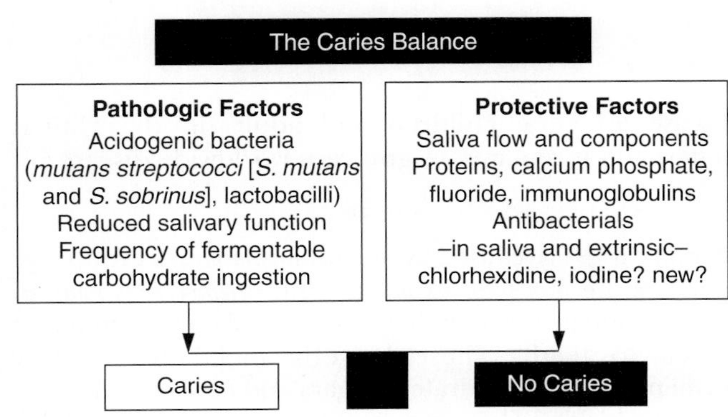

FIGURE 26–1 ✦ Schematic illustration of the "caries balance." *(Adapted from Featherstone; from the California Dental Jounal.)*

After the ingestion of fermentable carbohydrates stops, the pH gradually returns to neutral in 30 to 60 minutes. This drop in pH and the return to normal over time, initially reported by Stephan, is referred to as *Stephan's Curve*.[3] A variety of factors mediate the return to a neutral pH. Saliva plays a key role in that it neutralizes acids and provides minerals and proteins that protect the teeth (see Saliva's Beneficial Actions).

Demineralization and development of a white spot lesion relate to enamel surfaces. The demineralization process for cementum and dentin is similar to that described for enamel, except that the process does not typically result in an intact surface remaining over the body of the carious lesion.[2]

REMINERALIZATION. Once calcium and phosphate are lost from the tooth structure and the pH in the adjacent environment returns to neutral, the area experiences remineralization. Minerals in the saliva and minerals precipitated out of the tooth are available to redeposit on the tooth surface. This deposition of minerals into demineralized areas of tooth structure is *remineralization*, which repairs the initial carious lesion. This ongoing process of destruction and repair occurs with each carbohydrate challenge.

Whether or not an initial carious lesion progresses and develops into a frank carious lesion depends on a variety of factors. To prevent the lesion from progressing, there must be enough deposition of salivary minerals to repair and strengthen the area and provide support for the enamel surface. Minerals in the saliva initially enable the host to repair demineralized areas. Systemic and topical fluorides also play a role in the remineralization repair process and the overall prevention of carious lesions.

DENTAL CARIES RISK OVER THE LIFESPAN

Persons are at risk for developing dental caries beginning when they are infants and continuing for as long as they have their teeth. *Early childhood caries* (ECC), an infectious disease that affects children from birth to

Saliva's Beneficial Actions

Provides calcium and phosphate for remineralization
Carries topical fluoride around the mouth for remineralization
Neutralizes organic acids produced in plaque biofilm
Discourages growth of bacteria, inhibiting infection
Recycles ingested fluoride into the mouth
Protects hard and soft tissues from drying
Facilitates chewing and swallowing
Speeds oral clearance of food

From Eakle SW, Featherstone JDB: *Caries risk instruction*, Course Handout, San Francisco, 2002, University of California School of Dentistry.

2 years of age, rapidly destroys newly erupted teeth. Initially, ECC appears as bands of demineralized areas usually first seen on the primary maxillary incisors. These areas of demineralization quickly move onto yellow or brown cavitated areas.[5]

The cause of ECC is complex. The primary cause of demineralization in infants and toddlers involves the three factors of host, dental plaque, and diet. ECC involves:

Microbiologic Factors: Mothers and siblings are able to transmit *Streptococcus mutans* to infants and young children.

Local Factors: Frequent or prolonged feedings with bottled milk, formula, or human breast milk. Both cow's milk and formula contain fermentable carbohydrates. Also, breast milk is a poor buffer and becomes highly cariogenic in the presence of foods containing fermentable carbohydrates. Other local risk factors include lack of systemic fluoride and poor oral hygiene.

Physical Development: Birth weight of less than 5.5 pounds and dental defects.

Environmental Issues: The ingestion of lead or other heavy metals negatively affects salivary gland function, as does the ingestion of medications that may cause xerostomia.[5]

Based on ECC prevalence, the American Academy of Pediatric Dentistry recommends that children receive a dental examination as infants, prior to the age of 1 year. A parental interview, examination, education of parents/caregivers, and a demonstration of preventive measures can substantially decrease the risks for ECC.[5]

Dental caries is also an issue for the elderly. The degree of demineralization and its progression are mediated by a variety of contributing factors that occur throughout the client's life, such as medications, medical interventions (e.g., radiation), and gingival recession (resulting in root exposure and potential infection). As long as teeth are present, they are at risk for demineralization and ultimately frank carious lesions.[6]

DENTAL CARIES RISK ASSESSMENT

The term *caries risk* suggests the probability of an individual developing future dental caries. The goal of *caries risk assessment* is early identification of clients at risk for developing future caries and to implement interventions that address the remineralizing needs of the early carious lesions and/or prevent future caries. To date, the most consistent predictor of future caries is the presence of recent cavities. Other factors associated with caries include deep pits and fissures, poor oral hygiene, xerostomia, increased amounts of cariogenic bacteria, and poor diet (Table 26–1).

Caries Risk Assessment Guidelines

Caries risk assessment offers a valuable tool for clinical practice and can be tailored to specific client groups.

TABLE 26–1 CARIES RISK CLASSIFICATION GUIDELINES

	Age Category for Continued-Care Clients	
Risk Category	**Child/Adolescent**	**Adult**
Low	No carious lesions in last year Coalesced or sealed pits and fissures Good oral hygiene Appropriate fluoride use Regular dental visits	No carious lesions in last three years Adequately restored surfaces Good oral hygiene Regular dental visits
Moderate	One carious lesion in last year Deep pits and fissures Fair oral hygiene Inadequate fluoride White spots and/or interproximal radiolucencies Irregular dental visits	One carious lesion in last three years Exposed roots Fair oral hygiene White spots and/or interproximal radiolucencies Irregular dental visits
High	Two or more carious lesions in last year Orthodontic treatment Past smooth-surface caries Elevated *mutans streptococci* count Deep pits and fissures No/little systemic and topical fluoride exposure Poor oral hygiene Frequent sugar intake Irregular dental visits Inadequate saliva flow Inappropriate bottle feeding or nursing (infants)	Two or more carious lesions in last 3 years Orthodontic treatment Past root caries or large number of exposed roots Elevated *mutans streptococci* and/or lactobacilli count Deep pits and fissures Poor oral hygiene Frequent between-meal snacking or sugar intake Inadequate use of topical fluoride Irregular dental visits Inadequate saliva flow

Modified from American Dental Association, Council on Access, Prevention and Interprofessional Relations: Treating caries as an infectious disease, *Journal of the American Dental Association, Special Supplement* 126(suppl):1, 1995.

Table 26–1 outlines a classification guideline developed for children/adolescents and adults. Given that caries can progress at different rates, this classification designates a one-year time frame for children and three years for adults.[7] Evidence demonstrates that 70% of the population experience no caries per year, but 10% will experience one caries and 20% experience two or more caries per year.[8] On the basis of this evidence, a child with no new caries in a year and no significant modifying factors is classified as low risk. No caries and no modifying factors within a three-year period classifies an adult also as low risk. For moderate-risk groups, some significant modifying factors may be identified along with one caries per year for children, and one caries per three years for adults. High-risk groups may also have significant modifying factors and would include children with two or more caries per year and adults with two or more caries per three years.

Caries Risk Assessment Form[2a]

As described in the Caries Management Risk Assessment Consensus Statement in 2002[2a], Table 26–2 shows a caries risk assessment form for children 6 years of age and older and for adults (see www.cdafoundation.org for a caries risk assessment form for children 0 to 5 years of age). Questions 1 and 2 on the form shown in Table 26–2 relate to risk factors for dental caries. These questions are responded to with "yes" or "no" answers, and special notations are made such as the number of caries present, the number of restored caries in the past 3 years, the oral hygiene status, the type of fluorides used, the type and frequency of snacks consumed to determine the number and duration of acid challenges per day, and the names of medications that cause dry mouth used. Question 3 on the form relates to factors that protect tooth surfaces from caries such as fluoridation and topical fluoride use.

SALIVARY FLOW RATE TEST. Saliva neutralizes acids and provides minerals and proteins that protect the teeth from dental caries. Therefore it is essential for controlling dental caries. If visually inadequate saliva flow is noticed, or if the client reports having a dry mouth, then a saliva flow rate test should be conducted. This test is accomplished by having the client chew a paraffin pellet for 3 to 5 minutes and spit all saliva generated into a cup. The saliva is then measured in milliliters (ml) and divided by the amount of time it took to generate the saliva to determine the ml/minute of stimulated salivary flow. A flow rate of 1 ml/minute and above is considered normal; a level of 0.7 ml/minute is low; and a level of 0.5 ml/minute or less is considered dry, indicating a high-risk situation. The reason for the low salivary flow rate needs to be determined to plan for caries management. The client should be informed of the results and their implications for dental caries.[2a]

CARIES BACTERIA TESTING. If the answer is "yes" to question 1(a) or to any two questions from 1(b) to 1(g) on the form, bacterial testing is indicated. In the United States, at the time of writing, one readily available chairside test for cariogenic bacteria testing is the Caries Risk Test (CRT) marketed by Vivadent (Amherst, NY). This test allows a bacterial culture to be made from collected saliva and is sensitive enough to provide a level of low, medium, or high cariogenic bacterial challenge. The test kit comes with two-sided selective media sticks that assess *mutans streptococci* on the blue side and lactobacilli on the green side. Incubators suitable for a dental office also are sold by the company. Results are available after 48 hours.[2a] Directions for use of the test are as follows:

1. Remove the selective media stick from the culture tube. Peel off the plastic cover sheet from each side of the stick.
2. Pour the collected saliva over the medium on each side until it is wet.
3. Replace the media stick in the culture tube, screw the lid on, and label the tube with the client's name, registration number, and date. Place the tube in the incubator at 37° C for 48 hours.
4. Collect the tube after 48 hours and compare the densities of bacterial colonies with the pictures provided in the kit indicating relative bacterial levels. The dark blue agar is selective for *mutans streptococci* and the light green agar is selective for lactobacilli. Record the level of bacterial challenge in the client's record as low, medium, or high. The client should be informed of the results and their implications for caries risk and caries management.

Results of this bacterial test also can be used to motivate client compliance with recommended antibacterial regimens.[2a]

DETERMINATION OF CARIES RISK. To determine the caries risk for an individual, the clinician evaluates the number and severity of the risk factors. An individual with current caries or caries in the recent past is at risk for future caries. However, a client with low bacterial levels would need to have several other risk factors to be considered at moderate risk. The clinician also considers the existing protective factors and uses clinical judgment to determine risk.[2a]

CARIES MANAGEMENT

Caries management is aimed at restoring and maintaining a balance between protective factors and pathologic factors (Figure 26–1). Caries management involves:

- ✦ Suppressing bacteria that cause the infection
- ✦ Remineralizing early noncavitated carious lesions by enhancing salivary flow and using fluorides
- ✦ Protecting tooth surfaces by using sealants and fluorides
- ✦ Decreasing the frequency of sugar intake
- ✦ Surgically removing carious lesions that are beyond hope of remineralization and restoring the teeth with minimally invasive techniques and materials[2b]

TABLE 26–2

CARIES RISK ASSESSMENT FORM FOR CHILDREN 6 YEARS AND OLDER/ADULTS

Instructions on reverse

Patient Name:________________________ **I.D. #** ____________ **Age** ______ **Date** __________

Initial/baseline exam date________________________ **Recall/POE date**________________

Respond to each question in sections 1,2, and 3 with a check mark in the yes or no column			**Notes**
	Yes	**No**	
1. High Risk Factors**			
(a) Visible cavitation (carious) or caries into dentin by radiograph			
(b) Caries restored in past three years			
(c) Readily visible heavy plaque on teeth			
(d) Frequent (greater than three times daily) between-meal snacks of sugars/cooked starch			
(e) **Saliva-reducing factors:**			
1. Hyposalivatory medications			
2. Radiation to head and neck			
3. Systemic reasons, e.g., Sjögren's			
(f*) Visually inadequate saliva flow. (If yes, measure) less than 0.7 ml/min by test= low salivary flow or dry mouth			Amount:_________ ml/min
(g) Appliances present, fixed or removable, e.g., orthodontic brackets/bands/retainer or removable partial denture(s)			
2. Moderate Risk Factors			
(a) Exposed roots			
(b) Deep pits & fissures/developmental defects			
(c) Interproximal enamel lesions/radiolucencies			
(d) Other white spot lesions or occlusal discoloration			
(e) Uses recreational drugs			
3. Protective Factors			
(a) Lives/works/school in fluoridated community			
(b) Uses fluoride toothpaste daily			Type ____________
(c) Uses fluoride mouthwash/rinse/gel daily			Type ____________
(d*) Salivary flow visually adequate >1 ml/min by test			
(e) Uses xylitol gum or mints 4x day			Type ______ and % xylitol ______
(f) Mother/caregiver has no caries activity			Brand ____________ Frequency_______

****If yes to 1 (a) or any two of 1 (b)-(g), perform bacterial culture***	**High Count Date:**_____	**Moderate Count Date:**_______	**Low Count Date:** _______	
(a) Mutans streptococci				(Place a check in the box below the count)
(b) Lactobacillus				(Place a check in the box below the count)
Caries risk overall* (see over)	**High**	**Moderate**	**Low**	**Circle High, Moderate or Low**

Recommendations given: yes_____ **no** _______ Date given: ______ or Date follow up: ______

*Indicates that test descriptions for these procedures are on the following pages

Increasing protective factors involves strategies such as the use of fluorides, sealants, and agents to increase salivary flow; sugar-free gum, baking soda rinses, and baking soda gum; and other medications. Decreasing pathologic factors involves strategies such as client education, oral hygiene instruction, reducing the intake of fermentable carbohydrates, and the use of chlorhexidine rinse and/or xylitol gum.[2b]

After determining the caries risk of an individual, the clinician provides the client with educational material about the caries process (see www.cdafoundation.org for Patient Information Sheet on Tooth Decay) and makes recommendations based on test results, responses to questions, and clinical observation. Table 26–3 provides caries management strategies for low-, moderate-, and high-risk children and adults by risk assessment and age group. Also see Target Areas for Caries Management. The client's compliance with recommendations is assessed 3 to 6 months after the initial visit. If bacterial levels were moderate or high at the initial visit, repeat them to see if they have been reduced. Recommendations should be modified or reinforced based on bacterial results and patient compliance.[1]

FLUORIDE THERAPIES

Fluoride is a naturally occurring nutrient that in the right concentrations can decrease the likelihood of dental caries. As a preventive agent, fluoride may be delivered systemically or topically (Table 26–4).

Systemic fluoride products are ingested and delivered to the oral cavity via the bloodstream.

Topical fluoride products are utilized intraorally for variable amounts of time, provide fluoride to exposed crown and root surfaces, and are then expectorated.

Primary Mechanisms of Action

Fluoride inhibits demineralization when present in solution. Fluoride present on the tooth surface and in plaque

TARGET AREAS FOR CARIES MANAGEMENT

Target Area	Strategy
Tooth	Sealants and in-office and home fluorides
Diet	Controlled consumption and frequency of sugar intake
Acid in mouth	Baking soda rinses; enhanced saliva with salivary substitutes and sugarless gum (baking soda and xylitol)
Low saliva flow	Sugarless gum, drugs (e.g., 20 to 30 mg pilocarpine/day)
Bacteria	Good oral hygiene instruction; powered toothbrushes; chlorhexidine rinse

From Eakle SW, Featherstone JDB: Caries risk instruction, Course Handout, San Francisco, 2002, University of California School of Dentistry.

TABLE 26–3 CARIES MANAGEMENT BY RISK ASSESSMENT AND AGE GROUP

Risk Category	Child/Adolescent	Adult
Low	Educational reinforcement of good oral hygiene and use of fluoride dentifrice 1 year recall	Education about the caries process and reinforcement of good oral hygiene and use of fluoride dentifrice 1 year recall
Moderate	Dental sealants Educational reinforcement Dietary counseling Fluoride mouthrinse* Professional topical fluoride Sealants Brushing with fluoride dentifrice Fluoride supplements 6-month continued-care interval	Dental sealants Educational reinforcement Dietary counseling Fluoride mouthrinse Professional topical fluoride Sealants Brushing with fluoride dentifrice 6-month continued-care interval
High	Educational reinforcement Brushing with fluoride dentifrice Dental sealants Home fluoride (0.05% NaF mouthrinse/1.1% NaF gel custom trays at bedtime*) Professional topical fluoride at each visit Dietary counseling Monitoring of *mutans streptococci* and lactobacilli count Antimicrobial agents Fluoride supplements 3- to 6-month continued-care interval	Educational reinforcement Brushing with fluoride dentifrice Home fluoride (0.05% NaF mouthrinse/1.1% NaF gel custom trays at bedtime*) Professional topical fluoride at each visit Dietary counseling Monitoring of *mutans streptococci* and lactobacilli count Antimicrobial agents 3- to 6-month continued-care interval

* Not for children under 6 years of age.

Adapted from American Dental Association, Council on Access, Prevention and Interpersonal Relations: Treating caries as an infectious disease, *Journal of the American Dental Association, Special Supplement* 126(suppl):1, 1995; from Eakle SW, Featherstone JDB: Caries risk instruction, Course Handout, San Francisco, 2002, University of California San Francisco School of Dentistry.

TABLE 26–4 **FLUORIDE THERAPIES**

Fluoride Therapies	Available Preparations	Preeruptive Benefits	Posteruptive Benefits
Systemic	Community water fluoridation School water fluoridation Fluoride supplements Foods containing fluoride Salt	Incorporation of fluoride into the mineralizing structure during tooth development	Fluoride present in saliva enhances the mineralization of enamel during the enamel maturation phase. Systemic fluoride can have a crossover topical benefit as it passes through the oral cavity. As such, it inhibits demineralization and enhances remineralization (e.g., when fluoridated water passes over the teeth or when fluoride supplements are chewed or dissolved in the oral cavity prior to being swallowed).
Topical	Professionally applied fluoride agents (high potency products) Self-applied fluoride agents (lower potency products in the form of dentifrices, rinses, and gels)	Not the intended mechanism of action for topical agents Can only occur if topical agents are swallowed and then become systemic agents	Inhibits the action of acidogenic bacteria Inhibits demineralization Enhances remineralization

fluid inhibits acid demineralization by reducing the solubility of the tooth mineral.

Fluoride enhances remineralization. Fluoride accelerates the remineralization process by adsorbing to the tooth surface and attracting calcium ions. In addition, fluoride ions incorporate into the remineralizing tooth structure, resulting in the development of *fluorapatite crystals*. These crystals are less soluble than the original enamel mineral and make remineralized lesions less susceptible to future demineralization.

Fluoride inhibits plaque bacteria. Fluoride present in plaque is taken up by acid-producing bacteria and interferes with acid production.[4]

Fluoride is incorporated into the tooth mineral during tooth development (preeruptive). Some preventive benefit also is gained from systemic fluoride being incorporated into the developing tooth structure preeruptively. Recent research has questioned whether systemic fluoride incorporated into the tooth via this process is adequate to actually make the tooth more resilient to acid attack. Discussion and debate continue on this issue; a continuing review of the scientific literature enables the dental hygienist to evaluate this mechanism of fluoride action.[2,4,10]

Fluoride has posteruptive benefits. Fluoride is incorporated into the outermost layers of enamel during the enamel maturation period.[2]

Systemic Fluoride

Systemic fluorides are delivered via the community water supply or school-based water system, in the form of supplements (drops, lozenges, or tablets), and in foodstuffs (naturally occurring/added). In the United States the most common systemic fluoride delivery is via the community water supply. Approximately 62% of the U.S. population resides in communities where the water supply is fluoridated. This statistic reflects 70% of the U.S. cities with a population of over 100,000 and 42 of the 50 largest U.S. cities.[11]

COMMUNITY WATER FLUORIDATION. The notion of fluoridating the community water supply grew out of a need to address the prevalence of dental caries in the United States in the 1940s. At that time, the population was not exposed to the myriad of fluoride products that the population is exposed to today. Due to the dramatic drop in caries prevalence that occurred as a result of initial community fluoridation efforts (approximately 50%), some have "characterized community water fluoridation as one of the great disease prevention measures of all time…."[11]

Community water fluoridation is a nearly ideal public health measure. Community water fluoridation is a positive intervention because the system is:

- Inexpensive
- Effective
- Eminently safe
- Equitable (i.e., benefits the entire population)
- Not dependent on client compliance (cooperative effort)
- Beneficial over the client's lifespan as long as water consumption continues
- Instrumental in reducing costs for dental treatment
- Not dependent on the professional services of a licensed healthcare provider

As a public health measure, community water fluoridation calls for testing of the community water supply to determine the naturally occurring level of fluoride. The level of fluoride is then adjusted through fluoridation or defluoridation to the accepted level of 0.7–1.2 parts per million (ppm),[1] depending on the areas average climate. Defluoridation is necessary if the naturally occurring level of fluoride in the water exceeds the recommended level, putting the public at risk for dental fluorosis.

Although the benefits of community water fluoridation are well documented,[1,2,12] some individuals oppose this public health measure and actively seek to prevent or reverse water fluoridation programs. Antifluoridationists have a range of arguments for why community water supplies should not be fluoridated. They associate fluoride ingestion with an increased risk for certain systemic diseases and conditions (congenital anomalies, bone fractures, Alzheimer's disease, cancer, etc.), and view mandated fluoride ingestion as a conspiracy by the government, the healthcare industry, and others. These individuals cite a variety of other reasons for their antifluoride stance, including cost, freedom of choice, and a violation of individual and religious rights.[11] Antifluoridationists have been effective in blocking community fluoride programs in many areas.

BEVERAGES AND OTHER FOODSTUFFS. The public is exposed to a variety of foodstuffs that contain fluoride, and become part of the client's overall exposure to systemic fluoride. There is considerable variation in the amount of fluoride in products routinely ingested; thorough questioning is necessary to document this information during client assessment procedures (Chapter 9, Table 9–2 and Figure 9–3).

As infants, people primarily ingest breast milk, cow's milk, and milk-based and soy-based formulas. Fluoride levels are generally low in human breast milk (<0.01 ppm) and cow's milk (0.05 ppm). The amount of fluoride in milk-based formulas has varied over time. When the formula industry recognized that milk-based formula might be reconstituted with fluoridated water, many voluntarily reduced the fluoride content in powdered formula. Formula packaging should be consulted to determine fluoride levels in the prepared powder. Ready-to-use soy-based formulas have more fluoride than do milk-based products (0.30 ppm).[13]

Beverages prepared from natural ingredients may be a systemic source of fluoride. Raw tea leaves are high in fluoride content and contain as much as 400 ppm of fluoride. Brewed tea contains an average of 3 ppm of fluoride. This is a risk factor for dental fluorosis in cultures where children consume tea on a daily basis (e.g., Asian Indians and Asians).[13]

The fluoride level in processed beverages and bottled waters varies considerably. For example, fluoride content in fruit juices and carbonated beverages ranges from <0.1 to 6.7 ppm. The differences in fluoride content in processed beverages can be attributed to the variations in the fluoride levels of the water used to prepare these products.[13] Although there is also variation in the fluoride content of bottled waters, these beverages generally have low fluoride concentration. Bottled waters are marketed as distilled, drinking, mineral, or natural spring waters and may be carbonated or noncarbonated.[12] Given that consumption of tap water among U.S. children has declined and consumption of other beverages has grown, it is becoming increasingly difficult for healthcare providers to assess clients' fluoride exposure via fluid intake.[13]

Other foodstuffs such as seafood products, processed baby food, and chicken may also contain substantial levels of fluoride.[13] Increased utilization of prepared foods influences fluoride intake. Prepared foods are generally processed in urban areas with fluoridated water, and become additional sources of fluoride for individuals living in both fluoridated and nonfluoridated communities. Internationally, other foodstuffs are utilized as vehicles for delivering fluoride. In countries such as Switzerland, Jamaica, and France, fluoride is incorporated into table salt.[1]

PRESCRIPTION SUPPLEMENTS. Fluoride supplements in the form of drops, lozenges, or tablets, were developed as vehicles for providing systemic fluoride to children residing in *nonfluoridated communities* (community without water fluoridation or having well water with low/nondetectable levels of fluoride). The goal of supplementation was to have children in nonfluoridated communities reach a similar level of caries reduction as children living in *fluoridated communities.* Initial data reported in the 1960s and 1970s indicated that supplementation seemed to be achieving this goal.[2,14]

Beginning in the 1980s, fluoride supplementation underwent close scrutiny. Considerable debate remains regarding this issue because of the following factors:

- Studies indicate that fluoride supplementation results in an increased risk for dental fluorosis; the risk has increased over the years due to clients' exposure to multiple sources of fluoride[2]
- Clients' exposure to multiple sources of topical and systemic fluorides
- Improper prescriptive dosages of fluoride supplements, and supplements being prescribed inadvertently by both dentists and pediatricians
- Improper use of fluoride supplements in fluoridated communities
- Fluoride supplements being recommended for clients ingesting well water as their primary water source prior to the well water being tested to determine the naturally occurring level of fluoride
- Lack of compliance by clients/parents

After an evaluation of these issues, the American Dental Association Council on Scientific Affairs published a recommended supplementation schedule[14] (Table 26–5). Fluoride supplementation recommendations are based on client age and the level of fluoride in the primary water source. When supplementation is considered, assessment procedures should include questions about the client's primary water source (i.e., fluoridated community water supply, nonfluoridated community water supply, well water, filtered water, etc.), and exposure to other sources of systemic fluoride (see Chapter 9, section on dental history).

Should supplementation be recommended, it should be done in consultation with the child's pediatrician/primary medical care provider. This will prevent a child from receiving duplicate prescriptions for fluoride supplements. Given that many pediatric dentists are recommending that children be seen in general dental offices as infants, there is an increased risk that a child could be given prescriptions by more than one provider. Table 26–6 describes various types of fluoride supplements and recommendations for their use.

RISK OF CHRONIC FLUORIDE TOXICITY (DENTAL FLUOROSIS). *Dental fluorosis* is the hypomineralization of the enamel that results from the chronic ingestion of fluoride that exceeds optimal levels. This alteration in the enamel occurs during tooth formation and is therefore only a risk during the preeruptive stages of tooth development.[1,15] Dental fluorosis may be associated with chronic fluoride toxicity and can occur only as a result of systemic ingestion of fluoride (Figure 26–2).

TABLE 26–5 ADA/CDT GUIDELINES FOR PEDIATRIC SUPPLEMENT DOSAGE (1994)

	Level of Fluoride in Primary Water Supply		
Client Age	**<0.3 ppm Fl**	**0.3–0.6 ppm Fl**	**>0.6 ppm Fl**
Birth to 6 months	None	None	None
6 months to 3 years	0.25 mg	0	0
3 years to 6 years	0.50 mg	0.25 mg	0
6 years to at least 16 years	1.00 mg	0.50 mg	0

From Pendrys DG: Risk of enamel fluorosis in nonfluoridated and optimally fluoridated populations: Considerations for dental professionals, *Journal of the American Dental Association* 131:746, 2000.

Clients cannot develop fluorosis as a result of topical fluoride exposure, even if the topical exposure is excessive (high-concentration fluoride at frequent intervals). The only way a client can develop dental fluorosis from topical fluoride is by swallowing the product and changing the mechanism of fluoride action from topical to systemic. There is a particular fluorosis risk from the ingestion of low-concentration fluoride products such as dentifrices. These products are of concern because they are used unsupervised by young children, have an appealing taste and appearance, are often swallowed, and may be stored within reach of small children. The administration of professionally applied, high-concentration fluoride products may initially appear to be a risk factor for dental fluorosis. Scientific evidence confirms that fluoride ingestion occurs as the result of topical treatments and that plasma levels of fluoride are elevated after the treatment. Even though the concentration of fluoride in professional products is high, the infrequent

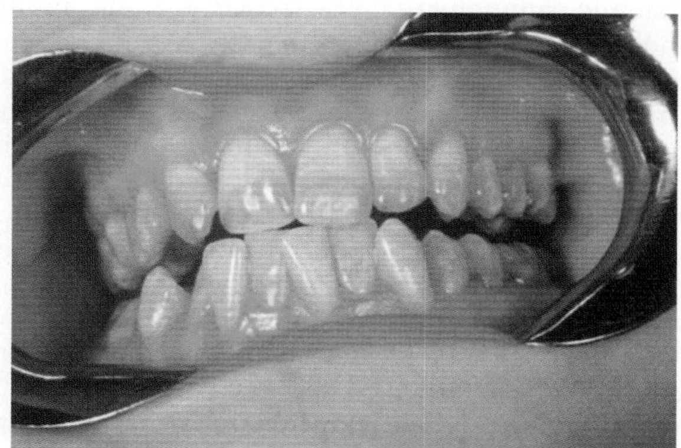

FIGURE 26–2 ✦ Dental fluorosis. *(From Ibsen OAC, Phelan JA:* Oral pathology for the dental hygienist, *ed 3, Philadelphia, 2000, WB Saunders.)*

TABLE 26–6 CONSIDERATIONS FOR THE USE OF PRESCRIPTION FLUORIDE SUPPLEMENTS*

Available Forms of Fluoride Supplements	Recommended Method for Ingestion	Indications for Use
Drops	Swallowed, then avoid milk products for one hour as calcium may interfere with the bioavailability of fluoride.	Children under 2 years of age who ingest nonfluoridated or under-fluoridated water and are at an elevated risk for dental caries. Infants who are solely breast fed and do not ingest a significant amount of prepared infant foods and/or cereals, etc. that are reconstituted with fluoridated water.
Tablets	Chewed, then avoid milk products for one hour as calcium may interfere with the bioavailability of fluoride.	Children from 2–16 years who ingest nonfluoridated and underfluoridated water and are at an elevated risk for dental caries.
Lozenges	Retained in oral cavity until dissolve, then avoid milk products for one hour as calcium may interfere with the bioavailability of fluoride.	Children from 2–16 years who ingest non/under-fluoridated water and are at an elevated risk for dental caries.

From Levy SM, Kiritsy MC, Warren JJ: Sources of fluoride intake in children, *Journal of Public Health Dentistry* 55(1):39, 1995; Newburn E: *Fluorides and dental caries,* Springfield, Ill, 1986 Charles C Thomas; Tate WH, Chan J: Fluoride concentration in bottled and filtered waters, *General Dentistry* 42(4):362, 1994.

application of these products does not result in enamel disturbances that are clinically evident.[7]

Dental fluorosis is detected by clinical evaluation and classified (Table 26–7). Mild dental fluorosis is often difficult to identify and requires careful assessment and good lighting. In its mildest form, dental fluorosis appears as faint white lines or streaks. Moderate to severe cases of fluorosis manifest as white mottling of the teeth (white lines coalesce into larger opaque areas) or brown staining or pitting of the enamel. Although some consider fluorosis primarily to be an aesthetic concern, in its most severe state the enamel may actually break down.[15]

SYSTEMIC FLUORIDE ISSUES FOR CONSIDERATION.

- Community water fluoridation remains a successful public health program and is the cornerstone of a fluoride protocol.[10] This systemic fluoride vehicle is available to all individuals residing in fluoridated communities, regardless of socioeconomic background or ability to access other types of fluoride.
- Debate continues regarding the need for additional systemic supplementation (based on the multiple sources of fluoride children receive from prepared foodstuffs, prepared beverages, and naturally occurring fluoride). Scientific literature provides the dental hygienist with evidence to support clinical decisions regarding supplementation.
- Many households use bottled waters as their primary water source. Bottled waters have low fluoride concentrations and typically do not indicate fluoride content.[12] Some bottled water manufacturers have addressed this issue by identifying fluoride content on product labels. Other companies are adding fluoride and using the added fluoride as a marketing tool (e.g., "nursery water with fluoride").
- It has become common for individuals to filter the community water supply by attaching water filtration devices to household water taps (reverse osmosis, bubbling ozone, activated charcoal, etc.). Many of these water filtration systems remove significant amounts of fluoride from the water.[12]

TABLE 26–7 CLASSIFICATION OF DEGREE OF DENTAL FLUOROSIS

Grade of Fluorosis	Description
Normal	None
Questionable	A few white flecks or white spots
Very mild	Small, opaque, paper-white areas involving less than 25% of the surface
Mild	White opacities are more extensive but do not involve as much as 50% of the surface
Moderate	All enamel surfaces affected; frequent brown staining
Severe	Discrete or confluent pitting; brown stains are widespread; all enamel surfaces affected

Newburn E: *Fluorides and dental caries,* Springfield, Ill, 1986, Charles C Thomas.

- Persons who use well water as their primary water sources should have the well water tested to determine its fluoride level.[15] Without this information, it is impossible to prescribe fluoride supplements. In addition, consideration may be given to how dental hygienists and other dental providers can facilitate water testing by providing clients with testing kits and submitting specimens for testing.
- Well water may contain water from various sources (with varying fluoride concentrations).
- Some water supplies are poorly monitored for optimum fluoride.
- There may be a systemic effect from topical fluoride preparations.
- Some topical preparations, especially dentifrices, may be swallowed, causing the client to receive both a topical and systemic exposure to fluoride. Children must be monitored when using fluoride products to decrease the risks for dental fluorosis.

Systemic fluoride delivery, especially community water fluoridation, has a track record of success in reducing caries incidence. A National Institutes of Health Consensus Conference on the Diagnosis and Management of Dental Caries (March 2001) did not evaluate the effectiveness of water fluoridation because "it is widely accepted as both effective and of great importance in the primary prevention of dental caries." Other issues surrounding the use of systemic fluorides and their impact on the client care will require continued monitoring. Just as with other client care decisions, the scientific literature provides evidence to substantiate changes in systemic fluoride protocols.

Topical Fluoride[1]

Topical fluorides are taken into the oral cavity in three primary forms:

- Self-applied by clients in the form of nonprescription products available over the counter
- Self-applied by clients in the form of prescription products
- Professionally applied prescription products

Typically, the topical fluoride agents available as *self-applied fluoride* agents for at-home use are lower in fluoride concentration than those that are applied professionally:

Low-concentration products are referred to as low potency and are usually applied more frequently.

High-concentration products are referred to as high potency and are typically applied less frequently.

Because carbohydrate challenges create daily opportunities for demineralization, it is prudent to recommend the frequent use of low-potency fluoride products for the daily management of this disease process (Table 26–8).

TABLE 26–8 VEHICLES FOR DELIVERING TOPICAL FLUORIDES

Vehicle	Fluoride Concentration	Typical Frequency of Application
Fluoride toothpaste	500–1500 ppm	Twice daily
Fluoride rinses	230–1000 ppm	Once daily
High-potency fluoride solutions	10,000 ppm	Typically biannually, but varies according to caries risk
Fluoride gels	4000–12,300 ppm	Varies with potency and caries risk
Fluoride vanishes	1000–22,600 ppm	Varies according to caries risk

Ten Cate JM, van Loveren C: Fluoride mechanisms, *Dental Clinics of North America* 43(4):713, 1999.

SELF-APPLIED DENTIFRICES. Other than the fluoride consumed in drinking water, *dentifrices* are the most widely used fluoride preparations. Dentifrices provide sufficiently large concentrations of fluoride to facilitate enamel remineralization.[10] Studies indicate that the routine use of fluoride dentifrices results in up to a 30% decrease in caries incidence.[16]

The majority of commercial dentifrices available in the United States contain 0.1% fluoride or 1000 ppm. Some manufacturers produce higher-strength dentifrices that contain 1500 ppm fluoride. Others have marketed a pediatric toothpaste with lower levels of fluoride ranging from 250 to 550 ppm.[2] Most dentifrices marketed in the United States contain:

- ✦ Sodium fluoride (NaF) formulated with a highly compatible, synthetic-silica base
- ✦ Sodium monofluorophosphate (NaMFP)

Comparisons between the two agents indicate superior caries reduction with the NaF system; these results are attributed to the rapid dissociation of sodium fluoride in NaF products.[2] Stannous fluoride dentifrices, also available, are currently advocated for the management of dentinal hypersensitivity and the antibacterial effects associated with the stannous ion (see Chapters 24 and 33). Figure 26–3 shows dentifrices that have received the ADA Seal of Acceptance.

One of the problems encountered in the manufacturing of dentifrices is the deactivation of fluoride that can occur as a result of its incompatibility with other ingredients in the dentifrice. Typically, the abrasive in the dentifrice deactivates the fluoride. It is important for the dental hygienist to recommend products that have undergone clinical evaluation and have documented caries-preventive ability.

Fluoridated dentifrices are designed for toothbrush application two to three times daily. Scientific literature provides clinical evidence to substantiate the use of a fluoridated dentifrice with this frequency. Studies done to compare caries reduction indicate that brushing once a day with a fluoridated toothpaste results in a 21% reduction in dental caries, whereas brushing three times a day resulted in 45% fewer caries.[2]

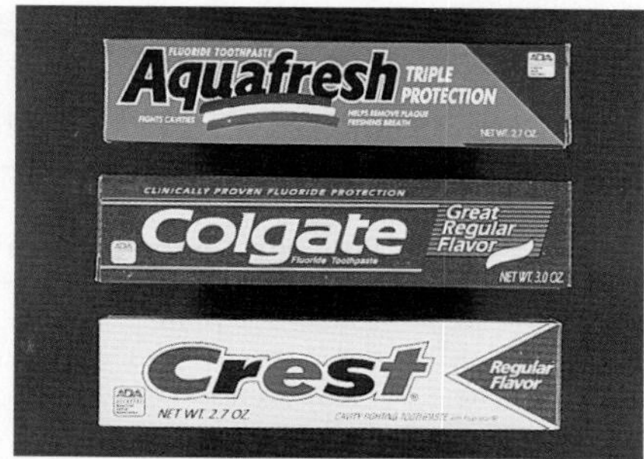

FIGURE 26–3 ✦ Sample dentifrices that have the ADA Seal of Acceptance for dental caries prevention.

Special consideration must be given when recommending fluoridated dentifrices for children under 6 years of age. The primary concern is that young children swallow dentifrices because they enjoy the taste, and are not capable of expectorating dentifrice remaining in their mouths. Clinical studies indicate that only 5% of children younger than 2½ years of age expectorate after brushing and only 32% of 2½- to 4-year-olds expectorate.[14] This inability to expectorate results in the ingestion of an agent designed for topical use and increases the risk for dental fluorosis. When recommending dentifrices for young children, it is important that the dental hygienist involve the client's parent or guardian and emphasize:

- ✦ Value of using a fluoridated toothpaste
- ✦ Importance of supervision when children are brushing their teeth
- ✦ Limiting the amount of toothpaste used to a pea-sized amount of paste or enough paste to cover one-quarter of the toothbrush
- ✦ How important it is for children to expectorate after brushing with a fluoridated dentifrice
- ✦ Avoidance of higher-concentration dentifrices and other fluoride products (children under 6 years of age)
- ✦ Storage of fluoridated dentifrices out of the reach of children[13]

Toothpaste is the most widely used at-home, topical fluoride vehicle, but a variety of other products are available for those clients whose caries activity or caries risk warrants the use of additional agents (Table 26–9). See Figures 26–4 to 26–6 for additional examples of products.

SELF-APPLIED MOUTHRINSES AND GELS. Fluoride rinses and gels may be used in addition to fluoride-containing dentifrice to manage dental caries. The majority of the rinses and gels are of low- to mid-range potency and as such are administered with higher frequency. The scientific literature indicates that these fluoride products reduce caries by 30% to 35%.[2] Table 26–9 identifies the various rinses and gels available to clients.

TABLE 26–9 TOPICAL FLUORIDES: SELF-APPLIED PASTES, RINSES, AND GELS

Fluoride Agent	Fluoride Concentration	Frequency of Application	Method of Delivery	Availability Examples of Products*
0.1% sodium fluoride (NaF) *or* 0.1 % sodium monofluorophosphate (MFP) dentifrices	1000–1500 ppm Some countries manufacture children's toothpaste at 250–550 ppm	Twice daily	Brush-on	OTC*
0.05% sodium fluoride (NaF) rinse	230 ppm	Once daily	Rinse	OTC examples: Act Fluorigard
0.2% sodium fluoride (NaF) rinse	910 ppm	Once weekly	Rinse; typically in a school-based program	Prescription examples: Fluorinse Nafrinse Point Two
0.4% stannous fluoride (SnF) gel	1000 ppm	Once daily	Brush-on after brushing with conventional dentifrice	OTC examples: Stop Gel-Kam Omni Gel
1.1% sodium fluoride (NaF) gel	5000 ppm	Once daily	Custom tray or brush-on after using conventional dentifrice	Prescription examples: Prevident 5000 Booster Karigel
0.05% acidulated phosphate fluoride (APF) gel	5000 ppm	Once daily	Custom tray or brush-on after using conventional dentifrice	Prescription

* *OTC,* Over the counter.
Warren DP, Chan JT: Topical fluorides: Efficacy, administration, and safety, *General Dentistry* 45(2):134, 1997.

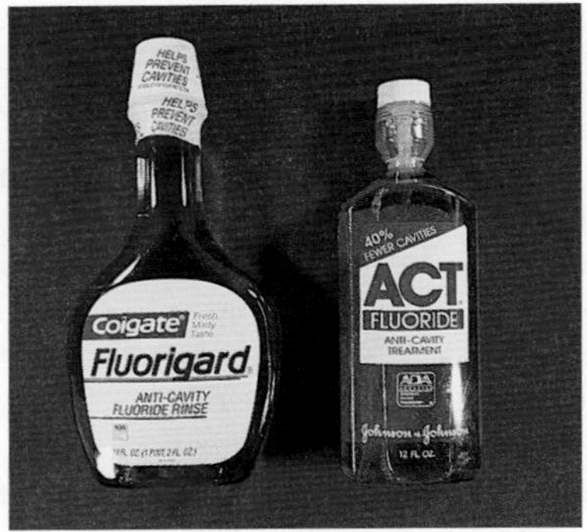

FIGURE 26–4 ✦ Sample of over-the-counter 0.05% sodium fluoride rinses with the ADA Seal of Acceptance.

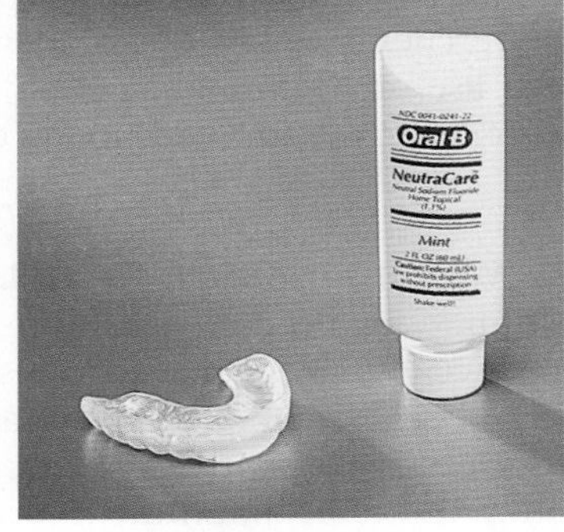

FIGURE 26–5 ✦ Tray method of fluoride gel application. *(Courtesy Oral-B Laboratories.)*

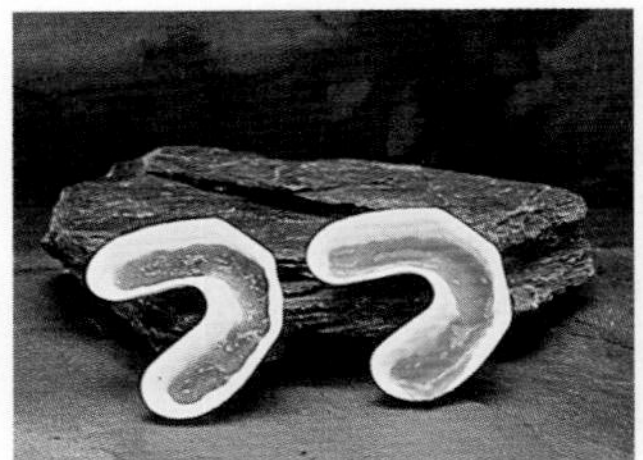
A

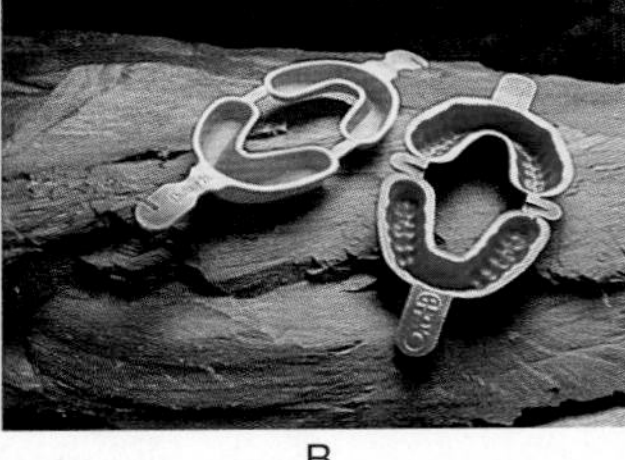
B

FIGURE 26–6 ✦ **A,** Single-arch trays. **B,** Dual-arch trays. *(Courtesy Dental Hygienist News, funded by educational grant from Procter and Gamble and published by Harfst Associates, Inc, Troy, Michigan.)*

Daily Fluoride Mouthrinses. Low-potency fluoride rinses are available as over-the-counter products; they have a fluoride concentration that equates to 230 ppm. These products are used as an adjunct to brushing with a fluoride dentifrice. Fluoride rinses (0.05%) are designed to be used daily. Clients should be educated to use ½ to 2 teaspoons of the rinse, to vigorously swish the rinse in the oral cavity, and then thoroughly expectorate the rinse. Because there is a risk for young children to swallow fluoride rinses, this product is not recommended for children under 6 years of age. For the same reason, fluoride rinses should be stored out of the reach of young children.[16]

Weekly Fluoride Mouthrinses. Sodium fluoride rinses (0.2%) are used for weekly rinsing, equate to 910 ppm,

TABLE 26–10 TOPICAL FLUORIDES: PROFESSIONALLY APPLIED GELS, FOAMS, SOLUTIONS, AND VARNISHES

Fluoride Agent	Fluoride Concentration	Frequency of Application	Method of Delivery	Availability Examples of Products
2.0% neutral sodium fluoride (NaF) gel or foam	9000 ppm	Twice annually or as caries incidence requires	Tray 4-minute application	Prescription
1.23% acidulated sodium fluoride (APF) gel or foam	12,300–12,500 ppm	Twice annually or as caries incidence requires	Tray 4-minute application	Prescription
8.0% stannous fluoride (SnF) solution	20,000–25,000 ppm	Rarely used due to its instability, bitter taste, and other adverse side effects (staining of teeth, gingival sloughing)	Rarely used	Prescription
Two-part fluoride rinses 0.31% APF 1.64% SnF	1500–3000 ppm	Not recommended due to lack of clinical evidence to warrant its use	2–4 minutes of rinsing	Prescription
5% sodium fluoride varnish	22,600 ppm	Depends on caries incidence and risk	Application with cotton tip applicator or syringe	Prescription examples: Duraphat Duraflor
1% difluorosilane fluoride varnish	1000 ppm	Depends on caries incidence and risk	Application with cotton tip applicator or syringe	Prescription examples: Fluor Protector

Sheehan JI: The fluoride decision, *RDH-The National Magazine for Dental Professionals* 21(4):20, 2001; Milgrom P, Reisine S: Oral health in the United States: The post-fluoride generation, *Annual Review of Public Health* 21:403, 2000; Warren DP, Chan JT: Topical fluorides: Efficacy, administration, and safety, *General Dentistry* 45(2):134, 1997; Beltran-Aguilar ED, Goldstein JW, Lockwood SA: Fluoride varnishes: A review of their clinical use, cariostatic mechanism, efficacy and safety, *Journal of the American Dental Association* 131:589, 2000.

and are typically used in school-based programs. These programs were originally designed to provide topical fluoride for children who did not reside in areas that had community water fluoridation.[11] School-based programs are effective because they are administered by school personnel, are closely supervised, are performed as part of a class schedule, and result in good compliance.

Daily Fluoride Gels. Fluoride gels are marketed as a stannous fluoride (SnF) product at 1000 ppm and neutral (NaF) and APF sodium products at 5000 ppm. These products are designed for daily use and are typically brushed on the teeth following toothbrushing with a conventional fluoride dentifrice. In cases in which increased duration of contact with the teeth is desired, the 5000 ppm products are used in custom trays. Because there is a risk for young children to swallow fluoride gels, these products are not recommended for children under 6 years of age. Although there are a very limited number of studies documenting their efficacy, the ADA Council on Scientific Affairs approved SnF gels. In addition, the Food and Drug Administration approved SnF gels for sale over-the-counter because they contain the same fluoride concentration as conventional dentifrices. Stannous gels do not contain abrasives and should not be substituted for dentifrices that achieve pellicle and stain removal.[16]

Neutral and acidulated sodium gels (5000 ppm) are used for clients with high caries risk due to the administration of radiation for head and neck cancers, those with systemic medical conditions, and those that routinely use medications that reduce salivary flow. These products are available as gels without abrasives and as gels with abrasives (marketed as prescription dentifrices). Although the 5000 ppm gels lack ADA Council on Scientific Affairs approval, these products have gained widespread use for clients with special needs. Careful client education is required when these products are recommended for unsupervised home use. The products should be used as directed in a custom tray or brushed on the teeth, swished in the oral cavity for one minute, and then expectorated. Clients should be reminded that these products are available by prescription due to their moderate levels of fluoride, and as such, should be carefully stored out of the reach of children.[16]

PROFESSIONALLY APPLIED FLUORIDE (IN-OFFICE ADMINISTRATION). The use of professionally applied topical fluorides solutions and gels dates back to the 1940s. In recent years, other professionally applied products (prescription agents) have been introduced into the market (Table 26–10). See Figures 26–6 and 26–7 for additional examples of products.

Solutions, Gels, and Foams. Professionally applied fluoride products are typically delivered using a tray technique, are one of the last procedures performed in the appointment sequence, and are administered by licensed dental professionals. Three high-potency topical fluoride systems have been approved by the FDA for in-office use. These systems

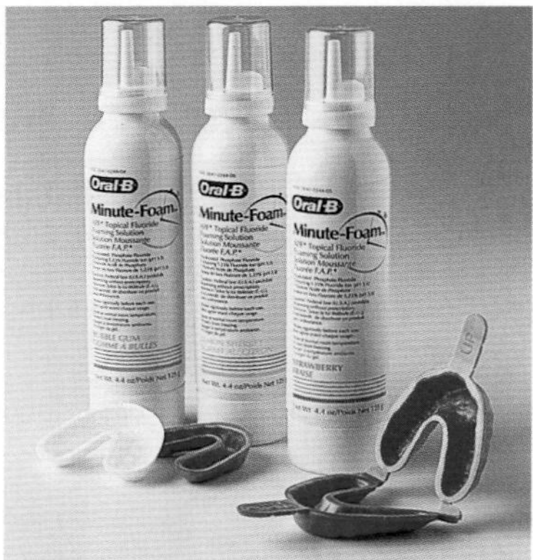

FIGURE 26–7 ✦ Fluoride foam. *(Courtesy Oral-B Laboratories)*

contain 9000 to 25,000 ppm of fluoride and are manufactured in the form of solutions, gels, or foams:

- 2.0% sodium fluoride
- 1.23% acidulated phosphate fluoride (sodium fluoride with hydrofluoric acid added)
- 8.0% stannous fluoride

These high-potency fluoride systems have a caries reduction rate of approximately 30%. Of the three products, the 1.23% APF system is the most widely researched and utilized. The 2.0% neutral sodium fluoride is the second most widely used and is recommended when it is inappropriate to use an acidulated product (when client has tooth-colored restoration and/or dentinal hypersensitivity). The 8.0% stannous fluoride system is rarely used due to its limited availability and lack of stability in aqueous solution. In addition, this product has poor client acceptance due to taste, tissue irritation, gingival sloughing, and staining.[2,16]

Client Selection. Client selection for professional topical fluoride application has changed significantly. When professional fluoride was first introduced, all clients treated in the clinical setting received fluoride treatments. Since the 1940s, the incidence of caries has decreased, the caries process is more fully understood, exposure to various sources of fluoride has increased, and dental hygienists have recognized the need to manage demineralization and remineralization more frequently with lower-potency products.

Although client selection criteria for this procedure will continue to evolve, the following issues must be considered when identifying clients who will benefit from this procedure:

- Demonstrated risk for developing caries. Client Selection for Professionally Applied Fluoride Treatments (Gel or Foam-Tray Technique) summarizes the caries risk factors that make children and adults candidates for a professionally applied topical fluoride treatments

Client Selection for Professionally Applied Fluoride Treatments (Gel or Foam-Tray Technique)

Caries risk factors that may indicate a need for a professionally applied topical fluoride:
- New carious lesions on previously sound surfaces
- Secondary lesions associated with restoration margins
- Wearing of orthodontic appliances

Compromised salivary flow
- Radiation therapy
- Prolonged use of medication that reduces salivary flow (e.g., antihistamines, sedatives, etc.)
- Age-related conditions
- Medical conditions (e.g., Sjögren's syndrome)

Ripa LW: Office fluoride gel-tray treatments: Current recommendations, *New York State Dental Journal* 58(2):47, 1992.

- Presence of newly erupted teeth (studies indicate that teeth are most susceptible to caries formation during the two years posteruption)
- Client's ability to tolerate a four-minute topical fluoride application
- Age of the client; extreme care should be used if in-office fluoride treatment is administered to a child under 6 years of age. Inadvertent swallowing of fluoride and the inability to effectively expectorate place the client at risk of ingesting high-potency fluoride. This could result in *acute fluoride toxicity*. Older adults may present the same risks as the child client.
- Physical or mental disabilities (e.g., inability to expectorate or understand the importance of refraining from swallowing, etc.)
- Fluoride level in the primary water supply
- Overall exposure to fluoride[2,7,13,17]

Tray Selection. Fluoride gel and foam products may be applied with a variety of techniques; however, the use of stock trays is the most widely used. The advantages of using the tray technique for professionally applied fluoride treatments are:

- Entire dentition can be treated simultaneously
- Effective contact between the agent and the teeth
- Little soft tissue contact
- Less dilution and contamination of the fluoride with saliva
- Client comfort
- Reduced potential for fluoride ingestion (also maximized with the use of a foam product)
- Time and cost effectiveness

Fluoride delivery trays are marketed by a number of dental product manufacturers. The design and fit of the tray are critical to optimize the anticaries efficacy of the treatment and prevent ingestion of these high-potency products. When selecting trays for fluoride delivery, the dental hygienist must consider the ability of the tray to create a distal dam to prevent flow of fluoride out the posterior border, anatomic arch fit, anterior vertical coverage, posterior vertical coverage, ease of use, and tray features that promote client comfort (Figure 26–6).[18]

Product Selection. Once it is determined that a client will benefit from a professionally applied topical fluoride treatment, the dental hygienist decides the type of high-potency fluoride that will be utilized for this procedure. There are several issues to consider when selecting a product:

- *Fluoride gel versus foam products.* Thixotropic gel products represent the evolution of in-office fluoride products from solutions to gels to thixotropic gels. Gels were initially developed because their viscosity made them easier to work with and facilitated the use of fluoride trays. The cellulose that was added to gels to increase viscosity had a negative effect on the ability of the fluoride to flow interproximally and into protected areas. To deal with this issue, thixotropic gels were developed; these gels flow under pressure, but remain viscous when they are not under pressure. Both professionally applied APF and neutral sodium products are available in thixotropic gels.[11]

  Professional-strength foam-based products were developed to address the risks associated with using high-potency fluoride products. The advantage of the foam products is that 75% less fluoride is needed; this dramatically reduces the risk of acute fluoride toxicity. Studies of APF foam products indicate that they deliver the same fluoride benefits as APF gels. Both professionally applied APF and neutral sodium products are available in foam-based products (Figure 26–7).[19]
- *APF versus neutral sodium products.* APF products are accepted by the American Dental Association Council on Scientific Affairs; their efficacy has been documented in controlled clinical trials.

  Neutral sodium fluoride gels that are routinely used for in-office fluoride treatment have not had their caries reduction abilities evaluated via scientific studies. The solution form of this concentration of neutral sodium fluoride has been evaluated and found to reduce caries incidence.

  Neutral sodium fluoride products were developed because of the concern that repeated exposure to APF products may result in the etching of the surfaces of porcelain crowns and other restorative and preventive materials that contain glass or similar filler particles (tooth-colored restorative materials, filled sealants).[7]

  To decide between APF sodium and neutral sodium products, the dental hygienist considers the client profile identified during assessment. Although APF is the most widely utilized professional fluoride product, the presence of restorative or preventive dental materials that may be damaged by APF products would contraindicate its use. When these materials are present intraorally, it is recommended that the dental hygienist select a neutral fluoride product. If a neutral sodium fluoride product is not available, then it is important to protect tooth-colored restorative material and other at-risk materials with petrolatum or a varnish prior to the fluoride treatment (Figure 26–8).
- *pH of APF products.* Fluoride uptake of APF products is influenced by the pH of the product. Evidence-based research indicates that a pH of 4.0 enhances fluoride uptake. Very slight elevations in the pH of APF products have a significant impact on the enamel-fluoride uptake. When APF products are used, it is the clinician's responsibility to check the pH level and determine if the product is effective.[19]

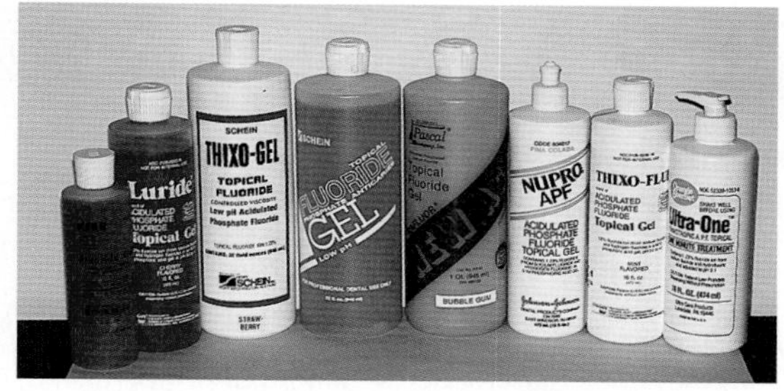

FIGURE 26–8 ✦ Topical fluoride gels for professional applications. *(Courtesy Oral-B Laboratories)*

Procedures for Application Using the Tray Technique. The procedural steps for administering a professional topical fluoride begin with the client and product selection processes outlined in the previous section of this chapter. The sequence for administering a professional topical fluoride using the tray technique is outlined in Procedure 26–1.

Varnishes. Fluoride varnishes are widely used in European countries and Canada for the purpose of caries control. These products provide an agent that is painted on the teeth to prolong fluoride exposure. In the United States, the FDA has approved these products as medical devices for use only as cavity liners and for the treatment of hypersensitive teeth. The FDA considers caries prevention a drug claim. To have the FDA consider approving varnishes as a caries prevention agent, manufacturers would have to conduct clinical trials and submit evidence that this product should be approved as a therapeutic, anticaries agent.[8,9,20]

Because of the numerous clinical studies and the successful use of fluoride varnishes in other countries, some U.S. dental professionals are using fluoride varnishes as off-label products. Some dental providers object to the use of varnishes for caries management, but others use varnishes in the following ways:

- For children and adults at risk for dental caries
- When longer fluoride contact is desired
- When the client cannot tolerate a professional fluoride treatment

Procedure 26-1 ADMINISTERING AN IN-OFFICE FLUORIDE TREATMENT (GEL OR FOAM)

EQUIPMENT

Mouth mirror	Timer
Cotton forceps	Saliva ejector
Fluoride tray(s)	2″ × 2″ gauze
Cotton rolls	Tissues
APF or NaF gel or foam	2 oz cup
Air syringe	Personal protective barriers and equipment barriers

STEPS	RATIONALE
1. Assemble equipment.	Promotes efficiency and infection control.
2. Seat client in upright position. Reiterate benefits and obtain informed consent.	Prevents gagging and accidental ingestion of fluoride gel/foam. Manages legal risk.
3. Try tray of appropriate size.	Trays must be pliable, comfortable, and deep enough to cover all surfaces.

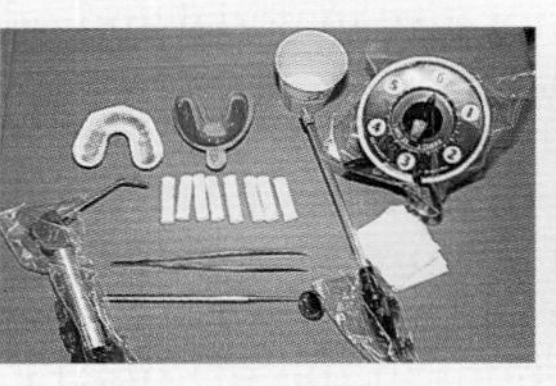
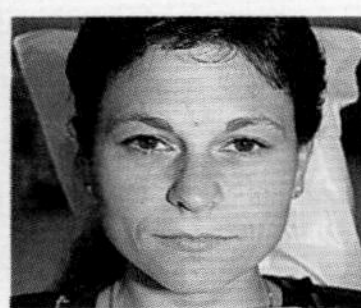
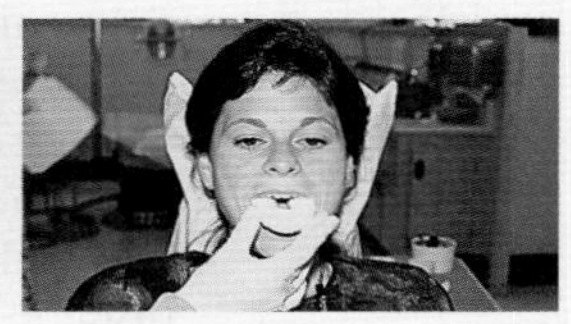

STEPS	RATIONALE
4. Load fluoride gel/foam into trays: 2 ml maximum for children, 2.5 ml maximum for adults.	Recommendations of the American Academy of Pediatric Dentistry; trays deliver fluoride to exposed tooth surfaces.
5. Isolate teeth with cotton rolls. Dry with air syringe.	A dry field maximizes fluoride uptake.

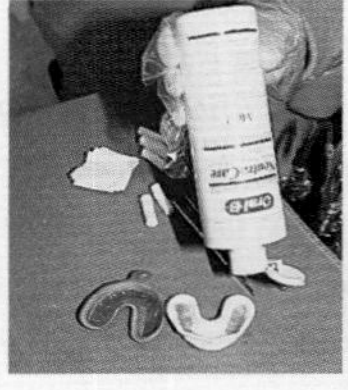
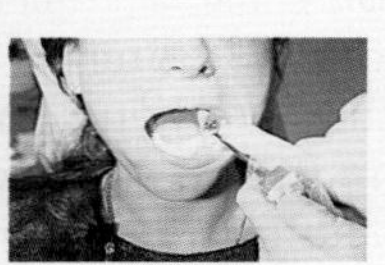

STEPS	RATIONALE
6. Insert mandibular tray.	Mandibular tray stays in place more easily than maxillary tray. Some trays connect both a mandibular and a maxillary arch into one tray designed for efficiency of insertion.
7. Press tray against teeth.	Ensures coverage into interproximal spaces.

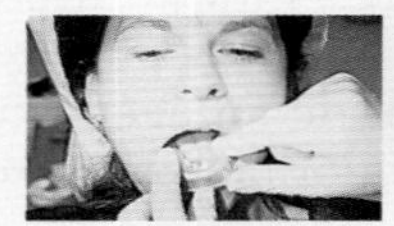
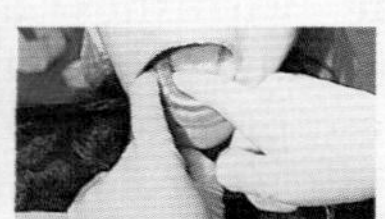

STEPS	RATIONALE
8. Air dry maxillary arch and insert maxillary tray.	A dry field maximizes fluoride uptake.
9. Press tray against teeth and ask client to close mouth and bite gently on trays or cotton rolls.	Slight pressure from biting helps force fluoride gel/foam around all surfaces.

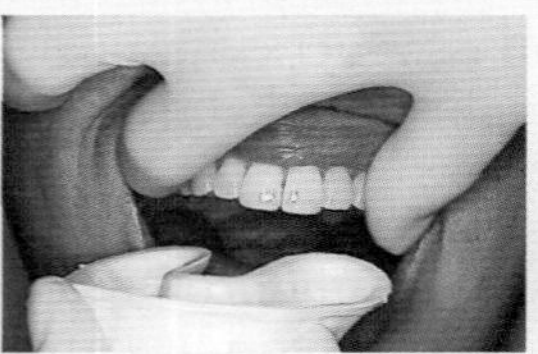
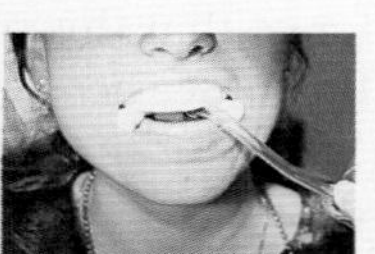

STEPS	RATIONALE
10. Place saliva ejector over mandibular tray. Set timer for 4 minutes. Never leave client unattended during procedure.	Prevents saliva from diluting fluoride. Maximum fluoride exposure requires 4 minutes. Supervision prevents accidental ingestion of fluoride response if gagging results.
11. Tilt chin down to remove trays.	Allows fluids to flow to anterior region of mouth.

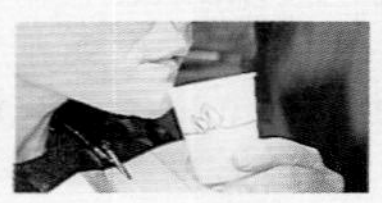
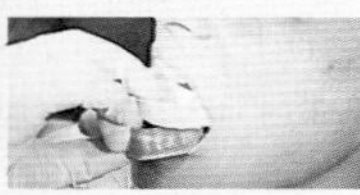

Procedure 26–1 ADMINISTERING AN IN-OFFICE FLUORIDE TREATMENT (GEL OR FOAM)—CONT'D

STEPS	RATIONALE
12. Ask client to expectorate; suction excess fluoride from the mouth with saliva ejector.	Prompt removal of fluoride gel/foam from mouth minimizes swallowing of excess gel/foam.
13. Instruct client not to eat, drink, or rinse for 30 minutes.	Allows residual fluoride to remain in contact with teeth.
14. Record service and type of fluoride used in the client's chart. Document in ink the completion of this service in the client's record under "Services Rendered" and date the entry (e.g., "Applied topical AFP fluoride foam to 32 existing teeth for 4 minutes. Use stock trays to apply approx 2–2.5 ml of 1.23% acidulated phosphate fluoride (insert brand name). The client agreed to this procedure; there were no complications/adverse reactions during the treatment.")	Documentation ensures continuity of quality care and risk management.

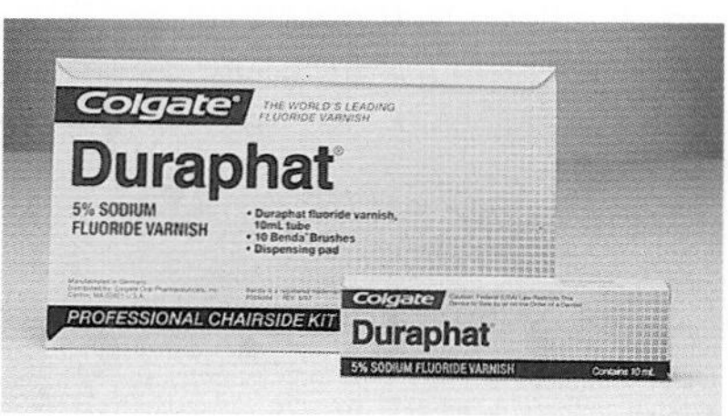

A

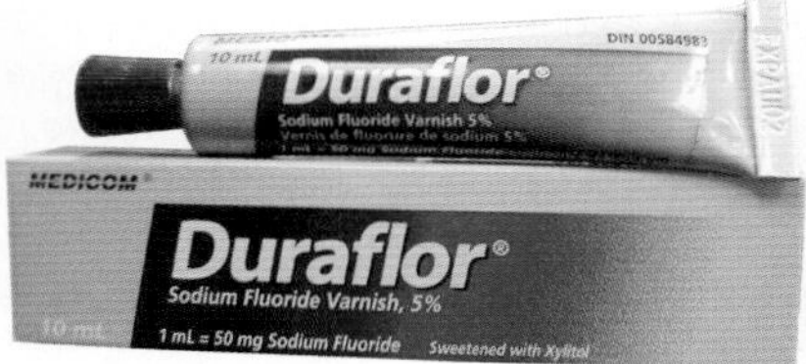

B

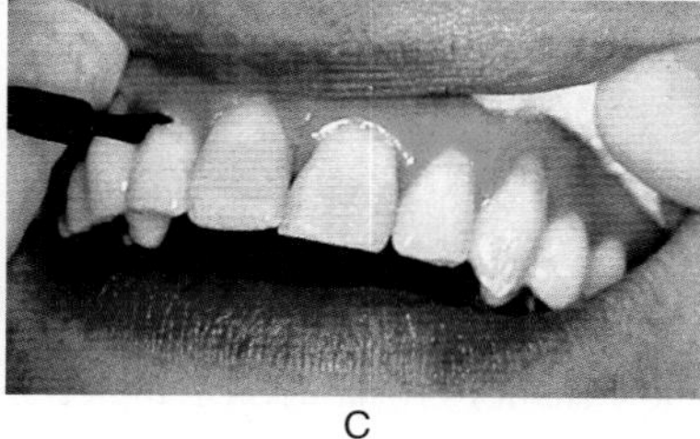

C

FIGURE 26–9 ✦ Fluoride varnish. **A,** Duraphat fluoride varnish. **B,** Duraflor fluoride varnish. **C,** Fluoride varnish on central incisors. *(Courtesy Colgate Oral Pharmaceuticals, 2001.)*

European studies that evaluated the ability of fluoride varnish to reduce caries on permanent teeth reported reductions of 18% to 77%. A preliminary U.S. study that assessed the ability of fluoride varnish to remineralize initial carious lesions in primary teeth reported an 80% reversal of lesions. In addition, the March 2001 National Institutes of Health Consensus Conference on the Management of Dental Caries endorsed the use of fluoride varnishes for caries control on permanent teeth. The Consensus Conference statement reported that evidence to support the use of fluoride varnish on primary teeth was inconclusive at the time of the conference.[8,9,20]

Several fluoride varnishes are available in the United States (Figure 26–9):

- ✦ 5% sodium fluoride (2.26% fluoride or 22,600 ppm; e.g., Duraphat and Duraflor)
- ✦ 1% difluorosilane (0.1% fluoride or 1000 ppm; e.g., Fluor Protector)

Some of the varnish products have a very high concentration of fluoride ion, raising concern regarding fluoride toxicity as a result of application procedures. To date there are no documented incidents of acute or chronic fluoride toxicity as a result of using fluoride varnish. The rapid drying that is characteristic of fluoride varnishes seems to prevent ingestion and minimize the risk for a toxic dose. The release of fluoride after placement peaks early and then drops dramatically. Plasma levels of fluoride following varnish applications are similar to those experienced after the use of a fluoridated toothpaste.[8,9,20]

The frequency of application for fluoride varnish has not been fully established. Some providers support a semiannual application, and others suggest that the frequency should be determined by the client's caries risk. Procedure 26–2 outlines the steps for placing fluoride varnishes.[8,9,20]

PROFESSIONALLY APPLIED FLUORIDES: ISSUES AND CONTROVERSIES. The scientific literature highlights issues and controversies regarding the use of professionally applied fluoride products. The following list identifies some of the key issues:

- ✦ *The use of a stannous-APF combination dual rinse system as a substitute for a professionally applied topical fluoride using the tray technique.* This two-part system is marketed as a 0.31% APF solution and a 1.64% stannous fluoride solution. The two solutions are used one at a time or are mixed together. The total recommended rinsing time is two minutes, and the fluoride exposure is 1500 to 3000 ppm. Many dental professionals utilize this procedure because it takes less time and equipment than the tray technique, is less labor intensive, and clients find it more tolerable than fluoride trays.

  Despite its use in some offices, this dual rinse protocol has come under criticism. To date, there are not any randomized, double-blind clinical studies to substantiate the use of a dual, sequential fluoride rinse system.[8,16,19] Contemporary standards of practice require that dental hygienists make client care

Procedure 26–2 ADMINISTERING A SODIUM FLUORIDE VARNISH TREATMENT

EQUIPMENT
Mouth mirror
Sodium fluoride varnish
Cotton-tip applicators or syringe applicator
Paper cup
Personal protective barriers and equipment barriers

STEPS	RATIONALE
1. Select fluoride varnish product and gather equipment/supplies for application.	Enhances time efficiency, ensures client comfort and safety, and promotes maintenance of infection control.
2. Provide client with information about procedure and reiterate benefits. Obtain informed consent.	Encourages client participation in care and manages risk.
3. Unless an oral prophylaxis has been performed at the same appointment, have client cleanse teeth with toothbrush.	Brushing is adequate preparation for placement of varnish.
4. Recline client to provide ergonomic access to oral cavity.	Ensures operator and client comfort.
5. Wipe application area with gauze or cotton rolls and insert a saliva ejector.	Varnish sets in contact with intraoral moisture, so drying with compressed air is unnecessary; removal of saliva will facilitate client comfort and cooperation.
6. Using a cotton-tip or a syringe-style applicator, apply 0.3–0.5 ml of varnish to teeth.	Varnish is not permanent; a thin layer will promote fluoride release and absorption.
7. Dental floss may be used to draw the varnish interproximally.	This procedure is optional because it must be done quickly as the varnish dries upon contact with moisture.
8. Allow client to rinse upon completion of procedure.	Varnish sets on contact; no need to avoid rinsing after application.
9. Remind client to avoid eating for 2 to 4 hours after application; avoid brushing teeth the night of the application.	Prevents premature removal of varnish and maximizes fluoride contact and release time.
10. Document in ink the completion of this service in the client's record under "Services Rendered" and date the entry, e.g., "Applied topical fluoride varnish to 28 existing teeth. Used a cotton-tip applicator to apply approx. 0.3 ml of 5% (22,600 ppm) sodium fluoride varnish (insert brand name) per tooth. The client agreed to this procedure; there were no complications/adverse reactions during the treatment."	Documentation is important for continuity of quality care and for risk management purposes.

Beltran-Aguilar ED, Goldstein JW, Lockwood SA: Fluoride varnishes: A review of their clinical use, cariostatic mechanism, efficacy and safety, *Journal of the American Dental Association* 131:589, 2000.

decisions based on evidence presented in the scientific literature. The SnF/APF combination dual rinse does not meet this standard.

✦ *The marketing and utilization of professionally applied APF gel and foam products for one minute, rather than four minutes.* Many manufacturers have successfully marketed one-minute 1.23% APF gel and foam products. These products have become popular among dental hygienists due to the reduced time required for administration. No clinical studies of caries inhibition substantiate leaving the gel in contact with the teeth for just one minute. Researchers concur that fluoride uptake by the enamel is limited when the fluoride contact is reduced to one minute.[7] In addition, there is no difference in the concentration of the products marketed as one-minute products versus those marketed as four-minute products. Currently, there is no scientific evidence to substantiate a reduction in fluoride exposure time.

✦ *Whether a professional fluoride treatment is required after coronal polishing procedures.* Many commercially available coronal polishing pastes contain fluoride. There is no existing clinical evidence to suggest that fluoride-containing pastes improve caries protection. These pastes should not be used in place of a professional fluoride treatment. Marketing of fluoride-containing pastes is supported by dental research. There is some clinical evidence to support that fluoride lost when enamel is removed during coronal polishing may be replaced by the fluoride in polishing pastes. Although this may be the case, researchers suggest additional studies to determine if the ingredients in polishing pastes restrict the bioavailability of the fluoride.[17] Prior to adjusting clinical protocols, dental hygienists should consult the literature for evidence that such a change is warranted.

✦ *The recommended frequency for applying fluoride varnishes.* In the United States, the use of fluoride varnish for caries prevention is an off-label use of this product. Until additional research is conducted, the frequency of application for dental caries prevention will depend on the clinical judgment of the practitioner.

RISK OF ACUTE FLUORIDE TOXICITY. Acute toxicity from a topical fluoride agent may range from a mild systemic reaction (stomach upset) to death. Many factors influence the toxicity of fluoride compounds (e.g., route of administration, age of the client, client weight, and rate of absorption). When fluoride is swallowed, it reacts with acids present in the stomach; the reaction product is hydrogen fluoride (HF). Hydrogen fluoride is very irritating and initial abdominal reactions can occur after swallowing a relatively small amount of higher concentration products.[21]

The initial symptoms of acute fluoride toxicity are nausea, gastrointestinal pain, and vomiting. If sufficient quantities of fluoride are ingested, these initial symptoms may be followed by muscular weakness and spasms that occur as a result of fluoride combining with blood calcium ions.[21] Toxic doses of fluoride affect the following body systems:

- *Gastrointestinal:* abdominal pain and cramps, nausea, vomiting, diarrhea
- *Neurologic:* paresthesia, tetany, central nervous system depression, and coma
- *Cardiovascular:* weak pulse, pallor, hypotension, shock, cardiac irregularities, and cardiac failure[16]

Management of Acute Fluoride Toxicity

Initial Emergency Response in the Oral Care Setting

Induce vomiting by administering an emetic, such as ipecac (this should occur only if the client has a gag reflex, is conscious, and is not convulsing)

This is followed by the oral administration of 1% calcium chloride or calcium gluconate; if these are not available, milk should be ingested

While the client is receiving attention, medical assistance is requested and transport to the medical emergency room should occur as soon as possible

Response by Emergency Personnel (emergency response is dependent on the severity of symptoms and may include the following options)

Inserting an endotracheal tube, followed by gastric lavage with a calcium-containing solution or activated charcoal

Establishing an airway

Establishing an intravenous line

Maintaining cardiovascular circulation

Hourly blood analysis for plasma fluoride levels and monitoring for hyperkalemia and hypocalcemia

Fluid replacement to reverse effects of vomiting and diarrhea and to maintain urine flow

Intravenous calcium replacement, glucose administration, oxygen, artificial respiration, or other supportive therapies

If the client responds favorably, continue supportive therapies until the following are in the normal range: mental alertness, vital signs, and serum chemistry profile

Ekstrand J, Fejerskov O, Silverstone LM: *Fluoride in dentistry,* Copenhagen, 1988, Munksgaard.

The goal of initial treatment for fluoride toxicity is to reduce the amount of fluoride available for absorption from the gastrointestinal tract. Depending on the amount of fluoride ingested, initial emergency response in the dental office should be followed by medical treatment.[22] Management of Acute Fluoride Toxicity outlines the treatment procedures for acute fluoride toxicity.

The amount of fluoride that will cause a toxic reaction or result in a lethal dose is difficult to determine because it is based on a variety of factors described earlier, including the client's body weight. Terms used to describe how much fluoride can be tolerated by a client are the *safely tolerated dose (STD)* and the *certainly lethal dose (CLD).* The CLD is the amount of fluoride that will result in patient death. The STD, the amount of fluoride that can be ingested without causing serious acute toxicity, is approximately one-quarter the CLD. Table 26–11 provides information regarding the safely tolerated dose and certainly lethal dose of fluoride; the data are based on client age and body weight.[17] Figure 26–10 outlines how to calculate the amount of fluoride ingested by a client; this calculation is based on the specific fluoride product utilized and the quantity administered during the treatment.

Although fluoride products have evident therapeutic benefits, their use and storage must be monitored. In the home setting, caution must be taken regarding the use and storage of even low-dose fluoride products. Oral care professionals must educate clients (and their parents or caregivers) regarding the safe use of fluorides. In addition, dental professionals must exercise extreme caution when using high-potency prescription products that contain the highest concentrations of fluoride available. To safely utilize professional-strength fluoride products in the dental treatment setting, it is essential that the dental hygienist carefully select clients for this procedure and know:

- The fluoride concentration of the products being used
- The amount of fluoride contained in the unit packaging (bottles, tubes, etc.)

TABLE 26–11 CERTAINLY LETHAL AND SAFELY TOLERATED FLUORIDE DOSES

Age	Body Weight (lb)	CLD (mg)	STD (mg)
2	22	320	80
4	29	422	106
6	37	538	135
8	45	655	164
10	53	771	193
12	64	931	233
14	83	1206	301
16	92	1338	334
18	95	1382	346

From Heifetz SB, Horowitz HS: The amounts of fluoride in current fluoride therapies: Safety considerations for children, *Journal of Dentistry of Children* 51:257, 1984.

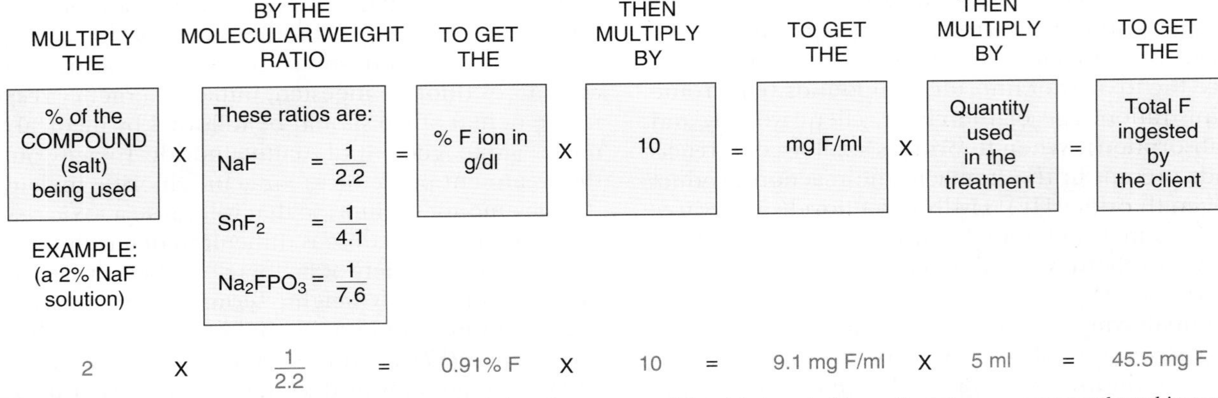

FIGURE 26–10 ✦ Flow chart depicts method for calculating the amount of fluoride ingested by a client from a compound used in professional care. *(Modified from Heifetz SB, Horowitz HS: The amounts of fluoride in current fluoride therapies: Safety considerations for children,* ASDC Journal of Dentistry for Children *51:257, July-August, 1984.)*

- ✦ The amount used in the treatment provided to the client
- ✦ How the amount provided relates to the CLD[22]

CHLORHEXIDINE AS AN ANTIBACTERIAL FOR DENTAL CARIES

Chlorhexidine gluconate is a broad-spectrum antibacterial agent that works by opening up the cell membranes of the bacteria. It is administered in the United States by prescription. In the United States, only 0.12 % chlorhexidine gluconate is available as a mouthrinse (Figure 26–11), and it is effective against *mutans streptococci.*[2a] Chlorhexidine gluconate has been used as an antibacterial in the dental treatment setting for the management of both dental caries and periodontal diseases.

The 2002 Caries Management Risk Assessment Consensus Statement[2a] recommends that 10 ml of 0.12 % chlorhexidine mouthrinse be used at bedtime for 1 minute, once daily for a 2-week period every 2 to 3 months. In high-bacterial–challenge individuals, this therapy needs to be continued for approximately 1 year and monitored by bacterial assessment. Problems associated with this compound are that it affects taste, and compliance is often poor.[2a]

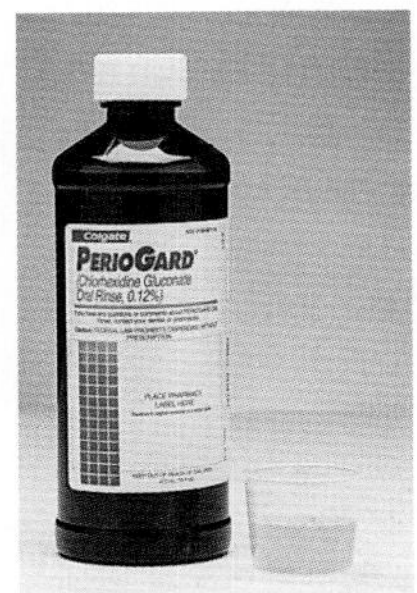

FIGURE 26–11 ✦ Chlorhexidine product: mouthrinse. *(Courtesy Colgate Oral Pharmaceuticals, 2001.)*

OTHER ANTIBACTERIAL THERAPEUTICS

Xylitol

Xylitol is a sweetener that looks and tastes like sucrose. It inhibits attachment and transmission of bacteria and can be delivered through chewing gum or lozenges as an effective anticaries therapeutic measure. Xylitol is not fermented by cariogenic bacteria.[2a]

Sodium Bicarbonate

Sodium bicarbonate (baking soda) neutralizes acids produced by acidogenic bacteria and has antibacterial properties. It can be delivered in toothpaste or in a solution for individuals with low saliva flow.[2a]

Fluoride and Chlorhexidine

For the dental hygienist to design a preventive treatment plan that will attempt to arrest existing white spot lesions and prevent new carious lesions, careful consideration must be given to the information gathered during the assessment phase of care. This information assists the dental hygienist in determining client risk for dental caries and recommending preventive strategies that will address client needs (Table 26–1).

An evaluation of the exposure to systemic fluoride will require careful questioning of the client. With young clients, the need for fluoride supplementation is based on an analysis of exposures to systemic fluoride and consultation with other dental and medical providers. As teeth erupt, the clinician must be alert to the presence of dental fluorosis. Should the dental hygienist identify even mild areas of fluorosis, every attempt should be made to determine the cause(s) of this enamel defect. Special attention should be paid to whether the client is receiving too much systemic fluoride or whether the client is ingesting topical fluoride and creating an additional systemic exposure.

Regardless of dental caries status, the use of a fluoridated toothpaste is the cornerstone of any caries prevention plan. The need for additional preventive measures is based on clinical judgment and presence of new demineralized areas. Should the client exhibit new demineralized areas, the dental hygienist must consider whether the continued-care interval is appropriate (if more frequent preventive visits are required), if the client is using a fluoridated dentifrice two to three times a day, and whether additional professionally applied or self-applied fluoride products are indicated.

Depending on the age of the client, number of caries risk factors, ability of the client to modify risk factors, and number of demineralized areas, the dental hygienist may decide that a modification in professional care is needed. This may involve more frequent preventive appointments, more frequent application of in-office fluoride gels/foams, or the application of fluoride varnish. An increase in the number of preventive dental visits is dependent on the client's compliance with this service.

The dental hygienist may also decide that an adjustment in self-applied fluoride products is the best approach for managing an increase in the number of demineralized areas. Self-applied products are less expensive, do not require a visit to the dental care setting, facilitate the delivery of low-dose fluorides on a more frequent basis, and address the demineralization dynamic on a daily basis. Table 26–9 identifies self-applied products that may be recommended in addition to a fluoridated dentifrice.

One approach may be to supplement the use of a fluoridated dentifrice with an additional fluoride vehicle, starting with a low-concentration product (e.g., 230 ppm/ 0.05% rinse). This adjustment would be followed by a reassessment visit in two to three months. Should additional demineralized areas be present, the dental hygienist may recommend a higher-concentration, self-applied product.

The use of 0.12% chlorhexidine mouthrinse is recommended for individuals with high caries risk, individuals with existing decay, and individuals with high levels of *mutans streptococci* in the mouth.[2a] The underlying rationale suggesting the use of chlorhexidine rinses for a 2-week period every 2 to 3 months in a caries-active client is to eliminate the microorganisms that initiate the caries process. The intent is to treat the infection as well as the result of the infection (which historically has been the placement of a restoration).

Client Education Issues

- ✦ Explain the caries process.
- ✦ Explain the role of diet, fluorides, plaque biofilm removal, saliva, antibacterial mouthrinses, and sealants as methods of preventing and controlling tooth decay
- ✦ Discuss that caries is an infection that can be transmitted from parent to child, or person to person.
- ✦ Emphasize the frequent use of low-dose fluoride-containing products (dentifrices and oral rinses) in the repair of demineralized areas.
- ✦ Explain how certain medications decrease salivary flow and increase dental caries risk.
- ✦ Explain that dental caries management is a life-long issue.
- ✦ Teach parents and caregivers that they are critical partners in the management of dental caries in children under 6 years of age.
- ✦ Explain that fluoride is an effective agent in caries management, and it must be safely used and stored.
- ✦ Explain that when well water is the primary water source, it should be tested to determine fluoride level.

Legal, Ethical, and Safety Issues

- ✦ Carefully analyze the client's overall fluoride exposure; take a fluoride history.
- ✦ Make recommendations based on the subjective and objective data collected during client assessment procedures.
- ✦ Emphasize the safe use of self-applied products, especially with children younger than 6 years of age.
- ✦ Document recommendations regarding self-applied products in the client record, including information regarding type of product, frequency of use, safe use and storage.
- ✦ Thoroughly document the administration of in-office products in the client's record.
- ✦ Safely store and manage professional-strength fluorides in the dental treatment setting.
- ✦ Work in collaboration with other oral care professionals to develop a response plan in the event of an acute fluoride overdose in the dental treatment setting.
- ✦ Have a clear understanding of the amount of professional-strength fluoride that is administered and how it relates to the CLD and SLD.
- ✦ Consult the professional literature regularly for current information and clinical evidence regarding strategies for managing dental caries.

Key Concepts

- The dental hygienist plays a key role in the management of dental caries over the client's lifespan.
- Dental caries involve an interaction among pathologic factors and protective factors. *Pathologic factors* include acidogenic bacteria (*mutans streptococci* and lactobacilli), low saliva flow due to salivary gland dysfunction or the use of many medications, and fermentable carbohydrates in the diet. *Protective factors* include calcium, phosphate, proteins, and fluoride in the saliva; normal salivary flow; and antibacterial agents if needed.
- Saliva plays a key role in that it neutralizes acids and provides minerals and proteins that protect the teeth.
- To determine caries risk, the dental hygienist evaluates the number and the severity of risk factors.
- After determining the caries risk of an individual, the clinician provides the client with educational materials about the caries process and makes recommendations based on test results, responses to questions, and clinical observation.
- Caries management is aimed at restoring and maintaining a balance between protective factors and pathologic factors.
- Caries management includes treatment of the bacterial infection that causes dental caries, rather than just treating the carious lesion.
- Caries management involves suppressing bacteria that cause the infection; remineralizing early noncavitated carious lesions by enhancing salivary flow and using fluorides; protecting tooth surfaces by using sealants and fluorides; decreasing the frequency of sugar intake, especially between meals; and surgically removing carious lesions that are beyond hope of remineralization and restoring the teeth with minimally invasive techniques and materials.
- Levels of cariogenic bacteria in the mouth can be assessed by selective media culturing in the dental office. Saliva that is stimulated by chewing can be used as a sampling to collect bacteria from the teeth and around the mouth.
- Chlorhexidine is used as a mouthrinse (10 ml once daily for a 2-week period every 2 to 3 months). In individuals with high bacterial challenge, this therapy will need to be continued for approximately 1 year and monitored by bacterial assessment.
- Demineralization and remineralization occur in the oral cavity on a daily basis.
- Saliva and fluoride are instrumental in the remineralization process.
- Demineralization is an issue from the time the primary dentition erupts into the oral cavity until death or the permanent teeth are prematurely lost.
- Systemic and topical fluoride delivery systems play key preventive roles.
- Community water fluoridation is the cornerstone of systemic fluoride delivery, and fluoridated dentifrices play a similar role in topical fluoride delivery.
- The incidence of chronic fluoride toxicity/dental fluorosis has increased and it is the dental hygienist's responsibility to assess systemic fluoride exposure.
- A variety of self-applied dentifrices, rinses, and gels are available, and the market continues to expand in this area.
- Use of professionally applied fluoride gels and foams has been documented in the literature; client selection has changed over time and is dependent on caries risk.
- Use of fluoride varnish is an emerging strategy for the management of dental caries.
- Acute fluoride toxicity is a risk, especially during the administration of professional-strength fluorides. The dental hygienist plays a primary role in the prevention of acute toxicity and is a member of the response team should a toxic overdose occur in the dental treatment setting.
- It is the dental hygienist's ethical responsibility to thoroughly document the use of and recommendations made regarding chemotherapeutic agents for the management of dental caries.
- It is the dental hygienist's ethical responsibility to read the scientific literature and utilize it to provide the evidence to substantiate professional decisions.

Critical Thinking Exercises

Sue works as a dental hygienist in a large group practice that employs a total of three full-time dental hygienists. This general practice is located in a town that has had community water fluoridation for the past 30 years; nearly all of the clients treated in the office reside in the town. Sue is providing a preventive appointment for a 5-year-old client. The client is new to the practice; her mother is waiting for her in the reception area. The client presents with the following dental history:

- Mixed dentition
- A healthy diet; infrequently ingests snacks containing fermentable carbohydrates
- Brushes two times a day using a fluoridated toothpaste; her mother monitors toothbrushing at bedtime
- Oral hygiene is fair to good
- Salivary flow appears normal
- No clinical evidence of demineralization
- No restorations present

The office policy is that professionally applied fluorides (tray technique) are administered to all children (3 to 16 years of age) two times annually. As Sue nears the end of her appointment, she explains to the client that she is going to administer a fluoride treatment; the client has never had this procedure before. Sue asks the client what flavor fluoride she would prefer: tooty-fruity, strawberry, or double chocolate. The client says that she loves chocolate, so she selects the double chocolate flavor.

Sue explains the four-minute tray application to the client, the use of the saliva ejector, and the need to avoid swallowing fluoride during the treatment. Sue selects a small, hinged fluoride tray and fills it two-thirds full with 1.23% APF. Sue then dries the teeth, inserts both trays concurrently, inserts the saliva ejector, and begins timing the treatment for four minutes. Sue remains chairside during the treatment and distracts the client by talking about her favorite sport.

As Sue removes the fluoride trays, the client immediately begins talking about how much she liked the taste of the double chocolate fluoride. Sue says that she is glad that the client enjoyed her first fluoride treatment and hopes she will look forward to the next appointment in six months.

Sue prepared to dismiss the client and return with her to the reception area to talk with the client's mother. As Sue and the client entered the reception area, the client reports to her mother that her stomach "does not feel good" and that she thought she might "be sick."

1. What aspects of the client assessment did Sue take into consideration when she decided to administer a professional fluoride application to this client?
2. Did Sue's administration technique impact the risk for a fluoride reaction?
3. Is Sue professionally and ethically bound to carry out the office policy regarding professionally applied fluoride applications? Are there any potential legal issues involved?
4. Is the office policy consistent with the evidence in the literature regarding professionally applied fluorides?
5. What should Sue and the mother do to assist the child?
6. How should this appointment be documented in the client record?

For References, Suggested Readings, and Related Websites, visit
http://evolve.elsevier.com/Darby/hygiene/

CHAPTER 27

PIT AND FISSURE SEALANTS

OBJECTIVES

Mastery of the content in this chapter will enable the student to:

- ✦ Define pit and fissure sealants and explain how they work
- ✦ Explain indications and contraindications for sealant placement
- ✦ Assess clients to determine their need for pit and fissure sealants
- ✦ Differentiate between filled, unfilled, and fluoride-releasing filled sealants
- ✦ Explain the difference between autopolymerized (self-cured) and photopolymerized (light-cured) sealants
- ✦ Explain to the client and/or guardian the importance of pit and fissure sealants as a caries preventive and/or therapeutic measure
- ✦ Place self cured and light-cured sealants
- ✦ Monitor the retention of pit and fissure sealants

KEY TERMS

Acid conditioning
Air abrasion
Air polishing
Articulating paper
Autopolymerization
Bis-GMA
Bonding
Bonding strength
Caries activity level of the client
Caries pattern of the client
Catalyst
Composite resin sealant
Curing light
Deficit in human need for biologically sound dentition
Deficit in human need for conceptualization and understanding
Deficit in human need for responsibility for oral health
Fluid-filled sealant
Glass ionomers
Hydrophilic primer
Incipient carious lesion
Monomer
Photopolymerization
Pit and fissure sealant
Preventive sealant
Therapeutic sealant
Unfilled sealant
Viscosity

Topically applied fluorides are most effective for preventing dental caries formation on the smooth surfaces of teeth and least effective in the pits and fissures. Consequently, the dental hygienist should consider the placement of pit and fissure sealants in planning dental hygiene care for the maximum prevention and control of dental caries. A *pit and fissure sealant* is a thin plastic coating of an organic polymer (resin) placed in the pits and fissures of teeth to act as a physical barrier (Figure 27–1).

The sealant bonds (mainly by mechanical retention) to the enamel surface of the tooth so that plaque bacteria cannot colonize within pits and fissures, thereby preventing dental caries. Research has shown that the incidence of caries can be reduced 17% to 54% by applying sealants to the occlusal surfaces of posterior teeth. Pit and fissure sealants along with fluoride therapy, oral hygiene instruction, modification of caries risk factors, and dietary counseling are integral components of any caries preventive program.

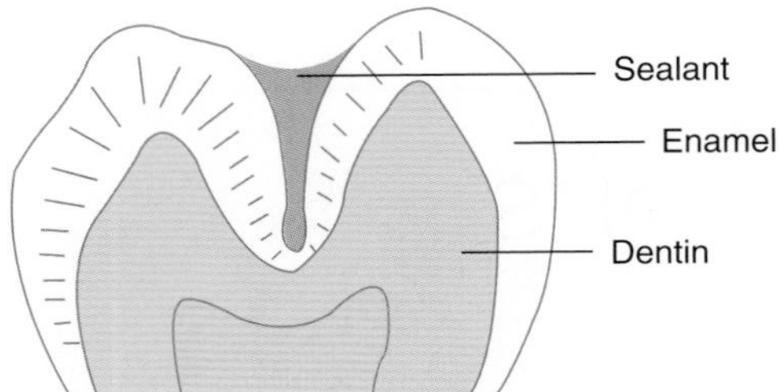

FIGURE 27–1 ✦ Sealant acts as a physical barrier. *(From* Preventing pit and fissure caries: A guide to sealant use, *Boston, 1986, Massachusetts Department of Public Health and Massachusetts Health Research Institute.)*

INDICATIONS FOR SEALANT PLACEMENT

Caries Risk Factors

During the assessment phase of the dental hygiene process, the dental hygienist assesses the client's risk factors for dental caries (see Chapter 26), and in consultation with the dentist makes a recommendation to the client to receive pit and fissure sealants. Clients with *incipient caries* (carious lesions limited to the enamel surface) and/or deep pits and fissures on the occlusal surfaces of their teeth that trap plaque biofilm can benefit from having sealants placed in their mouth. Sealants are indicated for clients of any age who are at risk for pit and fissure dental caries. This may include clients:

- ✦ With xerostomia
- ✦ Undergoing orthodontics
- ✦ Scheduled to undergo head and neck radiation therapy
- ✦ With incipient caries and with no radiographic evidence of caries on the proximal surface
- ✦ With infrequent professional preventive care
- ✦ With a high caries experience (i.e., other carious lesions in their mouth and a history of restored teeth)
- ✦ With newly erupted posterior teeth

Placement of a sealant by a dental hygienist is both a preventive and therapeutic intervention. *Preventive sealants* are those placed in caries-free teeth in an effort to prevent dental caries. *Therapeutic sealants* are those placed in teeth with incipient carious lesions in an effort to stop the decay process.

Tooth Assessment

An assessment of the tooth to be sealed involves identifying the pit and fissure morphology of the tooth. If the occlusal contour presents with deep and irregular pits and fissures and there is no radiographic evidence that the tooth has proximal dental caries, then a sealant should be placed. Primary second molars that demonstrate deep pits and fissures[1] also should be included in the sealant component of the dental hygiene care plan. Newly erupted teeth should be sealed as soon after eruption as possible. Retention rates of dental sealants are higher for fully erupted teeth than for partially erupted teeth.[2]

CONTRAINDICATIONS. If there is radiographic evidence of proximal dental caries, then sealant placement in occlusal pits and fissures is contraindicated and the client should be referred to the dentist to have the tooth restored. In addition, if the pits and fissures are well coalesced and self-cleansing, then sealants are contraindicated because such occlusal contours are at low risk for caries.

Teeth with deep plaque-retentive pits and fissures are at great risk for developing caries.[3] Research indicates that the first and second permanent molars are the teeth most at risk for pit and fissure caries.[4,5] Occlusal caries in the permanent dentition is five times more prevalent than caries found on mesiodistal surfaces, and 2.5 times more prevalent than caries found on the buccolingual surfaces.[6]

LEVEL OF CARIES ACTIVITY. The number of caries developed since the last dental visit (*caries activity level*) must be considered when deciding whether or not to place a sealant. Caries-free teeth should be considered for dental sealants if they have deep pits and fissures, if they are fully erupted, and if the client develops one or more carious lesions per year.[1] Carious lesions limited to the enamel surface of the teeth (incipient caries) should be sealed. A sealant placed over an incipient carious lesion can stop the caries from progressing to the dentin surface of the tooth, provided that the sealant remains intact.[7,8]

CARIES PATTERN. The *caries pattern of the client* reflects caries-prone tooth surfaces in a client's mouth. If the caries pattern indicates that an individual is predisposed to occlusal caries (i.e., developing one or more pit and fissure carious lesions per year), the remaining caries-free pit and fissure teeth are at great risk and should be sealed.[1] Figure 27–2 outlines the guidelines for making critical decisions about sealant use.

TYPES OF SEALANTS

Sealants are classified by their method of polymerization, their sealant content, and their color.

Classification by Polymerization Method

Sealants can be categorized by the method required to convert them from the liquid state to the solid state. The process by which sealants harden is known as *polymerization.* Polymerization can be accomplished by self-curing (*autopolymerization*), or light curing with a visible blue light *(photopolymerization).*

SELF-CURING/AUTOPOLYMERIZED SEALANTS. Autopolymerized sealants come in two components: a universal

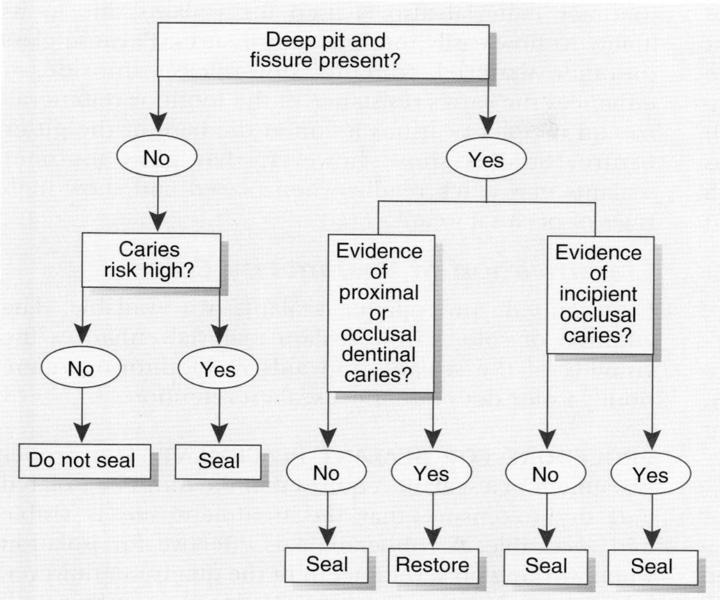

FIGURE 27–2 ✦ Guidelines for sealant placement decision making.

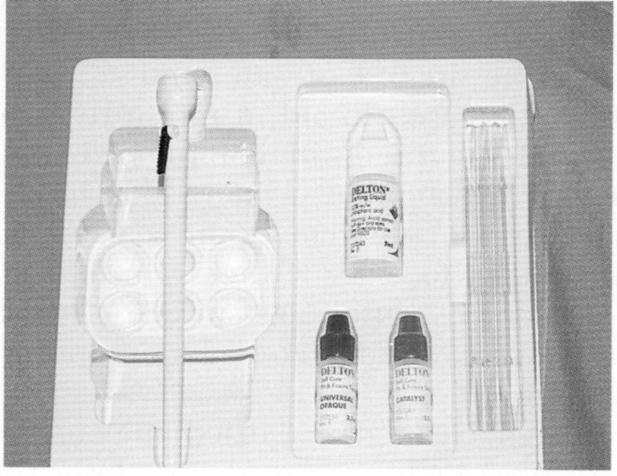

FIGURE 27–3 ✦ Universal liquid and catalyst vials shown with mixing wells and mixing stick.

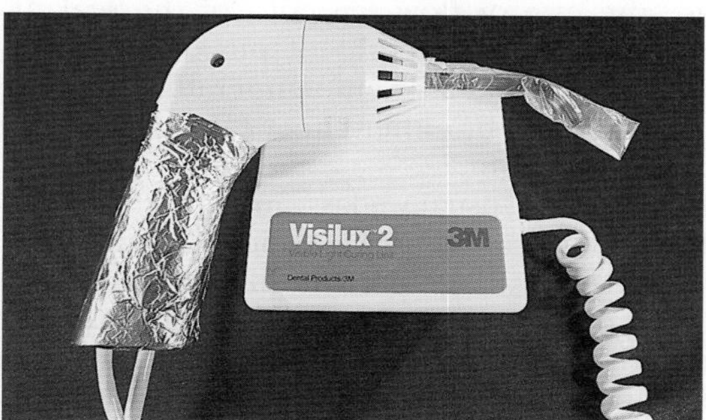

FIGURE 27–4 ✦ Curing light for photopolymerization.

liquid monomer and a catalyst (Figure 27–3). When the two components are mixed together, they harden (polymerize). Polymerization starts as soon as mixing begins and the material hardens within 60 to 90 seconds. Self-curing sealants are used in community health or school-based programs because there is no special equipment required.

PHOTOPOLYMERIZED/VISIBLE-LIGHT CURED SEALANTS. Photopolymerized sealants harden when exposed to a special curing light. Because no mixing time is required, the clinician controls the start of polymerization.

Today, handheld visible blue lights (curing lights) are commonly utilized (Figure 27–4) primarily for curing tooth-colored restorations. Using a curing light to polymerize sealants increases working time since the sealant will not harden until exposed to the curing light. Usual polymerization time is 20 to 60 seconds. Special lenses in eyeglasses or filters placed over protective eyewear are used to protect the clinician and client from potential retinal damage from the blue curing light (Figure 27–5).

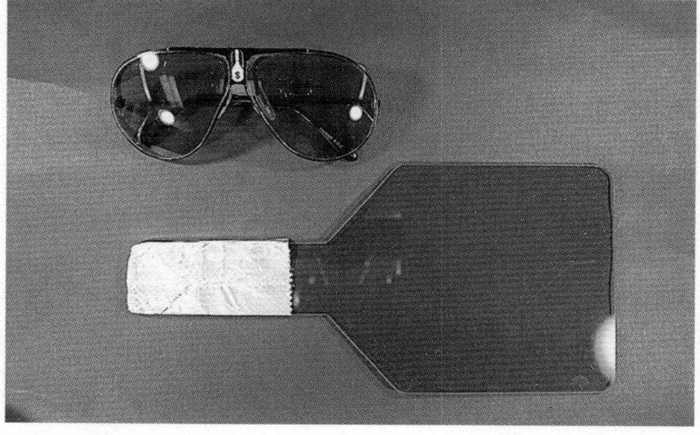

FIGURE 27–5 ✦ Protective glasses and shield used by the clinician for eye protection from the curing light.

These protective shields/glasses and the curing light incur additional costs.

Unlike self-cured sealant methods, the photopolymerized sealant method requires additional time for infection control. The curing light tip, a semicritical item, is in contact with mucous membranes, and therefore requires sterilization of the disposable tip or use of a plastic barrier. Plastic barriers, however, must not decrease the intensity of the light beam. If the output intensity of the curing light is less than 280 mW/cm^2, the polymerization process of the monomer will be incomplete and early loss of the sealant may occur. Research indicates the Sani-Shield barrier (DW Technology, Las Vegas, Nevada) to be the least likely to interfere with light output intensity. The intensity of the curing light can be measured by a dental radiometer.[9]

Classification by Sealant Content

The American Dental Association evaluates the effectiveness and safety of sealant materials. Most sealants are made of bisphenol a-glycidyl methylacrylate (*Bis-GMA*). The three types of sealants available based on content are filled, unfilled, and fluoride-releasing filled.

FILLED SEALANTS. Filled sealants are a mixture of resins, chemicals, and fillers. The resins contain monomers and chemicals to hold the filler particles together. The purpose of the filler is to increase *bonding strength* and resistance to abrasion and wear. In addition, fillers increase the rate of flow *(viscosity)* of the sealant, promoting flow into the depths of pits and fissures. The monomers are liquid at room temperature, and are activated or hardened by either chemical reactions or exposure to a curing light.

The fillers are usually glass and quartz particles of high hardness. Ground quartz (silicon dioxide) particles are categorized as large particle sized fillers, which give strength and hardness to the material. Silica particles are considered small particle sized fillers (microfill) and are less able to handle strong abrasive or occlusal forces. The ultimate combination of durability and strength in a composite sealant is with hybrid materials. This is a mixture of small and midsize particles that make up 50% to 70% of the total weight of the composite, and each filler particle is coated with saline to provide greater *bonding strength* between fillers and resins.[10]

Research indicates that filled sealants are twice as wear-resistant as unfilled sealants and that a 20- to 60-second light cure is all that is needed for the filled sealant to have adequate *bonding* to the enamel surface. Because of hardness and wear resistance, filled sealants must be checked after placement with *articulating paper* and adjusted with a dental handpiece and burr.

UNFILLED SEALANTS. Unfilled sealants are clear, making it difficult to see marginal deficiencies. Because unfilled sealants do not contain particles, they are less resistant to wear over the long term. Unfilled sealants are best used when the "high spots" in the occlusion cannot be adjusted with a dental handpiece. These sealants are most useful in school-based settings.

FLUORIDE-RELEASING SEALANTS (GLASS IONOMER SEALANTS). In restorative dentistry, *glass ionomers* are used as cavity liners or intermediary bases to occupy a small space between the tooth and the restoration. Glass ionomer material also is used for sealants due to its ability to flow easily into pits and fissures. Because glass ionomer material contains slow-release fluoride, it enhances the caries resistance of the tooth or remineralizes an incipient carious lesion at the base of the pit or fissure. Studies show, however, that glass ionomer sealants may crack readily when placed and show high rates of occlusal wear.[11,12]

Classification of Sealants by Color

Clear, tinted, and opaque sealants are available. The addition of color to the sealant material enhances the visibility of the sealant, and aids in monitoring retention.[13] Color does not affect sealant retention.

PROCEDURE FOR SEALANT PLACEMENT. The proper placement of a sealant requires that the tooth be isolated and dry to ensure that the treatment site is visible and accessible. A rubber dam is effective for isolation when working on several teeth in the quadrant; however, bibulous pads (e.g., Dri-Angles) placed over Stensen's duct and proper placement of cotton rolls in the vestibules and sides of the tongue are effective in promoting moisture control (Figure 27–6). It is critical to keep the working site free of water and saliva. The saliva ejector should be used to aid in moisture control, and the teeth should be dried with compressed air.

The use of hydrophilic primers aids in drying the enamel surface, which enhances the sealant attachment to the etched surface.[14,15] Other critical factors that influence sealant retention are surface cleanliness and the successful creation of etched micropores on the enamel surface.

Once isolated, cleaned, and dried, the enamel surface is ready for acid etching. An acid etching solution is applied to the tooth. The acid supplied by most manufacturers is 35% to 50% phosphoric acid in either liquid or gel form. Most common acids are at concentrations of 37%. The acid creates microscopic pores on the enamel to increase surface irregularities for sealant retention. The liquid acid is applied with a fine plastic-bristled brush using a continuous dabbing motion. The gel is placed on the tooth surface with a special syringe and left undisturbed (Figure 27–7). Many dental hygienists prefer to use gels because they are colored, making it easy to tell where the gel has been applied. Detailed methods for placement of light-cured and self-cured sealants are described in Procedures 27–1 and 27–2.

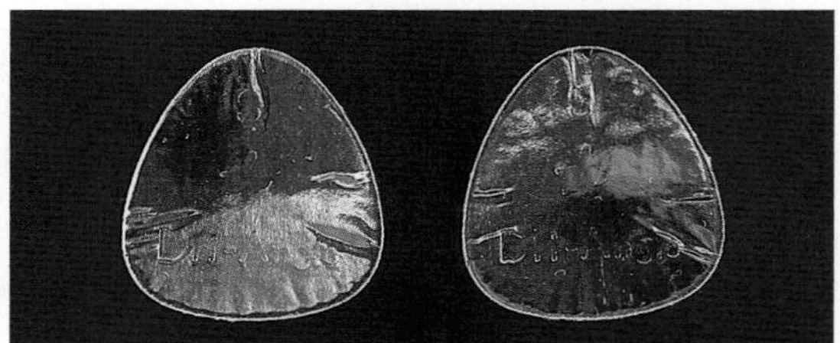

FIGURE 27–6 ✦ Dri-Angles for placement over Stensen's duct for isolation and moisture control.

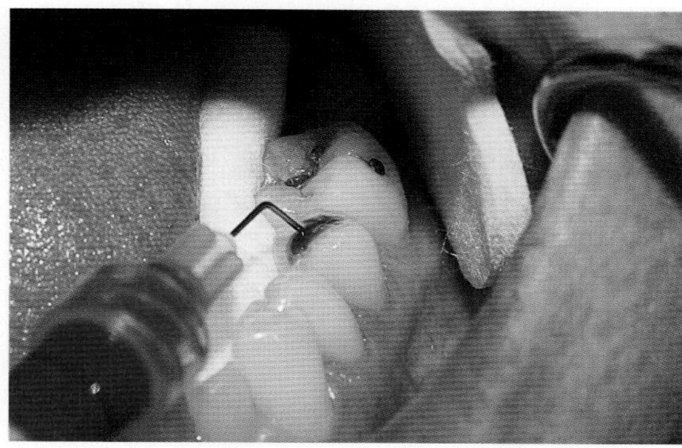

FIGURE 27–7 ✦ Acid etching solution in gel form.

Procedure 27–1 APPLYING LIGHT-CURED (PHOTOPOLYMERIZED) SEALANTS

EQUIPMENT

- Mouth mirror
- Explorer
- Cotton forceps
- Saliva ejector
- Sealant kit
- Cotton rolls/rubber dam
- Air/water syringe tip
- Dri-Angles
- High-speed evacuation tube
- Slow-speed handpiece
- Bristled brush
- Pumice
- Floss
- Protective shield
- Protective eyewear
- Personal protective equipment
- Light cure unit
- Finishing burrs
- Articulating paper

STEPS	RATIONALE
1. Provide client with protective eyewear with filter. Wear protective eyewear with filter.	To protect client and clinicians from potential retinal damage from the blue curing light. Eyeglasses are standard infection control procedures.
2. Polish the intended surface with a slurry of pumice and water. Use a bristled brush attached to a slow-speed handpiece. Rinse with water. 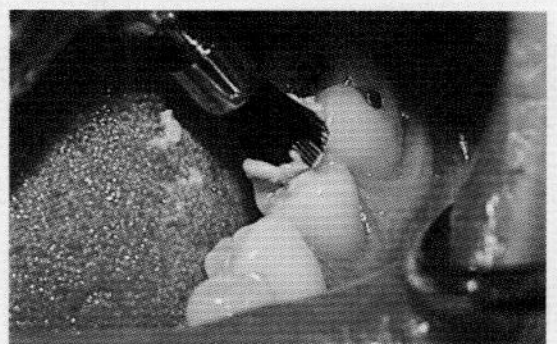 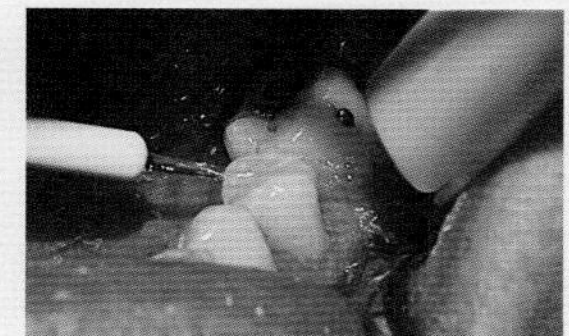	Surfaces to be sealed must be free of deposits and organic debris. Commercial pastes contain coloring and/or flavoring agents, glycerin, and/or fluoride, which may interfere with bonding. A bristled brush efficiently cleans the occlusal surface. Air abrasion units also are effective.
3. Isolate teeth with a rubber dam or cotton rolls. Place Dri-Angle over Stensen's duct. Insert saliva ejector into client's mouth.	Treatment site should be visible, accessible, and dry for proper sealant placement and retention.
4. Dry the site to be sealed with compressed air that is free of oil and moisture. 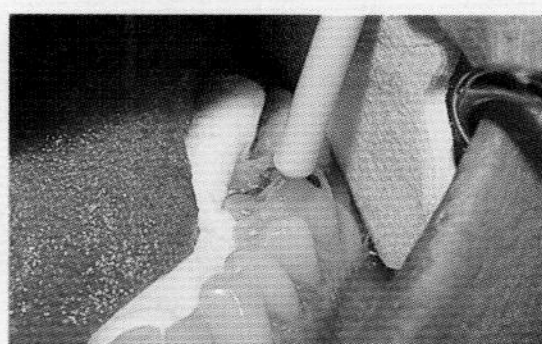	Presence of oil or moisture compromises bonding and retention.
5. Apply phosphoric acid to the clean, dry surface. Etch the tooth for 30 to 60 seconds. If using a liquid etch, apply it with a brush. If using a gel etch, apply it and leave undisturbed.	Acid etches the enamel to produce micropores into which the sealant flows and hardens, and is mechanically locked into place. Successful sealant retention depends on proper etching technique. Rubbing the gel acid burnishes the enamel surface and causes it to become smooth again, which decreases the retention and adversely affects bond strength.

Continued on following page

Procedure 27–1 APPLYING LIGHT-CURED (PHOTOPOLYMERIZED) SEALANTS—CONT'D

STEPS	RATIONALE
6. Rinse etched surfaces for 10 to 15 seconds using a water syringe and high-speed evacuation. If gel etch is used, rinse for an additional 30 seconds. 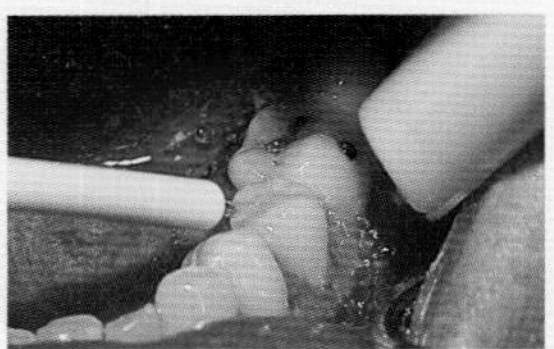	Rinsing removes the acid. If etched surface becomes contaminated with saliva, re-etch for 10 seconds.
7. Using cotton forceps, replace cotton rolls as they become wet. 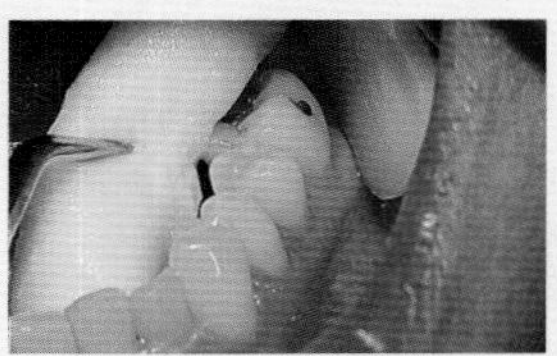	Moisture interferes with bonding and retention.
8. Dry the treatment site with compressed air for 10 seconds. Evaluate etched surface. 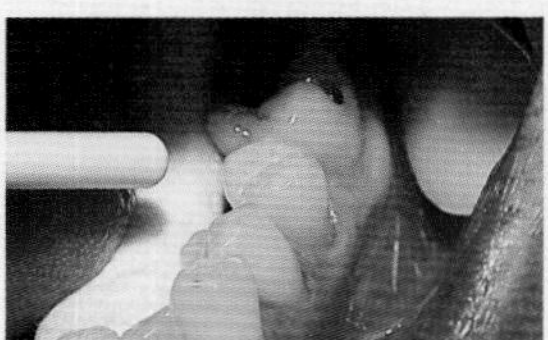	A properly etched area appears white, dull, and frosty.
9. Apply liquid sealant over the pits and fissures. Allow the sealant to flow into the etched surfaces. 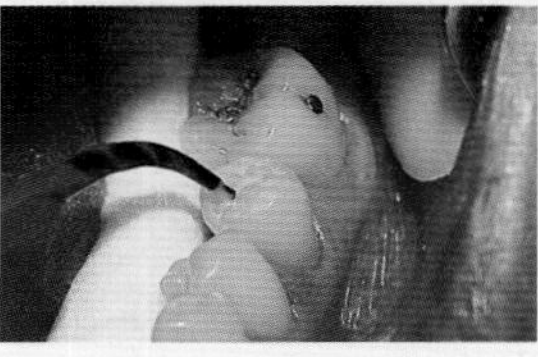	A low-viscosity sealant prevents air entrapment.
10. Apply light cure tip to each portion of the sealant. Place tip of light source 2 mm from sealant. Check manufacturer's instructions for time before advancing the light to another area. 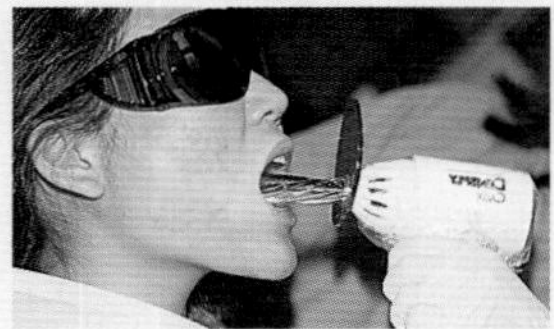	The curing process of the sealant is initiated by the light source. Time varies from 20–30 seconds. 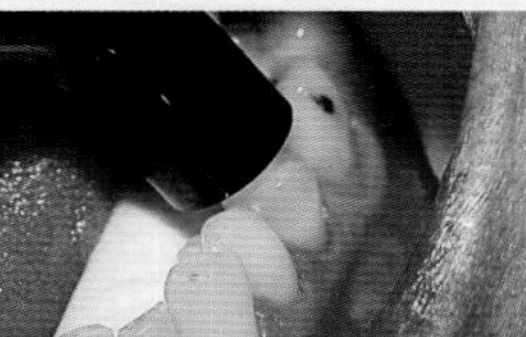

Procedure 27–1 APPLYING LIGHT-CURED (PHOTOPOLYMERIZED) SEALANTS—CONT'D

STEPS	RATIONALE
11. After the polymerization process, evaluate the sealant with an explorer and check for hard, smooth surface and retention. Set sealant appears as a thin, polymerized film.	A successful sealant feels hard and smooth and firmly bonded to the tooth. Air bubbles should not be present.
12. If imperfections are noted (e.g., incomplete coverage: air bubbles), re-etch tooth for 10 seconds; wash and dry teeth and apply additional sealant.	Air bubbles or a loose sealant do not provide effective caries prevention.
13. Check occlusion with articulating paper to detect high spot areas. Remove excess filled sealant material with a finishing burr.	High spot areas contain excess sealant material that interferes with normal occlusion. Minor discrepancies with an unfilled sealant are eliminated by normal masticatory processes.
14. Floss treated teeth. Scale away any residual sealant present.	This ensures that the sealant has not blocked contact between the teeth.
15. Apply topical fluoride.	Encourages remineralization of acid-etched surfaces.
16. Record type of sealant and teeth sealed in client's dental record.	Documentation allows for the proper monitoring of retention and serves as a legal document.
17. Evaluate sealants 3 months after application and at every continued care appointment.	If the site was contaminated from faulty technique, partial or complete loss of the sealant material occurs within 6 to 12 months. Early sealant loss exposes the tooth to dental caries. Complete retention of sealants has been documented up to 10 years.[16]

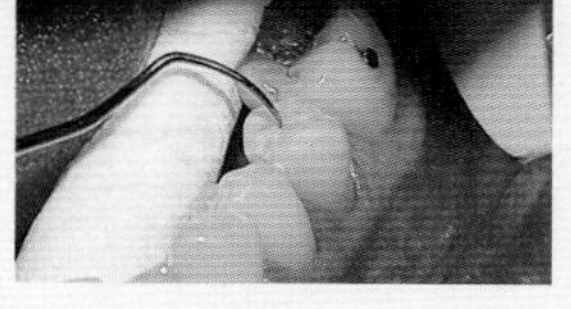

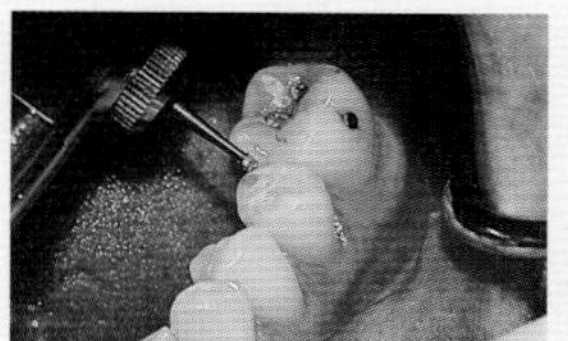

Photos courtesy Catrin Backlund, RDH.

Procedure 27–2 APPLYING SELF-CURED (AUTOPOLYMERIZING) SEALANTS

EQUIPMENT

- Mouth mirror
- Explorer
- Saliva ejector
- Self-cure sealant kit
- Gauze
- Cotton rolls/rubber dam
- Air/water syringe tip
- Dri-Angles
- High-speed evacuation tube
- Slow-speed handpiece
- Bristled brush
- Pumice
- Floss
- Face shield
- Protective eyewear
- Protective barriers

STEPS	RATIONALE
1. Follow steps 1 to 8 as described for light-cured sealants in Procedure 27–1.	
2. Mix one drop of Universal Liquid and one drop of Catalyst Liquid in mixing well. Follow manufacturer's directions, especially when sealing more than two teeth. 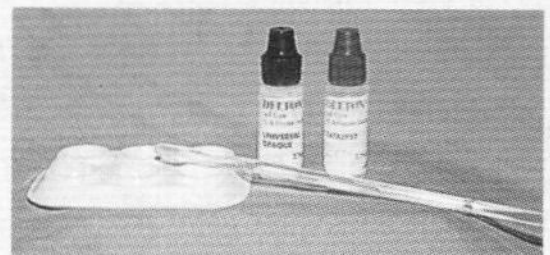	If a mix is prepared for more than two teeth, the mix sets prematurely and becomes thick and viscous. A viscous sealant does not allow for maximal flow into the pits and fissures. Bond strength and retention are compromised.
3. Mix for 10 to 15 seconds or as specified by manufacturer's directions.	Manufacturer's directions may vary.
4. Apply sealant with brush over pits and fissures. Working time: 45 seconds.	A low-viscosity sealant that flows over the etched surfaces prevents air entrapment.
5. Allow sealant to set for 60 to 90 seconds or according to manufacturer's instructions.	Do not disturb sealant. Allow specified time for the sealant to cure.
6. Follow steps 11 to 17 as described for light-cured sealants in Procedure 27–1.	

Client Education Issues

- Explain what a sealant is and why it is being placed.
- Explain that sealants can prevent the initiation and progression of dental caries and are a cost-effective component of any preventive oral healthcare program. Sealants are not permanent, and as such may need to be replaced.
- Explain that sealant placement does not eliminate the need for topical fluoride application, plaque control, or the limitation of sucrose in the diet. Sealants in combination with these other strategies are part of a total caries preventive program.
- Explain that sealants require cooperation from the client for optimal placement.

Legal, Ethical, and Safety Issues

- Care must be taken when using the acid-etch solution to avoid contact with any body tissues other than the tooth surface to be sealed.
- Clients must wear protective glasses as a barrier to the sealant chemicals and curing light.
- Clients must understand that sealants are not permanent, and may need to be replaced for continued protection against pit and fissure caries.
- It is legal for dental hygienists to place dental sealants in all 50 states.
- New Hampshire, New Jersey, Oregon, and Texas require special training for sealant placement by dental hygienists.
- In the state of Maine, dental hygienists can place sealants in schools or public health sealant programs without the diagnosis of a dentist.
- Louisiana, Maryland, Hawaii, and New Hampshire allow dental hygienists to place sealants under general supervision in settings outside the private dental office.
- Always follow manufacturers' instructions.

Key Concepts

- Dental sealants can be a preventive and/or therapeutic treatment for clients.
- Epidemiologic data reveal that dental caries are concentrated more on the occlusal surfaces than on smooth surfaces of the teeth.
- Clients' risk for developing dental caries is determined by identifying their caries experience, the frequency with which they use dental services, the type of dental care they have received in the past, and any medical conditions that might contribute to their caries experience. This information is integral to assessing their need for dental sealants.
- A dental hygiene diagnosis related to dental sealants is based on the client's deficits in the human needs for a biologically sound dentition, conceptualization and understanding, and responsibility for oral health.
- Composite resin sealants can be either filled or unfilled.
- Glass ionomer sealants release fluoride to provide a cariostatic benefit to the tooth.
- Filler particles in dental sealants enhance their wear resistance.
- Prior to placing a dental sealant, the tooth surface to be sealed must be cleaned, dried, etched, rinsed, and then dried again.
- Commercial pastes and fluoride interfere with bonding of sealants to the tooth surface.
- When placing a dental sealant it is important to allow the material to flow into the grooves of the tooth surface. This minimizes the presence of air bubbles.
- The process by which the sealant material hardens is called polymerization.
- Autopolymerization causes the sealant material to harden chemically by mixing an activator with a catalyst.
- Photopolymerization causes the sealant material to harden by use of a high-intensity blue light.
- The retention rate of dental sealants is enhanced by keeping the working area free from salivary contaminants, using a hydrophilic primer to dry the tooth surface, and thoroughly cleaning the tooth surface to be sealed.
- The retention rate of dental sealants should be evaluated at each continued-care visit.

Critical Thinking Exercises

Patient Profile: Sonia is a 15-year-old Hispanic female who presents to the dental office for an exam and oral prophylaxis.

Chief Complaint: "I am here today because I noticed black spots on the chewing surfaces of some of my back teeth, and my mouth always feels dry."

Medical History: Client reports that she suffers from allergies all year round. Her symptoms are relieved by taking Claritin once daily.

Dental History: She has not seen a dentist in 2 1/2 years. Her dental exam reveals the presence of three carious lesions: #18 MO, #30 DO, and #3 O. She has incipient carious lesions on the occlusal surfaces of #2, #14, #15, and #19.

Social History: She is single and lives at home with her parents. Sonia states that she drinks approximately three soft drinks a day to relieve her dry mouth.

Oral Self-care Assessment: The client states that she brushes her teeth with a fluoride toothpaste three times a day. However, her technique reveals that when brushing she covers only the facial surfaces of her maxillary and mandibular teeth. She uses no interdental aids.

Supplemental Notes: Client has gingival inflammation throughout, but very little calculus.

1. How would you use this information in planning dental hygiene care to meet the client's need for a biologic and functional dentition? What interventions would you plan and why?
2. Would pit and fissure sealants be beneficial for her? Where? Explain your response.
3. What would you say in educating Sonia about her caries prevention and treatment options during her dental hygiene care appointment?

For References, Suggested Readings, and Related Websites, visit

http://evolve.elsevier.com/Darby/hygiene/

CHAPTER 28

NUTRITIONAL COUNSELING

OBJECTIVES

Mastery of the content in this chapter will enable the reader to:

- Identify individuals in need of nutritional counseling
- Determine client compliance with *U.S. Dietary Guidelines*
- Assess a client's diet for adequacy of intake using the *USDA Food Guide Pyramid*
- Calculate ideal body weight, body mass index, and total energy expenditure
- Describe differences in nutritional requirements throughout the life span
- Provide nutritional counseling to control dental caries, promote postsurgical healing and tissue regeneration, reduce incidence of bone loss due to osteoporosis and osteopenia, or achieve optimal health

KEY TERMS

Basal energy expenditure (BEE)
Body mass index (BMI)
Dental health diet score
Diet history
Dietary Guidelines for Americans
Food frequency questionnaire
Ideal body weight
Nutrition assessment
Nutritional counseling
Nutritional rehabilitation
Osteoporosis/osteopenia
Primary nutritional deficiency
Secondary nutritional deficiency
Sugar exposure
Sweet score
Total daily acid production
Total daily energy expenditure
USDA Food Guide Pyramid

Nutritional counseling is a process used to help clients develop healthful behaviors that promote overall health. It is challenging because many factors influence an individual's selection of food, including:[1]

- Age and gender
- Ethnicity and culture
- Socioeconomic status (income, occupation, and educational level)
- Lifestyle (e.g., career, time, food, and preparation)

Diagnosis of a nutritional deficiency or metabolic disease is made by a physician after extensive data collection. Much of this information is outside of the scope of the dental hygienist and therefore precludes the dental hygienist from functioning in the role of nutrition professional. However, as the health professional most often seen by clients, the dental hygienist should be knowledgeable about nutrition, oral manifestations of nutritional deficiencies, and oral health (Figure 28–1).

NUTRITION ASSESSMENT

Nutrition assessment is the systematic collection of information to identify the need for nutritional counseling and make the appropriate recommendations and referrals. The client's personal history can reveal information regarding educational, cultural, financial, and environmental influences on food intake. The health and pharmacologic histories identify health factors and medications that interfere with an individual's ability to eat or the body's ability to absorb nutrients. The dental history provides information about caries susceptibility and use of fluoride; and the extraoral and intraoral examination may reveal the physical results of any nutritional excesses or deficiencies. These findings, along with a dietary assessment, direct the dental hygienist in the role of dietary counselor. Determining which clients need nutritional counseling involves analyzing information collected during the assessment phase of care. Every client

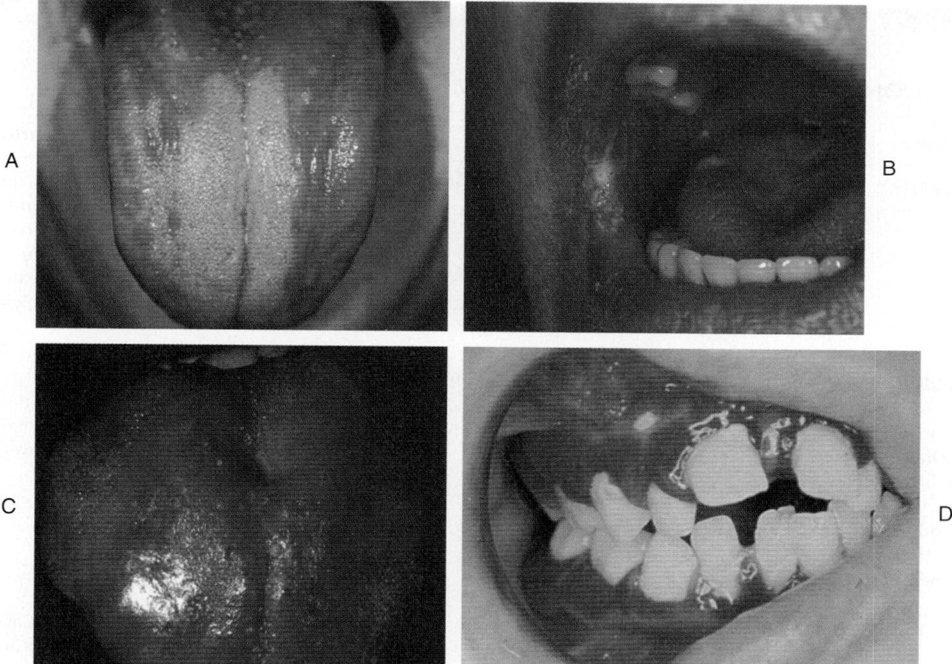

FIGURE 28–1 ✦ Some oral manifestations of nutritional deficiencies. **A,** Atrophy of the filiform and fungiform papillae on the dorsum of the tongue associated with iron deficiency anemia. **B,** Riboflavin deficiency characterized by erythema, maceration, and soggy white debris at the commissures of the mouth. **C,** Painful, beefy red, atrophic tongue often with ulceration as associated with niacin deficiency. **D,** Severe gingivitis associated with scurvy. *(From Eisen D, Lynch DP:* The mouth: Diagnosis and treatment, *St Louis, 1998, Mosby.)*

could benefit from nutritional counseling, but those most often targeted include clients:

- ✦ At risk for osteoporosis
- ✦ Diagnosed with osteopenia
- ✦ Undergoing oral maxillofacial surgery
- ✦ With dental caries or periodontal disease
- ✦ With oral manifestations of a possible nutritional deficiency.

Health and Pharmacologic Histories

Questions normally included in a comprehensive health history provide clues to nutritional status, lifestyle behaviors, and overall health (see Chapter 9, Figure 9–2 and Table 9–3). Conditions and medications that interfere with food digestion, absorption, and metabolism should be noted. The health history should always include anthropometric measurements of weight and height.

HEIGHT AND WEIGHT. Height and weight can be used to determine the client's body mass index. *Body mass index (BMI)* reflects weight in relation to height (Table 28–1); it is not a measure of lean body mass.

A BMI of 20 to 25 is considered within the normal range.

A BMI less than 20 is an indication of being underweight.

A BMI of 25 to 30 is in the overweight category.

A BMI of over 30 is considered obese.

Although a BMI measurement does not reflect how much of the weight is fat or where fat is located, it does give a measurement associated with health risks such as heart disease, hypertension, diabetes, and cancer. Another useful calculation is *ideal body weight* (Table 28–1).

EXERCISE PATTERNS. Activity levels ascertained during the health history interview may be used to calculate energy expenditure. An approximate daily caloric expenditure can be useful in planning for weight loss or weight gain. To accurately assess total daily energy expenditure, the basal energy expenditure must first be calculated.

Basal energy expenditure (BEE), the total energy output of a body at rest after a 12-hour fast in a room of comfortable temperature, is a measure of the amount of calories required to maintain body weight. To determine *total daily energy expenditure (TDE),* the BEE is multiplied by an activity factor (AF) (Table 28–1). Again, the calculation used in these formulas provides a calorie count required for maintenance of the body at its current weight. To lose or gain weight, the calorie count must be adjusted accordingly. Calculation of total daily caloric intake for periodontal and oral surgery clients can also be calculated by multiplying the total daily energy expenditure by an injury factor (IF) (see Calculation of Total Daily Calorie Intake for an Oral Surgery Client).

Assessment of the ingestion of vitamin and mineral supplements provides insight about such oral manifestations as xerostomia, lichenoid reactions, candidiasis,

TABLE 28–1 NUTRITION- AND EXERCISE-RELATED FORMULAS AND CALCULATIONS

Formula/Calculation	Definition	Use	Disadvantage
Body Mass Index (BMI) BMI = weight in pounds × 705 ÷ height in inches^2	Measurement of weight in relation to height	<20 underweight 20–25 normal 25–30 overweight >30 obese	Does not measure lean tissue in relation to fat (i.e., body builders may have a higher BMI due to a larger amount of lean tissue but are not overweight or obese).
Ideal Body Weight For men, 106 pounds for the first 5′ of height and 6 pounds for each inch after 5′; for women = 100 pounds for the first 5′ and 5 pounds for each inch after 5′.	Determines ideal body for height of individual	Useful in determining if client is underweight or overweight	Does not measure lean tissue in relation to fat. A client may be considered underweight but may still be "overfat."
Basal Energy Expenditure (BEE) For men, 66 + 13.7 (weight in kilograms) + 5 (height in cm) – 6.8 (age). For women, 655 + 9.6 (weight in kg) + 1.8 (height in cm) – 4.7 (age).	Determines the calories needed to maintain the client's body at current weight	Useful as a part of determining total daily energy expenditure	Does not account for the desire to lose or gain weight and must be adjusted accordingly in that case. A measurement of only the calories needed to keep a human body alive.
Total Daily Energy Expenditure (TDE) BEE × activity factor* (× injury factor†)	Determines the calories required per day to maintain the client's current weight while taking into account activity levels and, if necessary, calories expended due to illness or injury	Useful when used with weight loss, weight gain, or weight maintenance plans.	Most clients will overestimate their energy expenditure. Injury factors are used at the discretion of the clinician and may be over- or under-estimated.

* Activity factors include 1.5 = confined to bed, 1.3 = ambulatory, 1.5 to 1.7 = normally active, 2.0 = extremely active.
† Injury factors include 1.2 = minor surgery (1.35 = skeletal trauma, 1.44 = elective surgery), 1.6 to 1.9 = major sepsis, 1.88 = trauma plus steroids, 2.1 to 2.5 = severe thermal burns.

Calculation of Total Daily Calorie Intake for an Oral Surgery Client

A 35-year old female weighs 118 pounds and is 5 feet 6 inches tall. Her exercise includes walking 4 miles every evening. She has undergone oral and maxillofacial reconstructive surgery to correct her malocclusion.

Conversion of pounds to kg: divide pounds by 2.2.

Conversion of inches to cm: multiply inches by 2.4.

BEE: 655 + 9.6(54) + 1.8(158) – 4.7(35) = 1292 calories per day.

TDE: 1292 × 1.5 × 1.4 = 2713 calories per day postsurgery to promote healing without a resultant weight loss.

A registered dietitian should be the individual that adjusts specific nutrient values in the client's diet.

NOTE: The activity factor or injury factor may be adjusted to better describe the amount of activity or injury.

cheilitis, and glossitis. Table 28–2 lists drug and nutrient interactions that may produce oral side effects when combined with any of the 20 most commonly prescribed drugs in the United States.

DIET ASSESSMENT

Diet assessment is the identification of current dietary practices and diet requirements of the client. Diet assessment includes frequency of food intake, methods of food preparation, cultural or religious dietary considerations, and exercise or activity levels; it reflects the *Dietary Guidelines for Americans* and has some relation to the dental-related dietary recommendations of *Healthy People 2010*[2,3] (see Dietary Guidelines for Americans and *Healthy People 2010* Oral Health–Related Nutrition Objectives). Types of diet assessments include the diet history, a food frequency questionnaire, and a computer diet analysis.

TABLE 28–2 DRUG-NUTRIENT INTERACTIONS OF THE TOP TWENTY DRUGS PRESCRIBED IN THE UNITED STATES

Generic Drug Name (Trade Name)	Classification	Indication for Use	Drug-Nutrient Interaction
1. Conjugated estrogen (Premarin) (Wyeth-Ayerst Labs, Philadelphia, Pa)	Female sex hormone	Estrogen replacement; atrophic vaginitis; urinary incontinence secondary to estrogen deficiency; prostatic cancer; prevention of osteoporosis; inoperable breast cancer	Grapefruit juice may interfere with metabolic degradation of the conjugated estrogen, resulting in greater bioavailability of the drug
2. Levothyroxine (Synthroid) (Knoll Labs, Mt. Olive, NJ)	Thyroid hormone	Hypothyroidism, pituitary TSH suppressants (thyroid nodules, thyroiditis, thyroid cancer)	Absorption may be decreased by soybean products or iron
3. Atorvastatin (Lipitor) (Parke-Davis, Morris Plains, NJ)	Antihyperlipidemic	Adjunct to dietary therapy in hyperlipidemia	Grapefruit juice may increase serum levels of drug
4. Omeprazole (Prilosec) (Astra Zeneca, Wayne, Pa)	Antisecretory compound	Gastrointestinal reflux disease (GERD), peptic ulcer disease (PUD)	Decreases gastric secretions Inhibits solubilization of iron, calcium, magnesium, and zinc, thus decreasing absorption
5. Hydrocodone (Hydrocodone) (Watson Labs, Inc., Corona, Calif)	Narcotic analgesic	Management of moderate to severe pain	Alcohol consumption may result in potentiation of CNS depressant effect
6. Albuterol aerosol (Albuterol) (Watson Labs, Inc., Corona, Calif)	Adrenergic B2 agonist	Asthma; chronic obstructive pulmonary disease (COPD)	May cause a decrease in serum potassium levels, but does not usually require supplementation; may cause unusual taste or drying and irritation of the oropharynx
7. Amlodipine (Norvasc) (Pfizer Inc., New York, NY)	Calcium channel blocker	Angina; hypertension	Drug produces xerostomia; grapefruit juice may elicit severe hypotension
8. Loratadine (Claritin) (Schering Corp., Kenilworth, NJ)	Antihistamine	Perennial and seasonal allergic rhinitis; urticaria and other allergic symptoms	Grapefruit juice may enhance drug response; drug may increase appetite
9. Amoxicillin (Trimox) (Apothecon, New York, NY)	Antibiotic	Treatment of infections caused by susceptible bacteria	Absorption may be reduced or delayed by food
10. Fluoxetine (Prozac) (Eli Lilly & Co., Indianapolis, Ind)	Antidepressant	Mental depression; obsessive-compulsive disorder	Drug produces xerostomia; alcohol consumption may result in potentiation of CNS depressant effect
11. Sertraline (Zoloft) (Pfizer Inc., New York, NY)	Antidepressant	Mental depression; obsessive-compulsive disorder	Drug produces xerostomia; alcohol consumption may result in potentiation of CNS depressant effect
12. Metformin (Glucophage) (Bristol-Myers Squibb, Lawrenceville, NJ)	Hypoglycemic agent	Management of non–insulin-dependent diabetes mellitus	Shown to produce an anorectic effect in human obese subjects with subsequent loss of weight; shown to stimulate food intake in rat studies; bioavailability and peak concentration decreased when taken with food
13. Digoxin (Lanoxin) (GlaxoSmithKline, Research Triangle Park, NC)	Cardiac glycoside	Congestive heart failure; arterial dysrhythmias	Can affect sodium and potassium levels; bran may reduce drug absorption; drug may affect carbohydrate, vitamin, and mineral absorption; drug may cause nausea, vomiting, or anorexia; licorice-induced hypokalemia may enhance the action of digoxin to toxic levels
14. Conjugated estrogen (Prempro) (Wyeth-Ayerst Labs, Philadelphia, Pa)	Female sex hormone	Estrogen replacement; atrophic vaginitis; urinary incontinence secondary to estrogen deficiency; prostatic cancer; prevention of osteoporosis; inoperable breast cancer	Grapefruit juice may interfere with metabolic degradation of the conjugated estrogen
15. Paroxetine (Paxil) (GlaxoSmithKline Research Triangle Park, NC)	Antidepressant	Mental depression; obsessive-compulsive disorder	Drug produces xerostomia; alcohol consumption may result in potentiation of CNS depressant effect; may cause nausea, decreased appetite

Table continued on following page

TABLE 28–2 DRUG-NUTRIENT INTERACTIONS OF THE TOP TWENTY DRUGS PRESCRIBED IN THE UNITED STATES—CONT'D

Generic Drug Name (Trade Name)	Classification	Indication of Use	Drug-Nutrient Interaction
16. Azithromycin (Zithromax) (Pfizer, Inc., New York, NY)	Macrolide antibiotic	Broad spectrum antibiotic prescribed for respiratory tract, sinus, ear, and skin infections; also effective against chlamydia and certain other infections of reproductive tract	Should be taken on empty stomach; food may reduce or delay absorption
17. Lisinopril (Zestril) (Astra Zeneca, Wilmington, Del)	Angiotensin-converting enzyme (ACE) inhibitor	Hypertensive patients who have not responded to multidrug treatment; congestive heart failure, asymptomatic left ventricular dysfunction, diabetic nephropathy, idiopathic edema	Drug produces xerostomia; potassium supplements should be avoided as well as large amounts of foods containing potassium, such as bananas and orange juice; glycyrrhizic acid in natural licorice may induce hypokalemia and complicate antihypertensive therapy
18. Simvastatin (Zocor) Merck & Co. Inc., West Point, Pa)	Lipid lowering drug	Adjunct to dietary therapy in hyperlipidemia	Grapefruit juice may inhibit metabolism of drug, resulting in increased bioavailability/effectiveness of drug
19. Lansoprazole (Prevacid) (Tap Pharm, Lake Forest, Ill)	Gastric acid secretion inhibitor	Short-term treatment for healing and symptom relief of active duodenal ulcers	Bioavailability/effectiveness of drug decreases when taken with food or antacids
20. Amoxicillin/clavulanate (Augmentin) (GlaxoSmithKline, Research Triangle Park, NC)	Antibiotic	Treatment of infections caused by susceptible bacteria	Treatment with amoxicillin may alter intestinal flora, resulting in malabsorption of nutrients

Data from United States Pharmacopeia: *Drug information,* ed 19, Rockville, Md, 1999, US Government Printing Office.
Drug Information Handbook for Dentistry, ed 5, Hudson, Ohio, 1999–2000, Lexi-comp.

Healthy People 2010 Oral Health–Related Nutrition Objectives

Nutrition and Overweight Goal

Promote health and reduce chronic disease associated with diet and weight

Objectives

Increase the proportion of adults who are at a healthy weight.
Reduce the proportion of adults who are obese.
Reduce the proportion of children and adolescents who are overweight and obese.
Increase the proportion of persons aged 2 years and older who consume at least 2 daily servings of fruit.
Increase the proportion of persons aged 2 years and older who consume at least three daily servings of vegetables, with at least one third being dark green or deep yellow vegetables.
Increase the proportion of persons aged 2 years and older who meet dietary recommendations for calcium.
Increase the proportion of children and adolescents aged 6 to 19 years whose intake of meals and snacks at school contributes proportionally to good overall dietary quality.
Increase the proportion of work sites that offer nutrition or weight management classes or counseling.

Dietary Guidelines for Americans

Eat a variety of foods
Balance the foods you eat with physical activity; maintain or improve your weight
Choose a diet low in fat, saturated fat, and cholesterol
Choose a diet with plenty of vegetables, fruits, and grain products
Choose a diet moderate in sugars
Use salt and sodium only in moderation
Drink alcoholic beverages in moderation or not at all

From Report of the Dietary Guidelines Advisory Committee, Washington, DC, 1995, US Department of Agriculture, US Department of Health and Human Services.

Diet History

A *diet history* (Figure 28–2) may consist of a 24-hour or a 3-, 5-, or 7-day diet history in which the client records all foods and drinks consumed within the defined period. The diet history determines a client's usual intake over a period of time and is a screening tool to identify persons in need of nutritional counseling. A diet history is obtained by interview or self-administered questionnaire.

24-HOUR DIET FORM

Instructions to Client

1. List everything you eat and drink on an ordinary week-day, including snacks
2. Record when foods or snacks:
   (1) Were eaten
   (2) Amount ingested (examples: 4 oz tomato juice, 1 cup coffee with 1 tsp sugar, 3 oz chicken sandwich, 2 bread slices)
   (3) How food was prepared
   (4) Teaspoons of sugar added

Breakfast

Snacks

Lunch

Snacks

Dinner

Snacks

Instructions for Clinicians

1. Circle foods sweetened with added sugars or concentrated natural sweets (honey, figs, etc.), saturated fats, or alcohol
2. Place uncircled foods into one of the pyramid food groups on the form to calculate the dental health diet score
3. For each serving place a mark in food group block
4. Add number of checks and multiply by number shown
5. Add total and determine need for general nutritional counseling, then, complete steps for sugar evaluation and need for nutritional counseling for the prevention of dental caries

FIGURE 28–2 ✦ 24-hour diet form. *(From Nizel AE, Papas AS:* Nutrition and clinical dentistry, *ed 3, Philadelphia, 1989, WB Saunders.)*

Food models such as measuring cups and spoons help the client recall the amount of food consumed and should be used when possible. A 24-hour diet history usually requires 15 to 20 minutes of time and does not require the client to possess a long memory. If taken unannounced or with no prior indication, it minimizes the likelihood of socially acceptable responses. However, the 24-hour diet recall may not be representative of the person's usual food intake. For most people, workdays, weekends, or holidays influence food intake considerably.

An advantage of the 24-hour diet recall is that it serves as a teaching session. Accuracy as well as content of the history can be discussed during the session, and the technique can be applied to a 3-, 5-, or 7-day diet recall. The client and the dental hygienist determine the length of time the diet will be documented. The shorter the period, the less likely it is that the record will reveal usual eating patterns.

Food Frequency Questionnaire

A *food frequency questionnaire* (Figure 28–3) is similar to a 24-hour diet recall but specifically asks the client to record foods most frequently eaten within a stated timeframe (e.g., as short as a day or as long as a month). The 24-hour diet recall or food frequency questionnaire can be useful in assessing the cariogenic potential of the diet.

Computer Diet Analysis

All diet records have the potential for computer analysis. There are various programs available, and often the choice depends on the information obtained, its purpose, and the type of computer hardware available. Some programs are designed for research and provide everything from bar graphs to merging data for community-based programs. Most computer programs provide information on caloric intake as well as deficient or excess nutrient amounts. Some programs analyze sugar intake, including percentage of sugars in the diet (i.e., simple versus complex carbohydrates).

Diet Evaluation

A simple and practical client assessment includes:

- ✦ Daily sugar exposures
- ✦ Adequacy of food intake based on the five food groups/Food Guide Pyramid

Evaluation of the Cariogenic Potential of the Diet Using a Sweet Score

To assess the cariogenic potential of the diet, the client records a 24-hour diet that represents the client's typical eating patterns (Figure 28–2). Type and amount of each food eaten, food preparation, and time of day the food was eaten are reported. The 24-hour diet recall is then used to calculate the cariogenic potential of the diet. The sugar ingested reported on the 24-hour diet form is categorized according to liquid sugars, solid and sticky sugars, and slowly dissolving sugars. The frequency with which each sugar is ingested is tallied and multiplied by 5, 10, or 15 depending on the sugar source (Figure 28–4). A *sweet score* of 15 or more indicates that the individual is in need of nutritional counseling to reduce the cariogenic potential of his or her diet.

Evaluation of the Adequacy of the Diet Using a Dental Health Diet Score

The same 24-hour diet form used to calculate the cariogenic potential can be used to calculate the *dental health diet score.* Foods reported on the 24-hour dietary survey are placed into one of the pyramid food groups on the form used to calculate the dental health diet score (Figures 28–5 to 28–7). This information is useful in identifying individuals in need of general nutritional counseling. Nutritional requirements vary depending on the age, gender, and activity level of the individual. Because of these variations, a separate form should be used to calculate the dental health diet score for:

- ✦ Women and older adults (Figure 28–5)
- ✦ Most men, children, teen girls, active women (Figure 28–6)
- ✦ Teen boys and active men (Figure 28–7)

Directions for the dental hygienist: for assessing the frequency of food use, the following pattern of questions may be useful. Questions may need modification after learning information from the 24-hour recall. For instance, if the client has said he had a glass of milk yesterday, one wouldn't ask "Do you drink milk?" but rather "How much milk do you drink?" Record answers as 1/day, 1/wk, 2/mo, or as accurately as possible; also may be noted as "occasionally" or "rarely."

1. Do you drink milk?
   If so, how much?
   What kind? Whole Skim Low-fat
2. Do you use fat?
   If so, what kind?
   How much?
3. How often do you eat meat? Eggs? Cheese? Beans?
4. Do you eat snack foods?
   If so, which ones?
   How often? How much?
5. What vegetables do you eat (in each group)?
   How often?

a. broccoli
green peppers
cooked greens
carrots
sweet potatoes

b. tomatoes
raw cabbage

c. asparagus
beets
cauliflower
corn
cooked cabbage
celery
peas
lettuce

6. What fruits do you eat (in each group)?

a. apples or apple sauce
apricots
bananas
berries
cherries
grapes or grape juice
peaches
pears
pineapple
plums
prunes
raisins

b. oranges
orange juice
grapefruit
grapefruit juice

7. Bread and cereal products:

   a. How much bread do you usually eat with each meal?
      Between meals?
   b. Do you eat cereal (daily, weekly)?
      Cooked? Dry?
   c. How often to you eat foods such as macaroni, spaghetti, noodles, etc.?
   d. Do you eat whole-grain breads and cereals?
      If so, how often?
8. Do you use salt?
   Do you salt your food before tasting it?
   Do you cook with salt?
   Do you "crave" salt or salty foods?
9. How many teaspoons of sugar do you use per day (1 packet = 1 tsp)?
   (Be sure to ask client about sugar on cereal, fruit, and toast and in coffee, tea, etc.)
10. Do you eat desserts?
    If so, how often?
11. Do you drink sugar-containing beverages such as soda pop, bottled sports drinks, bottled juices, etc.?
    If so, how often?
12. Do you eat candy or cookies?
    If so, how often?
13. Do you drink water?
    How often during the day?
    How much each time?
    How much would you say you drink each day?
14. Do you use sugar substitutes in packet form or in drinks?
    If so, how often?
    What do you use?
15. Do you drink alcoholic beverages?
    If so, how often?
    How much? Beer? Wine? Liquor?
16. Do you drink caffeinated beverages?
    If so, how often?
    How much? How much per day?

FIGURE 28–3 ✦ Food frequency questionnaire.

Decay-promoting Potential

Form	Frequency	Points
Liquid: soft drinks, fruit drinks, cocoa, sugar and honey in beverages, nondairy creamers, ice cream, sherbet, gelatin dessert, flavored yogurt, pudding, custard, popsicles	_____ × 5 =	
Solid and Sticky: cake, cupcakes, donuts, sweet rolls, pastry, canned fruit in syrup, bananas, cookies, chocolate candy, caramel, toffee, jelly beans, other chewy candy, chewing gum, dried fruit, marshmallows, jelly, jam	_____ × 10 =	
Slowly Dissolving: hard candies, breath mints, antacid tablets, cough drops	_____ × 15 =	

TOTAL SCORE = _______

Sweet Score: _______
5 or less Excellent
10 Good
15 or more "Watch out" zone
* 15 or more—nutritional counseling needed for reducing sugar intake

FIGURE 28–4 ✦ Form to calculate the cariogenic potential of the diet from a 24-hour food diary. *(Modified from Nizel AE, Papas AS:* Nutrition and clinical dentistry, *ed 3, Philadelphia, 1989, WB Saunders.)*

Food Group	Recommended Servings	Portion Size Considered One Serving	Number of Servings	Points
Bread, cereal, rice, beans	6	1 slice of bread 1/2 C cooked rice or pasta 1 oz ready to eat cereal 1/2 C cooked cereal	____ × 4 =	______ (highest possible score = 24)
Vegetable group	3	1 C raw leafy vegetable 3/4 C vegetable juice 1/2 C other vegetable cooked or raw	____ × 8 =	______ (highest possible score = 24)
Fruit group	2	1 medium apple, orange or banana 3/4 C fruit juice 1/2 C chopped, cooked, canned fruit	____ × 12 =	______ (highest possible score = 24)
Milk, cheese, yogurt group	2	1 C milk or yogurt 1 1/2 oz natural cheese 2 oz process cheese	____ × 12 =	______ (highest possible score = 24)
Meat, poultry, fish, dry bean, egg, nut group	2 or 5 oz	2 to 3 oz lean meat, poultry, fish cooked 1 egg 1/2 C cooked dry beans 2 tbsp peanut butter	____ × 12 =	______ (highest possible score = 24)

Food Group Score _______
102–120 Excellent
92–101 Adequate
75–91 Barely adequate
0–74 Not adequate

TOTAL SCORE = _______
(highest possible score = 120)

* Score of 91 or less—nutritional counseling needed

FIGURE 28–5 ✦ Form to calculate the dental health diet score for women and older adults. *(Prepared by Lynn Tolle Watts, BSDH, MS, Gene W. Hirschfield School of Dental Hygiene, Old Dominion University; modified from Nizel AE, Papas AS:* Nutrition and clinical dentistry, *ed 3, Philadelphia, 1989, WB Saunders.)*

Food Group	Recommended Servings	Portion Size Considered One Serving	Number of Servings	Points
Bread, cereal, rice, beans	9	1 slice of bread 1/2 C cooked rice or pasta 1 oz ready to eat cereal 1/2 C cooked cereal	____ × 3 =	______ (highest possible score = 27)
Vegetable group	4	1 C raw leafy vegetable 3/4 C vegetable juice 1/2 C other vegetable cooked or raw	____ × 6 =	______ (highest possible score = 24)
Fruit group	3	1 medium apple, orange or banana 3/4 C fruit juice 1/2 C chopped, cooked, canned fruit	____ × 8 =	______ (highest possible score = 24)
Milk, cheese, yogurt group	2	1 C milk or yogurt 1 1/2 oz natural cheese 2 oz process cheese	____ × 12 =	______ (highest possible score = 24)
Meat, poultry, fish, dry bean, egg, nut group	2 or 6 oz	2 to 3 oz lean meat, poultry, fish cooked 1 egg 1/2 C cooked dry beans 2 tbsp peanut butter	____ × 12 =	______ (highest possible score = 24)

Food Group Score _______
106–123 Excellent
96–105 Adequate
80–95 Barely adequate
0–79 Not adequate

TOTAL SCORE = ______
(highest possible score = 123)

* Score of 95 or less—nutritional counseling needed

FIGURE 28–6 ✦ Form to calculate the dental health diet score for most men, children, teen girls, and active women. *(Prepared by Lynn Tolle Watts, BSDH, MS, Gene W. Hirschfield School of Dental Hygiene, Old Dominion University; modified from Nizel AE, Papas AS:* Nutrition and clinical dentistry, *ed 3, Philadelphia, 1989, WB Saunders.)*

Food Group	Recommended Servings	Portion Size Considered One Serving	Number of Servings	Points
Bread, cereal, rice, beans	11	1 slice of bread 1/2 C cooked rice or pasta 1 oz ready to eat cereal 1/2 C cooked cereal	____ × 2 =	______ (highest possible score = 22)
Vegetable group	5	1 C raw leafy vegetable 3/4 C vegetable juice 1/2 C other vegetable cooked or raw	____ × 5 =	______ (highest possible score = 25)
Fruit group	4	1 medium apple, orange or banana 3/4 C fruit juice 1/2 C chopped, cooked, canned fruit	____ × 6 =	______ (highest possible score = 24)
Milk, cheese, yogurt group	2	1 C milk or yogurt 1 1/2 oz natural cheese 2 oz process cheese	____ × 12 =	______ (highest possible score = 24)
Meat, poultry, fish, dry bean, egg, nut group	2 or 7 oz	2 to 3 oz lean meat, poultry, fish cooked 1 egg 1/2 C cooked dry beans 2 tbsp peanut butter	____ × 12 =	______ (highest possible score = 24)

TOTAL SCORE = ______
(highest possible score = 119)

Food Group Score ________
101–119 Excellent
91–100 Adequate
73–90 Barely adequate
0–72 Not adequate
* Score of 90 or less—nutritional counseling needed

FIGURE 28–7 ✦ Form to calculate the dental health diet score for teen boys and active men. *(Prepared by Lynn Tolle Watts, BSDH, MS, Gene W. Hirschfield School of Dental Hygiene, Old Dominion University; modified from Nizel AE, Papas AS:* Nutrition and clinical dentistry, *ed 3, Philadelphia, 1989, WB Saunders.)*

To calculate the dental health diet score, daily servings for each of the five food groups are tallied and multiplied by the number of servings represented on the form. A food group score is calculated for each of the five food groups, and summed to provide a total score ranked accordingly: excellent, adequate, barely adequate, and not adequate. A total score of 90 or less for women and older adults indicates that nutritional counseling is needed. Once an individual is identified for nutritional counseling, a more comprehensive dietary assessment must be completed. This assessment is accomplished by instructing the client to keep a 3-, 5-, or 7-day food diary and then evaluating the diary.

A food diary that includes a weekend is more likely to represent the individual's normal eating habits. All foods consumed in a 24-hour period should be recorded, including type of food eaten, manner in which it was prepared, exact amount of each food eaten, and time of day in which it was eaten (Figure 28–8). The client should be encouraged to adhere to his or her normal dietary regimen during assessment period.

Evaluation of the 3-, 5-, or 7-Day Food Diary

If the client's sweet score or dental health diet score indicates the need for nutritional counseling, the dental hygienist asks the client to complete a 3-, 5-, or 7-day food diary. Upon completion, the dental hygienist and client evaluate the diet for adequacy of intake from the five food groups (Figure 28–9). Foods consumed by the client are categorized into each of the five food groups. The average number of servings for a 3-, 5-, or 7-day period is calculated and recorded. Servings from the client's diet are compared to the daily servings recommended by the USDA Food Guide Pyramid (Figure 28–10), and deficiencies or excesses are noted.

In addition, the cariogenic potential of the diet also must be analyzed by calculating the amount of acid produced in the diet (Figure 28–11). Each *sugar exposure,* defined as any sweet or sugar-sweetened food or liquid, is circled in red. The total number of liquid and solid sugar exposures ingested over a 3-, 5-, or 7-day period is tallied and multiplied by the appropriate time interval. The number of liquid sugar exposures ingested over the period is multiplied by 20 minutes, and the number of solid sugar exposures ingested over the period is multiplied by 40 minutes. This figure is divided by the number of days assessed, and the resulting figure indicates the amount of time daily that the teeth are subjected to an acid exposure. The *total daily acid production* is calculated by adding the daily acid production from both liquid and solid sugars. Sugars consumed at the same time are considered one acid exposure (i.e., ice cream and cake eaten for dessert equals one acid exposure). Sweet foods or liquids eaten 20 minutes apart are recorded as two acid exposures. Calculating the number of acid exposures illustrates the cariogenic potential of the client's diet.

Instructions: Please record everything you eat or drink for a five-day period which includes either *a weekend or a holiday*. Don't forget to include all snacks, gum, candies, soft drinks, etc.

Be Specific! It is very important to write down the following:

Amount
- 1/2 cup string beans
- 1 tablespoon butter
- 6 ounces steak

How food was prepared
- 1/2 cup string beans—boiled
- 6 ounces steak—fried
- 1 orange—fresh
- 1 peach—canned

What was added to the food/drink
- 1 cup coffee—1 tsp milk
- 1/2 grapefruit—1 tsp sugar

Time of day
- Lunch—12:30 P.M.
- Snack—3:00 P.M.

Also include the order in which the solids or liquids are eaten.
If you want to use additional paper please feel free to do so.

____
Client Name

First Day		**Second Day**		**Third Day**	
Food	Quantity Prepared	Food	Quantity Prepared	Food	Quantity Prepared
Breakfast		Breakfast		Breakfast	
10:00 A.M.		10:00 A.M.		10:00 A.M.	
Lunch		Lunch		Lunch	
3:00 P.M.		3:00 P.M.		3:00 P.M.	
Dinner		Dinner		Dinner	
Extras		Extras		Extras	

Fourth Day		**Fifth Day**	
Food	Quantity Prepared	Food	Quantity Prepared
Breakfast		Breakfast	
10:00 A.M.		10:00 A.M.	
Lunch		Lunch	
3:00 P.M.		3:00 P.M.	
Dinner		Dinner	
Extras		Extras	

FIGURE 28–8 ✦ Five-day food diary form. *(Prepared by Lynn Tolle Watts, BSDH, MS, Gene W. Hirschfield School of Dental Hygiene, Old Dominion University; modified from Nizel AE, Papas AS:* Nutrition and clinical dentistry, *ed 3, Philadelphia, 1989, WB Saunders.)*

Instructions: For each food item, place a check mark (✓) in the appropriate block

Food Group	Portion Size Considered One Serving	1st Day	2nd Day	3rd Day	4th Day	5th Day	Average	Suggested Daily Amount: Women and Older Adults	Suggested Daily Amount: Most Men Children Teen Girls Active Women	Suggested Daily Amount: Teen Boys and Active Men	Difference
Bread, cereal, rice, pasta	1 slice bread 1/2 C cooked rice or pasta 1 oz cereal							6	9	11	
Vegetable group	1 C raw leafy vegetable 3/4 C vegetable juice 1/2 C other vegetable cooked or raw							3	4	5	
Fruit group	1 medium apple, orange, banana 3/4 C fruit juice 1/2 C chopped, cooked, canned fruit							2	3	4	
Milk, yogurt, cheese, group	1 C milk or yogurt 1/2 oz natural cheese 2 oz process cheese							2–3*	2–3*	2–3*	
Meat, poultry, fish, dry beans, egg, nut group	2 to 3 oz lean meat, poultry, fish cooked 1 egg 1/2 C cooked dry beans 2 tbsp peanut butter							2 total of 5 oz	2 total of 6 oz	3 total of 7 oz	
Fats, oils, sweets	1 tbsp margarine 1 tbsp salad dressing 1 can soft drink 1/2 C ice cream 1 slice cake							Sparingly	Sparingly	Sparingly	

* To age 24 need 3 servings; or if pregnant or breast feeding

FIGURE 28–9 ✦ Foundation foods. *(Prepared by Lynn Tolle Watts, BSDH, MS, Gene W. Hirschfield School of Dental Hygiene, Old Dominion University; modified from Nizel AE, Papas AS:* Nutrition and clinical dentistry, *ed 3, Philadelphia, 1989, WB Saunders.)*

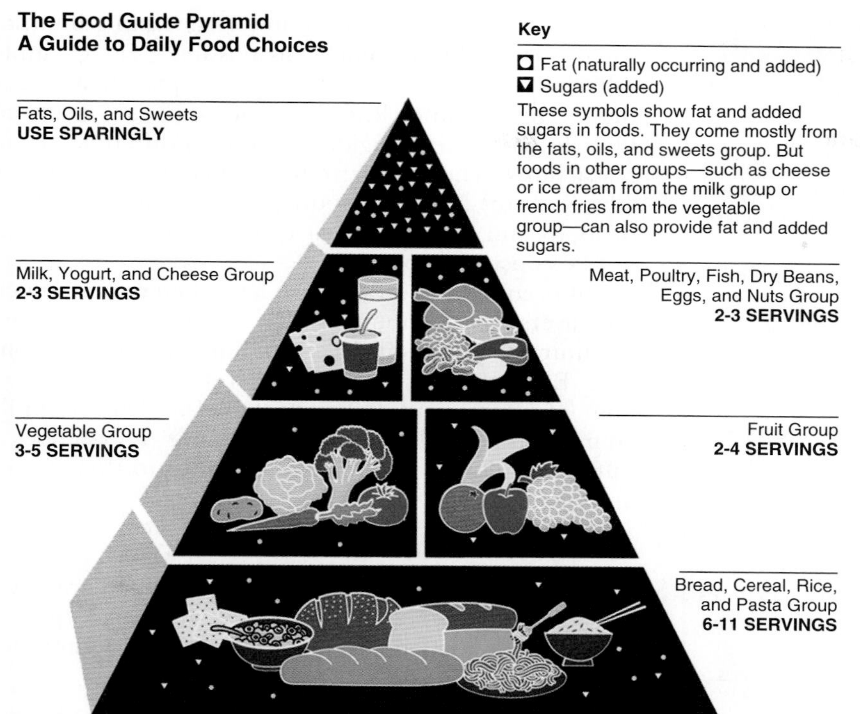

FIGURE 28–10 ✦ The USDA Food Guide Pyramid.

Form of Sugar		When Eaten	1st Day	2nd Day	3rd Day	4th Day	5th Day	Total
Liquid	(soda, sugar in coffee, etc.)	With meals						
		Between meals						
Solid	(cookie, candy)	With meals						
		Between meals						

Grand total = ______ (Sugar in liquid form)

Grand total = ______ (Sugar in solid form)

______ × 20 minutes / pH below 5.5 = ______ ÷ 5 DAYS = ______
Liquid Eposure — Acid Production — Daily liquid acid production

______ × 40 minutes / pH below 5.5 = ______ ÷ 5 DAYS = ______
Solid Eposure — Acid Production — Daily liquid acid production

Total daily acid production = ______ + ______ = ______
Liquid acid production total — Solid acid production total — Total time tooth is exposed to acid daily (demineralization)

FIGURE 28–11 ✦ Form to calculate the cariogenic potential of the diet from a 5-day food diary. *(Modified from Nizel AE, Papas AS:* Nutrition and clinical dentistry, *ed 3, Philadelphia, 1989, WB Saunders.)*

NUTRITIONAL COUNSELING

Using the information obtained from the health history and diet assessment, the dental hygiene clinician and client can now formulate a plan. Suggestions for Nutritional Counseling in the Oral Care Setting contains suggestions for nutritional counseling in oral care setting.

Cultural Sensitivity

Culture should be a part of every assessment and counseling session (see Chapter 5). Different beliefs and lifestyles exist in society and each should be accorded respect. The challenge for healthcare providers is to be culturally adaptable, to display cross-cultural communication skills, to remain aware of nonverbal cues that are

Suggestions for Nutritional Counseling in the Oral Care Setting

Maintain a separate space in the office for discussion of diet. This ensures that infection control is maintained and provides a more casual and relaxed atmosphere for discussion of nutrition issues.

Use plastic examples of foods to help client conceptualize size of portion.

Keep a set of measuring spoons and cups handy to help determine portion size.

Laminate an 11 × 14 picture of the Food Guide Pyramid to use as a teaching tool. Using a wipe-away marker, check marks can be placed in the appropriate section of the pyramid to illustrate dietary choices from a diet recall. The laminated picture also makes it easy to maintain infection control.

Have available brochures and information about the *U.S. Dietary Guidelines,* the Food Guide Pyramid, and dietary recommendations from the American Diabetes Association, American Heart Association, and American Cancer Society.

culturally based, and to move toward a trusting interpersonal relationship as quickly as possible.[4] For example, different religions often advocate unique dietary practices. Hindus and Buddhists advance a vegetarian lifestyle and other religions adhere to different dietary restrictions. The Jewish religion includes dietary laws (the Kashrut) about the source, fitness, and preparation of foods and describes what types of foods may or may not be consumed together.

Different ethnic groups also have dietary preferences and aversions. Although many internationals become acculturated, some still follow traditional dietary customs (see Examples of Dietary Preferences According to Some Cultural and Religious Beliefs.) The culturally competent dental hygienist maintains knowledge of different cultures and remains sensitive to their beliefs and practices.

Identifying Nutritional Deficiencies

Nutritional problems manifest themselves both orally and systemically (Table 28–3). A *primary nutritional deficiency* is caused by inadequate dietary intake of a nutrient.[4]

Examples of Dietary Preferences According to Some Cultural and Religious Beliefs

African American

Diet varies greatly according to region of country and lifestyle.

High incidence of lactose intolerance; low consumption of dairy products.

Most popular meat dishes include pork (variety cuts), fish, small game, poultry.

Frying and boiling are the most common preparation methods.

Primary grain product is corn.

Green leafy vegetables most popular, cooked with ham, bacon, lemon, broth.

Intake of fresh fruits and vegetables often low.

Dishes frequently seasoned with hot-pepper sauces. Onions and green pepper are common for flavoring.

Honey, molasses, and sugar products are preferred as snacks.

Asian

High incidence of lactose intolerance; traditional alternative sources of calcium include tofu, soy milk, small bones in fish and poultry.

Variety of protein-rich foods, often preserved by salting and drying.

Pastes of shrimp and legumes.

Wheat and rice are primary grain products.

Fresh fruits and vegetables, also pickled, dried, or preserved.

Buddhism

Vegetarianism with five pungent foods excluded: garlic, leek, scallion, chives, and onion.

Hinduism

Mostly vegetarian except in northern India where meat is eaten (except for beef).

Islam

No consumption of unclean foods (carrion or dead animals, swine).

No consumption of animals slaughtered without pronouncing the name of Allah or killed in manner that prohibits the complete draining of blood from their bodies.

No consumption of carnivorous animals with fangs, birds of prey, and land animals without ears (frogs, snakes).

Latino

High incidence of lactose intolerance; low consumption of dairy products.

Vegetable protein is more common in countries with large rural and urban poor populations.

Pork, goat, and poultry are common meats. Much of it is marinated, chopped, or ground. Often mixed with vegetables and cereals.

Principal bread is tortilla.

Foods are often heavily spiced.

Common fruits and vegetables include avocados, tomatoes, cactus, chiles, corn, jicama, guava, lemons, limes, banana, oranges, plantains.

Native American

High incidence of lactose intolerance; low consumption of dairy products.

Meat highly valued, mostly grilled, stewed, or preserved through drying and smoking.

Primary grain used is corn; wild rice also popular.

Preferred fruits and vegetables include indigenous plants, gathered or cultivated.

Orthodox Judaism

Prohibits consumption of swine, shellfish, and carrion eaters.

Ritual slaughtering of animals.

Ritual breaking of bread.

Meat and milk are prepared in separate dishes/utensils and containers and not cooked, served, or eaten together.

TABLE 28–3 VITAMINS AND MINERALS GROUPED ACCORDING TO FUNCTION, INCLUDING SOURCES, HUMAN DEFICIENCY/EXCESS SYNDROMES, AND ORAL IMPLICATIONS

Nutrient	Dietary Source	Deficiency Syndrome	Oral Implications of Deficiency	Excess/Other
Function: Structure and Calcification				
Vitamin A (fat soluble)	Vitamin A is present only in animal foods; beef liver is an excellent source. Beta carotene: carrots, melon, squash, sweet potato, spinach	Growth failure	Reduction in formation of ameloblasts and odontoblasts	Excess may cause headache, vomiting, severe liver damage, defect in long bone formation
Vitamin D (fat soluble)	Synthesized in skin exposed to sunlight	Rickets, osteomalacia	Enamel hypoplasia and loss of lamina dura	Excess may cause vomiting and diarrhea, hypercalcemia
Vitamin E (fat soluble)	Vegetable seed oils, widely distributed in foods	Anemia, neuropathy, myopathy	Loss of resistance to inflammation in periodontium	Excess may inhibit vitamin K functions, causing problems with blood clotting
Vitamin K (fat soluble)	Synthesized by intestinal bacteria: green leafy vegetables, soybeans, beef liver	Defective blood clotting	May be involved in bone formation	High doses of synthetic form may cause oxidation of membrane lipids, severe jaundice in infants
Vitamin C (water soluble)	Citrus fruits, papaya, cantaloupe, broccoli, potato, strawberries	Scurvy	Inhibition of formation of fibroblasts, osteoblasts, and odontoblasts	Overdose may cause diarrhea, kidney stones
Calcium	Milk and milk products, sardines, clams, turnip and mustard greens, broccoli	Rickets, osteomalacia, osteoporosis, scurvy, stunted growth	Tooth exfoliation due to osteoporosis in alveolar bone	Excess may cause constipation
Phosphorus	Meat, poultry, fish, eggs, milk products, chocolate	Rickets, osteomalacia	Possible failure of reparative dentin formation	Symptoms associated with excess are rare, problems appear to occur only when calcium to phosphorus ratios are altered significantly in infants
Magnesium	Nuts, legumes, cereal grains, chocolate, blackstrap molasses, spinach	Growth failure, neuromuscular dysfunction, personality changes, muscle spasms	Reduced formation of alveolar bone, hypoplasia of enamel, widening of periodontal ligament space, and gingival hyperplasia	Acute toxicity from excessive intravenous administration results in nausea, depression and paralysis
Fluoride	Mackerel, salmon, shrimp, meat, potatoes, wheat, sardines	Osteoporosis, osteosclerosis	Dental caries	Excess results in fluorosis
Function: Soft Tissue, Including Oral, Salivary, and Taste Function				
Vitamin B_1 thiamin (water soluble)	Pork, sunflower seeds, legumes	Beriberi, muscle weakness, tachycardia, enlarged heart, edema	Glossitis, gingival tissue discoloration	Excessive doses may cause headache, convulsion, cardiac arrhythmia, anaphylactic shock
Vitamin B_2 riboflavin (water soluble)	Beef liver, lean steak, mushrooms, ricotta cheese, milk	Photophobia, dermatitis, anemia	Cheilosis, glossitis, edema of pharyngeal and oral mucous membranes, angular stomatitis	No toxicity symptoms reported
Vitamin B_6 pyridoxine (water soluble)	Sirloin steak, navy beans, potato, banana	Dermatitis, convulsions, severe sensory neuropathy	Glossitis	Excess causes sensory and peripheral neuropathy. Minimal dosage at which toxicity occurs is not defined
Vitamin B_{12} (water soluble)	Meat, fish, shellfish, poultry, milk	Megaloblastic anemia, degeneration of peripheral nerves, skin hypersensitivity	Glossitis, eventual disappearance of the filiform and fungiform papillae	No effects from excessive doses have been reported
Niacin (water soluble B vitamin)	Tuna, beef liver, chicken breast, mushrooms	Pellagra, diarrhea, dermatitis, dementia	Stomatitis, atrophic changes of filiform and fungiform papillae, tongue smooth and shiny	Large doses used in the treatment of hyper-cholesterolemia. Excess may cause facial flushing, release of histamines which may be detrimental to asthmatics

Table continued on following page

TABLE 28–3 VITAMINS AND MINERALS GROUPED ACCORDING TO FUNCTION, INCLUDING SOURCES, HUMAN DEFICIENCY/EXCESS SYNDROMES, AND ORAL IMPLICATIONS—CONT'D

Nutrient	Dietary Source	Deficiency Syndrome	Oral Implications of Deficiency	Excess/Other
Folate (water soluble B vitamin)	Brewer's yeast, spinach, asparagus, turnip greens, lima beans, beef liver	Megaloblastic anemia, diarrhea, fatigue, depression, convulsions	Glossitis, chronic periodontitis, candida	Excess may cause insomnia, malaise, irritability, GI problems
Pantothenic acid (water soluble B vitamin)	Widespread in foods, egg yolk, liver, kidney	Deficiency very rare, numbness and tingling of hands and feet	May impair healing of oral tissues	Excess may increase niacin excretion
Biotin (water soluble B vitamin)	Synthesized in intestinal tract	Deficiency very rare, anorexia, nausea, depression, dermatitis	Glossitis, lingual and mucous pallor, papillae trophy	No effects from excessive doses reported
Vitamin C (water soluble)	See above	Scurvy	Poor collagen formation and oral wound healing	No effects from excessive doses reported
Vitamin A (fat soluble)	See above	Xerosis, keratomalacia	Decreased salivary secretion and xerostomia	No effects from excessive doses reported
Vitamin E (fat soluble)	See above	Anemia, neuropathy, myopathy	Loss of integrity in cell membranes of mucosa, atrophy of filiform papillae	No effects from excessive doses reported
Sodium	Table salt, meat, seafood, cheese, milk, bread, vegetables	Muscle atrophy, poor growth, weight loss	Thirst, dry, sticky tongue and mouth	High sodium intakes may affect calcium excretion
Potassium	Avocado, banana, dried fruits, wheat bran, eggs, dairy products	Muscular weakness, mental apathy, cardiac arrhythmias, paralysis, adrenal hypertrophy, decreased growth rate	None	Hyperkalemia is toxic, resulting in severe cardiac failure
Chloride	Table salt, seafood, eggs, meat, milk	Failure to thrive in infants, muscle weakness, hypokalemia, metabolic acidosis	None	No excess effects have been noted
Iron	Organ meats, clams, oysters, legumes, enriched and/or whole grain cereals and breads	Fatigue, palpitations on exertion, anemia, decreased resistance to infection	Sore tongue, angular stomatitis, dysphagia	Excess causes damage to tissues including liver, and other lorgans
Zinc	Wheat germ, oysters, beef liver, dark meat of poultry	Poor wound healing, subnormal growth, skin inflammation, anemia, retarded development of reproductive organs	Abnormal taste and smell	Acute toxicity produces metallic taste, nausea, vomiting, epigastric pain, abdominal cramps
Iodine	Iodized salt, saltwater shellfish, spinach, pumpkin, broccoli, chocolate	Enlargement of thyroid, myxedema, cretinism, increase in blood lipids, liver gluconeogenesis	Enlargement of thyroid gland	No adverse effects reported

From Dietary Guidelines Advisory Committee: *Dietary Guidelines for Americans, Washington, DC*, 1995, US Department of Agriculture, US Department of Health and Human Services.

Once identified, this type of deficiency can be corrected after dietary assessment followed by nutritional counseling that promotes proper selection and intake of nutrients. A *secondary nutritional deficiency* is caused by a systemic disorder that interferes with the ingestion, absorption, digestion, transport, and use of nutrients.[4] This type of deficiency is more complex, and referral to a physician and a nutritionist is necessary for treatment.

After dietary deficiencies and excesses are identified, the dental hygienist and client develop a dietary program. Four rules are adopted when making dietary modifications:[5]

✦ Maintain overall nutritional adequacy by conforming to the *USDA Daily Food Guide* for at least the recommended number of servings from each of the food groups.

- The diet should vary from the normal dietary pattern as little as possible.
- The diet should meet the body's requirements for essential nutrients as generously as the diseased condition can tolerate.
- The diet should accommodate the individual's cultural and religious beliefs and practices, likes and dislikes, food habits, and other environmental factors, as long as they do not interfere with the objectives.

The use of the *Dietary Guidelines for Americans* in conjunction with the USDA Food Guide Pyramid guides the necessary diet modifications. The Food Guide Pyramid stresses balance among all the food groups. The largest groups are those from which most of the daily servings of food should come. The bottom of the pyramid is the largest and includes bread, cereal, grains, and pasta; six to 11 servings should be chosen from this group. The vegetable group is next, with three to five servings, followed by the fruit group, with two to four servings. The milk group and the meat group each suggest two to three servings. Fats and oils should be used sparingly. All food groups contain some amount of fats or oils, depending on method of preparation, and this is depicted by the scattering of small triangles and circles throughout the Food Guide Pyramid. The portions shown in Food Groups and Serving Sizes are considered one serving size and can assist the client in recording a detailed food diary.

The dental hygienist also tailors recommendations to the client's lifestyle. Although most healthy clients have similar nutrient needs, stages within the life cycle may require special consideration, including pregnancy, infancy and childhood, and old age. Moreover, the dental hygienist considers the special nutritional needs of clients with caries risk, those undergoing periodontal and oral surgery, and those at risk for or with osteoporosis.

Food Groups and Serving Sizes

Grain Products (bread, cereal, rice, and pasta)
1 slice of bread
1 ounce of ready-to-eat cereal
½ cup of cooked cereal, rice, or pasta

Vegetables
1 cup of raw leafy vegetables
½ cup of other vegetables, cooked or chopped raw
¾ cup of vegetable juice

Fruits
1 medium apple, banana, orange
½ cup of chopped, cooked, or canned fruit
¾ cup of fruit juice

Milk (milk, yogurt, and cheese)
1 cup of milk or yogurt
1½ ounces of natural cheese
2 ounces of processed cheese

Meat and Beans (meat, poultry, fish, dry beans, eggs, and nuts)
2 to 3 ounces of cooked lean meat, poultry, or fish (about the size of a deck of cards)
½ cup of cooked dry beans or 1 egg can be substituted for 1 ounce of lean meat
2 tablespoons of peanut butter or ⅓ cup of nuts can be substituted for 1 ounce of meat

NUTRITIONAL NEEDS IN PREGNANCY

All stages of pregnancy require an increase in nutrients and energy intake, but the most relevant to fetal oral health may be the first and second trimesters when the development and calcification of teeth occur. Bone growth, which is equally important, occurs mainly in the second and third trimesters when most of the calcium essential for this process is transferred from mother to child. In most cases, the exception being an underweight or teenage pregnancy, the woman's energy requirement increases by approximately 300 kilocalories a day.[4] However, unlike energy needs, vitamin and mineral requirements nearly double (Figure 28–12). During pregnancy the woman may experience changes in taste and smell, food cravings, and food aversions that do not necessarily reflect real physiologic needs. These pregnancy-related experiences, along with varying levels of nausea, create a potential for nutrient imbalance. Fortunately, the developing fetus is usually not at risk during these short episodes because a healthy mother provides the essential nutrients from her own nutrient stores. However, a prolonged nutrient deficiency poses a problem.

The dental hygienist treating a pregnant woman should reinforce the recommendations of the obstetrician. Reinforcement of the importance of eating nutrient-dense foods along with meticulous oral hygiene will minimize the occurrence of pregnancy-associated gingivitis, pregnancy granulomas, and giving birth to premature, low-birthweight infants. Prenatal nutrient supplements recommended by the client's obstetrician help to ensure that the developing fetus receives adequate vitamins and minerals to promote healthy bone and tooth development.

NUTRITIONAL NEEDS IN INFANCY AND CHILDHOOD

Nutrient intake and food choices during infancy and childhood influence growth patterns. Undernutrition, overnutrition, or improper nutrient amounts can set the pattern for a life-long struggle with weight, developmental delays, or social discrimination.

Children often grow in spurts. Children are born with an innate sense of how much food they require. Parents who advocate completely finishing an entire meal may be causing the child to override his or her internal sense of

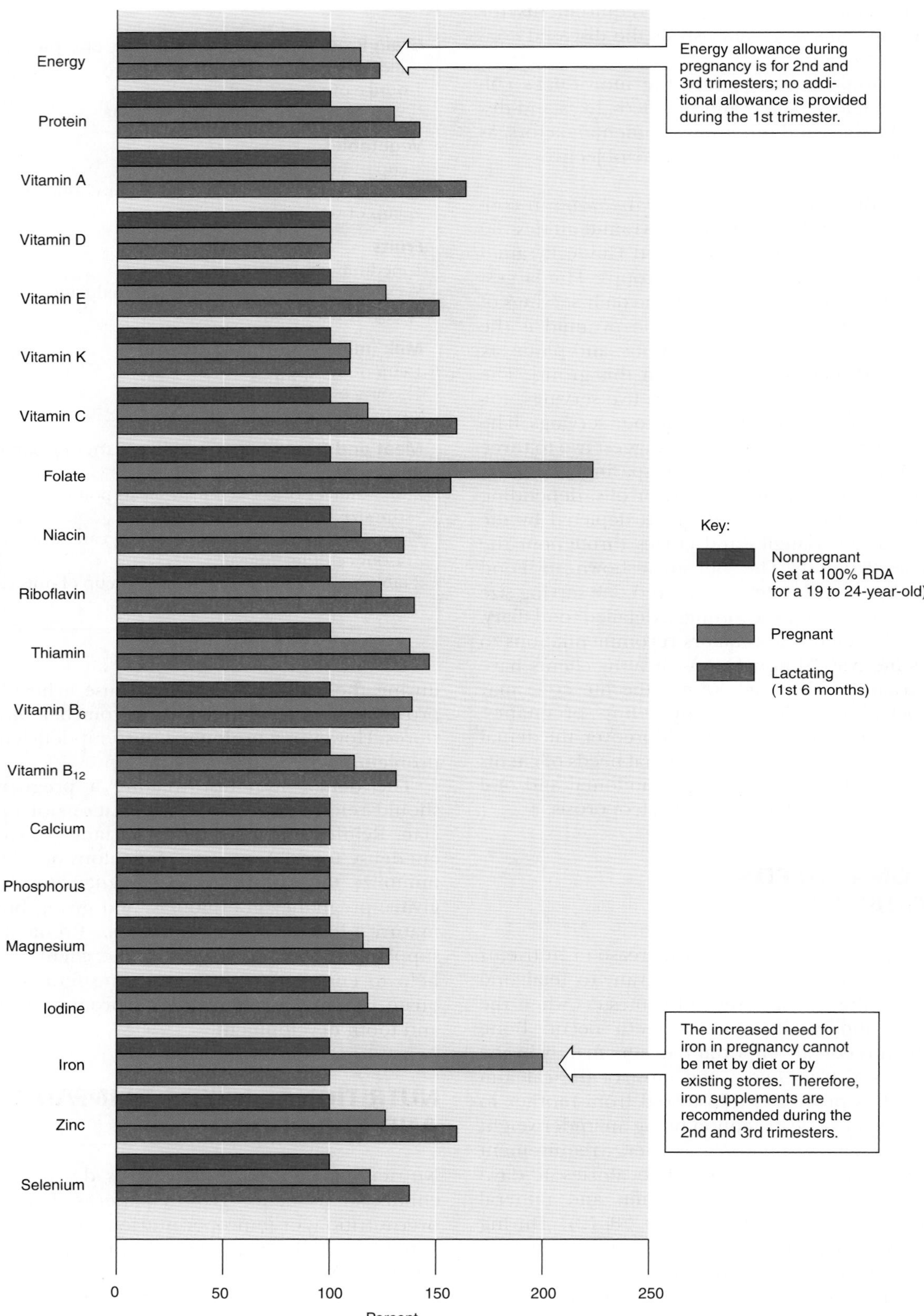

FIGURE 28–12 ✦ Comparison of nutrient RDA of nonpregnant, pregnant, and lactating women. *(Modified from Whitney EN, Rolfes SR:* Understanding nutrition, *St Paul, Minn, 1998, West.)*

TABLE 28–4 FOODS THAT PROVIDE APPROPRIATE ENERGY FOR VARIOUS AGE GROUPS IN CHILDREN

Age	Weight (kg)	Energy Needed (kcal)	Examples of Foods That Provide Appropriate Energy Intake
2 months	6	650	28 to 32 oz human milk or infant formula
6 months	7.5	750	28 oz human milk or infant formula 4 T dry infant cereal 4 oz fruit juice 5 T strained fruit
10 months	9	850	24 oz infant formula 8 T dry infant cereal 14 T junior fruit 8 T junior vegetable 4 T junior meat ½ slice toast 1 oz chopped chicken 1 T mashed green beans 1 small banana 2 T ice cream 1 graham cracker
4 years	20	1800	24 oz milk 6 to 8 oz fruit juice 3 slices bread ½ to ¾ c dry cereal 2 T peanut butter 1 t jelly 2 oz lean hamburger party ¼ c macaroni and cheese ¼ c green beans ⅓ c ice cream 1 graham cracker 1 medium apple 1 small banana

satiety. The simplest advice is the provision of nutrient-dense foods, regular meal times, and the achievement of a balanced diet over several days (Table 28–4).

The Centers for Disease Control and Prevention publish growth charts for children. The charts, used to determine a child's growth relationship to other same-age children, include a body mass index and are used to monitor growth. The CDC developed the charts in response to the facts that more than half of American adults are overweight, the number of obese adults has doubled in the past two decades, and the number of overweight children has increased significantly.[6]

Unless a child presents with extenuating medical circumstances, children should not ingest significant amounts of alternative sweeteners. Children need calories for growth and development. Artificial sweeteners should not be part of the diet of infants or children under 2 years of age. Although the anticariogenicity of alternative sweeteners may offer a desirable choice to most parents, good oral hygiene care, fluoridation, and healthy snack choices can reduce dental caries risk. Examples of appropriate snacks for children are listed in Healthy Snack Ideas for Children and Adults.

The focus of nutritional counseling for children in the oral care setting centers on caries control. Additionally, the importance of vitamins and minerals responsible for bone growth should be included in a discussion with the child and caregiver. As children age, their preference for a beverage often changes from milk and juices to carbonated beverages. This change may adversely affect the bone growth and tooth development of children and teenagers.[7] Dairy products, some of the best sources of calcium, phosphorus, and magnesium, are essential for adequate bone and tooth formation. Replacing dairy products with carbonated beverages eliminates the main source of these nutrients. A diet high in carbonated and caffeine-containing beverages may reduce bone density.[8]

NUTRITIONAL NEEDS IN ELDERLY CLIENTS

Significant nutritional issues in the elderly include a reduced energy requirement, an increased protein requirement, and an increased need for vitamins and minerals including the antioxidant vitamins A, C, E and minerals such as selenium and zinc (see Chapter 48). Most elderly people are not as active as younger people and therefore do not require the same amount of energy intake. The decrease in energy and increase in nutrient needs mean that the elderly client may need guidance in choosing nutrient-dense foods such as grains, breads, and pastas. Along with complex carbohydrates, fruits and vegetables are a natural source of the vitamins and

Healthy Snack Ideas for Children and Adults

Breads, Crackers, Grains
Cereal
Crackers
Toast (whole wheat)
Popcorn
Oatmeal (cookies)
Tortillas
Dried rice and corn cakes
Corn chips
Pizza

Vegetables
Raw and cut-up carrots, celery, broccoli, cauliflower
Cut-up raw vegetables served with cheese or peanut butter

Fruits
Apples, peaches, pears, plums
Bananas (with peanut butter)
Cut-up watermelon, cantaloupe, or other melon

Meat/Protein
Sandwiches containing lunch meat on whole wheat bread
Tuna on crackers
Bean and legumes
Hummus on crackers
Nuts (not recommended for young children because of choking hazard)

Milk and Dairy
Milk as a beverage with any snack
Yogurt
Cheese
Sugar-free pudding

Other
Sugar-free ice pops
Sugar-free candy and chewing gum
Sugar-free gelatin

minerals that promote tissue growth and regeneration. Due to a decrease in lean body per kilogram of body weight, elderly adults have a higher protein requirement. The current RDA for protein for adults is 0.8 g/kg of body weight.[9] A person who weighs 160 lb weighs approximately 67 kg and should have an intake of about 54 g of protein per day (54 grams is equivalent to about 2 ounces of protein). Protein intake in older adults should comprise approximately 12% to 14% of the total energy intake.[10] As an example, approximately 150 to 225 calories of an average 1500 calorie intake is about 10% to 15% of the total energy intake and is the amount of calories that should come from protein sources in elderly adults.

A factor that affects nutrient intake is lack of dental insurance. Many elderly people may be unable to afford dental care. Periodontal disease and carious teeth can be painful and restrict the elderly individual's ability to chew and swallow food. Hot or cold foods can aggravate oral disease conditions. Additionally, crisp or fibrous foods that require significant force when biting or chewing can also be painful. The aging process results in increased vulnerability to oral injury due to thinning of the oral tissues. For convenience, older adults may choose cakes, cookies, and breakfast cereals, which contribute to dental decay. Xerostomia also contributes to root caries and an inability to chew and swallow food adequately.

Providing quality nutrient sources that require only limited chewing should be a priority for the elderly with dental problems.[11] Sources of high-quality protein such as eggs, dairy products, well-cooked meats, chicken, and fish should be promoted as an important part of the diet. Protein also provides a good source of vitamin B_{12}, often deficient in the elderly. The decrease of intrinsic factor, a protein that aids in the absorption of vitamin B_{12} in the stomach, makes intramuscular injections of the vitamin necessary. Vitamins A, C, and B_6 can be obtained from a diet rich in cooked green vegetables and potatoes. Fresh fruit is also a good source of vitamins and minerals and can be tolerated if the fruit is ripe or peeled. Table 28–5 lists oral signs and symptoms of nutrient deficiencies in the elderly.

Finally, guidance should be given to the elderly to achieve optimum nutrition. Community-based services such as Meals on Wheels, congregate meal sites, and shopping assistance provide an opportunity for socialization and assistance for those who are disabled or who lack transportation. Also, modifications applied to oral hygiene aids for people with manual dexterity problems can be applied to eating utensils to increase the likelihood of adequate nutritional intake.

NUTRITIONAL NEEDS OF CLIENTS WITH DENTAL CARIES RISK

Nutritional counseling for dental caries prevention must emphasize decreasing the frequency with which sugar is consumed and replacing cariogenic foods with nutritionally sound foods. Although sugar consumption is an important factor in caries risk assessment[12,13] (see Chapter 26), three factors must be present for dental caries to occur:

- ✦ Acid-producing microorganisms (*Lactobacillus, Streptococcus mutans*)
- ✦ A fermentable carbohydrate
- ✦ A susceptible tooth surface

Nutritional counseling for dental caries prevention targets the elimination or reduction of fermentable carbohydrates from the diet. Frequent consumption of fermentable carbohydrates subjects the tooth enamel to repeated acid exposures. The demineralization process weakens the tooth and leads to the formation of dental caries. (See Chapter 13 for types of caries and Chapter 26 for a review of the caries process.) Table 28–6 illustrates the relative cariogenicity of certain foods. Foods with a

TABLE 28–5 POSSIBLE SIGNS OF NUTRITIONAL DEFICIENCIES IN THE ELDERLY

Clinical Signs	Possible Deficiency	Comments
Skin		
Edema	Protein, thiamin	Common in protein-calorie malnutrition as a result of aging
Poor tissue turgor	Water	Pellagra or hemochromatosis
Dermatitis	Protein	
Keratosis	Vitamin A, essential fatty acids	
Pigmentation	Niacin	Loss of lubrication or dryness of skin
Petechiae	Vitamin A, vitamin C	
Xerosis	Essential fatty acids	
Eyes		
Dull, dry conjunctiva	Vitamin A	Can lead to other eye problems including blindness
Keratomalacia	Vitamin A	
Bitot's spot	Vitamin A	
Corneal vascularization	Vitamin A	
Photophobia	Riboflavin Zinc	
Tongue		
Magenta tongue	Riboflavin	
Fissuring, raw	Niacin	May also be caused by food irritants, antibiotic administration, uremia
Glossitis	Pyridoxine, folacin, iron, vitamin B_{12}	Seen if anemia is not pronounced
Fiery red tongue	Folacin, vitamin B_{12}	
Pale	Iron, vitamin B_{12}	Seen in severe cases
Atrophic papillae	Riboflavin, niacin, iron	Also seen with ill-fitting dentures, food irritants, aging
Lips and Oral Structures		
Angular fissures, scars, or stomatitis	B-complex, iron, protein, riboflavin	Also seen with ill-fitting dentures
Cheilosis	B_6, niacin, riboflavin, protein	
Ageusia, dysgeusia	Zinc	Also seen with ill-fitting dentures, exposure to sun or cold
Swollen, spongy, bleeding gums	Vitamin C	Also associated with altered sense of smell, if not edentulous

cariogenic potential index in the 0.0 to 0.4 range are considered to have a low, noncariogenic potential. This information can be useful for suggesting foods for reducing the cariogenic potential of an individual's diet (see Dietary Recommendations for the Reduction of Dental Caries).

TABLE 28–6 CURRENT ESTIMATES OF CARIOGENICITIES AND CARIOGENIC POTENTIAL INDEX (CPI)

Food	Cariogenic Potential Index
Low Cariogenic Potential	
Gelatin dessert	0.4
Corn chips	0.4
Peanuts	0.4
Bologna	0.4
Yogurt	0.4
Moderate to High Cariogenic Potential	
Pretzels	0.5
Potato chips	0.6
Saltines	0.6
Natural snack (trail mix)	0.6
Rye crackers	0.7
Doughnut	0.7
Milk chocolate	0.8
Graham crackers	0.8
Sponge cake with filling	0.8
Bread	0.9
Sucrose	1.0
Granola cereal	1.0
French fries	1.1
Bananas	1.1
Cupcakes	1.2
Raisins	1.2

From Harris N, Madsen K: Nutrition and the plaque diseases. In Harris N, Christen A: *Primary preventive dentistry,* ed 5, East Norwalk, Conn, 1997, Appleton-Lange; Mundorff SA, Featherstone JBD, Bibby BG: Cariogenic potential of foods. I. Caries in the rat model, *Caries Research* 24:344, 1990.

Dietary Recommendations for the Reduction of Dental Caries

Limit the use of fermentable carbohydrates to mealtime. Foods other than carbohydrates serve as buffers to help neutralize plaque acids.

Omit sweet foods even with meals if the client is susceptible to caries.

Between-meal snacks should consist of protective, noncariogenic foods such as raw vegetables. Raw, unrefined foods in the vegetable and fruit group require chewing. The chewing action increases the salivary flow, thus aiding in the removal and dilution of sugars and their harmful by-products.

Use as few concentrated sweets in the preparation of foods as possible.

Do not eat sweets before bedtime unless the teeth are brushed. Salivary flow decreases at night and foods are not as readily cleared from the mouth as they are during waking hours. Acid left undisturbed remains in the mouth for 1½ to 2 hours.

Avoid natural sugars—they are as detrimental to the tooth surface as refined sugars.

Avoid sticky foods because they are retained in the mouth longer than nonsticky foods.

NUTRITIONAL NEEDS OF CLIENTS UNDERGOING SURGERY

In a healthy adult, creation of new proteins and breakdown of existing proteins closely balance one another. Any change in health status can cause a metabolic change in protein status. Many metabolic changes occur during the postsurgical period, including increased breakdown of body nutrient stores (e.g., protein and minerals from the body stores are used to remodel and repair oral structures). Protein breakdown most often exceeds synthesis. Other metabolic factors combine to cause a further increase in the breakdown of lean body tissues with a resultant weight loss. Depletion of protein mass is important because the body has no expendable protein reserves; therefore, any loss of protein adversely affects body function, leading to increased loss of lean body mass and the subsequent weight loss through metabolic processes. Periodontal and oral and maxillofacial surgical clients are often unable to consume an adequate amount of recommended nutrients due to loss of function. To minimize loss of lean body mass and to promote healing and overall health, clients should be instructed in proper postsurgical *nutritional rehabilitation*. Presurgical nutrition education includes:

- ✦ Discussion of the client's present status and recommended ranges for prevention of loss of lean body mass
- ✦ Review of adequate nutrients to enhance and facilitate the healing process

Calculations using the formula for basal energy expenditure multiplied by an activity factor provide an estimation of nutritional requirements. Postsurgically, the number will be multiplied by an injury factor to determine the increase in caloric needs. At this time, the RDA for daily protein needs for adults is set at 0.8 gram per kilogram of body weight. Postsurgically the increase in protein requirement can be as much as 1.2 to 1.5 grams per kilogram of body weight for mild to moderate stress. Need for increased protein may rise as much as 2.5 grams per kilogram of body weight for conditions accompanied by increased nitrogen excretion, such as burns, severe trauma, or presence of a fistula.[14] Table 28–7 illustrates the average energy and protein requirements of hospitalized patients.

In addition to caloric and protein requirement increases, there may also be an increase in select nutrient needs. It makes sense that B vitamin requirements would increase in conjunction with the increase in caloric intake. The primary function of the B vitamins is as a cofactor in energy metabolism. Catabolism and loss of lean body mass increase the loss of potassium, magnesium, phosphorus, and zinc. Fluid and electrolytes should be provided to maintain adequate urine output and normal serum electrolytes. The tendency is to prescribe a nutritional supplement in the form of a tablet, but it is always preferable to obtain nutrients through a food source. However, in cases in which the client is unable to adequately ingest the required nutrients, a liquid form of supplemental nutrition such as Ensure or Boost may be acceptable.

A practical education program for dental clients is accomplished using the USDA Food Guide Pyramid and *Dietary Guidelines for Americans.* Quick calculations and charts are used as visual aids to client education. Preprepared diets that incorporate caloric, protein, and other suggested nutrient needs postsurgically are an excellent resource in the private practice setting. The American Dietetic Association is an exceptional resource for examples of full liquid as well as mechanical soft diets designed to provide optimum calories and nutrients for surgical patients. Often it is easier to obtain compliance when clients are presented with an actual list of foods or meal plans to follow.

NUTRITIONAL NEEDS FOR CLIENTS WITH OSTEOPOROSIS[15–20]

Many factors affect mineralization of bone in the human body, including metabolic and dietary interactions and certain disease states. Improper bone mineralization can affect the dentition. Although several vitamins and minerals ultimately contribute to bone and tooth formation and preservation, calcium, phosphorus, and vitamin D directly support these processes. Calcium can be found throughout the body in bone, serum, and tissues. Approximately 98% of the calcium present in the human body is contained in bone and teeth. The balance of serum calcium is important in that it often causes the release or deposit of calcium from hard body tissues.

TABLE 28–7 AVERAGE ENERGY AND PROTEIN REQUIREMENTS OF CLIENTS

Metabolic Status	Energy Requirements (kcal/kg/day)	Protein Requirements (g/kg/day)	Related Condition
Normal	25 to 30	0.8 to 1.0	Normal, healthy client
Elective surgery	28 to 30	1.0 to 1.5	Periodontal surgery, impacted third molar extraction
Severe injury	30 to 35	1.5 to 2.0	Oral and maxillofacial reconstruction
Severe trauma/burn	45 to 55	2.0 to 2.5	Automobile accident resulting in severe facial trauma and other injuries

Phosphorus is equally important to bone growth and preservation. Approximately 85% of the phosphorus in the human body is found in combination with calcium in hydroxyapatite crystals of bones and teeth. Calcium and phosphorus are important components of bone and teeth, but vitamin D directs the use of these minerals in the body. The interaction of calcium, phosphorus, and vitamin D is required for adequate maintenance of bone growth and mineralization.

Osteopenia, a loss of mineralized bone tissue, regardless of its cause, is considered a precursor to osteoporosis. *Osteoporosis* is a disease characterized by low bone mass, microarchitectural deterioration of bone tissue leading to enhanced bone fragility, and consequent increase in fracture risk. Osteoporosis has become significant as a disease due to its relationship to mortality, morbidity, quality of life, and medical expense worldwide. Osteoporosis causes more than 1,300,000 fractures annually in the United States alone. Hip fracture is responsible for much of the mortality and morbidity of osteoporosis and is a leading cause of disability in the elderly. Risk Factors Associated with Osteoporosis identifies risk factors for osteoporosis. Osteoporosis may be a risk factor/risk indicator for periodontal disease, for tooth loss preceding dental implants, and in the prognosis of periodontal therapy (see Chapter 46).

When discussing the control of osteoporosis, the nutrient mentioned most often is calcium. The ideal calcium intake is difficult to determine. The current RDA is 800 mg/day. In recognition of the importance of calcium during the peak bone-forming years, the RDA for calcium has been raised to 1200 mg for young adults 19 to 24 years of age. An even higher calcium intake during adolescence and young adulthood may be needed to reach a genetically achievable peak bone mass. It has also been found that a calcium intake of at least the RDA can slow or prevent age-related bone loss and reduce the risk of fractures in postmenopausal women and the elderly.

The preferred source of calcium is food and dairy products. Bioavailability of calcium from dairy foods is good, especially when consumed with a meal (see Food Sources of Calcium). Emphasis also should be on vitamin D use to promote optimal calcium absorption. Table 28–8 provides a listing of the minerals and vitamins essential for calcified structures (see Chapter 46). Dietary calcium can also be augmented by drinking calcium-fortified orange juice and by taking calcium supplements such as calcium carbonate or calcium glycerophosphate.

TABLE 28–8 VITAMINS AND MINERALS REQUIRED FOR CALCIFIED STRUCTURES

Vitamin/Mineral	RDA (for adults)	Food Sources
Vitamin A (fat soluble)	1,000 mcg (men)/800 mcg (women)	Only found in animal foods: meats, milk, cheese, etc. Beta carotene found in orange fruits and vegetables (carrots, squash, pumpkin, sweet potato, apricots) and green leafy vegetables such as spinach
Vitamin D (fat soluble)	5 mcg	Sunshine, fortified milk
Vitamin E (fat soluble	10 mg (men)/8 mg (women)	Sweet potato, shrimp, sunflower seeds, canola oil, corn oil
Vitamin K (fat soluble)	80 mcg (men)/65 mcg (women)	Produced in the large intestine; cabbage, spinach, cauliflower, milk, eggs, garbanzo beans, beef liver
Vitamin C (water soluble)	60 mg	Citrus fruits such as oranges, grapefruit Vegetables such as potatoes, green pepper, broccoli, and Brussels sprouts
Calcium	800 mg	Dairy products such as milk, cheese. Sardines, almonds. Vegetables such as broccoli, turnip greens, cauliflower, kale, bok choy
Phosphorus	800 mg	Dairy products such as milk, cottage cheese. Meat and fish products such as salmon, sirloin steak
Magnesium	350 mg (men)/280 mg (women)	Vegetables such as black-eyed peas, spinach, baked potato. Other sources include oysters, dried figs, sunflower seeds
Fluoride	No RDA Estimated safe and adequate daily dietary intake = 1.5 to 4.0 mg	Fluoridated water
Copper	No RDA Estimated safe and adequate daily dietary intake = 1.5 to 3.0 mg	Shellfish, liver, nuts, seeds and legumes
Manganese	No RDA Estimated safe and adequate daily dietary intake = 2.0 to 5.0 mg	Legumes, whole-grain cereals, leafy vegetables
Molybdenum	No RDA Estimated safe and adequate daily dietary intake = 75 to 250 mcg	Legumes, whole-grain cereals, and vegetables
Selenium	70 mcg (men)/55 mcg (women)	Animal products such as meats and shellfish Vegetables and grains grown in selenium-rich soil (common in the U.S.)

Risk Factors Associated with Osteoporosis

Dietary Constituents
Alcohol abuse
Excessive antacid use
Low-calcium diet
Vitamin D deficiency
Caffeine use
High-fiber diet
High-protein diet
Excessive carbonated drink intake

Hormones
Surgical removal of ovaries
Chronic thyroid hormone use
Early menopause

Drugs
Chronic steroid use

Genetic Factors
Caucasian
Asian
Thinness
Family history of osteoporosis

Gender
Female

Other
Advanced age
Anorexia nervosa
Lack of weight-bearing exercise

Food Sources of Calcium

Excellent
Fish with bones (sardines)
Oysters
Molasses
Broccoli
Kale
Bok choy
Turnip greens
Mustard greens
Brussels sprouts

Good
Milk and milk products
Tofu (calcium set)
Soy milk
Orange juice enriched with calcium

Fair
Pinto beans
Sesame seeds
Almonds
Spinach

Client Education Issues

- ✦ Explain that a diet rich in nutrient-dense foods promotes oral health and overall health, and prevents osteopenia and osteoporosis in later life.
- ✦ Emphasize that decreasing the amount and frequency of simple sugars consumed promotes oral health, weight management, and systemic health.
- ✦ Explain that nutrient needs change during the life cycle, and at times of stress such as periodontal and oral surgery.
- ✦ Explain RDAs, nutrition labels on foods purchased, *Dietary Guidelines for Americans,* and the USDA Food Guide Pyramid as the basis for appropriate food choices.
- ✦ Discuss how healthy, nutrient-dense snack foods can be substituted for dental caries–promoting snacks.
- ✦ For clients undergoing oral and maxillofacial surgery, discuss present nutritional status and recommendations for prevention of loss of lean body mass; review those foods that will promote healing.

Legal, Ethical, and Safety Issues

- ✦ Dental hygienists should refrain from practicing nutrition assessment or counseling that is beyond the scope of their practice (e.g., weight management, metabolic disease control, eating disorders, etc.). Signs of nutrition-related diseases or deficiencies should be referred to a physician or nutritionist.
- ✦ Clients need to be alerted to potential signs and symptoms of nutritional deficiencies and referred to a physician for diagnosis.
- ✦ Information provided to the client during nutritional counseling for oral disease should be documented in the client's record.

KEY CONCEPTS

- ✦ Assessment of client nutritional status is part of comprehensive dental hygiene care.
- ✦ Nutritional counseling helps clients develop healthful eating behaviors.
- ✦ Diet assessment is the identification of current diet practices and diet requirements of the client. Diet assessment includes a diet history that may be gathered through a 1-, 3-, 5-, or 7-day recording of food intake. Diet assessment may provide clues to overall health through analysis of nutrient content
- ✦ Key factors influence an individual's selection of food, including age, gender, ethnicity and culture, income, educational level, and lifestyle.
- ✦ Cultural sensitivity is a part of every diet assessment and nutritional counseling session.
- ✦ Pregnancy, infancy and childhood, and aging require special consideration when the dental hygienist is counseling these clients or their caregivers on nutrition.
- ✦ The elderly often require increased amounts of protein but not calories.
- ✦ Diet assessment and nutrition counseling promote healing postoperatively in clients undergoing periodontal or oral and maxillofacial surgery.
- ✦ Minimizing the amount of sugar consumed and replacing cariogenic foods with nutrient-dense foods decrease dental caries risk.

CRITICAL THINKING EXERCISES

Two scenarios present clients with specific nutritional needs. Read each case and prepare a complete dental hygiene care plan for each (see Useful Calculations for Nutrition Assessment.) Do you agree or disagree with the nutritional plans presented? Is there anything you would do differently?

SCENARIO 1

ORAL AND MAXILLOFACIAL SURGERY CLIENT

Client: Mr. Xavier Rodriguez
Age: 32 years
Gender: Male
Height: 5′6″
Weight: 150 lb (63 kg)
Ethnicity: Hispanic

Health History: Family history of type-2 diabetes mellitus. In the past client has had abnormal glucose levels but recently has tested normal. Was considerably overweight and has worked hard to lose about 25 lb; cholesterol level is somewhere around 220.

Pharmacologic History: Allergic to penicillin. Postsurgically, Mr. Rodriguez will be taking Lortab for postoperative pain on a PRN basis and erythromycin for about 1 week postoperatively

Dental History:
Intraoral and extraoral exam findings show probing depths of 4–5 mm throughout his mouth.
Moderate amounts of plaque biofilm and moderate to heavy bleeding in the molar areas.
No carious lesions.
Currently undergoing orthodontic treatment and can expect to have limited use of his teeth and jaws for approximately 6 weeks postsurgically. Having trouble keeping his teeth clean since his orthodontic appliances were placed.

Mr. Rodriguez's surgeon has said that he probably won't have to worry about weight loss postsurgically as he could stand to lose a few more pounds. However, the surgeon mentioned that Mr. Rodriguez should try to eat more protein foods to support healing.

Chief Complaint: "I am scheduled to have oral surgery that will move my jaw and relieve my jaw pain. I want my surgery to go well so that I heal quickly."

Diet Assessment: After completion of a 24-hour diet history, the following is noted:
Caries risk is moderate.
Nutrient levels are within normal range except for calcium, which is only about 200 mg.
Daily nutrient values are approximately 40% carbohydrate, 45% fat, and 15% protein. The total amount of energy consumed is 1800 calories.
Allergic to dairy products.

Social History:
Daily exercise consists of a walk around the block 2 times a day with the family dog.
Moderately active on the weekends doing chores around the house.
Works as an accountant with normal hours except around tax time when he sometimes works 14-hour days.
Occasionally enjoys a beer after work.

Continued on following page

Critical Thinking Exercises—cont'd

ORAL AND MAXILLOFACIAL SURGERY CLIENT—CONT'D

Nutritional Risk Factors:

Most carbohydrate comes from rice and tortillas.
High-fat diet from the preparation of the foods he eats and the type of meat he consumes.
Drinks mostly iced tea and coffee.

Nutritional Counseling Plan: Recommendations for Mr. Rodriguez:

1. Decrease his amount of fat intake by 10 to 15% by starting with the following recommendations:
   - Gradually change food preparation to include monounsaturated fats.
   - Choose chicken breasts instead of thighs.
   - Choose beef cut from the loin or round.
   - Prepare eggs as soft-boiled, scrambled, or fried using a cooking spray.
   - Prepare beans as "borracho" or "charro" style instead of refried.
2. Make the following substitutions to increase nutrient content of meals:
   - Include a variety of grain products at each meal.
   - Choose brown rice instead of white.
   - Choose whole-wheat flour whenever possible.
   - Include more vegetables in diet.
   - Use tomato salsa or guacamole as a condiment with meals.
   - Include fresh fruits as a snack or dessert.
3. Postsurgically increase protein and caloric intake to promote remodeling and healing by consuming the following:
   - Frequent small meals that include high-protein foods.
   - Soft foods such as cooked beans, rice, eggs.
   - Include nutritional supplements such as Carnation Instant Breakfast, Ensure, and Boost. These products also help to increase caloric intake as well as vitamins and minerals.
   - A dairy choice such as Lactaid would provide needed protein and calcium but reduce the effects of lactose intolerance.
   - A soy product such as calcium set tofu is a good choice for increasing calcium intake for bone remodeling and providing protein for healing.

Continue with exercise patterns as time and healing permit. Increase walking distance by 1/2 mile per day.
Use the *USDA Food Guide Pyramid* to teach Mr. Rodriguez which groups he should choose most of his foods from.

Dental Hygiene Diagnoses:

Unmet need for protection from health risk due to high amount of fat in diet as evidenced by a high cholesterol level and evidence on the 24-hour diet history
Unmet need for skin and mucous membrane integrity of the head and neck due to impending oral and maxillofacial surgery as evidenced by low protein in diet on the 24-hour diet recall
Unmet need for freedom from head and neck pain due to malocclusion as evidenced by TMJ pain.

Goals:

Client will decrease fat intake to <30% of total kcal/day
Client will increase protein in diet to 126 g per day
Client will increase caloric intake to 2500 kcal per day
Client will undergo oral and maxillofacial surgery to correct his malocclusion

Mr. Rodriguez's 24-hour Diet History:

Breakfast
2 tortillas
3 breakfast sausage
2 eggs, fried
2 c. coffee

Lunch
8 oz. chicken (thigh) fajitas
2 c. rice
1 c. refried beans
2 tortillas
24 oz. iced tea, Sweet n Low

Snack
4 chocolate chip cookies

Dinner
12 oz. beef brisket, grilled
2 rolls with butter
12 oz. soft drink
1 c. potato salad
1 beer

Useful Calculations for Nutrition Assessment

IBW = 106 + 6 × 6 inches = 142 lb
BMI = 705 × 150 ÷ 66^2 = 24.3
BEE = 66 + 13.7(62.5) + 5(145) − 6.8(32) = 1429 kcal
TDD presurgically = 1429 × 1.5 = 2143.5 kcal
BEE × an activity factor of 1.5 (normally active person)
TDD postsurgically = 1429 × 1.4 × 1.35 = 2701 kcal
BEE × an activity factor of 1.4 (slightly less active postsurgically) × an injury factor of 1.35 (clients with skeletal trauma)

Critical Thinking Exercises—cont'd

SCENARIO 2

CLIENT WITH OSTEOPOROSIS

Client: Ms. Xi Tsing
Age: 50 years
Gender: Female
Height: 5′ 2″
Weight: 85 lb (38.6 kg)
Race: Asian American

Medical History: Client underwent early menopause, is lactose intolerant, and is currently being treated for irritable bowel disease.

Pharmacologic History: Medications include steroid treatment for her bowel problems and estrogen replacement therapy.

Dental History: Several carious areas. Radiologic exam shows moderate bone loss of the supporting structures and within her jaws. Suspect osteoporosis. Will discuss this with the dentist. Following dental treatment Ms. Tsing will be referred to her physician for evaluation and treatment of suspected osteoporosis.

Chief Complaint: "My teeth are hurting me."

Diet Assessment:

Food frequency questionnaire shows that Ms. Tsing follows a typical Asian diet pattern with fish and tofu as the main sources of protein.
Eats a variety of vegetables including green leafy vegetables such as spinach and green leaf lettuce, bean sprouts, bok choy, broccoli, and carrots.
Does not consume any dairy products due to her lactose intolerance.
Drinks tea.
Loves sweets and desserts and consumes candy regularly.
Diet consists of approximately 20% fat, 10% protein, and 70% carbohydrate.

Social History:

Client does not exercise and rarely goes outside during the day in an effort to avoid the sun and its damaging effects.
Worked as a seamstress for many years but is now retired.
Belongs to an informal social women's group and occasionally has the opportunity to meet for walks at the local mall.

Nutritional Risk Factors:

Asian descent
Underweight and of small stature
Long-term steroid treatment
Early menopause
Low exercise level

Nutritional Counseling Plan:

1. Using the *Food Guide Pyramid*, discuss the positive aspects of the client's diet including:
   - Calcium-rich foods such as bok choy, broccoli, and tofu
   - Herbal tea (green tea), no caffeine
   - Fish such as salmon or sardines that have a high level of calcium
2. Find solutions collaboratively with the client regarding:
   - Lack of dairy products
   - Large amount of simple sugars
   - Lack of weight-bearing exercise
   - No sun exposure for vitamin D
3. Recommendation of a vitamin D supplement or 5-10 minutes per day of early morning sunshine exposure.
4. A regular exercise plan can be recommended, starting with increasing walks at the mall.
5. Alternative sources of calcium or over-the-counter lactase enzymes or commercially available supplements such as Ensure or Boost. A dietitian should be consulted for the best sources of well-absorbed supplements.

Dental Hygiene Diagnoses:

Unmet need for protection from health risks due to lack of calcium-containing foods in diet as evidenced by osteoporosis.
Unmet need for biologically sound and functional dentition due to a combination of diet and oral hygiene care as evidenced by chief complaint of tooth pain.

Goals:

Increase amount of foods containing calcium in diet.
Increase nutrient values in diet to prevent osteoporosis and educate patient in proper oral hygiene care.

Continued on following page

Critical Thinking Exercises—cont'd

Scenario 3

CLIENT WITH RAMPANT DENTAL CARIES

Client: Kathleen Mulvaney
Age: 8 years
Gender: Female
Height: 3′ 10″
Weight: 55 lb (25 kg)
Race: Caucasian

Medical History: Client has experienced several childhood illnesses, including chicken pox, measles, and mumps and frequent sore throats and common cold symptoms. Client was injured on the school playground at age 6 years and underwent treatment for fractures of the right leg and arm.

Pharmacologic History: Because of frequent cold symptoms and sore throats, client regularly ingests over-the-counter cough drops. Her favorite flavors are cherry and honey lemon. These cough drops are not sugar free.

Dental History: Because of her medical history and subsequent treatment for illness and injury, Kathleen's parents have not taken her to the dentist often in an effort to avoid "overtraumatizing" her. Intraoral examination reveals rampant caries of remaining primary teeth with the largest lesions in the molar area. Radiographic exam shows decay throughout the mouth. Permanent tooth development appears to be normal. Erupted molars have incipient lesions with some surfaces requiring Class I restorations at this time.

Chief Complaint: "My friends at school make fun of my teeth because they are black. Sometimes it's hard to chew." Client does not appear to be experiencing pain at this time.

Diet History: Food frequency questionnaire indicates that client has a high intake of foods containing added sugars and appearing in the moderate- to high-cariogenic potential category.

On the Food Guide Pyramid, client can point out most foods from the base of the pyramid in her diet. Client also understands the concept of small triangles representing fats and sugars. Client indicates that she adds sugar to her breakfast cereals and on top of the fruit she eats with lunch.

Client loves raisins and dried fruit as a snack. She keeps a little bag in her desk at school in case she gets hungry during the day. Client's favorite snack is a bowl of chocolate ice cream, which she has every night before bed. Client drinks regular Coca Cola with each meal except breakfast.

Friends eat candy bars, but Kathleen prefers gummy bears, Dots, Sour Patch Kids, and other sticky fruit candies.

Social History: Client is the youngest child in a family of six. Parents both work outside the home. Family status is middle class with occasional financial challenges because of large family. Client stays after school until picked up by older siblings. Because of work and social obligations, parents have left most of the childcare responsibilities to older siblings.

Previous injuries and chronic illnesses have promoted special reward system at home of sweet desserts and ice cream before bed. Limited parental supervision has caused client to adopt diet and habits of older siblings who enjoy regular Coca Cola with meals instead of milk. Client appears to understand the importance of a healthy diet and appears receptive to adjusting habits "as long as my parents say it's OK."

Nutritional Risk Factors: Preferred snack foods have high concentration of added sugars and limited nutritional value. Snack habits (i.e., dried fruits available throughout the day) promote caries. Choice of beverage with meals unsatisfactory for promoting growth and development.

Limited parental supervision allows for poor food choices.

Dental Hygiene Diagnoses:

Need for biologically sound and functional dentition because of poor diet choice and poor oral hygiene care as evidenced by rampant decay.

Need for responsibility for oral health because of lack of parental supervision and infrequency of dental visits as evidenced by parental self-reports.

1. Given the history and dental hygiene diagnosis, develop a comprehensive overall dental hygiene care plan including: client goals, nutritional counseling plan, interventions, and evaluative measures. What factors would you use as motivators to change behavior? Share your approach to care with your peers.
2. Access the Internet. Find at least three sites that you could recommend for nutritional information appropriate for children, teens, adults, and senior citizens.
3. How might your nutritional counseling plan change if the client were Asian? Native American? Hispanic? African American?
4. Generate a list of healthy snacks that might be culture specific. Consider the culture represented in your community.

For References, Suggested Readings, and Related Websites, visit
http://evolve.elsevier.com/Darby/hygiene/

CHAPTER 29

TOBACCO CESSATION

OBJECTIVES

Mastery of the content in this chapter will enable the reader to:

- Describe the oral and systemic effects of tobacco use
- Describe the 5 A's approach to treating tobacco use and dependence
- Provide effective interventions to clients based on their readiness to quit tobacco use
- Describe the seven key elements of tobacco cessation counseling
- Describe action and thinking strategies for coping with the quitting process and for preventing relapse
- Describe available FDA-approved pharmacologic adjuncts that can facilitate client abstinence

KEY TERMS

Chewing tobacco
Dependence
Dip
Five A's approach
Free nicotine
Neuroadaptation
Nicotine addiction
Nicotine replacement therapy
Nitrosamines
Oral snuff
Relapse
Slip
Smoking tobacco
Spit (smokeless) tobacco
Stages of change theory
Tolerance
Withdrawal

Approximately 25% of adults in the United States smoke cigarettes.[1] An estimated10 million Americans smoke cigars and 12 million use *spit (smokeless) tobacco (ST)*.[1,2] Tobacco use in any form has the potential to profoundly alter a client's systemic and oral health and compromise dental hygiene care. Client tobacco use influences all phases of the dental hygiene process of care, and tobacco users often present with multiple unmet human needs. Because of the oral health effects associated with tobacco use, dental professionals are uniquely positioned to promote tobacco cessation and to encourage nonusers to remain tobacco free.

TOBACCO TOXICITY

All tobacco products contain hazardous chemicals that are damaging to human tissue. Nicotine leads to addiction, and other compounds found in tobacco such as *N*-nitrosamines, aromatic hydrocarbons, and polonium 210 are carcinogens (cancer-causing chemicals). *Nitrosamines* are very potent carcinogens known to cause cancer in over 30 species of animals. *Smoking tobacco* produces tar, carbon monoxide, and other chemically destructive by-products that are present in both mainstream and environmental tobacco smoke.[3] During the inhalation process, smoking tobacco users absorb nicotine through the lungs, where it is then distributed to tissues throughout the body. Human exposure to the chemicals contained in tobacco and the by-products of burning tobacco threaten the health of users and those around them. Over 450,000 Americans die annually from tobacco-related illness, yet tobacco use remains the most preventable cause of death in the United States.[4]

Spit (smokeless) tobacco (ST) use is predominantly associated with young white males and sporting activities. Approximately 20% of white male high school students use spit tobacco products.[4] The two main types of ST used are *oral snuff* (Figure 29–1) and *chewing tobacco* (Figure 29–2). Oral snuff is a finely ground tobacco leaf,

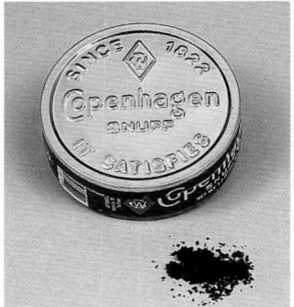

Figure 29–1 ✦ Example of an oral snuff product. *(Courtesy Dr. M. Walsh, University of California.)*

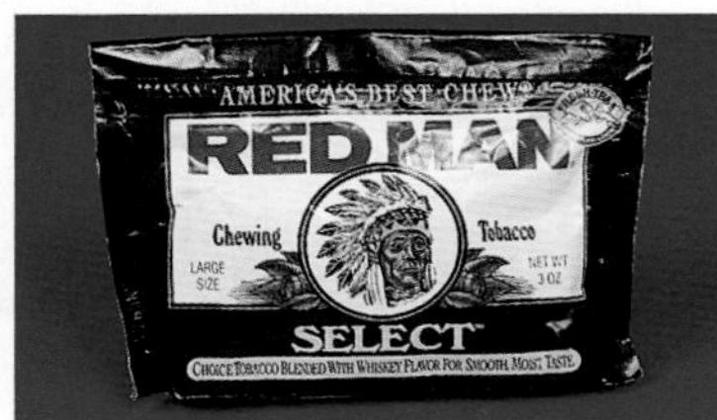

Figure 29–2 ✦ Example of a chewing tobacco product. *(Courtesy Dr. M. Walsh, University of California.)*

packaged either loose or in a tea bag–like sachet. Snuff users place a small amount or a *dip* between their cheek and gum. Chewing tobacco is a more coarsely shredded tobacco leaf. Tobacco chewers place a "chaw" of looseleaf tobacco, or a "plug" of compressed tobacco, in their cheeks. Both chewers and dippers suck on the tobacco and spit out the tobacco juices and saliva generated; sometimes they swallow them.

Spit tobacco products contain over 100 times the amount of nitrosamines legally allowed by the FDA in other consumable products.[5] Moreover, ST manufacturers control the amount of free nicotine available in their product for uptake into the body by controlling the pH of their products.

Free nicotine refers to ionized nicotine that passes rapidly through the oral mucosa into the bloodstream and into the brain. The higher the pH of the ST product, the more available free nicotine in the product. Brands of ST with high free nicotine are very addictive, making it difficult for individuals to quit, even if they are suffering from health problems.

Systemic Effects of Tobacco Use

- Cancer (mouth, pharynx, esophagus, stomach, bladder, lung, breast, and uterine)
- Cardiovascular disease (aortic aneurysm, atherosclerosis, chronic obstructive heart disease, and coronary artery disease)
- Hypertension, stroke
- Respiratory disease (emphysema, bronchitis, chronic obstructive lung disease, upper respiratory infection)
- Reproductive problems (miscarriage, preterm birth, low-birthweight babies, infants with cleft lip and palate, growth retardation and/or tooth malformation, early menopause, sudden infant death syndrome)
- Impotence
- Ulcers
- Osteoporosis
- Facial wrinkling
- Nicotine addiction

Oral Effects of Tobacco Use

- Cancers of the mouth, larynx, pharynx, esophagus, and lip
- Tooth abrasion
- Stain
- Calculus build-up
- Halitosis
- Impaired taste and smell
- Attrition
- Delayed wound healing/dry socket
- Hairy or coated tongue
- Increased risk of cleft palate/lip in newborns of mothers who smoke
- Increased risk of tooth anomalies and/or growth retardation in newborns of mothers who smoke
- Leukoedema
- Nicotine stomatitis
- Peri-implantitis
- Pre-cancerous lesions including leukoplakia, erythroplakia, dysplasia, hyperkeratosis
- Periodontal disease/gingival recession
- Sinusitis
- Tooth loss
- Xerostomia

ADVERSE HEALTH EFFECTS OF TOBACCO USE

Systemic Effects

There are numerous adverse systemic and oral health effects associated with tobacco use (see Systemic Effects of Tobacco Use and Oral Effects of Tobacco Use). Table 29–1 shows the related actual or potential unmet human needs of tobacco users.

Smoking increases the risk of cancer and cardiovascular, cerebrovascular, and pulmonary diseases.[1] Smoked tobacco is responsible for 87% of lung cancers and, on average, one-half of smokers lose 20 to 25 years of their life expectancies.[1] Spit tobacco use also can result in cancer, hypertension, and nicotine addiction. Client health history information must clearly document tobacco-related illness. Successful tobacco use interventions may be based on strategies that emphasize clients' systemic manifestations of their habit.

Oral Effects

The oral effects of tobacco use (see Oral Effects of Tobacco Use) range from the aesthetic (tooth staining) to

TABLE 29–1 THE TOBACCO-USING CLIENT AND THE HUMAN NEEDS MODEL

Human Needs	Actual or Potential Deficits*
1. Wholesome facial image	Tooth staining, halitosis, periodontal disease, missing teeth, facial wrinkling
2. Protection from health risks	Tobacco-related illness, e.g., heart disease, high blood pressure, cancer; delayed wound healing.
3. Biologically sound and functional dentition	Missing teeth, abrasion, erosion, chewing difficulties.
4. Skin and mucous membrane integrity of the head and neck	Oral lesions, oral cancer, attachment loss and pocket depths = 4 mm.
5. Freedom from anxiety/stress	Withdrawal due to nicotine addiction.
6. Responsibility for oral health	Oral health a low priority; inadequate ownership of personal oral hygiene
7. Conceptualization and understanding	Misconceptions and lack of knowledge about systemic and oral effects of tobacco use

* All unmet human needs can be addressed if efficient and effective tobacco interventions are implemented.

the life threatening (oral cancer). After conducting a thorough intraoral and extraoral examination of the tobacco-using client, the dental hygienist points out and discusses the visible effects of tobacco use and documents all relevant findings. For example, a smoker may have nicotine stomatitis (Figure 29–3) on the palate, and almost half of spit tobacco users have precancerous ST-associated oral mucosal lesions. These lesions are typically characterized as being white and wrinkled (Figure 29–4) and often disappear if ST use is terminated at an early enough stage. In addition, ST use is associated with periodontal recession at the site where the tobacco is held. All tobacco is associated with oral, pharyngeal, and esophageal cancer.

ORAL CANCER. Approximately 30,000 new cases of oral cancer are diagnosed each year, with an overall five-year survival rate of 50%.[1] The long-standing relationship between oral cancer and tobacco use is well documented. Concomitant use of alcohol with tobacco increases the risk of oral cancer ten-fold. Seventy-five percent of oral/pharyngeal cancers are attributed to tobacco and/or heavy alcohol use.[4] Consequently, during health history assessment, it is important to ask questions about alcohol use, tobacco use, and sun exposure, because they are all risk factors for head, neck, skin, and lip cancers. The extraoral and intraoral examination must be thorough and all tissue changes noted in the client's chart.

PERIODONTAL DISEASE. Periodontal disease is strongly associated with smoking. Smoking is a key risk factor for periodontal disease[6] and is associated with the following conditions:

- ✦ Early onset of periodontal disease

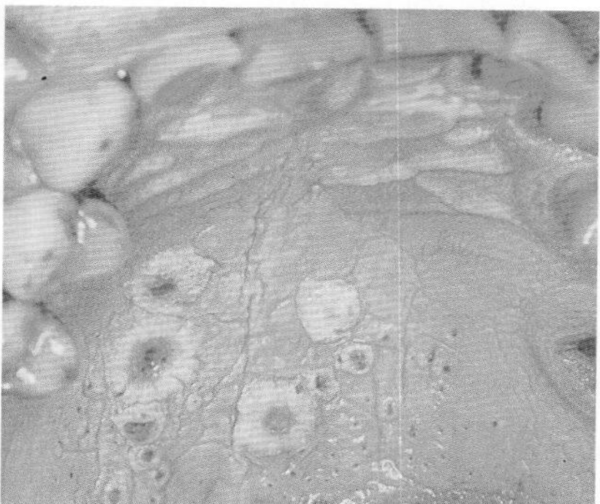

Figure 29–3 ✦ Nicotine stomatitis on the palate of a smoker. *(Courtesy Dr. M. Walsh, University of California.)*

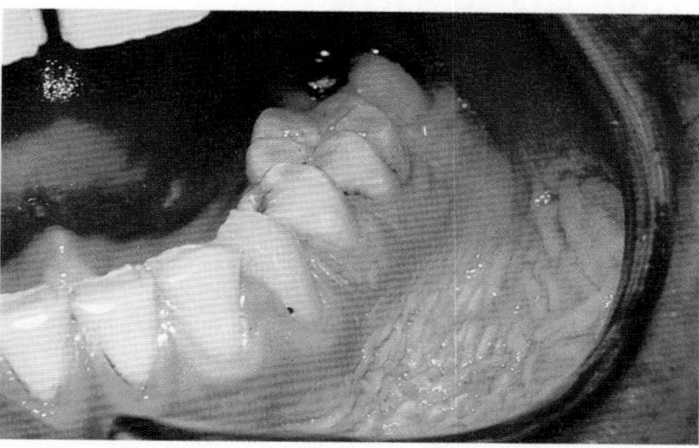

Figure 29–4 ✦ Spit tobacco-associated oral leukoplakia and gingival recession in the mouth of an oral snuff user. *(Courtesy Dr. M. Walsh, University of California.)*

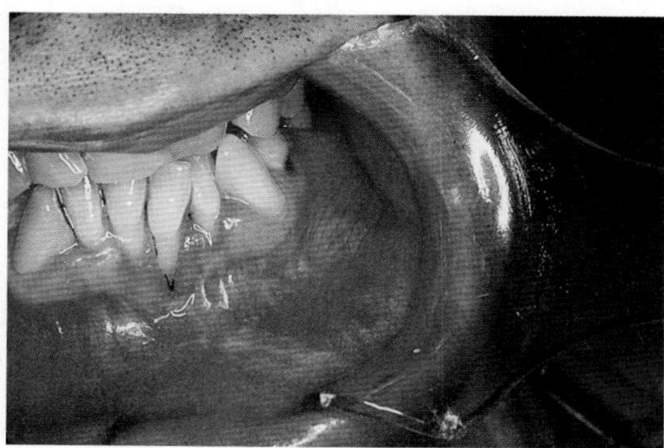

Figure 29–5 ✦ Gingival recession in a ST user. *(Courtesy Dr. M. Walsh, University of California.)*

- ✦ Rapid destruction of the periodontal tissues
- ✦ Persisting refractory status
- ✦ Delayed wound healing after periodontal surgery

Smokers are three to six times more likely than nonsmokers to develop periodontal disease. In addition, gingival recession is significantly associated with ST use (Figure 29–5). The clinical manifestations of tobacco-induced periodontal disease and their biologic bases are presented in Table 29–2.

TABLE 29–2 TOBACCO-INDUCED PERIODONTAL TISSUE CHANGES

Tissue Changes with Use	Biologic Bases for Changes	Tissue Changes with Abstinence
Paler tissue color	Increased vasoconstriction	Increased blood flow
Decreased bleeding	Oxygen depletion	Initially, more bleeding, erythema
Thickened fibrotic consistency; minimal erythema relative to extent of disease	Compromised immune response a. Fewer and impaired PMNS b. Reduced IgG antibody	Healthier consistency and anatomy
Gingival recession around anterior sextants	Increased collagenase production	
Greater probing depths, bone and attachment loss, furcation invasion	Reduction of bone mineral; impaired fibroblast function	Stabilization of attachment levels
Refractory status: continued use	Impaired wound healing	

NICOTINE ADDICTION

All forms of tobacco contain nicotine, a highly addictive substance. Most tobacco users find it difficult to quit because they are addicted to nicotine. Hallmarks for *nicotine addiction* are:

- Compulsive use
- Use despite harmful effects
- Pleasant (euphoric) effects
- Difficulty in quitting or controlling use
- Recurrent drug cravings
- Tolerance
- Physical dependence
- Relapse following abstinence

Nicotine acts on certain cholinergic receptors in the brain that cause the release of chemicals such as dopamine, norepinephrine, acetylcholine, vasopressin, serotonin, and beta-endorphins. The action of these chemicals in the brain causes the user to experience pleasure, arousal, memory improvement, appetite suppression, and reduction of anxiety and tension. These effects of nicotine make it difficult for individuals to stop their tobacco use.

TOLERANCE. With chronic exposure to nicotine, brain cells adapt to compensate for the actions of nicotine. This process is called *neuroadaptation. Tolerance* results from neuroadaptation, so that over time a given level of nicotine eventually has less of an effect on the brain and a larger dose is needed to produce the rewarding effects that lower doses formerly produced.

PHYSICAL DEPENDENCE. Even though the brain adapts to function normally in the presence of nicotine, it also becomes *physically dependent* on nicotine for that normal functioning. When nicotine is not available, the brain function becomes disturbed, resulting in *withdrawal* symptoms (Table 29–3).

Not all clients will experience withdrawal symptoms, and the degree of discomfort among abstainers also will vary. As blood level concentrations of nicotine fall, users reach for the next cigarette or dip of tobacco. Strategies recommended for coping with specific nicotine withdrawal symptoms and temptation to use are listed in Table 29–3. In general, the highly dependent tobacco user poses the greatest challenge to cessation efforts.

SOCIAL INFLUENCES. Social influences that pose challenges to abstinence include peer pressure, the influence of family members and significant others who use tobacco, and a social network that supports, accepts, and allows the habit. In addition, tobacco may by used as a diversion from a strife-filled existence.

HELPING CLIENTS BECOME TOBACCO FREE

In assisting clients in their efforts to stop tobacco use, physical, psychological, behavioral, and sensory aspects of nicotine addiction must be confronted and alternative coping strategies identified. Being supportive and assisting the client with problem solving are critical to promoting tobacco cessation.

5 A's Approach

A general framework for helping clients in the oral healthcare setting to become tobacco free is the 5 A's approach, a strategy developed by the National Cancer Institute and the Agency for Healthcare Research and Quality (AHRQ).[4] The *five A's approach* to tobacco cessation involves *asking* each client about tobacco use, *advising* users to quit, *assessing* their readiness to quit, *assisting* them with the quitting process either directly or by referral, and *arranging* follow-up to see how they are doing with the quitting process. The 5 A's approach serves as a usable model for brief, effective interventions that have been successfully implemented in both medical and dental care environments.[8,9] Each component of the 5 A's approach is described briefly in the following sections, and in detail in Table 29–4. Incorporating the 5 A's into the Dental Hygiene Process of Care relates the 5 A's to the dental hygiene process of care and provides sample assessment findings and suggested interventions.

TABLE 29–3 NICOTINE WITHDRAWAL SYMPTOMS AND SUGGESTED BEHAVIORAL COPING STRATEGIES

Symptoms	Mechanisms for Coping
Anger, irritability, depression	Professional counseling Support groups Exercise, deep breathing with slow exhalation Self-reward for abstinence
Restlessness/ insomnia	Relaxation exercises; go to bed later Getting up and moving around; avoiding caffeine Deep breathing Aerobic exercise but not within 2 hours of bedtime
Cravings	Realizing that cravings last 3–5 minutes; "waiting them out" Thinking responses, e.g., "I can do this and I will" Distraction techniques: carrying and reading list of reasons for stopping and/or inspirational poems Considering non-nicotine aspects of craving and using substitutions, e.g. oral stimulation: chewing gum; hand usage: doodling Avoiding triggers: people, places, or things associated with former habit; exercise
Tension/anxiety	Deep breathing Positive imaging Relaxation exercises Aerobic exercise
Loss of concentration	Recognition that symptom is short-lived Relaxation exercises Patience Deep breathing
Stomach/ intestinal problems	Mild OTC medications High-fiber diet Drink water Relaxation exercises
Hunger/weight gain	Aerobic exercise Healthy eating; drinking water; chewing sugarless gum/eating sugarless hard candy Support groups (e.g. Overeaters Anonymous, Weight Watchers) Restrictive dieting is not recommended; too much deprivation may be overwhelming

Modified from Severson H: *Enough snuff: A guide to quitting smokeless tobacco,* Point Richmond, Calif, 1997, Applied Behavior Science.

ASK. During the assessment phase of the dental hygiene process, the dental hygienist asks each client about tobacco use. A Tobacco Use Assessment Form such as the one presented in Figure 29–6 collects comprehensive information regarding the client's tobacco habits and is included in the client's record (Table 29–4, Strategy 1).

ADVISE. As a healthcare professional, it is important to advise clients that they should stop their tobacco use to protect their future health. Such advice should be clear, unequivocal, and related to something immediately relevant to the client. For example, the dental hygienist points out leukoplakias derived from ST use (Figure 29–4) to clients in their own mouths, describes these lesions as precancerous, and suggests them as a reason to stop their tobacco use. Brush biopsies should be performed (see Chapter 12) and, if indicated, a follow-up incisional biopsy. For clients exhibiting periodontal attachment loss, radiographic findings may enhance provider/client discussions. The dangers posed by tobacco-induced tissue changes must not be minimized. Personalizing cessation advice with findings visible to the client provides a "teachable moment"[10] that can motivate readiness to quit (Table 29–4, Strategies 2 and 3). Even sound advice coupled with demonstrating the damaging effects of tobacco use, however, may not move the client to a readiness that translates into taking action to quit tobacco use.

ASSESS. For all clients who state that they use tobacco, it is important to assess their readiness to quit. To assess readiness to quit, the dental hygienist simply asks clients if they are thinking about quitting their tobacco use in the next month. The concept of readiness to quit relates to the *stages of change theory.*[11,12] According to this theory, tobacco cessation (and any behavior change involving other health behaviors) involves movement through a series of five stages. These five stages of change range from no intention to change (precontemplation stage) to maintaining a changed behavior (maintenance stage). Definitions of each stage of change and implications related to tobacco cessation are discussed in Table 29–5. It is important to understand what occurs at the various stages of the change process to provide appropriate intervention. Consequently, for tobacco-using clients, it is important to assess their readiness to quit.

ASSIST. The manner in which the dental hygienist assists clients who use tobacco depends on their readiness to quit (Figure 29.7). For clients who are not ready to stop their tobacco use within the next month, the dental hygienist provides motivational material and discusses reasons to stop tobacco use (i.e., benefits of quitting) so that clients can consider the advantages and disadvantages of quitting. Also, it is helpful to remind clients that assistance is available when they feel ready to quit.

For clients who state they are ready to quit in the next month, there are multiple provider behaviors that can assist the client with abstinence. For the motivated user, these include providing relevant literature and behavior modification techniques, establishing a quit date, and recommending the use of pharmacologic adjuncts.

As individuals attempt to stop tobacco use, *relapse* (reverting to regular tobacco use) followed by recycling through the stages occurs frequently. When relapse occurs, the client will return to the contemplation or precontemplation stage before attempting to quit again. Relapse should be viewed as a learning opportunity because what is learned from relapse can be applied to the next quit attempt. It is important to understand what occurs at the various stages of the change process to provide appropriate intervention.

For clients who are ready to quit, the dental hygienist can either refer them to a tobacco cessation specialist in the community, or personally provide tobacco cessation counseling. Table 29–4, Strategy 3, suggests the paths tobacco intervention care plans take based on client readiness. For clients who need to be referred to a specialist, support groups are available through the American Cancer Society (ACS), the American Lung Association (ALA), other nonprofit organizations, and through select hospitals in most areas. A community list of group tobacco cessation programs offered should be developed for use in referral of clients.

ARRANGE. Follow-up must be arranged for all clients engaged in a tobacco cessation program. Behavior modification of any type necessitates follow-up. It is recommended that clients be telephoned or seen within one week of their quit date. At this juncture, not all clients will have abstained totally. For those who have, congratulations and reinforcement are warranted.

TABLE 29–4 THE 5 A's APPROACH: ASK, ADVISE, ASSESS, ASSIST, ARRANGE STRATEGIES[2]

Action	Strategies for Implementation
Strategy 1: Ask Implement an office-wide system that ensures that, for *every* client at *every* clinical visit, tobacco-use status is queried and documented.	Expand the vital signs to include tobacco use. Data collected by healthcare team. Implemented using preprinted progress note paper that includes the expanded vital signs, a vital signs stamp, or, for computerized records, an item assessing tobacco-use status. Alternatives to the vital sign stamp are to place tobacco-use status stickers on all client charts or to indicate tobacco use status using computer reminder systems.
Strategy 2: Advise In a *clear, strong,* and *personalized* manner, urge every tobacco user to quit.	Advice should be: *Clear:* "I think it is important for you to quit smoking now and I will help you." "Cutting down while you are ill is not enough." *Strong:* "As your dental hygienist, I need you to know that quitting smoking is the most important thing you can do to protect your current and future health." *Personalized:* Tie tobacco use to current health/illness, and/or the social and economic costs of tobacco use, motivation level/readiness to quit, and/or the impact of smoking on children and others in the household. Encourage clinic staff to reinforce the cessation message and support the client's quit attempt.
Strategy 3: Assess Ask every tobacco user if he or she is willing to make a quit attempt at this time.	If the client is willing to make a quit attempt at this time, provide assistance (see Strategy 4). If the client prefers a more intensive treatment or the clinician believes intensive treatment is appropriate, refer to interventions administered by a tobacco cessation specialist and follow up with the client regarding quitting. If the client clearly states he or she is not willing to make a quit attempt at this time, provide a motivational intervention and written information on reasons to quit.
Strategy 4: Assist Help the client with a quit plan.	Set a quit date. Ideally, the quit date should be within 2 weeks, taking client preference into account. A client's preparations for quitting: Inform family, friends, and co-workers of quitting and request understanding and support. Remove tobacco from environment. Prior to quitting, avoid using tobacco in favorite places (e.g., home, car). Review previous quit attempts. What helped? What led to relapse? Anticipate challenges to planned quit attempt, particularly during the critical first few weeks. These include nicotine withdrawal symptoms.
Recommend nicotine replacement therapy except in special circumstances.	Recommend the use of nicotine patch, nicotine gum, or bupropion hydrochloride therapy for tobacco cessation if not contraindicated.
Give key advice on successful quitting. Suggest action responses and thinking responses.	Abstinence: Total abstinence is essential. "Not even a single puff or dip after the quit date." Alcohol : Drinking alcohol is highly associated with relapse. Those who stop using tobacco should review their alcohol use and consider limiting/abstaining from alcohol during the quit process. Other tobacco users in the household: The presence of other tobacco users in the household, particularly a spouse, is associated with lower success rates. Clients should consider quitting with their significant others and/or developing specific plans to stay quit in a household where others still use tobacco.
Provide supplementary materials.	Sources: Federal agencies, including AHRQ; nonprofit agencies (e.g. American Cancer Society); or local/state health departments. Type: Culturally/racially/educationally/age appropriate for the client. Location: Readily available in every clinic office.

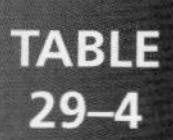

TABLE 29–4 THE 5 A's APPROACH: ASK, ADVISE, ASSESS, ASSIST, ARRANGE STRATEGIES—CONT'D

Action	Strategies for Implementation
Strategy 5: Arrange	
Schedule follow-up contact, either in person or via telephone.	Timing: Follow-up contact should occur soon after the quit date, preferably during the first week. A second follow-up contact is recommended within the first month. Schedule further follow-up contacts as indicated. Action during follow-up visit: Congratulate success. If tobacco use occurred, review circumstances and elicit recommitment to total abstinence. Remind client that a lapse can be used as a learning experience. Identify problems already encountered and anticipate challenges in the immediate future. Assess nicotine replacement therapy use and problems. Consider referral to a more intense or specialized program.

From U.S. Department of Health and Human Services: *Treating tobacco use and dependence,* U.S. Department of Health and Human Services Pub No 69-0692, Washington, DC, 2000, Government Printing Office.

Incorporating the 5 A's into the Dental Hygiene Process of Care

Assessment (ASK)

- Health history (see Tobacco Use Assessment Form, Table 29–4)
- Physical appraisal, extraoral head and neck exam, and potential tobacco-related findings
  - Skin lesions (e.g., nevi, crusted scabs, unhealed ulcerations)
  - Wrinkling
  - Swollen glands
  - Raised areas
  - Keratinized areas or unhealed lesions on lips
  - Body odors associated with smoke
  - Browned/yellowed fingers
- Intraoral exam and potential tobacco-related findings
  - Soft tissue
    - Keratotic areas, induration, raised borders, especially tongue
    - Raised white or red lesions, especially floor of mouth
    - Coated tongue, buccal mucosa
    - Presence of leukoedema, lichen planus
  - Hard tissue
    - Stain
    - Caries, with ST use
    - Attrition, with pipe use
    - Abrasion, with ST use
  - Aesthetics
    - Halitosis
    - Stain
    - Coated tongue
  - Periodontal Exam
    - Probe readings, generally greater
    - Attachment loss, generally greater
    - Recession, potentially greater
    - Tissue appearance, thickened, keratinized
    - Bleeding index, generally less
    - Furcations, generally more
- Radiographic exam and potential tobacco-related findings
  - Bone loss, generally greater
  - Tooth loss, generally greater
  - Calculus, generally more
- Exploring need satisfaction, i.e., why client uses tobacco
  - Habit
  - Stimulation
  - Relaxation
  - Hand usage
  - Oral gratification
  - Tension reduction
  - Craving
- Determining when client uses
  - Situational, environmental (after meals, when driving)
  - People-driven (friends, spouse)
  - Other triggers (alcohol)
- Helping client verbalize reasons for stopping
  - Personal self-esteem
  - Children, significant others
  - Cost
  - Health (oral and systemic)
  - New job, house, car
  - Other
- Establishing client's readiness to stop (ASSESS): "Are you interested in stopping smoking/chewing/pipe use/cigar use? If so, when?"

Dental Hygiene Diagnosis: Multiple Human Deficits Exist and Are Related to Tobacco Use

- Oral health analysis (derived from ASK)
  - Tobacco-associated periodontal disease
  - Aesthetic contraindications
  - Potential for oral cancer, precancerous lesions
  - Potential for increased caries (with ST use)
  - Greater risk for tooth loss
  - Potential for compromised dental and dental hygiene treatment outcomes
  - Potential for associated hard and soft tissue changes
- Tobacco habit analysis (derived from ASK)
  - Need satisfaction motivator(s)
  - Triggers/stimuli identification
  - Previous stop attempts
  - Level of addiction
  - Client readiness for abstinence

Continued on following page

Incorporating the 5 A's into the Dental Hygiene Process of Care—cont'd

Implementation/Dental Hygiene Care Plan (ADVISE, ASSIST)

Tobacco intervention care plan (implementation of Advise, Assist, Arrange)
Individualized plan based on assessment findings and analysis; must include oral cancer self-screening
Advising
- Includes "teachable moment," when relevant
- Must include firm, unequivocal advice: "As your dental hygienist and health professional, I must advise you to stop using tobacco. I care about your well-being and am available to assist you in your efforts to stop."
- Must provide relevant information about effects of tobacco

Assisting
- For the not-ready client:
  - Provide information on reasons to quit. The tobacco care plan ends and the door is left open for future readiness
- For the ready client:
  - Facilitate setting a quit date
  - Establish need for triage with client's physician, psychotherapist, pharmacist, and/or support group
  - Ascertain benefit of FDA-approved pharmacologic adjuncts

Instrumentation care plan
- Quadrant debridement depending on extent of deposit, disease
- Local anesthesia, desensitizing agents as needed
- Universal ultrasonic inserts for calculus and stain removal
- Slimline ultrasonic inserts and enhancement instruments for debridement in deeper pockets and furcation areas
- Polishing, if necessary, for further stain removal

Referral
- Periodontal, depending on disease status
- Pathology, if suspect lesions are present
- Physician, systemic concerns (e.g., high blood pressure)
- General dentist, caries, tooth loss, abrasion, erosion, attrition

Other Services
- Diet counseling
- Treatment for halitosis
- Oral hygiene instruction
  - Tongue scraper
  - Interdental cleaning aids as appropriate
  - Toothbrush, mechanical or manual

Evaluation/Follow-up (ARRANGE)

Responses to instrumentation interventions
- Tissue resolution
- Stain/calculus reformation
- Establishing appropriate recare interval
- Consultation with periodontist regarding further treatment

Tobacco intervention
- Contact client within 1 week of quit date
- Assess client's success
- Discuss withdrawal, slips, relapse/relearn
- Assess client's coping skills
- Reestablish quit date, if necessary
- Assess modification for pharmacologic adjuncts
- Consult other health care professionals, as needed
- Maintain contact with client on regular basis

Clients are to be commended if they have achieved abstinence for even one hour, one day, or two days. Strategies used to cope with problems and the need for nicotine replacement should be discussed. A subsequent follow-up contact with these clients is scheduled within a month, or sooner as needed.

For clients who have experienced a *slip* (use of tobacco but not a resumption of the previous habit), it is important to transform the event into a relearning/recycling situation. For example, clients may have learned that they really cannot be around friends who dip or that they need to focus on stress reduction techniques. The dental hygienist helps clients identify what caused their slip or relapse and what they can do to prevent a recurrence. If a full relapse has occurred (a resumption of the previous habit), a new quit date needs to be set. Ongoing support is critical, and referral to a more specialized program may be appropriate.

Relapse is a common phenomenon. It typically takes a user multiple attempts to achieve abstinence. The greatest number of users relapse during the first few weeks of abstinence. The key to relapse prevention is identifying high-risk situations in advance and planning what to do instead of using tobacco when the high-risk situation arises. Clients also need to eliminate all tobacco paraphernalia from their living and work environments. The more specific the relapse prevention, the greater the chance for abstinence.

Arranging follow-up, the fifth A, is comparable to the evaluation phase of the dental hygiene process of care (see Incorporating the 5 A's into the Dental Hygiene Process of Care, Evaluation/Follow-up [ARRANGE].). In follow-up, client success with abstinence is ascertained. Modifications (e.g., new quit date, other pharmacologic adjuncts, different coping mechanisms) may be introduced. New goals may be set.

Tobacco Cessation Treatment Plan by Appointment suggests how the 5 A's could be sequenced for appointment planning in the dental hygiene care plan, and Figure 29–7 provides a tobacco intervention flow chart.

FDA-APPROVED PHARMACOLOGIC ADJUNCTS

Clients who are nicotine dependent may need pharmacologic support to facilitate their quitting process.[9] The

Name ____________________

Date ____________

1. Do you use tobacco in any form? ☐ Yes ☐ No

1A. If no, have you ever used tobacco in the past? ☐ Yes ☐ No

How long did you use tobacco? _____ years _____ months

How long ago did you stop? _____ years _____ months

If you are not currently a tobacco user, no other questions should be answered. Thank you for completing this form.

Questions 2–10 are for current tobacco users only.

2. If you smoke, what type? (Check) How many? (Number)
☐ Cigarettes _____ Cigarettes per day
☐ Cigars _____ Cigars per day
☐ Pipe _____ Bowls per day

3. If you chew/use snuff, what type? How much?
☐ Snuff _____ Days a can lasts
☐ Chewing _____ Pouches per week
☐ Other (describe) ____________
Amount __________ per ____________

3A. How long do you keep a chew in you mouth?
_______minutes

4. How many days of the week do you use tobacco?
7 6 5 4 3 2 1

5. How soon after you wake up do you first use tobacco?
☐ within 30 minutes ☐ more than 30 minutes

6. Does the person closest to you use tobacco?
☐ Yes ☐ No

7. How interested are you in stopping your use of tobacco?
☐ not at all ☐ a little ☐ somewhat ☐ yes ☐ very much

8. Have you tried to stop using tobacco before? ☐ Yes ☐ No

8A. How long ago was your last attempt to quit?
_____ years _____ months

9. Have you discussed stopping with another physician, dentist, or dental hygienist? ☐ Yes ☐ No

10. If you decided to stop using tobacco completely during the next two weeks, how confident are you that you would succeed?
☐ not at all ☐ a little ☐ somewhat ☐ very confident

Thank you for completing this form

Client Tobacco Use Assessment Form			
Contact Record			
Date client contacted	Client asked Y/N	Advice given Y/N	Assist describe service

Figure 29–6 ✦ Tobacco use assessment form. *(Modified from* Tobacco effects in the mouth, *U.S. Department of Health and Human Services, NIH Pub No 94-3330, Bethesda, Md, 1992, US Government Printing Office.)*

extent of support the client needs, whether professional and/or pharmacologic, drives the tobacco cessation care plan. Although the prescribing of pharmacologic adjuncts may be the legal responsibility of the dentist, the dental hygienist must know about the various nicotine replacement therapies and other FDA-approved adjuncts. Many nicotine replacement therapies are available over-the-counter (OTC), and clients often ask for advice about particular products. Table 29–6 displays the different types of nicotine and nonnicotine replacement therapies, OTC or prescription status, and dosage information.

Clients need to be cautioned that no pharmacologic adjunct is a magic bullet. Such adjuncts are helpful in diminishing withdrawal symptoms, which allows the client to concentrate on action and thinking coping strategies to resist the temptation to use.

NICOTINE REPLACEMENT THERAPY

The key purpose of *nicotine replacement therapy* is to reduce or eliminate withdrawal symptoms while clients cope

TABLE 29–5

STAGES OF READINESS TO CHANGE[6,11]

Stage	Related Client Characteristics and Behavior	Dental Hygiene Intervention
Precontemplation	No thought of quitting in the next 6 months	Dispense educational material on reasons for quitting. Client may be defensive when confronted with the information
Contemplation	Thinking about quitting within the next 6 months	Dispense educational material & discuss pros and cons of quitting. Ambivalence may be present, but clients will more likely accept information as they are developing more belief in the value of change
Preparation	Willing to set a quit date in the next month and to make small changes in preparation for quitting in the next month	Client believes advantages outweigh disadvantages of behavior change. May need assistance in planning for the change. Implement cessation counseling
Action	Actively engaged in strategies to change behavior. This stage may last up to 6 months. May have stopped using tobacco, but for less than 6 months	Praise. Identify barriers and facilitators of change. Discuss relapse prevention
Maintenance	Has stopped using tobacco for more than 6 months. Sustained change over time. This stage begins 6 months after action has started and continues indefinitely	Praise. Discuss relapse prevention. Changes need to be integrated into the client's lifestyle
Relapse	Using tobacco again and many reach higher levels than before	Set new quit date and recycle

Modified from Prochaska JO, DiClemente CC: Stages of change in the modification of problem behaviors, *Progress in Behavior Modification* 28:184, 1992.

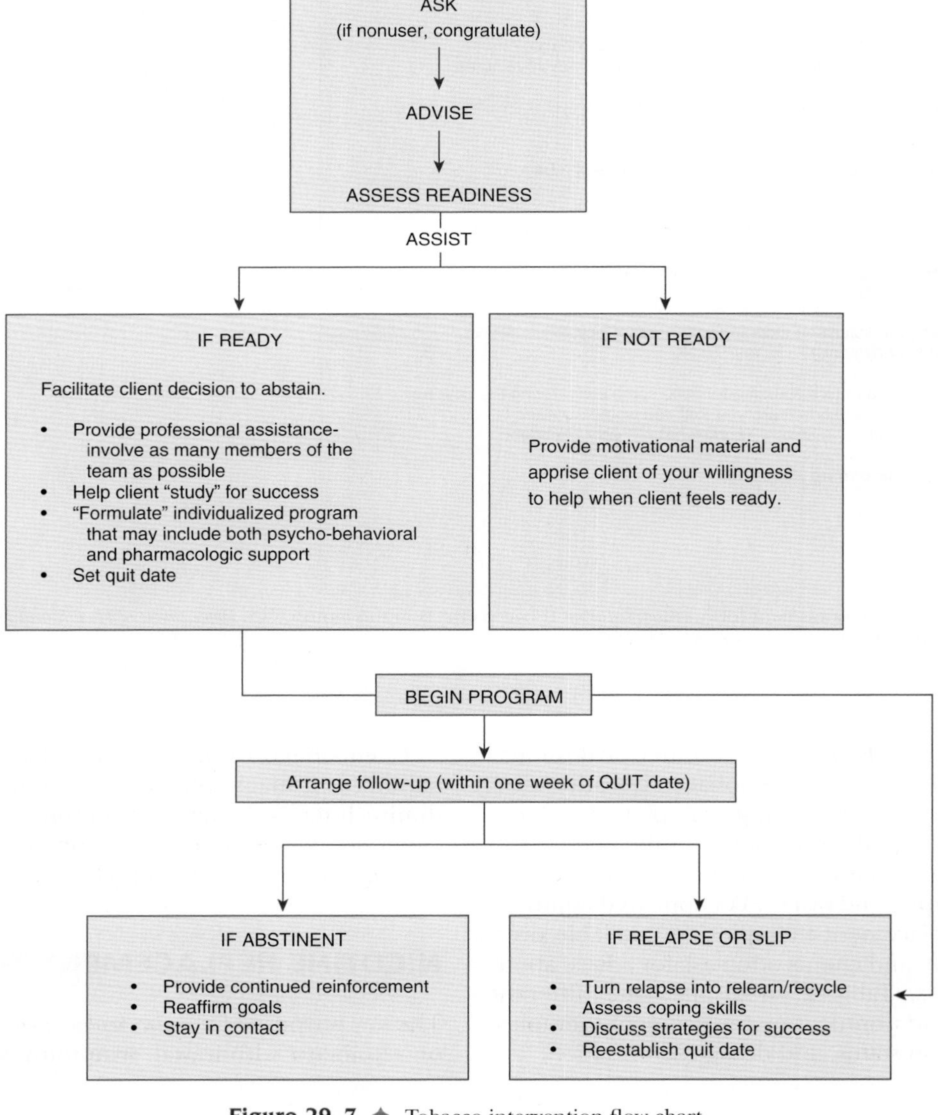

Figure 29–7 ✦ Tobacco intervention flow chart.

TABLE 29–6 FDA-APPROVED PHARMACOLOGIC AGENTS

Agent	Dosage	Side Effects	Comments	Contraindications
Nicotine Replacement Agents				
All nicotine replacement agents	Follow manufacturers' instructions	See below	Part of comprehensive behavioral cessation program to relieve withdrawal symptoms. Do not use with other tobacco products.	Hypertension Depression Asthma medication Stomach ulcers Diabetes Pregnancy Serious cardiac arrhythmias Severe or worsening angina pectoris Post heart attack Skin disorders
Nicotine transdermal patch OTC	7 to 21 mg/day Step-down dosing	Topical skin reaction, abnormal dreams, joint or muscle pain	Use 4 to 8 weeks Easy to use, disassociates cues from use, steady level of nicotine	
Nicotine polacrilex (gum) OTC	Available in 2- and 4-mg doses Average 9 to 12 pieces per day not to exceed 24 pieces	GI distress Mouth soreness Jaw ache Hiccups	Use on a fixed schedule throughout the day Provides an oral substitute to minimize weight gain Not to exceed 96 mg per day	TMJ problems Dentures Fixed bridge work Loose teeth
Nonnicotine Agent				
Bupropion HCi (Zyban) prescription	150 mg once daily in a.m. for 3 days then 150 mg twice daily (a.m. and p.m.) at least 8 hr apart for 7 to 12 weeks	Dry mouth Insomnia	Client should begin medication 7 to 14 days before stopping tobacco Use 1 to 2 weeks before "Quit Date" Increases dopamine levels in the mesolimbic system Dosage > 300 mg should not be used Easy to use Minimizes weight gain	History of head injury Seizure disorder Concomitant use of Wellbutrin, Wellbutrin SR Eating disorder Use of monoamine oxidase inhibitor in the past 14 days

Data from Dr. Robert Mecklenburg, Chair, National Dental Tobacco Free Steering Committee, National Cancer Institute, 12304 River's Edge Drive, Potomac, MD 20854.

with the psychosocial and behavioral aspects of dependence.[9,11] Nicotine transdermal patches, nicotine polacrilex gum, nicotine nasal sprays, and nicotine oral inhalers are the nicotine replacement products currently on the market. Transdermal nicotine patches and nicotine gum are available OTC and are the most widely studied nicotine replacement therapies. With transdermal patch use, nicotine is absorbed through the skin; with the gum, nicotine is released into the oral cavity during chewing and is absorbed via the oral mucosa. Both modalities enhance abstinence when used in conjunction[7] with psychosocial counseling. Choice of modality depends on client history, preference, and/or provider experience with a given product.

Transdermal Nicotine Replacement Therapy (Patch)

Transdermal nicotine patches are marketed for both 24-hour and 18-hour usage. Clients using the 18-hour patch receive no nicotine during sleeping hours. An advantage of the patch is that it delivers a constant dose of nicotine throughout its use. A small percentage of clients using the 24-hour patch have reported sleep interrupted by nightmares, an indication of nicotine toxicity. If this occurs, the dose of nicotine should be reduced or the patch removed during sleeping hours. Clients also may experience dermatitis as a side effect.

Directions for patches require the user to place a new patch each day on a nonhairy site of the upper trunk. No one site should be used again in less than a week. Used patches should be disposed of carefully, because residual nicotine could harm small children and animals. Patches work on a dosing-down principle until the client is eventually weaned off of nicotine. Each patch dose is generally of a two- to four-week duration, depending on client response. Small-framed or obese clients may require dose modification. Triage with the client's physician is advised, particularly if the client presents with systemic disease.

Nicotine Polacrilex (Gum)

In general, client compliance is easier to achieve with the patch than with the gum, because use of the gum requires more behavior modification. Once the patch is placed, a client needs to do no more. However, proper gum use requires clients to slowly chew the gum and then "park" it between their cheek and their gingiva. Overchewing can result in nicotine toxicity, in which the client may experience nausea, vomiting, and/or upset stomach. Success with nicotine gum also is greater when the client has a fixed dosing schedule (e.g., one piece of gum every hour throughout the day) rather than one that is ad lib, based on need. To avoid withdrawal and relapse, nicotine gum is sometimes used in the morning in combination with the 18-hour patch when the patch is first placed. This action enables the client to receive a quick boost of nicotine as the transdermally provided nicotine more slowly makes its way into the bloodstream.

Contraindications

Both the patch and gum are contraindicated for clients who experience hypertension, who take medication for asthma, and who have diabetes, cardiovascular disease, or stomach ulcers. Controversy surrounds pregnant women's use of the patch. However, some feel that the patch poses less risk to the mother and fetus than smoking, because transdermal nicotine is not inhaled and mainstream smoke effects are eliminated. Clients with fixed dental bridges, loose teeth, or loose restorations should not use nicotine gum. Side effects with nicotine gum include aphthous ulcers, jaw ache, and hiccups.[11]

Side Effects and Toxicity

Nicotine replacement products must be used according to manufacturers' instructions. Nicotine toxicity (overdose) can result if clients overuse nicotine replacement products. There may be, however, a period of trial and error to determine the optimum dosage of nicotine replacement to avoid withdrawal symptoms and at the same time avoid toxicity (Table 29–6).

Bupropion (Hydrochloride)

Some tobacco users achieve successful abstinence by using bupropion hydrochloride, a nonnicotine prescription antidepressant drug. The prescription initially allows users to continue their tobacco use while taking the medication. During the course of bupropion (Zyban) therapy, users report a lack of interest in tobacco and a lack of desire to use it.[14]

CONTRAINDICATIONS. History of head injury, seizure disorder, eating disorder, and/or use of monoamine oxidase inhibitors in the past 14 days precludes use of bupropion.

COMMUNICATION SKILLS

Communication skills are key when attempting to help an individual stop tobacco use (see Chapter 4). Tobacco users are apt to be sensitive about their habits; well-honed communication will help prevent client defensiveness. Effective Communication Strategies suggests useful communication approaches when interacting with tobacco-using clients.

Tobacco Cessation Treatment Plan by Appointment

This is a proposed appointment-by-appointment framework for a prototypical tobacco cessation treatment plan. Modifications will occur naturally, based on clients' individualized needs. This framework contains the desired components and is designed to guide the oral health professional. Fewer or more visits may be necessary.

Appointment 1: ASK, ADVISE (Assessment could be done in advance via self-administered survey.)

Ask client about use of tobacco.
Advise him or her to quit tobacco use.
Correlate oral findings with habit.
Suggest diary to monitor each time client uses tobacco (time of day, place, activity), to score the level of craving (1 to 10), and to identify mood state, why, with whom, and where.
Have client consider the idea of stopping.

Appointment 1 or 2: ADVISE

Determine extent of addiction and discuss with client.
Confirm client interest and elicit client reasons for wanting to stop.
Discuss benefits of stopping.
Have client consider triggers and coping strategies.
Discuss intervention options (counseling, nicotine replacement, pharmacologic adjuncts).
Suggest setting quit date.

Appointment 3: ADVISE, ASSIST (Could occur in fewer or more appointments.)

Address client concerns and questions.
Set quit date.
Discuss triggers and coping strategies.
Discuss withdrawal symptoms.
Discuss use of nicotine replacement and/or pharmacologic adjuncts.
Discuss need for follow-up and potential for slips/relapse.

Appointment 4: ASSIST

One or two days before quit date.
Review previous topics, e.g., withdrawal, coping strategies, triggers, slips, and relapse.
Provide reinforcement.
Congratulate client.

Appointment 5: ARRANGE FOLLOW-UP

Within a week of quit date, call client and schedule in-office visit.
Review progress, support mechanisms, and need for modifications.
Discuss withdrawal symptoms and coping strategies.
Continue follow-up as needed.
Address any prescription use modifications.

Effective Communication Strategies

Ask: Be direct, specific, thorough, nonjudgmental; listen well
Advise: Be empathic yet firm; provide an unequivocal "stop using/quit" message; be positive regarding benefits of cessation
Assess: Ask clients directly if they are interested in stopping; listen well; ask open-ended questions for clients who are uncertain
Assist: Offer concrete suggestions; be patient and nonjudgmental; address client-specific issues; be empathic
Arrange: Provide specific follow-up; consider triage, as indicated; be supportive

IMPLEMENTING A CLINICAL-BASED TOBACCO INTERVENTION PROGRAM[7]

Dental hygienists often are the strongest proponents of tobacco intervention activities in their employment settings. Three key steps are necessary to ensure successful incorporation of tobacco intervention programs into clinical settings: generating team support, designating a coordinator, and creating a tobacco-free environment (see Implementation of a Clinic-Based Tobacco Intervention Program).

DENTAL HYGIENIST'S ROLE IN THE COMMUNITY

The dental hygienist's role related to tobacco extends beyond the immediate clinical environment.[8] Given its magnitude as a public health issue, tobacco use commands dental hygienists' action at the professional and societal levels. Ethically, dental hygienists are committed to the health and well-being of society. Involvement with tobacco-related issues helps achieve that goal.

Professional and societal activities that dental hygienists can pursue within their professional associations and communities include the following:

- Endorse tobacco intervention policies within local, state, national, and international associations.
- Ensure that continuing education related to tobacco issues is on the agenda for professional conferences.
- Reinforce peer awareness of key tobacco information.
- Volunteer organizational support for tobacco-related events.
- Support existing policy that promotes a tobacco-free society.
- Advocate for tobacco-free children.
- Lobby for ordinances that encourage tobacco-free environments.
- Provide tobacco use education to children, sports teams, PTAs, and other relevant community groups.

Implementation of a Clinic-Based Tobacco Intervention Program

Establish the need for the program by providing staff members with information related to adverse effects of tobacco on health and on the outcome of dental and dental hygiene services
Facilitate support by:
- Educating team members about the 5 A's and tobacco intervention through staff meetings, reports from the literature
- Suggesting mechanisms for program incorporation into the oral healthcare setting
- Helping current team member tobacco users choose abstinence
- Researching available continuing education programs for all staff to attend

Designate a program coordinator who facilitates team involvement, publicizes the program to clients, orders literature, ensures client follow-up, and reinforces chart documentation
Create a tobacco-free environment by:
- Posting signs that promote tobacco-free lifestyles
- Ordering magazines that do not advertise tobacco products
- Ensuring that neither clients nor team members use tobacco in the oral healthcare setting
- Establishing a meaningful and efficient client tobacco user tracking system

Address reimbursement issues:
- Tobacco interventions that are brief and incorporated into routine service delivery do not constitute separate, billable charges
- If practices or clinical environments choose to provide more enhanced interventions, individual discretion should dictate acceptable charges. An ADA insurance code no. 01320 is designated for "Tobacco Counseling for the Prevention and Control of Oral Disease"
- In general, tobacco intervention activity should be viewed as an ethical and necessary component of the expected standard of care. Its worth is perhaps best measured by lives saved and improved quality of life, rather than by tangible practice income. A tobacco intervention program, in fact, may serve as a positive marketing tool for some practices

Client Education Issues

- Explain the adverse health effects of tobacco use and the benefits of stopping.
- Encourage nonusers to remain tobacco free.
- Offer cessation advice for users and show them the visible effects of tobacco use in their oral cavities.
- Teach skills to cope with the quitting process.
- Explain the addictive properties of tobacco.
- Explain how tobacco use will affect proposed dental hygiene and dental services.
- Teach clients the effects that secondhand smoke has on others.
- Learn about the pharmacologic and professional resources available in the practice setting and the community.

Legal, Ethical, and Safety Issues

- As oral healthcare providers, dental hygienists are ethically obligated to address a client's oral health and overall well-being.
- Tobacco use is a life-threatening habit. All tobacco-using clients must be informed of the deleterious effects of tobacco use and educated and guided toward abstinence.
- The linkage between tobacco use and oral cancer is undisputed. Clients who are diagnosed with oral cancer could potentially sue providers who have not informed them of the relationship between tobacco use, cancer, and periodontal diseases.
- With the current emphases on prevention, health promotion, and litigation, tobacco use interventions are a standard of care and are therefore expected behaviors of oral health professionals.

Key Concepts

- There are numerous adverse systemic and oral health effects of tobacco use.
- Nicotine addiction is a physical, psychological, behavioral, and sensory dependence: a compulsive use of tobacco that continues despite knowledge of adverse consequences.
- Five A's (5 A's) comprise a science-based approach to brief, effective practice-based tobacco use interventions; a methodology endorsed by the Agency for Healthcare Research and Quality (AHRQ) and the National Cancer Institute (NCI) for implementation for oral health and medical care teams in private practice and community settings.
- Providers should *ask* all clients about tobacco use; *advise* users to quit and *show* them the visible effects of tobacco use in their own mouths; *assess* their stage of readiness; offer *assistance* with the quitting process; and *arrange* follow-up on their cessation progress.
- Stages of readiness to change refer to progressive levels of mental readiness through which clients pass as they work to overcome an addiction; lengths of stay in each stage vary from client to client. When truly ready, a client takes action to abstain.
- The dental hygienist's role related to tobacco issues extends beyond the immediate clinic environment and commands action on professional and societal levels.
- A teachable moment is the opportunity to show clients the deleterious effects of tobacco use in their own mouths. The personalization of the client's habit can be the defining moment that facilitates readiness to quit tobacco use.

Critical Thinking Exercises

Client: Mr. Z

Profile: A 45-year-old white male presented to the dental clinic. He has been dipping snuff for 18 years. He drinks approximately three beers per day.

Chief Complaint: "My tooth hurts on the upper left back".

Dental History: Client erratically seeks care. He has not seen a dentist or dental hygienist in over 5 years.

Social History: The client is divorced and lives alone. He frequently travels abroad for business reasons. He is a full-time employee for a computer company.

Medical History: Client reports no use of medications. He broke his arm in a skiing accident two years ago. He reports no systemic disease.

Oral Health Behaviors Assessment: The client reports brushing one time per day with a hard brush. He does not rinse or floss. He uses no aids.

Supplemental Notes: Upon clinical examination, a 10 × 20 mm mixed leuko/erythoplakic lesion is found on the vestibular right labial mucosa of the maxilla, extending to the surrounding alveolar mucosa and attached gingiva. The client places his snuff in that area. He was unaware of the lesion, and the lesion was asymptomatic.

1. Will Mr. Z's lesion disappear if he abstains?
2. When assessing Mr. Z's habit, he reports that oral gratification is a key factor in his dependence. Based on this finding, what FDA-approved pharmacologic adjunct might be most beneficial for him?
3. Mr. Z states snuff use is safer than cigarette smoking. How would you respond?
4. Mr. Z also reports daily alcohol use. How would you use this information in educating Mr. Z?

Client: Ms. J

Profile: A 35-year-old female presents for a three-month recall appointment. The client reports smoking three packs of cigarettes per day.

Chief Complaint: "I am unhappy about the stains on my front teeth and the color of my fillings on my front teeth."

Dental History: Client makes regular dental visits although she is nine months overdue for her dental hygiene visit. She consistently has reported interest in tobacco cessation but has rejected the use of nicotine replacement. She states, "I want to do it on my own."

Social History: Client has been smoking for 25 years. She drinks six to eight cups of coffee/day. She is a recovering alcoholic. She is unmarried and lives with her father. Ms. J is weight conscious.

Medical History: Past history of depression. Ibuprofen p.r.n. for back pain from an injury sustained ten years ago.

Oral Health Behaviors Assessment: The client reports brushing three times/day with an electric toothbrush, flossing one time/day, and using a mouthrinse several times per day. She rarely exercises.

Supplemental Notes: Client presents with thick, heavy black stains generalized. She reports presence of xerostomia.

1. Which FDA-approved pharmacologic adjuncts might be most acceptable to Ms. J?
2. What message would best motivate Ms. J to stop smoking?
3. If Ms. J worries about weight gain with cessation, how should you advise her?

For References, Suggested Readings, and Related Websites, visit

http://evolve.elsevier.com/Darby/hygiene/

CHAPTER 30

Impressions, Study Casts, and Oral Stents

OBJECTIVES

Mastery in the content of this chapter will enable the reader to:

- Describe the types of dental impressions and their purposes
- Describe types of impression trays and their use
- Mix alginate impression material and make a dental impression
- Describe types of diagnostic casts, their use, and the materials used to create them
- Mix model plaster to make a diagnostic cast from a dental impression
- Mix dental stone to make a diagnostic cast from a dental impression
- Discuss reversible and irreversible treatments for bruxism
- Make dental impressions, wax-bite registrations, diagnostic casts, and EVA stents utilizing safety procedures

KEY TERMS

Alginate
Anatomic portion
Appliance therapy
Art portion
Biofeedback
Bruxism
Centric occlusion
Chemical change
Class I dental stone
Concussion
Dental impression
Dental stone
Diagnostic cast
Fast-set powder
Final impression
Imbibition
Irreversible hydrocolloid
Humidor
Hydrophilic
Mouthguard
Nightguard/Dayguard
Normal-set powder
Physical change
Plaster
Preliminary impression
Spatulation
Stents
Syneresis
Wax-bite registration

A *dental impression* is a negative imprint of the teeth and surrounding tissues. An impression is used to create an accurate three-dimensional reproduction of the teeth and surrounding tissues. This positive reproduction is called a model or a *diagnostic cast,* or a study cast. There are three main types of dental impressions used in dentistry: a preliminary impression, a final impression, and a bite registration. *Preliminary impressions* are used to make models for diagnosing, making *stents* (custom trays), documenting a client's dental arches as part of a permanent record, enhancing client education as a visual aid, and making a temporary crown or a removable dental appliance. *Final impressions* require more accurate detail of the tooth structures and surrounding tissues and are used by the laboratory technician to construct casted restorations such as crowns and bridges, partial or full dentures, and implants.

The dental hygienist often is responsible for making preliminary dental impressions.

This chapter provides an overview of concepts related to making dental impressions, pouring diagnostic casts, constructing bite registrations, and creating custom-made stents for such purposes as mouth protection, tooth whitening, and home fluoride application. The reader is advised to consult a text on dental materials for complete information on properties and manipulation of the different types of dental materials used.

DENTAL IMPRESSIONS

Impression Trays

Impression material is placed into the mouth in an impression tray. Because dental impressions are used in oral healthcare for many purposes, there are various types of impression trays. Impression trays are designed for different areas of the mouth and include quadrant trays, which cover half an arch, and full trays, which cover the complete maxillary or mandibular arch (Figure 30–1). The type of tray selected depends on the purpose of the impression. Metal, plastic, or Styrofoam trays are available in standard small, medium, and large sizes for children and adults. They may be perforated to promote a mechanical lock with the impression material. Guidelines for Proper Impression Tray Selections (See below) Procedure 30–1 describes the details of selecting the correct tray size and preparing it for use.

Alginate Impression Material

The impression material used most often in dentistry for preliminary and final impressions is hydrocolloid ("hydro" meaning water and "colloid" meaning gelatin). Because hydrocolloid is in a water suspension, the product is *hydrophilic,* meaning it loves water. Hydrocolloids can exist in a sol (solution) or a gel (solid) state. Depending on the type of hydrocolloid used, the physical change from sol to gel is either reversible (changed by thermal factors) or irreversible (changed by chemical factors).

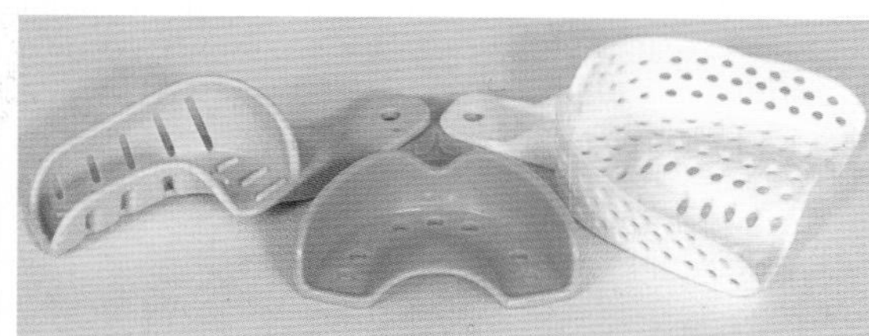

FIGURE 30–1 ✦ Types of impressions trays *(From Bird D, Robinson D:* Torres and Ehrlich: Modern dental assisting, *ed 7, Philadelphia, 2002, WB Saunders.)*

> **Guidelines for Proper Impression Tray Selections**
>
> Tray should feel comfortable to the client
> Tray should extend slightly beyond the facial surfaces of the teeth to enclose all teeth, musculature, and vestibule
> Tray should extend 2 to 3 mm beyond the most posterior tooth in the arch and include the retromolar or maxillary tuberosity area
> Tray should allow for a 2- to 3-mm depth of material beyond the biting surfaces/edges of the teeth
> Tray should be comfortable and minimize tissue trauma during insertion and removal

Gelation is the transformation from sol to gel. An *irreversible hydrocolloid* does not change its physical state after gelation. *Alginate* is an irreversible hydrocolloid powder impression material that changes from a sol to a gel state by means of a *chemical reaction* once cool water is added to the potassium alginate powder to produce a sol. The impression material reaches the gel state after the chemical setting reaction in the client's mouth. At this time, it is removed from the mouth.

PACKAGING AND STORAGE. Alginate impression material is available either in premeasured packages or in bulk canisters. The premeasured packages are more expensive, but they save time by eliminating the need to measure the powder. Because the powder deteriorates when exposed to elevated temperatures or water, it is important to store the powder in a tightly closed container in a cool, nonrefrigerated place. The individual premeasured packages should be used immediately upon opening to avoid water condensing on the powder from the humidity in the air. Properly stored alginate impression material has a shelf life of about one year.

Although an alginate impression does not change its physical state after gelation, it is subject to distortion as a result of slight changes in its physical surroundings. As a result, alginate impressions must be "poured up" within an hour of having been made. The potential for dimensional change is due to the fact that so much of the material is made of water. For example, if left exposed to the room environment unprotected, the impression may shrink due to *syneresis* (the loss of water) from evaporation, or swell due to *imbibition* (the uptake of water) in the presence of moisture. Moreover, if an alginate impression is stored in water or in a very wet towel, it will expand due to the absorption of water. It is recommended that a disinfected impression be wrapped in a slightly moistened towel and placed in a plastic biohazard bag, a condition that provides about 100% relative humidity and causes the least amount of distortion.

WATER/POWDER RATIO. When using alginate powder stored in canisters, a plastic scoop for dispensing the powder and a calibrated plastic cylinder for measuring the water are supplied (Figure 30–2). A mandibular

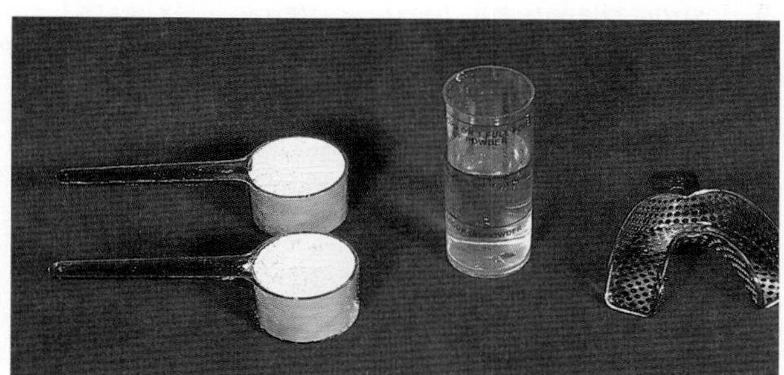

FIGURE 30–2 ✦ A plastic scoop and plastic cylinder are supplied with alginate. *(From Bird D, Robinson D:* Torres and Ehrlich: Modern dental assisting, *ed 7, Philadelphia, 2002, WB Saunders.)*

Procedure 30–1 SELECTING THE CORRECT TRAY SIZE AND PREPARING IT FOR USE

EQUIPMENT (Figure 30–3)

Protective barriers (safety glasses, mask, gloves, hair covering/bonnet)
Antimicrobial mouthrinse
Lubricating gel
Maxillary and mandibular impression trays
Mouth mirror
Utility wax

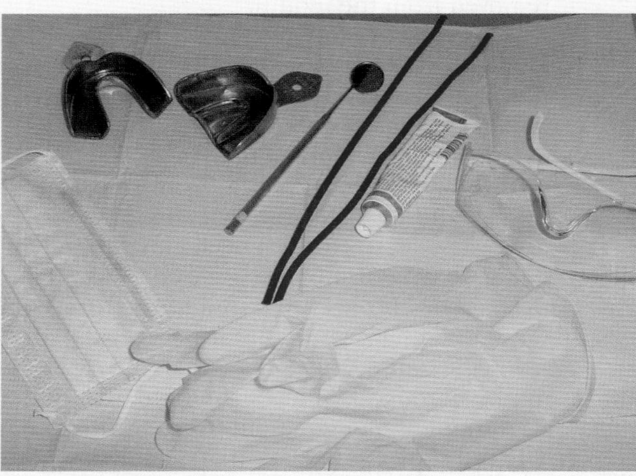

FIGURE 30–3 ✦ Equipment for selecting and preparing an impression tray. *(Courtesy Gwen Essex-Lancaster, RDH.)*

STEPS	RATIONALE
PREPARATION	
1. Gather all necessary supplies.	Prevents unnecessary interruptions to obtain supplies during the procedure.
2. Position self at side and front of client and seat the client in an upright position.	An upright position minimizes gagging. This positioning of clinician provides for good control of client and ease of insertion of tray.
3. Explain the procedure to the client. Have client remove any removable oral appliances.	The client who is familiar with the procedure is more manageable. Some may have had a negative experience; some may have a strong gag reflex.
4. Don personal protective equipment, safety glasses, mask, and bonnet. Wash hands and don gloves.	Necessary for infection control.
5. Place protective eyewear on the client.	Protective eyewear prevents injury to the client.
6. Provide preprocedural antimicrobial mouthrinse.	Decreases surface microorganisms and saliva. Aids in achieving an accurate impression, provides a satisfying feeling for the client and serves as a distraction.
7. Lubricate the client's lips with a small amount of lubricating gel.	Lubrication prevents the lips from cracking during impressions.
MANDIBULAR TRAY SELECTION	
8. Inspect client's mouth to estimate tray size. Note teeth out of alignment, tori, and length of dental arch that may require additional tray adaptation for client comfort.	A properly fitting impression tray will minimize tissue trauma and will hold an impression with all of the details of the mouth.
9. Instruct client to tilt chin down. Retract the client's lip and cheek with index and middle fingers of nondominant hand and at the same time turn the tray sideways and distend the lip and cheek on the opposite side of the mouth with the side of the tray to gain entry into the client's mouth. Insert the tray with a rotary motion (Figure 30–4).	Tilting the chin down minimizes gagging. Turning the impression tray sideways prior to insertion allows for the tray to be placed properly in the mouth with minimal tissue trauma.

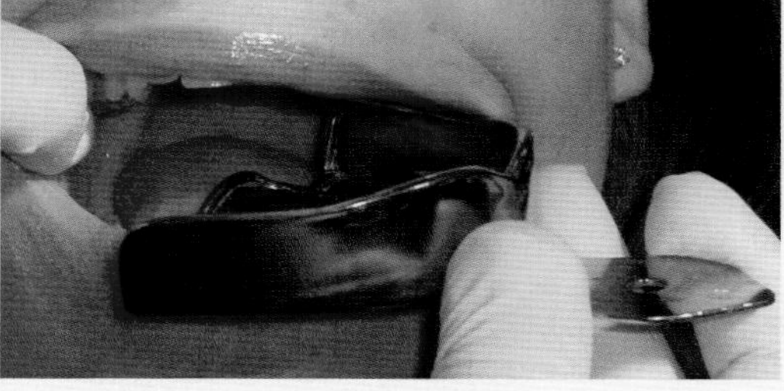

FIGURE 30–4 ✦ Inserting impression tray. *(Courtesy Gwen Essex-Lancaster, RDH.)*

Procedure 30–1 SELECTING THE CORRECT TRAY SIZE AND PREPARING IT FOR USE—CONT'D

STEPS	RATIONALE
10. Make sure the tray is centered over the lower teeth by placing the handle at the midline usually between the central incisors and in line with the center of the chin.	Ensures adequate fit for a symmetrical impression of the dental arch.
11. Instruct client to raise tongue. Lower the tray and at the same time retract the cheek to make certain the buccal mucosa is not caught under the rim of the tray.	Raising the tongue ensures that it can pass by the rim of the tray without interference. Catching the buccal mucosa under the tray rim is painful.
12. Check to be sure that the tray covers the teeth and soft tissue. Lift the front of the tray to make certain that posterior to the retromolar pad is covered and that there is enough room to allow for ¼ inch of impression material in the facial and lingual surfaces of the teeth. If necessary, adapt the tray borders with utility (beading) wax to extend into the depth of the vestibule or extend the posterior length of the tray (Figure 30–5).	The tray should fit to the depth of the vestibule and not impinge on the soft tissues.

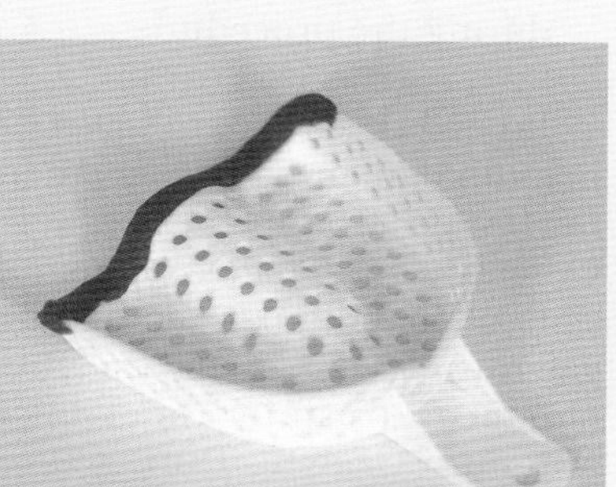

FIGURE 30–5 ✦ Extending impression tray with utility wax. *(From Bird D, Robinson D:* Torres and Ehrlich: Modern dental assisting, *ed 7, Philadelphia, 2002, WB Saunders.)*

STEPS	RATIONALE
13. Reselect larger or smaller tray as needed.	Trays must fit properly to obtain a satisfactory impression.
MAXILLARY TRAY SELECTION	
14. Repeat steps 8 and 9.	See rationales with preceding steps.
15. Center the tray by placing the handle between the central incisor in line with the center of the nose.	Ensures adequate fit for a symmetrical impression of the dental arch.
16. Bring the front of the tray about 1/4 inch anterior to the incisors.	Ensures room for impression material when fitting the tray to the anterior teeth.
17. Seat the tray first by lowering the handle toward the mandibular teeth.	Allows for viewing the access to posterior teeth and associated structures.
18. Make certain all the posterior teeth and soft tissue including the maxillary tuberosity are covered. Check that laterally there is enough room to allow for 1/4 inch space between the inside of the tray and the facial and lingual surfaces of the teeth.	Ensures proper fit to obtain adequate detail of all needed structures and that there is enough room for impression material on the facial and lingual surfaces of the teeth.
19. Retract the lip and raise the anterior portion of the tray into place. The tray should fit to the depth of the vestibule and not impinge on soft tissue.	Ensures proper and comfortable fit to obtain necessary detail of the anterior teeth and associated structures.
20. Reselect larger or smaller tray as needed.	Trays that are "tried" but not used must be sterilized prior to storage, or discarded.
TRAY PREPARATION	
21. Spray smooth trays with adhesive. Wait 15 minutes before use.	Smooth trays have no porous openings to create a mechanical lock. They require adhesive to hold the impression in the tray after gelation so that the impression material does not stay in the client's mouth. If the adhesive has not had time to dry, the impression will pull away from the tray and distort the impression.

impression generally takes two scoops of powder and two measures lines of water. A maxillary impression generally takes three scoops of powder and three measure lines of water.

SETTING TIME. The time needed to mix the impression material, load the tray, and seat it in the client's mouth is called the working time. The time required for gelation, after which the impression tray is removed from the client's mouth, is called setting time. Alginate impression material is available in *normal-set powder* (a working time of 2 minutes and a setting time of up to 4.5 minutes) and *fast-set powder* (a working time of 1.25 minutes and a setting time of 1 to 2 minutes). Currently, there are several brands of color-changing alginate available. When the alginate powder is mixed with water, it changes color from purple to pink or peach when it is time to place it into the mouth, and changes to white at gelation.

The alginate powder is mixed with room-temperature water (68° to 70° F or 20° to 21° C). The temperature of the water is measured with a thermometer prior to introducing the powder into the water. Powder is incorporated into the water to wet the powder completely, and then vigorously mixed until a smooth, creamy consistency is achieved. To allow the chemical reaction to proceed effectively, mixing time should be followed according to the manufacturer's instructions. Loading the tray and insertion should take no more than one minute. The objective is for the impression material to reach the gel state in the client's mouth. Procedure 30–2 describes the details for mixing alginate impression material. Table 30–1 presents factors that affect gelation and thus the success of the impression.

Impression Taking

Before taking the impression, the procedure should be explained to the client to enhance the client's comfort and cooperation. Specifically, clients should be informed that:

- ✦ The material will feel cold, will have or will not have a specific flavor, and will set quickly
- ✦ Breathing deeply through the nose during the procedure will help them to relax
- ✦ Refraining from talking after the tray has been placed will help make a good impression
- ✦ Raising their hand is best if they need to communicate during the procedure

Procedures 30–3 and 30–4 present details for making mandibular and maxillary dental impressions, respectively. See Mouth Areas to Precoat with Alginate and Criteria for a Quality Alginate Impression. The impression of mandibular teeth should be taken first, since gagging is less likely in the mandibular area and enhances trust in the clinician (see Guidelines to Minimize Gagging During Impression Taking for additional suggestions).

Text continues on page 615

TABLE 30–1 FACTORS THAT AFFECT GELATION

Factor	Comments
Water/alginate powder ratio	Manufacturer's directions must be followed carefully. The water/powder ratio must be exact. Too much water in the mix will make a weak impression that will tear easily during removal from the mouth due to tension. Too little water creates a grainy impression that will cause an inaccurate reproduction of the hard and soft tissues. If the container holding the alginate is not fluffed prior to measuring, too much powder will be dispensed, causing a grainy impression.
Water temperature	Water temperature affects gelation time. If the water is too warm, the product will gel at a faster rate, resulting in poor detail in the impression. If the water is cool, the product will gel at a slower rate and the final impression will be more accurate in detail. In hot, humid climates, it is recommended to use cooler water and to refrigerate the bowl and spatula.
Spatulation technique	Proper mixing (*spatulation*) will determine setting time. A mechanical device that automatically mixes the material can be used. Too much spatulation will decrease the strength of the impression material because the gel is broken as it forms. Too little spatulation decreases strength up to 50% and will cause a grainy impression that is inaccurate in details of the mouth.
Tray movement	Movement of the tray during gelation causes an inaccurate impression. It is important to hold the impression tray steady in the mouth during gelation.
Removal of impression	Premature removal of impression from the mouth also creates an inaccurate impression because the material has not fully gelled. The most frequent result of premature removal is inaccuracy of the incisor teeth. The elasticity of alginate increases with time. A better impression results from being patient. Rocking the tray back and forth to release it from the client's mouth may cause distortion of the impression.
Improper storage of impression	The impression should be poured within one hour. Leaving the impression unprotected to the environment can result in imbibition or syneresis. After disinfection, maintain the integrity of the impression, if it cannot be poured with a gypsum product, immediately by wrapping the impression in a wet towel or store it in a humidor. A *humidor* is a closed plastic container with a moist bottom layer of paper towels that create a humid environment. Before taking the maxillary impression, wrap the mandibular impression in a wet towel.

Procedure 30–2 MIXING ALGINATE

EQUIPMENT (Figure 30–6)

- Protective barriers (safety glasses, mask, gloves, hair covering/bonnet)
- Alginate powder
- Water
- Measuring scoop
- Vial for measuring water
- Wide-blade spatula
- Rubber mixing bowl
- Timer
- Thermometer

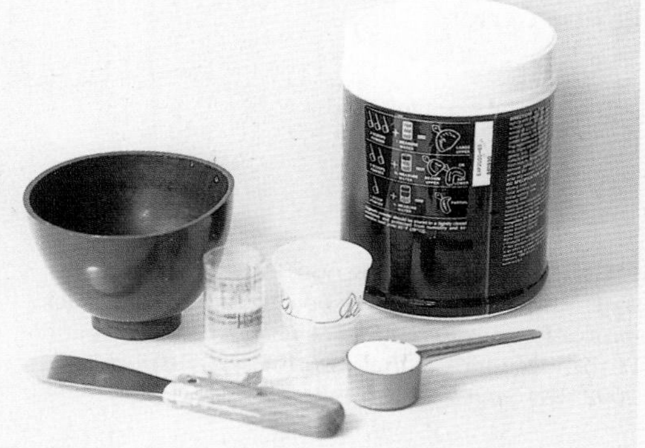

FIGURE 30–6 ✦ Equipment for mixing alginate impression material. *(From Bird D, Robinson D:* Torres and Ehrlich: Modern dental assisting, *ed 7, Philadelphia, 2002, WB Saunders.)*

STEPS	RATIONALE
1. Read the manufacturer's directions for the dispensing and manipulation of the alginate.	Following instructions will decrease the likelihood of errors in mixing and setting time.
2. Place one measure of room-temperature water into the mixing bowl for each scoop of alginate. Check temperature of water with thermometer.	Room-temperature water is important for proper setting time.
3. Shake or fluff the alginate by tipping the container two or three times.	It is essential to have correct measurements of alginate to obtain an accurate impression. Alginate tends to settle and pack down in the can. If the container holding the alginate is not fluffed prior to measuring, too much powder may be dispensed, causing a grainy impression.
4. Overfill the correct scoop with powder, tap the scoop with the side of the spatula. Scrape the excess from the scoop with the spatula.	Overfilling and tapping the scoop prior to scraping the excess from the scoop help to avoid air pockets to ensure a proper measure.
5. Sift the powder into the water, and stir with the spatula until all the powder has been moistened.	Moistening all powder facilitates adequate mixing.
6. Cup the rubber bowl in your hand with the mouth of the bowl next to the wrist. Firmly spread the alginate between the spatula and the side of the rubber bowl. Spatulate the mixture vigorously using a back and forth hand motion, spreading the material against the sides of the bowl. Use both sides of the spatula and turn the bowl with your fingers during spatulation (Figure 30–7).	This position stabilizes the bowl. Vigorous mixing and spreading of material against the sides of the bowl while turning the bowl facilitate the breakage of powder crystals.
7. Spatulate vigorously for 30 seconds and gather the material together. Use the spatula to crush the mixture and spread it out again. Repeat until a smooth, creamy consistency is achieved within the designated mixing time for either the normal-set or fast-set alginate.	Vigorous spatulation minimizes trapped air bubbles and promotes a smooth mix. A smooth mixture of alginate is important for an accurate impression.
8. Gather the material into one mass and wipe on the inside edge of the mixing bowl.	Positions the material for easy access to fill the tray.

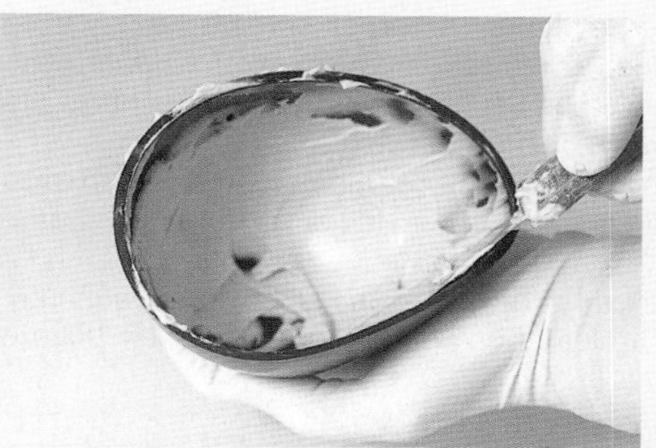

FIGURE 30–7 ✦ Proper consistency of mixed alginate impression material. *(From Bird D, Robinson D:* Torres and Ehrlich: Modern dental assisting, *ed 7, Philadelphia, 2002, WB Saunders.)*

Procedure 30–3 MAKING A MANDIBULAR PRELIMINARY IMPRESSION

EQUIPMENT (Figure 30–8)
Protective barriers (safety glasses, mask, gloves, hair covering/bonnet)
Antimicrobial rinse
OSHA-approved disinfecting solution
Alginate powder
Water
Measuring scoop
Vial for measuring water
Wide-blade spatula
Utility wax
Rubber mixing bowl
Selected mandibular impression tray
Saliva ejector

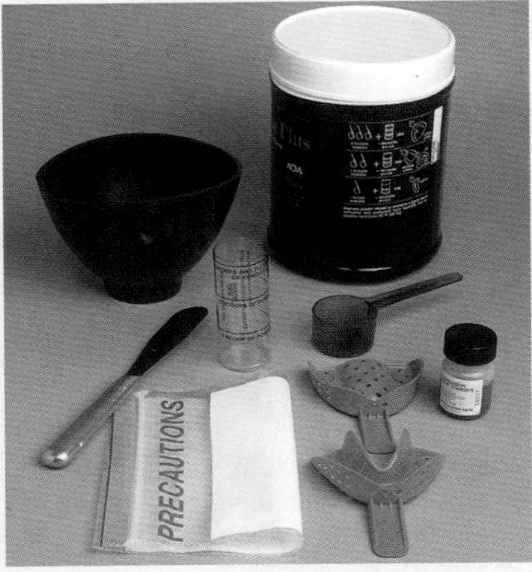

FIGURE 30–8 ✦ Scoop for alginate powder, water dispensers, mixing bowl, spatula, and stock impression tray. *(From Bird D, Robinson D:* Torres and Ehrlich: Modern dental assisting, *ed 7, Philadelphia, 2002, WB Saunders.)*

STEPS	RATIONALE
PREPARATION	
1. Gather all necessary supplies. Seat the client upright and explain the procedure. Have client remove any removable oral appliances.	Prevents unnecessary interruptions to obtain needed supplies. An upright position minimizes gagging. The client who is familiar with the procedure is more manageable. A removable oral appliance when left in place prevents an impression of all the anatomic details of the mouth.
2. If the client is at high risk for infectious endocarditis, check to be sure the client has taken antibiotic premedication.	Antibiotic premedication prevents the spread of oral bacteria to the heart in the high-risk client.
3. Don personal protective equipment, safety glasses, mask, and bonnet. Wash hands and don gloves.	Infection control procedures prevent the transmission of disease.
4. Place protective eyewear on the client.	Protective eyewear prevents injury to the client.
5. Provide preprocedural antimicrobial mouthrinse.	An antimicrobial mouthrinse decreases surface microorganisms and saliva. This aids in achieving an accurate impression, provides a satisfying feeling for the client, and serves as a distraction.
6. Lubricate the client's lips with a small amount of moisturizer.	Lubrication prevents the lips from cracking during impression making.
7. Dry the teeth with compressed air.	Drying the teeth removes saliva from the teeth, which can cause irregularities in the study cast.
8. Measure two measures of room-temperature water with two scoops of alginate and mix the alginate.	Initiates the chemical reaction.
LOADING THE TRAY	
9. Quickly gather half the alginate in the bowl onto the spatula. Wipe the alginate into one side of the tray from the lingual side, working from the posterior toward the facial. Fill to an area just below the rim. Quickly press the material down to the base of the tray.	Mandibular impression trays are loaded one half at a time to ensure complete filling of the impression tray. Pressing the material down to the base of the tray removes any air bubbles trapped in the tray.
10. Gather the remaining half of the alginate in the bowl onto the spatula and load the other side of the tray in the same way.	Loading one half of the tray at a time ensures proper fill of tray.
11. Moisten fingers with cold water and smooth over alginate. Make a slight indentation where teeth will insert (Figure 30–9).	Wiping the impression with wet fingers prior to insertion in the mouth smoothes the alginate and minimizes voids in the impression. Making slight indentations for teeth guides insertion of the tray.

Procedure 30–3 MAKING A MANDIBULAR PRELIMINARY IMPRESSION—CONT'D

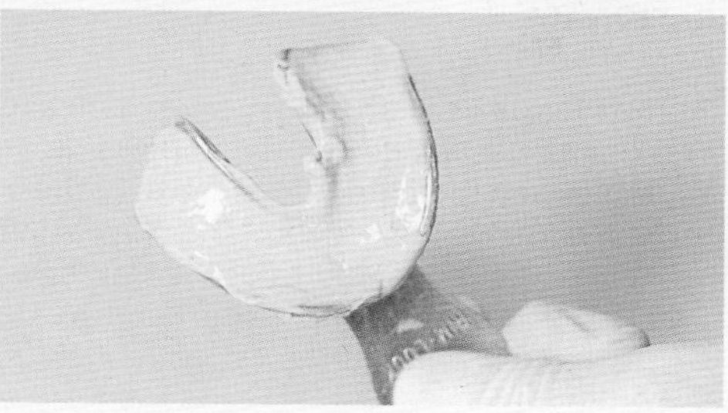

FIGURE 30–9 ✦ The mandibular impression tray is filled with alginate and is smoothed. *(From Bird D, Robinson D:* Torres and Ehrlich: Modern dental assisting, *ed 7, Philadelphia, 2002, WB Saunders.)*

STEPS	RATIONALE
LOADING THE TRAY—CONT'D	
12. Take a small amount of impression mixture from the spatula and quickly apply with a positive pressure to the occlusal surfaces of the teeth, undercut areas, and vestibular areas.	Pre-coating potential areas provides for accurate anatomy of the impression.
SEATING THE TRAY	
13. Place yourself at the 8 o'clock position (4 o'clock if left-handed) and ask the client to tilt the chin down.	Tilting the chin down minimizes gagging.
14. Turn the impression tray sideways.	Turning the impression tray sideways prior to insertion allows for the tray to fit through the lips comfortably.
15. Retract the client's lip and cheek with fingers of nondominant hand. Turn the tray sideways when placing it in the mouth, distending the lip and cheek on the opposite side of the mouth with the side of the tray.	Allows for insertion of tray with minimum discomfort to soft tissue.
16. Center the tray over the teeth and center the handle in line with the center of the client's chin.	Ensures symmetrical impression and adequate detail of anterior teeth, vestibule, and labial frenum.
17. Introduce the tray 1/4 inch anterior to the incisors. Press down the posterior portion of the tray first and then seat the anterior portion of the tray directly down with a slight vibratory motion from posterior to anterior. Instruct client to raise the tongue (Figure 30–10).	Seating the posterior border of the tray first forms a seal. Seating the tray in a posterior to anterior direction avoids triggering the gag reflex and moves the impression material forward, ensuring complete coverage of the oral structures with alginate. The vibratory motion helps to fill in all crevices and between the teeth. Asking the client to extend the tongue helps the clinician to be sure the mandibular tray is seated to the floor of the mouth and allows the alginate to make an impression of the lingual aspects of the alveolar process.

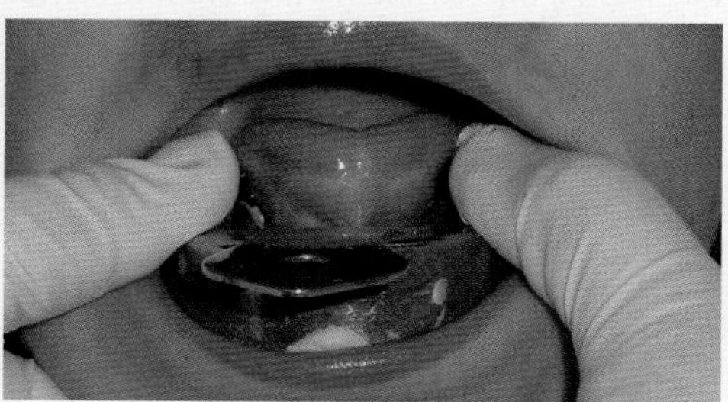

FIGURE 30–10 ✦ The mandibular impression tray is seated in the arch with the tongue out of the way. *(Courtesy Gwen Essex-Lancaster, RDH.)*

STEPS	RATIONALE
18. Instruct client to move the lips and to breathe normally.	Moving the lips ensures that the impression material flows into the depth of the vestibule. Breathing normally enhances client comfort and management.
19. Hold the tray steady in place until the material has gelled. Apply firm bilateral pressure with the middle fingers and use the thumbs to support the jaw (Figure 30–11).	Holding the tray steady prevents a double impression. Facilitates clear impression of structures.

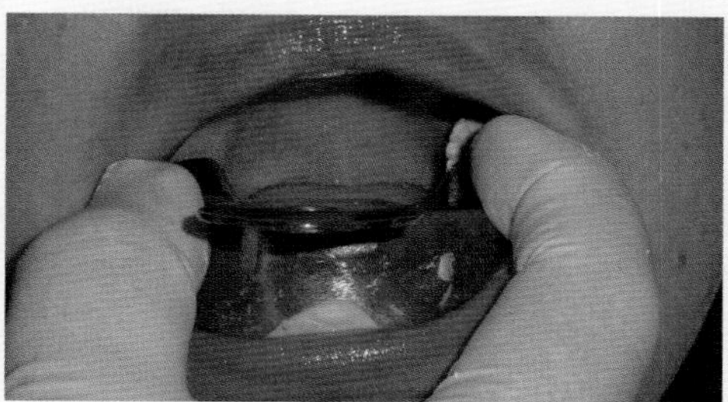

FIGURE 30–11 ✦ Holding the mandibular tray. *(Courtesy Gwen Essex-Lancaster, RDH.)*

Continued on following page

Procedure 30-3 MAKING A MANDIBULAR PRELIMINARY IMPRESSION—CONT'D

STEPS	RATIONALE
REMOVING THE IMPRESSION	
20. Place fingers of nondominant hand on top of the tray.	Protects maxillary teeth from damage during removal of the tray.
21. Move index finger of other hand inside the client's cheeks and lips to break the seal between the impression and the peripheral tissues. Then gently place that index finger under the posterior facial portion of the tray to break the seal between the impression and the teeth. Place the index finger of the nondominant hand on the incisal surface of the maxillary anterior teeth. Grasp the handle of the tray with the thumb and index finger of the dominant hand and use a firm lifting motion to break the seal.	Breaking the seal between the impression and the peripheral tissues and teeth prior to removal of the impression avoids injury to the impression. The finger/thumb grasp of the handle allows for control of the tray, and placement of the index finger of the opposite hand as described protects the anterior teeth in the opposite arch from being injured by the tray.
22. Remove the tray from the teeth with a straight snapping motion, turn it sideways, and remove it from the client's mouth.	The straight snapping motion promotes obtaining an intact impression, and turning it sideways facilitates tray removal from mouth.
23. Evaluate the impression for accuracy (Figure 30–12).	Determines need for re-making of the impression.

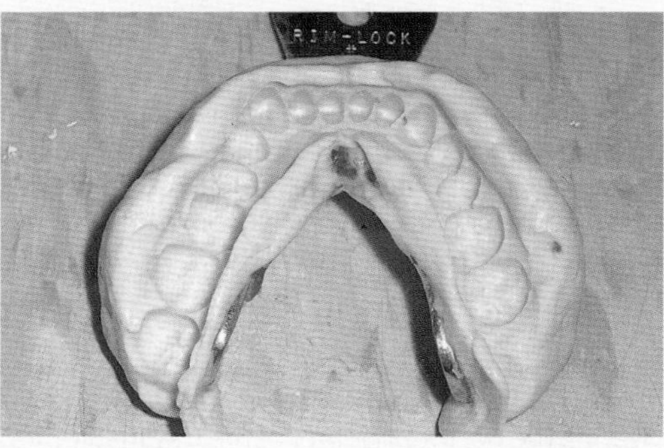

FIGURE 30–12 ✦ How a mandibular impression must look. *(Courtesy Gwen Essex-Lancaster, RDH.)*

STEPS	RATIONALE
POSTIMPRESSION CARE	
24. Have the client rinse with water.	Removes any excess alginate material from mouth; promotes client comfort.
25. Gently rinse the impression under cold water (Figure 30–13).	Rinsing the impression removes blood, saliva, and food debris that would interfere with the setting of the gypsum product.

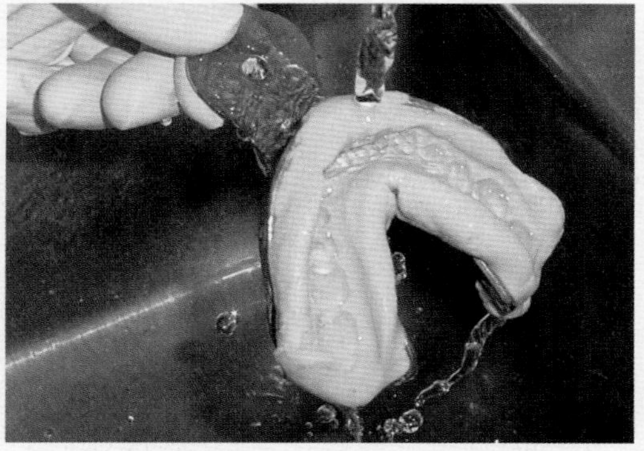

FIGURE 30–13 ✦ Rinsing the impression. *(From Bird D, Robinson D:* Torres and Ehrlich: Modern dental assisting, *ed 7, Philadelphia, 2002, WB Saunders.)*

STEPS	RATIONALE
26. Spray the impression with an approved disinfectant (e.g., 1:213 iodophor or 1:10 sodium hypochlorite) within 10 to 15 minutes. Follow the manufacturer's recommended procedure (Figure 30–14).	Use of approved disinfectants prevents disease transmission with no distortion of the impression. The procedure determined by the manufacturer must be followed to prevent distortion of the impression.
27. Wrap the impression in a slightly moistened paper towel and place in a biohazard bag before pouring it up (Figure 30–15) or in a humidor; label with client's name.	Prevents syneresis or imbibition.
28. Remove any remaining alginate from client's mouth with floss, scaler, or explorer.	Removes alginate from in between the teeth to prevent gingival inflammation.
29. Remove any alginate from client's face and lips.	Shows respect for client.

Procedure 30–3 MAKING A MANDIBULAR PRELIMINARY IMPRESSION—CONT'D

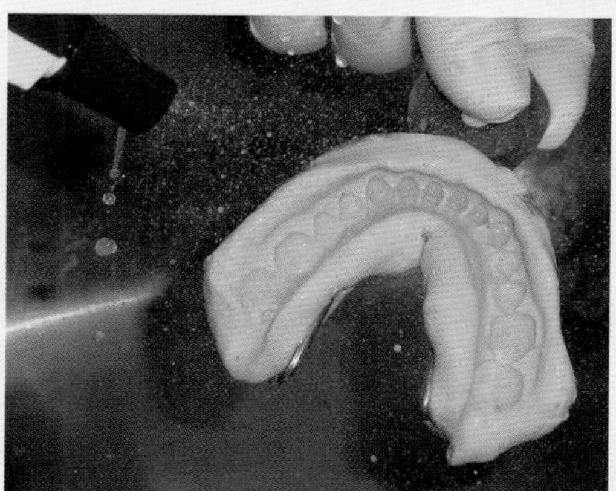

FIGURE 30–14 ✦ Spraying the impression. *(Courtesy Gwen Essex-Lancaster, RDH.)*

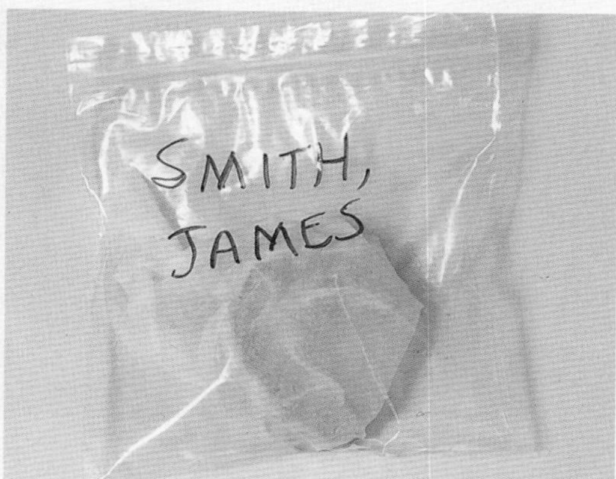

FIGURE 30–15 ✦ Impression in precaution bag with client name. *(From Bird D, Robinson D:* Torres and Ehrlich: Modern dental assisting, *ed 7, Philadelphia, 2002, WB Saunders.)*

STEPS	RATIONALE
POSTIMPRESSION CARE—CONT'D	
30. Return removable oral appliance to client.	Prevents client from leaving without it.
31. Document in ink the completion of this service in the client's record under "Services Rendered" and date the entry. For example, "9-1-02 Alginate impression for diagnostic casts."	Ensures the integrity of the client's record for both the client's health and the legal protection of the practitioner.

Procedure 30–4 MAKING A MAXILLARY PRELIMINARY IMPRESSION

EQUIPMENT

Protective barriers (safety glasses, mask, gloves, hair covering/bonnet)
Antimicrobial rinse
OSHA-approved disinfecting solution
Alginate powder
Water
Measuring scoop
Vial for measuring water
Wide-blade spatula
Bite registration wax (baseplate utility wax or wax wafer)
Rubber mixing bowl
Maxillary and mandibular impression trays
Saliva ejector

STEPS	RATIONALE
PREPARATION	
1. Gather all necessary supplies. Seat and prepare the client.	See Procedure 30–3, steps 1 through 7.
2. Measure three units of room-temperature water with three scoops of alginate and mix the alginate.	Initiates the chemical reaction.
LOADING THE TRAY	
3. Load the maxillary tray in one large increment. Load from the posterior end of tray. Use a wiping motion to bring the material forward with the spatula, being careful to place the bulk of the material in the anterior palatal area of the tray. Fill to an area just below the edge of the wax rim.	Maxillary impression trays are loaded from the posterior to prevent the formation of air bubbles in the material. Placing the bulk of the material in the anterior area of the tray prevents the alginate from overflowing into the throat when the tray is seated.
4. Be careful not to overfill the posterior portion of the tray that rests against the palate.	Overfilling the posterior portion of the tray will trigger the gag reflex.
5. Moisten fingers with water and smooth surface of the alginate (Figure 30–16).	Smoothing the surface with moistened fingers minimizes voids in the impression.

Continued on following page

Procedure 30–4 MAKING A MAXILLARY PRELIMINARY IMPRESSION—CONT'D

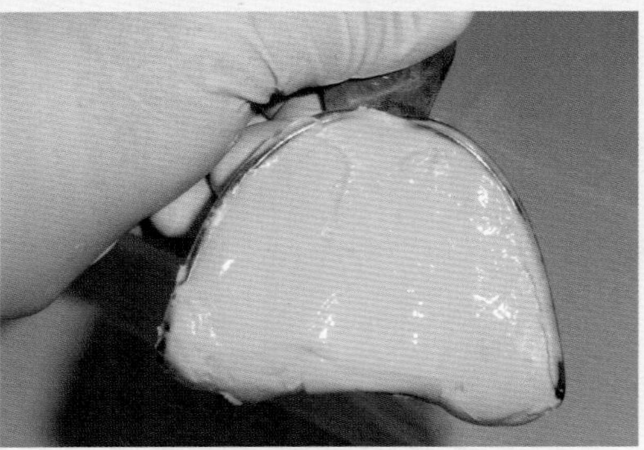

FIGURE 30–16 ✦ The maxillary impression tray is filled with alginate. The filled tray is smoothed on the alginate surface. *(Courtesy Gwen Essex-Lancaster, RDH.)*

STEPS	RATIONALE
SEATING THE TRAY	
6. Position yourself at the 11 o'clock position (1 o'clock if left-handed) and instruct the client to tilt head forward and chin down.	Tilting the head forward and the chin down minimizes gagging.
7. Retract the client's lips and cheek with fingers of non-dominant hand. With the dominant hand, turn the impression sideways and at the same time distend the lip and cheek on the opposite side of the mouth with the side of the tray.	Turning the impression tray sideways prior to insertion allows for the tray to be placed in the mouth with minimum impingement of soft tissue.
8. Center the tray over the client's teeth and center the handle at the midline in line with the center of the client's nose.	Centering the handle promotes a symmetrical impression.
9. Seat the back of the tray up against the posterior border of the hard palate to form a seal. Place the tray 1/4 inch or 6 mm anterior to incisors and seat posterior to anterior direction with a slight vibratory motion.	Seating the tray in a posterior to anterior direction avoids triggering the gag reflex, prevents the excess material from going toward the back of the mouth, and moves the impression material forward, ensuring complete coverage of the oral structures with alginate. The vibratory motion forces the material into crevices and proximal areas.
10. Gently move the client's lips out of the way as the tray is seated and instruct the client to move the lips (Figure 30–17).	Retracting the lips allows the impression material to flow into the vestibule. Moving the lips ensures that the impression material flows into the depth of the vestibule.
11. Place middle fingers over the premolar areas and hold the lip out with the index finger and the thumb.	This stabilization protects opposing teeth and promotes clear impression of structures.

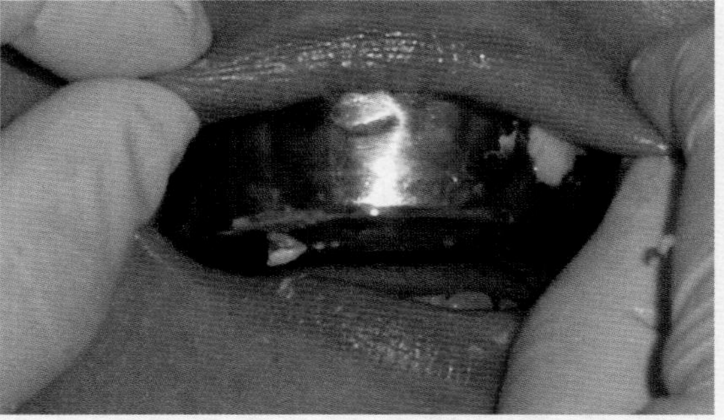

FIGURE 30–17 ✦ A maxillary alginate impression is placed in the arch. The maxillary lip is lifted and positioned outside of the tray. *(Courtesy Gwen Essex-Lancaster, RDH.)*

STEPS	RATIONALE
12. Instruct the client to breathe slowly through the nose and form an "O" with his or her lips.	Having the client form an "O" with the lips molds the impression material around the tray.
13. Hold the tray in place until the material has gelled.	Holding the tray steady prevents a double impression.
REMOVING THE IMPRESSION	
14. Place an index finger under the posterior facial portion of the tray to break the seal between the impression and the teeth.	Breaking the seal prior to removal of the impression avoids injury to the impression and the teeth.

Procedure 30–4 MAKING A MAXILLARY PRELIMINARY IMPRESSION—CONT'D

STEPS	RATIONALE
REMOVING THE IMPRESSION—CONT'D	
15. Grasp the handle of the tray with the thumb and index finger, and place the index finger of the other hand on the incisal surface of the mandibular anterior teeth.	This finger/thumb grasp allows for control of the tray. Placement of the index finger of the opposite hand as described protects the anterior teeth in the opposite arch from being injured by the tray during the tray removal process.
16. Remove the tray from the teeth with a straight snapping motion, turn it sideways, and remove it from the client's mouth.	The straight snapping motion promotes obtaining an intact impression, and turning it sideways facilitates tray removal from mouth.
17. Evaluate the impression for accuracy (Figure 30–18).	Determines need for retaking the impression.

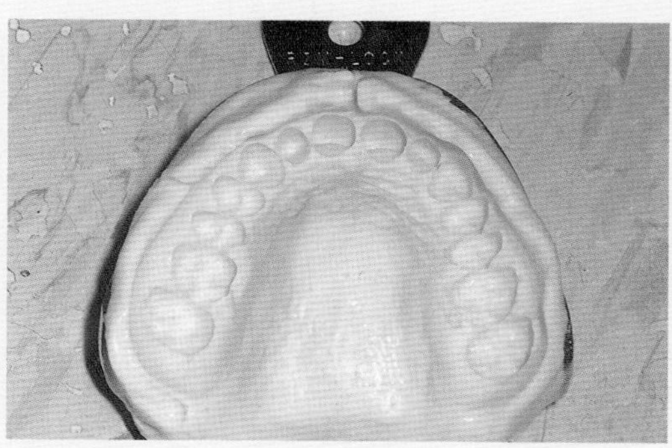

FIGURE 30–18 ✦ How a maxillary impression must look. *(From Bird D, Robinson D:* Torres and Ehrlich: Modern dental assisting, *ed 7, Philadelphia, 2002, WB Saunders.)*

STEPS	RATIONALE
POSTIMPRESSION CARE	
18. See Procedure 30–3, steps 24 through 31.	See Procedure 30–3, steps 24 through 31.

*If the same bowl and spatula are used that were used for the mandibular impression, they must be thoroughly cleaned and dried to prevent contamination of the maxillary mix (Figure 30–8).

Mouth Areas to Precoat with Alginate

Occlusal surfaces
Tooth surfaces adjacent to edentulous areas
Areas of erosion or abrasion
Vestibular areas

Criteria for a Quality Alginate Impression

No visible voids, tears, or debris
Clear and distinct detail of desired structures
Retromolar area or maxillary tuberosity present
Alginate material firmly attached to tray
Adequate peripheral roll

Guidelines to Minimize Gagging During Impression Taking

Seat maxillary tray from posterior to anterior to direct flow of impression material anteriorly away from soft palate
Avoid overfilling the tray with impression material. Fill to the level just below wax beading of tray rim
Seat client upright. During insertion of tray, instruct client to bend head forward with chin tilting down
Avoid using too large a tray
Use a calm, confident, yet gentle approach; work efficiently
Instruct clients to breathe slowly and deeply through the nose, to point toes, and/or to hold skin between index finger and thumb

Wax-Bite Registration

When an impression is made of both dental arches, the dentist and laboratory technician also need an accurate registration of the normal centric occlusion. *Centric occlusion* is the maximal stable contact between the occluding surfaces of the maxillary and mandibular teeth when the jaws are closed. This relationship is recorded as the *wax-bite registration.* The wax-bite registration is made at the time of the impression taking (see Procedure 30–5). It is used to articulate the models or diagnostic casts after the client has left the office. Articulated models can then be trimmed to ensure accurate articulation.

Baseplate wax and wax wafers are used to record the client's bite registration. Baseplate wax and wax

Procedure 30–5 MAKING A WAX-BITE REGISTRATION

EQUIPMENT (Figure 30–19)

Protective barriers (safety glasses, mask, gloves, hair covering/bonnet)
Antimicrobial rinse
Bite registration wax (baseplate wax or wax wafer)
Wide-blade laboratory knife
Heat source (warm water, Bunsen burner, or torch)
OSHA-approved disinfecting solution

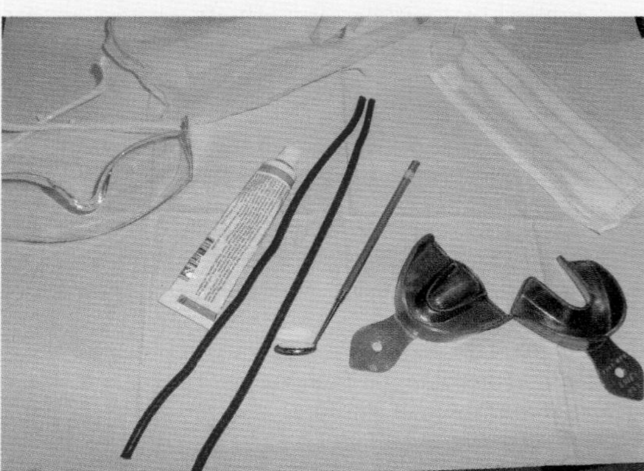

FIGURE 30–19 ✦ Supplies for taking a wax-bite registration. *(Courtesy Gwen Essex-Lancaster, RDH.)*

STEPS	RATIONALE
PREPARATION	
1. Gather all necessary supplies. Seat the client upright. Explain the procedure.	See Procedure 30–3, steps 1 through 7.
2. Reassure the client that the wax will be warm, not hot.	Reduces potential for client anxiety.
3. Measure the length of the wax needed by placing the wax over the biting surfaces of the teeth. If the wax extends past the last tooth, use the laboratory knife to shorten its length after removing the wax from the client's mouth.	This measurement ensures an accurate bite registration and client comfort.
4. Soften the bite registration wax in hot water or using another heat source (e.g., Bunsen burner or torch).	The softened wax allows the wax to make the bite registration.
SEATING	
5. Place the softened warm wax over the maxillary occlusal surfaces and instruct the client to bite together on posterior teeth, gently and naturally into the wax (Figure 30–20).	Ensures that the correct position will be recorded in the wax.

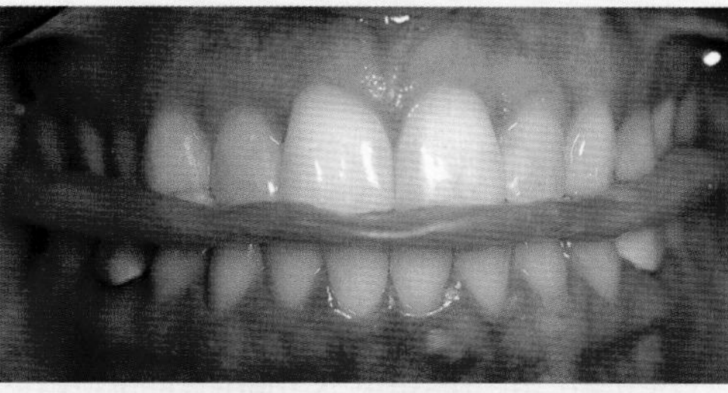

FIGURE 30–20 ✦ Wax-bite registration in client's mouth. *(From Bird D, Robinson D:* Torres and Ehrlich: Modern dental assisting, ed 7, Phila*delphia, 2002, WB Saunders.)*

STEPS	RATIONALE
6. Allow the wax bite to cool in the mouth. If necessary, air from the air/water syringe can cool the wax.	Cooled wax can be removed without distortion of the wax.

wafers are pliable waxes at room temperature. Baseplate wax is supplied in 1- to 2-mm-thick red or pink sheets, and wax bite wafers are horseshoe shaped. The most common technique used for obtaining a bite registration is to have clients close their teeth into softened wax.

DIAGNOSTIC CASTS

A *diagnostic cast* is an accurate three-dimensional model of the teeth and surrounding tissues of the client's maxillary and mandibular arches created from a dental impression. Gypsum products are used to make diagnostic casts.

Procedure 30–5 MAKING A WAX-BITE REGISTRATION—CONT'D

STEPS	RATIONALE
REMOVAL	
7. Remove the wax carefully when it has cooled.	Removing the bite wax carefully prevents distortion.
POST–WAX BITE CARE	
8. Inspect the wax to be sure it represents the client's bite (Figure 30–21). Chill in cold water until firm.	Chilling in cold water sets the registration.

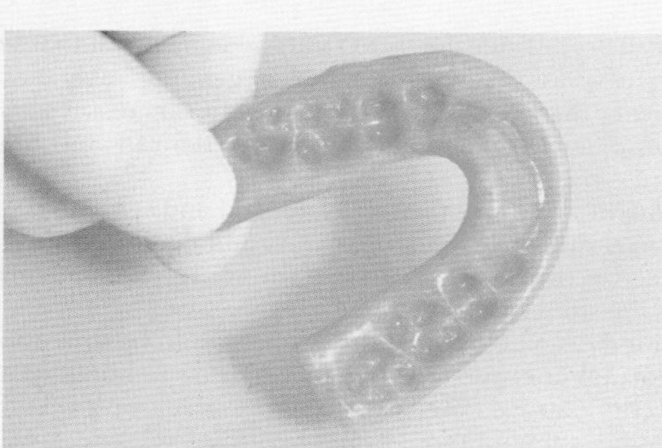

FIGURE 30–21 ✦ Wax-bite registration. *(From Bird D, Robinson D:* Torres and Ehrlich: Modern dental assisting, *ed 7, Philadelphia, 2002, WB Saunders.)*

STEPS	RATIONALE
9. Write the client's name on a piece of paper and keep it with the wax-bite registration.	This process will identify whose bite the wax-bite registration represents.
10. Store the wax-bite registration with the impressions or casts until it is needed for the trimming of the casts.	This storage will ensure that the wax-bite registration is available to articulate the client's models after the client has left the office.

Gypsum Products

Gypsum is a powdered hemihydrate, which means there is one-half part water to one part of calcium sulfate. When mixed with water, the hemihydrate crystals grow to form clusters of crystals that grow during the setting process. The more intermeshing of the crystals, the stronger and harder the final product. There are three types of gypsum products used in pouring up casts: model plaster, dental stone, and high-strength stone. These materials consist of hemihydrate crystals that vary in terms of size, shape, and porosity. These differences determine the characteristics of the product.

Plaster, a beta calcium sulfate hemihydrate (plaster of Paris), has very porous crystals that vary in shape. Because of its porosity, it requires the most water when mixing, compared to the other types of gypsum products. It is used for pouring preliminary impressions to construct models when strength is not critical but a detailed reproduction of the mouth is required (e.g., orthodontic models).

Dental stone, an alpha calcium sulfate hemihydrate, is stronger than plaster. Its crystals are uniform in shape and less porous than plaster. Dental stone is used when a stronger working diagnostic cast is needed to make dentures, orthodontic retainers, custom trays, nightguards, or a cast restoration. High-strength stone has very dense crystals and requires the least amount of water for mixing. High-strength stone has a hardness that makes it ideal to create casts used in the production of crowns, bridges, and indirect restoration. Both plaster and stone are mixed by hand with a spatula, or mechanically with a vacuum mixer, which eliminates trapping air into the mix.

Water/Powder Ratio

Each gypsum product has an optimal water-to-powder ratio specified by the manufacturer. The water/powder ratio effects the setting time and strength of the product. For one preliminary impression and its base, the commonly used water/powder ratio for plaster is 50 ml of water to 100 g of powder; for dental stone, it is 30 ml water to 100 g of powder; and for high-strength stone it is 24 ml of water to 1000 g of powder.

Setting Time

Time is another critical factor in the setting reaction of plaster and stone. There is working time immediately after mixing when the mixture will flow into the alginate impression. Initial setting time occurs when a semi-hard mass forms and is the point at which the mixture can no longer be poured into the impressions. For plaster, the initial setting time is 12 to 14 minutes; final setting time is 45 to 60 minutes. For stone, the initial setting time is 8–10 minutes; final setting time is 45 to 60 minutes. Final setting time occurs after the exothermic reaction (a chemical change accompanied by the liberation of heat) and the final product can no longer be manipulated without fracture. After final setting time (45 to 60 minutes), the preliminary alginate impression can be removed from the model or cast. Table 30–2 presents factors that affect setting time of plaster and stone.

TABLE 30–2 FACTORS THAT AFFECT SETTING TIME AND QUALITY OF CAST

Factor	Comment
Setting Time	
Type of gypsum	Dental stone sets more slowly than dental plaster
Water/powder ratio	The less water used, the faster the set. Follow manufacturer's proportions exactly. Too much water increases setting time and decreases strength. The resultant cast is smooth in appearance. Too little water decreases setting time and decreases strength. The resultant cast is grainy in appearance.
Water temperature	The warmer the water, the faster the set. Water that is too warm creates a cast that sets too fast, and water that is too cool, creates a cast that sets too slowly. In general, water should be at room temperature and no warmer than 70° F (21.1° C). Cool water increases setting time and warm water decreases setting time. On a humid day, the powder can absorb water, causing a slower set.
Mixing time	The longer and faster the spatulation, the faster the set. Prolonged and very rapid mixing shortens the setting time by increasing the chemical reaction and decreases the strength of the study model due to breakage of the crystals that are forming. Too little mixing also decreases strength and makes the study model grainy.
Improper storage of gypsum	Stone and scoop dispenser need to be kept clean and dry. Stone should be stored in a tight container that is closed immediately after use to eliminate exposure to humidity and problems with moisture (Procedure 30–2). Purchase gypsum products only when needed, because of possible contamination with moisture.
Quality of Cast	
Factors that affect setting time	See above.
Removal of the impression	Premature or improper removal of the alginate impression from the cast will break teeth or crack the cast.
Movement of tray or cast	Movement of the alginate impression or cast during the setting process will create a thin, flat base

Pouring the Cast

The cast consists of the anatomic portion and the art portion. The *anatomic portion* includes the teeth, oral mucosa, and muscle attachments. The *art portion* forms the base (Figure 30–22). The procedure for pouring the cast from a preliminary impression consists of two components: filling the impression with the mixed gypsum material to form the anatomic portion of the cast, and forming its base by mounding mixed gypsum on a smooth, nonabsorbent surface. These two parts are then connected by inverting the poured impression and seating it on the base. Procedure 30–6 provides details for pouring the cast from a preliminary alginate impression using dental plaster.

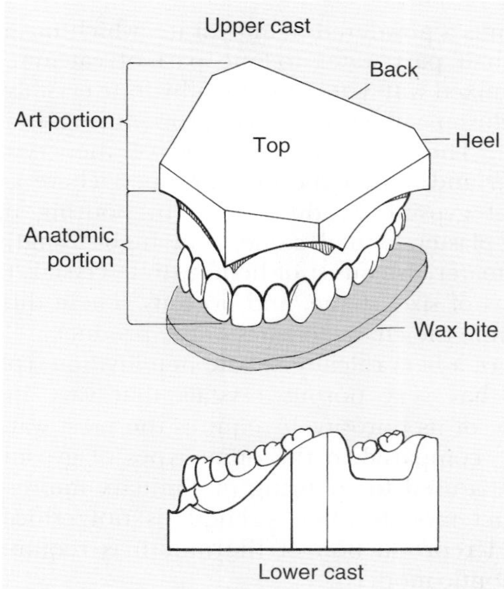

FIGURE 30–22 ✦ Anatomic and art portion of the diagnostic cast. *(From Bird D, Robinson D:* Torres and Ehrlich: Modern dental assisting, *ed 7, Philadelphia, 2002, WB Saunders.)*

Trimming and Finishing Casts

After the casts have set and the impression trays have been separated from them, the casts are trimmed to a geometric standard by using a model trimmer. The purpose of trimming is to produce attractive diagnostic casts for case presentation or for use as part of the client's permanent record. A model trimmer is a laboratory machine that has a circular abrasive wheel that is set to 90 degrees to the cast (Figure 30–32). The wax-bite registration is used to ensure that the teeth of the casts are in proper occlusion during the trimming process. The desired outcome of trimming is to make the bases parallel to themselves and the occlusal plane, and to make the base one-third and the anatomic portion two-thirds of the cast height (Figure 30–22). See Criteria for Evaluation of Study Models and Diagnostic Casts. The reader is advised to refer to a standard dental materials textbook for specific information on the trimming procedure and care of the trimming equipment.

Text continues on page 623

Procedure 30–6 POURING THE CAST AND THE BASE

EQUIPMENT (Figure 30–23)
Rubber bowl
#7 wax spatula
Scale
Room-temperature water
Dental plaster
2 Plexiglas squares
Laboratory spatula
Disinfected alginate impressions
Water measuring device
Plaster knife
Vibrator covered with plastic
OSHA-approved disinfectant

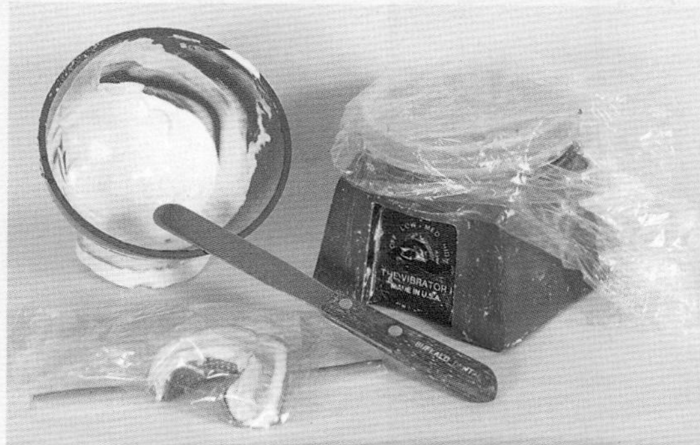

FIGURE 30–23 ✦ Supplies needed for pouring dental casts. *(From Bird D, Robinson D:* Torres and Ehrlich: Modern dental assisting, *ed 7, Philadelphia, 2002, WB Saunders.)*

STEPS	RATIONALE
PREPARATION	
1. Don personal protective equipment, safety glasses, and mask.	Safety procedures prevent injury and disease transmission to the clinician.
2. Rinse the OSHA disinfectant from the alginate impression with cool, running water. Shake the excess water in the sink and apply a gentle blast of compressed air.	A rinsed impression reduces the surface tension of the alginate and allows the gypsum product to flow. Overdrying could distort the impression.
3. Use the lab knife to remove any excess impression material that will interfere with the pouring of the model. For the mandibular arch, be sure to remove the excess material from the tongue area.	Excess impression material interferes with the pouring of the model. Removing the excess gypsum from the tongue area prevents having to scrape the area with a lab knife after hardening.
POURING THE MANDIBULAR IMPRESSION	
4. Measure 50 ml of room-temperature water and place it into a clean mixing bowl.	This is the recommended amount of mixing water for dental plaster. Clean equipment prevents a contaminated mix of gypsum.
5. Place a paper towel on a scale and make necessary adjustments. Obtain a measure of 100 g of dental plaster.	This is the recommended amount of dental plaster for mixing with 50 ml of water.
6. Add the powder into the water in steady increments and allow the powder to settle for 30 seconds.	Prevents the trapping of air bubbles.
7. Use the spatula to incorporate the powder slowly into the water. Use a wiping motion against the sides of the bowl. Spatulate 20 seconds to achieve a smooth, creamy mix (Figure 30–24).	Ensures a smooth mix of gypsum that is free of air bubbles and avoids spilling the powder.

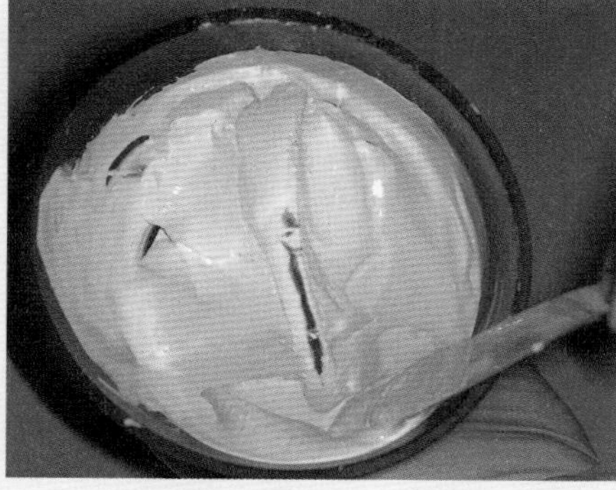

FIGURE 30–24 ✦ Smooth, creamy mix. *(From Bird D, Robinson D:* Torres and Ehrlich: Modern dental assisting, *ed 7, Philadelphia, 2002, WB Saunders.)*

STEPS	RATIONALE
8. Set the vibrator at low speed. Place the bowl on a vibrator and vibrate the material for 10 to 15 seconds. Lightly press and rotate the bowl on the vibrator.	Eliminates air bubbles in the mixture and in the final study model or diagnostic cast.
9. Gather the gypsum as a mass in the bowl. Remove bowl from vibrator (Figure 30–25).	Facilitates access for pouring the cast.
10. Hold the impression tray by the handle and press handle against the vibrator.	Positions the impression tray to begin to pour the impression.

Continued on following page

Procedure 30–6 POURING THE CAST AND THE BASE—CONT'D

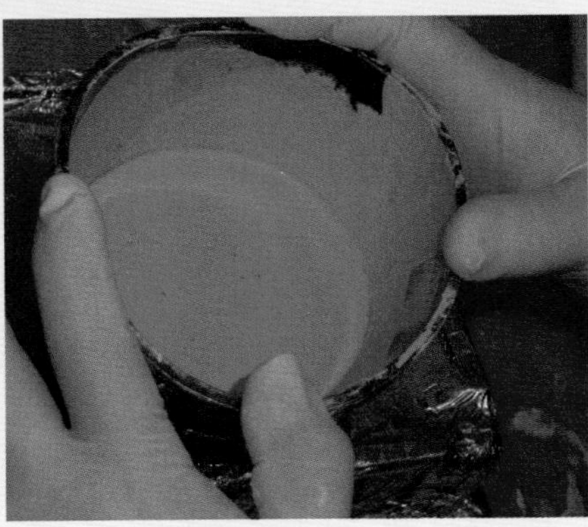

FIGURE 30–25 ✦ Mixing bowl on vibrator. *(Courtesy Gwen Essex-Lancaster, RDH.)*

STEPS	RATIONALE
POURING THE MANDIBULAR IMPRESSION—CONT'D	
11. Use the end of a wax spatula or laboratory knife to pick up about 1/2 teaspoon of mixed material. Allow mix to flow into the impression at the distal of the most posterior tooth while the impression is vibrated so that the material flows toward the anterior teeth. Turn the tray on its side to provide the continuous flow of material forward into each tooth. Tip the impression forward to make the gypsum mixture flow into the bottom of the alginate impression. Continue to add the gypsum product in small increments at the same place until the occlusal/incisal surfaces are filled. Vibrate continually (Figure 30–26).	The flowing of the material pushes out the air ahead of it and eliminates air bubbles. Adding small increments prevents trapping air in the occlusal/incisal areas of the impression, which would make the final outcome inaccurate. Filling all the occlusal/incisal areas first reduces the risk of trapped air.

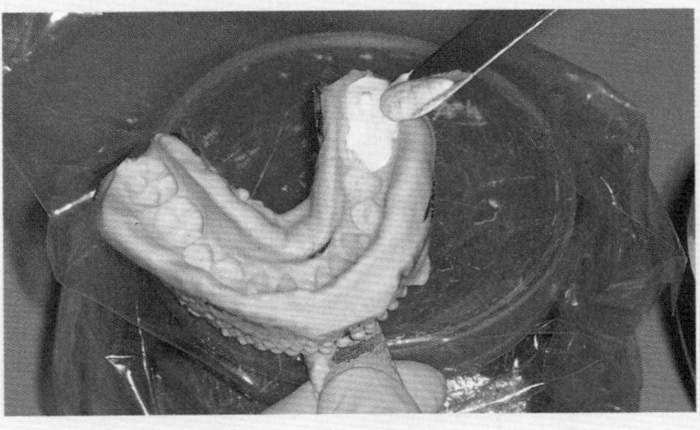

FIGURE 30–26 ✦ Initial placement of material in distal of most posterior tooth. *(From Bird D, Robinson D:* Torres and Ehrlich: Modern dental assisting, *ed 7, Philadelphia, 2002, WB Saunders.)*

12. When all tooth indentations are filled, use the laboratory spatula to add larger amounts of gypsum to fill the impression. Continue to vibrate until the entire impression is filled (Figure 30–27). Then, set the poured impression aside.	The laboratory spatula helps to adequately fill the depth of the vestibule area of the impression. Vibrating eliminates air bubbles.

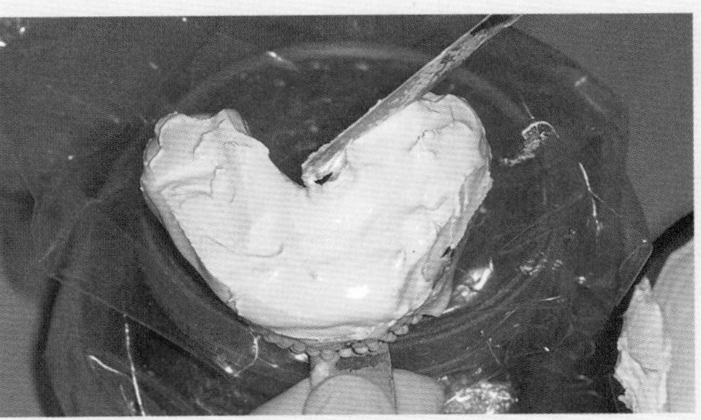

FIGURE 30–27 ✦ Impression filled with large amounts of gypsum. *(From Bird D, Robinson D:* Torres and Ehrlich: Modern dental assisting, *ed 7, Philadelphia, 2002, WB Saunders.)*

Procedure 30–6 POURING THE CAST AND THE BASE—CONT'D

STEPS	RATIONALE
POURING THE BASE FOR THE MANDIBULAR CAST	
13. Gather the remaining amount of mixed material together in the bowl.	The material flows and flattens, therefore mounding the gypsum product helps to ensure that a base 1 inch thick is constructed.
14. Place the mix in a mound on a Plexiglas square or tile. Shape the base to approximately 2 × 2 inches wide and 1 inch thick (Figure 30–28).	It is important to place the base on a smooth, nonabsorbent surface.

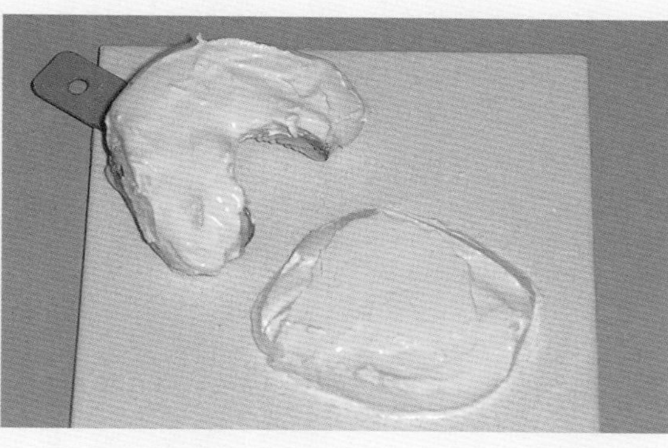

FIGURE 30–28 ✦ Filled impression tray and base on Plexiglas. *(From Bird D, Robinson D:* Torres and Ehrlich: Modern dental assisting, *ed 7, Philadelphia, 2002, WB Saunders.)*

STEPS	RATIONALE
15. Invert the firm, poured impression onto the firm base. Do not push the impression into the base.	The mix will flow out of the impression if inverted before the stone is firm.
16. Position impression tray on the base to provide a uniform thickness all around it. Position so the occlusal plane of posterior teeth is parallel with the table top, the midline (as judged by the handle of the tray) is at the center of the base.	This will provide for a symmetrical base.
17. Hold the tray steady and with the laboratory spatula or a moistened finger, smooth the sides around the base mix up onto the margins of the impression tray (Figure 30–29).	This will provide for a symmetrical base with uniform thickness.

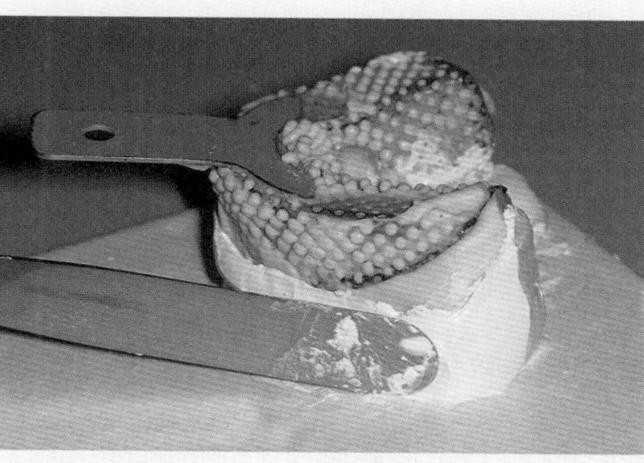

FIGURE 30–29 ✦ Smoothing the plaster base mix up into the margins of the tray. *(From Bird D, Robinson D:* Torres and Ehrlich: Modern dental assisting, *ed 7, Philadelphia, 2002, WB Saunders.)*

STEPS	RATIONALE
18. Remove excess stone/plaster above the edge of the tray rim.	A locked tray is very difficult to remove from the study model/diagnostic cast. Excess stone above the tray rim locks the tray in the model.
19. Allow the gypsum to reach the initial set before moving the Plexiglas squares.	Moving the Plexiglas before initial set will cause the base of the model/cast to flatten out, making the base too thin.
POURING THE MAXILLARY IMPRESSION AND BASE	
20. Repeat steps 2 through 19 above for the maxillary impression to create an anatomic and art portion of a dental cast. Use clean equipment for the fresh mix of plaster.	Remnants of material from the earlier mix or other debris will adversely affect setting time.

Continued on following page

Procedure 30–6 POURING THE CAST AND THE BASE—CONT'D

STEPS	RATIONALE
SEPARATING THE IMPRESSIONS FROM THE CASTS	
21. Wait 45 to 60 minutes after the base has been poured before attempting to separate the impression from the cast.	Final set occurs after the exothermic reaction has completed. The model/cast will feel cool to the touch. Separating after the final set occurs prevents damage to teeth.
22. Use a plaster knife to remove excess material from the edges of the impression tray and to gently separate the margins of the tray from the cast (Figure 30–30).	Removal of excess material frees the tray from the model.

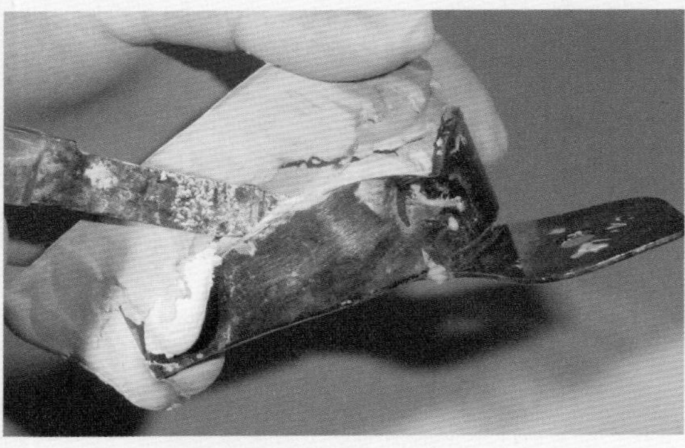

FIGURE 30–30 ✦ Plaster knife used to free tray from stone. *(Courtesy Gwen Essex-Lancaster, RDH.)*

STEPS	RATIONALE
23. If the teeth are in good alignment, remove tray and impression material together. First release the anterior portion by gently pulling downward and forward one time. Then make a firm, straight pull upward. Do not apply lateral pressure or rock the tray (Figure 30–31).	Forces created by lateral pressure and rocking of the tray may break teeth.

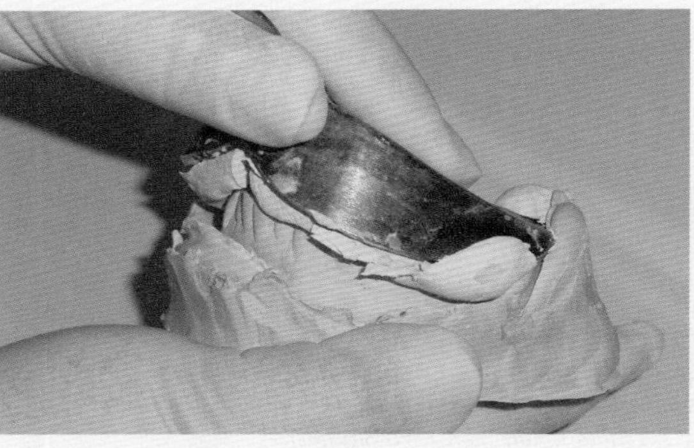

FIGURE 30–31 ✦ Removing impression from cast. *(Courtesy Gwen Essex-Lancaster, RDH.)*

STEPS	RATIONALE
24. If the tray does not separate, check to see where the tray may be locked by the stone. Use the plaster knife to free the tray from the stone.	Excess stone above the tray rim locks the tray in the model.
25. If teeth are malaligned, remove the tray first, then cut the impression material carefully along the occlusal line and gently peel off.	Prevents the accidental breakage of teeth on the cast.
POSTSEPARATION PROCEDURES	
26. Use a pencil or permanent marker to label the base (bottom) of the model/cast with the client's name. Keep the wax bite with the gypsum models/casts.	Proper labeling prevents unidentifiable models/casts.
27. Soak cast in water if it cannot be trimmed immediately.	Prevents distortion.
28. Remove gypsum material from the vibrator, spatula, and mixing bowl and clean with cool water.	It is easier to clean the equipment immediately, before the gypsum product sets up.

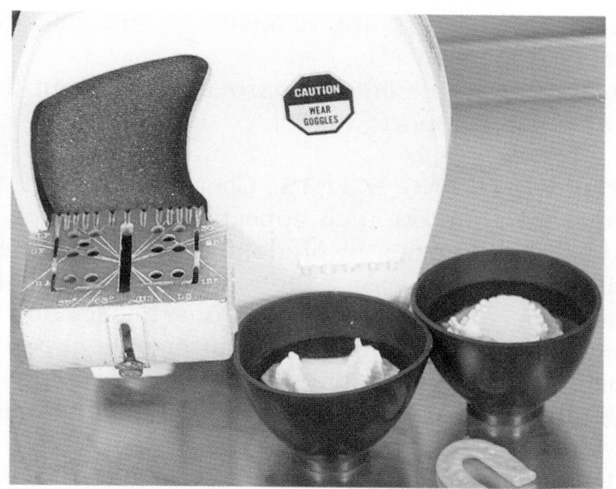

FIGURE 30–32 ✦ Model trimmer. *(From Bird D, Robinson D:* Torres and Ehrlich: Modern dental assisting, *ed 7, Philadelphia, 2002, WB Saunders.)*

Criteria for Evaluation of Study Models and Diagnostic Casts

No visible voids, air bubbles, fractures, or excess material
Surface is smooth and hard
Anatomic structures are visible and account for 2/3 of the cast
Base accounts for 1/3 of the cast; top and bottom of bases are parallel to the floor
Angles and cuts of base are accurate and symmetrical
Cast retains occlusion when placed on all sides
All oral landmarks are present

CUSTOM-MADE STENTS

Protective Mouthguards

A *mouthguard* is a protective appliance that covers the teeth and palate and fits to the depth of the vestibule. Mouthguards help meet the client's human need for protection from health risks. Wearing a mouthguard serves the following purposes:

- ✦ Protection of the teeth and oral tissues, the maxilla and mandible, the temporomandibular joint (TMJ), and the head and neck against intracranial pressure changes and bone deformation during contact sports. Blows transmitted to the TMJ during athletic competition can be absorbed and distributed throughout the mouthguard.
- ✦ Protection of the brainstem against shear stress in contact sports. A properly fitting mouthguard separates the mandible from the maxilla and thus reduces the force transmitted to the base of the brain at the TMJ.
- ✦ Prevention of tooth avulsion. Over 5 million teeth are avulsed yearly in the United States, the most frequent injuries occurring in 8- to 15-year-olds.

Types of Mouthguards

Stock Type
"One size fits all," purchased over-the-counter, inexpensive, offer the least protection

Boil and Bite
User formed, purchased over-the-counter, inexpensive, offer little protection

Custom Vacuum-Formed Single Layer
Fabricated in the dental office, custom fit, moderately expensive, provide good protection

Pressure Laminated Multiple Layer
Fabricated in the dental laboratory, custom fit, expensive, provide the best protection

- ✦ Prevention of facial bone fractures, TMJ injury, and head injuries.
- ✦ Providing an occlusal cushion against bruxism and clenching .
- ✦ Protection of the teeth during endotracheal anesthesia, bronchoscopy, tonsillectomy, and electric shock therapy.
- ✦ Containment of radon seeds in the radiation treatment of head and neck cancer.

Mouth protectors are made from natural or synthetic polymeric materials classified as thermoplastics or thermoset resins (see Types of Mouthguards).

ATHLETIC MOUTHGUARDS. The Academy of Sports Dentistry suggests a properly fitted mouthguard be worn while playing contact sports or participating in nonimpact sports. Nonimpact sports (e.g., weight lifting) require mouth protectors due to the clenching of teeth involved in these strenuous sports (see Sports Requiring that Participants Wear Mouth Protection). The Academy offers the following mouthguard guidelines:

- ✦ Adequate thickness in all areas to reduce impact forces.
- ✦ A fit that is retentive and does not dislodge on impact
- ✦ Full palatal coverage that equals the demands of the playing status of the athlete
- ✦ Construction with FDA-approved materials
- ✦ Life of mouthguard is limited to one season of play

In addition to preventing tooth avulsion, a full palatal coverage mouthguard worn during sports participation helps to prevent or moderate a variety of head injuries. *Concussion* is the alteration of consciousness and/or disturbance in vision and equilibrium caused by a direct blow to the head, rapid acceleration and/or deceleration of the head, or direct blow to the base of the skull from a vertical impact to the mandible. Symptoms of concussion include headaches, earaches, facial pain, photophobia, vertigo, and impaired speech.

Sports Requiring that Participants Wear Mouth Protection

Acrobatics	Motocross
Baseball	Racquetball
Basketball	Rugby
Boxing	Shot-put
Cycling	Skateboarding
Discus	Skiing
Equestrian sports	Skydiving
Field hockey	Soccer
Football	Squash
Gymnasticsw	Surfing
Handball	Tennis
Horseback riding	Trampoline
Ice hockey	Volleyball
In-line skating	Water polo
Lacrosse	Weight lifting
Martial arts	Wrestling

From American Academy of Sports Dentistry.

SINGLE LAYER MOUTHGUARDS. Thermoplastic polymers, physically vacuum-formed to make a single layer mouthguard, are called single layer mouthguards. They are made of one sheet of polyurethane or soft ethylene vinyl acetate (EVA) acrylic, are custom fit, allow for breathing and speech, and do not deform over time and use. They are the most commonly prescribed mouthguards in dental offices. These vacuum-formed mouthguards, custom fabricated by dental staff or laboratory technicians, are superior to the store-bought stock or boil and bite mouthguards. Strap attachments to helmets are easily adapted to the custom-made single layer mouthguard and the client can select the color and decorative pattern of the mouthguard (Procedure 30–7).

MULTIPLE LAYER MOUTHGUARDS (PRESSURE LAMINATED). Multiple layer mouthguards, made of EVA, are recommended for full-contact sports. They are pressure laminated in a dental laboratory by a technician and maintain their shape better than single layer mouthguards do. Two or three layers of EVA material are fused to achieve the necessary thickness. As a minimum, mouthguards should have a labial thickness of 3 mm, palatal thickness of 2 mm, and occlusal thickness of 3 mm. The mouthguard material should be biocompatible and last 1 to 2 years; however, mouthguard replacement is recommended after one season of play.

Several commercial laboratories fabricate pressure laminated mouthguards in the United States and Canada. Playsafe Mouthguards from Glidewell Laboratories are pressure-laminated mouthguards made from EVA material. One of the following four types of pressure-laminated mouthguards is recommended based on the client's degree of risk:

- ✦ Light (two layers approximately 2 mm thick)
- ✦ Medium (two layers approximately 5 mm thick)
- ✦ Heavy (two layers approximately 5 mm thick with power dispersion strips)
- ✦ Heavy Pro (three layers, approximately 5 mm thick, with a hard support)

TOOTH WHITENING STENTS. Clients often seek oral healthcare to improve their appearance. A focus on sexuality and self-image is predominant in the media. Because the smile speaks a thousand words, the appearance of one's teeth dominates our image-conscious society and is an important factor in meeting a person's human need for a wholesome facial image. Consequently, tooth discoloration and its removal are often the reasons individuals seek oral healthcare.

Many tooth whitening procedures require the use of a stent by the client. (See Chapter 22 for dentist dispensed/home-use and in-office tooth whiteners that carry the ADA Seal of Acceptance.) A stent is a custom-made tray constructed in the same manner as mouthguards are constructed, using EVA material. Stents are used for the target delivery of materials such as carbamide peroxide for tooth bleaching.

Not all teeth, however, will respond similarly to whitening procedures. Yellow teeth whiten the best, brown teeth less well, and gray teeth may not bleach well at all. Tetracycline stain and fluorosis may be treated with a combination of tooth whitening and restorative dentistry cosmetic procedures.

Some tooth whitening systems on the market do not require a stent for delivery. Tooth whitening strips containing carbamide peroxide are a viable option for clients with TMJ disorder who can't tolerate stents. Procedure 30–7 describes construction of a custom-made stent. See Chapter 22 for methods of in-office tooth whitening.

HOME FLUORIDE TRAYS. Stents also are used for the target delivery of topical fluoride for clients with high caries risk, such as individuals who have received radiation treatment for head and neck cancer.

NIGHTGUARDS AND DAYGUARDS. *Bruxism* is a subconscious habit of grinding, clenching, rubbing, or gritting of the teeth that usually occurs during sleep. Occlusion discrepancy between centric occlusion and centric relation is thought to be a cause of nocturnal bruxism. Stress, a major contributing factor in bruxism, may increase the frequency and intensity of bruxism. Central nervous system disorders such as Parkinson's disease and Huntington's disease can contribute to nocturnal bruxism. Many individuals experience bruxism, but the degree of bruxism determines the cause and effect sequelae. Sequelae of Bruxism lists the possible sequelae of bruxism.

Treatment of Bruxism. Treatment for bruxism is categorized as reversible and irreversible. Reversible treatment is conservative, noninvasive, and causes no permanent changes in the structure or position of the jaw or teeth.

Procedure 30–7 CONSTRUCTING A CUSTOM-MADE STENT (E.G., A SINGLE LAYER MOUTHGUARD, FLUORIDE TRAY, TOOTH WHITENING TRAY)

EQUIPMENT (Figure 30–33)

Protective attire (face mask, safety glasses, bonnet)
Petrolatum lubricant
Polyurethane (thermoplastic material)
Mouthguard 4 × 4 square
Long shank acrylic burr in a lab engine
Matches
Diagnostic casts
Crown and collar scissors
Hannau torch
Vacuum forming machine
Lab knife

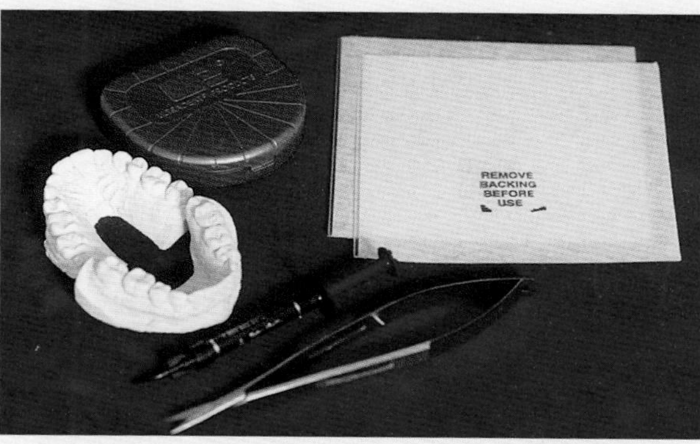

FIGURE 30–33 ✦ Supplies for constructing a custom-made stent. *(From Bird D, Robinson D:* Torres and Ehrlich: Modern dental assisting, *ed 7, Philadelphia, 2002, WB Saunders.)*

STEPS	RATIONALE
1. Don safety glasses, mask, and bonnet.	Safety glasses protect eyes from debris. The mask protects from breathing burning organic material and acrylic dust. The bonnet protects hair from fire and from getting caught in the machine.
2. Trim the diagnostic cast so that the base extends 3 to 4 mm past the gingival border and the vertical height is minimal. Spray the cast with silicone lubricant (Figure 30–34).	Casts made of stone must be used for stent manufacturing. Plaster casts are not strong enough to withstand the suction of the vacuum former. The smaller the base of the diagnostic cast, the more likely it is that the vacuum former can suck the material down around the cast. Lubricant helps in the removal of the stent.

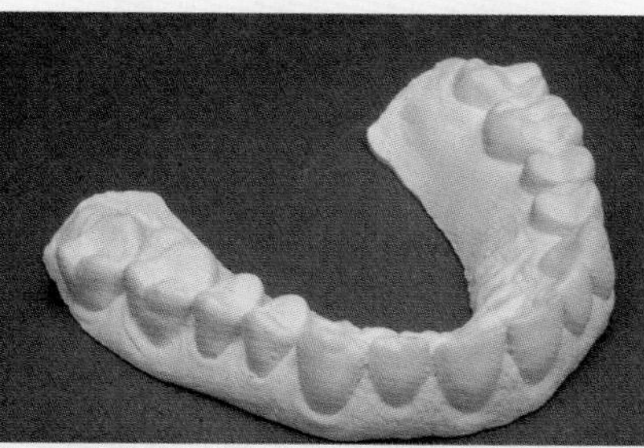

FIGURE 30–34 ✦ Trimmed diagnostic cast. *(From Bird D, Robinson D:* Torres and Ehrlich: Modern dental assisting, *ed 7, Philadelphia, 2002, WB Saunders.)*

STEPS	RATIONALE
3. Place the vacuum forming machine under a hood fan for control of organic emissions.	Constructing a stent involves the burning of organic material. OSHA safety regulations for the burning of organic compounds require that fumes be removed from the air by use of a hood fan.
4. Prepare the machine. The perforated vacuum plate and the sides of the hinged frame must be LIGHTLY sprayed with silicone lubricant.	Lubricating the vacuum former prevents the stent material from sticking when warm. Over-spraying will clog the suction holes.
5. Open the hinged frame and center the stent material onto the lower frame (Figure 30–35).	Holds the material securely in place.
6. Close the frame and secure the frame with the latch knob.	Ensures proper placement of material.
7. Grasp both handles of the locked, hinged frame and raise it until it clicks into position approximately 3 inches above the vacuum plate.	Ensures frame is locked into place.
8. Swing the heating unit to the center position and turn on the heating element switch at the base of the unit. The unit will require 3 minutes to preheat.	Ensures source of heat and proper distance of heating unit from material.
9. Center cast on the vacuum plate. Some units have extra holes at the front and back of the machine; place the cast between these holes.	Ensures proper placement of material over cast.

Continued on following page

Procedure 30–7 CONSTRUCTING A CUSTOM-MADE STENT (E.G., A SINGLE LAYER MOUTHGUARD, FLUORIDE TRAY, TOOTH WHITENING TRAY)—CONT'D

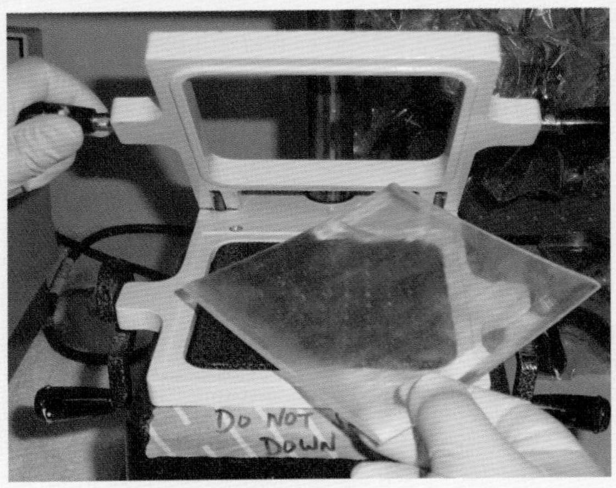

FIGURE 30–35 ✦ Opening hinge and placing mouthguard material. *(Courtesy Gwen Essex-Lancaster, RDH.)*

STEPS	RATIONALE
10. Do NOT leave the machine unattended. Watch the material as it heats for 1 to 2 minutes until it sags 1/2 inch below the hinged frame (Figure 30–36).	The material heats quickly and may be sucked into the motor if overheated.
11. Grasp both handles of the hinged frame and pull it down over the vacuum plate. The material will be draped over the cast (Figure 30–37).	Grasping with both handles allows for proper force.

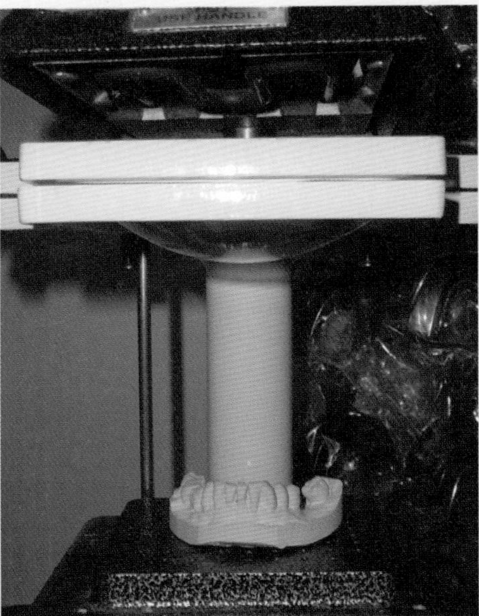

FIGURE 30–36 ✦ Sagging mouthguard material. *(Courtesy Gwen Essex-Lancaster, RDH.)*

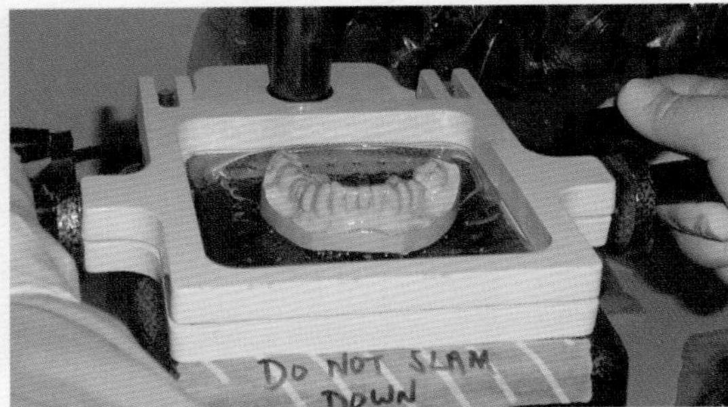

FIGURE 30–37 ✦ Hinged frame pulled over vacuum plate. *(Courtesy Gwen Essex-Lancaster, RDH.)*

STEPS	RATIONALE
12. Turn on the vacuum motor for 10 seconds.	Applying the vacuum adapts the material to the cast.
13. Swing the heating unit out of the way and turn the switch off.	There is no more need of the heating unit.
14. Turn off the vacuum switch. Release the hinged frame knob and open the frame and hold the stent by the edges to remove it from the vacuum plate.	Holding the polyurethane by the edges prevents getting fingerprints on the stent.
15. Hold the stent and cast under running, cold water for at least 30 seconds.	Cooling the stent hardens the thermoplastic material. The stent will become opaque in color.

Procedure 30–7 CONSTRUCTING A CUSTOM-MADE STENT (E.G., A SINGLE LAYER MOUTHGUARD, FLUORIDE TRAY, TOOTH WHITENING TRAY)—CONT'D

STEPS	RATIONALE
16. Cut gross excess material from the depth of the periphery of the stent to remove it from the cast (Figure 30–38).	Begins the tray trimming process. If the stent cannot be cut with the scissors, a hot instrument can melt through the material or a lab knife can be used to separate it from the cast.

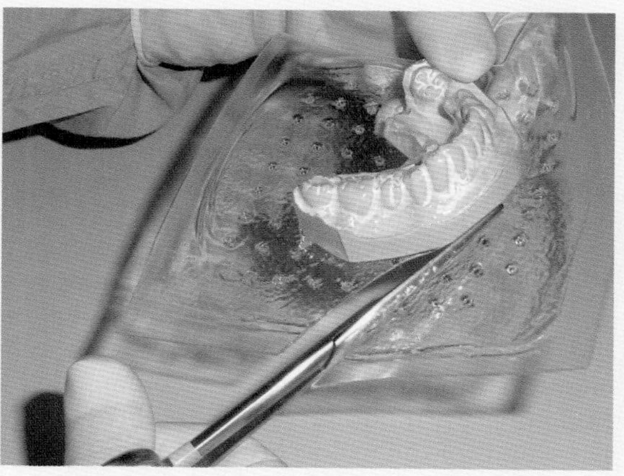

FIGURE 30–38 ✦ Cutting away gross excess material. *(From Bird D, Robinson D:* Torres and Ehrlich: Modern dental assisting, *ed 7, Philadelphia, 2002, WB Saunders.)*

STEPS	RATIONALE
17. Use small, sharp crown and collar scissors to trim the stent approximately 0.5 mm away from the gingival margin (Figure 30–39).	This trimming prevents the stent from irritating the client's soft tissues.

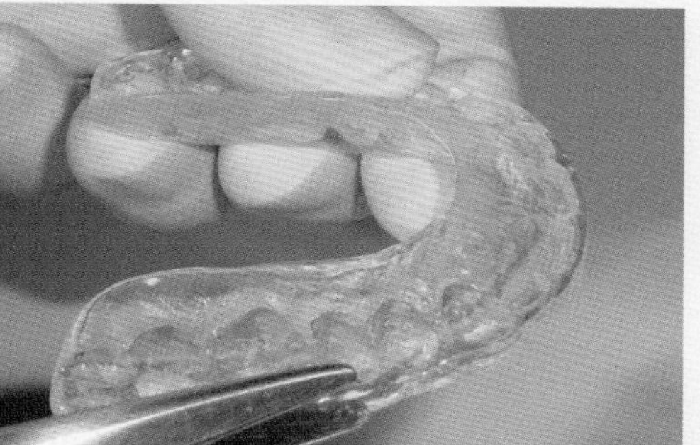

FIGURE 30–39 ✦ Trimming material away from the gingival margin. *(Courtesy Gwen Essex-Lancaster, RDH.)*

STEPS	RATIONALE
18. Place the stent back on the cast.	This replacement allows the checking of gingival extensions.
19. If necessary, place a thin coat of petroleum jelly on the facial surfaces of the stent. Use a low flame to gently readapt the margins of the stent so that they cover the entire tooth, but do not overlap the gingiva.	This readaptation of the margins of the stent to the model ensures complete coverage of client's teeth and comfort.
20. Wearing a mask, trim the stent with an acrylic burr in a lab engine (Figure 30–40).	This trimming smoothes the edges from the peripheral border. Acrylic dust created by trimming should not be inhaled.

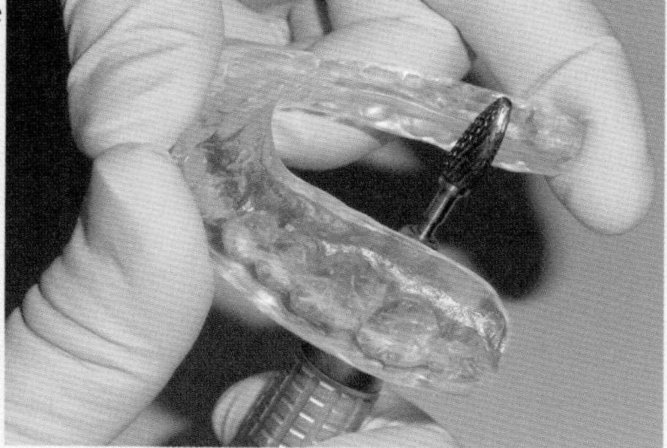

FIGURE 30–40 ✦ Trimming mouthguard with an acrylic burr. *(Courtesy Gwen Essex-Lancaster, RDH.)*

Enhances client comfort.

Sequelae of Bruxism

Abfraction lesions
Exostosis to support the teeth
Gingival recession
Headaches
Impaired hearing
Limited range of motion of mandible
Linea alba
Pain
Periodontal pockets
Tenderness of muscles of mastication
Tinnitus
TMJ disorders
TMJ noise with movement
Tooth fracture
Tooth mobility
Tooth sensitivity
Tooth wear facets (attrition)

Most therapy for bruxism starts with reversible interventions, but may progress to irreversible procedures. Irreversible treatment is invasive and causes permanent changes in the structure or position of the jaw or teeth.

Reversible Procedures. *Appliance therapy* is a generalized term that covers numerous designs of dental orthotics or splints used to relieve bruxism. Appliance therapy involves the use of nightguards or dayguards. Evidence suggests that wearing an appliance during sleep (e.g., nightguard) decreases damage to the oral structures due to bruxism.

Biofeedback uses electromyography (EMG) to record muscle activity. During treatment, the client has pairs of electrodes attached to the surface of the skin in contact with the muscles of mastication. The electrodes transmit muscle activity information to a computer monitor the client can see, to allow the client to consciously reduce the muscle tension. Sleep biofeedback therapy involves EMG-activated alarms, which sound during sleep to awaken the client to stop the bruxism. Sleep biofeedback using electrical stimulation to produce pain upon bruxing also awakens the client to stop the bruxism.

Drug therapy uses antianxiety, sedative, anti-inflammatory, and muscle relaxant drugs to control bruxism. Moreover, when the overuse of the muscles of mastication produces muscle fiber changes, Robaxin injected into muscle trigger points can provide relief. Over-the-counter medications such as ibuprofen and naproxen are recommended as nonsteroidal anti-inflammatory agents.

Exercise therapy using isokinetics and stretching of the muscles of mastication can be performed by the client. Reflex and relaxation exercises may also be useful.

Physical therapy procedures may be effective in restoring normal muscle function. Heat and cold therapy uses moist heat or ethylene chloride spray to break the muscle spasm and pain cycle. Mandibular relearning therapy helps the client to work on the opening and closing of the mouth.

Psychotherapy from an appropriate mental health professional may be indicated to reduce stress via relaxation, medication, and guided imagery. The antidepressant amitriptyline can be prescribed by the mental health professional. Other stress reduction strategies also may be recommended for the client to perform prior to sleep.

Irreversible Procedures. Equilibration therapy is used to adjust the occlusion of the teeth by recontouring occlusal enamel with dental burrs. The objective is to create a centric occlusion coincidental with centric relation.

Orthognathic surgery can be employed to improve a skeletal malocclusion. Splint therapy must first confirm the effectiveness of occlusal therapy in relieving the client's symptoms. Surgery is recommended only after preliminary orthodontics has eliminated the dental compensations of the malocclusion.

Nightguard/Dayguard Therapy. A *nightguard* or *dayguard* is a hard acrylic appliance that fits over the maxillary or mandibular teeth. If the appliance is worn during sleep it is referred to as a nigh guard. If the dentist prescribes the appliance to be worn throughout the day, it is called a dayguard. The purpose of these appliances is to:

- Reduce clenching or grinding of the teeth
- Minimize loss of tooth structure (attrition)
- Ease muscle hyperactivity
- Reduce pressure on the temporomandibular joint

There are several nightguard/dayguard designs:

- Partial coverage nightguards/dayguards are maxillary appliances that cover the palate and the lingual surfaces of the maxillary anterior teeth. The disadvantage of this appliance is that it covers only some of the teeth and the occlusal force may overstress those teeth covered by the acrylic. Subsequently, teeth that are not covered by the nightguard/dayguard may hypererupt or drift.
- Full occlusal coverage nightguards/dayguards, the appliances of choice, are acrylic appliances that cover the occlusal surfaces. A nightguard/dayguard that fully covers either the maxillary or mandibular teeth is the safest design because the dentist can adjust the occlusion on the appliance. The life span for full occlusal coverage nightguards/dayguards varies from three to ten years.
- A single layer athletic mouthguard is sometimes used as an inexpensive nightguard/dayguard to temporarily change the neuromuscular behavior and produce muscle relaxation. This appliance usually lasts less than one year. However, the occlusion cannot be adjusted and the mouthguard can create increased parafunctional clenching and related temporomandibular disorders.

The manufacture of nightguards and dayguards usually requires two dental appointments. At the first appointment, accurate alginate impressions are made. The alginate impressions are poured in *Class I dental stone* to create diagnostic casts. A centric relation bite registration is made to enable placement of the casts on an anatomic articulator so that they contact as if the TMJ is in the correct position. The articulated models are sent to the dental laboratory and the dental technician fabricates the appliance.

At the second appointment, the dentist adjusts the nightguard and the client receives postoperative instructions to wear the appliance either while sleeping or full-time. Part-time wear is intended to provide symptomatic relief and to protect the dental structures from parafunctional forces. Full-time wear is intended to establish an ideal centric relation position of the mandible in the joints. Professional evaluation occurs every two to three weeks until the client improves.

Client Education Issues

- ✦ Explain the purposes and importance of study casts/models.
- ✦ Explain the purpose of mouthguards and why they are recommended for use during contact sports.
- ✦ Explain the difference between layered mouthguards and store-bought stock or boil and bite mouthguards.
- ✦ Explain the rationale for recommending the use of multiple layer mouthguards made of ethylene vinyl acetate (EVA) by a dental technician for full contact sports.
- ✦ Explain the minimal acceptable dimensions of a mouthguard.
- ✦ Explain the need to replace mouthguards after one season of use.
- ✦ Explain the contributing factors in bruxism.
- ✦ Explain the difference between reversible and irreversible treatment of bruxism.

Legal, Ethical, and Safety Issues

- ✦ In some states, dental hygienists can legally make preliminary dental impressions. It is the legal responsibility of the dental hygienist to practice within the scope authorized by state law.
- ✦ Impression trays can be a source of cross-contamination. They are classified as semicritical instruments because they become contaminated by saliva and must be either discarded if disposable or sterilized for reuse.
- ✦ Impression trays, trial sized in the client's mouth but not used for the impression, are either discarded if disposable or sterilized for reuse.
- ✦ Anything that comes into contact with contaminated impression trays must be sterilized (e.g., spatulas, bowls, and measuring devices used for mixing alginate).
- ✦ Countertops are sprayed, wiped, and sprayed again with an OSHA-approved surface disinfectant after the impression procedure has been completed and the client has been dismissed (see Chapter 6).
- ✦ Product manufacturers are required to provide written handling instructions called Material Safety Data Sheets (MSDS) according to the Occupational Safety and Health Administration (OSHA) laws. MSDS warnings for alginate include eye irritation and congestion and irritation of throat, nasal passages, and upper respiratory system. Unnecessary exposure to alginate powder should be avoided.
- ✦ Health conditions aggravated by exposure to alginate powder include the lung diseases bronchitis, emphysema, asthma, and silicosis. Long-term exposure to alginate may produce silicosis due to the crystalline silica element of the diatomaceous earth ingredient. Dustless alginate powder is now available.
- ✦ After an alginate impression is removed from the mouth, it is a biohazardous material. Because they are contaminated with the blood and saliva of the client, alginate impressions must be disinfected according to the manufacturer's recommendations and labeled as biohazardous material prior to being sent to a dental laboratory.
- ✦ The protocol for disinfection of impressions is chemical sterilant immersion or spraying. Sterilization may be performed with bleach, iodophor, phenol, or glutaraldehyde sterilant immersion, or by spraying the impression with a disinfectant and wrapping it in a paper towel in a sealed plastic bag for ten minutes. Rinse the impression after disinfection and prior to pouring in a gypsum product.
- ✦ The hygienist is advised to always read the manufacturer's directions and Material Safety Data Sheets on gypsum materials.
- ✦ The dental hygienist must not inhale gypsum powder because it may be hazardous to health. Gypsum contains free crystalline silica (cristobalite quartz), and may cause delayed lung disease such as silicosis and pneumoconiosis.
- ✦ Study models need to be retained as part of the client's permanent record.

Key Concepts

- A dental impression is a negative imprint of the teeth and surrounding tissues.
- A dental impression is used to create an accurate three-dimensional reproduction of the teeth and surrounding tissues called a diagnostic cast, model, or study cast.
- There are three main types of dental impressions used in dentistry: a preliminary impression, a final impression, and a bite registration.
- Hydrocolloid impression materials that cannot return to the sol state after they become a gel are called irreversible hydrocolloids.
- Alginate is the irreversible hydrocolloid typically used in dentistry for making preliminary impressions.
- A mandibular impression generally takes two scoops of powder and two measure lines of water. A maxillary impression generally takes three scoops of powder and three measure lines of water.
- Loading and inserting the tray should take no more than one minute. The objective is for the impression material to reach the gel state in the client's mouth.
- The mandibular impression should be made first to enhance client confidence; discomfort and gagging are less likely in the mandibular area.
- A maxillary impression tray is seated in a posterior to anterior direction to avoid triggering the gag reflex, prevent the excess material from going toward the back of the mouth, and move the impression material forward, ensuring complete coverage of the oral structures with alginate.
- An impression is a contaminated item in the dental laboratory.
- Factors that affect setting of alginate impressions include water/alginate ratio, water temperature, spatulation time, removal of the impression, and storage of the impression.
- An alginate impression must be poured within an hour of being made. It must be properly stored if it cannot be poured immediately.
- Stone casts and plaster casts are made of gypsum products; stone casts are stronger than plaster casts.
- Safety precautions must be used when handling alginate and gypsum materials.
- When mixing gypsum material, powder is added to water.
- The gypsum material is placed beginning in the palatal area and at the most posterior tooth.
- Factors that affect setting time of a cast are: type of gypsum used, water/powder ratio, water temperature, mixing time, and storage of gypsum.
- Factors that affect quality of a cast are those that affect setting time, removal of the impression, and movement of the tray or cast during the setting process.
- Forty to 60 minutes should elapse before separating the cast from the impression tray.
- Baseplate wax and wax wafers are used for the bite registration procedures (interocclusal record).
- Mouthguards should be recommended to clients at risk for sports-related dentofacial injury. Tooth avulsion, facial bone fractures, TMJ injuries, and concussions can be reduced by using properly fitted professionally manufactured mouthguards.
- Signs and symptoms of bruxism include abfraction lesions, exostosis, gingival recession, headaches, impaired hearing, TMJ noise with movement, limited range of motion of jaw, linea alba, tenderness of muscles of mastication, pain, periodontal pockets, tinnitus, TMJ disorders, tooth fracture, tooth mobility, tooth sensitivity, and tooth wear facets (attrition).
- Bruxism is treated with reversible and irreversible therapies. Reversible therapies include biofeedback, drug therapy, appliance therapy, exercise therapy, physical therapy, heat and cold therapy, mandibular relearning therapy, and psychotherapy. Irreversible therapies include orthognathic surgery and occlusal equilibration.

Critical Thinking Exercises

1. Visit the local pharmacy and athletic store. Review the types of athletic mouth protectors available over-the-counter. What would you say to a client about these products?
2. Review the factors that affect alginate and gypsum materials. Manipulate the alginate and gypsum materials by purposefully using the factors in your procedure. What is the outcome in terms of quality?
3. What signs and symptoms are commonly associated with bruxism? Compare these signs and symptoms with those of students in your class who brux.

For References, Suggested Readings, and Related Websites, visit
http://evolve.elsevier.com/Darby/hygiene/

CHAPTER 31

Restorative Therapy

OBJECTIVES

Mastery of the content of this chapter will enable the reader to:

- Describe the rationale for restorative therapy
- Discuss the role of the dental hygienist in restorative therapy
- Discuss the continuous role of assessment in the delivery of restorative therapy
- Describe an acceptable technique for rubber dam application
- State the rationale for rubber dam isolation
- Describe the qualities of a properly placed rubber dam
- Describe the proper sequence of steps in the removal of a rubber dam
- State the function of the matrix
- Describe the qualities of a properly placed matrix
- Compare the advantages and disadvantages of restorative materials
- Describe the preparation, condensation, and carving of dental amalgam
- Describe an acceptable amalgam polishing technique
- List the procedures necessary for proper mercury hygiene in an oral care environment
- Describe the placement and finishing of resin composite
- Describe the preparation, placement, and finishing of glass ionomer cements
- Describe the rationale for using sealers, liners, and bases
- State the rationale for and function of temporary or interim restorations
- Describe the advantages and disadvantages of cements used as bases and luting agents
- Describe the tissue management technique for making impressions for indirect restorations

KEY TERMS

Bases
Bridges
Cavosurface margin
Crowns
Defective restorations
Dental amalgam
Direct restorations
Enamel bonding
Glass ionomer
Indirect restorations
Key punch
Line angles
Liners
Luting agent
Matrix
Mercury hygiene
Nomenclature
Occlusal adjustment
Point angle
Resin composites
Restorative therapy
Rubber dam
Sealers
Smear layer
Temporary (interim) restoration
Trituration (amalgamation)
Walls

Restorative therapy requires diagnosis and treatment planning by a licensed dentist. In some states and provinces, a range of restorative dental treatment may be legally delegated by the dentist to the licensed dental hygienist. Although the number of dental hygienists who perform the full range of restorative therapies presented in this chapter may be low, all dental hygienists conduct clinical assessments and provide educational information about restorative therapies. Therefore, it is important for dental hygienists to understand the rationale and goals of restorative therapy, the types of restorations, and the procedures involved in the restorative process.

RATIONALE FOR RESTORATIVE THERAPY

When a client's human need for a biologically sound and functional dentition is in deficit, it is necessary to intervene with therapies that restore the dentition to a state of health, support the maintenance of health and function, and provide aesthetic modification. *Restorative therapy* includes the restoration of damaged tooth structure, defective restorations, aesthetic inconsistencies, and anatomic and physiological abnormalities. In many cases, restorative therapy prevents tooth loss by halting disease progression.

Acquired Tooth Damage

Acquired tooth damage is one of the main reasons for restorative therapy. The types of acquired tooth damage are discussed in Chapter 13.

Defective Restorations

Defective restorations no longer restore the dentition to an acceptable state of form and function. Although restorations are referred to as being temporary or permanent, no restoration can be considered truly permanent. The physical properties of the available restorative materials make them susceptible to alteration and deterioration. Certain materials, however, have withstood the test of time and are more readily recognized for their longevity. When properly used, gold restorations are the most durable and compatible in the oral environment. Their resistance to corrosion, nonirritating chemistry, and similarity to enamel in texture and wear resistance are qualities that other materials often lack. Amalgam is the most commonly used restorative material in dentistry because of its versatility, workability, and clinical longevity. However, the forces generated through mastication and tooth-to-tooth contact eventually wear the occlusal margins of most amalgam restorations (Figure 31–1). Tooth-colored resin composite restorations abrade and wear, causing them to deteriorate more rapidly than metal restorations. Cement materials dissolve in the oral environment, resulting in the loosening of luted restorations or loss of form in restorations composed entirely of cement.

Defective restorations, however, may not always be related to the restorative material. Defective restorations also can be caused by the techniques used to place the restoration. Defects such as overhangs, open margins, poor contours, and open proximal contacts are the result of improper technique, poor judgment, and lack of attention to detail (Figures 31–2 and 31–3). These are avoidable defects and are not acceptable standards of care.

Aesthetic Appearance

Restorative therapy also is an important factor in meeting a person's human need for a wholesome facial image. Missing, broken, or obviously decayed teeth are often the reasons individuals seek oral healthcare.

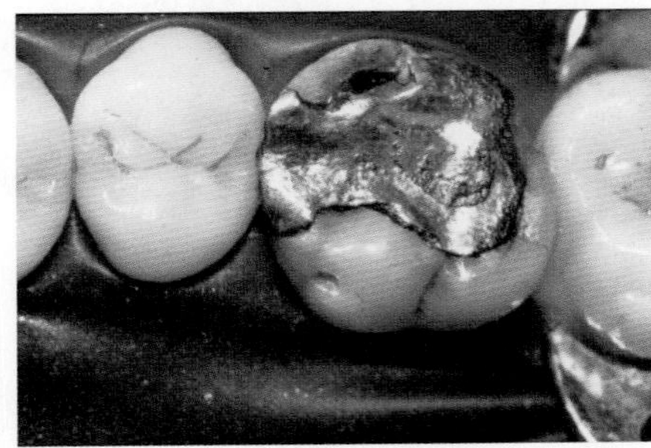

FIGURE 31–1 ✦ Large amalgam restoration, which has served for many years despite its poor design, exhibits defective margins.

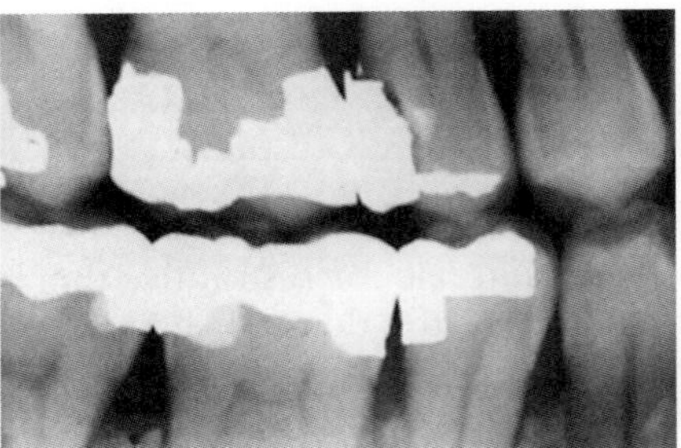

FIGURE 31–2 ✦ This radiograph shows poor proximal contour and a gingival overhang on the distal surface of the maxillary first molar. The maxillary second premolar exhibits amalgam fractures and dislodgement.

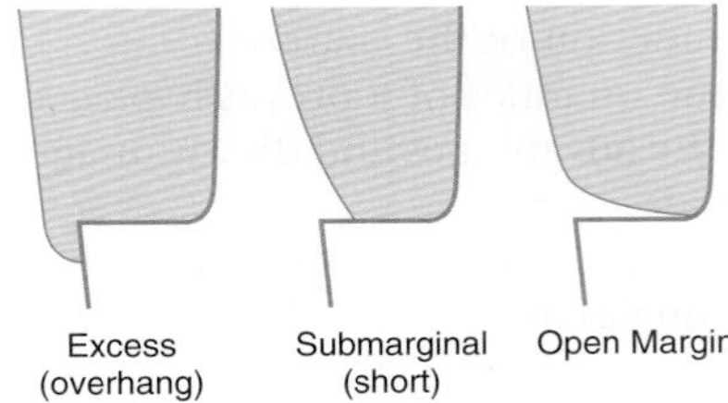

FIGURE 31–3 ✦ This illustration depicts possible defects at the gingival margins of restorations. It may be possible to remove an overhang without replacing the restoration; however, restorations with short and open margins require replacement.

Dental anomalies such as diastemas, mottled enamel, congenital tooth defects, and intrinsic tooth discolorations such as tetracycline staining also may require restorative interventions to improve appearance.

One of the main disadvantages of metallic restorations has been aesthetics (Figure 31–4). Because metals do not have the appearance of natural teeth, many clients object to their use. The relatively recent changes in consumer demands for natural-appearing restorations are the result of an unprecedented promotion and availability of tooth-colored restorative materials. These materials include resin composite, porcelain, castable ceramics, and glass ionomer cements. All of these materials have distinct limitations, but they can be an answer for the client who is motivated by appearance.

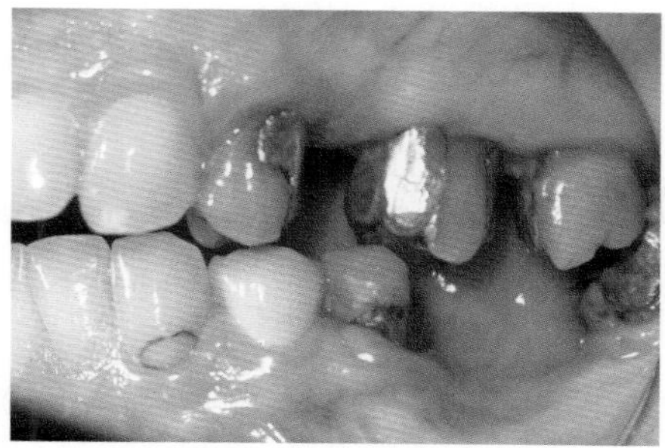

FIGURE 31–4 ✦ Tooth darkening due to the display of amalgam and associated internal staining.

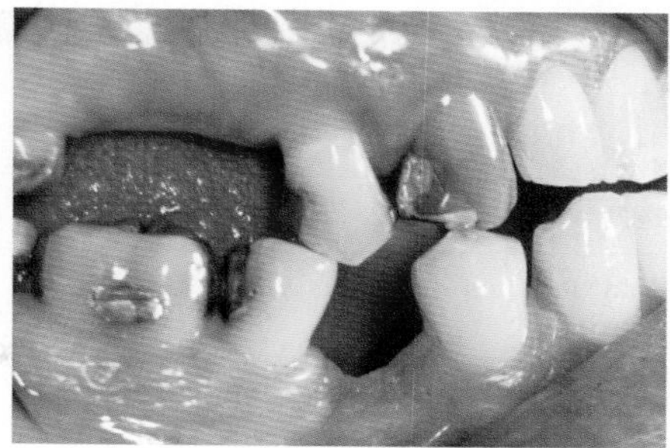

FIGURE 31–5 ✦ Tooth loss has resulted in pathologic occlusion from tooth movement (tip, drift, and extrusion).

Occlusion

The state of the occlusal relationship influences the function and health of the dentition. Various levels of restorative treatment can be provided to improve a person's occlusion. There are times when an *occlusal adjustment,* the selective reshaping or recontouring of the dentition by grinding, can improve the occlusion. This is especially true when previous restorations have been poorly shaped or contoured. When teeth become misaligned because of the loss of adjacent or opposing teeth, it may be necessary to recontour them to establish a stable, functional occlusion by realigning the vector of occlusal forces to be more parallel to the long axis of the teeth (Figure 31–5). Complex restorations are necessary if this recontouring results in substantial tooth crown removal. Complete coronal restorations (*crowns*) and even fixed partial dentures (*bridges*) are necessary to restore occlusion in badly damaged dentitions.

Mastication

The most basic function of teeth is to chew food and thus begin the process of digestion. A significant number of clients indicate inadequate chewing as their chief complaint. Often, frustration exists because certain favorite foods are difficult to chew. Therefore, a missing tooth, defective restoration, or carious lesion can compromise an individual's eating pleasure and nutrition.

CARIOUS LESIONS AND RESTORATIONS

Black's Classification System and the Complexity Classification System, presented in Chapter 13, are used most commonly to describe the type and location of dental caries and dental restorations. These classification systems are essential and expedite communication among the parties involved in the delivery of dental services.

Types of Restorations

Restorations are categorized by the technique required for placement of the restorative material. These placement techniques have been classified as direct and indirect. *Direct restorations* are placed and formed directly in the cavity preparation. These restorations are typically placed in increments, adapted closely to the cavity walls, and shaped to the desired contours. The shaping is done with carvers when the materials are still in a soft or unset state and with rotating instruments such as burrs and discs when the restorative materials are in a hard or set state. The materials used in direct restorations include moldable substances such as silver amalgam, resin composite, glass ionomer cement, and direct gold. The restorative procedures that have been legally delegated to dental hygienists fall within this direct restoration category. Table 31–1 outlines the uses, advantages, and disadvantages of direct restorative materials.

In contrast, *indirect restorations* are formed on reproductions (dies) of prepared teeth. The shaping of the restoration is done by preparing the desired form in wax and then casting this form in metal or ceramic. Porcelain restorations are formed by building the restoration to shape with porcelain powder and then solidifying the mass in a special "firing" oven. Gold inlays and porcelain crowns are typical indirect restorations. Because indirect restorations are rigid and solid objects, the cavity preparation must be specially designed (tapered) to allow complete seating of the restoration at the time of permanent cementation. Table 31–2 outlines the uses, advantages, and disadvantages of indirect restorative materials.

Cavity Preparation

A critical step in restoring the dentition is the preparation of the cavity. The intent of this section is not to discuss in detail the fundamentals of cavity preparation, but rather to present an overview of considerations essential to each member of the oral health team. Effective communication among team members supports the efficient delivery of oral health services. Essential to effective communication is a standardized nomenclature for cavity preparations. A basic understanding of the principles and instrumentation of cavity preparation supports the dental hygienist in the role of clinician, client advocate, and educator.

TABLE 31–1 DIRECT RESTORATIONS

Material	Primary Area of Use	Main Advantages	Main Disadvantages
Direct gold (foil, mat, and powder)	All Small cavities Avoid occlusal stress	Marginal seal Durability	High technical skill required Color
Silver amalgam	Posterior	Ease of placement Minimal leakage over time	Marginal breakdown Tarnish Color
Resin composite	All Avoid occlusal stress	Color Relative ease of placement	Occlusal wear Leakage
Glass ionomer cement	Class 5 (gumline cavities)	Ease of placement Bonds to enamel and dentin Fair color Releases fluoride	Easily abraded

TABLE 31–2 INDIRECT RESTORATIONS

Material	Primary Area of Use	Main Advantages	Main Disadvantages
Gold alloy	Posterior (inlays and crowns)	Durability Contours	Color High technical skill required
Porcelain	All (inlays, onlays, and crowns)	Color	Abrades opposing teeth Marginal seal High technical skill required
Castable ceramic	All (inlays, onlays, and crowns)	Color	Marginal seal High technical skill required
Porcelain fused to metal	All (crowns)	Color Strength Marginal seal	Abrades opposing teeth High technical skill required

Nomenclature

Nomenclature describes a cavity or a restoration according to basic rules that involve the combination of anatomic terms (see Chapter 13). Similar rules of nomenclature also are used to describe aspects of cavity preparations. Rules for describing the orientation of the features of a cavity preparation are as follows:

RULE #1. First, identify the tooth surfaces involved in the preparation. It is important to remember that involvement may not be limited to those surfaces exhibiting carious lesions. For example, a posterior tooth exhibiting a lesion on only the distal surface will likely require a cavity preparation involving the distal and occlusal surfaces. Following the basic rules of nomenclature described in Chapter 13, this cavity design is described as a disto-occlusal (DO) preparation. If the mesial surface is also involved, the cavity design becomes a mesio-occlusodistal (MOD) preparation. Similarly, a cavity design involving the facial, incisal, and lingual surfaces is a facioincisolingual (FIL) preparation.

RULE #2. All cavity preparations have walls, angles, and margins. *Walls* are vertical or horizontal surfaces within the cavity preparation. They are usually named according to the closest tooth surface or approximating dental tissue. A simple occlusal cavity preparation (Class I) on a mandibular molar has five walls:

- ✦ Mesial (M)
- ✦ Distal (D)
- ✦ Facial (F) or Buccal (B)
- ✦ Lingual (L)
- ✦ Pulpal (P)

The mesial, distal, facial, and lingual walls appear as vertical surfaces that closely approximate the corresponding tooth surfaces. The pulpal wall, named because of its proximity to the pulp, appears as a horizontal surface. Another term frequently associated with the pulpal wall is "pulpal floor." When visualizing a mandibular molar in a vertical position, it is easy to envision a floor surrounded by four walls. Another common area of reference is the long axis of the tooth. A wall aligned in the same general direction as the axis is termed an "axial wall." The axial wall appears as a vertical surface in keeping with the long axis of the tooth (Figure 31–6).

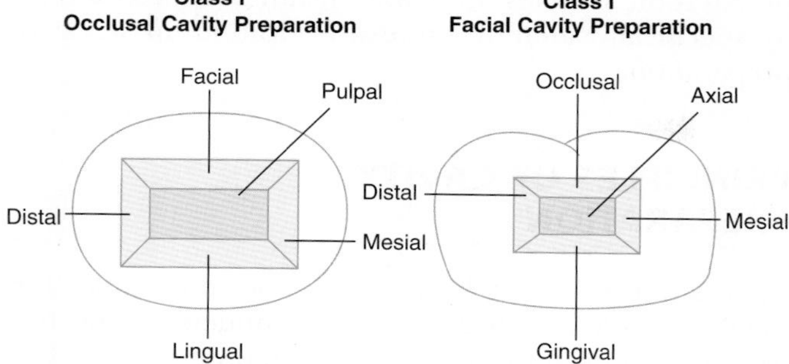

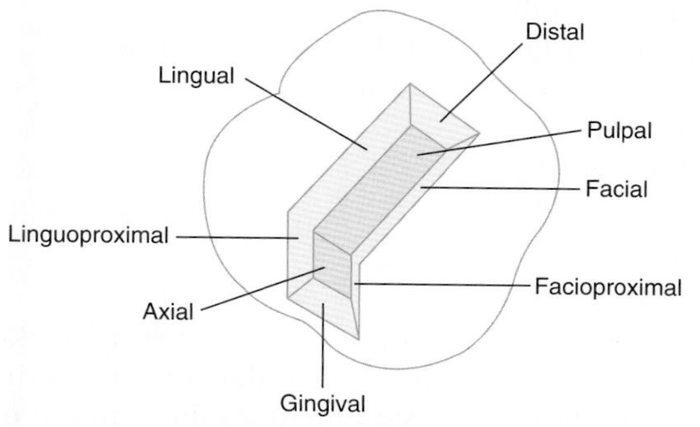

FIGURE 31–6 ✦ Schematic representation of the walls of Class I and Class II cavity preparations.

RULE #3. *Line angles* are formed by the meeting of two walls. They are usually named according to the walls involved. The naming of line angles follows the basic rules of cavity nomenclature. For example, the mandibular molar with a simple occlusal cavity preparation and five walls has eight line angles formed by the meeting of the vertical and horizontal walls (Figure 31–7). These line angles are named as follows:

- Mesiolingual (ML) line angle
- Distolingual (DL) line angle
- Mesiofacial (MF) line angle
- Distofacial (DF) line angle
- Mesiopulpal (MP) line angle
- Distopulpal (DP) line angle
- Faciopulpal (FP) line angle
- Linguopulpal (LP) line angle

The one exception to this rule for naming line angles is found in anterior proximal cavity preparations (Class III). Because the cavity form is typically a triangle, the line angle at the incisal junction of the facial and lingual walls can be called the faciolingual line angle. However, the more commonly accepted term is "incisal line angle" (Figure 31–8). The walls and line angles meet the unaltered tooth surface at the *cavosurface* (cavity-tooth surface) *margin.*

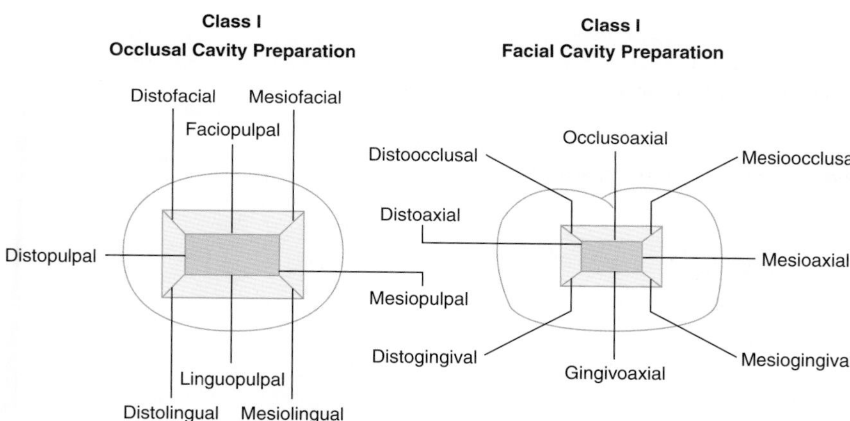

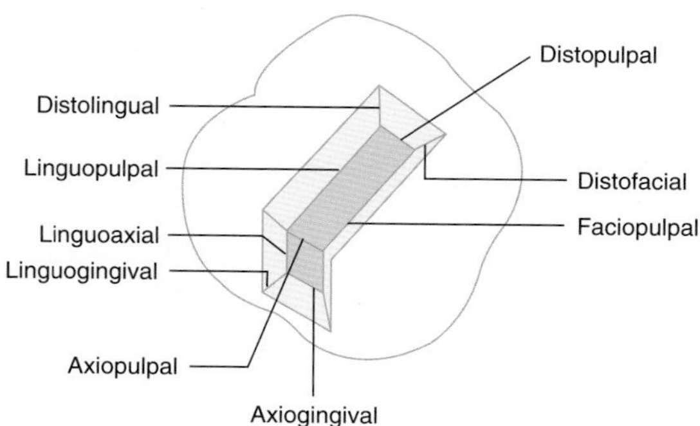

FIGURE 31–7 ✦ Schematic representation of the line angles of Class I and Class II cavity preparations.

RULE #4. The meeting of three walls results in a *point angle*. Point angles also are named according to the involved walls (Figure 31–9). The four point angles in the occlusal cavity preparation of the mandibular molar are as follows:

- Mesiolinguopulpal (MLP) point angle
- Distolinguopulpal (DLP) point angle
- Mesiofaciopulpal (MFP) point angle
- Distofaciopulpal (DFP) point angle

The application of the appropriate names of the walls, line angles, cavosurface margins, and point angles defines specific locations within the cavity preparation that are not open to multiple interpretations. The distofaciopulpal point angle can be only one location. Familiarity with these basic landmarks of a cavity preparation enables the oral healthcare professional to specifically identify an exact location in a cavity preparation.

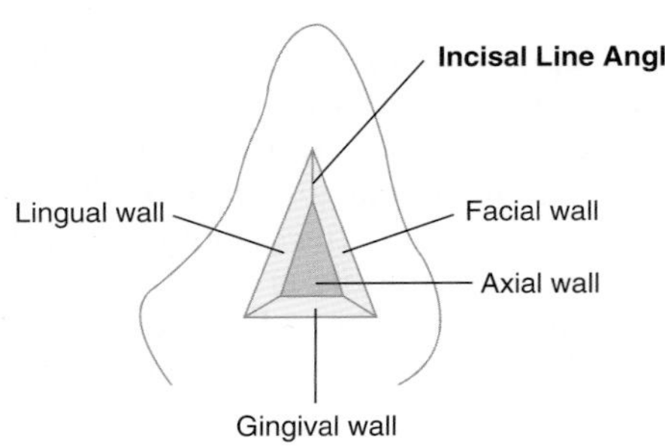

FIGURE 31–8 ✦ Schematic representation of the incisal line angle of a Class III cavity preparation.

PRINCIPLES OF CAVITY PREPARATION

Although the dental hygienist is not responsible for cavity preparation, there is value in understanding the systematic procedure of cavity preparation that is based on well-established biomechanical principles. Cavity preparation typically follows six steps:

1. Establish the outline form
2. Obtain the resistance and the retention form
3. Obtain the convenience form
4. Remove caries
5. Finish the enamel
6. Debride the cavity

Outline Form

The establishment of an outline form provides the framework from which the remainder of the cavity preparation develops. This step includes the removal of weak or undermined enamel and existing defective restorative materials. The preparation margins should extend laterally beyond the decay or defect into cleansable and sound tooth structure.

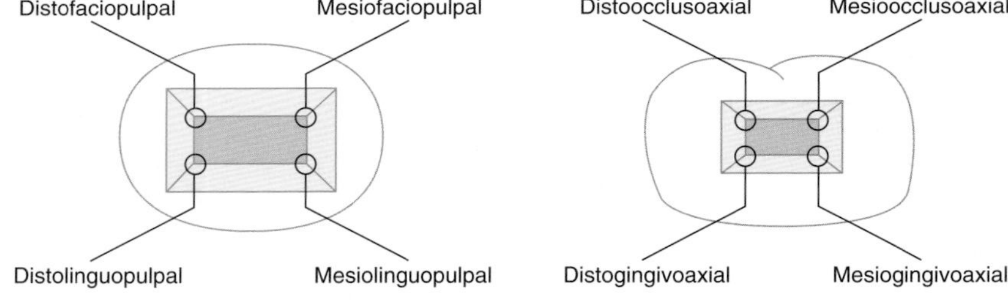

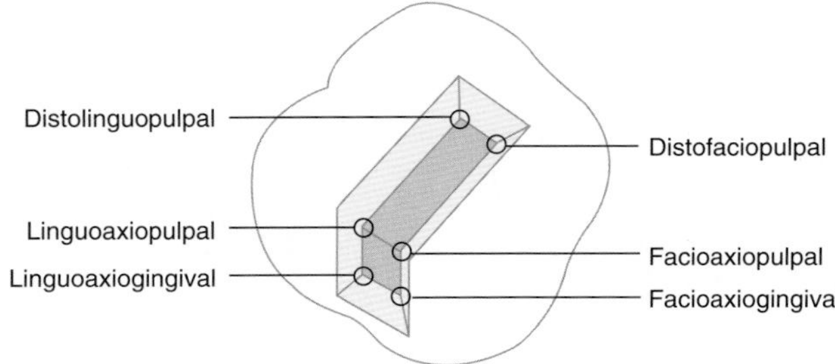

FIGURE 31–9 ✦ Schematic representation of the internal point angles of Class I and Class II cavity preparations.

Resistance and Retention Form

Obtaining the resistance and retention form involves the shaping of the internal aspects of the preparation to protect the tooth and restoration from forces that result in breakage or displacement. Primary concerns in this step are the extension and direction of cavity walls and the refinement of internal features. Retention form deals with the ability of the cavity preparation to retain the restoration, and resistance form is important for preventing lateral displacement in more complex restorations.

Convenience Form

In obtaining the convenience form, the operator enlarges and extends the cavity preparation to enable proper instrumentation for decay removal, thereby providing an optimal final result.

Caries Removal

Depending on the severity of the carious lesion, caries may have been removed in the previous steps. However, if carious dentin remains, it should be excavated to establish a disease-free environment. It is at this stage that protective agents such as sealers, liners, and bases are placed as needed.

Finish Enamel

At this stage, the operator smoothes the walls, sharpens the cavosurface margins, and removes any unsupported enamel from the margins. This process supports the desired marginal seal between the tooth structure and the restorative material.

Debridement

The final step in cavity preparation is the removal of debris and moisture that compromise the restoration. This is typically accomplished with the air–water syringe.

Each tooth and cavity presents a unique challenge to the practitioner. The severity of the carious lesion influences the complexity of the cavity preparation process. However, these fundamental steps in cavity preparation result in a preparation ready for restoration.

COLLABORATIVE ROLE OF THE DENTAL HYGIENIST

The participation of the dental hygienist in the delivery of restorative therapies affords a unique collaborative opportunity for enhancement of the dentist and dental hygienist partnership in oral healthcare delivery. The efficient use of the dentist, dental hygienist, and dental assistant allows all members of the team to contribute their expertise, assuring quality, cost-effective restorative treatment. Figure 31–10 illustrates the restorative care cycle that integrates the roles of the dentist and dental hygienist throughout the delivery of restorative care to the client.

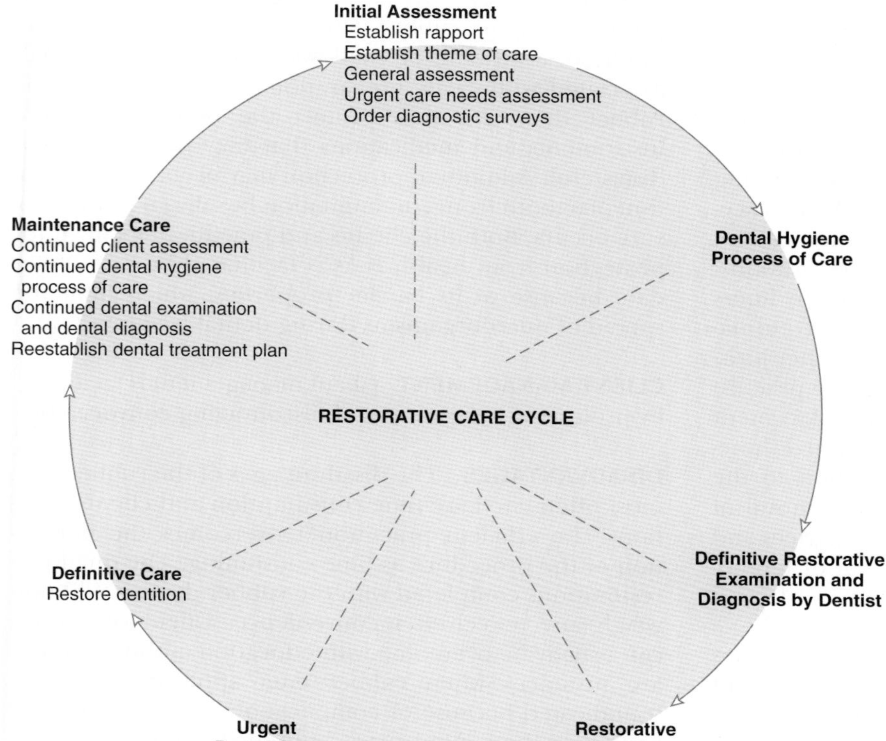

FIGURE 31–10 ✦ Comprehensive restorative care cycle.

The dentist is the oral healthcare professional responsible for the development of the restorative care plan. It begins with the client's chief complaint and integrates all information collected about the client and results in a dental diagnosis and a definitive restorative care plan. This plan outlines the steps to be followed for preventing and eliminating disease and for restoring and maintaining health. The restorative care plan, an essential component of the total care plan, is limited in that it focuses primarily on the restorative needs of the client.

Applying the dental hygiene process of care, the dental hygienist collaborates with the dentist to achieve effective restoration of the dentition. During the assessment phase of dental hygiene care, tooth damage and its cause may be identified and communicated to the dentist. In addition, based on assessment of the client's oral hygiene status and oral health behaviors, the dental hygienist plans, implements, and evaluates oral disease prevention and health promotion strategies for the client.

Originally, the dental hygienist chiefly was responsible for the prevention of oral disease, which explains why the dental hygienist today is recognized as an oral disease preventive and health promotion specialist. However, in the 1960s and 1970s it was further theorized that the dental hygienist could play a significant role in supporting the health of the dentition through the delivery of restorative therapies. It was at this time that the primary focus of the dental profession became improving the oral health of the public through the elimination and treatment of dental caries. Thus, the rationale for the initial delegation of restorative services was to provide a mechanism to respond to an expanding need and demand for dental care, and dental hygienists became responsible for expanded functions.

There is wide variability in the extent of delegation of restorative functions to the dental hygienist. In some jurisdictions, the dental hygienist is permitted to perform a broad range of restorative therapies including the placement and removal of the rubber dam; placement and removal of matrices and wedges; fabrication, placement, and removal of temporary restorations; placement of retraction cords; placement of cavity liners and bases; placement, carving, and finishing of permanent restorations; and amalgam polishing. In other jurisdictions the restorative scope of dental hygiene practice may be restricted to amalgam polishing and placement and removal of the rubber dam. The restorative functions most commonly permitted for delegation to the dental hygienist include the placement and removal of the rubber dam; placement and removal of matrices and wedges; fabrication, placement, and removal of temporary restorations; placement of retraction cord; and amalgam polishing.[1,2]

Because the scope of dental hygiene practice varies dramatically among states, provinces, and territories, not all educational programs prepare dental hygienists to practice in all locations. The procedures included in this chapter span a broad range of restorative interventions delegated to the dental hygienist. The dental hygienist has the legal and ethical responsibility to practice within the scope of the law at all times.

RUBBER DAM ISOLATION

Rationale

The primary purpose of the rubber dam is to improve the quality of restorative dental treatment. The effectiveness of the rubber dam is a result of four attributes:

- ✦ Moisture control
- ✦ Accessibility and visibility
- ✦ Client and operator protection
- ✦ Client management

MOISTURE CONTROL. The moisture-control property of the rubber dam ensures the essential dryness of the operating field and limits contamination by the oral fluids. Furthermore, the properties of the restorative material are preserved and protected in an environment free of moisture.

ACCESSIBILITY AND VISIBILITY. The *rubber dam* provides accessibility and visibility by retracting the gingival tissue surrounding the site of restoration, and by retracting the cheeks, lips, and tongue from the field of operation. The background of a dark rubber dam provides excellent contrast with the tooth structure and reduces glare from the moist surfaces of the tissues of the oral cavity.

CLIENT AND OPERATOR PROTECTION. The client is protected by the rubber dam because it limits the possibility of aspirating or swallowing debris and materials associated with cavity preparation and restoration. The rubber dam also may protect the oral tissues from instruments and medications that may be injurious or distasteful. Additional protection may occur in the isolation of a tooth from contamination by saliva if pulp exposure occurs. Both the client's and practitioner's need for protection from health risks is facilitated by the rubber dam because of its barrier properties, which limit the spread of microorganisms during dental treatment.

CLIENT MANAGEMENT. Client management is facilitated by promoting relaxation and discouraging conversation.

DISADVANTAGES. The disadvantages of the rubber dam most often cited are time consumption and client objection. The efficient practitioner overcomes the perception of the procedure as time-consuming. The quality of restorations completed with the rubber dam should outweigh any perceived inconvenience. Client objections can usually be overcome with education, although there are instances when rubber dam application is contraindicated because of complications such as cracks or fissures of the commissures, herpetic lesions, respiratory congestion, claustrophobia, asthma, and allergy to latex.

Rubber Dam Material

The features to be considered in the selection of rubber dam material are as follows:

- ✦ Size (in inches)
- ✦ Weight
- ✦ Color

The rubber dam material is typically marketed as a sheet of latex in a 5 × 5 inch child size or a 6 × 6 inch adult size. Rubber dam material is also available in rolls that may be cut to the dimensions desired by the operator. The available weights of rubber dam material are light, medium, heavy, extra heavy, and special heavy. The lighter weight, thinner dams are easier to apply because of their flexibility and comfort to the client, whereas the heavier weight, thicker dams provide better retraction of tissues and protection from revolving instruments. The medium and heavy weights are most commonly used for restorative procedures. The rubber dam material is available in an assortment of colors: black, gray, white, green, blue, and pastels. Although the color selection is based on operator preference, the main issues to consider in color selection are the contrast with the teeth and the comfort to the eye. Many of these materials now are pleasantly scented. Nonlatex rubber dam is available for clients allergic to latex.[3]

Rubber Dam Punch

The rubber dam punch, used to punch the tooth holes in the rubber dam material (Figure 31–11), typically has five to six hole sizes. The punch requires regular maintenance, which includes oiling of the movable parts and dry or chemical sterilization rather than autoclaving for infection control.

Rubber Dam Forceps

The rubber dam forceps are used to place the rubber dam retainer (clamp) on the anchor tooth (Figure 31–12). The instrument is a plierlike forceps that expands the rubber dam retainer for placement on the tooth. The beaks of the forceps are placed into the holes of the retainer, and by squeezing the handles of the forceps, the beaks are separated and the retainer expanded. The rubber dam forceps have a locking device that may be engaged by squeezing the handles, turning the forceps upside down, thus dropping the locking device into position, and allowing release at the handles without loss of the desired expansion.

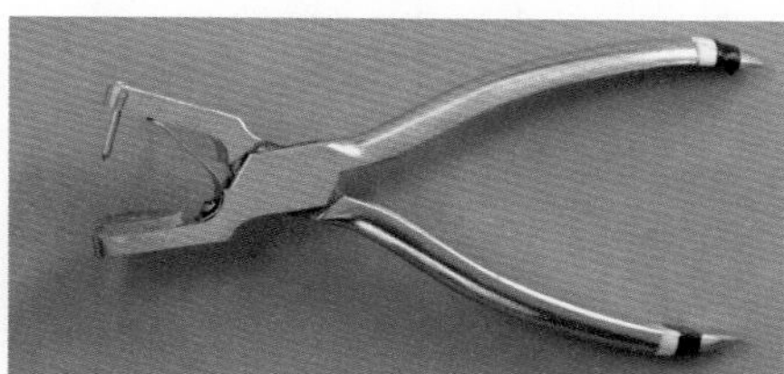

FIGURE 31–11 ✦ Rubber dam punch.

Rubber Dam Frame

The rubber dam frame is used to secure the extraoral rubber dam material (Figure 31–13). There are several styles of frames available to satisfy operator preference. However, the frames of choice must be sterilizable. The most commonly used rubber dam frame is a U-shaped stainless steel frame with small projections for securing the edges of the rubber dam sheet.

Rubber Dam Retainer

The rubber dam retainer provides the intraoral stabilization of the rubber dam material by anchoring the material securely in place. The rubber dam retainer is produced in winged and wingless designs. The parts of the rubber dam retainer include the jaws, prongs, bow, and forceps holes (Figure 31–14). The prongs of the retainer contact the clamped tooth, and the bow joins the two retainer jaws. The forceps holes are the insertion point for the rubber dam forceps during the placement and removal of the retainer.

Retainer designs are identified by number. Winged and wingless retainers of the same number are identical in shape; however, the letter "W" is used to designate the wingless retainer. The wings of a retainer provide addi-

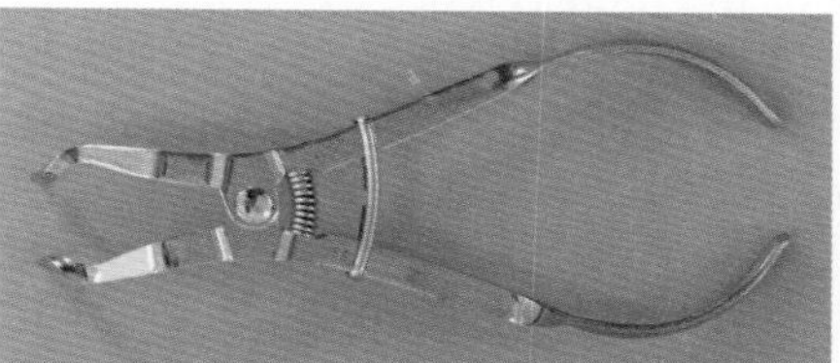

FIGURE 31–12 ✦ Rubber dam forceps.

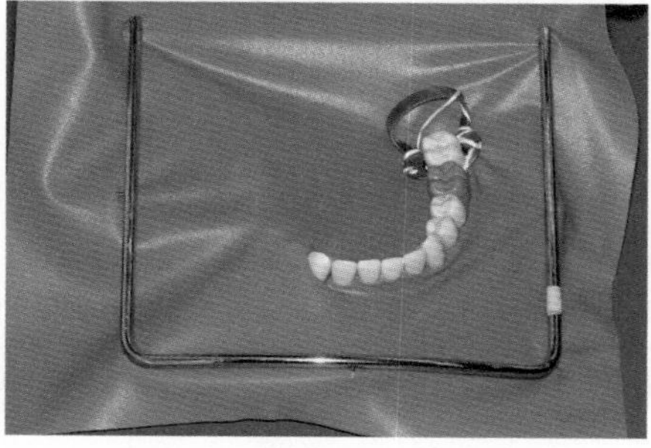

FIGURE 31–13 ✦ The rubber dam frame is used to secure the edges of the rubber dam.

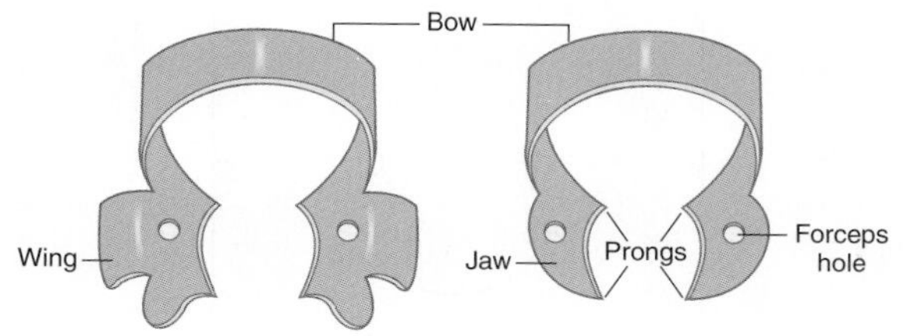

FIGURE 31–14 ✦ Rubber dam retainer basic design and parts.

tional retraction of the rubber dam material away from the retainer tooth. Retainers come in numerous shapes and sizes to take into consideration various factors such as the specific tooth to be retained (permanent or primary), the stage of eruption of the tooth to be retained, and the access needed for the operation (Figure 31–15). The success of the rubber dam isolation depends largely on the stability of the rubber dam retainer.

Rubber Dam Material Preparation

The operator is encouraged to custom punch the rubber dam for each client to best achieve the goals of isolation. The mandibular rubber dam should be divided into sixths by doing the following:

- Dividing the dam in half horizontally
- Dividing the dam into thirds vertically

The *key punch* (the hole that guides the placement of all remaining holes) for the mandibular posterior dam is the hole for the most distal tooth to be isolated. Figure 31–16 illustrates the placement of the key punch for first, second, and third molars. The key punch for the mandibular anterior rubber dam is for a mandibular central incisor. The placement is at the midsection of the lower half of the dam and 1.5 to 2.0 mm left or right of the center of the dam (Figure 31–17).

The maxillary rubber dam should be divided into fourths by doing the following:

- Marking the horizontal line approximately 1 inch below the top of the dam (when the rubber dam punch is positioned as seen in Figure 31–18, it is a handy guide for determining the location of the horizontal line)
- Dividing the dam in half vertically

The key punch for maxillary posterior and anterior rubber dams is the central incisor. Generally, there are 3 to 4 mm between the holes for the right and left central incisors, and they are placed at the center of the dam on the horizontal line (Figure 31–19).

Following the placement of the key punch, the remainder of the holes are placed according to tooth position and the following general guidelines.

The size of the hole should correspond with the size of the tooth. The number of holes in a rubber dam punch vary; however, the smallest hole is generally too small to be of value for any permanent tooth. A hole that is too small may tear during placement. On the other

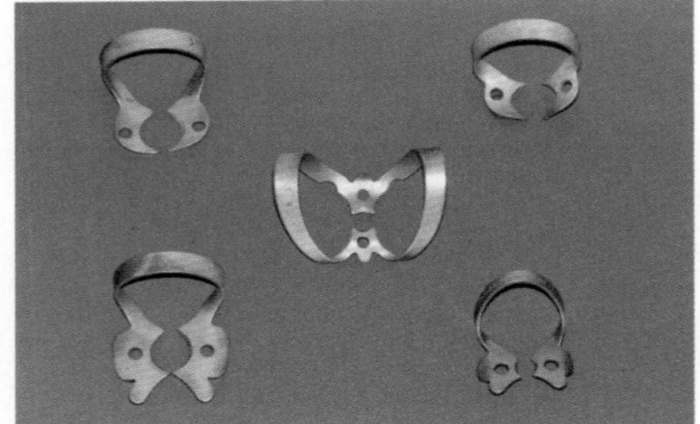

FIGURE 31–15 ✦ Rubber dam retainer variations: wingless molar retainers *(upper left and right)*, winged premolar retainer *(lower right)*, winged molar retainer *(lower left)*, and anterior retainer *(center)*.

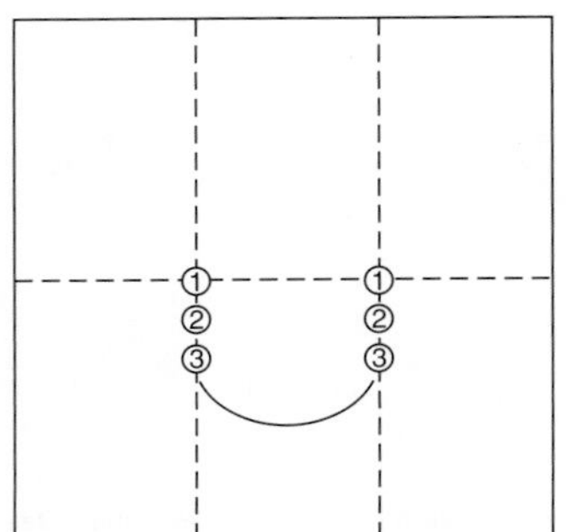

FIGURE 31–16 ✦ Key punch for the first molar (1), second molar (2), and third molar (3) in a mandibular posterior rubber dam.

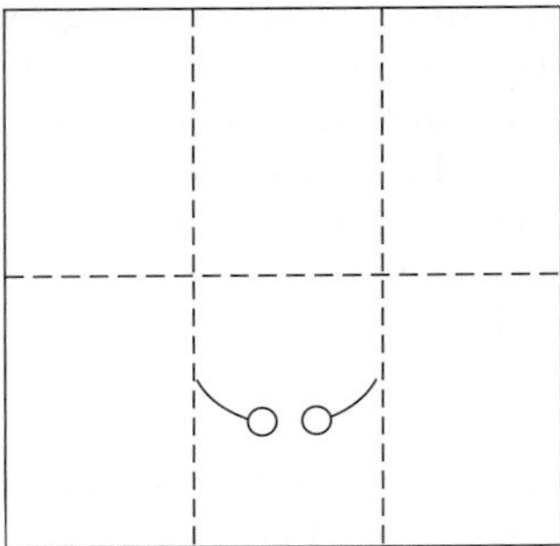

FIGURE 31–17 ✦ Key punch for the left or right central incisor in a mandibular anterior rubber dam.

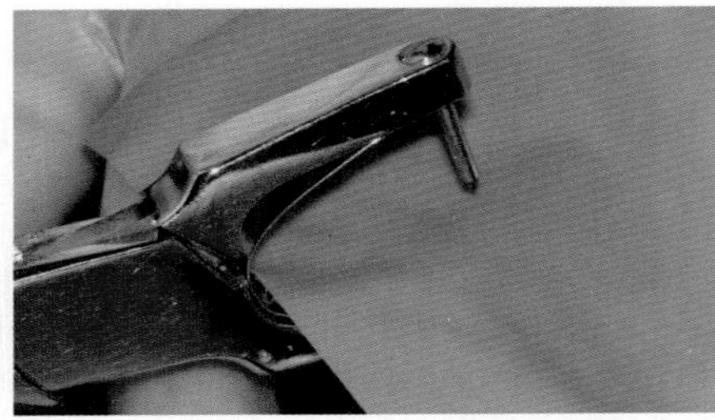

FIGURE 31–18 ✦ The rubber dam hole is being punched approximately 1 inch from the edge of the material.

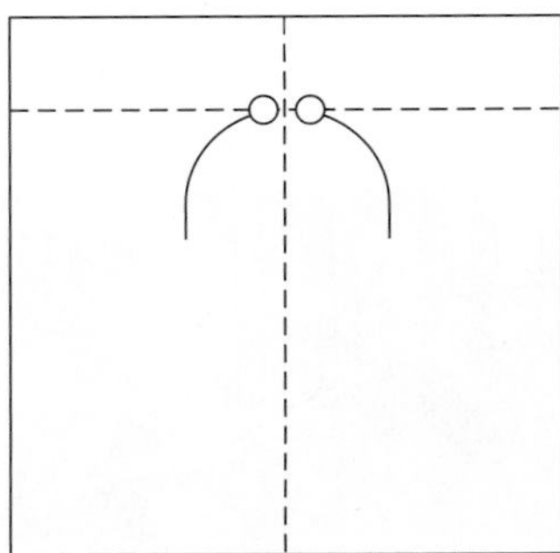

FIGURE 31–19 ✦ Key punch for the left or right central incisor in a maxillary posterior and anterior rubber dam.

hand, a hole that is too large may inadequately seal the tooth and may permit leakage.

The tooth to receive the retainer may require a double or triple hole. The holes must be punched precisely without leaving tags and tears. The presence of tags or tears indicates a weak area and facilitates tearing of the rubber dam when stretched over the involved tooth (Figure 31–20). To punch clean holes, the rubber dam punch must be well maintained and free of lodged rubber dam material. In addition, the action of punching the dam must be sharp and determined, not uncertain and hesitant.

When the dentition is normally spaced and aligned, 3 to 4 mm should be left between holes. Holes that are punched too close together cause stretching and inadequate seal around the tooth, whereas holes that are punched too far apart result in excess material and a bunching effect (Figure 31–21).

The placement of the holes should take into consideration the faciolingual positioning of the teeth. Additional space should be allowed for areas with missing teeth. This hole placement can be accomplished by measuring the space between the teeth adjacent to the edentulous area and adding 1 to 2 mm.

The arrangement of punched holes should correspond with the shape of the client's arch. Hole arrangements that are punched too straight or too curved produce folds and stretching that may hinder the operator's ability to attain an optimal seal. During the punching process it is also important that the punch device be centered directly above a hole to avoid damaging the instrument.

Retainer Selection

The selection of the rubber dam retainer is the next step in the application of the rubber dam. The anchor tooth is the tooth to be retained and is also the most distal tooth to be isolated. There are four points of consideration when selecting the retainer for the anchor tooth:

- ✦ The mesiodistal width between the prongs of the retainer jaws should be slightly narrower than the mesiodistal width of the anchor tooth at the cementoenamel junction (CEJ).
- ✦ The mesiodistal curvature of the retainer jaws must be greater than the mesiodistal curvature of the anchor tooth at the CEJ.
- ✦ The faciolingual width between the prongs of the retainer jaws should be narrower than the faciolingual width of the anchor tooth at the CEJ.
- ✦ The bow of the retainer must arch high enough to clear the occlusal surface of the anchor tooth when the retainer is appropriately seated.

These criteria are illustrated in Figure 31–22. Each of these criteria permits the correct and stable seating of the jaw prongs on the anchor tooth. Usually in the anterior aspects of the arches, the rubber dam can be successfully retained without the use of a retainer. Small pieces of rubber dam, or other devices such as wooden wedges and/or floss, can be inserted between teeth to hold the dam in position.

Rubber Dam Placement Technique

There are two techniques for the placement of the retainer and rubber dam material. The first technique involves a two-step process of placing the retainer and then the rubber dam material. The second technique combines the placement of the retainer and rubber dam material into a single step. This single-step method requires that the rubber dam material be placed over the bow of the retainer, and then carried into its ultimate location (Figure 31–23).

In a posterior application, the bow of the retainer is always positioned toward the distal aspect of the anchor

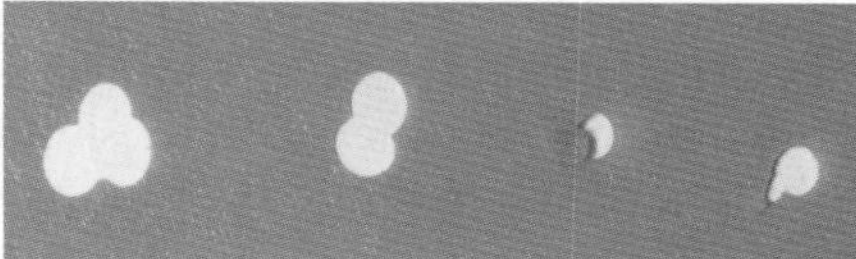

FIGURE 31–20 ✦ As pictured left to right, triple hole, double hole, tag, and tear.

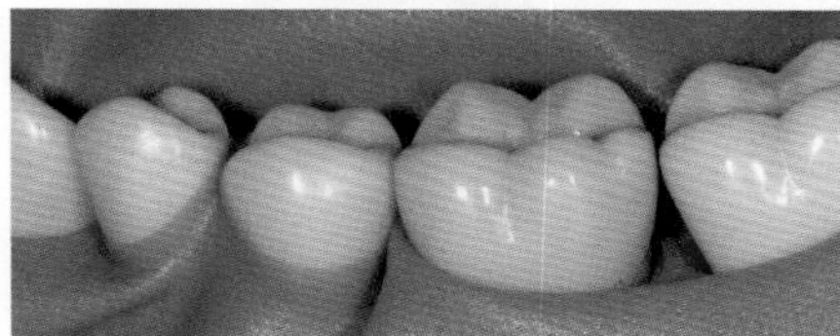

FIGURE 31–21 ✦ Rubber dam problems: dam not through proximal contact between no. 20 and no. 21; bunching of the dam between no. 19 and no. 20; and stretching of the dam exposing the gingiva between no. 18 and no. 19.

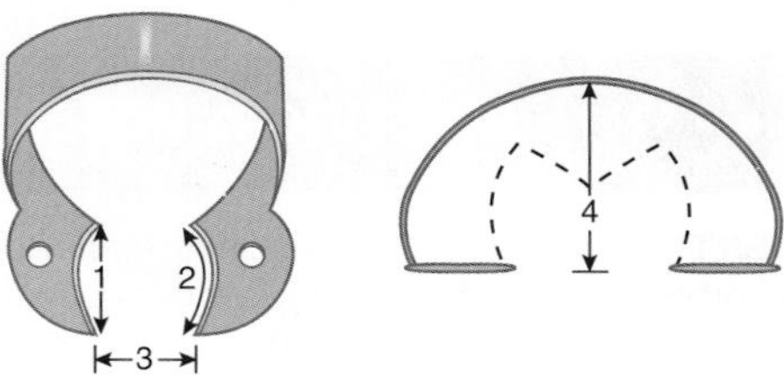

FIGURE 31–22 ✦ Retainer selection criteria: mesiodistal width of the retainer (1); mesiodistal curvature of the retainer (2); faciolingual width of the retainer (3); and height of the retainer (4).

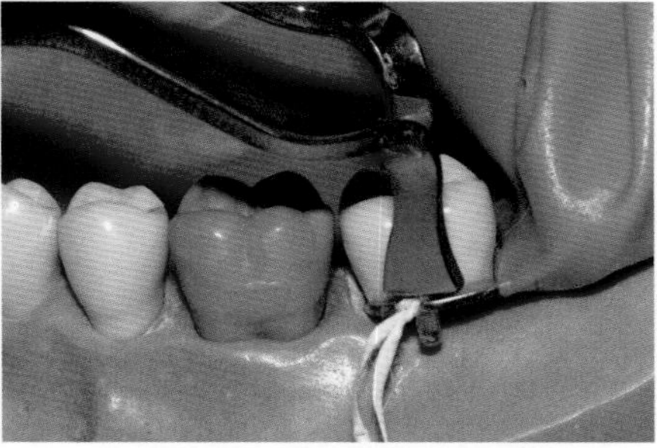

FIGURE 31–23 ✦ In a single step, the retainer is seated and the rubber dam carried in.

tooth. The seating of the retainer requires that the beaks of the rubber dam forceps be placed in the forceps holes. Using a palm grasp, the handles of the forceps are squeezed to separate the jaws of the retainer. The lingual jaw of the retainer is seated first, assuring that both prongs are in contact with the tooth below the height of contour (HOC). While continuing to squeeze the forceps to separate the jaws of the retainer, the facial jaw is rotated over the occlusal surface of the anchor tooth. The jaw is then seated apical to the HOC on the facial surface of the anchor tooth by releasing the pressure on the forceps handles (Figure 31–24). The seating of a stable retainer requires that all four prongs be in contact with the tooth. Having obtained this status, the rubber dam forceps are removed and the stability of the retainer checked by applying pressure to the bow and the lingual and facial jaws of the retainer. There should be no rocking or shifting of the retainer. Rocking and shifting is evidence that all four prongs of the retainer jaws are not in proper contact with the tooth. Two- or three-point contact by the prongs is unacceptable and encourages the retainer to pop off or the contacting jaw prongs to damage the tooth during treatment.

One advantage of the one-step procedure is the elimination of the necessity to stretch the rubber dam over the bow and risk dislodging the retainer from the anchor tooth. Another advantage is that if the retainer becomes dislodged, the rubber dam prevents it from entering the oral cavity and thus from being swallowed. On the other hand, the two-step procedure offers improved visibility when seating the retainer. The selection of a technique is best left to operator preference and experience. The remainder of the placement steps are identical for both techniques. The hole is then stretched to the lingual side and spread over the lingual jaw, then repeated for the facial side. The anchor tooth is now the only tooth isolated in the rubber dam (Figure 31–25). A piece of dental floss is often tied to the jaw of the retainer to facilitate retrieval should the retainer break or be dislodged. This is especially indicated for the two-step procedure. (See Procedure 31–1 for applying rubber dams and Procedure 31–2 for removing rubber dams.)

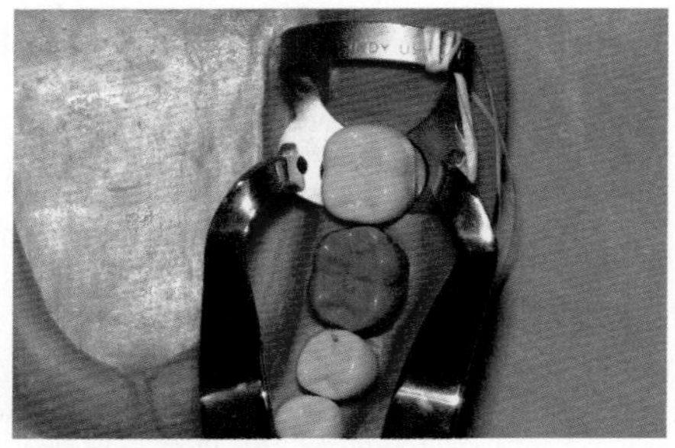

FIGURE 31–24 ✦ The retainer is positioned with rubber dam forceps.

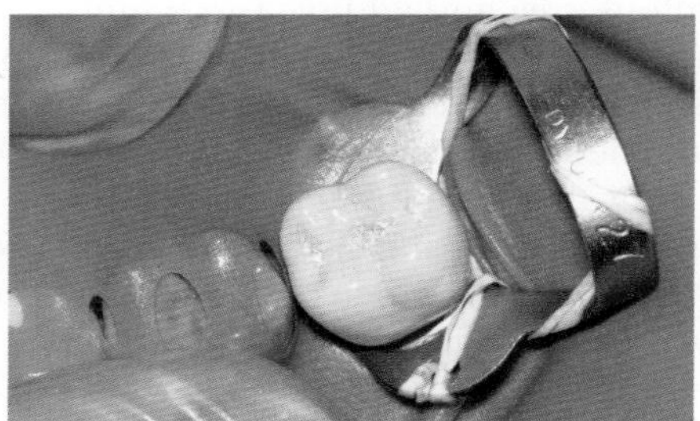

FIGURE 31–25 ✦ The rubber dam hole is stretched to enclose and isolate the retainer and anchor tooth.

Procedure 31–1 APPLYING A RUBBER DAM

EQUIPMENT

- Personal protective equipment
- Protective eyewear for client
- Rubber dam material
- Dental floss or tape
- Rubber dam punch
- Petrolatum
- Rubber dam retainers
- Water-soluble lubricant
- Rubber dam forceps
- Spoon excavator
- Rubber dam frame
- Air-water syringe
- Rubber dam napkin
- Mouth mirror
- Autoclave tape

STEPS	RATIONALE
1. Explain the procedure to the client. Instruct the client to breathe through the nose after application of the rubber dam and to maintain an open mouth after placement of the rubber dam retainer.	The client who is unfamiliar with the procedure is more apprehensive and unable to appreciate the value of the rubber dam to the ultimate success of the restorative treatment. One of the most threatening sensations produced by the rubber dam is the inability to breathe through the mouth. Also, maintaining an open mouth prevents biting on the bow of the retainer, which could cause it to become dislodged.
2. Use a bite block to support the jaws in maintaining an open position when individuals are unable to do this unassisted.	Using a bite block facilitates client comfort.
3. Put on protective eyewear and mask; wash your hands and put on gloves.	Infection control procedures prevent the transmission of microorganisms.

Continued on following page

Procedure 31–1 APPLYING A RUBBER DAM—CONT'D

STEPS	RATIONALE
4. Place protective eyewear on the client.	Protective eyewear prevents injury to the client by airborne objects.
5. Assess the condition of the client's dentition and soft tissues. Confirm the tooth or teeth to be restored. Floss all involved contacts with waxed floss.	These factors influence the operator's application of the rubber dam. Flossing before rubber dam placement lubricates the contacts, identifies difficult areas, and helps "loosen" contacts, making rubber dam placement easier.
6. Remove plaque biofilm, debris, and supragingival calculus.	The removal of oral debris simplifies the application process.
7. Lubricate the client's lips with petrolatum, especially the corners of the mouth.	This lubrication prevents the lips from becoming chapped during isolation.
8. If determined to be necessary, infiltrate a small amount of anesthetic solution adjacent to the area of retainer placement.	Routine injections for pulpal anesthesia may not anesthetize the areas where the retainer retracts the gingiva. Often, the lingual gingiva of maxillary molars and the facial gingiva of mandibular molars will require supplemental anesthesia. The anterior soft tissue is typically not a concern because anterior rubber dams can be successfully retained without retainers.
9. Select the correct size, color, and weight of rubber dam material for the procedure.	These features vary based on client dimensions and operator preference.
10. Mark the key punch for the rubber dam.	The key punch provides a general guide for the placement of all the remaining holes.
11. Mark the remainder of the holes based on the individual client specifications.	The individual placement of holes permits the operator to take into consideration factors such as missing teeth, extra teeth, tight contacts, and misaligned teeth.
12. Punch the holes as marked with a sharp and determined punching action.	It is essential to obtain clean holes free of tears and tags, which hinder the operator's ability to obtain the desired seal.
13. Lubricate the punched rubber dam with a water-soluble lubricant such as shaving cream.	The lubrication helps slip the dam through the contacts and prevents the dam from tearing during application.
14. Select the appropriate rubber dam retainer for the anchor tooth.	The placement of a stable rubber dam requires the selection of a retainer that securely adapts to the tooth.
15. Tie approximately 18 inches of dental floss to the retainer. Tie the floss through the lingual forceps hole, wrap it around the bow, and then tie it through the facial forceps hole.	This safety ligature ensures that both sides of the retainer are secured in the event of retainer breakage (Figure 31–26). It also permits the operator to recover the retainer in the event of dislodgment or breakage to prevent aspiration of the retainer.
16. Punch an additional hole in one of the upper corners of the dam.	This hole orients the dam, allowing the operator to properly align the holes to the respective teeth more quickly and to expedite proper placement of the rubber dam frame.
17. If using the "one-step" placement technique, fixate the anchor tooth hole over the retainer bow prior to placement in the oral cavity.	By carrying the retainer and rubber dam to the mouth in one piece, extra effort to stretch the rubber dam over the retainer is eliminated. Also, the risk of the retainer going down the client's throat is minimized.
18. If the anchor tooth has been restored with a gold or porcelain crown, cover the jaws of the retainer with a protective tape. (Autoclave tape is handy.)	The tape prevents scratching or gouging of the margins of the crown (Figure 31–27).
19. Seat the rubber dam and retainer on the anchor tooth with the rubber dam forceps.	A properly seated retainer has four prongs in contact with the anchor tooth and provides stabilization for the rubber dam. The retainer secures the rubber dam in place to expedite the placement of the remainder of the dam.

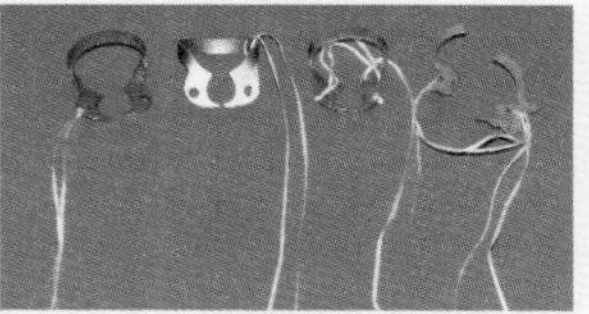

FIGURE 31–26 ✦ Retainer ligation progressing from lingual *(left)* to facial *(right)*, and a broken ligated retainer at far right.

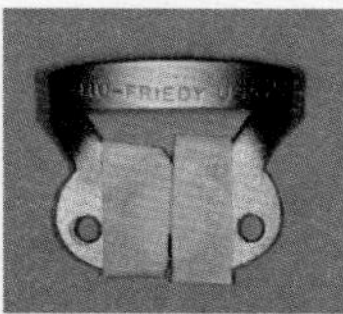

FIGURE 31–27 ✦ Jaws of a retainer covered with protective tape prior to being seated on a gold or porcelain crown.

Procedure 31–1 APPLYING A RUBBER DAM—CONT'D

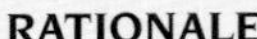

STEPS / **RATIONALE**

20. Reveal most forward tooth to be isolated through the appropriate hole (Figure 31–28). Use a piece of floss or dam to help seat the dam and secure the isolation (Figure 31–29).

This sequence ensures that the beginning and ending holes are appropriately placed and simplifies the isolation of the remaining teeth.

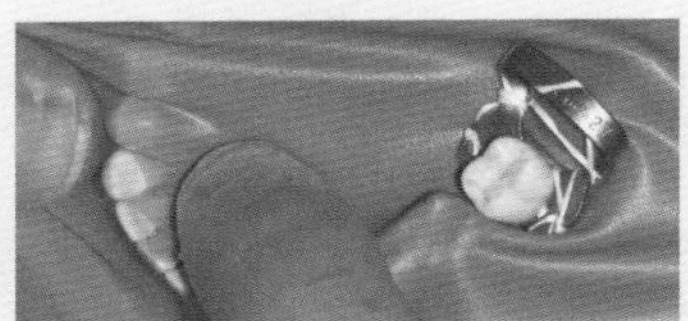

FIGURE 31–28 ✦ The rubber dam is stretched over the most forward tooth to be isolated.

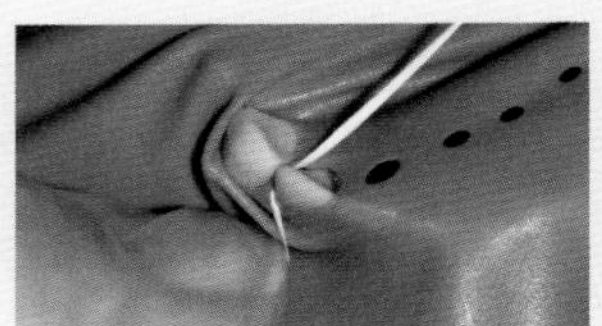

FIGURE 31–29 ✦ Dental floss is used to help seat the rubber dam around the most forward tooth.

21. Place the rubber dam napkin between the rubber dam material and the client's face.

The napkin enhances client comfort.

22. Place the rubber dam frame.

This removes the edges of the rubber dam from the isolation site.

23. Isolate the remainder of the teeth, working from front to back, through the holes. It is important to "tease" a small amount of rubber dam at a time through tight contacts.

This sequence provides an established regimen that provides for the isolation of the easiest teeth first.

24. Pass floss through the contacts using the double floss technique to assist in sliding the rubber dam material through the proximal contacts (Figure 31–30).

Double flossing not only facilitates faster rubber dam placement, but also enables movement of the rubber dam through tight contacts more effectively.

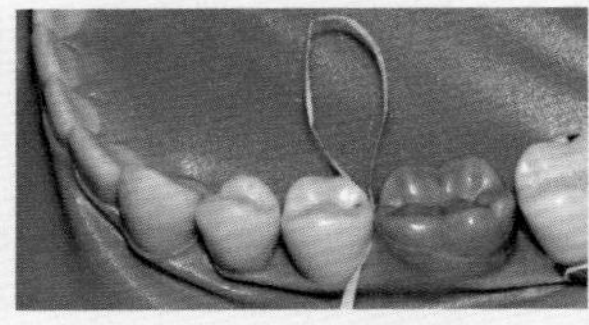

FIGURE 31–30 ✦ Dental floss is used to carry the septa between the teeth using the double flossing technique.

25. Invert rubber dam material when all teeth are completely isolated and the rubber dam is between all contacts. (Several instruments can be used to invert, or tuck, the dam; however, the spoon excavator is the instrument of choice.) Use an air stream to support the inversion process . When the teeth are properly isolated, secure the floss safety ligature to the frame or remove(Figures 31–31 and 31–32).

Inverting the rubber dam around all the teeth ensures a dry, isolated field in which to work.

A safety ligature that is not secured can get entangled in the handpiece and interfere with the operation.

Removal of the ligature is acceptable because the risk of the client swallowing the retainer after the rubber dam is in place is minimal.

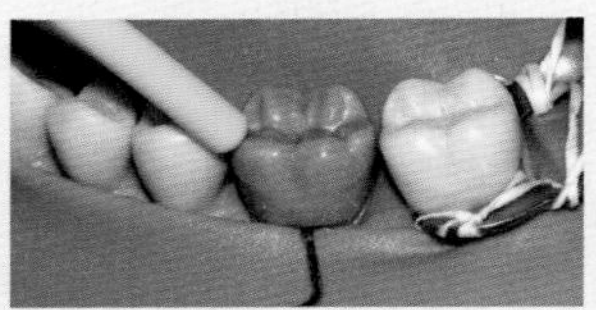

FIGURE 31–31 ✦ The spoon excavator is supported by an air stream to invert the dam and create a seal.

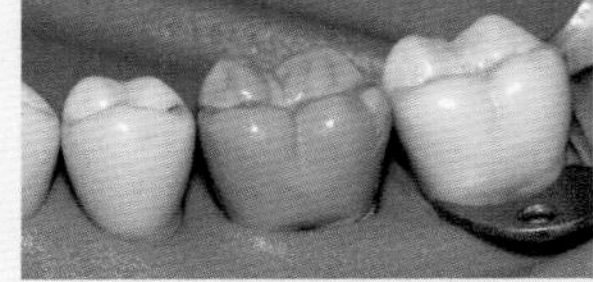

FIGURE 31–32 ✦ A well-sealed, properly inverted rubber dam.

26. Center the rubber dam frame on the client's face, with the upper lip covered and nose revealed. If the nose is inadvertently covered, fold or cut the rubber dam at the top of the frame to uncover the nose. If the client is experiencing nasal congestion or difficulty in breathing through the nasal passage, cut an incision in the rubber dam away from the surgical site to allow air passage.

A well-positioned dam and frame best isolate and facilitate access to the surgical site while still allowing the client to breathe comfortably.

27. Place a saliva ejector under the rubber dam if the client reports or exhibits signs of difficulty in swallowing.

The supplemental evacuation supports the client's efforts to remove saliva from the oral cavity.

Procedure 31–2 REMOVING A RUBBER DAM

EQUIPMENT

Personal protective equipment
Protective eyewear for client
Scissors
Rubber dam forceps
Dental floss or tape

STEPS	RATIONALE
1. Cut the safety ligature, if still present. Replace beaks of the rubber dam forceps in the retainer forceps holes, and spread the jaws of the rubber dam retainer. Raise the facial jaw of the retainer over the contour of the tooth and then raise the lingual jaw (Figure 31–33) to remove the retainer.	The removal of the retainer provides improved access to cut the septa.
2. Cut each septum between teeth with sharp, blunt scissors. On the mandibular arch, stretch the septa facially to improve access for cutting, while protecting the soft tissues by placing a finger under the dam (Figure 31–34). On the maxillary arch, stretch the rubber dam lingually to improve access for cutting.	Expedites the removal of the dam without concern for passage through the contacts.
3. Remove the dam, napkin, and frame together.	When possible, removal of the parts at one time is done for efficiency.
4. Wipe the client's lips to remove excess saliva and debris; rinse and evacuate the mouth.	Enhances client comfort.
5. Briefly massage the client's facial muscles.	This massage relieves the tension in the muscles from prolonged opening; many clients appreciate the show of concern for their comfort.
6. Examine the rubber dam to ensure the removal of all rubber dam fragments and septa.	Small fragments can go undetected and if left between teeth can produce discomfort, inflammation, and potential eventual tooth loss (Figure 31–35).
7. Floss dental contacts to remove any dam fragments as necessary.	Done if necessary to remove fragments.

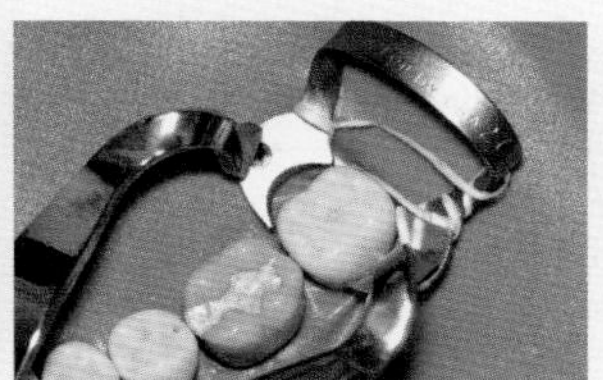

FIGURE 31–33 ✦ The retainer is removed from the tooth with forceps.

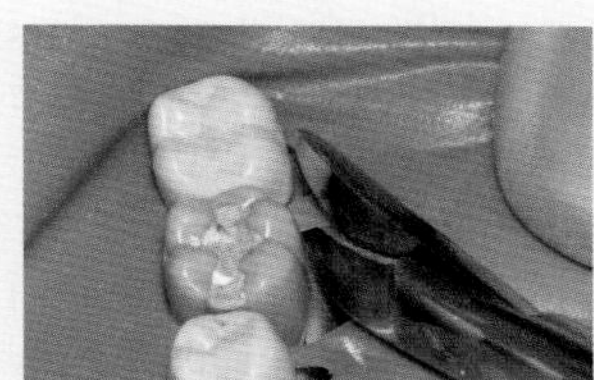

FIGURE 31–34 ✦ Rubber dam is stretched, and septa are cut with scissors.

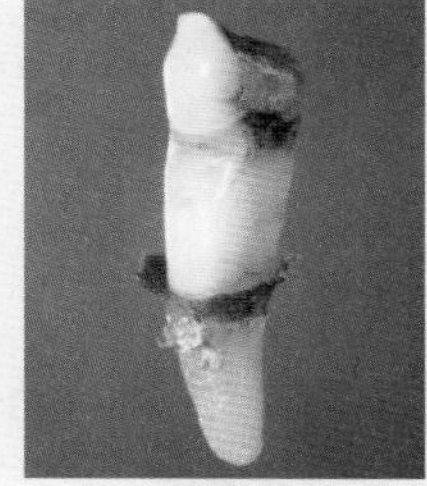

FIGURE 31–35 ✦ Tooth lost to undetected band of rubber dam left after dental treatment.

PERMANENT RESTORATIONS

Amalgam

RATIONALE. Dental amalgam remains the standard restorative material for posterior teeth.[4] Its reputation is based on decades of clinical evaluation during which it has proven to be a durable material even when placed in some highly compromised circumstances. Its longevity is directly related to proper cavity preparation and attention to basic principles of manipulation and condensation in a moisture-free environment.

MATERIAL. *Dental amalgam* is a compound of an alloy—a mixture of metals composed mainly of silver, copper, and tin—with mercury. The function of the mercury is to wet the alloy particles, causing the mass to undergo metallurgical changes. These changes result in a hardened metallic mass that functions well in the oral environment.

Early amalgams were unpredictable in their clinical longevity and were particularly subject to delayed expansion (creep), corrosion, and margin deterioration. Modern amalgam materials show marked improvement in stability, strength, and margin integrity. Amalgam alloy powders are available with spherical particle shapes or with a blend of spherical and lathe-cut particles. Spherical particle alloys handle differently when condensed into cavity preparations. These rounded particles do not resist condensation pressures as do the irregularly shaped, lathe-cut particles. Because the resulting amalgam restorations from both are quite similar, the selection of an alloy particle type is a matter of personal choice.

ARMAMENTARIUM. The following armamentarium is needed for the placement of an amalgam restoration:

Triturator. The triturator or amalgamator is the mechanical device used to mix the encapsulated alloy and mercury (Figure 31–36). It is adjustable for speed and time of trituration to achieve the correct amalgam mix.

Amalgam Well. The amalgam well is a small, heavy, stainless steel "dish" with a cuplike recess that confines the mixed amalgam to facilitate pick-up with the amalgam carrier (Figure 31–37). The mixed amalgam is transferred immediately from the amalgam capsule to the amalgam well after trituration.

Amalgam Carrier. The amalgam carrier is used to carry and dispense amalgam into the cavity preparation (Figure 31–37). Amalgam is loaded into the barrel (cylinder) by pressing the barrel tip into the amalgam mass contained in the amalgam well. When pushed, the instrument lever forces a plunger to dislodge the contained restorative material from the barrel.

Condensing Instruments. Condensing instruments are used to pack amalgam and other restorative materials firmly into a cavity preparation. There are numerous shapes and sizes of condensers (Figure 31–38). Noncutting hand instruments are similar in design to cutting instruments except that the nib replaces the blade and a face replaces the cutting edge (Figure 31–39). Selection of an instrument is based on the size and configuration of the cavity preparation and the amount of material to be condensed.

Carving Instruments. Carving instruments are used to remove excess restorative material and refine the margins of the restoration. All carvers are sharp, cutting instruments. There are numerous blade shapes and sizes that are selected for use based on the carving action to be completed and personal preference (Figure 31–40).

Tofflemire Matrix System. The Tofflemire matrix system is comprised of a Tofflemire retainer, matrix bands, and wedges. The Tofflemire retainer is a stainless steel mechanical device used to hold the matrix band. There are two styles of retainers:

- ✦ Straight (normally used for facial placement)
- ✦ Contra-angle (normally necessary when placed from the lingual)

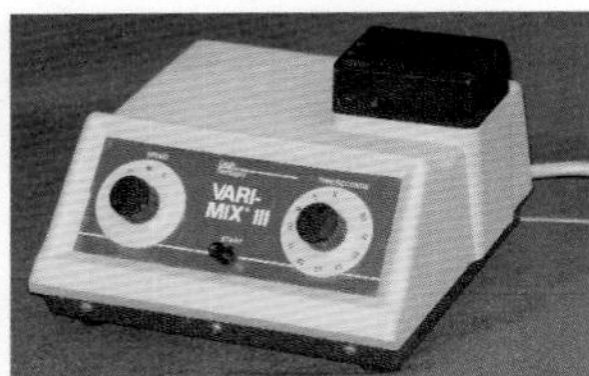

FIGURE 31–36 ✦ A typical amalgam triturator with dials for speed and time selection.

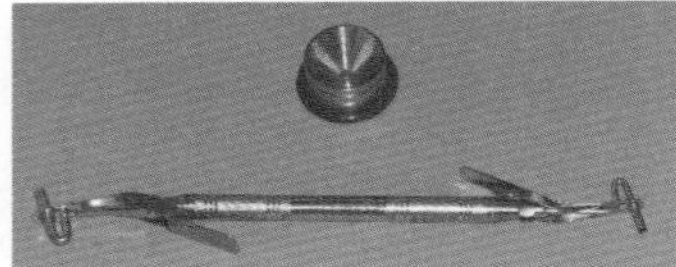

FIGURE 31–37 ✦ Amalgam well and carrier.

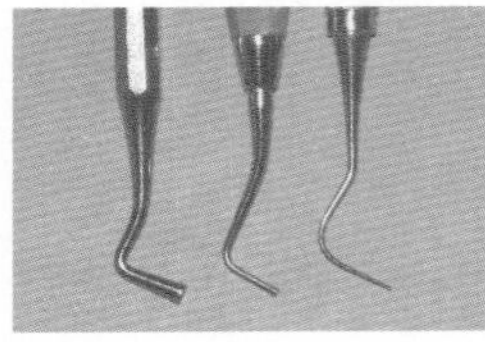

FIGURE 31–38 ✦ Large and small amalgam condensers.

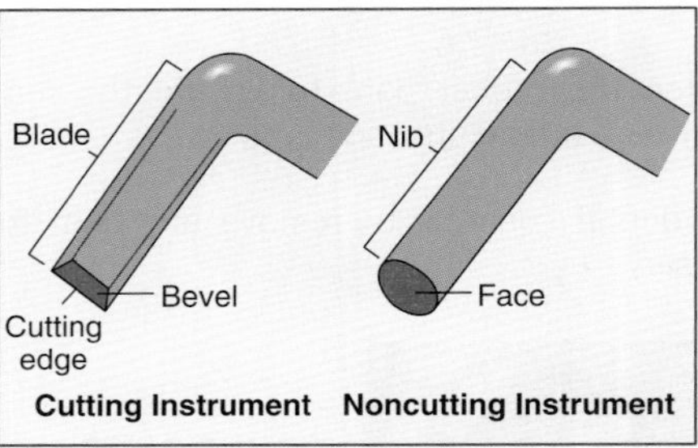

FIGURE 31–39 ✦ Comparison of the working end of a cutting hand instrument with a noncutting hand instrument.

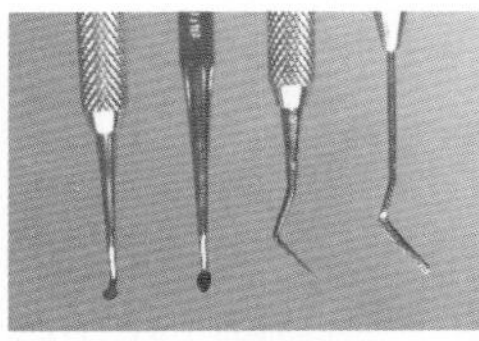

FIGURE 31–40 ✦ Common amalgam carvers. As pictured left to right, cleoid, discoid, 1/2 Hollenback, and Baum interproximal carver (IPC).

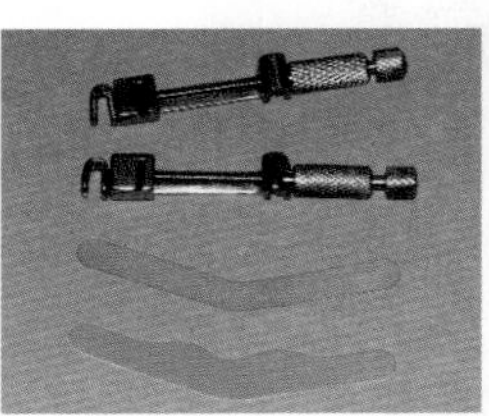

FIGURE 31–41 ✦ Tofflemire retainers and bands. As pictured top to bottom, contra-angle retainer, straight retainer, and modified bands that fit either retainer.

The matrix band is a stainless steel, boomerang-shaped strip that comes in various sizes and adaptations (Figure 31–41). The standard bands are 0.002 inch in thickness. However, contoured bands that are 0.0010 or 0.0015 inches thick often work better. Wedges are typically triangular (in cross section) pieces of wood that also come in numerous sizes and adaptations.

Occlusal Analysis and Tooth Preparation

An analysis of the occlusion is performed to help determine the final morphology of the planned restoration(s). In addition to examining wear facets, it may be useful to mark centric stops (tooth contacts in centric occlusion) and eccentric contacts (tooth contacts during mandibular movement) with articulating ribbon (Figure 31–42). The dentist may choose to modify the cavity shape based on occlusal contacts.

Following this analysis, anesthesia, rubber dam isolation, and cavity preparation are completed to the specifications previously outlined. The cavity preparation is then assessed for the need for sealer, liners, and/or bases. When any of these are determined to be necessary, placement is simplified if it precedes the positioning of the matrix band. A detailed discussion of sealer, liners, and bases is included in a separate section of this chapter.

Matrix and Wedge Placement

A *matrix* is an artificial wall that is needed whenever a lateral wall is missing in a cavity preparation. Typically, a mesial or distal wall is absent in complex posterior cavities. The matrix serves to:

- ✦ Confine the amalgam material during insertion, thereby allowing adequate condensation pressure
- ✦ Provide a framework for reconstruction and contouring of the missing tooth part
- ✦ Support the establishment of proper proximal contacts
- ✦ Prevent amalgam overhangs
- ✦ Burnish contact to make sure contact is obtained

For these reasons, the matrix must be rigid, contoured, and stable. Numerous matrix techniques are available, but by far the most popular and versatile is offered by the Tofflemire matrix system.

A wooden wedge is most often necessary to adequately form the gingival portion of the matrix band. It is usually placed from the lingual because the lingual embrasure is larger than the facial embrasure, thereby allowing a more complete wedge placement. (See Procedure 31–3 for placement of a Tofflemire matrix.) Numerous sizes of pretrimmed wedges are available for selection. The properly shaped and positioned wedge does the following:

- ✦ Gently displaces rubber dam and gingival papilla in an apical direction
- ✦ Supports the matrix band in the proximal space without encroaching on the contact area
- ✦ Adapts the band to the gingival cavity margin
- ✦ Provides slight tooth separation that supports the attainment of a positive proximal contact after the removal of the matrix band

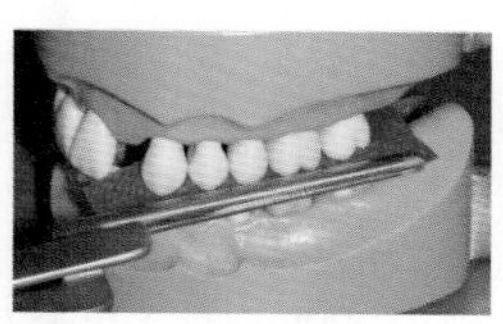

FIGURE 31–42 ✦ Occlusal contacts being registered with articulating ribbon.

Procedure 31–3 PLACING A TOFFLEMIRE MATRIX SYSTEM

EQUIPMENT

Personal protective equipment
Protective eyewear for client
Tofflemire retainer
Matrix bands
Wooden wedges
Metal cutting scissors
Cotton forceps
Modeling compound
Burnishing instrument

STEPS	RATIONALE
1. Evaluate the prepared tooth.	Helps to create a mental picture to aid in the selection of a matrix band.
2. Select a matrix band that (1) best encloses all lateral aspects of the cavity and (2) extends 1 to 2 mm above the adjacent marginal ridge and 1 mm beyond the gingival margin. Trim the band with metal-cutting scissors as necessary (Figure 31–43).	The selection of a band that needs little or no modification simplifies the procedure: (1) Class II cavities that have short proximal boxes can be enclosed with a standard band, (2) tall proximal boxes may require a band with gingival extensions, and (3) a single tall box may need a band with one gingival extension. In any case, all gingival margins must be sealed against the band and the band must extend occlusally high enough to enclose missing ridges and cusps.
3. Select a matrix retainer.	The contra-angle Tofflemire retainer fits most situations; its design allows it to be positioned from the lingual if necessary. The straight Tofflemire retainer is usually limited to facial applications.

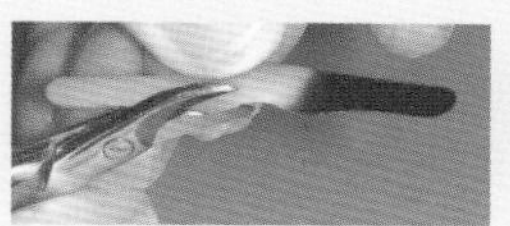

FIGURE 31–43 ✦ Metal-cutting scissors used to modify a matrix band.

Continued on following page

Procedure 31–3 PLACING A TOFFLEMIRE MATRIX SYSTEM—CONT'D

STEPS	RATIONALE
4. Loop the band in your fingers so that the ends are matched. The convergent opening (smaller) of the loop should be positioned next to the gingiva (rubber dam) (Figure 31–44).	The convergent opening is smaller and matches the converging area of the crown (CEJ).

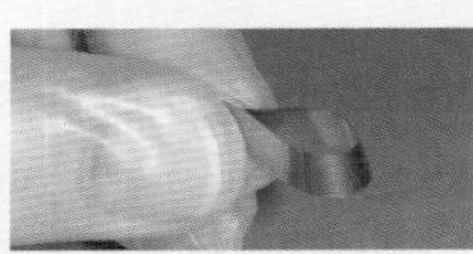

FIGURE 31–44 ✦ The ends of the band are placed evenly together to form a loop. The loop is tapered to permit adaptation at the gingival aspect.

STEPS	RATIONALE
5. Position the locking vise approximately 1/4 inch from the end of the retainer and free the locking screw (spindle) from the band slot in the locking vise (Figure 31–45).	This process prepares the retainer to receive the matrix band.

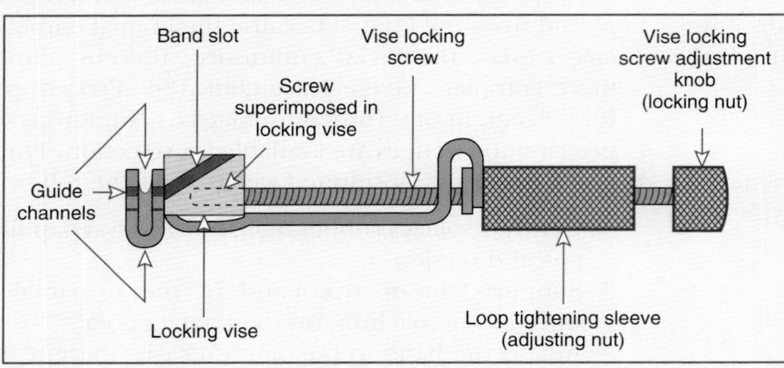

FIGURE 31–45 ✦ Diagram of the Tofflemire retainer.

STEPS	RATIONALE
6. Position the loop in the retainer (leading with the occlusal edge of the band). Insert the matched ends into the slots in the locking vise and the loop into the appropriate guide channel. When positioned, the guide channels of the retainer open toward the gingiva. The loop of the band should exit the guide channel to allow the loop to be positioned from the preferred side of the tooth (usually the facial side). Assuming that the seated retainer will be most commonly positioned on the facial aspect of the prepared tooth, use the left channel guide for dentition in the maxillary left and mandibular right, and use the right channel guide for dentition in the maxillary right and mandibular left. When inserting the band into the retainer, first insert the wider occlusal aspect of the band so that the retainer is seated with the slots of the retainer toward the gingiva (Figure 31–46).	The guide channel orientation allows the Tofflemire to be lifted occlusally when the matrix is being disassembled. If the Tofflemire is inverted (guide channels open occlusally) the retainer is trapped because it cannot be removed in a gingival direction. If this happens, the locking screw must be loosened and the Tofflemire totally removed before the band can be removed.

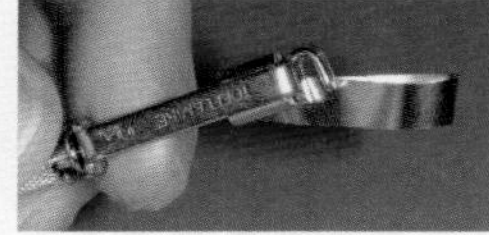

FIGURE 31–46 ✦ The initial placement of the band in the retainer slot with the occlusal aspect of the loop being inserted first.

STEPS	RATIONALE
7. Secure the matrix band by advancing the locking screw (Figure 31–47).	The band must be secured in the retainer or it may loosen during condensation, ruining the restoration.

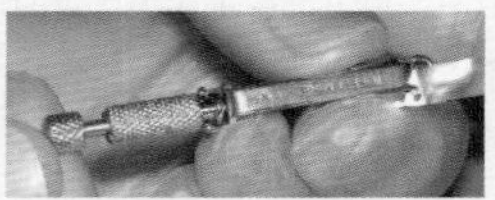

FIGURE 31–47 ✦ The locking nut is tightened to secure the band in the retainer.

STEPS	RATIONALE
8. Shape the matrix loop into a rounded form: (1) insert an instrument handle through the loop, (2) pinch the band between the instrument handle and your thumb, and (3) rotate your wrist as you pinch the band (Figure 31–48).	The opened loop slips over the tooth easily.

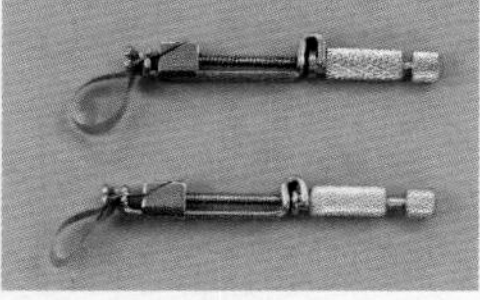

FIGURE 31–48 ✦ Inserted band before shaping *(bottom)* and band shaped to rounded form to facilitate placement *(top)*.

Procedure 31-3 PLACING A TOFFLEMIRE MATRIX SYSTEM—CONT'D

STEPS	RATIONALE
9. Position the loop around the tooth with the slots of the Tofflemire and the narrow aspect of the band toward the gingiva (Figure 31–49); brace the lingual aspect of the loop with the thumb of your opposite hand; gently tighten the band by rotating the adjusting nut. Examine the placement of the band to ensure that the band extends occlusally 1 to 2 mm beyond the adjacent marginal ridge; it should also extend apically approximately 1 mm beyond the gingival margin without impinging on the soft tissue.	The opposite thumb adapts the band against the lingual aspect of the tooth. Extreme tightening of the band tends to pull it away from the adjacent teeth, which could result in open proximal contacts.

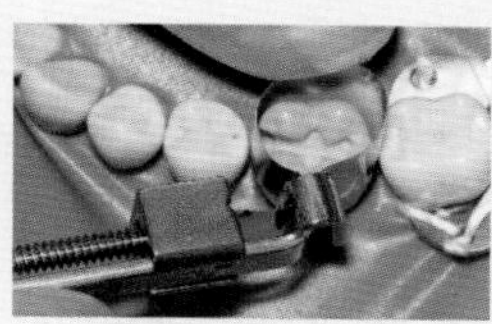

FIGURE 31–49 ✦ Initial placement of band over prepared tooth. Finger pressure supports the lingual aspect of the band.

STEPS	RATIONALE
10. Moisten the wedge(s) and then place it into the lingual embrasure between the band and the adjacent tooth, slightly beyond the gingival margin (Figure 31–50). Apply steady pressure on the base of the wedge to move it in a facial direction and to the desired position (Figure 31–51). Trim the wedge(s) as necessary. With a custom-trimmed wedge, trimming can be accomplished by removing the necessary height or width with a knife or rotary instrument (Figure 31–52). Numerous pretrimmed wedges are available for selection.	Wedges tend to be easier to position when moistened before being positioned. Moisture lubricates the wedge so that it will not stick to the rubber dam, thus making it easier to securely place. Wedge(s) adapt the band at the gingival margin(s); the wedge should not encroach on the proximal contact area, because (1) an open contact may result, or (2) the proximal surface will be undercontoured; these defects could result in food impaction and gingival irritation (Figure 31–53).

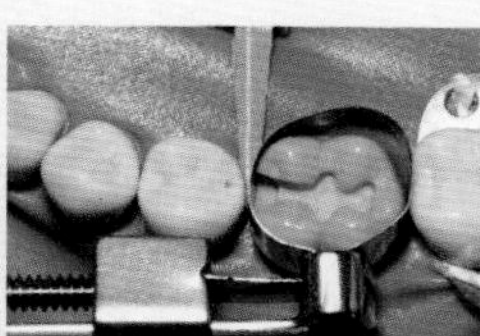

FIGURE 31–50 ✦ Wedge is inserted into the lingual embrasure between the band and the adjacent tooth using cotton forceps.

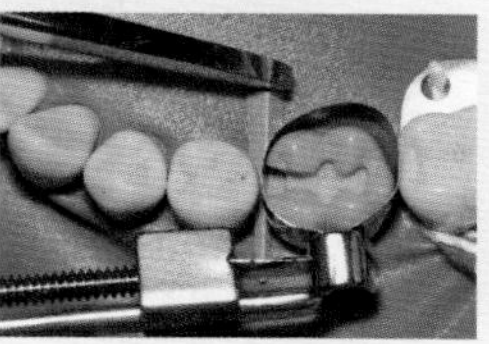

FIGURE 31–51 ✦ The handle of the cotton forceps is used to firmly position the wedge.

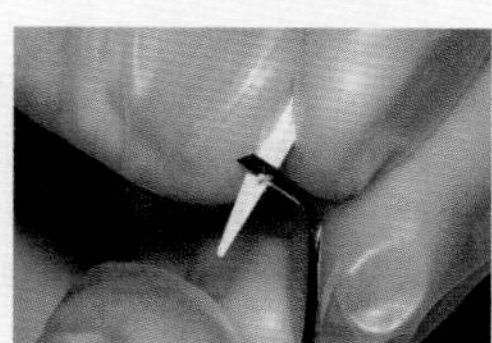

FIGURE 31–52 ✦ Trimming a wooden wedge with a gold knife.

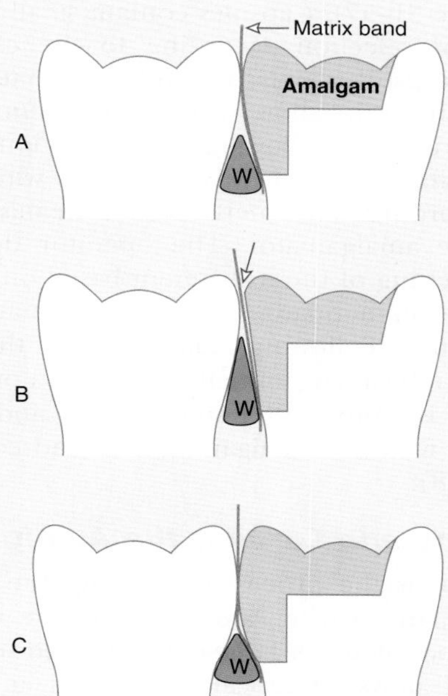

FIGURE 31–53 ✦ **A,** Proper selection and positioning of wedge *(W)* results in normal contour of the proximal surface amalgam. **B,** Untrimmed wedge encroaches on proximal contact area, causing flat, undercontoured surface. High wedge interferes with burnishing/contouring of the matrix band. Proximal contact is likely to be open, inviting food impaction *(arrow)*. **C,** Diminutive wedge may lead to overcontouring of proximal surface and gingival inflammation. The amalgam can be carved to contour, but with difficulty.

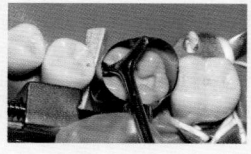

FIGURE 31–54 ✦ The band is firmly burnished against the adjacent tooth.

STEPS	RATIONALE
11. Burnish the internal aspect of the band against the adjacent tooth (teeth) with a thin but rigid instrument (Figure 31–54).	Burnishing facilitates achieving proximal contact(s) and proper proximal contour in the final restoration.

Continued on following page

Procedure 31-3 PLACING A TOFFLEMIRE MATRIX SYSTEM—CONT'D

STEPS	RATIONALE
12. Evaluate the matrix for stability; add warmed modeling compound to the outside of the band as necessary to enhance stability.	An insecure matrix is likely to move during condensation, resulting in fractures throughout the material. Thorough condensation of the amalgam is not possible against a flexible matrix; warmed compound can be easily applied against the band for support (Figure 31–55).
13. Conduct a final evaluation of the cavity preparation with the matrix system in place (Figure 31–56).	This evaluation verifies that the preparation for a quality restoration has been completed.

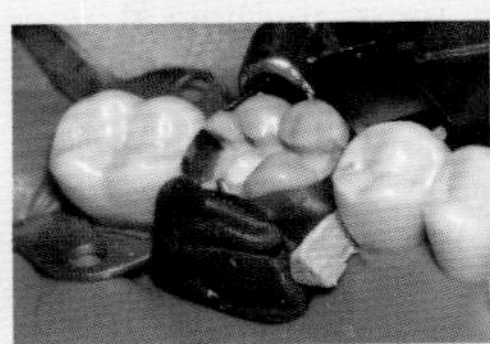

FIGURE 31–55 ✦ Modeling compound is used to stabilize the matrix in this complex cavity preparation.

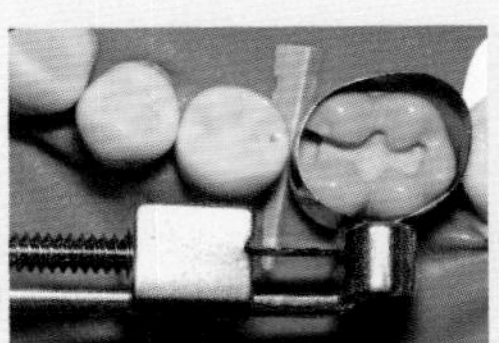

FIGURE 31–56 ✦ Final preparation and matrix system.

Trituration

Modern amalgam materials are preencapsulated to prevent mercury spills and provide consistent quality of mixes (Figure 31–57). Capsules contain small and large quantities for selection according to the cavity size. Within each capsule is a plastic diaphragm that separates the mercury from the alloy. At the start of *trituration,* the diaphragm ruptures, allowing amalgamation (trituration) to begin. Thorough mixing occurs within a few seconds, according to the metallurgy of the mass and the speed of the amalgamator. The operator determines the proper setting of the instrument based on the manufacturer's recommendation, the amalgam material, and the desired mix. Following amalgamation, the mass is transferred to the amalgam well. Generally, a proper mix of amalgam is shiny and homogeneous and is easily manipulated with the amalgam carrier and condensers (Figure 31–58).

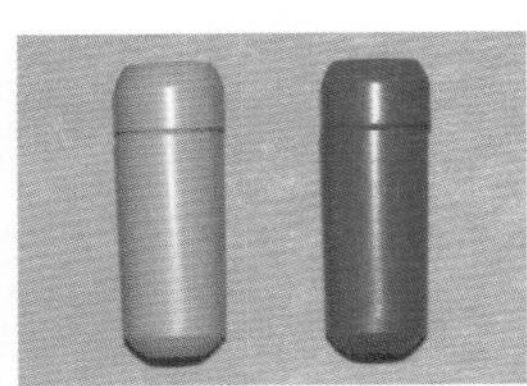

FIGURE 31–57 ✦ Common preencapsulated amalgam capsules.

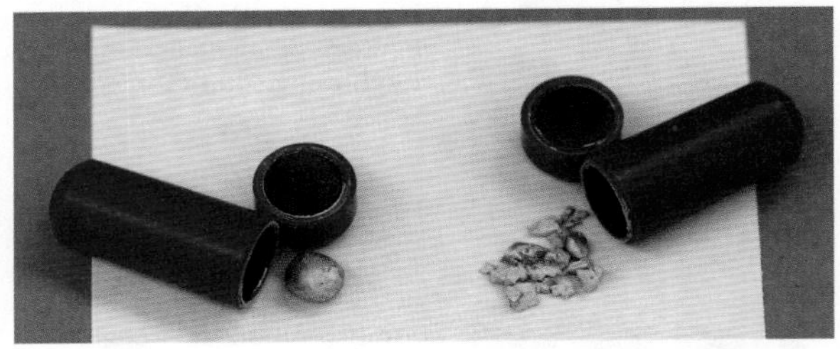

FIGURE 31–58 ✦ Soft, shiny proper amalgam mix *(left)* and dry, crumbly overtriturated mix *(right).*

Condensing and Carving the Amalgam

Condensation is the process of packing the amalgam into the prepared cavity. Adequate pressure is approximately 8 lb per inch^2 for lathe-cut alloys and slightly less for spherical alloys. Spherical particles make the alloy more fluid, which allows the use of a larger diameter condenser tip to achieve adequate condensation pressure. Lathe-cut particles, because of their irregular shape, offer more resistance to condensation. Therefore, a smaller diameter condenser tip and more condensation pressure should be used for adequate condensation. Carving is the process of using hand instruments to shape the freshly placed amalgam into the anatomic form that will restore the tooth to function. (See Procedure 31–4 for placing an amalgam restoration.)

Finishing and Polishing

Polished amalgam retains less plaque biofilm and resists tarnish and corrosion better than unpolished amalgam. After several hours, the amalgam hardens fully and can be polished to a high degree of smoothness. Obtaining a smooth surface is more important than achieving a high gloss on the metallic surface. The gloss is usually short-lived because of the scouring action of certain foods.

It is imperative in the polishing procedures that *undue heat is not generated* from rotating rubber cups and points as they contact the amalgam. Such heat can harm the pulp, leaving the tooth very sensitive. The metallurgy of the amalgam also can be adversely affected. Air coolant should be directed against the metallic surface whenever heat generation is a possibility.

Finishing and polishing procedures vary in materials and technique. However, the first step in the procedure is to recheck the occlusion to ensure that in polishing the operator does not destroy important occlusal contacts. If the carving has left a smooth amalgam, polishing proceeds simply and rapidly. In most cases, it is not realistic

Procedure 31–4 PLACING AN AMALGAM RESTORATION

EQUIPMENT

Personal protective equipment
Protective eyewear for client
Isolation materials
Triturator
Amalgam well
Amalgam carrier
Amalgam capsules
Condensing instruments
Tofflemire matrix system
Carving instruments
Articulating paper

STEPS	RATIONALE
1. Pretest access to the cavity by holding condenser nibs in the confined areas of the preparation to verify accurate condenser selection.	Condensers that are too large cannot adapt the amalgam to the internal aspects of the cavity.
2. Adjust triturator settings for speed and time of mix, according to manufacturer's recommendations.	Triturators vary in speeds; amalgam alloys also vary in composition and mixing requirements.
3. Secure the amalgam capsule in the triturator locking device and close the protective lid.	If not securely placed, the capsule may be propelled from the locking device, injuring someone or breaking open.
4. Mix the amalgam and remove the capsule; open it over a catch tray and dispense the mix into the amalgam well.	The tray catches loose fragments of amalgam; on occasion, amalgamation may not occur and free mercury could spill out when the capsule is opened.
5. Examine the mixed amalgam; note the time, or set a timer for 3 minutes.	The amalgam should be a soft, round, shiny ball of material. A dry, crumbly mix should be placed in the scrap container and a new mix prepared. Even proper mixes should be discarded after 3 minutes. Older amalgam cannot be properly condensed and will not produce a homogeneous mass.
6. Load the small end of the amalgam carrier; dispense a portion of this into the most confined area of the preparation (Figure 31–59).	Attempting to rapidly fill the cavity with large increments produces voids in critical parts of the restoration; voids at margins invite leakage, sensitivity, and recurrent caries.
7. Using small condensers and a stable hand position, firmly adapt the amalgam into all internal cavity features and over the margins (Figure 31–60).	Firm pressure with smaller condensers is less likely to produce voids in confined areas. Firm condensation is intended to (1) adapt the material intimately to cavity walls, (2) eliminate voids, and (3) express excess mercury from the mass.
8. Continue to add increments; gradually increase condenser size; remove any "mercury-rich" surface by lateral scooping motions of the condenser nib.	Firm condensation expresses mercury from the mass; its removal creates a dense, more durable restoration.
9. Triturate fresh amalgam as needed; continue to add increments and condense, to build a moderate excess over the cavity margins (Figures 31–61 and 31–62).	Larger cavities may require several mixes; if the mix begins to harden, discard it Overpacking ensures coverage of all margins and, when the material is heavily burnished, draws excess mercury to the surface so it can be readily carved away.
10. Rub and grossly shape the occlusal surface with a few firm strokes using a large ball of egg-shaped burnisher (Figure 31–63).	Excess mercury is brought to the surface for easy removal.
11. Carve and suction away all gross excess amalgam.	Removal of the mercury-rich amalgam leaves a dense, durable alloy.

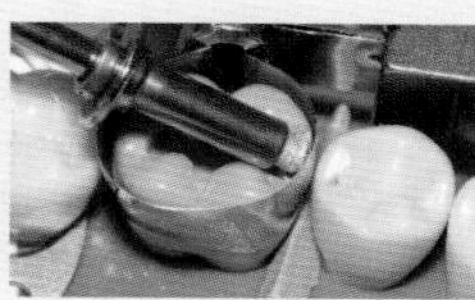

FIGURE 31–59 ✦ A small increment of amalgam is expressed into the proximal box of the cavity preparation.

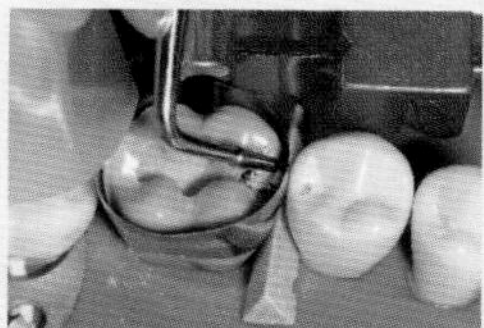

FIGURE 31–60 ✦ Initial condensation is begun with a small condenser in the proximal box.

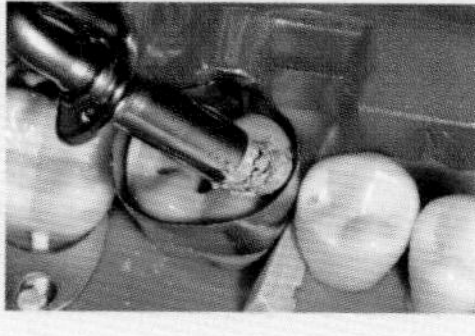

FIGURE 31–61 ✦ Additional increments of amalgam are carried to the cavity preparation.

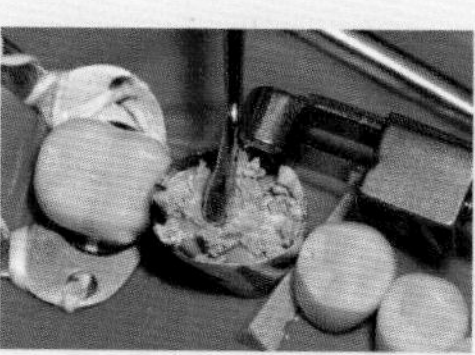

FIGURE 31–62 ✦ The cavity is overfilled with amalgam, and a large condenser is used to complete condensation.

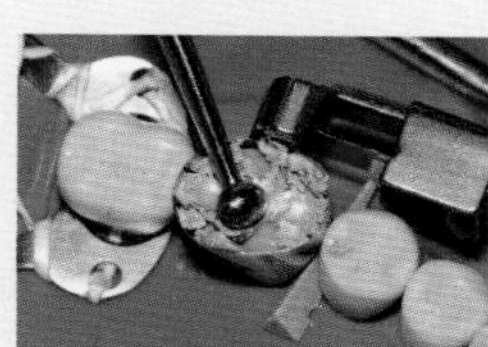

FIGURE 31–63 ✦ Burnishing of the overpacked amalgam.

Continued on following page

Procedure 31–4 PLACING AN AMALGAM RESTORATION—CONT'D

STEPS	RATIONALE
12. Establish the marginal ridge height and outer contours next to the matrix band by carving with an explorer or similar fine, sharp instrument. The excess amalgam is rapidly carved away, and occlusal margins are recovered (Figures 31–64 to 31–66).	Marginal ridge contours are the most difficult to form and so should be shaped while the amalgam is carvable and while the matrix is in place.
13. Release the matrix band from the retainer by loosening the band tightener and locking nut; remove wedges (Figure 31–67).	Removal of the matrix system en masse is difficult and may fracture the amalgam.
14. While maintaining gentle pressure on the marginal ridge with a large amalgam condenser, lift the matrix band from the unrestored proximal area first, then finally from the restored area (Figure 31–68).	The apically directed force of the condenser resists the occlusally directed removal of the matrix band, preventing marginal ridge fracture; removing the band from the unrestored area first reduces pressure on the restored proximal contact.
15. Explore the gingival margin for excess (overhang); carve away any excess with a fine-bladed instrument (such as an IPC carver) (Figures 31–69 and 31–70).	The gingival margin is the least accessible margin; it should be finalized before the amalgam becomes too hard.
16. Carve all proximal and outer contours to final form. Recover all margins. At the margins, all cutting strokes should be directed parallel to the margins to maintain a seal and to avoid overcarving. The tooth surface should be used as a guide by resting the carving edge on it as shaving strokes are made. Carve occlusal anatomy to general form, keeping pits and grooves shallow (Figure 31–71).	Steep anatomy in amalgam leads to marginal breakdown.
17. Remove the rubber dam; caution the client against biting at this time.	Inadvertent biting will likely fracture the amalgam because the occlusal surface has not yet been refined.
18. Wipe client's lips carefully and suction the mouth to remove saliva; isolate the operating site with cotton rolls.	Occlusal marking ribbon (articulation paper) does not mark well on wet surfaces.

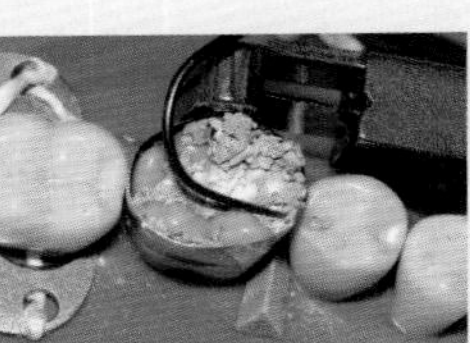

FIGURE 31–64 ✦ Marginal ridge height and outer contours are established with an explorer.

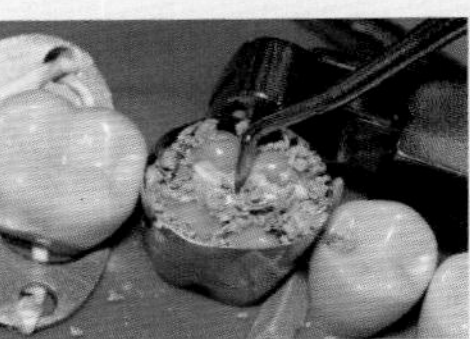

FIGURE 31–65 ✦ Excess amalgam is removed with a carver.

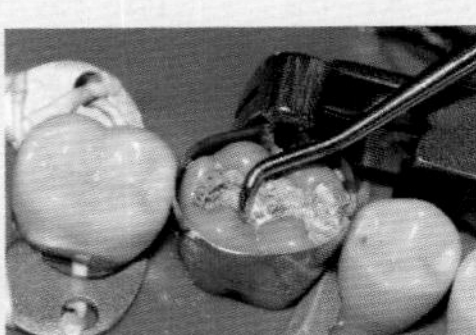

FIGURE 31–66 ✦ Occlusal margins are recovered.

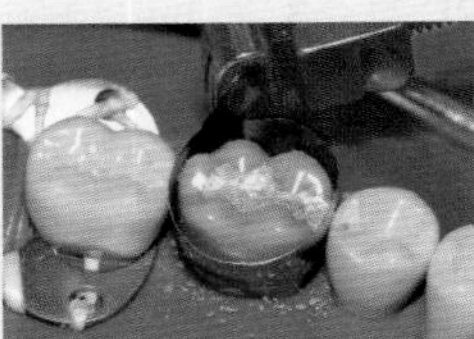

FIGURE 31–67 ✦ The wedge has been removed, and the retainer loosened from the band.

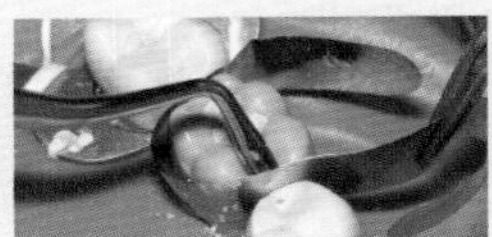

FIGURE 31–68 ✦ An amalgam condenser is used to stabilize the marginal ridge during the removal of the band.

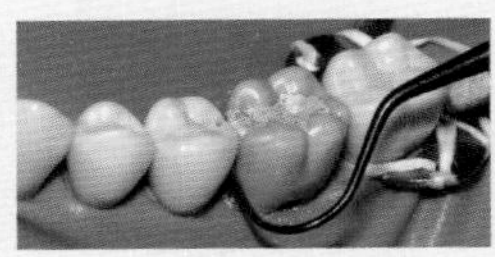

FIGURE 31–69 ✦ Gingival margin is checked for excess amalgam with an explorer.

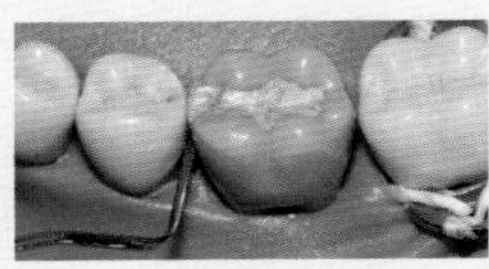

FIGURE 31–70 ✦ Excess amalgam at the gingival margin is carved away.

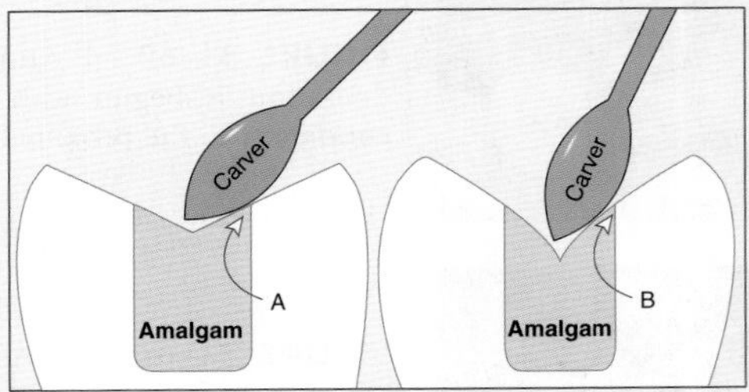

FIGURE 31–71 ✦ Amalgam anatomy should be carved to shallow form whenever possible. Doing so produces stronger margins *(A)*. Thin angles seen in *(B)* will eventually fracture from occlusal stress.

Procedure 31–4 PLACING AN AMALGAM RESTORATION—CONT'D

STEPS	RATIONALE
19. Insert articulating paper over the area and have the client "gently tap the back teeth together."	Forceful biting on fresh amalgam will cause fracture; tapping is done to examine centric occlusion.
20. Carve away marking spots on the amalgam until centric occlusion is reestablished as it was before the operation; re-mark the occlusion as necessary, carving away "high spots" each time with a carver or round burr, if the amalgam has set up (Figure 31–72).	Centric occlusion is reestablished by noting that wear facets on the remaining tooth structure as well as on adjacent and opposing teeth imprint even marks.
21. Insert the ribbon and have the client "gently grind the back teeth," making sure the client moves the teeth in all functional directions. Remove markings until presurgical contacts are restored.	Eccentric prematurities are removed.
22. Finalize the carving, rinse and suction away all debris, and caution the client not to chew on the restored tooth until the following day.	Amalgam requires several hours to achieve its maximal hardness.
23. After putting the client in an upright position, have the client "tap-tap-tap" again, then look at the new restoration for "shiny spots." Repeat the procedure; having the client grind his/her teeth for lateral movement. Adjust high spots as necessary.	A shift from the prone position of the dental chair to an upright position can produce a different bite pattern because the mandible changes position.
24. Caution the client that discernible "high spots" should be adjusted to avoid fracture.	The client may later be aware of a "high spot" when the anesthesia has worn off.

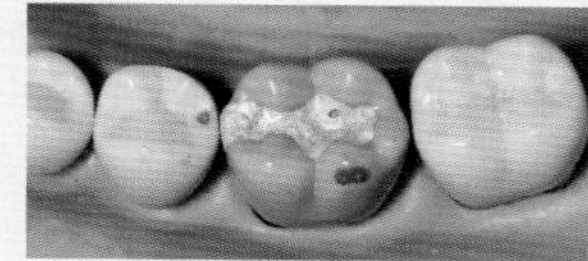

FIGURE 31–72 ✦ The occlusal markings show that the contact on amalgam, although present, is lighter than that on the natural tooth. As a result, the operator does not need to further reduce the occlusal contact.

to attempt a polish of the proximal surface. If it is smooth, it should be left alone except for a brief "shoeshine" using wet flour pumice and dental tape. Other areas can be finished with discs, brushes, and rubber cups and points. A flour of pumice slurry and other polishing powders are used by many operators. More recently, abrasives were incorporated into special rubber polishing cups and points. After the amalgam margins have been refined with a sharp carver or finishing burr, these polishing cups and points are excellent for producing a smooth metallic surface. Using a light intermittent touch and rotary speeds in the slow-to-moderate range, the operator can rapidly produce an excellent finish. A periodic reshaping of the rubber points, rounded from wear, against an abrasive disc enables the operator to properly polish grooves and fossae. (See Procedure 31–5 for finishing and polishing amalgam restorations.)

Mercury Hygiene

In dentistry, the care exercised in preventing bodily harm from mercury ingestion or inhalation is termed *mercury hygiene.* There is little question that disregard for mercury's potential to cause disease may produce injury. However, in decades of use, careful handling of mercury has made it and dental amalgam safe.[4,5] Practitioners may routinely restore teeth with amalgam with the assurance that, by exercising reasonable care, no harm will come to the professional staff or their clients. Alarmists have attempted to discredit not only the benefits of amalgam, but also the virtues of dentists who recommend amalgam. Many of their claims are based on half-truths and are motivated by reasons that are unclear.

The individuals primarily at risk from mercury exposure are dental personnel. In busy restorative practices, common sense provides a more than adequate margin of safety. This safety begins with work and storage spaces that are well ventilated. Special filters and detectors are available to monitor mercury vapors. In addition, a periodic monitoring service for mercury air levels is available through dental societies. Bulk stores of mercury are not recommended. Amalgam should be used as premeasured mercury and alloy and mixed in sealed capsules. Triturators are available that provide enclosed spaces for the capsules being triturated. All handling of amalgam mixes should be done over a deep tray to contain loose particles and promote easy cleanup of scrap amalgam. Carpeting in the work area is not recommended because periodic vacuuming of scrap amalgam may release mercury vapors. Scrap amalgam should be stored in airtight containers and covered with x-ray fixer (sulfide) solution or other inactivating solutions. Disposal of amalgam

Procedure 31–5 FINISHING AND POLISHING AMALGAM RESTORATIONS

EQUIPMENT

Personal protective barriers (safety glasses, mask, gloves, gown)
Isolation materials
Finishing burrs
Carving instruments
Handpiece
Rubber polishing cups and points (or flour of pumice and polishing powders)

STEPS	RATIONALE
1. Question the client regarding occlusion and tooth sensitivity since the operation.	Sensitivity may indicate premature centric and/or eccentric contacts; polishing should be delayed for very sensitive teeth.
2. Explain the value of polished versus unpolished restoration to the client.	The polished amalgam resists plaque biofilm retention, corrosion, and tarnish.
3. Isolate and dry the area.	For a simple polish, cotton roll isolation is adequate; several adjacent polishes or polishes in conjunction with new restorative treatment are best done under rubber dam isolation for improved visibility and control of polishing debris.
4. Examine the amalgam for burnish marks; adjust occlusion as necessary with a round finishing burr.	Burnish marks indicate occlusal contacts; large areas and areas on inclines should be reduced, consistent with the client's natural occlusion.
5. Refine the occlusal margins with a sharp discoid carver, drawn in shaving strokes parallel to the margins (Figure 31–73).	Minute excess amalgam is shaved flush with the margins, preventing fracture; parallel strokes reduce the possibility of enamel microfractures and overcarving the amalgam.
6. Using slow-to-moderate speeds and intermittent brief strokes, polish the amalgam with abrasive-impregnated rubber cups and points (Figures 31–74 and 31–75.) Begin with the most abrasive and end with the least abrasive; direct a gentle stream of air onto the amalgam during polishing procedures; avoid overpolishing established occlusal contacts.	Rotary rubber instruments rapidly generate heat due to friction; this can create pulpal sensitivity and damage the amalgam restoration. Once proper occlusal contacts are established, they should be maintained.
7. Remove isolation materials and rinse the mouth of debris.	Debris and excess saliva are annoying to the client.
8. Show the client the polished restoration(s) and reiterate the value of the procedure (Figure 31–76).	This helps to further instill confidence; clients may be motivated to take better care of their teeth; they appreciate professionalism and pride in extra effort.

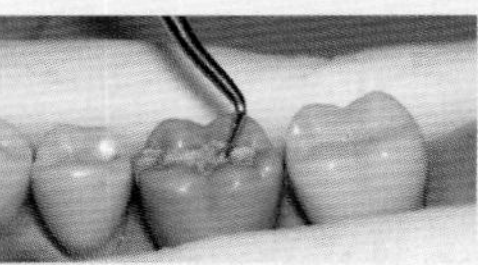

FIGURE 31–73 ✦ Using a stroke parallel to the margin, a sharp carver refines occlusal margins of the amalgam.

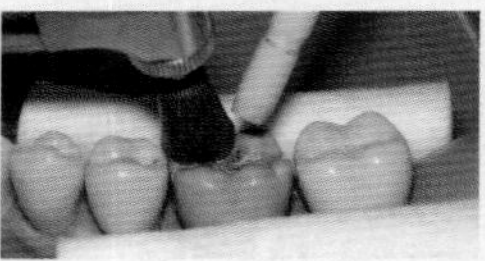

FIGURE 31–74 ✦ A rubber polishing cup is used to polish the marginal ridge and cusp slopes. An air stream is used as a coolant.

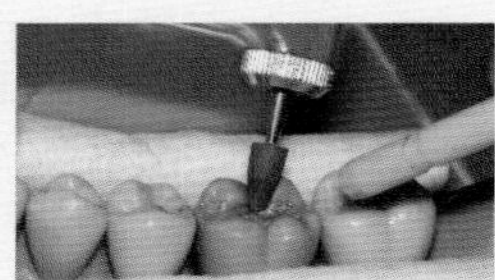

FIGURE 31–75 ✦ A rubber polishing point is used to polish pits and grooves.

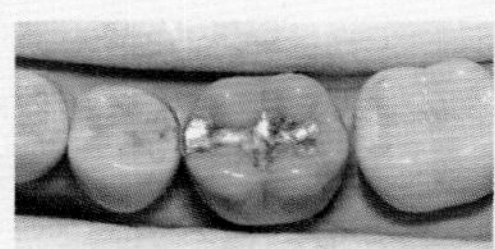

FIGURE 31–76 ✦ A polished amalgam.

capsules and other contaminated materials should be done in compliance with state and local environmental and safety policies. Careful examination and cleaning of trays, amalgam wells, chair seams, and other susceptible areas may reveal small scrap particles that should be recovered safely and stored. In addition, evacuation traps should be cleaned routinely and amalgam scrap properly stored. Amalgam carriers should be checked for residual amalgam. The practice of heating a carrier over a flame to soften and remove clogged amalgam should be avoided because the release of mercury fumes may be toxic.

Significant client exposure to mercury is negated by the brevity of the dental appointment and by controlled and clean placement of the amalgam. Rubber dam isolation provides the best control of the surgical site. All scrap is readily removed when the dam is in place. Careful and thorough suctioning of particles is recommended. The combining of the mercury with the alloy prevents the release of mercury in a significant quantity. The claim by a few individuals that dentists are poisoning their clients has not been demonstrated or proven scientifically. Except in cases of client allergy to mercury, which is rare, oral healthcare professionals may continue to render fine restorative care using amalgam.

Resin Composites

RATIONALE. *Resin composite* is tooth-colored restorative material made of complex organic resin that is hardened by chemical and/or light activation. Resin composite is the best material for conservative tooth-colored restorations. Its use has generally been limited to the anterior teeth and non–stress-bearing areas of posterior teeth. When clinically compared to amalgam, the wear resistance of tested resin composites is inadequate to justify their routine use in areas of high occlusal stress.[6] However, more and more posterior composites are being successfully placed because of the improved materials and techniques available.

MATERIAL. One of the great advances in operative dentistry was the development of a new, highly stable resin (BIS-GMA).[7] This complex organic resin has become the basis for the remarkable influx of new and steadily improving direct tooth-colored materials. The latest and best materials are activated and hardened by exposing the material to a special light. The light-activated materials are denser and more color stable than other resins. Dual-cure resin composites are also available for use in areas where light-curing is desirable but access to achieve a total curing of the material is compromised or doubtful. In these cases, the material will set up in spite of the inability to light-cure all the material. Incremental placement and curing overcomes much of the polymerization shrinkage common to bulk placement and allows the operator to develop the contours and shade blends of each restoration. Resin composite is often provided by manufacturers in handy dispensing devices (Figure 31–77).

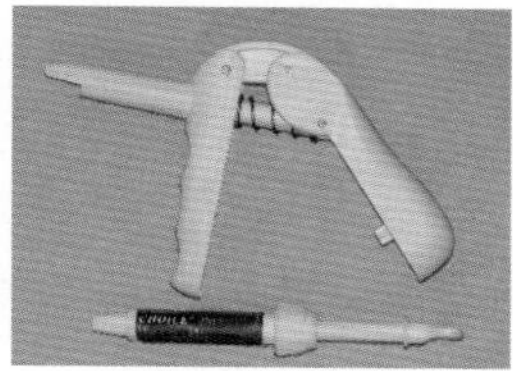

FIGURE 31–77 ✦ Two dispensing devices used to express limited quantities of resin composite. These containers are opaque to prevent polymerization due to exposure to sunlight.

Resin composite procedures and cavity design are unique. The research of Buonocore has provided a means for conserving tooth structure by his discovery that retention and resistance form for resins can be created on enamel.[8] This concept, known as *enamel bonding,* has become the basis for the routine placement of modern direct resin restorations and for such popular procedures as pit and fissure sealants and bonded veneers. As long as the prepared tooth presents an adequate enamel surface area, significant retention can be achieved via a careful technique. The enamel surface is shaped with instruments such as rotary burrs or diamonds to establish the desired design. Then, the controlled application of an acidic conditioning agent to the prepared enamel roughens the surface (acid etching). Thorough rinsing and forced-air drying displays the etched enamel (frosty appearance), which is ready to receive a primer and/or bonding resin and thereby retain a resin restoration. The bond attained in this manner is termed a micro-mechanical bond.

Compared to enamel bonding, dentin bonding is far less predictable. Lack of inorganic structure results in a weaker bond to organic collagen fibrils. The composition of dentin presents special challenges for those attempting to bond to it. Dentin is more organic than enamel and, when instrumented, leaves a surface covered with microscopically observable debris. This *smear layer* may interfere with strong bonding at the dentin–resin interface. In addition, a trace amount of moisture emanating from the vital pulp is present on the dentin surface. Because restorative resins are incompatible with moisture (hydrophobic), numerous adhesive systems (hydrophilic) have been developed to chemically unite the resin with the moist dentin surface. Most of these adhesives are tested in laboratory settings using extracted teeth. Oral health professionals have little assurance that they will be as successful when used clinically.

For many years, damage to a vital pulp from the toxic effects of dental materials was perceived to be the most important concern regarding dentin bonding. This concern centered around the cleansing or "conditioning" procedures that preceded the application of the bonding resin, because these procedures "opened" the dentinal tubules, exposing the vital pulp to insult. However, recent research has demonstrated that any inflammatory reaction to dental materials is transitory. In fact, adverse pulpal discomfort has been shown to be the result of invasion by bacteria and/or their toxins through inadequately sealed restorations.[9] Therefore, an optimal enamel and dentinal seal is of utmost importance. Shallow cavities limited to enamel can be acid-etched with impunity, because enamel is inert and virtually free of vital tissue. However, most cavities extend into dentin and it is the treatment of this tissue surface that is in question. The majority of manufacturers recommend the removal or modification of the dentinal smear layer by conditioning agents (usually acids). Current conditioning techniques utilize weaker acids and shorter exposure times. The trend in resin composite systems is also to combine the conditioning, priming, and bonding agents into one liquid for application. The reason for this combination of solutions is to facilitate enhanced permeation of the bonding agent into the dentinal tubules.

ARMAMENTARIUM. The following armamentarium is needed to place a resin composite:

Curing Light. The curing light is required to initiate polymerization of the resin matrix. The light is in the blue range and is transmitted from its electrical source via a fiberoptic bundle to the tip of a small wand that is positioned on the tooth surface (Figure 31–78). An intensity of 400 m Wcm^{-2} is considered adequate.[10]

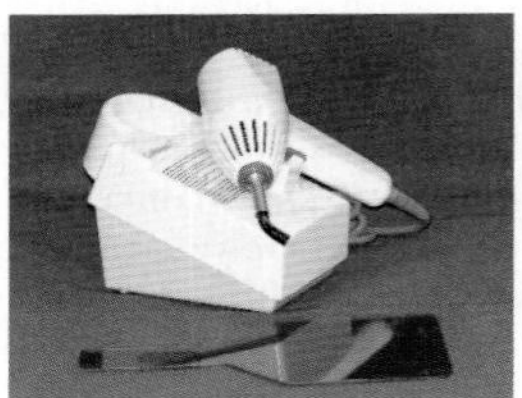

FIGURE 31–78 ✦ A light source for polymerization and a hand-held protective shield.

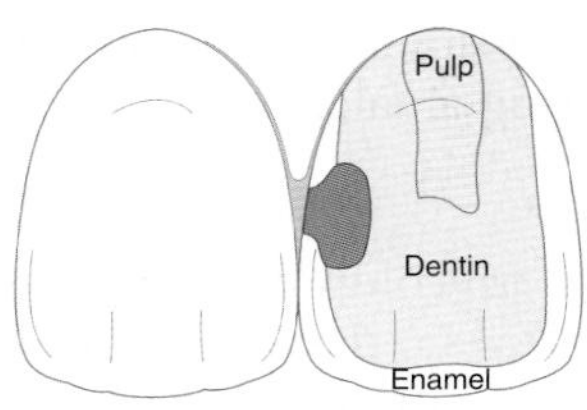

FIGURE 31–80 ✦ Class III carious lesion depicted. Caries is shown invading the dentin, but the cavity does not endanger the incisal corner.

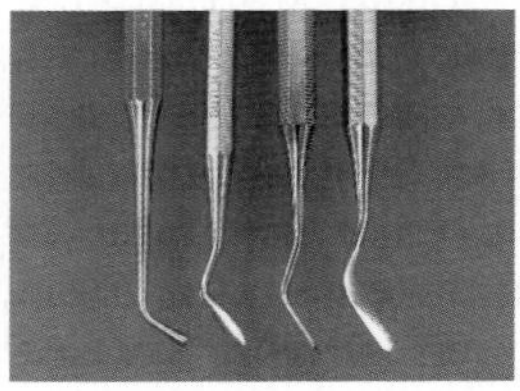

FIGURE 31–79 ✦ Common plastic instruments.

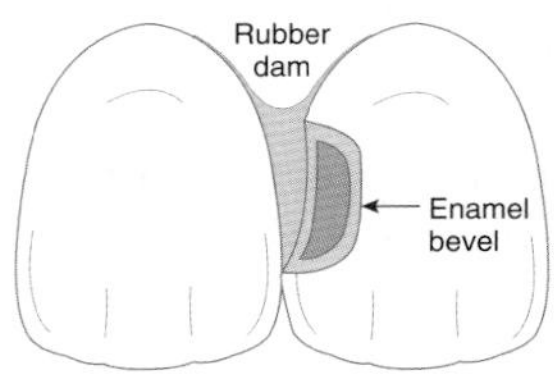

FIGURE 31–81 ✦ Lingual view of the completed Class III cavity preparation. The dentin is protected by a cavity liner, an enamel bevel has been placed, and the rubber dam retracts the gingiva to provide access.

Protective Shields. Protective shields are available to prevent eye injury and meet the human need for protection from health risks. The wavelengths produced by the curing light have been shown to damage the retina and must be screened to protect operator, assistant, and client. Protective shields may be hand-held, attached to the wand, or incorporated in specially made eyeglasses.

Plastic Instruments. Special composite placement instruments are conveniently designed to carry, shape, and mold soft (plastic) materials. They may be blunt-ended instruments or flat blades not intended for firm condensation or cutting (Figure 31–79). Selection of instruments is based on the location of the cavity preparation and personalized preference. Anodized instruments have been specifically developed to facilitate placement of sticky, tooth-colored materials without adhering to the instrument.

Class III Restoration Placement and Finishing

Before applying the rubber dam, small samples of resin composite should be placed on the tooth surface and cured for 20 to 30 seconds. Matching the tooth shade before it becomes dry (and lighter in shade) under isolation ensures a closer shade match in the final restoration. Resin also tends to change slightly in shade after curing. Removal of this sample resin by "popping" it off is simple because the tooth surface has not been etched.

A typical Class III carious lesion is illustrated in Figure 31–80. The preparation is made to satisfy all principles but with emphasis on conservatism in outline form. The plastic nature of the resin material allows it to be placed under virtually no force, and specially designed delicate instruments are available for placement and finishing. In the maxillary anteriors, access is usually from the lingual direction and care is taken to preserve the marginal ridge whenever possible. In deep restorations, dentin coverage with a glass ionomer cement helps decrease microleakage and the possibility of sensitivity by bacterial invasion. An enamel bevel enhances mechanical retention by exposing the ends of enamel rods, which are highly susceptible to etching (Figure 31–81; Procedure 31–6).

Class V Restoration Placement and Finishing

One of the most perplexing problems in restorative dentistry is the course and treatment of lesions at the gingival margin. Abrasion, erosion, dental caries, or combinations of these can create defects that are difficult to properly restore. They often require isolation with special rubber dam retainers, because they frequently extend into the gingival sulcus. The most durable material for restoring these lesions is direct gold; amalgam is a satisfactory compromise. But these metals are often unacceptable to the client because of their unnatural color. Resin composite is a reasonable alternative, offering a natural appearance with fair longevity.

Shade selection is accomplished prior to the rubber dam placement. The rubber dam is placed in a routine manner. To properly isolate the lesion, it may be necessary to retract the free gingiva to expose the gingival margin of the cavity. Several rubber dam retainers work well for this purpose. Perhaps the most versatile is the Ivory 212 retainer, which was specifically designed to gain access for Class V cavities. It should be stabilized with modeling compound to prevent it from moving during the operation. The lingual jaw of this retainer often needs to be bent upward to facilitate its fit. This is done by heat treating the jaw until it can be adequately bent. Another option is to use the Ivory 212-SA retainer, which has already been heat treated to allow bending without heating. If a 212 retainer is used, the hole for that tooth in the rubber must be punched 3 to 5 mm facial to its normal position using the largest punch hole. This distance allows the proper retraction of the gingival tissue without having open gaps and seepage between the interproximal rubber dam and the tooth.

Enamel, again, is the key to retention and margin seal. Because enamel is absent on the root, the dentist may place a supplemental retention groove in the gingival wall. Deep areas within the cavity may be covered with

Procedure 31–6 PLACING AND FINISHING A RESIN COMPOSITE RESTORATION

EQUIPMENT

Personal protective equipment
Protective eyewear for client
Isolation materials
Glass ionomer cavity liner/sealer as needed
Conditioning agent (acid gel)
Priming agent
Bonding resin
Resin composite
Resin surface coating
Matrix system
Dispensing syringe
Curing light and protective shields
Plastic instruments
Finishing burrs and discs
Spoon excavator
Articulating paper

STEPS	RATIONALE
1. Query the client regarding expectations, and explain the nature of resin composites.	All restorative materials have limitations; resin composites may stain and fracture, resulting in the need for replacement in time; shades may not be perfect.
2. Select the composite shade, place a small amount of material on the tooth near the lesion and cure it; involve the client in the shade selection.	Cured resin may have a slight shade difference from the shade guide (one to two shades), and client preapproval is always a good idea, especially where aesthetics is concerned.
3. Place the rubber dam.	A dry operating field is essential.
4. Following cavity preparation, apply cavity liner/sealer, and/or base as needed.	Deep preparations close to the pulp should be protected from undue irritation caused by the operating procedure.
5. Position a clear, plastic matrix strip between the preparation and the adjacent tooth.	This prevents acid from etching the adjacent tooth surface.
6. Dry the tooth and apply etchant to the peripheral, beveled enamel or on the entire cavity surface according to manufacturer's instructions Rinse with an air–water spray for at least 15 seconds; dry with forced-air drying. Reposition the matrix as necessary and position a wedge interproximally.	Enamel etching is the primary retentive feature of most resin composite cavity preparations. However, depending on the etching system used, total etching of both enamel and dentin is often recommended. Times vary from 10 seconds to 60 seconds. The wedge stabilizes the matrix and adapts it to the gingival margin, preventing overhangs.
7. Inspect the peripheral etched pattern.	A chalky appearance over the entire bevel and enamel surface identifies adequate etching; if not present, repeat the etching procedure.
8. Apply thin coats of the primer to the etched surfaces according to manufacturer's instructions, and lightly dry.	Some systems combine the etchant and primer, others combine the primer and bonding agent or all three agents, and others keep all separate. Following manufacturer's instructions is considered mandatory to achieve maximum bonding.
9. Apply a thin coat of bonding resin to the primed surface; spread the resin over the etched enamel with a small brush or sponge and a gentle stream of air (Figure 31–82).	The fluid resin flows into the minute irregularities of the enamel. The stream of air evenly spreads the resin over the preparation, prevents pooling of the resin, and ensures a more uniform coating.
10. Place a special protective eyeshield on operator, assistant, and client to avoid eye damage during the curing that is about to start.	The eyes must be protected from the damaging effects of the blue curing light.
11. Polymerize the bonding resin with the curing light for 15 to 20 seconds; light wand should be as close as possible without direct contact. Careful inspection of the cured bonding resin will reveal a slightly tacky surface. This very thin layer of resin is unable to completely polymerize because of the influence of air. It will rapidly polymerize once covered by resin composite or a matrix strip and reexposed to the curing light.	Establishes the bond of resin composite to enamel. For systems using separate steps, light-curing is not done until application of the bonding resin. For systems combining the primer with bonding resin, curing is done after placement. The surface layer is called the "air-inhibited" layer and is responsible for facilitating bonding to the resin composite restorative material.

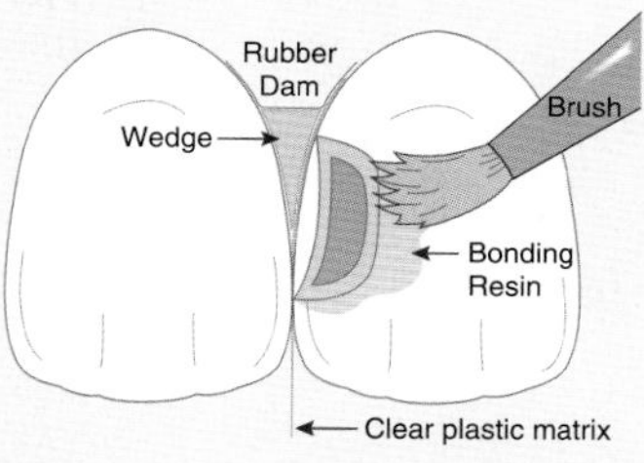

FIGURE 31–82 ✦ The etched enamel receiving a coating of bonding resin. A matrix separates the cavity from the adjacent tooth and is contoured and stabilized by a wedge placed interproximally.

Continued on following page

Procedure 31–6 PLACING AND FINISHING A RESIN COMPOSITE RESTORATION—CONT'D

STEPS	RATIONALE
12. Remove the cap from the resin composite dispensing device and express a small amount of the selected resin composite onto a small paper pad; replace the cap . Many systems are "preencapsulated," so only need to be mixed (triturated) for the specified time.	The pad is convenient for loading the placing instrument. It can also be covered with an opaque lid to protect the resin from sunlight; replacing the cap prevents the material in the dispensing device from polymerizing.
13. With a plastic instrument, or preencapsulated mixture placed in dispensing gun, place an increment of resin (no more than 2 mm thick) in the preparation and adapt it to the walls and margins; cure this first increment for 20 to 30 seconds (Figure 31–83).	Careful adaptation eliminates voids and enhances retention and marginal seal; larger increments and use of dark shades of composite require longer curing times to ensure penetration of the light waves into the mass.
14. Continue to add and cure increments, building the form to a slight excess in contour. In small cavities final form may be achieved by firmly wrapping the clear matrix against the tooth and curing through it (Figure 31–84). Remove the wedge and matrix.	Slight overcontouring allows finishing without leading to undercontouring.
15. Contour the restoration with finishing burrs and discs, exercising care to avoid tooth damage (Figures 31–85 and 31–86).	Rotary instruments can rapidly remove tooth structure while removing excess composite material.
16. Remove the rubber dam and check for occlusal prematurities on the restoration. Lingual high spots can be carefully reduced with a large, round finishing burr or a football-shaped fine diamond.	In particular, lingual aspects of maxillary Class III restorations may require occlusal adjustment.
17. Polish all accessible parts of the restoration with polishing discs; examine the gingival sulcus and remove debris.	Polishing enhances oral hygiene and reduces plaque biofilm accumulation.
18. Condition the restoration surface with conditioning agent.	Cleans and prepares surface for the final resin surface coating.
19. Apply the resin surface coating with a cotton pellet or foam applicator; cure for 10 seconds.	Resin surface coating fills any rough surfaces or voids in the resin composite.
20. Show the client the restoration; explain shade discrepancies (Fig. 31–87).	Teeth isolated by the dam appear lighter because of their being dry; as moisture returns they appear more natural, blending with the new resin restoration.

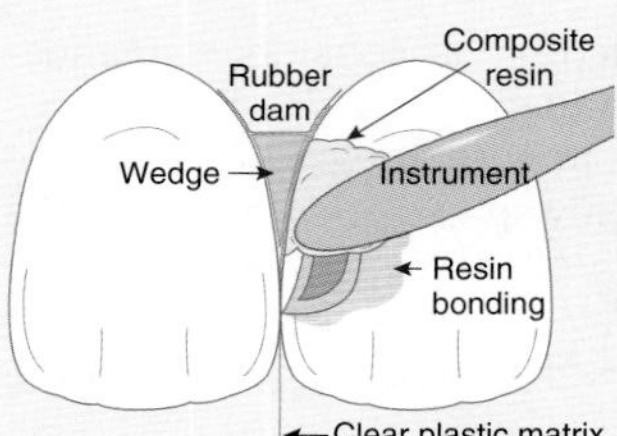

FIGURE 31–83 ✦ The placement of increments of resin composite into the preparation. The resin must be adapted into the recesses of the cavity and built against the matrix and cavity walls.

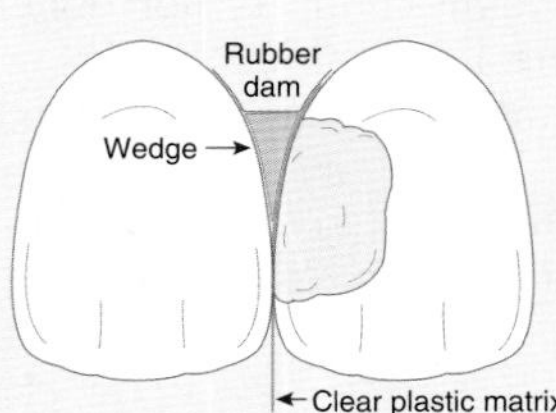

FIGURE 31–84 ✦ The cavity filled to slight excess, cured and prepared for finishing.

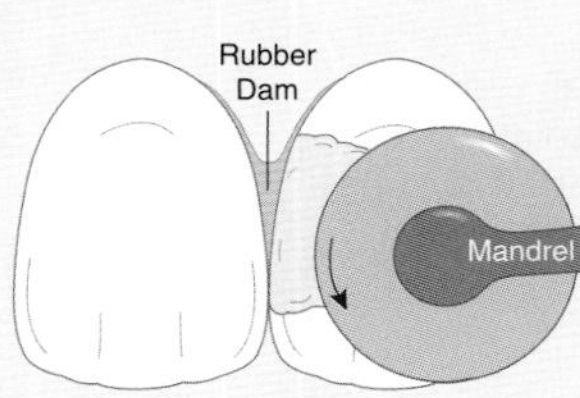

FIGURE 31–85 ✦ Contouring the resin composite with a disc to achieve the final form. The wedge and matrix have been removed.

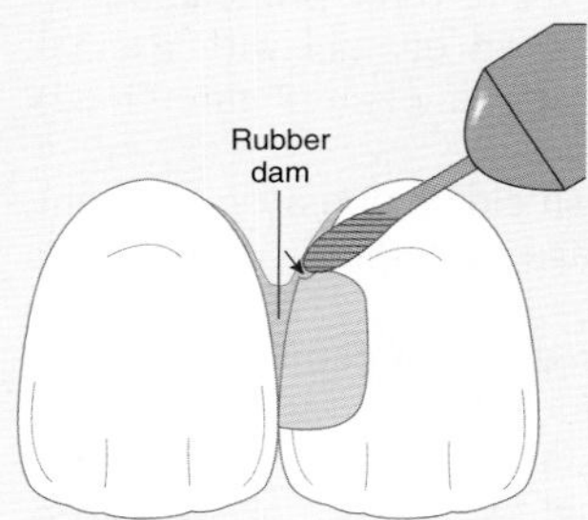

FIGURE 31–86 ✦ Damage to the tooth structure occurs if due caution is not exercised with the use of a burr in the finishing procedure.

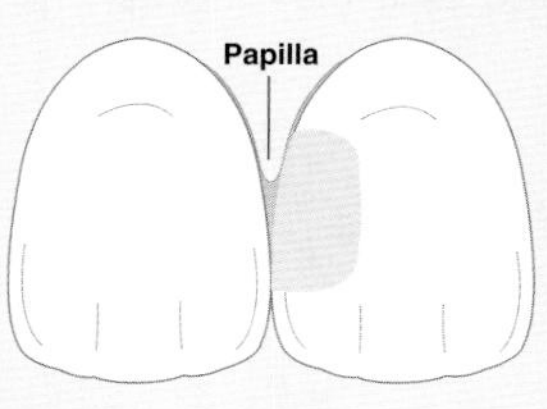

FIGURE 31–87 ✦ Finished Class III resin composite restoration.

a protective liner such as calcium hydroxide or glass ionomer cement. An enamel bevel is created with a rotary instrument and is then etched with an acid gel conditioning agent. After etching, rinsing, and drying, following the manufacturer's instructions, the preparation is coated with one or more coats of a priming agent and lightly air-dried. Then, the bonding resin is spread gently over the internal surface, lightly air-dried, and cured for 15 seconds. This is followed by incremental placement and curing of the resin composite. Contour can be developed by tamping the final increments into place with an instrument tip that has been dipped in bonding resin to prevent sticking to the composite. This procedure produces a smooth, contoured surface that requires a minimum of finishing. Cleansing the resin composite surface with the conditioning agent, then washing, drying, and applying a surface coating of unfilled resin liquid (Fortify) has gained popularity for providing a smooth-looking surface. This is then light-cured for 20 seconds. Although this coating may not last long, it is useful for filling voids, including marginal gaps. After final curing, careful shaping and polishing are accomplished with finishing burrs and discs. The gingival sulcus should be cleansed of any debris and surface coating material before dismissing the client.

Class I (Occlusal) and Class II Restorations

Clients' demands for natural-looking teeth have also resulted in the use of resin composites for restoring posterior teeth. However, these materials have not found acceptance for all such cases. Wear-resistance properties have vastly improved and are almost adequate when compared with dental amalgam, the time-honored standard. Accordingly, the use of resin composites in posterior teeth should be limited to small lesions and conservative preparations, to minimize wear and direct occlusal contact. As these materials are improved, their use may become routine for more complex restorations.

Class II composite restorations have an additional drawback: marked technique sensitivity. In addition to the need for very careful isolation and moisture control, manipulation of the matrix is critical. Establishing a positive proximal contact that is physiologically contoured is one of the biggest challenges facing the operator. Because resin composite cannot be forcibly condensed against the matrix (as with amalgam), developing the proximal contact necessary to prevent food impaction and tooth drift is difficult. The placement, curing, and finishing of resin composites for other than the simplest posterior restorations demand the utilization of four-handed dentistry at its best.

Glass Ionomer Cements

RATIONALE. These cements have been improved in recent years and are available as cavity liners as well as definitive restorative materials. Like all cements, they undergo dissolution when exposed to saliva. However, these restorative cements dissolve slowly after their initial set and release fluoride ions in the process. As a result, recurrent caries is rarely seen at the margin of a glass ionomer cement restoration. *Glass ionomer* cements are composed of aluminosilicate glass (powder) and polyalkenoic acid (liquid) that set through an acid–base reaction between the filler and the resin (Figure 31–88). A great benefit of this material is that it apparently truly adheres (chemical bonding) to prepared tooth structure.[11] Glass ionomer restorative cements are brittle and should not be used in areas of direct occlusal stress.

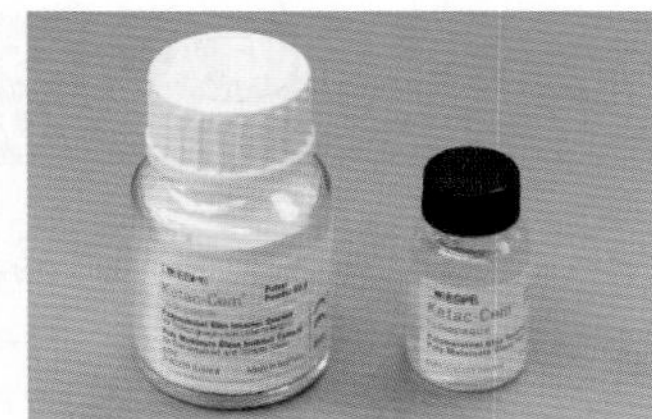

FIGURE 31–88 ✦ A typical glass ionomer cement product.

Root caries is one of the more perplexing decay patterns, often presenting as nearly impossible restorative challenges. Access and detailed cavity design can be extremely difficult. In these cases, caries excavation and restoration with glass ionomer cement can provide the solution. As compared to amalgam, which requires specific retention design and a rigid matrix to withstand condensation, glass ionomer cements adhere to the tooth and flow into the recesses of the cavity. Another excellent use of glass ionomer cements is for the restoration of gingival Class V abrasion and erosion (gingival margin) lesions. Resin-modified glass ionomer cements have been developed that offer enhanced aesthetics, less solubility, and greater strength than glass-ionomer materials, but retain some of their fluoride release characteristics. In addition, these materials are dual-cure restorations, characterized by utilizing the acid–base reaction critical to curing of true glass ionomers, and supplementing this with light-activated polymerization. This type of cure increases the ease of placement over original glass ionomer materials.

Class V (Abrasion Lesion) Placement and Finishing

Because surgery of the teeth is not necessary in many abrasion lesions, it is possible to accomplish these restorations without anesthesia unless the lesion is substantially below the gingival margin. If these lesions are not carious, and therefore require no operative preparation, restoration can be completed at the oral prophylaxis appointment. Once placed, care should be taken at subsequent appointments to prevent dehydration of the glass ionomer cement restorations. Resin composite restorations are not as sensitive to dehydration as are the glass ionomer or resin-modified glass ionomer materials. (See Procedure 31–7 for placing and finishing glass ionomer cement restorations of Class V abrasion lesions.)

Procedure 31–7 PLACING A GLASS IONOMER CEMENT RESTORATION OF CLASS V ABRASION LESIONS

EQUIPMENT

Personal protective equipment
Protective eyewear for client
Isolation materials
Glass ionomer cement
Polyacrylic acid
Flour of pumice
Polishing cup
Plastic instruments
Carving instrument
Bonding resin
Special protective varnish
Curing light and protective shields
Matrix system

STEPS	RATIONALE
1. Examine the lesions and assess the need for local anesthetic.	Nonsensitive, noncarious lesions that are easily accessible may not require anesthetic.
2. Select the shade of restorative material to be used; involve the client in the selection.	Client preapproval is always a good idea, especially where aesthetics are concerned.
3. Place the rubber dam (Figure 31–89).	The rubber dam is the best device to control contamination of the cavity.
4. Briefly, debride the cavity and adjacent tooth structure with nonfluoridated flour of pumice and water slurry in a rubber polishing cup; rinse thoroughly and dry (Figure 31–90).	Plaque biofilm and debris compromise the adherence of the restorative material. Residual fluoride may inhibit or decrease bonding.
5. Select a matrix that matches the tooth contour in the cervical area.	A cervical matrix greatly facilitates the management of runny glass ionomer systems.
6. According to the manufacturer's instructions, apply polyacrylic acid to the abrasion lesion (approximately 15 seconds); rinse thoroughly for 15 seconds with a strong air-water spray, and dry lightly, ensuring a moist surface, but do not desiccate (Figure 31–91).	Brief exposure to polyacrylic acid removes microscopic debris (smear layer) without opening dentinal tubules; desiccation of the dentin causes collapse of the tender collagen fibrils, decreasing bonding strength of the cement. The cement is also very sensitive to moisture changes.
7. According to the manufacturer's directions, prepare a creamy mix of restorative cement (Figure 31–92).	Directions should be followed closely because ratios of powder and liquid, as well as mixing times, are critical.
8. Rapidly fill the cavity to slight excess, using a plastic instrument to place the material (Figure 31–93); position the cervical matrix over the cavity to hold the cement against the tooth (Figure 31–94); light-cure as indicated by the system using protective shields.	The cement may begin to harden, so expeditious placement is important. The matrix prevents the material from slumping or running out of the cavity; it also prevents the material from drying out and crazing as it hardens. Protective shields prevent eye injury that is possible from the wavelengths.

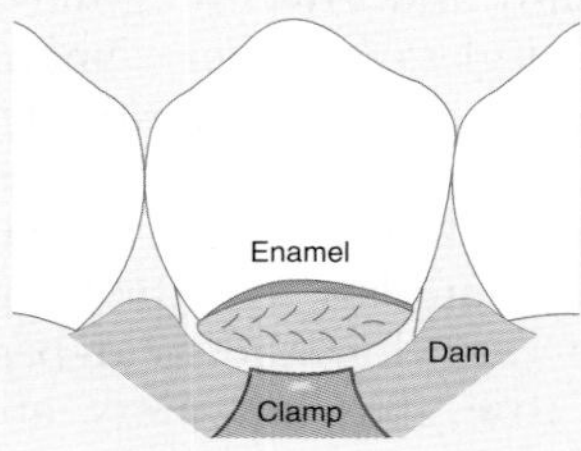

FIGURE 31–89 ✦ A typical abrasion lesion isolated with a rubber dam and retracting retainer.

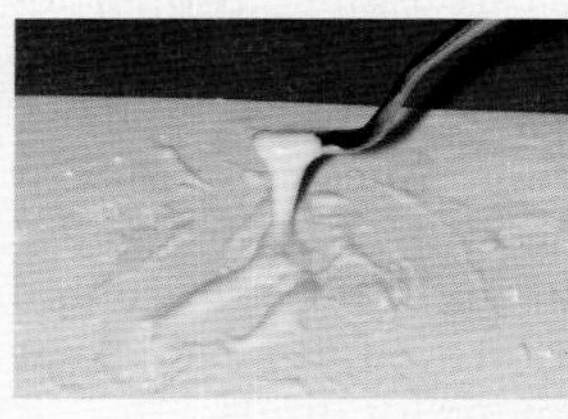

FIGURE 31–92 ✦ A proper mix of glass ionomer cement.

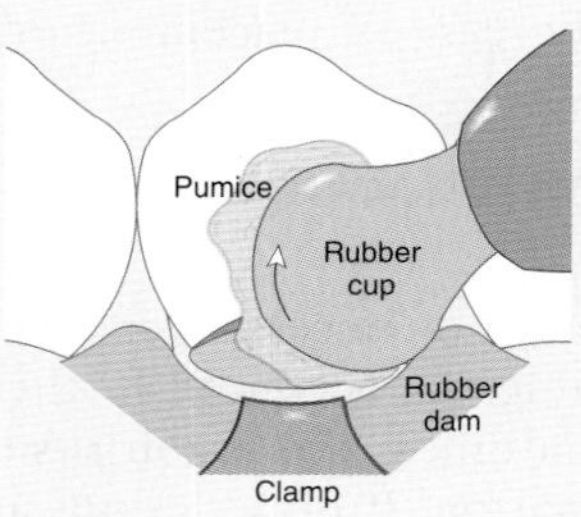

FIGURE 31–90 ✦ The debridement of the lesion with a flour of pumice slurry and rubber cup.

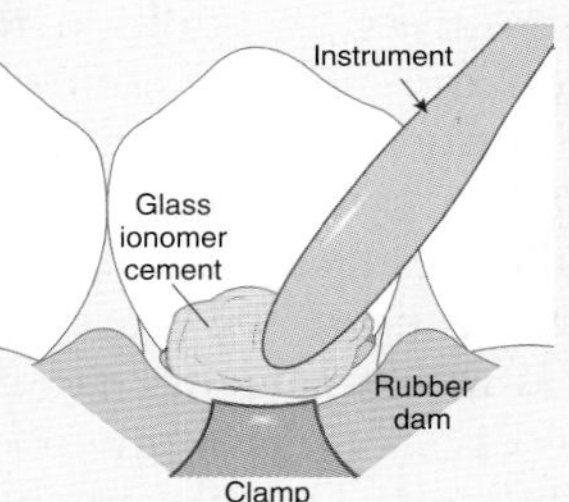

FIGURE 31–93 ✦ The placement of the glass ionomer cement to slightly overfill the cavity.

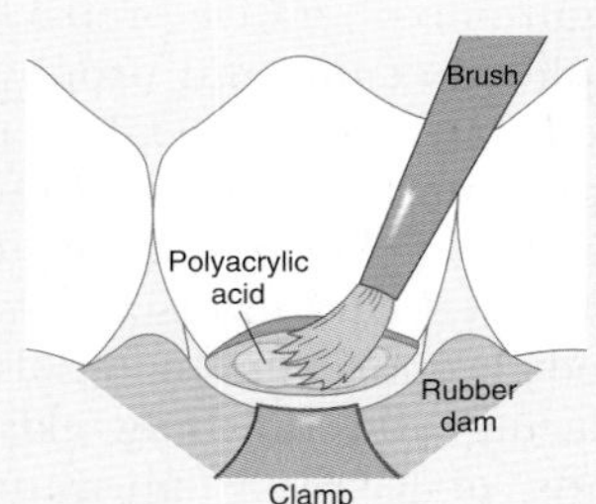

FIGURE 31–91 ✦ The application of polyacrylic acid to cleanse the dentin.

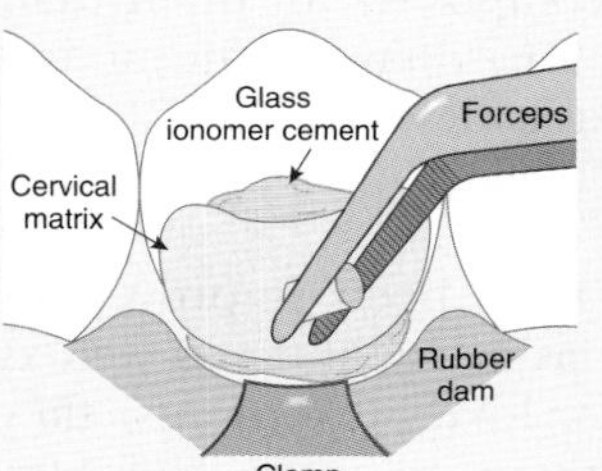

FIGURE 31–94 ✦ The positioning of the clear cervical matrix over the cavity and expressing excess glass ionomer cement at the edges of the matrix.

Procedure 31–7 PLACING A GLASS IONOMER CEMENT RESTORATION OF CLASS V ABRASION LESIONS—CONT'D

STEPS	RATIONALE
9. If it is stable, pressure on the matrix may be released after 1 minute or immediately after light-curing if appropriate for the system; coat the excess cement at the matrix periphery with bonding resin or special protective varnish.	The coating of bonding resin prevents dehydration of the cement. Glass ionomer is very soluble until it gets its final set; protection against external moisture is important.
10. After 4 to 5 minutes, remove the matrix; shave off the gross excess cement with a sharp, chisel-like instrument or scalpel with #12 blade (Figure 31–95); recoat with bonding resin or special varnish; cure the bonding resin for 15 seconds.	The cement can still be shaped easily. Final contouring is delayed until it has fully hardened; it is not necessary to cure the resin to protect against dehydration of the cement, but uncured resin is messy.
11. After approximately 10 more minutes, contour the restoration with finishing burrs and discs (Figure 31–96); take care to avoid damage to the tooth root.	Most glass ionomer cement restorations can be finished after this length of time. Rotary instruments can rapidly score the root (Figure 31–97).
12. Apply a thin coat of bonding resin to the cement restoration surface and cure the resin for 15 to 20 seconds.	The cured resin coating will protect the cement from excess moisture or drying for several hours.
13. Remove the rubber dam; examine the gingival sulcus and remove debris.	Cured bonding resin debris is very difficult to see because it is transparent.
14. Show the final result to the client (Figure 31–98).	This helps to further instill confidence; clients may be motivated to take better care of their teeth; they appreciate pride in one's work.

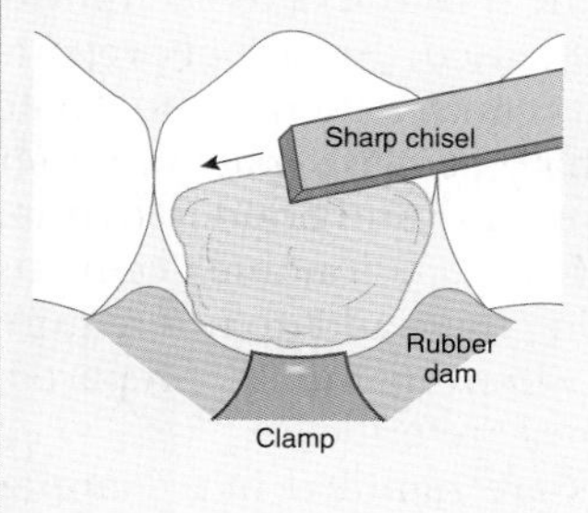

FIGURE 31–95 ✦ The trimming of the gross excess with a sharp instrument such as a chisel.

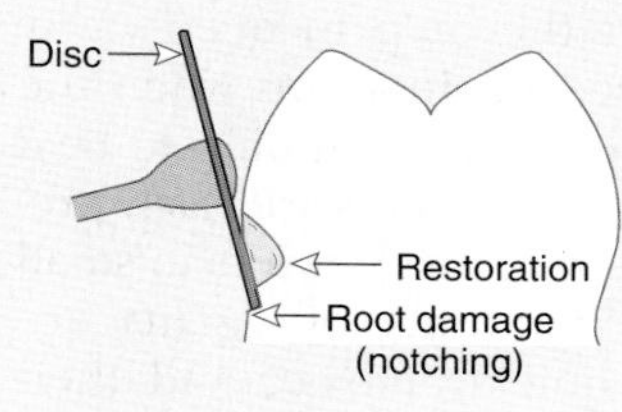

FIGURE 31–97 ✦ Root damage from improper discing.

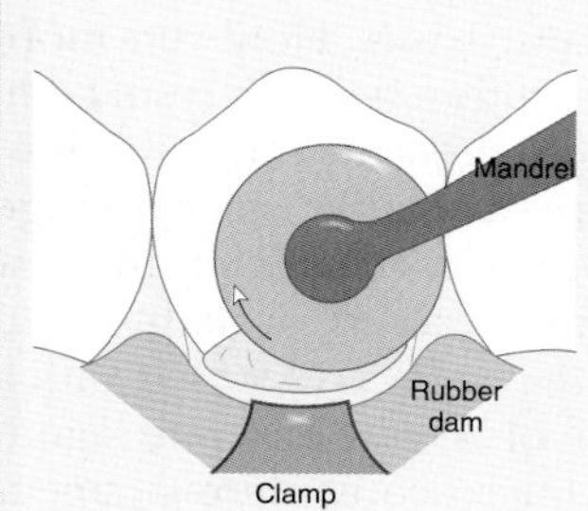

FIGURE 31–96 ✦ The final contouring of the restoration with a disc.

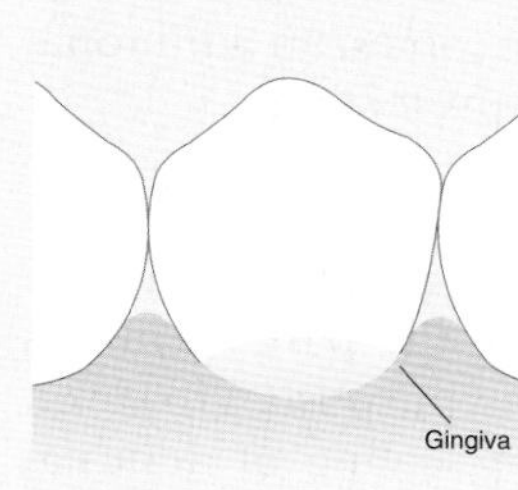

FIGURE 31–98 ✦ The finished glass ionomer cement restoration.

SEALERS, LINERS, AND BASES

Rationale

Preserving and protecting the dental pulp are concerns in every restorative procedure on vital teeth. Some pulps seem to survive numerous insults whereas others degenerate and die from what appears to be minor trauma. The insults of dental caries followed by drilling procedures, chemical and thermal shock, and microleakage around restorations, individually or collectively, can cause pulpal damage and discomfort to the client. It should be the goal of each therapist to perform procedures in the most atraumatic manner possible so as to promote pulp protection.

Vital dentin is a dynamic tissue. The tubules of which it is constituted connect with the pulp and contain fluid and cellular components that are adversely affected by surgical procedures. At a microscopic level it is easy to understand how a gentle stream of air may be injurious to a delicate pulp that is covered by a paper-thin thickness of dentin. Deep cavities in particular must be treated to protect the pulp from further insult. Liners and bases are intended to provide such protection.[12]

Liners

Liners are liquidlike materials applied in thin coatings (< 0.5 mm) that act as cavity sealers and provide expanded beneficial functions such as fluoride release, adhesion to

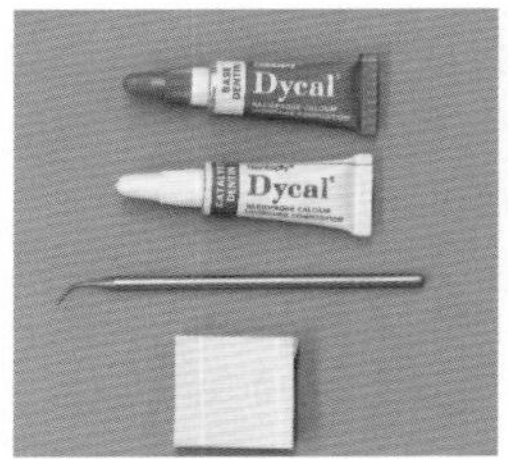

FIGURE 31–99 ✦ A popular calcium hydroxide product, an applicator, and a mixing pad.

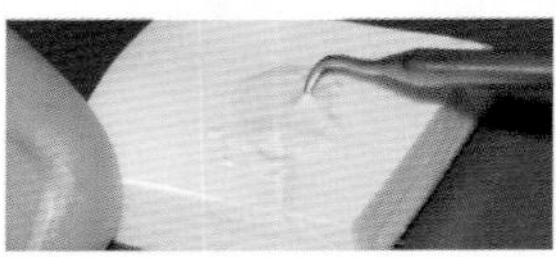

FIGURE 31–100 ✦ Equal amounts of the calcium hydroxide base and catalyst have been mixed.

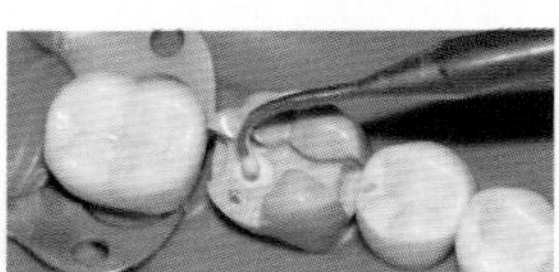

FIGURE 31–101 ✦ Placement of the mixed calcium hydroxide in the deeper areas of the cavity preparation.

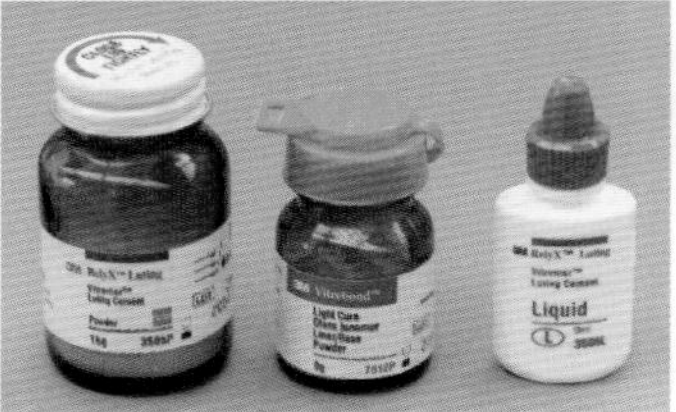

FIGURE 31–102 ✦ A popular dental liner.

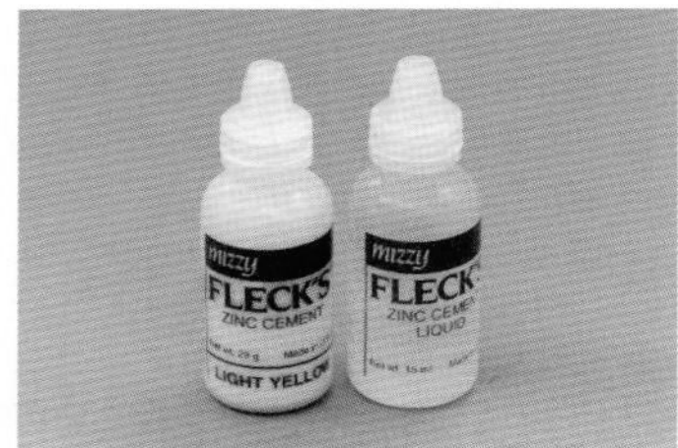

FIGURE 31–103 ✦ A popular zinc phosphate cement.

tooth structure, and/or antibacterial action that promotes the health of the pulp.[12] Calcium hydroxide preparations are commonly used to protect the pulp in deep cavity preparations. They also are used in situations when the pulp has been exposed to stimulate the vital pulp to heal if the wound is small and clean. These liners are easily prepared and are usually supplied by manufacturers in small tubes (Figure 31–99). Equal amounts of agents are expressed onto a small pad, quickly mixed, and then specifically placed on the dentin or over the pulp exposure (Figures 31–100 and 31–101). Because these materials typically do not resist compressive forces, an additional hard base material is often used for protection.

Sealers

Cavity *sealers* are used to seal dentinal tubules to protect the pulp from chemical irritation. In the past, varnishes were the material of choice for this purpose. However, recent research has shown superior sealing of dentinal tubules by bonding resins or liners.[12] Dentin bonding agents provide a micro-mechanical bond formed between the restorative material and the tooth structure (hybrid layer) that has been found to better seal tubules and provide some retentive strength for resin composites where used (Figure 31–102).

Bases

Bases are materials placed to provide thermal insulation and support under metallic restorations. They must be strong enough to resist occlusal forces and, in the case of amalgam, resist firm condensation. This category includes zinc phosphate, glass ionomer cements, and resin composites.

Bases of zinc phosphate cement have served dentistry well, providing dependable support and insulation under metallic restorations (Figure 31–103). The rationale for its use in preventing sensitivity, however, has become questionable in recent times. Currently, gaining a seal of the dentinal tubules to prevent microleakage is felt to be far more important in controlling postoperative sensitivity than is physical insulation. When used, the proper preparation of zinc phosphate cement requires attention to detail.

Compared to zinc phosphate cement, glass ionomer cements require less time to prepare and bond to dentin, achieving a desirable seal. Most glass ionomer cements are available in a self-dispensing form and do not require manual mixing. However, when manually prepared, mixing and manipulation times are critical.

Resin composite materials are handled in a manner similar to glass ionomer cement bases. However, more care is required in ensuring retention because resin composites adhere only by micro-mechanical retention. However, most of them are available in cartridge (compule) form and can be mixed mechanically in a few seconds. These may be chemical-cured or light-cured materials. For best adhesion, the cavity is cleansed with a 10- to 20-second application of a conditioning agent (polyacrylic acid) to remove microscopic debris (smear layer). Following rinsing and gentle drying of the cavity, the mixed cement is injected into the cavity and molded with a suitable instrument to the desired form while it is in a gel state. If chemical-cured, the material hardens in a few minutes, at which time it should be coated with a special varnish provided with the resin composite system to prevent moisture loss or gain. If light-cured, the operator has time to mold the material before light-activating it. Depending on the specific product, amalgam can be condensed on the set base within 4 to 10 minutes.

GINGIVAL RETRACTION

Rationale

The essential first step for the fabrication of an indirect restoration is the making of an accurate impression. Gingival tissue management is important for ensuring that the margins of the preparation are appropriately captured in the impression. Gingival retraction, through the use of retraction cord around the preparation, is a critical step in achieving the desired impression. Retraction cord relaxes the gingival tissue, thereby "opening" the gingival sulcus and enabling impression material to be injected into the gingival crevice to capture the gingival margins of the preparation.

Armamentarium

RETRACTION CORD. Many types and sizes of retraction cord are available. Use of knitted gingival retraction cords has been found to work better than twined cords.[13]

RETRACTION CORD HEMOSTATIC AGENT. Retraction cord is soaked in a hemostatic agent to lubricate the cord for placement into the sulcus and minimize bleeding during the impression procedure.[14]

RETRACTION INSTRUMENTS. Placement of the retraction cord is best achieved using a periodontal probe and explorer. Other popular retraction instruments include the IPC carver, Thompson #4, and Stellate 1-2.

Gingival Tissue Management

For any preparation for impression, the depth of the gingival margin of the preparation must be evaluated in relation to the gingival sulcus. In addition, the health and flexibility of the free gingival tissue must be assessed. Normal, healthy tissue does not require pretreatment prior to the tissue retraction procedure. Hemorrhagic tissue, however, may require treatment prior to retraction or postponement of the retraction and impression procedures. Hemorrhaging may be controlled using an astringent/coagulation liquid such as Monsel's solution (15% ferric subsulfate) or AstringedentX (20% ferric subsulfate).

Retraction Cord Placement

Tissue retraction can be accomplished using a one-cord or two-cord retraction technique. The two-cord technique is preferred unless the depth of the sulcus or "tightness" of the free gingival tissue, especially on the facial surface, does not permit placement of the second cord.[15] The bottom cord, which should be smaller in diameter, acts to control seepage and promote slight lateral displacement of the sulcular base. This cord is left in place during the impression procedure; therefore, placement apical to the gingival margins of the preparation is critical. The top cord, which should be larger in diameter, provides enhanced lateral displacement of the gingival tissue and is removed prior to the impression procedure. Adequate tissue retraction is achieved within 8 to 10 minutes. Each layer of cord is placed using the same technique. There are times when a small amount of anesthetic is needed for tissue retraction, such as for lingual areas of maxillary teeth. In an effort to avoid a potentially painful lingual injection, the retraction cord can be soaked in a mixture of 12.5 g of aluminum chloride crystals with 50 cc of 4% lidocaine (Procedure 31–8).

Procedure 31–8 PLACING RETRACTION CORD

EQUIPMENT

Personal protective equipment
Protective eyewear for client
Exam kit (mouth mirror, explorer, periodontal probe, cotton pliers)
Dappen dish
Scissors
2″ × 2″ gauze
Cotton rolls or "dry aids"
Retraction cord hemostatic agent
Retraction cord of various sizes
Astringent/coagulation liquid

STEPS	RATIONALE
1. Estimate the circumference of the preparation; cut a piece of bottom cord (e.g., Deknatel #00, 0, 1, 2, or 3) to encompass the preparation margins.	This ensures complete coverage of the preparation with a single piece of bottom retraction cord. The appropriate cord size is dependent on the status of the gingival tissue.
2. Cut a piece of top cord that is approximately 1/2 inch longer than the bottom cord and thicker in diameter.	The top cord is longer and thicker than the bottom cord because it provides the primary lateral tissue displacement necessary for satisfactorily allowing injection of the impression material.
3. Soak the bottom and top cords in hemostatic agent; place the cord on a dry 2″ × 2″ gauze to remove excess solution.	The hemostatic agent serves as a lubricant during placement of the cord into the sulcus, minimizing damage to the friable gingival tissues. The hemostatic agent also minimizes hemorrhagic seepage during the impression procedure, which could distort the final impression.
4. Isolate the site of the preparation(s) with cotton rolls and/or "dry aids."	Having a moist but not wet environment is critical to achieving the necessary replication of the tooth preparation margins.

Procedure 31-8 PLACING RETRACTION CORD—CONT'D

STEPS	RATIONALE
5. Using the bottom cord, lasso the tooth having the loop around the lingual of the tooth (Figure 31–104).	The cord approximates its ultimate location on the tooth and simplifies the placement process.
6. Start placement of the bottom cord in one of the interproximal areas using a periodontal probe; while the periodontal probe holds the packed cord in place, the side of the explorer rotates the cord into place in the sulcus (Figure 31–105). Cord placement is achieved by gently rolling the cord down the tooth into the gingival sulcus and below the gingival margin of the preparation. Avoid forceful apical pressure of the cord.	The small area of the explorer offers excellent control, and following along with the periodontal probe to hold down the cord that has just been packed ensures a methodical retraction with minimal necessity to repack. The explorer easily locates the gingival margin of the preparation so the operator receives immediate feedback on whether the cord is correctly placed apical to the margin. Many of the other retraction instruments have rounded ends that encourage cord movement in the wrong direction if not carefully monitored (Figure 31–106). The bottom cord will remain in place during the impression procedure. Excess apical pressure could traumatize the tissue, causing bleeding and gingival recession.
7. Proceed in a methodical manner around the tooth, ending on the facial surface. Work from one end of the cord to the other and avoid skipping around. Excess cord should be cut at this point to avoid overlapping.	Ensures adequate placement of the retraction cord.
8. With the bottom cord in place, take the top cord and lasso the tooth having the loop around the lingual of the tooth.	The cord approximates its ultimate location on the tooth and simplifies the placement process.
9. Start placement of the top cord in one of the interproximal areas and proceed with the placement technique described in Steps 6 and 7. Depending on the gingival status, the top cord placement may not be below the gingival margin of the preparation. A small end of the top cord will extend out of the sulcus after it has been placed around the circumference of the tooth (Figure 31–107).	The top cord will be removed prior to the impression procedure. The small end of the top cord facilitates removal when the impression material is ready for injection.

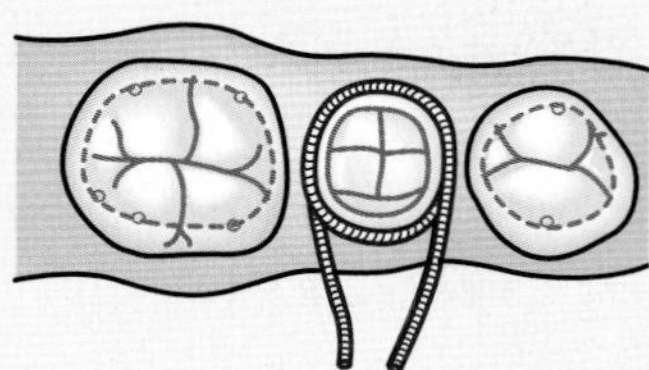

FIGURE 31–104 ✦ The retraction cord is looped around the lingual of the prepared tooth.

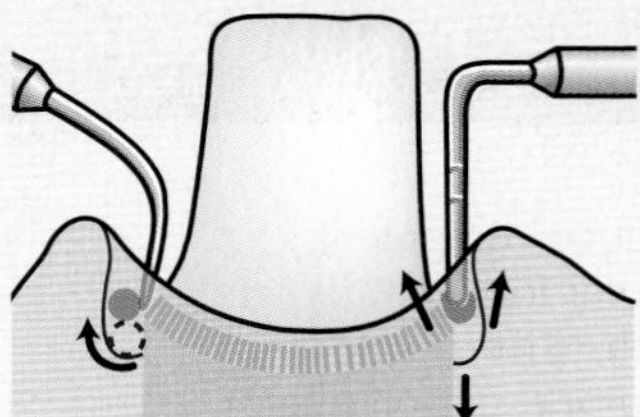

FIGURE 31–106 ✦ The explorer on the left properly permits the cord to roll into place but the round-ended instrument on the right permits the cord to improperly pop up on the sides.

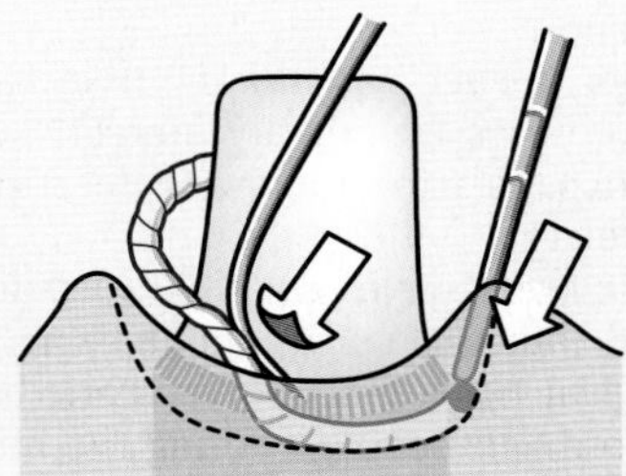

FIGURE 31–105 ✦ The periodontal probe holds the packed cord in place while the side of the explorer rotates the cord into place in the sulcus.

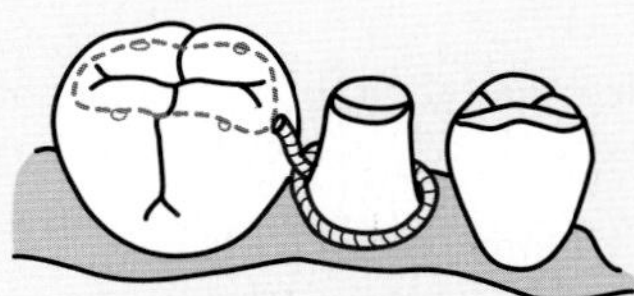

FIGURE 31–107 ✦ A small end of the top cord extends out of the sulcus.

TEMPORARY OR INTERIM RESTORATIONS

Rationale

Frequently, a significant span of time elapses between the initial or final tooth preparation and the restoration placement. The reasons for this lapse in time vary, but may include the need to prepare or cast the final restoration, the desire to allow the tooth to respond to a medication, or the lack of time in a given appointment to complete a procedure. In these situations, protection of the prepared tooth and associated dentition may be imperative to prevent client discomfort and technical complications. *Temporary restorations* can provide the protective function required during this interim phase in restorative treatment. The primary factors to be considered when determining the need for temporary restorations include the following:

- Client comfort
- Tooth protection
- Gingival protection
- Tooth movement

CLIENT COMFORT. Vital, freshly cut dentin is very sensitive to thermal and chemical insults. As a result, all vital dentin should be covered and sealed from salivary and bacterial contamination. This protection also prevents the pulp from being exposed to undue insults that may threaten the vitality of the tooth. The temporary restoration also can permit the individual to chew normally.

TOOTH PROTECTION. The protection of cusps and cavity margins from fracture after the final tooth preparation is extremely important. The unprotected tooth may break irreparably. Even small fractures to a cavity preparation may require that the tooth be reprepared prior to the placement of a final restoration. A proper temporary restoration protects the prepared tooth from mechanical insult prior to the placement of the final restoration.

GINGIVAL PROTECTION. Unsupported gingival papillae and free gingival margins tend to grow into open, unprotected cavity preparations. It is difficult for the client to maintain a bacterial plaque-free environment with the presence of gingival overgrowth. These factors result in gingival irritation and bleeding that may compromise the quality and success of the final restoration. A restoration must provide proper contour and proximal contact to support the gingiva and prevent food impaction and plaque biofilm retention that can injure the periodontium and cause discomfort to the client. The temporary restoration can provide this necessary anatomic form for an interim period.

TOOTH MOVEMENT. Without a temporary restoration or unless the temporary restoration is durable and properly contoured, the prepared tooth may drift or move slightly in a mesial or distal direction. The prepared tooth may also extrude or move in an occlusal (incisal) direction. In addition, adjacent teeth may drift toward the prepared tooth, and opposing teeth may extrude. These situations may complicate the fabrication of a successful permanent restoration. The temporary restoration prevents the occurrence of tooth movement and maintains the occlusal relationship.

Temporary Materials and Placement Techniques

TEMPORARY STOPPING. Temporary stopping is a thermoplastic compound that is quickly and easily prepared and placed (Figure 31–108). It is best used to seal small, shallow cavities requiring temporary restoration for periods of not more than 2 weeks. Temporary stopping rapidly develops leakage because of expansion and contraction in response to thermal changes, limiting its use to short durations.

The placement of the temporary stopping requires that the end of a stick of material be slowly warmed over an alcohol flame until it softens. It is then allowed to cool until it can be handled by the operator. Small increments are rapidly molded in the fingers and positioned on the tip of a placing instrument (Figure 31–109). These increments are rapidly and firmly packed into the cavity until the material fills the preparation. The criterion for determining the amount of material required to fill a cavity preparation is that the margins be secured and sealed. Minor shaping of the restoration, to restore the tooth as closely as possible to the original occlusion or anatomy, is done with a warm, not hot, instrument tip.

REINFORCED ZINC OXIDE WITH EUGENOL. Reinforced zinc oxide with eugenol readily restores intermediate-size cavities that require a more durable material. It is prepared with a mixture of zinc oxide powder and eugenol liquid (Figure 31–110). The insulating properties of the hardened zinc oxide mass and the obtundent

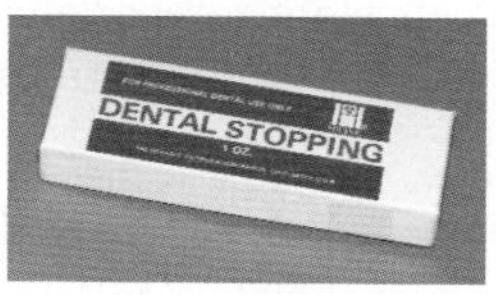

FIGURE 31–108 ✦ A popular temporary stopping product.

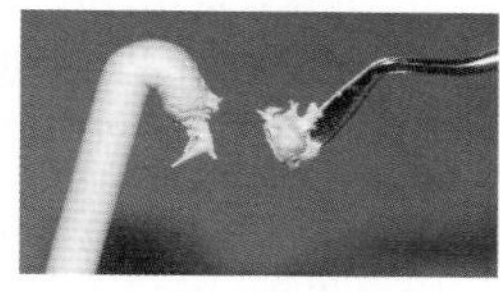

FIGURE 31–109 ✦ Temporary stopping material has been warmed over an alcohol flame until soft and then positioned on the tip of a placing instrument.

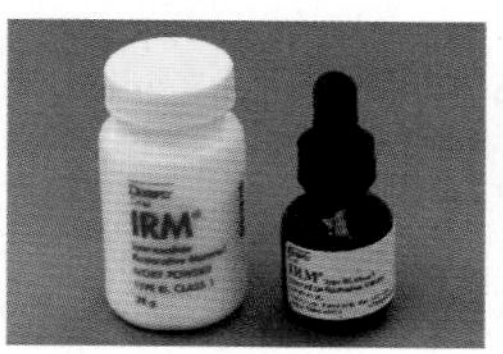

FIGURE 31–110 ✦ A popular reinforced zinc oxide with eugenol material.

effect of the eugenol result in a material that dependably protects the vital pulp against chemical and thermal insults. Reinforced zinc oxide with eugenol is relatively easy to prepare and place and is reliable for interim periods of a few months.

The powder and liquid are mixed on a nonabsorbent pad according to the manufacturer's instructions. Firm pressure on the spatula is needed to thoroughly mix the material. When properly mixed, the consistency of the material is thick and claylike. The material is then rolled with the fingertips (on the pad) into a cylindrical form. Increments can be pinched off the end of the mass with a placing instrument and firmly packed into the preparation until it is full (Procedure 31–9).

Procedure 31–9 PREPARING REINFORCED ZINC OXIDE AND EUGENOL TEMPORARY RESTORATIONS (CLASS II CAVITY PREPARATION)

EQUIPMENT

- Presonal protective equipment
- Protective eyewear for client
- Isolation materials
- Tofflemire matrix system
- Petrolatum
- Reinforced zinc oxide and eugenol
- Nonabsorbent mixing pad
- Plastic instruments
- Cotton pellets and rolls
- Finishing burrs
- Carving instruments
- Articulating paper

STEPS	RATIONALE
1. Isolate operating site as appropriate.	Isolation varies, depending on goals of therapy. Cotton roll isolation may be sufficient.
2. Prepare a Tofflemire matrix system. Apply a thin coat of petrolatum, with a cotton pellet or cotton swab, on the inside of the matrix band; position the matrix, secure it, and place interproximal wedges as needed.	A matrix is useful to contain the material in the cavity preparation because the walls are missing. The petrolatum prevents the material from sticking to the band. Excess material may be expressed into the gingival sulcus if the band is not supported interproximally.
3. Review the manufacturer's instructions for measuring and mixing.	Products vary.
4. Prepare the mix; when the material has reached the consistency of firm clay, carry an ample amount to the cavity with a plastic instrument. Firmly adapt the rubbery material to all walls of the cavity with a placement instrument (Figures 31–111 and 31–112).	If the material is too soft, it will not adapt well and it will stick to the instrument; if the material is too firm, it will not condense adequately to prevent voids and will result in leakage.
5. Fill the cavity to slight excess; shape the occlusal anatomy by using a moist cotton pellet in cotton forceps to create a general anatomic form.	Excess material ensures margin coverage; moisture hastens the set of zinc oxide–eugenol materials. Detailed anatomy is not needed.
6. When the material has hardened, remove wedge(s), retainer, and matrix band; apply pressure apically on the temporary restoration to counteract the removal of the band.	Removing the band before the material has set may break the marginal seal and dislodge the temporary restoration.
7. Check the proximal and gingival margins for excess material and remove with a sharp, narrow-bladed carving instrument.	Excess material at the gingival margins (overhang) could result in gingival irritation and hinder the client's ability to maintain a plaque-free environment.
8. Remove isolation materials; evaluate premature occlusion on the temporary restoration with articulating paper and adjust as necessary with a large, round bur and carving instruments (Figure 31–113).	Premature occlusion is very likely to fracture the temporary restoration.
9. Examine the gingival sulcus for debris and remove as necessary; excess material at the gingival margin can be removed using a bladed instrument such as the 1/2 Hollenback or IPC carver.	Debris from the restorative procedure can irritate the gingival tissues.

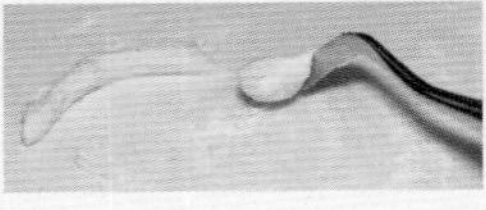

FIGURE 31–111 ✦ Properly mixed reinforced zinc oxide with eugenol ready for placement.

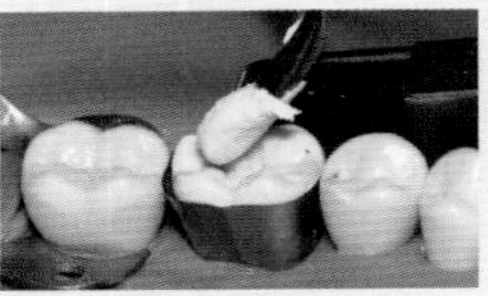

FIGURE 31–112 ✦ Reinforced zinc oxide with eugenol being placed in cavity preparation.

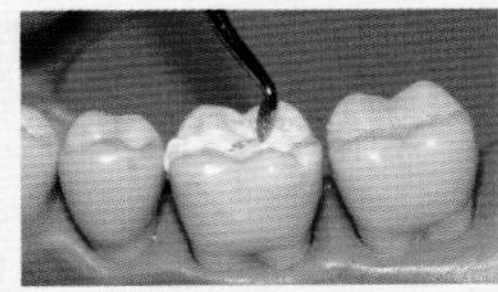

FIGURE 31–113 ✦ Final adjustment to the occlusal aspect of the temporary restoration with a carver.

CUSTOM-MADE ACRYLIC RESIN. The custom-made acrylic resin temporary restoration is recommended for complex restorations such as inlays and partial or complete veneer crowns. The main advantage of this type of temporary restoration is that the technique permits the reproduction of the client's tooth anatomy. The material used in the construction of this temporary restoration is an autopolymerizing acrylic resin. The acrylic is composed of a liquid (monomer) and a powder (polymer) that are mixed together and polymerize through a chemical reaction, resulting in a hardened resin mass. Because of the numerous steps involved in the preparation of a custom-made acrylic resin restoration, the main disadvantage of this type of restoration is the time required for production. A limitation of this technique is the requirement that the tooth be restored or be intact enough to allow adequate retention of the temporary restoration. However, the final product is durable, smooth, and comfortable and can serve for several months.

Bis-acryl resin (e.g., Integrity) provisional restorations are gaining in popularity because of their ease of use, low heat release, and minimal shrinkage on seating. However, they have only moderate strength because they are brittle, lack a putty stage, require some form of matrix to form the restorations, and are more costly than the conventional methylmethacrylate temporary materials.

PREFORMED STOCK CROWN (METAL OR POLYCARBONATE). Preformed stock crowns make handy and useful temporary crowns. These crown forms are readily trimmed and modified for fit and provide a satisfactory alternative to the custom-made acrylic crown previously discussed. The final product is extremely durable; however, it is a compromise in both form and shape. These temporary crowns are usually comfortable for the client, but on occasion, the metal crowns present an objectionable metallic taste. This technique is useful primarily for complete veneer crowns.

A suitable crown form is selected after the completion of the tooth preparation. Preformed stock crowns come in an assortment of sizes for each tooth within the dentition. The size of the desired temporary crown is based on the space present in the area of the preparation.

Luting Agents

RATIONALE. Indirect restorations are fabricated in the dental laboratory on dies made from impressions of prepared teeth. These restorations include crowns and inlays made of rigid substances such as metal, cast ceramic, or porcelain. When these restorations are completely seated, all margins should intimately fit. However, between the restoration and the cavity walls exists a minute space. This space is filled with a *luting agent* (cement) that, when set, prevents the indirect restoration from loosening. Dislodging forces of occlusion and mastication are resisted by this firm interface of cement. Without a proper luting agent, castings leak and loosen and therefore fail.

ZINC PHOSPHATE CEMENT. Zinc phosphate is the oldest of the luting agents. It has stood the test of time and remains the standard for cementation of most indirect restorations, especially for partial coverage castings and full crown metal restorations. Because it is quite acidic, vital pulps are often protected by a varnish barrier between the cement and dentin. Research has shown, however, that any dentinal sensitivity caused by the cement acidity is only transient, disappearing within 90 days postoperatively. When properly mixed, the set is extended, allowing the operator ample time to adapt and seal the margins of the restoration.

GLASS IONOMER CEMENT. The chemical adhesion of this material to the tooth surface and relative ease in handling have led to its increasing popularity as a luting agent. To gain this adhesion, no protective varnish is used to coat the dentin. When compared to zinc phosphate, it is less acidic and more compatible with the dental pulp and it inhibits recurrent caries through the slow release of fluoride. The mixing and working times for the chemical-cured glass ionomer cement are quite short, and thus the dental team must exercise expediency when luting restorations with glass ionomer cement. Most cements of this type can be prepared on a nonabsorbent paper pad, in accordance with manufacturer's instructions. The luting cement is mixed to a much less viscous state than the glass ionomer cement base material or restorative material previously described.

RESIN CEMENTS. Resin cements have become a valuable part of the dental practice as new materials and techniques have advanced. Chemical-cured cements are needed when strength of bonding is needed and light activation is not possible, (e.g., cementation of cast post and cores and Maryland bridges). The bond strength of resin cements is much greater than that of other cements, but handling characteristics are more sensitive, coupled with a shorter working time. The modified resin cements are also useful for cementation of complete metal or metal ceramic crowns to be placed on tooth preparations with minimal retentive features. Dual-cured resin cements are the cementing agents of choice for all porcelain/ceramic restorations (veneers, inlays, onlays, complete veneer crowns).

ZINC OXIDE AND EUGENOL. The primary materials for temporary cementation of restorations are preparations of zinc oxide with eugenol. These materials vary in their hardness and retaining abilities and should be selected accordingly. Temporary cements are most commonly contained in small tubes and have a fluid-paste consistency. Equal amounts of base and catalyst are expressed onto a small pad and rapidly mixed. The cement is applied to cover the inside of the restoration (usually a temporary restoration), which is then seated and held in place until the cement has hardened. The excess, hard cement is removed carefully with an appropriate instrument such as a periodontal curet or an explorer. Finally, smudges can be wiped away with a cotton pellet moistened in alcohol or orange solvent. The gingival sulcus should be examined carefully and all debris removed. Contact with moisture accelerates the set.

EVALUATION

The continuity of the restorative care cycle demands an ongoing assessment and evaluation regimen. The appropriateness of treatment must be judged from the perspectives of both the professional and the client. The professional must be responsible for paying attention to detail and evaluating the technical qualities of the restoration, whereas the client is best prepared to address issues such as comfort, function, and acceptance.

DOCUMENTATION

All restorative treatment must be accurately documented in the client's record. The documentation must include all procedures in the delivery of restorative treatment and may include, but is not limited to, the teeth and locations of restoration, anesthetic agents and medications, tooth isolation procedures, restorative materials, complications, and client education. When restorative treatment may dictate special precautions for future treatment, specific details should be provided in the record. For example, lesions restored with glass ionomer cement should be protected against dehydration. When these lesions require prolonged rubber dam isolation that results in dehydration, a special varnish can be used to prevent damage to the restoration. However, unless specifically noted, this preventive measure could go unaddressed. A special section in the client record can be designed to summarize restorative treatment precautions for all members of the oral health team. When establishing mechanisms of documentation, it is imperative that the impact of restorative therapies on the delivery of comprehensive care is considered and recordkeeping practices are appropriately designed to address the needs of all members of the oral healthcare delivery team.

MAINTENANCE OR CONTINUED CARE

Assessment is an ongoing element in the delivery of restorative care. For example, the dental hygienist may have primary responsibility for the maintenance care programs. During the maintenance care appointment, the dental hygienist thoroughly reviews the health and personal status of the client, assesses the outcomes of dental hygiene care and dental treatment, and evaluates the client's current tooth and oral health status. These assessments, when regularly communicated to the dentist, support a continued plan of care.

Client Education Issues

- Advise clients of the importance of bacterial plaque control in maintaining the integrity of dental restorations.
- Explain the advantages and disadvantages of the various dental restorations.
- Explain that restorations treat the signs of dental caries, but not the etiology of caries.
- Explain that a restored mouth takes more time and effort to maintain.
- Explain that professional maintenance care, on a regular basis, is necessary to monitor the status of the restorations and oral health.
- Explain that poor oral hygiene may manifest itself at the margins of restorations and result in the necessary replacement and extension of existing restorations.
- Explain that the maximum strength of amalgam occurs many hours after placement; therefore, care is required when chewing with force on newly placed amalgam restorations.
- Explain that for best aesthetics, whitening of teeth should be done before restoration because tooth-colored restorations are not affected by the whitening procedure.
- Explain that the use of stannous fluoride can result in staining of tooth-colored restorations.
- Explain that food and other substances that are known for staining (e.g., coffee, tea, wine, fruit juices, medications, and tobacco) can stain tooth-colored restorations.
- Explain that temporary restorations are placed only for the short-term, interim comfort of the client and protection of the cavity preparation. Permanent follow-up treatment is necessary.
- Explain that temporary restorations are easily broken or removed and do not fit as well as permanent restorations; therefore, special care is required. Caution should be taken with regard to sticky and hard food consumption (e.g., caramels and peanuts) and oral habits (e.g., gum chewing).
- Explain that any change in the client's occlusion (e.g., high spots) after dental treatment should be reported immediately to the dentist for follow-up assessment.

Legal, Ethical, and Safety Issues

✦ It is the legal responsibility of the dental hygienist to practice within the scope authorized by state law.
✦ Carefully check statutes to determine scope of practice in restorative dental procedures.
✦ Overhangs, open margins, short margins, poor contours, and open proximal contacts are avoidable defects and are not acceptable standards of care.
✦ The final plan of restorative treatment must reflect an agreement between the dentist and an educated client. In cases when the dentist is unable to render the restorative service of choice, there is an ethical obligation to refer the client to a dentist who has the necessary skills and expertise.
✦ All restorative plans are subject to change as a result of the development of unknowns; the principle of informed consent should be applied and clients should be informed about possible modifications to the restorative care plan.

Key Concepts

✦ Restorative therapies restore the dentition to a state of health, support the maintenance of health, and provide aesthetic modifications to the dentition.
✦ A cavity nomenclature is a system for communicating the features of a cavity preparation.
✦ The rubber dam is an isolation technique used to control moisture, improve accessibility and visibility, provide for the protection of the client and operator, and manage the client.
✦ Dental amalgam is a common, durable, and safe restorative material for posterior teeth.
✦ Resin composite is a tooth-colored restorative material commonly used in anterior restorations.
✦ Glass ionomer cements release fluoride ions and are well suited for restoration of root caries and Class V abrasion and erosion lesions.
✦ Cavity sealers, liners, and bases preserve and protect the dental pulp against insult.
✦ Gingival retraction is essential for making an accurate impression of the gingival margins of an indirect restoration.
✦ Temporary or interim restorations ensure client comfort, provide tooth and gingival protection, and prevent tooth movement during the period between initial and final tooth preparation and restoration placement.
✦ Luting agents are used to cement indirect restorations and to prevent the restoration from leaking and loosening.

Critical Thinking Exercises

Client 1: Ms. G.

Profile: A very well-groomed 53-year-old professional woman has what appears to be root caries on teeth numbers 29, 28, 8, 9, and 27. She has lost an MOD amalgam on tooth number 30 and an MO amalgam on tooth number 20. She states she has some concerns about putting any more mercury in her mouth and wonders if the new tooth-colored fillings are as good as silver fillings.

Chief Complaint: "My teeth have become very sensitive, and I have lost two fillings. I can't decide if I should have silver fillings put back in or if I should go with white fillings."

Dental History: Her radiographic and clinical dental evaluation reveal no additional dental caries; however, the clinical dental hygiene evaluation reveals generalized gingivitis and moderate plaque, calculus, and tobacco stain.

Social History: Client is single and lives alone.

Health History: Client is in excellent general health. She currently takes no medications, and her blood pressure is within normal limits.

Oral Health Behavior Assessment: Client states that she brushes her teeth once a day, does not use floss, and visits the dentist once every 2 years.

Supplemental Notes: She has dental insurance, demonstrates a sincere interest and motivation to maintain her teeth, but states she would prefer to not have to wear one of those pieces of rubber when the dentist fills her teeth.

1. Use the assessment data to arrive at a dental hygiene diagnosis, set client goals, and plan dental hygiene interventions.
2. How would you respond to Ms. G's question about the relative benefits of amalgam fillings versus "tooth-colored" fillings?
3. How would you respond to Ms. G's concern about mercury exposure?
4. How would you respond to Ms. G's desire not to wear a rubber dam?

Acknowledgment

The authors of this chapter wish to acknowledge James R. Clark for the photography provided for this chapter.

For References, Suggested Readings, and Related Websites, visit

http://evolve.elsevier.com/Darby/hygiene/

SECTION 6

Pain and Anxiety Control

CHAPTER 32

BEHAVIORAL MANAGEMENT OF PAIN AND ANXIETY

OBJECTIVES

Mastery of the content in this chapter will enable the reader to:

- Describe the prevalence of dental fear and anxiety in the United States
- Explain the stress response and its relationship to pain
- Differentiate dental fear, dental anxiety, and dental phobia signs and symptoms
- Apply assessment tools for determining the degree of dental fear or anxiety
- Apply behavioral options for managing dental fear and dental anxiety
- Identify the legal and ethical implications of behavioral management of fear and anxiety

KEY TERMS

Behavioral effect
Behavioral modeling
Deep breathing
Dental anxiety
Dental fear
Direct conditioning
Distraction
Guided imagery
Hypnosis
Pain threshold
Pain tolerance
Phobia
Progressive relaxation
Social phobia
Somatoform disorders
Specific phobia
Stimulus generalization
Systematic desensitization

Managing the client who is fearful, anxious, or phobic is a skill used daily when practicing dental hygiene. Almost half of the U.S. population report significant subclinical dental fear, while approximately two-thirds experience some degree of apprehension when considering upcoming dental treatment.[1] Surveys done in Britain, China, Sweden, Norway, and Australia corroborate these figures as a transcultural phenomenon (see Chapter 5).

Clinically significant dental fear is termed *phobia*. *Specific phobia* is a persistent fear in which an object or situation is avoided or endured with intense anxiety or interferes with normal routines. Examples of specific phobias in the oral healthcare setting are the sight of the syringe needle, and the sound of the dental drill.

Dental fear is defined as an unpleasant mental, emotional, or physiologic sensation derived from a specific dental-related stimulus, while *dental anxiety* is nonspecific unease, apprehension, or negative thoughts about what may happen during a dental or dental hygiene appointment. The source of the unease is often unknown to the individual. Although it is a normal reaction to anything threatening, excess anxiety interferes with efficient functioning of the individual. Dental fear and anxiety may be distinguished from dental phobia by the degree of avoidance. Individuals who are dentally fearful or anxious can cope with the intensity of the feelings they experience and obtain oral healthcare, whereas dental-phobic individuals usually are not able to cope to the degree required to attend appointments.

An array of behavioral options exists for managing dental fear and anxiety. The purpose of this chapter is to identify the physiologic, psychologic, and behavioral components of the dental fear response and introduce behavioral techniques to manage client fear, and help control or reduce perceived pain.

EFFECTS OF FEAR ON THE BODY

Understanding the physiology and psychology of the individual who experiences dental fear will help dental hygienists empathize, effectively communicate with, and ultimately treat their fearful clients.

Physiologic Effects

The effects of stress on body physiology evokes the *stress response.* This response includes a basic core of integrated neuroendocrine processes that occurs to support the fight-or-flight response when an individual is exposed to an acute stressor. The fear response is initiated in the hypothalamus of the brain, during which hypothalamic neurons stimulate the adrenal cortex to produce cortisol, and the adrenal medulla and the sympathetic free nerve endings to produce epinephrine. Cortisol is a steroid that regulates carbohydrate, protein, fat, and water metabolism, maintains vascular reactivity, affects the sensitivity of the nervous system, and regulates blood cell numbers. Epinephrine, or adrenaline, is a catecholamine chemical transmitter that effects bronchodilation and cardiac stimulation. If the production of these chemicals continues for some time in response to emotional stress (anxiety and fear), various medical complications follow: decrease in the body's immune system, elevated blood pressure, elevated blood cholesterol, elevated blood glucose, increased heart rate and respiration, and irritation to the lining of the stomach and intestinal tract (see Effects of Fear on the Body). Prolonged exposure to high-stress situations will eventually cause fatigue and disease as the body tries to maintain the elevated actions of these responses. Studies indicate that clients who are fearful of dental treatment experience elevated blood pressure, heart rate, and salivary cortisol levels immediately before dental checkups and treatment.[2–5]

Effects of Fear on the Body

Adrenal cortex produces cortisol to:

Inactivate lymphoid tissue
Stimulate glucose production
Stimulate kidney to produce renin
Irritate gastrointestinal tract lining

Adrenal medulla and sympathetic nerve endings produce epinephrine to:

Dilate pupils
Decrease salivation
Increase respiration
Increase blood pressure
Increase heart rate
Increase blood glucose
Irritate gastrointestinal tract
Increase blood cholesterol

Behavioral Effects

How a person acts during a significant fearful episode is his or her *behavioral effect.* Examples of behavioral effects of fear are impulsiveness, accident proneness, nervous laughter, emotional outbursts, excessive drinking or smoking, and changes in eating habits. For children, behavioral effects are acting out, crying, screaming, and holding on to the parent/guardian.

Psychological Effects

How an individual feels emotionally during periods of stress causes irritability, guilt, anger, or anxiety. These effects may also lead to lowered self-esteem, depression, and a feeling of loneliness. Symptoms of stress can also be seen when a person is sensitive to constructive criticism. In fearful dental hygiene clients, behavioral and psychological signs of distress may add synergistically to physiologic symptoms and manifest extreme dental fear.

When an individual is fearful of oral healthcare, regardless of the reason, his or her pain perception is altered. Although not completely understood, researchers are in general agreement that the *pain threshold,* the point at which an uncomfortable stimulus is perceived as painful, and *pain tolerance,* that amount of pain that is the most the individual can bear, decrease when an individual is fearful of the treatment.[4] Anxiety not only lowers one's pain threshold, but may also lead to the perception that a normally nonpainful stimulus is painful. If the state of tension is reduced, then the client's pain threshold is elevated and treatment is tolerated more readily.

ETIOLOGY OF DENTAL FEAR AND ANXIETY

Surveys have shown that 50% to 85% of dental-anxious individuals reported dental fear onset during their childhood or adolescence, while the remainder became fearful of dental care during adulthood.[6] Negative dental experiences lead to dental fear regardless of age of onset. Childhood fear onset has been shown to occur in families with a history of dental anxiety. Individuals who became fearful as children are more likely to fear specific dental objects, procedures, and smells. Dental fear and anxiety are barriers to good oral health (Figure 32–1). Regardless of the age of onset, dental fear can be learned through a variety of personal and nonpersonal experiences and can be associated with personality traits.[6]

Personal Experience

When a child is brought to the dental office for a first appointment, fear of the unknown is an overriding concern. Specific objects and instruments, procedures, smells, and the oral healthcare providers are new and foreign. When the treatment procedures are accomplished, simple physiologic pain may occur, and the child may show behavioral and psychological signs of pain and fear. Such an experience is an example of *direct conditioning.* At a future appointment, the child may remember

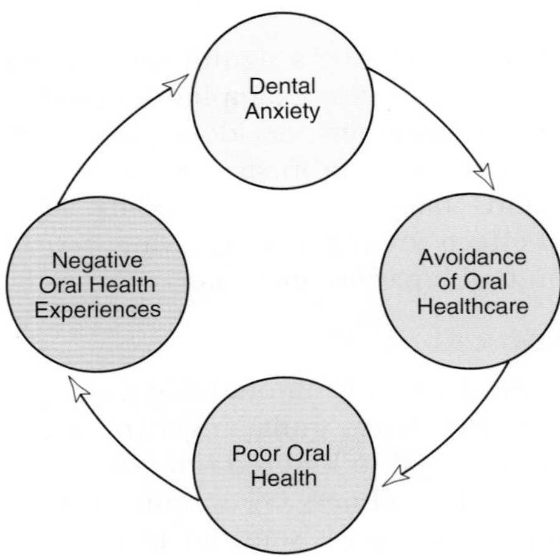

FIGURE 32–1 ✦ Theoretical model relating dental anxiety, oral healthcare, and oral health. *(From Ronis D:* Journal of Dental Hygiene *68(5): 229, 1994.)*

only the fear he or she experienced then, rather than attributing the procedure's pain as the reason for the fear.

Extending the direct conditioning of the dental appointment itself, fear of specific stimuli may become generalized from one healthcare setting to all healthcare settings. Both children and adults may have had negative medical experiences that caused them to fear the dental setting. For example, a history of hospitalization or emergency room visit may lead an individual to associate injury, pain, and fear with white walls and uniforms. When the fearful child or adult enters the oral healthcare environment and finds white walls and a staff dressed in white, the tendency is to recall the hospital experience, and the fearful response to professional oral care is intensified. Such a phenomenon is termed *stimulus generalization.*

The entire realm of oral local anesthesia provokes fear in many individuals—both children and adults. Initially, a procedure that elicits a degree of true pain may become a phobia for some individuals. Inadequate anesthesia with previous dental care that caused pain or discomfort may be associated with all oral care in the individual's mind. An incident of adverse reactions to local anesthetics (e.g., pallor, dizziness, nausea, sweating, and fainting) may lead to adverse psychological reactions when the client is confronted with the thought of future appointments. Additionally, rough, uncomfortable injections performed during childhood immunizations may be remembered and generalized to the dental injection. For approximately half of the population, direct conditioning was the cause of their dental fear.

Emotional distress appears to sensitize individuals to interactions with the oral healthcare provider. Such vulnerability heightens any negative perception, leading to the attitude by the client that oral healthcare providers' comments or behaviors "made things worse."

Examples of interactions that could increase dental anxiety are:

- Condescending remarks or rejection
- Perceived powerlessness
- Dominating personality
- Being too busy
- Continuing to treat when the individual felt pain
- Not talking or explaining things to the individual

A person with extreme dental anxiety may be suffering from a social or specific phobia. *Social phobia* is persistent fear in one or more social situations in which fear of embarrassment or humiliation is avoided. Those individuals who are socially phobic may feel:

- They cannot escape
- Embarrassed about dental treatment
- That help might not be available when they need it
- Unable to take pauses
- Unable to be heard
- Unable to be understood
- Not taken seriously or accepted by dental practitioners

The resulting feelings of powerlessness and embarrassment in dental situations lead to phobic avoidance. Prevention of phobic avoidance highlights the importance of social acceptance in the oral care environment.

Nonpersonal Experience

Learning to be fearful of dental treatment may occur before the individual experiences the first dental appointment. Such learning is termed *vicarious,* or felt by sharing in the experience of another. Vicarious learning takes place when role models, peers, and society influence individuals before their first-hand experience. Observing others, listening to embellished experiences, viewing or reading sensational material—all can negatively sensitize individuals to dental appointments. Parents who experience dental anxiety often pass along such feelings to their children. Indirect suggestion by others and identification of another's pain by the individual damage the chances for healthy, cooperative dental experiences.

Personality Traits

Dental fear and anxiety are correlated with several individual personality traits, such as hostility, neuroticism, and psychological and somatic lack of well-being. Somatic complaints are often reflected in the client's health history.

Somatoform disorders are recurrent and multiple chronic somatic complaints, where no physical disorder can be found with medical examination. These can be unreasonable body image problems or mind/body reactions that result in psychogenic-like pains, tachycardia, fainting, hypochondriasis, gagging, or other similar complaints.[7] In the absence of psychogenic pains and hypochondria, which are unlikely to be offered by the client during health history assessment, conditions such as stomach ulcers, gastric reflux, and ulcerative colitis, in addition to elevated heart rate and blood pressure, may be cited. Such signs may indicate a nervous nature underlying the anxiety of the dental procedures. Cues such as these may give the oral healthcare practitioner insight into the anxiety level of the client.

ASSESSMENT

In order to employ a comprehensive approach to fear management, strategies need to be tailored to each client's human needs. Such an approach to care includes assessing human needs related to fear (freedom from anxiety, stress, and pain), and then setting related goals to modify care as needed. Measurement of fear may be accomplished via physiologic, psychological, and behavioral assessments.

Physiologic Assessment

Physiologic changes attributed to fear may be easily assessed through accurate performance and recording of vital signs (see Chapter 10). Autonomic nervous system activation causes blood pressure, heart rate, and respirations to increase in response to the epinephrine. Additional effects of epinephrine are dilation of pupils and decrease in salivary flow.

A thorough health history review may identify other physiologic signs of a nervous disposition, such as somatoform disorders. When the dental hygienist has identified elevated vital sign readings and/or a history of digestive and cardiovascular signs for which no physiologic explanation is appropriate, dental anxiety may be suspected, and the dental hygienist will question the client regarding past oral healthcare experiences and degree of anxiety. An additional tool for determining the potential existence and degree of dental fear or anxiety is the psychological assessment survey.

Psychological Assessment

Psychological assessment of dental fear is accomplished mainly through surveys or questionnaires completed by the client. A rating scale applied to the responses provides an indication of degree of fear and, in some instances, specific feared objects or situations. Two widely used scales to assess dental fear are the revised Corah Dental Anxiety Scale and the Dental Fear Survey.

CORAH DENTAL ANXIETY SCALE (DAS). The revised version of the Corah Dental Anxiety Scale (DAS-R) consists of four questions dealing with feelings and physiologic reactions in different oral healthcare situations, with the total score ranging from 4 to 20.[8] A score of 13 to 14 suggests a dentally anxious person, while 15 or higher suggests a highly anxious client. This easy-to-use scale provides limited information on narrow or specific areas of fear reactions (see Revised Dental Anxiety Scale). Data confirm the high reliability and validity of the DAS-R.[9,10]

DENTAL FEAR SURVEY (DFS).[11] This survey assesses a broad range of dental fear components across three different dimensions: avoidance and anticipatory anxiety, autonomic or physiologic arousal, and fear of specific objects or situations (e.g., fear of seeing and feeling an injection needle and fear of the drill). Twenty items are rated on a high (5) to low (1) intensity of reactions, giving a score range of 20 to 100. Severe dentally fearful individuals have been shown to have scores from 75 and above. The DFS has been used in epidemiology research to measure the prevalence of dental fear and in clinical trials to measure effects of dental fear treatment (see Dental Fear Survey).

Revised Dental Anxiety Scale (DAS-R)

Please circle the number of the most appropriate answer to each question:

If you had to go to the dentist tomorrow, how would you feel about it?
1. I would look forward to it as a reasonably enjoyable experience.
2. I wouldn't care one way or another.
3. I would be a little uneasy about it.
4. I would be afraid that it would be unpleasant and painful.
5. I would be very frightened of what the dentist might do.

When you are waiting in the dentist's office for your turn in the chair, how do you feel?
1. Relaxed
2. A little uneasy
3. Tense
4. Anxious
5. So anxious that I sometimes break out in a sweat or almost feel physically sick

When you are in the dentist's chair waiting while he gets the drill ready to begin working on your teeth, how do you feel?
1. Relaxed
2. A little uneasy
3. Tense
4. Anxious
5. So anxious that I sometimes break out in a sweat or almost feel physically sick

You are in the dentist's chair to have your teeth cleaned. While you are waiting and the dentist or hygienist is getting out the instruments, which will be used to scrape your teeth around the gums, how do you feel?
1. Relaxed
2. A little uneasy
3. Tense
4. Anxious
5. So anxious that I sometimes break out in a sweat or almost feel physically sick

DAS summary score is the sum of the four individual scores = ______________

Corah NL: Development of a dental anxiety scale, *Journal of Dental Research* 48:596, 1969.

Behavioral Assessment

Because young children are not able to complete the DAS-R or DFS described previously, close observation of their behavior provides information on their degree

Dental Fear Survey (DFS)

Please rate your feeling or reaction on these items using the following scale:

1	2	3	4	5
never	once or twice	a few times	often	nearly every time

1. Has fear of dental work ever caused you to put off making an appointment? ___________
2. Has fear of dental work ever caused you to cancel or not appear for an appointment? ___________

When having dental work done: (use the following scale)

1	2	3	4	5
not at all	a little	somewhat	much	very much

3. My muscles become tense. _________
4. My breathing rate increases. _________
5. I perspire. _________
6. I feel nauseated and sick to my stomach. _________
7. My heart beats faster. _________

Using the scale above, please rate how much fear, anxiety, or unpleasantness each of the following causes you:

8. Making an appointment for dentistry _________
9. Approaching the dentist's office _________
10. Sitting in the waiting room _________
11. Being seated in the waiting room _________
12. The smell of the dentist's office _________
13. Seeing the dentist walk in _________
14. Seeing the anesthetic needle _________
15. Feeling the needle injected _________
16. Seeing the drill _________
17. Hearing the drill _________
18. Feeling the vibrations of the drill _________
19. Having your teeth cleaned _________
20. All things considered, how fearful are you of having dental work done? _________

Kleinknecht RA, Klepac RK, Alexander LD: Origins and characteristics of fear of dentistry. *American Dental Association Journal* 86:842, 1973.

of fear. Children are more behavioral in their display of dental fear and anxiety, and in most instances, the dental hygienist is readily able to discern their degree of fear. Clinging or uncooperative behavior and crying are actions that depict fear. For young children who may not be talking, determining what object or situation is inciting a fearful response is often a challenge.

Adults, although usually more in control of their bodies than children, display fearful behaviors in several ways. As a result of activation of the autonomic nervous system, muscular activity may be increased. Increased startle reflex, nervous tics, fidgeting, hand clenching, gripping the armrests of the chair, and breath holding are all behaviors that indicate stress.

MANAGEMENT OF FEAR AND ANXIETY

The behavioral management of anxious and fearful clients employs a caring approach to care and helps clients learn skills to cope with their fear. When the fear is specific, regarding the needle or related to anesthesia, options are clear and focused; however, when the anxiety is generalized, or when no specific fear is identifiable, a more empathetic, intuitive approach is needed. Factors to consider in the behavioral management of fear and anxiety are described as follows.

Reception and Treatment Area

Correctly assessing the client upon reception and using the CARE approach to client interaction (Comfort, Acceptance, Responsiveness, and Empathy, see Chapter 4) can prevent or manage clients' anxiety and assist them with having a positive experience. A primary consideration in managing clients' anxiety is assisting them in feeling as comfortable as possible within the dental environment. Individuals whose fears regarding dental procedures and their context are acknowledged and understood may experience lower levels of anxiety because of the empathetic attitude of the caregiver. Sensory cues in the office that may elicit negative perceptions must be minimized to the extent possible. Consider the senses of sight, hearing, smell, and touch when planning office lighting and furniture, wall and window treatments, background music, and potential odors from

Dental Office Design for the Fearful Client

Reception Area

Situate reception area away from treatment areas to minimize noises, smells, and traffic.

Create a comfortable "family room" or "living room" ambience: consider soft-colored walls and furniture and subdued lighting.

Music in Reception Room

Consider classical largos or adagios with a 60 beats per minute pace, which approximates a human heartbeat.

In Treatment Area

Consider headsets with compact disc or audiocassette players, with client selecting from in-office music libraries or bringing their own music.

Smell

Mask medicinal, especially eugenol, smells as much as possible via optimum venting and aromatherapy.

Personnel

Dress casually but professionally. Avoid all-white attire.

treatment and clean-up areas. Planning for individual comfort demonstrates staff concern and sensitivity (see Dental Office Design for the Fearful Client).

In the treatment areas, instruments should be kept out of client sight until the dentist or hygienist is ready to use them. Local anesthetic syringes should be passed behind the individual's head so that the needle—a prime visual object of fear—is not seen. For individuals who are fearful of the sound of the handpiece, ultrasonic scalers, or air abrasive polishers, using portable headsets and compact disc or audiotape players with self-selected music can help to diminish their anxiety. Studies have shown that eugenol smells elicit emotional responses from dentally fearful individuals;[12] therefore, medicinal smells and chemical odors should be managed using optimum ventilation, exhaust fans, and masking to the extent possible. A pleasant room freshener, aromatic candle, or other similar scenting device creates a more comforting, less sterile atmosphere. Attention to detail when planning the reception and treatment areas combined with a friendly, empathetic staff may engender an environment of support.

Positive Communication and Rapport

Positive and frequent communication by office staff is of vital importance in alleviating anxiety. Treatment should be explained fully in sensory terms: how treatment will sound, feel, and look. Information about the procedure, including showing the instruments to be used and describing in clear terms how they will be used and any discomfort that may be experienced, is often enough to alleviate fear. Unseen fears regarding radiation, infection control, or mercury or nitrous oxide exposure may be alleviated via accurate information.

Fear of being unable to afford optimum care often deters individuals from seeking treatment. Costs for treatment should be dealt with empathetically. Any flexible payment schedules should be fully discussed with the client, providing ample time for questions. Condescending remarks or appearing to be too busy should be avoided.

By relating to the feelings of the client, staff members display empathy and concern. Asking how they are feeling and genuinely listening to the response convey the message that what the individual relates is important. Such a climate may foster trust and openness and begin the process of relearning the dental experience. Valuing the individual's time by minimizing waiting and occupying the individual by helping him or her choose music and complete forms may correspondingly decrease anticipatory anxiety.

The gentle manner of an empathetic staff should carry into the treatment area in the form of a subtle but definite attitude of caring. Positive communication, in which words are carefully chosen, helps to describe exactly what the procedure entails. Additionally, phrases used to lead the client to a positive mental outcome are another example of reducing anxiety. For example, consider phrasing such as, "It is possible that you may feel a swelling or sponginess in your gums tonight and tomorrow, as if your teeth were floating in your tissues. When you bite, they may feel like they float up and down in their sockets. You may also feel as if your gums are itchy. These feelings are perfectly normal. You may not experience any aftereffects from our scaling; most people don't, especially when they use their saltwater rinses to decrease the swelling in their tissues." The client now knows what to expect in sensory terms. Additionally, the idea was conveyed that if the client used saltwater rinses, most likely even those sequelae would not occur.

Clients are often mistrustful or hostile because of past bad experiences. Emotionally, they may be ill-prepared for a dental hygienist who may be brusque, too busy to listen, or uncaring of their comfort. Even though the care may be technically excellent, the dental hygienist may have unknowingly created fearful, avoidant behavior in the person he or she is trying to help. Respectful treatment of individuals includes inquiring about client comfort level and stopping if pain is felt to alleviate discomfort. Consider providing individuals of all ages with a means of controlling the pace of treatment and honor it. When the individual must stop treatment for whatever reason, a signal such as raising the hand or similar action demonstrates the dental hygienist's caring attitude. An anxious client may often respond to such a show of respect and empathy, so that other behavioral management techniques are unnecessary (see Communication Strategies for Managing Dental Anxiety).

Treatment Sequencing

Depending on the level of anxiety, beginning treatment with a less-involved procedure may be the optimum sequence to help an anxious, fearful individual feel more

Communication Strategies for Managing Dental Anxiety

Practice the tell-show-do technique
Full disclosure of "unseen fears"
Radiation
Infection control
Mercury exposure
Nitrous oxide exposure

Provide full disclosure of financial matters
Costs of procedures per procedure
Prioritizing as finances dictate
Payment options
Consider payment plans and financing options

Minimize waiting time in reception and treatment rooms
Occupy client by asking for form completion.
Choose treatment room music carefully.
Consider offering refreshments.

Offer respectful treatment that gives client some control
Inquire into comfort: Stop and alleviate pain/discomfort.
Offer contracted pauses.
Encourage client to use stop signal (e.g., raising hand or other device).

Treatments for Dental Anxiety and Pain Management

Behavioral Treatments
Tell-show-do
Distraction
Relaxation therapy
Deep breathing
Guided imagery
Progressive relaxation
Systematic desensitization
Hypnosis

Pharmacologic Treatments
Local application (topical sprays/rinses: Cetacaine)
Systemic oral sedation (e.g., benzodiazepines: diazepam, temazepam, midazolam, triazolam)
Nitrous oxide–oxygen analgesia
Intravenous conscious sedation (e.g., midazolam)
General anesthesia

successful and in control of his or her dental hygiene experience. As the appointments transition into more difficult procedures, the trust, control, and confidence in not only the dental hygienist's abilities and manner, but also the level of confidence in the client's own capacity to endure the treatment, may transition a perceived nightmare into a bearable procedure.

Specific Behavioral Management Techniques

As the degree of fear and anxiety become more overt, specific behavioral management techniques may be necessary to augment positive communication and assist the individual in coping with the procedure. Such techniques include behavioral modeling, distraction, relaxation therapy (deep breathing, guided imagery), progressive relaxation training, systematic desensitization, and hypnosis (see Treatments for Dental Anxiety and Pain Management). These techniques are safe, free from adverse effects when judiciously used, and give the individual a sense of control.

BEHAVIORAL MODELING. The strategy of *behavioral modeling*, frequently used to modify children's behavior, can produce significant and stable changes.[12] With modeling, the child watches another individual undergo a procedure, either live or in video format, and then is encouraged to behave as that person did. An example of behavioral modeling may occur when an older sibling is undergoing dental hygiene care while his or her younger sibling watches. Care must be exercised in choosing the individual to be watched because he or she must exhibit the desired behaviors.

DISTRACTION. Some individuals are not interested in a full disclosure of the treatment to be accomplished, but prefer instead to be distracted by some pleasurable image or interesting activity. *Distraction* involves engaging the client's mind actively at something other than attending to the dental treatment. Distraction works well for activities of a short duration, such as exposing radiographs, timing topical fluoride treatments, and waiting for alginate impressions to set. Effective distractions include picking out as many items of a particular set as possible on a mounted poster, mentally reciting one's multiplication tables, or holding one foot in a position while doing another action with the other foot. Imagination is the only limitation to suitable distractions.

Allowing the fearful client to listen to self-selected music using a headset or to watch an absorbing program on a television monitor mounted in viewing range of the dental chair is a type of distraction that can provide audio or video analgesia. Such methods of anxiety and pain management are unpredictable in their anxiety management and may not work consistently for the same client. Additionally, a barrier against effective communication may be created because of the individual not attending to professional actions and conversation.[12]

RELAXATION THERAPY. Relaxation therapy includes a variety of techniques used to elicit the relaxation response, as a protective mechanism against stress that decreases heart rate, lowers metabolism, decreases respiratory rate, and decreases muscle tension. Before instructing the individual in any type of relaxation therapy, however, the client should be prepared with a full explanation and the option to decline the therapy (Procedure 32–1).

Procedure 32–1 MONOLOGUE FOR PREPARING THE CLIENT FOR RELAXATION THERAPY

The dental hygienist should not begin relaxation therapy without thoroughly explaining the process to the client and obtaining informed consent.

STEPS	RATIONALE
1. "If you would like to feel more relaxed during dental procedures, I can help you focus on feelings other than how tense you are."	Phrasing the concept permissively gives clients control of the situation. They must give their consent to proceed with the relaxation therapy.
2. "It may help you feel better."	Positive phrasing contributes to the idea that clients will be helped if they participate.
3. "With your permission, I'll help you focus on how your muscles are feeling now and guide you into relaxation. Since tension and relaxation cannot exist at the same time, you will slowly become accustomed to feeling a warm heaviness in your arms and legs and a sense of well-being. You will be in control of yourself at all times."	Cooperation is needed for clients to be helped. If clients give their consent, you may proceed with the progressive relaxation. If they do not, you may offer other strategies. Explaining the process eliminates the fear of the unknown and validates clients' knowledge that they are in control of the experience.
4. "Several methods are perfectly suited for the dental situation. One focuses on mentally touching your muscles to target tension; one allows you to take a 'mental vacation.' Which one do you prefer?"	Explaining the different scenarios for relaxation allows the individual a choice.

Procedure 32–2 MONOLOGUE FOR TEACHING DEEP BREATHING TO A FEARFUL CLIENT

STEPS	RATIONALE
1. "Place your hands on your stomach."	When clients are very anxious, they sometimes clench the armrests of the dental chair or wring their hands. Holding their hands on the stomach will draw their attention to what their hands are doing.
2. "Take a slow, deep breath in through your nose."	Breathing through the nose diminishes hyperventilation and helps normalize blood gases.
3. "As you inhale, feel your stomach expand. You should be breathing from your diaphragm rather than your chest. Push your abdomen out as you inhale."	Focusing on breathing from the diaphragm corrects a shallow and potentially inadequate oxygen exchange.
4. "Hold the breath for the count of 4."	Diverts clients' attention from the dental experience.
5. "Exhale through your mouth very slowly, pushing out tension that you feel."	Gives clients the capability of helping rid themselves of tension.
6. "Repeat the exercise 4 or 5 times, or until you feel more relaxed."	Continues to normalize blood gases and rid body of excess tension. Provides a mental focus.

One of the easiest relaxation therapies to learn and teach is *deep breathing*. Occasionally, fearful individuals are not aware that they are holding their breath or breathing in a shallow manner. When the breath is held unnecessarily or when inhalations are shallow and tense, the muscles of the back and abdomen begin to tense, narrowing alimentary and respiratory passages. Such tensions can by themselves produce a state of anxiety. Deep breathing promotes increased oxygen to the brain and muscles and a sense of calm (Procedure 32–2).

Following completion of dental hygiene care, awakening from relaxation must always be performed to assure that the client is fully alert before dismissal. The wakening procedure follows every relaxation therapy session (Procedure 32–3).

GUIDED IMAGERY. *Guided imagery* is a therapeutic technique for relieving pain or discomfort in which the person is encouraged to concentrate on an image that helps relieve pain or discomfort. In guided imagery, individuals "think in mental pictures," creating for themselves a sense of calmness and security in a setting of their choice. Many clients are enthusiastic about "leaving" the treatment room for a mental vacation, guided by a person they trust. When asked if they could go anywhere and do anything, fearful clients often clearly and unambiguously reveal their imaginary locations and activities. During the appointment, the provider, guided by the client's suggestions, verbally constructs a scenario for the client to visit mentally. The suggestion that the individual concentrate on the mental scene with closed eyes helps block visual fear-inducing stimuli. The dental hygienist converses throughout treatment, building details into the scenario to keep the client's attention in the scene and not on the dental hygiene care (Procedure 32–4).

Procedure 32–3 MONOLOGUE FOR AWAKENING THE CLIENT

STEPS	RATIONALE
1. "Now that we have completed treatment, I'd like for you to begin the process of coming back from relaxing so well."	Alerts clients that treatment is complete and the relaxation session is terminating.
2. "As you begin to waken, do so at your own pace. You may find that a few deep breaths will arouse you, with lots of oxygen getting to your body."	Deep breaths will arouse clients.
3. "When you are ready, you may open your eyes, feeling completely refreshed. Retain as much of the relaxation as you choose as you continue your day."	Permissive phrasing allows clients to pace their awakening and alerts them that they may feel more relaxed than when they began their appointment.

Procedure 32–4 MONOLOGUE FOR HELPING THE CLIENT RELAX WITH GUIDED IMAGERY

STEPS	RATIONALE
1. "Now that you know more about relaxation therapy, I'd like to help you deal with dental hygiene appointments. You may also apply the techniques when receiving dental treatment."	Uses positive phrasing regarding outcome; provides a tool for the client to use for future appointments.
2. "To begin, allow yourself to ease into a comfortable position in the chair. You don't need to be in a rigid or tense position."	Permits the client to move around and settle in, before initiation of care.
3. "If you were able to go anywhere and do anything you choose to relax, where would you go and what would you do?"	Asks the client to become introspective and think about how he relaxes. Depending on response, the dental hygienist begins to construct a mental scene based on information offered by the client.
For purposes of this exercise, we will assume that the client verbalized that he enjoys lying in the sand at the beach.	
4. "You may find it easier to imagine the beach if you close your eyes to block out external sights, but that is entirely up to you. We will just talk quietly for a few minutes before doing any work."	Provides the client with the option of keeping his eyes open if he is mistrustful of closing them. Informs the client of what to expect.
5. "Picture in your mind's eye, your favorite beach, what you're wearing, what you are sitting or lying on, and what the sand looks like."	Focuses the client's attention on visual cues of the beach. Since he chose the scene, he can begin constructing the setting. Since most individuals are visually oriented, these details are easy to imagine.
6. "Now look at the water. Notice what color it is, and what the waves look like: their height, where they break, how far they roll up the beach toward you."	Deepens the client's attention on visual cues.
7. "Now feel the ocean breeze blow across your skin. Is it cool or warm, harsh or soft? Notice the sand now. Is it hot, warm, or cool? Is the sand powdery, coarse, or pebbly?"	Focuses the client's attention on the sense of temperature and touch.
8. "Try to pick up on the scents of the ocean: the salty tang in the air, the whiff of seaweed, the freshness of the breeze."	Focuses the client's attention on the sense on smell.
9. "Now look at the horizon and sky. Pick out a cloud if there are any present and allow yourself to float like it is. Allow the breeze to carry you softly and safely until you feel like you're floating."	Deepens relaxation by suggesting a floating sensation.
10. "Now as you continue relaxing, allow yourself to become more and more a part of the scene, blending into the scene more and more with every breath. As you continue relaxing, I will begin my treatment. You may find that your jaw slackens and your mouth opens while you stay just as deeply relaxed as you are now."	Deepens relaxation for mouth to open and for treatment to begin.

PROGRESSIVE RELAXATION. *Progressive relaxation* is based on the theory that if a muscle is relaxed, it cannot be tense at the same time. This physiologically active technique involves alternate tensing and relaxing of skeletal, forehead, eye, and vocalizing muscles to induce physical and mental relaxation. The dental care provider guides the client through tensing then relaxing the extremities first, adding the facial muscles only if needed. This strategy may work with individuals who require a more active method of relaxing. Although

Procedure 32–5 MONOLOGUE FOR GUIDING THE CLIENT INTO PROGRESSIVE RELAXATION

STEPS	RATIONALE
1. "Rest comfortably against the back of the chair; let your hands rest in your lap or on the armrests."	Helps clients focus on how their body feels; begins introspection.
2. "If you would like to close your eyes, feel free. If you'd rather keep them open, that's fine, too."	Gives clients control over how the experience will begin.
3. "As you settle back into the chair, in your mind's eye, focus on your feet as they rest against the chair."	Heightened awareness of the feet moves attention from the dental procedures.
4. "Try to feel every muscle. Feel each toe. Feel the way your shoes cradle and hold your feet securely. Allow them to become warm and relaxed. Allow them to feel limp and heavy."	Suggesting feelings and sensations helps clients to create the relaxation.
5. "Now allow that feeling of limp, heavy warmth to move up into your calves and lower legs. Just let them feel like cooked spaghetti noodles (or other similar metaphors)."	Working from the extremities confines the sensation and gives clients a chance to develop deeper levels of relaxation so that when the head and inner organs are approached, the phenomenon is noticeable.
6. "And now let the feeling of loose, limp relaxation move into your hips and lower back. Allow yourself to be supported by the chair. Let it push up against you to hold you in calm quietness."	Constant use of metaphors provides cues to how clients should feel. Reinforcement of the relaxed state should happen frequently.
7. "As the calmness flows up your back, vertebra by vertebra can soften and ease into the chair, to be cradled and supported as you go even deeper into relaxation."	"Softening" the back reinforces the suggestion that relaxation cannot coexist with tension.
8. "Allow that limp, warm relaxation to flow up into and across your shoulders. Go deeper and deeper into relaxation with every breath."	Suggestions allow clients to feel more profound relaxation and sense of well-being as additional muscle groups are targeted.
9. "Now let the feeling of warm, limp muscles ease up the back of your neck into the base of your skull. Let your head rest comfortably into the headrest."	Same as above.
10. "As your neck and head rest even more deeply into the chair, allow that sense of tranquility to ease into your scalp and forehead. Allow your jaw to slacken and your tongue to relax. You may notice that your eyelids are getting heavier and heavier as you breathe evenly and deeply."	Same as above. Using verbiage phrased permissively, such as "you may notice," not only guides the attention of the subjects but also suggests in an optional manner what they might feel.
11. "Now turn your attention inward to your heart, diaphragm, stomach, and intestines. Your brain is able to tell your organs to slow down, to become smooth, calm, stress-free, yet retain healthy functioning."	Using many synonyms allows a choice of words to cue the subjects. Wording for one subject may not work for another.
12. "Just take a few moments now to scan your body for any pockets of tension. Your brain knows what to do to find them. Focus on them now and allow warmth and relaxation to soften and release them. Breathe out the tension. Get rid of it and become even more peaceful, tranquil, warm, and cozy. Feeling more relaxed than you ever thought possible."	This last suggestion acknowledges that the first pass over the body may not have relieved all of the tension. Clients may now return to be certain or continue deepening their state of relaxation. The scanning of the body for residual tension should take 30 to 60 seconds.
13. Now, if you could stay that relaxed and keep scanning your body, permit your jaw to slacken so that I can look in your mouth."	The suggestion for clients to open their mouth is combined with jaw relaxation as a transition into treatment.
14. "You're doing very, very well. Please continue relaxing and softening as we begin to work. Allow that feeling of well-being to intensify the longer we work. You're doing so well."	Always reinforce any positive behavior to encourage its continuance.

tensing and relaxing muscles involves covert muscular movement, such actions do not typically interfere with treatment and may be carried out in conjunction with dental hygiene care (Procedure 32–5).

Progressive relaxation is usually preceded by deep breathing and guides the client into deeper relaxation, focusing progressively on different muscle groups. Suggestions by the dental hygienist to begin with the feet and to progress toward the head draws attention from the head and dental procedures.

For the dental hygienist beginning to use the progressive relaxation technique, audiotaping the script ahead of time and listening to it to relax yourself is an excellent way to learn and hone the technique. Practicing will lead to comfort and ease of application. When you have customized your phrasing, voice tone, and modulation, and feel confident of yourself, try the technique on a friend or colleague. Before implementing progressive relaxation into a dental hygiene care plan, the client's extent of anxiety or fear must be assessed.

ADVANCED BEHAVIORAL TECHNIQUES

Advanced behavioral techniques include systematic desensitization and hypnosis. Because of the complexity of these techniques, they should be provided only by dental hygienists, dentists, and mental health professionals who are trained in their use. Information regarding systematic desensitization and hypnosis is provided to facilitate accurate education of the fearful client regarding more advanced behavioral management strategies. Dental hygienists and dentists with training in systematic desensitization and hypnosis may be found by calling the local dental society.

When referred to a mental health professional, clients may not feel that the additional expense of involving a second healthcare professional in their dental treatment is justified; however, the benefits are distinct and desirable. The advantage of such behavioral therapy over more expedient pharmacologic options is that the behavioral change is permanent, versus pharmacologic methods that must be used for each future appointment.

Systematic Desensitization

Systematic desensitization employs a hierarchy of fearful stimuli constructed by the subject to gradually address his or her fears in ascending order. The concept of gradual exposure from the least fear-arousing aspects of an object or behavior to the most fear-arousing situation is used to mentally address fears while in a deep state of relaxation. The individual begins the desensitization process by developing a list of fear-invoking stimuli, with the least noxious at bottom, graduating up to the most painful, fearful stimulus. A sample hierarchy to desensitize for fear of the dental drill might begin with making an appointment, going to the dental office, sitting in the reception area, and gradually progress to entering the treatment area, sitting in the chair, seeing the dentist, hearing noises, receiving an injection, and receiving the drilling.

When practicing relaxation, the client is asked to imagine confronting the least noxious stimulus, and simultaneously scan the body for any sign of tension. Clients are instructed to substitute relaxation for their anxiety response at each level of the hierarchy, which can be either experienced or imagined. As the client becomes more adept at relaxing while imagining the stimulus, he or she can begin to work up the chart, addressing the increasingly aversive stimuli. The client stays at one level until completely relaxed when confronting the experience, before progressing to the next level.

Hypnosis

Hypnosis is a state of mental relaxation and restricted awareness in which individuals are engrossed in their inner experiences, such as feelings and imagery, are less analytical and logical in their thinking, and have an enhanced capacity to respond to suggestions in an automatic and disassociated manner. The appropriately trained dental professional serves as a guide to clients, leading them to concentrate on internal feelings or pleasant images. As clients become less analytical in their thinking, they more easily accept suggestions for their comfort and well-being. Active therapeutic suggestions may be given that benefit both client and oral care professional by:

- Increasing the amount of cooperation by the client
- Producing analgesia
- Controlling bleeding
- Lessening postoperative discomfort and speeding healing
- Controlling salivation
- Controlling gagging
- Controlling habits such as bruxism, thumbsucking, and tongue-thrusting

Client Education Issues

- Explain that when clients are relaxed, they feel less pain.
- Explain that behavioral management techniques are safe, effective, and do not require drugs.
- Explain that it is possible for clients to relearn to receive dental treatment. They will not always be fearful or anxious when approaching dental care.
- Explain that dental hygienists who attend formal education or training are legally qualified within the scope of dental hygiene practice to provide advanced behavioral management techniques.
- Provide skills related to behavioral management techniques, such as progressive relaxation and guided imagery, to be used to relax during any stressful period.
- Explain that behavioral management treatments were developed to help all clients become more comfortable. All clients can benefit from these strategies.

Legal, Ethical, and Safety Issues

- Behavioral management techniques taught within formalized educational programs and practiced under supervision are part of a comprehensive dental hygiene care plan.
- Client rights and confidentiality should be strictly maintained.
- Adequate, routine precautions need to be taken for each client, such as maintaining continuous oversight of the client to prevent any claims that the client was unattended in a time of need.
- Document in the treatment record that the client was informed of relaxation therapy options to manage pain and anxiety and gave his or her consent. Entries should include which therapy was performed, the client's response, and the fact that the client was fully alert when dismissed.
- An effective care plan includes a behavioral management component to promote a sense of control and to optimize client cooperation and comfort.[13]
- Dental hygienists wishing to use hypnosis must be instructed through a dental school curriculum on anesthesia and pain management or attend formalized instruction offered through the American Society of Clinical Hypnosis.
- Legal aspects of hypnosis can be separated into two divisions: (1) there are laws that pertain to the practice of dentistry and dental hygiene, and (2) there are laws that pertain to conduct as a citizen outside of the professional role. As long as dental hygienists use hypnosis within the context of their professional roles, their usual insurance that includes malpractice will cover them. A rider to the policy including the specific use of hypnosis is generally not needed; however, individual state dental practice acts should be reviewed.

Key Concepts

- Dental fear or anxiety affects approximately three-fourths of the total world population.
- There are physiologic, psychological, and behavioral cues to identifying a client who is fearful or anxious of dental treatment.
- Pain threshold and pain tolerance are lowered in the presence of fear or anxiety.
- The etiology of dental fear or anxiety may be either through direct personal experience or through vicarious nonpersonal experience.
- Behavioral management techniques can effectively lower pain perception.
- Behavioral management techniques used to control pain and anxiety include behavioral modeling, distraction, relaxation therapy (deep breathing, guided imagery, progressive relaxation), systematic desensitization, and hypnosis.
- Dental hygienists wishing to use hypnosis and systematic desensitization must receive formal instruction in these strategies.

Critical Thinking Exercises

Client: Ms. D

Profile: Ms. D, age 35, is scheduled for nonsurgical periodontal therapy with the dental hygienist. She is a new patient and has not been seen for dental care in more than two years. As you enter the reception room to announce Ms. D's name, you notice a woman flipping through a magazine and sitting on the edge of her chair. She looks up quickly as you say her name, and she gives you a hesitant smile.

Chief Complaint: "I am in pain from a back left lower tooth."

Medical History: Ms. D's vital signs are pulse: 92, respirations: 25, temperature: 99 degrees, and supine blood pressure: 140/80. She admits to having gastric reflux and prefers to sit back partially rather than supine. She smokes approximately one-half pack of cigarettes per day.

Social History: Ms. D is single and lives alone.

Dental History: As you seat her in your treatment room, she admits that the last time she attended a dental office was more than two years ago. Ms. D. said the dentist did not numb her tooth enough to take the pain away and began a root canal in a lower left molar. She never went back for the completion of the endodontic therapy, and now the tooth is bothering her. Intraorally, Ms. D's gingival tissues are erythematous along the margins, and the interdental papillae are bulbous. Her gingival tissues are smooth, with generalized bleeding

Continued on following page

Critical Thinking Exercises—cont'd

on probing. You notice the tooth in question, #19, has a large opening on the occlusal surface. In addition to the incomplete endodontic treatment, Ms. D has two other carious areas on interproximal surfaces.

Oral Health Behavior Assessment: Her home care consists of brushing once per day with a soft brush and trying to floss once per week. She realizes she could do more, but states that she "doesn't have time."

Supplemental Notes: Ms. D grips the armrests of the chair upon periodontal probing. After numerous stops and starts, she admits that she is terrified of dental treatment—no matter who performs it—and has been fearful of dentistry since a child.

1. What interventions would you plan to meet the client's need for freedom from stress?
2. Using the above information, role play with a student partner one of the following relaxation strategies to manage the client's pain and anxiety:
   - ✦ Deep breathing
   - ✦ Progressive relaxation
   - ✦ Guided imagery

For References, Suggested Readings, and Related Websites, visit
http://evolve.elsevier.com/Darby/hygiene/

CHAPTER 33

DENTINAL HYPERSENSITIVITY MANAGEMENT

OBJECTIVES

Mastery of the content of the chapter will enable the reader to:

- Describe dentinal hypersensitivity, its prevalence, etiology, and treatments
- List teeth most likely to experience dentinal hypersensitivity
- Explain the hydrodynamic theory
- Identify risk factors contributing to dentinal hypersensitivity
- Explain factors that reduce dentinal hypersensitivity
- Distinguish between dentinal hypersensitivity and other sources of tooth pain
- Describe active ingredients available to treat hypersensitivity and mechanisms of action
- Identify self-applied and professional (in-office) interventions for dentinal hypersensitivity

KEY TERMS

Abfraction
Abrasion
A-delta fibers
Attrition
Dentinal hypersensitivity
Dentinal sclerosis
Dentinal tubule
Erosion
Frenal pull
Hydrodynamic theory
Nerve hyperpolarization
Smear layer

DENTINAL HYPERSENSITIVITY

Tooth pain and sensitivity are common client complaints in the oral care environment. Several conditions may elicit a pain response, but the nature and extent of the pain vary substantially. Therefore, it is critical to assess oral sites of sensitivity to identify and manage the problem correctly. *Dentinal hypersensitivity* is characterized by short, sharp pain arising from exposed dentin that occurs in response to stimuli, typically thermal (both hot and cold), evaporative, tactile, osmotic, or chemical, and that cannot be ascribed to any other form of dental defect or pathology.[1,2]

Etiology and Nature of Dentinal Hypersensitivity

Tooth development results in the following cementum-to-enamel relationships:

- Cementum overlaps the enamel (14% of time)
- Cementum and enamel meet without overlap (76% of time)
- Cementum and enamel do not meet (10% of time) but with no exposed dentin (see Chapter 21)

Histologically, dentin reflects thin, numerous tubules that transverse from the pulp to the outer dentin surface. Three types of sensory nerve fibers within the *dentinal tubules* extend from the pulpal side of the dentinal tubule, 10% to 15% of the distance to the dentinoenamel junction. Stimulation of these sensory nerve fibers manifests as tooth pain. The transient type of pain is a result of the stimulation of the *A-delta fibers*—small, myelinated fibers that evoke a sensation of well-localized sharp pain. Activation of the A-delta fibers is responsible for dentinal hypersensitivity. Similarly, the A-beta fibers are susceptible to the same types of stimuli but respond more sensitively to electrical stimulation. In contrast to the A-delta and A-beta fibers, stimulation of the unmyelinated C-fibers results in a dull, poorly localized, aching type of pain usually associated with pulpal pain. Thus the activation of specific fibers results in different types of tooth pain.

Hypersensitive dentin has the following characteristics:

- ✦ Dentinal tubules open to the oral cavity
- ✦ Large and numerous dentinal tubules
- ✦ Thin, poorly calcified or breached *smear layer* (a deposit of salivary proteins, debris from dentifrices and other calcified matter)

In nonsensitive dentin, the smear layer covers the opening of the dentinal tubules, or mineral compounds occlude the tubules, reducing the ability of stimuli to induce fluid flow. Hence, the loss or removal of a smear layer may result in a pain response. Moreover, fewer dentinal tubules at the surface are present than in sensitive dentin.[3]

Hydrodynamic Theory

Brannstrom was the first to provide evidence to support the widely accepted *hydrodynamic theory* explaining the pain of dentinal hypersensitivity. The hydrodynamic theory proposes that stimuli (i.e., thermal, tactile, or chemical) are transmitted to the pulp surface via movement of the fluid or semifluid materials in the dentinal tubules. Fluid movement acts as the transducing medium for conveying peripheral stimuli to free nerve endings of A-delta fibers near the odontoblastic layer by the pulp-dentin interface. This reaction results in a pain response (Figure 33–1).

For dentinal hypersensitivity, dentin must be exposed and dentinal tubules must be open at the dentin surface and open to vital pulp. Dentin exposure is a result of gingival recession or enamel loss. When gingival recession occurs, cementum is exposed. The layer of cementum is thin and labile and is easily abraded or eroded away, thus offering little protection against sensitivity.[4] Scanning electron photomicrographs verify that hypersensitive dentin has eight times as many open dentinal tubules and twice the diameter of open tubules as nonsensitive dentin. These findings serve as the basis for treatment options.

Causes of Gingival Recession

- ✦ *Anatomy of the labial plate of the alveolar bone.* A thin, fenestrated, or absent labial alveolar bone is a major predisposing factor to recession.[5,6] Tooth anatomy[7] and tooth position[8] also affect the thickness of the labial plate. For example, orthodontic treatment may move the tooth through the buccal plate to predispose it to recession.
- ✦ *Oral hygiene status.* Poor oral hygiene results in plaque-induced gingival disease. Hence, it would make sense that poor oral hygiene would lead to gingival recession; however, research reveals that more recession occurs with meticulous oral hygiene.[9]
- ✦ *Acute or chronic trauma.* Gingival trauma and injury caused by toothbrushing are significant risk factors.[10–12] The technique, frequency, duration, and force of brushing and toothbrush filaments have been implicated in recession.[13–15] Injury to the gingiva caused by foreign objects[16] or damaging habits such as fingernail scratching also may cause recession.
- ✦ *Frenal attachment at the gingival margin.* Progressive recession may occur when the fibers of the frenum insert near the gingival margin and cause a tight *frenal pull* on the gingival tissues. Tissue movement resulting from speech and mastication pull the gingiva from the cementoenamel junction (CEJ), resulting in gingival recession.[17]
- ✦ *Occlusal trauma.* Occlusal trauma that results in the movement of teeth can alter the attachment of the gingiva to the tooth.[18]

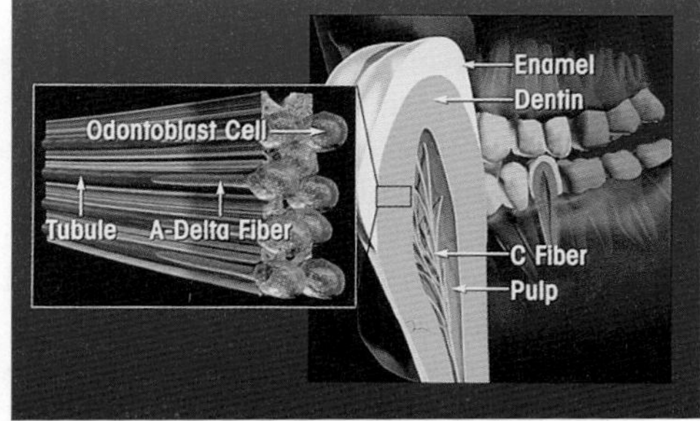

FIGURE 33–1 ✦ Structure of dentinal tubules. *(Courtesy Osprey Communications.)*

Causes of Enamel Loss

- ✦ *Attrition.* Sites of tooth structure wear are commonly found on the incisal or occlusal surfaces of teeth caused by the masticatory forces. Unless malocclusion is involved, it is highly unlikely that attrition is observed at the buccal sites.
- ✦ *Abrasion.* Toothbrush variation (stiffness and configuration of the bristles), coupled with force, method, frequency, and duration of brushing, results in tooth structure loss. Toothbrushes in conjunction with dentifrices produce measurable enamel loss, implicating the abrasiveness of the toothpaste. In comparison, enamel loss is considerably less than loss of dentin or cementum that had been brushed with toothpaste. For example, dentin abrades 25 times faster than enamel, while cementum abrades 35 times faster than enamel.
- ✦ *Erosion.* Erosion—tooth structure loss caused by a chemical process—is most responsible for enamel loss. *Intrinsic erosion* is caused by acid regurgitation associated with medical and psychological disorders (e.g., bulimia, morning sickness). *Extrinsic erosion* is a result of dietary factors that contribute to a highly acidic oral environment (e.g., the frequent consumption of acidic, carbonated, or fruit drinks, or frequent sugar consumption).[19]
- ✦ *Abfraction.* The ongoing flexion, tension, and compression forces exerted in the cervical area of a tooth from mastication and occlusal trauma can result in cracking and eventual loss of cervical tooth structure.

The effects of abrasion and erosion suggest that the loss of enamel and dentin by toothpaste abrasion is considerably increased if there is prior exposure to low-pH fluids such as juices.[19,20] Thus loss of enamel can occur at an accelerated rate under the combined conditions of abrasion, erosion, and abfraction, resulting in exposed dentin.

Prevalence and Distribution of Dentinal Hypersensitivity

Dentinal hypersensitivity has been reported during the early teens to 70 years of age;[21] however, peak incidence occurs at 20 to 40 years of age and is consistent with the incidence and progression of gingival recession.[22] As an individual ages, prevalence of dentinal hypersensitivity decreases because of an increase in reparative dentin formation; reduction in pulpal chamber size, vascularity, and pulpal nerve fibers; and *dentinal sclerosis* (reduction of the dentinal tubule lumen as a result of the deposition of intratubular dentin). Hence, with age, dentinal hypersensitivity often decreases.

Dentinal hypersensitivity is more prevalent in females than in males.[2,22,23] The difference between females and males may be attributed to the better oral hygiene of females than of males, specifically at the buccal sites.[24]

Dentinal hypersensitivity is most prevalent on the buccal cervical regions of teeth.[2,22,25] Similarly, these same sites have a predilection for gingival recession and are the area where the enamel is the thinnest. Thus gingival recession and loss of enamel appear to be related to the initiation of dentinal hypersensitivity.

The teeth most commonly affected in order of frequency are canines and first premolars, incisors and second premolars, and molars.[21–23] Epidemiologic data show that dentinal hypersensitivity is negatively correlated with plaque scores.[26] Buccal cervical plaque scores on canines and premolars tend to be lower than at other buccal sites.

Persons with moderate to severe sensitivity exhibit hypersensitivity at the same tooth sites, and there is a greater frequency of left-sided tooth sensitivity in comparison to their right contralateral tooth types. Hence, individuals who are right-handed tend to clean their left sides more vigorously than their right-sided teeth, contributing to unilateral hypersensitivity.

Diagnosis

Many oral conditions exhibit symptoms similar to dentinal hypersensitivity. Conditions such as chipped or fractured teeth, dental caries, pulpal pathology, or leaking, fractured, or failing restorations require completely different treatment from dentinal sensitivity. Hence, a thorough clinical and radiographic examination must be conducted to exclude these conditions and arrive at a differential diagnosis of dentinal hypersensitivity (see Characteristics of Hypersensitive Versus Nonsensitive Dentin). For a diagnosis of dentinal hypersensitivity to be made, specific clinical and radiographic criteria must be present:

Clinical criteria

- ✦ Sensitivity or pain when a stimulus is applied
- ✦ Presence of bacterial plaque biofilm
- ✦ Exposed dentin at the site of sensitivity
- ✦ No clinical signs of dental caries
- ✦ No evidence of fracture lines in tooth structure
- ✦ Restoration margins flush with tooth structure

Radiographic criteria

- ✦ Radiolucency may be present at the cervical third of the tooth where pain is reported, but must be confirmed clinically to exclude dental caries
- ✦ No pulpal inflammation or apical pathology
- ✦ Absence of distinct fracture lines
- ✦ No radiolucent areas under restorations

MANAGEMENT OF DENTINAL HYPERSENSITIVITY

In managing dentinal hypersensitivity, it is essential to identify the cause and risk factors of dentinal hypersensitivity (see Factors that Contribute to Dentinal Hypersensitivity). Without addressing etiology and risk factors associated with dentinal hypersensitivity, little success will be gained in long-term management of the condition.

Characteristics of Hypersensitive Versus Nonsensitive Dentin

Hypersensitive Dentin

Ends of dentinal tubules open to the oral cavity

Tubules larger and more numerous than in nonsensitive dentin

Smear layer is thin, poorly calcified, or breached

Nonsensitive Dentin

Fewer dentinal tubules at tooth surface are present than in sensitive dentin.

Either a smear layer is present or tubules are occluded by mineral compounds

Factors that Contribute to Dentinal Hypersensitivity

Factors that may expose dentin or opening tubules that are already blocked or sealed:

- Gingival recession
- Loss of enamel
- Toothbrush abrasion
- Erosion
- Abfraction
- Acidic foods
- Periodontal surgery
- Occlusal hyperfunction
- Cusp grinding
- Instrumentation (root planing, scaling, extrinsic stain removal)
- Cosmetic tooth whitening (see Chapter 22)

After identifying cause and risk factors, the client is educated about behaviors that exacerbate symptoms of dentinal hypersensitivity. If necessary, behavior modification may be discussed (e.g., dietary choices such as avoiding carbonated beverages and extremes in hot and cold foods; use of a daily fluoride mouthrinse and a low-abrasive, fluoride dentifrice for sensitive teeth) to arrest the hypersensitivity.

Treatment options include self-applied (at-home) care or professionally applied (in-office) desensitizing procedures. Desensitizing agents used in treatment are classified by mode of action (Table 33–1): inactivation of the nerve membrane (hyperpolarization) or occlusion of the open dentinal tubules.

- ✦ *Nerve hyperpolarization.* Intradental nerves are hyperpolarized by raising their extracellular potassium ion concentration. The sustained hyperpolarized state reduces nerve excitation, and the nerves become insensitive to further stimulation. An example is potassium nitrate.
- ✦ *Dentinal tubule occluding.* Examples include oxalate compounds, strontium chloride, calcium hydroxide, fluorides, silver nitrate, and hydroxyethyl methacrylate (HEMA).

Without effective daily plaque biofilm control, the desensitizing effects of these agents are limited.

Self-Applied Desensitizing Agents

(Table 33–2 and Figure 33–2)

Self-applied desensitizing agents should be recommended to manage mild dentinal hypersensitivity. These agents are cost effective, noninvasive, and simple to use, and can be applied at home for convenience. Regular and continuous application is necessary to manage sensitivity. Clients may apply a range of desensitizing agents in the form of dentifrices, gels, or rinses as part of their daily self-care regimen at home.

Potassium nitrate is the most common desensitizing agent in dentifrices. At a concentration of 5%, potassium nitrate in conjunction with sodium or monofluorophos-

TABLE 33–1 DESENSITIZING AGENTS AND THEIR MODE OF ACTION

Nerve inactivator	Potassium nitrate
Tubule obtundent	Fluorides
	Oxalates
	Calcium compounds
	Sodium citrate
	Strontium chloride
Protein precipitant	Strontium chloride
	Silver nitrate
	Formaldehyde
	Glutaraldehyde

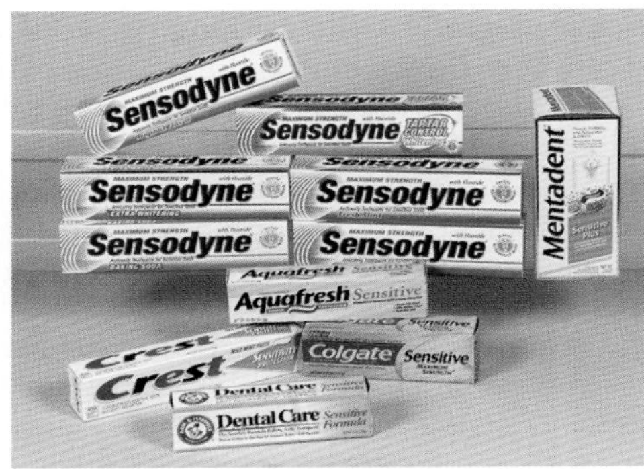

FIGURE 33–2 ✦ Some desensitizing dentifrices. *(Courtesy GlaxoSmithKline.)*

TABLE 33–2 SOME DESENSITIZING DENTIFRICES

Product	Manufacturer	Active Agent	Mechanism of Action	Comments
Sensodyne Original	GlaxoSmithKline	Potassium nitrate	Inactivates nerve	NaF, does not contain sodium lauryl sulfate
Sensodyne Cool Gel	GlaxoSmithKline	Potassium nitrate	Inactivates nerve	NaF, does not contain sodium lauryl sulfate
Sensodyne Fresh Mint	GlaxoSmithKline	Potassium nitrate	Inactivates nerve	NaF
Sensodyne Baking Soda	GlaxoSmithKline	Potassium nitrate	Inactivates nerve	NaF
Sensodyne Tartar Control + Whitening	GlaxoSmithKline	Potassium nitrate	Inactivates nerve	NaF
Sensodyne Extra Whitening	GlaxoSmithKline	Potassium nitrate	Inactivates nerve	Na MFP
Dental Care Sensitive	Arm & Hammer	Potassium nitrate	Inactivates nerve	
Crest Sensitive	Procter & Gamble	Potassium nitrate	Inactivates nerve	NaF
Colgate Sensitive	Colgate-Palmolive Company	Potassium nitrate	Inactivates nerve	SnF, dual-chamber delivery
Colgate Sensitive + Whitening	Colgate-Palmolive Company	Potassium nitrate	Inactivates nerve	SnF, dual-chamber delivery
Mentadent Sensitive	Chesebrough-Ponds Co	Potassium nitrate	Inactivates nerve	NaF
AquaFresh Sensitive	GlaxoSmithKline	Potassium nitrate	Inactivates nerve	NaF

phate fluoride in the toothpaste significantly reduces symptoms within two weeks. Potassium ions penetrate the length of the dentinal tubule and block repolarization of the nerve ending. Increasing the extracellular potassium ion concentration depolarizes nerve fiber membranes and renders them unable to repolarize. Frequent application of a potassium nitrate dentifrice is necessary to avoid recurrence of symptoms, maintain a high abundance of extracellular potassium ions, and maintain the intradental nerves in a hyperpolarized state. Therefore, application via a dentifrice is ideal. Moreover, clients can be instructed to dab very small amounts of sensitivity-protection dentifrice on the sensitive area of the tooth at bedtime and leave it there overnight.

Self-applied desensitizing agents also are marketed in gels and rinses. The active agents for these products are various fluoride compounds, such as sodium fluoride, sodium silicofluoride, and stannous fluoride. Although fluoride compounds in dentifrices have the American Dental Association (ADA) Seal of Acceptance for caries prevention, they have not been approved for treatment of dentinal hypersensitivity. Application of fluoride to exposed dentin leads to the formation of calcium fluoride and other precipitates, reducing the functional radius of the dentinal tubules or blocking the dentinal tubules. Hence, some relief is provided by the use of fluoride-containing gels and rinses.

Professionally Applied Desensitizing Agents (Table 33–3 and Figure 33–3)

Although mild hypersensitivity may be managed by using a sensitivity-protection toothpaste twice daily, moderate to severe dentinal hypersensitivity must be treated professionally. Professionally applied agents include varnishes and precipitants, primers containing HEMA, and polymerizing agents. In severe cases, loss of cervical tooth structure often requires restoration to control hypersensitivity.

Before any desensitizing treatment, hard and soft deposits should be removed from the tooth surfaces. Therapeutic scaling may cause considerable discomfort, in which case teeth should be anesthetized before mechanical treatment.

VARNISHES

- ✦ *5% sodium fluoride varnish.* Fluoride varnishes temporarily occlude dentinal tubules because the material is lost over time. This desensitizing agent is effective for relief of dentinal hypersensitivity (see Chapter 26, section on Topical Fluorides, Professionally Applied Varnishes).

TABLE 33–3 SOME PROFESSIONALLY APPLIED DESENSITIZING AGENTS

Product	Manufacturer	Active Agent	Mechanism of Action	Comments
Gel-Kam Oral Care Rinse	Colgate Oral Pharmaceuticals	0.63% stannous fluoride	Remineralization	May cause staining
Gel-Kam DentinBloc	Colgate Oral Pharmaceuticals	1.09% sodium fluoride, 0.4% stannous fluoride, 0.14% hydrogen fluoride	Obturation of dentinal tubules	Preprocedural (before scaling and root planing)
Protect Drops	Sunstar Butler	Monohydrogen-monopotassium oxalate	Combines with calcium ions in dentinal fluid to form insoluble calcium oxalate complex, which occludes dentinal tubules	Dispensed in single ampules or dropper bottle
Duraphat	Colgate Oral Pharmaceuticals	5% sodium fluoride varnish	Obturates dentinal tubules	Postprocedural
Zarosen Desensitizing	Cetylite Industries, Inc.	6.9% copal resin, 0.146% strontium chloride	Seals dentinal tubules, cavity varnish	After scaling, before and after extrinsic stain removal, after cavity preparation, and before any crown and bridge cementation, and pin and post seating
HemaSeal G Desensitizing Solution	Germiphene Corporation	35% HEMA, 5% glutaraldehyde	Binds with proteins to seal dentinal tubules	
HurriSeal	Beutlich	Benzalkonium chloride, HEMA, 0.5% sodium fluoride, water	HEMA seals the dentinal tubules to produce a physiologic barrier for desensitizing, while benzalkonium chloride acts as an antimicrobial	Used in conjunction with bonding adhesive systems and crown and bridge luting agents
Gluma Desensitizer	Heraeus Kulzer	HEMA, glutaraldehyde, water	Seals dentinal tubules	No mixing or curing involved, strong smell and taste

PRECIPITANTS

- *Oxalates.* The efficacy of oxalate-containing agents is unclear. Comparison of the clinical evidence fails to objectively demonstrate the efficacy of oxalate-containing agents because of various experimental designs.
- *Calcium phosphate compounds.* Burnishing of calcium phosphate into areas of sensitive dentin significantly relieves discomfort. The mechanism of action involves the occlusion of dentinal tubules by forming a calcium phosphate precipitate.

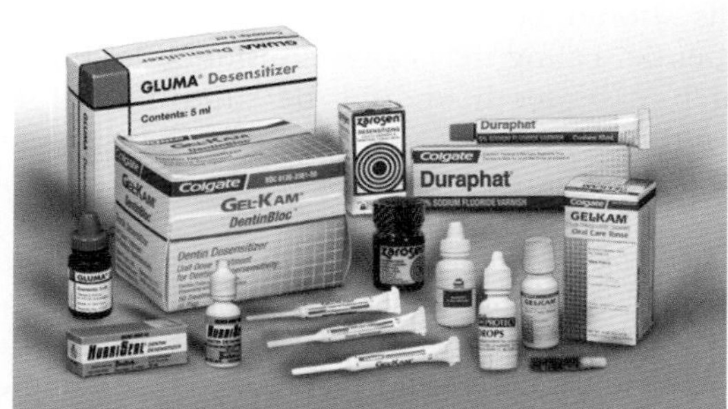

FIGURE 33–3 ✦ Some professionally applied desensitizing agents. *(Courtesy GlaxoSmithKline.)*

- *Calcium hydroxide.* This desensitizing agent has been used to block dentinal tubules and promote peritubular dentin formation. It also is effective in reducing the permeability of acid-etched dentin and smear layers.

PRIMERS CONTAINING HEMA. Although few controlled clinical trials have been conducted on the efficacy of HEMA-containing primers, desensitizing agents containing either 5% glutaraldehyde and 35% HEMA in water or 35% HEMA in water alone are popular.

- *5% glutaraldehyde, 35% HEMA in water.* One study demonstrated that the primer containing 5% glutaraldehyde and 35% HEMA in water is effective in reducing dentinal hypersensitivity; however, sensitivity was only measured once, 14 days after crown preparation. Another study of HEMA-containing desensitizing agents showed reductions in sensitivity that lasted for the entire six-month trial.[27]

POLYMERIZING AGENTS

- *Glass ionomer cements (GICs).* GICs are used in cervical abrasions and abfractions for treatment of dentinal hypersensitivity. The cervical areas of a tooth are etched with 50% citric acid for 30 to 45 seconds, rinsed with water, and dried before GIC placement.

Procedure 33–1 ADMINISTRATION OF DESENSITIZING AGENTS

EQUIPMENT

Isolating materials (cotton rolls, gauze, etc.)
Cotton applicators
Dappen dish
Personal protective equipment

STEPS	RATIONALE
1. Assemble armamentarium for desensitization.	Preparation results in less chair time and greater comfort for the client.
2. Explain rationale, procedure, and limitations of desensitizing agent to the client.	Dispels any confusion regarding consent, purpose, extent, duration, and consequences of treatment. Client is actively involved in the decision-making process.
3. Identify sensitive sites requiring desensitization treatment.	Site-specific application of desensitizing agent is prudent and acceptable.
4. Remove plaque biofilm and debris from tooth surfaces before desensitizing agent is applied.	Allows for greater retention and effectiveness.
5. Isolate area with cotton rolls and dry dentin surface by blotting with gauze.	Prevents the flow and ingestion of the product and maximizes uptake where needed.
6. Dispense desensitizing agent and apply according to manufacturer's instructions.	Different products will require different application procedures. Note instructions for maximum effectiveness.
7. Evaluate treated areas for success and reapply if necessary.	Reapplication may be necessary to achieve adequate amounts of the active agent at specific sites in order to overcome pain threshold.
8. Discard materials according to infection control procedures.	Prevents cross-contamination.
9. Record treatment in services-rendered section of client record, including tooth number, region of treatment, agent used, and client response.	Manages legal risks and facilitates evaluation at next appointment.
10. Educate client about supplementary procedures for controlling sensitivity.	Prevents further incidences of hypersensitivity and manages the problem over the long term.

GICs are effective in treating hypersensitivity if they cover the affected area.

- *Adhesive resin primers.* Adhesive resin primers decrease dentin permeability by occluding the open dentinal tubules. Resin primers come in a two-bottle system that requires mixing. The mixed product is gently rubbed on the hypersensitive dentin for approximately 30 seconds and then air-dried.

IONTOPHORESIS. Iontophoresis involves the delivery of sodium fluoride by passing an electrical current through the cervical dentin. This procedure is based on the principle that similar electromagnetic charges repel each other. When the negative fluorine ions contact the negatively charged electrode and a current is passed through the tooth to the other electrode (which is held by the client, completing the circuit), fluoride ions are pushed into the dentinal tubules, where they react with ions in the hydroxyapatite. Fluorapatite precipitate, an insoluble compound, is formed, thus occluding the tubules.

This technique-sensitive procedure has been supported by Gangaros, Kerns, and Christiansen to treat hypersensitive dentin.[28-31] Lack of efficacy reported by others may be the result of the inadvertent passage of current through adjacent gingival tissue rather than through cervical dentin.[32] Mild cases of dentinal hypersensitivity may only require a single treatment, whereas in more severe cases, two or three applications one week apart may be necessary. The procedure requires a special apparatus.

LASERS. Laser therapy is relatively quick, and one treatment drastically reduces or eliminates sensitivity by sealing the dentinal tubules. Dentin treated with laser is harder than untreated dentin. Laser therapy is based on the coagulation and precipitation of plasma proteins in dentinal fluid[33] by using a neodymium:yttrium-aluminum-garnet (Nd:YAG) laser to treat cervical sensitivity; however, producing uniform laser treatment on irregularly shaped cervical areas of the tooth is difficult. Use of lasers to treat dentinal hypersensitivity is not well documented in the literature.[34,35] Clinical results do not yet justify the high cost for the apparatus.

RESTORATIONS. Desensitizing agents either occlude the open tubule or inactivate the nerve. Restorations may be placed to cover exposed dentin and restore tooth anatomy, especially where aesthetics are important. In extreme circumstances, it may be necessary to remove the pulp and perform root canal therapy, or extract the tooth. These last two options will be indicated for other reasons, additional to the dentinal hypersensitivity, such as inability to restore the tooth, severe periodontal destruction, overeruption, or aesthetics.

Client Education Issues

- Explain the multifaceted causes of dentinal hypersensitivity and risk factors that can be managed by the client.
- Discuss dietary information to monitor acidic/sugary fruits and beverages that might contribute to hypersensitivity.
- Explain the significance of proper toothbrushing; low-abrasive, fluoride dentifrices for sensitive teeth; and interdental cleaning.
- Explain the use of an ultrasoft toothbrush without the application of a toothpaste.[36]
- Suggest dabbing a sensitivity-protection dentifrice on the most sensitive areas of the tooth at bedtime.

Legal, Ethical, and Safety Issues

- Proper assessment of client's hypersensitivity is essential to rule out alternative causes of pain.
- Document in the client record the problem, product recommendation, instructions provided, and client's response to care (e.g., compliance, product success, or adverse effects).
- Evaluate the clinical outcome following treatment to ensure effectiveness of therapy.
- Comply with the State Practice Act regarding dental hygienists' scope of practice in terms of product recommendation, use, and clinician application.

Key Concepts

- ✦ Assessment of etiology and risk factors is critical in accurately identifying dentinal hypersensitivity.
- ✦ Hypersensitive dentin has the following characteristics: dentinal tubules open to the oral cavity, large and numerous dentinal tubules, and thin, poorly calcified, or breached smear layer (a deposit of salivary proteins, debris from dentifrices and other calcified matter).
- ✦ Abfraction is the ongoing flexion, tension, and compression forces exerted in the cervical area of a tooth from mastication and occlusal trauma. It results in cracking and eventual loss of cervical tooth structure.
- ✦ Dentinal hypersensitivity is characterized by short, sharp pain arising from exposed dentin that occurs in response to stimuli, typically thermal (both hot and cold), evaporative, tactile, osmotic, or chemical, and that cannot be ascribed to any other form of dental defect or pathology.
- ✦ The hydrodynamic theory proposes that stimuli (i.e., thermal, tactile, or chemical) are transmitted to the pulp surface via movement of the fluid or semifluid materials in the dentinal tubules.
- ✦ Desensitization measures are incorporated into the client's care plan and daily self-care regimen.
- ✦ Most persons experiencing dentinal hypersensitivity can be treated with self-applied desensitizing dentifrices; however, if the sensitivity persists, professionally applied tubule-occluding desensitizing agents and other restorative interventions can reduce sensitivity.
- ✦ Dental hygienists have a role in the management of dentinal hypersensitivity. This includes staying informed of current research and new products, selecting treatments that meet the clients' needs, and educating clients about effective self-care habits.

Critical Thinking Exercises

Use Figure 33–4 and the following information to answer the questions on this case.

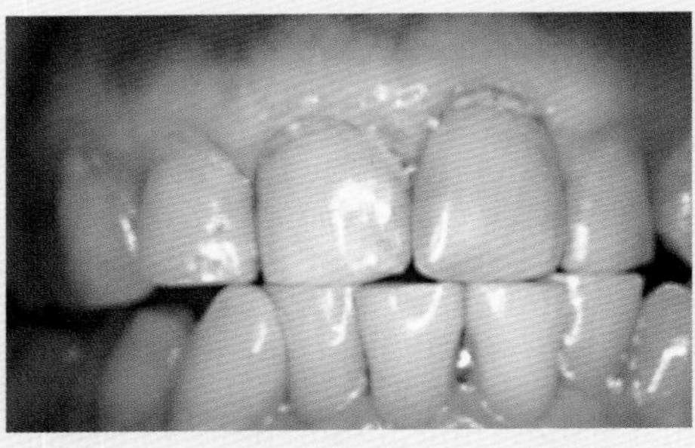

FIGURE 33–4 ✦ Intraoral photo of a young woman. Note accumulation of bacterial plaque biofilm, gingival recession, cervical abrasion, and attrition. *(Courtesy GlaxoSmithKline.)*

Client Profile:

- ✦ 32-year-old female
- ✦ Single mother of two boys (ages 2 and 4)
- ✦ Occupation: Emergency room nurse

Chief Complaint: "My teeth are very sensitive when I eat or drink cold foods and beverages."

Health History: No significant findings

Pharmacologic History: Client taking the following medications:

- ✦ Ortho Tri-Cyclen (norgestimate/ethinyl Estradiol)
- ✦ Wellbutrin SR (Bupropion HCl 100 mg)
- ✦ Imitrex (Sumatriptan succinate 50 mg)

Dental History:

- ✦ Regular 6-month continued-care appointments
- ✦ History of frequent aphthous ulcers
- ✦ Brushes twice daily
- ✦ Flosses once daily

Clinical Examination:

- ✦ Absence of soft tissue pathology
- ✦ Absence of clinical carious lesions
- ✦ Light to moderate calculus
- ✦ Localized attrition along anterior incisal and canine surfaces
- ✦ Localized recession and cervical abrasion evident on teeth numbers 6, 7, 8, 9, 22, 23, 24, 25, 26, 27, 28, and 29
- ✦ There appears to be a hairline fracture on the labial of number 9.

Radiographic Findings:

- ✦ Incipient enamel lesions (distal of 3, mesial of 15, distal of 19)
- ✦ Linear radiolucent areas along the CEJ of 28 and 29 premolar teeth, consistent with the clinically observed posterior cervical abrasion

Questions: Given the client profile, chief complaint, and examination findings, answer the following questions:

1. What client characteristics indicate that she is at risk for dentinal hypersensitivity?
2. What are some common explanations for gingival recession?
3. What dental conditions must be considered to arrive at a differential diagnosis?

Critical Thinking Exercises—cont'd

4. Based on the differential diagnosis determined by you and the dentist, what are the treatment options?
5. What special self-care instructions will relieve the client's symptoms of sensitive teeth? What specific products may reduce the occurrence of aphthous ulcers?
6. Explain the potential significance of the hairline fracture on number 9.

For References, Suggested Readings, and Related Websites, visit

http://evolve.elsevier.com/Darby/hygiene/

CHAPTER 34

LOCAL ANESTHESIA

OBJECTIVES

Mastery of the content in this chapter will enable the reader to:

- ✦ Describe nerve conduction
- ✦ Describe each of the anesthetic agents and vasoconstrictors used in dentistry and discuss the rationale behind the selection of a particular agent when providing dental hygiene care
- ✦ Calculate the maximal safe dose of each local anesthetic agent and vasoconstrictor for each client
- ✦ Assess each client's health history to determine his or her suitability to receive local anesthetics or vasoconstrictors.
- ✦ Assemble, disassemble, and properly maintain the armamentarium required for the administration of local anesthetic agents
- ✦ Identify the anatomic landmarks on both a skull and a client for the following injections: supraperiosteal, anterior superior alveolar nerve block, infraorbital nerve block, middle superior alveolar nerve block, posterior superior alveolar nerve block, greater palatine nerve block, nasopalatine nerve block, inferior alveolar nerve block, lingual nerve block, buccal nerve block, mental nerve block, incisive nerve block
- ✦ Identify which nerves, teeth, and soft tissue structures are anesthetized with each of the preceding injections
- ✦ Identify the local complications that may result from the administration of anesthetic agents and the proper management of these complications

KEY TERMS

Absolute contraindication
Amide anesthetics
Anterior superior alveolar nerve
Aspiration
Buccal nerve
Epinephrine
Ester anesthetics
Field block
Greater palatine nerve
Hemostasis
Incisive nerve
Inferior alveolar nerve
Infraorbital nerve
Lingual nerve
Local anesthesia
Local infiltration
Maximal safe dose
Mental nerve
Middle superior alveolar nerve
Mylohyoid nerve
Nasopalatine nerve
Needle
Nerve block
Posterior superior alveolar nerve
Relative contraindications
Supraperiosteal
Syringe
Topical anesthetic
Trigeminal nerve
Vasoconstriction
Vasodilation

Local anesthesia is the loss of sensation in a circumscribed area of the body as a result of the depression of excitation in nerve endings or the inhibition of the conduction process in peripheral nerves.[1] Local anesthetic agents used in clinical practice today prevent both the generation and conduction of a nerve impulse. Essentially, the local anesthetic agent provides a chemical roadblock between the source of the impulse (e.g., a periodontal abscess) and the brain. The impulse is unable to reach the brain and is thus not interpreted as pain or discomfort by the client.

Not all individuals require local anesthesia. Clients receiving a preventive oral prophylaxis or even periodontal maintenance care may experience little or no discomfort; however, local anesthetic administration usually is required if the dental hygiene care plan includes therapeutic scaling and root planing or gingival curettage, or if a client is simply experiencing undue tooth or soft tissue sensitivity. Additionally, a dental hygienist working in collaboration with a dentist may be called on to anesthetize individuals for the dentist in preparation for them to receive restorative or periodontal therapy.

The purpose of this chapter is to discuss the physiology of nerve conduction, the properties of local anesthetic agents and vasoconstrictors, the preanesthetic client evaluation, the armamentarium, the procedures for a successful injection, the injection techniques, and the prevention and management of local and systemic complications.

PHYSIOLOGY OF NERVE CONDUCTION

To understand how local anesthetic agents work, the dental hygienist needs to be familiar with the physiology of nerve conduction. Two principal ions are needed for nerve conduction: potassium (K^+) and sodium (Na^+). Because these two molecules are positively charged, they normally exist in equal concentration across a membrane; however, in a nerve cell this equilibrium does not exist (Figure 34–1, phase 1). Because of a sodium pump located within the cell membrane, the positively charged sodium molecules are forced outside the nerve cell. As the sodium leaves the intracellular fluid, a state of negativity is created inside the nerve cell. At the same time, the extracellular fluid, which has received the sodium, becomes positive. Once the sodium ion is transported out of the cell, it is not able to diffuse back into the intracellular fluids because of the relative impermeability of the nerve membrane to this ion. Although the nerve membrane is freely permeable to the potassium, this ion remains within the nerve cell because the negative charge of the nerve membrane restrains the positively charged ion by electrostatic attraction. The nerve is polarized or in a resting state or at resting potential when this balance exists between positive sodium ions on the outside of the nerve membrane and negative potassium ions on the inside of the membrane. Polarization of the membrane continues as long as the nerve remains undisturbed.

A stimulus, which may be chemical, thermal, mechanical, or electrical in nature (such as pain), produces excitation of the nerve fiber and thus a change in the ion balance (Figure 34–1, phase 2). During this phase, referred to as *depolarization,* the nerve membrane becomes more permeable to the sodium ion. Consequently, the positive sodium ions move rapidly across the nerve membrane to the inside of the nerve cell. During this influx of sodium, the potassium ions diffuse from the inside to the outside of the nerve membrane. Thus during depolarization the ion balance of the nerve cell reverses. The interior of the nerve membrane contains the positive sodium ions, whereas on the exterior of the nerve cell are the potassium ions. The inside of the nerve is now electrically positive compared to the outside of the nerve.

Immediately after depolarization, the permeability of the membrane to the sodium ion once again decreases (Figure 34–1, phase 3). This is referred to as *repolarization.* During this phase, the sodium pump actively transports the sodium ion out of the nerve cell, while potassium ions diffuse and are pumped to the inside of the nerve cell. Thus the nerve's resting potential is reestablished, whereby the interior of the nerve cell is negative, while the exterior of the nerve cell consists of the positive sodium ions. This rapid sequence of changes, depolarization and repolarization, is termed *action potential.*

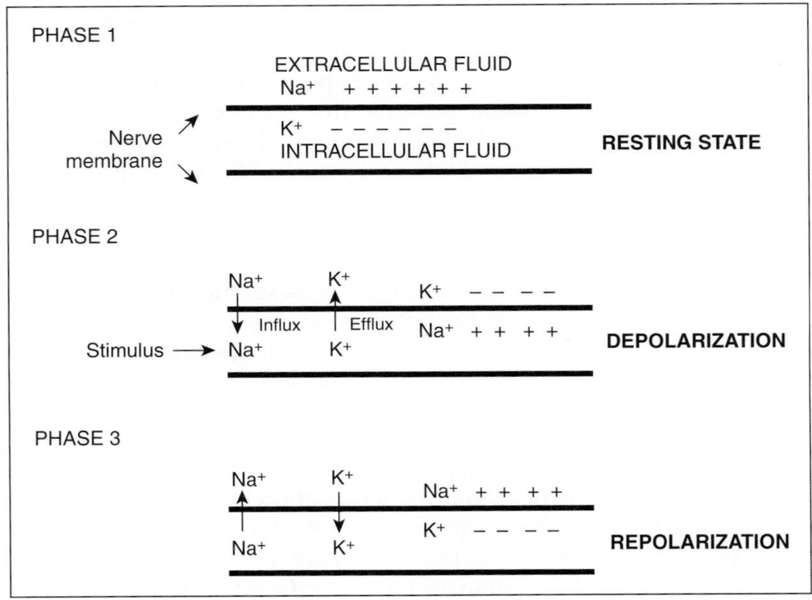

FIGURE 34–1 ✦ Action potential.

Once the resting potential of the nerve membrane is disrupted by a stimulus, such as pain, and depolarization occurs, the impulse must be transmitted along the nerve fiber. This impulse propagation is achieved when the ion changes during depolarization produce a new electrical equilibrium (the interior of the cell changing from negative to positive, the exterior of the cell changing from positive to negative). This in turn produces local currents that flow from the depolarized segment of the nerve to the adjacent resting area. As a result of this electrical current flow, depolarization begins in this previously resting area and continues propagating itself along the entire length of the nerve fiber. Thus the depolarization step begins a chain reaction that continues the action potential along the nerve. In this manner, the impulse is propelled along the nerve fiber to the central nervous system.

MECHANISM OF ACTION OF LOCAL ANESTHETIC AGENTS

Although there are several theories on how local anesthetics work, it has been established that the primary action of these drugs is in reducing the nerve membrane permeability to the sodium ions (Na^+). The nerve membrane remains impermeable to the sodium ions despite the introduction of a stimulus to the nerve. Because the sodium ions remain on the outside of the nerve cell and are unable to enter the nerve membrane, an action potential never occurs. The nerve cell remains in a polarized state (*resting state*) because the ionic movements responsible for the action potential do not develop. Thus the action of depolarization that is required to initiate or to continue nerve impulse transmission (*propagation*) is blocked. An impulse that arrives at the blocked nerve segment is unable to be transmitted to the brain and is, therefore, not interpreted as pain or discomfort by the client.

LOCAL ANESTHETICS

Chemical Properties

Chemically, all injectable local anesthetic agents (Figure 34–2) used in oral healthcare today have three components:

- ✦ Aromatic lipophilic group
- ✦ Intermediate chain
- ✦ Hydrophilic amino group

The lipophilic group, composed of the aromatic ring structure, ensures that the anesthetic agent is able to penetrate the lipid-rich nerve membrane where impulse conduction is blocked. The hydrophilic portion, when combined with hydrochloric acid, allows the anesthetic to diffuse through the interstitial fluid in the tissues to reach the nerve.

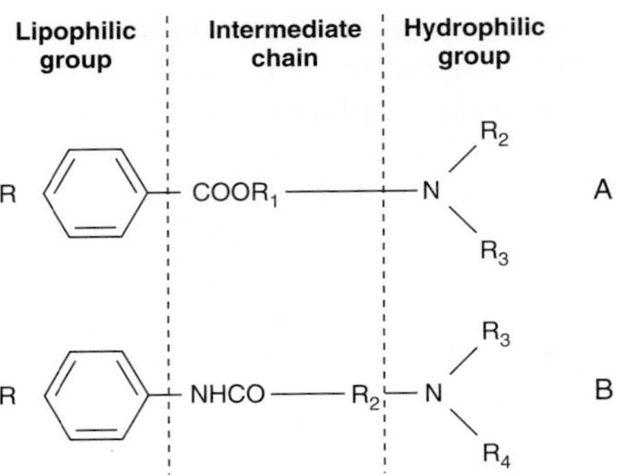

FIGURE 34–2 ✦ Typical local anesthetic. **A,** Ester type. **B,** Amide type. *(From Malamed SF:* Handbook of local anesthesia, *ed 3, St Louis, 1990, Mosby.)*

The third component of the chemical structure of local anesthetics is the intermediate chain linkage. This linkage determines whether the local anesthetic agent is classified as an ester or an amide. The nature of the intermediate linkage is important in defining several properties of the local anesthetic, including possible allergic response (discussed in the later section, Preanesthetic Client Assessment) and metabolism (biotransformation).

Metabolism (Biotransformation) and Excretion

The mechanism by which local anesthetic agents are metabolized is important because the overall toxicity of an agent depends on the balance between the agent's rate of absorption into the bloodstream at the injection site and the rate of the agent's removal from the blood through the processes of tissue uptake and metabolism. An important difference between the two classifications of local anesthetic drugs—ester and amide—is the process by which they are metabolized. *Ester local anesthetics* are metabolized by hydrolysis (splitting of the compound into fragments by the addition of water) (Table 34–1). The hydrolysis process occurs primarily in the plasma and to a lesser extent in the liver, and is activated by the enzyme pseudocholinesterase. Concern about the metabolism of ester local anesthetics arises regarding persons with genetically determined atypical plasma cholinesterase, which is found in approximately 1 of every 2800 individuals. These individuals have an increased potential for toxicity because they are unable to inactivate the ester agents at the normal rate and, therefore, develop high blood levels of the anesthetic (see later sections, Preanesthetic Client Assessment and Systemic Complications).

Amide local anesthetics undergo biotransformation in the liver by microsomal enzymes (Table 34–2). Therefore, the liver function of a client influences the rate of biotransformation of an amide drug. Those clients with impaired liver function are unable to metabolize amide local anesthetics at a normal rate, thereby leading to excessive levels of the agent in the blood, which increases the potential for toxic overdose (see later sections, Preanesthetic Client Assessment and Systemic Complications).

TABLE 34–1 ESTER LOCAL ANESTHETICS

Generic Name	Proprietary Name
Procaine	Novocain
Propoxycaine	Ravocaine
Benzocaine (topical)	
Tetracaine (topical)	

TABLE 34–2 AMIDE LOCAL ANESTHETICS

Generic Name	Proprietary Name
Articaine	Septocaine
Bupivacaine	Marcaine
Etidocaine	Duranest
Lidocaine	Xylocaine, Alphacaine, Octocaine
Mepivacaine	Carbocaine, Arestocaine, Isocaine, Polocaine
Prilocaine	Citanest

The metabolic products of both the ester and amide local anesthetics are almost entirely excreted by the kidneys. In addition, a small amount of a given dose of local anesthetic agent is excreted unchanged in the urine. Because the esters are metabolized almost completely in the plasma, this agent appears in only small amounts in an unchanged form in the urine. Because of their more complex process of biotransformation, amides are usually excreted in their original form in larger amounts than the esters. Despite this difference, only small concentrations of the amides are found unchanged in the urine. Clients with significant renal impairment or those undergoing renal dialysis may be unable to efficiently remove the unchanged form of the local anesthetic compound or its breakdown products from their blood, leading to elevated local anesthetic levels and an increased potential for toxicity (see later sections, Preanesthetic Client Assessment and Systemic Complications).

VASOCONSTRICTORS

All local anesthetic agents presently used in dentistry produce *vasodilation.* After their injection into the tissues the following reactions occur:[2]

- ✦ Increased blood flow to the injection site as the local anesthetic agents dilate the blood vessels
- ✦ Accelerated rate of absorption of the local anesthetic into the bloodstream, causing the anesthetic to be carried away from the injection site
- ✦ Higher amounts of local anesthetic in the blood, with the attendant greater risk for an overdose reaction
- ✦ Decreased duration of action and decreased effectiveness of the local anesthetic because it diffuses away from the site of administration more rapidly
- ✦ Increased bleeding at the injection site because of the increased blood flow to the area

To counteract the vasodilating properties of the local anesthetic agents, vasoconstrictors are added to the local anesthetic solution. These drugs constrict the blood vessels, and thus control bleeding in the area of the injection. This *vasoconstriction* in turn leads to:

- ✦ Decreased blood flow to the injection site as the vasoconstrictors constrict the blood vessels
- ✦ Slowed rate of absorption of the local anesthetic into the bloodstream, thus keeping it at the injection site longer and producing lower levels in the bloodstream
- ✦ Lower amounts of local anesthetic in the blood, thereby decreasing the risk for an overdose reaction (or reducing the potential for systemic toxicity)
- ✦ Increased duration of action and increased effectiveness of the local anesthetic as higher concentrations of the agent remain in and around the nerve for a longer period
- ✦ Decreased bleeding at the injection site (*hemostasis*) from the decreased blood flow to the area

Vasoconstrictors are an important addition to a local anesthetic solution because they decrease the potential toxicity of the anesthetic solution while increasing the duration and effectiveness of pain control. For example, the addition of 1:100,000 or 1:200,000 epinephrine to 2% lidocaine increases the duration of pulpal and hard tissue anesthesia from approximately 10 minutes to 60 minutes. Dental hygiene appointments are frequently 45 to 60 minutes in length, and thus vasoconstrictors are necessary to provide a pain-free state for clients during completion of dental hygiene care.

Moreover, dental hygiene care often involves soft tissue manipulation, and hemorrhage is a frequent result, especially when inflammation is present. The use of local anesthetics without vasoconstrictors is problematic because the vasodilating properties of the anesthetic actually increase bleeding at the site of the injection. Vasoconstrictors are added to the anesthetic solution to counteract this unwanted action, and thus they prevent or minimize bleeding during dental hygiene care.

For pain control, nerve blocks, such as the posterior superior alveolar or inferior alveolar nerve blocks, are frequently the technique of choice when providing dental hygiene care. To derive the benefits of bleeding control from the vasoconstrictor, however, the drug must be administered, via local infiltration, directly into the area where the bleeding is occurring or is expected to occur. For example, to provide pain control to the maxillary molars and the buccal tissue over these teeth, a posterior superior alveolar nerve block is administered. The anesthetic agent is deposited posterior and superior to the posterior border of the maxilla, some distance from the area being anesthetized. If hemostasis is needed on the buccal tissue over any of the molars, however, the administration of a local infiltration into the area is necessary even though the anesthesia may be profound.

Fortunately, only small volumes of solution are required (approximately 1 ml) for hemostatic purposes.

Mechanism of Action

The sympathetic nervous system component of the autonomic nervous system, in addition to other functions, controls the dilation and constriction of various blood vessels throughout the body. Adrenalin, also known as *epinephrine*, is one of the naturally occurring agents responsible for sympathetic nervous system activity.[3] The vasoconstrictors used with local anesthetics are chemically identical to or very similar to adrenalin produced naturally during sympathetic nervous system stimulation. Thus, because the actions of the vasoconstrictors so closely mimic the action of the sympathetic autonomic nervous system, they are referred to as *sympathomimetic* or *adrenergic agents*.

Throughout the tissues of the body, adrenergic receptors are found that are stimulated by the chemicals released by the sympathetic nervous system or a sympathomimetic agent (drug). These receptor sites are divided into two major categories: alpha and beta. Activation of the alpha (α) receptors by a sympathomimetic agent (drug) results in contraction of the smooth muscle in blood vessels. This contraction produces a constriction of the vessels referred to as *vasoconstriction*. The primary reason sympathomimetic agents are added to local anesthetic solutions is to produce this desirable vasoconstriction.

Activation of the beta (β) receptors by a sympathomimetic agent (drug) produces smooth muscle relaxation and cardiac stimulation. Beta receptors have been further characterized as $beta_1$ and $beta_2$. Activation of $beta_1$ receptors increases cardiac rate and force, whereas $beta_2$ receptors are responsible for bronchodilation and vasodilation. Those changes resulting from beta-receptor stimulation are undesirable side effects of sympathomimetic drug incorporation into local anesthetic solutions. These beta effects are potentially hazardous.

Concentrations

Vasoconstrictor concentrations are most often expressed as a ratio, such as 1 part per 100,000. This ratio appears as 1:100,000 in a written format. Table 34–3 lists the vasoconstrictors and their concentrations that are incorporated into dental local anesthetic solutions in the United States.

Whereas a variety of vasoconstrictors are used presently in oral healthcare, epinephrine is the most potent and widely employed, and is the standard by which all other vasoconstrictors are compared. Epinephrine 1:100,000 is the most commonly used concentration; however, it is thought that the optimal concentration for prolongation of pain control is 1:200,000[4] or even 1:250,000.[5] *The use of 1:50,000 epinephrine for pain control is neither necessary nor recommended.*[6] The 1:50,000 dilution contains twice the epinephrine per milliliter as a 1:100,000 dilution and four times that contained in a 1:200,000 concentration, and does not increase the quality or duration of pain control. Although the 1:50,000 dilution may be more effective in the control of bleeding, effective hemostasis also may be obtained with concentrations of 1:100,000 epinephrine. Because there is always concern about the systemic effects, it is recommended that the less concentrated solution be used, particularly with clients known to be cardiovascularly compromised.[7] (Refer to later section, Preanesthetic Client Assessment, for further guidelines.)

Levonordefrin and norepinephrine (levarterenol) also are proven effective vasopressors. Levonordefrin is approximately one-sixth (15%) as potent a vasoconstrictor as epinephrine, and as such is used in a greater concentration of 1:20,000. At this concentration, levonordefrin possesses the same clinical capabilities as epinephrine 1:100,000. Similarly, norepinephrine is approximately 25% as effective a vasopressor as epinephrine and is used clinically in a 1:30,000 dilution.

Epinephrine is the preferred agent for hemostasis. Levonordefrin is thought to be less effective in providing hemostasis, and norepinephrine can cause tissue ischemia, leading to necrosis and sloughing, particularly on the palate. Therefore, norepinephrine should not be considered for vasoconstricting purposes. Many authorities recommend that it be excluded from all local anesthetic agents.[7]

SELECTION OF A LOCAL ANESTHETIC AGENT

As detailed in Table 34–1 and Table 34–2, several local anesthetic agents are available to the dental hygienist when he or she is providing pain control. Table 34–4 lists those local anesthetics and the combinations of vasoconstrictors that are currently available in the United States and Canada.

TABLE 34–3 VASOCONSTRICTORS USED IN DENTAL LOCAL ANESTHETIC SOLUTIONS

Generic Name	Proprietary Name	Concentrations
Epinephrine	Adrenalin	1:50,000; 1:100,000; 1:200,000
Levonordefrin	Neo-Cobefrin	1:20,000
Norepinephrine (levarterenol)	Levophed	1:30,000

The dental hygienist must weigh the following factors when determining the appropriate anesthetic agent to use during dental hygiene care:

- ✦ The duration of action of the local anesthetic agent and the length of time that pain control is needed
- ✦ The need for pain control after treatment
- ✦ The health status of the client
- ✦ Current medications being taken by the client
- ✦ A local anesthetic allergy

Both duration of action and length of time that pain control is needed and the requirement for pain control after treatment are discussed here. Those remaining factors influencing the dental hygienist's choice of a local anesthetic agent are reviewed in the section on preanesthetic client evaluation.

Duration of Action and Length of Time That Pain Control Is Needed

An important consideration when selecting a local anesthetic agent for pain control during dental hygiene care is the approximate duration of action of the local anesthetic agent, coupled with the length of time that pain control is needed. Table 34–4 lists the local anesthetic agents and their approximate duration of pulpal and soft tissue anesthesia. The anesthetics are categorized as:

- ✦ Short-duration local anesthetics that provide approximately 30 minutes of pulpal anesthesia
- ✦ Intermediate-duration local anesthetics that provide approximately 60 minutes of local anesthesia
- ✦ Long-duration local anesthetics that provide approximately 90 minutes or more of local anesthesia

These times are approximations, and the actual duration of clinical anesthesia may vary. In addition to the presence or absence of a vasoconstrictor (see later section, Selection of a Vasoconstrictor), several other factors may affect both the duration and depth of the anesthetic agent's action either increasing or, more commonly, decreasing the drug's effectiveness, including:[7]

1. *Variation of the individual's response to the agent administered.* Although most individuals respond predictably to an anesthetic agent (e.g., the duration of pulpal anesthesia after administering 2% lidocaine with epinephrine 1:100,000 is approximately 60 minutes), some clients exhibit either a longer or shorter duration of action than anticipated. This variation in response is normal and is simply a variation in the individual's reaction to the anesthetic agent.
2. *Accuracy of the administration of the agent.* This factor becomes significant when a substantial amount of soft tissue must be penetrated to reach the nerve to be anesthetized. For example, the inferior alveolar nerve block involves advancing through 20 to 25 mm of soft tissue before reaching the nerve, thereby influencing the accuracy of the injection. When injecting where it is not necessary to penetrate a large amount of tissue to block the nerve, however, such as with an infiltration, accuracy is seldom a problem.
3. *Condition of the soft tissues at the site of drug deposition.* Anesthetic duration is increased in areas of decreased

TABLE 34–4 LOCAL ANESTHETIC AGENTS AND DURATION OF PULPAL AND SOFT TISSUE ANESTHESIA

		Duration (Approx. Minutes)	
Agent	**Category**	**Pulpal**	**Soft Tissue**
Short Duration			
Lidocaine 2%	Amide	5–10	60–120
Prilocaine 4% (infiltration)	Amide	5–10	90–120
Mepivacaine 3%	Amide	20–40	120–180
Intermediate Duration			
Procaine 2%, propoxycaine 0.4%, Levonordefrin 1:20,000	Ester	30–60	120–180
Lidocaine 2%, epinephrine 1:50,000	Amide	60	180–240
Lidocaine 2%, epinephrine 1:100,000	Amide	60	180–240
Mepivacaine 2%, levonordefrin 1:20,000	Amide	60	180–240
Prilocaine 4% (block)	Amide	60	120–240
Articaine 4%, epinephrine 1:100,000	Amide	75	180–300
Prilocaine 4%, epinephrine 1:200,000	Amide	60–90	120–240
Long Duration			
Bupivacaine 0.5%, epinephrine 1:200,000	Amide	>90	240–540
Etidocaine 1.5%, epinephrine 1:200,000	Amide	>90	240–540

Short-duration agents provide pulpal anesthesia for 30 minutes or less; intermediate-duration agents for approximately 60 minutes; long-duration agents for longer than 90 minutes. The classification of duration is approximate. Variations may be noted.
Modified from Malamed SF: *Handbook of local anesthesia*, ed 3, St Louis, 1990, Mosby.

vascularity. Conversely, the presence of inflammation or infection often decreases the anesthetic agent's duration of action due to more rapid absorption of the anesthetic agent, resulting from the increased vascularity.

4. *Anatomic variation.* The injection techniques described in this chapter are based on a "normal" anatomy. Of course, anatomic variations from this "norm" exist and can decrease the duration of local anesthetic action. Those variations in the maxilla that may account for failed effectiveness and duration include:

   - Extra dense alveolar bone
   - Palatal roots of maxillary molars that flare more than normal to the midline of the palate, thus affecting the anesthetic's action on these roots
   - An unusually low zygomatic arch common in children, thereby preventing anesthesia or lessening its duration in the first and second molars

   Those anatomic variations in the mandible that are cause for concern include,[4,7,8]

   - The height of the mandibular foramen
   - A wide, flaring mandible
   - A wide ramus in the anterior-posterior direction
   - A long ramus in the superior-inferior direction
   - Bulky musculature or excess adipose tissue
   - Accessory innervation to the mandibular teeth

   Suggestions for overcoming these variations in anatomy when administering anesthetic solution are discussed in the section on injection techniques.

5. *Type of injection administered.* For any anesthetic solution administered, both pulpal and soft tissue anesthesia are sustained for a longer period when a nerve block rather than a supraperiosteal/infiltration injection is administered. For example, if administering 2% lidocaine with 1:100,000 epinephrine, a posterior superior alveolar nerve block provides approximately 60 minutes of pulpal anesthesia, whereas a supraperiosteal injection allows only 40 minutes' duration. In order to achieve the desired duration, the recommended minimal volume of anesthetic must be administered.

Need for Pain Control After Treatment

Although the need for pain control after dental hygiene care may be limited, the dental hygienist should be advised that long-duration agents may be administered if posttreatment discomfort is a factor. Anesthetic agents, such as 4% prilocaine with 1:200,000 epinephrine, can provide 5 to 8 hours of soft tissue anesthesia, whereas 0.5% bupivacaine or 1.5% etidocaine with 1:200,000 epinephrine can alleviate posttreatment discomfort for 8 to 12 hours. These agents can be administered before beginning dental hygiene care or even at the end of the care to allow for maximal posttreatment anesthesia. These drugs should not be given to children or to people who are mentally or physically disabled because these individuals may accidentally chew or bite their lip or tongue.

MAXIMAL SAFE DOSES

Local Anesthetics

All drugs, if administered in excess, are capable of producing an overdose reaction. The exact dosage or the blood level at which a toxic reaction occurs is impossible to predict because biologic variability greatly influences how individuals respond to a drug; however, maximal dosages can be calculated to serve as a guideline for the dental hygienist. A *maximal safe dose* is the maximal amount of a drug that can be safely administered to a healthy individual. Maximal doses of injectable local anesthetics should be determined after consideration of the following factors:[2]

- *Client's age.* Individuals on both ends of the age spectrum (i.e., the young child or the elderly adult) may be unable to tolerate normal dosages. Therefore, the dosage of local anesthetic should be decreased accordingly.
- *Client's physical status.* The calculated dosage must be adjusted for clients with compromised health. For example, a client with significant liver or renal dysfunction may be given a reduced dosage of local anesthetics.
- *Client's weight.* The larger the individual (within limits), the greater the drug distribution. When administering a normal dosage of local anesthetic to a large individual, the blood level of the drug is lower than that in a small person. Thus a larger dose can be safely given. Although this rule is generally true, there may be exceptions, and care must always be exercised.

Table 34–5 lists the recommended maximal safe dose and the milligrams of local anesthetic per cartridge of available local anesthetic agents. It is important to note that the maximal dosages are expressed in terms of milligrams per pound of body weight. Therefore, the dental hygienist must be familiar with the relationship between solution percentage and the number of milligrams contained in that solution.

A 1% solution of local anesthetic contains 10 mg/ml of solution. A 2% solution contains 20 mg/ml, 3% contains 30 mg/ml, 4% contains 40 mg/ml, and so on. The number of milligrams of anesthetic in a cartridge is derived by multiplying the number of milligrams per milliliter of solution (e.g., 20 in a 2% solution) and the amount of solution (1.8 ml in a dental cartridge). The computation $20 \times 1.8 = 36$ gives the dental hygienist the number of milligrams of anesthetic in the dental cartridge.[7] Table 34–5 provides the computed number of milligrams of local anesthetic per cartridge for anesthetic agents.

Table 34–6 provides recommended maximal doses based on body weight for more commonly used local anesthetic agents. The guidelines provided in Tables 34–5 and 34–6 are helpful when working with healthy clients. Unfortunately, there are no set guidelines to determine the amount of dosage reduction needed for an elderly adult or medically compromised individual. It is suggested that the dental hygienist carefully assess the client's dental

TABLE 34–5 RECOMMENDED MAXIMAL SAFE DOSES FOR AVAILABLE LOCAL ANESTHETICS

Local Anesthetic Agent	Anesthetic Dose per Cartridge (mg)	Maximal Safe Dose: Mg/lb of Body Weight	Maximal Safe Dose: Maximum (mg)
Articaine 4%	72	3.2 (adults) or 2.3 (children)	500
Bupivacaine 0.5%	9	0.6	90
Etidocaine 1.5%	27	3.6	400
Lidocaine 2% with or without vasoconstrictor	36	2	300
Mepivacaine 2% or 3% with or without vasoconstrictor	2% = 36; 3% = 54	2	300
Prilocaine 4% with or without vasoconstrictor	72	2.7	400
Propoxycaine 0.4% + Procaine 2%	43.2	2.7	400 mg of total amine (propoxycaine + procaine)

TABLE 34–6 RECOMMENDED MAXIMAL SAFE DOSES OF COMMONLY USED LOCAL ANESTHETICS* (BASED ON BODY WEIGHT)

	Lidocaine 2% with/without Vasoconstrictor, 2 mg/lb, 300 mg Max		Mepivacaine 2% or 3%, 2 mg/lb, 300 mg Max			Prilocaine 4% with/without Vasoconstrictor, 2.7 mg/lb, 400 mg Max		Articaine 4% with Vasoconstrictor: Adult 3.2 mg/lb, 500 mg Max		Articaine 4% with Vasoconstrictor: Child 2.3 mg/lb, 500 mg Max	
Client Weight (lb)	mg	No. of Cartridges	mg	No. of Cartridges (2%)	No. of Cartridges (3%)	mg	No. of Cartridges	mg	No. of Cartridges	mg	No. of Cartridges
20	40	1.1	40	1.1	0.8	54	0.75	64	0.9	46	0.6
40	80	2.2	80	2.2	1.5	108	1.5	128	1.8	92	2.3
60	120	3.3	120	3.3	2.0	162	2.25	192	2.7	138	1.9
80	160	4.4	160	4.4	3.0	216	3.0	256	3.6	184	2.5
100	200	5.5†	200	5.5	3.5	270	3.75	320	4.4	230	3.0
120	240	6.5	240	6.5	4.0	324	4.5	384	5.33		
140	280	7.5	280	7.5	5.0	378	5.0	448	6.2		
160	300	8.0	300	8.0	5.5	400	5.5	500	7.0		
180	300	8.0	300	8.0	5.5	400	5.5	500	7.0		
200	300	8.0	300	8.0	5.5	400	5.5	500	7.0		

* These are for normal, healthy patients. They should be decreased for debilitated or elderly persons.
† The limiting factor for 1:50,000 epinephrine is the 0.2 mg dose.
From Malamed SF: *Handbook of local anesthesia*, ed 3, St Louis, 1990, Mosby.

hygiene care needs and formulate a care plan that takes into account that individual's requirement for a decreased dose of local anesthetic at each appointment.

Fortunately, it is not likely that the dental hygienist will need to approach the maximal doses listed, especially in adult clients. If the dental hygiene care plan involves scaling and root planing a quadrant, the administration of one to two cartridges often suffices. There is seldom a need to administer more than four cartridges during any appointment involving dental hygiene care.

In addition to considering the recommended maximal safe doses, the dental hygienist must follow other procedural guidelines to increase safety during administration of local anesthetics and prevent an overdose reaction. These include:

- ✦ Careful evaluation of the client's health history
- ✦ Use of a vasoconstrictor whenever possible
- ✦ Aspiration before deposition
- ✦ Slow injection
- ✦ Use of the smallest amount of drug necessary

A more detailed discussion of these guidelines can be found in the later section, Procedures for a Successful Injection and Systemic Complications.

TABLE 34–7 **RECOMMENDED MAXIMAL SAFE DOSE OF VASOCONSTRICTOR FOR HEALTHY AND CARDIAC CLIENTS**

Agent	Concentration	Mg/ml	Mg per Cartridge (1.8 ml)	Maximal Dose (mg)	Max. Number of Cartridges
Epinephrine	1:50,000	0.02	0.036	Healthy adult client 0.2 Cardiac client 0.04	5 1
Epinephrine	1:100,000	0.01	0.018	Healthy adult client 0.2 Cardiac client 0.04	10 2
Epinephrine	1:200,000	0.005	0.009	Healthy adult client 0.2 Cardiac client 0.4	20 4
Levonordefrin (Neo-Cobefrin)	1:20,000	0.5	0.09	Healthy adult client 1.00 Cardiac client 0.2	10 2
Norepinephrine/ levarterenol (Levophed)	1:30,000	0.034	0.06	Healthy adult client 0.34 Cardiac client 0.14	5 2

Adapted from Malamed SF: *Medical emergencies in the dental office*, ed 4, St Louis, 1993, Mosby.

Vasoconstrictors

Currently, vasoconstrictors commonly are used in local anesthetic solutions. Epinephrine has proven to be the most effective agent and is most frequently employed. Overdose reactions, although possible, are uncommon with vasoconstrictors other than epinephrine because of the lesser potency of these agents.[7] Table 34–7 outlines the recommended maximal safe doses in milligrams and number of cartridges per appointment of epinephrine, levonordefrin, and levarterenol for healthy clients and for clients with significant cardiovascular impairment. (Refer to later sections, Selection of a Vasoconstrictor and Preanesthetic Client Assessment, for further discussion.)

It is important to note that in any local anesthetic solution containing a vasoconstrictor, the maximal safe dose of the solution may be determined by either the anesthetic agent or the vasoconstricting agent. For example, the maximal safe dose for 2% lidocaine may be reached before the maximal safe dose of the 1:100,000 epinephrine, included in the solution, is reached. Thus the anesthetic agent limits the total amount of solution to be administered. Conversely, the maximal safe dose for epinephrine 1:50,000 may be reached before the maximal safe dose of the 2% lidocaine in which it is incorporated. In this case, the epinephrine limits the total amount of solution to be administered. Therefore, the dental hygienist must be familiar with the maximal safe doses of both the local anesthetic agent and the vasoconstricting agent to determine which drug limits the total amount of solution that can be administered to a client.

PREANESTHETIC CLIENT ASSESSMENT

To meet the human need for protection from health risks, an evaluation of the client's health history and current health status is an essential prerequisite to dental hygiene care. The dental hygienist must ascertain if any conditions represent contraindications or require alterations to the dental hygiene care plan to eliminate or decrease the risk presented to the client. The administration of local anesthetic and vasoconstricting agents provides an additional rationale for a thorough health history and health status review. Local anesthetics and vasoconstrictors, like all drugs, exert actions on multiple body systems. It is important to evaluate, through the health history, the client's ability to physically tolerate the administration of a local anesthetic or vasoconstrictor, a history of allergic responses, and current medications. Collection of these data guides the dental hygienist in determining the appropriateness of administering a local anesthetic or vasoconstrictor, of seeking medical consultation, and of modifying the dental hygiene care plan. Thus a thorough preanesthetic client assessment helps prevent or minimize complications and emergencies.

Contraindications to local anesthetics and vasoconstrictors are divided into two categories: absolute and relative.

Absolute contraindications require that the offending drug not be administered to the individual under any circumstances.[2] The administration of such a drug is contraindicated in all situations because it substantially increases the possibility of a life-threatening risk for the client. An example is a documented local anesthetic allergic reaction.

Relative contraindications signify that it is preferable to avoid administration of the suspected drug because there is the increased possibility that an adverse reaction may occur; however, if an acceptable substitute is not available, the drug may be used judiciously (i.e., administration of a minimal dose that still produces sufficient pain control).

Health Status of the Client

Although local anesthetics and vasoconstrictors are considered relatively safe drugs when administered properly, certain health conditions require limiting or eliminating their use. Table 34–8 summarizes those health conditions

TABLE 34–8 HEALTH CONDITIONS THAT REQUIRE SPECIAL CONSIDERATION WHEN ADMINISTERING LOCAL ANESTHETICS

Health Condition	Reason for Modification	Recommended Action
Hyperthyroidism	Possible exaggerated response to vasoconstrictors	Avoid or limit use (uncontrolled) of vasoconstrictors; use 3% mepivacaine or 4% prilocaine.
Atypical plasma cholinesterase	Toxic overdose to esters	Use amide anesthetic agents.
Methemoglobinemia	Potential for cyanosis-like state, respiratory distress, and lethargy in response to prilocaine and articaine	Use other anesthetic agents.
Malignant hyperthermia	Life-threatening syndrome caused by administration of certain drugs in combination with amide agents	Use amides or esters in normal doses; seek medical consult.
Significant liver dysfunction	Difficulty metabolizing amide agents, potential for overdose	Seek medical consult; use amide agents judiciously.
Significant renal dysfunction	Difficulty excreting local anesthetic agents, potential for overdose	Seek medical consult; use anesthetic agents judiciously.
Pregnancy	Potential for complications with pregnancy	Avoid elective treatment during first trimester; use local anesthetics judiciously.

that may affect the selection of a local anesthetic or vasoconstrictor and appropriate actions that the dental hygienist may follow. Those conditions include:

- ✦ Hyperthyroidism
- ✦ Atypical plasma cholinesterase
- ✦ Methemoglobinemia
- ✦ Malignant hyperthermia
- ✦ Significant liver dysfunction
- ✦ Significant renal dysfunction
- ✦ Pregnancy

Few health conditions are absolute contraindications to vasoconstrictors in the concentrations found in local anesthetic solutions used in oral healthcare, such as documented allergy; however, the dental hygienist must carefully consider the benefits versus the risks of administering a vasoconstrictor to clients with a history of hypertension, cardiovascular disease, or hyperthyroidism because often the benefits outweigh the risks.

Current Medications Being Taken by the Client

A drug interaction occurs when one drug modifies the action of another drug. A drug may potentiate or diminish the action of another drug and may alter the way in which another drug is absorbed, metabolized, or eliminated from the body.[9] Although local anesthetics and vasoconstrictors exhibit few interactions with other drugs, the dental hygienist should consult the *Physicians' Desk Reference* or another comparable reference when a client reports being treated with any medication. This practice enables the clinician to assess both the drug's activity and the drug-to-drug interactions between the local anesthetic and vasoconstrictor and the prescribed medication, and thereby meet the client's human need for protection from health risks. If further questions remain regarding the use of a local anesthetic or vasoconstrictor while a prescribed medication is being taken, the dentist or the individual's physician should be consulted.

Table 34–9 summarizes those medications that may affect the selection of a local anesthetic or vasoconstrictor and appropriate actions the dental hygienist may choose.

Local anesthetics have proven to have few interactions with other prescribed drugs. Procaine has been cited as interfering with the action of antiinfective sulfonamide drugs.[5] When central nervous system (CNS) depressants or cardiovascular system (CVS) depressants are being taken by an individual, it is recommended that doses of local anesthetics be kept to a minimum because they may cause further depression.[2]

There are many conflicting reports of drug-to-drug interactions between vasoconstrictors and prescribed medications, but it is recommended that the dental hygienist proceed cautiously when administering a vasopressor to a person who is being treated with any of the following groups of drugs:

- ✦ Tricyclic antidepressants
- ✦ Phenothiazines
- ✦ Beta-receptor blockers
- ✦ Adrenergic neuron blockers

Currently, none of these drugs (described as follows) poses an absolute contraindication to the administration of a vasoconstrictor; however, it is recommended that the dental hygienist exercise caution by administering the smallest dose that is clinically effective (such as that recommended for persons at cardiovascular risk) or eliminating the vasopressor entirely. If the dental hygienist is uncertain about the inclusion of a vasoconstrictor in the local anesthetic solution, consultation with the client's physician is advisable.

- ✦ *Tricyclic antidepressants.* Tricyclic antidepressant medications have been cited as possibly potentiating the

TABLE 34–9 MEDICATIONS THAT AFFECT THE SELECTION OF LOCAL ANESTHETIC AGENTS OR VASOCONSTRICTORS

Medication	Type of Contraindication	Drugs to Avoid	Potential Problem(s)	Action/Alternative Drug
CVS depressants CNS depressants	Relative	Large doses of local anesthetics	Increased depression of CVS or CNS	Minimize dose of local anesthetic
Tricyclic antidepressants	Relative	Large doses of vasoconstrictors	Potentiate the action of epinephrine and increase blood pressure	Epinephrine concentrations of 1:200,000 or 1:100,000 used judiciously or mepivacaine 3% or prilocaine 4%
Phenothiazines	Relative	Large doses of vasoconstrictors	Potentiate the action of epinephrine and increase blood pressure	Epinephrine concentrations of 1:200,000 or 1:100,000 used judiciously or mepivacaine 3% or prilocaine 4%
Beta-receptor blockers	Relative	Large doses of vasoconstrictors	Potentiate the action of epinephrine and increase blood pressure	Epinephrine concentrations of 1:200,000 or 1:100,000 used judiciously or mepivacaine 3% or prilocaine 4%
Adrenergic neuron blockers	Relative	Large doses of vasoconstrictors	Potentiate the action of epinephrine and increase blood pressure	Epinephrine concentrations of 1:200,000 or 1:100,000 used judiciously or mepivacaine 3% or prilocaine 4%
Sulfonamides	Relative	Esters	Esters inhibit action of sulfonamides	Amides

TABLE 34–10 CLIENT ALLERGIES THAT AFFECT THE SELECTION OF LOCAL ANESTHETIC AGENTS OR VASOCONSTRICTORS

Reported Allergy	Type of Contraindication	Drugs to Avoid	Potential Problem(s)	Alternative Drug
Local anesthetic allergy, documented	Absolute	All local anesthetics in same chemical class (esters vs. amides)	Allergic response, mild (e.g., dermatitis, bronchospasm) to life-threatening reactions	Local anesthetics in different chemical class (esters vs. amides)
Sulfa	Absolute	Articaine	Allergic response	Non–sulfur-containing local anesthetic
Sodium bisulfite/ metabisulfite	Absolute	Local anesthetics containing a vasoconstrictor	Severe bronchospasm, usually asthmatics	Local anesthetic without vasoconstrictor

action of epinephrine and norepinephrine and resulting in an increase in blood pressure.[10] Phenothiazines such as prochlorperazine are categorized as antipsychotic drugs but also are often prescribed for treatment of nausea. There is concern that these drugs, when combined with vasoconstrictors, may cause an exaggerated response to the vasopressor.

- ✦ *Beta-receptor blockers.* Beta-receptor blockers such as propranolol decrease systolic and diastolic blood pressures.[3] When combined with epinephrine from a local anesthetic injection, however, significant increases in blood pressure may result.
- ✦ *Adrenergic neuron blockers.* Adrenergic neuron blockers such as guanethidine and reserpine also are used to lower blood pressure through the interference in the normal release of norepinephrine.[3] When these drugs are combined with a vasoconstrictor, the effects of the vasopressor may be exaggerated, resulting in an increase in blood pressure.

Allergies

An allergy is a hypersensitive reaction acquired through exposure to a specific substance (allergen); reexposure to the allergen increases one's potential to react. Approximately 1% of all reactions that occur during local anesthetic administration are true allergic reactions.[5] A documented local anesthetic allergy, however, represents an absolute contraindication and must be investigated for authenticity. Table 34–10 summarizes allergies that affect the selection of a local anesthetic agent or vasoconstrictor and appropriate alternative drugs the dental hygienist may choose.

One of the breakdown products of the ester local anesthetics is para-aminobenzoic acid (PABA). This substance induces allergic reactions in a small percentage of the population.[2] Allergic reactions that occur in response to ester local anesthetics are probably not reactions to the ester local anesthetic agent itself but rather to the PABA.

Allergic response to ester local anesthetics is well documented; however, substantiation of a true allergic response to a *pure* amide drug is extremely rare. The potential for a true allergic reaction to amides may exist; however, a verifiable occurrence is virtually nonexistent.

Allergic reactions are specific to the two chemical classifications of local anesthetic agents: amides and esters.[5] An individual who is allergic to an ester local anesthetic should not be allergic to an amide drug, and vice versa. Therefore, if a client reports a previous allergic response to a local anesthetic, it is imperative that the dental hygienist determine the specific agent responsible for the allergic response and the chemical group to which it belongs (see later section, Systemic Complications).

Allergic reactions have been documented for various contents of the dental cartridge. Sodium bisulfite and metabisulfite are antioxidants that are incorporated into local anesthetic solutions to act as a preservative for the vasoconstrictor. In addition to their use in local anesthetic cartridges, these agents are often sprayed on fruits and vegetables to keep them appearing fresh. They also are included in a variety of canned foods. Allergy to the bisulfites has been reported.[11,12] Clients with a history of asthma may be particularly susceptible to an allergic response. The Food and Drug Administration (FDA) estimates that 5% of the 9 million allergy sufferers in the United States may be hypersensitive to sulfites.[13,14] The FDA has recently enacted regulations limiting the use of bisulfites on food. If a client reports a history of sulfite sensitivity, the dental hygienist should be alerted to the possibility of a similar response if a sulfite is included in the dental cartridge. Although sodium bisulfite or metabisulfite is found in all dental cartridges containing a vasoconstrictor, these agents are not included in solutions in which there is no vasopressor. Thus it is recommended that the dental hygienist administer local anesthetics containing no vasoconstrictor to clients with a history of sulfite sensitivity.[15]

ARMAMENTARIUM

The equipment essential for the administration of a local anesthetic agent are the following:

- ✦ Syringe
- ✦ Needle
- ✦ Cartridge of local anesthetic agent
- ✦ Supplementary armamentarium

Syringe

The *syringe* is that component of the local anesthetic armamentarium that holds the needle and cartridge of anesthetic (thus allowing the solution to be delivered to the client). Several types of syringes may be used for local anesthetic administration.[2,5]

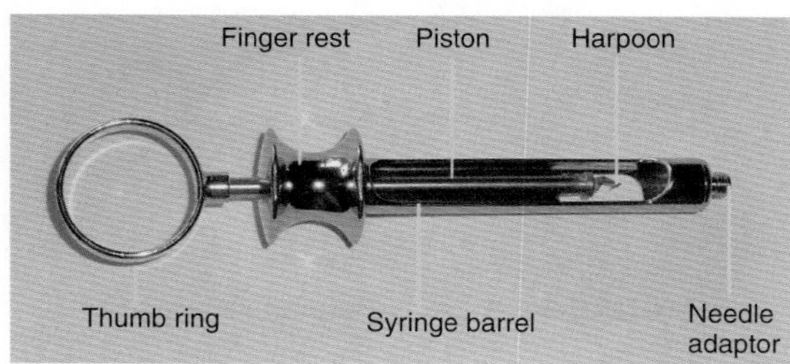

FIGURE 34–3 ✦ Breech-loading, metallic, cartridge-type aspirating syringe.

1. Reusable
   a. Breech-loading, metallic, cartridge-type
      1. Aspirating
      2. Nonaspirating
      3. Self-aspirating
   c. Computer-controlled anesthetic delivery system
   d. Pressure-type
   e. Jet injector
2. Disposable

Those syringes most often employed in oral healthcare are the reusable aspirating syringe and the self-aspirating syringe.

REUSABLE BREECH-LOADING, METALLIC, CARTRIDGE-TYPE ASPIRATING SYRINGE. This is the most commonly used syringe for administration of an intraoral local anesthetic agent (Figure 34–3). The needle is affixed to the threaded portion (or needle adaptor) at one end of the syringe. At the other end, a thumb ring and finger rest provide the dental hygienist with a means to grasp and control the syringe. The body of the syringe holds the cartridge of anesthetic solution. The aspirating syringe is characterized by a barbed piston also referred to as the *harpoon.* The harpoon engages the rubber or silicone stopper of the cartridge of anesthetic. The harpoon allows the dental hygienist to exert negative pressure on the thumb ring to assess the location of the lumen of the needle, a procedure referred to as *aspiration.* If the needle lumen rests within a blood vessel, blood appears in the cartridge after applying negative pressure to the thumb ring. If this should occur, the dental hygienist needs to withdraw the needle, replace the cartridge of anesthetic solution, and repeat the procedure. Positive pressure on the thumb ring injects the anesthetic solution into the tissues.

REUSABLE BREECH-LOADING, METALLIC, CARTRIDGE-TYPE NONASPIRATING SYRINGE. This syringe does not have a harpoon on the end of the piston, and thus the dental hygienist is unable to aspirate before depositing the anesthetic solution (Figure 34–4). It is impossible for the dental hygienist to ascertain the precise location of the needle tip with a nonaspirating syringe, and thus this

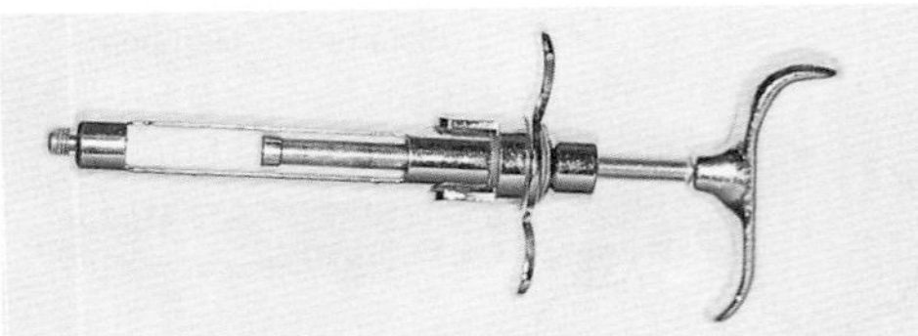

FIGURE 34–4 ✦ Nonaspirating syringe.

type of instrument should *never* be employed when administering local anesthetic during dental hygiene care.

REUSABLE BREECH-LOADING, METALLIC, CARTRIDGE-TYPE, SELF-ASPIRATING SYRINGE. The importance of aspirating before injecting an anesthetic solution is widely accepted, and the self-aspirating syringe was developed to aid the oral healthcare provider in completing this important step. This type of syringe achieves the negative pressure necessary for aspiration via the elasticity of the rubber diaphragm in the cartridge of anesthetic. When the cartridge is placed in the syringe, the diaphragm rests against a metal projection inside the syringe; this projection also directs the needle into the cartridge (Figure 34–5). Pressure exerted by the dental hygienist on the thumb disc (Figure 34–6) or on the plunger by way of the thumb ring moves the cartridge slightly toward the metal projection, thereby stretching the rubber diaphragm. When the pressure is released, the cartridge rebounds slightly, thus producing enough negative pressure within the cartridge to achieve aspiration. Therefore, the dental hygienist does not need to pull back on the thumb ring to aspirate, as is necessary with an aspirating syringe.

As noted, there are two methods to achieve aspiration with the self-aspirating syringe. First, the dental hygienist need only depress and release the thumb ring (and thus the plunger). This way, aspiration is achieved whenever the dental hygienist stops applying positive pressure to the thumb ring. A second method involves moving the thumb off the thumb ring and onto the thumb disc (Figure 34–6). Pressure is applied to the thumb disc, thereby increasing the pressure within the cartridge. Pressure on the thumb disc is then released and aspiration is accomplished. At this point the thumb is placed back into the thumb ring to deliver the anesthetic solution. This is the best technique to ensure satisfactory aspiration with the self-aspirating syringe, but adequate aspiration also may be obtained by the first method of simply pressing and releasing the thumb ring.[2]

COMPUTER-CONTROLLED LOCAL ANESTHETIC DELIVERY. The CompuDent (formerly known as the WAND) is a computer-controlled local anesthetic delivery system that can be used instead of the traditional breech-loading aspirating syringe. The CompuDent has several unique features. The handpiece is light and ergonomic; it is held in a pen grasp instead of a palm grasp, allowing a higher level of comfort and control for the clinician. The handpiece is also good for use with fearful clients

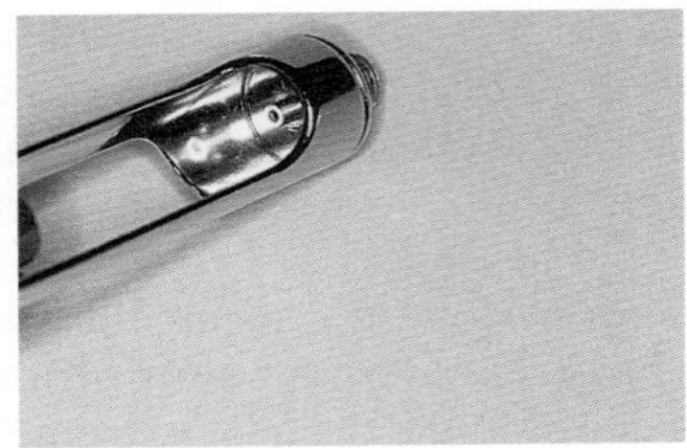

FIGURE 34–5 ✦ Metal projection of a self-aspirating syringe that directs the needle into the cartridge and depresses the cartridge diaphragm.

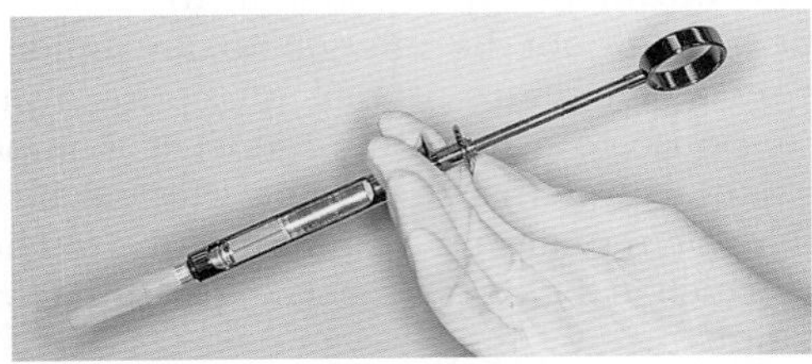

FIGURE 34–6 ✦ Pressure exerted on the thumb disc (as shown in illustration), or the thumb ring increases pressure within the cartridge. Aspiration occurs when the pressure is released.

because it looks nothing like the traditional syringe, and therefore is much less threatening. The local anesthetic delivery is controlled by a computer that regulates the flow rate of the agent and the pressure of the deposition. The computer-controlled rate allows for creation of an anesthetic pathway immediately in front of the needle, as it moves through the soft tissues, resulting in a high level of comfort for the client. Particularly with administration of palatal injections, the CompuDent can greatly increase client comfort and acceptance of local anesthetic procedures.

To initiate anesthetic delivery and aspiration, the clinician controls the computer via a foot pedal. The pedal allows for two levels of deposition: (1) a slow rate—one drop of anesthetic every 2 seconds, and (2) a fast rate—a steady stream of anesthetic. Removing their foot from the pedal, clinicians can initiate a 5-second aspiration cycle. By allowing the clinician to control the needle with the fine muscles of the hand rather than the large muscles required to operate a traditional syringe, the clinician can penetrate the soft tissues by gently rotating the needle back and forth between the thumb and fingers (bidirectional rotation) rather than the typical linear penetration. This technique has two advantages: (1) by allowing the bevel to cut into the tissues by rotating, there is no tearing of the tissue on penetration; (2) the bidirectional rotation results in less needle deflection as the tissue is penetrated. The lessened needle deflection can increase the effectiveness of the injection because the needle is more likely to be at the desired deposition site.

PRESSURE-TYPE SYRINGE. Another type of syringe that the dental hygienist may encounter is a pressure-type syringe (Figure 34–7). This type of instrument is presently

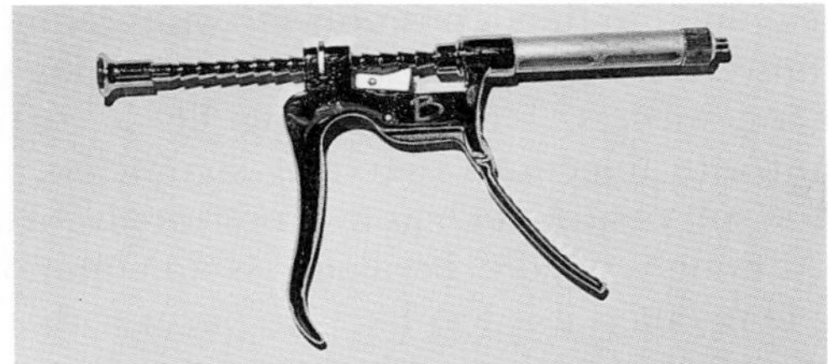

FIGURE 34–7 ✦ Pressure-type syringe.

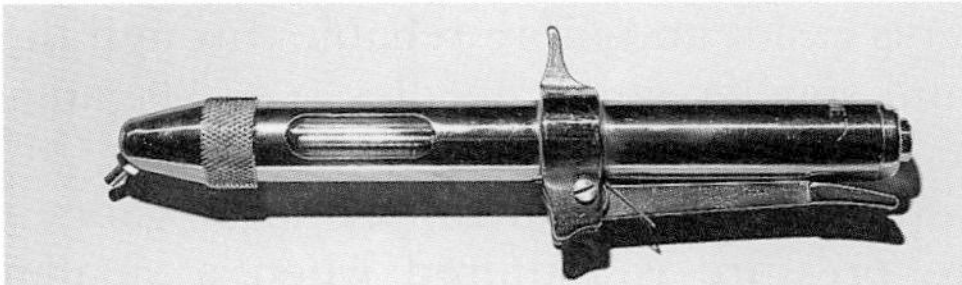

FIGURE 34–8 ✦ Jet injector syringe.

used when administering a periodontal ligament (PDL) or intraligamentary injection (ILI), which provides pulpal anesthesia to one tooth on the mandible. A standard aspirating syringe can be used for this type of injection, but the pressure-type syringe is equipped with a trigger mechanism that delivers a measured dose (0.2 ml) of anesthetic solution and allows the administrator to more easily express the solution despite significant tissue resistance. This type of syringe permits easy administration of the solution; however, the dental hygienist must take care to slowly inject even this small measured dose of anesthetic agent. If deposition of the agent is done too rapidly, client discomfort may ensue during the injection and after the anesthesia has worn off.

JET INJECTOR SYRINGE. The jet injector syringe delivers 0.05 to 0.2 ml of anesthetic agent to the mucous membranes at a high pressure (2000 psi) via small openings called *jets* (Figure 34–8). The jet injector is used primarily to obtain topical anesthesia before insertion of a needle or to achieve soft tissue anesthesia of the palate. To acquire complete anesthesia, nerve blocks or supraperiosteal injections also must be administered with a conventional syringe and needle. With the jet injector, the anesthetic solution is delivered without the use of a needle, hence it becomes a needleless injection. Clients may dislike the jolt of the jet injection, however, and postinjection discomfort may follow. Properly applied topical anesthetics accomplish the same objectives as the jet injector.

DISPOSABLE SYRINGE. Disposable plastic syringes are most often used for intramuscular or intravenous drug administration, but they may be employed during intraoral injections. These syringes do not accept standard dental cartridges, and thus it is necessary to insert the attached needle into a vial or cartridge of local anesthetic drug and eject the appropriate amount of solution. Furthermore, because these syringes have no thumb ring, aspiration is difficult and may require two hands. Because the disadvantages of the disposable syringe far outweigh the advantages, this type of syringe is not recommended for routine use.

CARE AND HANDLING OF THE SYRINGE. Recommendations for the care of reusable syringes used for local anesthetic administration follow:[2,5]

- The syringe should be sterilized after each use following the appropriate infection control protocol. Deposits resembling rust may accumulate on the syringe and interfere with function and appearance. Such deposits may be removed by ultrasonic cleaning or scrubbing (see Chapter 6).
- After several autoclavings, the hygienist should dismantle the syringe and lubricate all the threaded joints.
- The piston and harpoon may be replaced if the harpoon loses its sharpness and fails to engage the rubber stopper of the cartridge.

PROBLEMS WITH THE SYRINGE

- *Bent harpoon.* The syringe harpoon must be sharp and straight to embed the rubber stopper of the cartridge. If the harpoon becomes bent, it may fail to engage the rubber stopper of the cartridge accurately. Consequently, aspiration may be unreliable.
- *Disengagement of the harpoon from the rubber stopper of the cartridge during aspiration.* Disengagement may ensue if the harpoon is dull or if the dental hygienist applies excessive pressure to the thumb ring during aspiration. With regard to aspiration, only a gentle retraction of the thumb ring is needed; forceful action is not required.
- *Difficulty aspirating because of practitioner's hand size.* When using an aspirating syringe, the dental hygienist must be able to stretch her or his fingers and thumb to retract the thumb ring of the syringe. If this cannot be done effectively, reliable aspiration does not occur. Thus it becomes important that the syringe fits the practitioner's hand. Most syringes are similar in their dimensions, but variations do exist. Therefore, when selecting an aspirating syringe, it is beneficial to hold the syringe and test your ability to aspirate efficiently. If this is not possible, other syringes should be tested so that aspiration is easy to perform. A practitioner with small hands may use a self-aspirating syringe and thus avoid the step of pulling back on the thumb ring.

Needle

The *needle* is that component of the armamentarium that delivers the anesthetic agent from the cartridge to the tissues surrounding the needle tip. Virtually all needles used in oral healthcare today are made of stainless steel, are presterilized by the manufacturer, and are disposable.

PARTS OF THE NEEDLE. Needles used for local anesthetic administration have several components (Figure 34–9, *A*).

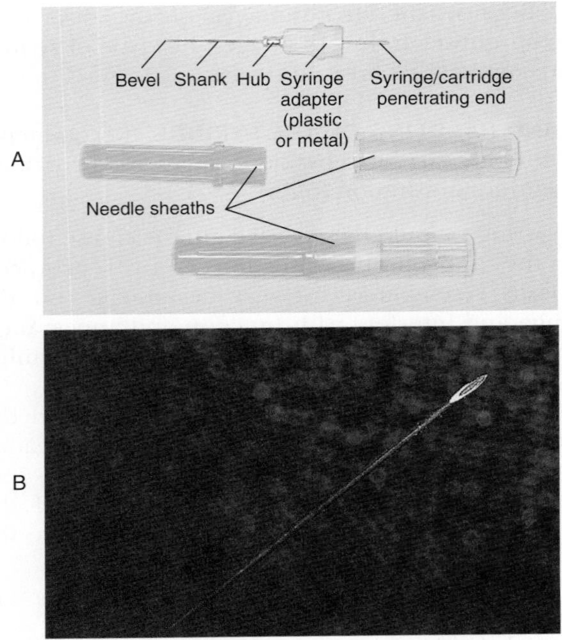

FIGURE 34–9 ✦ **A,** Parts of the needle. **B,** Bevel of the needle.

The *bevel* (Figure 34–9, *B*) is the angled surface of the needle point that is directed into the tissues. The *shank* refers to the length of the needle from the point to the hub. The *hub* or *syringe adaptor* is a plastic or metal piece that attaches the needle onto the syringe. The interior surface of metallic syringe adaptors is prethreaded. Plastic syringe adaptors are not prethreaded. Consequently, to attach a plastic-hubbed needle to a syringe, the dental hygienist must concurrently push and screw the needle onto the syringe. The syringe/cartridge-penetrating end enters the needle adaptor component of the syringe and engages the rubber diaphragm of the local anesthetic cartridge. This sterile needle is packaged in a plastic encasement consisting of two protective shields. A colored shield protects the part of the needle that is inserted into the tissues, and a clear or white shield covers the syringe and cartridge end of the needle.

GAUGE. *Gauge* is the diameter of the lumen of the needle. The higher the gauge number, the smaller the diameter of the lumen. Thus a 30-gauge needle has a smaller internal diameter than a 27-gauge needle. The most commonly employed needles in oral healthcare are the 25-, 27-, and 30-gauge.

A common assumption is that a larger-diameter needle (e.g., 25-gauge) is more uncomfortable to the client upon insertion than a smaller-diameter needle (e.g., 30-gauge); however, this assumption is untrue. Research suggests that people cannot distinguish between a 25-, a 27-, or a 30-gauge needle when injected with each.[2]

Actually, larger-gauge needles (i.e., 25-gauge) have several advantages over smaller-gauge needles. Less deflection occurs when the larger-gauge needle passes through the tissues. Because it is larger and more rigid, it can be guided to the deposition site with minimal deviation, thus ensuring greater accuracy and a higher rate of injection success. This needle rigidity is particularly important with injections requiring significant penetration of the soft tissues, such as the inferior alveolar nerve block. Although needle breakage is uncommon with disposable needles, it is less likely to occur with a larger-gauge needle. Another advantage of larger-gauge needles is the ability to aspirate and thereby reduce the possibility of intravascular injections.

Opinions vary, but many authorities conclude that aspiration is easier and more reliable through the larger lumen, and smaller-gauge needles (i.e., 30-gauge) have diameters too narrow to adequately aspirate.[2,5,16] Blood may be aspirated through a 25-, 27- or 30-gauge needle, but more pressure is required when a smaller-gauge needle is employed. This difficulty in aspirating may decrease the reliability of the aspiration and increase the likelihood of the harpoon of the aspirating syringe becoming disengaged from the rubber stopper. Therefore, it is recommended that the dental hygienist use a 25-gauge needle for those injections that pose a high risk for aspiration or when a significant depth of soft tissue must be penetrated (e.g., inferior alveolar, posterior superior alveolar, or mental/incisive nerve blocks). The 27-gauge needle may be used for all other injections, provided the possibility of aspiration and the depth of tissue penetration are minimal. The 30-gauge needle is not recommended.

LENGTH. The most common needle lengths used in oral healthcare are the short (approximately 1 inch or 25 mm) and the long (approximately 1 5/8 inches or 40 mm), as measured from the hub to the needle tip. Choice of needle length depends on accessibility of the area to be anesthetized. Long needles are preferred for those injections that require penetration of a significant thickness of soft tissue (e.g., inferior alveolar nerve block). Short needles are indicated for injections in which smaller amounts of tissue are to be entered.

CARE AND HANDLING OF THE NEEDLE. Recommendations for the care and handling of disposable needles used for local anesthetic administration follow:[2]

- Never use a needle for more than one client.
- The needle should be changed after the administration of approximately three to four injections on the same client. The stainless steel becomes dull after several injections, causing each succeeding tissue penetration to be potentially traumatic and causing postinjection soreness.
- The needle should be covered with a protective sheath when it is not being used—both before the injection and immediately upon completion of the injection.
- The position of the uncovered needle tip should be watched at all times to prevent needle injury to both the client and the operator.

✦ Needles should be disposed of in an approved sharps container. These rigid, puncture-proof, leak-resistant containers should be disposed of in accordance with federal, state, and local regulations (see Chapter 6).

PROBLEMS WITH THE NEEDLE. The following are problems the dental hygienist may encounter with the needle when administering local anesthetic agents:

✦ *Pain on insertion.* Clients may experience discomfort of the tissues during insertion if the needle is dull; therefore, the clinician should change the needle after three or four insertions if reinjection is necessary.
✦ *Pain on withdrawal.* Client discomfort may occur when the needle is being withdrawn from the tissues if any barbs are on the needle tip. Barbs may be a result of the manufacturing process; however, they are more likely to occur if the needle tip contacts bone or any hard surface with too much force. To check for needle sharpness during preparation of the armamentarium, the needle tip may be drawn backward across a sterile piece of gauze. A needle barb snags the gauze, indicating the need for replacement with a new needle. Additionally, a needle should never be pushed forcefully against bone.
✦ *Needlestick exposure to the administrator.* To prevent an accidental needlestick injury, the needle should remain capped with a protective shield before being used and immediately on termination of the injection. Should a needlestick exposure occur, follow the percutaneous exposure protocol and postexposure evaluation outlined in Chapter 7.
✦ *Needle breakage.* Refer to the later section, Local Complications.

Cartridge

The cartridge is that component of the armamentarium that contains the local anesthetic drug in addition to other ingredients. The local anesthetic cartridge is often referred to as a *carpule* by oral health professionals; however, this term is a registered trademark name for the anesthetic cartridge manufactured by Cook-Waite Laboratories.[2]

PARTS OF THE CARTRIDGE. The cartridges used for local anesthetic administration have four components (Figure 34–10):

1. The *rubber stopper/plunger* is located on one end of the cartridge and is the part in which the harpoon of an aspirating syringe is embedded. This component is pushed into the glass cylinder by pressure on the thumb ring of the syringe, thereby ejecting the local anesthetic solution through the needle. During manufacturing, the rubber stopper is often treated with silicone to allow it to transverse the glass cylinder without sticking. In an unused local anesthetic cartridge, the end of the rubber stopper is slightly indented from the rim of the glass cylinder. Cartridges that do not exhibit this characteristic should not be used because it is an indication that the solution has been contaminated. This topic is discussed more fully under the later section, Problems.

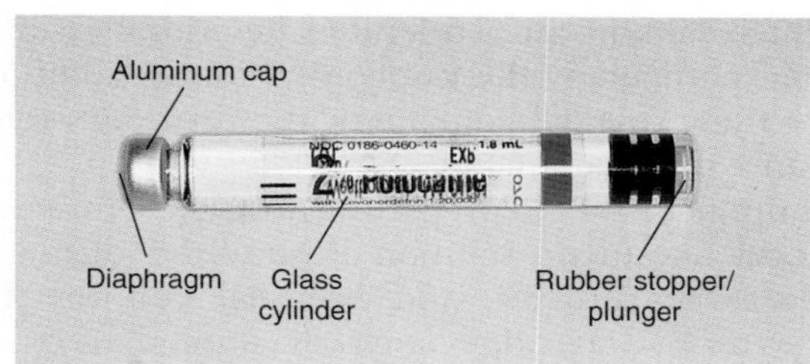

FIGURE 34–10 ✦ Components of the local anesthetic cartridge.

2. On the opposite end of the cartridge is a *diaphragm* into which the needle penetrates. The diaphragm is made of a semipermeable material, usually rubber, that allows solutions to diffuse into the cartridge if it is stored improperly.
3. An *aluminum cap* fits securely around the neck of the cartridge, holding the diaphragm in place.
4. The *glass cylinder* makes up the body of the cartridge on which the contents of the cartridge, the amount of solution, and the manufacturer's name are imprinted. Also, several manufacturers now place a color-coding band around the glass cylinder to aid in identification of the drug.

INGREDIENTS. Several ingredients collectively form the anesthetic solution. The local anesthetic drug or combination of drugs is, of course, the primary reason for the dental cartridge. The local anesthetic molecule is stable and can withstand being boiled or processed in an autoclave without breaking down. Unfortunately, other ingredients and components of the dental cartridge are more fragile.

A vasoconstricting drug in various concentrations is included in some anesthetic cartridges. This component increases the safety and duration of action of the local anesthetic agent. Those cartridges that include a vasoconstrictor also contain a preservative for the vasoconstrictor. The agent most often employed is sodium bisulfite, which prevents biodegradation of the vasoconstrictor by oxygen.

Sodium chloride is added to the dental cartridge to make the solution isotonic with the body tissues. Finally, distilled water is incorporated into the anesthetic solution to produce a sufficient volume of solution in the cartridge. Cartridges available in the United States contain a total of 1.8 ml of solution.

CARE AND HANDLING OF THE CARTRIDGE. Local anesthetic cartridges are packaged either in a vacuum-sealed metal canister containing 50 cartridges or in boxes that include 10 sealed units of 10 cartridges each, referred to as a blister pack. Regardless of how the cartridges are packaged, it is recommended that the cartridges be stored in their original container at room temperature in a dark place. Exposure to prolonged heat or direct sunlight results in an accelerated deterioration of the solution, particularly the vasoconstrictor. In addition, if kept in these original containers, the cartridges remain clean and uncontaminated.

It is not necessary to prepare a cartridge before usage. The local anesthetic solution is sterilized during the manufacturing process, and bacterial cultures taken from exterior cartridge surfaces immediately after opening a container usually fail to produce bacterial growth.[2] If the oral healthcare provider is concerned about the exterior of the cartridge, however, all components may be wiped with a disinfectant approved by the American Dental Association (ADA) and Environmental Protection Agency (EPA). Plastic cartridge dispensers are also available to aid in disinfecting cartridges. They can hold one day's supply of cartridges with the diaphragm/aluminum cap placed downward. Gauze moistened with a disinfectant is placed in the center. When assembling the armamentarium for local anesthetic administration, the oral healthcare provider may wipe the diaphragm end of the cartridge against the moistened gauze.

Cartridges should never be immersed in liquid disinfectant or sterilant. These solutions may diffuse through the semipermeable material of the diaphragm and contaminate the contents of the cartridge or may corrode the aluminum cap. In addition, local anesthetic cartridges should not be processed in the autoclave. Neither the labile vasoconstrictor nor the seals of the cartridge can withstand the extreme temperatures.

Cartridge warmers that bring the local anesthetic solution to body temperature to promote client comfort during administration are commercially available; however, they are neither necessary nor recommended.[2,5] Local anesthetics stored and injected at room temperature are not uncomfortable to clients. Indeed, an overheated cartridge may cause a burning sensation during the injection and may destroy the heat-sensitive vasoconstrictor, thus producing a shorter duration of anesthesia.

Each box or canister is marked with an expiration date by the manufacturer. This expiration date also appears on the individual cartridges. Cartridges should not be used beyond the expiration date because injection with an outdated local anesthetic solution may result in client discomfort and unreliable anesthesia.

A product identification package insert is placed in all local anesthetic containers. It includes important information about the local anesthetic agent, including dosages, contraindications, warnings, care and handling, and more. It is imperative that the dental hygienist be familiar with this material to ensure client safety and comfort.

PROBLEMS. Problems are seldom encountered with cartridges, but the following may be noted:[2,5]

- *Bubble in the cartridge.* Small bubbles (1 to 2 mm in diameter) may at times be seen in a cartridge: It is nitrogen gas that was bubbled into the anesthetic solution during the manufacturing process to preclude oxygen, which destroys the vasoconstrictor, from being trapped in the cartridge. These bubbles are harmless and may be ignored. A larger bubble (larger than 2 mm) in the cartridge, however, is an indication that the solution has been frozen. This may be accompanied by a stopper that extends beyond the end of the cartridge (extruded). Because sterility of the solution is no longer guaranteed, the cartridge should not be used.
- *Extruded stopper.* As noted previously, an extruded rubber stopper accompanied by a large bubble in the cartridge is an indication the solution has been frozen. Having a stopper that extends beyond the rim of the glass cylinder with no bubble present is often a sign that the cartridge was stored in a disinfectant and the solution has diffused through the diaphragm into the cartridge. When this occurs, the contents are contaminated and the cartridge should be discarded.
- *Sticky stopper.* A sticky stopper does not advance smoothly through the glass cylinder when pressure is applied to the thumb ring of the syringe. Because rubber stoppers are more frequently being treated with silicone during manufacturing, this has become less of a problem. If, however, paraffin is being employed by the manufacturer, difficulty may be encountered. To minimize the problem, cartridges should be stored at room temperature. If the problem persists, the healthcare provider should consider using only cartridges that have a silicone-treated stopper to facilitate a smooth, even deposition of solution.
- *Corroded cap.* Corrosion of the aluminum cap may be observed if it has been immersed in quaternary compounds such as benzalkonium chloride. If disinfecting the cartridge is necessary, an ADA/EPA-approved disinfectant is recommended. Cartridges exhibiting corrosion should not be used.
- *Rust on the aluminum cap.* The presence of rust signifies that a cartridge has broken or leaked in the metal container. The metal container rusts, and deposits appear on the cap of the cartridge. A cartridge that has a rust deposit should not be used, and each cartridge in the container should be carefully inspected.
- *Broken cartridge.* Cartridge breakage may occur if the cartridge has been fractured during handling. Damaged containers should be returned to the supplier. Before being used, each cartridge should be checked for signs of cracked or chipped glass. The area surrounding the stopper and the cylinder/cap interface need to be carefully examined. If a fractured cartridge is subjected to the pressure of an injection, it may shatter. Fortunately, the introduction of the color-coding band around the glass cylinder has minimized such an occurrence by reinforcing the glass.

A broken cartridge may result if excessive force is used when the dental hygienist engages the harpoon of an aspirating syringe. The harpoon is engaged by gently pressing the thumb ring and piston into the rubber stopper. If it is necessary to use more pressure to embed the harpoon, the dental hygienist should use one hand to cover the glass cartridge.

Pressure on the thumb ring of the syringe may cause the cartridge to break if the syringe harpoon is bent or the needle is bent and not perforating the cartridge diaphragm. Thorough examination and proper preparation of the armamentarium before use prevent this problem from occurring. One should never apply excessive pressure on the dental cartridge if significant resistance is met.

✦ *Leakage during injection.* An off-center perforation of the needle into the diaphragm of the cartridge produces an oval-shaped puncture. When positive pressure is applied to the plunger, anesthetic solution may leak through the perforation. It is important to carefully insert the needle into the cartridge diaphragm so a centric perforation occurs and leakage during the injection is prevented.

✦ *Burning on injection.* Refer to the later section, Local Complications.

Supplementary Armamentarium

In addition to the syringe, needle, and cartridge, other items are needed to effectively administer local anesthetics. These include topical antiseptic, topical anesthetic, applicator sticks, gauze, and hemostat or cotton pliers.

TOPICAL ANTISEPTICS. Topical antiseptics may be applied to the surface of the mucosa at the injection site to reduce the risk of introducing surface microorganisms into the tissue, which could result in inflammation and infection. Betadine (povidone-iodine) and Merthiolate (thimerosal) are agents commonly used for this purpose.[2] A small quantity of the agent is placed at the site of the injection for 15 to 30 seconds before placement of the topical anesthetic and the initial needle penetration. The use of sterile gauze for wiping the surface has been suggested as an adequate alternative, with topical antiseptic application as an option for further microbe reduction.[2] Because postinjection infections may occur, however, the use of a topical antiseptic should be considered, especially when administering local anesthetic agents to individuals who may be immunosuppressed.

TOPICAL ANESTHETIC AGENTS. *Topical anesthetic* agents are applied to the mucous membrane before the initial needle penetration to anesthetize the terminal nerve endings, and thus promote client comfort during the injection procedures. For maximal effectiveness, the topical anesthetic agent should be placed at the penetration site, on dried tissue, for 1 to 2 minutes.

The concentration of agents used for topical application is high to facilitate diffusion of the drug through the mucous membranes (usually 2 to 3 mm). Therefore, only small amounts applied to a limited area should be used to avoid toxicity. Both ester and amide topical anesthetic agents are available. They are prepared in the form of gels, ointments, solutions, or sprays. Topical anesthetic sprays that, when activated, deliver a continuous stream until deactivated may potentially deliver a very high dose of the anesthetic agent and are therefore not recommended. Those sprays that deliver a measured dose limit the amount that can be expelled and are much preferred.

COTTON-TIPPED APPLICATOR STICKS. Cotton-tipped applicator sticks are needed for topical antiseptic and anesthetic agent application. They also may be used to apply pressure to the tissue before and during palatal injections.

GAUZE. Gauze is used to wipe the tissue at the injection site before applying the topical antiseptic and anesthetic agents and again before inserting the needle. This procedure removes the saliva and debris from the injection site. It also may serve as a suitable, although not as effective, replacement for the topical antiseptic (see preceding Topical Antiseptic section). In addition, the gauze aids in retraction, visibility, and stability during the injection procedures.

HEMOSTAT, FORCEPS, COTTON PLIERS. Hemostat, forceps, or cotton pliers should be a component of the armamentarium in the unlikely event a needle breaks during administration and must be retrieved from the soft tissues.

PREPARATION OF ARMAMENTARIUM

Loading the Syringe

Proper loading of the syringe is essential to prevent complications associated with the syringe, cartridge, and needle, and to ensure client safety and comfort during local anesthetic administration (Procedure 34–1).

Unsheathing and Resheathing the Needle

A needle should be covered with a protective shield when it is not being used. Concerns regarding the possibility of a needlestick exposure have led to the formulation of guidelines for resheathing needles. Oral healthcare providers are most often injured with needles when the needle is being resheathed after an injection.[17] At this time the needle is contaminated with blood, saliva, and debris, and the potential for disease transmission exists. A variety of techniques have been suggested, but currently a one-handed "scoop" technique for sheathing the needle is recommended. Procedure 34–2 describes each step for unsheathing and resheathing the needle using the one-handed "scoop" procedure.

Mechanical devices such as shields and needle sheath props are available to aid in preventing an accidental needlestick exposure (Figure 34–15). Dental hygienists should be familiar with the devices available and determine which technique or mechanical device is most acceptable to them. The one-handed resheathing technique or an approved mechanical device should be consistently used by the dental hygienist regardless of whether the needle has been contaminated.

Procedure 34–1 LOADING THE SYRINGE

EQUIPMENT

Syringe
Needle gauze
Anesthetic cartridge
Protective barriers

STEPS	RATIONALE
1. Inspect each component of the armamentarium before assembly.	Ensures armamentarium is free of defects and in proper working order.
2. Retract the piston of the syringe by pulling back fully on the thumb ring (Figure 34–11).	Allows room for the cartridge to fit into the syringe.
3. Insert the cartridge, rubber stopper end first, while continuing to retract the piston (Figure 34–12). The cartridge should lie flat within the barrel of the syringe.	Cartridge fits into the syringe without being damaged.
4. Release the piston of the syringe.	Secures the cartridge in the barrel of the syringe.
5. Engage the harpoon by gently pressing on the thumb ring until the harpoon is embedded into the rubber stopper of the cartridge. Excessive force is not necessary (Figure 34–13). This step is unnecessary when loading a self-aspirating syringe.	The harpoon must engage into the rubber stopper for the dental hygienist to aspirate. Too much force on the thumb ring of the syringe may cause the cartridge to break.
6. Attach the needle to the syringe by removing the clear or white plastic cap from the syringe end of the needle and screwing the needle onto the syringe (Figure 34–14). Needles with a plastic hub need to be pushed and screwed onto the syringe. Metal hub needles have threading. Do not dispose of the cap because it will be needed when unloading the syringe. *Safety Note*: The sequence of inserting the cartridge and engaging the harpoon (of an aspirating syringe) before attaching the needle is preferred. This prevents having to hit the thumb ring and piston with force to engage the harpoon when the needle is already attached. This may lead to a broken cartridge or to anesthetic solution leaking from the needle before the injection. The sequence described also prevents the needle from being bent when perforating the diaphragm of the cartridge	Secures the needle onto the syringe.

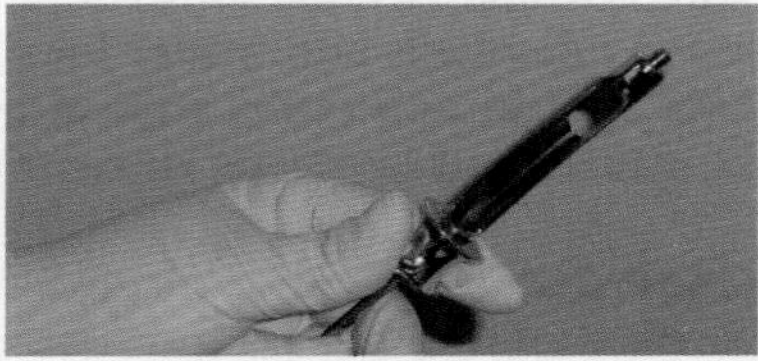

FIGURE 34–11 ✦ Retract the piston of the syringe.

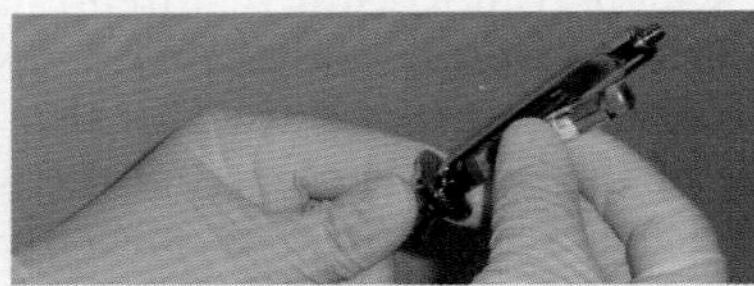

FIGURE 34–12 ✦ Insert the cartridge while continuing to retract the piston.

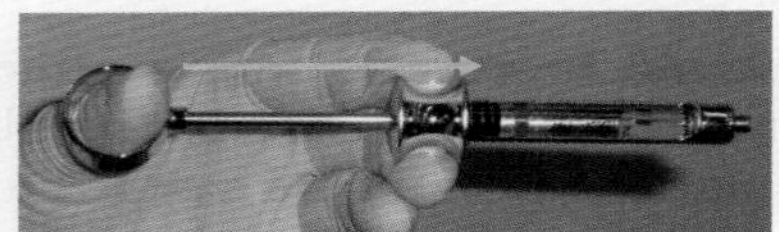

FIGURE 34–13 ✦ Engage the harpoon with gentle finger pressure (*arrow*).

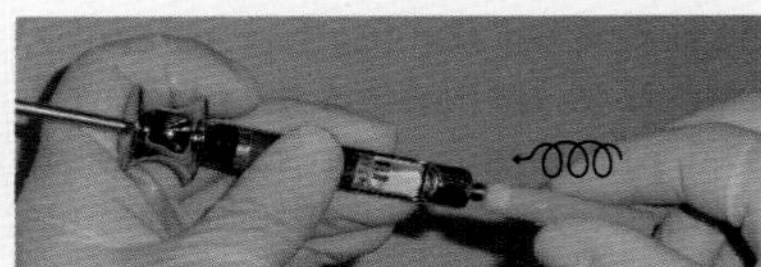

FIGURE 34–14 ✦ Attach the needle to the syringe. A plastic needle must be screwed onto the syringe while being pushed onto the metal hub (*arrow*).

STEPS	RATIONALE
7. Check for needle sharpness by removing the colored plastic cap from the needle and drawing the needle tip across sterile gauze (optional). A needle barb would snag the gauze and the needle should be replaced. Secure the needle onto the syringe.	Checks for needle sharpness to ensure an atraumatic insertion and withdrawal.
8. Expel a few drops of anesthetic solution.	Ensures the syringe, needle, and cartridge are properly prepared and functional.
9. Resheath the needle using a one-handed "scoop" technique or an approved mechanical device for needle capping (Figure 34–15).	Keeps the needle in a sterile field and prevents needlestick exposure.

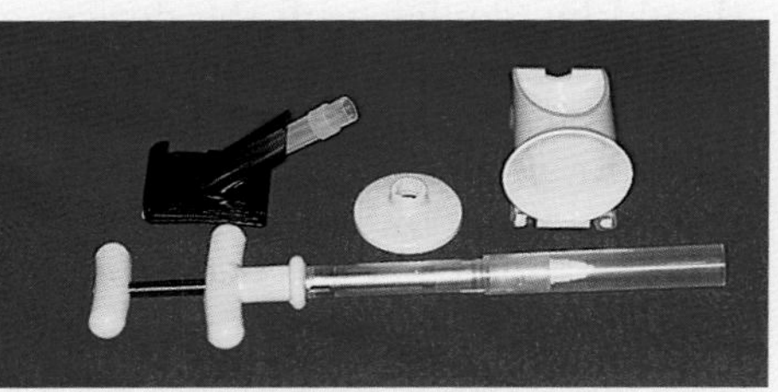

FIGURE 34–15 ✦ Shields and needle sheath props are available to prevent needlestick exposure.

Procedure 34–2 UNSHEATHING AND RESHEATHING THE NEEDLE: ONE-HANDED "SCOOP" TECHNIQUE

EQUIPMENT
Syringe
Anesthetic cartridge
Needle gauze
Protective barriers

STEPS	RATIONALE
UNSHEATHING THE NEEDLE	
1. Disengage the colored plastic cap while directing the needle away from the body or hand.	Decreases the likelihood of a puncture injury.
2. Keeping the hand at the needle hub, gently loosen the cap (Figure 34–16). Avoid disengaging the cap while holding onto the needle tip end of the plastic sheath.	Removing the cap by pulling on the needle tip end may cause the hand to "bounce back," leading to a needlestick exposure.
3. Let the cap slide off the needle and onto a piece of sterile gauze lying on the instrument tray (Figure 34–17).	Minimizes the likelihood of a puncture injury.

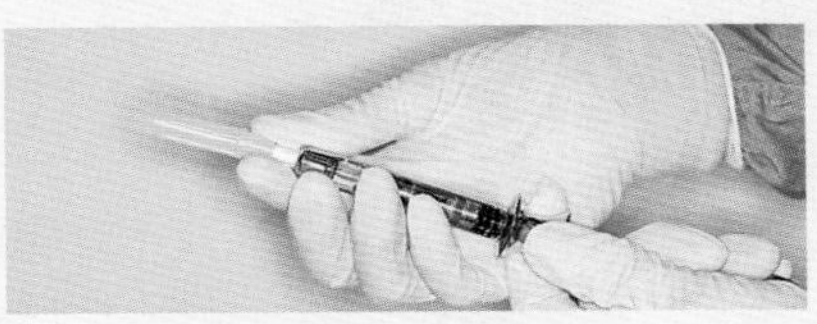

FIGURE 34–16 ✦ Directing the needle away from the body, keep the hand at the needle hub and loosen the cap.

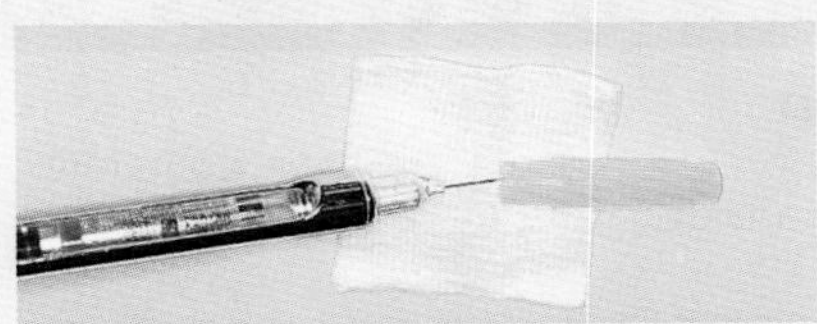

FIGURE 34–17 ✦ Let the cap slide off the needle and onto a piece of sterile gauze.

STEPS	RATIONALE
RESHEATHING THE NEEDLE: ONE-HANDED "SCOOP" TECHNIQUE	
1. Hold the syringe with one hand and glide the needle into the colored plastic cap lying on the instrument tray (Figure 34–18). Never attempt to hold cap with other hand. As an alternative, forceps may be used to hold cap on tray. This provides more control over cap and keeps dental hygienist's hand a safe distance from needle.	Prevents the dental hygienist from self-inflicting a puncture wound.
2. Tilt the syringe upward to allow the cap to slide down to the hub and cover the needle. If the cap starts to slip off the needle, do not attempt to stop it with the other hand because this may lead to an accidental needlestick exposure. Instead, let the cap fall on the instrument tray and begin the process again.	Prevents the dental hygienist from an exposure incident.
3. Secure the cap to the hub of the needle.	Creates a barrier between the outside environment and the contaminated needle.
4. When removing the needle from the syringe, the colored plastic cap should remain on the needle. The syringe end of the needle should be resheathed using the one-handed "scoop" technique or an approved mechanical device for needle capping (Figure 34–18).	Prevents an accidental needlestick exposure.

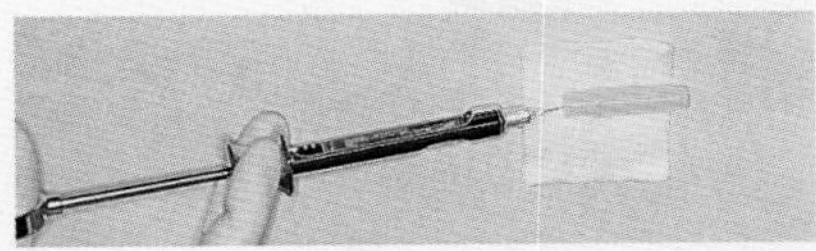

FIGURE 34–18 ✦ "Scoop" technique for recapping the needle after injection.

Dismantling the Armamentarium

At the completion of the dental hygiene care appointment, the local anesthesia armamentarium needs to be dismantled. Procedure 34–3 describes the sequence of properly unloading the syringe and the rationale for each step.

TRIGEMINAL NERVE

The *trigeminal nerve* is the fifth and largest of the 12 cranial nerves (Figure 34–22, *A*). The three divisions of the trigeminal nerve include the ophthalmic (V_1), the maxillary (V_2), and the mandibular (V_3). The ophthalmic and maxillary divisions are completely sensory; the mandibular division is sensory and also carries the motor root to the muscles of the mandible.

Ophthalmic Division (V_1)

The ophthalmic nerve, the first and smallest division of the trigeminal nerve, branches off the trigeminal (semilunar or gasserian) ganglion and forms three branches: the nasociliary nerve, the frontal nerve, and the lacrimal nerve. This division of the trigeminal nerve innervates tissues superior to the oral structures, including the eye, nose, and frontal cutaneous tissues. It has only sensory

Procedure 34–3 UNLOADING THE SYRINGE

EQUIPMENT

Syringe
Anesthetic cartridge
Needle
Sharps container
Protective barriers

STEPS	RATIONALE
1. Resheath the needle utilizing the one-handed "scoop" technique or an approved mechanical device for needle capping (Procedure 34–2).	Prevents a needlestick exposure while unloading the syringe.
2. Retract the piston of the syringe by pulling back fully on the thumb ring.	Allows room for the cartridge to be disengaged from the syringe.
3. While retracting the piston, remove the cartridge by pulling it away from the needle and disengaging the rubber stopper from the harpoon (Figure 34–19). Turn the window of the syringe downward to aid in removal. With a self-aspirating syringe, there is no harpoon disengagement.	Frees the cartridge from the barrel of the syringe. 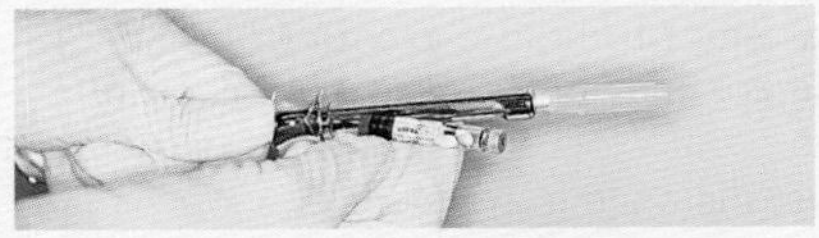 FIGURE 34–19
4. Unscrew and remove the needle from the syringe (Figure 34–20). 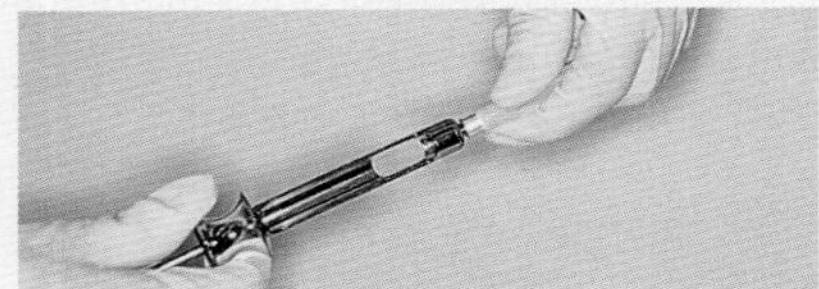 FIGURE 34–20	Frees the needle from the syringe
5. Resheath the syringe end of the needle using the one-handed "scoop" technique or an approved mechanical device for needle capping (Procedure 34–2).	Protects the dental hygienist from needlestick exposure during disposal.
6. Directly dispose of the needle and cartridge in a sharps container (Figure 34–21). *Safety Note:* Needles should not be bent, broken, or cut before disposal in a sharps container. This minimizes the possibility of a needlestick exposure.	Used needles and cartridges are considered infectious. Sharps must be discarded in a rigid, puncture-proof, leak-resistant container (see Chapter 6). 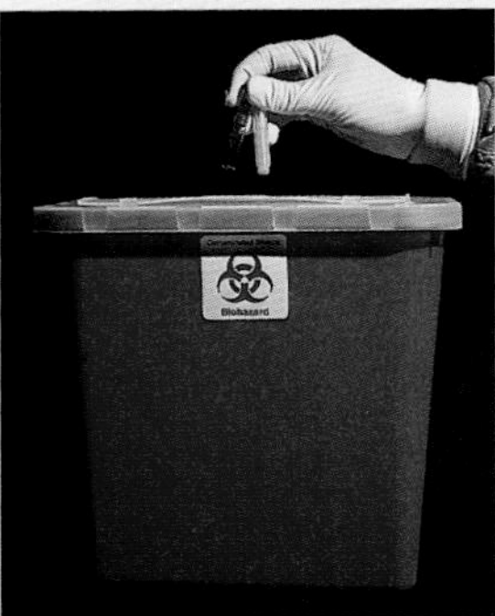 FIGURE 34–21
7. The syringe should be sterilized following the appropriate protocol.	Syringe is available for subsequent utilization.

function. Of the three divisions of the trigeminal nerve, the ophthalmic is the least important to intraoral local anesthetic administration.

Maxillary Division (V_2)

The maxillary division of the trigeminal nerve, which is entirely sensory in function, arises from the trigeminal (semilunar or gasserian) ganglion, exits the cranium via the foramen rotundum, and then passes into the pterygopalatine fossa, where it gives off several branches (Figure 34–22, *B* and *C*). Only those branches pertinent to intraoral local anesthesia are discussed.

PTERYGOPALATINE NERVES. Two branches pass through the pterygopalatine ganglion and form the greater (anterior) palatine nerve and the nasopalatine nerve (Figure 34–22, *B*). The *greater palatine nerve* enters the oral cavity on the hard palate via the greater palatine foramen and innervates the palatal soft tissues and bone of the posterior teeth. The *nasopalatine nerve* leaves the pterygopalatine ganglion and passes forward and downward, entering the oral cavity through the incisive foramen. This nerve provides sensory innervation to the lingual bone and soft tissues in the premaxilla (canine to canine).

POSTERIOR SUPERIOR ALVEOLAR NERVE. The *posterior superior alveolar nerve* (PSA) (Figure 34–22, *C*) descends from the main trunk of the maxillary nerve just before it enters the infraorbital canal. Most often there are two PSA branches that pass downward on the posterior surface of the maxilla. An internal branch enters the posterior superior alveolar foramen located on the superior portion of the maxillary tuberosity. This branch provides sensory innervation to the pulpal and osseous tissues and the periodontal ligaments of the maxillary third, second, and first molars (usually with the exception of the mesiobuccal root of the first molar). An external branch of the posterior superior alveolar nerve remains on the outer surface of the maxilla and continues downward to innervate the facial gingiva of the maxillary molars and the adjacent vestibular mucosa.

BRANCHES OF THE INFRAORBITAL NERVE. The maxillary nerve continues anteriorly after having given off the posterior superior alveolar nerve and enters the infraorbital canal. At this point the maxillary nerve is referred to as the *infraorbital nerve* (Figure 34–22, *C*). Two branches may descend from the infraorbital nerve: the middle superior alveolar and the anterior superior alveolar nerves.

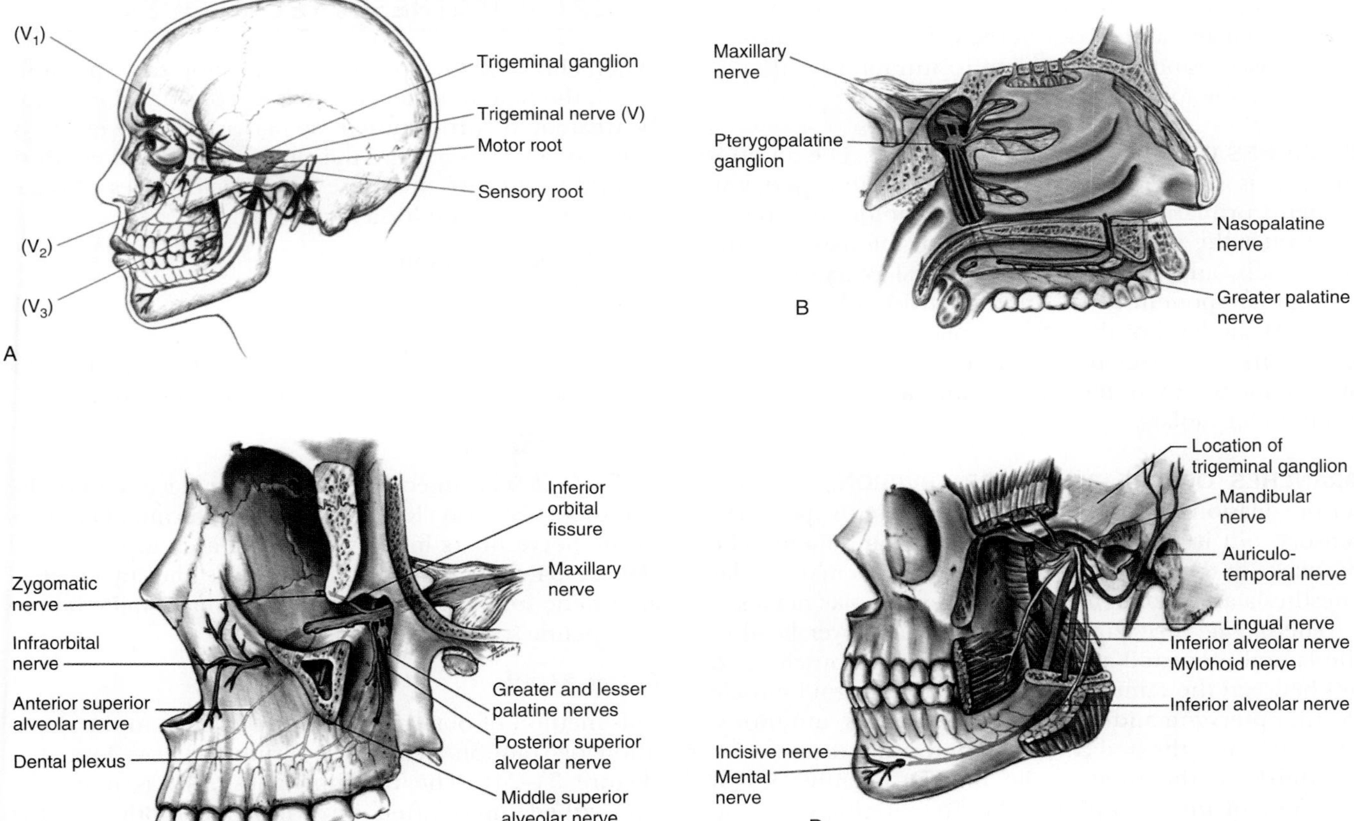

FIGURE 34–22 ✦ **A,** Trigeminal nerve distribution. **B,** Palatal branches of the maxillary division (V_2). **C,** Distribution of the maxillary division (V_2). **D,** Distribution of the mandibular division (V_3). (*A to* D *from Fehrenbach MJ:* Illustrated anatomy of the head and neck, *Philadelphia, WB Saunders, [in press].*)

The *middle superior alveolar nerve* (MSA) branches off the infraorbital nerve within the infraorbital canal. This nerve provides sensory innervation to the maxillary premolars, the mesiofacial root of the first molar, the periodontal tissues, and the facial soft tissue and bone in the premolar area. The MSA nerve is not present in approximately 60% of individuals.[18] In its absence, these areas are innervated by the posterior superior alveolar nerve, or more commonly, the anterior superior alveolar nerve.

The *anterior superior alveolar nerve* (ASA) descends from the infraorbital nerve just before the latter's exit from the infraorbital foramen. The ASA nerve provides innervation to the central and lateral incisors, the canine, the periodontal tissues, and facial soft tissue and bone over these teeth. In those individuals without an MSA nerve, the ASA nerve most often provides innervation to the premolars and possibly the mesiofacial root of the first molar.

Mandibular Division (V_3)

The mandibular nerve, the third and largest division of the trigeminal nerve, both has a sensory root and carries the motor root for the trigeminal nerve (Figure 34–22, *D*). The sensory root arises from the trigeminal ganglion, after which it is joined by the motor root. Both roots emerge from the cranium via the foramen ovale, and at this point, they unite to form the main trunk of the mandibular nerve. The trunk then divides into an anterior branch and a posterior branch. Those nerves arising from these branches that relate to intraoral local anesthesia are the following:

BRANCHES OF THE ANTERIOR DIVISION. The anterior division is smaller than its posterior counterpart and contains primarily motor fibers. The motor component innervates the muscles of mastication: the masseter, the temporalis, and the lateral and medial pterygoid. The sensory component of the anterior division is the *buccal nerve.* At the level of the occlusal plane of the mandibular molars, it crosses the anterior border of the ramus and branches to innervate the buccal gingiva of the mandibular molars.

BRANCHES OF THE POSTERIOR DIVISION. The posterior division of the mandibular nerve is primarily sensory, but it also has a small motor component. The branches of the posterior division related to mandibular anesthesia are the lingual and inferior alveolar nerves.

The *lingual nerve* emerges between the lower head of the lateral pterygoid and medial pterygoid muscles and lies between the ramus and the medial pterygoid muscle in the pterygomandibular space. It turns anteriorly, where it enters the oral cavity and innervates the anterior two-thirds of the tongue, the mucous membranes of the floor of the mouth, and the lingual gingiva of the mandible.

The *inferior alveolar nerve* runs posterior and parallel to the lingual nerve within the pterygomandibular space, where it enters the mandibular foramen. Within the mandible the inferior alveolar nerve travels in the mandibular canal and innervates the pulpal and osseous tissues of the mandibular teeth in the quadrant and facial soft tissues anterior to the first molar. Throughout its course the inferior alveolar nerve is accompanied by the inferior alveolar artery and vein.

As the inferior alveolar nerve reaches the mental foramen, it divides into two terminal branches. The *incisive nerve* is a direct extension of the inferior alveolar nerve, continuing anteriorly within the mandibular canal. It innervates the pulpal and osseous tissues of the mandibular first premolar, canine, lateral and central incisors, and the facial periodontal tissues of the teeth.

The *mental nerve* branches from the inferior alveolar nerve and exits the mandible via the mental foramen and provides sensory innervation to the mucous membranes and skin of the lower lip and chin.

The *mylohyoid nerve* branches from the inferior alveolar nerve before the latter enters into the mandibular foramen. It advances downward and forward in the mylohyoid groove on the medial side of the ramus and provides motor innervation to the mylohyoid and anterior digastric muscles. In some individuals the mylohyoid nerve may supply accessory sensory innervation to the mandible in the premolar and molar area.

LOCAL ANESTHESIA TECHNIQUES

When choosing the appropriate injection to be administered, the dental hygienist needs to consider the area to be treated, the procedure to be performed, the extent of anesthesia necessary, and the client's needs and comfort. In oral healthcare there are three major types of injections used to obtain local anesthesia:

- Local infiltration
- Field block
- Nerve block

These are differentiated by the site of anesthetic solution deposition relative to the area to receive treatment.

Local Infiltration

A *local infiltration* injection refers to the placement of the anesthetic solution close to the smaller terminal endings of the nerve fibers in the immediate area to be treated (Figure 34–23). An example would be the injection of anesthetic solution into an interproximal papilla before therapeutic scaling and root planing.

Field Block

This method of obtaining anesthesia refers to the deposition of solution near large terminal nerve branches (Figure 34–24). The resulting anesthesia is more circumscribed, most often involving one tooth and the tissues surrounding the tooth. Treatment is away from the site of the injection. The deposition of anesthetic solution above the apex of a maxillary tooth, such as the maxillary right central incisor, is an example of a *field*

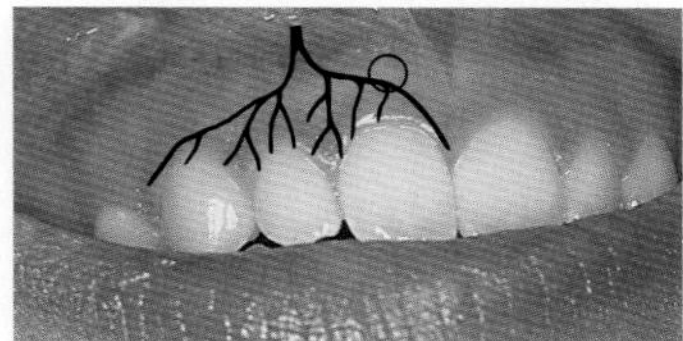

FIGURE 34–23 ✦ Local infiltration. The local anesthetic is placed in the immediate area to be treated.

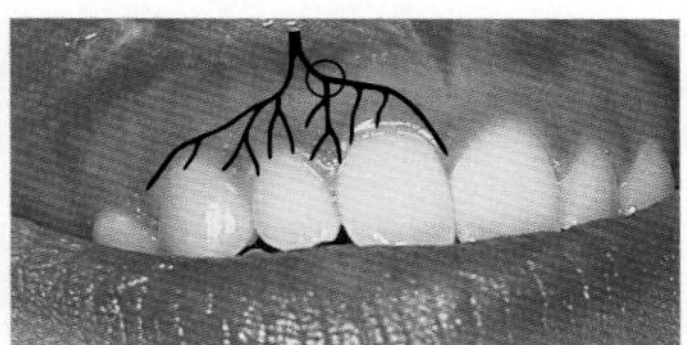

FIGURE 34–24 ✦ Field block. The local anesthetic is deposited near the larger terminal nerve endings. Treatment is away from the site of the injection.

block. In oral healthcare a field block is often incorrectly referred to as a *local infiltration*.

Nerve Block

The *nerve block* refers to the deposition of anesthetic solution close to a main nerve trunk, often at some distance from the treatment area (Figure 34–25). This type of injection most often anesthetizes a larger area than that of a field block. Examples include a posterior superior alveolar nerve block and an inferior alveolar nerve block.

Thus, when providing dental hygiene care in a small, isolated area, infiltration anesthesia may be the best choice, whereas a field block is the injection of choice when one or two teeth are to be treated. When the dental hygiene care plan involves a sextant or quadrant, nerve block anesthesia is recommended.

The term *anesthesia* is often preceded by either the word *local* or *regional*. Either phrase is correct; each indicates that a specific area is anesthetized and that the client is conscious, unlike general anesthesia, in which the client is unconscious. Thus the use of either term is appropriate, and they can be used interchangeably, although *local anesthesia* appears to be more commonly used.

PROCEDURES FOR A SUCCESSFUL INJECTION

The goal for each administration of local anesthetic is, of course, to give a safe, comfortable injection for control and elimination of painful sensations during and after dental hygiene care. It is ironic, however, that a procedure meant to control pain for clients is often reported to be the most dreaded. Although the prospect of receiving an intraoral injection provokes fear and apprehension for many individuals, local anesthetic agent administration need not be painful. The dental hygienist strives to make all dental hygiene care free from pain and stress, especially when administering intraoral local

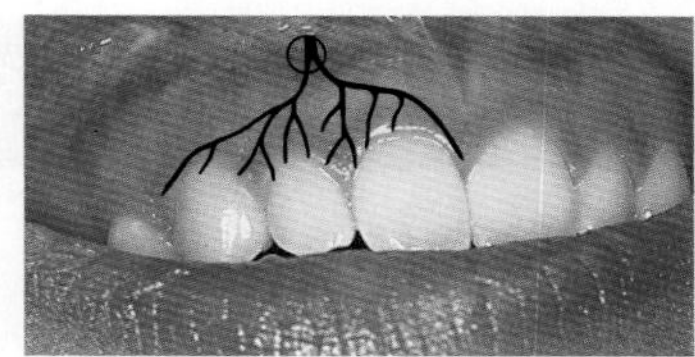

FIGURE 34–25 ✦ Nerve block. The local anesthetic is deposited near a main nerve trunk, often located some distance from the site of treatment.

anesthetics. Such techniques as using a topical anesthetic before needle insertion, depositing a few drops of anesthetic solution and waiting 5 seconds before cautiously advancing the needle, and slowly depositing the anesthetic solution help minimize or eliminate discomfort.

Strategies used to minimize anxiety include communicating with the client about the progress of the procedure. Keeping clients informed of the procedures in a calm manner and using nonthreatening language helps minimize apprehension and promote trust and cooperation. For example, telling clients "I'm applying the topical anesthetic to the tissue so the remainder of the procedure is more comfortable" or, "I don't expect you to feel this" when inserting the needle into the tissue places a positive idea in the client's mind regarding the injection and keeps the client informed of the impending procedure. Taking the extra time results in a more comfortable procedure for the client, thus meeting the human needs for freedom from pain and stress.

Procedure 34–4 presents steps to ensure comfort, safety, and success common to all injections. Although each injection is unique with regard to anatomic considerations, these steps should be employed regardless of the injection being administered. Not every injection is successful and totally free of discomfort because the reactions of clients and the skills of hygienists vary; however, if the steps in Procedure 34–4 are followed, the client and the dental hygienist will enjoy the benefit of the safest and least traumatic injection possible.

INJECTION TECHNIQUES FOR THE MAXILLARY TEETH AND FACIAL HARD AND SOFT TISSUES

The injection techniques available to anesthetize the maxillary teeth and the facial hard and soft tissues include supraperiosteal injection, anterior superior alveolar nerve block (ASA), middle superior alveolar nerve block (MSA), infraorbital nerve block, and posterior superior alveolar nerve block (PSA).

Supraperiosteal Injection (Local Infiltration)

A *supraperiosteal* injection, more commonly referred to as a *local infiltration*, involves depositing anesthetic solution near the apex of a single tooth, thus providing anesthesia of the tooth and the immediate surrounding area.

Text continues on page 727.

Procedure 34–4 GIVING A SUCCESSFUL INJECTION

EQUIPMENT

Health history form
Sphygmomanometer
Stethoscope
Gauze
Topical anesthetic agent
Cotton-tipped applicator
Syringe
Anesthetic cartridge
Needle
Protective barriers

STEPS	RATIONALE
1. Assess the health history data.	Assists the dental hygienist in determining if the client is physiologically and psychologically able to tolerate the proposed treatment and local anesthetic administration, and in modeling approach to care, if necessary, to decrease risks and prevent subsequent medical emergencies.
2. Take vital signs. Minimal examination should include blood pressure, heart rate (pulse), and respiratory rate.[7]	Following guidelines for dental management of clients according to blood pressure level, heart rate, and respiratory rate minimizes medical complications.
3. Confirm care plan.	Verifies with the client the dental hygiene care indicated.
4. Check armamentarium.	Ensures that all materials are properly assembled, prepared, and functional so the procedure is efficient.
5. Load the syringe and determine the syringe window and needle bevel orientation.[7]	The large window of the syringe should face the operator so she or he is able to see the amount of anesthetic being administered and detect a positive aspiration. The bevel of the needle should face the bone; thus, if the needle contacts bone, the bevel deflects over the periosteum, minimizing discomfort and trauma. If the bevel faces away from the bone, the point of the needle may tear the sensitive tissues, causing discomfort both during and after the injection.
6. Check needle sharpness by pulling the needle tip across sterile gauze, and watching for snags (optional).[7]	A sharp needle free of barbs does not snag gauze and provides an atraumatic insertion and withdrawal.
7. Check the flow of solution.	Ensures the syringe, needle, and cartridge are properly prepared and functional so the procedure is efficient.
8. Place the client in a supine position.	Placing the client in a supine position provides better accessibility and visibility for the clinician and reduces the likelihood of syncope for the client. Position may vary with client's health status or clinician's preference.
9. Communicate with the client. Do not use words with a negative connotation, such as *shot, injection, pain,* or *hurt.* Instead, speak in less-threatening terms such as "administer the local anesthetic."[7]	Keeping clients informed of the procedures helps them anticipate the operator's actions. A calm approach minimizes client anxiety.
10. Position self (clinician) appropriately.	Provides optimal accessibility and visibility for the clinician relative to the specific injection being administered.
11. Visualize or palpate to locate the penetration site.	Accurate injection of anesthetic requires insertion in correct site.
12. Dry the penetration site with gauze.	Removes saliva and debris from the penetration site, reducing the risk of infection.
13. Apply topical antiseptic to the penetration site (optional).	Decreases microorganisms at the penetration site, reducing the risk of infection.
14. Apply topical anesthetic to the penetration site for 1–2 minutes.	Application of topical anesthetic results in a more comfortable penetration.
15. In the case of palatal injections, when placing topical anesthetic on the injection site, apply considerable pressure with the cotton swab for a minimum of 1 minute before the injection. Move the swab immediately adjacent to the penetration site and maintain pressure at this site during the injection.	Injections into the dense, tightly attached palatal tissue can be extremely painful to the client. Pressure anesthesia provides for a more comfortable procedure by producing ischemia and blocking pain impulses arising from the needle penetration.[7]
16. Redry the penetration site.	Removes the saliva and excess topical anesthetic from the injection site.
17. Make the tissue taut at the penetration site by retracting it (except the palate), utilizing sterile gauze.	Gauze is used to aid in retraction and stability. Stretching the tissue tight at the penetration site provides maximal visibility and allows the needle to enter the tissue with minimal resistance and discomfort. Avoid jiggling the soft tissues or pulling the lip over the needle tip, which may impair visibility of the penetration site.

Procedure 34–4 GIVING A SUCCESSFUL INJECTION—CONT'D

STEPS	RATIONALE
18. Keep syringe and needle out of the client's line of vision.	Minimizes client anxiety.
19. Place the needle at the penetration site.	Accurate injection of anesthetic agent requires insertion in the correct site.
20. Use a handrest (Figure 34–26).	Provides stability and control during the injection, thus ensuring greater client safety and comfort.
21. Gently insert the needle into the mucosa until the bevel is completely under the tissue.	Initiates needle penetration with minimal discomfort.
22. Observe and communicate with the client. Watch for any signs of discomfort or distress.	Keeping clients informed of the procedures helps them anticipate the operator's actions and minimizes anxiety. Careful observation of the client alerts the clinician to a potential behavioral problem or medical emergency.
23. Deposit a few drops of anesthetic solution and pause for 5 seconds and then advance the needle a few millimeters. Repeat process as you slowly advance to the deposition site.	Anesthetizes the tissues in front of the needle before its advancement, thus minimizing discomfort. Pausing for several seconds allows the anesthesia to develop.

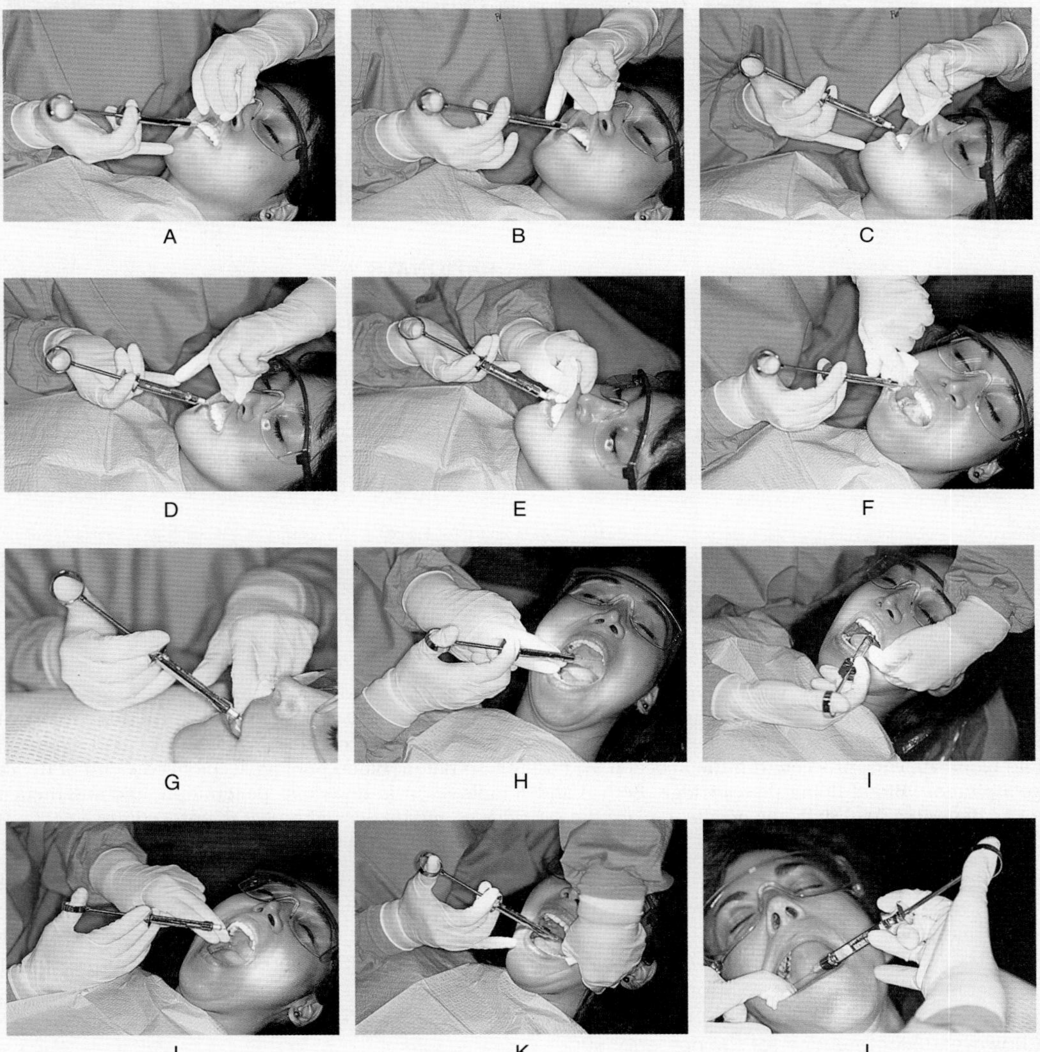

FIGURE 34–26 ✦ Handrests. **A** to **E,** Handrests that may be used for a maxillary supraperiosteal injection, anterior superior alveolar, and middle superior alveolar nerve blocks. *A* and *E* may be used for the infraorbital nerve block. **F** and **G,** Handrests for a posterior superior alveolar nerve block. **H** and **I,** Handrests for a greater palatine nerve block. **J,** Handrest for the nasopalatine nerve block. **K** and **L,** Handrests for the inferior alveolar and lingual nerve blocks.

Continued on following page

Procedure 34-4 GIVING A SUCCESSFUL INJECTION—CONT'D

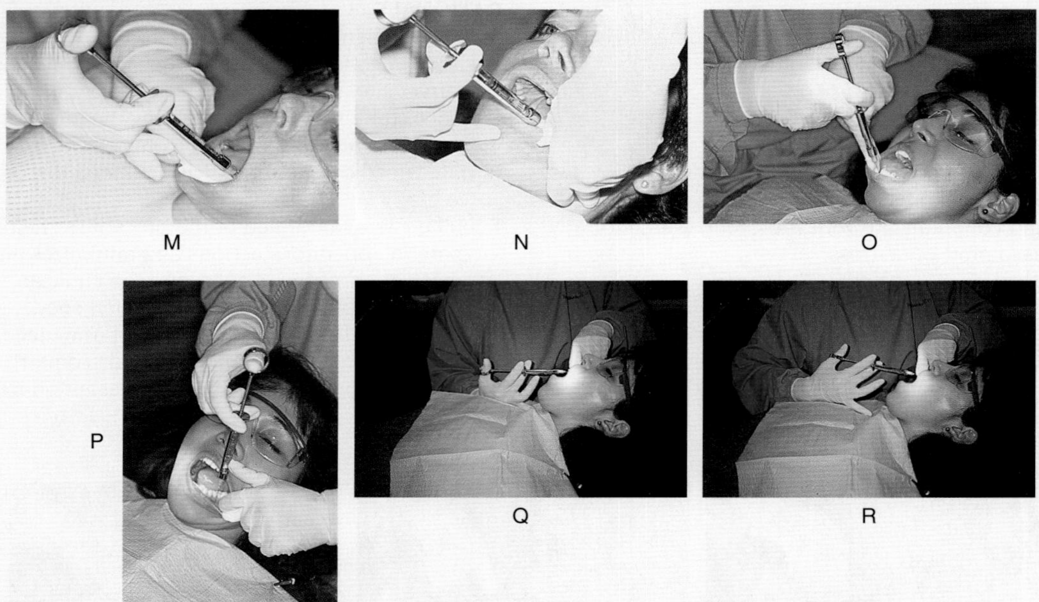

FIGURE 34–26, CONT'D ✦ **M** and **N,** Handrest for the buccal nerve block. **O** and **P,** Handrests for the mental and incisive nerve blocks. **Q,** When possible, hold the arms close to the body to increase stabilization. **R,** Do *not* use the client's arm or chest as a handrest.

STEPS	RATIONALE
24. Inject solution drop by drop in advance of the needle.	At this point, aspiration is not necessary because of the small amount of solution being deposited over a changing injection site.
25. Aspirate on arrival at the deposition site.	Minimizes the possibility of an intravascular injection by ascertaining if the needle tip is located within a blood vessel. Aspiration of blood into the cartridge indicates intravenous placement of the needle (Figure 34–27) and the need to replace the cartridge and repeat the procedure.

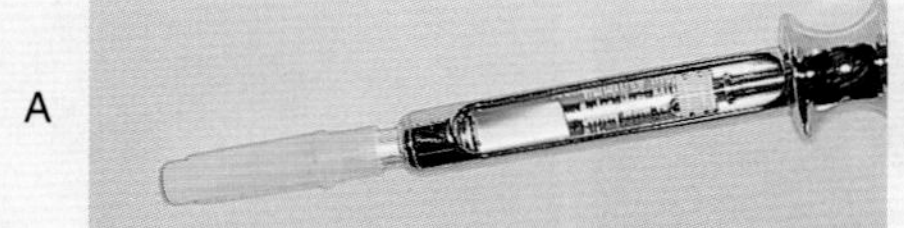

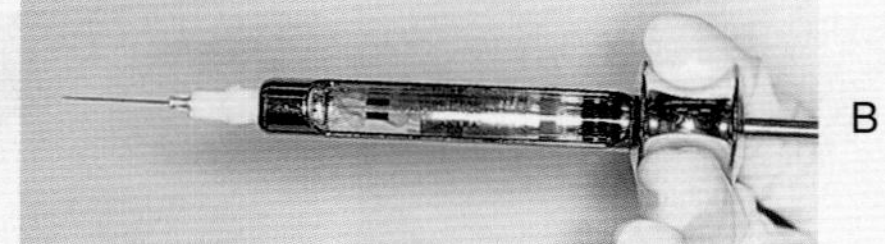

FIGURE 34–27 ✦ Before injecting anesthetic solution at the deposition site, with an aspirating syringe, gently pull back on the thumb ring without moving the needle tip. With a self-aspirating syringe, stop applying pressure (pushing forward) on the thumb ring, or apply pressure to the thumb disc. Observe the needle end of the cartridge for signs of blood entering the cartridge. If no blood appears, proceed with the injection. **A,** Positive aspiration. Blood pooling at the needle end of the cartridge. **B,** Positive aspiration. Blood filling the cartridge. Both *A* and *B* indicate an intravascular penetration, and anesthetic solution should not be deposited. Withdraw the needle, replace the cartridge of anesthetic, and repeat the procedure.

STEPS	RATIONALE
26. Perform multiple aspirations as indicated. a. Rotate the syringe slightly (approximately 1/4 turn) between the index and third fingers. b. Reaspirate. c. Return the syringe to its original position. d. Reaspirate. (Optional; however, recommended for the posterior superior alveolar nerve block, inferior alveolar nerve block, and mental/incisive nerve blocks because of high percentage of positive aspirations)	False-negative aspiration may occur if the needle bevel is occluded by the inner wall of the blood vessel. Multiple aspirations with the needle bevel in different planes prevent this potential problem (Figure 34–28).

Procedure 34–4 GIVING A SUCCESSFUL INJECTION—CONT'D

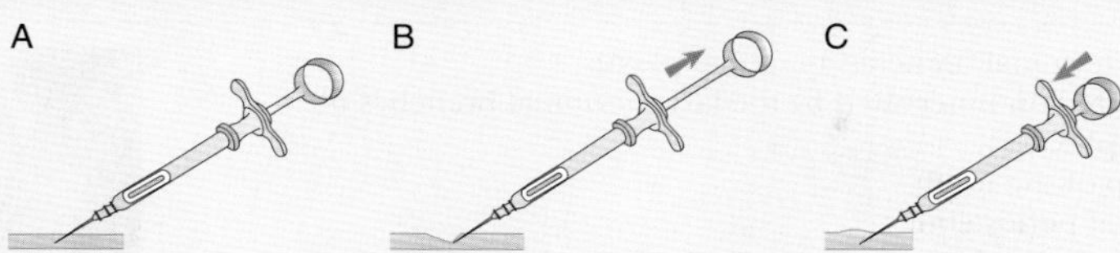

FIGURE 34–28 ✦ Intravascular injection of local anesthetic. **A,** Needle is inserted into lumen of blood vessel. **B,** Aspiration test is performed. Negative pressure pulls vessel wall against bevel of needle; therefore, no blood enters syringe (negative aspiration). **C,** Drug is injected. Positive pressure on plunger of syringe forces local anesthetic solution out through needle. Wall of vessel is forced away from bevel, and anesthetic solution is deposited directly into lumen of blood vessel. *(From Malamed SF:* Medical emergencies in the dental office, *ed 4, St Louis, 1993, Mosby.)*

STEPS	RATIONALE
27. Slowly deposit the anesthetic solution over the indicated number of seconds. Solution should be introduced into the tissues at a rate of 1 ml/min or approximately 2 minutes for a full cartridge.	Aspirating several times while injecting helps the operator to slow down the deposition rate and reaffirms extravascular position of the needle tip. Slow deposition reduces the risk/severity of an overdose reaction in case of inadvertent intravascular injection and prevents tearing and necrosis of the tissue and subsequent discomfort. If, despite slow introduction of the solution, blood levels of anesthetic become elevated, the severity and duration of the toxic reaction will be reduced. Slow injection of the anesthetic solution is critical to preventing an adverse drug reaction.
28. Observe and communicate with the client. Watch for any signs of discomfort or distress; Reassure the client with statements such as, "I'm depositing the solution slowly so this procedure is comfortable for you."	Keeping the clients informed of the progress of the procedures helps them to anticipate the operator's actions and minimizes anxiety.
29. When the indicated amount of anesthetic has been deposited, slowly withdraw the needle.	Concludes the injection with minimal discomfort.
30. Replace the needle sheath utilizing the "scoop" technique (Procedure 34–2).	Prevents inadvertent needlestick injury with a contaminated needle to the hygienist and other oral healthcare personnel.
31. Observe the client.	Most adverse reactions, such as syncope, occur either during the injection or within 5–10 minutes after completion of administration, thus remaining with the client following the injection is imperative.[7]
32. Rinse the client's mouth.	Washes out any anesthetic solution that may have dripped into the client's mouth.
33. Massage the tissue over the injection site when indicated.	Gives the client a sense of well-being.
34. Test for anesthesia by touching the rounded back of an explorer to both the area anesthetized and an area not anesthetized. The client should have little or no sensation in the anesthetized area.	Ensures that proper anesthesia is obtained before commencing treatment.
35. Reassure the client that numbness, tingling, and a sense of swelling or the tooth feeling different are normal responses.	Gives the client a sense of well-being.
36. Record the injection(s) in the client's chart, including: a. Area anesthetized and specific injection(s) given b. Type of anesthetic used and type of vasoconstrictor and its concentration (ratio) c. Total amount of solution administered (in milliliters and/or total cartridges) d. Client reaction	Accurate documentation provides a reference for future appointments and essential information if the client exhibits any negative reactions and provides your best line of defense if a client challenges the care received.[19]

This injection is most often used to anesthetize maxillary teeth. The rather thin, porous nature of the bone in the maxilla facilitates diffusion of the anesthetic solution from the deposition site to the apex of the tooth to be treated. By contrast, the mandible consists of much denser bone, which prevents diffusion of the anesthetic agent to the apices of the posterior teeth, therefore precluding the supraperiosteal injection in this area. A supraperiosteal injection may be used to anesthetize the central and lateral teeth in the mandible because the bone in this area is thinner and nutrient canals may be present.

TABLE 34–11 SUPRAPERIOSTEAL INJECTION (LOCAL INFILTRATION)

Nerves anesthetized	Large terminal branches of dental plexus
Areas anesthetized	Entire region innervated by the large terminal branches of the plexus: Pulp of the tooth Facial periosteum Connective tissue Mucous membranes overlying the tooth (Figure 34–29)
Needle gauge/length	25- or 27-gauge short
Operator position	8 or 9 o'clock
Penetration site	Height of the mucobuccal fold above the apex of the target tooth (Figure 34–30)
Landmarks	Mucobuccal fold Crown of tooth Root contour of tooth
Syringe orientation	Parallel to the long axis of the tooth (Figure 34–31)
Handrests	Client's chin Forefinger, or wrist of operator's opposite hand (Figure 34–26)
Deposition site	Apical region of the target tooth
Penetration depth	Usually only a few millimeters, no more than 5 mm or ¼ of a short needle
Amount of anesthetic to be deposited	0.6 ml, or ⅓ of a cartridge
Length of time to deposit	Approximately 30–60 seconds

Potential Problems	Technique Tips
Anesthetic deposition below apex of target tooth, resulting in insufficient pulpal anesthesia	Increase depth of penetration so the needle is at the apical region of the target tooth.
Needle too far from bone, and thus solution deposited into buccal tissue	Redirect needle closer to periosteum.
Dense bone may cover apices. Most often occurs on permanent maxillary first molars in children because the apex is located under the dense zygomatic bone. May occur on central incisors where the apex lies beneath the nose.	Administer a nerve block.
Pain on insertion with the needle against the periosteum	Withdraw the needle and reinsert farther away (laterally) from the periosteum.

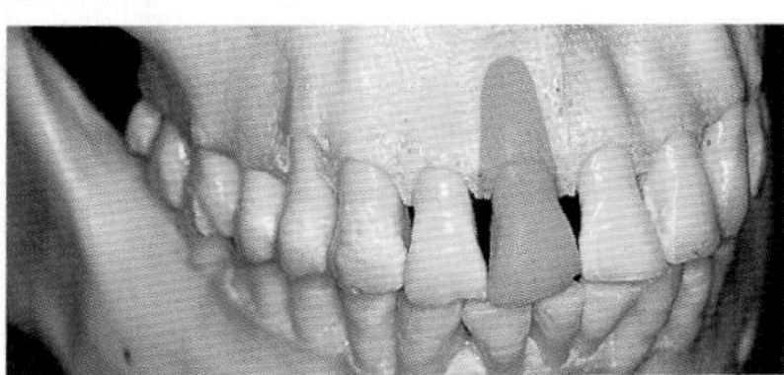

FIGURE 34–29 ✦ Area anesthetized with a local infiltration of a maxillary central incisor. The deposition site is at the apical region of the target tooth.

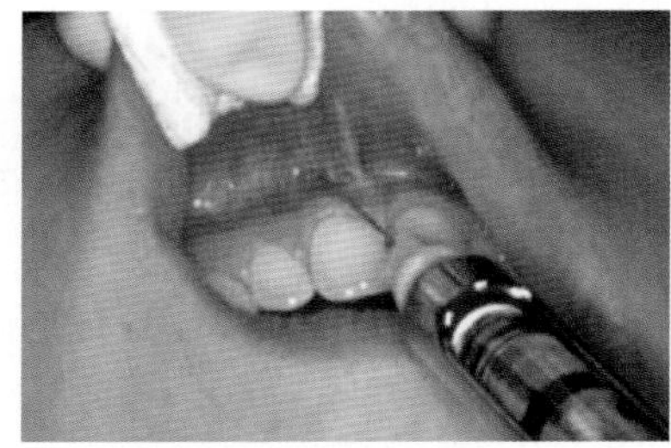

FIGURE 34–30 ✦ Penetration site for a supraperiosteal injection of the maxillary right central incisor.

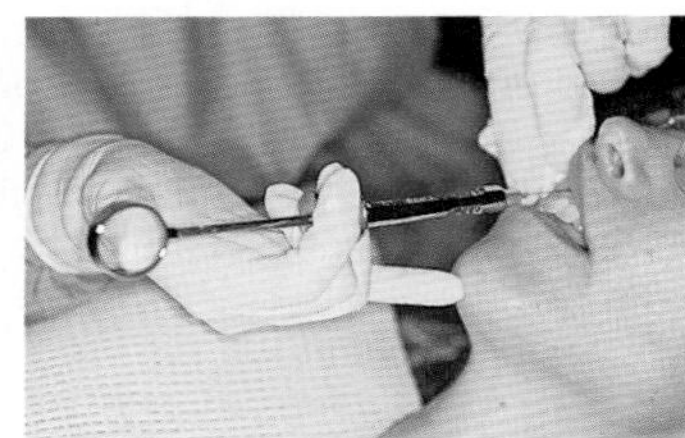

FIGURE 34–31 ✦ Syringe orientation and handrest for a local infiltration of the anterior maxilla.

Indications for this injection include the need for pulpal anesthesia of maxillary teeth when only a limited number of teeth are to be treated and for soft tissue procedures to be performed on a circumscribed area. Because the anesthetic and vasoconstrictor are deposited so near the area to be treated, this injection provides effective hemostasis, which is often needed during dental hygiene care. Conversely, if there is infection or severe inflammation in the area, administration of the anesthetic solution at a distance from the area of inflammation (i.e., nerve block) provides better and safer pain control because of the presence of more normal tissue conditions at the deposition site. Furthermore, if a large area involving several teeth needs to be treated, the supraperiosteal injection is not suitable because of the need for multiple needle insertions and the necessity of administering large volumes of anesthetic solution.

Table 34–11 summarizes the criteria pertinent to a supraperiosteal injection and provides tips for success. Procedure 34–4, Giving a Successful Injection, should be referred to for those procedures common to all intraoral injections to ensure comfort, safety, and success.

Anterior Superior Alveolar Field Block

The anterior superior alveolar nerve block (ASA) is recommended for management of pain when treatment is to be done only on the maxillary anterior teeth. Table 34–12 describes the criteria specific to the anterior superior alveolar nerve block.

Middle Superior Alveolar Field Block

The middle superior alveolar nerve block (MSA) is the injection of choice when treatment involves only the premolars or if the infraorbital nerve block fails to provide pain control distal to the maxillary canine. Research indicates that the MSA nerve is present in only 28% to 40% of the population, in which case this area is most often innervated by the ASA nerve.[18,20] Regardless of its pres-

TABLE 34–12 ANTERIOR SUPERIOR ALVEOLAR FIELD BLOCK (ASA)

Nerves anesthetized	Anterior superior alveolar
Areas anesthetized	Pulpal tissue of the following maxillary teeth unilaterally: Central incisor Lateral incisor Canine Facial periodontal tissues and bone of these same teeth (Figure 34–32)
Needle gauge/length	25- or 27-gauge short
Operator position	8 or 9 o'clock
Penetration site	Height of the mucobuccal fold just mesial to the canine (Figure 34–33)
Landmarks	Mucobuccal fold Canine and canine eminence
Syringe orientation	Parallel to the long axis of the canine (Figure 34–34)
Handrests	Client's chin Forefinger, or wrist of operator's opposite hand (Figure 34–26, *A* to *E*)
Deposition site	Apical region of the canine
Penetration depth	Usually only a few millimeters, no more than 5 mm or ¼ of a short needle
Amount of anesthetic to be deposited	0.6–0.9 ml, or ⅓ to ½ of a cartridge
Length of time to deposit	Approximately 30–60 seconds

Potential Problems	Technique Tips
Anesthetic deposition below apex of target tooth, resulting in insufficient pulpal anesthesia	Increase depth of penetration so the needle is at the apical region of the canine.
Needle too far from bone, and thus solution deposited into buccal tissue	Redirect needle closer to periosteum.
Pain on insertion with the needle against the periosteum	Withdraw the needle and reinsert farther away (laterally) from the periosteum.
Persistent sensitivity at mesial of central incisor due to cross innervation	Infiltrate contralateral central incisor.

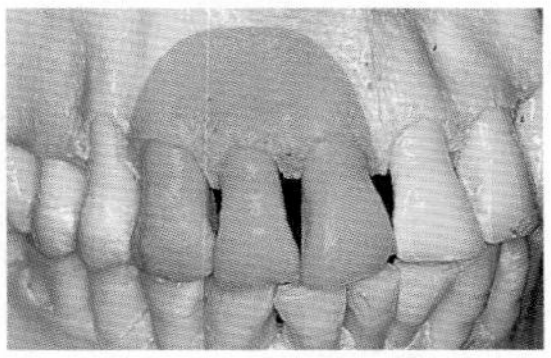

FIGURE 34–32 ✦ Area anesthetized with the anterior superior nerve block.

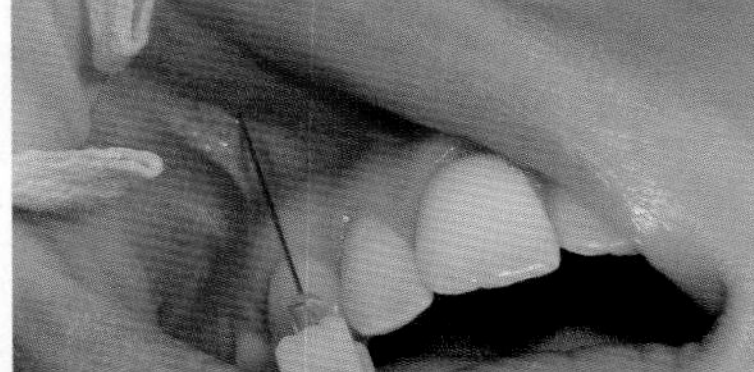

FIGURE 34–33 ✦ Penetration site for the anterior superior nerve block.

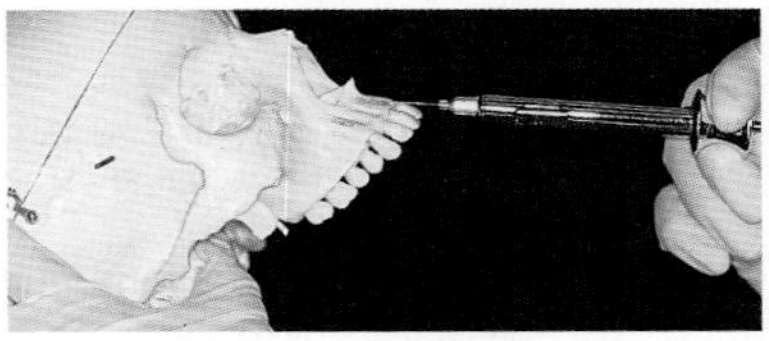

FIGURE 34–34 ✦ Syringe orientation for the anterior superior nerve block.

ence or absence, this area can be anesthetized easily by means of the MSA technique described in Table 34–13. This table provides the guidelines for administering an MSA nerve block and suggestions to ensure success.

Infraorbital Nerve Block

While the ASA (Table 34–12) and the MSA (Table 34–13) nerve blocks can be employed by oral healthcare professionals when they are anesthetizing the maxillary anterior and premolar teeth, the infraorbital nerve block is the injection of choice by many authorities when providing pain control to this area.[2,5] The infraorbital nerve block provides both pulpal and facial soft tissue anesthesia of the maxillary central incisor through the premolars in approximately 60% of individuals.[18] Thus one injection of 0.9 to 1.2 ml of solution provides pain control in a relatively large area, effectively minimizing needle penetrations and volume of solution administered. Despite these advantages, this injection is not used as often as indicated because many operators are fearful of injuring the client's eye. This fear, however, is unfounded, and when the appropriate procedures are followed, this injection is highly effective and safe. Table 34–14 describes the criteria applicable to the infraorbital nerve block and includes directions for locating the infraorbital foramen and directing the needle and anesthetic solution to the nerve.

Posterior Superior Alveolar Nerve Block

The posterior superior alveolar nerve block (PSA), employed to anesthetize the maxillary molars, is preferred to supraperiosteal (infiltration) injections because it minimizes both the number of injections required and the volume of anesthetic solution administered. Also, because the anesthetic solution is deposited into an area of soft tissue with no bony landmarks (hence no bone contact), it is a comfortable injection for the client. Complete pulpal anesthesia is obtained in the first, second, and third molars in at least 60% of persons.[18] Dissection studies reveal, however, that the MSA nerve, when present, may supply sensory innervation to the mesiobuccal root of the first molar, therefore necessitating either a supraperiosteal injection, an MSA nerve block, or an infraorbital nerve block to anesthetize the remainder of this tooth. Furthermore, if access is difficult or if the third molar is missing and treatment is limited to only the first and second molars, supraperiosteal injections may be substituted.

TABLE 34–13 MIDDLE SUPERIOR ALVEOLAR NERVE BLOCK (MSA)

Nerves anesthetized	Middle superior alveolar
Areas anesthetized	Pulpal tissue of the following maxillary teeth unilaterally: First premolar Second premolar Mesial root of first molar Buccal periodontal tissues and bone of these same teeth (Figure 34–35)
Needle gauge/length	25- or 27-gauge short
Operator position	8 or 9 o'clock
Penetration site	Height of the mucobuccal fold above second premolar (Figure 34–36)
Landmarks	Mucobuccal fold Second premolar
Syringe orientation	Parallel to the long axis of the second premolar (closer to vertical than in the anterior maxilla) (Figure 34–37)
Handrests	Client's chin Client's cheek Forefinger, or wrist of operator's opposite hand (Figure 34–26)
Deposition site	Above the apical region of the second premolar
Penetration depth	Usually only a few millimeters, no more than 5 mm or ¼ of a short needle
Amount of anesthetic to be deposited	0.9–1.2 ml, or ½ to ⅔ of a cartridge
Length of time to deposit	Approximately 60–90 seconds

Potential Problems	Technique Tips
Anesthetic deposition below apex of target tooth, resulting in insufficient pulpal anesthesia	Increase depth of penetration so the needle is at the apical region of the second premolar.
Needle too far from bone, and thus solution deposited into buccal tissue	Redirect needle closer to periosteum.
Pain on insertion with the needle against the periosteum	Withdraw the needle and reinsert farther away (laterally) from the periosteum.
Dense bone of the zygomatic arch at the injection site prevents diffusion of anesthetic solution	Administer an infraorbital block instead of the MSA.
Buccal frenum present at preferred penetration site	Penetrate slightly mesial to the frenum.

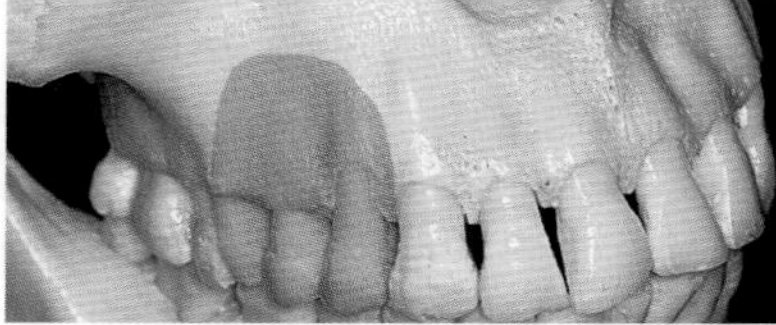

FIGURE 34–35 ✦ Area anesthetized by a middle superior alveolar nerve block.

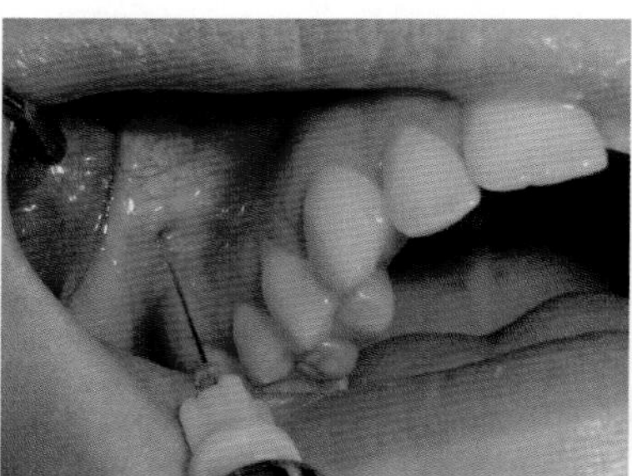

FIGURE 34–36 ✦ Penetration site for a middle superior alveolar nerve block.

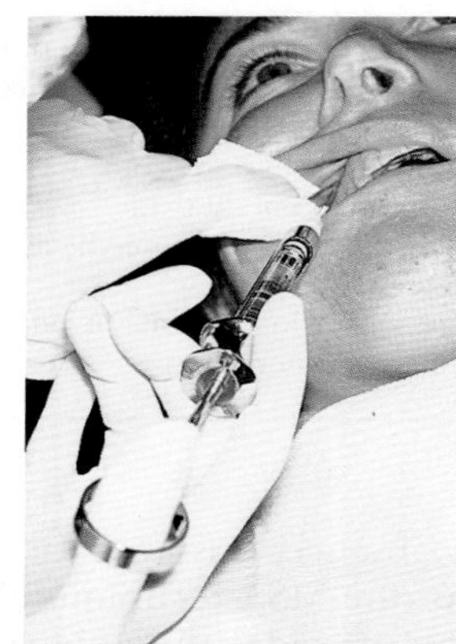

FIGURE 34–37 ✦ For a middle superior alveolar nerve block, the syringe is lined up parallel to the long axis of the maxillary second premolar.

Other considerations are safety and needle length. A long 25-gauge needle is often recommended for this injection. Problems associated with needle length, however, may result in an increased risk of hematoma formation. There are no anatomic safety features to prevent inadvertently inserting the needle too far posteriorly into the pterygoid plexus of veins and the facial artery, thereby causing a hematoma. Therefore, to minimize the risk of hematoma formation following the PSA nerve block, a short 25- or 27-gauge needle is recommended. Although depth of insertion with the long needle is 16 mm, or one-half of its length, the short needle is inserted three-fourths of its length. Thus the risk of overinsertion and hematoma formation decreases when using a short needle. Regardless of the needle length used, multiple aspirations and slow anesthetic deposition are imperative to ensure a safe injection.

Table 34–15 provides the essential criteria for a PSA nerve block. Of particular significance to this injection is the syringe orientation of 45 degrees to the maxillary occlusal plane and 45 degrees to the midsagittal plane. This angulation, maintained throughout the injection, advances the needle around the maxillary tuberosity to reach the deposition site.

INJECTION TECHNIQUES FOR THE PALATAL HARD AND SOFT TISSUES

When dental hygiene care involves the hard and soft tissues of the palate, such as during therapeutic scaling,

TABLE 34–14 INFRAORBITAL NERVE BLOCK (IO)

Nerves anesthetized	Infraorbital Anterior superior alveolar Middle superior alveolar Inferior palpebral Lateral nasal Superior labial
Areas anesthetized	Pulpal tissue of the following maxillary teeth unilaterally: Central incisor Lateral incisor Canine First premolar Second premolar Mesial root of first molar Buccal periodontal tissues and bone of these same teeth Lower eyelid Lateral aspect of the nose Upper lip (Figure 34–38)
Needle gauge/length	25- or 27-gauge short (in rare instances a long needle may be preferred)
Operator position	8 or 9 o'clock
Penetration site	Height of the mucobuccal fold above first premolar (Figure 34–39)
Landmarks	Infraorbital notch Infraorbital ridge Infraorbital foramen Mucobuccal fold First premolar (Figure 34–40, *A*)
Syringe orientation	Parallel to the long axis of the first premolar, follow the angle of the maxilla to the infraorbital foramen (Figure 34–41)
Handrests	Client's chin Client's cheek Forefinger, or wrist of operator's opposite hand (Figure 34–26)
Deposition site	Upper rim of the infraorbital foramen, the needle should gently contact bone prior to deposition (Figure 34–42)
Penetration depth	16 mm or ¾ of a short needle
Amount of anesthetic to be deposited	0.9–1.2 ml, or ½ to ⅔ of a cartridge
Length of time to deposit	Approximately 60–90 seconds

Technique Notes

1. Locate the infraorbital foramen: With your forefinger, palpate across the zygomatic arch; the foramen lies at the area of concavity directly below the medial border of the client's iris when the client gazes straight ahead (Figure 34–40, *A* and *B*).
2. Maintain finger pressure over the foramen throughout the injection and for 1 to 2 minutes after deposition. This will aid in directing the needle to the foramen and assist in directing the anesthetic solution to the foramen (Figure 34–41).

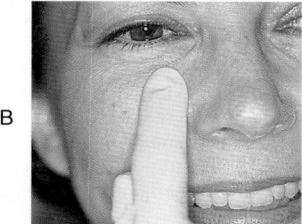

Potential Problems	Technique Tips
Needle contacting bone below the infraorbital foramen; anesthesia of the lower eyelid, nose, or upper lip with little or no pulpal anesthesia	Keep needle in line with the infraorbital foramen during penetration; line the syringe up with your finger over the foramen.

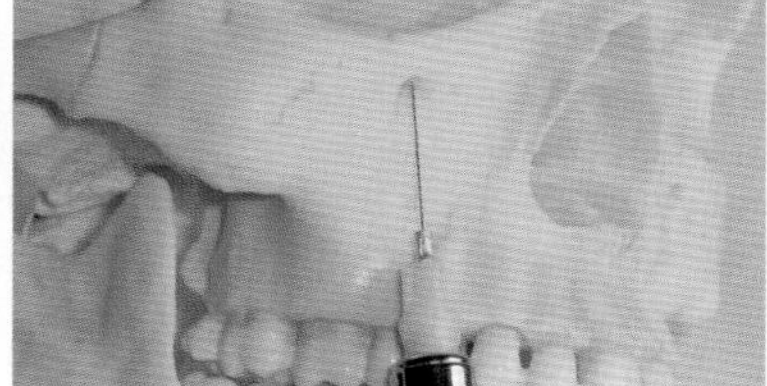

FIGURE 34–42 ✦ Position of the needle tip before deposition of local anesthetic at the infraorbital foramen.

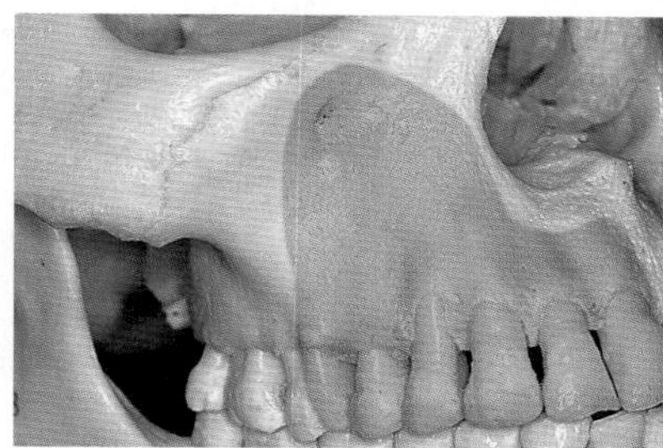

FIGURE 34–38 ✦ Area anesthetized by an infraorbital nerve block in approximately 60% of individuals.

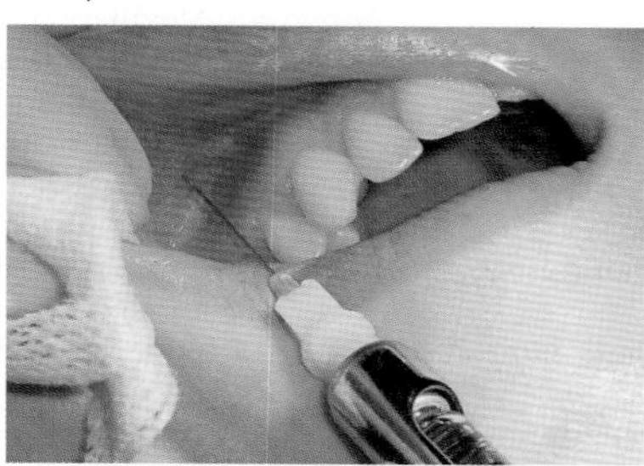

FIGURE 34–39 ✦ Penetration site for the infraorbital nerve block.

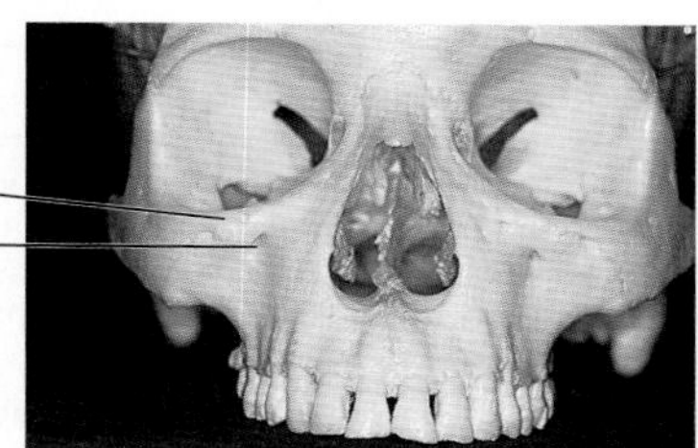

FIGURE 34–40 ✦ **A,** Location of the infraorbital notch and infraorbital foramen. **B,** Palpate to locate the infraorbital notch and foramen.

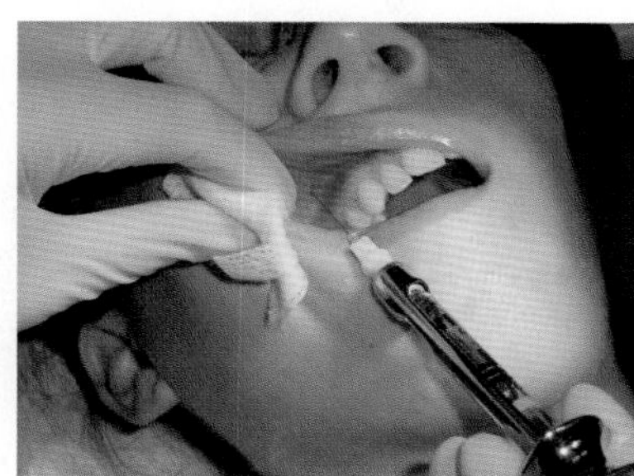

FIGURE 34–41 ✦ Syringe orientation for the infraorbital nerve block. During the injection, keep a finger over the infraorbital foramen while retracting the lip.

TABLE 34–15 POSTERIOR SUPERIOR ALVEOLAR NERVE BLOCK (PSA)

Nerves anesthetized	Posterior superior alveolar
Areas anesthetized	Pulpal tissue of the following maxillary teeth unilaterally: Third molar Second molar Distal buccal and palatal root of first molar (in 60% of clients the first molar is entirely anesthetized) Buccal periodontal tissues and bone of these same teeth (Figure 34–43)
Needle gauge/length	25- or 27-gauge short (in rare instances a long needle may be preferred)
Operator position	8 or 9 o'clock
Penetration site	Height of the mucobuccal fold posterior and superior to the last molar present (Figure 34–44)
Landmarks	Mucobuccal fold Maxillary tuberosity Maxillary occlusal plane Midsagittal plane Maxillary molars
Syringe orientation	45 degrees to the maxillary occlusal plane and 45 degrees to the midsagittal plane (Figure 34–45)
Handrests	Forefinger, or thumb of opposite hand as it retracts client's buccal tissue (Figure 34–26, *F* and *G*)
Deposition site	Posterior and superior to the posterior border of the maxilla at the PSA nerve foramina (Figure 34–46)
Penetration depth	16 mm or ¾ of a short needle
Amount of anesthetic to be deposited	0.9–1.8 ml, or ½ to 1 cartridge
Length of time to deposit	Approximately 60–120 seconds

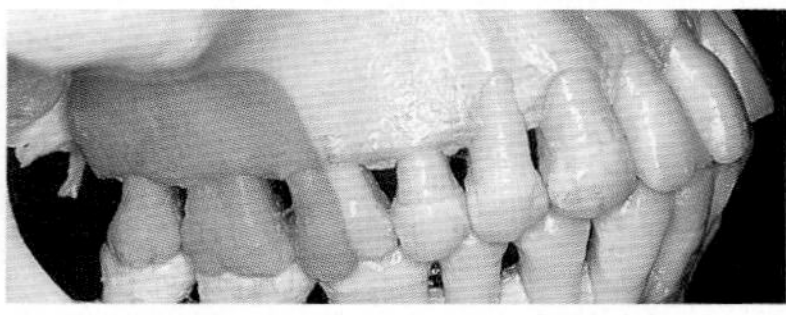

FIGURE 34–43 ✦ Area anesthetized with the posterior superior alveolar nerve block.

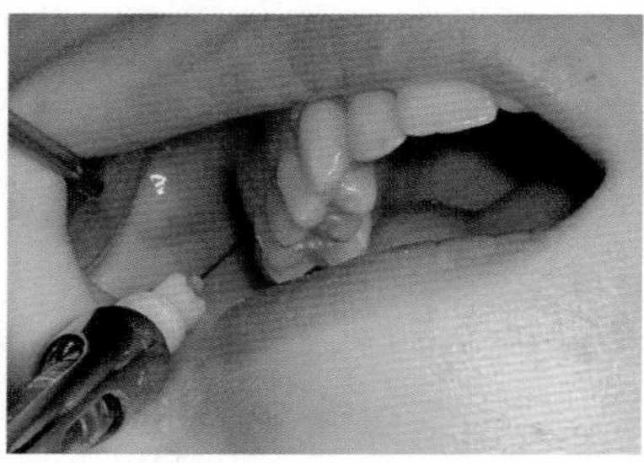

FIGURE 34–44 ✦ Penetration site for the posterior superior alveolar nerve block.

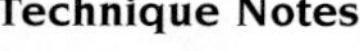

Technique Notes

1. Due to the high vascularity of the deposition site for the PSA, a triple aspiration is recommended to ensure that the needle bevel is not against the interior wall of a vessel, thus providing a false-negative aspiration (Figure 34–28). To aspirate in multiple planes, perform a single aspiration as usual, then rotate the body of the syringe toward you slightly, reaspirate, then rotate the body of the syringe back to the original position and perform a final aspiration. If all three aspiration tests are negative, it is safe to administer the anesthetic solution.

Potential Problems	Technique Tips
Bone is contacted when the angle of needle is too great in regard to the midsagittal plane	Withdraw the needle and bring the syringe closer to the midline.
Mandibular anesthesia: The mandibular division of the trigeminal is lateral to the PSA nerves	Review landmarks and syringe orientation so as not to deposit lateral to the PSA nerves.

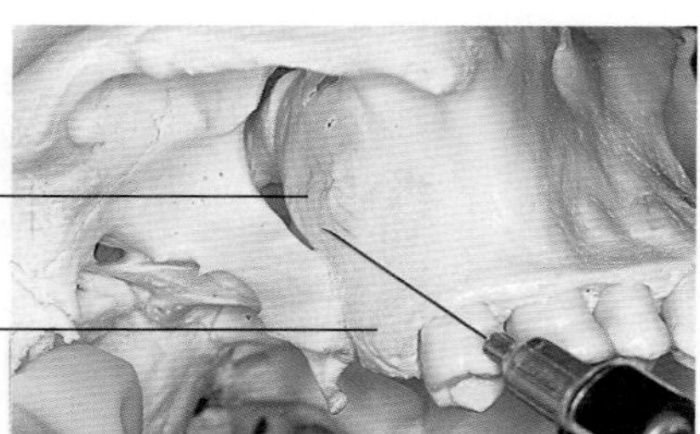

FIGURE 34–46 ✦ Deposition site for the posterior superior alveolar nerve block.

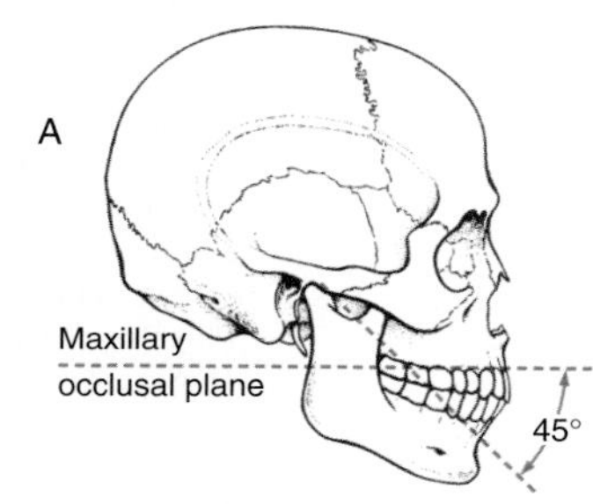

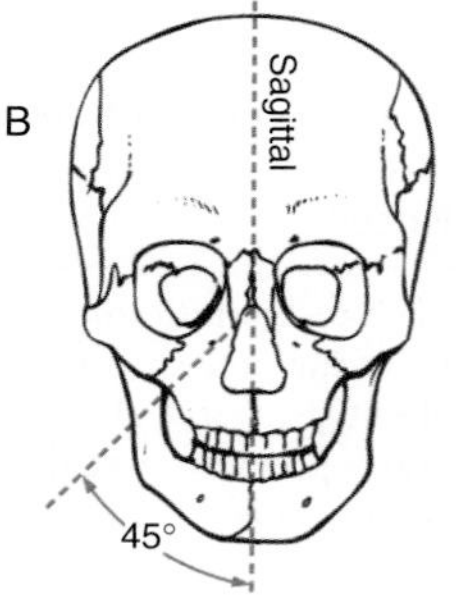

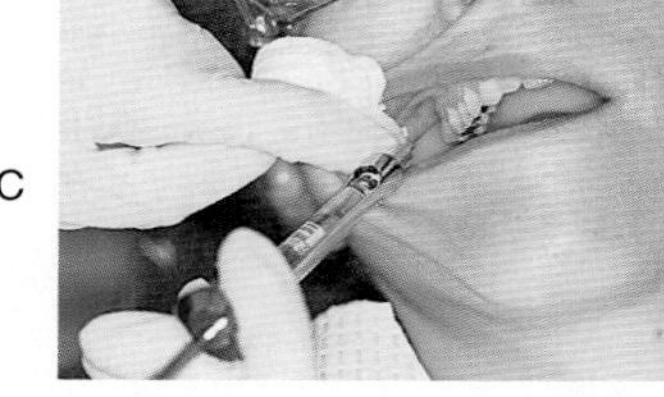

FIGURE 34–45 ✦ **A,** Forty-five degrees to the maxillary occlusal plane. **B,** Forty-five degrees to the midsagittal plane. **C,** Orientation of syringe during a posterior superior alveolar nerve block.

root planing, and soft tissue curettage procedures, anesthesia of the palatal tissue may be needed. Unfortunately, for many clients these injections are traumatic, but palatal injections need not be painful if appropriate techniques are followed. Especially important to facilitate comfort during palatal injections are the following tasks:

- Provide pressure anesthesia with a cotton swab at the penetration site both before and during the injection because topical anesthetics have limited value on keratinized tissues such as the palate.
- Deposit the solution slowly to avoid tearing the palatal tissue, which is dense and firmly attached to the bone.
- Be confident that you, the dental hygienist, will administer the injection with minimal discomfort to the client.
- Utilize a triple injection technique whenever possible when administering the nasopalatine nerve block to minimize client discomfort (this technique is described in the following discussion of the nasopalatine nerve block.)

Injection techniques used to anesthetize the palatal hard and soft tissues are the greater palatine nerve block and the nasopalatine nerve block.

Greater Palatine Nerve Block

The greater palatine nerve block is used to anesthetize the hard and soft palatal tissues overlying the molars and premolars; no pulpal anesthesia is obtained. This nerve block provides anesthesia to a large area, thereby minimizing the number of needle penetrations and total amount of anesthetic solution needed; however, the greater palatine nerve can be blocked at any point after it emerges from the foramen and passes anteriorly between the hard and soft tissues. As a result, anesthesia

TABLE 34–16 GREATER PALATINE NERVE BLOCK (ANTERIOR PALATINE) (GP)

Nerves anesthetized	Greater palatine
Areas anesthetized	Hard palate and overlying soft tissue unilaterally from the maxillary third molar to the first premolar (Figure 34–47)
Needle gauge/length	25- or 27-gauge short
Operator position	8 or 9 o'clock
Penetration site:	Just anterior to the greater palatine foramen (Figure 34–48)
Landmarks	Greater palatine foramen Junction of alveolar process and palatine bone Maxillary second molar
Syringe orientation	Approaches from opposite the side being injected with the needle at a right angle to the penetration site (Figure 34–48)
Handrests	Back of opposite hand Corner of client's mouth (Figure 34–26, *H* and *I*)
Deposition site	Just anterior to the greater palatine nerve foramen
Penetration depth	3 to 6 mm, often only the bevel is inserted
Amount of anesthetic to be deposited	0.45 ml, or ¼ cartridge; determine by development of blanching of palatal tissues
Length of time to deposit	Approximately 20–30 seconds

Technique Notes

1. To locate the greater palatine foramen, palpate the posterior palate with a cotton-tipped applicator or your forefinger at the junction of the hard palate and the alveolar process near the second molar until a depression is felt.
2. Topical anesthetics have very limited action on keratinized tissue such as the palate. To ensure client comfort, pressure anesthesia with a cotton-tipped applicator is recommended for a minimum of 1 minute before injection and throughout deposition (Figure 34–49).

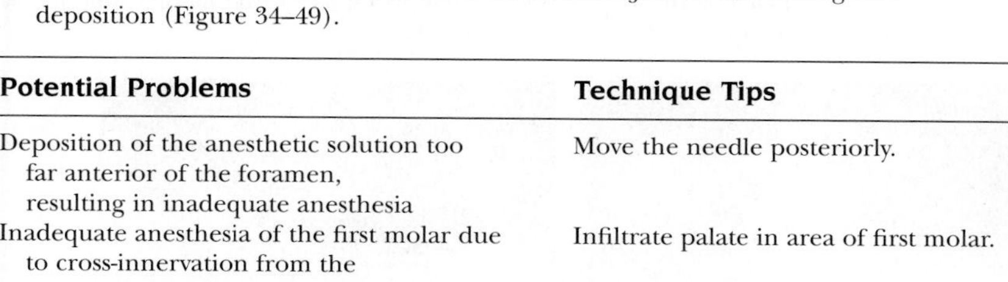

Potential Problems	Technique Tips
Deposition of the anesthetic solution too far anterior of the foramen, resulting in inadequate anesthesia	Move the needle posteriorly.
Inadequate anesthesia of the first molar due to cross-innervation from the nasopalatine nerve	Infiltrate palate in area of first molar.

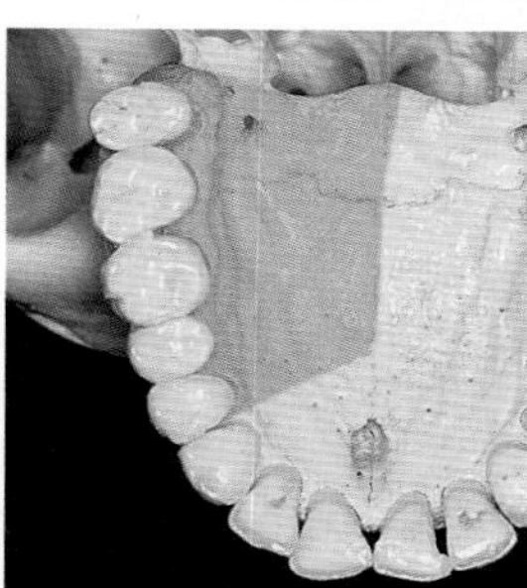

FIGURE 34–47 ✦ Area anesthetized with the greater palatine nerve block.

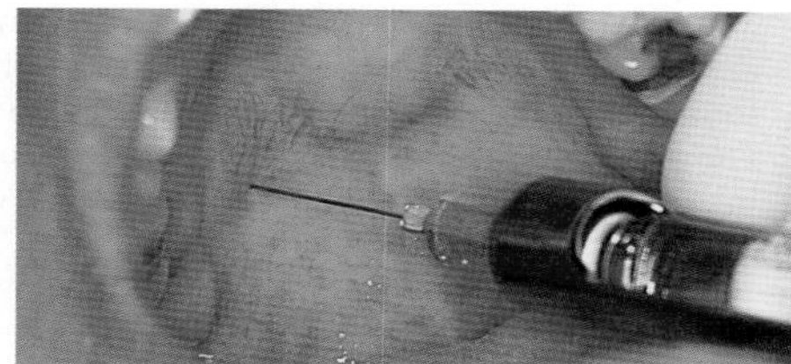

FIGURE 34–48 ✦ Syringe orientation and penetration site for a greater palatine nerve block.

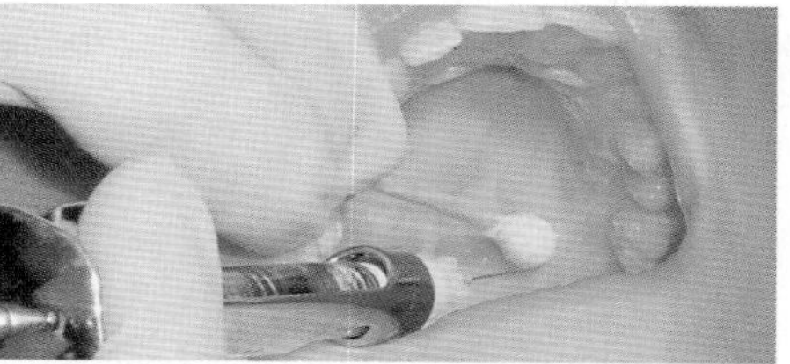

FIGURE 34–49 ✦ Pressure anesthesia applied with a cotton-tipped applicator to increase client comfort during the greater palatine nerve block.

is obtained only anterior to the site of the injection. For example, if treatment is limited to the first molar and premolars, the injection site should be slightly posterior to the first molar along the greater palatine nerve path. This practice ensures that the areas to be treated are anesthetized, but the posterior region of the palate is not unnecessarily anesthetized.

Table 34–16 provides the criteria pertinent for the administration of a greater palatine nerve block and includes suggestions for locating the greater palatine foramen and maximizing client comfort.

Nasopalatine Nerve Block

The nasopalatine nerve block anesthetizes the palatal hard and soft tissues from the mesial aspect of the right premolar to the mesial aspect of the left premolar. As with the greater palatine nerve block, a minimal number of needle penetrations and a small amount of anesthetic solution are needed to anesthetize a wide area. Because the soft tissue is dense, firmly attached to the bone, and very sensitive, however, this nerve block is potentially the most painful of all the injections unless the protocol for an atraumatic injection is closely followed.

Two techniques are available when giving this injection. The first involves only one needle penetration on the lateral side of the incisive papilla. The second technique includes giving three sequential injections, one between the maxillary central incisors followed by a second penetration into the papilla between these same teeth. In some cases these two injections provide suffi-

TABLE 34–17 NASOPALATINE NERVE BLOCK (NP)

Nerves anesthetized	Nasopalatine
Areas anesthetized	Hard palate and overlying soft tissue bilaterally from the maxillary canine to canine (Figure 34–50)
Needle gauge/length	25- or 27-gauge short
Operator position	8 or 9 o'clock
Penetration site	Just lateral to posterior portion of the incisive papilla (Figure 34–51)
Landmarks	Central incisors Incisive papilla
Syringe orientation	Approaches from canine/premolar region at a 45-degree angle to the incisive papilla (Figure 34–51)
Handrests	Finger of opposite hand Syringe can be stabilized against the corner of the client's mouth (Figure 34–26, *J*)
Deposition site	Incisive foramen, beneath incisive papilla
Penetration depth	3 to 6 mm, often only the bevel is inserted
Amount of anesthetic to be deposited	0.45 ml, or ¼ cartridge; determine by development of blanching of palatal tissues
Length of time to deposit	Approximately 20–30 seconds

Technique Notes

1. Topical anesthetics have very limited action on keratinized tissue such as the palate. To ensure client comfort, pressure anesthesia with a cotton-tipped applicator is recommended for a minimum of 1 minute before injection and throughout deposition (Figure 34–52).
2. For greatest client comfort, the nasopalatine nerve block is best administered in a triple injection sequence as follows: infiltration of a central incisor, papillary infiltration of tooth numbers 8 and 9, and then the nasopalatine. Each injection anesthetizes the area of the subsequent injection, resulting in an atraumatic procedure for the client (Figure 34–53).

Potential Problems	Technique Tips
Unilateral anesthesia due to deposition of anesthetic solution to one side of incisive foramen	Reinsert the needle until it is directly over the incisive foramen.
Inadequate anesthesia of canine or first premolar due to cross-innervation from the greater palatine nerve	Infiltrate the palate at the area of the canine or first premolar.

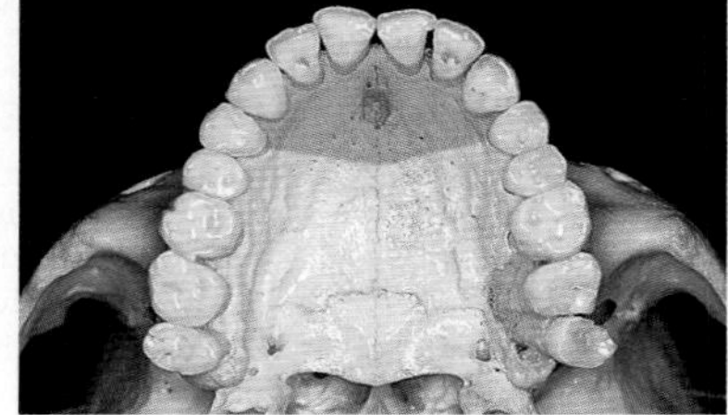

FIGURE 34–50 ✦ Area anesthetized with the nasopalatine nerve block.

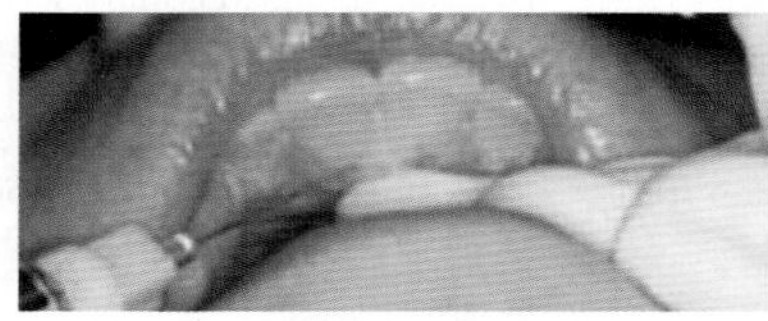

FIGURE 34–51 ✦ Syringe orientation and penetration site for the nasopalatine nerve block.

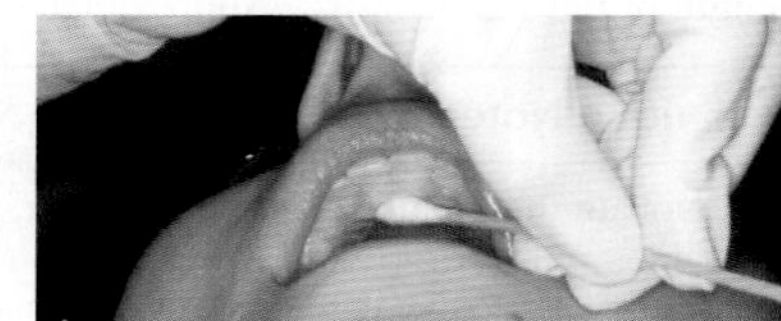

FIGURE 34–52 ✦ Pressure anesthesia with a cotton-tipped applicator to increase client comfort for the nasopalatine nerve block.

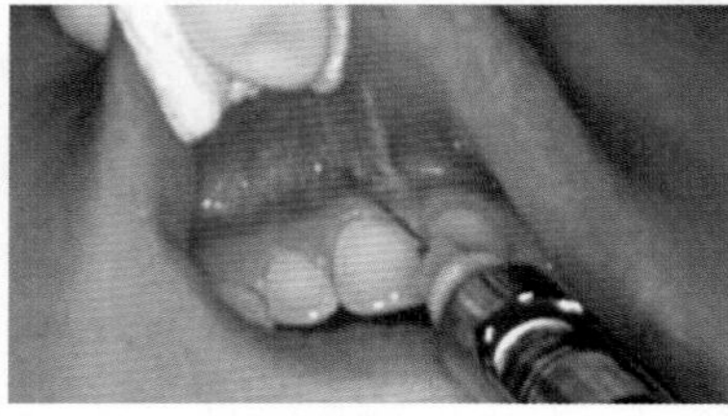

A

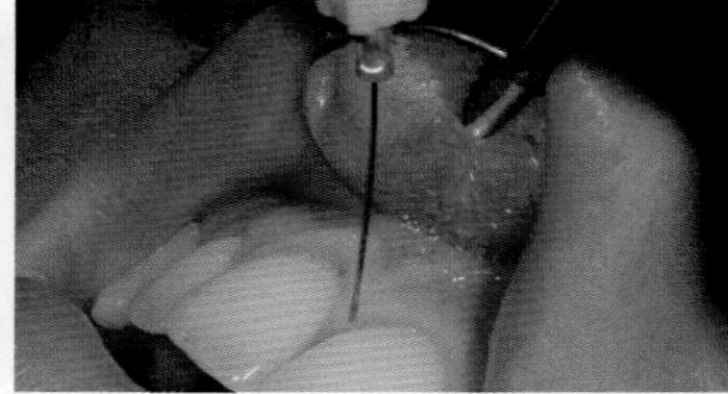

B

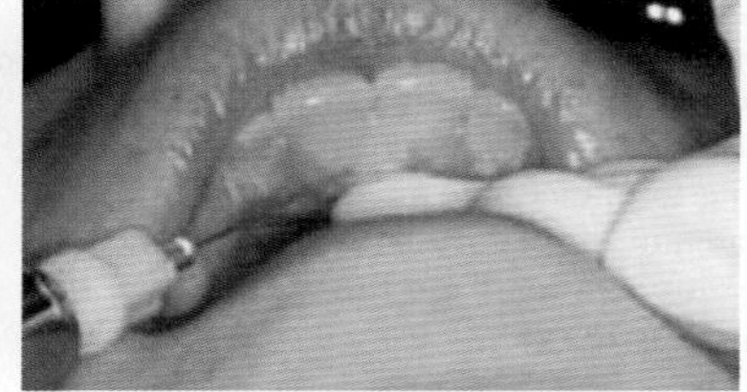

C

FIGURE 34–53 ✦ Triple injection technique for the nasopalatine nerve block. **A,** First injection infiltration of the central incisor, or labial frenum. **B,** Second injection into interdental papilla of centrals. **C,** Third injection at incisive papilla (traditional nasopalatine injection.)

cient pain control for dental hygiene care. If not, an injection is made into the partially anesthetized palatal tissues on the lateral side of the incisive papilla to complete the nasopalatine nerve block. Each approach is acceptable, and dental hygienists should select the procedure they feel most comfortable with and that provides the most atraumatic injection possible for the client (Table 34–17).

INJECTION TECHNIQUES FOR THE MANDIBULAR TEETH AND HARD AND SOFT TISSUES

The dense bone of the mandible that covers the apices of the teeth eliminates the possibility of supraperiosteal injections into the posterior teeth. In addition, because of mandibular bone density, anesthetic solution must be deposited within 1 mm of the target nerve to obtain pulpal anesthesia.

The injection techniques available to anesthetize the mandibular teeth and hard and soft tissues include the inferior alveolar, lingual, buccal, mental, and incisive nerve blocks. Of these, only the inferior alveolar and incisive nerve blocks obtain pulpal anesthesia.

Inferior Alveolar Nerve Block and Lingual Nerve Block

The inferior alveolar and lingual nerve blocks are often employed when dental hygiene care involves the mandible. The biggest advantage is that one penetration anesthetizes the entire quadrant, with the exception of the facial soft tissue over the molars. The disadvantages, however, are formidable, and the success rate of the inferior alveolar nerve block is considerably lower than that of many other injections. Reasons for lack of success are as follows:

- ✦ The anatomic variations with regard to the height of the mandibular foramen on the medial side of the ramus
- ✦ Accessory innervation by means of the mylohyoid nerve or a bifid inferior alveolar nerve
- ✦ The considerable depth of soft tissue penetration needed to reach the nerve

In addition, the inferior alveolar nerve block has the highest rate of positive aspiration of all the intraoral injections.[2] Table 34–18 describes the criteria essential

TABLE 34–18 INFERIOR ALVEOLAR AND LINGUAL NERVE BLOCK (IA/Li)

Nerves anesthetized	*IA:* Inferior alveolar Incisive Mental *Li:* Lingual
Areas anesthetized	*IA:* Mandibular teeth unilaterally to midline Body of mandible Inferior portion of the ramus Facial tissue anterior to the first molar Lower lip to midline *Li:* All lingual gingival tissue unilaterally to midline Anterior 2/3 of the tongue Floor of the mouth unilaterally (Figure 34–54)
Needle gauge/length	25- or 27-gauge long
Operator position	8 or 9 o'clock
Penetration site	Middle of the pterygomandibular triangle (formed by the pterygomandibular raphe medially and the internal oblique ridge laterally) at the height of the coronoid notch, 6–10 mm above the mandibular occlusal plane (Figure 34–55)
Landmarks	Anterior border of the ramus External oblique ridge Coronoid notch Internal oblique ridge Pterygomandibular raphe Pterygomandibular triangle Mandibular occlusal plane (Figure 34–56)
Syringe orientation	Approaches from contralateral premolar area, parallel to the occlusal plane (Figure 34–55)
Handrests	Small finger on client's chin (Figure 34–26)
Deposition site	*IA:* Superior to the mandibular foramen *Li:* Withdraw needle 1/2 way after deposition for IA

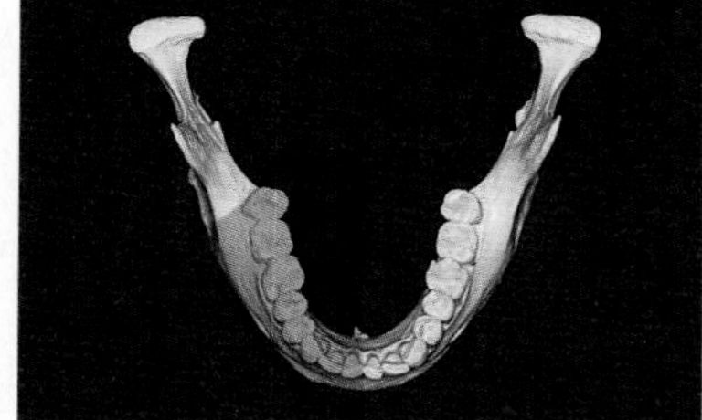

FIGURE 34–54 ✦ Area anesthetized with the inferior alveolar and lingual nerve blocks.

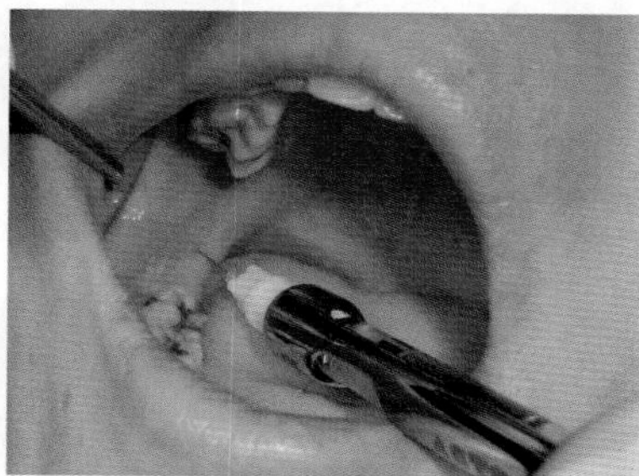

FIGURE 34–55 ✦ Syringe orientation and penetration site for the inferior alveolar and lingual nerve blocks; needle shown advanced to deposition site.

Table continued on following page

TABLE 34–18 INFERIOR ALVEOLAR AND LINGUAL NERVE BLOCK (IA/Li)—CONT'D

Penetration depth	*IA:* Until bone is gently contacted (Figure 34–57) Approximately 20–25 mm or ⅔ to ¾ of needle (withdraw 1 mm prior to deposition) *Li:* Withdraw needle ½ way after deposition for IA
Amount of anesthetic to be deposited	*IA:* 0.9–1.8 ml or ½ to 1 cartridge *Li:* 0.45 ml or ¼ cartridge
Length of time to deposit	*IA:* 60–120 seconds *Li:* 10–15 seconds

Technique Notes

1. To locate the pterygomandibular triangle, place your thumb or index finger on the greatest depression on the anterior border of the ramus; this is the coronoid notch. Roll your finger medially to locate the internal oblique ridge. The point of penetration is between the internal oblique ridge and the pterygomandibular raphe (in the pterygomandibular triangle), 6–10 mm above the mandibular occlusal plane (Figures 34–55 and 34–56, *B*). While inserting, advancing, and withdrawing the needle, it is important to place the thumb or index finger on the internal oblique ridge and at the same time grasp the posterior border of the mandible with the remainder of the hand. This technique provides stabilization and control in the event the client moves unexpectedly during the procedure.
2. Due to the high vascularity of the deposition site for the IA, a triple aspiration is recommended to ensure that the needle bevel is not against the interior wall of a vessel, thus providing a false-negative aspiration (Figure 34–58). To aspirate in multiple planes, perform a single aspiration as usual, then rotate the body of the syringe toward you slightly and reaspirate, then rotate the body of the syringe back to the original position and perform a final aspiration. If all three aspiration tests are negative, it is safe to administer the anesthetic solution.
3. If bone is contacted prematurely, before half of the needle length has entered the tissues, it is likely that the needle is too far anterior and has contacted the lingula, which covers the mandibular foramen (Figure 34–58, *A*). To correct: Withdraw the needle half-way, but do not remove from the tissues. Bring the body of the syringe over the mandibular anterior teeth and reinsert past the depth previously penetrated. Redirect the body of the syringe back over the contralateral premolars and continue to penetrate until bone is contacted (Figure 34–58, *B*).
4. If bone is not contacted and the penetration depth is nearing the hub of the needle, it is likely that the needle is too far posterior (Figure 34–59, *A*). To correct: Withdraw the needle half-way but do not remove it from the tissues. Redirect the syringe further over the contralateral molars and continue insertion until bone is contacted (Figure 34–59, *B*).

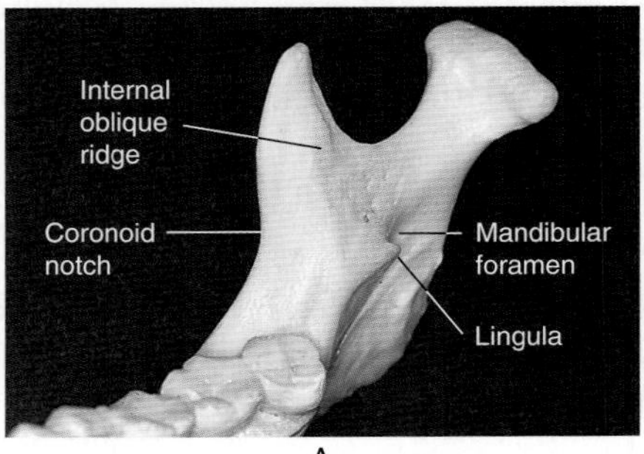

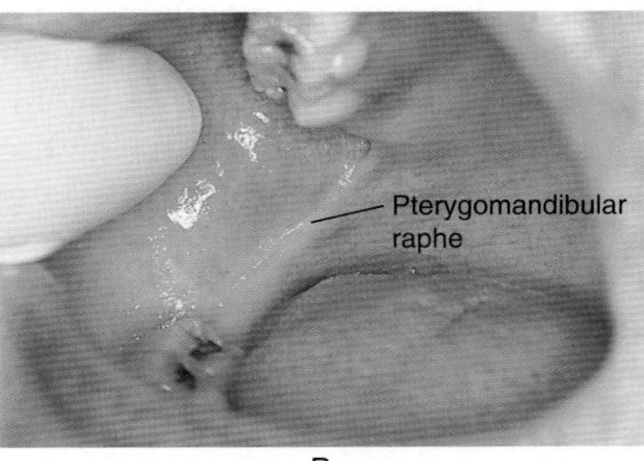

FIGURE 34–56 ✦ **A,** Landmarks on the mandible for the inferior alveolar and lingual nerve blocks. **B,** Intraoral landmarks, for inferior alveolar and lingual nerve blocks.

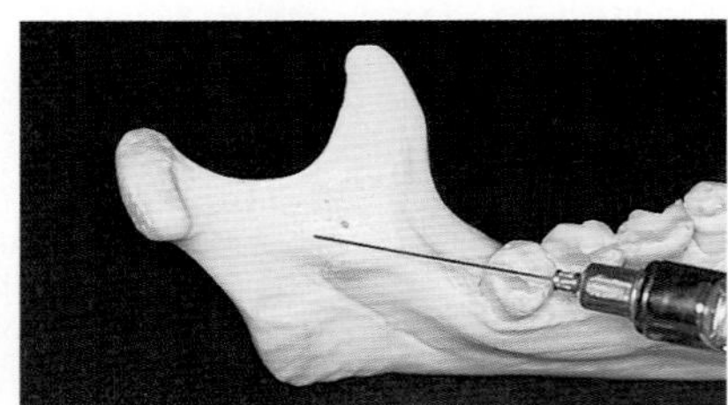

FIGURE 34–57 ✦ Deposition site for the inferior alveolar nerve block.

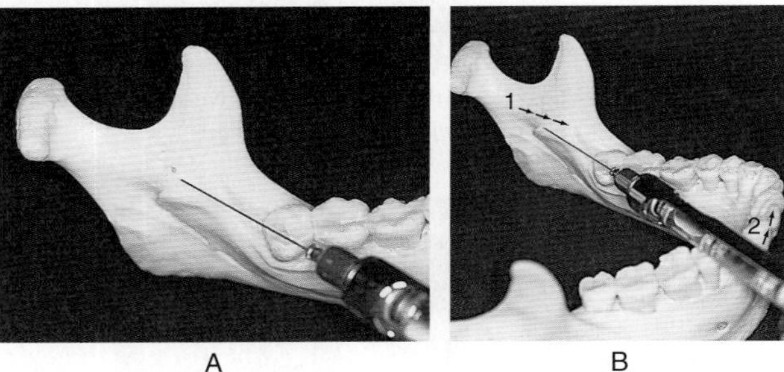

FIGURE 34–58 ✦ **A,** Premature bone contact on the lingula. **B,** Path of syringe orientation to correct for premature contact of bone.

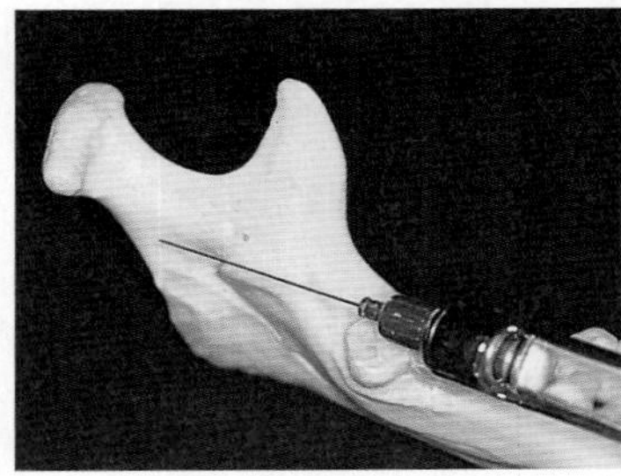

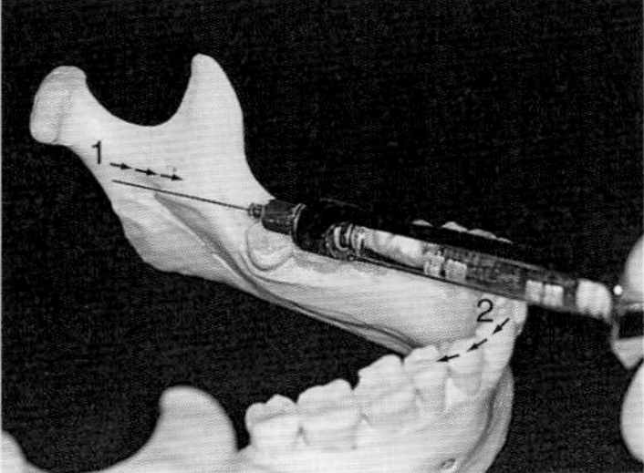

FIGURE 34–59 ✦ **A,** The needle is too far posterior, no bone is contacted. **B,** Path of syringe orientation to correct needle position.

TABLE 34–18 INFERIOR ALVEOLAR AND LINGUAL NERVE BLOCK (IA/Li)—CONT'D

Potential Problems	Technique Tips
Deposition of anesthesia below the mandibular foramen	Reinject at a higher penetration site.
Deposition of anesthetic too far anterior on the ramus, indicated early bone contact, with less than 1/2 the needle length inserted	See technique note 3.
Incomplete pulpal anesthesia of the molars (often mesial of the first molar) or premolars. Theorized that the mylohyoid nerve, which is not blocked by the IA, provides accessory innervation to these areas	Using a 27-gauge long needle, direct syringe from opposite corner of mouth and penetrate the apical region of the tooth just distal to the unanesthetized tooth. Advance 3–5 mm and deposit 0.6 ml or ⅓ of a cartridge over 20 seconds (Figure 34–60).
Incomplete anesthesia of the central or lateral incisors. May be due to cross-innervation from the opposite side inferior alveolar nerve	Using a 27-gauge short needle, infiltrate the mucobuccal fold and advance to the apical region of the unanesthetized tooth. Deposit 0.6 ml or ⅓ of a cartridge over 20 seconds (Figure 34–61).

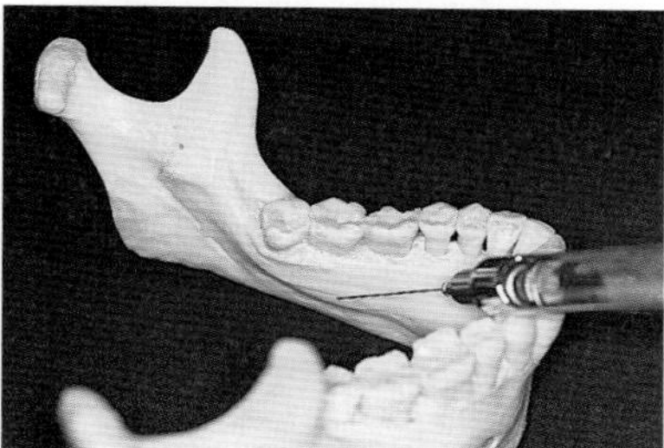

FIGURE 34–60 ✦ Direct the needle tip below the apical region of the tooth immediately posterior to the tooth in question.

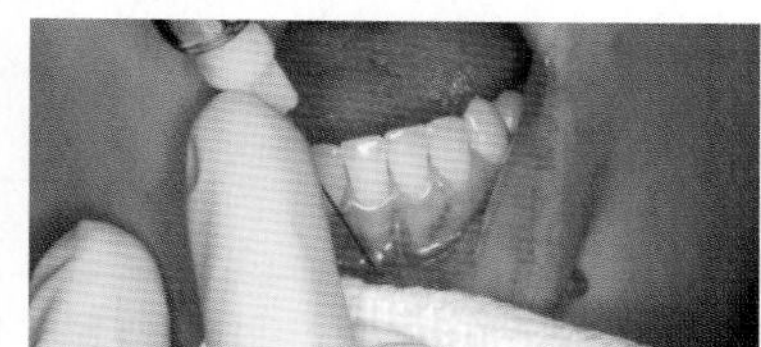

FIGURE 34–61 ✦ Local infiltration of the mandibular incisors.

for administering the inferior alveolar and lingual nerve blocks. It is important to carefully follow the guidelines regarding the landmarks for the penetration and deposition sites to ensure a successful injection and minimize or eliminate complications.

Appropriate care planning is important when anesthetizing the mandible. Bilateral inferior alveolar and lingual nerve blocks should be avoided. Such a procedure produces anesthesia of the client's entire tongue and lingual soft tissues, resulting in an inability to swallow and enunciate, and a lack of sensation. Thus anesthetizing the entire mandible has a high risk of client self-injury to the soft tissues and is not recommended. The optimal care plan is to anesthetize only the right side or only the left side at one appointment. Another alternative is to administer the inferior alveolar nerve block to that side, which requires the most treatment (particularly involving lingual tissue) or has the greatest number of teeth, and administer the incisive nerve block (Table 34–21) on the opposite side. Because the incisive nerve block does not provide pain control to the lingual tissues, a lingual infiltration may be given, if necessary.

In many instances the deliberate deposition of anesthetic solution to anesthetize the lingual nerve is unnecessary because solution deposited for the inferior alveolar nerve block diffuses and anesthetizes the lingual nerve; however, a separate technique for a lingual nerve block is described in Table 34–18 in the event that deliberate deposition of anesthetic solution is needed.

Buccal Nerve Block

The buccal nerve block provides pain control to the soft tissues buccal to the mandibular molars. This injection, along with the inferior alveolar and lingual nerve blocks, anesthetizes the entire quadrant in which it is given. If dental hygiene care involves manipulation of the buccal tissues of the molars, such as therapeutic scaling, root planing, and soft tissue curettage, this injection is indicated. If treatment does not include these tissues, however, the dental hygienist may simply forgo this injection. Unlike the other injections needed to anesthetize the mandible, the buccal nerve block is easy to administer and has a high success rate (Table 34–19).

Mental Nerve Block

At or near the apices of the premolars, the mental nerve exits the mental foramen and innervates the facial soft tissues anterior to the foramen, the lower lip, and the chin on the side of the injection. Because of the easy access of the anatomic landmarks, the mental nerve block is simple to administer, has a high success rate, and is usually atraumatic.

Although this injection has limited application in restorative dentistry, it may be used more commonly by dental hygienists doing gingival curettage in the anterior portion of the mandible. Because the mental nerve block does not provide pain control to the lingual tissues, a lingual infiltration may be needed.

Table 34–20 presents essential criteria for administration of the mental nerve block, including suggestions for locating the mental foramen.

TABLE 34–19 BUCCAL NERVE BLOCK (LB)

Nerves anesthetized	Buccal
Areas anesthetized	Soft tissues buccal to the mandibular molars unilaterally (Figure 34–62)
Needle gauge/length	25- or 27-gauge long
Operator position	8 or 9 o'clock
Penetration site	In the vestibule, distal and buccal to the most distal molar at the height of the occlusal plane (Figure 34–63)
Landmarks	Mandibular molars Buccal vestibule Mucobuccal fold
Syringe orientation	Parallel to the mandibular occlusal plane on the buccal side of the teeth (Figure 34–63)
Handrests	Client's cheek or chin Back of operator's opposite hand (Figure 34–26)
Deposition site	Buccal nerve as it passes over the anterior border of the ramus
Penetration depth	1 to 4 mm, often only the bevel is inserted
Amount of anesthetic to be deposited	0.3 to 0.45 ml, or ⅛ to ¼ cartridge
Length of time to deposit	Approximately 10–20 seconds

Technique Notes

1. The buccal nerve block can be administered immediately following the IA/Li. Thus the penetration sites can be prepared simultaneously with topical.

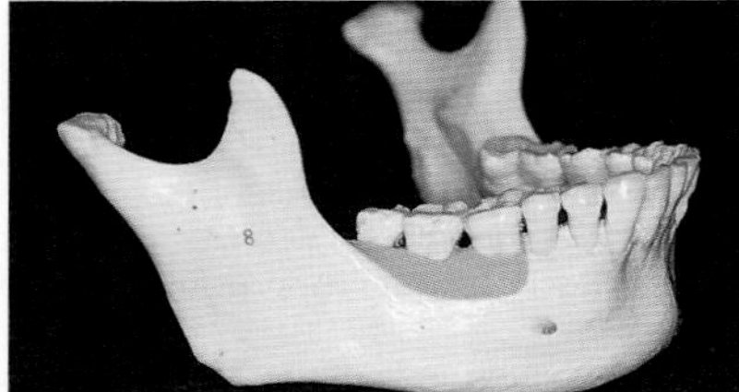

FIGURE 34–62 ✦ Area anesthetized with the buccal nerve block.

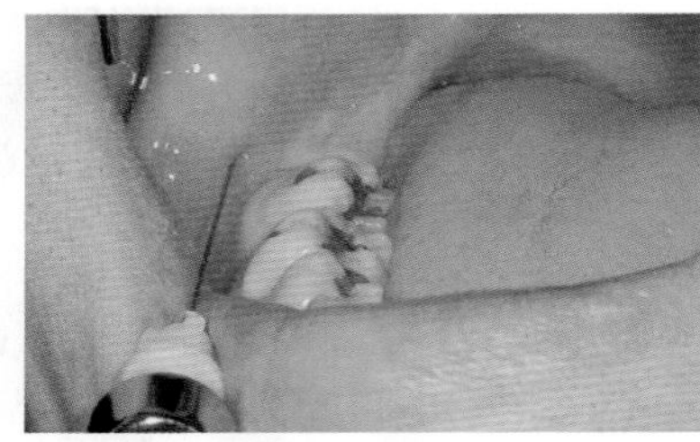

FIGURE 34–63 ✦ Syringe orientation and penetration site for the buccal nerve block.

TABLE 34–20 MENTAL NERVE BLOCK

Nerves anesthetized	Mental (terminal branch of inferior alveolar)
Areas anesthetized	Facial soft tissues unilaterally from the mental foramen anterior to midline Lower lip Skin of chin (Figure 34–64)
Needle gauge/length	25- or 27-gauge short
Operator position	8 or 9 o'clock or 11 or 1 o'clock
Penetration site	Mucobuccal fold directly over the mental foramen (Figure 34–65)
Landmarks	Mucobuccal fold Mandibular premolars Mental foramen
Syringe orientation	Directed toward the mental foramen
Handrests	Client's chin Back of operator's opposite hand or wrist (Figure 34–26)
Deposition site	Directly over the mental foramen, between the apices of the premolars
Penetration depth	5 to 6 mm, or 1/4 the needle length (do not enter the mental foramen)
Amount of anesthetic to be deposited	0.6 mL, or 1/3 of a cartridge
Length of time to deposit	Approximately 30–60 seconds

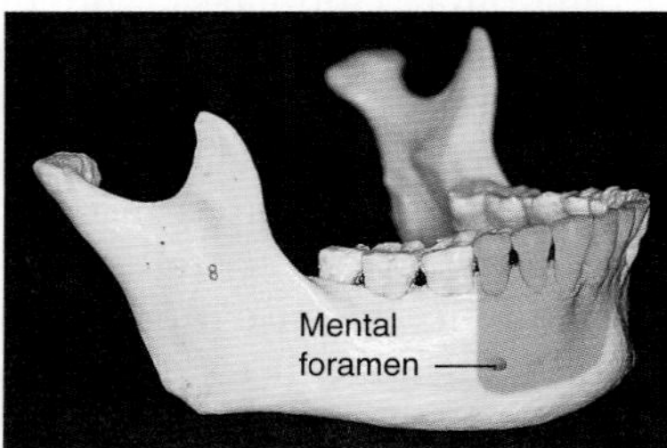

FIGURE 34–64 ✦ Area anesthetized with the mental nerve block.

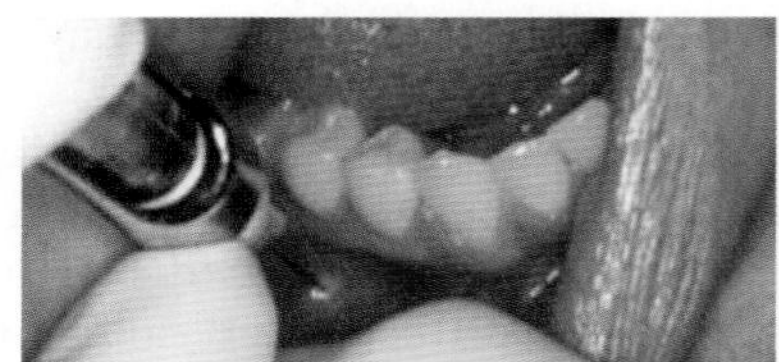

FIGURE 34–65 ✦ Penetration site for the mental and incisive nerve blocks.

TABLE 34–20 MENTAL NERVE BLOCK—CONT'D

Technique Notes

1. To locate the mental foramen, place your forefinger in the mucobuccal fold against the body of the mandible near the first molar. Palpate anteriorly until a depression is felt or the bone feels irregular. This is the mental foramen, which is most often found between the apices of the first and second premolars (Figure 34–66).
2. Use radiographs to assist you in finding the mental foramen (Figure 34–67).

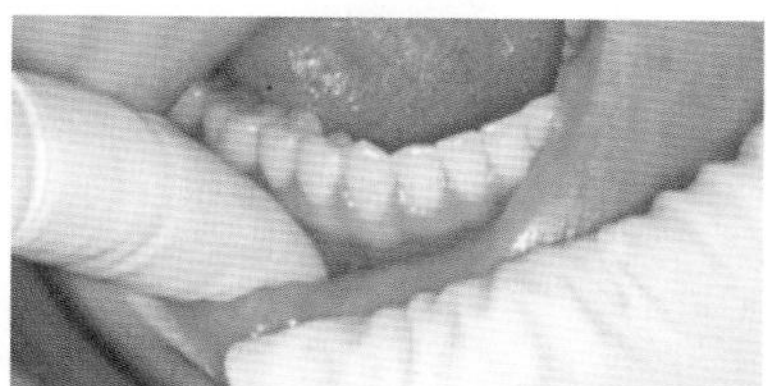

FIGURE 34–66 ✦ Locate the mental foramen by palpating the vestibule at the premolars.

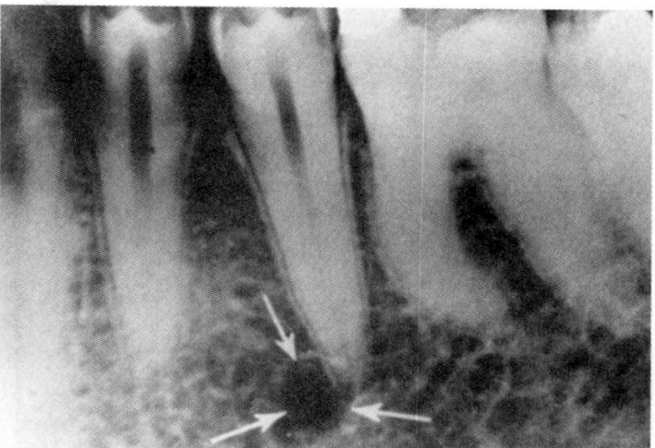

FIGURE 34–67 ✦ Radiographs can assist in locating the mental foramen.

Incisive Nerve Block

The incisive nerve originates at the mental foramen and innervates those teeth anterior to the foramen. As a terminal branch of the inferior alveolar nerve, the incisive nerve is anesthetized when an inferior alveolar nerve block is successfully given. The incisive nerve block, however, may be the injection of choice in several instances. Because bilateral inferior alveolar and lingual nerve blocks are contraindicated as a result of client discomfort, an alternative may be to administer the inferior alveolar and lingual nerve blocks to the side needing the most treatment or having the greatest number of teeth, and to administer the incisive nerve block on the other side. The incisive nerve block also may be used concurrently on both the right and left sides when dental hygiene care requires anesthesia on only the anterior portion of the mandible. An infiltration of the lingual tissues may be needed because this area is not anesthetized by the incisive nerve block.

Table 34–21 presents the criteria necessary for administration of the incisive nerve block and suggestions for locating the mental foramen. Although some authorities recommend penetrating the needle into the mental foramen to reach the incisive nerve, anesthesia can be obtained much more easily and safely by depositing the solution outside the foramen and using digital pressure over the site to direct the anesthetic into the foramen.[5]

LOCAL COMPLICATIONS

Despite careful preanesthetic client assessment and adherence to the recommended procedures for local anesthetic administration, the following local complications may develop.

Needle Breakage

The introduction of disposable stainless steel needles has significantly reduced the incidence of needle breakage; however, virtually all needle breaks are preventable. When breakage does occur, it is primarily caused by a sudden, unexpected movement by the client during needle insertion or by poor injection technique.[2] If a needle does break during insertion and can be retrieved without surgical intervention, no emergency exists. Those needles that are not retrieved most often remain in place and become encased by scar tissue. Leaving the needle in the tissue often produces fewer difficulties than the surgery required for its removal.

To prevent needle breakage:

- ✦ Inform the client about the local anesthetic procedure both before and during the injection. Effective communication helps the individual anticipate the dental hygienist's actions and control anxiety.
- ✦ Use long, large-gauge needles (e.g., 25-gauge) when penetrating significant tissue depth. These are less likely to break than smaller needles.
- ✦ Never bend the needle, because it weakens the metal.
- ✦ Advance the needle slowly. A forceful contact with bone may break the needle or may precipitate a quick movement by the client because of associated pain.
- ✦ Never force a needle against firm resistance such as bone.
- ✦ Do not change the direction of the needle while it is almost completely within the tissues. If it is necessary to redirect the needle, first withdraw almost completely out of the tissue and then modify the direction.
- ✦ A needle should not be inserted into the tissues all the way to the hub. This juncture at the needle shaft and hub is the weakest part of the needle and is vulnerable

TABLE 34–21 INCISIVE NERVE BLOCK

Nerves anesthetized	Incisive Mental (terminal branches of inferior alveolar)
Areas anesthetized	Mandibular second premolar to central incisor unilaterally Facial soft tissues unilaterally from the mental foramen anterior to midline Lower lip Skin of chin (Figure 34–68)
Needle gauge/length	25- or 27-gauge short
Operator position	8 or 9 o'clock or 11 or 1 o'clock
Penetration site	Mucobuccal fold directly over the mental foramen (Figure 34–65)
Landmarks	Mucobuccal fold Mandibular premolars Mental foramen
Syringe orientation	Directed toward the mental foramen
Handrests	Client's chin Back of operator's opposite hand or wrist (Figure 34–26)
Deposition site	Directly over the mental foramen, between the apices of the premolars
Penetration depth	5 to 6 mm, or ¼ the needle length (do not enter the mental foramen)
Amount of anesthetic to be deposited	0.6 to 0.9 ml, or ⅓ to ½ of a cartridge
Length of time to deposit	Approximately 30–60 seconds

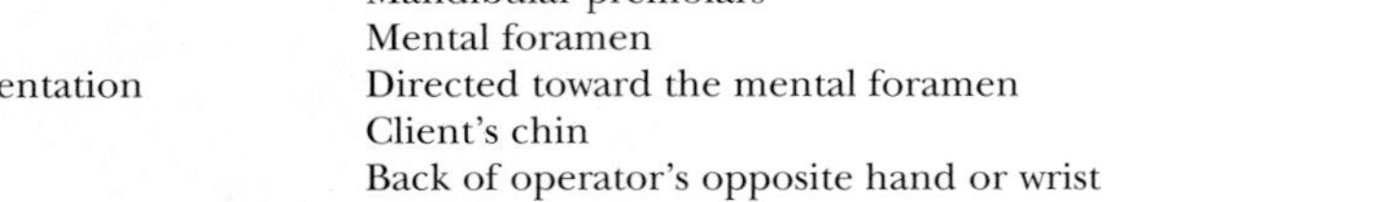

FIGURE 34–68 ✦ Area anesthetized with the incisive nerve block.

Technique Notes

1. The incisive nerve block is administered in the same manner as the mental, differing only in the application of pressure over the deposition site to direct the anesthetic solution into the mental foramen, resulting in pulpal anesthesia.
2. To locate the mental foramen, place your forefinger in the mucobuccal fold against the body of the mandible near the first molar. Palpate anteriorly until a depression is felt or the bone feels irregular. This is the mental foramen, which is most often found between the apices of the first and second premolars (Figure 34–66).
3. Use radiographs to assist you in finding the mental foramen (Figure 34–68).
4. Maintain pressure over the mental foramen with your finger for 1–2 minutes following the injection. This aids the flow of solution into the foramen, providing the pulpal anesthesia.

Potential Problems	Technique Tips
Incomplete anesthesia of the central or lateral incisors. May be due to cross-innervation from the opposite side inferior alveolar nerve	Using a 27-gauge short needle, infiltrate the mucobuccal fold and advance to the apical region of the unanesthetized tooth. Deposit 0.6 ml or ⅓ of a cartridge over 20 seconds (Figure 34–61).
Incomplete pulpal anesthesia	Redirect needle toward mental foramen and maintain pressure over the deposition site.

to breakage. If needle breakage occurs at this point, a portion of the shaft must be exposed in order for the needle to be retrieved without surgery.

When a needle breaks:

- ✦ Remain calm; do not panic.
- ✦ Instruct the client not to move. Do not remove your hand from the client's mouth and keep the client's mouth open. If possible, place a bite block in the client's mouth.
- ✦ If the needle fragment is protruding, attempt to remove it with cotton pliers or a hemostat.

If the needle is not visible and cannot be readily retrieved:

- ✦ Calmly inform the client; attempt to alleviate fears and apprehension.
- ✦ Refer the client to an oral and maxillofacial surgeon for consultation.
- ✦ Document the incident and the client's response in the client's chart. Keep the remaining needle fragment. Inform your insurance carrier immediately.

When a needle breaks, surgical removal should be considered:

- ✦ If it is superficial and easily located through radiologic and clinical examination, removal by an oral and maxillofacial surgeon is possible.
- ✦ If, despite the superficial location, retrieval is unsuccessful, it is prudent to abandon the attempt and allow the needle fragment to remain in the tissue.
- ✦ If the needle is located in deeper tissues or is difficult to locate, permit it to remain without an attempt at removal. There is considerable precedent to justify the retention of a broken needle if removal appears difficult.

Pain During the Injection

Pain during local anesthetic agent administration may be attributed to several factors: a careless injection technique and callous attitude toward the client; a dull needle from multiple injections; a barbed needle from hitting bone; or rapid deposition of the anesthetic solution. It is not possible to ensure that every injection is totally free from discomfort because the reactions of clients vary; however, the dental hygienist should take every precaution to prevent pain during the injection or prevent its recurrence.

To prevent pain during injection:

- Adhere to the proper techniques of administration as described in Procedure 34–4 and Tables 34–11 to 34–21.
- Deposit a few drops and then wait 5 seconds before advancing the needle 2 to 3 mm. Repeat the process until the deposition site is reached.
- Use sharp, disposable needles.
- Apply topical anesthetic before insertion of the needle.
- Use sterile anesthetic agents.
- Inject the anesthetic agent slowly.
- Store anesthetic solutions at room temperature and avoid using cartridge warmers.

Burning During the Injection

A burning sensation reported by the client during deposition of the local anesthetic agent may be caused by a local anesthetic with a vasopressor that is more acidic than the tissue in which it is deposited. The burning sensation, which lasts only a few seconds, disappears as anesthesia develops and is unapparent when the anesthesia fades. A more acute burning may occur, however, if the local anesthetic solution is contaminated from improper storage of the cartridge in a chemical disinfectant; if the cartridge is overheated in a cartridge warmer; if the expiration date of the solution has lapsed; or if the solution is deposited too rapidly, particularly on the palate. When burning occurs as a result of these factors, the tissue is damaged and subsequent postanesthetic trismus, edema, or possible paresthesia may develop.

To prevent burning during the injection:

- Store the cartridges in a dark place at room temperature in the original container. Avoid storing cartridges in chemical disinfectants or using cartridge warmers.
- Check the expiration date of each cartridge before usage. Anesthetic solution that has exceeded the expiration date should be discarded.
- Inject the anesthetic solution slowly.

Most often, burning during an injection is a temporary condition and needs no specific treatment.

Hematoma

A *hematoma* is a swelling and discoloration of the tissue resulting from the effusion of blood into the extravascular spaces (Figure 34–69). Hematomas occur subsequent to an inadvertent puncture of a blood vessel, particularly an artery, during local anesthetic administration. They appear most often after the administration of a posterior superior alveolar or inferior alveolar nerve block because the tissues associated with these injections are less dense and readily accommodate large volumes of blood. Bleeding continues until extravascular pressure exceeds intravascular pressure or until clotting occurs. A hematoma is less likely to develop after a palatal injection because of the density of the tissue in this area.

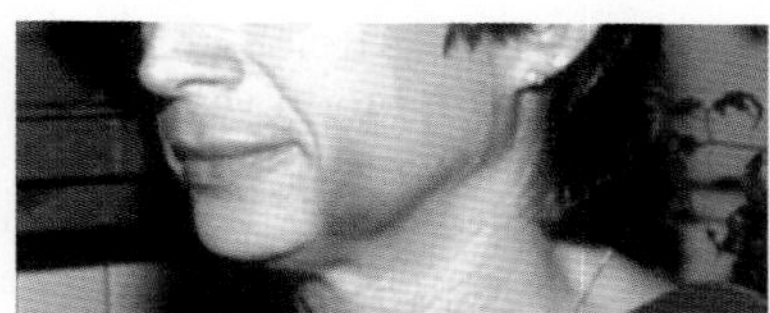

FIGURE 34–69 ✦ Hematoma resulting from administration of left mental block.

A hematoma that ensues following a posterior superior alveolar nerve block is the largest and most visible. The bleeding occurs in the infratemporal fossa, and swelling and discoloration appear on the side of the face. Clinical manifestations of a hematoma following an inferior alveolar nerve block include intraoral tissue discoloration and swelling on the lingual aspect of the ramus. Other than the bruise, which may or may not be visible extraorally, a hematoma may be accompanied by trismus and pain.

To prevent a hematoma:

- Be attentive to anatomic detail involved in each injection.
- Modify the injection technique as indicated by the client's anatomy. For example, the depth of needle penetration for a posterior superior alveolar nerve block may be shallower for a client with small anatomic features.
- Use a short needle for the posterior superior alveolar nerve block to minimize the risk of overinsertion and the potential for hematoma formation.
- Minimize the number of needle insertions.
- Observe the appropriate techniques for local anesthetic administration.

Management includes the following:

- If swelling appears, immediately apply direct pressure to the site of the bleeding for at least 2 minutes. For an inferior alveolar nerve block, the pressure point is the medial side of the ramus. For the mental or incisive nerve blocks, pressure is applied over the mental foramen. If hematoma formation follows an infraorbital nerve block, the pressure point is the skin over the infraorbital foramen. Unfortunately, it is difficult to apply pressure directly to the site of bleeding after a posterior superior alveolar nerve block because the vessels are located posterior, superior, and medial to the maxillary tuberosity. Pressure may be applied to the tissues of the mucofacial fold as far distally as the client can tolerate.

- Apply ice to the region when hematoma formation begins. Ice constricts the blood vessels, minimizes the size of the hematoma, and acts as an analgesic.
- Inform the client about the possibility of soreness and limitation of movement. If soreness develops, analgesics may be taken. Beginning the next day, warm, moist towels may be applied to the affected region for 20 minutes every hour. This provides comfort and helps blood resorption. Heat therapy should not commence for at least 4 to 6 hours after hematoma formation, however. Before this time, heat may produce further vasodilation and an even larger hematoma.
- Advise the client that the swelling and discoloration will gradually disappear over 7 to 14 days.
- Dismiss the client when the bleeding has stopped. Avoid further dental hygiene care in the area until signs and symptoms of the hematoma have disappeared. Document the incident and the client's response in the client's chart.

Facial Nerve Paralysis

Facial paralysis is a loss of motor function of the facial expression muscles. Unilateral facial nerve paralysis occurs when the local anesthetic solution is inadvertently deposited into the parotid gland, located on the posterior border of the ramus, during an inferior alveolar nerve block.

The loss of motor function is temporary and subsides in a few hours; however, during this time, the client is unable to control these muscles and the face appears lopsided. It also may be impossible for the client to voluntarily close the eye on the affected side. Fortunately, the corneal reflex is functional, and tears continue to lubricate the eye.

To prevent facial nerve paralysis:

- Adhere to the techniques recommended for the inferior alveolar nerve block.
- The needle should contact bone (medial aspect of the ramus) before deposition of the local anesthetic solution.
- If bone is not contacted, withdraw the needle almost entirely out of the tissue, bring the barrel of the syringe more posterior (thereby directing the needle more anterior), and readvance the needle until bone is contacted.
- Following these steps precludes deposition of the solution into the parotid gland.

Within a short time after deposition of the anesthetic solution into the parotid gland, the client senses a weakening of the facial muscles on the affected side. The inferior alveolar nerve is not anesthetized. Management includes the following:[7]

- Reassure the client. Explain that the paralysis lasts only a few hours and resolves with no residual effects.
- Instruct the client to remove contact lenses.
- Ask the client to close the eyelid manually to keep the cornea lubricated.
- There are no contraindications to proceeding with treatment at this time, but it may be advisable to reschedule the client.
- Document the incident and the client's response in the client's chart.

Paresthesia

Prolonged anesthesia or paresthesia is a condition wherein the client experiences numbness for many hours or days after a local anesthetic injection. Paresthesia may be the result of irritation to the nerve after injection of an anesthetic agent that has been contaminated with alcohol or a disinfectant. The ensuing edema places pressure on the nerve, leading to paresthesia. Persistent anesthesia also may result from trauma to the nerve sheath caused by the needle contacting the nerve during an injection. Clients often report the sensation of an electric shock when this occurs. Finally, hemorrhage into or around the neural sheath may create pressure and subsequent paresthesia.

A complication of paresthesia is the client inadvertently precipitating a biting, thermal, or chemical injury from the diminished sensation in the area.

To prevent paresthesia:

- Store dental cartridges properly. Avoid placing cartridges in disinfectants.
- Follow the proper injection protocol as recommended in Procedure 34–4 and Tables 34–11 to 34–21.

Most often paresthesia involves the lingual nerve or the inferior alveolar nerve. The sensory deficit usually is minimal and rarely is accompanied by permanent nerve damage. Fortunately, most incidents resolve within 8 weeks. Recommendations for the management of a client with paresthesia follow:[7]

- Reassure the client. The client usually contacts the dental office the day after treatment to report continuing numbness. Explain that paresthesia following local anesthetic administration is not uncommon.
- Arrange for an examination of the client by the dentist, who will determine the location and extent of paresthesia. Explain to the client that paresthesia often continues for 2 months and may last longer.
- Arrange to have the client examined every 2 months until cessation of the paresthesia. Consultation with an oral and maxillofacial surgeon is advisable if paresthesia persists after 12 months or sooner if the client and dentist consider it appropriate.
- Record the incident, conversations with the client, and all clinical findings in the client's chart. Inform your liability carrier of the circumstances.
- Dental and dental hygiene care may continue. Avoid injecting into the area of the traumatized nerve and employ alternative pain control techniques.

Trismus

Trismus, a spasm of the muscles of mastication that results in soreness and difficulty opening the mouth, most often occurs as a result of trauma to the muscles in the infratemporal space after intraoral injections. This trauma may be the result of multiple needle insertions, administration of an anesthetic solution contaminated with a disinfectant, injection of large amounts of local anesthetic solution into a restricted area causing distention of the tissues, hemorrhage that leads to muscle dysfunction as the blood is resorbed, or a low-grade infection.

To prevent trismus:

- ✦ Store the local anesthetic cartridges properly. Avoid immersing the cartridges in a disinfectant.
- ✦ Use sharp, sterile, disposable needles.
- ✦ Follow appropriate infection control protocol. Needles that become contaminated should be replaced.
- ✦ Use minimal effective amounts of local anesthetic solution and deposit the solution slowly.
- ✦ Adhere to the recommended techniques of local anesthetic administration as outlined in Procedure 34–4 and Tables 34–11 to 34–21. Observe anatomic landmarks and strive to improve administration techniques. Each of these recommendations facilitates atraumatic injections and prevents repeated needle insertions.

Clients often complain of soreness and difficulty in opening the mouth the day after the administration of an inferior alveolar or a posterior superior nerve block. Recommendations for management of clients with trismus follow:[2,5]

- ✦ Arrange for an examination of the client by the dentist.
- ✦ Start heat therapy immediately. Place moist, hot towels on the affected area for 20 minutes every hour. Analgesics may be recommended to manage the discomfort. Codeine and muscle relaxants may be prescribed by the dentist if needed.
- ✦ Direct the client to open and close and move the mandible from side to side (lateral) for 5 minutes every 3 to 4 hours. This exercise may be accomplished by chewing gum.
- ✦ Continue steps 1 to 3 until the client is free of symptoms. Improvement is often reported within 48 hours, and symptoms diminish gradually over several days.
- ✦ If symptoms continue after 48 hours, the possibility of an infection exists. Antibiotic therapy (prescribed by the dentist) should be added to the recommended care regimen.
- ✦ If severe pain and dysfunction continue despite therapy, refer the client to an oral and maxillofacial surgeon for consultation.
- ✦ Record the incident, conversations with the client, the results of clinical examinations, and care recommended in the client's chart.
- ✦ Avoid elective dental hygiene care until symptoms resolve and the client is more comfortable.

Infection

Infection from local anesthetic administration occurs rarely with the introduction of sterile disposable needles and glass cartridges; however, postinjection infection may be precipitated by contamination of the needle before the injection, improper handling of the local anesthesia armamentarium, or improper tissue preparation before the injection. When a contaminated needle or local anesthetic solution is introduced into the deeper tissues, infection may occur. If infection is not recognized and treated, trismus may ensue.

To prevent infection:

- ✦ Use sterile, disposable needles.
- ✦ Sheath the needle before use and resheath it after use to prevent it from coming in contact with nonsterile surfaces.
- ✦ Use appropriate infection control protocol when handling the anesthetic cartridges. Store the cartridges in their original container, and, if necessary, wipe the diaphragm of the cartridge with a disinfectant before syringe assembly.
- ✦ To reduce microorganisms at the penetration site, wipe the tissue with gauze and apply a topical antiseptic before the initial needle insertion.

When infection occurs, the client often reports pain and dysfunction, similar to trismus, a few days after dental hygiene care. At this point signs and symptoms of infection often are not obvious, and immediate treatment includes procedures for managing trismus (e.g., heat therapy, physiotherapy, analgesics, and muscle relaxants). If the client does not respond to therapy within 3 days, an infection most likely exists, and antibiotic therapy should be prescribed by the dentist or physician. Document the recommended therapy and client progress in the client record.

Edema

Edema, a swelling of the tissues, is a clinical sign of a complication. It may be caused by trauma during the injection, administration of contaminated solutions, hemorrhage, an infection, or an allergic response. Most often edema manifests as localized pain and dysfunction. In the most severe case, edema precipitated by an allergic response may produce airway obstruction and represents a life-threatening emergency.

To prevent edema:

- ✦ Follow appropriate infection control protocol when storing and handling components of the local anesthesia armamentarium.
- ✦ Observe the guidelines for administering atraumatic injections, as described in Procedure 34–4.
- ✦ Conduct an adequate preanesthetic client assessment before local anesthetic administration.

The course and treatment of edema depend on its etiology.[7] When produced by the administration of a contaminated anesthetic solution or traumatic injection, edema usually subsides in 1 to 3 days without treatment. Analgesics may be recommended. If edema is caused by hemorrhage, the tissue appears discolored and should be managed in the same manner as a hematoma. Resolution of the edema may take 7 to 14 days as the blood is resorbed into the tissues. Edema produced by infection often becomes progressively worse. If the pain and dysfunction do not subside in 3 days, antibiotic therapy may be instituted by the dentist or physician. The treatment of edema caused by an allergic reaction depends on the degree and location of the tissue swelling. If there is no airway obstruction, treatment involves the administration of intramuscular and oral antihistamines and consultation with an allergist/physician. If the edema occurs in an area where it compromises the airway, the recommendations outlined in the section on systemic complications should be followed.

Tissue Sloughing

Surface layers of epithelium may be lost because of tissue irritation caused by the application of topical anesthetic for an extended period or a client's heightened sensitivity to the local anesthetic. A sterile abscess—a form of tissue sloughing most frequently occurring on the hard palate—may develop after prolonged ischemia induced by the inclusion of a vasoconstrictor in the local anesthetic agent.

To prevent tissue sloughing:

- Use topical anesthetics appropriately. Apply a limited amount of topical anesthetic to the tissue for 1 to 2 minutes to minimize irritation and maximize effectiveness.
- When using vasoconstrictors for hemostasis, avoid using high concentrations. Epinephrine 1:50,000 and norepinephrine (Levophed) 1:30,000 are the agents most likely to cause prolonged ischemia leading to a sterile abscess.

Tissue sloughing usually requires no treatment and disappears within a few days. A sterile abscess resolves in 7 to 10 days. Analgesics may be recommended for discomfort and topical ointment can be applied to minimize irritation. Document the progress and response of the client in the client's record.

Soft Tissue Trauma

Lip, tongue, or cheek trauma results when the client inadvertently chews or bites these tissues while they are still anesthetized. Trauma—most often observed in children or in mentally or physically disabled individuals—may lead to swelling and significant discomfort when the anesthesia subsides.

To prevent soft tissue trauma:

- Select a local anesthetic agent with appropriate duration for the length of the dental hygiene appointment.
- Warn the client not to eat, drink, or test the anesthetized area by biting until normal sensation has returned. The client's guardian also should be advised of the potential for injury.
- If anesthesia is still present on dismissal, place a cotton roll between the teeth and soft tissues. The cotton roll can be held in position with dental floss wrapped around the teeth.
- Warning stickers may be placed on children to serve as a reminder to the child and the guardian to be careful.

Management of soft tissue trauma includes the following:

- Coat the lip with petrolatum to minimize irritation and discomfort.
- Recommend warm saline rinses to help decrease swelling.
- Recommend analgesics for pain.
- If infection occurs, the dentist or physician may prescribe antibiotic therapy.

Postanesthetic Intraoral Lesions

Intraoral lesions, such as those from aphthous stomatitis or herpes simplex virus, may develop after the administration of local anesthesia or trauma to the intraoral tissues. Aphthous stomatitis occurs on tissue not attached to bone, such as the mucofacial fold or inner lip. Herpes simplex virus lesions (see Chapter 12) may develop intraorally on tissues attached to bone, such as the hard palate, or extraorally. Trauma to the area by a needle or any equipment used during the dental hygiene care appointment may activate herpetic recurrence.

Preventing the development of postanesthetic intraoral lesions is impossible in susceptible clients; however, minimizing trauma during procedures for local anesthetic administration is advisable.

Approximately 2 days after the dental hygiene care appointment, the client reports ulcerations and intense pain, usually near the injection site(s). If the discomfort is tolerable, no management is necessary. If the pain is acute, topical anesthetic solutions or protective pastes, such as Orabase, may provide relief. The lesions last for 7 to 10 days. Reassure the client and document the occurrence of the lesion in the client's record.

SYSTEMIC COMPLICATIONS

Client assessment is a key factor in preventing systemic complications associated with local anesthetic administration. It is estimated that a comprehensive health assessment will prevent approximately 90% of potential life-threatening situations.[21] The remaining 10% occurs despite all preventive efforts.

The dental hygienist should be able to recognize the signs and symptoms of an adverse drug reaction and properly manage the emergency that may develop. To be adequately prepared for an emergency, the dental hygienist, as well as all members of the oral health team, should be able to recognize and manage medical emergencies, monitor vital signs, administer oxygen, and perform basic life support procedures. By establishing an airway and performing basic cardiopulmonary resuscitation, the dental hygienist administers care to reverse the emergency or to sustain the client until advanced life support systems arrive (see Chapter 7).

Local Anesthetic Overdose

A drug overdose reaction or toxic reaction is defined as those signs and symptoms that result from overly high blood levels of a drug in various organs and tissues.[7] Normally, the drug is continually absorbed from its site of administration into the circulation. Concurrently, the drug is being removed from the blood as it undergoes redistribution and biotransformation. When this equilibrium exists, high blood levels of the drug seldom occur. If this equilibrium is altered, however, the elevation of the blood level of the drug may be sufficient to produce an overdose reaction.

Many factors influence the rate at which a local anesthetic drug level is elevated and the length of time it remains elevated. The presence of one or more of these factors predisposes the client to the development of an overdose reaction. These factors are divided into predisposing client factors and drug factors. Client factors modify the response of an individual to the usual drug dosage. Drug factors involve the drug and its site of administration. Table 34–22 describes how each of these factors influences the potential for an overdose reaction.

CAUSES AND PREVENTION. High blood levels of local anesthetics may occur in one or more of the following ways:[2,5]

- Biotransformation of the anesthetic is unusually slow.
- Elimination of the anesthetic from the body through the kidneys is unusually slow.
- The total dose administered is too large.
- Absorption of the anesthetic from the site of injection is unusually rapid.
- The anesthetic is inadvertently administered intravascularly.

The first two potential causes of an overdose—delayed biotransformation and elimination of the anesthetic agent—relate to the health of the client. Therefore, it is imperative that the dental hygienist carefully assess the client's health status, obtain medical consultation if necessary, and modify the dental hygiene care plan as indicated to prevent drug-related complications.

The three remaining causes of an overdose reaction—excessive dose, rapid absorption, and intravascular injection—may be prevented through adherence to proper technique of local anesthetic agent administration. Thus careful assessment of the client before dental hygiene care and proper administration technique minimize the risk of a local anesthetic overdose.

Biotransformation and Elimination of the Anesthetic. Ester anesthetics are biotransformed primarily in the blood by the enzyme pseudocholinesterase, which causes the drug to undergo hydrolysis to para-aminobenzoic acid. Clients with a familial history of atypical pseudocholinesterase may be unable to detoxify ester anesthetic agents at the usual rate. As a result, high blood levels of anesthetic may develop. Amide anesthetics may be administered to these individuals without an increased risk of overdose.

Biotransformation of amide anesthetics occurs in the liver. A history of liver disease may indicate some hepatic dysfunction, and the ability of the liver to biotransform

TABLE 34–22 PREDISPOSING FACTORS TO LOCAL ANESTHETIC OVERDOSE REACTION

Predisposing Factors	Causal Factors
Client Factors	
Age	Biotransformation may not be fully developed in younger age groups and may be diminished in older age groups.
Body weight	Lower body weight increases risk.
Genetics	Genetic deficiencies may alter response to certain drugs (e.g., atypical plasma cholinesterase).
Disease	Presence of disease may affect the ability of the body to biotransform the drug into an inactive substance (e.g., hepatic or renal dysfunction, cardiovascular disease).
Mental attitude and environment	Psychological attitude affects response to stimulation; anxiety decreases seizure threshold.
Gender	Very slight risk increase during pregnancy.
Drug Factors	
Vasoactivity	Vasodilation increases risk.
Drug dosage	Higher dose increases risk.
Route of administration	Intravascular route increases risk.
Rate of injection	Rapid injection increases risk.
Vascularity of injection site	Increased vascularity increases risk.
Presence of vasoconstrictors	Decreases risk.
Other medications	Concomitant medications may influence local anesthetic drug levels.

Modified from Malamed SF: *Medical emergencies in the dental office,* ed 4, St Louis, 1993, Mosby.

amide anesthetics may be compromised. Clients with a history of liver disease who are ambulatory may still receive amide local anesthetics; however, only small amounts should be injected because average amounts may produce an overdose reaction.

Both ester and amide anesthetics are eliminated to some degree through the kidneys. Renal dysfunction may delay elimination of the local anesthetic from the blood, precipitating accumulated levels of local anesthetic and increased potential for an overdose. Those clients who have significant renal impairment or who require renal dialysis should receive the minimal amount of local anesthetic needed for effective pain control.

Excessive Total Dose of Anesthetic. If an excessive total dose of local anesthetic is administered to a client, toxic effects develop. Responses to drugs vary considerably, but guidelines exist for the dental hygienist to calculate maximal safe doses of local anesthetic agents based on body weight (Tables 34–5 and 34–6). The dental hygienist also needs to factor in the client's age and physical status and adjust the dosage accordingly. A more detailed discussion can be found under the earlier section, Maximal Safe Doses of Local Anesthetics.

Rapid Absorption of Anesthetic into the Circulation. The addition of a vasoconstricting drug in the local anesthetic solution reduces the systemic toxicity of the anesthetic agent by slowing its absorption into the cardiovascular system. Therefore, unless specifically contraindicated because of health status or limited duration of dental hygiene care, local anesthetic solutions containing a vasoconstrictor should be employed. A vasoconstrictor minimizes the potential for an overdose reaction and subsequently increases client safety.

Topical anesthetic agents applied to the oral mucosa are absorbed rapidly into the circulation. The concentration of these topical agents is much greater than that of injectable anesthetic solutions. When small amounts are used in a localized area, there is little chance of complications developing. If applied over a large area such as a quadrant or whole arch, however, a significant increase in blood level may occur, precipitating an overdose reaction.[7] To prevent complications with topical anesthetics, it is recommended to limit the area of application and avoid topical anesthetic aerosol sprays because of lack of dosage control and sterility concerns.

Intravascular Injection. The introduction of a local anesthetic solution directly into the bloodstream via an intravascular injection (intravenous or intraarterial) may produce an overdose response. An intravascular injection may result with any intraoral injection; however, it is more likely to occur during a nerve block, particularly an inferior alveolar, mental, incisive, or posterior superior alveolar nerve block.[22]

Fortunately, an overdose reaction from an intravascular injection can be prevented by having a complete knowledge of the anatomic features of the area to be anesthetized and by adhering to careful injection technique. This includes using an aspirating syringe, a 25- or 27-gauge needle, aspirating in two planes before deposition, and slowly administering the anesthetic agent.

CLINICAL MANIFESTATIONS AND MANAGEMENT. The onset, intensity, and duration of a local anesthetic toxic reaction may vary depending on the original cause of the overdose. Table 34–23 compares the various patterns of local anesthetic overdose reactions.

Table 34–24 describes the clinical signs and symptoms that may occur during an overdose reaction (during minimal-to-moderate and moderate-to-high blood levels of anesthetic) and the procedures for managing a local anesthetic overdose response. Management of an overdose response depends on the severity of the reaction. Most often, the reaction is mild and transitory, with little or no specific treatment need.[2,5] A severe or longer-duration reaction necessitates prompt recognition and immediate care.

Epinephrine Overdose

Although several vasoconstrictors are currently used in oral health care (Table 34–3), epinephrine is the most potent and most widely employed. Consequently, overdose reactions occur more often with epinephrine than with other vasopressor agents because the latter agents are weaker and are used less frequently.

CAUSES AND PREVENTION. An epinephrine overdose reaction is more likely to develop if concentrations of epinephrine greater than 1:100,000 are administered. Some authorities state that a concentration of 1:250,000 epinephrine provides adequate duration of action for dental procedures and minimal toxicity. Therefore, the use of a 1:50,000 concentration of epinephrine for pain control is unwarranted. The only benefit this concentration may have over lesser concentrations is its ability to control bleeding. If epinephrine is to be used for hemostasis, only small quantities of solution need be infiltrated into the immediate area. Overdose reactions under these circumstances are rare. Therefore, to avoid an epinephrine overdose reaction, it is recommended that the dental hygienist use the lowest effective concentration of epinephrine needed to produce the desired effect and carefully observe dosage guidelines (Table 34–7).

Clients with cardiovascular disease have a greater potential for epinephrine overdose. An increased workload on an already compromised cardiovascular system may precipitate further cardiac distress. Therefore, the total dose of vasoconstrictor must be reduced to avoid systemic complications (Tables 34–7 and 34–8).

An intravascular injection may also produce an epinephrine overdose reaction.[4] Recommendations for prevention of an intravascular injection may be found in the preceding Local Anesthetic Overdose section.

CLINICAL MANIFESTATIONS AND MANAGEMENT. Clinically, the signs and symptoms of epinephrine toxicity

TABLE 34–23 COMPARISON OF PATTERNS OF LOCAL ANESTHETIC OVERDOSE

Factors Related to Overdose	Rapid Intravascular	Too Large a Total Dose	Rapid Absorption	Slow Biotransformation	Slow Elimination
Likelihood of occurrence	Common	Most common	Likely with "high normal" dosages if no vasoconstrictors are used	Uncommon	Least common
Onset of signs and symptoms	Most rapid (seconds); intraarterial faster than intravenous	3–5 minutes	3–5 minutes	10–30 minutes	10 minutes to several hours
Intensity of signs and symptoms	Usually most intense	Gradual onset with increased intensity; may prove quite severe		Gradual onset with slow increase in intensity of symptoms	
Duration of signs and symptoms	2–3 minutes	Usually 5 to 30 minutes; depends on dose and ability to metabolize or excrete		Potentially longest duration because of inability to metabolize or excrete agents	
Primary prevention	Aspirate, slow injection	Administer minimal doses	Use vasoconstrictor; limit topical anesthetic use or use nonabsorbed type (base)	Adequate pretreatment physical assessment of client	
Drug groups	Amides and esters	Amides; esters only rarely	Amides; esters only rarely	Amides and esters	Amides and esters

From Malamed SF: *Medical emergencies in the dental office*, ed 4, St Louis, 1993, Mosby.

TABLE 34–24 CLINICAL MANIFESTATIONS AND MANAGEMENT OF A LOCAL ANESTHETIC OVERDOSE REACTION

Signs/Symptoms	Management
Minimal to Moderate Blood Levels (Mild Overdose Reaction)	
Confusion	Terminate procedure.
Talkativeness	Reassure client.
Apprehension	Position client comfortably.
Excitedness	Administer oxygen.
Lightheadedness	Provide basic life support, as indicated.
Dizziness	Monitor vital signs.
Ringing in ears (tinnitus)	Summon medical assistance, if needed.
Headache	Allow client to recover and discharge.
Slurred speech	
Generalized stutter	
Muscular twitching and tremor of face and extremities	
Blurred vision, unable to focus	
Numbness of perioral tissues	
Flushed or chilled feeling	
Drowsiness, disorientation	
Elevated blood pressure	
Elevated heart rate	
Elevated respiratory rate	
Loss of consciousness	
Moderate to High Blood Levels (Severe Overdose Reaction)	
Tonic-clonic seizure, followed by:	Terminate procedure.
CNS depression	Position client supine, legs elevated.
Depressed blood pressure, heart rate, and respiratory rate	Summon medical assistance.
Unconsciousness	Manage seizure: protect client from injury.
	Provide basic life support, as indicated.
	Administer oxygen.
	Monitor vital signs.
	Administer an anticonvulsant (prolonged seizure).
	Transport client to hospital after stabilization.

Some data from Malamed SF: *Medical emergencies in the dental office*, ed 4, St Louis, 1993, Mosby.

resemble the fight-or-flight response. Table 34–25 identifies signs and symptoms of an epinephrine overdose reaction and procedures for management. Most cases of epinephrine overdose are of short duration and need little or no definitive management. If a prolonged reaction occurs, however, the dental hygienist must be prepared to respond accordingly.

Allergy

Allergic reactions are the result of an antigen-antibody response to a specific agent. Exposure to an initial dose of a medication causes an immunologic response. The drug acts as an antigen, prompting antibodies to be produced. As a result, administration of a subsequent dose causes the client to develop an allergic response to the drug, its chemical preservative, or a metabolite.[9] Once clients manifest a specific drug allergy, they remain allergic to that drug indefinitely.[5]

CAUSES. Allergic reactions to local anesthetics occur most often in response to ester-type anesthetic agents (Table 34–1). The incidence of such responses is extremely rare with the amide-type local anesthetics (Table 34–2). As a result of their nonallergenic nature, amides are now used almost exclusively for pain control during dental and dental hygiene procedures.

Allergic responses to other contents of the dental cartridge have been demonstrated. Reports of allergy to sodium bisulfite and metabisulfite are numerous.[11-15] Bisulfites are incorporated in all dental cartridges containing a vasoconstrictor; however, they are not included in cartridges that contain no vasopressor. These agents are also sprayed on fruits and vegetables to prevent discoloration. A client with a history of bisulfite allergy (e.g., asthmatic clients) should alert the dental hygienist to the possibility of a similar reaction if a local anesthetic containing a vasoconstrictor is administered. See the earlier section on Preanesthetic Client Assessment/Allergies for further discussion.

PREVENTION. The preanesthetic client assessment is the primary measure for prevention of an allergic reaction. A client who has multiple allergies (e.g., asthma, hay fever, allergy to foods) has an increased potential for allergic reactions to medications.[2,5,21] Thus the dental hygienist must proceed cautiously when considering administration of local anesthetics to these clients.

If the client reports that he or she has experienced an allergic reaction to local anesthetics, it is important that the dental hygienist assume that the client is truly allergic to the local anesthetic in question until proven otherwise. Unfortunately, any adverse drug reaction is often labeled an allergy by clients when in fact overdose reactions occur much more frequently than allergic reactions.[23] Thus it is imperative for the dental hygienist to seek as much information as possible from the client so that the exact nature of the reaction can be determined. A dialogue history is used, whereby the dental hygienist asks the client a series of questions to ascertain the validity of the allergy[2] (see Dialogue to Evaluate an Alleged Allergic Reaction to a Local Anesthetic). It is important that the anesthetic agent or any closely related agent to which the client claims to be allergic *not* be used until the allergy is disproved.

If, after the dialogue history, questions remain about the cause of the reaction, the dental hygienist should consult with the dentist and the client's physician, and referral for allergy testing should be considered. Dental hygiene care requiring local anesthetics (topical or injectable) should be delayed until an evaluation of the client is complete. Dental hygiene procedures not requiring anesthesia may be performed during the interim.

For those clients who have a confirmed allergy to local anesthetics, management varies according to the nature

TABLE 34–25 CLINICAL MANIFESTATIONS AND MANAGEMENT OF A CLIENT WITH AN EPINEPHRINE OVERDOSE REACTION

Signs/Symptoms	Management
Fear, anxiety	Terminate procedure.
Tenseness	Position client upright.
Restlessness	Reassure client.
Throbbing headache	Provide basic life support, as indicated.
Tremor	Monitor vital signs.
Perspiration	Summon medical assistance, if needed.
Weakness	Administer oxygen, if needed.
Dizziness	Allow client to recover and discharge.
Pallor	
Respiratory difficulty	
Palpitations	
Sharp elevation in blood pressure, primarily systolic	
Elevated heart rate	
Cardiac dysrhythmias	

Some data from Malamed SF: *Medical emergencies in the dental office*, ed 4, St Louis, 1993, Mosby.

Dialogue to Evaluate an Alleged Allergic Reaction to a Local Anesthetic

Describe exactly what occurred.
What treatment was given?
What position were you in during the injection?
What was the time sequence of events?
What drug was used?
What amount of drug was administered?
Did the drug contain a vasoconstrictor?
Were you taking any other medications at the time of the incident?
What is the name and address of the doctor (dentist, physician, hospital) who was treating you when the reaction occurred?

Adapted from Malamed SF: *Handbook of local anesthesia*, ed 3, St Louis, 1990, Mosby.

of the allergy. Table 34–10 describes alternative drugs that may be employed in place of those agents that cause an allergic response.

CLINICAL MANIFESTATIONS AND MANAGEMENT. The amount of time that elapses between exposure to an allergenic agent and manifestation of signs and symptoms is important. As a rule, the more rapid the onset of signs and symptoms following exposure, the more severe the ultimate reaction.[24] Conversely, the greater the time between exposure and onset of signs and symptoms, the less severe the reaction. This time factor helps the dental hygienist determine the appropriate management of the reaction.

The most common allergic reaction associated with local anesthetics is a dermatologic reaction. A skin reaction that appears alone or after a considerable lapse of time (60 minutes or more) is usually not life-threatening; however, if a skin reaction develops rapidly, it may be the first indication of an ensuing generalized reaction.

An allergic reaction may manifest solely in the respiratory tract or may accompany other systemic responses. In slowly evolving generalized allergic reactions, respiratory distress follows skin and gastrointestinal reactions, but occurs before cardiovascular signs and symptoms.

Generalized anaphylaxis is the most life-threatening allergic reaction. Most reactions develop quickly, reaching maximum intensity within 5 to 30 minutes of exposure, although delayed responses have been reported.[7]

Table 34–26 describes the signs and symptoms and the management of clients with dermatologic and respiratory reactions and generalized anaphylaxis. The reaction types are further defined as delayed and immediate.

TABLE 34–26 CLINICAL MANIFESTATIONS AND MANAGEMENT OF AN ALLERGIC REACTION

Type of Allergic Response	Signs/Symptoms	Management
Delayed		
Skin	Erythema Urticaria (hives) Pruritus (itching) Angioedema (localized swelling of extremities, lips, tongue, pharynx, larynx)	Administer antihistamine. Obtain medical consultation.
Respiration	Bronchospasm Distress Dyspnea Wheezing Perspiration Flushing Cyanosis Tachycardia Anxiety	Terminate procedure. Position client semierect. Reassure client. Provide basic life support, as indicated. Summon medical assistance, if needed. Administer epinephrine. Monitor vital signs. Administer antihistamine. Allow client to recover and discharge.
Laryngeal edema	Swelling of vocal apparatus and subsequent obstruction of airway Respiratory distress Exaggerated chest movements High-pitched sound to no sound Cyanosis Loss of consciousness	Terminate procedure. Position client supine. Summon medical assistance. Administer epinephrine. Maintain airway. Administer oxygen. Additional drug management: antihistamine, corticosteroid. Cricothyrotomy, if needed. Transfer client to hospital.
Immediate Anaphylaxis		
Skin	Pruritus (itching) Flushing Urticaria (face and upper chest) Feeling of hair standing on end Conjunctivitis, vasomotor rhinitis	Terminate procedure. Position client supine, legs elevated. Provide basic life support, as indicated. Summon medical assistance. Administer epinephrine. Administer oxygen. Monitor vital signs. Additional drug management: antihistamine, corticosteroid. Transport client to hospital.
Gastrointestinal/genitourinary	Abdominal cramps Nausea, vomiting Diarrhea	Same as management of anaphylaxis related to skin.

Table continued on following page

TABLE 34–26 CLINICAL MANIFESTATIONS AND MANAGEMENT OF AN ALLERGIC REACTION—CONT'D

Type of Allergic Response	Signs/Symptoms	Management
Immediate Anaphylaxis—cont'd		
Respiratory	Substernal tightness or chest pain Cough, wheezing Dyspnea Cyanosis of mucous membranes, nail beds Laryngeal edema	Same as management of anaphylaxis related to skin.
Cardiovascular	Pallor Lightheadedness Palpitations, tachycardia Hypotension Cardiac dysrhythmias Unconsciousness Cardiac arrest	Same as management of anaphylaxis related to skin.

Client Education Issues

- ✦ Explain the advantages of receiving local anesthetic during dental hygiene procedures that may produce discomfort
- ✦ Explain measures taken to ensure comfortable local anesthetic delivery
- ✦ Explain normal, anticipated sensations associated with local anesthesia, including areas that will be anesthetized and the anticipated duration of the anesthesia
- ✦ Explain the importance of following postoperative instructions to minimize the possibility of self-inflicted soft tissue injury

Legal, Ethical, and Safety Issues

- ✦ It is the legal responsibility of the dental hygienist to practice within the scope authorized by state law concerning local anesthetic delivery.
- ✦ It is imperative that the dental hygienist carefully evaluate the client's health history to determine suitability for local anesthetic procedures.
- ✦ The client treatment record must accurately reflect any local anesthetic procedure completed, including complete drug name and amount delivered.

Key Concepts

- ✦ Local anesthesia is the temporary loss of sensation in a circumscribed area brought about by the reduction of nerve membrane permeability to sodium ions. When sodium ions are blocked, the nerve cell cannot depolarize, stopping transmission of a stimulus to the brain.
- ✦ Local anesthetic agents are classified chemically as either amides or esters, which differ in how they are metabolized: esters are metabolized in the blood by pseudocholinesterase, and amides are metabolized in the liver.
- ✦ Local anesthetic agents produce vasodilation. For the maximum anesthetic effect, vasoconstrictors are often combined with local anesthetics to slow down absorption, reduce hemorrhage, and increase the length of time the anesthesia is effective.
- ✦ Many local anesthetic drugs are available. The clinician must choose the best agent for the circumstance considering each of the following: the health of the client, medications taken by the client, possible client allergies, the amount of time anesthesia is desired, the areas being anesthetized, the planned procedure/injections, the client's past response to anesthesia, and the possible need for hemostasis.
- ✦ There is a maximum amount of local anesthetic agent and vasoconstrictor that can safely be administered to a client at one time. This amount varies with the client's weight, the client's age, and the specific agent administered.
- ✦ A thorough health history evaluation before local anesthetic delivery is crucial. Many medications influence a client's response to local anesthesia. There are also several systemic conditions that require modifications of local anesthetic delivery, such as pregnancy, hyperthyroidism, liver dysfunction, renal dysfunction, allergies to sulfa or bisulfite, atypical plasma cholinesterase, methemoglobinemia, and malignant hyperthermia.

KEY CONCEPTS—CONT'D

- The local anesthetic armamentarium includes a syringe, a needle, local anesthetic agent, topical anesthetic, cotton-tipped applicators, gauze, cotton forceps, and a mouth mirror.
- Oral anesthetic procedures involve the maxillary and mandibular branches of cranial nerve V, the trigeminal nerve.
- There are three categories of local anesthetic procedures: local infiltration, field block, and nerve block. These differ in the relationship between the area anesthetized and the area of delivery of the anesthetic agent, and in the scope of the area anesthetized; nerve blocks are delivered further from the treatment site and anesthetize a larger area when compared to local infiltrations, which are delivered directly at the apex of the target tooth and only anesthetize one to two teeth.
- The attitude and demeanor of the clinician have a significant impact on the comfort of the client and the overall success of the local anesthetic injection.
- Local anesthetic procedures for maxillary anesthesia include local infiltration, anterior superior alveolar field block, middle superior alveolar field block, infraorbital nerve block, posterior superior alveolar nerve block, greater palatine nerve block, and nasopalatine nerve block.
- Local anesthetic procedures for mandibular anesthesia include inferior alveolar nerve block, lingual nerve block, buccal nerve block, mental nerve block, and incisive nerve block.
- Local anesthetic delivery has the potential to cause both local and systemic complications. Potential local complications include needle breakage, pain during injection, burning during injection, hematoma, facial nerve paralysis, paresthesia, trismus, infection, edema, tissue sloughing, soft tissue trauma, and postanesthetic intraoral lesion. Potential systemic complications include local anesthetic overdose, epinephrine overdose, and allergy. Most of these potential complications can be avoided with proper preanesthetic client assessment, careful selection of anesthetic agent, conscientious delivery techniques, and proper postoperative instructions.

CRITICAL THINKING EXERCISES

Scenario: Ms. S

Client Profile: 45-year-old female who lives alone

Chief Complaint: Wants periodontal maintenance scheduled at 4-month intervals. Indicates discomfort during previous scaling throughout the maxillary bilaterally.

Dental History: Past history of orthodontic treatment. Received four quadrants of scaling and root planing three years ago, with a very good result. Third molars removed. Low caries rate. Clinically, client exhibits extensive maxillary buccal recession.

Social History: Limited social drinking, nonsmoker, exercises regularly

Health History: Noncontributory; weighs 123 lb.

Oral Health Behaviors: Client is compliant with home-care regimen and maintains appropriate recare schedule.

Assessment: Client requires local anesthetics to allow for comfortable periodontal maintenance.

Exercises:

1. Review the previous client profile and make the following determinations:
   - Client suitability for local anesthetic administration
   - Preferred local anesthetic agent
   - Preferred injection/injections
   - Maximum dose of local anesthetic
2. Record the local anesthetic as would be necessary in the client treatment record.

For References, Suggested Readings, and Related Websites, visit
http://evolve.elsevier.com/Darby/hygiene/

CHAPTER 35

Nitrous Oxide–Oxygen Analgesia

OBJECTIVES

Mastery of the content in this chapter will enable the reader to:

- Discuss the indications and contraindications for use of nitrous oxide–oxygen (N_2O–O_2) sedation
- Discuss the advantages, disadvantages, and complications associated with its use
- Discuss the signs and symptoms of the baseline level N_2O–O_2 sedation
- List safety features associated with gas cylinders and the gas machine
- Calculate the percentage of nitrous oxide and the percentage of oxygen from the tidal volume
- Safely administer nitrous oxide oxygen sedation by using titration to induce the proper level of sedation, monitoring the client during analgesia, and oxygenating the client at the completion of the sedation period

KEY TERMS

Analgesia stage
Baseline
Conscious sedation
Cylinders
Delirium
Diffusion hypoxia
Excitement phase
Flowmeter
Gas hose
Hypoxia
Inhalation sedation
Nitrous oxide
Psychosedation
Pressure gauge
Quick-coupling outlet
Relative analgesia
Reservoir bag
Scavenger system
Sign
Surgical anesthesia
Surgical anesthesia with respiratory paralysis
Symptom
Tidal volume
Titration
Yokes

Nitrous oxide (N_2O) delivered in combination with oxygen (O_2) is an inhalation method of conscious sedation known as *nitrous oxide–oxygen analgesia* (N_2O–O_2). This conscious sedation method can significantly enhance the clinician's ability to meet the client's need for freedom from pain and stress in a safe and effective way. When used as the sole sedative, N_2O–O_2 suffices to relax individuals who are mildly apprehensive about the dental or dental hygiene experience and provides pain control for procedures that are only slightly or moderately painful. Such procedures include scaling hypersensitive root surfaces, removing periodontal sutures, cementing crowns or inlays, irrigating under an inflamed operculum, or administering a local anesthetic. If significant pain is anticipated during a dental or dental hygiene procedure, then N_2O–O_2 is accompanied by local anesthesia. Nitrous oxide–oxygen is used in combination with other general anesthetics, such as Halothane and Demerol, by oral surgeons to achieve surgical anesthesia. When used alone, N_2O–O_2 is a very weak anesthetic but an intense analgesic.[1] This pharmacologic property of N_2O–O_2 makes it ideal for use in dental hygiene care because clients often are mildly apprehensive and require minor pain control, but also must remain conscious and responsive.

Several synonyms refer to N_2O–O_2 analgesia, including the following:[1]

- Conscious sedation
- Inhalation sedation

✦ Nitrous oxide psychosedation
✦ Relative analgesia

Conscious sedation refers to the fact that during the administration of N_2O–O_2 the client is always awake and able to respond to verbal commands, breathe automatically, and cough so that aspiration is avoided.[2] *Inhalation sedation* reflects that the nitrous oxide and oxygen gases are inhaled through the nose. Nitrous oxide *psychosedation* refers to the fact that nitrous oxide acts on the psyche or the central nervous system in such a way that pain impulses are not relayed to the cerebral cortex or their interpretation is altered.[3] *Relative analgesia* refers to the state of sedation produced, that alters mood and increases the pain reaction threshold, but does not totally block pain sensations.[4]

This chapter presents the principles and techniques of N_2O–O_2 analgesia, highlighting indications, contraindications, advantages, and disadvantages of its use as a sedation modality. Initially, however, a brief overview is presented of the chemistry, pharmacology, and physiology of N_2O–O_2, and the stages of anesthesia.

CHEMISTRY

Nitrous Oxide

Nitrous oxide is a colorless, tasteless, sweet-smelling agent that supports combustion.[5] It is stored as a liquid at 650 to 900 pounds per square inch (psi) in a blue compressed-gas cylinder (Figure 35–1). Although it is stored as a liquid and vapor (gas) in equilibrium, it is delivered as a gas to the client. The pressure within the cylinder, indicated by the needle reading on the pressure gauge, reflects the pressure created by the nitrous oxide gas in the cylinder (Figure 35–2).

As long as one-eighth of the liquid nitrous oxide is present in the cylinder to convert to the gaseous state, the reading on the pressure gauge of 650 to 900 psi remains constant. Consequently, clinicians use their nitrous oxide for a considerable amount of time before the pressure gauge reads 500 psi. Once the pressure reading drops to 500 psi, the pressure gauge precipitously drops, indicating that the cylinder is empty. Because the amount of nitrous oxide in the cylinder cannot be determined by the pressure gauge reading until it is almost empty, it is important for the operator to keep a close eye on the nitrous oxide pressure gauge of portable gas machines. This monitoring allows the clinician to detect when the pressure begins to fall and to substitute a full nitrous oxide cylinder before the original cylinder is empty. In addition, each nitrous oxide cylinder should be marked with the date the full tank was opened and the dates and lengths of subsequent use to facilitate the monitoring process and to prevent the clinician from running out of nitrous oxide before the client care procedure is completed.

The blood/gas solubility coefficient of nitrous oxide is 0.47, meaning that 100 ml of blood dissolves 47 ml of nitrous oxide. This blood/gas solubility coefficient accounts for the rapid onset and rapid recovery from the analgesic effects of nitrous oxide sedation. Because nitrous oxide is 15 times more soluble in blood than nitrogen, it displaces nitrogen in the blood. It does not compete with oxygen and carbon dioxide for combination with the hemoglobin molecule.[1,6]

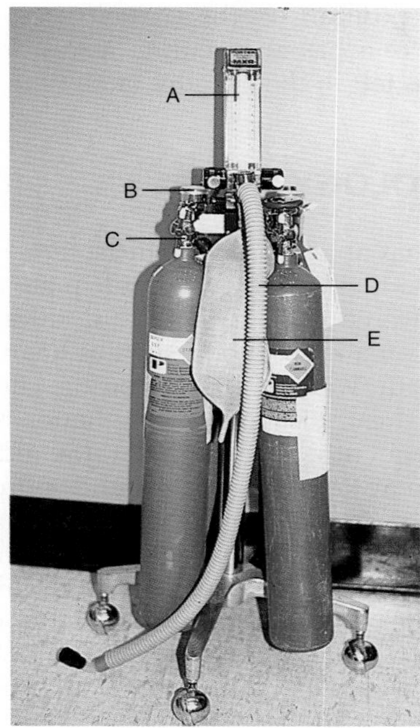

FIGURE 35–1 ✦ A portable gas machine with a green cylinder containing oxygen and a blue cylinder containing nitrous oxide, stored directly on the gas machine. **A,** Flowmeter. **B,** Pressure gauge. **C,** Yoke. **D,** Gas hose. **E,** Reservoir bag.

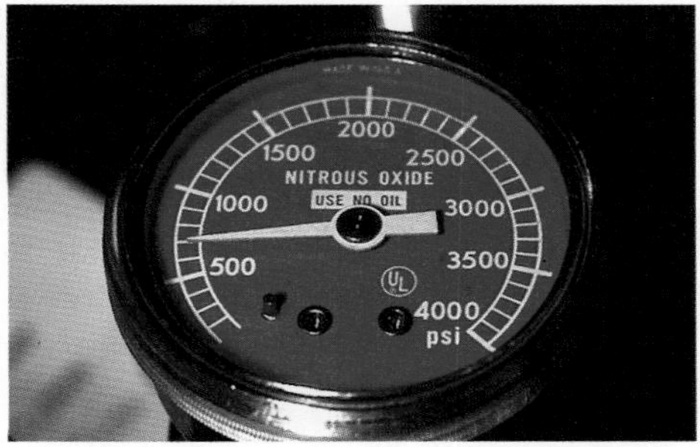

FIGURE 35–2 ✦ Pressure gauge for a nitrous oxide cylinder.

Oxygen

Oxygen is stored as a gas in green compressed-gas cylinders and is delivered as a gas (Figure 35–1). The contents of the oxygen cylinder can be determined by the reading on the pressure gauge. A full tank of oxygen is reflected by a pressure gauge reading of 2100 psi (Figure 35–3). As the oxygen is depleted in the cylinder as a result of use, the pressure falls correspondingly, as indicated by the needle position on the oxygen pressure gauge. Consequently, one has an accurate assessment of how much oxygen is left in the cylinder at all times.

PHARMACOLOGY

Nitrous oxide has no effect on the heart rate, blood pressure, liver, or kidney as long as an adequate amount of oxygen is delivered concurrently.[2,7] It does, however, have an effect on all sensations, such as hearing, touch, pain, and warmth. With regard to hearing, clients report that they can hear distant sounds, better than close sounds. Consequently, clients under the influence of nitrous oxide may key in to background sounds such as music or the conversation in the next room rather than to what the clinician is saying. In addition, nitrous oxide reduces the gag reflex, but does not eliminate it. Therefore, if a client tends to gag, this sedation modality should be considered for use.[1]

PHYSIOLOGY

Nitrous oxide acts to depress the central nervous system. Specifically, it affects the cerebral cortex, thalamus, hypothalamus, and reticular activating system. The exact mechanism of action is unknown; however, it results in either altering the relay of nerve impulses to the cerebral cortex or causing them to be interpreted differently.[3] As a result, the individual experiences reduced anxiety and increased pain tolerance. Pain perception is not blocked, however, and $N_2O–O_2$ must be used in combination with a local anesthetic for many procedures. Nitrous oxide does not combine with any body tissues, and it is the only anesthetic used that is not metabolized. The nitrous oxide molecule enters the blood through the lungs, where it displaces nitrogen and eventually exits unchanged through the lungs.[1]

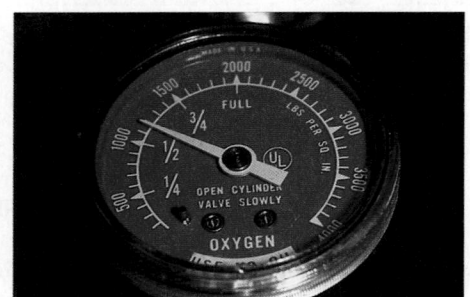

FIGURE 35–3 ✦ Pressure gauge for an oxygen cylinder.

Nevertheless, there are toxic reactions associated with oversedation with nitrous oxide. *Hypoxia* (lack of oxygen to the tissues), characterized by a headache and nausea, is associated with receiving too much nitrous oxide and lack of a subsequent oxygenation period. In addition, bone marrow depression and white blood cell depression have been reported after prolonged administration of 2 to 4 days.

STAGES OF ANESTHESIA

The four stages of anesthesia are depicted in Figure 35–4.

- Stage I is the *analgesia stage.* In analgesia, the person feels pain, but does not care. The analgesia stage of anesthesia has three planes. The first two planes are relative analgesia, and these are the planes appropriate for dental hygiene care.
- Stage II is the *delirium* or *excitement phase* of light anesthesia. This stage of anesthesia is characterized by hyperresponsiveness to stimuli, exaggerated inspirations, and loss of consciousness. For individuals receiving dental hygiene care, the immediate treatment of entry into the excitement stage of anesthesia is to increase the percentage of oxygen immediately to 100% and to turn the nitrous oxide off.
- Stage III is *surgical anesthesia,* and it has four planes. Oral and maxillofacial surgeons take their patients to this level of anesthesia, and it is acceptable; dental hygienists never need to provide this level of anesthesia for their clients. Loss of consciousness by an individual receiving dental hygiene care indicates oversedation, and the immediate treatment is to increase the percentage of oxygen immediately to 100% and to turn the nitrous oxide off. The 0.47 blood/gas solubility coefficient for nitrous oxide promotes rapid recovery of the individual.
- Stage IV anesthesia is *surgical anesthesia with respiratory paralysis.* This level of anesthesia is reserved for use when a person undergoes major surgery in a hospital setting.

Nitrous oxide produces intense analgesia, but it is a very weak anesthetic. In fact, usually one would need to give more than 80% nitrous oxide to achieve surgical anesthesia.[1] This pharmacologic property makes $N_2O–O_2$ a good pain and anxiety control modality for use in dental hygiene care.

Stage I			Stage II	Stage III				Stage IV
Analgesia Stage			Delirium (Excitement)	Surgical Anesthesia				Respiratory Paralysis
Plane 1	Plane 2	Plane 3		Plane 1	Plane 2	Plane 3	Plane 4	

FIGURE 35–4 ✦ Stages of anesthesia.

INDICATIONS FOR USE

$N_2O–O_2$ analgesia is recommended for use in the following situations:[1,2,4,5,8]

- ✦ Mild apprehension
- ✦ Allergy to local anesthetics
- ✦ Refusal of local and general anesthesia
- ✦ Hypersensitive gag reflex
- ✦ Intolerance for long appointments
- ✦ Cardiac conditions
- ✦ Hypertension
- ✦ Asthma
- ✦ Cerebral palsy
- ✦ Mental retardation

Mild Apprehension

Individuals who are fearful of, or mildly anxious about, the oral healthcare experience are good candidates for $N_2O–O_2$ because it relaxes them and takes the edge off their apprehension.

Allergy to or Refusal of Other Anesthetics

Individuals who are allergic to all types of local anesthetics, those who refuse a local or general anesthetic for other reasons, or those who are unable to experience good local anesthesia because use of a vasoconstrictor is medically contraindicated are good candidates for $N_2O–O_2$ analgesia.

Hypersensitive Gag Reflex

Individuals who are prone to gagging easily during oral healthcare procedures, such as those having impressions taken or their third molars scaled, are good candidates for $N_2O–O_2$ because this analgesic reduces the gag response.

Inability to Tolerate Sitting for Long Periods

Nitrous oxide–oxygen analgesia is recommended for persons with back problems or other conditions that make them unable to tolerate sitting in the dental chair for long periods. This recommendation is based on the fact that $N_2O–O_2$ makes one perceive that time is passing quickly.

Cardiovascular Disease and Hypertension

Individuals who have cardiovascular disease or hypertension are good candidates for $N_2O–O_2$ because it decreases stress and exposes the individual to more oxygen than is normally available. For example, even at a gas ratio of 50:50, the client is receiving 50% oxygen compared with the 22% oxygen available in room air. This oxygen enrichment coupled with stress reduction is a major advantage of $N_2O–O_2$ sedation for these medically complex clients.

Asthma

Individuals who have asthma are candidates for $N_2O–O_2$ because during sedation they receive more oxygen than normally is available to them. This oxygen enrichment facilitates breathing and decreases stress.

Cerebral Palsy and Mental Retardation

Persons with cerebral palsy and mental retardation are candidates for $N_2O–O_2$ because they are sometimes difficult to manage in the oral healthcare setting, and this analgesic relaxes them. The client, however, must be able to communicate with the operator, breathe through the nose, and cooperate by leaving the mask in place.

CONTRAINDICATIONS TO USE

There are no absolute medical contraindications to use of $N_2O–O_2$ analgesia, but there are some relative contraindications that make it a poor choice for certain clients. The following conditions contraindicate the use of nitrous oxide–oxygen sedation:[1,2,4,5,9]

- ✦ Pregnancy
- ✦ Communication difficulty
- ✦ Nasal obstruction
- ✦ Emphysema
- ✦ Multiple sclerosis
- ✦ Emotional instability
- ✦ Epilepsy
- ✦ Negative past experience

Pregnancy

$N_2O–O_2$ analgesia is not recommended for individuals who are pregnant. Although there is no evidence that sufficient nitrous oxide crosses the placenta to produce depression of the fetal central nervous system, it is better to err on the side of caution with pregnant women given that long-term exposure to nitrous oxide is associated with spontaneous abortion.[1] In general, all unnecessary drugs are avoided during pregnancy, especially during the first trimester.

Communication Barrier

Individuals who have a language barrier or with whom communication is difficult should not be given $N_2O–O_2$ because communication between the client and the operator is essential for success with conscious sedation. The operator must question the client during the administration of $N_2O–O_2$ to determine the appropriate level of sedation and the client's response to the drug. Communication barriers make it difficult or impossible for this monitoring to occur.

Nasal Obstructions

Individuals who have a cold, allergy, or other type of nasal obstruction are not good candidates for $N_2O–O_2$ because the gas is inhaled. Nasal obstruction prevents the client from obtaining the benefit of the drug. Also, respiratory infections contaminate the tubing and reservoir bag.

Chronic Obstructive Pulmonary Disease

The respiratory systems of persons with emphysema, multiple sclerosis, or chronic bronchitis function on less oxygen than those of healthy individuals because these diseases affect the lung's capacity to exchange air. Consequently, they depend on a lowered blood oxygen level to stimulate respiration. The increased oxygen saturation of the blood made available with $N_2O–O_2$ removes the stimulus of the lowered oxygen blood level and may indicate to the brain that the individual need not perform as many inspirations, thus producing apnea.[8]

Emotional Instability

$N_2O–O_2$ is contraindicated for individuals who are emotionally unstable. Because this type of sedation causes a distortion of one's perception of reality, it can precipitate problems for clients with a history of schizophrenia or alcoholism. Moreover, individuals who have recently experienced the death of a loved one or who are going through a painful divorce often go through a period of emotional instability. It is, therefore, not recommended to use $N_2O–O_2$ sedation because unpleasant feelings may surface under the influence of this drug and cause the client to cry uncontrollably.

Epilepsy

$N_2O–O_2$ analgesia may trigger epileptic seizures in individuals with epilepsy. Therefore, its use is not recommended for clients with a history of epilepsy.

Fear of Nitrous Oxide–Oxygen Sedation

Individuals who are fearful of having $N_2O–O_2$ or those with compulsive personalities who must always be in control may suddenly tear off the sedation mask from fear of the unknown or of becoming unconscious. In the dental hygiene care setting, a good rule of thumb is never to talk someone into being sedated with nitrous oxide. Individuals should be willing and wanting to try this sedation method.

ADVANTAGES OF USE

The following are advantages associated with $N_2O–O_2$ analgesia:

- It is an excellent choice of sedation for the high-risk person with a history of cardiovascular disease.
- It is a simple, relatively safe procedure to perform and not requiring the service of special personnel such as an anesthetist.
- Equipment is not cumbersome and requires little maintenance.
- Restraining straps and pharyngeal airways are not required.
- Individual is awake and responsive at all times, and the depth of sedation can be controlled moment to moment.
- Onset and recovery are nearly always rapid.
- Most adults being sedated do not have to be accompanied to their appointment by another responsible adult.
- No need for preoperative laboratory tests or for food intake to be restricted before sedation, as is the case before having a general anesthetic.
- No need for a special recovery room, or to monitor the person for a long time after recovery.

DISADVANTAGES OF USE

The following are disadvantages associated with $N_2O–O_2$ analgesia:

- Production of vertigo, nausea, or vomiting may occur if too much nitrous oxide is given or if the operator fluctuates the levels of nitrous oxide too much during administration of the agent. (Aspiration is not a problem, however, because the client is awake and the gag reflex is not eliminated.)
- Individuals with extremely difficult behavior problems cannot always be managed.
- When instrumenting teeth in the maxillary anterior region, the mask gets in the way.

SIGNS AND SYMPTOMS OF NITROUS OXIDE–OXYGEN SEDATION

A *sign* is something that can be directly observed. A *symptom* is something that must be reported to one person by another. Thus signs of $N_2O–O_2$ sedation are observed objectively by the operator and symptoms of $N_2O–O_2$ sedation are reported subjectively by the client.

Signs

Objective signs that clients have reached a desirable level of $N_2O–O_2$ sedation are that they are awake but drowsy and relaxed in appearance (e.g., feet pointing out and hands limp). They have reduced reaction to painful stimuli, and respiration is normal and smooth. In contrast, if a client demonstrates hyperresponsiveness to stimuli and exaggerated inspirations, these are signs of oversedation (i.e., entry into the excitement stage of anesthesia) and of the need to give 100% oxygen to the person and discontinue the nitrous oxide altogether.

Other signs that clients have reached a desirable level of $N_2O–O_2$ sedation are that their blood pressure and pulse, eye reaction, and pupil size are observed to be normal.[2,7] Little or no gagging or coughing is observed.

Signs of N_2O–O_2 Analgesia Appropriate for Dental Hygiene Care

Client awake
Lessened pain reaction
Drowsy, relaxed appearance
Eye reaction and pupil size normal
Respiration normal
Blood pressure and pulse normal
Minimal movement of limbs
Flushing of skin
Perspiration
Lacrimation
Little or no gagging or coughing
Speech infrequent and slow

The client's speech is slow and tends to be guttural.[1] There may be some perspiration and tearing. Heavy perspiration and lacrimation, although possibly reflecting appropriate sedation for oral surgery treatment, are inappropriate for dental hygiene care and indicate a need to turn down the nitrous oxide. Likewise, uncontrollable laughing by the client indicates a need to turn down the nitrous oxide level. See Signs of N_2O–O_2 Analgesia Appropriate for Dental Hygiene Care.[1]

Symptoms

Subjective symptoms of N_2O–O_2 sedation can be determined by direct questioning of the client as well as by observation. For example, asking "How do you feel?" or "Do you feel relaxed?" elicits desired information. If clients report that they are relaxed, that sounds seem distant, and if they indicate an indifference to their surroundings, these are symptoms that the desired level of sedation for dental hygiene care has been achieved. For instance, if the operator says to the client, "Shall I go ahead and numb up this area?" and the client replies "I don't care," indifference is apparent. Other desirable symptoms are client reports of lessened pain awareness during, for example, probing a previously sensitive tooth; and of feeling tingling, lightheadedness, a floating sensation, or waves of warmth over the entire body. A tingling sensation in the fingers and toes and then in the arms and the legs is usually one of the first symptoms reported, indicating a desirable level of sedation. The operator may begin by asking the client, "Do you feel any tingling in your fingers or toes or in your arms and legs?"

Reported feelings of heaviness in the chest or of vibration or spinning, although reflecting appropriate sedation for oral surgery treatment, are not symptoms of appropriate sedation levels for dental hygiene care. Instead, they indicate a need to turn down the nitrous oxide. If the client does not respond to questioning, this indicates that he or she has sunk below the desirable level of sedation. The operator should immediately decrease the liter flow of nitrous oxide and increase the oxygen by 2 L. If this does not produce a client response, 100% oxygen should be given.

Symptoms of Baseline Level of N_2O–O_2 Analgesia

Mental and physical relaxation
Indifference to surroundings and passage of time
Lessened pain awareness
Floating sensation
Drowsiness
Warmth
Tingling or numbness
Sounds seem distant

The point at which a relaxed state of floating sensation is reported can be taken as the baseline level of sedation. *Baseline* is the term used to designate the ideal minimal amount of nitrous oxide with oxygen needed to relax the client. Once baseline is obtained, the person should then be maintained at a slightly reduced nitrous oxide level by reducing the nitrous oxide level by 1 to 2 L and increasing the oxygen level by 1 to 2 L. See Symptoms of Baseline Level of N_2O–O_2 Analgesia.

The percentage of nitrous oxide delivered to the lungs determines the sedative effect on the central nervous system. Although individual reactions at any given concentration of nitrous oxide may vary greatly from individual to individual, a range of responses may occur at given concentrations, as summarized in Table 35–1.

EQUIPMENT

Cylinders

Nitrous oxide and oxygen[1] are dispensed in steel containers called *cylinders,* which are colored green for oxygen and blue for nitrous oxide (Figure 35–1). Cylinders should always be returned to the appropriate vendor for refilling. It is hazardous to refill a small cylinder from a larger one, and this should not be attempted by oral healthcare personnel. For quality control, cylinders are tested usually every 5 years by the manufacturer. The date of the test is permanently stamped on the cylinder. Cylinders should be stored in an upright position, away from a heat source, and chained to the wall to prevent them from falling on their cylinder valve stem, which could cause the cylinder to explode. In addition, at high pressures, oxygen and nitrous oxide can form an explosive mixture in the presence of grease or oil. Therefore, grease or oil should never be used on cylinder valves and gauges on the gas machine.

Cylinders may be stored directly on the gas machine (Figure 35–1) or in an area away from the gas machine (Figure 35–5). When cylinders are stored in an area away

TABLE 35–1 SIGNS AND SYMPTOMS IN RESPONSE TO NITROUS OXIDE AND OXYGEN CONSCIOUS SEDATION

Concentration N_2O	Response
10% to 20%	Body warmth
	Tingling of hands and feet
20% to 30%	Circumoral numbness
	Numbness of thighs
20% to 40%	Numbness of tongue
	Numbness of hands and feet
	Droning sounds present
	Hearing distinct but distant
	Dissociation begins and reaches peak
	Mild sleepiness
	Analgesia (maximum at 30%)
	Euphoria
	Feeling of heaviness or lightness of body
30% to 50%	Sweating
	Nausea
	Amnesia
	Increased sleepiness
40% to 60%	Dreaming, laughing, giddiness
	Further increased sleepiness, tending toward unconsciousness
	Increased nausea and vomiting
50% and over	Unconsciousness and light general anesthesia

From Bennett CR: *Conscious sedation in dental practice*, ed 2, St Louis, 1978, Mosby.

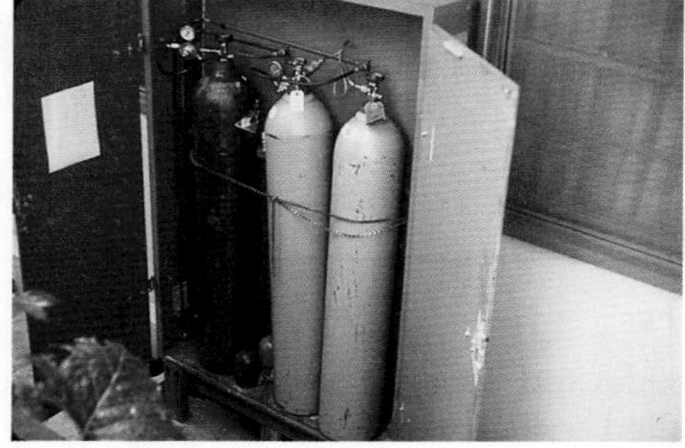

FIGURE 35–5 ✦ N_2O and O_2 cylinders stored in an area away from the gas machine.

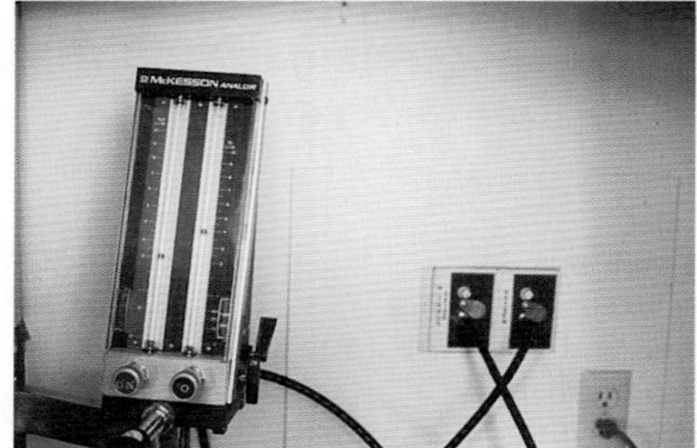

FIGURE 35–6 ✦ A quick-coupling type of outlet.

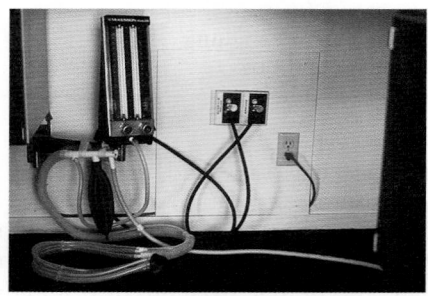

FIGURE 35–7 ✦ Gas machine with gas cylinder stored in an area away from the gas machine. Also shows quick-coupling outlet, reservoir bag, flowmeter, and gas hose.

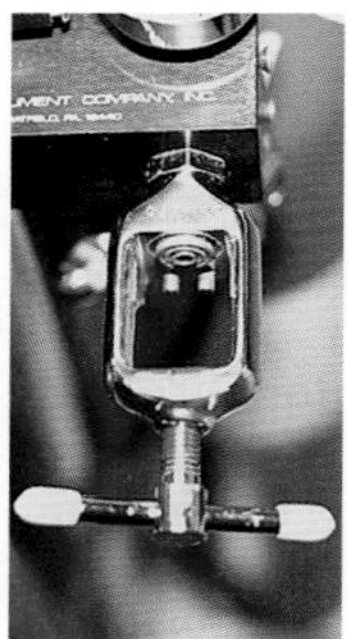

FIGURE 35–8 ✦ Yoke to hold cylinders in contact with gas machine. Note prongs that will insert into the valve stem of the gas cylinder.

from the gas machine, regulation copper tubing with a 3/8-inch outside diameter is fed through drilled holes in the wall to a quick-coupling type of outlet. A *quick-coupling outlet* is ideal because it permits rapid hookup and disengagement of the machine (Figure 35–6).

Gas Machine

N_2O–O_2 gas machines are available as a portable (Figure 35–1) or as a central system (Figure 35–7). Components of gas machines are yokes, control valves, flowmeters, pressure gauges, a reservoir bag, and a gas hose. *Yokes* hold the cylinders in contact with the gas machine (Figure 35–8). From each yoke, gas goes through an automatic pressure-reducing valve and then to a fine-control valve that allows the gas to be delivered to the client at 50 psi.

The *flowmeter* indicates the rate of flow of the gas. A small ball floats in the stream of gas that flows upward through a tapered tube. The greater the flow of volume of the gas used, the higher the ball rises. Separate color-coded flowmeters are used for nitrous oxide and oxygen, and each is calibrated to measure the volume of gas delivered (Figure 35–9). Flowmeters show the exact volume and proportions of gas output from the gas machine.

The *pressure gauge* indicates the pressure of the cylinder contents (Figures 35–2 and 35–3). The *reservoir bag* (Figure 35–7) is attached to the gas machine and is the site where the gases (nitrous oxide and oxygen) are mixed and stored so that the client has a plentiful supply upon which to draw for breathing. The *gas hose* delivers the gas mixture from the reservoir bag to the client's mask continually at the volumes and proportions set by the clinician on the flowmeter (Figure 35–7).

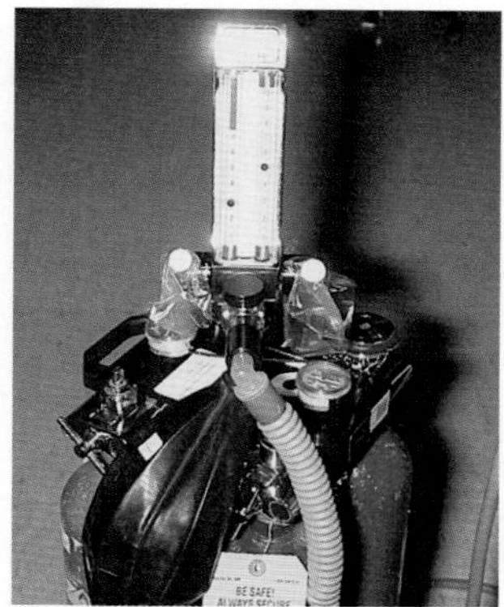

FIGURE 35–9 ✦ Flowmeter.

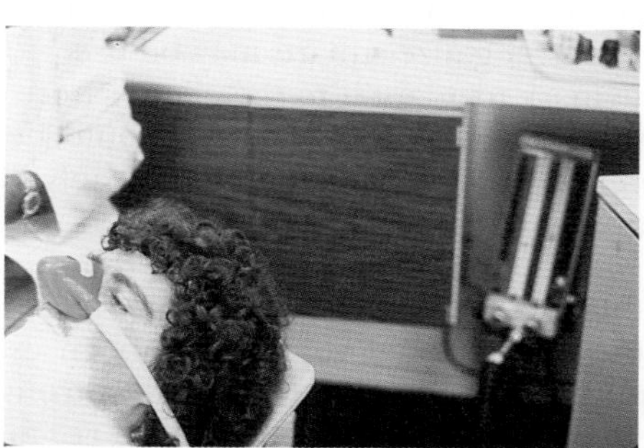

FIGURE 35–10 ✦ Mask with only one hose coming off each side of it, indicating there is no scavenger system in place.

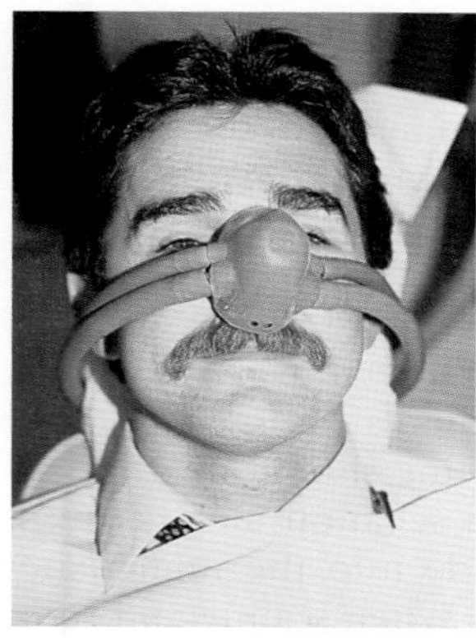

FIGURE 35–11 ✦ Mask with two hoses coming off each side of it, indicating that there is a scavenger system in place.

Mask

The mask is the nasal inhaler through which the client breathes the $N_2O–O_2$ analgesic. Masks come with and without a scavenger system. If there is no scavenger system in place, the mask has only one hose coming off each side of it (Figure 35–10). These two tubes carry the $N_2O–O_2$ to the client. If there is a scavenger system in place, the mask has two hoses coming off each side of it (Figure 35–11). One pair of hoses delivers the $N_2O–O_2$ and the other carries away the exhaled nitrous oxide–oxygen into the suction system. The purpose of a *scavenger system* is to reduce the nitrous oxide exhaled into the air by the client and thus breathed by the operator. Scavenger systems reduce the amount of nitrous oxide breathed into the environment from 900 parts per million (ppm) to 30 ppm. The ideal, maximal amount of $N_2O–O_2$ allowable in the healthcare environment is 50 ppm.

SAFETY MEASURES

Safety features are built into cylinders and gas machines to prevent the inadvertent delivery of nitrous oxide when one is intending to deliver oxygen to the client. These fail-safe mechanisms are listed and explained as follows:[2,5,9]

- Color-coded tanks
- Pin index system
- Diameter index system
- Audible alarm system
- Automatic turnoff
- O_2 automatically maintained at 2 to 3 L
- O_2 flush

Color Coding

Cylinders, quick-coupling tubing, outlets, and pressure gauges are color coded according to the gas they contain and monitor. Green indicates oxygen and blue indicates nitrous oxide.

Pin Indexing System

Prongs (pins) on the yoke that hold the oxygen cylinder and the corresponding holes on the oxygen cylinder head are placed a specific distance apart, which is different from their counterparts on the nitrous oxide yoke and cylinder (Figures 35–8 and 35–12). Thus the nitrous oxide cylinder does not fit in the yoke that is to hold the oxygen cylinder and vice versa. Also, to prevent delivering nitrous oxide to an individual in the mistaken belief that oxygen is being delivered, the connection for the cylinders and hoses for nitrous oxide does not fit to the oxygen hookups, and vice versa.

Diameter Indexing System

The diameter of the hole at the top of the oxygen cylinder and the corresponding diameter of the cylinder head that is inserted into the hole are different from the diameter of their counterparts on the nitrous oxide cylinder and cylinder head. Consequently, a cylinder head for a nitrous oxide cylinder does not fit into an oxygen cylinder. Thus a diameter indexing system prevents an override of the pin indexing system, and is another protective mechanism for assuring that an adequate supply of oxygen always is delivered to the client.

Indicators That Oxygen Is Depleted

Many gas machines have an alarm that goes off when the oxygen runs out. Other machines simply turn off automatically when the oxygen is depleted. These features prevent the operator from administering 100% nitrous oxide to the client.

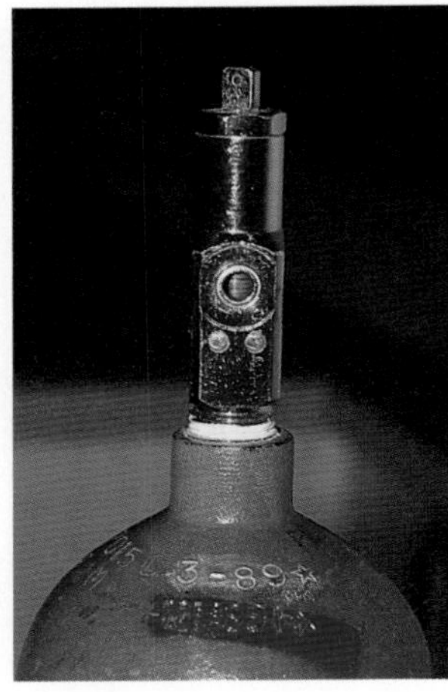

FIGURE 35–12 ✦ O_2 cylinder head, with holes placed at a specific distance apart to fit the prongs on the yoke that holds the O_2 cylinder.

Automatic Maintenance of Minimal Oxygen Levels

On most gas machines, the oxygen flowmeter cannot go below 2 to 3 L of oxygen. When the machine is turned on, the oxygen volume automatically goes to 2 to 3 L. This constant flow of oxygen is provided at all times when the gas machine is on, thus preventing the possibility of providing 100% nitrous oxide to the client.

Oxygen Flush Button

All machines have an oxygen flush button that, when pushed, fills the reservoir bag with 100% oxygen and enables a high flow rate of oxygen to the client very quickly, if needed.

TECHNIQUE OF ADMINISTRATION

Administration of $N_2O–O_2$ includes inducing the appropriate level of analgesia, monitoring the individual during the sedation period, and oxygenating the individual for the appropriate amount of time upon completion of treatment.

The office should have a quiet atmosphere throughout the sedation period. All oral healthcare personnel who interact with clients should have experienced personally the sensations produced by $N_2O–O_2$ sedation so that they can relate these feelings to the client. Preparation of armamentaria should be completed before seating the client. Upon seating clients, ask them if they need to visit the restroom. If they wear contact lenses, ask them to remove them because sometimes gas escaping from the mask can dry out the cornea and increase the risk of corneal abrasion.

After reviewing the health history and vital signs, the operator explains to the client what is about to happen and describes the sensations of warmth and tingling that will be experienced. For example, the operator tells clients that they will feel very relaxed, as if they have had a couple of alcoholic drinks. The dental hygiene operator assures clients that they are in complete control in the sense that if they feel they are receiving too much $N_2O–O_2$ sedation, they just need to inform the operator, who will turn down the nitrous oxide and turn up the oxygen.

The client's tidal volume is estimated. *Tidal volume* is the amount of air a person needs for one respiration cycle. For an average adult, it could be from 6 to 8 L, depending on the size and metabolic rate of the individual. A flow of oxygen is introduced based on the estimated tidal volume. For example, if the tidal volume is estimated to be 8 L, the oxygen flowmeter is set to 8 L of oxygen and the nose mask is placed over the nose and centered on the face snugly to prevent leakage at the edges of the mask. If the mask is too big and gas is escaping at its edges, a gauze square may be used to contour around the mask to adapt it to the client's nose and plug some of the leakage spaces. Clients should be asked if they have enough air to breathe comfortably. If they do not, the tidal volume should be increased. If the air is reported to be blowing up their nose, the tidal volume should be decreased.

Once the correct tidal volume has been established and documented in the client's record, nitrous oxide is introduced at the rate of 1 L per minute (L/min) while decreasing the oxygen flow at a similar rate. A 1- to 2-minute pause is made between each adjustment until the baseline state is reached. Generally, for dental hygiene care, 50% nitrous oxide or less is effective for achieving baseline. Once baseline is reached, the operator should drop back on the nitrous oxide flow about 0.5 to 1 L, because with time the intensity of the sedation increases. This *titration* technique minimizes the risk of overshooting baseline and causing a problem by carrying the person too deeply into the excitement stage of general anesthesia.

Once baseline is reached, the dental hygienist works efficiently and quietly, asking clients periodically how they are doing. Unnecessary talking should be avoided to allow clients to relate to the sedation and because their talking expels nitrous oxide into the immediate environment of the practitioner. When scaling and root planing are completed, the nitrous oxide should be turned off and the oxygen increased to maintain the tidal volume. For every 15 minutes of exposure to nitrous oxide, the client must receive 5 minutes of 100% oxygen. Thus, if clients receive 45 minutes of $N_2O–O_2$ sedation, they should receive 15 minutes of 100% oxygen. If clients are sedated for less than 5 minutes, they still should be oxygenated for a minimum of 5 minutes. This oxygenation period is essential to prevent tissue hypoxia, characterized by headache and upset stomach, upon completion of the sedation procedure.

The tidal volume, the time baseline was reached, and the amount or percentage of gases administered should be recorded in the client's chart. To calculate the percentage of gases administered, the flow rate of a specific gas is divided by the tidal volume and multiplied by 100.

For example, if the client's tidal volume (TV) is 7 L/min, the oxygen flow is 5 L/min, and the nitrous oxide flow rate is 2 L/min, the percentage of nitrous oxide delivered is $2/7 \times 100$, which is 29% of total flow, and the percentage of oxygen delivered is $5/7 \times 100$, which is 71%. Notation for documentation would be:

TV = 7 L
N_2O = 2/7 or 29%
O_2 = 5/7 or 71%

In addition to the tidal volume and the percentages of gases used, the duration of sedation, the length of the oxygenation period, the client's response, and the dental hygiene care delivered should all be documented in the client's chart (Figure 35–13).

The specific techniques for N_2O–O_2 administration are presented in Procedure 35–1.

Health Hx and vital signs WNL; TV = 7 L; N_2O = 2 L (29%); O_2 = 5 L (71%) for 45 minutes. Oxygenation period = 15 minutes. Client did well. Probing WNL scaled and polished. Excellent oral hygiene, no gingival inflammation observed throughout. Continued care interval 6 months.

FIGURE 35–13 ✦ Sample entry into client's record.

Procedure 35–1 ADMINISTRATION OF NITROUS OXIDE–OXYGEN ANALGESIA

EQUIPMENT

Personal protective equipment
Gas machine
Sterilized mask
Gauze
Saliva ejector

STEPS	RATIONALE
1. Prepare the gas machine and related armamentaria before seating the client. Select appropriate sterilized nasal mask for size and attach it to mask tubing.	Preparation of equipment when the client is seated may raise the anxiety level of the client.
2. Open gas cylinder valves and check on gas supply. Open oxygen tank slowly, then the nitrous oxide tank. (Centralized systems are turned on at the beginning of the day.)	This check enables the operator to replenish the gas supply to ensure that adequate gas is available for the procedure.

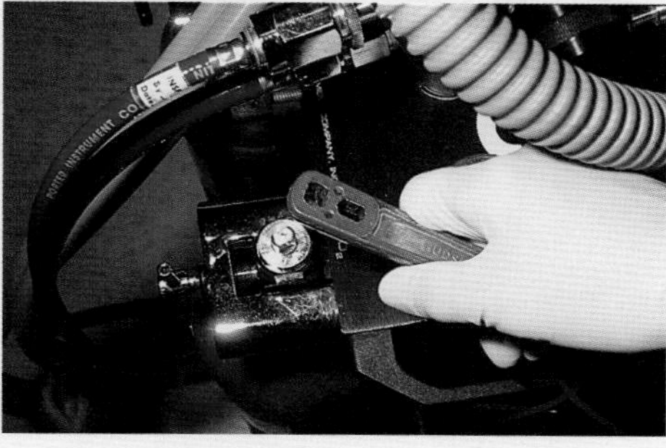

FIGURE 35–14 ✦ Opening gas cylinder valves.

STEPS	RATIONALE
3. Adjust scavenger system. Obtain suction calibrator.	Adjusting the suction calibrator allows the operator to obtain the optimal level of suction for the scavenger system.

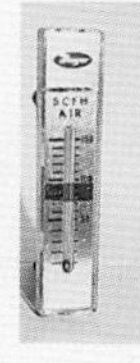

FIGURE 35–15 ✦ Suction calibration.

STEPS	RATIONALE
4. Attach the suction calibrator to the high-speed vacuum system and adjust the suction until the steel ball in the calibrator is made to float in the clear zone of the calibrator's window.	Calibrating the degree of suction in the high-suction vacuum system ensures that the suction removes the exhaled nitrous oxide–oxygen at an appropriate rate—not so fast that gas is removed before air has been inhaled, and not so slow that gas overaccumulates in the mask and leaks into the breathing zone of the operator.

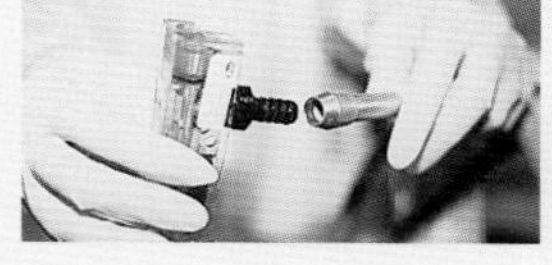

FIGURE 35–16 ✦ Connect suction calibrator to high-speed vacuum.

Continued on following page

Procedure 35–1 ADMINISTRATION OF NITROUS OXIDE–OXYGEN ANALGESIA—CONT'D

STEPS	RATIONALE
5. Remove the suction calibrator from the high-speed suction system and tape the button used to adjust the suction in place.	Taping the suction adjustment button in place prevents it from being moved and altering the degree of suction available.
6. The sterilized nose mask connects to two hoses coming off each side of it.	One pair of hoses delivers the $N_2O–O_2$ to the client and the other pair carries away the exhaled $N_2O–O_2$ into the suction system, thus providing a scavenger system.

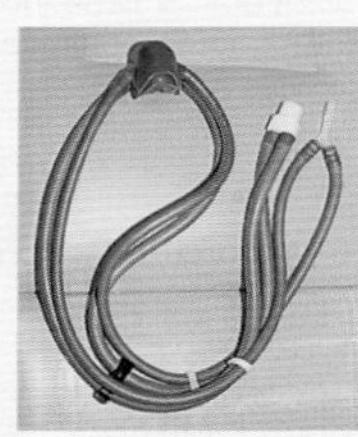

FIGURE 35–17 ✦ Nose mask with two pairs of hoses.

Each pair of hoses is joined by an adaptor. The larger adaptor connects to the gas machine. The smaller adaptor connects to the high-speed suction system.

STEPS	RATIONALE
7. Attach the smaller adaptor on the nose mask to the calibrated high-speed vacuum system.	This connection allows the exhaled $N_2O–O_2$ to be suctioned from the airway, ensuring that nitrous oxide concentration breathed by the operator is reduced to 30 to 50 ppm from 900 ppm.

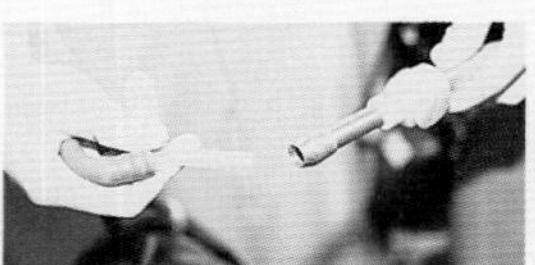

FIGURE 35–18 ✦ Attaching adaptor on nose mask to high-speed suction to provide for the scavenging system.

STEPS	RATIONALE
8. Attach the larger adaptor of the sterilized nose mask to the gas machine. Turn on the gas machine.	This connection carries the gas mixture (of proportions preset by the clinician) to the client from the reservoir bag.

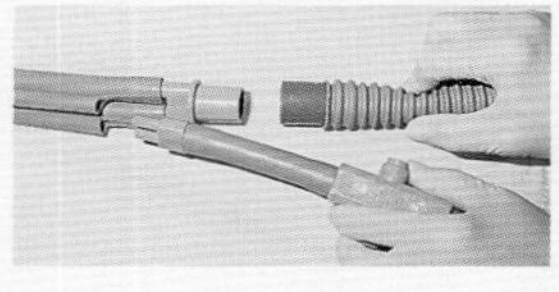

FIGURE 35–19 ✦ Attaching the larger adaptor of the sterilized nose mask to the gas machine.

STEPS	RATIONALE
9. Seat the client; check and record the health history, blood pressure, and pulse.	To meet clients' human need for safety, it is essential that their health and vital signs are within normal limits before providing dental hygiene care.

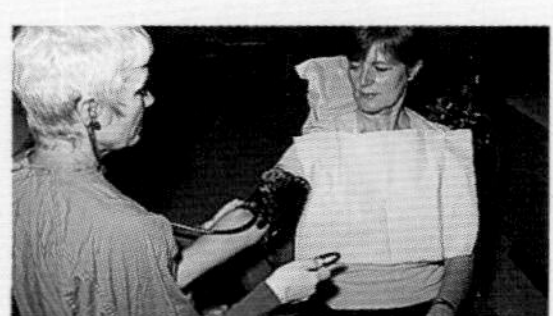

FIGURE 35–20 ✦ Checking client's blood pressure.

STEPS	RATIONALE
10. Familiarize client with procedures; discuss nasal breathing and nose mask, and describe sensations of warmth and tingling that will be experienced; reaffirm the relaxing, comfortable feeling the client will experience. Assure clients that they will be aware of and in control of their actions.	Informing clients about what they can expect to experience with nitrous oxide–oxygen sedation helps prevent behavior problems based on the fear of the unknown, of going unconscious. In addition, studies report that providing information to individuals receiving a drug increases pain thresholds and tolerance of pain. These findings suggest that influencing the thought process in conjunction with giving analgesia can increase the depth of sedation.

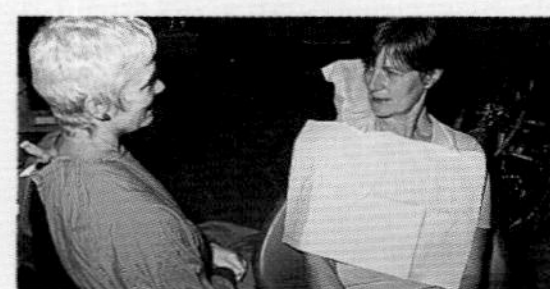

FIGURE 35–21 ✦ Familiarizing client with procedures.

Procedure 35–1 ADMINISTRATION OF NITROUS OXIDE–OXYGEN ANALGESIA—CONT'D

STEPS	RATIONALE
11. Start oxygen flow at estimated tidal volume (6 to 8 L/min).	This estimate provides a reasonable amount of oxygen as a basis for determining the exact tidal volume.

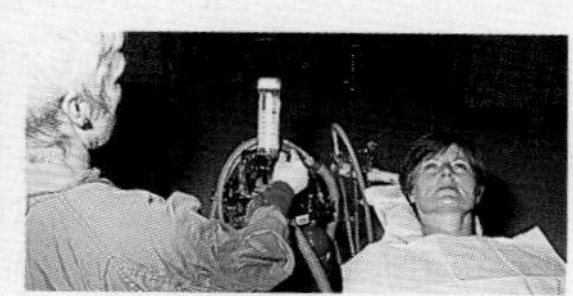

FIGURE 35–22 ✦ Starting oxygen flow at estimated tidal volume.

STEPS	RATIONALE
12. Activate oxygen flush valve to fill the reservoir bag with oxygen.	Filling the reservoir bag with oxygen ensures that there is enough oxygen available for the client's first couple of breaths.

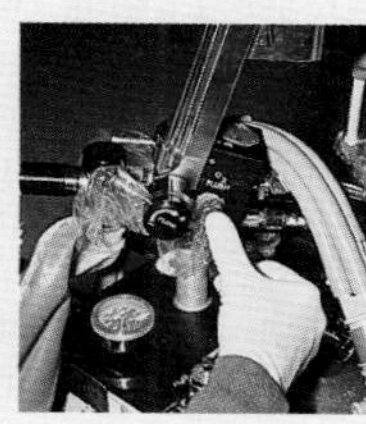

FIGURE 35–23 ✦ Activating O_2 flush.

STEPS	RATIONALE
13. Have client seat the nose mask on him- or herself and adjust it so it is comfortable. Then, operator should adjust nose mask tubing to hold the mask in place, and confirm comfortable fit with the client.	Personal placement and adjustment of the mask by the client ensure a comfortable fit; adjustment of mask tubing holds nose mask in place and ensures a minimum amount of gas leakage from the mask.

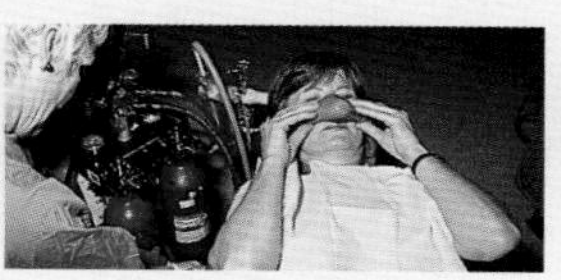

FIGURE 35–24 ✦ Client seating nose mask.

STEPS	RATIONALE
14. If mask is impinging on a sensitive area on the face or if the mask is too big, place a gauze square under the edge of the mask.	The gauze square makes the mask feel more comfortable if there is a sensitive area and closes any leakage if the mask is too big.

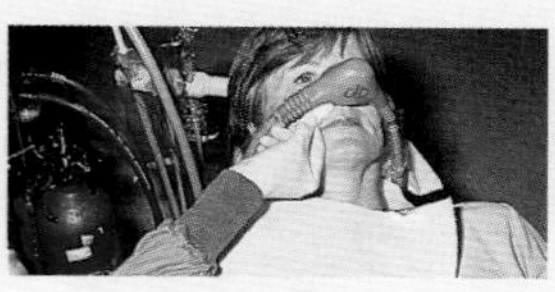

FIGURE 35–25 ✦ Placing gauze square.

STEPS	RATIONALE
15. Determine exact tidal volume by asking the client if he or she has enough air to breathe comfortably. Adjust volume of oxygen as per client response.	This determination provides the client with an adequate and comfortable amount of gas per respiration.

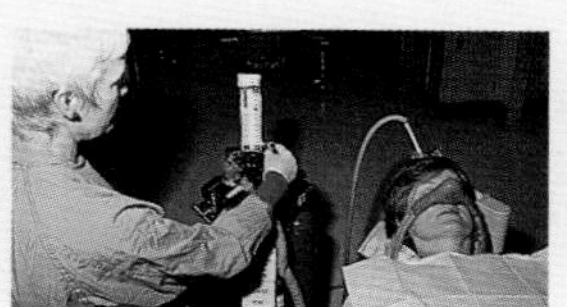

FIGURE 35–26 ✦ Determining tidal volume.

STEPS	RATIONALE
16. Introduce nitrous oxide in increments of 0.5 to 1 L/min and reduce oxygen by a corresponding amount.	Slow introduction of nitrous oxide allows the operator to find the baseline for the individual and ensures that the client is not oversedated. Decreasing the oxygen the same amount that nitrous oxide is increased maintains the established tidal volume.

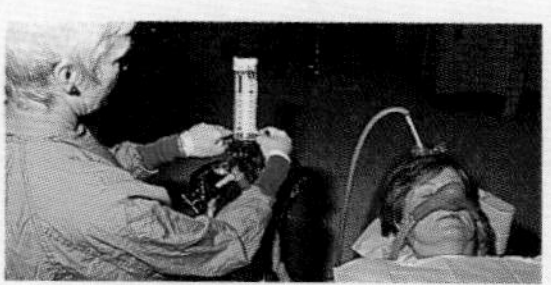

FIGURE 35–27 ✦ Introducing nitrous oxide.

Continued on following page

Procedure 35–1 ADMINISTRATION OF NITROUS OXIDE–OXYGEN ANALGESIA—CONT'D

STEPS	RATIONALE
17. Repeat step 14 at 60-second intervals until a baseline level is established. (This is called titration.)	There is a great deal of individual variation as to the amount of nitrous oxide one needs to achieve baseline. Usually the optimal concentration of nitrous oxide does not exceed 35%.
18. Determine client's baseline level using subjective symptoms and objective signs and document baseline nitrous oxide and oxygen volumes (or concentrations) as well as the time that baseline is established in the client record.	Documenting baseline levels provides a reference for future nitrous oxide–oxygen sedation procedures. Noting time baseline is necessary to determine oxygenation period before dismissing the client.
19. Monitor client and reassure as necessary; comment on how comfortable and relaxed the client seems.	Checking with clients periodically about their comfort level allows the operator to reduce or increase nitrous oxide concentration as needed. The client should never be left alone while under nitrous oxide–oxygen sedation in case the level of sedation needs to be lowered or in case of emergency. Persons under nitrous oxide–oxygen sedation are very suggestible.
20. If nausea, sleepiness, dreaming, vertigo, repeated closing of the mouth, a rigid mandible, or restlessness is observed by the operator or reported by the client, reduce the percentage of nitrous oxide by 2 L/min to lighten the level of sedation.	These signs and symptoms indicate that the concentration of nitrous oxide is too high and the client is no longer comfortable.
21. When baseline is achieved, proceed with the care plan.	At this level of sedation, the client is relaxed and comfortable.
22. Near the end of the appointment (e.g., during tooth polishing), discontinue the nitrous oxide and increase the oxygen concentration to 100%. Oxegenate 5 minutes for every 15 minutes of exposure to N_2O–O_2.	Oxygenating clients 5 minutes for every 15 minutes of nitrous oxide exposure prevents diffusion hypoxia.
23. Remove the nose mask and slowly bring the client to an upright position.	Bringing the client to an upright position in an abrupt manner may cause syncope.

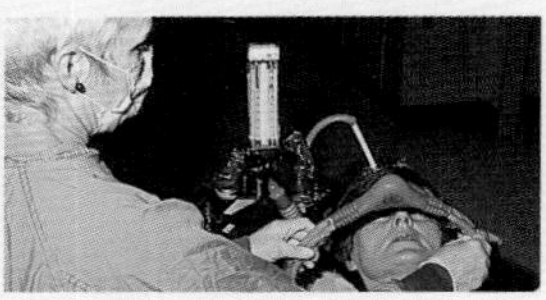

FIGURE 35–28 ✦ Removing nose mask.

STEPS	RATIONALE
24. If the client feels normal, discharge him or her.	After the appropriate oxygenation period, there is no additional recovery time needed if the individual states that he or she feels normal.

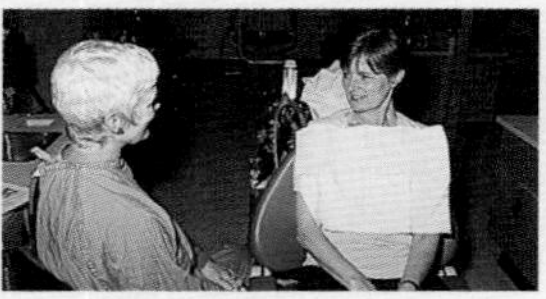

FIGURE 35–29 ✦ Assessing if client feels normal before discharging him or her.

STEPS	RATIONALE
25. Document the experience in the client's record. Note vital signs, concentrations of nitrous oxide and oxygen administered, length of time of sedation and oxygenation, the care provided, and the client's response to the sedation.	This documentation provides a legal record of care and serves as a reference for future care and administration of nitrous oxide–oxygen conscious sedation.

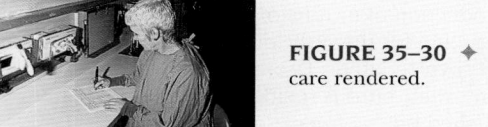

FIGURE 35–30 ✦ Documenting care rendered.

POTENTIAL COMPLICATIONS[1]

Complications associated with $N_2O–O_2$ can be mitigated by carefully selecting candidates based on their health and personal history, and by adopting the technique described in Procedure 35–1 for the administration of this sedation modality. Specifically, inducing clients to an individualized baseline level by the process of titration and oxygenating them for an appropriate amount of time facilitate the avoidance of some complications with this somewhat innocuous agent. The following is a list and individual description of the possible complications associated with $N_2O–O_2$ sedation:[1]

- Diffusion hypoxia
- Head injury during expectoration
- Nausea
- Vomiting
- Corneal irritation
- Behavior problems
- Airway obstruction
- Repeated closing of the mouth
- Rigid mandible
- Reluctance to awaken
- Emotional reaction
- Excessive perspiration

Diffusion Hypoxia

Diffusion hypoxia, a lack of oxygen to the tissues, is characterized by headache, grogginess, nausea, and what generally may be described as a "hungover" feeling after exposure to $N_2O–O_2$ analgesia. This complication is related to not being oxygenated for an appropriate period following the completion of the sedation procedure.

Head Injury During Expectoration

Sedated clients are at risk for bumping their heads on the cuspidor if they attempt to expectorate while under sedation. Consequently, a saliva ejector or high-vacuum suction should be used in place of allowing the client to rinse or expectorate into a cuspidor. If such expectoration cannot be avoided, however, the clinician should place her or his hand on the client's forehead to guide the client to the cuspidor and prevent possible injury.

Nausea and Vomiting

Nausea and vomiting are associated with giving the client too much $N_2O–O_2$ sedation, although it also may occur when the client consumes a heavy meal before the dental hygiene care appointment. In addition, nausea can be brought on by fluctuating the nitrous oxide levels back and forth during the titration process. For example, giving a client 3 L of nitrous oxide then increasing the amount to 5 L and decreasing it back down to 4 L and then back up to 6 L in a short period can produce nausea. If a client indicates nausea (either verbally by self-report or nonverbally by holding the stomach), the nitrous oxide should be turned down by 2 L and oxygen should be increased by 2 L. If the nausea persists, nitrous oxide should be discontinued and the client should be given 100% oxygen for an appropriate oxygenation period.

If vomiting occurs, the nitrous oxide must be turned off immediately, the mask removed, and the client's head tipped forward over the cuspidor to facilitate emesis. A high-vacuum suction may be used to facilitate removal of vomitus. Give the client a cool, wet towel to clean up, and clean the treatment area as quickly as possible. Reassure the individual that he or she will feel better after breathing 100% oxygen.

Corneal Irritation

Leakage of gas from the mask can dry out the eyes and cause corneal abrasion in individuals wearing contact lenses. This problem can be prevented by having clients remove their contact lenses before administering the $N_2O–O_2$ sedation to them.

Behavioral Problems

Several types of behavioral problems can be associated with $N_2O–O_2$ sedation. Repeated closing of the mouth and a rigidity of the mandible are usually signs of too much nitrous oxide. Turning the nitrous oxide down by 2 L and increasing the oxygen by 2 L eliminates the problem.

Individuals who do not like to give up control are often threatened by the tingling and floating feelings characteristic of this mode of sedation. As a result, they may respond by suddenly sitting forward and taking off the mask because of fear of the unknown or of becoming unconscious. This problem can be prevented by carefully screening candidates for this sedation method, thoroughly explaining what they can expect to experience, and never talking clients into having it unless they express a desire for this type of anxiety and pain control.

Individuals who are going through a period of emotional instability may be prone to crying under the influence of $N_2O–O_2$ sedation. If this occurs, the nitrous oxide should be discontinued and 100% oxygen should be given for an appropriate oxygenation period. Careful screening of candidates before offering this sedation modality prevents this problem, which can be embarrassing to both client and clinician.

Sexual fantasies and attempts at amorous behavior have been reported in individuals who have been given nitrous oxide concentration greater than 50% and who were sedated without an assistant as a witness in the room.[10] Decreasing the amount of nitrous oxide by at least 2 L and increasing the oxygen by a corresponding amount may solve the problem. If not, the nitrous oxide should be discontinued and 100% oxygen given to the client for an appropriate amount of time. Individuals who respond with this type of behavior problem should not be judged harshly because they have placed themselves in the care of the clinician and have allowed their sense of reality to be altered based on the trust and confidence they have in the clinician. It is the responsibility of the clinician to protect the client while the client is under the clinician's care.

Equipment Malfunction

Contaminated nitrous oxide cylinders can contain nitrogen dioxide and on administration may produce nitric acid with serious consequences to a client. Valves on the nitrous oxide cylinders must be kept closed when not in use to prevent this dire circumstance from occurring.[1]

Hazards to Personnel

The effects of chronic exposure to nitrous oxide (1000 to 15,000 ppm) reported in animal[11] and human studies of operating room personnel and of oral surgeons and others who used nitrous oxide in their practice[12-15] include the following:

- Spontaneous abortion
- Birth defects
- Bone marrow depression
- Anemia
- Hepatic and renal diseases
- Cancer

Hazardous concentrations of nitrous oxide in the oral healthcare setting can be reduced from 900 ppm to 30 ppm using a combination of the following methods:

- Using a nitrous oxide scavenging system
- Fitting the nasal mask to the client as well as possible
- Discouraging client conversation and mouth breathing
- Venting the suction machine containing the exhaled gases outside the building
- Using a fan to direct the nitrous oxide away from the breathing zone of the operator
- Maintaining the anesthetic equipment, testing for leakage, and inspecting the connectors at frequent intervals
- Monitoring nitrous oxide in the oral healthcare environment; a badge can be worn to detect nitrous oxide levels in the operator's breathing zone
- Opening a window in the treatment area to improve air circulation or using a nonrecycling air conditioning system
- Limiting the duration of nitrous oxide exposure for clients
- Shutting off and securing the equipment at the end of each day that it is used

Client Education Issues

- Explain what N_2O–O_2 analgesia is and what it does
- Explain the sensations that will be experienced and describe them in positive terms (e.g., warmth, tingling).
- Explain that clients are in control and responsive at all times. If they feel they are receiving too much sedation, they just need to say so and the hygienist will turn down the N_2O and turn up the O_2.
- Advise no heavy meals, alcohol, or fasting before the appointment.
- Explain the importance of contact lens removal to avoid extreme drying of the eyes resulting from gas leaks around the mask, which could lead to corneal abrasion.

Legal, Ethical, and Safety Issues

- It is the legal responsibility of the dental hygienist to practice within the scope authorized by state law concerning N_2O–O_2 analgesia administration.
- It is important to gain informed consent.
- It is imperative that the dental hygienist carefully evaluate the client's health history to determine suitability for N_2O–O_2 sedation.
- It is the responsibility of the dental hygienist to protect the client while the client is under the influence of N_2O–O_2 sedation during dental hygiene care.
- The dental hygienist must completely document the provision of N_2O–O_2 sedation in the client's record, including the client's condition upon leaving the dental hygiene care setting.

KEY CONCEPTS

- Nitrous oxide delivered in combination with oxygen is an inhalation method of conscious sedation known as $N_2O–O_2$ analgesia. It relaxes individuals who are mildly apprehensive about the dental or dental hygiene experience and provides pain control for procedures that are only slightly or moderately painful.
- Oxygen is present in a compressed-gas cylinder in a gaseous state.
- Nitrous oxide is present in a compressed-gas cylinder in a liquid and gaseous state.
- The treatment of entry into the excitement stage of analgesia is increasing the percentage of oxygen immediately to 100%.
- Light anesthesia rather than relative analgesia may be indicated by the patient becoming hyperresponsive to stimuli and producing exaggerated inspiration.
- Subjective symptoms of relative analgesia include heaviness of limbs, floating sensation, tingling, decreased fear, decreased pain memory, desire to maintain that state, feeling of warmth, and decreased awareness of time.
- Objective signs of a desired level of sedation are normal eye reaction and pupil size, normal blood pressure and pulse, ability to answer questions, and relaxation of hands, fingers, and mandible.
- Headache, grogginess and a "hangover" feeling after $N_2O–O_2$ are symptoms of diffusion hypoxia.
- Relative contraindications to $N_2O–O_2$ include breathing difficulties, communication problems, epilepsy, and emotional instability.
- $N_2O–O_2$ sedation may be particularly useful for clients with a history of hypertension, asthma, and cardiovascular disease.
- Nausea following $N_2O–O_2$ exposure may be easily induced by fluctuating the nitrous oxide delivery.
- Oversedation with nitrous oxide may be manifested by loss of consciousness.
- Following the administration of $N_2O–O_2$ analgesia, oxygen alone should be given for a minimum of 3 to 5 minutes before releasing the client.
- When adjusting the proportions of nitrous oxide and oxygen to achieve the desired level of analgesia, each adjustment should be at the rate of 1/2 to 1 liter nitrous oxide for at least 1 minute.
- A scavenger system incorporated into the $N_2O–O_2$ units takes out nitrous oxide that is exhaled through the mask.
- The ideal maximum room air concentration of nitrous oxide is 50 parts per million.
- The effects of chronic exposure to nitrous oxide may include spontaneous abortion, birth defects, bone marrow depression, anemia, hepatic and renal diseases, and cancer.
- To reduce nitrous oxide exposure, the dental hygienist uses a scavenging mask system, discourages unnecessary client talking, and has all the equipment leak-tested regularly.
- Before placing the mask on the client, a predetermined mixture of nitrous oxide and oxygen should *never* be established.
- The nitrous oxide blood/gas solubility coefficient of 0.47 accounts for rapid onset and rapid recovery of nitrous oxide sedation.
- The ideal minimal amount of nitrous oxide needed for a client is referred to as the baseline.

CRITICAL THINKING EXERCISES

1. You administer 3 L of N_2O and 3 L of O_2 for 30 minutes to a client. Just as you are finishing the scaling procedure, the client complains of nausea. You oxygenate the client for 15 minutes and after determining the client is fine, dismiss him. What *exactly* would you write in the treatment record?
2. List five client symptoms that would indicate to you, the operator, to decrease the amount of N_2O at least 2 liters and increase the oxygen by the same amount.
3. The flowmeters indicate that the client is receiving 4 L of nitrous oxide and 6 L of oxygen. What is the tidal volume and the proportion of nitrous oxide that is being delivered?
4. Scenario:

Client: Ms. G

Profile: A 35-year-old female presents for dental hygiene care. She wears contact lenses.

Chief Complaint: "My teeth really need to be cleaned. I have finally got up my courage to come in and have it done."

Dental History: Client makes regular dental visits, but she is 12 months overdue for her dental hygiene care appointment. She reports her teeth are sensitive.

Social History: Client is single and lives with her mother.

Continued on following page

CRITICAL THINKING EXERCISES—CONT'D

Medical History: Client's blood pressure is 140/90. She reports she is trying to control it with diet and exercise and is under the care of her physician.

Oral Self-care Assessment: Client reports brushing once a day, but does not floss or use any other interdental cleaning device.

Supplemental Notes: Client presents with moderate subgingival calculus and gingival inflammation throughout. Mesial and distal probing depths of 4 to 5 mm are in all posterior teeth.

A. How would you use this information in planning dental hygiene care to meet the client's need for freedom from stress? What interventions would you plan and why?

B. Would N_2O–O_2 be beneficial for her? Explain your response.

C. What would you say in educating Ms. G about her stress-control options during her dental hygiene care appointment?

For References, Suggested Readings, and Related Websites, visit

http://evolve.elsevier.com/Darby/hygiene/

SECTION 7

Dental Hygiene Care for Individuals with Special Needs

CHAPTER 36

PERSONS WITH DISABILITIES

OBJECTIVES

Mastery of the content of this chapter will enable the reader to:

- Identify barriers to healthcare for clients with disabilities
- Explain how stereotypes and public attitudes affect the acceptance of physically and mentally challenged persons
- Design a dental hygiene care facility that meets the federal barrier-free design standards for accessibility
- Contrast *disability* and *handicap* by definition and example
- Identify positive and negative portrayal issues associated with persons with special needs
- Distinguish between congenital, developmental, and acquired disabilities
- Describe assistive devices for activities of daily living
- Assess range of motion, grip strength, and finger closure when designing oral hygiene assistive devices
- Stabilize a client during wheelchair transfers and professional care
- Advocate for clients with special needs

KEY TERMS

Acquired disability
Activities of daily living (ADLs)
Assistive devices
Autonomic dysreflexia
Barrier-free design
Decubitus ulcers
Deinstitutionalization
Dependency
Developmental disability
Discrimination
Disability
Functional status
Handicap
Independence
Mainstreaming
Mouthstick
Normalization
Range of motion
Transfer belt
Transfer board
Transfer techniques (one person, two person, and semidependent)
Universal strap
Wheelchairs

LEGISLATION FOR DISABLED PERSONS

Disabled individuals face obstacles that limit their access to healthcare, education, and employment opportunities. Access to these services is essential for persons to function at an acceptable level of health and wellness and maintain as much *independence* as possible. Other barriers include limited financial resources, lack of transportation, inadequate housing, poor environmental design of existing facilities, and limited access to personal and vocational rehabilitation services.

Normalization is a process that enables mentally challenged citizens to engage in normal patterns of everyday life. The outcome is *mainstreaming,* which means incorporating special needs persons into conventional activities. This concept promotes *deinstitutionalization* of mentally challenged persons capable of living and functioning independently with little or no assistance from a caregiver. Mainstreaming is the goal of long-term care providers and educators assisting people with disabilities.

Mainstreaming disabled people created a host of problems—problems that demanded immediate attention and resources, most of which were either unavailable or nonexistent. Groups of individuals with disabilities (e.g., disabled veterans) organized cooperative efforts to address the needs of specific population groups. Many of these organizations grew into nationwide networks. Their efforts greatly influence standards to ensure equal opportunities for the disabled.

In 1975, the *Education for All Handicapped Children Act (Public Law 94-142)* was passed to ensure all disabled children the right to an adequate education. This law, which is the culmination of years of advocacy via state and national legislation, mandated diagnostic testing to determine the extent of the child's disability, that the test be given in the native language of the child, that the child has the right to attorney representation for protection, and that the parents or legal guardians of the child have access to all information obtained through diagnostic testing. Because there are certain societal stigmas to classifying a child as *handicapped* within the school system, classification and diagnostic standards are built into this law to promote accurate confirmation of a diagnosis of a learning or mental disability. In addition, the diagnostic process must lead to the categorization of the child's disability to enable the child to be eligible for state and federal aid. It is unethical to classify a child as *disabled* without providing an educational opportunity to assist with his or her development.

Discrimination in the Workplace

The *U.S. Vocational Rehabilitation Act of 1973, Section 503,* requires all employers with federal contracts over $2500 to take affirmative action in employing and advancing qualified disabled employees. This law helps prevent *discrimination* against hiring a disabled individual by enforcing the removal of job-related criteria that prohibit employing a disabled person and by demanding that the workplace be architecturally accessible.

Section 504 of the *Rehabilitation Act of 1973* and the *Americans with Disabilities Act of 1992* resulted in the most significant and lasting effects in removing barriers for the disabled, by guaranteeing that:

> No otherwise qualified person shall, by reason of his/her handicap, be discriminated against in the areas of education, employment, or social services including healthcare.

Physical Barriers to Independent Living

The *Americans with Disabilities Act of 1992* mandated universal changes nationwide, perhaps most notably the barrier-free design, which enabled wheelchair accessibility to public buildings. This law strengthened existing legislation for improved telecommunication systems for sensory-impaired people and the development of closed-captioned television programs, which were first developed under *Section 504* of the *Rehabilitation Act of 1973.*

Barrier-free design enables a person to function independently both within and outside of the home environment. Barrier-free oral healthcare environments facilitate the disabled person's human needs for responsibility and freedom from health risks. Furthermore, such settings are an indication that healthcare providers who staff the facility appreciate the needs of the disabled, respect them as human beings, and value them as clients.

The concept of *continuous sequence* is used when constructing these facilities, meaning that all aspects of the design are interrelated without limiting the use of any parts of the facility. For example, a building that contains elevators and accessible restrooms is not considered truly barrier-free if there are no ramps or electronically operated doors to gain entrance to the building.

Specific building codes and architectural standards for a barrier-free facility are available from federal and state resources. These guidelines are applicable to all types of buildings, whether in public or private domain (see Basic Design Characteristics for a Barrier-Free Facility).

Barriers to Transportation

One aspect of accessibility that is frequently overlooked is mass transportation services. Subways, buses, rail systems, and airplanes provide only limited assistance to the disabled, despite federal regulations that require modifications for greater ease of use by disabled people. The *Urban Mass Transportation Act of 1974, Section 16,* states that disabled and elderly people have the same rights as others to use mass transportation facilities and services. This law also requires that federal programs providing assistance in mass transportation support these rights by building accessible transportation services.

Many stations and transportation vehicles remain inaccessible today, partly because the ratio of disabled persons to nondisabled persons is low, and efforts required to renovate are costly. When modifications are made, renovation expenses are passed along to passengers, driving transportation costs upward. The expense of traveling then becomes an additional barrier to disabled people, who are usually on fixed incomes and unable to afford transportation services anyway. These persons often rely on others for transportation to and from their homes, which may not always be convenient for the driver or for the disabled person.

Public transportation services can be difficult and frustrating for everyone. Interpreting the schedule, finding the exact fare, waiting at a boarding stop during inclement weather, boarding the right vehicle, and tracking the number of stops can be extremely difficult for someone with a physical or mental impairment. Not surprisingly, many disabled people do not use mass transportation, but choose to remain at home rather than risk travel.

BARRIERS TO HEALTHCARE

Cost

Even though federal mandates have increased availability of services to disabled people, cost remains the primary barrier to most services. Financial resources are needed to obtain an education, to participate in rehabilitative programs, to train for a job, to find adequate housing, to utilize basic transportation services, and just to survive. State and federal funds fail to cover the costs of everyone's needs, forcing many disabled people to prioritize

Basic Design Characteristics for a Barrier-Free Facility

Parking. One space per 25 spaces should be allotted for those who are disabled. Space width must be a minimum of 96 inches wide, and should be clearly marked with a sign posted 5 feet above street level. Spaces should be located closest to the nearest accessible ramp and/or building entrance.

Ramps. Ramps should be located at all curbs and should be close to the building entrance. Ramp elevation should not exceed 36 inches, with a slope not to exceed 1:12 inches. A minimum of one handrail should be present at a height of 32 inches and should extend for the length of the rampway. No lip should be present at the junction of the ramp with the platform or sidewalk. If outside, a nonskid surface must be used, preferably with a snow-melting device.

Doors. At least one accessible doorway with access to elevators should be present. Doors should be made of a clear material to permit viewing of the approach. Doorways must be a minimum of 32 inches wide to permit clear wheelchair passage, preferably with an additional 4 to 8 inches to limit bumping against the doorframe. Doorframes should be flush with the floor. Door weight should not exceed 8 pounds. Electronically operated doors are preferred, and may be constructed with either a sensing device that causes doors to open automatically, or with a wall-mounted button to operate the opening. Closure of the doors should be timed for adequate clearance through the doorway. Lever handles, as opposed to doorknobs, should be no higher than 48 inches above the floor.

Stairs. Outside stairs should have a nonskid surface, with a handrail height at 32 inches. Riser height should not exceed 6 inches. Inside stair design is the same, although riser height may be as great as 7 inches. All stairwells should be clearly marked and lighted. No protrusions that may cause tripping should extend beyond the riser.

Elevators. Elevators must be installed in all buildings with two or more floors. The minimum size of the elevator cab is 5 feet deep and 5 1/2 feet wide. Doors should allow for maximal clearance of a wheelchair, and should have a sensing device for safety of entering passengers. Buttons should be clearly marked and at a height no more than 4 feet from the floor. Controls should be marked with Braille for blind clients and should have voice-activated announcements upon arrival at each floor.

Corridors. Hallways must be a minimum of 48 inches wide, preferably 64 inches wide to accommodate two passing wheelchairs. Adequate space should be available to allow a 360-degree turn in a wheelchair without bumping into the wall. Hallways should be clearly marked with signs no higher than 5 feet above the floor, and should always be lighted.

Signs. Signs should be easily read, and should contain bright, contrasting colors. Signs should be posted no higher than 5 feet above the floor. Braille and/or raised lettering is needed for blind clients. Alarms should contain both a visual and an audible warning announcement to accommodate both hearing and visually impaired clients.

Restrooms. Stall sizes should be a minimum of 3 feet wide by 5 feet deep, with an out-swinging door of 32 inches clearance. Toilets should be wall-mounted, with the seat no higher than 17 inches. Grab bars should be wall-mounted for easy access throughout the stall. Sinks should be wall-mounted, with a 27-inch minimal clearance from the floor. Faucets should be of a lever type or have buttons with a slow, timed release of water. Soap and towel dispensers should be no more than 4 feet above the floor. Automatic sensors are available for toilet flushing and for water dispensing in the sink.

Floor coverings. Floors should be covered in a nonskid surface. Seamless linoleum floors are preferred; however, if carpeting is present, it should be a smooth, low pile to prevent snagging of wheels or other devices. Area rugs and doormats should be eliminated.

Water fountains. Fountains should be wall-mounted, with a minimal clear space of 27 inches above the floor. Controls should be located at the front of the fountain with a push-plate or lever to operate.

Telephones. Telephones should not be placed in booths and should have a clearance of 27 inches above the floor. Controls should be located between 3 and 4 feet from the floor. Devices for raising and lowering the volume should be available for hearing-impaired people.

their spending, often at the expense of basic needs. Most disabled people rely on state and federal support (e.g., Social Security payments) to cover daily living expenses. Those individuals who are able to work earn low wages, and unemployment rates remain relatively high.

Without adequate funds for daily expenses, healthcare is often neglected. Most cannot afford private healthcare insurance and rely on Medicare and Medicaid reimbursement for financial assistance. For those on a limited income without insurance, money for healthcare services is an out-of-pocket expense; healthcare is often sought on an episodic basis, specifically for emergencies or pain control. For those living in an institution, medical and limited dental services may be provided, but high fees may be associated with these services, the cost of which is passed on to either family or state. If a severely disabled person needs to be institutionalized, costs to the family may drain their financial resources. Many families choose to care for a severely disabled individual at home because the cost of long-term care is too great a burden for the family.

The fact that more disabled persons now live outside of institutional settings means that more of them need to be treated within the private sector. Some private practitioners choose not to treat disabled individuals because reimbursement for services through Medicare and Medicaid is often not equivalent to the fee schedules charged in the area. In fact, eligibility requirements for Medicare and Medicaid may actually limit access to oral care services for mainstreamed residents that otherwise would have been provided in an institutional setting. In addition, extra time is often needed to treat these individuals, so that time for and income from treating others is lost.

Attitudes of Health Professionals

The attitudes of some practitioners pose a significant barrier to care. Fear of interacting with a disabled person and conflicting personal values about the disabled may make an individual avoid treating such a person. It may be argued that disabled Americans have been "shut out" from access to dental services as a result of failure on the part of the medical and dental communities to provide comprehensive healthcare to this population.

Client Factors

Oral care holds significance in that it is frequently the lifeline for the disabled client. The mouth is important for mastication, speaking, expressing personality, using telecommunicative devices, working at a job, and portraying a positive self-image. A healthy, well-functioning mouth implies that the individual values health and physical appearance. This positive portrayal of the person contributes to the client's acceptance into society, as well as to his or her self-worth, self-esteem, and facial image.

Self-esteem is an essential component of the disabled client's sense of self-concept. All people have periods of achievement that build confidence and periods of disappointment that lower confidence, and the disabled client copes with these normal life events with the same behaviors as the nondisabled individual; however, disabled clients experience barriers that interfere with how others may view them, which in turn affects how they view themselves.

Physical positioning of the disabled person may cause feelings of intimidation or self-consciousness in proximity to others. For example, people who use wheelchairs are physically lower than those who do not use wheelchairs, hence others look down on them while conversing. People who use assistive devices, such as canes, braces, or walkers, may be viewed as inept because they are unable to ambulate on their own. People who are hearing or visually impaired may have difficulty participating and following a conversation, and therefore may be excluded from the group. People with tremors or other muscular disorders may take a longer time to speak and may be viewed as mentally impaired by those unwilling to listen.

Counseling and group discussions may benefit the disabled client in promoting self-worth by providing an opportunity to discuss frustrations and a forum for objective self-evaluation. Disabled clients are individuals who have their own personal capabilities and limitations, and they adapt to life experiences in much the same way as others cope with these challenges. Therefore, clients should not be viewed as stereotypically different from their counterparts, but rather as individuals who can contribute despite their disabilities and who have needs similar to others.

Defining Disabilities

Disability describes a condition that is either permanent or semipermanent and that interferes with an individual's ability to do something independently. This term can be used either as a noun or as an adjective (e.g., as in *the disabled* or *disabled clients*). An individual who has a disability is different from a "normal" person in some way because of trauma, birth defects, accidents, or disease. These differences may be physical, mental, or psychological manifestations of the individual's ability to function.

Handicap describes the feeling a person may have regarding adequacy of performance either generally or under a particular circumstance. For example, when a person uses a computer for the first time, lack of computer skills may handicap the person in the ability to adequately operate the computer. An individual who is unable to bend at the knees may be handicapped by stairs or by street curbs that are too high. Everyone is handicapped at some point or another, regardless of functional status. Clearly, this term is not synonymous with disability, and care should be taken when utilizing the word.

Negative Portrayals

When describing or interacting with persons with disabilities, remember several key points:

- A person is not a disability; the client is a person who has a disability. Therefore, it is inappropriate to say, "She is my multiple sclerosis case." It is more appropriate to say, "This is my client, Mrs. Jones. She has multiple sclerosis."
- Presence of a disability does not override all other characteristics of the client; therefore, the disability should be addressed only when necessary or relevant to the situation. Emphasizing the disability without reason should be avoided.
- Clients with disabilities are not superhuman; learning to function as a person despite a disability is survival, not a unique act that requires special talents or gifts. Sensationalizing goal attainment by disabled people is a common reaction, such as "he triumphed over his inability to walk," implying that the client was a victim of the disability.
- Sensationalizing terms that draw on emotions, such as "relies on a cane" or "bound to a wheelchair," are inappropriate and imply a false level of *dependency* on the part of the client.
- People with disabilities are not necessarily sick, regardless of whether the disability was caused by an illness. It is inappropriate to describe a disabled client as a "patient" or a "case" unless that person is actively under medical care.

Other negative portrayal issues are encountered through personal contact or mass media. For example, people may express pity for a disabled person without knowing the individual, or disbelief when seeing a disabled person enjoying himself "despite his disability." Healthcare professionals who work with disabled clients are often viewed as having special motivation or as "truly patient." Television portrayals often treat the disabled adult like a child or an inferior. A disabled adult may be addressed by first name or with a surname when the situation dictates a more formal title. Other examples include speaking for the disabled person as if he or she was not there and assuming that the individual cannot make decisions independently. Negative portrayals should be corrected to lay the foundation for a positive therapeutic relationship.

Classification of Disabilities

Several methods are used to categorize individuals with disabilities. Government classification standards are based on criteria delineated in *Section 504* of the *Vocational Rehabilitation Act of 1973*. These criteria state that an individual with a disability is one who:

- Has a physical or mental impairment that substantially limits one or more life activities such as caring for oneself, performing manual tasks, walking, seeing, hearing, speaking, breathing, learning, and working
- Has a record of such an impairment that limits major life activities
- Is regarded as having such an impairment

These criteria are used to determine eligibility for federal assistance under the *Section 504* legislation. These definitions can be further delineated into developmental and acquired disabilities.

DEVELOPMENTAL DISABILITIES. A *developmental disability* is one that occurs congenitally or during the developmental period of the child, a period that lasts from birth to age 22 years. Developmental disabilities are generally chronic in nature, continue throughout the life of the person, and appear as mental, physical, or combined impairments. Individuals with developmental disabilities may experience difficulties with many functions and may be limited in their abilities to care for themselves, communicate effectively, learn new concepts, ambulate, or live independently.

ACQUIRED DISABILITIES. An *acquired disability* occurs after the age of 22 years, or is caused by a disease, trauma, or injury to the body. Common acquired disabilities include spinal cord paralysis from sports or motorcycle accidents, limb amputation because of disease, and limitations in range of motion from arthritis.

A second classification system groups types of disabilities into several major divisions, clustering impairments with similar manifestations together for ease of reference (Table 36–1). These categories are useful when studying a group of disorders or when attempting to classify the condition of a client who presents with oral pathology associated with a known disorder. This system mainly categorizes a person according to medical status, however, and provides little information about how well an individual can compensate for limitations in daily function.

Evaluating functional status is perhaps the most useful method for categorizing disabilities because each disabled person presents with different abilities and limitations, regardless of medical diagnosis or degree of system involvement. *Functional status* describes how well the client can conduct his or her *activities of daily living (ADLs)* (i.e., eating, speaking, bathing, dressing, toileting, and ambulation). The dental hygienist who is able to optimize the client's oral health behaviors also increases the client's functional status and quality of life.

Impairments can affect five aspects of function: communication, movement, mental ability, medical health, and sensory perception. These aspects of function are limited, however, in that they do not address the degree of severity or extent of involvement of the impairments, which may cause varying degrees of functional limitations. Table 36–2 illustrates how functional limitations are related to the severity of impairment, according to four levels of involvement.

Many clients present with complex oral care needs associated directly with their conditions or with medications taken to stabilize or control the symptoms of their conditions. In addition, clients may require special assistance in accomplishing self-care behaviors necessary for oral health and awareness.

ASSISTIVE DEVICES

The client's disability dictates the need for *assistive devices*, tools used to achieve independence in daily functions and communication. Many devices are available through area pharmacies and agencies; others are professionally or self-designed, specifically tailored for the client. It is important for the dental hygienist to be familiar with these devices because their use may affect client goals and decisions in the process of care.

Walking Devices

A variety of devices are available to assist the client who has difficulty with ambulation. Canes, leg braces, crutches, and walkers are all devices that assist the client by bearing the weight of the body during motion (Figure 36–1, *A* and *B*). These devices replace function either unilaterally or bilaterally, greatly increase mobility, increase mobility for ambulation, and support the individual while moving from bed or chair. *The walking device should remain close to the client for access when needed.* For example, if the dental hygienist moves the device from the treatment area, the client must be informed of its location to avoid feeling trapped. The dental hygienist retrieves the device when needed or at the client's request, and hands the device directly to the client for use. The anxious client may prefer to hold the device on his or her lap as a measure of security. Although not ideal, this behavior may be tolerated as long as the device does not interfere with care.

Wheelchairs are devices that assist clients who have limited or no mobility in the legs for ambulation. Wheelchairs increase mobility for those who may other-

TABLE 36–1 CLASSIFICATIONS OF DISABILITIES

Disability	Characteristics
Developmental Disabilities	
Mental retardation	Includes Down syndrome and reflects difficulties with learning, critical thinking, and skill development
Cerebral palsy	Nonprogressive disorder caused by brain damage either at birth or before the central nervous system (CNS) reaches maturity
Epilepsy	Caused by a chemical imbalance in the brain; associated with head injury, infection, and developmental disorders
Autism	Lifelong neurologic disability; associated with mental retardation
Sensory Impairments	
Visual impairments	Ranges from changes in visual acuity to blindness
Hearing impairments	Varying degrees of hearing loss to deafness
Orthopedic Disorders	
Paralysis	Most commonly associated with stroke
Spinal cord injury	Most commonly associated with accidents or injury
Missing extremities	Most commonly associated with injury or diabetes
Medical Disabilities	
Cardiovascular diseases	Hypertension, congestive heart disease, stroke, valvular disease
Arthritis	Lupus, gout, Sjögren's syndrome, scleroderma, rheumatoid arthritis, and osteoarthritis
AIDS	
Cancer	
Diabetes	
Respiratory diseases	
Renal disease	
Blood disorders	Bleeding disorders, platelet disorders, sickle cell anemia, other anemias
Alcoholism	
Drug abuse	
Cognitive Impairments/Mental Illness	
Anorexia and bulimia	
Depression	
Alzheimer's disease	
Dementia	
Cerebrovascular accident (CVA, stroke)	
Degenerative Nervous System Disorders	
Alzheimer's disease	Neuronal degeneration in the cerebral cortex, resulting in loss of memory, critical thinking, and reasoning ability
Parkinson's disease	Degeneration of deep cerebral nuclei, resulting in loss of control of voluntary movements; tremors, slowness of movement (bradykinesia); gradual onset of dementia
Huntington's disease	Autosomal-dominant disorder that causes degeneration of the deep nuclei, cauda, and putamen; behavioral problems and constant muscle movement (chorea)
Cerebellar ataxias	Normal mental status; changes in gait and coordination
Motor neuron disease and amyotrophic lateral sclerosis (ALS)	Cell death in the motor neurons of the spinal cord and cerebral cortex; progressive muscle atrophy leading to respiratory failure; no loss of mental or sensory functions
Multiple sclerosis (MS)	Muscle weakness characterized by cyclical nature of progression
Myasthenia gravis	Muscle involvement around the eyes and throat; difficulty in swallowing
Neurofibromatosis	Genetic autosomal dominant disease; multiple benign tumors
Communication Disorders	
Dysarthria	Speech disorder from muscle weakness caused by damage to central or peripheral nervous system or both; slurred speech patterns; associated with Parkinson's disease, amyotrophic lateral sclerosis, multiple sclerosis, and cerebrovascular accident
Apraxia	Speech disorder caused by a lesion within the CNS; impaired capacity to position muscles to form speech; stuttering
Aphasia	Language disorder caused by neurologic damage; inability to put thoughts into words or to comprehend words

wise be confined to bed or chair. Because of improvements in building design, many facilities are completely accessible to wheelchairs, thus enabling clients to move freely without being inhibited by physical limitations in ambulation. Clients may be treated in the wheelchair or transferred to the dental chair for care (see section and procedures on wheelchair transfer techniques later in this chapter). Most clients prefer to operate the wheelchair themselves; *assistance should be provided only at their specific request.*

Prosthetic Devices

Prosthetic devices enhance client appearance and improve function. Fitted after amputation, prosthetic legs improve

TABLE 36–2 **FUNCTIONAL LEVELS FOR CATEGORIZING DISABILITIES BASED ON ABILITY TO CONDUCT ACTIVITIES OF DAILY LIVING**

Level of Impairment	Communication	Movement	Mental Ability
Level I Near-normal function	May be difficult for the practitioner to understand the client and vice versa.	Client may walk more slowly than normal.	Extra effort for explanations and reassurance to client
Level II Simulation of normal function with adaptive equipment, medication, or methods	Client may use communication board, writing, or gesturing instead of speech.	Office may need to be wheelchair accessible and have furniture rearranged to allow room for movement. Client may need to make special arrangements for transportation. Possible assistance getting into treatment chair	Client may be using medications to maintain emotional equilibrium or need special approach to accept dental and dental hygiene care in office.
Level III Simulation of normal function with aid of third party	Deaf person may need interpreter. Client may bring friend, parent, or attendant to assist in communication. Client consent may be needed to give information to third party.	Attendant or other caregiver may be responsible for dental hygiene. Obtain client consent to give information and education to third party. Will need assistance getting into treatment chair.	Client may have legal guardian. If so, practitioner should have guardian's consent and proof of guardianship.
Level IV Simulation of normal function not possible	Client will have legal guardian. Practitioner should have guardian's consent and proof of guardianship for care. Residential caregiver responsible for dental hygiene should be given information and education.	Home visit required for routine dental and dental hygiene care. If practitioner cannot make one, refer to appropriate resource.	Client will have legal guardian. Must have guardian's consent and proof of guardianship for care.

Modified from Shaffer S, Margon C, Stiefel DJ: *Principles of rehabilitation* (Project DECOD), Seattle, 1985, University of Washington School of Dentistry.

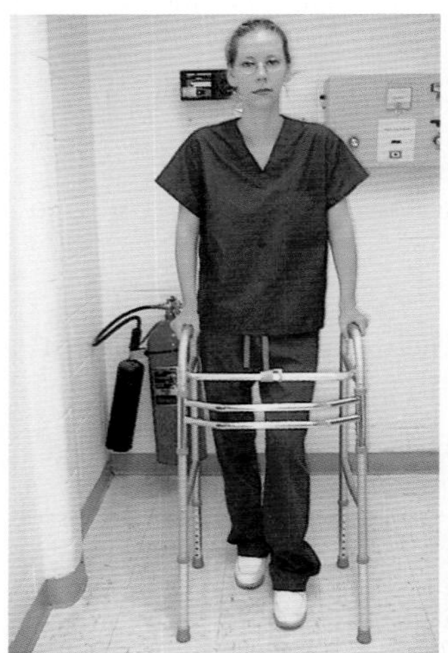

A

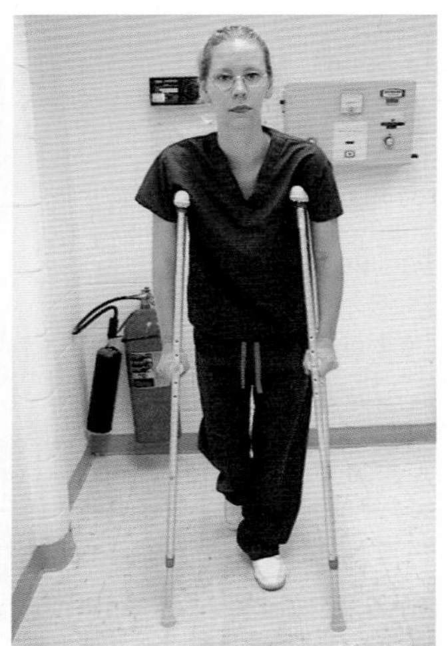

B

FIGURE 36–1 ✦ Walking devices. **A,** Use of a walker greatly increases client's mobility. **B,** Crutches assist client by bearing the weight of the body during motion. *(Courtesy Marye J. McLanahan, BSDH, Gene W. Hirschfield School of Dental Hygiene, Old Dominion University, Norfolk, Va.)*

ambulation, prosthetic arms increase reach and range of motion, and prosthetic hands improve grasp. Other devices may replace structures or organs because of congenital anomalies or that were removed because of pathology or trauma. Prosthetic devices may be permanently fitted through surgical implantation or may be removable and worn only when needed for functional or cosmetic purposes. Clients with removable devices such as those designed for loss of facial structure may feel more comfortable when the prosthesis is in place; therefore, removal should occur only during assessment or when indicated during care. All devices should be replaced immediately after completion of the procedure to ensure client comfort and ease. Privacy must be maintained when the prosthetic device is removed, preferably in a closed area or examination room. Prophylactic antibiotic premedication may be indicated for the client with a prosthetic joint replacement or prosthetic device before dental hygiene care (see Chapter 9, section on antibiotic premedication).

Assistive Listening Devices

Assistive listening devices, for clients with hearing deficits, detect sounds and assist with understanding speech. *Hearing aids* amplify sounds and are effective only when some hearing capacity exists. Hearing aids may be worn in the outer ear to improve sound conduction or behind the ear for inner ear conduction. Because many people deny hearing loss, some clients may own a hearing aid but choose not to wear the device out of self-consciousness or embarrassment. These clients may appear unresponsive to questions or conversation. Such behaviors should alert the dental hygienist to possible hearing impairment, and the client should be asked about the use of a hearing device.

The oral care environment can create annoyances for persons with hearing aids. Close operator proximity or incorrect placement of the hearing aid may cause it to squeal. High-pitched noises from dental handpieces or ultrasonic devices initiate this reaction. *The dental hygienist should instruct the client to turn down the hearing aid during some phases of care.* Clients adapting to a new hearing aid often turn down the aid because "everything seems so noisy." Because all sounds are amplified, these clients may become aware of sounds they never heard before or have not heard in a long time, especially if the hearing loss was gradual and untreated. Most environments contain background noise, and clients may turn off the hearing aid before coming for their appointments.

Other assistive listening devices are available to those with hearing impairments. Amplifiers can be used on telephones, televisions, and radios to increase sound volume for those with partial hearing loss. Closed-captioned television programs assist the hearing-impaired client with lip reading. Telecommunication devices for telephones reproduce sounds from a caller and convert them into written type that can be read from a monitor. A typed response transmits a message back to the caller.

Aids for the Visually Impaired

Clients who are visually impaired usually wear *corrective lenses* to improve vision and augment communication. If oral healthcare instructions are given to a client who has forgotten his or her glasses, instructions should be supplemented with written material to read after the appointment. These materials should contain large print with adequate contrast. Clients who are blind frequently wear dark glasses to protect the eyes from light sensitivity. Blind clients require guidance, especially if new to the environment, and depend on tactile stimulation to understand the environment:

- ✦ A blind client can be greeted by the grasping hands of the hygienist.
- ✦ To assist the client to the treatment area, the client's nondominant hand should be placed under the elbow of the hygienist, and the client should be asked to stand next to, but slightly behind, the hygienist.
- ✦ Specific directions guide the client (e.g., "Take three steps forward, then turn to the right. We're going to step down onto a smooth floor. There is only one step.").
- ✦ When arriving in the treatment area, the client should be told about the location of objects in the room (e.g., "The chair is directly in front of you, about one foot away from where you are standing now."). Allow the client to feel the location and direction of the chair by placing the client's hands onto the chair while giving verbal instructions. It is reassuring if the dental hygienist remains close with a hand resting on the client's shoulder to ensure comfort and concern while the client is getting settled into the chair.

Blind clients may use a *cane* or a *guide dog* during ambulation and prefer these aids to assistance by another individual. Guides dog are permitted to remain in the treatment area and should be directed by the client to sit close within clear view of the client. Guide dogs should never be left alone in another area; they may become extremely anxious in the absence of their owners.

Assistive Speaking Devices

Assistive speaking devices recreate sounds that mimic normal speech patterns for persons who have had surgical removal of the larynx and cannot make sounds from the throat. *Electronic speech devices* held against the throat detect vibrations of air passing through the throat as the person mimics normal speech. The device reproduces a noise that resembles an automated, robot-like speech. Use of this device enhances verbal communication. Speech therapists train clients with laryngectomies to expel air from the esophagus for sound formation to produce altered speech. When treating this type of client, the dental hygienist must listen carefully and repeat the message given by the client to ensure accuracy in understanding. With practice, it becomes relatively easy to understand and communicate with these clients.

Assistive Devices for Paralyzed Persons

ELIMINATION DEVICES. Clients paralyzed below the waist experience difficulty with normal waste elimination and may use a *catheter* for assistance with urination. Care must be taken when moving a client with a catheter so that it does not become kinked or dislodged. Also, clients may have a bowel and bladder routine to regulate their waste elimination. Clients should be questioned regarding their waste elimination schedule so that appointment modifications can be made.

COMMUNICATION DEVICES. Clients paralyzed below the neck use a variety of devices to accomplish ADLs, most of which are designed by occupational therapists. The mouth is needed to operate many of these devices, which alters the health and function of oral structures. The most common device used by quadriplegic clients is the *mouthstick*, a simple plastic or balsa wood rod with a rubber tip held in place by the teeth and lips (Figure 36–2).

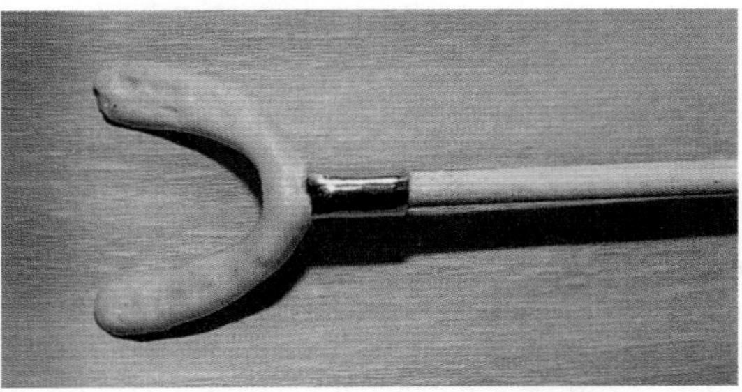

FIGURE 36–2 ✦ Custom-fabricated mouthstick for persons with quadriplegia. *(From Daniel SJ, Harfast SA:* Dental hygiene concepts, cases and competencies, *St Louis, 2002, Mosby.)*

Mouthsticks are used mainly for communication, such as typing on a keyboard or pressing the buttons to dial a telephone. Mouthsticks are also used to turn pages in a book, operate a computer, and operate appliances such as microwave ovens and remote-controlled television sets.

Teeth may be subjected to occlusal trauma from the mouthstick, which, in the presence of inflammation and risk factors, may result in rapid periodontal destruction and tooth loss. A biologically sound dentition and skin and mucous membrane integrity are of great significance to these clients, because without healthy teeth and supporting structures, they may not be able to hold the stick and therefore lose the ability to communicate and function independently.

Mouthsticks may contribute to muscle fatigue, oral tissue trauma from inserting the stick, difficulty with insertion without assistance by a caregiver, unpleasant taste, temporomandibular joint (TMJ) discomfort, and gagging. Considerations in the fabrication of mouthstick appliances are listed in Key Considerations in the Fabrication of a Mouthstick Appliance.

In manufacturing a mouthstick, an impression is taken of both arches for the fabrication of study casts. Next, an acrylic mouthguard is made to fit over the mandibular study cast. The mouthguard is adjusted in the client's mouth for fit and occlusal stability. A hole is made within the appliance and adapted for the mouthstick. The occupational therapist assists the prosthodontist with final evaluation of the length and design of the stick based on client needs. Before insertion of the appliance, oral inflammation should be eliminated. Careful monitoring of the fit and use of the appliance minimizes periodontal trauma and ensures optimal benefit for the client.

Assistive Devices for Protection and Oral Function

Assistive devices for protection and oral function (i.e., *custom mouth protectors*) are used to prevent self-inflicted trauma by clients with behavioral problems (see Chapter 30, section on mouth protectors). The custom mouth protector:

- Prohibits the client from chewing the lips and biting the tongue.
- Provides a protective function by allowing traumatized tissues to heal without further injury.
- Trains the client to stop injuring the oral tissues with uncontrolled chewing habits.

Key Considerations in the Fabrication of a Mouthstick Appliance

Should minimize occlusal trauma by equally distributing the biting forces across as many teeth within arch as possible to decrease periodontal destruction and muscle fatigue.

Should not cause tooth movement; should be stable when held in place.

Should be relatively inexpensive to make and easy to clean.

Should be designed to hold a variety of implements to best meet client's needs.

Should be comfortable; should not inhibit speech or swallowing; stick should be out of client's line of vision.

The devices should be used only in consultation with a behavioral specialist.

Clients with neuromuscular disorders such as Parkinson's disease and stroke or who have had surgery in which a portion of the throat or palate has been removed may experience difficulty in speaking and swallowing and require a device to assist with oral function. *Palatal lifts, palatal augmentation devices,* and *obturators* are all devices that improve function by recreating normal physiologic movement of the oral tissues. The dental hygienist caring for the client with this type of device must monitor changes in speaking patterns, swallowing ability, and cleanliness of the device. If adjustment of the device is needed, the client should be referred to a prosthodontist.

DESIGNING ORAL SELF-CARE DEVICES

Although many devices facilitate ADLs, few existing devices help the client carry out oral self-care behaviors independently. Creative alternatives to traditional oral hygiene devices are designed for those with limitations in function. These devices should adapt to the client's needs, skill level, and functional status.

Client Assessment

The dental hygienist assesses the client's physical and mental limitations that affect how the client adapts to using a device.

- *Range of motion.* The client's ability to reach the oral cavity with the arms and hands is determined. The extent of *range of motion* dictates the length of the device required to accommodate physical limitations in reaching the mouth. For example, a client with a muscular impairment may be able to reach halfway across his or her body, yet elevate the arm only to heart level. This client needs an extended length to compensate for the limited motion of reaching above heart level. Similarly, the client who is unable to bend at the elbows or wrists may have difficulty reaching certain areas of the oral cavity and may need an angled device for improved reach to fit in all areas of the mouth.

- *Grip strength.* Clients with arthritis or neuromuscular disorders experience difficulty holding a device that is too narrow or small (Figure 36–3). To assess grip strength, have the client grasp various sizes of balls to determine the extent of finger closure around the ball. Tennis balls, softballs, and golf balls are helpful with this exercise. Another measure of grip strength includes assessing the client's ability to retain finger closure for an extended length of time. Grasp the client's hand gently, and ask the client to squeeze with as much force as possible and hold this position for one minute. This assessment determines the strength needed to hold the device for a given length of time. If the client is unable to keep the fingers closed for 1 minute, a Velcro strip may be needed for holding the device.
- *Skill level.* Watching the client simulate the motion used to brush the teeth, or watching the client actually brush the teeth with his or her current technique enables the hygienist to assess skill level. The client should be prompted to perform certain skills such as reaching into the upper right quadrant, brushing the tongue, cleaning the lingual surfaces, and brushing the facial surfaces of anterior teeth. It is important to note what the client is capable of performing with relative ease and which behaviors present the most difficulty or confusion.
- *Ability to understand and follow directions.* This is evaluated during the grip strength assessment. The hygienist asks a sufficient number of questions to determine whether the client is capable of responding accurately to verbal commands and instructions. For example, the client who is cognitively impaired may have difficulty in producing a response on command and may require a device such as a powered toothbrush that accomplishes the task with little effort.
- *Perception about what seems easy or difficult.* Direct client feedback is essential for a complete assessment, in that the client's perceptions may influence compliance with any device, whether well adapted for his or her needs or not. The client should understand his or her role in the design of the device—a motivational strategy that promotes ownership of the responsibility for oral self-care behaviors.
- *Current oral status and self-care techniques, the range of opening of the mouth, and the activity of the oral musculature, especially the tongue.* Intraoral assessment provides information about existing oral conditions that may dictate the need for certain device design characteristics.

A comatose or semicomatose person in a hospital or extended-care facility may benefit from toothbrushes such as the Plak-Vac Oral Suction Brush (Trademark Medical Corporation), which is a specially designed toothbrush that can be connected to a bedside suction (Figure 36–4).

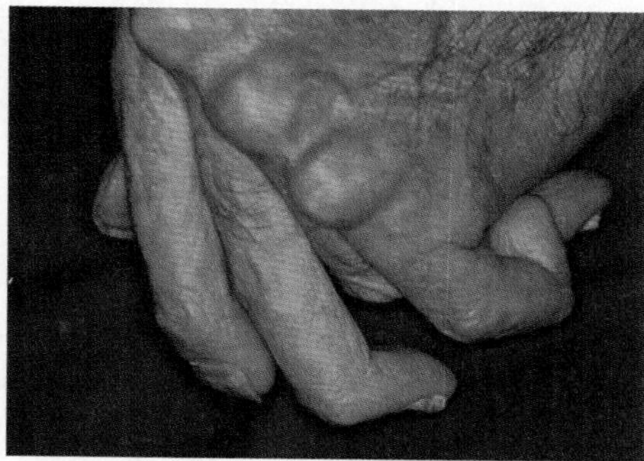

FIGURE 36–3 ✦ Persons with neuromuscular disorders may have difficulty in holding an oral self-care aid. A modified oral self-care aid or powered toothbrush or interdental cleaner is indicated. *(From Babbush CA:* Dental implants: The art and science, *Philadelphia, 2001, WB Saunders.)*

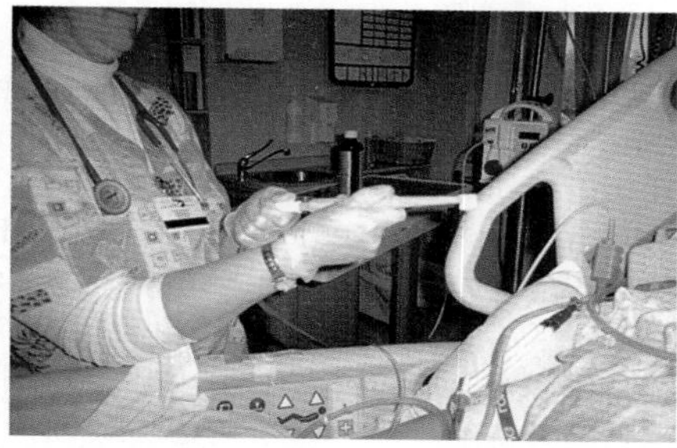

FIGURE 36–4 ✦ Plak-Vac Oral Suction Brush being connected to the bedside suction in a critical care unit. *(Courtesy Michelle Bopp, BSDH, MS, Gene W. Hirschfeld School of Dental Hygiene, Old Dominion University, Norfolk, Va.)*

These assessment measures work well with clients who are mentally and physically capable of learning new self-care techniques; however, some clients may not be able to move their upper extremities at all and therefore rely on a primary caregiver to perform daily care. Caregiver interviews are important to assess the willingness of the individual to provide daily oral care, to determine the existing skill level of the caregiver, and to identify concerns that the caregiver may have.

Customizing Oral Self-Care Devices
(Figure 36–5)

For clients with a limited range of motion, extended handles are needed to access the mouth. Plastic rulers and plastic rods are available from most hardware stores. They can be attached to toothbrushes and floss holders with heavy electrical tape. The added length of the handle facilitates reach but may make placement of the working end of the device in the mouth difficult. To compensate for this problem, a toothbrush with a compact head size may be used for better intraoral fit. The existing plastic handle of the toothbrush can be bent to angu-

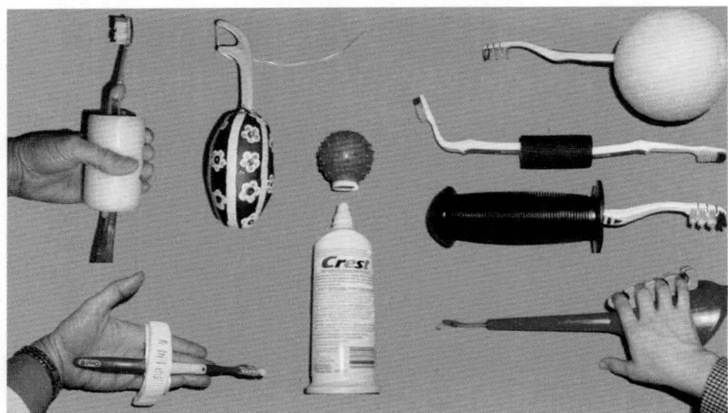

FIGURE 36–5 ✦ Customized oral care aids for persons with physical disabilities. *(Courtesy Kathleen Muzzin, RDH, MS, Assistant Professor, Department of Dental Hygiene, Baylor College of Dentistry, An Institution of the Texas A & M System.)*

late the brush bristles against the curve of the arches. To bend the handle of a toothbrush, gently heat the handle above a flame or simply hold the handle under very hot tap water until it becomes pliable.

To assist the client with weak grip strength, the handle of the device can be built up with a variety of materials to fit the client's finger closure capability. For the client with limited finger closure, a wide, bulky handle is needed to assist with grip. Bicycle grips, tennis balls, Styrofoam molds, and arts-and-crafts compounds as alternative handles greatly improve the client's ability to hold the device. Toothbrushes and floss holders can be inserted into these items easily and changed when necessary. The disadvantage of tennis balls and Styrofoam molds is that they retain water and become damaged and dirty with time. In addition, Styrofoam molds break easily for the client with a clumsy but strong grip because the material is weak and porous. Clients who have difficulties with coordination may find that a lightweight handle is hard to manage and that a weighted end may be easier to find and hold. Plastic bicycle grips are preferred because they are available in a variety of sizes, textures, and weights; are inexpensive; and are easily cleaned after use.

The dental hygienist is responsible for making these devices initially, but the caregiver should be trained to construct them thereafter. Custom-made devices should be brought to every appointment to assess design, usage, and need for replacement.

Clients with poor dexterity and coordination, and/or limited gripping ability, benefit from powered toothbrushes with large handles that are easily used on the client by a caregiver (see Chapter 18).

Several manufacturers market manual toothbrushes that can be bent by hand without heating to promote better angulation and access into the client's mouth. Floss holders and toothbrushes with wide handles or with specific handle designs all promote improved grasping ability by the client. Toothpaste containers with alternative dispensers, such as flip-top lids and levers, should be recommended to clients with limited finger motion because minimal grip strength is needed to dispense the toothpaste. Oral irrigation devices are excellent supplementary aids for self-care and local delivery of antimicrobial agents (see Chapters 18, 19, and 24).

For clients who are unable to hold devices on their own, a *universal strap* may be used for assistance. The strap, with Velcro adhesive on which various implements can be attached, fits around the arm or wrist and acts as a splint for stabilization. Universal straps may be adapted for use with oral physiotherapy aids. The dental hygienist should consult with an occupational therapist when treating a client who could benefit from use of a universal strap for oral home care devices.

The hygienist considers several design characteristics of the device:

- ✦ Made of a lightweight, readily available, inexpensive material and easily constructed; plastics are preferred because they resist water damage and can be easily cleaned, rinsed, and dried.
- ✦ Interchangeable parts (e.g., a constructed alternative handle on a device should adapt easily to changing worn-out toothbrushes without having to replace the handle)
- ✦ Ease of use and minimal setup time

CLIENT POSITIONING AND STABILIZATION

Disabled clients frequently have problems with support and balance; therefore, a physical assessment before care determines whether adaptations are needed to treat the client safely. A list of client stabilization and supportive devices is found in Table 36–3.

Clients with neuromuscular problems, such as tremors, muscle spasms, or hyperflexive responses, may require the use of a physical restraint, such as a seatbelt, to help remain in an upright and stable position. Other restraints, such as wraps, are available to use with clients who have extreme spasticity or severe behavioral problems, but these restraints should not be considered for routine use because they promote distrust in the client and may actually make the problem worse (Figure 36–6). In addition, *physical restraints* have been associated with bruising, respiratory compromise, aspiration pneumonia, and cellulitis from limb restraint. Pillows or rolled towels may be placed underneath the knees and neck of the client to prevent muscle spasms and to provide additional support during treatment. Restraint or *support devices* should be used with caution with a seizure-prone client because these devices must be removed quickly in the event of a seizure.

Clients with involuntary muscle spasms or clients who exhibit aggressive behavior during a procedure require minimal restraint for the protection and safety of both the healthcare provider and the client. To prevent injuries during care, a dental assistant or caregiver may hold the client's arms and legs in a comfortable position. A dental assistant can easily rest the arm closest to the

TABLE 36–3 CLIENT POSITIONING AND STABILIZATION DEVICES

Item	Manufacturer	Telephone
Mouthprops	McKesson/MDT Biologic	714-630-7637
	Specialized Care Co.	800-722-7375
Stabilizers/ safe holding devices	AliMed	800-225-2610
	J.T. Posey	800-447-6739
	Specialized Care Co.	800-722-7375
	Humane Restraint Co.	800-356-7472
Portable dental equipment/ mobile dental units	A-Dec, Inc.	800-549-1883
	Aseptico, Inc.	800-426-5913
	DNTL Works Equipment Corp.	800-847-0694
	Dodgen Mobile Technologies	515-332-3755
	E.F. Brewer Company	800-558-8777
	M-DEC	800-321-MDEC
	Pro-Dentec	800-228-5595

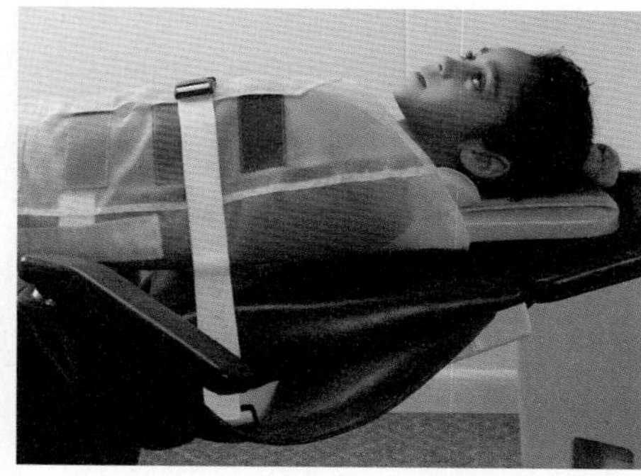

FIGURE 36–6 ✦ Physical restraint used to maintain the disabled client in a stable, safe position. *(Courtesy Specialized Care Co., Hampton, NH.)*

TABLE 36–4 BEHAVIORAL MANAGEMENT TECHNIQUES

Technique	Description
Explanation and exposure (desensitization)	Use of graduated exposure to the oral healthcare setting instills familiarity with the environment and others.
Familiarization visit	Introducing the client to the oral healthcare environment before the initiation of care reduces anxiety and fear of unknown.
Demonstration (tell-show-do)	Use of demonstration exercises reinforces verbal instructions.
Modeling	Use of a live or videotaped model aids in skill development by demonstrating a proper or desired behavior or technique.
Feedback	Providing immediate feedback improves client learning and skill development through evaluation of progress and performance.
Negative consequences (punishment)	Use of negative feedback decreases the likelihood of repeating an undesired behavior; most effective when used as an early intervention strategy in cases of undesired behavior.
Positive consequences (reward)	Use of rewards strengthens behavior and encourages the repetition of a behavior; includes praise, special privileges, token systems, and material goods.
Distraction	Use of other audiovisual stimuli, such as listening to music through headphones or watching a videotape, decreases uncooperative behavior by providing stimuli on which the client can focus during dental hygiene care.
Communication	Choosing words and phrasing that reflect empathy, respect, and warmth enhances client and provider interaction and builds trust.
Hand signals	Allowing the fearful client to raise his or her hand as a sign to stop treatment promotes the client's feelings of safety and security.
Touch	Use of a reassuring touch displays warmth and understanding toward the anxious client.
Relaxation, hypnosis, sedation	Use of additional techniques that require counseling or drugs may be needed for clients who demonstrate extreme levels of anxiety, fear, or uncooperative behavior.

client across the client's chest, with the client's arms tucked underneath, so that in the event of a muscular reflex, the client's arms are prevented from moving into the working area. In the case of the disabled child who is difficult to keep still while in the dental chair, the child may lie on top of the parent, with the parent's arms around the child's body. This practice should be discontinued early in the course of care after behavioral management techniques and trust exercises have been conducted with the child (Table 36–4). Clients who are unable to remain still in the dental chair may be indicated for sedation.

The dental hygienist may find the need for additional head support and stabilization for the client during care. Sitting at the 12 o'clock position, the dental hygienist should wrap her or his nondominant arm around the head and under the chin of the client. The hand may be used to gently but firmly cup the client's chin for stabilization. Small pillows also may be placed on either side of the client's head for additional support, as may a neck roll or a rolled bath towel.

Seatbelts and handles are commonly used on wheelchairs to help keep the client positioned correctly in the chair. Cushions are helpful with paralyzed clients to provide additional support and to minimize the occurrence of pressure sores *(decubitus ulcers* or *decubiti).* Removable headrests and neck and back supports are available for wheelchair adaptation.

If a client is uncooperative and resists sitting in a chair, parents and caregivers can have the client lie on the floor, with the client's head in the caregiver's lap, so that improved visual and physical access into the mouth may be obtained.

Caregivers must be cautioned not to apply dentifrice or topical agents when the client is supine because of the risk of aspiration. The disabled person with neuromuscular or behavioral problems may use ingestible toothpaste as a safe alternative.

During professional care, it is essential to use good evacuation with the aid of a dental assistant, especially when increased salivation is present. Rubber dams should be used for dental sealant placement, amalgam recontouring, and placement of temporary restorations to further prevent aspiration of dental materials.

Use of a mouth prop is recommended for treating most disabled clients, especially for those who are seizure prone, have muscle weakness, or experience muscle spasms, to prevent closure of the mandible onto the operator's fingers. The mouth prop should be attached to the napkin clips around the client's neck via a piece of dental floss or string so that in the event of an emergency, the mouth prop can be readily pulled from the mouth (Figure 36–7).

The client is usually the best source of advice on how to approach positioning and movement. Ideally, all clients should be treated in the dental chair, but on occasion a client in a wheelchair may be too weak to transfer into the dental chair. Regardless of the reason, the client in a wheelchair may be treated from the chair position if treatment areas are wide enough for positioning of the client either alongside or behind the dental chair. Clients who remain in the wheelchair need additional head support during care, which can be obtained by using a portable headrest or by turning the client around in the wheelchair so that the head is leaning against the back of the dental chair's headrest. Treating multiple clients from this position may cause musculoskeletal problems (see Chapter 8); therefore, clients who cannot be transferred should be treated early in the day while the hygienist is well rested. After providing care from a compromised operator position, the hygienist should break for adequate rest and muscle stretching before treating another client.

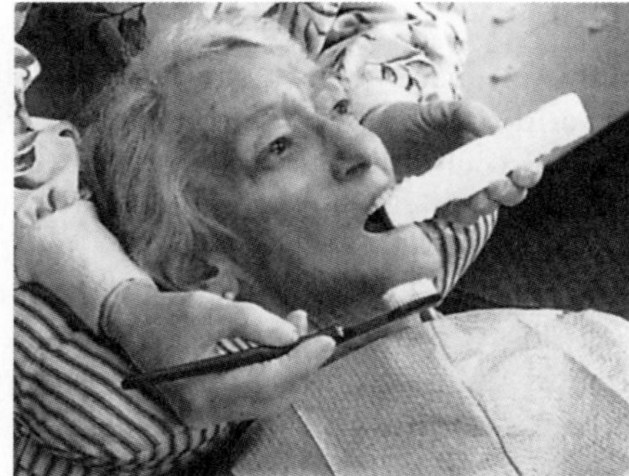

FIGURE 36–7 ✦ Clinician using the Open Wide disposable mouth prop on an adult. *(Courtesy Specialized Care Company, Hampton, NH.)*

WHEELCHAIR TRANSFER TECHNIQUES

Transferring from Wheelchair to Dental Chair

The health history must be carefully assessed to determine the client's current health status, the nature of the condition that dictates the use of a wheelchair, existing physical strength, risk of inducing muscle spasm, and areas of the body that could possibly become injured if moved incorrectly. In addition, the client should be questioned regarding the use of urinary appliances, such as catheters and collecting bags, which may become dislodged during transfer. A kinked catheter may result in inadequate drainage of the bladder, causing an accumulation of toxic waste, and thus trigger an emergency situation. It is important to ask the client about the use of urinary appliances so that proper care can be taken not to dislodge the appliance during the transfer. The client's physician should be consulted about specific medical concerns raised during the health history review before attempting any transfer movement.

The client's physical ability to participate with the transfer should be assessed. Many clients who have undergone physical therapy for their condition may be accustomed to transfer techniques, especially if they have been taught to transfer at home by themselves. Some clients have the ability to assist with the transfer, although they may be unfamiliar with the actual procedural steps involved. Still other clients may perceive that they have the physical strength and skills needed to assist the dental hygienist with the transfer, when actually they do not possess these abilities. Misconceptions about abilities to transfer may be dangerous if the transfer is attempted without verifying whether the client's perceptions and abilities are realistic. Also, the client's willingness to transfer is essential for the dental hygienist to know; it is important to remember that during any transfer procedure there is a certain level of dependency on the practitioner by the client, especially during lifting from the wheelchair. An uncooperative client who overestimates or underestimates his or her abilities or a client who resists transfer attempts poses significant management challenges for the hygienist, as well as increased risk for injury to both the client and the practitioner.

The client's level of coordination and balance determines the need for assistance with the transfer process. Assistance may be required from another operator, or may be obtained with the use of a transfer belt or transfer board:

- ✦ *Transfer belts* are straps secured around the client's waist to provide a place to hold the client in the event that the person begins to slip or fall during the transfer process. Transfer belts are especially useful with clients who have little to no upper body strength, such as quadriplegics.
- ✦ *Transfer boards* are used to assist the client with good upper body strength by helping him or her slide out of the wheelchair across the board and into the dental chair. The wheelchair must be positioned beside the dental chair, and the arms to both chairs must be removed to accommodate the board. One end of the board is placed underneath the client and the other end is laid across the dental chair. The client uses upper arm and body strength to pull the body across the board, while the board provides support from underneath the client's legs. Transfer boards also are useful with clients who are overweight or are otherwise too big for one person to safely move alone. Transfer belts may be used as an added precaution during a sliding transfer with a board.

In addition to client safety, the operator's safety should be ensured:

- ✦ The operator should never attempt to transfer a client alone. Although the one-person transfer technique requires only one individual to maneuver the client, an additional person must always be available to provide assistance if needed. The presence of an additional person greatly reduces the risk of falling or injury to the client during a transfer.
- ✦ The operator should never attempt alone to transfer a client who is very tall or heavy, especially those clients who have no upper body strength. These clients have a much greater chance of falling because of their lack of coordination and balance, and they may injure both themselves and the operator.
- ✦ All transfer movements performed by the operator should be done with the feet separated for good balance and with the knees bent to protect against back strain.
- ✦ All lifting procedures should be performed with the legs, while keeping the back straight and slightly bent forward at the waist to prevent muscular back injury to the operator.
- ✦ The operator should never twist the back while lifting the client out of the wheelchair and into the dental chair; twisting may cause severe muscular back strain and injury. Instead, the operator should move with small steps to position the client.

Before beginning the transfer procedure, the hygienist explains the steps to reduce client anxiety and to answer questions. If the client is expected to assist with the transfer, he or she is informed of how and when assistance is needed. A simulation is helpful before performing the actual procedure, especially for clients who have never been transferred previously. Preparation for a wheelchair transfer is explained in Preparation for a Wheelchair Transfer.

Some clients are able to transfer themselves into and out of the dental chair with little to no assistance. These transfer techniques are called *semidependent transfers*, and the dental hygienist is used only to provide support and assistance on an as-needed basis. Each client has a different level of need; there are no strict guidelines to follow when assisting a client. The hygienist remains readily available to ensure the safety of the client during the transfer process. The main transfer techniques used for dependent clients are the *one-person* and *two-person transfer lifts* (see Procedures 36–1 and 36–2). Each lift contains specific safety criteria to follow.

Preparation for a Wheelchair Transfer

1. Position wheelchair parallel to dental chair with seats aligned. Dental chair should be slightly lower than wheelchair.
2. Position wheelchair wheels facing forward and lock wheels. This steadies the chair and prevents tipping or slipping during the transfer.
3. Remove footrests from chair or fold them back so that client's feet do not become caught during the transfer. Client's feet are *gently* placed on floor to prevent spasm and to position feet for the transfer.
4. Remove arms of both wheelchair and dental chair. If arm of dental chair is not removable, then position it as far back as possible so that it does not interfere with the transfer (Figure 36–8).
5. Check area for any sharp edges, hazards, obstacles, or cords that could cause injury during the transfer.
6. Unfasten client's safety belt. After belt is removed, operator must support client to prevent falling.
7. Transfer any special padding underneath the client to the dental chair. Gently rock client forward while an assistant removes the padding from wheelchair and places it onto dental chair.

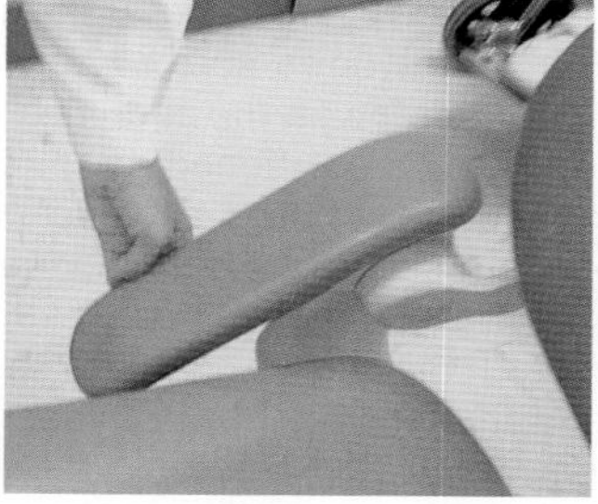

FIGURE 36–8 ✦ Lowering of dental chair armrest in preparation for transfer. *(From Steifel DJ: Wheelchair transfers in the dental office: Dental Education in Care of the Disabled (DECOD) Program,* Dental Hygienist News, *Seattle, University of Washington.)*

*For images and additional information on wheelchair transfers in the dental office, visit http://www.dentalcare.com/soap/journals/dh_news/dhn0804/dn01n09.htm

Procedure 36–1 TRANSFERRING CLIENT FROM WHEELCHAIR TO DENTAL CHAIR USING A ONE-PERSON LIFT

STEPS	RATIONALE
1. Position transfer belt around client's waist just below ribcage.	Ensures client safety.
2. Insert your hands underneath the client's thighs, and gently slide the client forward in wheelchair seat so that client's buttocks are positioned on front portion of seat.	Brings client's center of gravity closer to operator, facilitating transfer.
3. Place client's feet together and hold them in place on either side by your feet. Close your knees on the client's knees, thus supporting and stabilizing the client's legs, which allows the client to bear some of his or her own weight during the lift.	Helps prevent client from falling forward onto the operator during the lift.
4. Place client's arms over your shoulders, and instruct client to rest his or her head on your left shoulder.	Allows operator to see behind client and to clearly view the dental chair.
5. Grasp client around waist and hold transfer belt securely between both hands. If there is no transfer belt available, use an overlapping wrist grasp for greater stability.	Overlapping the arms to grasp the belt is recommended to provide added stability.
6. Rock gently backward onto your heels and, using your leg muscles, lift client off seat. (Client is now resting against you, the operator.)	Provides momentum and minimizes operator back injury in the transfer.
7. Pivot on your foot closest to the dental chair, and maneuver client over seat of dental chair. This should be done in a smooth motion.	Pivoting maximizes the clinician's strength and minimizes the energy required for the transfer.
8. Lower client onto dental chair by bending at your knees. Do not release transfer belt around client until client is securely placed into chair.	Bending at knees reduces the risk of operator injury. Maintaining hold of the transfer belt ensures client safety.
9. Release your right hand to lift client's legs onto chair while still holding transfer belt with your left hand. Reposition armrest of dental chair for client safety.	Repositioning the armrest establishes client stability and safety.

Procedure 36–2 TRANSFERRING A CLIENT FROM WHEELCHAIR TO DENTAL CHAIR USING A TWO-PERSON LIFT

STEPS	RATIONALE
1. The first operator stands behind the client and reaches around the client's torso underneath the client's armpits. The operator crosses her or his arms in front of the client, and grasps the client's hands at the wrists with the opposite hands (right over left, left over right). The operator then slides her or his arms down so that arms are positioned under the client's ribcage on the abdomen.	The stronger of the two operators is placed behind the client to support the majority of the client's weight. For images and additional information on wheelchair transfers in the dental office, visit http://www.dentalcare.com/soap/journals/dh_news/dhn0804/dn01n09.htm
2. The second operator is positioned on the right side of the wheelchair at the client's legs and feet. Bending at the knees, the operator slides one arm underneath the client's thighs slightly above the knees, while the other arm is placed underneath the client's ankles to support the feet.	The second operator provides support for the client's lower extremities during transfer.
3. Client is lifted simultaneously by both operators. The lift is done at a prearranged signal, such as at the end of a count ("1, 2, 3, lift"). One person should coordinate the lift, preferably the operator who is supporting the client's torso—the operator who is lifting the most weight.	Use of a prearranged signal eliminates the risk of loss of client support by one or both operators during the lift. Loss of client support places the client and the operators at risk for injury.
4. The client is lifted in one smooth motion and is placed into the dental chair.	This maximizes the operators' strength and minimizes the energy required for the transfer.
5. The operator holding the legs releases the grasp on the client and repositions the client in the chair. The other operator does not release the client until the client is stabilized and the arm of the dental chair is replaced.	Repositioning the client establishes client stability and safety.

Complications in Wheelchair Transfer

Several risks are associated with wheelchair transfers.

MUSCLE SPASMS. Movement may stimulate muscle spasms, and the hygienist must be prepared to protect the client from injury if spasms occur. Continuous spasms may be reduced by gently massaging the affected area or simply by waiting until the muscle relaxes. Use of supportive pillows may reduce the incidence of spasms induced by movement. Anxiety can also contribute to spasms; therefore, the hygienist talks to the client to reduce fear and to address any concerns before initiating the transfer.

DECUBITUS ULCERS (PRESSURE SORES). Individuals who use wheelchairs are prone to developing decubitus ulcers. Decubiti form in areas where there is blood pooling, such as on the buttocks and on the backs of the thighs. Decubiti can be extremely painful and become easily infected. The dental hygienist questions the disabled client during the health history review about the presence of decubiti. To prevent decubiti from occurring, clients must perform *weight shifts* every 20 minutes to relieve pressure from the skin. When clients are transferred into the dental chair, supportive devices and weight shifts must be incorporated into the client's appointment plan. Changes in skin integrity are monitored carefully and brought to the attention of the client's physician.

BOWEL AND BLADDER ELIMINATION SCHEDULES. Clients who are transferred into the dental chair may need to be reminded of the time so that they may adhere to their bowel and bladder elimination program. Adequate time must be allotted to transfer the client back into the wheelchair if the client needs to use the restroom during an appointment. The client's elimination schedule should be documented in the dental record.

AUTONOMIC DYSREFLEXIA. Any of these aforementioned complications poses a significant risk for the development of *autonomic dysreflexia*, a severe condition that can be fatal if left untreated. The presence of noxious stimuli, such as urinary backflow or pain from decubitus ulcers, leads to the development of dysreflexia, manifested by a variety of signs and symptoms. The client may appear disoriented and flushed and exhibit profuse sweating and goosebumps. The most characteristic manifestation of dysreflexia is an extremely elevated blood pressure, which ultimately results in stroke. The practitioner who is alerted to any of these clinical signs must stop work immediately, check the client's blood pressure, and begin to look for the cause of the reaction. Usually, treatment of the cause produces an immediate, favorable response, such as when a kinked catheter is straightened. Any suspicion of dysreflexia is treated as a severe medical emergency, and assistance must be summoned immediately. Because of the nature of this risk, it is imperative that *no client who is transferred to the dental chair be left unattended.*

Transferring from Dental Chair to Wheelchair

When the appointment is completed, the client must be transferred from the dental chair back into the wheelchair. The same procedures are conducted to move the client, with special attention given to replacing the padding and supports underneath the client before seating him or her in the wheelchair. The wheels of the chair must always be locked when transferring the client back into the wheelchair.

Transfer techniques require practice to perform safely and successfully. Routinely practicing these techniques, especially for those who conduct actual client transfers infrequently, ensures competence in performing transfer procedures. The assistance of physical therapists in training and practice can help hygienists who are unfamiliar with providing dental care for clients in wheelchairs. Transfer techniques, when used in daily practice, enable hygienists to treat a variety of clients who may otherwise not receive oral healthcare.

HEALTH PROMOTION AND ADVOCACY

The hygienist develops and implements programs that focus on early detection and intervention that enable the client to achieve oral wellness. Dental hygienists also promote wellness by encouraging proper oral healthcare behaviors, by participating in educational programs such as health fairs, and by volunteering for community service.

The hygienist supports disabled clients not only in the healthcare arena but also by promoting the rights of these clients as contributing members of society. Opportunities abound to work to improve access to dental hygiene services (e.g., participation on councils, local boards, and in area support groups; holding leadership positions in organizations; initiating community programs; and contributing to both lay and professional communities via speaking engagements and publications).

Client Education Issues

- Teaching begins at the initial client contact and is used while assessing the client's needs related to dental hygiene care, designing and evaluating self-care programs, and monitoring client progress throughout the person's lifetime.
- Work with caregivers, physicians, nurses, physical and occupational therapists, and dietitians in identifying needs, setting goals, and planning client health programs; help other healthcare providers understand oral health as it relates to systemic health.
- Clarify information and maximize the roles of family and caregivers as healthcare providers for the disabled client.
- Demonstrate methods for modifying and using oral care devices to achieve optimal oral health.

Legal, Ethical, and Safety Issues

- Clients with disabilities undergo long-term care with multiple providers, so oral care interventions must complement other health services for the client. If the client is ambulatory, fully functional, and without cognitive impairment, consent to speak with other caregivers and providers, as well as permission to proceed with care, must be obtained directly from the client.
- If the client is under the care of a legal guardian, the guardian must provide informed consent for planned interventions and consultations with other providers.
- Information obtained from other care providers and original copies of written correspondence are maintained in the client's dental record.
- Care must be taken to ensure client stability during positioning and transfer; clients should never be left unattended.
- The client should be an active participant in all conversations with caregivers who attend the appointment.
- Some individuals with disabilities may become victims of violence, abuse, or neglect. The hygienist is ethically obliged to report suspected cases of abuse and neglect to the proper authorities.

Key Concepts

- Human needs, such as the need for wholesome facial image, freedom from health risks, conceptualization and understanding, responsibility for oral health, and freedom from anxiety and pain are often unmet in clients with special needs.
- Access to healthcare, education, and employment opportunities is essential for the client to achieve an acceptable level of health and wellness and to maintain as much independence as possible.
- Oral care is significant for disabled clients because the mouth is used not only for mastication and speaking, but also for expressing personality, using telecommunicative devices, working at a job, and portraying a positive self-image.
- A disability is a permanent or semipermanent condition that interferes with an individual's ability to function independently.
- A handicap is the feeling a person perceives regarding adequacy of performing either generally or under a particular circumstance.
- Developmental disabilities occur congenitally or during the developmental period of the child and are generally chronic in nature, continue throughout the life of the individual, and appear as mental, physical, or combined impairments.
- Acquired disabilities occur in early adulthood, from disease or some type of trauma or injury to the body.
- Assistive devices are used to achieve independence in daily functions and communication.
- The hygienist assesses the client's degree of cognitive awareness, ability to ambulate with or without an assistive device, ability to communicate and interpret information, and need for assistance by a caregiver.
- The dental hygienist develops specialized oral self-care devices to promote better oral health among those with limitations in function.
- Caregiver interviews are important to assess willingness to provide daily oral care for the client, determine the existing skill level of the caregiver, and identify concerns in performing oral care procedures.
- Most disabled clients can be transferred safely and easily into the dental chair if proper procedures are followed.
- Autonomic dysreflexia, a life-threatening medical emergency, can be prevented.
- Dental hygienists work closely with lay and professional communities to improve the quality of life for citizens with special needs.

CRITICAL THINKING EXERCISES

1. Form groups of three to practice wheelchair transfers and client positioning and stabilization techniques. Alternate roles as clients and practitioners. Practical exercises should include one-person and two-person lifts, and when possible, include practice using a transfer board. Consider utilizing the assistance of a physical therapist or physical therapy students for a collaborative learning experience.
2. Assume the role of a disabled person for several hours, and complete a set of exercises designed to enhance one's appreciation of the difficulties associated with conducting normal activities of daily living. Randomly draw from a list of disabilities, including hearing impairment, visual impairment, inability to speak, blindness, limited mobility (arm, leg, both legs). Assemble the necessary equipment and assistive devices for use during these activities (e.g., canes, dark glasses, safety glasses coated with petroleum jelly, ear plugs, crutches, wheelchairs, splints, slings, shoe lifts). Consult with a physical therapist or physical therapy students for assistance. Exercises for completion while "disabled" may include completing a health history form in the clinical setting, riding in elevators, visiting another building to retrieve a newspaper or beverage, obtaining signatures from faculty in other departments, or obtaining something from the campus bookstore. Following completion of the exercises, discuss the experiences. (*NOTE:* Extreme caution and care must be taken to plan activities that will not place the student in danger while "impaired." Students should not be permitted to cross roadways or other high-traffic areas to prevent accidental injury. Consideration should be given to severely "impaired" students who may benefit from pairing with a buddy for assistance or safety. Always inform campus officials when students will be completing this exercise to help ensure student safety and participation by others.)
3. Select a medical condition associated with disability, and prepare a dental hygiene care plan tailored to meeting the needs of clients with this type of condition. Use the care plan approach presented in Chapter 17. In addition, include information on population affected, age of onset, rate of onset, rate of change or disease progression, need for assistive devices, related medical conditions, medications used to manage this condition, oral manifestations of the condition, and special clinical considerations for providing dental hygiene care. Prepare oral presentations about the care plans, and provide copies of all care plans to peers, as a guide for practice.
4. Design oral self-care devices for the following client conditions: inability to grasp and hold; inability to raise hand; inability to move forearm in a back-and-forth motion.
5. Visit the following website at the University of Florida College of Dentistry: www.dental.ufl.edu/Faculty/Pburtner/disabilities/index.htm. Work independently through the entire online materials for the course titled *Oral Health Care for Persons with Disabilities.*

For References, Suggested Readings, and Related Websites, visit
http://evolve.elsevier.com/Darby/hygiene/

CHAPTER 37

PERSONS WITH AUTOIMMUNE DISEASES

OBJECTIVES

Mastery of the content in this chapter will enable the reader to:

- Recognize signs and symptoms of each of the following autoimmune diseases:
  1. Cicatricial pemphigoid (benign mucous membrane pemphigoid)
  2. Pemphigus
  3. Erythema multiforme
  4. Immune-mediated (Type 1) diabetes mellitus
  5. Hashimoto's thyroiditis
  6. Rheumatoid arthritis
  7. Sarcoidosis
  8. Systemic sclerosis (scleroderma)
  9. Sjögren's syndrome
  10. Lichen planus
  11. Systemic lupus erythematosus
- Develop a dental hygiene care plan appropriate for persons with autoimmune disease
- Identify human needs related to each of the above autoimmune diseases and describe their implications for dental hygiene care

KEY TERMS

Autoimmune disease
Bullae
Chronic cutaneous lupus erythematosus
Cicatricial pemphigoid (benign mucous membrane pemphigoid)
Discoid lupus erythematosus
Erythema multiforme major (Stevens-Johnson syndrome)
Hashimoto's thyroiditis
Lichen planus
Nikolsky sign
Pemphigus
Pemphigus vulgaris
Raynaud's phenomenon
Rheumatoid arthritis
Sarcoidosis
Sjögren's syndrome
Subacute cutaneous lupus erythematosus
Systemic lupus erythematosus
Systemic sclerosis (scleroderma)
Toxic epidermal necrolysis (Lyell's disease)

As the population of aging persons continues to increase, so will the incidence of treating individuals with *autoimmune diseases.* Many autoimmune diseases manifest after the age of 30. In these diseases, the immune cells either become confused and attack normal cells (self) or normal cells become altered antigenically and are no longer recognized as self by the person's immune system. In any case, the immune system is stimulated to destroy normal cells. This chapter describes select autoimmune diseases (Table 37–1), manifestations of each, and dental hygiene interventions necessary to manage clients successfully.

PEMPHIGUS

Pemphigus represents four related diseases of an autoimmune etiology: pemphigus vulgaris, pemphigus vegetans, pemphigus erythematosus, and pemphigus foliaceus. Of the four diseases, only the first two affect the oral mucosa with any degree of frequency, pemphigus vegetans being the rarer of the two.[1]

Pemphigus vulgaris (*vulgaris* Latin for "common"), although the most common of these disorders, is not seen very often. Annually, only one to five cases per million population are diagnosed. If untreated, the result is often death. Oral lesions are often the first sign of the disease, and they are the most difficult to resolve with therapy. Blistering is often present because of an abnormal production of autoantibodies directed against an epidermal cell surface glycoprotein, resulting in a split in the epithelium and subsequent blister formation.[1,2]

Clinical Features

Initial manifestations often involve the oral mucosa. Average age at diagnosis is 50 years; childhood cases are rare. No gender predilection has been observed; however, the condition is more common in persons of Jewish ancestry. Intraorally, superficial "ragged" erosions and ulcerations are distributed haphazardly on the oral mucosa. The disease may affect any oral mucosal location but is most commonly found on the palate, labial and buccal mucosa, ventral surface of the tongue, and gingivae. Almost 50% of affected individuals have oral mucosal lesions before the onset of cutaneous lesions, sometimes by as much as a year or more. Eventually, however, nearly all affected persons have intraoral involvement.

Extraorally, skin lesions appear as flaccid vesicles ("without tone") and *bullae* (blisters) that rupture quickly (usually within hours to a few days), leaving an erythematous, denuded surface. A characteristic feature of this disease is the induction of a bulla on otherwise normal-appearing skin if firm lateral pressure is exerted. This is known as a positive *Nikolsky sign.* Without proper treatment and control, both oral and skin lesions tend to persist and progressively involve more surface area.

Treatment and Prognosis

Medical diagnosis should be made as early as possible because control is generally easier to achieve at that time. Treatment consists primarily of systemic corticosteroids (usually prednisone), often in combination with other immunosuppressive drugs, such as azathioprine, a steroid-sparing agent.[2] Side effects with long-term use of systemic corticosteroids are significant and include diabetes mellitus, adrenal suppression, weight gain, osteoporosis, peptic ulcers, severe mood swings, and increased susceptibility to infections. Pemphigus rarely undergoes complete resolution, although remissions and exacerbations are common. If pemphigus vulgaris is left untreated, it is inevitably fatal.

Before the development of corticosteroid therapy, mortality was as high as 60% to 80%. Death was primarily a result of infections and electrolyte imbalances. Today, even with the use of corticosteroids and other immunosuppressive drugs, the mortality rate of pemphigus vulgaris is in the range of 5% to 10%. These deaths are usually the result of complications from long-term systemic corticosteroid use.[1]

CICATRICIAL PEMPHIGOID (BENIGN MUCOUS MEMBRANE PEMPHIGOID; MUCOUS MEMBRANE PEMPHIGOID)

Cicatricial pemphigoid is a "chronic, blistering, mucocutaneous autoimmune disease in which tissue-bound autoantibodies are directed against one or more components of the basement membrane."[1] The precise incidence of the disease is not known, but most authors believe that it is at least twice as common as pemphigus vulgaris.[1] The term *pemphigoid* is used in naming this disease because clinically it appears similar to pemphigus. Prognosis and microscopic features of pemphigoid, however, are very different from pemphigus. *Cicatricial* is derived from the word *cicatrix,* meaning "scar." When the conjunctival mucosa of the eye is affected, the scarring that results is serious because it will result in blindness unless the disease is promptly recognized and treated. Oral lesions, however, often do not exhibit a tendency for scar formation.[1]

Clinical Features

Cicatricial pemphigoid usually affects older adults; the average age of onset is 60 years. Females are more frequently affected than males (ratio of 2:1). Oral lesions are most common, but other sites may be involved, including conjunctival, nasal, esophageal, laryngeal, and vaginal mucosa, as well as the skin.

Oral lesions begin as either vesicles or bullae that may occasionally be evident clinically. In pemphigus, however, such blisters are rare. Eventually, the oral blisters rupture, leaving large areas of superficial, ulcerated, and denuded mucosa (Figure 37–1). The lesions are usually painful and persist for weeks to months if left untreated. They are often seen diffusely throughout the mouth but may be limited to certain areas, namely the gingiva. Gingival involvement is usually termed *desquamative gingivitis.* This clinical reaction pattern may also be seen in other conditions, such as erosive lichen planus, or much less frequently, pemphigus vulgaris.[1]

The most significant complication of cicatricial pemphigoid is ocular involvement. This occurs in approximately 25% of persons with oral involvement. One eye may be affected before the other. The earliest ocular

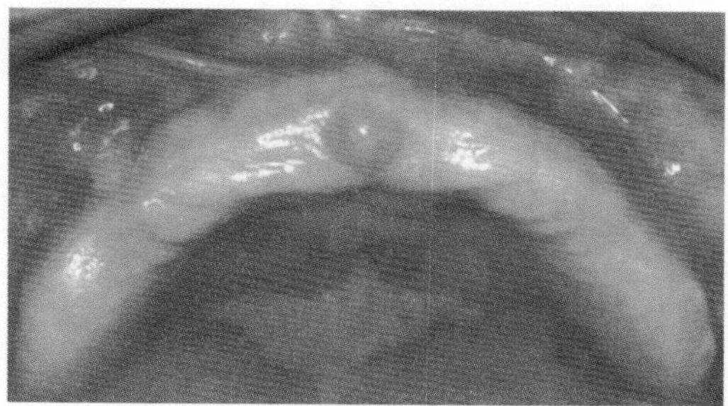

FIGURE 37–1 ✦ Large, irregular oral ulcerations after the initial bulla ruptures in a person affected with cicatricial pemphigoid. Similar ulcerations are seen in persons with pemphigus vulgaris and erosive lichen planus.

Text continued on p. 786.

TABLE 37–1 SUMMARY TABLE OF AUTOIMMUNE DISEASES

Disease	Oral Manifestation(s)	Systemic Signs and Symptoms	Dental Hygiene Interventions	Pharmacologic Treatment
Cicatricial Pemphigoid	Vesicles or bullae that rupture, leaving large areas of superficial, ulcerated, and denuded mucosa; lesions are painful; may persist for weeks or months if untreated	Involvement of other mucosal sites: conjunctiva, nose, esophagus, larynx, and vagina	Client education: practice of meticulous oral hygiene may decrease severity of lesions; demonstration on use of flexible mouthguard as a medicine carrier	Topical corticosteroids Systemic corticosteroids Immunosuppressive agents (cyclophosphamide)
Pemphigus	Superficial "ragged" erosions and ulcerations; haphazard distribution; most common areas: palate, labial mucosa, buccal mucosa, ventral surface of the tongue, and gingivae	Skin lesions: flaccid vesicles ("without tone") and bullae that rupture quickly, producing erythematous, denuded surface Positive Nikolsky sign Lesions persist and involve more surface area (without treatment)	Referral to physician and/or dermatologist is necessary Client education: side effects of long-term systemic corticosteroids on oral cavity and systemic health	Systemic corticosteroids Other immunosuppressive agents
Erythema Multiforme	Erythematous patches that undergo epithelial necrosis; become large, shallow erosions and ulcerations with irregular borders; lesions emerge quickly; very painful; diffuse distribution; hemorrhagic, crusted lips common; gingivae and hard palate lesions rare	Diffuse sloughing and ulceration of entire skin and mucosal surfaces (in its severe form) Prodromal period: fever, malaise, headache, cough, and sore throat Skin lesions (50% of cases): variety of lesions present ("many forms"); early lesions flat, round, "dusky-red"; and appear on extremities; may evolve into bullae with necrotic centers; "target lesions" may develop (highly characteristic of disease)	Referral to physician and/or dermatologist as necessary Client education: side effects of systemic or topical corticosteroid therapy	Topical corticosteroid syrups or elixirs Topical anesthetic agents (for painful oral lesions) Intravenous rehydration (in severe forms of disease) Systemic corticosteroids
Immune-mediated (type 1) Diabetes Mellitus	(In poorly controlled diabetes): Cheilosis Xerostomia Glossodynia Enlarged salivary glands Increased glucose in saliva Fungal infections (candidiasis) Commonly: Gingivitis Periodontitis Dental caries	Sudden onset: Constant urination Excessive thirst Extreme hunger Dramatic weight loss Irritability Obvious weakness and fatigue Nausea and vomiting	Immediate referral to physician necessary Client education: caries and diet; importance of recall frequency; periodontal disease and diabetes connection; blood sugar monitoring and regular insulin dosing; meticulous oral home care	Fluoride therapy Salivary replacement therapy Antimicrobial subgingival irrigation of periodontal pockets Antifungal therapy (if necessary)
Hashimoto's Thyroiditis	Thickened lips Enlarged tongue	Lethargy, weakness, fatigue; dry coarse skin; swelling of face and extremities; huskiness of voice; constipation; slow heart rate (bradycardia); reduced body temperature (hypothermia)	Client education: referral to physician if suspected; stress importance of thyroid replacement therapy	Thyroid replacement therapy
Rheumatoid Arthritis	TMJ involvement (75% of cases)	Swelling, stiffness, and pain (usually in joints of extremities); joint deformity; disability	Client education: risk for TMJ involvement; regular panoramic radiographs to assess mandibular condylar wear and TMJ Premedication when indicated before dental services	Antiinflammatory agents

Sarcoidosis	Chronic, violaceous (of violet color) indurated lesions on lips; enlarged salivary glands; xerostomia; mucoceles may occur (oral manifestations are uncommon). Occasionally: submucosal mass, isolated papule, or area of granularity; may be normal in color, brownish-red, violaceous, or hyperkeratotic; bony involvement may mimic periodontal disease Radiographically: widened PDL spaces	Dyspnea, dry cough, chest pain, fever, malaise, fatigue, arthralgia, and weight loss 20% have no symptoms Granulomatous inflammation of skin (25%) Erythema nodosum (scattered, nonspecific, tender, erythematous nodules) may occur on lower legs Xerophthalmia	Referral to physician if necessary Client education: xerostomia's effects on teeth and tissues; increased risk of dental caries; salivary substitute; fluoride regimen (at home)	Case dependent
Systemic Sclerosis (Scleroderma)	Microstomia Limited opening of the mouth Loss of attached gingival mucosa and generalized recession Difficulty swallowing Firm, hypomobile tongue	Raynaud's phenomenon Skin develops a diffuse, hard texture Fibrosis of organs (may lead to organ failure): Lungs, heart, kidneys, GI tract	Client education: augmentation of oral hygiene regimen in cases of limited manual dexterity	Immunosuppressive agents
Sjögren's Syndrome	Erythematous oral mucosa Xerostomia Difficulty swallowing Altered taste Difficulty wearing dentures Fissured tongue; atrophy of papillae	General malaise, fatigue Dry skin Xerophthalmia Rheumatoid arthritis Diffuse, firm enlargement of major salivary glands (usually bilateral), may be nonpainful, tender, or intermittent Retrograde bacterial sialadenitis	Referral to physician/ ophthalmologist if necessary Client education: Daily fluoride application at home to prevent xerostomia-induced dental caries Daily fluoride regimen Use of artificial tears and saliva Antifungal therapy for secondary candidiasis Sugarless gum and candy to stimulate salivary flow	Sialagogues (pilocarpine) Evoxac (cevimeline hydrochloride)
Lichen Planus	White, interlacing lines over erythematous areas (Wickham's striae) Sites of involvement: primarily bilateral posterior buccal mucosa, but may be found on lateral and dorsal of tongue, the gingivae, and the palate	Skin lesions are purple, pruritic, polygonal papules; located on flexor surfaces of extremities; itch and are painful; may exhibit Wickham's striae on surface of papules Other sites affected: glans penis, vulvar mucosa, and the nails	Referral to physician if necessary Client education: meticulous oral hygiene may lessen severity of gingival involvement	No treatment for reticular type Antifungal therapy needed if secondary candidal infection present Erosive lesions: topical corticosteroids (e.g., fluocinonide gel); follow-up for 3 months required (small chance of malignant transformation)
Systemic Lupus Erythematosus (SLE)	Oral lesions (5% to 25% of patients) Location of lesions: palate, buccal mucosa, gingivae May appear lichenoid, may look nonspecific or granulomatous Ulceration, pain, erythema, hyperkeratosis	Fever, weight loss, arthritis, malaise Characteristic "butterfly rash" over malar area and nose (40% to 50%) Kidneys affected (40% to 50%); may lead to kidney failure Cardiac involvement common: warty vegetations on heart valves	Referral to physician if necessary Client education: meticulous oral hygiene; analgesic rinses when necessary; avoid excessive sun exposure	Systemic corticosteroids Other immunosuppressive agents
Chronic Cutaneous Lupus Erythematosus (CCLE)	Painful lesions are practically identical to lesions of erosive lichen planus	Skin lesions: discoid lupus erythematosus (scaly, erythematous patches frequently on sun-exposed skin; head and neck areas)	Referral to dermatologist/ physician if necessary Client education: Avoid exposure to acidic or salty foods if painful intraoral lesions are present; avoid excessive sun exposure	Systemic corticosteroids Antimalarial drugs may be effective
Subacute Cutaneous Lupus Erythematosus	Features intermediate between SLE and CCLE	Arthritis or musculoskeletal problems Photosensitivity Features intermediate between SLE and CCLE Skin lesions most prominent feature	Referral to dermatologist/ physician if necessary Client education: Avoid excessive sun exposure	Systemic corticosteroids Antimalarial drugs may be effective

change is subconjunctival fibrosis. As the disease progresses, the conjunctiva becomes inflamed and eroded. Scarring (during the healing process) occurs between the bulbar (lining the globe of the eye) and palpebral (lining the inner surface of the eyelid) conjunctiva; adhesions result (*symblepharons*). Without treatment the inflammatory changes become more severe. Eyelids may turn inward (*entropion*) from severe scarring. Eyelashes may then rub against the cornea and globe (*trichiasis*). Scarring may close the openings of the lacrimal glands, resulting in loss of tears and extremely dry eyes. The cornea then will produce keratin as a protective mechanism, but this is detrimental because keratin is an opaque material, and blindness soon results. In end-stage ocular involvement, adhesions may occur between the upper and lower eyelids.[1]

Other mucosal sites may be involved. In female patients, vaginal mucosal lesions may be considerably painful. Although fairly uncommon, laryngeal lesions may be serious because of the possibility of airway obstruction by the bullae that form. Patients who experience "a sudden change in vocalization or who have difficulty breathing" should receive an examination with laryngoscopy.[1]

Treatment and Prognosis

If only oral lesions exist, the disease may be controlled with application of one of the more potent topical corticosteroids to the lesions several times each day. Once controlled, the applications may cease; however, lesions are certain to return. Sometimes alternate-day application minimizes disease activity.[1]

Clients with only gingival lesions should practice good oral hygiene measures to help decrease severity of the lesions and reduce the amount of topical medication required. Sometimes a flexible mouthguard (used as a medication carrier) may aid in treating gingival lesions.

If topical corticosteroids are unsuccessful, systemic corticosteroids plus other immunosuppressive agents (e.g., cyclophosphamide) are used if the individual has no medical contraindications. Aggressive treatment of this nature is a necessity when ocular involvement is severe. Surgical correction of ocular lesions must take place when the disease is under control. Occasionally an alternative therapy, dapsone, is used, which may produce fewer serious side effects. Dapsone is a sulfa drug derivative, so it is contraindicated for use in those with allergy to sulfa drugs.[1]

ERYTHEMA MULTIFORME

Erythema multiforme (EM) is a blistering, ulcerative mucocutaneous condition of uncertain etiology. In one study, however, 50% of the individuals with EM either had a preceding infection, such as herpes simplex or *Mycoplasma pneumoniae*, or had been exposed to any one of a variety of drugs, particularly antibiotics or analgesics.[1]

Clinical Features

With EM, there is acute onset, but the disease may present with a wide spectrum of clinical disease. At the mild end of the spectrum, ulcerations develop that primarily affect the oral mucosa. In its severe form, diffuse sloughing and ulceration of the entire skin and mucosal surfaces may be seen. The severe form is known as *toxic epidermal necrolysis*, or *Lyell's disease*. Patients are usually first diagnosed in their twenties and thirties; men are affected more often than women.

EM has a prodromal period, with individuals experiencing fever, malaise, headache, cough, and sore throat one week before onset of characteristic clinical symptoms. The disease is self-limiting, usually lasting 2 to 6 weeks; however, 20% of those affected experience recurrent episodes, usually in the spring and autumn.

Erythematous skin lesions occur in 50% of cases. A variety of appearances of these lesions may be present (*multiforme* means "many forms"). Early lesions are flat, round, and dusky-red and appear on the extremities. The lesions may become slightly elevated and may evolve into bullae with necrotic centers. Occasionally, concentric circular erythematous lesions resembling a target or bull's eye (target lesions) develop that are highly characteristic of the disease (Figure 37–2).

Intraorally, erythematous patches undergo epithelial necrosis and become large, shallow erosions and ulcerations with irregular borders. The lesions emerge quickly and are very uncomfortable. There is a diffuse distribution, but the most common areas affected are the lips, labial mucosa, buccal mucosa, tongue, floor of the mouth, and soft palate. Hemorrhagic, crusted lips are also common (Figure 37–3). The gingivae and hard palate are seldom affected.[1]

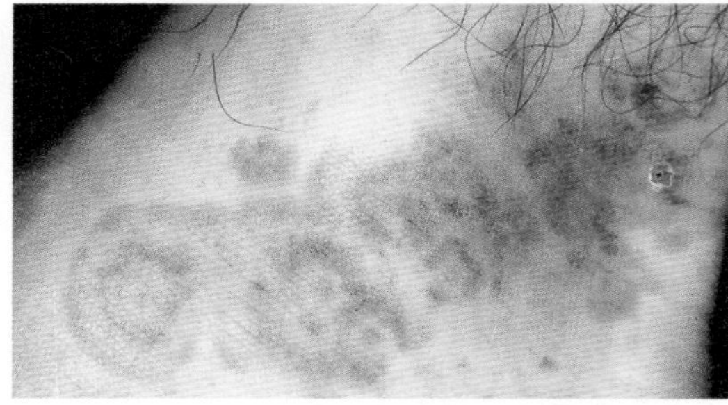

FIGURE 37–2 ✦ Target lesions of erythema multiforme. *(Courtesy Dr. Donald Cohen and Dr. Indraneel Bhattacharyya.)*

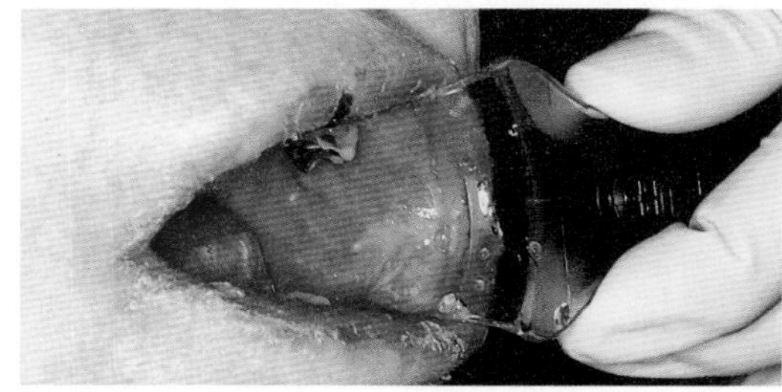

FIGURE 37–3 ✦ Crusted lips of erythema multiforme. *(Courtesy Dr. Donald Cohen and Dr. Indraneel Bhattacharyya.)*

A severe form of EM, known as *erythema multiforme major* or *Stevens-Johnson syndrome*, is usually triggered by a drug reaction rather than an infection. Ocular, genital, oral, and skin lesions are present. There are approximately five cases per million persons every year.

The most severe form of EM, toxic epidermal necrolysis, is almost always triggered by drug exposure. The disease presents as diffuse sloughing of a significant portion of the skin and mucosal surfaces, similar to a bad scalding. Although fairly rare, this form tends to occur in older people and is more common in females. If a patient survives, the cutaneous lesions resolve in 2 to 4 weeks, but oral lesions may take longer to heal. Half of patients affected present with significant ocular damage. There is approximately one case per million people annually.

Treatment and Prognosis

EM can be managed with systemic corticosteroids. Minor forms of the disease may be managed effectively with topical corticosteroid syrups or elixirs. Topical anesthetic agents are effective in decreasing oral discomfort. With more severe forms of the disease, intravenous rehydration may be necessary. EM is not life-threatening except in its most severe forms. Mortality rates with toxic epidermal necrolysis and Stevens-Johnson syndrome are 34% and 2% to 10%, respectively.[1]

IMMUNE-MEDIATED (TYPE 1) DIABETES MELLITUS

See Chapter 41, "Persons with Diabetes Mellitus."

HASHIMOTO'S THYROIDITIS

Hashimoto's thyroiditis, a form of hypothyroidism characterized by decreased levels of thyroid hormone, is caused in adults by autoimmune destruction of the thyroid gland or by iatrogenic factors (induced by the treatment itself), such as radioactive iodine therapy or surgery for the treatment of hyperthyroidism.[1]

Thyroid hormone is necessary for normal cellular metabolism. Therefore, many clinical signs and symptoms of hypothyroidism can be related to the decreased metabolic rate in these patients. The most common signs and symptoms include those listed in Table 37–1.

Treatment for hypothyroidism usually consists of thyroid replacement therapy, most commonly with levothyroxine, and the prognosis is generally good for adults. If recognized early in children, the prognosis is also good; if not identified early, permanent damage to the central nervous system may occur, resulting in mental retardation. Fortunately in children, thyroid replacement therapy often results in a dramatic resolution of the condition.[1]

RHEUMATOID ARTHRITIS

Rheumatoid arthritis (RA), a chronic, possibly autoimmune disorder characterized by a nonsuppurative inflammatory destruction of the joints, is of unknown etiology in most cases. It affects 3% of the U.S. population, and 200,000 new cases are diagnosed yearly. The disease begins as an attack against the synovial membrane (synovitis). Subsequently, enzymes such as collagenases and other proteases destroy the cartilage and underlying bone. Attempted remodeling by the exposed bone results in a characteristic deformation of the joint.[3]

Clinical Features

RA affects women three times more frequently than men; however, men are diagnosed at a somewhat younger age than women (25 to 35 versus 35 to 45 years). Onset and course of the disease are extremely variable, regardless of gender. For many people, no more than one or two joints are involved and significant pain or limitation of joint motion may never develop. In others, the disease rapidly progresses to debilitating *polyarthralgia* (pain in several joints).[3]

Signs and symptoms tend to become more severe over time. Symptoms are listed in Table 37–1. Bilateral involvement of the small joints of the hands and feet is almost always present, but it is not unusual for knees and elbows to be affected. The hip joint is least affected by RA. Twenty percent of patients also have firm, partially movable, nontender rheumatoid nodules beneath the skin near the affected joint. The temporomandibular joint (TMJ) eventually becomes involved in 75% of cases, although this is usually clinically insignificant. Radiographically, involved TMJs demonstrate a flattened condylar head with irregular surface features, an irregular temporal fossa surface, and anterior displacement of the condyle.[1]

Treatment and Prognosis

There is no cure for RA. Current treatment strives to only suppress the disease process as much as possible. With early and mild cases of RA, nonsteroidal anti-inflammatory drugs (NSAIDs) are prescribed, with occasional corticosteroid injections into the joint as needed. Injections are used sparingly because they have been associated with additional degenerative changes and fibrous ankylosis. Second-line medications include systemic corticosteroids, gold injections, penicillamine, cyclophosphamide, and methotrexate. All of these drugs, however, are associated with significant side effects. Iron supplementation may also be necessary because some patients may have mild anemia, discovered during blood work to detect levels of rheumatoid factor (RF), which is used in diagnosis.[1,3] Extended use of corticosteroids may warrant antibiotic prophylaxis before dental hygiene care.

SARCOIDOSIS

Sarcoidosis, a multisystem granulomatous disorder of unknown cause, is more commonly recognized in the developed world. In North America, blacks are affected 10 times more frequently than whites. Females are affected slightly more frequently than males, with age at onset between 20 and 40 years. The disorder presents acutely over a period of days to weeks, and the symptoms are variable.

Approximately 20% of patients have no symptoms, and the disease is discovered on routine chest radiographs. When present, common clinical symptoms include dyspnea, dry cough, chest pain, fever, malaise, fatigue, arthralgia, and weight loss. Pulmonary symptoms are most common.[1,4]

Although any organ may be affected, the most common sites are the lungs, lymph nodes, skin, eyes, and salivary glands. Lymphoid tissue is almost always involved. Twenty-five percent of persons experience granulomatous inflammation of the skin, which can best be described as chronic, violaceous (of violet color), indurated lesions often on the nose, ears, lips, and face (Figure 37–4). Bilateral, elevated, indurated, purplish plaques also are seen commonly on the limbs, back, and buttocks. Frequently, scattered, nonspecific, tender, erythematous nodules, known as *erythema nodosum,* occur on the lower legs. In 25% of cases, ocular involvement affects the lacrimal glands, causing dry eyes.[1,4]

Salivary glands may be affected, resulting in clinical enlargement and xerostomia. Any major or minor salivary gland may be involved, and sometimes it is necessary to remove intraoral mucoceles that occur. It is important to note that salivary gland enlargement, xerostomia, and dry eyes can combine to mimic Sjögren's syndrome. If salivary gland and lymph node involvement are excluded, clinically evident oral manifestations in sarcoidosis are uncommon.

Any oral mucosal site may manifest lesions such as a submucosal mass, an isolated papule, or an area of granularity. These may be normal in color, brownish-red, violaceous, or hyperkeratotic. Bony involvement is rare, but when present, may mimic periodontal disease.[1]

Prognosis is varied. With 60% of patients, prognosis is excellent because symptoms resolve spontaneously within two years without treatment. Twenty percent of patients can be treated successfully with corticosteroids; 10% to 20% do not respond to treatment. Approximately 4% to 10% of patients die of pulmonary, cardiac, or central nervous system complications.[1]

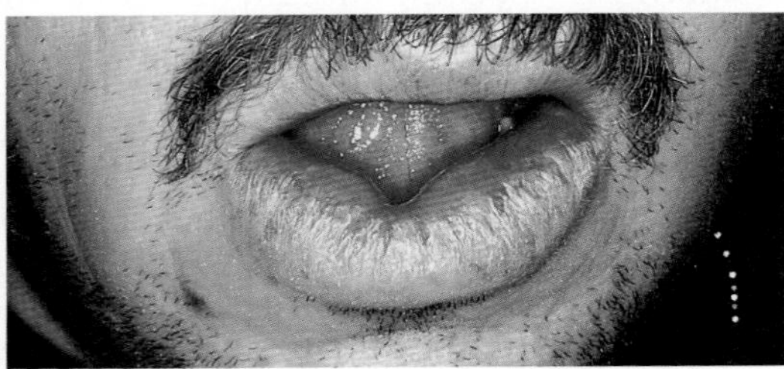

FIGURE 37–4 ✦ Indurated lip lesions characteristic of sarcoidosis. *(Courtesy Dr. Donald Cohen and Dr. Indraneel Bhattacharyya.)*

SYSTEMIC SCLEROSIS (SCLERODERMA)

Systemic sclerosis, or *scleroderma* (also referred to as hidebound disease), is a relatively rare condition that probably has an immune-mediated component. For unknown reasons, dense collagen is deposited in the body tissues in extraordinary amounts. The most dramatic effects are seen in the skin; however, the disease is often serious because most organs of the body can be affected.[1]

Clinical and Radiographic Features

Scleroderma affects approximately 19 persons per million population each year, affecting women three times more frequently than men. Most patients are adults. Cutaneous (relating to the skin) changes are the first symptoms to manifest, often bringing the condition to the person's attention.

One of the first signs of the disease is often *Raynaud's phenomenon,* a vasoconstrictive condition often triggered by emotional distress or exposure to cold. Resorption of the terminal phalanges and flexion contractures results in clawlike fingers (Figure 37–5). Vasoconstriction and abnormal collagen deposition sometimes lead to ulcerations on the fingertips. As a result of these phenomena, the skin develops a diffuse, hard texture (*sclero* means "hard"; *derma* means "skin"). The surface of the skin is also usually smooth. Facially, smooth, taut skin results in a mask-like appearance. Sometimes the alae of the nose become "pinched-in."[1]

Involvement of other organs may be insidious, but the results are more serious. Organ fibrosis may include the lungs, heart, kidneys, and gastrointestinal tract, leading to organ failure. Pulmonary fibrosis is a primary cause of death for patients affected.[1]

The oral cavity is affected to varying degrees. *Microstomia* (smallness of the oral aperture, or opening) often develops as a result of collagen deposition in perioral tissues. In 70% of persons afflicted, a tight, purse-string appearance of the lips causes a limitation in mouth opening. Intraorally, loss of attached gingival mucosa and generalized recession may occur. Difficulty in swallowing

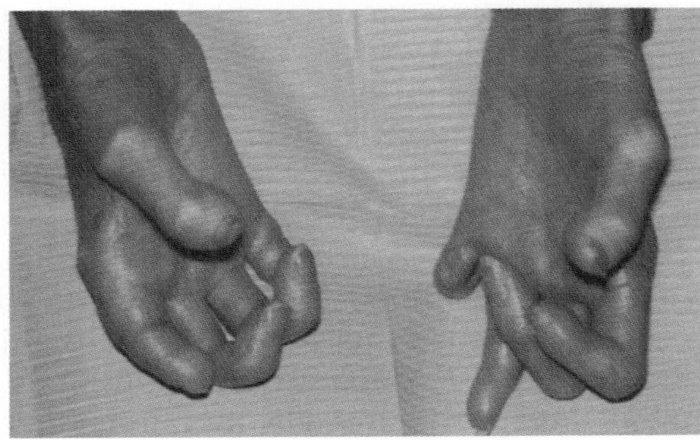

FIGURE 37–5 ✦ Clawlike finger position characteristic of systemic sclerosis.

from deposition of collagen in the mucosa of the lingual and esophageal areas is further hindered by a firm, hypomobile tongue and an inelastic esophagus.[1]

Radiographically, generalized widening of the periodontal ligament space may be subtly apparent or dramatic (Figure 37–6). In 20% of patients, there are varying degrees of resorption of the posterior ramus of the mandible, the coronoid process, and the condyle.[1]

A mild form of this condition, known as *localized scleroderma,* usually affects only a small patch of skin. The lesions often look like scars, hence the name *coup de sabre,* or "strike of the sword" (Figure 37–7). This is primarily a cosmetic issue and is rarely life-threatening.

Treatment and Prognosis

The management of scleroderma is difficult. D-penicillamine or other systemic medications may be prescribed in an effort to inhibit collagen production. Unfortunately, corticosteroids have proven to be of little benefit.

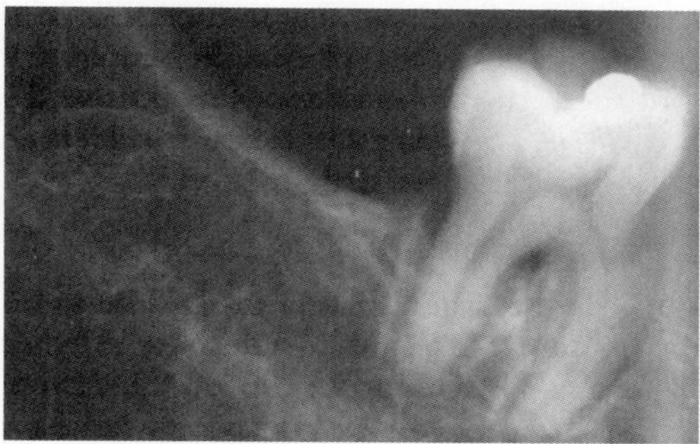

FIGURE 37–6 ✦ Widening of the periodontal ligament space characteristic of systemic sclerosis.

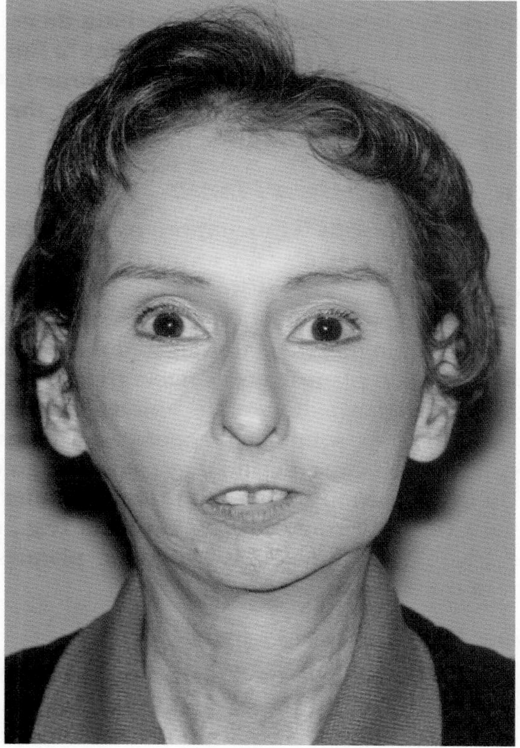

FIGURE 37–7 ✦ Localized scleroderma of the face presenting a scarlike appearance (coup de sabre).

Other treatments are aimed at controlling symptoms. Esophageal dilation is often performed to correct the dysphagia. Nifedipine (Procardia) helps increase peripheral blood flow and decrease symptoms of Raynaud's phenomenon.[1]

Persons afflicted who wear removable prostheses may develop problems because of the microstomia and inelasticity of the mouth. Patients may also have problems performing adequate oral hygiene resulting from a decreased ability to handle a toothbrush because of sclerosis of the fingers and hands. In some cases, resorption of the mandible may become so severe that a fracture results.[1]

Although the overall prognosis is poor, it is better for patients with limited cutaneous involvement than for those with systemic involvement. Approximately 80% of patients survive two years following diagnosis, but the survival rate drops off with time. Fifty percent survive eight years; the survival rate drops to 30% at 12 years.[1]

SJÖGREN'S SYNDROME

Sjögren's syndrome, a chronic, systemic autoimmune disorder that principally involves the salivary and lacrimal glands, results in xerostomia and xerophthalmia (dry eyes). In primary Sjögren's syndrome, a patient presents with xerostomia and xerophthalmia, but no other autoimmune disorder is present; in secondary Sjögren's syndrome, a patient presents with the aforementioned symptoms in addition to another associated autoimmune disease.

Although the cause of Sjögren's syndrome is unknown, there is evidence of a genetic influence. Relatives of affected patients have an increased frequency of other autoimmune diseases. Furthermore, there is speculative evidence that viruses, such as Epstein-Barr virus, play a role in disease onset.[1]

Clinical Features

Although Sjögren's syndrome is not a rare condition, the exact prevalence is unknown. It has been estimated to occur in 0.5% of the U.S. population. Eighty to ninety percent of cases occur in middle-aged females, and they rarely occur in children.

The most common associated disorder is rheumatoid arthritis. Fifteen percent of patients with RA have Sjögren's syndrome. Secondary Sjögren's syndrome may also develop in 30% of patients with systemic lupus erythematosus.[1,5]

Patients with Sjögren's syndrome and its associated xerostomia may complain of difficulty swallowing, altered taste, or difficulty wearing dentures. Fissured tongue and atrophy of papillae are common. Along with xerostomia, the oral mucosa may be red and tender, usually resulting from secondary candidiasis. Denture sores and angular cheilitis are also common. Furthermore, lack of salivary cleansing action increases patient risk for dental caries, especially cervical caries.[1]

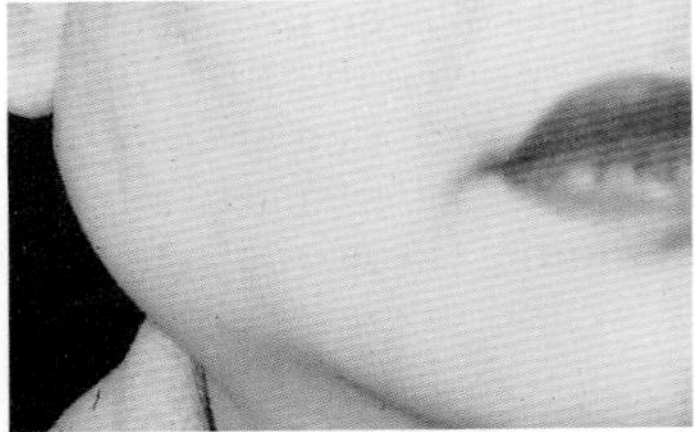

FIGURE 37–8 ✦ Enlargement of parotid gland in Sjögren's syndrome. *(Courtesy Dr. Donald Cohen and Dr. Indraneel Bhalla.)*

One-third to one-half of patients have diffuse, firm enlargement of the major salivary glands during the course of their disease (Figure 37–8). The swelling is usually bilateral, may be nonpainful or slightly tender, and may be intermittent or persistent. Usually, the greater the severity of disease, the greater the likelihood of salivary gland enlargement. Furthermore, reduced salivary flow places persons with Sjögren's syndrome at an increased risk for retrograde bacterial sialadenitis.[1,5]

The eyes may be affected as well. Patients often complain of a scratchy, gritty sensation or the perceived presence of a foreign body in the eye. Vision may become blurred, and sometimes there is an aching pain. Ocular problems are least severe in the morning on wakening and become more pronounced as the day progresses.[1]

Other body tissues are affected by the inflammatory process. The skin and the nasal and vaginal mucosae may also become dry. General malaise or fatigue is also fairly common and depression sometimes occurs. Other possible associated problems include lymphadenopathy, primary biliary cirrhosis, Raynaud's phenomenon, interstitial nephritis, interstitial lung fibrosis, vasculitis, and peripheral neuropathies.

Treatment and Prognosis

Treatment is mostly supportive in nature. Dry eyes are best managed by occasional use of artificial tears. Artificial salivas, sugarfree gum, and sugarless candy are available for the xerostomia. Sialagogues, for example pilocarpine, can be helpful to stimulate salivary flow if enough functional salivary tissue still remains. Because of an increased risk of dental caries, daily fluoride applications may be indicated in dentulous patients. Antifungal therapy may be needed to treat secondary candidiasis. Patients with Sjögren's syndrome have up to a 40 times higher rate of lymphomas (predominantly non-Hodgkin's B-cell lymphomas) than the normal population. Close follow-up is necessary with the client's physician of record if symptoms persist or if the condition appears to worsen.[1,5]

LICHEN PLANUS

Lichen planus is a "relatively common, chronic dermatologic disease that often affects the oral mucosa." The name of the disease comes from the words for primitive plants composed of algae and fungi (lichens) and the term *planus*, which is Latin for "flat." Although the name suggests a flat, fungal condition, current evidence indicates that it is an immunologically mediated mucocutaneous disorder.[1]

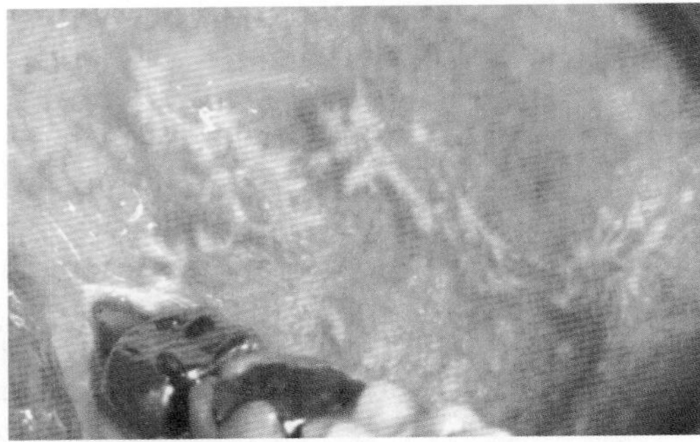

FIGURE 37–9 ✦ Reticular lichen planus. The white interlacing lines typical of reticular lichen planus are present on the posterior buccal mucosa. *(Courtesy Dr. William Bruce.)*

A variety of medications may induce lesions that are clinically identical to lichen planus (lichenoid drug reactions), but the terms *lichenoid mucositis* (mucosal involvement) or *lichenoid dermatitis* (skin involvement) are names for lesions that are drug-related.[1]

Clinical Features

Most patients with lichen planus are middle-aged adults. Children are rarely affected. Women are affected more often than men, usually by a ratio of 3:2. About 1% of the population experiences cutaneous lichen planus. The prevalence of oral lichen planus is between 0.1% and 2.2%.[1]

Skin lesions are purple papules (circumscribed solid elevations). They usually affect the flexor surfaces of the extremities. The lesions itch, but scratching them is very painful. The surface of the papules exhibits "a fine, lace-like network of white lines" (Wickham's striae). Other extraoral sites that may be involved include the glans penis, the vulvar mucosa, and the nails.[1]

Reticular Oral Lichen Planus

Reticular lichen planus is much more common than the erosive form. The reticular form usually does not cause symptoms and involves the posterior buccal mucosa bilaterally. Other sites may include the lateral and dorsal surfaces of the tongue, the gingivae, and the palate.

Reticular lichen planus gets its name from the characteristic white interlacing lines of the lesions (Figure 37–9). These white lesions sometimes appear as papules. The lesions are not usually static and may come and go over a period of weeks or months. Also, the reticular pattern may not be as evident in some sites as in others (e.g., dorsal tongue lesions may appear as "keratotic plaques with atrophy of the papillae").[1]

Erosive Oral Lichen Planus

Erosive lichen planus, even though not as common as the reticular form, is more significant because the lesions—erythematous areas with central ulceration—are usually symptomatic. The edge of the lesions exhibit the fine, white, radiating striae characteristic of the

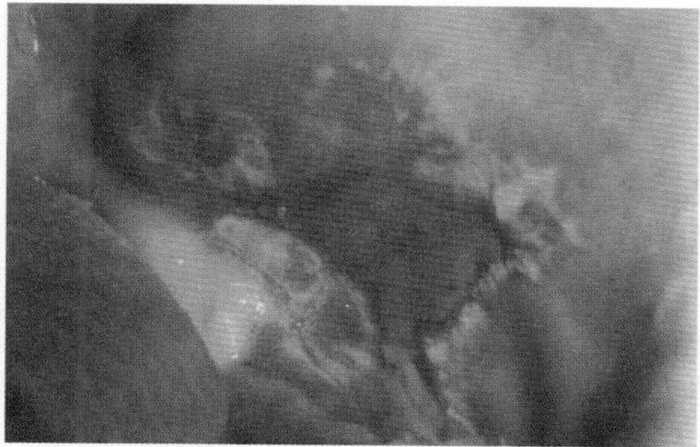

FIGURE 37–10 ✦ Erosive lichen planus. Ulceration of the buccal mucosa shows peripheral radiating keratotic striae, characteristic of oral erosive lichen planus.

disease (Figure 37–10). When the ulcerations are limited to the gingival mucosa, this is termed *desquamative gingivitis.* When confined to the gingiva, biopsy is indicated to rule out cicatricial pemphigoid and pemphigus vulgaris because they may appear similarly in gingival areas.[1]

Treatment and Prognosis

Treatment for reticular lichen planus is usually not needed because there are no symptoms. Occasionally, patients may have a concurrent candidiasis infection for which antifungal therapy is prescribed. Erosive lichen planus, however, requires treatment for the open sores in the mouth. Corticosteroids are often prescribed. A topical corticosteroid (e.g., fluocinonide gel) may be applied several times each day to the most severe lesions to induce healing. Follow-up every 3 months is recommended because there is the potential for malignant transformation.

LUPUS ERYTHEMATOSUS

Lupus erythematosus is a classic example of an immunologically mediated condition. There are several forms: systemic lupus erythematosus, chronic cutaneous lupus erythematosus, and subacute cutaneous lupus erythematosus.[1]

Systemic Lupus Erythematosus (SLE)

Systemic lupus erythematosus is a serious multisystem disease with a variety of cutaneous and oral manifestations. Although the precise cause is unknown, genetic factors probably play a role. Difficult to diagnose in its early stages, SLE often presents in a nonspecific, vague fashion, with periods of remission or disease inactivity. Women are affected 8 to 10 times more frequently than men. The average age at diagnosis is 31 years.[1]

CLINICAL FEATURES. Common systemic symptoms include fever, weight loss, arthritis, and malaise. In 40% to 50% of afflicted persons, there is a characteristic "butterfly rash," which develops over the malar area and the nose (sunlight often makes the rash worse), and kidneys are affected (Figure 37–11). Typically, the most significant aspect of the disease is kidney failure. At autopsy, nearly 50% of persons display warty vegetations affecting the heart valves. The significance is debatable, however; some may develop a superimposed subacute bacterial endocarditis.[1]

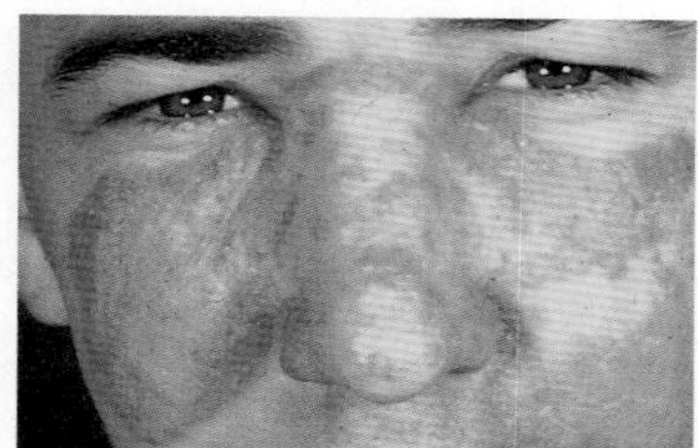

FIGURE 37–11 ✦ Malar rash seen in systemic lupus erythematosus. *(Courtesy of Dr. Donald M. Cohen and Dr. Indraneel Bhattacharyya.)*

Oral lesions develop in 5% to 40% of these patients. Lesions usually affect the palate, buccal mucosa, and gingivae. Sometimes they appear as lichenoid areas or look nonspecific or somewhat granulomatous. Varying degrees of ulceration, pain, erythema, and hyperkeratosis may be present.

Criteria for making an SLE diagnosis have been established by the American Rheumatism Association and include both clinical and laboratory findings (Table 37–1).[1,6,7]

Chronic Cutaneous Lupus Erythematosus (CCLE)

Chronic cutaneous lupus erythematosus primarily affects the skin and oral mucosa and has a good prognosis. Patients usually have few or no systemic signs or symptoms. Skin lesions that erupt are known as *discoid lupus erythematosus.* They begin as scaly, erythematous patches, that are frequently distributed on sun-exposed skin, especially in the head and neck area. The healing process usually results in cutaneous atrophy with scarring and hypopigmentation or hyperpigmentation of the resolving lesion.

Intraorally, the lesions appear practically identical to the lesions of erosive lichen planus; however, the lesions of CCLE rarely occur in the absence of skin lesions. The ulcerative and atrophic oral lesions may be painful, especially when exposed to acidic or salty foods.[1,7]

Subacute Cutaneous Lupus Erythematosus (SCLE)

Subacute cutaneous lupus erythematosus has clinical features intermediate between those of SLE and CCLE. Skin lesions are the most prominent feature of this variation. Most patients have photosensitivity, accompanying arthritis, and musculoskeletal problems.[1,7]

Treatment and Prognosis

For all forms of lupus erythematosus, the patient must avoid excessive sunlight exposure because ultraviolet light may precipitate disease activity. With acute episodes of disease, systemic corticosteroids are generally indicated, sometimes supplemented with other immunosuppressive agents. Antimalarial drugs may be effective, usually more so for the CCLE or SCLE types. If oral lesions are present, they typically respond to the systemic therapy.[7]

Prognosis for the patient with SLE varies. For patients in treatment, the 5-year survival rate is approximately 95%. By the 15-year mark, survival rate falls to 75%.[1] Prognosis depends on which organs are affected and how frequently the disease is reactivated. The most common cause of death is renal failure caused by kidney involvement. For reasons that are poorly understood, the prognosis is worse for men than for women. Furthermore, for patients with CCLE, prognosis is considerably better than that for those with SLE. Transformation to SLE may be seen in approximately 5% of CCLE patients. About 50% of CCLE cases resolve after several years.[1]

DENTAL HYGIENE PROCESS OF CARE FOR PERSONS WITH AUTOIMMUNE DISEASE

Assessment

During the assessment phase, it is of utmost importance to obtain a thorough health and dental history from the client. If there are indications that the client is not well or that referral to a physician is needed immediately, dental hygiene care must be postponed until a time approved by the physician of record. If pain is reported by the client during the assessment phase, the first course of action would be referral to the physician for pain management.

Diagnosis

Human needs assessments will differ depending on the autoimmune disease(s) of the client. All eight human needs may pertain to an individual with erythema multiforme, whereas only a few may pertain to the individual with rheumatoid arthritis. The dental hygiene diagnosis is highly dependent on the signs observed by the clinician and the symptoms reported by the client at the assessment phase.

Planning

The planning phase may be complicated by medical attention needed by the client at the time of dental hygiene care. Consultation with the client's physician to establish goals and communication is helpful in determining how to coordinate dental hygiene care with concurrent medical care. An example of a goal might be: "Client will report a decrease in oral discomfort at next appointment."

Implementation

The implementation phase of the dental hygiene process includes client education, periodontal debridement, tissue evaluation, and referral back to the physician if warranted. Depending on the severity of oral symptoms, clients may need specialized care from a specialist, oral pathologist, or periodontist. Client education must include disease pathophysiology, effects on the oral cavity, palliative treatments for oral discomfort, and preventive oral therapies where appropriate (see Topical Analgesic Agents Prescribed by the Dentist for Palliative Management of Oral Discomfort).

Evaluation

Clients with autoimmune disease must be placed on 2- to 3-month maintenance intervals because of their compromised immune system. Furthermore, it is important that after initial therapy is completed, an evaluation appointment be scheduled to assess the client's host response to dental hygiene care and to reinforce self-care.

At each subsequent appointment, the client's overall health, as well as oral health, is reassessed. Continued communication between the dental hygienist, dentist, and physician is extremely important when making changes in planned professional care.

The dental hygienist must be able to relate the human needs of the client to the factors that are contributing to the problem(s). The diagnostic statements and goals are used to guide clinical decisions regarding appropriate dental hygiene interventions so that oral health can be achieved. Whether signs and symptoms first documented are still evident at the evaluation appointment will determine if the goals were met, partially met, or not met. Further treatment and referral may be necessary, depending on outcomes.

Topical Analgesic Agents Prescribed by the Dentist for Palliative Management of Oral Discomfort

Diphenhydramine HCl (without alcohol) mixed with Kaopectate, Maalox, AlternaGEL, or Carafate suspension; or

Viscous lidocaine, 2%; or

Dyclonine HCl

CLIENT EDUCATION ISSUES

- ✦ Explain that daily self-care and 2- to 3-month maintenance care are necessary to control and/or prevent oral manifestations of autoimmune diseases.
- ✦ Explain that regular evaluation by the physician's of record and reporting of those findings to the oral healthcare team are important to maintain coordinated, comprehensive health care.
- ✦ Explain that strict adherence to the physician and dentist's and/or dental hygienist's recommendations will ensure that adequate care is rendered. Client's must not self-medicate, stop medications, or ignore preventive practices recommended by the healthcare team.

Legal, Ethical, and Safety Issues

- The dental hygienist should thoroughly update the client's medical and dental histories and document any updates or changes in health status.
- If concern exists that the client is at risk for harm by proceeding with care, the dental hygienist must inform the dentist so that a prompt referral to the physician of record is made.
- The dental hygienist must document any adverse reaction or occurrence during the provision of care. This information must be shared with the dentist and physician of record.

Key Concepts

- The incidence of encountering individuals with autoimmune diseases in the oral care environment will increase as the percentage of aging persons increases.
- The dental hygienist must be able to recognize typical signs, symptoms, and manifestations of autoimmune diseases.
- Some autoimmune diseases affect the head and neck area only, whereas others can affect almost any organ system of the body.
- Autoimmune diseases compromise clients' immune systems and put them at risk for periodontal disease.
- Some autoimmune diseases can be effectively managed with medication.
- Some autoimmune diseases warrant antibiotic prophylaxis before beginning any invasive care.
- Scleroderma may affect a client's ability to perform adequate oral self-care measures.
- Use of salivary substitutes, sugarless candy, and sugarless gum may help manage xerostomia in those with Sjögren's syndrome.
- Referral and consultation with the client's physician are helpful to coordinate dental hygiene care with concurrent medical care.

Critical Thinking Exercises

Client: Mrs. M

Profile: Mrs. M., age 40, who has not been to a dentist for three years, was scheduled for care with the dental hygienist.

Chief Complaint: "I have a very dry mouth. Also I cannot eat spicy foods because they irritate the skin inside my mouth. I haven't been able to really taste my food for some time."

Medical History: Besides the slight discomfort from her inflamed tissues, she believes her health is satisfactory.

Social History: Married with two children

Dental History: Intraorally, her probing depths range from 4 to 6 mm, with generalized, moderate-to-severe bleeding on probing. The gingivae and oral mucosa are moderately inflamed and erythematous. The tissues are smooth without stippling, and the tongue is fissured with atrophic papillae. She has Class II periodontitis, with generalized, moderate calculus deposits and heavy cervical bacterial plaque. Six Class V carious lesions were identified.

Oral Health Behavior Assessment: She brushes her teeth two times per day, but admits that she does not floss.

Supplemental Notes: There is obvious facial swelling bilaterally in the area of the parotid glands; however, she does not report any injury to the head and neck.

1. Use the assessment data to arrive at a dental hygiene diagnosis, set client goals, and plan dental hygiene interventions.
2. What should the dental hygienist do if the client's response to therapy is poor and her periodontal disease continues to progress?

For References, Suggested Readings, and Related Websites, visit
http://evolve.elsevier.com/Darby/hygiene/

CHAPTER 38

Persons with Neurologic and Sensory Disabilities

OBJECTIVES

Mastery of the content in this chapter will enable the reader to:

- Describe fundamental characteristics of the more common neurologic disorders, including dysfunctions of the motor system, sensory disorders, developmental disorders, peripheral neuropathies, spinal cord dysfunctions, demyelinating disorders, seizures, disorders of higher cortical function, and vascular insufficiencies
- Describe the oral clinical findings frequently observed in clients with each of the more common neurologic deficits
- Describe specific considerations needed to deliver dental hygiene care to clients with specific neurologic deficits
- Describe communication techniques for clients with sensory and mental deficits
- Describe oral self-care instructions individualized for clients with each of the more common neurologic deficits

KEY TERMS

Alzheimer's disease
Amyotrophic lateral sclerosis
Basal ganglia
Bell's palsy
Central nervous system
Cerebellum
Cerebral hemispheres
Cerebral palsy
Cerebrovascular accident
Cranial nerves
Epilepsy
Huntington's disease
Hydrocephalus
Multiple sclerosis
Muscular dystrophies
Myasthenia gravis
Neuron
Parkinson's disease
Poliomyelitis
Spina bifida
Spinal cord injury
Trigeminal neuralgia

The nervous system makes each of us unique. It senses and evaluates the internal and external environment, controls our body, and is responsible for our abilities, intellect, and personality. These characteristics are the result of complex interactions within the nervous system, and any structural damage or physiologic change to a component of this system may cause a loss of function and create a variety of neurologic deficits. The incidence and prevalence of some of the more common neurologic diseases or conditions, which will be discussed in this chapter, are listed in Table 38–1.

While each neurologic deficit has a unique etiology and pathology, the clinical manifestations may be similar. In these situations the oral clinical findings, special considerations for dental hygiene care, and oral self-care instructions would also be similar, and so will first be described in general terms. The more specific descriptions, unique to a particular neurologic disorder, will be discussed in the section on that disorder.

ORAL CLINICAL FINDINGS

Many clients with neurologic deficits exhibit extensive accumulations of plaque biofilm, food debris, and supragingival and subgingival calculus, dental caries, and inflammation of the gingiva, possibly extending to the periodontal attachment. The major factors contributing to this poor oral health are the clients' inability to perform adequate self-care because of impaired motor

TABLE 38–1 EPIDEMIOLOGY OF NEUROLOGIC DISEASES

Disease or Condition	Incidence*	Prevalence†
Cerebrovascular disease	200	650
Seizures and epilepsy	120	650
Peripheral neuropathy	100	No data
Dementia	50	250
Parkinson's disease	20	200
Primary tumors	15	65
Spinal cord disorders	13	90
Trigeminal neuralgia	4	40
Multiple sclerosis	3	60
Motor neuron disease	2	6
Muscular dystrophies	1	8
Hereditary degenerative disorders	1	20
Huntington's disease	0.4	5
Myasthenia gravis	0.4	4

Adapted from Collins R: *Neurology*, Philadelphia, 1997, WB Saunders.
*New cases/100,000 population/year
†Number of cases in existence at any one point in time per 100,000 population

coordination, inadequate sensation, or generalized muscle weakness and fatigue. Further debilitation may necessitate dependence on their caregiver, who may be overwhelmed with the number of responsibilities. Access to care may be an additional problem because of limited finances, problems with mobility/transportation to dental care, and the attitudes of oral health care practitioners. This issue was addressed in Chapter 36.

Disturbances of the oral musculature, observed in many of these clients, interfere with the self-cleansing mechanisms of the tongue, cheek, and lip and, consequently, the oral clearance of plaque biofilm and food debris. The client may have lost sensation and not be aware of the debris collecting in the vestibule. This retention around the teeth and oral mucosa is accentuated by the consumption of a soft, carbohydrate-rich diet, which the client chooses because of problems with mastication and swallowing.

Oral effects of the client's medications will also be observed, the most common being xerostomia or dry mouth. Xerostomia in turn causes susceptibility to oral infections such as candidiasis, taste dysfunction, difficulty in swallowing, and dental caries. Phenytoin and Dilantin, drugs used to control seizures, may cause severe gingival enlargement or overgrowth (see Figures 39-5 and 39-6). Dilantin alters the metabolism of the gingival fibroblasts, so that the cells produce excessive amounts of collagen. This drug-induced overgrowth, which occurs in approximately half of these clients, may be disfiguring and may interfere with mastication and speech.

SPECIAL CONSIDERATIONS FOR DENTAL HYGIENE CARE

Frequent recall appointments are usually needed to achieve and maintain optimal oral health, especially in clients whose deficit may limit their ability to perform oral self-care. Frequent visits are useful to monitor oral health and hygiene and to reinforce preventive self-care procedures for both client and caregiver. Weakness and fatigue increase during the day, so appointments are usually best scheduled early in the morning. Sufficient appointment time should be allowed so that the client does not feel rushed, in terms of both communication and physical movements.

Clients may be ambulatory, but using assistive walking devices, or be confined to a wheelchair. Their needs for assistance will vary; certain clients will do better without assistance because they have developed their own coping mechanisms; others will need aid in seating and rising from the dental chair or in being transferred to and from the wheelchair. Wheelchair transfer techniques have been described in Chapter 36. Depending on the client's condition, some may be more easily treated in the wheelchair.

During the appointment, clients with difficulty in swallowing and a diminished gag reflex may need to be seated in a more upright position to avoid choking and aspiration of water and foreign substances. Optimal suctioning and limiting the amount of water also help prevent airway obstruction. Mouth props or bite blocks may be useful for clients with impaired oral reflexes, muscle weakness, and tremors, and for those easily fatigued; however, extended use of these devices may create problems with their temporomandibular joint apparatus. Instrument fulcrums may need additional stabilization. To prevent injury to the clinician, in situations of the client's mouth closing without warning, a finger guard, such as a metal tailor's thimble, may be helpful.

In many clients, maintenance of stability is a great concern. The client may need to be secured in the dental chair with restraint or support devices, such as soft ties, belts, or pillows, although the caregiver holding the client may be the best, less restrictive means. The rationale for the use of assistance should always be explained to the client and/or caregiver as being facilitative for treatment, rather than as restraint. The client's head can be supported by the clinician sitting or standing at the 12 o'clock position and cradling the client's head with the clinician's nondominant arm. Further suggestions for stabilization are described in Chapter 36.

ORAL SELF-CARE INSTRUCTIONS

Instructions for individualized self-care depend on the client's level of energy and motor coordination (i.e., hand strength, abilities to grasp and to manipulate a toothbrush). All clients should be encouraged to be as self-sufficient as possible in maintaining their own oral health. The client's capabilities should be assessed, so that devices may be recommended or created to satisfy physical limitations. Toothbrush handles with a larger diameter are easier to grip. They can be enlarged with a bicycle grip, rubber or sponge ball, or modeling clay, as illustrated in Chapter 36. Powered toothbrushes usually have larger handles and do not require the client to produce a brushing stroke; however, supporting and controlling the weight of a powered brush may be more difficult than holding a manual toothbrush with both hands. A client may need to prop his or her elbows and arms during brushing to maintain motor control and minimize fatigue. For the client who wears dentures, a denture brush secured to the sink by suction would facilitate cleaning the prosthesis with one hand.

Other adaptations to assist plaque control are pump dispensers for toothpaste, toothpaste tubes with flip-top caps, and floss holders. The use of dental floss may be too difficult to master, so another interdental aid may be more appropriate. Respiratory problems may contraindicate a foamy toothpaste, so a brand without the detergent sodium lauryl sulfate may be suggested. Only clients with adequate ability to control gagging and swallowing can safely use fluoride and chlorhexidine rinses at home. Those suffering from severe oral motor dysfunction may be harmed by ingesting those products, so alternate preventive procedures, such as brush-on fluoride gels and fluoride trays, may be suggested.

Clients who are experiencing difficulties in mastication and swallowing may be consuming soft, carbohydrate-rich foods, so noncariogenic and nutritious foods should be recommended. The discomforts from xerostomia may be alleviated by the use of saliva substitutes (see Chapter 43). Fluoride mouthrinses and brush-on gels may also be recommended to xerostomic clients to protect their teeth from dental, especially root, caries, which are prevalent in this population. Because alcohol further dries out the oral mucosa, alcohol-containing mouthrinses would be contraindicated.

For those clients requiring assistance with their self-care, their caregivers should be instructed in effective plaque control procedures (see Chapters 18, 19, and 36), as well as client positioning for maximal stability and access. The parent or caregiver may need to sit or stand behind the person or wheelchair. For the client with uncontrollable movements, a second person may be needed to stabilize the client.

Powered toothbrushes may be easier for caregivers to use. Also, the use of a floss holder allows one hand of the caregiver to prop the mouth open, while the other hand is grasping the floss holder. If a mouth prop is necessary to keep the mouth open, an inexpensive one can be made by securing five or six tongue depressors together with adhesive tape. Written as well as oral instructions should be provided to both the caregiver and client so the information can be reviewed at home.

DYSFUNCTIONS OF THE MOTOR SYSTEM

Motor actions require the integration of several central nervous system (CNS) and peripheral nervous system (PNS) components. To review, the *central nervous system* is composed of the brain and the spinal cord (Table 38–2), and the PNS is composed of the spinal, cranial, and autonomic nerves and ganglia. In both systems the nerve cell or *neuron* is the basic functional unit (Figure 38–1) and has the specialized properties of excitation and impulse conduction. Except in rare situations, neurons do not divide after birth. Therefore, when there is injury or death of neurons, function is compromised or lost. Lesions in one or more of the motor neuron pathways lead to problems with motor strength or control.

TABLE 38–2 OVERVIEW OF THE MAJOR SUBDIVISIONS OF THE CENTRAL NERVOUS SYSTEM

Structure	Primary Function(s)
Brain	
CEREBRAL HEMISPHERES	
Lobes:	
Frontal lobe	Voluntary motor control, including speech
Parietal lobe	Somatic sensations
Occipital lobe	Vision
Temporal lobe	Hearing; memory
Limbic lobe	Drives, emotions, memory
Basal ganglia	Motor control
DIENCEPHALON	
Thalamus	Reciprocal connections with cerebral cortex
Hypothalamus	Integrative control of autonomic functions
Subthalamus	Motor control
CEREBELLUM	Control of range and force of movement and acquisition of motor skills
BRAINSTEM	
Midbrain	Control of motor and sensory functions; substantia nigra
Pons	Motor relay from hemispheres to cerebellum
Medulla	Control of vital autonomic functions
Spinal Cord	Integration of sensory and motor information from body and control of body movements

Lesions of the Cell Bodies of Motor Neurons

Motor neurons transmit nerve impulses away from the brain or spinal cord to or toward muscle or glandular tissue. The upper motor neurons (UMNs) are in the cerebral cortex or brainstem and descend to synapse primarily with motor neurons in the brainstem and spinal cord. The lower motor neurons (LMNs) have their cell body in the brainstem or spinal cord, and the axon exits as the motor division of the cranial and spinal nerves. Lesions to UMNs interrupt smooth motor control. A lesion anywhere from the cell body of the LMN to a muscle will produce a decrease in strength or weakness of the muscle and atrophy (degeneration) of muscle fibers.

POLIOMYELITIS OR POLIO. *Poliomyelitis* is an acute, highly contagious infectious disease caused by one of three types of polioviruses that attack the lower motor neurons of the spinal cord. Current poliomyelitis vac-

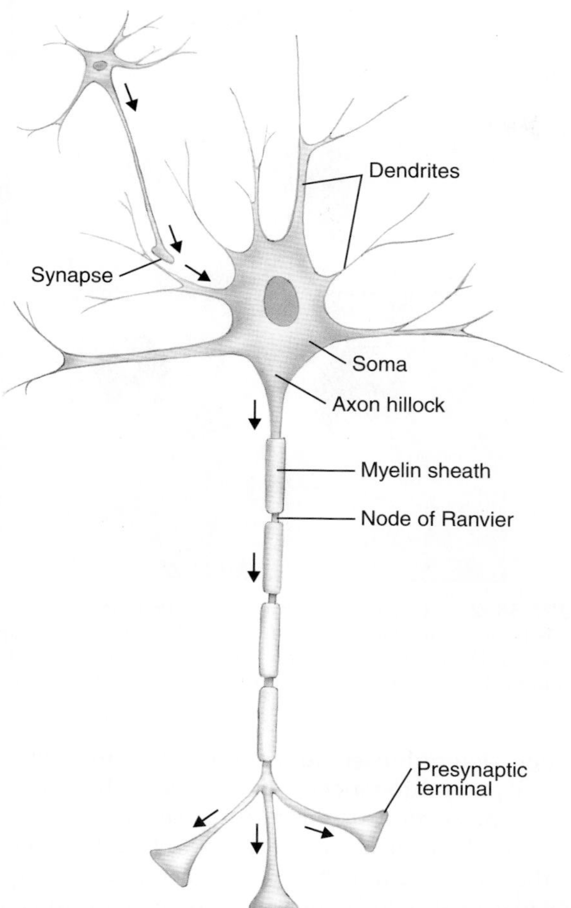

FIGURE 38–1 ✦ Principal parts of a typical neuron. The multiple dendrites receive input from other cells, the cell body (soma) processes the input, and a single axon with its presynaptic terminal contacts another neuron, gland, or muscle cell by way of a synapse. *(Modified from Lundy-Ekman L:* Neuroscience: Fundamentals for rehabilitation, *Philadelphia, 1998, WB Saunders.)*

cines, using a live, attenuated virus, have almost eliminated the disease.

Characteristics. Damage to LMNs in the spinal cord and brainstem causes a flaccid paralysis with loss of reflexes associated with the involved muscle or glandular cells. Initially there is fever, painful muscles, nausea, and vomiting, which in a few days is followed by stiffness of the neck and weakness of muscles supplied by the spinal and cranial nerves. Paralysis is usually maximum within this time. The pattern of weakness is highly variable—from a few muscles to almost complete paralysis. The most common muscles involved are those associated with the lower extremities, lungs, pharynx, and face.

Treatment and Prognosis. Treatment is purely supportive and symptomatic, with pain management and physical therapy. Sometimes mechanical ventilation may be required. Many patients recover completely, and most improve considerably. Those muscles with lasting motor neuron damage remain weak or paralyzed and atrophic.

AMYOTROPHIC LATERAL SCLEROSIS (ALS). *Amyotrophic lateral sclerosis* is a chronic degenerative disease consisting of signs and symptoms related to damage to the cell bodies of both the UMNs and the LMNs. The etiology is unknown, although some cases are familial. It generally appears between the ages of 50 and 70.

Characteristics. ALS usually presents with progressive painless weakness in a limb or progressive cranial nerve involvement. It may present with one of four characteristic forms, depending on the location of the involved motor neurons: the spinal cord, the lower brainstem, the motor cortex of the cerebrum, or the cranial nerves.

Treatment and Prognosis. Treatment is multidisciplinary, including psychological support. Although most patients die from respiratory failure or infection within 3 years of diagnosis, about 20% of patients have a more benign course and live several years.

Disorders of the Neuromuscular Junction

Communication among neurons, or between neurons and glands or muscle, occurs at specialized sites called *synapses.* Presynaptic terminals of axons contain vesicles, which store neurotransmitters (Figure 38–1). When an impulse arrives at the synapse, the neurotransmitter is released and interacts with receptors on another neuron, muscle, or gland cell in order to transmit the nerve impulse. A major neurotransmitter is acetylcholine, which is released at neuromuscular junctions.

MYASTHENIA GRAVIS (MG). *Myasthenia gravis* is an autoimmune disorder involving the production of antibodies against the acetylcholine receptors and, thus, impairing nerve impulse transmission at the neuromuscular junction. Women are affected twice as often as men. The peak for women is in their twenties and thirties, contrasted to a peak for men in their fifties and sixties.

Characteristics. The hallmark of MG is fluctuating or fatigable weakness, which worsens with exercise and improves with rest. Ocular symptoms are common, including ptosis (drooping eyelid) and diplopia (double vision). Other presenting symptoms include dysarthria (impaired speaking) or dysphagia (impaired swallowing), leg weakness with impaired walking, and generalized weakness.

Treatment and Prognosis. Mild weakness is treated with cholinesterase inhibitors (CEIs). The thymus is removed in patients younger than age 55 with moderate to marked weakness. The long-term natural course is variable. Some patients have spontaneous remission and some continue to have only ocular symptoms.

Dental Hygiene Care. Weakness of muscles of mastication and of the face and tongue leads to disturbed swallowing and mastication. Generalized muscle weakness and fatigue contribute to the client's inability to perform adequate self-care. Adaptations to problems in muscle weakness and ambulation have been previously described. In addition, an assistant may be needed for clients with serious respiratory complications to monitor vital signs and maintain the airway.

The dental office should be prepared for a myasthenic crisis in which the marked weakness of the respiratory and pharyngeal muscles may lead to an abrupt inability to swallow, speak, or maintain a patent airway. This crisis is best avoided by the elimination and prevention of infection and precipitating factors, such as excitement, surgery, alcohol intake, and loss of sleep.

Disorders of Muscle (Myopathies)

Myopathies include a variety of diseases of the skeletal muscles involving the muscle cells or connective tissue components. The more common myopathies include the *muscular dystrophies,* idiopathic inflammatory myopathies, viral inflammatory myopathies (HIV infection, Reye's syndrome), and parasitic inflammatory myopathies.

DUCHENNE'S MUSCULAR DYSTROPHY. The most important chronic, progressive, hereditary myopathies are the X-linked dystrophies, which include Duchenne's. Almost all patients with dystrophies are male. The disease is already present in utero, as muscle necrosis and serum enzyme elevation are found in neonates.

Characteristics. Motor developmental delay is noticeable after the first year, and onset of walking is usually delayed until after 15 months of age. Lower extremities and lower trunk are affected first, and children develop hyperlordosis (excessive forward curvature of the spine) with a prominent abdomen and enlarged calves. They often walk on their tiptoes, and in order to stand up from the floor they use their hands to walk up their legs, called a Gowers' maneuver (Figure 38–2). Progression is rapid, and many patients become wheelchair-bound by the age of 10; by the midteens they lose upper extremity function. Mental retardation occurs in about 10% of patients.

Treatment and Prognosis. Physical therapy is given to preserve mobility, prevent contractures, and maintain maximum function. Respiratory therapy maintains function and decreases respiratory infections. The disease is usually fatal by the end of the second decade because of respiratory failure, pulmonary infections, cardiomyopathy, or gastrointestinal complications.

Prevention includes carrier detection, genetic counseling, and prenatal diagnosis. Although one-third of cases do not have a family history, a known carrier has a 50% chance of giving birth to a Duchenne's male or a carrier female.

Dental Hygiene Care. The generalized muscle deterioration is also evident in the orofacial region and contributes to poor oral hygiene. The type and stage of the disorder determine modifications of dental hygiene care. Adaptation for specific problems, such as stabilization and protection of the airway, has been previously discussed. The procedure may need to be interrupted so that the client can expectorate accumulated mucus. Safety glasses should be provided to clients who cannot close the eyelids tightly because of muscle weakness.

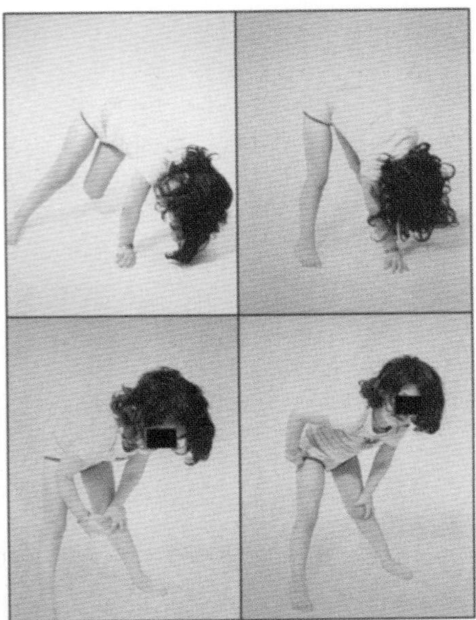

FIGURE 38–2 ✦ Gowers' maneuver in a child with Duchenne's muscular dystrophy. The child gets up from the floor by walking up his thighs with his hands due to weakness of the thigh muscles. *(From Perkin G:* Mosby's color atlas and text of neurology, *London, 1998, Mosby-Wolfe.)*

Abnormalities of Movement, Coordination, Tone, and Posture

Several regions of the brain are involved in the control of voluntary movement and in motor responses to sensory stimuli, particularly the motor region (frontal lobe) of the cerebral cortex, the cerebellum, and the basal ganglia. The outline of the CNS in Table 38–2 and the diagram of the brain in Figure 38–3 demonstrate the relationship of these specific regions to other components of the CNS. The *basal ganglia* refers to clusters of neuron cell bodies (gray matter) embedded deep within the forebrain and midbrain of the CNS. Although not evident in Figure 38–3, it is diagramatically represented in Figure 38–4. Disorders affecting cells of the *cerebellum* and basal ganglia, which project to the motor regions of the cerebral cortex, disturb movements and produce abnormalities of muscle tone, abnormal posturing, and tremors. There may be hyperkinesis (increase in movement), hypokinesis (lessening of muscular movement), a decrease in associated movements (e.g., arm swing when walking), or abnormal involuntary movements. Degenerative, metabolic, or vascular diseases; toxins; infections; trauma; or neoplasms may cause these abnormalities.

PARKINSON'S DISEASE (PARKINSON'S SYNDROME, PARALYSIS AGITANS). *Parkinson's disease* is rather

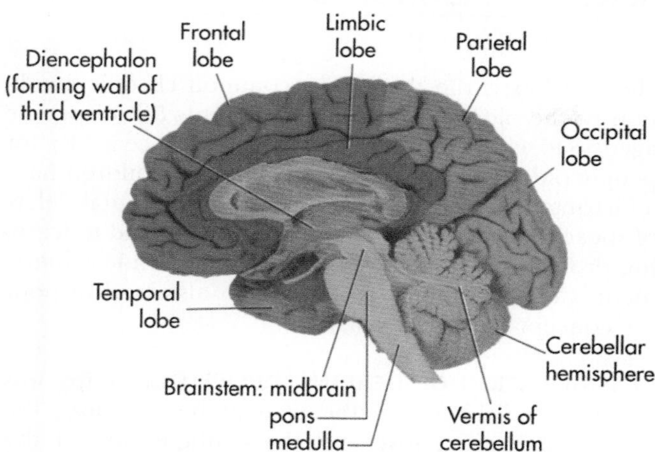

FIGURE 38–3 ✦ Major regions of the brain, as observed in a midsagittal view. Lobes of the cerebral cortex, diencephalon, brainstem, and cerebellum are illustrated; the regions of the basal ganglia are not evident in this view. *(Modified from Nolte J:* The human brain, *ed 4, Philadelphia, 1999, Mosby.)*

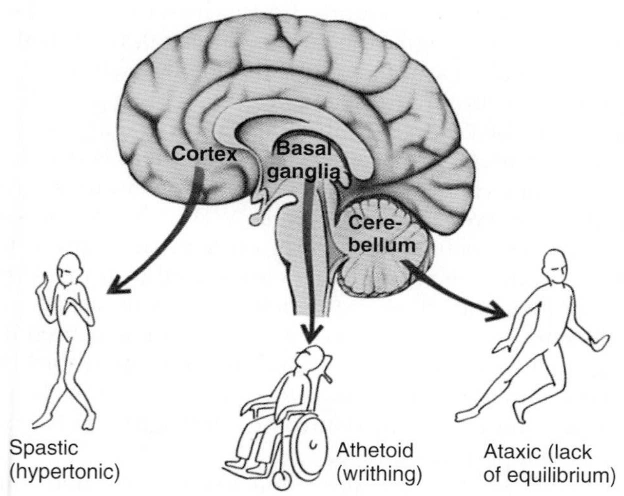

FIGURE 38–4 ✦ Parts of the brain affected in the major types of cerebral palsy. The types of the movement disorders depend on the part of the brain that has been damaged. *(Modified from Nowak AJ:* Dentistry for the handicapped patient, *St Louis, 1976, Mosby.)*

common in middle and old age, with the peak of onset in the sixth decade. Several conditions may present a clinical picture similar to that of Parkinson's disease (e.g., reaction to certain drugs), but the most common type has an unknown cause. The incidence is higher among Caucasians than African-Americans and Asians.

Pathologically, the disorder is characterized by the progressive loss of dopamine-synthesizing neurons in the substantia nigra of the midbrain of the brainstem (Figure 38–3). Dopamine, a neurotransmitter, is released from axons that originate from the cell bodies in the substantia nigra and terminate in the basal ganglia, where it serves as a neurotransmitter. A deficiency of dopamine at this site interferes with the conduction of nerve impulses related to muscle activity.

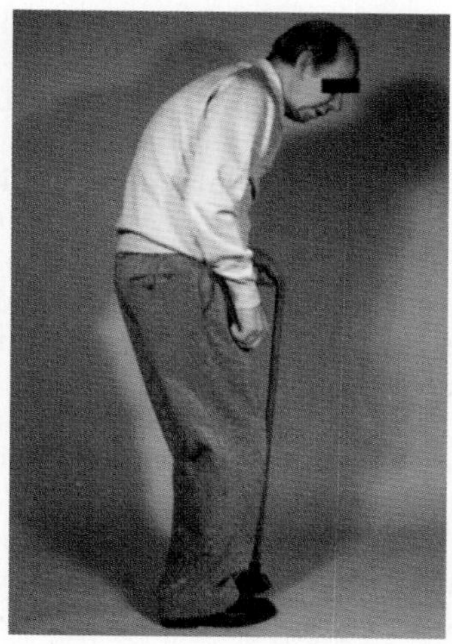

FIGURE 38–5 ✦ A man with an advanced case of Parkinson's disease. His stance demonstrates the typical flexed or stooped posture and general stiffness of these patients. *(From Trend P, Swash M, Kennard C:* Neurology: Color guide, *Edinburgh, 1998, Churchill Livingstone.)*

Characteristics. The cardinal manifestations of Parkinson's disease are rigidity, akinesia (impaired muscle movement), and tremor, although the absence of tremor does not exclude the diagnosis of the disease. Rigidity of the muscles is felt in all passive movements. Akinesia leads to an expressionless face, infrequent blinking, disturbances of gait and posture, and bradykinesia (slowness of movements). Other symptoms include a soft, barely audible voice and monotony of pitch, dysphagia (impaired swallowing), drooling, and progressive difficulty with writing, which is often extremely small. The tremor is rhythmic, seen at rest, usually involves primarily the hands, and has been given the name pill-rolling tremor. The tremor usually stops during intended movements.

Patients often have great difficulty rising from a sitting position and trying to turn from one side to the other in the recumbent position. Patients usually stand in a slightly stooped posture with the arms flexed (Figure 38–5). When attempting to walk, they may have great difficulty getting started and when they finally succeed, steps are short and arm swing is decreased or absent. When turning, the normal fluid movements become replaced by turning the body as a whole, and they may have difficulty stopping immediately. Depression is common, and dementia is sometimes present.

Treatment and Prognosis. Most patients significantly improve on levodopa therapy. Early institution of this therapy may prolong the patient's quality of life. Because of its unpleasant peripheral side effects (e.g., nausea, vomiting, low blood pressure), other medications are also prescribed.

Dental Hygiene Care. One of the first noticeable signs of Parkinson's disease is a lack of facial expression and animation, also known as "masked face." The characteristic tremors also occur in the tongue, lips, and neck. Common manifestations are the "fly-catcher" tongue,

tongue thrusting, and lip pursing. In the later stages of the disease, the muscles used in swallowing may work less efficiently. Food and saliva may collect in the mouth and back of the throat, which can cause choking or drooling. On the other hand, xerostomia often results from medications. Some clients experience a pulsating, burning pain involving the anterior tongue, hard palate, lip, and alveolar ridge, termed burning mouth syndrome.

The client's involuntary muscle movements create a safety concern for the clinician, and methods to address this problem have been discussed previously. In severe cases, it may be necessary to refer the client to be treated under general anesthesia. In addition, the client may be susceptible to orthostatic hypotension and dizziness caused by low blood pressure induced by the medications. Thus the clinician should be cautious when adjusting the dental chair. As tremors and postural instability become more pronounced, clients with Parkinson's disease have more difficulty performing their own oral hygiene care and become more dependent on their caregiver (see Chapter 36).

HUNTINGTON'S DISEASE. This dominantly inherited disorder affects the basal ganglia and cerebral cortex. *Huntington's disease* presents with progressive dementia and chorea. Choreiform movements are characterized by quick, purposeless, small-amplitude movements usually involving the distal parts of the extremities, as well as the tongue and lips. Either dementia or chorea may be the initial manifestation, but eventually both are present. The disorder usually manifests itself in the third and fourth decades of life. Pathologically, there is loss of neurons and proliferation of astrocytes (cells of the supporting tissue) in the basal ganglia.

Characteristics. Initially, the choreiform movements are subtle and are often interpreted as restlessness. As the disease progresses, the movements become more obvious, and the patient may appear to be dancing. There is no known therapy. All patients become totally dependent, and most die within 15 to 20 years.

TREMORS. Tremors are involuntary rhythmic repetitions or oscillations of movement at regular intervals. They may be physiologic, postural, static (resting), or intentional, and there are multiple causes. Intentional tremor is the most common tremor and the most common movement abnormality. It may start at any age, but most commonly in the third or fourth decade. The etiology and pathology are unknown. The tremor is most prominent during volitional movements, particularly skilled movements such as writing, and is aggravated when the patient is tense or after caffeine use. Tremor of the head and voice is common and is often confused with the tremor of Parkinson's disease; however, essential tremor is faster, is not present during rest, and is not accompanied by other neurologic symptoms or signs. Alcohol, phenobarbital, and diazepam are effective in suppressing the tremor temporarily.

SENSORY DISORDERS

Hearing Loss

Hearing loss is the third most common chronic condition in the older population. While only 5% of people aged 18 to 44 have a deficiency, the prevalence is 54% for people older than age 65. Five percent of children have a hearing loss. This loss can cause developmental delays of speech and language. Language deficits lead to learning problems, which cause decreased academic achievement. Communication problems can also lead to poor self-concept and social isolation.

CLASSIFICATION OF HEARING DEFICITS. Hearing loss can be subdivided into the type of hearing loss, the degree of hearing loss, and the configuration of the hearing loss. It can also be classified on the basis of what part or where in the auditory system there is damage.

Conductive hearing loss occurs when sound is not efficiently conducted through the outer and middle ears (ear canal, eardrum, bony ossicles) to the cochlea or inner ear. It usually involves a decrease in volume or the inability to hear faint sounds. Causes include ear wax or presence of a foreign body in the ear canal, fluid in the ear from a cold, ear infections (otitis media), allergies, or a poorly functioning eustachian tube. This type of loss can usually be corrected with medication or surgery.

Sensorineural hearing loss occurs when there is damage to the inner ear (cochlea) or to nerve pathways in the auditory nerve (cranial nerve VIII) (Table 38–3) between the cochlea and the brainstem. In addition to loss of volume, nerve damage is associated with high-frequency loss, and there are deficits in hearing clearly or understanding speech. This type of loss can be caused by drugs that are toxic to the auditory system (aspirin), viruses, diseases, birth injury, noise exposure, head trauma, tumors, genetic syndromes, and aging. This type results in a permanent loss.

Central auditory processing disorders occur when the central auditory processing center (the temporal lobe of the cerebral hemisphere) (Figure 38–3) is damaged by tumors, diseases, infarcts, heredity, or unknown causes. This type of loss involves problems with sound localization, auditory discrimination, temporal aspects of sound, auditory pattern recognition, and the ability to hear decreasing or competing acoustic signals.

DESCRIPTIONS OF HEARING LOSS. The severity of hearing loss is described as the lowest value (decibels or dB) of sound heard at three different frequencies. The normal range is 10 dB to 15 dB, and values progressively increase with greater impairment. For example, the range of severe loss is 71 dB to 90 dB. Configuration of hearing loss is the extent of hearing loss at the different frequencies, such as a high-frequency loss (with good hearing in the lower frequencies). Hearing loss can also be described as bilateral versus unilateral, symmetrical versus asymmetrical, and progressive (such as caused by a growing tumor) versus sudden (such as the result of head trauma).

TABLE 38–3 CRANIAL NERVES AND THEIR FUNCTIONS

Number	Name	Function (s, m, or p)/Location
I	Olfactory	s: from superior nasal cavity
II	Optic	s: from retinae of eyes
III	Oculomotor	m: to eye-movement and eyelid muscles p: smooth muscle of eyeball
IV	Trochlear	m: to eye-movement muscle
V	Trigeminal	
	Ophthalmic	s: from forehead, eye, superior nasal cavity
	Maxillary	s: from inferior nasal cavity, face, upper teeth and mucosa
	Mandibular	s: from lower teeth and mucosa; anterior tongue m: to muscles of mastication
VI	Abducens	m: to eye-movement muscle
VII	Facial	m: to facial muscles of expression and cheek muscle p: lacrimal and salivary glands s: taste to anterior two-thirds of tongue
VIII	Vestibulocochlear	s: from equilibrium and auditory sensory organs
IX	Glossopharyngeal	s: from pharynx and posterior tongue including taste to posterior one-third of tongue m: to superior pharyngeal muscles p: to parotid gland
X	Vagus	s: from viscera of thorax and abdomen m: to larynx and middle and inferior pharyngeal muscles p: heart, lungs, digestive system
XI	Accessory	m: to neck muscles
XII	Hypoglossal	m: to extrinsic and intrinsic muscles of tongue

s, Sensory; *m*, motor; *p*, parasympathetic.
Modified from Guyton A: *Basic neuroscience*, ed 2, Philadelphia, 1991, WB Saunders.

NOISE LEVELS AND HEARING LOSS. Both the length of exposure time and the amount of noise determine effects on hearing loss. Sounds greater than 80 dB are potentially dangerous. Hair cells of the inner ear can be damaged by brief intense sounds, like an explosion, or by continuous or repeated noise exposure. See Noise Levels of Some Common Sounds.

Noise can disturb digestion and cause ulcers; increase blood pressure and breathing rate; intensify the effects of alcohol, drugs, aging, and carbon monoxide; disturb the developing fetus; and possibly contribute to premature birth. Noise can also reduce efficiency and attention to tasks, increase fatigue, and cause feelings of irritability, anger, and frustration.

NOISE LEVELS OF SOME COMMON SOUNDS

Noise Level	Decibel Level	Examples of Noise Level
Faint	30 dB	Quiet library, whisper
Moderate	50 dB	Medium rainfall
Very loud	60 dB	Dishwasher, conversation
	70 dB	Vacuum cleaner, busy traffic
	80 dB	Alarm clock
Extremely loud	90 dB	Shop tools, subway
	110 dB	Rock music
Painful	120 dB	Car stereo, jet plane takeoff
	140 dB	Firearms, jet engine
	150 dB	Peak rock music

ORAL CLINICAL FINDINGS. No specific oral clinical findings are associated with hearing deficits; however, the overall oral health of deaf or hearing-impaired clients may be compromised because of their limited access to dental care and information.

SPECIAL CONSIDERATIONS FOR DENTAL HYGIENE CARE. Communication is the major challenge in achieving and maintaining optimal oral health in clients with hearing deficits. Scheduling and confirming appointments for both deaf and hearing-impaired clients should be conducted by mail, either regular or electronic. Suggestions for facilitating communication with clients with impaired hearing are listed in Techniques for Communicating with Clients with Impaired Hearing.

Each communication mode has advantages and disadvantages. For each deaf client, the preferred mode of communication initially needs to be established.

- *Lipreading* or *speech reading* is difficult to learn and use. Only about 30% of sounds in the English language are visible on the lips. Many sounds appear the same on the lips and others are not visible at all. Speaking should occur at a natural pace without exaggerated lip movements. Any exaggeration distorts the visible pattern for the lip reader. Although most deaf people

Techniques for Communicating with Clients with Impaired Hearing

Get the client's attention. Do not startle the client when entering the room. Do not approach a client from behind.

Face the client and stand or sit on the same level. Be sure your face and lips are illuminated to promote lipreading. Keep hands away from mouth. Remove mask.

If the client wears a hearing aid, make sure it is in place and working.

If the client wears glasses, be sure they are on so that your gestures and face can be seen.

Speak slowly and articulate clearly. Older adults may take longer to process verbal messages.

Use a normal tone of voice and inflections of speech.

Do not shout. Loud sounds are usually higher pitched and may impede hearing by accentuating vowel sounds and concealing consonants. If it is necessary to raise your voice, speak in lower tones.

When you are not understood, rephrase rather than repeat the conversation.

Use visible expressions. Speak with your hands, your face, and your eyes.

Talk toward the client's best or normal ear.

Use written information to enhance the spoken word.

Modified from Potter PA, Perry AG: *Fundamentals of nursing*, ed 5, St Louis, 1993, Mosby.

can lipread to some extent, few will rely on this method alone.

- *American Sign language* (ASL) is the primary means of interpersonal communication for persons who have had a hearing loss since early life. ASL consists of its own vocabulary, idioms, grammar, and syntax, distinct from written and spoken English. Body gestures and facial expressions help convey meaning. The knowledge of a few specific signs may be beneficial for health professionals. ASL classes are widely available, offered at community colleges, universities, and Red Cross chapters.
- *Finger spelling* (American manual alphabet) is the manual reproduction of English using the hands and fingers. It is tiresome and time-consuming; therefore, it is used primarily to supplement ASL for proper names and for words that do not have a present sign.
- *Use of an interpreter* to translate the spoken words into sign language is costly and limits the client's privacy; however, according to the Americans with Disabilities Act, the dental office, being a place of public accommodations, must retain and pay for an interpreter if one is needed to achieve equally effective communication. When using an interpreter, focus still should be directed at the client.
- *Writing* is probably the best method of communication when the speaker does not know sign language; however, it is time-consuming and tiring. Some deaf persons do not read or write beyond the fifth-grade level, so your notes need to be kept simple and easy to read. Paper and pencil should be conveniently located and disposed after the visit to prevent cross-contamination. Laminated cards of expressions and phrases commonly used during treatment are also useful.
- *Electronic aids* are available to facilitate communication. Teletypewriters (TTY) and telecommunications devices (TDD), containing an alphanumeric keyboard and an LCD screen, function to send text messages back and forth by telephone; however, both parties must have the equipment. In recent years, electronic mail probably has assumed that function as computers and Internet access are more widely available. Clients with limited hearing also may prefer this mode of communication.

Hearing-impaired clients who wear hearing aids require specific adaptations in the dental environment. While most hearing aids amplify all sounds, some of the newer ones do have a directional microphone to decrease extraneous sounds. In either case, all extrinsic noise should be eliminated or reduced to minimize the client's discomfort. Background music should be turned off, as should the saliva ejector and suction, when not in use. Unnecessary instrument rattling should be avoided. The hearing aid should be turned down or removed when ultrasonic scalers or dental handpieces are used, but turned on again for oral hygiene instruction.

ORAL SELF-CARE INSTRUCTIONS. Correct brushing and flossing techniques should be demonstrated, step-by-step, on the client while he or she is watching in the mirror. Disclosing agents help identify plaque biofilm, and visual aids, such as pictures and diagrams, are useful to discuss the disease process. Written instructions and pamphlets or brochures on brushing, flossing, and causes of gum disease will assist clients' understanding of plaque control and the importance of preventing gingivitis and periodontitis.

Deficits in Vision

Common visual problems are blurring of vision and loss of vision in one eye or loss of part of a visual field. Deficits can occur anywhere from the eye via the optic nerve (cranial nerve II) (Table 38–3) to the visual region (occipital lobe) of the cerebral cortex (Figure 38–3). Some common terms used to describe visual deficits are defined in Descriptive Terms for Visual Deficits. There are about 10 million blind and visually impaired individuals in the United States, and about 1.3 million of them are legally blind. About 5.5 million individuals 65 years or older are blind or visually impaired.

MOST COMMON CAUSES OF AGE-RELATED VISION LOSS

- *Macular degeneration* (age-related macular disease) is the leading cause of vision impairment and legal blindness in individuals 50 years and older. There is

Descriptive Terms for Visual Deficits

Low vision: Vision that cannot be improved with corrective aids or surgery

Legal blindness: A field of vision 20 degrees or less in its widest diameter, or central visual acuity for distance 20/200 or less in the better eye with correction

Functional blindness: No useful vision

Myopia (nearsightedness): Blurred vision caused by focusing light in front of the retina, usually because the eyeball is elongated

Hyperopia (farsightedness): Blurred vision caused by focusing light behind the retina, usually because the eyeball is too small or short

Astigmatism: Distortion of the focus of light caused by an irregularly curved cornea

Presbyopia: Loss of accommodation or eye's ability to focus and adjust the eye on the distance between the object and the individual. Decreased elasticity of the lens with age, with a progressive loss of focusing ability for near vision

Sighted Guide Techniques to Assist a Blind Person

Offer the blind person your assistance.

If assistance is accepted, brush your arm against his or her arm or tap the back of your hand against his or her hand. The person will then grasp your arm just above the elbow. Children will grasp your wrist or hold your hand.

Walk at a normal pace, staying one step ahead of him or her. Continually describe changes in terrain, as well as stairs, narrow spaces, and so on.

When approaching a narrow area, such as a doorway, move your forearm and hand so that they rest against the lower portion of your back. The blind person will take this cue and move directly behind you at an arm's length.

To assist seating, guide the patient to the back of the chair. Guide his or her hand over the back, arm, and seat portion of the chair, and then allow him or her to seat him- or herself.

Adapted from *Sighted guide techniques,* Braille Institute, 741 N. Vermont Ave., Los Angeles, CA 90029

damage to the central visual area, the macula, which is responsible for the ability to see central vision and detail.

- *Glaucoma* is the leading cause of blindness among African-Americans, and the second most common leading cause of blindness in the United States. It is caused by a buildup of pressure in the eye, with resultant optic nerve damage. Side vision is affected before central vision. It cannot be prevented, but can usually be controlled with medication.
- *Diabetic retinopathy* is a complication of diabetes, caused by damage to retinal blood vessels. There are effective surgical treatments, so early detection is important to prevent visual loss.
- *Cataract* is a clouding of the lens preventing light from passing through the lens and thus causing vision to become blurred or hazy. Surgical removal of the lens, and replacement with an intraocular human-made lens, is safe and successful.

ORAL CLINICAL FINDINGS. Oral abnormalities would not be expected to occur at a greater rate than in the sighted population, unless a blind or visually impaired person has other medical conditions or disabilities. There may be a greater incidence of poorer oral hygiene and the subsequent gingivitis and periodontitis because of the client not being able to see her or his oral hygiene efforts and possibly from not having received effective oral hygiene instructions.

SPECIAL CONSIDERATIONS FOR DENTAL HYGIENE CARE. Minor adaptations in client management need to be made to effectively accommodate clients with visual impairments, mostly increased verbal descriptions of surroundings and procedures. When a blind or visually impaired person arrives in the dental office, he or she should be greeted by someone who acclimates him or her to the layout of the reception area, especially the location of furniture and available chairs. When clinicians greet the client in the reception area, they should introduce themselves each time. If at the initial appointment the clinician describes him- or herself, the client is better able to form an image of the clinician as a person. Other office staff should be introduced so that the client can recognize their voices whenever they speak because the client will be hearing the noises, movements, and conversations of others in the background.

Techniques described in Sighted Guide Techniques to Assist a Blind Person should be used when leading the client to the treatment room. All obstacles should have been previously cleared away. The client should be informed of how the operatory is set up, and for returning clients, any changes, especially new furniture arrangements, should be described. Guide dogs are permitted to remain in the treatment area so they can be kept close to their master at all times. The dog should not be distracted or touched, but led to a close-by, but out-of-the way, corner.

For clinical procedures, each step should be described in detail before proceeding, as well as all instruments and materials and their application. The client can be allowed to handle instruments, but assistance would be required when exploring ones with sharp ends. A second set of sterilized instruments can be used for the actual care. Also, the client can be allowed to feel a moving prophy cup on his or her fingernail. The flavors, taste, and feeling of each dental material should be described. The mirror and explorer can be tapped together so the client gets a sense of what these objects sound like when they come in contact with each other. Informing the client first will avoid surprising him or her with sounds, such as the evacuator, and with movements, such as of the chair, instruments, air, water, or power-driven instruments. Maintaining contact of a finger on a tooth or through retraction, while changing instruments, avoids repeated orientation. The client should always be told when the clinician is leaving and reentering the room to avoid embarrassment.

ORAL SELF-CARE INSTRUCTIONS. Oral hygiene instruction for blind clients can be approached in several ways, all involving clear verbal, step-by-step descriptions of the technique. One method begins with the client demonstrating his or her current brushing technique in his or her own mouth. Deficiencies can be refined and corrected by the clinician placing her or his own hand on the client's hand to guide hand position and movements, while concurrently verbally describing the technique. Another way of demonstrating the proper brushing technique is by the clinician performing the task inside the client's mouth. To help a child become aware of a clean feeling in the mouth, he or she can be taught to feel his or her teeth with the tongue. Flossing can be approached in a similar manner. All clients can be told that they should hear the teeth squeak with the floss when the tooth surface is clean. Audiotapes or materials prepared in Braille can be provided to supplement verbal explanations of plaque biofilm and the oral disease processes.

When oral hygiene instructions are given to the visually impaired client, the following factors should be considered. The client should be positioned for the best view and be wearing his or her eyeglasses before instructions are started. The client should not be expected to be able to see fine detail, such as on a radiograph. Written instructions and educational materials in large print can be provided for the client to take home and read at his or her own pace.

DEVELOPMENTAL DISORDERS

Cerebral Palsy

Cerebral palsy (CP) is the second most common neurologic impairment in childhood, mental retardation being the first. It is a chronic disorder caused by damage to mainly motor areas of the immature brain, primarily affecting the ability to control posture and movement. Most cases are caused by factors occurring before birth, although some are caused by factors perinatally or during the first few years, such as from traumatic brain injury, child abuse or neglect, and infections such as meningitis.

CHARACTERISTICS. The symptoms of CP vary from mild, with only an awkwardness of movement or difficulty with fine motor skills, to severe, which may completely incapacitate the child. There may be associated conditions such as hearing and vision problems, communication problems, impairment of other senses, epilepsy, and mental retardation.

Cerebral palsy is classified into four broad categories according to the type of movement disorder, and subdivided based on the number of limbs involved: monoplegia affects one limb; diplegia, two limbs and usually both legs; triplegia, three limbs; and quadriplegia, four limbs. Hemiplegia affects both limbs on one side of the body. The types of movement disorder are classified on the basis of motor activity and the part of the brain that had been damaged (Figure 38–4).

Most CP patients are of the spastic type, which is characterized by spasticity in the muscles leading to stiffness, resistance to movement, and contractures (Figure 38–6). The sudden, involuntary contractions of muscles or spasms result from damage to the motor area (frontal lobe) of the cerebral cortex (Figure 38–4).

Athetoid or dyskinetic cerebral palsy is characterized by slow, writhing, uncontrolled movements, which usually affect the hands, feet, arms, or legs, and sometimes the face, causing drooling and grimacing. The movements may increase with emotional stress and disappear during sleep. Children with CP may have dysarthria (difficulties with articulation), caused by problems in coordination of speech muscles. People often think that children with CP have a mental or emotional problem because of their awkward movements, although this form of CP usually involves only the motor centers, resulting from damage to the basal ganglia (Figure 38–4).

Ataxic cerebral palsy presents with problems associated with balance, coordination, and depth perception, caused by damage to the cerebellum (Figure 38–4). The affected patients have poor coordination, walk with a wide-based gait, and may have difficulty with quick or precise movements. Mixed forms of CP are a combination of symptoms, such as spastic-athetoid.

TREATMENT AND PROGNOSIS. Many types of therapy are used to help each child reach his or her optimum capabilities: physical and occupational therapy, speech and language therapy, biofeedback, orthopedic devices, and medications. Some children die in infancy, but most

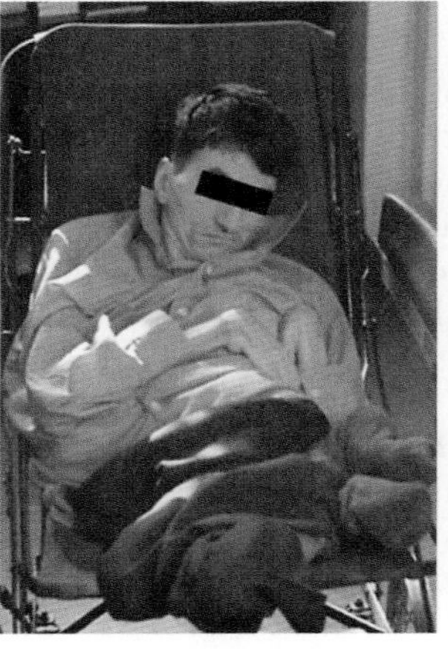

FIGURE 38–6 ✦ A man with the spastic type of cerebral palsy. The spasticity of his antigravity muscles has caused his limbs to assume a severe flexed posture. *(From Porter SR et al:* Medicine and surgery for dentistry, *Philadelphia, 1999, Churchill Livingstone.)*

grow to adulthood. The main causes of death are respiratory and heart diseases.

ORAL CLINICAL FINDINGS. Most of the oral clinical findings in CP clients are related to disturbances of the oral musculature. Abnormal functioning of the tongue, lips, and cheeks can make oral clearance of food difficult, which is accentuated by the consumption of a soft, carbohydrate-rich diet. Those who have an associated convulsive disorder may be being treated with phenytoin and, thus, be susceptible to gingival overgrowth.

Fractures of the maxillary anterior teeth are common because of the uncoordinated ambulation and seizures that lead to frequent falls and the lack of lip protection to the protrusive teeth. Signs of attrition and bruxism result from severe involuntary grinding of the teeth. The teeth of children who are born with CP may exhibit enamel hypoplasia. This enamel defect may be related to the time of cerebral injury. Malocclusion commonly results from the abnormal functioning of the facial, masticatory, and lingual musculature, in conjunction with oral habits, such as tongue thrusting, mouth breathing, and faulty swallowing. Drooling, caused by impaired swallowing and hypotonic lip muscles, is frequently observed.

SPECIAL CONSIDERATIONS FOR DENTAL HYGIENE CARE. The client's involuntary muscle movements create a safety concern for the clinician, and methods to address this problem have been discussed previously. Abnormal muscle responses or reflexes are often triggered by changing the position of the head or neck of the client in the dental chair. The clinician may be able to control the tonic labyrinthine and asymmetric tonic reflexes, as indicated in Table 38–4. Informing the client when lowering, raising, or tilting the dental chair also may prevent a startle reflex.

Hydrocephalus

In *hydrocephalus*, which is one of the most common developmental disorders, there is an increase in the volume of cerebrospinal fluid (CSF) in the ventricular system of the brain. The ventricular system contains the specialized tissue that produces the CSF and the interconnecting spaces through which CSF flows. The location of one of the ventricles is indicated in Figure 38–3. Hydrocephalus usually results from a blockage somewhere along the flow of CSF, causing a buildup of CSF, enlargement of the involved regions of the ventricular system, and resultant compromise to neural tissue. Before the cranial sutures have closed, the increased pressure can cause the skull to enlarge.

CHARACTERISTICS. Clinical signs and symptoms, when present, depend on the brain region being compromised. They may include unexplained vomiting, increasing headaches, frequent crying, irritability, developmental delay, unsteady gait or increased tone in the legs, disinterest in the environment, endocrine dysfunction, or ophthalmologic signs.

TREATMENT. The main treatment for hydrocephalus is the surgical placement under the scalp of a ventriculoperitoneal shunt for CSF with pressure-controlled valves under the scalp. Shunting may reverse some preexisting neurologic deficits.

Neural Tube Defects

Some of the most common major malformations are neural tube defects, resulting from incomplete neural tube formation. Etiology is unknown but is believed to be a combination of genetic and environmental factors.

Spina bifida is a developmental defect in the vertebral column in which there is a failure of the vertebral ring around the spinal cord to fuse, resulting in a posterior gap in the ring and a vertebra that is bifid (divided into two parts). The gap may occur in one or more vertebrae, but is most common around waist-level. There are three main types of spina bifida: spina bifida occulta, which rarely causes disability and is usually not visible; meningocele, in which there is a saclike protrusion containing the meninges (fibrous covering of the brain) but little or no disability; and myelomeningocele.

TABLE 38–4 REFLEX RESPONSES OF CEREBRAL PALSY CONDITIONS AND THEIR MANAGEMENT

Condition	Tonic Labyrinthine Reflex	Asymmetric Tonic Neck Reflex
Stimuli	Tilting head backward, so neck loses support	Turning head to one side, away from midline
Response	Body into full extension Arms and legs extend and stiffen	Arm and leg on face side extend Opposite arm and leg flex
Prevention	Keep head supported and flexed Maintain chair in upright position Hands folded at midline	Use rear operating position Stabilize head in midline position
Management	Bring arms forward Separate legs Massage shoulders	Place face in midline Help flex extended arm and leg

Modified from DeBiase CB: Treating the patient with cerebral palsy, *Dental Hygienist News* 5:13, 1987.

TABLE 38–5 FUNCTIONAL SIGNIFICANCE OF SPINAL CORD LESIONS

Level	Intact Sensation and Motor Ability	Deficit*	Functional Potential and Independence	Required Aids
C4	Head and upper neck	1, 2, 3, 4	None	WC,† ventilator, tracheotomy
C5	Lateral upper arm‡	1, 2, 3, 4	Minimal	Electric WC
C6	Lateral forearm and hand‡	1, 2, 3, 4	Sitting, eat with devices	Manual WC, handsplints
C7	Middle finger‡	1, 2, 3, 4	Personal self-care with devices	Manual WC
C8-T1	Medial hand and forearm‡	1, 2, 3, 4	Personal self-care, WC self-transfers	Manual WC
T1-T6	Upper trunk‡	2, 3, 4, 5	Complete, WC self-transfers	Manual WC, leg braces
T11-L2	Torso, anterior thigh‡	3, 5	Complete, limited walking	Manual WC, leg braces
L4-L5	Medial and lateral leg, dorsal foot‡	3, 5	Complete	Foot braces, crutches
S2-S4	Posterior thigh, calf, lateral foot‡	4, 6	Complete	Catheter
S5	Complete except ring around anus	None	Complete	None

* 1 = Quadriplegia; 2 = Impaired respiration; 3 = Some reflex control of pelvic organs (bowel, bladder), sexual function; 4 = Impaired autonomic reflexes, poor thermoregulation, orthostatic hypotension; 5 = Paraplegia; 6 = Lack of control of pelvic organs.

† *WC,* Wheelchair.

‡ Plus regions at preceding levels.

Myelomeningocele (meningomyelocele) is the most common and most serious defect because the sac contains the spinal cord and/or the spinal nerves. The spinal cord may be damaged or not completely developed. The amount of disability depends on the vertebral/cord level defect and the amount of cord and nerve damage (Table 38–5). There may also be an associated hydrocephalus.

TREATMENT AND PROGNOSIS. The spinal defect is usually closed within the first 24 to 48 hours, with concurrent shunting if there is coexisting hydrocephalus. Primary prevention has focused on dietary folate replacement around the time of conception.

DENTAL HYGIENE CARE. Clients with spina bifida are at a high risk for latex hypersensitivity because of their frequent exposure to latex products during multiple medical surgeries and treatment. The clinician should avoid all latex-containing products and schedule the client's appointment early in the day, before the air is contaminated with glove powder.

PERIPHERAL NEUROPATHIES

Peripheral neuropathies are abnormalities that affect the PNS. Normally, the dendrites of peripheral sensory cranial and spinal nerves receive input (i.e., pain, temperature, touch, pressure, vision, hearing) from the body or external environment, and the axon transmits this information to cells in the CNS (Figure 38–1). Cells in the CNS process this information and respond via motor nerves to the muscle or internal organs. The conduction of nerve impulses is accelerated by some axons having a myelin (lipid) sheath. Damage to the nerve cell may occur in the axon, the myelin sheath of the axon, or the connective tissue and vasculature surrounding the nerve.

Neuropathic Symptoms and Conditions

Pain is the most upsetting symptom to the patient and the hardest to treat. It can be described in several ways, including burning, constant pain; short jabbing pain; tight or bandlike pressure pain; cold, frostbitelike pain; and painful, sunburnlike hypersensitivity to touch. Other symptoms include paresthesias (prickles or "pins and needles"), loss of sensation, unstable balance, sensory loss, or weakness, especially in the lower extremities.

Specific neuropathic conditions are associated with alcoholism (Chapter 45), diabetes (Chapter 41), and HIV infection (Chapter 44). See specific chapters for details.

Common Cranial Nerve Mononeuropathies

Of the 12 *cranial nerves,* some are both sensory and motor (V, VII, IX, X), while some are only sensory (I, II, VIII) and some mainly motor (III, IV, VI, XI, XII) (Table 38–3).

FACIAL NEUROPATHY OR BELL'S PALSY. *Bell's palsy* is one of the most common neurologic disorders affecting the cranial nerves and is the most common cause of an acute facial paralysis. The cause is generally unknown; however, research supports a viral cause. It is thought that the virus triggers edema and inflammation in the nerve, leading to infarction and damage to the facial nerve (cranial nerve VII). Herpes simplex virus is believed to be the most likely causative virus. Temporary or permanent facial paralysis may be iatrogenically caused from damage to nerves during intraoral local anesthetic injection or during oral surgery procedures.

Characteristics. Patients may describe an abrupt functional impairment, their face becomes distorted, and they think they have had a stroke (Figure 38–7). Other

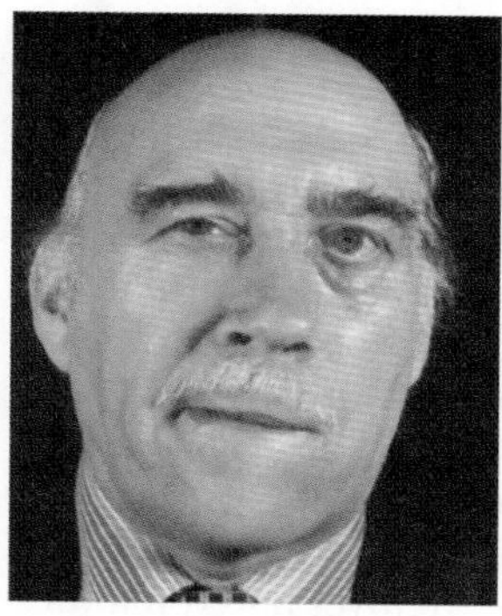

FIGURE 38–7 ✦ A man with Bell's palsy on the left side. On his attempt to smile, there is a lack of movement of the entire left face and forehead muscles. *(From Trend P, Swash M, Kennard C:* Neurology: Color guide, *Edinburgh, 1998, Churchill Livingstone.)*

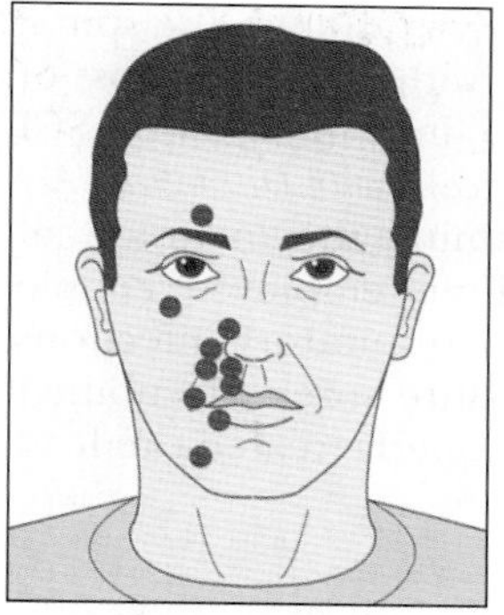

FIGURE 38–8 ✦ Distribution of trigger zones for trigeminal neuralgia. Pain is triggered by irritation of cranial nerve V. *(From Perkin G:* Mosby's color atlas and text of neurology, *London, 1998, Mosby-Wolfe.)*

common symptoms include pain behind the ears, drooling, altered taste, tearing from the eyes, numbness or paralysis on the affected side of the face, and a recent viral syndrome and/or upper respiratory infection.

Treatment and Prognosis. Treatment includes steroids and sometimes antiviral agents, and protection of the eyes with lubricants, artificial tears, and eye protection. Other treatments include surgical decompression of the seventh nerve and galvanic stimulation of paralyzed facial muscles. Most patients recover without cosmetically obvious deformities. With incomplete motor regeneration, patients may have nasal obstruction, excessive tearing, or problems with oral musculature. Incomplete sensory regeneration may result in loss or impairment of taste and disagreeable or impaired sensations.

Dental Hygiene Care. Adaptations for the client's problems with his or her impaired oral musculature have been previously discussed. In addition, the client should wear protective eyewear to prevent foreign material, such as prophylaxis paste, from entering the eye because the client's eyelids may not close on the affected side of the face.

TRIGEMINAL NEURALGIA OR TIC DOULOUREUX. *Trigeminal neuralgia* is a common cause of mononeuropathy of the trigeminal nerve (cranial nerve V) (Table 38–3). It is usually caused by a compression of the nerve by crossing arteries, benign tumors, or vascular malformations. The condition is seen more often in females, with a mean onset of 50 years.

Characteristics. It is characterized by sudden, brief, severe lancinating (shooting or sharp stabbing) pains occurring in the distribution of one or more of the branches of the trigeminal nerve. The symptoms are usually unilateral, occur most often in the third or mandibular division, and present more often on the right side of the face. The pain usually lasts less than a minute and can be triggered by speaking, eating, cold temperatures, or touching the face in specific sites (Figure 38–8). Remission of pain may last months or years, but eventually becomes chronic. Neurologic examination is usually normal; however, there may be areas of hypesthesia (impaired sensation) in some patients.

Treatment and Prognosis. The first treatment of choice is drug therapy. Surgical procedures are tried if drug treatment is not tolerated or is ineffective.

OCULOMOTOR, TROCHLEAR, AND ABDUCENS NEUROPATHIES. A lesion of cranial nerves III, IV, or VI (Table 38–3) will produce a disorder of ocular motility, causing the client to complain of double vision (diplopia). If cranial nerve III is lesioned, there may also be drooping eyelid (ptosis) and pupillary enlargement. Dysfunction in these nerves is usually caused by vascular lesion, tumors, or trauma, but sometimes the cause is unknown (idiopathic).

SPINAL CORD DYSFUNCTION

Spinal Cord Injury (SCI)

The spinal cord lies within the vertebral column and is the lowest level in the hierarchy of complexity in the CNS. It receives sensory impulses brought in from the periphery, integrates reflex activity, sends motor impulses out to the viscera and skeletal muscles, and/or passes information on to higher CNS structures for synthesis and integration. Connected to the spinal cord are 31 pairs of nerves, which are numbered according to the level of the spinal column at which they emerge from the spinal cavity: 8 cervical, 12 thoracic, 5 lumbar, 5 sacral, and 1 coccygeal. All spinal nerves are both sensory and motor.

Spinal cord injury (myelopathy) may occur from trauma or from diseases such as spina bifida, polio, multiple sclerosis, and cancer. The major causes of SCI are motor vehicle accidents, acts of violence, falls, and sports, especially from diving. Most victims are males between the ages of 16 and 30, resulting in some loss of function in arms and legs (quadriplegia) more commonly than in only trunk and legs (paraplegia). Most victims have some other systemic or head injury.

CHARACTERISTICS. The effects of SCI depend on the level and type of injury. The extent of motor function at various levels and the person's potential for independence are indicated in Table 38–5. Clients with SCI may also have problems with temperature and/or blood pressure control, chronic pain, and inability to sweat below the level of the injury.

TREATMENT AND PROGNOSIS. Even though the spinal cord remains intact, most people with SCI have a loss of function. Only in rare cases do individuals with SCI recover all functioning. The *Americans with Disabilities Act* (ADA) has promoted mainstreaming the inclusion of people with SCI, but most are still not employed. People who use ventilators are at risk for respiratory infections and pneumonia. Cutaneous pressure sores (decubitus) are a major concern, and if not properly treated can lead to death.

DENTAL HYGIENE CARE. The oral clinical findings and subsequent special considerations for dental hygiene care and oral self-care instructions all depend on the level and type of spinal cord injury. Adaptations for specific problems have been previously described in this chapter and in Chapter 36.

For clients without the use of their hands, the mouth and teeth play a critical role in performing a variety of tasks. Figure 36–2 in Chapter 36 illustrates a mouthstick for use by quadriplegic persons. The use of mouth-held appliances assists the client in grasping, stabilizing, and opening objects and contributes to the client's maintenance of independence. The design, manufacture, and problems of mouthsticks are described in Chapter 36. Briefly stated, the appliance should be designed so that it does not harm the oral tissues. The occlusal forces need to be distributed throughout the mouth to prevent trauma to the periodontal supporting structures. Cleaning the mouthpiece portion of the appliance should be an integral part of the oral self-care regimen. Compliance with these procedures to prevent oral disease and subsequent tooth loss is important because edentulousness severely affects the use of these appliances.

DEMYELINATING DISEASES

The demyelinating disorders are a broad category of diseases of the CNS in which there is destruction of the myelin sheath of specific axons. The lipid composition of the myelin sheath provides insulation for the axon (Figure 38–1), so the degeneration of the sheath causes interference in the transmission of nerve impulses. Demyelinating diseases result from a variety of causes, such as viral infections, vaccines, and certain genetic disorders.

Multiple Sclerosis (MS)

Multiple sclerosis is the only demyelinating disorder that is frequently encountered, and the most common progressive and disabling neurologic condition affecting young adults. It typically begins in early adulthood, with a mean age of onset being 33 years. White women are more frequently affected, and it is more common in the cold and temperate climates of the higher latitudes in both hemispheres, predominantly affecting individuals of northern European ancestry.

CHARACTERISTICS. Current theories favor an immunologic pathogenesis of MS caused by a fundamental defect in the host, with or without the presence of a triggering viral agent. No two patients with MS are exactly alike, and the clinical manifestations in a particular individual are related to the distribution of lesions within the CNS. Lesions may be found virtually anywhere within the white matter regions, termed that because of the white appearance of the myelinated axons located there. The *cerebral hemispheres*, brainstem, cerebellum, and spinal cord are particularly vulnerable (Figure 38–3 and Table 38–2). The pathology consists of discrete demyelinated plaques that range in size from a few millimeters to several centimeters and are often around veins and the lateral ventricles of the brain. In fresh plaques an abundance of macrophages and perivenous cuffs of lymphocytes and mononuclear cells is present.

Motor symptoms are common and include muscular weakness and spasticity caused by lesions of the nerve fibers from the motor cortex of the cerebrum to the motor neurons of the spinal cord. Lesions in the cerebellar white matter or cerebellar pathways may produce prominent gait and extremity incoordination (ataxia) and a halting or scanning quality of speech. Severe intention tremor of the upper extremities may make the simplest self-care tasks impossible, and severe ataxia of gait may prevent effective ambulation even when muscular strength is adequate.

Visual disturbances (e.g., impaired visual acuity, impaired color vision, visual field deficits, double vision, optic neuritis, and pain in or behind the eye) are common and may be the first symptom. Other sensory symptoms include numbness, tingling, impairment of temperature sensation, and abnormal sense of limb position. Complaints of severe fatigue are common, and exhaustion may frequently be disabling after an ordinary day's activities.

TREATMENT AND PROGNOSIS. The natural progression of MS is unpredictable. Trauma, infection, and surgery have all been associated with worsening of MS. Fever, heavy physical exertion, hot weather, a hot shower or bath, and exposure to sunlight may all cause a transient and reversible worsening of existing symptoms. In most MS patients the disease is initially exacerbating-remitting, and after several years there is a transition to a slow and relentless chronic progression. In some patients the disease maintains an exacerbating-remitting course, and in others the course is benign, with the patient suffering only one or two mild exacerbations and no permanent functional disability.

The management of MS includes treating the acute exacerbation with medications and preventing and treating associated medical and psychological complications.

ORAL CLINICAL FINDINGS. Clients suffering from MS exhibit extraoral complications. They often experience facial pain and temporomandibular joint and muscle dysfunction, and sometimes trigeminal neuralgia. With progression of MS, as the client loses muscular coordination, oral hygiene care is difficult, and the involvement of the tongue and facial muscles interferes with the self-cleansing mechanisms in the oral cavity. Medications may induce xerostomia or gingival overgrowth.

SPECIAL CONSIDERATIONS FOR DENTAL HYGIENE CARE. Relapses in disease symptoms may be stimulated by various types of infections. Frequent recall appointments will help prevent oral infections and thus prevent exacerbations of the disease process. Short appointments scheduled in the morning may minimize fatigue, and a comfortable, quiet, relaxed environment may reduce stress. The client may be sensitive to heat, so the room temperature should be kept cool. Clients may have incontinence problems, so frequent bathroom breaks should be allowed.

Adaptations for problems in ambulation, muscle weakness, and tremors have been previously discussed. Disturbances in the client's visual acuity need to be considered in discussions of oral health maintenance.

Causes of Seizures

Genetic: Inborn errors of metabolism
Congenital abnormalities: Maldevelopment of brain
Perinatal: Anoxia, ischemia, hemorrhage
CNS infections: Encephalitis, meningitis, abscess
Trauma: Penetrating wound, closed head injury, surgery
Neoplastic: Primary gliomas, metastatic
Vascular: Infarction, hemorrhage, arteriovenous malformations
Toxic: Alcohol or cocaine use, alcohol and sedative drug withdrawal
Metabolic: Hypoglycemia, hypocalcemia, high fever
Degenerative: Alzheimer's disease, Creutzfeldt-Jakob disease

Adapted from Collins R: *Neurology*, Philadelphia, 1991, WB Saunders.

SEIZURE AND EPILEPSY

Seizure

A seizure is a brief (less than 2 minutes) disturbance of cerebral function caused by excessive abnormal neuronal discharge. Seizures are common, and during one's lifetime there is a 6% chance of having one and a 3% chance of having more than one. About 1% of children younger than 5 years of age will have at least one seizure, usually associated with a high fever. Seizures result from primary CNS dysfunction or an underlying systematic or metabolic disorder. Characteristics include one or more of the following: a loss or altered state of consciousness, abnormal or cessation of motor activity, abnormal sensory perceptions, and/or loss of bowel and bladder control.

Epilepsy

When seizures are recurrent, the condition is referred to as *epilepsy* or a seizure disorder. The specific underlying brain dysfunction causing the seizure disorder can be found in approximately half of both childhood-onset and adult-onset seizures. See Causes of Seizures. When a specific cause cannot be determined, it is called idiopathic.

CHARACTERISTICS. There are many types of seizures. Only three of the common ones are described here.

Tonic-clonic seizures are the most common type and can be divided into several phases, beginning with vague prodromal symptoms (aura) that occur hours to days before the convulsion. A series of brief, bilateral muscle contractions may precede the tonic phase. Tonic (stiffening) contractions begin in the trunk and progress, including contraction of abdominal muscles, producing forced expiration across the spasmodic glottis and causing the characteristic vocalization. The clonic phase begins after generalized extension, with tonic contractions alternating with loss of muscle tone, causing rhythmic jerking of all four extremities, until contractions cease. Autonomic dysfunction (loss of bowel and bladder control) often occurs during the tonic and clonic phases. Persons experiencing seizures may bite their tongue or break their bones as a result of the violence of the jerking during the clonic phase. Afterward the individual may enter a deep sleep or experience headaches, muscle aches, and stiffness.

Typical absence (petit mal epilepsy) seizures are familial and occur almost exclusively in childhood between the ages of 3 and 12 years. The seizures consist of brief (less than 15 seconds) episodes of altered states of consciousness during which the child has a vacant stare, and, sometimes, eyelid blinking. After the seizure the child goes on with normal activities and has no recollection of the seizure.

Generalized status epilepticus is defined as a single seizure lasting for at least 20 minutes or recurrent generalized seizures without regaining consciousness between the seizure episodes. This is a life-threatening medical emergency and requires prompt and intensive therapy.

TREATMENT OF SEIZURES. Anticonvulsant medications, such as phenytoin or Dilantin, are effective in preventing most seizures. Several are available, but sometimes the side effects are worse than the disorder (e.g., when a person has one seizure a year at night), so medication is not used.

ORAL CLINICAL FINDINGS. Seizures and epilepsy themselves do not produce oral changes, but the medications to treat the condition and the accidents resulting during the seizures may. As previously discussed, phenytoin or Dilantin may cause severe gingival enlargement or overgrowth. Scarring of the lips, buccal mucosa, and especially the tongue may be indicative of past injury to the oral cavity during a seizure. Teeth also may have been injured—fractured from the forceful biting that frequently occurs during a grand mal seizure.

SPECIAL CONSIDERATIONS FOR DENTAL HYGIENE CARE. The major considerations in management of the epileptic client are prevention of seizures in the dental chair and preparation for managing seizures if they occur. When a client responds positively to seizures on a medical history form, further information should be obtained. Examples of questions one could ask are listed in Chapter 9. Based on the client's responses, one may choose to postpone treatment for fear of triggering a seizure in the dental chair. Nitrous oxide sedation is known to elicit seizures in epileptics, so it is not recommended for them. Likewise, fatigue can induce seizures, so appointments should be made early in the day. Despite all preventive measures, seizures may still occur. Management should focus on preventing injury and maintaining adequate ventilation. Steps to follow are outlined in Management of Generalized Tonic-Clonic (Grand Mal) Seizures.

Recall intervals should be established on the basis of the presence or severity of gingival overgrowth, induced by phenytoin. Other medications, frequently prescribed to control seizures, also may have negative side effects. For example, valproic acid affects blood coagulation and prolongs bleeding time.

ORAL SELF-CARE INSTRUCTIONS. Frequent maintenance visits, along with immaculate self-care, have been shown to diminish the drug-induced gingival changes, so it is imperative that oral hygiene instruction be stressed at every appointment.

Management of Generalized Tonic-Clonic (Grand Mal) Seizures

1. Terminate procedure.
Remove instruments and dental appliances from client's mouth

2. Position the client supine with legs elevated.
Turn client onto his or her side to minimize aspiration of secretions
Nothing placed in mouth, between teeth
Loosen tight clothing

3. Summon medical assistance.

4. Assess and perform, when necessary, basic life support.
Head-tilt/chin lift to maintain airway
Protect client from injury

5. After seizure, reassure client and allow him or her to recover.
Assess oral cavity for injury to teeth and tissues

6. Discharge client to hospital, physician, or home with a responsible adult.

Modified from Malamed FS: *Medical emergencies in the dental office*, ed 4, St Louis, 1993, Mosby.

DISORDERS OF HIGHER CORTICAL FUNCTION

Dementia

Dementia is characterized by a progressive intellectual decline that eventually leads to deterioration of occupational, social, and interpersonal functions. Onset is usually insidious, with disturbances of memory frequently attributed to the normal aging process. Sooner or later other areas of cognition become impaired: orientation, language, perceptions, ability to learn new skills, calculation, abstraction, and judgment. Consciousness is preserved until terminal stages, and other neurologic signs usually do not develop until the syndrome is well established.

Even though dementia may occur at all ages, the incidence of most dementias, including Alzheimer's disease, rises substantially with increasing age. Dementia may be caused by the following factors: metabolic disorders, anemia, hypoxia and anoxia, brain tumor, trauma, infections, deficiency diseases, toxins, and medications.

CHARACTERISTICS. In early stages, patients often complain of diminished energy and enthusiasm, show less interest in subjects they previously cherished, and may show emotional instability and heightened anxiety levels because of the awareness of failing mental functions. As the disease progresses, the patient becomes increasingly self-absorbed, anxiety increases, and the recognition of personal failure may lead to depression. At this stage, there may be pronounced mood swings and poor judgment, followed by diminished drive and feeling. As the mental deterioration progresses, anxiety and depression disappear and are replaced by complete flatness of mood. Personal cleanliness deteriorates and patients will do little, if anything, spontaneously. At this stage, other neurologic dysfunctions, such as hemiparesis (one-sided weakness) and seizures, may develop. Lower-level cerebral functions usually remain intact until very late. Once the patient has reached the point of complete flatness of mood, inability to communicate, and total dependence on others, even treatable dementias are usually irreversible.

OLD AGE VERSUS DEMENTIA. In old age mental processes become slowed, but the older healthy person still retains a firm grasp on reality, is oriented, can reason, has good judgment, and can continue to lead an active and self-supporting life. Most aged individuals will show a decrease in speed of performance on mental tasks and less endurance. Previously learned material is usually well retained, but learning of new material becomes more difficult and takes longer. The primary senses become somewhat less sharp, but are still adequate. Speech may become a bit slow, and there may be some awkwardness in skilled movements; a slight intention tremor may develop. Gait becomes more deliberate, and general stability may be impaired partly because of vestibular dysfunction, impaired vision, and loss of peripheral sensory receptors. Like all other organs and biologic systems, the brain ultimately will fail in old age. Severe disturbances of higher cortical functions do not occur until weeks to months before death.

Alzheimer's Disease

Alzheimer's disease (AD) is the most common form of dementia, affecting 10% or more of those older than 65 years and maybe 50% of those older than age 85. It is a degenerative disorder of the brain that gradually destroys the ability to remember, reason, learn, and imagine. The affected neurons develop abnormal clumps (called *senile plaques*) and irregular knots (called *neurofibrillary tangles*), which destroy the areas of the brain associated with intellectual functions (Figure 38–9). Risk factors include family history, aging, genetics, and Down syndrome.

CHARACTERISTICS. The stages are described in Chapter 48, Table 48-4. In the early and middle stages of AD, affected individuals may be painfully aware of their intellectual decline, and it is important to support their emotional and mental health with affection and warmth. In the beginning there is simple forgetfulness, especially of directions to familiar places or recent events. There may also be personality changes such as restlessness, increased stubbornness, distrust, and poor judgment and impulse control, and increased difficulty with activities requiring planning and decision making. The affected individuals may begin to withdraw socially. As the disease progresses, the ability to perform daily living tasks is lost, and there may be trouble recognizing everyone except the person's closest daily companions. Communication becomes difficult as written and spoken language decline. In the last stages of the disease, patients with AD become bedridden, unable to recognize themselves or their closest family members.

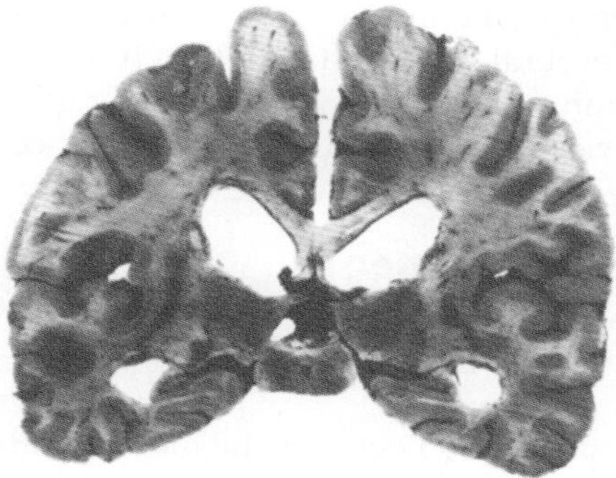

FIGURE 38–9 ✦ Coronal section of the brain from a patient with Alzheimer's disease. The degeneration of the cerebral cortex neurons leads to the thinning of the cortex and secondary enlargement of the lateral ventricles. *(From Perkin G:* Mosby's color atlas and text of neurology, *London, 1998, Mosby-Wolfe.)*

TREATMENT AND PROGNOSIS. Because there is no cure for AD, treatment is aimed at prevention, slowing progression of the disease, and improving quality of life for the patients. Some of the dying neurons use acetylcholine for a neurotransmitter, so acetylcholine drugs are used to improve cognition, although the effects are not permanent. The time from the earliest symptoms to death has an average duration of 8 years. Death results from a secondary illness such as urinary tract infection or pneumonia.

ORAL CLINICAL FINDINGS. Clients with Alzheimer's disease have more gingival disease and caries than the normal elderly population, mainly because of poor oral hygiene from significant neglect. Clients forget to brush, forget how to brush, may not want to brush, or may be resistant to a caregiver brushing their teeth. Medications, such as phenytoin to control seizures, may cause gingival overgrowth, and many induce salivary gland dysfunction.

SPECIAL CONSIDERATIONS FOR DENTAL HYGIENE CARE. Frightening and frustrating the client may lead to uncooperative, even combative, behavior, so clients with Alzheimer's disease are managed best by a caring and understanding approach. Suggested ways of achieving this approach are listed in Techniques for Communicating with Clients with Alzheimer's Disease. Appointments should be scheduled early in the day and preferably when the office is not busy. The office environment should be as free of unnecessary noise, people, and physical clutter as possible. The caregiver should accompany the client to discuss special client management issues, as well as oral care procedures.

ORAL SELF-CARE INSTRUCTIONS. In the early stages of Alzheimer's disease the client should be encouraged to be self-sufficient. Toothbrushing instructions should be given slowly, step-by-step, in simple, concrete language.

Techniques for Communicating with Clients with Alzheimer's Disease

Use a calm, soft voice pattern.
Be cheerful and reassuring.
Speak slowly and clearly, in short sentences.
Allow ample time for comprehension.
Explain procedures before treatment.
Repeat instructions and explanations in exactly the same words.
Tell clients what you need them to do, instead of giving them a choice.
Distract clients who are uncooperative or argumentative by changing the activity or take advantage of their forgetfulness by leaving the room for a few minutes and then returning and cheerfully trying the same activity again.
Use supportive body posture and facial motion, such as direct eye contact and smiling.

As the disease progresses, the client becomes more dependent on his or her caregiver for oral home care, so the caregiver needs to be familiar with these procedures. While a powered toothbrush may be easier for a caregiver to use on the client, electrical appliances are known to disturb or be a safety concern to some individuals with Alzheimer's disease. Mouthrinses are not usually recommended because the client may not understand that it would be harmful to swallow.

Disorders of Speech and Language

Speech or vocalization is the mechanical aspect of oral communication. It is produced by the coordination between the respiratory muscles, vocal cords, soft palate, tongue, and lips. Speech abnormalities can result from dysfunction in any of these structures. Speech disorders result in dysphonia, a disturbance in phonation, or dysarthria, which is a dysfunction in articulation. Almost all speech abnormalities result from peripheral, brainstem, and/or cerebellar dysfunction.

Language is a cognitive function using abstract symbols to communicate (comprehend, read, write, repeat, and converse). Language depends on central processing to either comprehend or to formulate the sounds and symbols. Dysfunction of language is termed *aphasia* and includes disturbances in comprehension and expression of spoken or written language. It affects the ability to express oneself through speech, writing, and gesture, and to understand the speech, writing, and gestures of others.

CEREBROVASCULAR DISEASE

Cerebrovascular accident (CVA) or stroke is the third most frequent cause of death in the United States, heart disease and cancer being the first and second. Approximately one-half million patients per year in the United States are expected to suffer from strokes of all etiologies. It is the major cause of serious disability in adults.

Risk factors for stroke are listed in Risk Factors for Stroke. The major factor is hypertension. Because hypertension is in most instances a treatable condition, the single most important measure in preventing strokes is detection and treatment of hypertension. A transient ischemic attack (TIA) is a transient neurologic deficit that persists for less than 24 hours and is followed by complete clinical recovery. Most TIAs do not last longer than 10 to 20 minutes.

Risk Factors for Stroke

Common Risk Factors
Transient ischemic attack
Recent stroke
Hypertension
Cigarette smoking
Cardiac diseases
Diabetes mellitus

Uncommon Risk Factors
Inflammatory disorders
Hematologic disorders
Coagulation disorders
Drug abuse

Possible Risk Factors
Oral contraceptives
Obesity
Physical inactivity
Alcohol
Pregnancy

Modified from Collins R: *Neurology*, Philadelphia, 1997, WB Saunders.

Characteristics

Loss of blood (ischemia) to the brain results from diminished blood flow into the brain tissues from embolism (occlusion of artery), atherothrombosis (fatty clot within blood vessel), or systemic hypoperfusion (e.g., from cardiac pump failure). The ischemia leads to infarction (necrosis or death) of brain tissue supplied by the affected artery or arteries. Hemorrhage, or rupture of a brain vessel, causes leakage of blood into the brain tissue, ventricles, or into the space between the brain and skull. The resultant hematoma exerts pressure on brain tissue, causing ischemia of adjacent tissue. Occlusion of a blood vessel to the brain with subsequent infarction accounts for most stroke cases.

Regardless of the underlying etiology, in the development of a stroke a certain part of the brain does not receive an adequate blood supply for a period of time. If brain tissue is deprived of blood supply for 10 to 20 minutes, infarction will occur. Occlusion of a given artery does not necessarily imply infarction of brain tissue in the perfusion territory of that blood vessel because adequate collateral circulation may exist. If adequate blood supply is restored to the brain within time, there will be total resolution of the neurologic deficit.

The right and left hemispheres specialize in different functions, and the two sides of the brain are interconnected. Sensory and motor axons cross on their way to or from the cerebral cortex, so that the left side of the brain controls motor and sensory input for the right side of the body and vice versa. Thus the side of the face and body affected is opposite to that of the brain injury.

Common Impairments

Signs and symptoms depend on the involved region of the brain, but the following are the more common ones:

- ✦ *Motor impairments.* These are the most common deficits and usually involve face, arm, and leg, alone or in combination on the same side. Motor functions affected include cranial nerve functions to muscles of the head and neck, reflexes, gait, balance, and coordination. Often there is apraxia (the inability to perform purposeful movements), although no muscular paralysis or sensory disturbance is present.

- *Sensory deficits.* Impairments range from loss of primary senses (e.g., vision, pain, temperature, touch) to more complex losses of perception.
- *Language and cognition.* There is often dysphasia after a stroke, manifest by disturbances in comprehension, repetition, naming, fluency, reading, or writing. Strokes can cause deficits in memory, calculation abilities, attention, and orientation.
- *Depression.* This is the most common affective disturbance after a stroke. Symptoms of depression include lack of interests, loss of energy, insomnia, and loss of appetite. Stroke patients may also display instability of emotions.

Treatment

Occupational and physical therapy can help the stroke patient learn new ways of perfoming activities of daily living, sometimes with the aid of assistive devices such as braces, wheelchairs, and special utensils.

Oral Clinical Findings

The specific oral findings of a CVA survivor depend on the areas of the brain affected and the type of CVA, as well as the resultant dysfunction. Effects of motor dysfunction have been previously described. Many of the prescribed medications cause xerostomia. Periodontal disease has been demonstrated to be associated with the risk of stroke, as well as heart disease. While invasion of the periodontal pathogens into the periodontium is able to induce a bacteremia and systemic inflammatory response, a causal relationship has not been established.

Special Considerations for Dental Hygiene Care

It is recommended that the stroke survivor not undergo any elective dental care within 6 months of the episode. A positive response to stroke on the health history form should elicit several follow-up questions, which are listed in Chapter 9. This information will determine the need for treatment modifications. A client who has had a stroke or TIA is at a greater risk for having another one, so prevention of a recurrence is of utmost concern. Factors such as pain and anxiety add to the risk and so need to be managed by creating a safe and comfortable environment. Efforts should be made to minimize fatigue and optimize energy and patience for both clinician and client. Adaptations for these clients' problems in ambulation and muscle weakness have been previously described.

Blood pressure should be carefully monitored because marked deviations in blood pressure increase the risk of recurrent CVAs. Blood pressure of 200 mg systolic and/or 115 mg diastolic and higher warrants immediate medical consultation before dental treatment is initiated. Many CVA and TIA survivors receive anticoagulant therapy, which predisposes a client to excessive bleeding. Consultation with the physician is strongly recommended to determine whether the therapy should be altered. The physician may also be consulted regarding whether prophylactic premedication is necessary. The presence of oral infections may cause changes in blood coagulation factors, which may trigger a repeat CVA. The minimum amount of a local anesthetic with vasoconstrictor should be used.

Oral Self-Care Instructions

During the immediate post-stroke phase, the caregiver needs to perform all the daily hygiene functions; thus, he or she will need demonstrations and instructions of proper brushing and/or maintenance of prosthesis so that he or she can perform these tasks until the client has relearned them. Even during the rehabilitation phase, clients with residual physical deficits may need assistance performing oral hygiene procedures. Special adaptations that foster the stroke survivor's self-sufficiency have been described previously.

The discomfort from xerostomia can be alleviated by saliva substitutes and associated products. Fluoride therapy is beneficial to prevent root caries.

Client Education Issues

- Individualize recommendations and expectations for self-care based on evaluating the physical and mental condition of the client.
- Encourage clients to maintain their own oral health for as long as their physical condition allows.
- Facilitate the client's self-sufficiency by modified oral hygiene aids: toothbrushes with adapted handles, powered toothbrushes, toothpaste tubes with flip-top caps or pump dispensers, and floss-holders.
- Educate caregivers should be educated about the importance of disease prevention, as well as plaque control procedures and client positioning for maximal stability and access.
- Provide written and oral instructions to both the client and caregiver so the information can be reviewed at home.

Legal, Ethical, and Safety Issues

- The dental hygienist should not refuse to care for persons with disabilities because Title III of the *Americans with Disabilities Act* "makes it illegal to discriminate against persons with disabilities, and those with whom they associate, in the provision of services in places of public accommodation."
- The dental hygienist should obtain informed consent from all clients or their legal caregivers for the performance of all procedures.
- The dental hygienist should be prepared to manage medical emergencies, such as a generalized tonic-clonic seizure, a stroke, or airway obstruction.
- The dental hygienist should be prepared to safely assist the client in walking and in transferring a wheelchair-confined client to the dental chair.
- The dental hygienist should carefully assess vital signs and medications to determine the safety of delivering dental hygiene care to the client.
- The operatory should be clear of all obstacles to prevent accidents from happening to visually or physically impaired clients.
- The dental hygienist should be aware that clients with spina bifida are more likely to have latex allergies.

Key Concepts

- Poor oral hygiene is frequently observed in clients with neurologic deficits because of the following reasons: their poor muscle coordination limits their ability to perform self-care; disturbances in tongue and facial muscles interfere with self-cleaning mechanisms; and when completely debilitated, they must depend on caregivers, who may be overwhelmed.
- Xerostomia often results from medications, which leads to susceptibility to oral infections and root caries, taste dysfunctions, and difficulty in swallowing.
- Malocclusion results from abnormal functioning of the musculature, in conjunction with oral habits such as tongue thrusting, mouth breathing, and faulty swallowing.
- Medications, such as phenytoin or Dilantin to control seizures, may cause gingival enlargement or overgrowth. Immaculate self-care and frequent maintenance appointments may diminish this condition.
- Disturbances in musculature cause impaired swallowing and gag reflexes. Good suctioning techniques and possibly an upright position may prevent choking and aspiration of water and foreign substances.
- Stabilizing the client is a concern with clients who have impaired motor control. The head and jaw can be supported by physically cradling the head and using mouth props. Body movements may need to be limited, preferably by the caregiver restraining the client, but physical restraints, such as belts, may be used if necessary.
- Communication with clients with impaired hearing is facilitated by reducing all extraneous noise and articulating clearly. Deaf clients may prefer a specific mode of communication.
- Enhanced verbal descriptions of surroundings and procedures are necessary to care for clients with visual deficits.
- Communicating with clients who have impaired mental function is facilitated by speaking slowly, with direct commands.
- Powered toothbrushes or toothbrushes with adapted handles may be easier to maneuver when muscle strength or range of motion is impaired and also when used by a caregiver.
- Caregivers must be educated about the importance of disease prevention, as well as plaque control procedures and client positioning for maximal stability and access.

Critical Thinking Exercises

Client: Mrs. M.

Profile: Mrs. M, a new client in your dental office, inquires whether you are able and would be willing to deliver dental hygiene care to her 6-year-old daughter, Lisa.

Chief Complaint: "I recently noticed large amounts of plaque on Lisa's front teeth and am worried about the possibility of dental decay."

Medical History: Lisa has been affected by cerebral palsy since birth.

Dental History: Mrs. M apprehensively explains that she has not previously brought Lisa to a dental office because she assumed that there would be difficulties in caring for Lisa.

Social History: Lisa lives with her parents and is confined to a wheelchair.

Oral Behavior Assessment: Mother reports Lisa uses an electric toothbrush once a day.

Supplemental Notes: Mother reports Lisa has dental insurance and is somewhat fearful of coming to the dental office for care.

1. What questions could you ask Mrs. M that would help you prepare for Lisa's appointment so that you can deliver optimal dental hygiene care?
2. What factors, inherent to cerebral palsy, would place Lisa at risk for oral health problems?
3. What barriers to care had Mrs. M anticipated that would have prevented her daughter from receiving optimal dental and dental hygiene care?
4. What type of fear management would you suggest for Lisa?

For References, Suggested Readings, and Related Websites, visit
http://evolve.elsevier.com/Darby/hygiene/

CHAPTER 39

Persons with Mental Retardation

OBJECTIVES

Mastery of the content in this chapter will enable the reader to:

- Discuss etiologies of mental retardation, Down syndrome, and autism
- Describe general characteristics of persons with mental retardation, Down syndrome, or autism
- Plan educational interventions for a client with mental retardation, Down syndrome, or autism
- Outline instructional strategies to overcome communication barriers with an autistic client
- Describe medical conditions that may accompany Down syndrome and their effect on dental hygiene care
- Recognize oral manifestations seen in the client with mental retardation, Down syndrome, or autism
- Plan an oral hygiene program based on individual needs

KEY TERMS

Atlantoaxial subluxation
Autism
Behavior modification
Brushfield spots
Chronologic age
Differential reinforcement of incompatible behavior (DRI)
Differential reinforcement of other behavior (DRO)
Down syndrome
Echolalia
Epicanthal folds
Hirschsprung's disease
Hypotonia
Hypoxemia
Keratoconus
Kernicterus
Mental age
Mental retardation (MR) (mild, moderate, severe, and profound)
Mosaicism
Phenylketonuria
Scoliosis
Self-injurious behavior (SIB)
Translocation
Trisomy 21

MENTAL RETARDATION

Mental retardation (MR) is a significantly subaverage general intellectual functioning accompanied by significant limitations in adaptive functioning in at least two of the following skill areas: communication, self-care, home living, social/interpersonal skills, use of community resources, self-direction, functional academic skills, work, leisure, health, and safety. Onset must occur before the age of 18.[1] Mentally retarded persons usually have an intelligence quotient (IQ) below 70 and impairments in communicative, social, and daily living skills.

Etiology

MR can stem from genetic biologic factors (chromosomal and genetic disturbances), nongenetic biologic factors (prenatal, perinatal, postnatal causes), and psychologic factors (caregiving environment). Genetic biologic factors include disorders evident at conception. Approximately 15% of persons with MR fall into this category. These include chromosomal disturbances (10%), as in Down syndrome, or a metabolic disorder, such as in *phenylketonuria* (5%), which causes an abnormal accumulation of phenylalanine that is toxic to the brain.

Nongenetic biologic etiologies of MR are grouped as prenatal, perinatal period, and postnatal causes. Approximately 32% of cases of MR occur in the prenatal period, 11% in the perinatal period, and 4% in postnatal period.[2] Prenatal causes can result from infection such as rubella, toxoplasmosis, syphilis (dental signs: Hutchinsonian incisors, mulberry molars, microdontia), cytomegalovirus and HIV; maternal-fetal blood incompatibilities; drug and alcohol consumption; maternal-fetal irradiation; and chronic maternal health problems such as hypertension and diabetes. Perinatal refers to the time immediately before, during, and after the birth. Prematurity, *hypoxemia* (intracranial hemorrhage), head trauma, infection (HIV, herpes), and *kernicterus* (toxic accumulation of bilirubin in the brain) are perinatal causes of mental retardation. Because of advances in medicine, the likelihood of MR as a result of perinatal causes is unlikely. Postnatal factors are infections of the brain (encephalitis, meningitis), cerebral trauma (head injury, brain tumor, accident), poison, environmental toxins, and dietary protein deficiency. Psychologic causes include an environment void of sensory and intellectual stimulation during growth and development.

Levels of Mental Retardation

MR is categorized as mild, moderate, severe, and profound. Persons with *mild MR* have an IQ of approximately 50 to 70. This group represents the largest population of mentally retarded persons (about 85%). These clients are designated as educable and are able to learn some academic skills. Persons with mild retardation can learn simple skills in detail, but their attention spans and memories are short. For clients with mild retardation, dental hygienists should explain and demonstrate oral hygiene instructions and teach activities instead of concepts. Clients with mild MR require public recognition, praise, and reward for progress. Mildly retarded individuals typically live either independently or in supervised settings.

Moderate MR is defined as an IQ of approximately 35 to 55. Persons with moderate MR can learn self-care behaviors, social adjustment, and economic usefulness but very few academic skills past the second-grade level. Poor hand and finger coordination may be evident; therefore, clients should be taught only the fundamental skills by employing the show-and-tell method. Additional skills may be taught, depending on client progress. Every successful step performed during therapy and oral hygiene instruction should be rewarded with both tangible and verbal praise. Oral hygiene instructions should be reviewed at each appointment because of the short memory and attention span of clients. Moderately retarded individuals typically live in group settings where the primary caregiver can supervise the daily oral hygiene regimen to ensure that optimal home care is practiced.

Severe MR is evident in persons with an IQ of approximately 20 to 40. Persons with severe retardation can be trained in elementary self-care skills; therefore, the client can acquire some oral care skills with supervision. These clients learn by habit training, which consists of repeating procedures and movements continuously so that the client can grasp the procedures. It is important to set realistic client goals and to include the caregiver when teaching oral hygiene behaviors to clients with severe MR. Depending on the environment, all successfully performed skills should be rewarded by the dental hygienist or the caregiver. See Table 39–1 for suggested awards. Severely retarded individuals typically reside at home with their families or in group homes.

Profound MR is characterized as having an IQ below 20. These clients are incapable of total self-care, social skills, or economic usefulness and require continued supervision and care from the primary caregiver. Some self-care may be achievable in a highly structured environment when appropriate training is provided by the caregiver. The caregiver is responsible for the client's general and oral hygiene care; therefore, there is a need to educate the caregiver.[1] The hygienist must realize that the caretaker's task is challenging and that oral care may not be a top priority.

General Characteristics

Some common traits characterize MR, many of which are consistent with the specific type of MR. Dental hygienists should avoid the overgeneralization and instead consider individual needs, abilities, and circumstances.

HEALTH. Persons with MR usually have a decrease in physical stamina compared to the general population, delayed physical development and speech, and physical challenges such as poor motor coordination, vision, and hearing. It is not uncommon to see persons with MR who are overweight or underweight as a result of environmental factors such as inadequate parental or institutional care, or from genetic and metabolic factors such as phenylketonuria. Also, persons with MR may have poor oral health as a result of nutritional deficiency, limited self-care capabilities, economic barriers to care, and limited access to care. Therefore, during assessment, the dental hygienist considers the client's diet, possible

TABLE 39–1 REWARDS THAT CAN BE USED TO REINFORCE POSITIVE BEHAVIOR FOR CLIENTS WITH MENTAL RETARDATION

Types of Rewards	Examples of Rewards
Social rewards	Attention, smiles, hugs, praise, and other signs of approval and affection
Activity rewards	Any activity a person enjoys: watching television, playing a game, going to a party
Material rewards	An item that a person can use, play with, wear, or consume: toys, money, food, clothing

chewing or swallowing difficulties, and the possibility of dietary restrictions.

MENTAL AND MOTOR ABILITIES. Mentally retarded persons usually have short memories, an inability to concentrate, limited speech, and a lack of adaptive, associative, or organizational skills. They may have an inability to see differences or likenesses between objects. Success for a mentally retarded person usually occurs from concrete rather than abstract experiences, and therefore, these persons are more adept in manual skills than academic skills. Depending on the level of MR, some clients may be able to render their own oral hygiene care.

SOCIAL AND EMOTIONAL ABILITIES. Persons with MR are viewed as followers rather than leaders, (i.e., they tend to imitate others). Mentally retarded persons frequently show behavioral problems to gain attention or release emotion. Some maladaptive behaviors may be destructive, including aggressiveness directed toward others, property destruction, and self-injury. These persons have an awareness of not fitting in, and become discouraged easily. Criticism is not taken positively and there is an inability to learn through experience.

SELF-INJURIOUS BEHAVIOR. Clients with MR may exhibit *self-injurious behavior (SIB)* including head banging, self-biting, striking themselves, or teeth grinding. Figure 39–1 shows an autistic child who has bitten his own hands. SIB has been viewed as an early developmental stress response that disappears in "normal" children, but remains in clients with mental retardation. Self-injury can be used by a client as positive reinforcement to get something he or she wants such as attention or a certain food. SIB can also be used to receive negative reinforcement, such as escape from undesired situations (dental experience) or from certain demands. These behaviors can intimidate caregivers to the point that the client gets his or her demands. If the client is allowed this power, he or she becomes difficult to manage.

To prevent SIB, the dental hygienist initiates fact finding with the caregiver to identify SIB triggers and antecedents. Most commonly used behavioral treatment is *differential reinforcement of other behavior (DRO)*. The goal of DRO is to reinforce any behavior other than the SIB. Good results have been shown when DRO and *differential reinforcement of incompatible behavior (DRI)* have been used simultaneously.[3] For example, if a client strikes himself in the mouth with his hands, give the client something to assemble or hold with his hands. Another example would be to let the client hold a piece of cotton or mirror until needed. Strategies for managing self-injurious behavior are listed in Table 39–2.

ORAL MANIFESTATIONS. Persons with MR often exhibit specific oral manifestations (see Some Oral Manifestations Observed in Clients with MR). Lips of clients are sometimes larger than those of the general population, and tooth anomalies such as microdontia and delayed eruption patterns are usually present as a result of develop-

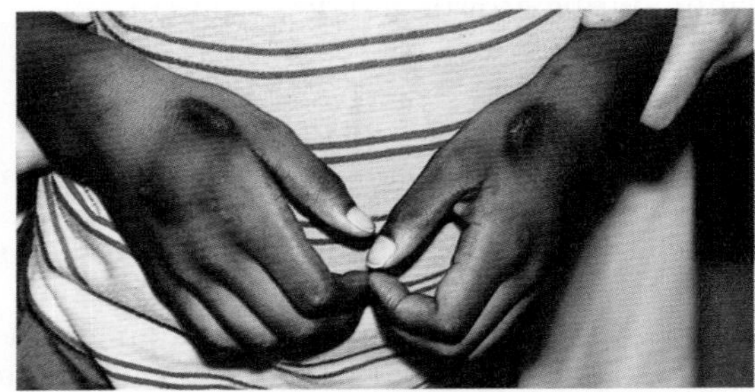

FIGURE 39–1 ✦ Physical outcome of self-injurious behavior in a child with mental retardation. *(Courtesy Dr. F.T. McIver, Department of Pediatric Dentistry, University of North Carolina School of Dentistry.)*

TABLE 39–2 NINE STRATEGIES FOR MANAGING SELF-INJURIOUS BEHAVIOR IN DENTAL HYGIENE CLIENTS

Strategy	Defined	Examples
Differential reinforcement	Reinforcement of any behavior other than the self-injurious behavior	Draw interest away from injurious behavior
Positive reinforcement	Used in order for a person to repeat a desired behavior	Praise: "you really did well"; "good job"
Ignoring unwanted behavior	Refusing to take notice of behavior	Consciously ignoring a negative behavior
Positive reinforcement of wanted behavior	Reinforcement when the wanted behavior is directly addressed	"You really brushed those back teeth well"
Psychoactive medication	Medication that alters one's psychologic state	Neuroleptics, antidepressants, psychostimulants
Restraint	Confinement of a person physically	Papoose board, Velcro straps
Counseling	Professional guidance of a person using psychologic methods	Offer support, positive reinforcement, and trust
Application of consequences after behavior	Punishment after the unwanted behavior to reinforce the idea that the behavior was unacceptable	Time out, not allowing a reward after treatment
Overcorrection	Correction requiring duties above and beyond the specific unwanted behavior	Joe colors on the wall, he should clean more of the wall than where he colored

mental abnormalities. Tooth surface wear from bruxism has been observed, which seems to be linked to anxiety and emotional distress.

Consequences of bruxism can include dental attrition, functional problems such as temporomandibular joint disorders, and eventually sensitivity and pain. Wear is usually seen in the incisors and canines and increases with age. By 30 to 49 years of age, wear becomes so significant that restorative measures may be needed. Bruxism may be the result of a lack of personal contact and may be a type of self-stimulation. Before treatment can be given for these problems, assessment must be completed to reveal the origin and chronicity of the behavior.

Periodontal disease in persons with MR is attributed to lack of professional care, lack of funds to support care, increased susceptibility, and poor oral hygiene. Mentally retarded persons usually depend on someone else to facilitate their access to oral healthcare, and a layperson's assessment of need is likely to differ from that of a dental professional.

Management of Clients with Mental Retardation

Most (89%) mentally retarded persons treated in the oral healthcare environment are mildly retarded. A smaller percentage (6%) is moderately retarded, and 4.5% is severely or profoundly retarded.[4] When developing client oral hygiene skills and behaviors, the dental hygienist teaches based on the client's *mental age* (MA) (age reflected in the level of functioning), not *chronologic age* (true age of the person). A client's MA can be determined by the following formula, where CA represents chronologic age and MA represents mental age:

$$\text{Estimation of MA} = \text{CA} \times \text{IQ} \div 100$$

Mental age can be further estimated with the following formulas:

Mild MR	$\frac{2}{3} \times$ CA
Moderate MR	$\frac{1}{2} \times$ CA
Severe MR	$\frac{1}{3} \times$ CA
Profound MR	less than $\frac{1}{4} \times$ CA

Some Oral Manifestations Observed in Clients with MR

Self-biting
Bruxism
Thick, flaccid lips
Microdontia
Malocclusion
Delayed tooth eruption
Dental attrition and sensitivity
Temporomandibular joint disorder
Periodontal disease
Poor oral hygiene

As with any client, a humanistic approach is used, coupled with a care plan designed according to the individual's assessed abilities and human need deficits related to dental hygiene care. Once this is accomplished, the hygienist begins instructions with familiar activities, praises small accomplishments, and uses a gentle but firm demeanor. Extra instructional time may be required for conveying new information. If problems occur (e.g., crying, frustration), the dental hygienist repeats an earlier achievement level to meet the client's need for freedom from stress. Effective communication with the client leads to a trusting relationship, which in turn allows the oral healthcare experience to be successful for both the client and clinician.[4] Approaches to form this trusting relationship are listed in Strategies for Establishing a Trusting Relationship.

When providing care to clients with MR, the dental hygiene process can increase the likelihood that the visit will be successful. During assessment, the dental hygienist also collects data about the self-care status of the client (e.g., toilet training, oral hygiene habits, developmental level, eating habits). The client's primary caregiver may be able to suggest behavior guidance to facilitate a pleasant dental experience. Factors to consider include the client's diet and ability to chew, the client's oral hygiene potential, client interests, parent's/caregiver's interests and values, client's and parent's/caregiver's level of cooperation, cost of care, and access to care. See Figure 39–2 for a sample dental hygiene care plan.

Strategies for Establishing a Trusting Relationship

At first appointment, help client become familiar with surroundings.

Schedule time for oral healthcare team to meet client; alleviate anxieties by getting to know client and by client getting to know the team.

Keep first appointment short and nonthreatening.

Give explanations slowly, with one instruction at a time.

Use tell-show-do technique when teaching oral hygiene instructions; teach one technique at each appointment to avoid overwhelming client.

Make sure client understands instructions; have client perform the procedure (i.e., brushing or interdental cleaning).

Reward client often for positive behavior.[3] Rewards might include verbal positive reinforcement such as "good job," tangible reinforcement such as a toy or special outing arranged by the caregiver, and public recognition such as a certificate that can be displayed in the client's home or work setting.

If client can read, provide handouts, designed at the appropriate level of reading comprehension, that can be taken home.

Jill is an 18-year old female who resides with her parents. She is mildly retarded with good-fair psychomotor skills. She presents with dental caries and bleeding gingiva. Her plaque index is 75%. She receives public assistance and has not received dental care in several years.

Dental Hygiene Diagnosis	Due To or Related To	As Evidenced By	Client Goal	Evaluative Statements
Biologically Sound and Functional Dentition	Inadequate oral care by caregiver Inadequate self-care Lack of resources	Signs of caries, defective restorations and missing teeth Report of oral pain	Reduce caries index score Seek dental treatment for caries and defective restorations	Reduced caries index score at 3-month continued-care interval Completed restorative treatment by 3-month continued-care interval
Skin & Mucous Membrane Integrity of the Head & Neck	Inadequate care by caregiver Inadequate self-care Lack of resources	Presence of numerous gingival bleeding points Attachment loss of 4-7 mm	Decrease gingival bleeding by 50% Stop progression of attachment loss Find additional resources to enable client to receive needed care, e.g. CHIP program	Decrease gingival bleeding on probing by 50% Attachment loss remains stable Client enrolled in CHIP program
Freedom from Head and Neck Pain	Inadequate care by caregiver Inadequate self-care	Signs of caries Verbal indicators of pain	Seek dental treatment for pain relief and caries	All carious lesions restored No evidence of oral pain
Responsibility for Oral Health	Impaired mental ability Impaired motor coordination Low value placed on oral health	Presence of plaque, bleeding & caries Reports no previous dental care and fails to report to appointments	Demonstrate self-care with follow up by caregiver Seek dental care Verbalizes a commitment to having a healthy mouth	Perform oral hygiene with minimal supervision Reports for scheduled dental visits Verbalizes that she likes the way her teeth feel and look
Conceptualization and Understanding	Knowledge deficiency in the oral disease process	Inability to verbalize that bacterial plaque contributes to bleeding gums and tooth decay	Client and caregiver verbalize the relationship between plaque, bleeding gums & caries	Client and caregiver verbalize the role of plaque in oral disease Client and caregiver use disclosing agent to evaluate their oral hygiene

Dental Hygiene Interventions

- Assess Jill's mental level and oral health knowledge.
- Provide education on the role of plaque in causing dental disease.
- Provide education to Jill and the caregiver on toothbrushing (powered toothbrush due to limited psychomotor skills) and flossing (by caregiver); a powered interdental cleaner may also be appropriate.
- Communicate the importance of at-home fluoride therapy for dental caries control.
- Provide periodontal debridement and prescribe an antimicrobial rinse (prescription written by dentist).
- Teach Jill and the caregiver to evaluate their oral hygiene for progress (i.e., less bleeding points, use of disclosing agent.)
- Apply fluoride varnish.
- Apply dental sealants.
- Provide nutritional assessment and counseling.
- Introduce procedures slowly based on Jill's mental age.
- Provide rewards for oral health and healthy behavior.
- Use techniques for establishing a trusting relationship.

FIGURE 39–2 ✦ Sample dental hygiene care plan: Client with mental retardation.

DOWN SYNDROME

Down syndrome is the most common and frequently observed chromosomal abnormality in the human race. This syndrome, first observed by Langdon Down (1866) in a group of mentally handicapped individuals, occurs in all socioeconomic levels, geographic regions, ethnic groups, and cultures. Down syndrome occurs 1 in approximately every 800 to 1,000 live births; therefore, approximately 5,000 Down syndrome babies are born each year. More than 350,000 people in the United States have Down syndrome. Because of the prevalence of Down syndrome, dental hygienists are likely to provide care for clients with this condition.

Etiology

Down syndrome affects chromosome number 21 and results in a defined set of physical characteristics and

MR. Three manifestations of chromosomal abnormality can occur: trisomy 21, translocation, or mosaicism. About 95% of people with Down syndrome manifest the effects of trisomy 21. *Trisomy 21* is a failure of a pair of number 21 chromosomes to segregate (nondisjunction) during the formation of either an egg or sperm before conception. Trisomy 21 is not inherited and has no known etiology. The incidence is correlated with increased maternal age. For example, mothers younger than 30 years of age have a 1 in 1,000 chance of giving birth to an infant with Down syndrome; those 35 years of age have a 1 in 400 chance; those 40 years of age have a 1 in 110 chance; and women older than 45 have a 1 in 35 chance.[5]

Translocation is hereditary and occurs when a piece of chromosome in pair 21 breaks off and attaches to another chromosome, usually chromosome 14, 21, or 22. Translocation occurs in approximately 4% to 5% of children with Down syndrome. *Mosaicism,* which occurs in only 1% of children with Down syndrome, is a result of an error in one of the first cell divisions shortly after conception. Regardless of the specific chromosomal anomaly, the presence of three number 21 chromosomes is responsible for the specific physical characteristics and mental deficiencies observed in persons with Down syndrome.

General Characteristics

Approximately 50 different physical characteristics have been observed in infants with Down syndrome; however, not every infant with Down syndrome manifests all 50 characteristics. Only the most common characteristics are discussed in this chapter.

The skull of a child with Down syndrome usually appears small and is shortened in anterior to posterior diameter (from forehead to the crown). A hypoplasia of midfacial bones also is apparent. There is an upward slant to the eyes, the nose is recessed, and the mouth and ears are small. Eyes present with prominent *epicanthal folds*—folds of skin extending from the root of the nose to the median end of the eyebrow. The iris of the eye is speckled with marks called *Brushfield spots.* The nose is reduced in size, nostrils are upturned, and the nasal bridge is depressed. Deviations in the nasal septum also are common. Because of the flat nasal bridge and the underdevelopment of the midfacial region, the face of a Down syndrome person appears flat. This flat facial profile is the most frequently observed characteristic of Down syndrome.

Figure 39–3 depicts the facial features of a person with Down syndrome. The ears of a person with Down syndrome may appear small and abnormal in structure. In most cases the ears have a lack of distinct contour, which results in a round or square appearance; the hands may appear short and broad, with nails that are hyperconvex (Figure 39–4). Persons with Down syndrome tend to be short and overweight.

Persons with Down syndrome usually score in the IQ range 20 to 85. Despite IQ limitations, most children with Down syndrome develop into happy and, in some cases, self-reliant individuals.

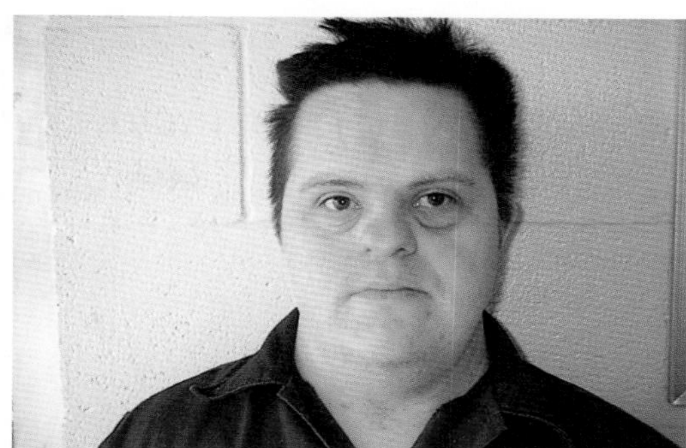

FIGURE 39–3 ✦ Facial characteristics of a Down syndrome client. *(Courtesy Marye J McClanahan, Gene W Hirschfield School of Dental Hygiene, Old Dominion University, Norfolk, Va.)*

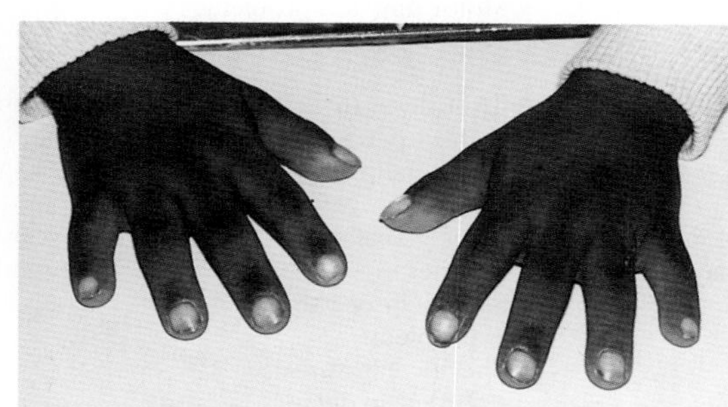

FIGURE 39–4 ✦ Hands of a Down syndrome client. *(Courtesy Dr. F.T. McIver, Department of Pediatric Dentistry, University of North Carolina School of Dentistry.)*

Medical Considerations

Life expectancy for persons with Down syndrome is approximately 55 years of age. Lives of these people can be lengthened by quality healthcare and healthy lifestyle behaviors. Persons with Down syndrome may have various medical problems that affect the dental hygiene process of care (Table 39–3). Knowledge of the potential health problems and the care modifications indicated, awareness of community services and resources, presence of good client and family and/or caregiver rapport, and use of a collaborative approach in meeting the client's healthcare needs are required to achieve oral health and wellness. Knowledge of resources available to families and oral healthcare professionals can aid in meeting client needs beyond the scope of dental hygiene (see Resources for Clients with Mental Retardation and Autism). Specific organizations may not be in the immediate geographic location but may be able to supply information, referral, and support. The yellow or blue pages of the telephone directory under Social Services, Disabilities, or Mental Retardation can supply local assistance.

CONGENITAL HEART DISEASE (see Chapter 40). Congenital heart disease is the most common and serious

TABLE 39–3 MEDICAL AND DENTAL HYGIENE CONSIDERATIONS FOR CLIENTS WITH DOWN SYNDROME

Concern	Clinical Expression	When Seen	Dental Hygiene Care Implications/Management Issues
Congenital heart disease	Endocardial cushion defect Septal defects Tetralogy of Fallot Valvular defects Pulmonary artery hypertension	Newborn or first six weeks	Increased susceptibility to infection Prevention of infective endocarditis via antibiotic premedication before dental hygiene care Susceptible to infective endocarditis Secondary concerns: cardiac dysrhythmias and congestive heart failure Review health history to confirm status and need for prophylactic coverage Assess symptoms of secondary concerns
Hypotonia	Reduced muscle tone Increased range of joint movement Motor function problems	Throughout life Improvement with maturity	Important to address client's comfort while in the dental chair Limited neck movement and pain Motor function problems making oral hygiene care difficult May exhibit spastic movements Considerations with client positioning Alterations in oral hygiene aids
Delayed growth	Typically at or near the third percentile of general population	Throughout life	Evaluate mental age Nutrition assessment and counseling During assessment may see delays in tooth development and facial growth
Developmental delays	Some global delay, degree varies Specific processing problems Specific expressive language delay	First year, monitor Throughout life	Assess client's mental age to appropriately plan oral hygiene instruction Utilize the caregiver to communicate with client when needed
Hearing problems	Otitis media Small ear canals Conductive impairment	Assess by 6 months Review annually	May need to speak loudly and use visual aids Thorough medical history to identify hearing problems Involve the caregiver to determine what mode of communication would work best with the client
Ocular problems	Refractive errors Strabismus Cataracts	Eye exam in early months Regular follow-up	Tactile communication important Assist client with seating to prevent injury Thorough health history to identify ocular problems Involve the caregiver to determine the severity of the problem When giving oral hygiene instruction, be in clear view Adjust oral hygiene based on client's need (i.e., don't expect client to see small anatomy on a radiograph) Avoid glare of the dental light into the eyes
Cervical spine problem	Atlantoaxial subluxation Skeletal cervical anomalies Possible spinal cord compression	X-ray by 3 years	May require shorter appointments for comfort Aid client in walking to the treatment area if needed Place the client in a position that is comfortable for treatment
Thyroid disease	Hypothyroidism (rarely hyper-) Decreased growth, activity	Some congenital, most second decade or older Check by age 1, repeat	Be cognizant of room temperature for client comfort May be cold and require a blanket Assess use of thyroid medication During assessment may see swelling of the tongue Create a low-stress environment Stress good oral hygiene to prevent infection Gingiva may appear spongy
Obesity	Excessive weight gain	Especially 2–3 years, 12–13 years, and in adult life	May require a large blood pressure cuff size Nutritional counseling If client is in a group home, may consider doing an in-service program on nutrition and oral health with a dietician
Seizure disorder	Primarily generalized (grand mal) Also, myoclonic, hypsarrhythmia	Any time	Validate that client has taken seizure medication Minimize stress Avoid flashing dental light into client's eyes Assess health history for anticonvulsive medications May see gingival enlargement caused by medications Stress need for good oral hygiene because of gingival effects of medications Avoid stress-inducing situations Dental sealants and fluoride beneficial If gingival enlargement is present, more frequent continued care may be needed

TABLE 39–3 MEDICAL AND DENTAL HYGIENE CONSIDERATIONS FOR CLIENTS WITH DOWN SYNDROME—CONT'D

Concern	Clinical Expression	When Seen	Dental Hygiene Care Implications/Management Issues
Emotional problems	Inappropriate behavior, depression	Mid- to late childhood, adulthood	Praise client to build self-esteem and cooperation Treat client with respect and concern Assess client's frame of mind with the caregiver before the appointment Assess health history for medications
Premature senescence	Behavior changes; functional losses	Fifth decade and older	Evaluate mental age Treat client with respect and concern Assess client's frame of mind with the caregiver before the appointment Assess health history for medications

Also, variable occurrence of congenital gastrointestinal anomalies, *Hirschsprung's disease* (an extreme dilation of the colon), leukemia, hepatitis B carrier state, *keratoconus* (conical protrusion of the center of the cornea), dry skin, hip dysplasia, diabetes, mitral valve prolapse.
Modified from Crocker AC: The spectrum of medical care for developmental disabilities. In Crocker AC, Rubin IL, eds: *Developmental disabilities: Delivery of medical care for children and adults*, Philadelphia, 1989, Lea & Febiger.

Resources for Clients with Mental Retardation and Autism

National Down Syndrome Congress
7000 Peachtree-Dunwoody Rd. NE
Lake Ridge 400 Office Park Bldg. #5, Suite 100
Atlanta GA 30328
1-800-232-NCDC
email: NDSCcenter@aol.com

American Association on Mental Retardation
444 North Capital St. NW, Suite 846
Washington DC 20001-1512
1-800-424-3688
website: aamr.org

Autism Society of America
7910 Woodmont Ave., Suite 300
Bethesda, MD 20814-3015
1-800-3AUTISM x150
website: autism-society.org

National Down Syndrome Society
666 Broadway, 8th Floor
New York, NY 10012-2317
1-800-221-4602
email: info@ndss.org

medical condition in persons with Down syndrome. Most cardiovascular malformations associated with Down syndrome are acutely or chronically life-threatening. Cardiac problems are present in 40% to 50% of newborns with Down syndrome; heart defects are major causes of high mortality during the first 2 years of the infant's life.[6] Additionally, persons with Down syndrome have increased susceptibility to infection, which continues to be a major cause of morbidity and mortality.

Two of the common heart defects are atrial septal defects (45%) and ventricular septal defects (35%) for the Down syndrome population with congenital heart disease. The most common congenital heart defects, detected by echocardiogram, are endocardial cushion defects. Endocardial cushions are ridges in the developing fetal heart. These cushions are involved in the formation of the septum that separates the right and left ventricles, formation of the septa that separates the right and left atria, and formation of the two valves between the atria and ventricles. Symptoms of these heart defects are defective heart valves, severe heart failure, frequent pneumonia, and poor growth. Also frequently seen in Down syndrome is pulmonary artery hypertension, characterized by constriction of the blood vessels in the lungs, which causes back pressure and overload on the right ventricle. Pulmonary artery hypertension is often a consequence of the increased flow to the lungs caused by the heart defects.

Multiple cardiac abnormalities exist in approximately 30% of persons with Down syndrome. Medical care depends on the severity of the symptoms. When providing care for a Down syndrome client, it is imperative to obtain a detailed health history to determine cardiac abnormalities present. Prophylactic antibiotic premedication is prescribed when congenital heart defects are present because defective heart valves are at risk for infective endocarditis from dental hygiene care (see Chapter 9 on prophylactic antibiotic premedication).

ORTHOPEDIC CONCERNS. Orthopedic problems are usually a result of *hypotonia* (low muscle tone).

✦ *Atlantoaxial subluxation*, a cervical spine instability, is characterized by an abnormal increase in mobility within the joint between the first two cervical vertebrae in the neck.[7] Most children have no symptoms of atlantoaxial subluxation, but if symptoms are present (i.e., neck pain, change in gait, extremity weakness, spasticity, and limited neck movement), they are related to spinal cord compression.

- *Scoliosis* (curvature of the spine) is frequently detected in Down syndrome but is usually mild. Persons with Down syndrome usually have excessive external rotation and abduction of the hip. As a result, a wide-angled gait and widespread legs when sitting are evident. Persons with mild scoliosis may not be aware that they have a problem with their spine, but it is still important to ensure client comfort during care.

OTHER DISORDERS (see Chapter 38)

- *Thyroid disorders* are common in persons with Down syndrome. In older persons with Down syndrome, as many as 50% have thyroid disorders, with hypothyroidism being the most common.[8] Classic symptoms of hypothyroidism include delayed growth, short stature, obesity, lethargy, and dry skin.
- *Hearing impairments*, either unilateral or bilateral, are present in 40% to 75% of persons with Down syndrome. Hearing loss is usually mild to moderate and is often caused by persistent fluid in the middle ear. Ear infections also are common. Cataracts occur in 12% to 54% of persons with Down syndrome, but do not affect vision or require surgery.
- *Seizure activity* in infants and young children with Down syndrome occurs at the same rate as in the general population; however, at age 20 to 30 grand mal seizures are seen more frequently in persons with Down syndrome. Gingival enlargement caused by medications taken to control seizure activity is of particular significance. Phenytoin (dilantin), which is often prescribed to control epileptic seizures, causes various degrees of gingival enlargement (Figures 39–5 and 39–6). Effective plaque control reduces the extent of drug-influenced gingival enlargement; therefore, daily self-care must be effective before use of phenytoin.

Adults with Down syndrome often demonstrate neuropathologic changes similar to those seen in individuals diagnosed with Alzheimer's disease. Anatomic changes of Alzheimer's disease appear to be almost universal in adults with Down syndrome older than 40 years, most of whom do not show behavioral signs of Alzheimer's disease.[7] The relationship between Alzheimer's disease and Down syndrome is under investigation.

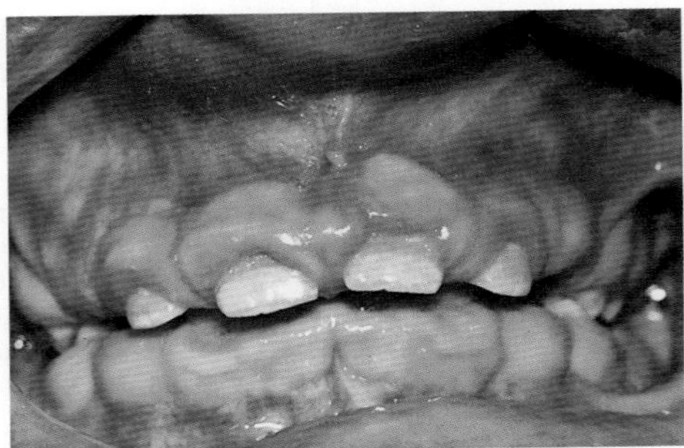

FIGURE 39–5 ✦ Moderate drug-influenced gingivitis associated with Dilantin (phenytoin) therapy for seizure control in a client with Down syndrome. *(Courtesy Dr. F.T. McIver, Department of Pediatric Dentistry, University of North Carolina School of Dentistry.)*

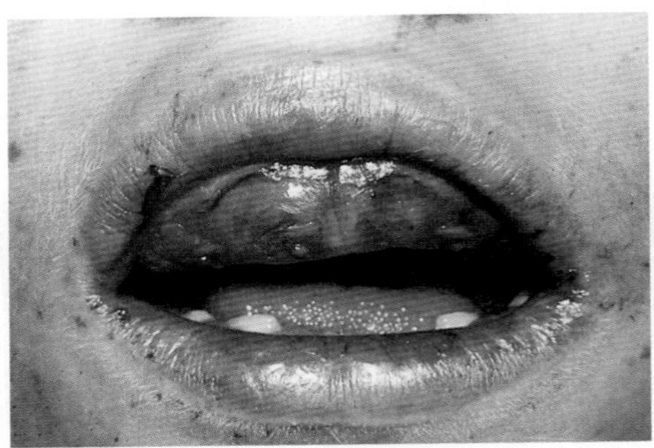

FIGURE 39–6 ✦ Severe drug-influenced gingivitis associated with Dilantin (phenytoin) therapy for seizure control in a client with Down syndrome. *(Courtesy Dr. F.T. McIver, Department of Pediatric Dentistry, University of North Carolina School of Dentistry.)*

Oral Manifestations (see Some Oral Manifestations Observed in Clients with Down Syndrome)

Some Oral Manifestations Observed in Clients with Down Syndrome

Mouth open with protruding tongue
Underdeveloped maxilla
Narrow palate with broadened alveolar ridges
Congenitally missing teeth
Malocclusion
Enamel hypoplasia
High rate of tooth loss caused by periodontal disease
Shortened roots
Enlarged tonsils and adenoids
Fissured tongue
Enlarged vallate papilla on tongue
Microdontia
Tetracycline staining
Periodontal diseases
Poor oral hygiene
Low caries risk

TONGUE. A person with Down syndrome often has his or her mouth open and tongue protruding. The tongue seems enlarged as a result of an underdeveloped maxilla, mandibular prognathism, a narrow palate with broadened alveolar ridges, and enlarged tonsils and adenoids, all of which produce a small oral cavity. Fissuring of the tongue and enlargement of the vallate papillae are observed in 37% to 60% of persons with Down syndrome. Because of this finding, it is imperative that these patients receive thorough oral hygiene instructions, including tongue brushing to reduce bacterial counts and halitosis.

TOOTH MORPHOLOGY. The teeth are commonly found to be small (microdontia) in persons with Down syndrome. Maxillary teeth are generally more affected in size than mandibular teeth. All teeth except for the maxillary first molars and mandibular incisors are reduced in size, but root formation, although roots are shortened, is complete.[7] The most frequently affected permanent teeth in the maxillary arch are the second molars (52%), lateral incisors (42%), canines (41%), first molars (40%), and central incisors (35%). In the mandibular arch the first and second premolars are most commonly affected (63% and 48%). Tetracycline staining and hypoplastic enamel may be evident as a result of the significant number of early childhood infections requiring antibiotic therapy experienced by persons with Down syndrome.

MISSING TEETH AND MALOCCLUSION. Congenitally missing teeth and delayed eruption occur in persons with Down syndrome at a much higher rate than that in the general population. The increased incidence of congenitally missing permanent teeth (25% to 50%) is probably related to ectodermal dysplasia, local inflammation that damages the tooth germ, or other medical infections. The most frequently missing permanent teeth in persons with Down syndrome are the mandibular second premolar (3.4%) followed by the lateral incisor (2.2%). Within each quadrant it is common to find the most posterior tooth to be missing more than the most anterior tooth. Malocclusion also is seen frequently, with mandibular overjet and posterior crossbite occurring in virtually all persons with Down syndrome.[7] Correction of malocclusion is usually not indicated. If crossbites are corrected, an earlier tissue breakdown may occur as a result of the underdeveloped maxilla and its relation to basal bone. Lingual movement of mandibular teeth is difficult because of the tendency of persons with Down syndrome to have large, protruding tongues.

As a result of an increase in the number of persons with Down syndrome working and living in the community, dental professionals have observed an increase in clients with Down syndrome seeking extensive dental care. With evidence of cognitive functioning for most of these individuals, there is an increase in self-esteem and self-image. Healthcare professionals must assess the client to determine if he or she could tolerate extensive treatment. If orthodontic treatment is not chosen for a Down syndrome client, the dental professional employs creative strategies to meet individual oral hygiene needs. Clients with Down syndrome are given the same treatment options as other clients. Therefore, treatment objectives should not be limited simply because the client has Down syndrome. Care plans are adapted to the individual's conditions, but overall the goal is to provide comprehensive care.

PERIODONTAL DISEASE. Individuals with Down syndrome have a high incidence of periodontal disease. Type and severity of periodontal disease are both functions of immunodeficiency and impaired host defense rather than poor oral hygiene alone. Periodontal disease has been reported to begin as early as age 6 years, and by adulthood nearly all people with Down syndrome are affected.[7,9]

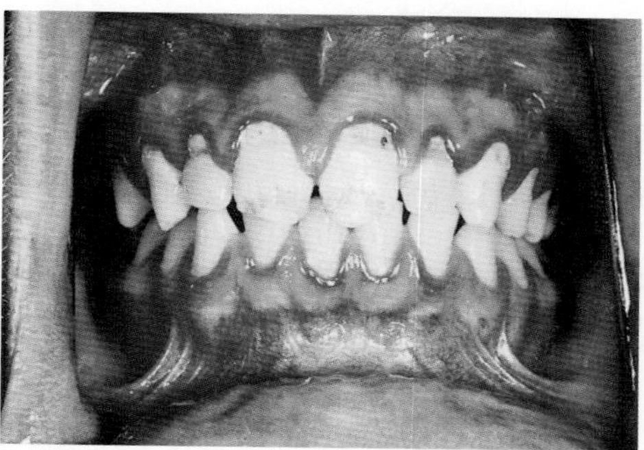

FIGURE 39–7 ✦ Plaque-induced marginal gingivitis and enamel hypoplasia in an individual with Down syndrome. *(Courtesy Dr. F.T. McIver, Department of Pediatric Dentistry, University of North Carolina School of Dentistry.)*

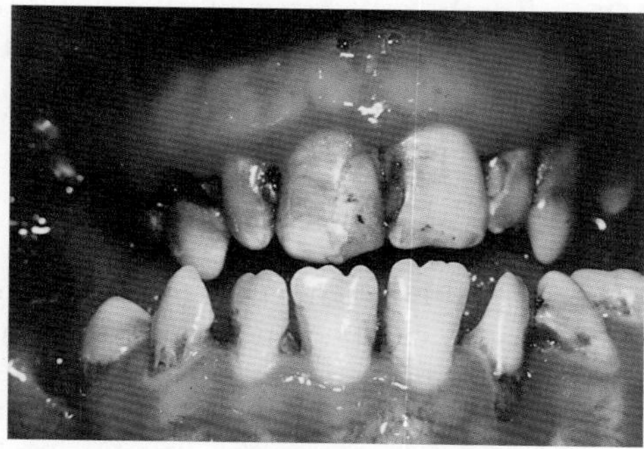

FIGURE 39–8 ✦ Severe chronic periodontal disease in a Down syndrome client. *(Courtesy Dr. F.T. McIver, Department of Pediatric Dentistry, University of North Carolina School of Dentistry.)*

Figure 39–7 depicts a Down syndrome client with marginal gingivitis and enamel hypoplasia. Figure 39–8 shows more severe periodontal problems in a Down syndrome client. Periodontal disease is more common in individuals living in institutions as compared to individuals living in the community. This finding may be the result of the lack of education given to the healthcare providers in these institutions, diet, and inadequate daily oral health behavior. In individuals with Down syndrome living in the community, the level of oral hygiene practiced and the extra care given by their caregivers may be sufficient to slow down disease progression.

POOR ORAL HYGIENE. Maintaining optimal oral hygiene is very difficult for persons with Down syndrome; therefore, dental hygienists educate caregivers and stress the importance of close supervision during oral hygiene procedures and diet habits that promote oral health and wellness. If oral healthcare professionals can incorporate effective oral hygiene care as a part of the client's daily routine, gingival and periodontal conditions may be prevented or controlled. Oral hygiene instructions must be presented to the client and a family member or primary caregiver in a clear and concise manner. It is important to communicate directly to the client in order to build trust. It may be necessary to determine what motivates the client and agree on an award system to ensure cooperation.

Persons capable of performing their own self-care should be encouraged to do so. Powered toothbrushes may enable persons with minimal motor control to independently perform oral self- care, thereby facilitating the human need for responsibility for oral health. If persons can perform their own self-care, they own the task and are likely to perform the behavior regularly. Persons with Down syndrome learn better from visual teaching than from auditory teaching; therefore, instruction should be augmented with visual materials such as pictures, models, and diagrams.

TOOTH LOSS. Tooth loss occurs in about 50% of individuals with Down syndrome, which may be attributed to the high prevalence of periodontal disease in this population.[10]

Management of Clients with Down Syndrome

Generally, persons with Down syndrome are content and affectionate, but they can become aggressive if confused or disoriented. Although speech patterns are retarded, most adults speak intelligently with a husky quality of voice. It is important to assess the mental level of the client mathematically (see formula discussed at the beginning of the chapter) or by observing behavioral patterns, evaluating responses during conversation, and questioning the caregiver. More likely, the client does not comprehend the need for care or that it is beneficial. Everything related to care should be introduced slowly, explained, and shown if possible. Humanistic behavior should be used to calm the client's fears. Some Down syndrome clients with higher IQs (mild and slightly moderate MR) can become involved and appreciate the attention given to them during dental hygiene care.

If these clients are unmanageable, it is usually because they are frightened or have had a previous traumatic dental experience or because their mental limitations do not allow them to comprehend the procedure. Preoperative medications and general anesthesia can be prescribed and administered if necessary. When care requires a general anesthetic agent, a thorough health history review is imperative and all possible needs should be met while the person is anesthetized. A sample dental hygiene care plan for the client with Down syndrome is presented in Figure 39–9.

AUTISM

Autism is a developmental disorder and lifelong disability characterized by a persistent aloneness. Other names have been used to describe autism, including Kanner's syndrome, early infantile autism, primary autism, infantile or childhood autism, and childhood psychosis. Individuals with autism relate poorly to people and would rather spend quality time with objects. For most dental hygienists, the provision of care for an autistic person is likely because statistics indicate that autism and its associated behaviors have been estimated to occur in as many as one in 500 individuals. Males have a four to five times higher incidence than females.[1]

Etiology

The etiology of autism is unknown. Several theories exist, including psychogenic, genetic, biochemical deficits, and neurophysiologic theories. No single theory has been completely accepted. The care of clients with autism is consistent with the theory held by the healthcare provider. Types of treatment include psychotherapy, educational intervention, communication therapy, special education, medications, and behavioral therapy. The most commonly prescribed medications include tranquilizers such as methylphenidate, thioridazine, diphenhydramine, and anticonvulsants such as phenytoin and carbamazepine.

General Characteristics

Autistic children are unable to relate in an ordinary manner to people and situations from the beginning of life. Children with autism are sometimes described as "self-sufficient," "living life in a shell," "happiest when alone," "acting as if people were not there," and "giving the impression of silent wisdom." From the beginning of life, the child desires an extreme autistic aloneness that ignores, disregards, and shuts out anything that comes from outside of the child. The child has an all-powerful need for being left undisturbed. Everything and anything that changes his or her external environment is looked on as an intrusion. The first characteristic sign of autism is the lack of posture on being picked up and the failure to adjust the body to that of the person holding the child. Many children with autism come from highly intelligent families. For a person to be diagnosed as autistic, delays or abnormal functioning must be seen in at least one of the following before age 3: social interaction, language used for social communication, or symbolic or imaginative play. Approximately 75% of these clients have diagnosed MR, commonly of the moderate range.[1]

COMMUNICATION. Autistic children are usually devoid of speech or have abnormal language. Their language consists mainly of naming nouns and adjectives that identify objects, and indicating colors and numbers that represent nothing specific. This type of language is referred to as excellent *rote memory*. Language becomes a valueless or grossly distorted memory exercise with no use for communication. In other words, autistic children meaninglessly parrot what they hear (*echolalia*). When sentences are formed, they are mostly parrotlike repetitions of word combinations that have been heard. For the autistic child, words become inflexible and cannot be used with any other reference but the original acquired meaning. Autistic children repeat and use personal pro-

James Pardue is a 41-year-old client with Down syndrome. His health history reveals a mitral valve prolapse. He is currently taking Zyprexa. His father reveals James' fear of being reclined in the dental chair. Intraoral assessment reveals dental caries at the gingival margin and a significant amount of plaque along the same area. The father verbalizes that James likes to play "Let's Make a Deal," which is very helpful in coercing James to perform a specific behavior.

Dental Hygiene Diagnosis	Due To or Related To	As Evidenced By	Client Goal	Evaluate Statements
Protection from Health Risks	Mitral value prolapse	Need for premedication as reported by father	Client takes appropriate premedication	No medical emergency
Biologically Sound & Functional Dentition	Inadequate home care and diet	Signs of caries at the gingival margin	Obtain restorative care Alter diet to exclude cariogenic foods/beverages	No evidence of caries activity in 6 month period
Skin & Mucous Membrane Integrity of the Head and Neck	Inadequate daily home care	Numerous gingival bleeding points	Performance of successful oral hygiene by the caregiver & client	Demonstrates successful oral hygiene at 3-month continued-care interval Decrease gingival bleeding points by 50%
Freedom from Anxiety & Stress	Fear of the dental chair	Client will not sit in the chair while it is moving	Sits in chair without disruptive behavior	Demonstrates comfort level with the dental setting
Responsibility for Oral Health	Lack of caregiver supervision Too much autonomy for self-care by the client Skill deficiency	Plaque accumulation Signs of caries	Reduce deposit accumulation by next continued-care interval Decrease plaque index score by 1 point by next appointment Client cleans his own teeth then caregiver follows up Both caregiver & client demonstrate effective oral hygiene techniques	Decrease calculus classification from a Class III to a II. Decrease plaque index by 1 point at continued-care interval
Conceptualization & Understanding	Oral disease knowledge deficiency of caregiver	Inability to explain disease process & etiology	Caregiver can explain disease process & etiology Caregiver can see a difference in James' gingival tissues Caregiver verbalizes the value of oral disease prevention	Client and caregiver report that they evaluate oral hygiene and oral health at least once monthly in the home environment

Dental Hygiene Interventions

- Determine if the client has taken the appropriate prophylactic antibiotic premedication for mitral valve prolapse.
- Address concerns with the medication Zyprexa:
  Monitor vitals
  Assess salivary flow
  Consider a semi-supine position
  Have client sit for 2 minutes before standing
- Conduct nutritional counseling for caries control.
- Discuss the value of daily fluoride treatment for caries control.
- Assess the need and apply dental sealants if indicated.
- Instructions for caregiver:
  Etiology of disease
  Reasoning for plaque index
  Use of oral hygiene devices
  Techniques for successful patient management
  How to look for improvements in the tissue
  Importance of recalls
- Place the dental chair into supine position, then have James get into the chair.
- Introduce procedures slowly based on James' mental age.
- Give the client positive reinforcement. Use the techniques for forming trusting relationships described in the chapter.
- Complete periodontal debridement and apply fluoride varnish.
- At the 3-month continued-care interval, reevaluate the homecare.
- Modify the plan if needed. Keep open communication between the caregiver and other healthcare providers.
- Refer to the dentist for restorative procedures.

FIGURE 39–9 ✦ Sample dental hygiene care plan: Client with Down syndrome.

nouns just as they are heard. For example, if an autistic child desires milk, he may say, "Are you ready for your milk?" Children with autism slowly learn to speak of themselves in the first person and of the person addressed in the second person; this occurs around the age of 6 years. Also, it is noted that children with autism avoid eye-to-eye contact, facial expressions, and any other form of nonverbal communication.[1]

BEHAVIOR. An autistic child is controlled by the obsession for sameness that no one can disrupt but the child. Living monotonously repetitious lives makes them feel secure. These clients exhibit restricted, repetitive, and stereotypical patterns of behavior, interests, and activities.

Food is the first intrusion that an autistic infant has to face. Babies with autism may find eating difficult, which may result in vomiting. Their unsuccessful struggle against the intrusion of food leads to a limited selection of food choices.[1] If food selection includes regular sucrose intake, dental caries may be a major concern.

An inflexible adherence to specific, nonfunctional routines or rituals is evident in these clients. Despair and confusion can be caused by minor changes in routine, everyday tasks, and furniture arrangement. Autistic children also react to loud noises and moving objects with horror. Noise, or motion of an object or person, is not feared by the child, but rather the disturbance may threaten the child's aloneness. Another characteristic of autism is stereotypical body movements such as rocking, spinning, sniffing, hand clapping, and swaying. A range of behaviors is evident, including hyperactivity, short attention span, impulsivity, aggressiveness, and self-injurious behaviors.[1]

PHYSICAL CHARACTERISTICS. Persons with autism are usually normal physically, although autism may occur along with other conditions such as metabolic disturbances (i.e., phenylketonuria, Tay-Sachs disease), Down syndrome, and epilepsy. Some autistic persons acquire skill in fine muscle coordination, whereas others have a clumsy gait or poor gross motor performance.

INTERPERSONAL RELATIONSHIPS. Children with autism are more interested in objects than people because objects rarely change in appearance or position. The sameness of objects does not threaten the child, allowing the child to have undisturbed power and control. Autistic children are not afraid of people but of the objects they acquire. For example, an autistic child is scared of a pin pricking his body, not the person doing the pricking. Dental hygienists should try to alleviate a fear of dental instruments by explaining each procedure and the use of each instrument to the client.

The children are not interested in surrounding conversation. When addressed, autistic children respond quickly to "get it over with" so they can continue their activity, or they may not respond at all. Family members derive the same response as a casual acquaintance. Similarly, autistic children are very interested in pictures of people but not in people themselves. The pictures of people cannot disturb their environment.

PROGRESS. By the age of 5 or 6 years, language becomes more communicative because the autistic child has experienced several patterns. Food is accepted, noises and motions are tolerated, and panic tantrums subside. The children also experience increased contact with people, especially people who satisfy their needs, answer their questions, and help them do things (such as reading). By the age of 6 or 8 years, autistic children play alongside other children (parallel play) but never with a group. They also acquire reading skills quickly at this age. As autistic children grow older, several changes begin to occur. They are still in their world of aloneness and sameness, but they emerge from solitude to varying degrees. Some people are accepted into their life because they finally compromise and gradually extend feelers into a world to which they have been total strangers. Other behaviors exhibited by autistic persons at various age periods are shown in Table 39–4. Only a small percentage of clients with autism will live and work independently.[1]

Oral Manifestations

Persons with autism exhibit no specific oral findings, although particular circumstances may increase the risk and prevalence of caries and periodontal disease. Oral care may have been neglected as a result of language difficulties, anxiety, and lack of social contact. Psychotropic medications may be used as adjuncts to other treatments, causing decreased salivation. The client may benefit from a saliva substitute and at-home fluoride therapy. Persons with autism also may have epilepsy requiring oral medication such as phenytoin (Dilantin) that produces drug-influenced gingival enlargement, especially when the individual has poor bacterial plaque control.

Individuals with autism often have nutritional needs because of dietary fixation, preference for soft or sweet foods that require little chewing, and lack of tongue coordination. Autistic people are known to pouch their food (hold in their mouth, for example, in their cheeks) instead of swallowing. Therefore, these persons may have poor dietary habits and heavy accumulations of materia alba and plaque. Because of the eating habits of autistic clients, nutritional counseling and rigorous plaque control interventions may be needed.

Management of Clients with Autism

Management of clients with autism incorporates two approaches: communication techniques and pharmacologic therapies. To choose the best approach, the dental hygienist interviews the caregiver to gather information about the client's peculiarities, behaviors, and communication skills.

Communication includes the caregiver, client, and the dental staff. An autistic client may require conditioning before dental hygiene care. To accomplish this goal,

TABLE 39–4

POSSIBLE BEHAVIORS EXHIBITED BY AUTISTIC PEOPLE

Age Period	Response to Environment	Social/Play Skills	Language Communication Skills	Feeding/Eating	Motor Development
Infancy	"Good": The infant is quiet and placid, seldom cries, and is fascinated by lights. "Irritable": The infant screams and may quiet only with vigorous rocking or car rides. Fights washing, dressing, and feedings. Stiff, hard to cuddle. Body rocks, head bangs.	Unresponsive to parents' presence Poor response to social games Little eye contact No reaching or pointing No interest in baby toys May enjoy roughhousing	Ignores speech Ignores loud sounds Is fascinated with soft sounds Has decreased verbalizations	Poor sucking Refusal to eat lumpy foods Does not cry when hungry	On schedule or uneven May bypass a motor stage, such as creeping
Toddler	Self-stimulating behaviors, rocking, head banging Sleep patterns irregular Resists changes in routine Disturbances in response to stimuli: Is fascinated with some sounds Uses touch, taste, and smell to extremes Ignores objects of usual childhood interest. Zeros in on details Uses peripheral vision Recognizes parents by outline rather than by features Does not respond to painful stimuli	Inappropriate use of an attachment to objects Stereotypic, repetitive play May be extremely passive May be destructive, aggressive, and self-injurious Difficult to manage Frequent tantrums	Unresponsive to voice, tone, or name Echolalia: delayed or immediate Screams Leads adult by the arm Responds to simple commands	Likes pureed foods Will eat only a limited variety of foods Does not recognize foods in other forms, such as a banana without the peel	Prolonged cruiser Tiptoe walks May be normal May be hyperactive
Preschool	Toddler responses continue	Aloof and expressionless Delayed toilet training More affectionate Socially embarrassing behaviors Tantrums continue Stereotypic, repetitive play continues Passivity may continue	Echolalia may develop Meaningful speech is produced with effort: poor pronunciation and voice control Unable to understand most speech Can understand short, concrete sentences Confusion with pronouns, similar-sounding words, and word order Uses and understands limited gestures	Food jags	May be normal May jump, spin, flap arms/hands May be graceful or clumsy Fine motor ability may differ from gross Difficulty with copying movements May walk with elbows bent, hands together, and wrists dropped May be earthbound Hyperactivity may continue
School Years	Behaviors (tantrums) decrease Sleep irregularities may continue Continues to have disturbances in response to stimuli	Increased affection Increased social skills May help with simple household chores	Language skills may increase Same problems as preschooler may continue	Food jags continue May begin trying new foods	Increased motor skills Unusual walk Earthbound behavior continues Splinter skills may develop May pace, jump, spin
Adulthood	Same as school years	Increased affection Increased social skills	Language skills continue to increase	Diet broadens Food jags continue	Motor skills continue to increase Earthbound behavior continues Relatively self-sufficient

the caregiver is encouraged to bring the client to the office to familiarize the client with upcoming care. Rehearsals at home can be advantageous. The caregiver practices commands that the dental professional may use such as "hands down," "open your mouth," and "look at me." The reception area should be quiet with as few people as possible. The client should not wait for extended periods because of the possibility of heightened fear and stress. The dental hygiene procedure is kept short and organized. *Behavior modification* techniques that consist of tell-show-do, and immediate, frequent positive and negative reinforcement are used with short, clear commands (see Steps in Behavioral Modification for the Individual with Autism).

Caregivers are encouraged to be present during treatment to provide a familiar face and particularly if immobilization is needed for behavior control. Many methods, including those mentioned earlier, can be used for behavior control (e.g., holding the client's hands down, the use of a papoose board—only indicated when a safe working environment is not attainable—and mouth props). If the client needs to return, the appointments should remain the same weekday and time, with the same dental professionals. The procedure/routine should remain constant as much as possible.

Pharmacologic therapies are needed if all other methods fail. The most commonly prescribed medications include nitrous oxide–oxygen analgesia, diazepam, hydroxyzine, chloral hydrate, meperidine, and promethazine. Pharmacologic therapies may be administered in various combinations and dosages depending on each client's individual needs. See Figure 39–10 for a sample dental hygiene care plan for a client with autism.

Steps in Behavioral Modification for the Individual with Autism

Use extensive positive social reinforcement to put the client at ease.

Use a very simple reward system and explain the system to the client. For example, the client could be given a toy if good behavior is exhibited throughout the appointment. If the client is an adult, a trip to a favorite restaurant may be appropriate. The reward should be suited to the individual client.

Give constant positive social reinforcement throughout each appointment.

Following each desired behavior, provide verbal praise immediately and precisely.

Give instructions in a reassuring manner with each desired behavior.

Do not discuss dental treatment needed during dental hygiene care.

Make sure that points earned during the appointment for desired behavior always entitle the person to a prize at the end.

Conclude each session with excessive praise.

EDUCATING MENTALLY CHALLENGED CLIENTS

Oral hygiene for mentally challenged individuals requires modifications because of the physical, cognitive, and behavioral challenges they might have. The client's cognitive and physical limitations and abilities, oral and systemic disease risk, systemic and oral health status, level of deposit accumulation, medications, diet, and ability to cooperate are assessed so dental hygiene care can meet the client's human needs.

Cognitive Limitations

Cognitive level affects the client's oral self-care potential. Clients with mild or moderate MR can usually learn to brush. Successful teaching methods include using pictures, tell-show-do, and modeling. A consistent challenge these clients face is brushing long enough; therefore, an egg timer could be used to lengthen brushing time. Oral irrigators, interdental cleaning aids, and disclosing tablets can be used by clients with mild MR. Moderately retarded clients require repetitive training but can usually manipulate a powered toothbrush. With severe MR clients, emphasis is on as much self-care as possible, with the caregiver following up to ensure thorough plaque control. Normally these clients are limited to a push-pull stroke and often isolate brushing to one side. Profound MR clients depend on caregivers for oral cleansing. Emphasis is on acceptance of oral hygiene procedures, which is accomplished through nonverbal communication and desensitization techniques.

Physical Limitations

In addition to the physical limitations (already discussed), communication may be a challenge if the client has visual or hearing limitations. Visual cues work best with persons with hearing impairments; tactile and auditory cues are used with visually impaired clients. A severe gag reflex may be managed by placing the client in a semisupine position and/or eliminating the use of toothpaste to reduce gagging and provide better vision for the caregiver or dental professional. Water, a flavorful mouthwash, or an ingestible dentifrice can be used in place of toothpaste. NASA Dent dentifrice, produced by Scherer Laboratories, is nonfoaming and safe for ingesting. Dental professionals and caregivers may need to use a mouth prop to allow access during oral care. When working with severe and profoundly mentally retarded clients, using a toothbrush designed for a suction attachment can prevent aspiration (see Chapter 36, Figure 36–4).

Selection of Oral Hygiene Aids

Oral hygiene aids should be selected based on a thorough assessment of the client. Brush recommendations are the same as for other clients, except the handle should be longer to facilitate reaching posterior areas and the brush head size should be selected based on the client's oral cavity size and ability to open. Existing toothbrushes can be altered according to client need

Ben Brown, age 28, is a client with autism. He has come to the dental office for examination and treatment. Ben is accompanied by his sister, who is his caregiver. Ben displays ritualistic behaviors such as slow, thought-out walking and tapping. He has limited verbal skills, is sensitive to high-pitched noises, and is taking Zoloft. Ben presents with mild dental caries, cervical tooth abrasion, and light supragingival deposits on the mandibular anterior lingual teeth.

Dental Hygiene Diagnosis	Due To or Related To	As Evidenced By	Client Goal	Evaluate Statements
Biologically Sound & Functional Dentition	Inadequate home care Inadequate diet	Signs of dental caries	Obtain restorative treatment Alter diet to exclude cariogenic foods	Decrease plaque index score by 1 point Report ingestion of noncariogenic snacks
	Harmful toothbrushing technique	Signs of cervical abrasion	Reduce amount of pressure when toothbrushing	No additional abrasion evident
Skin & Mucous Membrane Integrity of the Head and Neck	Medication (Zoloft)	Signs of xerostomia	Use of saliva substitutes & fluoride therapy	Less xerostomia observed and reported
	Inadequate home care	Supragingival soft and hard deposits	Caregiver and client to demonstrate thorough oral hygiene	Reduction of deposit accumulation at continued-care visit
Freedom from Anxiety & Stress	Sensitivity to high-pitched noises	Verbal & nonverbal indicators of stress	Respond positively to the use of equipment which typically causes unpleasant sensation in the ears	Client appears comfortable & cooperative during treatment
	Client carefulness & not being sure of his environment	Tapping Well thought-out (deliberate) walking	Decrease behaviors that interfere with treatment	Tapping and deliberate walking behaviors decreased by 50%
Responsibility for Oral Health	Lack of caregiver supervision Too much autonomy for self-care by the client Skill deficiency	Plaque accumulation Signs of supragingival deposits	Decreased plaque accumulation by 50% at continued-care appointment Caregiver reports that client cleans his own mouth daily and it is followed up by caregiver. Both caregiver & client demonstrate appropriate oral hygiene techniques	PI score decreases by 50%
Conceptualization & Understanding	Knowledge deficiency of caregiver & client	Inability to explain disease process & etiology	Caregiver can explain disease process & etiology Caregiver can see a difference in client's gingival tissues	Caregiver verbalizes that a difference is observed in Ben's oral health as a result of the home care

Dental Hygiene Interventions

Addresses concerns with the medication Zoloft:
- Monitor vitals
- Assess salivary flow
- Consider a semi-supine position
- Have client sit for 2 minutes before standing

Conduct nutritional counseling

Instructions for caregiver:
- Etiology for disease
- Rationale for plaque index
- Use of oral hygiene devices
- Use less pressure when toothbrushing
- Use a soft toothbrush
- Techniques for successful client management
- How to look for improvements in the gum tissue (i.e. bleeding points)
- Importance of frequent continued-care appointments

Communicate the value of at-home fluoride therapy for caries control
Discuss the use of sugarless gum, frequent water or saliva substitutes for managing xerostomia
Avoid the use of equipment with high-pitched noises
Give verbal commands for desired behavior. Allow Ben time to process the command and wait for a response
Incorporate behavior modification techniques and techniques for forming a *trusting relationship*
Give Ben positive reinforcement for appropriate behavior
Complete periodontal debridement and apply fluoride varnish
Refer to a dentist for restorative procedures
After 3 months, re-evaluate home care and oral health status
Modify care plan if needed; maintain communication between caregiver and other healthcare providers

FIGURE 39–10 ✦ Sample dental hygiene care plan: Client with autism.

(e.g., motor ability and grip problems) (see Chapter 36, Figure 36–5). Some companies manufacture modified toothbrushes for special needs clients. The Collis Curve by Collis Curve, Inc. and the Action 2 by Oranamics, Inc. are powered toothbrushes that are excellent for clients with grip problems and limited fine motor control.

Flossing may be extremely difficult for clients and caregivers, but some interdental cleaning is better than none. If only the anterior teeth can be reached and/or tolerated, then this should be encouraged. Interdental cleaning devices with long handles are recommended to protect fingers from inadvertent or intentional biting and to reach posterior areas. Holders must be easy to thread and use to ensure compliance. Oral irrigators are not generally recommended for this population except to deliver prescribed antimicrobial agents. Chlorhexidine mouthrinse is commonly prescribed for clients with disabilities because of the potential for higher plaque and gingivitis prevalence. It can be administered via an oral irrigator, a spray, or a swab. (*Note*: Chlorhexidine is absorbed through the gastrointestinal system; therefore, no harm is caused by swallowing a small amount of the agent.) Other antimicrobial agents may be indicated for these clients: Listerine, stannous fluoride gels and mouthwashes, povidone iodine (Betadine) mouthwashes, and similar products. These products are often less expensive and do not stain teeth or alter taste like 0.12% chlorhexidine gluconate. If cooperation is high, home fluoride application is commonly done with a toothbrush after toothbrushing.[11]

Client Education Issues

- Begin with the caregiver's personal oral health in order to evaluate and form positive attitudes and habits toward oral health and hygiene.
- Ensure that caregiver has knowledge and equipment to perform effective oral hygiene on the client.
- Clients with mild MR are educable; therefore, explain and demonstrate oral hygiene instructions based on activities instead of concepts.
- Clients with moderate MR should be taught fundamental skills by employing the show-and-tell method.
- Discuss preventive therapies (e.g., diet counseling, dental sealants, fluoride therapy, and frequent continued-care intervals) and their feasibility with caregiver.
- Provide verbal and written instructions so caregiver can have a reference if needed.

Legal, Ethical, and Safety Issues

- The 1992 Title III of the *Americans with Disabilities Act* "makes it illegal to discriminate against persons with disabilities, and those with whom they associate, in the provision of services in 'places of public accommodation.'"
- Many dental practices do not treat mentally challenged clients based on a lack of knowledge, lack of equipment, and inadequate compensation of services rendered. Many disabled persons rely on Medicaid and other government-funded sources. Therefore, access to care is a problem for this population.
- The ADHA *Code of Ethics* states that clients should be treated without discrimination. Dental hygienists who are ill-prepared to treat these clients should seek continuing education opportunities and/or refer the client so that quality care can be rendered.
- Close supervision is required of mentally challenged clients when professional care is being provided.

Key Concepts

- ✦ Etiologies of MR are grouped into three categories: prenatal, at birth, and postnatal causes.
- ✦ Level of MR determines if the client is capable of giving informed consent for care. Consultation with the client's physician, social worker, or caregiver is necessary to determine the level of MR.
- ✦ When planning oral hygiene interventions for the severe and profound MR clients, the caregiver should be included. Severely retarded clients can learn by habit training, but need follow-up by the caregiver.
- ✦ Persons with MR may have poor oral health as a result of malnutrition, limited self-care capabilities, economic barriers to care, and limited access to care.
- ✦ Oral manifestations observed in mentally retarded clients often coincide with a specific type of syndrome.
- ✦ Lips of MR clients are sometimes larger than those of the general population, and tooth anomalies such as microdontia and delayed eruption patterns are usually present as a result of developmental abnormalities. Tooth surface attrition from bruxism is often seen as a result of anxiety and/or stress.
- ✦ Prevalence of periodontal disease in the MR population is attributed to lack of professional care, lack of funds to support care, increased susceptibility, and poor oral hygiene.
- ✦ When developing oral hygiene skills in a client with MR, the dental hygienist should teach based on the client's mental age, not chronologic age.
- ✦ Down syndrome is the most common and frequently observed chromosomal abnormality in humans.
- ✦ Congenital heart disease is the most common and serious medical condition in persons with Down syndrome; therefore, the dental hygienist must determine need for prophylactic antibiotic premedication.
- ✦ Individuals with Down syndrome have a high incidence of periodontal disease.
- ✦ Autism is a developmental disorder and disability characterized by a persistent aloneness. The etiology is unknown.
- ✦ Stereotypical body movements such as rocking are characteristic of autism.
- ✦ Many autistic clients take psychotropic medications that cause decreased salivation; therefore, saliva substitutes may be prescribed.
- ✦ Behavior modification is the recommended technique when working with autistic clients.
- ✦ When educating clients with MR, their cognitive and physical limitations and abilities, level of periodontal health and caries risk, level of deposit accumulation, medications, diet, and ability to cooperate should be assessed.
- ✦ When choosing toothbrushes, the handle should be long and brush size should be selected based on the client's ability to open and size of the oral cavity. Powered toothbrushes are excellent for limited fine motor control (see Chapters 18 and 36).
- ✦ Floss holders are recommended to reach posterior areas and protect the fingers from inadvertent or intentional biting (see Chapter 19).
- ✦ When formulating a care plan for MR clients, the dental hygienist must be empathetic and realistic, especially if a caregiver is responsible for the client's daily care.

Critical Thinking Exercises

1. Arrange to visit a sheltered workshop in the community. Invite the workers to receive dental hygiene care in the dental hygiene care facility. After the clients have completed treatment, share the challenges experienced with peers. How were you able to overcome the challenges faced? What strategies were successful? What strategies were unsuccessful?
2. Arrange to visit a school for severely and profoundly retarded persons. Based on your observations and discussions with the teachers there, what would you do to improve the oral health status of the persons at the school? What recommendations would you have for the teachers?
3. Read each of the dental hygiene care plans (Figures 39–2, 39–9, and 39–10). Are other interventions needed to achieve the client goals and therapeutic outcomes? Assuming that the goals are met, what future goals might move these clients to higher levels of oral health and wellness?

For References, Suggested Readings, and Related Websites, visit
http://evolve.elsevier.com/Darby/hygiene/

CHAPTER 40

PERSONS WITH CARDIOVASCULAR DISEASE

OBJECTIVES

Mastery of the content in this chapter will enable the reader to:

- Discuss cardiovascular disease in terms of risk and protective factors, and links to periodontal disease
- Identify signs and symptoms of rheumatic heart disease, infective (bacterial) endocarditis, valvular heart defects, cardiac arrhythmias, hypertension, coronary heart disease, congestive heart failure, and congenital heart disease
- Discuss the oral complications associated with cardiovascular disease
- Develop a dental hygiene diagnosis and care plan for a client with cardiovascular disease
- Determine need for emergency medical care in a client with coronary heart disease

KEY TERMS

Angina pectoris (stable and unstable)
Angioplasty
Atherosclerosis
Atrial-septal defect
Bradycardia
Cardiac dysrhythmias/arrhythmias
Cardiovascular disease (CVD)
Congenital heart disease
Congestive heart failure (CHF)
Coronary heart disease (CHD) (coronary artery or ischemic heart disease)
Heart murmur (organic, inorganic, functional, nonfunctional)
Hypertensive cardiovascular disease (HCD)
Infective (bacterial) endocarditis (IE)
Mitral valve prolapse (MVP)
Myocardial infarction
Patent ductus arteriosus
Rheumatic heart disease (RHD)
Tachycardia
Tetralogy of Fallot
Valvular heart defects (VHDs)
Ventricular septal defect

CARDIOVASCULAR DISEASE

The major structures of the heart and their basic functions are found in Figure 40–1. Normal cardiovascular structure and physiology establish the baseline for a discussion of cardiac pathology.

Cardiovascular disease (CVD) is an alteration of the heart and/or blood vessels that impairs function. Although CVD is the number-one cause of death in developed countries, mortality rates have declined as a result of the increased management of CVD risk factors.[1] Risk factors associated with poor cardiovascular health are displayed in Table 40–1.

A link exists between CVD and periodontal disease. Persons with periodontal disease have a 1.5- to 2.0-fold greater risk of incurring fatal CVD than clients without periodontal disease.[2] It is believed that bacterial byproducts such as lipopolysaccharide increase a client's inflammatory response, which in turn exacerbates the process of atherogensis.[3-5] Some believe that platelet-aggregating bacteria, such as *Porphyromonas gingivalis* and *Streptococcus sanguis*, enter the bloodstream and increase the risk for thrombosis, leading to myocardial infarction and stroke.[3,4,6,7] Changing risk-related behavioral patterns assists in decreasing the risk and prevalence of heart disease in the population (Table 40–1).

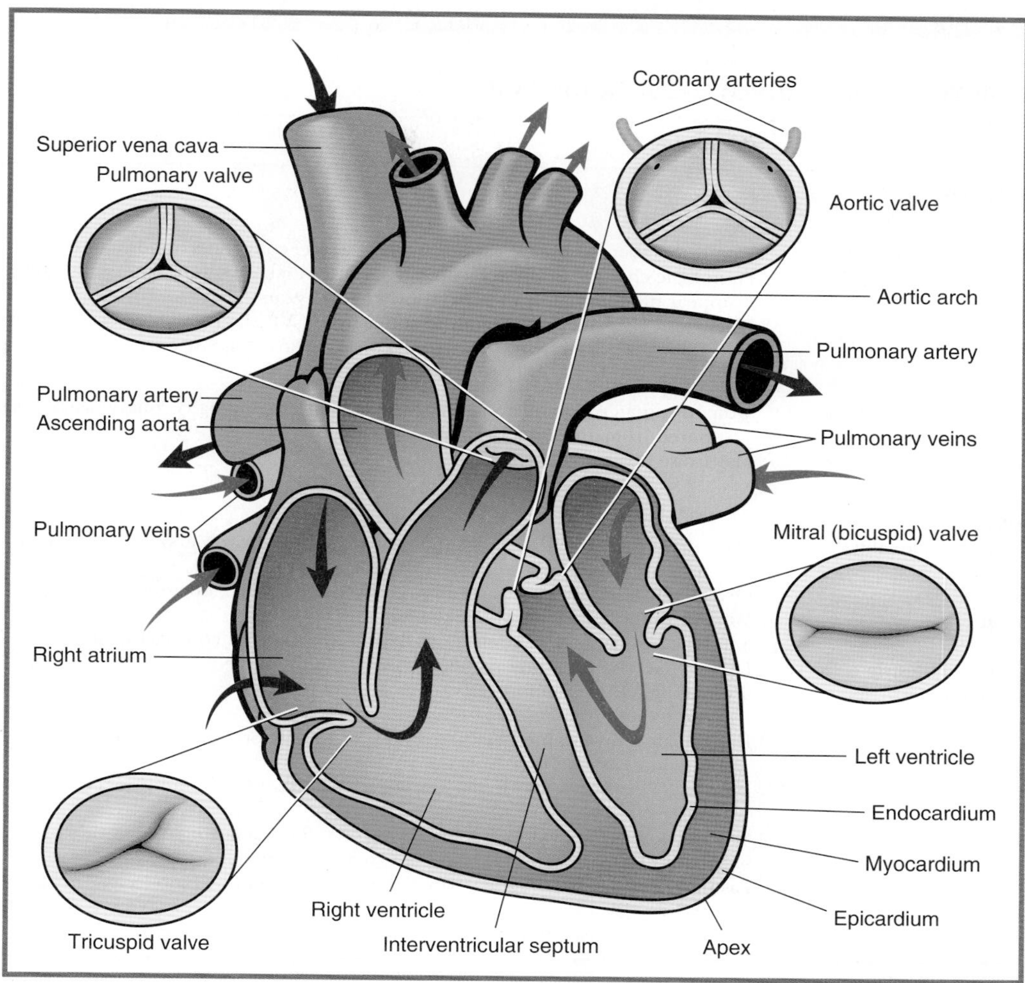

FIGURE 40–1 ✦ Diagram of the heart. *(From Kinn ME, Woods MA, Derge EF:* The medical assistant: Administrative and clinical, *ed 7, Philadelphia, 1993, WB Saunders.)*

Rheumatic Heart Disease

Rheumatic heart disease (RHD) is the cardiac manifestation of rheumatic fever. Persons with a history of rheumatic fever often have valvular heart damage that is detrimentally affected by the assault of microorganisms in the bloodstream, often occurring during dental hygiene care. Persons with a history of rheumatic heart disease are at risk of infective endocarditis (see Chapter 9).

ETIOLOGY. Rheumatic fever is an acute or chronic systemic inflammatory process characterized by attacks of fever, polyarthritis, and carditis. The latter may eventually result in permanent valvular heart damage.

RISK FACTORS. Persons who have suffered a beta-hemolytic streptococcal pharyngeal infection (strep throat) may develop rheumatic fever within 2 to 3 weeks after initial infection. Persons with a history of rheumatic fever are predisposed to rheumatic heart disease because of the involvement of the heart muscles, resulting in cardiac valve damage.

DISEASE PROCESS. The most destructive effect of rheumatic fever is carditis, an inflammation of the cardiac muscle that is found in most individuals exhibiting signs and symptoms of rheumatic fever. Carditis may affect the endocardium, myocardium, pericardium, or heart valves. Valvular damage is responsible for the familiar *organic* or *nonfunctional heart murmur* associated with rheumatic fever or rheumatic heart disease. *(Note that* inorganic *or* functional *heart murmurs are not related to rheumatic heart disease, and clients with this type of murmur do not need to be premedicated).* The *heart murmur* is an irregularity of the auditory heartbeat caused by a turbulent flow of blood through a valve that has failed to close. Valves most commonly affected are the mitral valve and the aortic valve. Damaged valves are susceptible to infection that may lead to infective endocarditis. Severe rheumatic carditis may cause difficulty in breathing, elevation of the diastolic blood pressure, and increasing signs of heart failure (see Basic Types of Heart Murmurs and Dental Implications).

TABLE 40–1 RISK FACTORS FOR CARDIOVASCULAR DISEASE

Factors	Examples
Nonmodifiable Risk Factors	
Personal Factors	
Genetic predisposition/family history	Family members who have cardiovascular disease; congenital abnormality
Age	Pathologic changes within the coronary arteries that are severe enough to cause symptoms appear predominantly in persons over age 40 years
Race	Blacks and Hispanics more likely to suffer from CVD than whites or Pacific Islanders
Gender	Men four times as likely to suffer from coronary heart disease as women up to age 40 years
Disease Patterns	
History of anorexia nervosa or bulimia	Women younger than 40 are at increased risk of developing coronary heart disease if they have suffered from an eating disorder
Past use of fen-phen (fenfluramine and phentermine)	May cause heart valve damage
Modifiable Risk Factors	
Personality traits (type A personality)	Hard-driving, competitive individuals who worry excessively about deadlines and who consistently overwork
Professional stresses	Occupations that impose tremendous responsibility (e.g., doctors, executives)
Oral contraceptive use	Women younger than 40 who take oral contraceptives
Tobacco use	Smoking two packs of cigarettes per day increases risk of coronary heart disease four-fold
Sedentary occupation and lifestyle	Lack of exercise promotes mental depression and obesity
Diet high in calories, cholesterol, fat, and sodium	Overeating and consuming fatty foods promote obesity, lipid abnormalities, and diseases; high-sodium diet promotes hypertension
Hypertension	Individuals with sustained blood pressure of 160/95 or higher double their risk of myocardial infarction
Obesity	Weight 30% or more above that considered standard for an individual of a certain height and build
Lipid abnormalities	Serum cholesterol of higher than 200 mg/100 ml or a fasting triglyceride of higher than 250 mg/100 mL; abnormal level of C-reactive protein
Diabetes mellitus	Fasting blood sugar of higher than 120 mg/dl or a routine blood sugar of 180 mg/dL increases risk
Periodontal disease	Periodontal disease increases risk of fatal cardiovascular disease by 1.5 to 2.0.

BASIC TYPES OF HEART MURMURS AND DENTAL IMPLICATIONS

Type	Abnormal Sound Heard from Heart and Associated Large Blood Vessels	Implications
Organic heart murmur (nonfunctional murmur)	Attributed to cardiac pathology	Require prophylactic antibiotic premedication before invasive dental or dental hygiene care
Inorganic heart murmur (functional murmur)	Occurs in the absence of cardiac pathology	*Does not* require prophylactic antibiotic premedication before invasive dental or dental hygiene care

PREVENTION. RHD prevention requires early diagnosis and treatment of streptococcal pharyngeal infections that may lead to rheumatic fever. Clients need to be informed of the importance of early medical diagnosis and treatment for prevention of this disease.

DENTAL HYGIENE CARE. The client with RHD is susceptible to infectious endocarditis as a result of dental hygiene procedures that cause a transient bacteremia. To protect clients from health risks, the care plan must include recommended prophylactic antibiotic premedication regimens (see Tables 9–5, 9–6, and 9–7 in Chapter 9) and meticulous bacterial plaque control. Oral health stability must be maintained by the client to reduce the possibility of developing a self-inflicted bacteremia that can occur when toothbrushing or interdental cleaning in a mouth with periodontal disease.

APPOINTMENT GUIDELINES (see Table 9–8). When a client is taking the prescribed prophylactic antibiotic regimen, appointment scheduling is affected. It is *not* in the client's best interest to prolong treatment procedures.

If therapeutic scaling and root planing are necessary, appointments should be scheduled in longer periods and as close together as possible. The interval between antibiotic coverage should be 9 to 14 days.[8] If possible, a combination of procedures should be planned within the same appointment. For example, if a client has been classified as case type II periodontal disease, a care plan may divide invasive procedures (therapeutic scaling and root planing) into an organized sequence that allows for 9- to 14-day periods off prophylactic antibiotic premedication. The client's human need for protection from health risks is met by dividing the invasive treatment appointments into two separate intervals with a lag time separating each interval. Sample Dental Hygiene Care Plan for a Client Taking Prophylactic Antibiotic Premedication provides a sample dental hygiene care plan.

Sample Dental Hygiene Care Plan for a Client Taking Prophylactic Antibiotic Premedication

Dental Hygiene Diagnosis

Protection from Health Risks: Potential for developing a resistance to prescribed antibiotic if taken over a period of time

Skin and mucous membrane integrity of the head and neck

Client Goals

Schedule invasive dental hygiene treatment so that appointments are 9–14 days apart

Reduce gingival bleeding by 9/03

Reduce periodontal probing depths by 9/03

Expected Outcomes

Complete chart of periodontal probing depths

Dentition and periodontium free from soft and hard deposits

Root surfaces debrided and tissue healing observed

Bleeding index score reduced by 50%

Periodontal probing depths reduced by at least 1 mm

Dental Hygiene Interventions

Schedule treatment into three appointments

Appointment 1, probe entire mouth, scale and debride maxilla; bacterial plaque biofilm control with toothbrush and interdental cleaning device

Plan for host response time, no treatment (9–14 days)

Appointment 2, evaluate tissue state of maxilla; scale and debride mandible; bacterial plaque biofilm control continued

Plan for host response time, no treatment (9–14 days)

Appointment 3, One month after treatment, evaluate overall outcome

Infective Endocarditis

Infective or bacterial endocarditis (IE) is an infection of the endocardium, heart valves, or cardiac prosthesis resulting from microbial invasion.

ETIOLOGY. IE is caused by the formation of a bacteremia—the presence of microorganisms in the bloodstream. Endocarditis is characterized by the formation of vegetative growths of *Staphylococcus aureus, Staphylococcus epidermidis, Streptococcus viridans,* and, the most prevalent, alpha-hemolytic streptococci on the heart valves or endocardial lining. Although staphylococci and streptococci are found in most cases, yeast, fungi, and viruses also have been identified, hence the term *infective* rather than bacterial. If left untreated, endocarditis is usually fatal, but with proper antibiotic treatment, recovery is possible.

RISK FACTORS. During dental and dental hygiene therapy, a transient bacteremia is produced. Tissue trauma from instrumentation coupled with periodontal disease status determines the severity of infection. Additionally, a client may self-induce a bacteremia as a result of mastication and daily oral hygiene care. Risk factors for IE include clients with rheumatic heart disease, valvular heart defects, prosthetic heart valves, and previous episodes of IE. Table 9–5 in Chapter 9 delineates risk categories associated with cardiovascular diseases.

DISEASE PROCESS. There are two types of IE:

- *Acute bacterial endocarditis (ABE)* is a severe infection with a rapid course of action usually caused by pathogenic microorganisms such as *S. aureus* and *S. epidermidis* that are capable of producing widespread disease.
- *Subacute bacterial endocarditis (SBE)* is a slow-moving infection with nonspecific clinical features. Clients usually exhibit a continuous low-grade fever, marked weakness, fatigue, weight loss, and joint pain. Dental and dental hygiene procedures that involve the manipulation of soft tissue may be responsible for the development of SBE. As endocarditis progresses, the circulating microorganisms attach to the damaged heart valves or other susceptible areas and proliferate in colonies. The result of this invasion includes cardiac failure from continued valvular damage and embolization (vessel obstruction) due to fragmentation of the colonized microorganisms.

PREVENTION. Clients with conditions that increase their susceptibility to IE, such as cardiac abnormalities and prosthetic heart valves, require preventive antibiotic therapy before procedures that produce bacteremias (see Tables 9–5, 9–6, and 9–7 in Chapter 9).[8]

DENTAL HYGIENE CARE. To prevent IE:

- Identify high-risk individuals by accurately reviewing the health history and questioning the client during assessment.
- Ensure that preventive antibiotic coverage is administered 1 hour before dental or dental hygiene procedures that produce bacteremias, so optimal blood

levels are established (see Tables 9–6, 9–7 and 9–8 in Chapter 9).

- Direct the client to use a preprocedural antimicrobial rinse before tissue manipulation.
- Prevent unnecessary trauma during intraoral procedures to reduce the severity of the bacteremia.
- Help the client maintain optimal oral health to reduce oral microorganisms and the presence of disease.

APPOINTMENT GUIDELINES. Same as for Rheumatic Heart Disease.

Valvular Heart Defects

Valvular heart defects (VHDs) result in cardiovascular damage from malfunctioning heart valves such as the mitral valve, the aortic valve, or the tricuspid valve (Figure 40–1). *Mitral valve prolapse (MVP)* is one of the most frequently occurring VHDs. When the left ventricle pumps blood to the aorta, the mitral valve flops backward (prolapses) into the left atrium, resulting in MVP. Other names for MVP are "floppy mitral valve syndrome" and the "click murmur syndrome," referring to the sound the valve makes when it flops backward (Figure 40–2).

ETIOLOGY. VHDs are commonly associated with rheumatic fever but may also be caused by congenital abnormalities or develop after IE.

DISEASE PROCESS. Valvular malfunction can occur by stenosis, an incomplete opening of the valve, or regurgitation, a backflow of blood through the valve because of incomplete closure. When malfunction occurs, the left ventricle hypertrophies to compensate for the increased amount of blood. This, in turn, causes the left atrium to hypertrophy, leading to pulmonary congestion and right ventricular failures. The person ultimately develops congestive heart failure if the condition is left untreated.

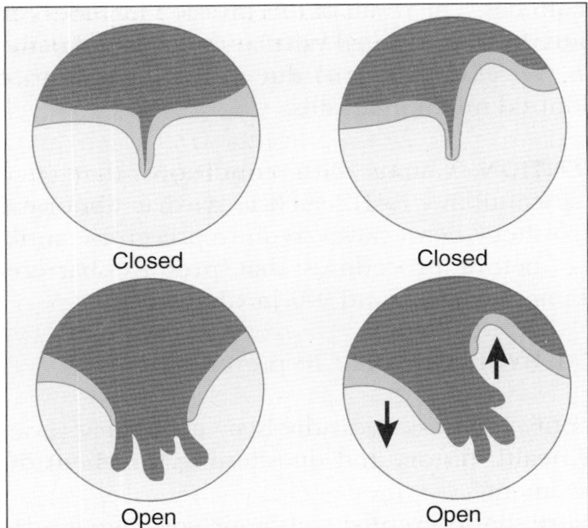

FIGURE 40–2 ✦ Diagram of a normal and a prolapsed mitral valve. *(Courtesy Mid-Island Hospital, Bethpage, NY.)*

An echocardiogram, used by the physician, determines the presence of a valvular heart defect. Ultrasound (sound waves) evaluates the heart size, as well as chamber and valve function, during an echocardiogram.

MEDICAL TREATMENT. Corrective surgery is done for most VHDs. If the valve cannot be repaired, in most cases prosthetic valves are available to replace the defective valves. For clients with MVP, surgical treatment is not always necessary and is aimed at alleviating symptoms such as palpitations, chest pain, nervousness, shortness of breath, and dizziness. Medications are given to control chest pain, slow the heart rate, reduce palpitations, and/or lower anxiety.

DENTAL HYGIENE CARE. Prophylactic antibiotic premedication is needed before care, and consultation with the client's physician is recommended to validate the client's current health status. The client with RHD is susceptible to IE as a result of dental hygiene procedures that cause a transient bacteremia. Care plan considerations to protect the client from health risks include the recommended prophylactic antibiotic premedication regimens (see Tables 9–5, 9–6, and 9–7 in Chapter 9) and a comprehensive daily plaque control program. Oral health stability must be maintained to reduce the possibility of developing a self-inflicted bacteremia that can occur when toothbrushing or interdental cleaning in a diseased mouth.

APPOINTMENT GUIDELINES (see Table 9–8). Prophylactic antibiotic premedication requirements are the same as for a client with RHD. Sample Dental Hygiene Care Plan for a Client Taking Prophylactic Antibiotic Premedication illustrates a sample dental hygiene care plan. VHDs present in the client require no care plan modifications unless the client has an underlying cardiovascular condition or is on anticoagulant drug therapy. The frequently prescribed anticoagulants—heparin, warfarin (Coumadin), and indanedione derivatives—affect the dental hygiene care plan if scaling or root planing procedures are indicated or if the gingiva bleed spontaneously. Consultation with the client's physician is recommended to validate the client's current health and medication status.

When damaged heart valves are replaced by prosthetic valves, the new valves are susceptible to IE and the client must be protected from health risks. Care plan modifications should follow the standard prophylactic antibiotic protocol and regimen listed in Tables 9–5, 9–6, and 9–7 in Chapter 9.

When the client is taking anticoagulant therapy, the client's physician is consulted to determine if a reduction should be made in the dosage of anticoagulant medication or if it is safer for the client to maintain the prescribed dosage. The reduction in medication dosage should increase the prothrombin time by 2 seconds. *Normal prothrombin time varies between 10 and 16 seconds; optimal prothrombin time for dental hygiene therapy in persons taking anticoagulants should be between 20 and 32 seconds on the day of the scheduled procedure.*[9] When treating a client on anticoagulant medication:

- ✦ Consult the client's physician to verify prothrombin time.
- ✦ Scale one area at a time to manage bleeding.
- ✦ Begin in the least inflamed area so that bleeding will be minimal.
- ✦ Periodically check for clotting; discontinue therapy if there is a long delay in clotting.
- ✦ Emphasize the importance of daily oral self-care for the reduction of disease and associated bleeding during professional treatment.

Hypertensive Cardiovascular Disease

Hypertensive cardiovascular disease (HCD) or *hypertension* is a persistent elevation of the systolic and diastolic blood pressures at or above 140 mm Hg and 90 mm Hg, respectively (see Chapter 10). Half of the 60 million hypertensive people in the United States are thought to be undiagnosed. Many diagnosed cases of hypertension are not treated or inadequately treated, leaving the client in an uncontrolled state and at risk for other serious diseases.

ETIOLOGY. Hypertension is not considered a disease but rather a physical finding or symptom. A sustained elevation of the blood pressure affects the heart and leads to HCD, resulting in heart failure, myocardial infarction, cerebrovascular accident (stroke), and kidney failure.

RISK FACTORS. Risk factors for hypertension include family history, race, stress, obesity, a high dietary intake of saturated fats or sodium, use of tobacco or oral contraceptives, fast-paced lifestyle, and age. Hypertension is three times more common in obese persons than in normal-weight persons.[10] There is a higher incidence of hypertension among African-Americans than American whites.

DISEASE PROCESS. Two major types of hypertension include the following:

- ✦ *Primary hypertension*, also known as essential idiopathic hypertension, with etiology unknown, is the most common type; it is characterized by a gradual onset or an abrupt onset of short duration.
- ✦ *Secondary hypertension* is the result of an existing disease, such as those of the cardiovascular system, renal system, adrenal glands, or neurologic system.

Because hypertension usually follows a chronic course, the client may be asymptomatic. Early clinical signs and symptoms are occipital headaches, vision changes, ringing ears, dizziness, and weakness of the hands and feet. As the condition persists, advanced signs and symptoms can include hemorrhages, enlargement of the left ventricle, congestive heart failure, angina pectoris, and renal failure. The dental hygienist refers clients for medical diagnosis if a hypertensive disorder is suspected.

PREVENTION. Early identification of hypertensive clients minimizes the occurrence of medical emergencies, helps meet the client's human need for protection from health risks, and proves life-saving for individuals who are unaware of their condition. Blood pressure measurement during assessment can identify individuals with hypertensive heart disease (see Chapter 10).

MEDICAL TREATMENT. Treatment of hypertension is based on lifestyle changes to reduce risk factors, antihypertensive drug therapy, and/or correction of the underlying medical condition in the case of secondary hypertension. The goal is to reduce and maintain the diastolic pressure level at 90 mm Hg or lower. Some clients need only to watch their dietary consumption of sodium and saturated fats, whereas others must reduce their daily stress level and alter their lifestyle (Table 40–2). When a client needs drug therapy, periodic monitoring is essential. Some drugs may stabilize the condition temporarily and then an elevation can occur, indicating that an alternative drug selection is needed.

Drugs used for hypertension vary in their method of action. Some are diuretics that promote renal excretion of water and sodium ions; others modify sympathetic nerve activity and are called *sympatholytic agents;* others are vasodilators that increase blood vessel size and facilitate blood flow. Clients receiving hypertensive drug therapy may experience fatigue, gastrointestinal disturbances, nausea, diarrhea, cramps, xerostomia, orthostatic hypotension with dizziness, and/or depression (Table 40–3).

DENTAL HYGIENE CARE. Care for the hypertensive individual is planned according to the client's actual or potential unmet human need. If the individual's hypertension is uncontrolled, treatment procedures are postponed until the disorder is regulated. If the client is being treated with antihypertensive agents and if clinical blood pressure evaluations are within normal limits, care can continue; however, stress and anxiety reduction strategies and local anesthetic drug modification are implemented to reduce the potential for medical emergencies. Drug considerations for the use of local anesthetics in clients with hypertensive heart disease are based on the avoidance of vasopressors (such as epinephrine), which are in some local anesthetic agents to constrict blood vessels, concentrate the anesthetic in the desired area, and prevent its dissipation. A side effect of vasopressors is an elevation in blood pressure. In the normal person, a slight elevation in blood pressure is harmless; however, with vasopressors, hypertensive individuals are at increased risk of cerebrovascular accident, myocardial infarction, and congestive heart failure. *Therefore, anesthetic agents that contain vasopressors are contraindicated in clients with a history of hypertension* (see Chapter 34 on Local Anesthesia).

TABLE 40–2 ALTERNATIVE FOOD CHOICES BASED ON THE CHOLESTEROL–SATURATED FAT INDEX (CSI) FOR CLIENTS AT RISK FOR CORONARY HEART DISEASE

		Choices/Alternatives (Scale 1–4) 1 = Best Choice, 4 = Worst Choice			
Food Item	**Avoidances**	**1**	**2**	**3**	**4**
Meats			Poultry	Lean beef	Fatty beef
Fish		Snapper Perch, sole	Salmon	Shellfish	
Poultry		Chicken (no skin)	Turkey (no skin)		
Beef		10% fat ground sirloin Flank steak	15% fat ground round	20% fat ground chuck Pot roast	30% fat ground beef
Pork					Pork
Lamb					Lamb steaks, chops Roasts
Eggs		Egg whites	Egg substitutes	Whole egg	
Fats	Coconut oil, palm oil Cocoa butter	Vegetable oil	Soft margarine	Soft shortening	Butter
Cheeses		Pot cheese Low-fat cottage cheese	Cottage cheese	Part-skim mozzarella	Cheese spreads
Frozen desserts	Ice cream	Water ice Sorbet	Sherbet Frozen yogurt	Ice milk	Ice cream

TABLE 40–3 COMMONLY PRESCRIBED CARDIOVASCULAR MEDICATION

Brand Name	Generic Name	Indications for Use	Oral Implications
Glycosides			
Lanoxin	Digoxin	CHF, atrial fibrillation	Excessive salivation, sensitive gag reflex
Diuretics			
Dyazide	Triamterene	CHF, hypertension	Decreased salivary flow
Maxzide	Hydrochlorothiazide		
Lasix	Furosemide		
Beta-Blockers			
Tenormin	Atenolol	Hypertension, angina	Xerostomia
Inderal	Propranolol		
Lopressor	Metoprolol		
Calcium Channel Blockers			
Cardizem	Diltiazem	Hypertension, angina	Decreased salivary flow, gingival enlargement
Procardia	Nifedipine		
Calan	Verapamil		
ACE (Angiotensin Converting Enzyme) Inhibitors			
Capoten	Captopril	Hypertension	Xerostomia, taste impairment, oral ulceration
Vasotec	Enalapril		
Vasodilators			
Nitroglycerin	Nitroglycerin	Angina	Burning under tongue

APPOINTMENT GUIDELINES (see Table 9–8). Care plan considerations for the individual with controlled hypertension focus on stress and anxiety reduction strategies (see Chapter 32) and local anesthetic drug modification to reduce the potential for medical emergencies (as discussed in previous section). Cases of Clients with Various Hypertensive Conditions and Appropriate Dental Hygiene Actions displays four situations based on initial blood pressure measurement and family history information. Each situation demonstrates the appropriate dental hygiene care modification necessary to meet a specific human need.

Coronary Heart Disease

Coronary heart disease (CHD), also known as *coronary artery disease* and *ischemic heart disease,* is the result of insufficient blood flow from the coronary arteries into the heart or myocardium. Disorders associated with this con-

Cases of Clients with Various Hypertensive Conditions and Appropriate Dental Hygiene Actions

No History of Hypertension, Elevated Blood Pressure
During assessment, client reports no history or symptoms of hypertension; however, a blood pressure reading of 160/100 mm Hg was obtained. One dental hygiene diagnosis may be an unmet need for protection from health risks caused by a potential for heart attack or stroke as evidenced by an elevated blood pressure of 160/100 mm Hg. The dental hygiene care plan may include repeated blood pressure measurements during the assessment phase, approximately 10 minutes apart. If, after repeated measurements, the diastolic pressure is still above 100 mm Hg, the appointment should be limited to assessment and planning; no treatment should be implemented. The client must be referred to the physician of record for medical consultation and diagnosis. After medical evaluations have been completed, if the client is classified as nonhypertensive, it can be inferred that anxiety concerning dental hygiene care was the reason for the elevated blood pressure. Blood pressure must be monitored at each appointment thereafter and strategies implemented to minimize stress.

Client Under Treatment for Hypertension
During assessment, client indicates that he is hypertensive and under the care of a physician. The hygienist must obtain information on the client's medications and verify at each visit that the prescribed medication has been taken. Client may have an unmet need for freedom from stress. To meet this need, the care plan may include the administration of nitrous oxide–oxygen analgesia to reduce client anxiety. The client's blood pressure should be monitored at each visit and periodically recorded throughout the appointment.

Client Noncompliant with Hypertension Treatment
Client indicates that she is hypertensive and has discontinued her recommended medical treatment program. Rather, she takes the medication irregularly based on her symptoms. This client has uncontrolled hypertension and a need for protection from health risks. Dental hygiene care is stopped after assessment until her hypertension is stabilized. Client should be referred to her physician for further medical evaluation and treatment. Although care for client is postponed, remaining appointment time can facilitate the client's need for protection from health risks via educational strategies directed toward the importance of controlling hypertension and possible lethal effects if left uncontrolled. The client's blood pressure is monitored and periodically recorded throughout the appointment.

Client with Hypertension and Acute Symptoms
During assessment, client demonstrates hypertension with diastolic readings above 110 mm Hg and symptoms (e.g., headache, dizziness, restlessness, decreased level of consciousness, blurred vision, palpitations) indicative of HCD. To meet the client's need for protection from health risks, client should be directed to his physician for immediate medical consultation and evaluation. Dental hygiene care should be delayed until the HCD is under control. Because hypertension can be related to anxiety and stress, the dental hygienist must determine if client needs stress control and, if affirmative, reduce the apprehension associated with therapy. Some stress control strategies may include encouraging client to express fears and concerns, encouraging client participation in goal setting and care plan development, explaining procedures completely, obtaining informed consent, demonstrating humanistic behaviors, and discussing apprehensions directly.

dition are arteriosclerotic heart disease, angina pectoris, coronary insufficiency, and myocardial infarction.

ETIOLOGY. The major cause of CHD is *atherosclerosis*, a narrowing of the lumen of the coronary arteries, thereby reducing the volume of blood flow. Narrowing of the lumen is accomplished by the deposition of fibro-fatty substances containing lipids and cholesterol. Deposits thicken with time and eventually close the vessel (Figure 40–3). Atherosclerosis usually develops in high-flow, high-pressure arteries and has been linked to many risk factors. Other causes of CHD are congenital abnormalities of the arteries, changes in the arteries due to infection, vascular changes from autoimmune disorders, and coronary embolism (blood clot).

RISK FACTORS. CHD is influenced by age, gender, race, diet, lifestyle, and environment. Individuals who are obese, anorexic, bulimic, limit their amount of physical exercise, or smoke increase their risk of developing CHD. Additional predisposing factors can be found in Table 40–1.

- ✦ Age is associated with CHD after age 40. Pathologic changes in the arteries are noticeable with age, usually producing symptoms of disease.
- ✦ Gender increases the risk of developing CHD, demonstrating that men are four times as likely to suffer from the disease as are women up to age 40; however, after age 40 years the prevalence of CHD among women and men is the same. Women younger than 40 years are at an increased risk of developing CHD if they are taking oral contraceptives or have a history of anorexia nervosa or bulimia.
- ✦ Race may be associated with the development of CHD. White men and nonwhite women are at a higher risk for the disease than nonwhite men and white women. Researchers are trying to determine which genetic factors are involved; however, a familial connection between the disease and family members is suspected.

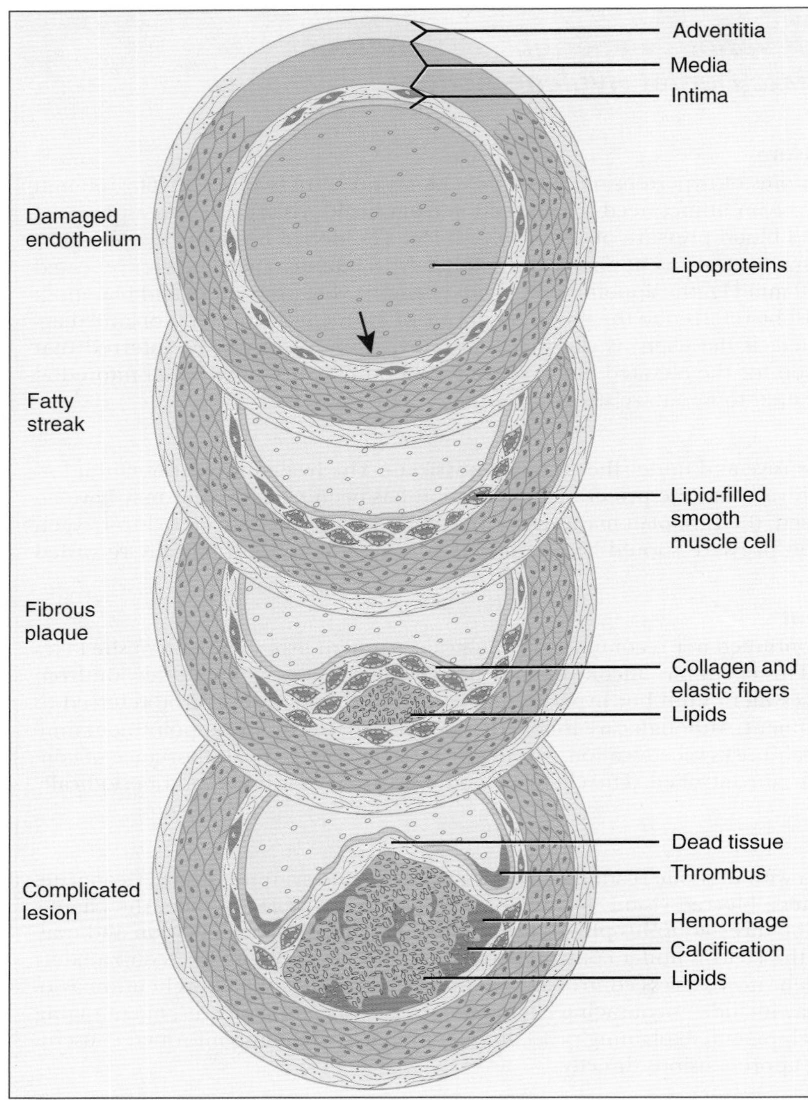

FIGURE 40–3 ✦ Types of atherosclerotic lesions. *(From Debakey M, Grotto A:* The living heart, *New York, 1977, David McKay.)*

- Populations consuming a low-cholesterol, low-fat diet have little CHD, whereas populations whose diet consists of foods rich in cholesterol and saturated fat have a very high rate of CHD.
- Social and economic environments contribute to an individual's chance of developing CHD. The disease is seven times more prevalent in North America than in South America, and urban populations are at a higher risk than rural dwellers. Cigarette smoking and stressful job situations increase an individual's chance of developing CHD at an early age.
- Research also supports a relationship between periodontal disease and CHD. The exact relationship is unclear but points to a link between host response and bacteremia from chronic periodontal disease.

DISEASE PROCESS. Three basic manifestations of CHD are angina pectoris, myocardial infarction, and sudden death.

Angina Pectoris. *Angina pectoris* is the direct result of inadequate oxygen flow to the myocardium, manifested clinically as a burning, squeezing, or crushing tightness in the chest that radiates to the left arm, neck, and shoulder blade. The person typically clenches his fist over his chest or rubs his left arm when describing the pain. When sudden attacks of angina pectoris follow physical exertion, emotional excitement, or exposure to cold, and the symptoms are relieved by administration of nitroglycerin, they are classified as *stable angina.* Conversely, *unstable angina* may occur at rest or during sleep, and pain is of longer duration and not relieved readily with nitroglycerin.

Medical treatment for angina pectoris has two goals: (1) reduce myocardial oxygen demand and (2) increase oxygen supply. The method of therapy consists primarily of physical rest to decrease oxygen demand and the administration of nitrates, such as nitroglycerin, to provide more oxygen.

Nitroglycerin (glyceryl trinitrate), a vasodilator, increases blood flow (oxygen supply) by expanding the arteries. Administration can be sublingual for immediate absorption or by nitroglycerin pads and patches for time-released medication absorbed by the skin and incorporated into the bloodstream. Obstructive lesions that do not respond to drug therapy may need surgery.

Myocardial Infarction. *Myocardial infarction,* the second manifestation of CHD, is a reduction of blood flow through one of the coronary arteries, resulting in an infarct. An infarct is an area of tissue that undergoes necrosis because of the elimination of blood flow. A myocardial infarction is also known as a heart attack, coronary occlusion, and coronary thrombosis.

Symptoms associated with a myocardial infarction are similar to those experienced with angina pectoris; however, the pain usually persists for 12 or more hours and begins as a feeling of indigestion. Other manifestations include a feeling of fatigue, nausea, vomiting, and shortness of breath.

Treatment includes combination therapy to reduce cardiac workloads and increase cardiac output. Cardiac workload reduction therapies include bedrest, morphine for pain reduction and sedation, and oxygen if necessary. To increase cardiac output, therapy associated with the control and reduction of cardiac dysrhythmias is recommended. Medical treatment may include antiarrhythmic drugs and possibly a cardiac pacemaker. Nitroglycerin is indicated to relieve chest pain and increase cardiac output by intensifying the blood flow and redistributing blood to the affected myocardial tissue. Anticoagulants may be used to thin the blood in an effort to increase blood flow and reduce the possibility of another myocardial infarction.

Sudden Death. Sudden death, the last manifestation of CHD, occurs during the first 24 to 48 hours after the onset of symptoms. Most sudden cardiovascular deaths are caused by ventricular fibrillation. For example, ventricular fibrillation results in ventricular standstill (cardiac arrest) if insufficient blood is pumped into the coronary arteries to supply the myocardium with oxygen. Biologic death results when oxygen delivery to the brain is inadequate for 4 to 6 minutes. Therefore, CPR must be administered to maintain enough blood oxygen to sustain life. Transportation to the hospital for emergency medical care is necessary.

PREVENTION. Seven lifestyle behaviors are associated with the prevention of CHD:

1. Regular checkups
2. Prudent diet
3. Regular exercise
4. Avoidance of stress
5. Avoidance of tobacco
6. Controlling high blood pressure
7. Prevention of periodontal disease

Knowledge of the warning signs of a heart attack is also associated with preventing CHD. These behaviors practiced consistently can reduce the risk of CHD.

A reduction of saturated fat and cholesterol in the diet, recommended by the American Heart Association, has gained public attention. Many people are making food choices based on this recommendation. Major food companies are introducing foods that are low in cholesterol and saturated fats, and restaurants are expanding their menu options for diet-conscious patrons.

Food choices to control dental diseases and improve oral health are part of comprehensive dental hygiene care. Factors associated with CHD must be taken into consideration when providing nutritional counseling to a client. In facilitating the client's human need for protection from health risks, the dental hygienist recognizes the importance of dietary choices related to coronary heart disease and incorporates that knowledge into the nutritional education session. Table 40–2 lists food choices and avoidances for the client at risk for coronary heart disease.

In response to the evidence that periodontal disease is a risk factor for coronary heart disease, clients will have a need to grasp this relationship and make sound decisions about their oral health. Therefore, educational sessions should emphasize the link between oral disease and systemic disease. By stressing the importance of oral disease prevention, the dental hygienist will be able to promote active self-care by the client. Interventions to assist the client in achieving success include teaching self-care behaviors to maintain oral wellness, encouraging active participation in formulating goals for dental hygiene care, and facilitating choices and decision making by the client.

DENTAL HYGIENE CARE. The client with coronary heart disease is susceptible to angina pectoris and myocardial infarctions.

Angina Pectoris. The client with angina pectoris should be treated in a stress-free environment to meet the client's human need for protection from health risks and freedom from stress. Considerations associated with angina pectoris include identification of the client's condition and frequency of angina attacks. Suggested health history–related questions to ascertain the stability of the client's angina condition include the following:

1. Do you have pain in your chest on exertion?
2. Do you have pain in your chest at rest?
3. How frequent are your attacks?
4. Is the pain in your chest relieved promptly with nitroglycerin?
5. How long are your periods of discomfort?

If the client reports that his or her angina condition has gradually worsened and that the painful episodes occur more frequently and not only during exertion, then the client's condition is classified as unstable angina. These clients should be referred to their physician of record, and dental hygiene care should be postponed.

For clients with stable angina, appointments should be short and preferably scheduled for the morning. The atmosphere should be friendly and conducive to relaxation. If the client becomes fatigued or develops significant changes in pulse rate or rhythm, termination of the appointment is suggested.

Before initiating care for a client with a history of angina pectoris, the client's supply of nitroglycerin should be placed within reach of the dental hygienist. Potency of nitroglycerin is lost after 6 months outside of a sealed container; consequently, fresh supplies should be available in the oral care environment. If an emergency develops, dental hygiene treatment should be stopped and the client placed in an upright position. The client should be reassured and given nitroglycerin sublingually. The emergency medical service (EMS) should be activated if the client continues to experience pain after the administration of nitroglycerin. Vital signs must be monitored and the results recorded on the client's record.

Myocardial Infarction. Clients who have a history of myocardial infarction do not require a change in care plan procedures unless the myocardial infarction has occurred within 6 months of the appointment. In this case dental hygiene therapy should be postponed until the individual is 6 months or more post-infarction with no complications. The client's medical status should be confirmed with the cardiologist of record during the assessment phase of care.

The drugs used to treat myocardial infarctions are anticoagulants, digitalis, and antihypertensive agents. These drugs necessitate care plan alterations. Anticoagulant drugs increase bleeding time and may have to be stopped several days before dental hygiene or surgical treatment that involves tissue manipulation. Some cardiologists believe that it is more dangerous to take the individual off the anticoagulant than it is to keep the individual on the drug and provide care; therefore, confirmation from the client's cardiologist is recommended.

Digitalis is a drug that increases the contractility of the heart. The improvement in force makes the heart more efficient as a pump, increasing its volume in relation to cardiac output. This type of drug, botanical in origin, is classified as a glycoside. The most commonly prescribed digitalis drug is digoxin (Lanoxin).

Oral health professionals may detect early signs of digitalis toxicity in clients that include anorexia, nausea, vomiting, increased salivation, and lower facial pain resembling the type associated with trigeminal neuralgia.[11] If digitalis toxicity is not detected early, cardiac irregularities can develop. These irregularities include arrhythmias that can progress to ventricular fibrillation and sudden death.

Antihypertensive agents used to control myocardial infarctions are similar to those used to control hypertension. These agents do not influence the care plan unless the underlying condition is uncontrolled.

Clients with coronary heart disease may experience fear, depression, and disturbances in body image, associated with a change in lifestyle (e.g., dietary restrictions, exercise, and maintaining low stress). The dental hygienist needs to be aware of the client's psychological condition influencing human needs to motivate a change in oral health.

Emergency situations associated with myocardial infarction should be managed by an emergency medical team. Oral health professionals are responsible for monitoring vital signs, administering nitroglycerin, and performing cardiopulmonary resuscitation (CPR) if the client experiences cardiac arrest. Certification in basic life support (BLS) should be maintained by all oral health professionals (see Chapter 7).

APPOINTMENT GUIDELINES. For an individual with CHD:

- ✦ Clarify the stability of the client's angina. If uncontrolled, do not treat. If stable, continue treatment with caution.
- ✦ Schedule short morning appointments to help control environmental stress.
- ✦ Use nitrous oxide–oxygen analgesia to reduce stress if no contraindications to the drug exist.
- ✦ Select interventions designed to address the client's need regarding lifestyle changes and periodontal disease status.

Cardiac Dysrhythmias/Arrhythmias

Cardiac dysrhythmias/arrhythmias are dysfunctions of the heart rate and rhythm that manifest themselves as heart palpitations. The terms *dysrhythmia* and *arrhythmia* are used interchangeably. Dysrhythmias may develop in both normal and diseased hearts. In healthy hearts the arrhythmia may be associated with physical and emotional stresses (e.g., exercise, emotional shock). These arrhythmias usually subside in direct response to stimulus reduction. Diseased hearts develop dysrhythmias directly associated with the cardiovascular disease present, most commonly rheumatic heart disease, arteriosclerotic heart disease, and coronary artery heart disease. In some cases, a cardiac dysrhythmia may develop in response to drug toxicities and electrolyte imbalances.

ETIOLOGY. Dysfunction of heart rate and rhythm arises from disturbances in nerve impulse formation or nerve impulse conduction and is categorized according to the part of the heart in which it originates. Common dysrhythmias include bradycardia, tachycardia, atrial fibrillation, premature ventricular contractions (PVCs), ventricular fibrillation, and heart block.

All cardiac dysrhythmias are medically diagnosed using an electrocardiogram (ECG) and/or a Holter monitoring system. The ECG is a graphic tracing of the heart's electrical activity. It can determine the heart rate, rhythm, and size. Each dysrhythmia is associated with a specific graphic pattern indicating a definitive medical diagnosis.

RISK FACTORS. See Table 40–1.

DISEASE PROCESS

Bradycardia. *Bradycardia* is defined as slowness of the heartbeat, as evidenced by a decline in the pulse rate to less than 60 beats per minute. Naturally this occurs during sleeping; however, severe bradycardia can lead to fainting and convulsions. If a client presents with an episode of bradycardia following a normal pulse rate of 80 beats per minute, emergency medical treatment is necessary. This individual may be encountering the initial symptoms of an acute myocardial infarction (heart attack). Emergency medical treatment would include discontinuance of the dental hygiene appointment, administration of oxygen, and activation of the EMS.

Tachycardia. Increased heartbeat is termed *tachycardia.* This arrhythmia is associated with an abnormally high heart rate, usually above 150 beats per minute. Tachycardia can increase the individual's chance of developing angina pectoris, acute heart failure, pulmonary edema, and myocardial infarction if not controlled. These diseases are directly related to the amount of work the heart is doing and its decreased cardiac output. Treatment consists of antiarrhythmic drug therapy to control tachycardia and reduce the potential of recurrence.

Atrial Fibrillation. Atrial fibrillation, a condition of rapid, uneven contractions in the upper chambers of the heart (atrium), causes an irregularity in ventricular beats. Atrial fibrillation is the result of inconsistent impulses through the atrioventricular (AV) node transmitted to the ventricles at irregular intervals. The lower chambers (ventricles) cannot contract in response to the impulses, the contractions become irregular, and this results in a decreased amount of blood pumped through the body. During assessment, the pulse rate may appear consistent, with periods of irregular beats. Medical treatment is focused on the causative factors, not on the condition itself. Congestive heart failure, mitral valve stenosis, and hyperthyroidism may be linked to atrial fibrillation.

Premature Ventricular Contractions (PVCs). PVCs are easily identified as pauses in an otherwise normal heart rhythm. The pause develops from an abnormal focus of the ventricle, allowing the ventricle to be at a refractory (resting) period when the impulse for contraction arrives. The feeling of the heart skipping a beat is PVC; these increase with age and are associated with fatigue, emotional stress, and excessive use of coffee, alcohol, or tobacco.

Recognition of PVCs has significance in the client with cardiovascular disease. *If five or more PVCs are detected during a 60-second pulse examination, medical consultation is strongly recommended.* Individuals who are distressed and who have five or more detectable PVCs per minute may be undergoing an acute myocardial infarction or ventricular fibrillation. To protect the client from health risks, the following actions are taken:

1. Terminate dental hygiene care.
2. Place client on oxygen.
3. Activate EMS.

Ventricular Fibrillation. Ventricular fibrillation, one of the most lethal dysrhythmias, is characterized as an advanced stage of ventricular tachycardia with rapid impulse formation and irregular impulse transmission. The heart rate is rapid and disordered, and contains no rhythm. The immediate medical treatment for ventricular fibrillation is precordial shock or use of electric current to halt the dysrhythmia. The electric current depolarizes the entire myocardium at the time of shock, allowing the cardiac impulses to gain control of the heart rate and rhythm. This should reestablish cardiac regulation. Following precordial shock, the person is placed on drug therapy to maintain regulation of the cardiac rate and rhythm. *Without immediate medical attention (advanced cardiac life support), blood pressure will fall to zero, resulting in unconsciousness; death may occur within 4 minutes.*

Heart Block. Heart block is a dysrhythmia caused by the blocking of impulses from the atria to the ventricles at the AV node. It is an interference with the electrical impulses controlling the heart muscle. There are three forms of heart block. Each form is dangerous; however, third-degree heart block presents the greatest danger, that of cardiac arrest.

- *First-degree heart block* is usually associated with coronary artery disease or digitalis drug therapy. The individual usually is asymptomatic with a normal heart rate and rhythm.
- In *second-degree heart block,* the atrial and ventricular rates are disordered. Impulses from the AV node are fully blocked in irregular patterns.
- *Third-degree heart block* is the blocking of all impulses from the atria at the AV node, resulting in atrial and ventricular dissociation. The ventricles begin beating in response to their biologic pacemaker cells, producing an independent heartbeat from the atrium.

MEDICAL TREATMENT. The cardiac pacemaker, an intracardiac device, is an electronic stimulator used to send electrical currents to the myocardium to control or maintain the heart rate. The pacemaker may be designed to control one or both of the heart chambers. There are two types of pacemakers:

1. *Temporary pacemaker* is used in emergency situations to correct ventricular standstill or arrhythmias that are not responding to other forms of treatment.
2. *Permanent pacemaker* is inserted into the body, and electrodes are transvenously placed in the endocardium and used for 5 to 10 years before battery replacement is necessary. Two general methods of cardiac pacing

for the permanent pacemaker are fixed-rate pacing and demand or standby pacing.

- *Fixed-rate pacing* systems are based on a preset or fixed impulse.
- *Demand* or *standby pacing* systems operate only when needed to stimulate ventricular contraction. These systems contain mechanisms that sense when the client has an independent heartbeat and stimulates the heart only when the rate deviates from normal. This pacing system is most commonly used and is replacing the fixed-rate pacing system because of its increased sensitivity to the body's natural metabolic requirements.

Pacemakers vary in their sensitivity to electrical interferences that may alter or cease their function. Newer models are bipolar and have a special shield to protect against interference and *do not* require any special consideration during dental hygiene care. The older unipolar pacemaker models are less protected from electrical interference and can be negatively affected by mechanized dental instruments and equipment. When in doubt, the dental hygienist should consult with the client's cardiologist.

DENTAL HYGIENE CARE. During assessment, the dental hygienist determines the type of pacemaker a client has and whether it is shielded from electrical interference. Dental devices that apply an electrical current directly to the client are most likely to cause interference in unshielded pacemakers (e.g., ultrasonic scaling systems, electrodesensitizing equipment, pulp testers, powered toothbrushes, and electrosurgery equipment). Care must be modified with respect to these devices because the use of such equipment, even in proximity of the client, is contraindicated with unshielded pacemakers. Care plans should incorporate nonelectrical procedure alternatives to reduce the possibility of functional interference (e.g., hand instrumentation, tooth desensitization with a nonelectronic apparatus, and pulp testing performed by tooth percussion). Additional protection of the pacemaker can be accomplished by placing a lead apron on the client to interrupt electrical interferences generated by standard dental equipment such as the air-abrasive system, slow- or high-speed hand piece, and computerized periodontal probe. Care should be taken in an open clinical setting where electrical dental equipment may be used for an adjacent client. Coordination between clinicians must take place if a client has an unshielded pacemaker.

Moreover, the physician of record is contacted to verify clients' needs for prophylactic antibiotic premedication before dental hygiene care. Premedication is usually recommended for the first 6 months following the implantation of the pacemaker. Care plans should denote a standard prophylactic antibiotic regimen when necessary to prevent IE.

Care plan development for the individual with a cardiac pacemaker also can be affected by the drugs used to treat the client's underlying medical condition—anticoagulants and antihypertensive agents. The monitoring and assessment of drug therapy provide information necessary to modify treatment.

If the cardiac pacemaker fails or malfunctions during the dental hygiene appointment, the client may experience difficulty breathing; dizziness; a change in the pulse rate; swelling of the legs, ankles, arms, and wrists; and/or chest pain. When this situation arises:

1. Turn off all sources of interference.
2. Activate the EMS.
3. Prepare to administer BLS (see Chapter 7, Procedure 7–1).

APPOINTMENT GUIDELINES. Individuals wearing cardiac pacemakers may be susceptible to IE, and the unshielded pacemaker can be affected by electrical interference in the oral healthcare setting. Some care planning considerations follow:

- If necessary, recommend prophylactic antibiotic premedication before dental hygiene care to reduce the possibility of IE (see Chapter 9).
- Use a lead apron to interrupt electrical interferences generated by standard dental equipment.
- Use manual rather than mechanized procedures to reduce the possibility of interference created by dental equipment such as ultrasonic scalers and electronic pulp testers.
- Monitor the client for signs of interference and be prepared to administer BLS (see Chapter 7).

Congestive Heart Failure

Congestive heart failure (CHF) is a syndrome characterized by myocardial dysfunction that leads to diminished cardiac output or abnormal circulatory congestion. The weakened heart develops compensatory mechanisms to continue to function (i.e., tachycardia, ventricular dilation, and enlargement of the heart muscle).

CHF can occur as two independent failures, termed left-sided and right-sided heart failure; however, because the heart functions as a closed unit, both pumps need to be functioning properly or the heart's efficiency is diminished.

ETIOLOGY. Causative factors associated with CHF are arteriosclerotic heart disease, hypertensive cardiovascular disease, valvular heart disease, pericarditis, circulatory overload, and coronary heart disease. These factors contribute to the gradual failure of the heart by reducing the inflow of blood to the heart, increasing the inflow to the heart, obstructing the outflow of blood from the heart, or damaging the heart muscle itself.

RISK FACTORS. See Table 40–1.

DISEASE PROCESS. Clients who have left-sided heart failure have difficulty receiving oxygenated blood from the lungs. The result is an increase of fluid and blood in the lungs, causing dyspnea on exertion, shortness of breath on lying supine, cough, and expectoration. These clients tend to require extra pillows to sleep and cannot be placed in a supine position.

Right-sided heart failure is associated with the blood return from the body, resulting in systemic venous congestion and peripheral edema. Clients with right-sided heart failure have edema in the feet and ankles and often complain of cold hands and feet.

MEDICAL TREATMENT. Medical treatment of CHF is directly related to the removal of the cause. Usually the corrective therapy associated with the underlying disease eliminates the presence of CHF. Some cases require additional methods of rehabilitation, such as dietary control, reduced physical activity, and drug therapy. Drugs most frequently used for the control of CHF include diuretics to reduce the retention of salt and water and digitalis to strengthen myocardial contractility.

DENTAL HYGIENE CARE. Individuals with CHF who are closely monitored by a physician do not require a change in conventional dental hygiene care; however, factors associated with the cause of CHF should be considered in the care plan. Alterations are based on the causative factors (e.g., hypertension, valvular heart disease, congenital heart disease, and myocardial infarction) in association with the individual's current medical status.

Clients taking digitalis are prone to develop nausea and vomiting during dental procedures. Therefore, procedures that may promote gagging should be performed with extra care. In addition, the dental hygienist should be aware of any underlying heart conditions that are responsible for the CHF. These conditions must be evaluated and appropriate precautions taken.

Alterations in the care plan for a client with left-sided CHF are related to the human needs for protection from health risks and for freedom from stress. Client–operator positioning needs to be adjusted to an upright position that supports breathing. Care should be taken to observe clinical symptoms of distress, and educational sessions should reinforce the need for a reduced-sodium diet to alleviate fluid retention.

If an emergency arises with a client who has CHF, medical assistance should be obtained. The client is usually conscious and demonstrating difficulty breathing. The mode of treatment is to:

1. Position the person upright to facilitate breathing.
2. Administer oxygen if necessary.
3. Monitor vital signs.

APPOINTMENT GUIDELINES. When treating clients with CHF:

- ✦ Position the client in an upright position to decrease collection of fluid in the lungs.
- ✦ Limit use of ultrasonic instrumentation so that unnecessary fluid does not back up in the oral cavity. This will minimize client anxiety and facilitate breathing.

Interventions that include nutritional counseling should decrease the amount of sodium intake and fluid retention.

Congenital Heart Disease

Congenital heart disease affects approximately 1% of live births and constitutes 3% of all cases of heart disease after infancy.[9] Commonly observed congenital heart malformations are the ventricular septal defect, the atrial septal defect, and the patent ductus arteriosus.

ETIOLOGY. The etiology of congenital heart disease is generally unknown; however, genetic and environmental factors have been attributed to poor intrauterine development. Genetic conditions are related to heredity and are apparent in some situations. The environmental factors are based on the health of the mother. Rubella (German measles) and drug addiction have produced delayed fetal development and growth retardation associated with the cardiovascular structure.

RISK FACTORS. See Table 40–1.

DISEASE PROCESS AND MEDICAL TREATMENT. Congenital heart disease is the result of various heart defects that dictate the disease process:

Ventricular Septal Defects. A *ventricular septal defect*—a shunt (opening) in the septum between the ventricles—allows the oxygenated blood from the left ventricle to flow into the right ventricle (Figure 40–4). Small defects that close spontaneously or are correctable by surgery have a good prognosis. Larger defects that are left untreated or are irreparable usually result in death from secondary cardiovascular complications. The ventricular septal defect can be detected by a characteristic heart murmur audible at birth.

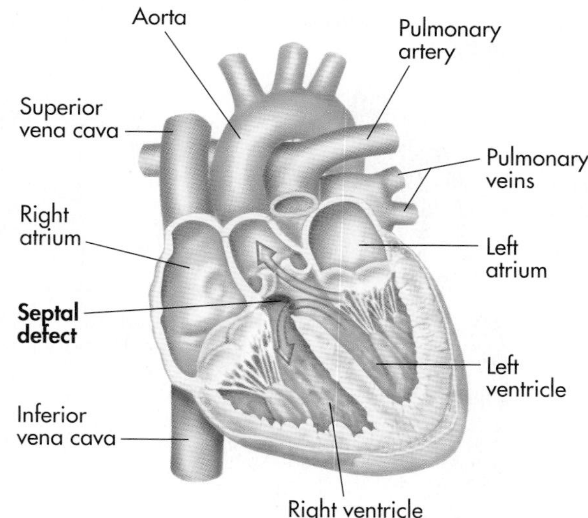

FIGURE 40–4 ✦ Ventricular septal defect. *(From Bleck E, Nagel D: Physically handicapped children: A medical atlas for teachers, ed 2, Needham Heights, Mass, 1982, Allyn & Bacon.)*

Clinical manifestations vary with the size of the defect, infant age, and the effect of the deviated blood passage on the cardiovascular structure. Large ventricular septal defects cause hypertrophy of the ventricles, resulting in congestive heart failure.

Atrial-Septal Defect. The *atrial-septal defect,* a shunt (opening) between the left and right atria, is responsible for approximately 10% of congenital heart defects. The blood volume overload eventually causes the right atrium to enlarge and the right ventricle to dilate (Figure 40–5).

Clinical manifestations are few. Usually, the client is asymptomatic and the defect goes undetected; however, in adults, clinical symptoms become more pronounced. The client is easily fatigued and becomes short of breath after mild exertion. Treatment includes cardiovascular repair surgery, observance of developing atrial arrhythmias, and monitoring of vital signs.

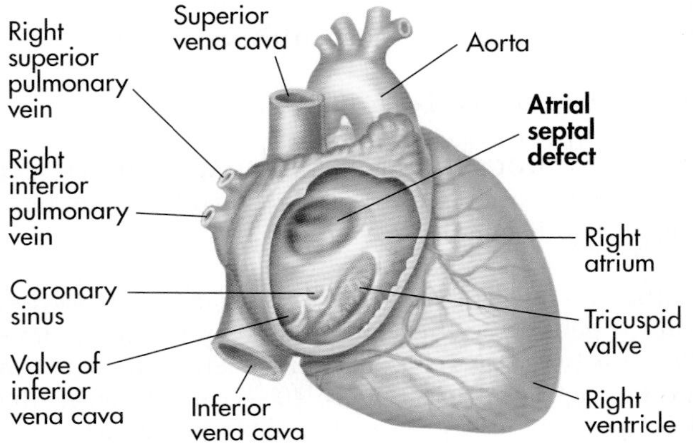

FIGURE 40–5 ✦ Atrial septal defect. *(From Bleck E, Nagel D:* Physically handicapped children: A medical atlas for teachers, *ed 2, Needham Heights, Mass, 1982, Allyn & Bacon.)*

Patent Ductus Arteriosus. *Patent ductus arteriosus* is the most common congenital heart defect found in adults. During development, the fetal heart contains a blood vessel called the ductus arteriosus. This vessel connects the pulmonary artery to the descending aorta. Normally following birth, the vessel closes. If the vessel fails to close, a congenital heart defect forms. Failure to close is associated with premature births and thus failure of the vessel's contracture necessary for closure. Patent ductus arteriosus has been linked to the rubella syndrome.

Shunting of blood in a patent ductus arteriosus defect is from the aorta to the pulmonary artery (Figure 40–6). This type of blood flow results in the recirculation of oxygenated blood through the lungs. Thus the left atrium and ventricle have an increased workload from increased pulmonary blood return, which can result in congestive heart failure. If left untreated, severe obstructive pulmonary vascular disease may develop.

Clinical manifestations include respiratory distress, susceptibility to respiratory tract infections, and slow motor development. Treatment consists of surgical correction and the elimination of symptoms associated with secondary complications.

Tetralogy of Fallot. *Tetralogy of Fallot* is a rare and complex congenital heart defect, generally associated with cyanosis. The defect is composed of four congenital abnormalities: ventricular septal defect, pulmonary stenosis, right ventricular hypertrophy, and malposition of the aorta. The blood shunts right to left through the ventricular septal defect, permitting unoxygenated blood to mix with oxygenated blood resulting in

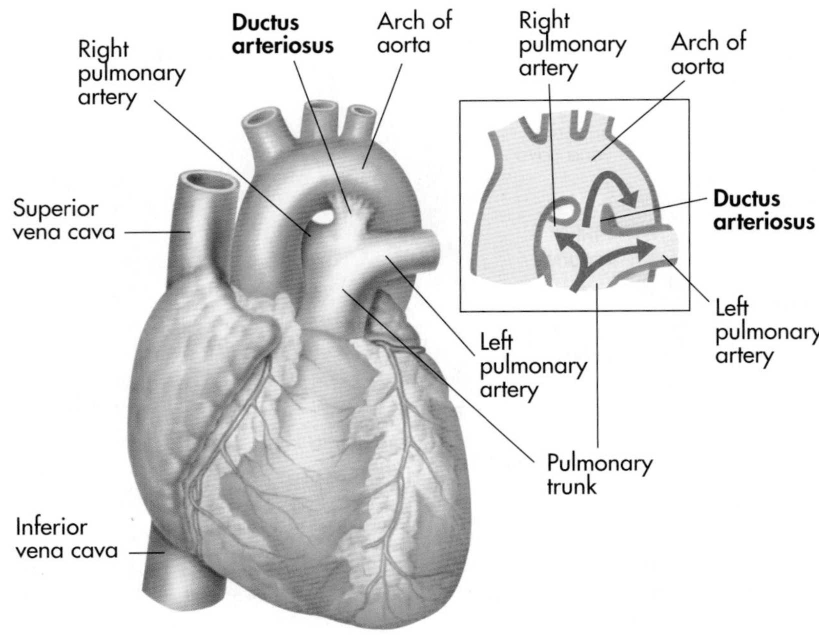

FIGURE 40–6 ✦ Patent ductus arteriosus defect. *(From Bleck E, Nagel D:* Physically handicapped children: A medical atlas for teachers, *ed 2, Needham Heights, Mass, 1982, Allyn & Bacon.)*

cyanosis. Treatment of this defect includes measures to relieve cyanosis and palliative and corrective surgery.

DENTAL HYGIENE CARE. The individual with congenital heart disease does not require extensive alterations in care. Because of susceptibility to IE, these individuals are administered standard prophylactic antibiotic regimens similar to those required by individuals with RHD or artificial heart valves. Even those clients who have had surgery to correct congenital defects are susceptible to endocarditis during the healing phase. Secondary concerns focus on the management of cardiovascular complications, such as CHF and cardiac dysrhythmias, resulting from the congenital defect.

Dental hygiene care includes medical consultation to confirm drug usage and the current medical status, prophylactic antibiotic medication to prevent IE, and assessment of symptoms secondary to the disease that may indicate treatment alteration. If the individual develops CHF, then care plan considerations should follow those outlined.

CARDIOVASCULAR SURGERY

Cardiovascular surgery revolutionized medical treatment for individuals with certain cardiovascular diseases. Heart transplants, repair of congenital heart lesions, and diseased heart valve replacements are commonplace.

Open-heart surgery is necessary for complex procedures that need direct visualization of the heart while being performed (e.g., heart transplants, heart valve replacements, and coronary bypass surgery). Open-heart surgery is always performed with the use of a heart-lung machine that completely controls cardiopulmonary function, enabling surgeons to operate for long periods without interfering with the individual's metabolic needs. Closed-heart surgery is usually associated with cardiac catheterization.

Types of Cardiovascular Surgery

ANGIOPLASTY. The most common type of closed-heart surgery, *angioplasty* involves the use of a catheter (a long, slender tube) with a tiny balloon at the end that is inserted into the coronary artery. Specifically, the balloon is inserted into places where the artery narrows, inflated to flatten fatty deposits, and deflated to allow the increased blood flow to compress and redistribute the atherosclerotic lesion. This procedure is used in individuals who have a small atherosclerotic lesion constricting blood flow. If the lesion cannot be corrected by the angioplasty procedure, bypass surgery may be necessary.

CORONARY BYPASS SURGERY. Coronary bypass surgery, a common procedure to replace blocked arteries, is performed by removing part of the leg vein or chest artery and then grafting it onto the coronary artery, thereby creating a new passageway for the blood. This type of surgery can be done for more than one artery at a time and is named accordingly (double-bypass, triple-bypass). The benefits of coronary bypass surgery include relief from angina, increased tolerance to exercise, improved quality of life, and extended life span. A person who has had a bypass operation has no contraindications to dental hygiene therapy.

VALVULAR DEFECT REPAIR. Valvular defect repair or replacement is performed frequently. Prosthetic cardiac valves for valve replacement have been available for 25 years, and outcomes have steadily improved. Persons with artificial heart valves are especially susceptible to infections and bacterial endocarditis. Individuals who have artificial heart valves must be premedicated with an antibiotic before dental hygiene care (see Tables 9–5 and Sample Dental Hygiene Care Plan for a Client Taking Prophylactic Antibiotic Premedication).

HEART TRANSPLANTATION. Heart transplantation is a viable option for individuals with end-stage heart disease in which no other therapeutic intervention is considered effective. Although about 120 hospitals in the United States perform cardiac transplantation, the dilemma is finding donors.

Future goals and implications of heart transplantation include the development of a safe, reliable, permanent, totally implantable artificial heart device. Ideally, the artificial heart should allow a recipient to carry out normal activities. The development of such a device may increase availability of this life-saving procedure for eligible recipients who at this time await donors.

DENTAL HYGIENE CARE

Client Who Has Had Closed-Heart Surgery. No contraindications are associated with dental or dental hygiene treatment unless the individual is taking anticoagulant medication. As in all cardiac-associated situations, consultation with the client's cardiologist is recommended.

Client After Open-Heart Surgery. No dental hygiene procedures relate uniquely to the individual who has had cardiovascular surgery. When in doubt, the cardiologist is consulted; however, prosthetic valvular heart replacements and those cardiac surgeries that make the client susceptible to infection require prophylactic antibiotic premedication (see Chapter 9, Table 9–5).

The complications from dental hygiene care observed in clients who have had cardiovascular surgery are associated with the drug therapy used rather than the surgery itself. Most post-surgical clients are placed on medication to increase healing, suppress immune response, reduce infection, and/or decrease clot formation. Careful evaluation of drug contraindications and reactions is necessary.

Client Who Has Had a Heart Transplant. A major concern of the heart transplant patient is infection and transplant rejection. Before care, consultation with the client's cardiologist is highly recommended to determine if additional premedication is indicated. Most transplant patients are on long-term preventive antibiotic therapy to control systemic bacteremias. They are also placed on immunosuppressant medications such as Sandimmune to reduce the possibility of rejection.

If possible, dental hygiene care should be performed before cardiac surgery to eliminate the presence of active oral infection and to control dental diseases over the remaining life span. Such an approach not only meets the client's human need for skin and mucous membrane integrity but also empowers the individual with responsibility for her or his oral health status, which is particularly important at a time when control over cardiac health is impossible.

ORAL MANIFESTATIONS OF CARDIOVASCULAR MEDICATIONS

(see Chapter 11 and Table 40–3)

Some medications used in cardiovascular disease therapy have a profound effect on the oral cavity. These medications typically include those that treat hypertension, heart transplant stabilization, and CHD. Persons taking cardiovascular medications should seek regular dental hygiene care to balance their increased vulnerability to dental and periodontal diseases.

Most medications for the treatment of hypertension have the side effect of xerostomia, increasing the individual's risk of developing dental caries and periodontal disease. In addition, individuals with exposed root surfaces are at risk of root surface caries and dentinal hypersensitivity. Self-administered fluoride therapy and the use of saliva substitutes should be incorporated into the individual's daily self-care regimen to meet the client's needs (see Chapter 26). Some calcium channel blockers may alter taste perception, cause gingival enlargement, and create salivary gland pain. Immunosuppressants used for the stabilization of heart transplants increase the individual's risk of developing periodontal disease or may exaggerate a preexisting condition, leading to an unmet need in skin and mucous membrane integrity.

Another dental hygiene diagnosis to consider is a need for protection from health risks because immunosuppressants place the individual at risk for developing opportunistic infections such as candidiasis, herpes simplex, herpes zoster, and necrotizing ulcerative gingivitis, and drug-influenced gingival enlargement. In addition to regular professional dental hygiene care, these individuals should be instructed to use antimicrobial mouthrinses as part of their self-care regimen to reduce the threat of disease.

Persons with a history of heart attack or cerebrovascular accident are placed on blood thinners (anticoagulants) to increase blood flow. The side effects are prolonged bleeding and spontaneous oral bleeding in the presence of infection. These individuals must maintain a healthy periodontium to reduce the possibility of periodontal disease.

PREVENTING AND MANAGING A CARDIAC EMERGENCY

The individual with a CVD, symptom, or defect is considered high risk—one whose life may be threatened by daily activities. High-risk clients have a need for protection from health risks because of their increased potential for an emergency in the oral care setting. The most common physical pain encountered is chest pain accompanied by difficulty breathing. If the client complains of physical pain that cannot be alleviated, referral to the physician is recommended. If the pain is associated with dental hygiene procedures, alterations in the care plan are necessary.

For individuals with angina pectoris, hypertension, previous myocardial infarctions, and CHF, the risk for life-threatening medical emergencies rises as a result of an increase in anxiety, fear, and stress.

Assessing past responses in oral healthcare situations and monitoring the client's reactions to dental hygiene procedures are important. Muscular tenseness, excessive perspiration, and verbal cues are indications of a potential emergency and indicate that the client's need for protection from health risks is not being met.

Individuals with CVD may not take responsibility for their oral health and give dental hygiene care low priority. Understandably, these individuals fail to relate their life-threatening medical condition with oral disease; however, by increasing a client's conceptualization and understanding that the presence of periodontal disease increases the severity of his or her systemic condition, the dental hygienist may change the client's value system, alter his or her oral health behavior, and improve his or her systemic health. An accurate assessment of the client's personal beliefs, behaviors, and values can identify motivators (needs) that can lead to a commitment to therapeutic goals and priorities. Table 40–4 illustrates sample dental hygiene diagnoses for a client with CHD.

Planning prevents emergencies and ensures that client needs are the focus of therapeutic interventions. When developing a care plan, attention should be given to drug therapies to ensure that no contraindications are present and that side effects are identified (Table 40–3). Tables 40–5 and 40–6 can be used when developing care plans for clients with a CVD.

Implementation of care takes into consideration the possibility of a medical emergency (see Chapter 7). The most life-threatening emergency situation is cardiac arrest. In an emergency, the basic responsibilities of the dental hygienist are to:

1. Contact the EMS or 911.
2. Monitor vital signs and state of consciousness.
3. Administer oxygen.
4. Provide BLS.

Other medical emergencies associated with cardiovascular disease are attacks of angina pectoris and myocardial infarctions. Basic Steps in a Cardiac Emergency Situation lists basic steps to take in the event of an emergency.

TABLE 40–4 SAMPLE DENTAL HYGIENE DIAGNOSIS FOR A CLIENT WITH CORONARY HEART DISEASE

Dental Hygiene Diagnosis	Related to	As Evidenced by
Protection from health risks: Potential for myocardial infarction	Stress Anxiety Recent life-threatening medical diagnosis	Pain in chest, jaw, neck, throat, interscapular area, and left arm Agitation
Responsibility for oral health	Low value ascribed to oral health	Client reports a lack of interest in performing daily oral hygiene care
Potential for health risks: Potential for infection	History of mitral valve prolapse	Client self-reports condition on health history questionnaire
Biologically sound and functional dentition	Drug therapy (diuretics) taken by client	Xerostomia Root caries
Biologically sound and functional dentition	Dietary restrictions of cholesterol, saturated fat and sodium	Client self-report of overweight and high cholesterol blood values

TABLE 40–5 QUICK REFERENCE TO THE SIGNS, SYMPTOMS, AND TREATMENT OF INDIVIDUALS WITH CARDIOVASCULAR DISEASES

Disease	Signs and Symptoms	Medical and Surgical Treatment
Rheumatic heart disease	Carditis, polyarthritis, chorea, erythema marginatum, subcutaneous nodules, fever	Bedrest and medications associated with manifestations
Bacterial endocarditis	Initial high fever, cardiac decompensation, heart murmur	Antibiotic therapy
Valvular heart defects	Fatigue, shortness of breath, and pulmonary edema If left untreated, congestive heart failure will develop	Valvular repair or replacement with a prosthetic heart valve
Mitral valve prolapse	Palpitations, chest pain, nervousness, shortness of breath, dizziness	Treatment is not always necessary and is aimed at alleviating symptoms
Cardiac dysrhythmias/arrhythmias	Bradycardia: pulse rate less than 60 beats/minute Tachycardia: pulse rate above 150 beats/minute	Antiarrhythmic drug therapy or cardiac pacemaker
Hypertension	Headache, fatigue, diminished exercise tolerance, shortness of breath	Antihypertension drug therapy and dietary control of sodium
Coronary "ischemic" heart disease	Angina pectoris, discomfort in jaw, neck, throat, interscapular area, and left arm	Bedrest and administration of nitroglycerin
Congestive heart failure	Fatigue, weakness, dyspnea, cough, anorexia	Treatment is directed at the underlying etiology
Congenital heart disease	Dependent on type of defect	Surgery to correct defect

Basic Steps in a Cardiac Emergency Situation

Make certain the client is comfortable, loosen restricting garments, and position the client so the head is slightly elevated.

Angina Pectoris

Immediately administer nitroglycerin sublingually and 100% oxygen with a face mask or nasal cannula to prevent disease transmission.

Monitor vital signs.

Myocardial Infarction

Transfer client to an emergency facility as soon as possible.

Be prepared to administer CPR if necessary.

Stay with the client until he or she is transferred to the care of a physician or emergency medical technician (EMT).

Oral care professionals evaluate the current health status of the client in light of the established client goals. By reviewing the assessment data, dental hygiene diagnoses, care plan, and intervention used, one can determine where less than desirable outcomes occurred and modify care if necessary. Table 40–7 illustrates an evaluation of dental hygiene interventions for the care plan in Sample Dental Hygiene Care Plan for a Client Taking Prophylactic Antibiotic Premedication.

TABLE 40–6 QUICK REFERENCE TO DENTAL HYGIENE CARE IMPLICATIONS FOR INDIVIDUALS WITH CARDIOVASCULAR DISEASE

Disease	Implications for Dental Hygiene Care	Dental Hygiene Care Precautions
Rheumatic heart disease	When carditis is present, the client is susceptible to bacterial endocarditis and requires antibiotic premedication prior to invasive dental hygiene therapy Special attention should be given to home care practices because self-inflicted bacteremias may occur when oral disease is present	Careful manipulation of soft tissues during instrumentation to reduce the presence of a transient bacteremia
Bacterial endocarditis	Client susceptible to reinfection in the presence of a transient bacteremia Prophylactic antibiotic premedication is indicated for invasive dental hygiene procedures	Invasive dental hygiene procedures should include careful manipulation of soft tissue
Valvular heart defects	Bacterial endocarditis may occur following dental hygiene procedures that cause transient bacteremias Clients receiving anticoagulant medication may have a prolonged bleeding time	If anticoagulant medication is being used and scaling procedures are planned, the dosage of anticoagulant medication should be discussed with the client's cardiologist
Mitral valve prolapse	Prophylactic antibiotic premedication given as a precaution	Careful manipulation of soft tissue during invasive dental hygiene procedures
Cardiac dysrhythmias/ arrhythmias	Electrical interferences can cause pacemaker malfunction	Usage of dental hygiene equipment that interferes with pacemaker function is contraindicated
Hypertension	Stress and anxiety associated with dental hygiene treatment may increase blood pressure	If blood pressure is uncontrolled, dental hygiene care is contraindicated Implement stress and anxiety-reducing strategies; create atmosphere conducive to relaxation
Coronary "ischemic" heart disease	Stress and anxiety associated with dental hygiene treatment may precipitate an angina attack	Nitroglycerin should be available during dental hygiene treatment Implement stress- and anxiety-reducing strategies; create atmosphere conducive to relaxation
Congestive heart failure	None if patient is under appropriate medical care	Client should be treated in upright position to decrease fluid in the lungs

TABLE 40–7 SAMPLE EVALUATION OF DENTAL HYGIENE INTERVENTIONS

Client Goals	Evaluative Measures	Expected Outcomes
Complete invasive dental hygiene therapy so that antibiotic coverage occurs with a 9- to 14-day interval between coverage	Review treatment appointment scheduling for appropriate time intervals	Dentition and periodontium free from soft and hard deposits
By 9/03, reduce gingival bleeding	Document client's periodontal condition for treatment results using periodontal probing depths and a gingival bleeding index	Minimal to no gingival bleeding
By 12/03 reduce periodontal probing depths	Document client's periodontal condition for treatment results using periodontal probing depths	Periodontal probing depths reduced by at least 1 mm

Client Education Issues

- Explain that prophylactic antibiotic premedication must be taken 1 hour before the scheduled appointment to achieve optimal blood levels and reduce the possibility of IE (see Chapter 9, Table 9–6).
- Discuss how maintenance of good oral health helps to reduce self-induced and professionally induced transient bacteremias for the prevention of IE.
- Explain that reducing gingival inflammation with daily plaque biofilm control practices to minimize unnecessary bleeding during instrumentation is important when taking anticoagulant medication.
- Explain that good oral health reduces the possible occurrence of a myocardial infarction. Periodontal disease increases one's risk for CHD because it increases the development of blood clots in the arteries. The formation of blood clots and atheromas is enhanced by the presence of specific bacteria associated with periodontal disease and an increase in the body's inflammatory response toward periodontal disease.
- Discuss how some forms of cardiovascular diseases are preventable by reducing the classic risk factors; however, lifestyle changes are required in most cases. A low-sodium, low-fat, and low-cholesterol diet decreases potential risks, supplemented by daily exercise, reduced stress, and no tobacco use.

Legal, Ethical, and Safety Issues

- The client with cardiovascular disease poses a potential malpractice threat if treatment procedures fail to follow the standard of care. The following legal issues confront the healthcare professional as a result of a medical emergency.[12]
- The original "incident" may subject the practitioner to liability for causing additional harm (even death), resulting from (1) later negligent care and treatment addressed to the original injury, (2) later care and treatment (not negligent), or (3) later care and treatment, when an inherent risk (e.g., infection) is the aftermath.
- If a client with CVD develops chest pain and begins to feel anxious, the provider should (1) stop dental hygiene care; (2) alert the dentist, and (3) together with the dentist, manage the immediate emergency situation, which may include BLS.
- If dental hygiene care is continued and the client undergoes a myocardial infarction, liability charges may be brought against the practitioner.
- If dental care is performed on a client who was not appropriately interviewed about his or her health history and that status is not documented on an acceptable health history form, the practitioner could be held responsible for any damage resulting from care.
- If a client reports on the health history that he or she has a cardiac condition that requires an antibiotic premedication regimen and he or she is not premedicated, then the practitioner is liable for the risk of infection and complication thereof following treatment. Medical emergency situations must be prevented and properly managed or malpractice could arise.

Key Concepts

- Review of the health history, pharmacologic history, and risk factors for systemic and oral disease is a standard of care; consultation with the client's physician or cardiologist also may be required.
- Periodontal disease increases one's risk for CVD because bacteria found in periodontal disease (e.g., *Porphyromonas gingivalis*) assist in platelet aggregation, and the inflammatory process associated with periodontal disease increases the potential for thrombosis development.
- Prevention of IE requires prophylactic antibiotic premedication and maintenance of periodontal disease.
- Hypertension, which is often unnoticed, can be detected by routinely measuring blood pressure as a part of the dental hygiene assessment.
- Unstable angina pectoris indicates that a client has increasing chest pain at rest and during sleep. Clients with unstable angina present with a possible medical emergency and should not be treated.
- The drug of choice for a client experiencing angina is nitroglycerin, which is usually administered sublingually.
- Dental hygiene care should be postponed if a client has had a myocardial infarction within 6 months of his or her scheduled appointment.
- Cardiac dysrhythmias/arrhythmias are dysfunctions of the heart rate and rhythm and may be detected during assessment by evaluation of the client's pulse rate.

Continued on following page

Key Concepts—cont'd

- ✦ Unshielded cardiac pacemakers are susceptible to interferences generated by some dental equipment (e.g., ultrasonic scalers, pulp testers, electrodesensitizing equipment, air-abrasion systems, computerized periodontal probes, slow- or high-speed hand pieces).
- ✦ Clients with CHF experience difficulty breathing in a supine position.
- ✦ Clients with a history of CVD should not be given local anesthetic agents that contain epinephrine.
- ✦ Anticoagulant medications increase bleeding time. Clients on this medication need a medical consultation before dental hygiene care.
- ✦ Clients on immunosuppressant medication for a heart transplant and calcium channel blockers for hypertension are at risk for drug-influenced gingival enlargement.
- ✦ The prevention of CVD requires lifestyle changes, such as a reduction in saturated fat, cholesterol, and sodium; increased exercise; decreased stress; no tobacco use; and control of hypertension.

Critical Thinking Exercises

Case 1: Client with a history of myocardial infarction taking anticoagulant medication

During the assessment phase, the client reports that he has had a myocardial infarction 2 years ago and is taking Coumadin, twice daily. The client has case type II periodontal disease.

1. What are the implications of the myocardial infarction and anticoagulant medication on dental hygiene care?
2. What unmet human needs does this client present with?
3. Should this client be treated? Why or why not?
4. If the client is treated, should the dental hygiene care plan be altered?
5. What educational issues need to be incorporated into the care plan?

Case 2: Documentation of health history for a client with CHD

A well-documented health history decreases the possibility of a medical emergency occurring. The following case presents a medical profile of a client with CVD.

Medical Profile: Mrs. J, age 56, was last examined by her physician in September 2002. Upon completion of the medical history, you note that Mrs. J has responded "yes" to some questions concerning CHD. She indicated that she gets pain in her chest and carries nitroglycerin with her. She claims that the nitroglycerin usually helps, but she sometimes needs to take two doses. All other responses were insignificant.

1. What additional questions would you want to ask Mrs. J concerning her condition?
2. What unmet human needs does this client have?
3. Does her condition have any implications for dental hygiene care? Explain.
4. Would you alter the care plan? If so, how?
5. What medical emergency is this client at risk for, based on the medical profile?

For References, Suggested Readings, and Related Websites, visit
http://evolve.elsevier.com/Darby/hygiene/

CHAPTER 41

Persons with Diabetes Mellitus

OBJECTIVES

Mastery of the content in this chapter will enable the reader to:

- Describe the differences between type 1 and type 2 diabetes mellitus in terms of prevalence, symptoms, and medications used to control the disease.
- Describe the chronic complications of diabetes mellitus.
- Identify appropriate prophylactic antibiotic premedications to prescribe for the diabetic client.
- Recognize a diabetic emergency and take appropriate action for management.
- Appreciate lifestyle adjustments required by the individual with diabetes.
- Understand the link between control of the diabetic condition and control of oral infections.
- Develop client-centered dental hygiene care plans for individuals with diabetes.
- Recognize oral complications of diabetes mellitus: salivary and oral changes, periodontal changes, infection and wound healing, tongue changes, and opportunistic changes.
- Apply the dental hygiene process of care to the individual with diabetes mellitus.
- Suspect the diabetic condition when oral tissues fail to respond to traditional treatment.

KEY TERMS

Advanced glycation end products (AGE)
Control of diabetes
Diabetes mellitus
Dyslipidemia
Gestational diabetes mellitus (GDM)
Glucose
Glucosuria
Hyperglycemia
Hypoglycemia
Impaired fasting glucose
Impaired glucose tolerance
Insulin (rapid-acting, intermediate, long-acting)
Ketoacidosis
Ketonemia
Ketonuria
Lipolysis
Microangiopathy
Neuroglycopenia
Neuropathy
Polydipsia
Polyphagia
Polyuria
Sulfonylureas
Type 1 diabetes mellitus
Type 2 diabetes mellitus

Diabetes mellitus, one of the most widespread diseases, affects 15.7 million people, or 5.9% of the U.S. population. Approximately 5.4 million are unknown or undiagnosed cases. These numbers are increasing substantially. Individuals with diabetes face shortened life spans and the probability of developing acute and chronic health complications. Only heart disease and cancer kill more Americans than diabetes and its complications.

Diabetes mellitus is actually a group of disorders characterized by the following:

- Relative or absolute lack of insulin or improperly functioning insulin

- Impairment in the body's ability to metabolize carbohydrates, fats, and protein
- Resulting abnormalities in the structure and function of blood vessels (*microangiopathy*) and nerves (*neuropathy*)

The result of diabetes is *hyperglycemia,* a condition of abnormally increased blood *glucose.*

CLASSIFICATION OF DIABETES AND CATEGORIES OF GLUCOSE REGULATION

Most cases of diabetes fall into two broad categories, type 1 and type 2 diabetes. However, in understanding diabetes, it is essential to separate the disease into four major clinical types:

- Type 1 diabetes mellitus
- Type 2 diabetes mellitus
- Gestational diabetes mellitus[1]
- Other specific types, including diabetes mellitus associated with certain conditions and syndromes (see Categories of Diabetes Mellitus and Glucose Regulation)

A description of all four categories follows; a comparison of the characteristics of type 1 and type 2 disease is presented in Table 41–1.

Type 1

Type 1 diabetes mellitus, which involves about 15% of the diabetic population, commonly occurs in childhood and adolescence but can strike at any age. An absolute deficiency of insulin secretion is characteristic in this type, and treatment requires regular lifelong administration of insulin by injection to prevent ketosis and sustain health.

Type 1 diabetes mellitus results from autoimmune destruction of the β-cells of the pancreas with an abrupt onset of symptoms in children and slow onset in adults. Genetic predisposition related to the presence of certain human leukocyte antigens (HLAs) that influence immune activity directed against islet cells is essential for

Categories of Diabetes Mellitus and Glucose Regulation

Diabetes Mellitus

TYPE 1

β-cell destruction usually leading to absolute insulin deficiency

A. Immune mediated

B. Idiopathic

TYPE 2

Insulin resistance with relative insulin deficiency or insulin secretion defect with insulin resistance.

Other Specific Types

Other types of diabetes associated with certain conditions or syndromes: pancreatic disease, endocrinopathies, infections, chemical- or drug-induced disease, genetic defects, genetic syndromes, insulin-receptor abnormalities, and others.

Gestational Diabetes Mellitus

Any degree of glucose intolerance with onset or first recognition during pregnancy.

Impaired Glucose Tolerance (IGT) and Impaired Fasting Glucose (IFG)

Metabolic stages intermediate between normal glucose homeostasis and diabetes.

TABLE 41–1 CHARACTERISTICS OF TYPE 1 AND TYPE 2 DIABETES MELLITUS

Factor	Type 1	Type 2
Age at onset	Usually young, but may occur at any age	Usually in persons older than 40 years of age, but may occur at any age
Type of onset	Usually abrupt	Insidious
Genetic susceptibility	HLA-related DR3, DR4, and others	Frequent genetic background; not HLA-related
Environmental factors	Virus, toxins, autoimmune stimulation	Obesity, nutrition
Islet-cell antibody	Present at outset	Not observed
Endogenous insulin	Minimal or absent	Stimulated response is (1) adequate but delayed secretion, or (2) reduced but not absent
Nutritional status	Thin, catabolic state	Obese, or may be normal
Symptoms	Thirst, polyuria, polyphagia, fatigue	Frequently none, or mild
Ketosis	Prone, at onset or during insulin deficiency	Resistant, except during infection or stress
Control of diabetes	Often difficult, with wide glucose fluctuation	Variable, helped by dietary adherence
Dietary management	Essential	Essential, may suffice for glycemic control
Insulin	Required for all	Required for about 40%
Sulfonylurea	Not efficacious	Efficacious
Vascular and neurologic complications	Seen in majority after 5 or more years of diabetes	Frequent

type 1 diabetes. Environmental factors, still poorly defined, are postulated to play an etiologic role in genetically predisposed individuals. Individuals who develop type 1 diabetes mellitus are rarely obese.

Results of twin studies suggest a genetic difference between type 1 and type 2 diabetes, a concept further supported by HLA presence and family studies. More than 95% of persons with type 1 diabetes possess certain HLAs, compared with only 40% of type 2 and nondiabetic individuals.[2] A predisposition to type 1 diabetes seems to be inherited because approximately 50% of nondiabetic individuals have the HLAs in question, yet only 0.1% of that population develop type 1 diabetes.

Type 2

Type 2 diabetes mellitus is recognized as a heterogeneous disorder that results from insulin resistance and insulin secretory defect. People with type 2 diabetes constitute approximately 80% to 85% of the diabetic population. The risk of developing type 2 diabetes increases with age, obesity, lack of physical activity, history of gestational diabetes mellitus, hypertension, and *dyslipidemia* (abnormal amounts of lipids in the blood). Frequency of type 2 diabetes varies in different racial and ethnic groups. Most individuals with type 2 diabetes are obese, and obesity itself causes some degree of insulin resistance. Individuals who are not obese by traditional weight criteria may have an increased percentage of body fat distributed in the abdominal region. Ketoacidosis seldom occurs in type 2 diabetes, or when present, is associated with infection. Type 2 diabetes usually goes undiagnosed for years because hyperglycemia develops gradually without classic symptoms. Nevertheless, the risk of developing macrovascular and microvascular complications (problems in the large and small blood vessels) is high. Symptoms may be gradual, and weight loss is uncommon.

Persons with type 2 diabetes often respond to weight reduction, dietary management, exercise, and oral hypoglycemic agents (sulfonylurea medications). Persons with type 2 diabetes may require insulin therapy to achieve good control or during illness, which is an important distinction between insulin-dependent and insulin-treated individuals.

Predominantly, type 2 diabetes is genetically inherited and has no association with autoimmune β-cell destruction. In research studies, type 2 diabetic twins are 91% concordant (both twins have the disease).[3] If nongenetic or environmental factors were important in the development of type 2 diabetes, discordance in twins (only one twin is affected) would be common.

Gestational Diabetes Mellitus (GDM)

Gestational diabetes mellitus (GDM) occurs in 4% of pregnancies in the United States.[1] GDM represents 90% of all pregnancies complicated by diabetes. Clinical characteristics include glucose intolerance that has its onset or recognition during pregnancy. Thus, diabetics who become pregnant are not included in the GDM classification. High-risk individuals include women with the following:

- ✦ Marked obesity
- ✦ Previous GDM
- ✦ Strong family history for diabetes
- ✦ Glucosuria (glucose in the urine)

Even in the nondiabetic individual, normal pregnancy affects both fetal and maternal metabolism, and exerts a diabetogenic effect. GDM generally reverts following birth because the condition is a consequence of the normal antiinsulin effects of pregnancy hormones and the diversion of natural glucose to the developing fetus.

GDM increases the risk of perinatal morbidity and mortality. Maternal complications include increased rate of cesarean delivery and chronic hypertension. Furthermore, women with a history of GDM are at increased risk of developing diabetes 5 to 10 years later. Six weeks or more after pregnancy ends, the woman with GDM should be reclassified into one of the following categories:

- ✦ Diabetes
- ✦ Impaired glucose tolerance or normoglycemia
- ✦ Impaired fasting glucose

Other Types of Diabetes Mellitus

The clinical category *other specific types* is heterogeneous in nature and includes diabetes in which the etiologic relationship is known (e.g., genetic defects of the β-cells, pancreatic disease, endocrine disease, chemical-induced agents, and genetic syndromes). In other diabetic disorders such as genetic syndromes associated with glucose intolerance, an etiologic relationship is suspected. Rare and highly specific causes of diabetes and insulin resistance include defects in insulin receptors located on the cell membrane and conditions such as systemic lupus erythematosus in which insulin-receptor antibodies may develop. In addition to the presence of the specific condition or syndrome, diabetes mellitus also is present. A partial listing of disorders that constitute this clinical category of diabetes is given in Other Types of Diabetes Mellitus: Disorders and Syndromes.

Impaired Glucose Tolerance and Impaired Fasting Glucose

The designations *impaired glucose tolerance (IGT)* and *impaired fasting glucose (IFG)* refer to a metabolic stage intermediate between normal glucose homeostasis and diabetes. Impaired glucose tolerance is a risk factor for future diabetes and cardiovascular disease. Impaired glucose tolerance can be determined only by an oral glucose tolerance test (OGTT) consisting of a standard glucose challenge followed 2 hours later by measurement of venous plasma glucose concentration. Disease management includes dietary control of obesity, treatment of hypertension and hyperlipidemia (high amounts of fat in the blood), and elimination of smoking, if present.

*Other Types of Diabetes Mellitus: Disorders and Syndromes**

Pancreatic Disease
Pancreatitis, carcinoma, cystic fibrosis, hemochromatosis, pancreatectomy

Hyperendocrinopathy
Cushing's syndrome, pheochromocytoma, glucagonoma, aldosteronoma, acromegaly

Chemical- or Drug-Induced Disease
Glucocorticoids, most thiazide diuretics, phenytoin, oral contraceptives, phenothiazines, tricyclic antidepressants, clonidine, lithium

Certain Genetic Syndromes
Hyperlipidemia, Turner's syndrome, myotonic dystrophy, leprechaunism, Prader-Willi syndrome

Insulin-Receptor Abnormalities
Type A: altered receptor response
Type B: receptor antibodies

Other Types
Diabetes associated with malnourished populations

* For additional examples of secondary forms of diabetes, see Gavin et al (2000) in *References* and *Suggested Readings* at this book's website: http://evolve.elsevier.com/Darby/hygiene/

Signs and Symptoms of Ketoacidosis

Common Cardinal Symptoms
"Fruity" acetone breath
Frequent urination
Excessive thirst
Unusual hunger
Weight loss
Weakness
Nausea
Dry skin and mucous membranes
Flushed facial appearance
Abdominal tenderness
Rapid, deep breathing
Depressed sensory perception

Other Symptoms
Recurrence of bedwetting
Repeated skin infections
Malaise
Drowsiness
Headache
Marked irritability

PATHOPHYSIOLOGY OF DIABETES

To use glucose, the body must produce insulin. A person with diabetes produces too little insulin or a type of insulin that cannot be used. *Insulin,* an anabolic hormone (used to build up the body), stimulates entry of glucose into the cell and enhances fat storage. The presence of insulin, therefore, prevents the body from breaking down fat. Without insulin, glucose remains in the bloodstream (hyperglycemia) rather than being stored or used by cells to produce energy.

Insulin Deprivation

The net effect of insulin deficiency is that blood glucose concentration rises (*hyperglycemia*). Without insulin, the glucose derived from a meal cannot be utilized or stored. When the blood glucose level rises above 150 mg/dl, the kidney tubules become incapable of resorption. Glucose appears in the urine (*glucosuria*), taking with it a large amount of fluid, thus raising the volume of urine (*polyuria*) and necessitating frequent urination. Dehydration follows, leading to excessive thirst (*polydipsia*).

Ketoacidosis may follow hyperglycemia (see Signs and Symptoms of Ketoacidosis) when blood glucose levels rise to above 400 mg/dl. Impaired carbohydrate metabolism, which the body interprets as energy starvation, necessitates use of fats and proteins (hyperglycemia progressively glycates body proteins) to satisfy energy requirements. Ketoacids and ketone bodies (acetone) are produced as a result of catabolism of fatty acids (*lipolysis*). Ketones accumulate in the tissues, are excreted in the urine (*ketouria*), and circulate in the blood (*ketonemia*), causing a drop in the pH of the blood and leading to diabetic coma.

Clinical Signs and Symptoms

Diabetes is characterized by hyperglycemia. In type 1 diabetes mellitus, the predominant problem is impaired insulin production, whereas in type 2 diabetes mellitus the predominant problem is the inability to use the insulin produced by the body. A considerable overlap exists, however, in clinical features of the two forms of diabetes. The deficiency of insulin action leads to derangements of the intermediary metabolism of carbohydrates, protein, and lipids. In clinical practice, the suspicion of diabetes is gleaned from history and physical findings (see Warning Signs of Diabetes).

The following symptoms are indications of probable diabetes mellitus:

- Polydipsia
- Polyuria
- Unexplained weight loss

Symptoms of marked hyperglycemia also include *polyphagia* (eating extreme amounts of food) and blurred vision. Impairment of growth and susceptibility to certain infections may also accompany chronic hyperglycemia. A family history of diabetes, obesity, GDM, premature atherosclerosis, and neuropathic disorders also are indications of probable diabetes mellitus (see Criteria for Testing for Diabetes in Asymptomatic, Undiagnosed Individuals).

Warning Signs of Diabetes

Type 1 Diabetes Mellitus is Characterized by the Sudden Appearance of:
Constant urination
Excessive thirst
Extreme hunger
Dramatic weight loss
Irritability
Weakness and fatigue, nausea and vomiting

Type 2 Diabetes Mellitus is Characterized by Slow Onset and Includes Any of the Type 1 Symptoms and/or:
Recurring or hard-to-heal skin, gum, or bladder infections
Fatigue
Blurred vision
Tingling or numbness in hands or feet
Itching

Modified from the American Diabetes Association: *Know the warning signs of diabetes: Who We Are, What We Do,* Alexandria, Va, 1991, American Diabetes Association.

Criteria for Testing for Diabetes in Asymptomatic, Undiagnosed Individuals

Testing for diabetes should be considered in all individuals at age 45 years and above and if normal should be repeated at 3-year intervals.

Testing should be considered at a younger age or be carried out more frequently in individuals who:

- Are obese (≥120% desirable weight or a BMI ≥27 kg/m^2)
- Have first-degree relatives with diabetes
- Are members of a high-risk ethnic population (e.g., African American, Hispanic American, Native American, Asian American, Pacific Islander)
- Have delivered a baby weighing >9 lb or have been diagnosed with GDM
- Are hypertensive (≥140/90)
- Have an HDL cholesterol level ≤35 mg/dl (0.90 mmol/L) and/or a triglyceride level ≥250 mg/dl (2.82 mmol/L).
- On previous testing, had IGT or IFG

The oral glucose tolerance test (OGTT) or fasting prandial glucose (FPG) test may be used to diagnose diabetes; however, in clinical settings the FPG test is greatly preferred because of ease of administration, convenience, acceptability to clients, and lower cost.

Chronic Complications

People with both types of diabetes mellitus show a tendency for severe, multisystem, long-term complications, including the following:

- ✦ Microvascular and macrovascular disease
- ✦ Diabetic retinopathy with potential loss of vision
- ✦ Nephropathy leading to renal failure
- ✦ Peripheral neuropathy with risk of foot ulcers, amputation, and neuropathic joint disease
- ✦ Autonomic neuropathy causing gastrointestinal genitourinary and cardiovascular symptoms and sexual dysfunction

TABLE 41–2 COMPLICATIONS OF DIABETES MELLITUS

Affected Area	Complications
Eyes	Retinopathy Cataracts Glaucoma
Kidneys	Glomerulonephritis Nephrosclerosis Pyelonephritis
Mouth	Gingivitis Dental caries Periodontitis
Reproductive system	Stillbirths Miscarriages High-birthweight babies Congenital defects Neonatal deaths
Skin	Xanthoma diabeticorum Pruritus Furunculosis Limited joint mobility
Vascular system	Arteriosclerosis Microangiopathy Large-vessel disease Myocardial infarction
Peripheral nerves	Earliest recognized complication Somatic neuropathy Autonomic neuropathy

The mechanisms thought to cause tissue damage in diabetics are glycation of tissue proteins[4–6] and excess production of polyol compounds from glucose. Individuals with diabetes have an increased incidence of atherosclerotic, cardiovascular, peripheral vascular, and cerebrovascular disease. Hypertension, abnormalities in lipoprotein metabolism, and periodontal disease are found in people with diabetes. The emotional and social impact of diabetes and the demands of therapy cause significant unmet human needs in individuals with diabetes and their families[1] (Table 41–2). All complications affect clients with both type 1 and type 2 diabetes, although clinical manifestations and consequences differ greatly. Generally, kidney and eye diseases predominate in type 1 diabetes, atherosclerotic disease predominates in type 2 disease, and neuropathy occurs in both.

Diabetes as a Risk Factor for Periodontal Disease

See Chapter 15, section on modifiable risk factors.

DIABETIC EMERGENCIES (also see Chapter 7)

An individual with uncontrolled diabetes increases the risk of emergency situations such as:

- ✦ Coma
- ✦ Hypoglycemia
- ✦ Ketoacidotic hyperglycemia

- Nonketotic hyperosmolar hyperglycemia
- Lactic acidosis
- Uremia
- Nondiabetic coma
- Infection
- Myocardial infarction
- Stroke
- Emergency surgery

The occurrence of stupor or coma in diabetes may be due to several causes. The diabetic condition may be undiagnosed, or the person with type 1 disease may not have followed the required insulin regimen. Stress, infection, and increased level of activity contribute to an emergency situation.

Hypoglycemia

Hypoglycemia, the most common metabolic emergency in persons with type 1 diabetes mellitus, is a condition resulting from an excess of insulin and a deficiency of glucose in the body. It is defined as a blood glucose concentration below 50 mg/dl (80 to 120 mg/dl is normal). Severe episodes occur in one of five individuals annually. Minor episodes occur every 2 weeks on average in each insulin-treated person. In clients with type 2 disease treated with sulfonylurea agents, hypoglycemia is more common than is generally recognized, and may be severe, especially in older persons treated with longer-acting agents.[7] Signs and symptoms of hypoglycemia result from a lack of glucose in the brain and compensation by the nervous system for this lack of glucose (see Signs and Symptoms of Hypoglycemia). The main causes of hypoglycemia in persons with type 1 disease are shown in Table 41–3.

Individuals with diabetes can manage mild hypoglycemia themselves by ingesting glucose, sweet drinks, or milk. Between 10 and 20 g of glucose (about the amount in an 8-ounce glass of 2% fat milk, a 4-ounce glass of orange juice, three pieces of hard candy, or eight Lifesavers candies) is generally adequate, although many persons take considerably more because they fear prolonged hypoglycemia. More severe hypoglycemia also can be treated by oral ingestion of carbohydrates, but friends or relatives may have to administer it. If the person is unconscious, treatment requires intravenous dextrose solution or an intramuscular injection of 0.5 to 1.0 mg glucagon, followed on awakening by oral complex carbohydrate with a protein source (i.e., small meat or cheese sandwich, or cottage cheese and fruit).

Hyperglycemic Ketoacidotic Coma (Diabetic Coma)

Although the percentage of all diabetic deaths caused by *hyperglycemia ketoacidotic coma* has decreased dramatically from more than 60% in pre-insulin days to 1% at present, it is still considerable, especially in younger individuals. Prevention is the best treatment; however, emergency treatment requires hospitalization to correct fluid and electrolyte imbalances (Table 41–4).

Signs and Symptoms of Hypoglycemia

Lack of Glucose to the Brain (Neuroglycopenia)
Confusion
Blurred vision
Paresthesia (tingling in arms and legs)
Fatigue
Stupor
Convulsions
Unconsciousness (coma)
Irritability
Impaired concentration
Headache
Somnolence (sleepiness or drowsiness)
Psychiatric disorders (stupor)
Transient sensory or motor defects (weakness, slurred speech)

Nervous System Compensations (Adrenergic Discharge)
Anxiety
Sweating
Pallor
Tachycardia
Palpitations
Hunger
Restlessness
Excitability
Trembling
Headache
Nausea
Dizziness

TABLE 41–3 CAUSES OF HYPOGLYCEMIA IN TYPE 1 DIABETES MELLITUS

Type	Cause
Insulin	Inappropriate insulin regimens
	Day-to-day variability in absorption
	Insulin antibodies
	Inappropriate site rotation
	Factitious hypoglycemia
	Renal failure
Food	Delayed intake
	Decreased intake
Exercise	Increased energy requirements
	Increased insulin absorption
Other	Impaired counterregulation
	Liver disease
	Hypoendocrine states
	Alcohol
	Potentiating drugs
	Hypoglycemic unawareness (absence of signs and symptoms, long-standing diabetes, autonomic neuropathy)

Coma resulting from absolute insulin deficiency is found in persons with acute-onset type 1 diabetes in whom diagnosis was unknown or delayed and in individuals with known diabetes who discontinued or decreased their insulin dose for some reason. Coma from a tempo-

TABLE 41–4

HYPOGLYCEMIA COMPARED WITH HYPERGLYCEMIA

Signs and Symptoms	Hypoglycemia 40–50 ml/dl	Hyperglycemia 400–600 ml/dl
Onset	Rapid (minutes)	Slow (days/weeks)
Thirst	Absent	Increased
Nausea and vomiting	Absent	Frequent
Vision	Double	Dim
Respirations	Normal	Difficult, hyperventilation
Skin	Moist, pale	Hot, dry, flushed
Tremors	Frequent	Absent
Blood pressure	Normal	Hypotension

Causes of Hyperglycemic Ketoacidotic Coma

Absolute Insulin Deficiency

Newly presenting type 1 diabetes with β-cell depletion
Incorrect insulin dosage (omitted or decreased)

Relative Insulin Deficiency

Stress states
Infection
Myocardial infarction
Trauma
Cerebrovascular accident

Drugs and Endocrine Disorders

Steroids
Adrenergic agonists
Hyperthyroidism
Pheochromocytoma
Thiazide diuretics

rary insulin deficiency may be caused by infection or stressful situations in which there is an increase in secretion of antiinsulin hormones (i.e., glucagon, cortisol, and catecholamines; see Causes of Hyperglycemic Ketoacidotic Coma). Failure to eat, therefore mistakenly decreasing the person's insulin dose, often compounds the situation. Infection is the most common precipitating factor and is present in more than 50% of all persons with diabetic ketoacidotic coma.

A series of biochemical events explains the basis of severe ketoacidosis, and signs and symptoms are presented in Table 41–5. Clear guidelines on maintaining control should be provided to the diabetic client with intercurrent infection to clear the infection early (see Guidelines for Maintaining Glycemic Control in Persons with Diabetes Mellitus).

Treatment of diabetic ketoacidosis requires hospitalization to restore the disturbed metabolic fluid and electrolyte state to normal. Fluid (salt and water) rehydration, insulin, potassium, broad-spectrum antibiotic therapy, and treatment of precipitating factors are the main elements of diabetic coma treatment.

TABLE 41–5

PRESENTING FEATURES OF SEVERE DIABETIC KETOACIDOSIS

Features	Possible Causes
Symptoms	
Thirst	Dehydration
Polyuria	Hyperglycemia, osmotic diuresis
Fatigue	Dehydration, protein loss
Weight loss	Dehydration, protein loss, catabolism
Anorexia	*
Nausea, vomiting	Ketones,* gastric stasis, ileus
Abdominal pain	Gastric stasis,* ileus, electrolyte deficiency*
Muscle cramps	Potassium deficiency*
Signs	
Hyperventilation	Acidemia
Dehydration	Osmotic diuresis, vomiting
Tachycardia	Dehydration
Hypotension	Dehydration, acidemia
Warm, dry skin	Acidemia (peripheral vasodilation)
Hypothermia	Acidemia-induced peripheral vasodilation (when infection is present)
Impaired consciousness or coma	Hyperosmolality
Ketotic breath	Hyperketonemia (acetone)
Blood Chemistry	
High blood glucose	Insulin deficiency
High blood ketone bodies (glycosuria, ketonuria)	
Low arterial blood pH	Ketone bodies
Low arterial pCO_2	Metabolic acidosis
Normal or low arterial pO_2	Pulmonary arteriovenous shunting*
Low plasma bicarbonate	Metabolic acidosis
Low plasma sodium	Hyperglycemia
Variable plasma potassium	Loss through diuresis, acidemia, dehydration
Leukocytosis	Raised ketone bodies

* Indicates speculated cause or unknown cause.
From Alberti K, Phil D: Diabetic emergencies. In Galloway JA, Potrin JH, Shuman CR, eds: *Diabetes mellitus*, ed 9, Indianapolis, 1988, Lilly Research Laboratories.

Guidelines for Maintaining Glycemic Control in Persons with Diabetes Mellitus

Increase self-monitoring of blood glucose (or urine glucose if blood-monitoring equipment is not available) to four times daily (fasting, before lunch, before evening injection, bedtime).

Test for urine ketones twice daily.

If not eating normally, replace carbohydrate content of meals and snacks with sugar-containing drinks or milk; ensure adequate fluid intake (2 to 3 L/day).

If two preceding blood tests show glucose level greater than 200 mg/dl (11.1 mmol/L), increase the next insulin dose by 4 units (2 short-acting, 2 intermediate).

If two preceding blood tests show glucose levels greater than 200 mg/dl (11.1 mmol/L), increase the next insulin dose by 4 units (2 short-acting, 2 intermediate). If, in addition, the ketone test is positive, increase by 6 units (2 short-acting, 4 intermediate); continue this with each injection.*

If vomiting supervenes or blood glucose is greater than 300 mg/dl plus positive ketones for more than 24 hours, call for urgent medical advice.

* Alternatively, the total daily dose can be given as four equal divided doses of short-acting Regular insulin with carbohydrate taken after each injection. This allows flexibility for increasing insulin, but is necessary only for seriously uncontrolled diabetes with infections.

DISEASE MANAGEMENT

Diet Therapy

Diet remains the hallmark of diabetes therapy, despite therapeutic advances in insulin formulations, delivery systems, and oral medications. Diabetic diets are designed to provide appropriate quantities of food at regular intervals, supply daily caloric requirements to aid in achieving or maintaining desirable body weight, and reduce fat intake to correct an unfavorable lipid profile conducive to atherosclerosis.

In type 2 diabetes, reduction in hyperglycemia is correlated with weight loss. In type 1 diabetes mellitus, nutritional strategies involve monitoring the percentage of carbohydrate (55% to 60% of total calories) to protein (12% to 20% of total calories) intake. Meal planning for diabetics is based on the food exchange lists system of the American Diabetes Association.

Blood-Glucose Monitoring

The most important clinical advance in the management of diabetes mellitus is self-monitoring of blood glucose with small, automated devices. Blood glucose levels can be monitored as needed; however, four times per day is generally recommended. Monitoring is done by placing a small drop of blood on a reagent strip, which is then inserted into the meter. The meter analyzes the glucose concentration and displays a measurement of glucose in millimeter per deciliter of blood. Glycosylated hemoglobin (HbA_{1c}) laboratory tests are used by the physician to determine if long-term (3-month) glycemic control has been attained.

Insulin Therapy

The person with type 1 diabetes has essentially no pancreatic insulin, is unresponsive to oral sulfonylurea hypoglycemic agents, and is ketosis-prone, and therefore, dependent on lifelong administration of exogenous insulin. Approximately 40% of people with type 2 diabetes use insulin to control hyperglycemia, 49% use oral medications, and 10% use a combination of insulin and oral medications.

There are three types of insulin, categorized by time of action:

- Rapid-acting
- Intermediate
- Long-acting

Insulin may be injected subcutaneously with an insulin syringe or a penlike device. Insulin pumps are widely used to deliver a programmed, steady drip of insulin (basal rate) under the skin 24 hours a day. A push of a button on the pump delivers a bolus dose to respond to the number of carbohydrate grams consumed at a meal. Table 41–6 illustrates insulin types that may be used alone or in combination. Dosages, frequency, and times of administration are dependent on several factors:[8]

- Prescribed treatment program
- Lifestyle
- Exercise
- Food intake
- Dietary habits
- Certain medications
- Trauma
- Infection
- Physical stress
- Emotional stress
- Pregnancy
- Hyperthyroidism
- Hyperpituitarism[8]

Various factors influence insulin treatment regimens:

- Client's ability to detect and counter-regulate hypoglycemia
- Client's capacity to comply with diet, exercise, self-monitoring of blood glucose, and insulin regimen guidelines
- Client's educational level, lifestyle, and home support system
- Client's endogenous insulin secretory status, including type of diabetes (type 1 or type 2)
- Client's age and weight (including degree of ponderosity [weight] and growth status)
- Concurrent medical conditions, including pregnancy
- Client's pharmacodynamic response to or ability to use specific types of insulin or insulin prescriptions
- Availability of competent professional supervision

TABLE 41–6 TYPES OF INSULIN PREPARATIONS

Type	Onset of Action	Peak Effect (hr)	Duration (hr)
Rapid			
Regular or crystalline	15 min	2–3	5–7
Semi lente	30 min	3–6	12–16
Intermediate			
NPH	3 hr	6–10	18–24
Globin zinc	3 hr	8–12	18–24
Lente	3 hr	8–12	18–24
Prolonged			
Protamine zinc (PZI)	3.5 hr	14–20	30–36
Ultra lente	3.5 hr	16–18	36

Oral Drug Therapy

When type 2 control of hyperglycemia is not achieved with diet and exercise, oral drug therapy is prescribed by the physician:

- *Sulfonylureas* such as glyburide or glipizide stimulate the pancreas to increase insulin production and, therefore, may cause weight gain and hypoglycemia.
- Metformin (Glucophage) decreases the amount of glucose secreted by the liver. Hypoglycemia is not a side effect, but this medication usually decreases appetite. Metformin is contraindicated with several other medications commonly prescribed for diabetic conditions.
- Acarbose (Precose) inhibits enzymes in the small intestines, which are responsible for the digestion of starchy food, thus delaying carbohydrate metabolism.
- Thiazolidinedione (Actos, Avandia) is used for individuals with type 2 diabetes treated with insulin whose hyperglycemia is not adequately controlled. These drugs, sometimes referred to as "insulin reducers," make the body more sensitive to insulin. Target cell response to insulin is improved, thus reducing insulin dosages.[9] Liver problems associated with Rezulin, now off the market, are not associated with Actos and Avandia.
- Repaglinide (Prandin) helps to put more insulin into the bloodstream. It is prescribed for persons taking Glucophage who still do not have good diabetic control.

DENTAL HYGIENE PROCESS OF CARE

Well-controlled diabetes occurs when the client's blood glucose is within the normal range as a result of a careful balance of medication, diet, and exercise. Clients with well-controlled diabetes can be treated safely, provided that their daily routine is not affected. Diabetics with well-controlled disease have a reduced incidence of dental caries.

Infections of any type can cause a profound disturbance of glycemic control, potentially leading to ketoacidosis and diabetic coma. When infection is present, counter-regulatory hormone secretion increases (specifically, that of cortisol and glucagon), leading to hyperglycemia and increased ketogenesis. Infection is the most common precipitating factor for severe ketoacidosis. In the client with poorly controlled diabetes, phagocytic function is impaired and resistance to infection decreased.[10] Prevention of oral diseases and infections is critical to the diabetic control of the client, and poor diabetic control may aggravate the oral disease status.

Several unmet human needs relate to dental hygiene care for individuals with diabetes. For example, emotional stress induced by a dental appointment causes the release of epinephrine, which mobilizes glucose from glycogen stored in the liver. Stress, therefore, can contribute to a hyperglycemic condition becoming ketoacidotic. Periods of waiting and treatment time should be minimized to meet the client's need for freedom from stress.

Diabetes in people on intensive regimens of multiple insulin injections and daily self-monitoring of blood glucose may abruptly become uncontrolled as a result of an active periodontal infection. When unrecognized, the periodontal infection may cause the human needs for skin and mucous membrane integrity and protection from health risks to become compromised. Table 41–7 reflects some unmet human needs and their effect on outcomes of self-monitoring of blood glucose. Figures 41–2 and 41–3, which occur later in the chapter, show clinical examples of periodontal disease in diabetics.

Assessment

HEALTH HISTORY. In taking the health history, the dental hygienist questions the client regarding the signs and symptoms of ketoacidosis (see Warning Signs of Diabetes) to determine an undiagnosed diabetic condition.[11] High-risk factors for developing diabetes include the following:

- Age over 45 years (incidence of diabetes increases with age)
- Diabetic family members (parent, brother, or sister)
- Seriously overweight for age group
- Females who have had high-birthweight babies (i.e., 9 or more pounds)
- Little or no daily exercise
- African-American, Hispanic-American, Pacific Islander, or Native-American ethnicity
- Impaired glucose tolerance
- Symptoms of an expanding waistline, elevated levels of triglycerides, and tendency toward hypertension

Among the aging, classic symptoms do not usually manifest. Rather, clinical findings are related to chronic complications of the disease, such as vascular disorders or neuropathic syndromes.

TABLE 41–7 SOME UNMET HUMAN NEEDS OF PERSONS WITH DIABETES AND THE EFFECT ON OUTCOMES OF SELF-MONITORING OF BLOOD GLUCOSE

Unmet Human Need	Client's Feeling	Example: Client's Behavioral Response
Protection from health risks	I want to be 100% okay.	Seeking perfection; therefore, records results as 100% okay.
Responsibility for oral health	I want you to be pleased, proud.	Seeking approval; therefore, "I'll give you information that makes you pleased or proud."
	I want to be in charge.	Seeking independence; therefore, "I'll give you records that show what I want you to see."
	I don't want you to punish me.	Avoiding punishment; therefore, "I'll give you records so that you think I don't deserve punishment."
	I don't want you to question or accuse me.	Avoiding confrontation and criticism; therefore, "I'll give you records that encourage you to leave me alone."
Conceptualization and understanding	I don't want to hear if I'm good or bad.	Avoiding judgment; therefore, "I'll give you records that you won't have to comment about."
	I don't have diabetes.	Expressing denial; therefore, "I'll need no test."
Freedom from anxiety/stress	I don't want to pay attention to diabetes and feel sad.	Avoiding depressions; therefore, "I won't test so that I won't have to face sadness."
	I hate diabetes, or I hate how you make me deal with diabetes.	Expressing resentment or anger; therefore, "I won't do what you ask me to do."
	I cheated.	Expressing guilt; therefore, "I'll hide it."

Adapted from Skyler JS, Reeves ML: Intensive treatment of type I diabetes mellitus. In Olefsky JM, Sherwin RS, eds: *Diabetes mellitus: Management and complications,* New York, 1985, Churchill Livingstone.

If the person is a known diabetic, the client and health history interview should address the following:

- ✦ Date of onset of diabetes
- ✦ Type of diabetes
- ✦ Regularity of appointments with a physician
- ✦ Methods for controlling diabetes (medication, diet, and exercise)
- ✦ Date of last insulin reaction
- ✦ Method of testing diabetic control (blood or urine)
- ✦ Results of testing (trends and day of appointment)
- ✦ Results of last HbA_{1c} test
- ✦ Medication schedule and dosages
- ✦ Complications from diabetes such as diabetic retinopathy or kidney disorders

ORAL ASSESSMENT. Intraoral examination may reveal conditions common in poorly controlled diabetes (Table 41–8):

- ✦ Cheilosis
- ✦ Xerostomia
- ✦ Glossodynia
- ✦ Enlarged salivary glands
- ✦ Increased glucose in saliva
- ✦ Fungal infections such as candidiasis (thrush)
- ✦ Dental caries
- ✦ Periodontal diseases

Diabetes has long been considered an important factor that influences the risk of periodontal diseases. How diabetes affects periodontal health is under investigation.[12] The prevalence and severity of periodontal diseases are increased in individuals with both type 1 (insulin deficient) and type 2 (insulin resistant) forms of diabetes, as compared with nondiabetics. Well-controlled diabetics, as measured by their blood glycated hemoglobin (HbA_{1c} levels less than 9%) levels, have less severe periodontal disease than poorly controlled diabetics (HbA_{1c} greater than 9%). The presence of hyperglycemia contributes to enhanced periodontal inflammation and alveolar bone loss in diabetes. Hyperglycemia progressively glycates body proteins, forming *advanced glycation end products (AGE)*, which stimulate phagocytes to release inflammatory cytokines. These cytokines in turn aggravate inflammatory tissue destruction by activating B or T lymphocytes and producing oxygen-free radicals, which directly damage the tissues (Figure 41–1). Periodontal disease is therefore the sixth complication of diabetes.[13–15] Control of periodontal infection in individuals with diabetes reduces the level of advanced glycation end products in the blood. Periodontal infection control is an integral part of diabetic control (Figure 41–2).[16–19]

Uncontrolled diabetes increases dental caries risk as a result of reduced saliva secretion and increased glucose content of saliva. Other oral complications associated with diabetes may affect nutrition by causing the person to select foods that are easy to chew but nutritionally inadequate.

Diagnosis and Planning

A dental hygiene care plan focuses on the client's unmet human needs and allows the clinician to manage the risks of potential diabetic emergencies, thereby protecting the client from health risks. Appointments should be brief to minimize anxiety and stress and avoid interference with medication and meal or snack schedule. Morning appointments are ideal because most people with diabetes are under best control at this time. An hour to an hour

TABLE 41–8 **ORAL COMPLICATIONS OF DIABETES MELLITUS**

Clinical Signs and Symptoms	Pathophysiology
Salivary and Oral Changes	
Xerostomia	Increased fluid loss
Bilateral, asymptomatic parotid gland swelling with increased salivary viscosity	Increased fatty acid deposition Increased salivary glucose levels Compensatory hypertrophy due to a decrease in saliva production
Increased dental caries, especially in the cervical region	Secondary to xerostomia
Unexplained odontalgia and percussion sensitivity (acute pulpitis)	Pulpal arteritis from microangiopathies
Lingual erosion of anterior teeth*	Complications of anorexia nervosa and bulimia
Periodontal Changes	
Periodontal diseases†	Induction and accumulation of advanced glycation end products (AGE)
Tooth mobility	Degenerative vascular changes
Rapidly progressive pocket formation	Microangiopathies
Gingival bleeding	Local factors
Yellow, soft, rapidly forming calculus	Local factors Decreased granulocytosis
Subgingival polyps	Etiology unknown
Infection and Wound Healing	
Slow wound healing (including periapical lesions after endodontics) and increased susceptibility to infection	Hyperglycemia reduces phagocytic activity Ketoacidosis may delay chemotaxis of granulocytes Vascular changes lead to decreased blood flow Abnormal collagen production
Oral ulcers refractory to therapy, especially in association with a prosthesis	Microangiopathies Neuropathies
Increased incidence and prolonged healing of dry socket	Degenerative vascular changes Postextraction infection
Tongue Changes	
Glossodynia	Neuropathic complications Xerostomia Candidiasis
Flabby tongue and indented lateral borders	Neuropathies leading to decreased muscle tone
Median rhomboid glossitis (glossal central papillary atrophy)	*Candida albicans*
Other Changes	
Opportunistic infections: *Candida albicans* and mucormycosis	Repeated use of antibiotics Compromised immune system
Acetone or diabetic breath (seen when the person is close to a diabetic coma)	Ketoacidotic state
Increased incidence of lichen planus (as high as 30%)	Diabetes mellitus, hypertension, and lichen planus have been called the Grinspan syndrome‡

* Although not a complication of diabetes per se, this pattern is seen when the person wants to maintain the weight-loss aspect of diabetes while ignoring or tolerating the hyperglycemic side effects. The client may not be taking the proper insulin doses and may not be truthful when asked about this.
† This disease is seen in up to 40% of diabetic patients. Adequate periodontal therapy may result in decreased insulin requirements.
‡ This syndrome has been the subject of controversy (Smith MJA: Oral lichen planus and diabetes mellitus: A possible association, *Journal of Oral Medicine* 32(4):110, 1977).
Adapted from Skoczylas LJ et al: Dental management of the diabetic patient, *Compendium of Continuing Education in Dentistry* 9:394, 1988.

and a half after breakfast is best for appointments to avoid the peak action time of medication. Regular (fast-acting) insulin, often taken in the morning or at each meal, peaks within 2 to 3 hours after the injection. Oral hypoglycemic agents do not cause peaks, as does injected insulin.

Therapeutic scaling and periodontal debridement is contraindicated for people in the uncontrolled diabetic condition (Figure 41–3). Clients should be treated in consultation and referred to the physician of record for systemic evaluation. Dental hygiene care should not begin until the diabetic condition is controlled. When planning care, the dental hygienist considers interventions such as:

- Nutritional and dietary analysis (see Chapter 28)
- Fluoride therapy (see Chapter 26)
- Salivary replacement therapy
- Systemic doxycycline therapy prescribed by the dentist[17,18] (see Chapter 24)
- 3-month continued-care intervals[18]
- Collaboration with the physician and certified diabetes educator

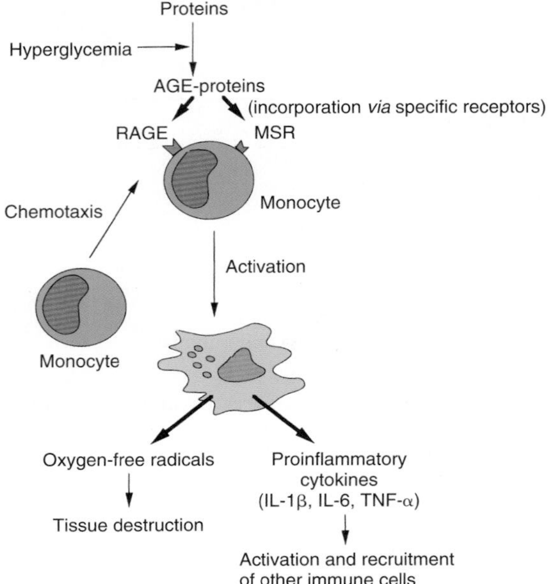

FIGURE 41–1 ✦ Hypothetical model of inflammatory tissue destruction induced by advanced glycation end products in diabetic patients. When body proteins are exposed to a high concentration of glucose for a long time in vivo, they are nonenzymatically glycated and structurally modified. These modified proteins are termed advanced glycation end products (AGE). Monocytes are chemotactic to AGE and take up this protein via specific receptors termed RAGE or MSR. Monocytes thus activated produce oxygen-free radicals that are destructive to tissues and proinflammatory cytokines, which further exaggerate inflammatory tissue destruction. *(From Nishimura F et al:* Periodontal disease as a complication of diabetes mellitus, *Annals of Periodontology 3(1):20, 1998.)*

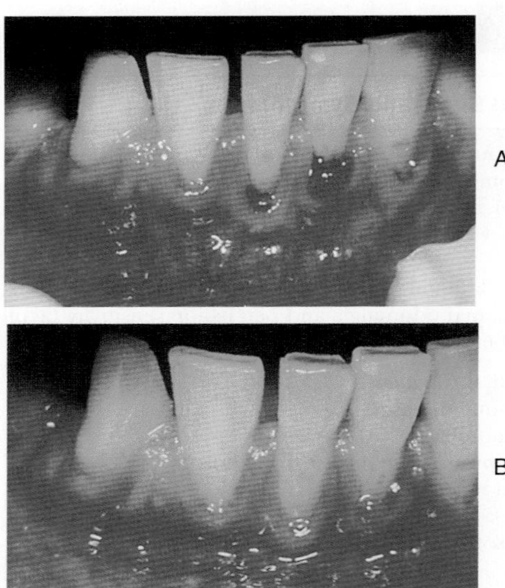

FIGURE 41–2 ✦ Diabetes and periodontal disease. **A,** An adult with diabetes (blood glucose level of 400 mg/100 ml). Note gingival inflammation, spontaneous bleeding, and edema. **B,** Same patient after 4 days of insulin therapy (glucose level less than 100 mg/100 ml). Gingivae have improved in the absence of professional mechanical therapy. *(From Newman MG, Takei, HH, Carranza FA:* Carranza's clinical periodontology, *ed 9, Philadelphia, 2002, Saunders.)*

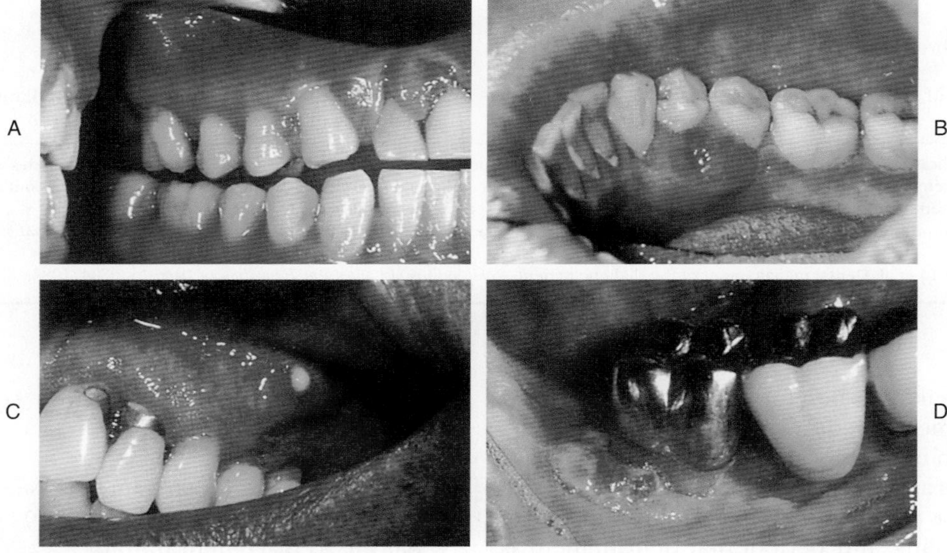

FIGURE 41–3 ✦ Uncontrolled diabetes and periodontal therapy. **A,** An adult with uncontrolled diabetes. Note enlarged, smooth red gingiva with initial enlargement in the anterior area. **B,** Same patient. Note the inflamed, enlarged area around teeth nos. 27–30. **C,** Suppurating abscess, facial or maxillary cleft area in a person with uncontrolled diabetes. **D,** Delayed healing around no. 31 in an adult with uncontrolled diabetes 7 weeks after surgery. *(From Newman MG, Takei HH, Carranza FA:* Carranza's clinical periodontology, *ed 9, Philadelphia, 2002, Saunders.)*

Alterations in Dental Hygiene Care of Older Adults with Diabetes

Potential Risk Relating to Dental Hygiene Care
In uncontrolled diabetic older adult:
- Infection
- Poor wound healing

In older adult treated with insulin:
- Insulin reaction

In diabetic older adult:
- Early onset of complications relating to cardiovascular system, eyes, kidney, nervous system, angina, myocardial infarction, cerebrovascular accident, renal failure, peripheral neuropathy, blindness, hypertension, congestive heart failure

Prevention of Medical Complications
Detection by:
- Health history
- Clinical findings
- Screening blood sugar

Referral for medical diagnosis
Older adult receiving insulin:
- Prevent insulin reaction
- Advise older adults to eat normal meals before appointments
- Schedule appointments in morning or midmorning
- Advise older adults to inform you of any symptoms of insulin reaction when they first occur
- Have sugar in some form to give in case of insulin reaction

Older adults with diabetes being treated with insulin who develop oral infection may require increase in insulin dosage; consult with physician in addition to local and systemic aggressive management of infection
Drug considerations
- Insulin: insulin reaction
- Hypoglycemic agents: on rare occasions, aplastic anemia, etc.
- In severe diabetics, avoid general anesthesia

Dental Hygiene Care Plan Modifications
In well-controlled diabetic older adults, no alteration of dental hygiene care plan is indicated unless complications of diabetes are present, such as:
- Hypertension
- Congestive heart failure
- Myocardial infarction
- Angina
- Renal failure

Oral Complications
Accelerated periodontal disease
Periodontal abscesses
Oral ulcerations and opportunistic infections
Numbness, burning, or pain in oral tissues
Xerostomia
Glossodynia
Prolonged healing

Data from Little JW, Falace DA: *Dental management of the medically compromised patient,* ed 4, St Louis, 1993, Mosby; prepared by Pamela P Brangan, BSDH, MPH, MS.)

A sample dental hygiene care plan is in the Critical Thinking Exercises section. Other management concerns are shown in Alterations in Dental Hygiene Care of Older Adults with Diabetes.

Implementation

THERAPEUTIC SCALING AND PERIODONTAL DEBRIDEMENT. Gingival and periodontal diseases associated with systemic factors, as found in persons with diabetes, may not respond well to subgingival scaling, periodontal debridement, and bacterial plaque biofilm control. However, removal of hard and soft deposits and toxic elements from crown and root surfaces of teeth is critical in the prevention of periodontal infection in people with diabetes. Unnecessary tissue manipulation and trauma should be avoided to promote healing and minimize risk of postoperative infection.

Severe periodontitis is associated with increased risk of poor glycemic control; therefore, severe periodontitis may be a risk factor in the progression of diabetes. Also, evidence suggests that antimicrobial treatment, specifically systemic tetracycline, has the potential to reduce glycated hemoglobin levels in diabetic clients. Doxycycline should be considered in lieu of tetracycline because it is not metabolized in the kidney, which can be problematic in some diabetics.

The increase in the glucose content in GCF may result in altered plaque microflora influencing the development of periodontal disease and dental caries. The short-term response (i.e., probing depths, attachment levels, subgingival microbiota) of diabetics to nonsurgical periodontal therapy (NSPT) appears to be equivalent to the response of nondiabetic clients; however, poorly controlled diabetic clients have more rapid recurrence of deep pockets and a compromised long-term response. At five years after nonsurgical and surgical periodontal treatment in combination with regular periodontal maintenance therapy, diabetic clients who were well controlled had clinical attachment levels similar to those of nondiabetic clients.[10] (See the AAP position paper for a more comprehensive review of periodontal disease and diabetes mellitus).

A well-controlled diabetic with no evidence of infection does not require prophylactic antibiotic premedication.[20,21] In fact, antibiotic use in diabetic persons may lead to oral or systemic fungal infections. If an infection is present, preoperatively or postoperatively, antibiotic therapy is mandatory. Prophylactic antibiotic premedication prior to periodontal instrumentation should be considered following consultation with the client's physician (see Chapter 9).

Diabetic microangiopathy causes blindness and kidney disease. Therefore, a client exhibiting eye disorders also may suffer from kidney disease. Medications that are excreted renally may be retained in the body of the diabetic client with kidney disease, causing toxic effects. When administering local anesthetics, minimal use of vasoconstrictors is required because epinephrine is capable of raising blood glucose.

Evaluation

The periodontal tissues of the client with well-controlled diabetes respond positively to nonsurgical periodontal therapy. Delayed healing, however, may indicate hyperglycemia, which decreases the normal healing actions of leukocyte phagocytosis, chemotaxis, and adherence properties.

Client Education Issues

- ✦ Relate the diabetic's greater risk of infection and increased healing times to the need for good oral hygiene.
- ✦ Teach the client to use daily subgingival irrigation for target delivery of antimicrobial agents to reduce potentially pathogenic microorganisms.
- ✦ Inform clients about the maintenance of the dentition for chewing good foods, because diet and nutrition are essential in the control of diabetes.
- ✦ Emphasize that individuals with diabetes may not tolerate dentures well because of oral conditions.
- ✦ Stress meticulous oral home care as a method to control oral disease progression and diabetes. Outcomes of dental hygiene care contribute significantly to the long-term systemic health of the diabetic client.

Legal, Ethical, and Safety Issues

- ✦ Collaboration with the physician should follow periodontal instrumentation when healing is delayed. The oral health educator/promoter may find a very receptive and interested co-therapist in the certified diabetes educator (CDE) or health education consultant. Many hospitals interested in marketing via a community service are developing diabetes centers. The dental hygienist can provide these centers with expertise in oral disease prevention, client education, and oral health screenings and referrals to reduce the threat that infection poses to the individual with diabetes.
- ✦ Therapeutic scaling and periodontal debridement are contraindicated in persons with uncontrolled diabetes mellitus.
- ✦ When administering local anesthetics, minimal use of vasoconstrictors is required because epinephrine is capable of raising blood glucose.
- ✦ A well-controlled diabetic with no evidence of infection does not require prophylactic antibiotic premedication.

Key Concepts

- ✦ Many people with diabetes do not know they have the condition.
- ✦ Type 1 diabetes involves about 15% of the diabetic population. These individuals need to take insulin injections.
- ✦ The presence of certain human leukocyte antigens (HLAs) creates a genetic predisposition for the autoimmune cause for type 1 diabetes mellitus.
- ✦ Type 2 diabetes involves about 85% of the diabetic population. These individuals usually respond to weight reduction, dietary management, exercise, or oral medications.
- ✦ Insulin resistance or a defect in insulin secretion is the cause of type 2 diabetes. The risk of developing type 2 diabetes increases with age, inactivity, history of gestational diabetes mellitus (GDM), hypertension, and dyslipidemia.
- ✦ GDM occurs in 4% of pregnancies. Those at high risk include women with obesity, family history of diabetes, and previous GDM.
- ✦ GDM usually disappears after birth because the condition is a consequence of the normal antiinsulin effects of pregnancy hormones and the diversion of natural glucose to the child.
- ✦ Without insulin, glucose remains in the blood (hyperglycemia) rather than being stored or used by the cells to produce energy. The suspicion of diabetes is gleaned from the history of symptoms: glucosuria, polyuria, polydipsia, weight loss, polyphagia, and blurred vision.
- ✦ Diabetes mellitus causes severe multisystem, long-term complications. Kidney and eye diseases predominate in type 1 diabetes mellitus; atherosclerosis predominates in type 2; peripheral nerve disease occurs in both.
- ✦ Hypoglycemia, the most common emergency in persons with type 1 diabetes mellitus, results from an excess of insulin and a deficiency of glucose.
- ✦ Hyperglycemic ketoacidosis requires hospitalization to correct fluid and electrolyte imbalances.
- ✦ Infection (oral infection) is the most common precipitating factor of hyperglycemic ketoacidosis.
- ✦ Well-controlled diabetes occurs when the individual's blood glucose is within the normal range as a result of a careful balance of medication diet and exercise.
- ✦ Emotional stress (induced in the oral healthcare setting) causes a release of epinephrine, which mobilizes glucose in the body, contributing to a hyperglycemic condition becoming ketoacidotic.
- ✦ Strict application of oral care protocols will increase the chances of achieving good clinical outcomes for the individual with diabetes.

Critical Thinking Exercises

1. Use the Internet to find information on the link between periodontal disease and diabetes that can be used to educate clients with diabetes mellitus.
2. Review the emergency kit in your oral care facility. What in the emergency kit would you use if the diabetic client you were treating became disoriented and confused, and reported that he took his insulin but did not have time to eat breakfast?
3. Go to the local pharmacy and purchase glucose tablets that can be kept in the treatment areas. When might these glucose tablets be used?
4. Read the following scenario and dental hygiene care plan. Use this information to answer the questions that follow it.

Dental Hygiene Care Plan: Client with Diabetes

Bettie Douman is a 40-year-old professional secretary at a large university. She has had type 1 diabetes mellitus for 20 years. Bettie has been using the insulin pump for 2 years, which has greatly lowered her blood glucose levels. Her 24-hour blood sugar test results average 180 ml/dl and 3-month HgA_{1c} was 8%. Bettie walks the family dog at a fast pace every evening for 30 minutes. She is embarrassed that she has not been as careful about eating a nutritionally balanced diet in the last year and a half. On examination, the dental hygienist notes low risk for dental caries, generalized moderate gingival bleeding on probing, with localized 4- and 5-mm pocket depths in the molar areas.

What changes would you make, if any, in this overall dental hygiene care plan?

What emergency would you most likely prepare for when treating this client? What steps would you take to prevent this emergency?

Develop a detailed self-care plan for this client.

Dental Hygiene Diagnosis	Goal/Expected Behavior
Unmet need for conceptualization and understanding	By 12/1, client explains the role of bacterial plaque biofilm in causing periodontal disease. By 12/1, client verbalizes the role of oral infection in glycemic control.
Unmet need for responsibility for oral health	By 1/1, client decreases bleeding points by 75%. Client reports improvement in hyperglycemia through the control of periodontal disease.

Dental Hygiene Interventions

1. Present “bleeding gums” as an indicator of a bacterial infection that further complicates glycemic control; explain diabetes as a risk factor for periodontal disease.
2. Demonstrate bacterial plaque biofilm control measures.
3. Demonstrate value of oral antimicrobial agents for control of inflammation and technique for application.
4. Scale, root debride with ultrasonic instrumentation.
5. Consult with dentist regarding possible systemic doxycycline therapy.
6. Monitor oral health behavior through frequent evaluation.
7. Schedule follow-up evaluation of tissue response.

Evaluative Statements

1. Client explains the interrelationships of diabetic control and periodontal/gingival infection.
2. Client demonstrates oral health behavior congruent with the maintenance of glycemic control.
3. Client decreases gingival bleeding by 75% to enhance glycemic control.

Dental Hygiene Diagnosis	Goal/Expected Behavior
Unmet need for skin and mucous membrane integrity of the head and neck (undernutrition and increased frequency of carbohydrate consumption)	By 2/1, client verbalizes the need for adequate nutrition. By 2/1, client participates in dietary counseling. By 4/1, client increases nutrients in diet.

Dental Hygiene Interventions

1. Relate nutritional needs in terms of both diabetes control and integrity of periodontium.
2. Relate frequency of meals and snacks to need for bacterial plaque biofilm control.
3. Relate importance of healthy dentition and periodontium to optimal diet consumption and glycemic control.
4. Design bacterial plaque biofilm control measures consistent with frequency of carbohydrate consumption.
5. Referral to certified diabetes educator for design of a dietary prescription and meal planning.

Evaluative Statements

1. Client reports normal blood glucose levels.
2. Client indicates compliance with individual dietary prescription and meal plan.

For References, Suggested Readings, and Related Websites, visit
http://evolve.elsevier.com/Darby/hygiene/

CHAPTER 42

PERSONS WITH RESPIRATORY DISEASES

OBJECTIVES

Mastery of the content in this chapter will enable the reader to:

- Identify the risk factors, signs and symptoms, related medications, and dental hygiene care implications for the following respiratory diseases: asthma, chronic bronchitis, emphysema, and tuberculosis
- Explain the oral/systemic link between periodontal disease and respiratory conditions

KEY TERMS

Asthma
Blue bloater
Candidiasis
Cavitation
Chronic bronchitis
Chronic obstructive pulmonary disease (COPD)
Dyspnea
Emphysema
Nosocomial pneumonia
Pneumonia
Status asthmaticus
Tuberculosis

Respiratory diseases are common among the general population and can compromise dental and dental hygiene care. To properly manage this group of clients, it is important for the dental hygienist to understand respiratory diseases, medications used in their treatment, their link with periodontal health and oral hygiene, and their implications for dental hygiene care.

The most frequently encountered respiratory diseases are asthma and chronic obstructive pulmonary disease (COPD), including emphysema and chronic bronchitis. In addition, tuberculosis, a disease that has afflicted mankind for centuries, continues to be a worldwide problem. The emergence of multidrug resistant strains of tuberculosis poses yet another infection control and treatment challenge to healthcare providers.[1,2]

RESPIRATORY DISEASES

Asthma

Asthma is a chronic inflammatory respiratory disease characterized by an increased responsiveness of the airways to various stimuli. Asthma is classified as mild, moderate, or severe based on the severity and occurrence of airflow obstruction symptoms, tolerance to exercise, and nighttime symptoms.[3]

ETIOLOGY. Various substances or environmental factors can precipitate an asthmatic attack, including specific antigens such as pollen, ragweed, molds, and house dust mites. Chemical irritants such as tobacco smoke and house sprays may trigger an asthmatic attack. Other nonspecific stimulators—environmental pollutants and irritants, exercise, cold air, and emotional stress—also can cause an attack. Generalized narrowing of bronchi and bronchioles caused by mucosal inflammation, increased secretions, and smooth muscle contraction produce asthmatic symptoms.[4,5]

SIGNS AND SYMPTOMS. Clinical manifestations of asthma include periodic wheezing, *dyspnea* (difficulty in breathing), coughing, and chest tightness. These and other signs and symptoms are listed in Signs and Symptoms of an Acute Asthmatic Attack. The onset of an asthmatic attack usually begins with mild wheezing and coughing, progressing to increased difficulty in breathing. As the attack

Signs and Symptoms of an Acute Asthmatic Attack

Wheezing
Cough
Nasal flaring
Dyspnea
Feeling of pressure or tightness in the chest
Need to sit upright or lean forward
Increased anxiety and apprehension
Perspiration
Respiratory rate of more than 30 rpm
Increased pulse rate of more than 120 bpm
Rise in blood pressure (particularly in severe attacks)
Confusion
Agitation

develops, the individual may experience a sense of pressure or tightness in the chest and a feeling of suffocation. A severe asthmatic attack that does not respond to treatment with an adequate dosage of commonly used bronchodilators is referred to as *status asthmaticus*. This condition may produce bronchospasms for hours or days without remission, and often requires hospitalization.

IMPLICATIONS FOR DENTAL HYGIENE CARE. To prevent an acute asthmatic attack and to address the unique needs of the asthmatic client, the dental hygienist should do the following:

- Assess the frequency, time of onset, and type (mild, moderate, or severe) of asthmatic attacks experienced; their management, including the type of medication used and precipitating factors; and whether an attack has warranted emergency treatment.[6, 7]
- Seek a medical consultation in cases of moderate to severe asthma, or reported symptoms suggesting poorly controlled asthma. Document if the client is taking systemic corticosteroids, such as prednisone, for chronic asthma. The physician may want to increase the regular dose of prednisone to prevent an adrenal crisis during a particularly stressful dental appointment.[8]
- Note the precipitating factors reported by the client and avoid these factors during professional care.
- Instruct clients to bring the medical inhalers prescribed by the physician to every appointment for use in case of an acute attack, or for use prophylactically when chronic moderate to severe disease is present.
- Note that some medications used by asthmatics cause xerostomia (dry mouth) and unpleasant taste sensation after inhalation use. Consequently, the asthmatic client may be more prone to dental caries and gingivitis. Children in particular may increase their sucrose intake to combat the unpleasant taste from the inhalant. Table 42–1 describes drugs commonly used in the treatment of asthma.
- Instruct the client to avoid drugs listed in Table 42–2 such as aspirin-containing medications, nonsteroidal anti-inflammatory drugs, barbiturates, and narcotics because they can precipitate an attack.
- Avoid use of the air polisher, a power-driven polisher, or an ultrasonic scaler (Table 42–3).
- Use a local anesthetic agent without epinephrine or levonordefrin because some asthmatics are sensitive to the sulfite preservatives present in these anesthetic solutions.[6]
- Make the oral care environment as stress free as possible because anxiety can induce an asthmatic attack for many people, particularly children (see Chapter 32).
- Use nitrous oxide–oxygen analgesia and/or small doses of diazepam, as prescribed by the dentist, to reduce stress if indicated.[6]
- Convey a calm, caring, and compassionate attitude to relax the client and to reduce stress-induced asthmatic attack.
- Evaluate children carefully for malocclusion; many asthmatic children are mouth breathers and a correlation has been observed between posterior cross-bite incidence and mouth-breathing in children.[9]
- Observe any asthmatic symptoms during and after dental procedures, because decreased lung function can be triggered by anxiety, supine positioning, tooth enamel dust, and aerosols commonly created by dental procedures.
- Take prompt action to manage symptoms of an acute asthmatic episode (Procedure 42–1).[10–12]
- Set goals with the client to achieve meticulous home care to combat negative effects of medication and mouth breathing on oral health.

Chronic Obstructive Pulmonary Disease

Chronic obstructive pulmonary disease (COPD) is a general term used to describe pulmonary disorders characterized by chronic irreversible obstruction of airflow from the lungs.[4] The two most common diseases classified as COPD are chronic bronchitis and emphysema. Although these two conditions can be described individually, due to the difference in the basis for the obstructed airflow, they often coexist and represent the progression of the disease. Because of the progressive nature of COPD, quality of life is greatly compromised in severe cases.[13]

ETIOLOGY. Cigarette smoking has been identified as the major risk factor in COPD. Air pollutants and industrial dust and fumes may contribute to COPD for cadmium or silica miners, furnace workers, metal molders, and grain farmers.[14,15] Underlying respiratory disease, severe respiratory infection in early childhood, and genetic tendencies can all be risk factors for COPD.[4,16]

Chronic Bronchitis

Bronchitis is as an inflammation of the lining of the bronchial tubes. These tubes or bronchi connecting the

TABLE 42–1
DRUGS COMMONLY USED IN THE TREATMENT OF ASTHMA

Action	Indication	Generic Name	Brand Name	Drug Classification
Anti-inflammatory agents	Inhibit release of agents that trigger asthma by inflammatory cells; taken on a daily basis to achieve and maintain control of asthma	Beclomethasone dipropionate Triamcinolone Flunisolide	Beclovent, Vanceril Azmacort Aerobid	Inhaled synthetic corticosteroids
	Used to speed resolution of airway obstruction and reduce rate of reccurrence of symptoms	Methylprednisolone Prednisone	Medrol Apu-Prednisone, Orasone	Systemic corticosteroids
	To prevent acute bronchospasms	Cromolyn sodium Nedocromil sodium	Intal, Nasalcrom Tilade	Inhaled antiasthmatic, mast cell stabilizer
Bronchodilators	Temporarily dilate or relax the muscles surrounding the bronchial tubes that tighten during an asthma attack	Albuterol Metaproterenol Bitolterol mesylate	Ventolin, Proventil Alupent Tornalate	Short-acting inhaled beta$_2$ adrenergic agonists
	Relax bronchial smooth muscles and inhibit release of mast cell inhibitors	Salmeterol	Serevent Diskus, Glaxo Wellcome	Long-acting beta$_2$ adrenergic agonists
	Provide maintenance regulation of airway smooth muscle tone; may be used instead of beta$_2$ adrenergic agonists when not well tolerated by patient	Ipratropium bromide	Atrovent	Anticholinergic, long-acting bronchodilator
Oral sustained-release tablet/capsule	Used as adjunct to inhaled corticosteroids for prevention of night-time symptoms; relaxes smooth muscles of respiratory system	Theophylline	Slo-Bid, Respbid, Theovent	Methylxanthine
Nonsteroidal preventive therapy	Long-term control and prevention of symptoms in cases of mild persistent asthma in those 12 years or older	Montelukast Zafirlukast Zileuton	Singulair Accolate Zyflo	Selective leukotriene receptor antagonist
Combined medication	Drugs used simultaneously to treat both inflammation and bronchoconstriction (Haveles)	Salmeterol xinafoate and fluticasone propionate	Advair Diskus	Inhaled corticosteroid (salmeterol xinafoate) and long-acting beta$_2$ agonist (fluticasone propionate)

Data from Haveles EB: Advances in the treatment of asthma hold much promise, *Drug Topics* 4S(suppl):11S, 2000; and Gage TW, Pickett FR: *Mosby's dental drug reference*, ed 4, St Louis, 1999, Mosby.

TABLE 42–2
CONTRAINDICATED DRUGS FOR THE INDIVIDUAL WITH ASTHMA

Drugs	Rationale
Aspirin-containing medications	Ingestion of aspirin is associated with precipitating attacks in some clients
Nonsteroidal anti-inflammatory drugs (NSAIDs)	Ingestion of NSAIDs may precipitate asthma attack in some individuals
Barbiturates and narcotics	Association of these drugs with precipitation of asthma attacks
Erythromycin and ciprofloxacin in clients taking theophylline	May result in toxic blood level of theophylline

trachea with the lungs become inflamed and/or infected. As a result, less air is able to flow to and from the lungs and heavy mucus or phlegm is expectorated.[14] Chronic bronchitis is associated with the presence of a mucus-producing cough with expectoration for at least three months of the year for more than two consecutive years, without other underlying disease to explain the cough.[6] Smokers may dismiss symptoms of chronic bronchitis as a "smoker's cough" and avoid medical care. Consequently, the individual may be in danger of developing serious respiratory problems or heart failure. Chronic bronchitis is consistently more prevalent in females than in males and can affect people of all ages, but is usually higher in those over 45 years old.[14]

SIGNS AND SYMPTOMS. Chronic bronchitis symptoms appear gradually, but intensify in individuals who smoke

TABLE 42–3 TECHNIQUES TO BE AVOIDED IN INDIVIDUALS WITH CERTAIN RESPIRATORY DISEASES

Disease	Techniques Contraindicated or Used with Precautions	Rationale
Asthma	Use of air polisher	Aerosols created by air polisher may precipitate asthma attack
	Use of power-driven polisher	Polisher may exacerbate existing breathing problems
	Use of ultrasonic scaler	Pathogens found in bacterial plaque and periodontal pockets may be aspirated into the lungs
COPD: Chronic bronchitis and emphysema	Avoid use of rubber dam	Rubber dam may cause more breathing difficulties
	Use of power-driven polisher	Polisher may exacerbate existing breathing problems
	Use of ultrasonic scaler	Pathogens found in bacterial plaque and periodontal pockets may be aspirated into the lungs
	Nitrous oxide–oxygen analgesia	May produce cessation of respiration (apnea)
Tuberculosis	Use of air polisher	Airborne pathogens of communicable diseases may be transmitted by aerosols emitted by air polisher
	Use of ultrasonic scaler	Airborne pathogens of communicable diseases may be transmitted by aerosols emitted by ultrasonic instrumentation

Procedure 42–1 **MANAGEMENT OF AN ACUTE ASTHMATIC EPISODE**

STEPS	RATIONALE
1. Terminate the dental procedure and remove all materials from client's mouth immediately.	Client may inhale materials during asthma attack.
2. Place the client in a comfortable position as soon as symptoms are apparent—usually sitting with the arms thrown forward over the back of a chair.	This positioning allows for most comfort during acute attack.
3. Try to calm client and allay apprehension.	Anxiety can exacerbate symptoms, producing a "vicious cycle."
4. Evaluate A-B-C (airway-breathing-circulation) and monitor vitals.	Client remains conscious and breathing in most attacks; client usually has increased blood pressure and heart rate.
5. Definitive care:	
a. Administration of bronchodilator (client's prescribed medication preferred).	Bronchodilators are drugs used to manage the bronchospasm of an acute attack.
b. If attack persists, administer oxygen.	Clinical signs of low oxygen levels (confusion, anxiety, cyanosis, hypertension, hypotension, headache) warrant use of supplemental oxygen.
c. Call for emergency assistance if bronchodilators fail to resolve bronchospasm.	Emergency personnel may be needed to transport client to hospital if attack not controlled.
d. Administration of epinephrine if necessary (available in pre-loaded syringe).	Epinephrine may be needed if bronchodilator does not arrest attack.
6. Discharge of the client: alone, escorted, or with emergency personnel, depending on severity of attack.	Client may not be able to leave office without an escort or may need hospitalization if attack is severe.

Adapted from Malamed SF: *Medical emergencies in the dental office,* ed 5, St Louis, 2000, Mosby.

or when atmospheric concentrations of sulfur dioxide and other air pollutants increase. A cough producing large amounts of sputum may linger for several weeks after a winter cold seems to be cured. With time, upper respiratory infections become more serious, and coughing and expectoration of phlegm continue for longer periods after each episode.[14] *Dyspnea* (difficulty breathing) initially is mild and is brought on only by exercise or exertion. Eventually, breathing difficulty becomes more frequent and is brought on with less effort. At this point, other symptoms of respiratory failure will be evident.[4] As the disease progresses and becomes more obstructive, there may be evidence of prolonged expiration and wheezing. Acute attacks of breathing distress with rapid, labored breathing, intensive coughing, and bluish skin can occur; hence, the term *blue bloater* has been used to describe an individual with these symptoms.[16] Heart failure is a common result of advanced chronic bronchitis.[4,16]

Emphysema

Emphysema is a chronic pulmonary disorder in which there is over-inflation of structures in the lungs known as alveoli or air sacs. This over-inflation is caused by a breakdown of the walls of the alveoli, resulting in decreased respiratory function, and often, dyspnea.[14] More prevalent among older men, emphysema is rapidly increasing among women primarily due to tobacco use.[14]

SIGNS AND SYMPTOMS. Emphysema can be localized or generalized. Individuals with localized emphysema may have no symptoms. At the early stage, symptoms of chronic bronchitis with cough and expectoration will predominate. As with chronic bronchitis, dyspnea occurs only with exertion, but gradually over time intensifies in severity and frequency. Some may experience rapid progression of dyspnea and disability, and others will experience a slower progression. Chronic coughing with expectoration, wheezing, recurrent respiratory infection, and fatigue may also be present. In later stages, severe dyspnea, cyanosis, and other signs of respiratory failure may be evident.[4] As with chronic bronchitis, individuals may experience periods of exacerbation of symptoms usually related to infections or other complications.

Physical findings may be normal in cases of mild or localized emphysema. However, in more advanced cases there is usually weight loss and a "barrel-chest" appearance.[4,6] The client may appear short of breath and use accessory respiratory muscles. Many may find it easier to breathe in a sitting position, bent over and resting their elbows on their thighs. Usually, the expiration phase of respiration is prolonged and the client may be breathing against pursed lips. With some individuals, wheezing may be heard on expiration. In advanced stages of emphysema, cyanosis may be evident along with other signs of respiratory failure such as a change in mental state, headache, weakness, and muscle tremor or twitching.[4]

DRUGS COMMONLY USED IN THE TREATMENT OF COPD. Although there is no cure for COPD and medications cannot alter disease progression, they can improve airflow, relieve symptoms, and enhance the quality of life.[13] Antibiotics are often prescribed during the acute attack of symptoms, particularly if there is a bacterial infection present. Bronchodilators such as those used by asthmatics have been commonly used as treatment. These drugs, particularly the $beta_2$ agonists, are fast acting, and in addition to relaxing the bronchial tubes, improve mucous clearance.[4] However, recent studies question the effectiveness of inhaled corticosteroids with COPD clients.[13,15]

Advanced cases of COPD are often treated with a combination of medications. A $beta_2$ agonist along with an anticholinergic may be followed by theophylline as an add-on therapy for clients who have insufficient relief of symptoms. At this stage, many individuals are also on long-term oxygen therapy at home.

Acute exacerbations of COPD may occur every one to two months for some clients, but occur rarely for others. Indications of acute exacerbations include increased coughing, increased quantity or change in the character of the sputum, and increased shortness of breath.[13] Often, fever, an indication of infection, is present. Immediate medical care must be given in these situations and hospitalization may be necessary.[13]

IMPLICATIONS FOR DENTAL HYGIENE CARE. To meet the specialized needs of the individual with chronic obstructive pulmonary disease, the dental hygienist should do the following:

- ✦ Seat the client in a semi-supine or upright chair position.
- ✦ Plan short appointments to decrease stress if client does not tolerate sitting in dental chair for long periods of time.
- ✦ Assess severity, frequency of symptoms, and conditions that exacerbate symptoms.
- ✦ Review the health history for evidence of concurrent heart disease; take appropriate precautions if heart disease is present (see Chapter 40).
- ✦ Assess for ineffective salivary flow related to medication-induced xerostomia.
- ✦ Set goals with the client to initiate a smoking cessation program if applicable.
- ✦ Monitor periodontal status; client is at increased risk for disease if a smoker.
- ✦ Be especially observant of the potential for oral lesions if client is a smoker.
- ✦ Avoid use of a rubber dam if possible, as this may further obstruct respiration. Also avoid use of a power-driven polisher or an ultrasonic scaler (Table 42–3).
- ✦ Offer low-flow (2 to 4 L/min) supplemental oxygen if needed.
- ✦ Avoid nitrous oxide–oxygen inhalation sedation with emphysema (Table 42–3).
- ✦ Suggest low-dose oral diazepam or other benzodiazepine, as prescribed by the dentist, if needed to reduce stress.
- ✦ Be aware that clients taking steroids may need supplementation.
- ✦ Instruct the client to avoid erythromycin, macrolide antibiotics, and ciprofloxacin if client is taking theophylline.
- ✦ Inform clients that outpatient general anesthesia is contraindicated.

Tuberculosis

Tuberculosis (TB), an airborne communicable disease, primarily affects the lungs, but also can attack other organs and tissues.[5,14] TB is one of the oldest diseases known to strike humans and still remains one of the most widespread ailments in the world.[4]

ETIOLOGY. Tuberculosis is caused by *Mycobacterium tuberculosis.* Close contact with persons having TB increases the incidence of disease transmission to others. The following groups are at greatest risk for contracting tuberculosis:

- ✦ Those infected with HIV
- ✦ IV drug abusers
- ✦ Residents and employees of shared habitation settings: prisons, nursing homes, mental institutions, shelters
- ✦ Healthcare workers who care for high-risk individuals

- Immigrants from countries that have a high occurrence of TB
- Medically underserved persons
- High-risk racial or ethnic minority populations

SIGNS AND SYMPTOMS. The diagnosis of tuberculosis is made via an evaluation of several assessments, including a Mantoux tuberculin skin screening, commonly called a PPD (purified protein derivative) test, chest radiograph, sputum culture, and clinical symptoms.[5] TB is usually a chronic infection with various clinical manifestations, depending on the stage and duration of the disease.[4] Persons with primary pulmonary infection often have no clinical evidence of the disease. They test positive on a tuberculin skin test, but do not have active TB and are not infectious. When symptoms are present, they are usually mild, with a low-grade fever, listlessness, loss of appetite, and occasional cough. The most common obvious symptom of active TB is a chronic cough. Other symptoms of disease progression include fever, night sweats, weight loss, central pulmonary necrosis (death of lung tissue) and *cavitation* (hollow spaces in the lungs).[5]

TREATMENT. The treatment of tuberculosis is dependent on whether an individual has active TB or only primary TB infection. Those persons who test positively for TB but do not have the disease may be treated with a preventive therapy. This treatment usually involves a daily dose of isoniazid (also called INH) for six months to a year.[17] Treatment for individuals with active TB may include a short hospital stay along with the concurrent administration of several drugs prescribed for six to nine months. Isoniazid remains the primary drug of choice for these patients along with at least two others that may include rifampin, ethambutol, pyrazinamide, and streptomycin.[5] Multidrug-resistant TB is a dangerous form of tuberculosis often due to low patient compliance. A treatment referred to as "directly observed therapy," which involves observing patients as they take each dose of medication, has been successful in some cases to remedy this problem.[1] It is imperative for patients on a tuberculosis drug therapy regimen to be vigilant about taking medication as it has been prescribed even if symptoms have subsided.[5,6,17]

IMPLICATIONS FOR DENTAL HYGIENE CARE. When considering treatment options for the individual with tuberculosis, the major concern is the risk of disease transmission.[1] Tuberculosis may be transmitted from clients to dental professionals; conversely, if the clinician is infected, clients and other staff members may contract the disease. To prevent disease transmission and meet the needs of the client with tuberculosis, the dental hygienist does the following:

- Judiciously uses universal infection control precautions, keeping in mind that many clients with infectious diseases such as tuberculosis may not be identified during assessments[6]
- Is aware of signs and symptoms of tuberculosis when gathering data through the client's health history
- Questions a client who reports a history of tuberculosis or a positive skin test for tuberculosis, concerning dates and results of chest radiographs, sputum cultures, and physical examinations by his/her physician
- Has a thorough understanding of the type of tuberculosis that the client has reported and determines the current health status of the individual
- Obtains a physician's consultation to determine if it is safe to treat the client outside of a hospital setting; a client with active tuberculosis should be treated in a hospital setting under strict infection control conditions[6]
- During treatment, the clinician should minimize aerosol contamination; use of a rubber dam is recommended
- Avoids use of an air polisher or an ultrasonic scaler (Table 42–3)

RELATIONSHIP BETWEEN PERIODONTAL DISEASE AND RESPIRATORY CONDITIONS

Evidence suggests a relationship between oral infections and lower respiratory conditions.[2] Lower respiratory infections commence when microorganisms from the inner surfaces of the nose and mouth are aspirated or inhaled into the respiratory tract.[18] Bacteria found in the oral cavity can be released from plaque biofilm into the saliva. These salivary secretions also are inhaled, allowing oral bacteria common to respiratory infections to travel (translocate) into the lungs.[2]

Periodontitis is a localized chronic inflammatory disease that results in destruction of supporting bone and connective tissues. In untreated periodontitis, oral pathogens continuously stimulate cells of the oral tissues and periodontium to release a variety of cytokines and other biologically active molecules.[16,19] Cytokines are immune system proteins that act as chemical messengers to stimulate inflammation in the respiratory epithelium. As seen in Figure 42–1, cytokines produced by epithelial and connective tissue cells in response to these bacteria include IL-6, IL-8, and TNF.[19] This release of cytokines increases a person's susceptibility to colonization by respiratory pathogens.[2] Weakened host defense mechanisms allow these bacteria associated with periodontitis to proliferate in the lung, resulting in infection and tissue destruction. Daily oral hygiene reduces the amount of oral bacteria available for translocation and may prevent lower respiratory infection such as pneumonia.[2]

Pneumonia is an acute inflammation of the gas-exchanging units of the lungs. These units include respiratory bronchi, alveolar ducts, alveolar sacs, and alveoli.[4] Bacterial pneumonia can be broadly categorized into two types: community-acquired pneumonia

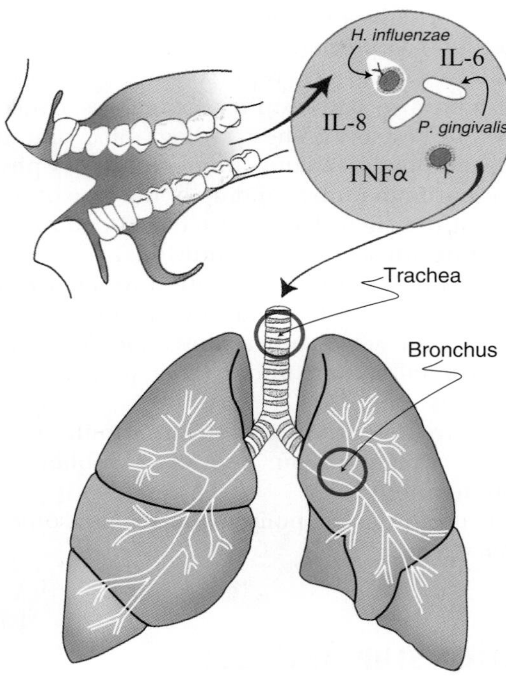

FIGURE 42–1 ✦ Oral bacteria, oral infection, and pneumonia. Bacteria that colonize the supragingival or subgingival dental plaque are shed into the saliva. The saliva is aspirated into the lower respiratory tract (bronchus), where an infection can ensue. Cytokines from periodontally diseased tissues that enter the saliva from the gingival crevicular fluid may be aspirated to stimulate local inflammatory processes that contribute to the initiation or progression of infection in the lung. *(From Scannapieco FA:* Role of bacteria in respiratory infection, *Journal of Periodontology 70:793, 1999.)*

and hospital-acquired pneumonia, also called *nosocomial pneumonia.*[20] Community-acquired pneumonia is most often associated with pathogens that normally reside on the oropharyngeal mucosa, such as *Streptococcus pneumoniae, Haemophilus influenzae, Mycoplasma pneumoniae, Chlamydia pneumoniae, Legionella pneumophila, Candida albicans,* and anaerobic species.[2] In contrast, hospital-acquired pneumonia is caused by a very different spectrum of organisms. These bacteria are not normally found in the oropharynx, but enter this region from the environment. Gram-negative bacilli, including *Escherichia coli, Klebsiella pneumoniae, Serratia* species, *Enterobacter* species, *Pseudomonas aeruginosa,* and *Staphylococcus aureus,* are the most prevalent.[2] Nosocomial pneumonia frequently prolongs hospital stays, increases healthcare costs, and causes death, especially in the elderly and the immunocompromised.[17]

Poor oral health also has been associated with chronic obstructive pulmonary disease, particularly during periods of exacerbation. Some exacerbations are thought to be provoked in part by bacterial infection.[21] Chronically ill patients who are hospitalized or in nursing homes often are unable to carry out proper oral self-care. The lack of attention to oral self-care results in an increase in amounts and complexity of dental plaque biofilm. Researchers have concluded that the teeth and periodontium may serve as reservoirs for respiratory infection.[2]

CLIENT EDUCATION ISSUES

- ✦ Explain that rinsing the mouth with water after using an inhaler will decrease the risk of oral *candidiasis* and dental caries.
- ✦ Explain that the use of a spacer attached to a metered dose inhaler may prevent *candidiasis* in asthmatics.
- ✦ Explain that if the client experiences xerostomia and/or an unpleasant taste following inhalant therapy, the use of sugarless chewing gum will increase salivary flow, minimizing the risks of dental caries and gingivitis.
- ✦ Explain to clients undergoing drug therapy for tuberculosis (primary or active) the importance of compliance. Inconsistent or incomplete therapy may result in multidrug-resistant tuberculosis and/or a longer recovery period.
- ✦ Explain that smoking cessation therapy is one necessary strategy for managing clients with respiratory diseases.

LEGAL, ETHICAL, AND SAFETY ISSUES

- ✦ Acute asthma attacks may occur before, during, and after dental procedures. Dental hygienists must be knowledgeable in the management of such an attack. Avoidance of precipitatory factors is the best risk-management strategy.
- ✦ Clients reporting a history of asthma must have their bronchodilators at each dental appointment for immediate administration if necessary.
- ✦ Clients with active tuberculosis should be treated in a hospital setting to minimize risk of disease transmission to personnel or other clients.

Key Concepts

- Asthma is a respiratory disease characterized by an increased responsiveness of the airways to various stimuli, which causes periodic wheezing, dyspnea, coughing, and chest tightness.
- An asthma attack may be triggered by allergens, anxiety, cold air, or exercise, or no apparent irritant may be involved.
- Many asthma medications have side effects, including oral candidiasis and xerostomia.
- Two major diseases categorized as chronic obstructive pulmonary disease (COPD) are emphysema and chronic bronchitis.
- COPD is most often caused by cigarette smoking, but chronic exposure to occupational and environmental pollutants is also a risk factor contributing to COPD.
- The major risk associated with treating clients with active tuberculosis is disease transmission; clients with active tuberculosis should be treated in a hospital setting only for emergency dental care.
- Patient compliance problems during lengthy drug therapy for tuberculosis have contributed to the problem of multidrug-resistant strains of tuberculosis.
- Recent research has discovered a link between periodontal disease and systemic illnesses such as lower respiratory tract infections.
- Pathogenic bacteria found in dental plaque biofilm may be aspirated into the lungs of a seriously ill patient. These bacteria, along with epithelial changes in lung tissue associated with the inflammatory process, may increase the client's susceptibility to a lower respiratory tract infection.
- Effective daily oral hygiene care reduces the amount of oral bacteria available for aspiration into the lungs and may prevent lower respiratory tract infection such as pneumonia.

Critical Thinking Exercises

Client: Mr. G

Profile: A 5′10″, 18-year-old Caucasian male weighing 175 lb presents for dental hygiene care.

Chief Complaint: "My gums bleed, particularly around my upper front teeth, and I have a dry mouth most of the time, which is very uncomfortable."

Health History: Client's vital signs are: blood pressure of 112/64 mm Hg, pulse rate of 70 bpm, and respiration rate of 14 rpm. Client reports history of asthma for past 10 years, exacerbated by exposure to cats, pollens, and dust. Currently sees physician for acne and a chiropractor for lower back pain. Currently takes doxycycline 100 mg daily for acne and Alupent 650 μg aerosol inhaler (one puff as needed for asthma attack).

Social History: Client is single and lives with parents. He appears very quiet and reserved.

Dental History: Suspected carious lesions on occlusal surfaces of teeth # 2, 3, 15, & 31

Gingival evaluation reveals slight gingival enlargement and rolled margins throughout with moderately enlarged, erythematous gingiva and bulbous papillae in the maxillary anterior facial region. Pocket depths 3 mm or less throughout, except in maxillary anterior and posterior molar regions where some 4–5 mm pockets were noted.

Oral Health Behavior Assessment: Client brushes twice daily but does not floss. Moderate plaque biofilm throughout on the gingival third of teeth and interproximal surfaces.

Supplemental Notes: Smokes one pack of cigarettes per week.

1. What are the dental hygiene diagnoses for this client?
2. Develop a dental hygiene care plan for this client that includes goals and interventions.
3. What client education issues should be addressed?
4. What factors could be contributing to this client's periodontal health?
5. Are there any contraindications to this client's care?
6. What measures should be taken during treatment to prevent an asthmatic attack?

For References, Suggested Readings, and Related Websites, visit
http://evolve.elsevier.com/Darby/hygiene/

CHAPTER 43

PERSONS WITH CANCER

OBJECTIVES

Mastery of the content in this chapter will enable the reader to:

- Discuss cancer risk factors.
- Identify the general signs and symptoms of cancer.
- Describe the psychological responses related to cancer.
- Discuss the benefits of oral hygiene care prior to cancer therapy.
- List reasons for an oral evaluation prior to cancer therapy.
- List the common signs of oral cancer.
- Describe the types of oral cancer treatment and the management of the oral complications.
- Develop a dental hygiene care plan for clients before, during, and after cancer therapy.

KEY TERMS

Allogeneic bone marrow transplant
Benign tumor
Bone marrow–blood transplantation
Cancer
Carcinogenic
Chemotherapy
Dysphagia
End-stage disease
Erythroplakia
Graft versus host disease
Immunosuppression
Leukoplakia
Malignant neoplasm
Metastasize
Mucositis
Myelosuppression
Neurotoxicity
Oncologist
Oncology
Osteoradionecrosis
Peripheral blood stem cells
Radiation caries
Radiation therapy
Simulation appointment
Squamous cell carcinoma
Telangiectasia
Thrombocytopenia
Xerostomia

Cancer is not a single disease, but a broad classification of more than one hundred types of disease. The common element in *cancer* is the abnormal and unrestricted growth of cells that can invade and destroy surrounding normal body tissues, sometimes spreading to other parts of the body. The difference between a malignant and a benign neoplasm is that a *benign tumor* is usually circumscribed and encapsulated, usually grows slowly, and is composed of cells that resemble the tissue from which it arises. A *malignant neoplasm* or cancer not only infiltrates locally but also has the potential to *metastasize* or spread to distant sites. The cells are usually atypical or dysplastic and may not resemble the parent tissue.

CANCER

Incidence

Figure 43–1 lists the leading sites of new cancer cases and deaths according to the American Cancer Society 2001 Estimates.[1] Estimates for cancers of the oral cavity, pharynx, and larynx by site and sex were 28,200 for men and 11,900 for women. Of these, 8200 men and 3600 women were expected to die from these cancers.

Although cancer is rare in children, it is the chief cause of death by disease in children under age 15.[1] The most common sites include the blood and bone marrow (leukemia), bone, lymph nodes (lymphoma), brain, sympathetic nervous system (neuroblastoma), kidneys

Leading Sites of New Cancer Cases* and Deaths—2001 Estimates

Cancer Cases by Site and Sex: Male	Cancer Cases by Site and Sex: Female	Cancer Deaths by Site and Sex: Male	Cancer Deaths by Site and Sex: Female
Prostate 198,100 (31%)	Breast 192,200 (31%)	Lung and bronchus 90,100 (31%)	Lung and bronchus 67,300 (25%)
Lung and bronchus 90,700 (14%)	Lung and bronchus 78,800 (13%)	Prostate 31,500 (11%)	Breast 40,200 (15%)
Colon and rectum 67,300 (10%)	Colon and rectum 68,100 (11%)	Colon and rectum 27,700 (10%)	Colon and rectum 29,000 (11%)
Urinary bladder 39,200 (6%)	Uterine corpus 38,300 (6%)	Pancreas 14,100 (5%)	Pancreas 14,800 (6%)
Non-Hodgkin's lymphoma 31,100 (5%)	Non-Hodgkin's lymphoma 25,100 (4%)	Non-Hodgkin's lymphoma 13,800 (5%)	Ovary 13,900 (5%)
Melanoma of the skin 29,000 (5%)	Ovary 23,400 (4%)	Leukemia 12,000 (4%)	Non-Hodgkin's lymphoma 12,500 (5%)
Oral cavity 20,200 (3%)	Melanoma of the skin 22,400 (4%)	Esophagus 9,500 (3%)	Leukemia 9,500 (4%)
Kidney 18,700 (3%)	Urinary bladder 15,100 (2%)	Liver 8,900 (3%)	Uterine corpus 6,600 (2%)
Leukemia 17,700 (3%)	Pancreas 15,000 (2%)	Urinary bladder 8,300 (3%)	Brain 5,900 (2%)
Pancreas 14,200 (2%)	Thyroid 14,900 (2%)	Kidney 7,500 (3%)	Stomach 5,400 (2%)
All sites 643,000 (100%)	All sites 625,000 (100%)	All sites 286,100 (100%)	All sites 267,300 (100%)

*Excludes basal and squamous cell skin cancers and in situ carcinomas except urinary bladder.

FIGURE 43–1 ✦ American Cancer Society incidence and deaths by site and sex, 2001 estimates. *(From the American Cancer Society:* Cancer Facts and Figures, 2000, *2001, American Cancer Society.)*

(Wilms' tumor), and soft tissues (rhabdomyosarcoma). Mortality rates have declined by 57% since the early 1970s due to improved diagnostics and advances in treatment and supportive care.

The branch of medicine that studies and treats cancer is called *oncology,* and the physician specialist is an *oncologist.* When cancers are left untreated, they result in significant morbidity and death. In the United States, only heart disease causes more deaths in adults.[1]

Risk Factors

Carcinogenic, or cancer-causing, influences may be both environmental and genetic. The National Cancer Institute implicates tobacco as the single major cause of preventable cancer deaths. Other environmental carcinogenic agents are alcohol, chemicals, radiation, sunlight, hormones, and asbestos. There is evidence that certain viruses are linked to the development of cancers, especially cancers of the liver, nasopharynx, cervix, and lymphatic system.

Common Signs and Symptoms

In early stages, most cancers exhibit no symptoms. Early Signs and Symptoms of Cancer lists the most common presenting signs and symptoms of early cancer, which vary depending on the type of cancer.

Pain is not often a symptom in early stages of cancer. A person who has one of the seven common signs of cancer for longer than two weeks should see a doctor promptly.

Psychosocial and Developmental Responses to a Cancer Diagnosis

A medical diagnosis of cancer immediately presents a major disruption of life and threat of loss: loss of life from the disease, and loss of control, self-esteem, and

Early Signs and Symptoms of Cancer

Change in bowel or bladder habits
A sore that does not heal
Unusual bleeding or discharge
Thickening or lump in breast or elsewhere
Indigestion or difficulty in swallowing
Obvious change in a wart or mole
Nagging cough or hoarseness

From the American Cancer Society.

function from the treatment of the disease. The acute emotional reaction is one of turmoil, shock, and disbelief. Concerns about trauma to the family, loss of work, and drain on finances cause additional anxiety.

Individuals with cancer enter a grieving process with manifestations not unlike those of a person undergoing bereavement, grieving for loss of their own lives and lifestyles. Common psychological manifestations resulting from a cancer diagnosis include denial, anger, anxiety, depression, and hopelessness. Some of these stages are an important part of the person's coping mechanism. Denial can initially serve to save and protect psychological integrity. Anger often is a signal that the individual desires to fight to stay alive and is attempting to regain the control that was lost with the initial diagnosis. These reactions must be respected by the healthcare professional and allowed to surface and to be expressed at appropriate levels.

Persons in all stages of the life cycle experience the aforementioned stages, but different age groups may have varied reactions. Older adults sometimes are resigned to a life-threatening diagnosis and may resist treatment. Some enter a significant depression because of the fear that they will become a physical and financial burden on their loved ones. Adult men may resent their loss of control and the loss of their role as caretaker and provider; this may be the first time in their adult lives when someone else assumes care of their needs, which produces guilt and loneliness. Younger persons may express more anger and resentment than older people express, and may feel threatened by loss of career, sexuality, and family. Children have varied responses according to their age. Children younger than 5 years of age fear abandonment or separation. From ages 6 to 10, the greatest fear is that of bodily harm; children in this age group have some awareness of death. The greatest fear for children older than 10 years of age is fear of death. Coupled with this fear may be difficult communication with adults.[2]

Treatment

The choice of cancer treatment is dependent on the type and stage of cancer. It may include surgery, chemotherapy, radiation, bone marrow and blood transplantation, and/or immunotherapy. Some cancers respond to a single mode of treatment, whereas others require multimodal treatment strategies. The goal of cancer treatment is to totally remove or destroy the malignant cells from the body. Unfortunately, treatments available today are not able to target only the cancer cells, and normal healthy cells must sometimes be destroyed during the treatments. This may result in significant psychological stress and physical morbidity or death.

The goals of multidisciplinary care are to cure the disease and prevent and palliate the side effects of therapy. Ideally, a care plan is developed at a conference or tumor board attended by members of the oncology team. The care plan includes not only the initial therapy protocol, but also the management of the side effects of the treatment, and a plan for reconstruction and rehabilitation.

Oral side effects from cancer treatment can be so debilitating that patients may tolerate only lower, less-effective doses of cancer therapy, or may delay or discontinue scheduled treatments. Preventing and managing oral complications helps support optimal cancer treatment, and enhances patient survival and quality of life. The National Institutes of Health formally recognizes the critical role that dentists and dental hygienists play in the overall care of the individual with cancer.[3] Dental hygiene care is critical to the prevention or amelioration of the oral complications associated with cancer treatment.

Who Has Oral Complications?

All patients receiving radiation for head and neck malignancies, more than 75% of recipients of bone marrow transplants, and almost 40% of patients receiving chemotherapy for any malignancy have oral complications. Risk for oral complications varies with the treatment regimen (see Risk Levels for Oral Complications).

Some oral complications occur only during cancer therapy, while others, such as *xerostomia* (client complaint of dry mouth) and salivary gland dysfunction may be lifelong. The dental hygienist plays a key role in helping clients with cancer understand that good oral hygiene care prevents or reduces oral complications, which in turn improves clients' quality of life and the likelihood that they will be able to tolerate optimal doses of cancer treatment (see Benefits of Good Oral Hygiene Care Before and During Cancer Therapy). For example, the dental hygienist collaborates with the client to establish an oral self-care regimen to protect mouth tissues and to minimize oral complications. To that aim, the dental hygienist reviews toothbrushing and interdental cleaning techniques and other approaches such as the use of antimicrobial and fluoride mouthrinses and fluoride gel to keep the mouth as moist and clean as possible to reduce risk of dental caries, oral infection, and pain. The importance of the role of the dental hygienist in enhancing quality of life and potential survival cannot be overemphasized.

Importance of Oral Evaluation Before Cancer Treatment

A pretreatment oral evaluation, conducted by a dental professional, includes a thorough examination of hard and soft tissues, and radiographs to detect possible

Risk Levels for Oral Complications

Low Risk

Patients receiving mildly myelosuppressive chemotherapy (mildly decreases the immune system)

Moderate Risk

Patients receiving single agent or outpatient therapy

High Risk

Patients undergoing head and neck radiation for oral and pharyngeal cancer

Patients receiving stomatotoxic chemotherapy resulting in prolonged myelosuppression

Adapted from U.S. Department of Health and Human Services National Institutes of Health: *Oral complications of cancer treatment: What the oncology team can do,* Pub No 99-4360, Bethesda, Md, US Department of Health and Human Services National Institutes of Health.

Benefits of Good Oral Hygiene Care Before and During Cancer Therapy

Reduces risk and severity of oral complications

Improves the likelihood that the client will tolerate optimal doses of cancer treatment

Prevents oral infections that could lead to potentially fatal systemic infections

Prevents or minimizes complications that can compromise nutrition

Prevents or reduces oral pain

Prevents or reduces incidence of bone necrosis in radiation clients

Preserves oral health

Improves quality of life

Adapted from U.S. Department of Health and Human Services National Institutes of Health: *Oral complications of cancer treatment: What the oncology team can do,* Pub No 99-4360, Bethesda, Md, US Department of Health and Human Services National Institutes of Health.

sources of infection. Reasons for an Oral Evaluation Before Cancer Treatment lists the benefits of an oral evaluation by the dental professional before treatment for oral cancer begins.

ORAL CANCER

Each year there are approximately 30,100 new cases of oral/pharyngeal cancer (hereafter referred to as oral cancer) and an expected 7,800 deaths yearly—more than the number from skin cancer and cervical cancer.[1] The overall five-year survival rate for oral cancer is 50%, a mortality rate unchanged for 50 years. The public often does not comprehend the serious nature of oral cancers,

Reasons for an Oral Evaluation Before Cancer Treatment

Identification and treatment of existing infections and problem teeth

Elimination of potential sites of infection and trauma (e.g., exfoliating teeth in children, partially erupted third molars, orthodontic bands, ill-fitting dentures, fractured teeth/restorations)

Construction of oral stents to be worn during radiation therapy to the head and neck area

For clients scheduled for head and neck radiation, extraction of teeth that may pose a future problem (for prevention of posttherapy osteoradionecrosis)

Construction of custom fluoride gel trays and instruction on use

Instruction on oral hygiene, nutrition, and tobacco cessation

Provision of professional mechanical dental hygiene care (oral prophylaxis, periodontal maintenance, or nonsurgical periodontal therapy) to reduce periodontal infection and promote periodontal health

perhaps because it associates disease in the mouth with dental care that is not life threatening.

Approximately 9 of every 10 oral malignancies are *squamous cell carcinomas.* Most occur in persons older than 40 years of age, but all persons should have a routine oral cancer screening by dental professionals, especially those in high-risk categories (see Oral Cancer Risk Factors). The use of all tobacco products (cigarettes, smokeless/spit tobacco, cigars, and pipes) and alcohol is associated with an increased risk of oral cancer. This risk is higher with increased product use. Individuals who use tobacco and drink alcohol heavily are at 10 times greater risk for developing oral cancer than persons who do not smoke or drink.

The prognosis for a specific oral cancer, however, is highly variable and depends on the stage and location of the disease when it is first diagnosed. National Cancer Institute data collected between the years 1973 and 1984 demonstrated that persons with a small, localized oral squamous cell cancer had a 72% five-year survival rate, compared with only 34% for a late-stage oral cancer.[4] Early detection is the key to survival. The most common presenting signs of squamous cell carcinomas of the oral cavity, pharynx, and larynx are listed in Common Signs of Oral Cancer.

The most common intraoral sites for squamous cell cancer are the lateral borders and ventral surfaces of the tongue, floor of the mouth, and the oropharynx. Any of the signs and symptoms that persist for longer than two weeks after removal of potentially irritating factors and/or application of therapeutic measures must be considered a cancer until proven benign by biopsy (surgical removal of all or part of the lesion) and microscopic evaluation.

Histologically, squamous cell carcinoma is assessed by the pathologist according to the similarity of appearance

Oral Cancer Risk Factors

Use of tobacco
Prior oral cancer lesion
Use of alcohol
Older age
Frequent sun exposure
Low consumption of fruits and vegetables
Human papillomavirus

From the American Cancer Society.

Common Signs of Oral Cancer

Swelling, lump, growth, or area of induration or hardness anywhere in or about the mouth or neck, which is usually painless
Erythroplakia patch (velvety, deep red)
Leukoplakia patch (white or red/white patch)
Any sore (ulcer, irritation) that does not heal after two weeks
Repeated bleeding from the mouth or throat
Difficulty in swallowing or persistent hoarseness

of the cancer cells to the cells from which it was derived. Cells that appear like the parent cells are classified as "well-differentiated' or "moderately differentiated." If they do not resemble the original cells, they are classified "undifferentiated" or "anaplastic." The less differentiated cells generally indicate a more aggressive cancer.

Histologic studies demonstrate that 90% of red or combined red and white oral mucosal lesions and only 20% of white lesions are dysplastic or carcinomatous. Red or combined red and white lesions therefore should be considered to be more dangerous than white lesions and should be evaluated carefully. Other cancers less frequently found in the oral cavity include adenocarcinomas of salivary gland origin, lymphomas, melanomas, and bone and soft tissue sarcomas. Cancers that begin in other parts of the body may metastasize to or exhibit manifestations in the oral cavity. The most common metastases are from tumors in the lung, breast, colon, and kidney. Manifestations of leukemia, lymphomas, and multiple myeloma may also be present within the oral cavity.

TREATMENT

Choice of treatment for oral squamous cell cancer depends on the stage of disease at the time of diagnosis. A small lesion of less than 1 cm may require only surgery or radiation therapy. Larger cancers, especially those that have spread to the lymph nodes in the neck, may require surgery, radiation, and chemotherapy. Chemotherapy is not a curative treatment for oral squamous cell cancer, but it may be used as an adjunct prior to surgery, concurrently with radiation therapy to enhance the ability of radiation to reduce the size of the tumor, or as a palliative treatment for recurrent and advanced tumors.

SURGICAL TREATMENT OF ORAL CANCER

Surgery is chosen as primary treatment when oral cancer is small; is completely excisable without complication; is not sensitive to radiation therapy; when lymph nodes, salivary glands, or bone are involved; or when there is a recurrence of tumor in an area that has already received a therapeutic dose of radiation. The disadvantage of surgery is the sacrifice of important functional oral structures.

Potential Complications

PHYSICAL. Acute physical complications after head and neck surgery may include infection; airway obstruction; fistula formation; necrosis in the surgical site; impairment of swallowing, hearing, vision, smell, and speech; and compromised nutritional status. Long-term complications include speech impairment, malnutrition from the inability to swallow foods, drooling, malocclusion, temporomandibular disorders, facial deformity, and chronic pain in the shoulder muscles.

PYSCHOSOCIAL. There may be significant psychosocial problems associated with surgery of the head and neck because the results of the cancer and its treatment are often visible and humiliating and can be psychologically devastating. Physical impairments cannot be completely disguised by clothing, prostheses, or cosmetics. These surgical defects may result in long-term disability, but these problems may be short-term when reconstructive surgery and rehabilitation are available. In today's society, self-image is often equated with body image. As a result, some individuals experience depression, withdrawal and social death, anger, and stigmatization. Some who are heavy smokers and drinkers experience guilt because of the association of these habits with oral cancer.

MANAGEMENT. The person who has surgery for oral cancer often requires a long postoperative hospital course. To assist with postoperative management, a dental hygienist working in a hospital can do the following:

- Provide in-service programs for nursing staff on oral assessment and oral hygiene care during cancer therapy
- Act as a liaison between the surgical and dental teams
- Facilitate ongoing prosthodontic and oral surgery consultations
- Teach clients to insert, remove, and clean their surgical prosthesis
- Assess the oral tissues for irritation and comfort
- Teach the client to maintain the oral cavity and all remaining teeth in optimal condition with frequent gentle cleansing and hydration. This cleansing and

hydration is usually accomplished with irrigation bag or bulb syringe saline rinses and gentle debridement with large cotton-tipped applicators, sponge swabs, or gauze. Care must be taken when cleansing and suctioning not to disrupt new granulation tissue

✦ Encourage clients who have been cleared to take food by mouth by the surgeon to use a spoon to place small bites of food on the unaffected side of the mouth and as far back as possible. Forks should be avoided until incisions heal. (Note: Immediately after surgery, a client may not be able to take food and drink by mouth, at which time a tube is placed in the stomach for liquid nutritional supplement.)

A client who has had a recent surgical procedure to the head and neck may be in the process of accepting the facial deformity and functional alterations. Encouragement to talk about these issues aids the client in moving toward acceptance of the new body image. It is important for the dental hygienist to listen empathetically to the client's concerns and fears. Taking time to do so decreases client stress and promotes cooperation with recommendations. It is important to remember that although the surgical treatment may have removed head and neck tissue, it did not remove the person of the client. The client, as a whole person, has human needs related to oral health and disease. It is very important to actively listen to the client, communicate respectfully with good eye contact, and interact directly about ways to promote oral health and cope with the challenges that the surgery has presented.

Prosthetic Rehabilitation

Planning for rehabilitation of the person with head and neck cancer by the dentist begins at the time of medical diagnosis. When a surgical resection creates facial defects and oral dysfunction, the client must be assured that there is a plan to restore at least partial function and improve cosmetic appearance. The oral and maxillofacial surgeon, the maxillofacial prosthodontist, the general dentist, and the dental hygienist all may play a role in the initial care planning.

Maxillary defects result in unintelligible speech because of nasal voice quality, difficulty in eating, thickened nasal and sinus secretions, and facial disfigurement. Optimal management begins at the time of surgery when the prosthodontist may place a surgical obturator (a temporary prosthetic device) to help correct these problems. Approximately 3 to 4 months after surgery, if no complications arise, a permanent prosthesis is fabricated. This prosthesis usually allows the most effective restoration for the client because speech, swallowing, mastication, and facial contour all can effectively be restored with a prosthesis instead of reconstructed with plastic surgery.

Mandibular defects are often created during surgery for oral cancers. Immediate reconstruction is sometimes possible. Following extensive intraoral surgery, the client may need additional surgical procedures to release the tongue from the floor of the mouth, to graft skin, to create a vestibule for saliva pooling, and to allow for extension of denture flanges. These procedures also aid in speech, mastication, and swallowing.

Following surgical and radiation therapy to the oral cavity (see following sections), clients who are partially or fully edentulous require conservative prosthetic management. The thinned and friable tissue, scarring and fibrosis from surgery, and lack of lubrication and protective qualities of the saliva from radiation treatment make denture placement difficult and place the client at risk for soft tissue breakdown and osteoradionecrosis. Some clients are never able to wear dentures. Detailed education, close professional supervision, and client acceptance of recommendations are necessary for successful prosthetic rehabilitation.

RADIATION TREATMENT OF ORAL CANCER

Radiation therapy employs the use of ionizing radiation, either from external beams or from internally implanted sources. Radiation therapy may be used by itself for the treatment of oral squamous cell carcinoma when the lesion is small and superficial and when a surgical procedure would result in significant functional or cosmetic morbidity. Radiation also may be used in combination with chemotherapy to enhance its ability to reduce the tumor, or with surgery, postoperatively to eliminate residual disease, or preoperatively to reduce the size of the tumor. Radiation therapy also may be used in the treatment of other cancers of the head and neck, including lymphomas and salivary gland tumors.

Radiation damage to some normal cells may be acute and resolve after completion of therapy (e.g., taste buds). Other normal cells affected may not have the capacity to repair themselves, resulting in long-term complications (e.g., salivary gland cells). After the first week of radiation, the client begins to experience some of the acute side effects (e.g., loss of taste and dry mouth), whereas other complications may not become evident until later in radiation therapy.

Radiation Mask and Oral Prosthetic Devices

When external radiation is planned, the client is first scheduled for a *simulation appointment.* At this time the exact field of radiation is planned and a radiation mask (Figure 43–2) is custom fit. The mask is used at all radiation therapy appointments to immobilize the head to ensure a precise treatment field. Following the simulation appointment, the client returns for daily treatments. The number of treatments varies from 15 to 37, depending on the type of malignancy (e.g., lymphomas and some solid tumors are more radiosensitive and require less radiation than squamous cell carcinoma). If claustrophobia due to the mask is a problem, clients may be given an oral sedative prior to their treatments to help them cope with the experience.

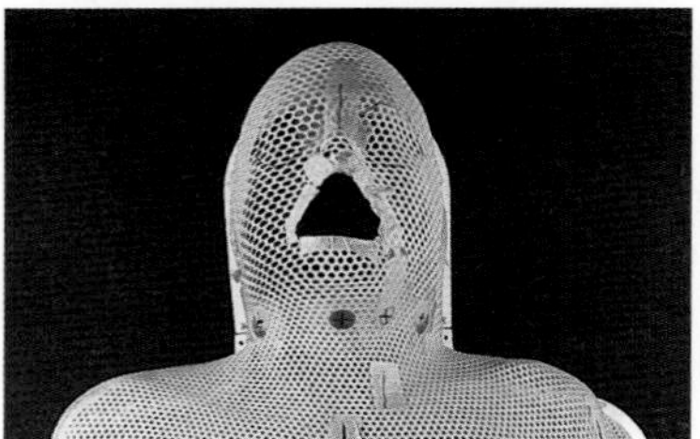

FIGURE 43–2 ✦ A radiation mask.

Potential Complications of Radiation to the Head and Neck Area

Acute

Xerostomia
Loss of taste
Mucositis
Dysphagia
Secondary infection
Trismus
Impaired nutrition (from xerostomia, pain, and dysphagia)
Hearing loss
Fatigue

Chronic

Xerostomia/salivary gland dysfunction
Taste alteration from preradiation status
Telangiectasia, friable mucosa
Continued fungal infections due to the lack of saliva
Osteoradionecrosis/soft tissue necrosis
Rampant caries
Muscle fibrosis, temporomandibular disorder, and trismus
Altered tooth and jaw development in children

Adapted from U.S. Department of Health and Human Services National Institutes of Health: *Oral complications of cancer treatment: What the oncology team can do,* Pub No 99-4360, Bethesda, Md, US Department of Health and Human Services National Institutes of Health.

Clients may require an oral prosthetic device (stent, splint, shield, or carrier) to facilitate the delivery of radiation therapy. Upon referral of a client for a preradiation dental evaluation, and prior to the simulation appointment, it is important for the dental professional to communicate with the radiation oncologist about the need for a custom oral device. This inquiry will ensure that the client has the appropriate devices prior to the simulation appointment.

One oral device used to stabilize the teeth during the treatment of nasopharyngeal cancer is similar to a custom-fitted acrylic bleaching or fluoride tray. These stents are easily made by the dental professional to fit snugly over the client's teeth. For other types of oral cancer, the radiation oncologist may request a more complex oral device to displace or shield normal tissue from the effects of the radiation, or to position radioactive materials adjacent to a tumor site. In these cases, referral of the client to a prosthodontist for fabrication of the device is indicated.

Side Effects/Complications

The complications associated with radiation to the head and neck will vary among clients, depending on the field and treatment and total dose of radiation required. Only the tissues in the direct field of radiation are affected. For example, a client undergoing treatment for lymphoma may receive only 20 radiation treatments and involve only a portion of the salivary glands and cervical lymph nodes, and will thus experience fewer complications than a client who is undergoing treatment for a squamous cell carcinoma in the oral cavity. To avoid unnecessarily alarming the client, and to be able to offer sound advice, the dental professional must establish good communication with the radiation oncologist to understand the anticipated radiation side effects.

The client undergoing radiation therapy to the oral cavity and salivary glands begins to experience some side effects after the first week of therapy. Throughout therapy, it is important to support the client with suggestions to prevent and reduce side effects or complications of radiation therapy. These complications are summarized in Potential Complications of Radiation to the Head and Neck Area and are described in the following paragraphs.

XEROSTOMIA/SALIVARY GLAND DYSFUNCTION. Exposure of the salivary glands to radiation is unavoidable when treating tumors of the oral cavity and neck because they are in close proximity to the lymphatic system and cannot be shielded. Ionizing radiation induces fibrosis and atrophy of the salivary gland tissue. Clients begin to experience a change in their saliva after the first week of radiation. They first complain of a thickened and ropy saliva, and as the treatments progress their mouths become drier. The degree of dryness is dependent on the dose of radiation and the extent of salivary tissue within the radiation field. One study at M.D. Anderson Cancer Center demonstrated that persons undergoing high doses of radiation therapy to all of the major salivary glands experience a 67% decrease in saliva after 1 week of radiation, a 76% loss after 6 weeks, and a 95% loss 3 years after completion of radiation.

Xerostomia due to thickened, reduced, or absent salivary flow compromises speaking, chewing, and swallowing and increases risk of impaired nutrition due to an inability to eat all foods. Persistent dry mouth also increases the risk of dental caries and other oral infections. Because the irradiated salivary glands are permanently damaged, the change in both the quality and the quantity of saliva remains, although the client may over time perceive a partial return in salivary flow. Clients often complain bitterly about the complications associated with xerostomia.

Management. Clients who undergo radiation therapy to the neck involving the submandibular and sublingual salivary glands with only partial inclusion of the parotid glands complain mostly of a thick, ropy saliva. These clients benefit greatly from baking soda and saline water rinses. A baking soda solution is mucolytic, which aids in cleansing and refreshing the mouth. A prescribed medication such as pilocarpine can be provided by the oncologist or dentist to help stimulate residual salivary gland tissue to produce saliva. Also, commercial saliva substitutes are available as over-the-counter products. Although the latter may be palliative, they do not contain the protective proteins and mucoproteins found in saliva, and some clients do not feel the cost is justified for the limited relief. In addition, the lips should be lubricated with a moisturizing lip balm or cream recommended by the radiation oncologist, not pure petrolatum, which provides only an occlusive agent and does not moisturize the perioral tissues. These and other suggestions for management of a dry mouth are listed in Recommendations for Clients with Xerostomia.

Recommendations for Clients with Xerostomia

Carry bottled water and sip often
Use liquids to soften or thin foods
Use sugarless gum or sugar-free hard candies to help stimulate saliva flow
Use OTC saliva substitutes (Table 43–1)
Rinse frequently with $\frac{1}{4}$ tsp baking soda, $\frac{1}{8}$ tsp salt, and 8 oz of water
Let ice chips melt in the mouth
Suck on sugar-free popsicles
Humidify rooms with cool-mist humidifiers
Avoid highly seasoned foods, tobacco, and the drying effects of alcohol and alcohol-containing products
Ask the dentist or oncologist to prescribe a saliva stimulant
Lubricate lips with a moisturizing lip balm or cream, not pure petrolatum

Adapted from U.S. Department of Health and Human Services National Institutes of Health: *Oral complications of cancer treatment: What the oncology team can do,* Pub No 99-4360, Bethesda, Md, US Department of Health and Human Services National Institutes of Health.

ALTERATION OF TASTE. When the tongue is in the field of radiation, the client experiences partial or full taste loss. Loss of taste is an acute effect, and usually occurs following the first few treatments. Taste returns a few months following the completion of radiation therapy, but may be altered from preradiation status. Taste loss is a significant side effect that makes radiation therapy almost intolerable. Eating becomes a chore; clients complain that all food tastes like mush or straw. Eating ceases to be a pleasurable activity and clients must force themselves to eat only to maintain nutritional status.

Management. Clients are helped by having someone listen to their complaints. They should be assured that taste dysfunction is a normal side effect of radiation and that taste will return several months after treatment. In addition, clients should be encouraged to continue eating. Use of nutritional liquid substitutes such as Ensure and/or referral for nutritional counseling may be necessary to avoid weight loss and medical complications. If patients do not maintain adequate nutrition during the treatment process, then a stomach tube is surgically placed for liquid feeding at home.

MUCOSITIS/STOMATITIS AND INFECTION. If all nonsurgical dental or dental hygiene procedures have not been accomplished prior to initiation of radiation, they should be done within the first 2 weeks of therapy before the onset of mucositis. Usually, by the third week of radiation the client begins to experience mucosal inflammation and pain. The mucosa first becomes edematous and inflamed. Later the tissue becomes thinned, pseudomembranes form, and the tissue becomes denuded. This inflammation and ulceration of the oral mucous membranes is called *mucositis.* As the treatments progress, small ulcerations may enlarge to a confluent and pseudomembranous mucositis. Oncologists sometimes schedule a short interruption of therapy to allow regeneration of normal cells. Mucositis can increase the risk of severe pain, oral and systemic infection, unpleasant odors, difficulty in talking, and nutritional compromise. Lack of saliva increases the risk of ulceration and bleeding. Also, the patient may experience *dysphagia* (the inability to swallow) as a result of salivary gland dysfunction and painful ulcerated tissue within the radiation field.

Because of mucositis, secondary infections of the oral mucosa are common and may intensify the mucosal irritation. The fungal organism *Candida albicans* is most often implicated, but any organism may be responsible for infection when the tissues are severely compromised from xerostomia, mucositis, altered nutrition, and inadequate oral hygiene. Early detection and treatment of an oral infection are imperative to prevent exacerbation of mucositis that may require interruption of cancer therapy. Following completion of all radiation treatments, gradual resolution of the mucositis can be expected, although the epithelium undergoes permanent fibrosis and the tissue may be thin and fragile, and may show evidence of *telangiectasia* (a vascular lesion of dilated small blood vessels).

Management. Managing Mouth Pain from Mucositis summarizes ways to help clients with mouth pain from mucositis. *A clean, well-hydrated mouth during radiation therapy reduces the severity of mucosal ulceration and risk of oral infection.* Toothbrushes are available that are supersoft and nonabrasive. Once the client begins to experience mucositis, it is necessary to modify oral hygiene procedures to be nonirritating and atraumatic but adequate to remove plaque biofilm and thickened saliva. Toothbrushes should be extra soft and may be further softened in hot water. Use of commercial toothpastes with strong flavoring agents may have to be temporarily discontinued and replaced with a paste made of baking

TABLE 43–1 ORAL HYGIENE PRODUCTS USED DURING CANCER THERAPY

Product	Description	Indication/Rationale/Use	Precautions
Toothbrushes	Several are available with extra-soft or super-soft bristles: Rx Ultra Suave, PHB, Inc. 1-800-553-1440, or Biotene Supersoft, Laclede Inc. 1-800-922-5856 Child-size brush may be helpful for clients with limited opening. Some brushes are available with suctioning capability.	Plaque biofilm removal after meals when not severely compromised from surgery, chemotherapy, or bone marrow transplantation. Tongue must be brushed, especially in clients on soft or liquid diets.	Beware of inexpensive hospital-supplied hard, unpolished bristled toothbrushes. Benefit vs. risk of brushing may need to be assessed in clients with severely compromised condition.
Floss	Unwaxed or waxed	Important for plaque biofilm removal at least 1 time/day.	Assess client's dexterity. Assist if necessary. Discontinue only when client is at high risk of bleeding and bacteremia.
Dentifrices	Commercial without strong flavoring agents. Paste made from baking soda and water is an alternative.	Aid in plaque biofilm removal.	Strong flavoring agents may intensify mucositis. Fully rinse baking soda residue from oral cavity.
Foam or Sponge-sticks	Alternative to toothbrushes available from medical supply companies. Some are impregnated with cleansing agents.	Use to cleanse oral cavity only when client cannot use manual toothbrush because of pain from ulcerated tissues or when platelet count is below 20,000/mm^3. If used, the sponge should be dipped in a chlorhexidine solution for greatest efficacy. May also be used to apply topical medications.	Does not adequately remove plaque biofilm. Do not soak in solution; sponge top may fall off stick and client could aspirate it. May abrade friable tissue. Do not use lemon-glycerin swabs because they are acidic and drying to the tissues.
Gauze	Alternative to toothbrush. Use 2 × 2 or 4 × 4 squares.	Use to cleanse oral cavity only when toothbrushing is not possible due to pain from ulcerated tissues or when toothbrushing precipitates bleeding. Moisten in water, saline 0.9% (1 tsp NaCl to 16 oz H_2O), or baking soda solution. Wrap around finger and cleanse teeth, tongue, and tissues.	Does not adequately remove plaque biofilm.
Baking Soda/Saline Rinse	Mucolytic cleansing solution of $\frac{1}{2}$ tsp baking soda, $\frac{1}{4}$ tsp salt, 16 oz water.	An alkaline soothing rinse used to cleanse mouth every 2 to 4 hours for clients with mucositis, xerostomia, thick secretions, or after emesis. May be used in irrigation bag to assist in rinsing painful mouth. Rinse with plain water after use.	High sodium content. Instruct client not to swallow solution. Not to be used by clients on sodium-restricted diet.
Topical Anesthetics	Palliative agents. OTC products include alcohol-free Benadryl mixed in equal parts with a coating agent such as Maalox to create a rinse. Other agents that are helpful are topical Orabase with benzocaine or Orabase Sooth-n-Seal (1-800-225-3756) or UlcerEase Rinse (1-800-334-4286) (available OTC through pharmacies).	Used to control pain associated with mucosal ulcerations.	Topical anesthetics may decrease the gag reflex, resulting in aspiration of food. These OTC agents/rinses may not provide adequate relief from severe oral ulcerations. The client's oncologist may prescribe analgesics or narcotics.
Saliva Replacement and Xerostomia Palliation	Saliva substitutes include OTC rinses/gels such as Oral Balance Gel (Laclede Inc, 1-800-922-5856) or Moi-Stir (Kingswood Labs, 1-800-968-7772). Dietary guidelines should encourage high-moisture foods, oily foods, and sugar/acid-free foods. Saliva stimulants include pharmacologic prescription drugs (pilocarpine) for systemic stimulation of functional salivary gland tissue, or mechanical stimulation with sugar-free chewing gum or candy.	For palliation of xerostomia and dysphagia.	Clients may find saliva substitutes to be unacceptable in taste and expensive. Clients should be discouraged from using tobacco products, excessive alcohol and alcohol-containing mouthwash because they promote dry mouth.
Chlorhexidine Gluconate 0.12%	Bactericidal mouthrinse.	Prophylactic or therapeutic mouthrinse to reduce plaque biofilm and oral microbes. Rinse for 30 seconds with 1 capful b.i.d.	Products available in United States are prepared with alcohol, and may be irritating. This should be used only when mechanical plaque control is inadequate. May cause staining, which is removable with dental prophylaxis. May alter taste perception.
Commercial Mouthwashes	Dilute heavily with water.	May serve as mouth freshener.	Most commercial mouthwashes have a high concentration of alcohol or phenol, which are very drying and irritating to tissues unless diluted heavily with water. Flavoring agents may intensify mucositis Alcohol-free mouthwashes are available (Biotene and Clear Choice).

Managing Mouth Pain from Mucositis

Early detection and treatment of oral infection
Good oral hygiene, including tongue brushing, to prevent further infection
Frequent irrigation with 1 tsp baking soda, ½ tsp salt, and 32 oz of water
Frequent rinsing with sodium bicarbonate mouthrinses and nonalcoholic mouthrinses (e.g., Biotene and Clear Choice
Daily cleaning of dentures and changing of soaking solution; denture removal while sleeping
Use of prescribed topical anesthetics with caution to avoid anesthetizing the soft palate, which could cause food aspiration; excessive use may potentiate mucositis
Use of OTC or prescribed systemic analgesics if necessary
Avoidance of irritating or rough-textured foods
Use of perioral moisturizers directed by the radiation oncologist

Adapted from U.S. Department of Health and Human Services National Institutes of Health: *Oral complications of cancer treatment: What the oncology team can do,* Pub No 99-4360, Bethesda, Md, US Department of Health and Human Services National Institutes of Health.

soda and water. If tooth brushing becomes impossible because of painful tissues, the teeth, gingiva, and tongue may be swabbed with gauze moistened in warm water. Dental flossing should be continued as long as possible and resumed as soon as the mucositis resolves.

Sponge-tipped swabs are supplied for oral care to hospitals through medical supply companies and are not effective in plaque biofilm removal. However, if their use is necessary due to ulcerated tissue, they should be dipped in a nonalcoholic antimicrobial solution for greatest efficacy. A suction toothbrush is available commercially, or one can be made by drilling a hole in the back of the head of a toothbrush and attaching suction tubing. When nondisposable products are used, they must be rinsed well and kept dry. Rinsing in an antimicrobial solution may be advisable.

All commercial mouthwashes with alcohol or phenol should be avoided because of their drying and irritating effects. Although half-strength peroxide and water solutions are sometimes used in hospitals to remove encrusted secretions or for acute infections, they are not recommended for long-term use because they are acidic and may alter the normal oral flora. Frequent mouth rinses with baking soda and saline water should be suggested. When the mouth is too sore to swish the mouthrinse, gentle irrigation of the mouth is useful. A disposable enema or irrigation bag is hung over a sink and filled with a solution of 1 tsp of baking soda, $\frac{1}{2}$ tsp of salt, and 32 oz of water. The solution is directed throughout the mouth with the hose and is allowed to flow out into the sink to avoid swallowing.

Chlorhexidine gluconate mouthrinse has not been shown conclusively to be beneficial in reducing oral infections and severity of mucositis during cancer therapy. Such a rinse, when prepared with alcohol, should be evaluated for its antimicrobial benefit versus the irritating effect of the alcohol.

Topical anesthetics and coating agents in addition to the soothing bland rinses (Table 43–1) give temporary relief. However, all clients, especially children and their parents, should be cautioned that topical anesthetic agents may anesthetize the soft palate and epiglottis, potentially causing aspiration of food. Excessive use also may potentiate mucositis. Some clients may require systemic analgesics and sometimes even narcotics to control the pain of mucositis.

During radiation therapy, care of the perioral tissues should be directed by the radiation oncologist. Some lip lubricants can potentiate the effects of the radiation and cause significant radiation dermatitis. Physicians order their preferred product for skin care during therapy.

Client's whose condition is not compromised should be scheduled for regular preventive oral healthcare. The role of the dental hygienist in providing professional mechanical oral hygiene care and supportive patient education is important to prevent mucositis and oral infection. Clients with dentures should be instructed to leave the dentures out of their mouths as often as possible. If the field of radiation encompasses all of the oral tissues, it may be impossible for the client to wear dentures because of significant oral tissue changes from edema and inflammation. The client should keep the dentures as clean as possible and should store them in a soaking solution that is changed daily to avoid microbial contamination. These clients often eat a soft or liquid diet and the tongue becomes coated and infected. Therefore, keeping the mouth well cleansed and the tongue brushed are extremely important.

TRISMUS/TISSUE FIBROSIS/TEMPOROMANDIBULAR JOINT DYSFUNCTION. Limited ability to open the mouth (trismus) may result from loss of elasticity of masticatory muscles or temporomandibular joint ligaments after a high dose of radiation. Trismus usually occurs within 3 months after therapy and remains a lifelong problem. It can result in significant discomfort and can interfere with eating, talking, and posttreatment examination.

Management. The client receiving radiation therapy to the muscles of mastication should be placed on an exercise program to prevent trismus. The jaw should be exercised three times a day by opening and closing the mouth, 20 times, as wide as possible without causing pain.

RADIATION CARIES/DEMINERALIZATION. Rampant caries and demineralization of the tooth structure usually begin within the first year following radiation therapy unless intensive oral hygiene and preventive measures are instituted. Figure 43–3 shows the typical pattern of this demineralization process. Demineralization of the enamel (loss of minerals without decay)

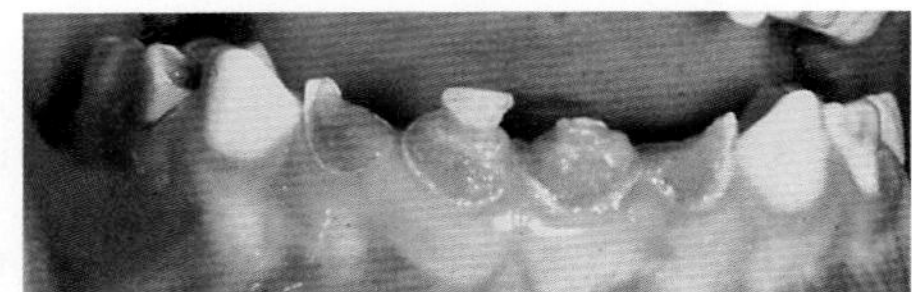

FIGURE 43–3 ✦ Radiation caries.

and/or rapid decay is a result of changes in both the quality and quantity of saliva following cancer treatment. The decreased salivary flow limits the availability of calcium and phosphate in the saliva to prevent the natural remineralization of the tooth structure and to buffer acids produced by cariogenic bacteria in the plaque biofilm. With dry and friable tissues, these clients may change to a soft, high-carbohydrate diet, adding to the lifelong risk of rampant dental decay.

Management. All clients receiving cancericidal doses of radiation therapy to any of the salivary glands must have custom fluoride trays made for daily application of a 1.1% neutral-pH sodium fluoride gel to aid in prevention of rampant tooth demineralization. The dental hygienist may be responsible for making impressions for study models to fabricate the custom tray. Impressions may be sent to a dental laboratory or the trays may be made in the dental clinic using a vacuum unit. The fluoride trays are made from a soft, vinyl mouthguard material. They should be adapted to extend slightly above the cervical line of the teeth, with full coverage of all teeth. The tray edges must be absolutely smooth and nonirritating to the client's oral tissues to prevent soft tissue breakdown.

The client begins use of the fluoride trays at the initiation of therapy. Clients are instructed to first brush and floss their teeth and then place a thin ribbon of 1.1% neutral-pH sodium fluoride gel in each of the trays. They place the trays on their teeth and leave them in place for 5 to 10 minutes. Upon removal, they rinse the trays well with water, but do not rinse the mouth or eat anything for 30 minutes. This must be done once each day. It is important to let the client decide on a time of day when cooperation with the routine is most likely. Many clients feel it is easiest to use the trays when they are bathing or showering. In this way, the procedure is incorporated into a regular daily routine.

There may be a period of time during therapy when severe mucositis prevents fluoride application with trays. During this time, the client is encouraged to use nonalcohol and bland fluoride rinses, increase hydration of tissues, and resume the daily fluoride gel application as soon as the mucositis resolves.

In addition, dietary habits and daily food intake should be discussed to assess the intake of sugar, acidic juice, or soda pop (diet included). The dental hygienist plays a critical role in helping clients prevent radiation caries by educating them about the importance of daily fluoride application, good nutrition, and oral hygiene.

ALTERED TOOTH AND JAW DEVELOPMENT. The latent effects of therapeutic radiation therapy to children with cancers of the oral cavity and associated structures vary with radiation dose and field, and stage of growth and development. Radiation has the potential to alter or arrest craniofacial growth and tooth development. Older children who receive minimal doses may experience only slightly altered root development, whereas younger children treated at an age when their jaws and teeth are under development may experience gross malformation of the dentition and may suffer significant skeletal deformities.[3]

SOFT TISSUE NECROSIS AND OSTEORADIONECROSIS. Radiation therapy may irreversibly injure the vascularity of soft tissue and bone, resulting in decreased ability to heal if traumatized and in increased susceptibility to infection.[5] *Osteoradionecrosis* is defined as exposed bone that does not respond to treatment over a 6-month period of time. There is a higher risk of osteoradionecrosis as the dose of radiation and the volume of irradiated bone and tissue increase. Nonhealing soft tissue or bone may become secondarily infected and the client may eventually experience intolerable pain and jaw fracture. The mandible appears to be more susceptible than the maxilla because of its dense bone and limited blood supply. Clients who are at the greatest risk are those who have surgery or trauma to irradiated tissue and bone, or clients who have dental infection in close proximity to bone compromised by radiation. Prevention of osteoradionecrosis by preradiation therapy dental evaluation and treatment is mandatory. Following radiation, the teeth and periodontium must be professionally managed at intervals to ensure excellent oral hygiene, early intervention, and minimal disease. The dental hygienist is an extremely important member of the professional team to manage this potentially very serious problem.

HEARING LOSS AND FATIGUE. As treatment progresses, the client becomes more easily fatigued and may require daytime naps. In addition, the client may report partial or total loss of hearing in the ear on the side of the head being irradiated.

Management. Due to fatigue, clients may need to cut back on their work schedule and obtain plenty of rest. After radiation therapy is completed, hearing and physical energy usually return.

CHEMOTHERAPY

Chemotherapy is the use of drugs for the treatment of cancer. Combinations of chemotherapeutic agents have resulted in significant improvement in cure rates for some cancers. Other cancers are not cured by chemotherapy alone, but the drugs are used in combination with surgery and/or radiation to destroy cancer cells that may have spread systemically. Sometimes chemotherapy is used by itself for a period of time to control a tumor that cannot be eradicated.

Chemotherapy alone is not a curative treatment for oral squamous cell carcinoma, but it is sometimes used as an adjunct to surgery and radiation, or may be used to palliate advanced tumors. Prior to surgery, it may be given to reduce the size of very large tumors. All chemotherapy protocols for oral squamous cell carcinoma are under investigation, with improvement in long-term survival rates still to be assessed.

Chemotherapy is not only physically demanding but also stress-producing. Persons undergoing cancer therapy need support from family, friends, and caregivers who are good listeners, who allow a full range of emotions, and who encourage hope. Chemotherapy for cancers of the head and neck, as well as malignancies in other parts of the body, may result in oral complications.

Potential Complications

The most common overall complication of chemotherapy is infection as a result of *myelosuppression* (decreased immune response). Oral infections may spread systemically, leading to sepsis and death. Other complications of chemotherapy include electrolyte imbalances, bleeding and hemorrhage, and acute toxicity from the drugs, including nausea and vomiting, photosensitivity, central nervous system dysfunction, alopecia (hair loss), and poor nutritional status. Drugs are available for the control of nausea and vomiting.

Oral Complications

Not all chemotherapy protocols result in oral manifestations, but many have either a direct or indirect effect on the mouth (see Oral Complications of Chemotherapy). Most of these oral problems are similar to those discussed in the section on radiation therapy; however, they will be discussed in the following sections in the context of chemotherapy.

Approximately 40% of persons treated for non–head and neck malignancies experience oral complications.[6] Oral problems related to myelosuppression may be significantly and favorably affected through aggressive preventive dental hygiene interventions. The oral manifestations of chemotherapy listed in Oral Complications of Chemotherapy and described in the following sections are not permanent, but the client will be at risk for these complications throughout the entire period the drugs are being administered.

MUCOSITIS. Some chemotherapeutic drugs are toxic to the oral mucosa and cause edema, inflammation, and ulcerations within 7 to 10 days following the administration of the drug. Ulcerations usually appear individually, but may progress to diffuse and confluent lesions. If the tissues do not become secondarily infected, the ulcerated tissue will heal within a few weeks of the drug delivery. The lesions are often very painful, causing difficulty in eating and talking.

Oral Complications of Chemotherapy

Mucositis
Neurotoxicity
Infection
Bleeding/hemorrhage
Xerostomia/salivary gland dysfunction
Dental caries/demineralization
Altered tooth development

Adapted from U.S. Department of Health and Human Services National Institutes of Health: *Oral complications of cancer treatment: What the oncology team can do,* Pub No 99-4360, Bethesda, Md, US Department of Health and Human Services National Institutes of Health.

Management. Mucositis may be prevented or lessened in severity by dental hygiene interventions that create a clean and well-hydrated oral environment, good nutritional status, and control of secondary infection. The client should be encouraged to rinse frequently with sodium bicarbonate/saline water rinses and alcohol-free mouthrinses. These rinses soothe and hydrate the inflamed tissues, aid in bacterial plaque removal, and neutralize pH if the client is vomiting. Pain management begins with mild topical anesthetics and may progress to systemic analgesics and even narcotics.

NEUROTOXICITY. Some chemotherapeutic agents derived from plant alkaloids (such as vincristine) are toxic to nerve tissue and may cause severe, deep, and often bilateral odontogenic-like pain. When no dental pathology can be found, the drug may be implicated. The pain subsides within a few days after administration of the drug.

INFECTION. Some chemotherapeutic agents suppress the bone marrow, resulting in immunosuppression and bleeding problems. During these periods, the client will be at risk for developing oral infections (fungal, viral, and bacterial) that may increase the risk for a systemic infection, especially if there is a break in the mucosal integrity allowing organisms to enter the blood. Oral infections can result in significant morbidity for the client undergoing chemotherapy. Oral infections not only intensify mucositis, but with a breach in the oral mucosa, oral infections may lead to septicemia and death in clients with profound *immunosuppression* (decreased immune response).[3] Inappropriately timed dental and dental hygiene procedures can result in a bacteremia causing sepsis and death.

Management. The final decision regarding the safest time to schedule oral healthcare appointments is made by the oncologist. If necessary, the oncologist may recommend antibiotic prophylaxis prior to dental and dental hygiene care.

Another reason for antibiotic prophylaxis prior to dental treatment exists when the client has an indwelling

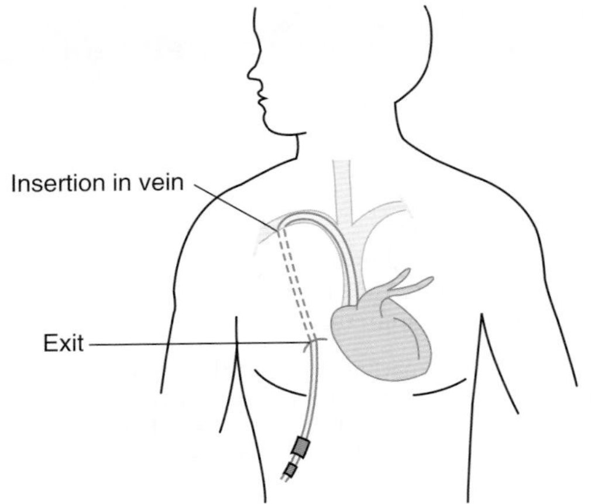

FIGURE 43–4 ✦ Placement of an indwelling central venous catheter.

central venous catheter for delivery of chemotherapy (Figure 43–4). Some individuals begin chemotherapy without a central venous catheter, but have one placed later during therapy. Therefore, each time a client is seen it is necessary to ask if a catheter has been placed since the last appointment, because it may become colonized with oral organisms following a dental or dental hygiene procedure. Although no data are currently available to document the absolute need for prophylactic antibiotics in this patient population prior to dental procedures, the current American Heart Association endocarditis prophylaxis regimen is generally recommended (see Chapter 9 for antibiotic premedication). Again, the oncologist should be consulted as to what antibiotics are necessary.

Some cancer centers have clients discontinue tooth brushing and flossing during severe myelosuppression. This practice is controversial, however, because there is evidence that toothbrushing and flossing during immunosuppression are not detrimental, and a decrease in plaque biofilm and local infection reduces the risk of potentially life-threatening systemic infection.

Clients with dentures should be evaluated frequently and encouraged to call the dental office whenever necessary to seek early intervention for an oral complication or dental-related sources of pain, irritation, or dental trauma. Oral tissues may change significantly during chemotherapy from edema, inflammation, ulceration, and/or weight loss. Clients should understand that when denture irritation occurs, the prosthesis should be removed from the mouth to avoid further trauma. Persons with oral infections may reinfect their mouths with poorly cleansed dentures. It is important for the client to clean and disinfect the dentures daily and keep them out of the mouth while sleeping. Denture soaking solutions must be changed daily and the soaking container cleansed and rinsed thoroughly.

BLEEDING. Myelosuppression from chemotherapy may result in *thrombocytopenia,* reduction of clotting factors. Clients with platelet counts under 50,000/mm^3 may experience oral bleeding during invasive dental and dental hygiene procedures. The occurrence of spontaneous gingival bleeding increases with a platelet count below 20,000/mm^3. When there is a disruption of the mucosal integrity and/or periodontal disease, clients are at greater risk of bleeding. This fact emphasizes the need for early soft tissue management and periodontal maintenance care.

Management. When scheduling a client undergoing chemotherapy for a dental hygiene appointment, it is imperative to consult the oncologist regarding the status of the client's blood counts and clotting factors to avoid potential bleeding problems associated with chemotherapy. Generally, a platelet count of at least 50,000/mm^3 is recommended prior to invasive dental or dental hygiene procedures. If a dental or dental hygiene procedure is absolutely necessary during periods of thrombocytopenia, platelet support therapy may be given by the oncologist. Adequate bleeding times are dependent on the extent of the oral procedure. The client also should be warned that trauma from improper toothbrushing or a poorly fitting dental prosthesis may initiate bleeding when platelets are low.

SALIVARY GLAND DYSFUNCTION. Not all persons on chemotherapy experience xerostomia or ropy saliva. Some clients, however, complain of a dry mouth, thickened secretions, or excessive drooling during chemotherapy. Studies are inconclusive as to the drugs' effects on salivary glands; however, persons who complain about salivary dysfunction should be offered palliative measures such as adequate hydration (Table 43–2) to help manage this debilitating and uncomfortable side effect and to prevent further exacerbation of other oral complications.

DENTAL CARIES. Rampant tooth decay is not directly caused by the toxicity of chemotherapeutic drugs. However, clients with chronically dry mouths or persons who increase their intake of high-carbohydrate foods because of eating problems may experience an increase in caries development. For example, children who are chronically ill may be given nighttime bottle feedings and/or diets high in sugar. During periods of stress, parents and caregivers may allow an unbalanced diet to avoid additional stress from confrontation. Such eating patterns may increase dental caries.

Management. Depending on the severity of this problem, various preventive regimens may be prescribed. A fluoride rinse or brush-on 1.1% sodium fluoride gel may be adequate. If, however, there is evidence of demineralization and if dryness continues over months, the client may require custom-fit gel trays for daily gel application. Additionally, in-office fluoride varnish applications may be beneficial. The dental hygienist educates about the importance of daily fluoride application, good nutrition, and oral hygiene. The dental hygienist also counsels

TABLE 43–2 MANAGEMENT OF ORAL MANIFESTATIONS OF CANCER THERAPIES

Manifestation	Prevention	Palliative Measures and Management	Dental Hygiene Care Guidelines
Mucositis/stomatitis (related to direct effect of radiation therapy and cytotoxic chemotherapy)	Caused by toxicity of the cancer therapy. Early onset and severity can be minimized by consistent hydration and excellent bacterial plaque control. Gentle tooth and gingival brushing with extra-soft toothbrush. Discontinue toothpastes with strong, irritating flavoring agents and replace with baking soda and water paste. Discontinue alcohol-based rinses, full-strength peroxide, and irritating foods.	Increased hydration with water, saliva substitutes, ice chips, or sugar-free popsicles. Cool-mist humidifiers may be helpful, especially in dry environments. Baking soda/water rinses (1 tsp baking soda, $\frac{1}{2}$ tsp salt, and 16 oz water) may be used as a rinse or placed in disposable irrigation bag (let solution flow through mouth to gently rinse). Topical anesthetics (Table 43–1).	Do not schedule dental hygiene procedures while client is experiencing oral ulcerations and pain.
Salivary gland dysfunction/xerostomia (related to direct radiation damage to salivary gland tissue and possible indirect effect of chemotherapeutic agents. Salivary gland dysfunction is permanent following radiation therapy, whereas function usually returns after chemotherapy.)	Eliminate use of products with alcohol and irritating agents. Diminish caffeine intake. Discontinue tobacco use. Humidify air with cool-mist humidifier. Consult with oncologist for salivary gland stimulant prescription.	Suggest OTC saliva substitutes. (See Recommendations for Clients with Xerostomia.) Stimulate functional salivary gland tissue by chewing sugar-free gum or wax bolus. Consult physician for salivary gland stimulant prescription. Lubricate lips with balm or cream (not pure petrolatum). Increase hydration with water, ice chips, or high-moisture foods. Thin food with liquids. Recommend cool-mist humidifier, especially while client is sleeping. Suggest baking soda and water rinsing for ropy saliva (see details under Mucositis)	To prevent rampant caries, encourage improved oral hygiene measures, diet low in sucrose, and fluoride supplementation (e.g., daily use of 1.1% neutral-pH sodium fluoride gels for 5 to 10 minutes in customized fluoride trays for home use).
Infection: fungal, viral, and bacterial (related to chemotherapy-induced immunosuppression. Oral infections may not present with typical signs and symptoms. Candidiasis is common during radiation therapy.	Frequent and consistent oral hydration with water, ices, and/or saliva substitutes. Increase bacterial plaque control. Oral infections may be unrelenting when the client is severely immunosuppressed during chemotherapy.	Oral microbiologic culturing and assessment. Alert oncologist at first signs of oral infection. Encourage antifungals that are sugar-free.	Do not proceed with dental hygiene procedures while a client has an acute oral infection. Schedule dental hygiene procedures when the client's absolute neutrophil count is $>1000/mm^3$. If the client has a central venous catheter, the American Heart Association antibiotic prophylactic protocol should be followed for invasive dental hygiene procedures, including dental prophylaxis.
Bleeding (related to chemotherapy-induced myelosuppression)	Bleeding is not preventable, but bacterial plaque can exacerbate the complication if not consistently removed.	Refer to oncologist for management.	Dental hygiene procedures should be delayed until the client has a platelet count over $50,000/mm^3$ or has a blood transfusion.

Table continued on following page

TABLE 43–2 MANAGEMENT OF ORAL MANIFESTATIONS OF CANCER THERAPIES—CONT'D

Manifestation	Prevention	Palliative Measures and Management	Dental Hygiene Care Guidelines
Rampant dental caries/demineralization (related to therapy-induced salivary gland dysfunction)	Bacterial plaque control. Frequent oral hydration with water, ices, or saliva substitutes. Daily 5- to 10-minute application of 1.1% sodium fluoride gel in custom gel carriers (soft vinyl trays adapted to extend beyond the cervical line of the teeth) or topical fluoride. In-office application of fluoride varnish to exposed cementum. Dietary guidelines to discourage frequent snacking on cariogenic foods, sugared beverages, or acidic beverages (diet sodas with citric or phosphoric acid). If there is evidence of dental decay despite daily fluoride application, place client on 2-week chlorhexidine regimen and in-office fluoride varnish application.	Same as prevention measures.	Encourage participation of client in planning oral hygiene home care and ensure strict adherence by frequent monitoring. Establish a 2- to 3-month continued care interval until client demonstrates ability to care for teeth and acute side effects of therapy have resolved.
Trismus/TMD (related to direct effect of radiation on muscles of mastication and/or TMJ)	Daily exercise for muscles of mastication: instruct client to open and close mouth 20 times without causing pain to the TMJ. This exercise should be repeated 3 times a day.	Same as prevention. Also instruct client to encourage further opening of the mouth by placing increasing numbers of tongue blades between posterior teeth for several minutes a day.	Dental hygiene procedures may need to be altered for clients with trismus to avoid exacerbating the associated pain (e.g., shortened appointments or sedation).
Soft tissue and osteoradionecrosis (related to direct effect of radiation on tissue and bone. Tissue becomes hypovascular, hypoxic, and hypocellular. Damage to the bone/soft tissue is permanent)	All teeth within the field of radiation that have a poor lifelong prognosis should be extracted 14 to 21 days prior to the initiation of radiation therapy. Avoid all surgical insult to irradiated bone throughout the client's lifetime.	Referral to an oral surgeon for possible hyperbaric oxygen therapy and surgical management of the necrotic tissue and bone.	Frequent and regular dental hygiene continued-care interval to ensure prevention of periodontal disease and adherence to oral hygiene home care protocol.

clients and primary caregivers about cariogenic foods and behaviors and suggests alternatives.

ALTERED TOOTH DEVELOPMENT. Studies have shown that some chemotherapy drugs given before the age of 10 years, and especially before the age of 5 years, may alter root development.

BONE MARROW AND BLOOD TRANSPLANTATION

Bone marrow and blood transplantation (BMT) is a therapeutic procedure used to treat a variety of hematologic diseases including aplastic anemia, leukemias, lymphomas, neuroblastoma, and immunodeficiency diseases. It is also used to treat some solid tumors.

Bone marrow and blood transplantation begins with the donation of normal bone marrow or *peripheral blood stem cells.* The individual with cancer then goes through a "conditioning phase" when super-lethal doses of chemotherapy and sometimes total body irradiation (TBI) are administered. The goal is to destroy all of the malignant cells and suppress the immune system to permit engraftment of the normal bone marrow. After clients have been conditioned, the marrow or peripheral blood stem cells are intravenously infused into their blood. If engraftment takes place, the cells begin to reproduce new marrow within 2 to 4 weeks.

A significant problem that exists for clients who receive marrow or peripheral blood stem cells from another individual *(allogeneic bone marrow transplant)* is *graft-versus-host disease (GVHD).* This disease results from an immunologic reaction wherein the donor cells react against the host tissue antigens. If this occurs within the first 100 days after transplant it is called acute GVHD and is characterized by dermatitis, enteritis, and hepatitis. If it occurs after the first 100 days, it is termed chronic GVHD with manifestations similar to those of autoimmune disorders. These may include skin diseases, keratoconjunctivitis, oral mucositis, salivary gland dysfunction/xerostomia, esophageal and vaginal strictures, pulmonary insufficiency, intestinal problems, and chronic liver disease. Both forms of GVHD can result in fatal infections. To prevent GVHD, various types of immunosuppressive therapy are used.

The other major problem after transplant is decreased immunologic function, making the transplanted individual susceptible to opportunistic infections. After the first year, most recover their immune function unless they have developed chronic GVHD.

Oral Complications

During the first 30 days of transplantation, the client experiences cytotoxic and immunosuppressive oral manifestations from the chemoradiotherapy conditioning. These may include severe mucositis, ulceration, hemorrhage, infection, and salivary gland dysfunction. Infections during the first 30 days intensify the mucositis and ulcerations, opening a portal of entry for organisms into the blood.

During the next several months, the client's acute manifestations begin to resolve unless GVHD develops. Common complaints with GVHD are xerostomia and mucositis. Also, there may be evidence of lichen planus–like or lupuslike lesions, sometimes becoming erosive. Generalized atrophy of the mucosa and changes consistent with scleroderma may be seen. Viral infections, including herpes simplex virus and fungal infections, are common.

After the first 100 days after transplant, persons with no evidence of GVHD usually do not have any oral complaints other than varying degrees of xerostomia. Those persons with persistent xerostomia may develop rapid demineralization of the tooth structure and oral infections. Patients who are scheduled for bone marrow or blood transplantation should undergo a thorough oral and dental evaluation and necessary treatment prior to transplant. All potential sources of infection and irritation should be treated because chronic, nonsymptomatic oral infections may become acute during immunosuppression and/or GVHD and may lead to sepsis and even death.

DENTAL HYGIENE PROCESS OF CARE

The dental hygienist, either as a member of a hospital oncology team or as a clinician in consultation with the oncologist, has the opportunity to prevent and/or ameliorate many of the oral and systemic complications associated with cancer treatment by designing a dental hygiene care plan that promotes a clean and healthy oral cavity. Prior to the initial dental hygiene care appointment, consultation must be sought with other oncology team members involved in the care of the person with cancer. Open and continuous communication with physicians and nurses reduces the risk of providing care that compromises the client's condition. Figure 43–5 provides a dental consultation referral form to demonstrate important information to seek from the oncologist.

Assessment

The dental hygienist collaborates with the dentist to identify sources of infection that may delay postoperative healing for a client scheduled for surgery to the oral cavity. In addition, the pretherapy assessment also is critical for a client scheduled for radiation therapy to the oral cavity and/or salivary glands. Any part of the maxilla and/or mandible that will be irradiated is at lifelong risk for the development of osteoradionecrosis. Therefore, all infections and teeth that cannot be maintained for the client's lifetime should be identified for removal. Teeth to be extracted include not only those with gross caries and refractory periodontal disease, but also those that potentially may not be maintained because of the client's lack of personal motivation, physical or mental ability, and/or financial resources.

Oncology Dental Support Clinic
University of Missouri-Kansas City
School of Dentistry
650 E. 25th, Kansas City, MO 64108

______________________________ is referred for an oral/dental evaluation and treatment.

This adjunctive medical care is essential so that the patient may complete cancer therapy.

______________________________ Physician's Signature ______________ Date

Diagnosis: ______________________________

Proposed therapy: ______________________________

If therapy includes radiation to the salivary glands or oral cavity, please indicate field of therapy: ______________________________

If therapy is myelosuppressive, please give current:

absolute granulocyte count ______________

platelet count ______________

Does the patient have a central venous catheter?
______ (yes) ______ (no)

Does the patient need antibiotics prior to dental treatment?
______ (yes) ______ (no)

Additional important medical information: ______________________________

To schedule an appointment, contact the Special Patient Care Clinic at 235-2160 or the Oncology Dental Support Clinic Coordinator, Ms. Gerry Barker (RDH, MA), at 235-2300.

APPOINTMENT DATE: ______________ **TIME:** ______________

FIGURE 43–5 ✦ Oncology dental consultation and referral form.

Because intraoral infection may spread through the bloodstream and result in sepsis and possibly death during immunosuppression, all potential sources of irritation that may potentiate mucositis also must be identified and eliminated. Assessment of a potential BMT recipient should identify any oral problem that may arise within the first year following the transplant when the client is in an immunosuppressed condition.

CLIENT INTERVIEW. The client interview provides critical information that influences future oral hygiene care and dental treatment. Social support of the person with cancer is an important part of the treatment process. Therefore, those closest to the individual should be involved in the client interview and education whenever possible. Clients who have had a laryngectomy or those with a surgical speech defect should be provided a pad of paper and pencil to assist in answering questions. If they use a communicative assistive device (e.g., an electro-larynx), the dental hygienist should encourage its use. It is difficult to understand a client who is just beginning to use the device, but time and patience increase the client's self-confidence, thus promoting mutual trust and respect. It is important for the dental hygienist to verify what clients understand about their cancer diagnosis and medical treatment prior to discussing the dental hygiene component of care. This approach facilitates the person's human need for conceptualization and understanding. Physicians employ different strategies for telling clients about their disease. Most doctors feel it is their ethical and legal responsibility to disclose fully the consequences of a cancer diagnosis and complications associated with treatment. Some doctors, however, tell the client only what the client seems able to comprehend at the time of initial diagnosis, and have not completed the educational process when the person is referred for dental consultation. Even when a physician offers a full explanation to the person and the family, emotional factors often prevent a clear understanding of all information.

Ethically, it is inappropriate to give a judgmental opinion about the client's medical care plan. It is appropriate and important, however, to offer empathy and listen to the client's fears. Taking time to listen to the client's perceptions decreases client and family stress, promotes consistency, encourages cooperation among members of the oncology team, and assists the dental hygienist in assessing the client's human needs that shape the dental hygiene process of care.

The client's current oral status and health and dental histories are reviewed, including frequency of care, dental experiences that were unpleasant or painful, oral self-care habits, and current attitude and knowledge about the teeth and mouth. This information assists the dental hygienist in planning dental hygiene care. The interview also reveals the client's socioeconomic status, and cultural and ethnic influences that may affect perceptions of cancer, health beliefs, coping strategies, social support system, dietary habits, and ability to adhere to the supportive care.

Other important information includes history of tobacco use and alcohol intake. Amount used, duration of use, and attempts to quit should be documented. The dental hygienist should determine if the client understands the association of tobacco and alcohol to oral cancer, and if there is a desire to quit these habits.

During the interview, the dental hygienist also is sensitive to the client's mood. One of the most common psychological responses to cancer is depression. Signs of depression include a loss of interest in daily activities, lack of motivation, loss of energy and appetite, insomnia or hypersomnia, feelings of worthlessness, diminished ability to think, psychomotor agitation or retardation, and suicidal thoughts. Some clients appear to accept their diagnosis, but actually are repressing their fears and anxiety, which can lead to depression. When the dental hygienist suspects a client is experiencing depression, the client's physician should be consulted to identify ways to manage it. Most chemotherapeutic agents do not have any direct psychological effects, but a few may cause confusion, depression, delirium, lethargy, and fatigue.

Diagnosis

Dental hygiene diagnoses identify human needs related to direct dental hygiene care prior to initiation of cancer therapy, during therapy, and after the client has completed all proposed therapy. As therapy progresses and the client moves through various physical changes and psychosocial stages related to the cancer, the dental hygiene diagnoses change and the care plan is continually revised.

Planning

The client undergoing cancer therapy or in *end-stage disease* requires a care plan directed toward meeting actual or potential needs associated with the oral and systemic complications of cancer therapies.

Initially, when clients are faced with a life-threatening cancer diagnosis, they are unable to conceptualize the importance of care beyond their most basic physiologic and survival needs. As these needs appear to be no longer at imminent risk, the client often begins to accept the diagnosis and may be capable of participating in supportive care. A client in the dental office with a previous positive attitude about the teeth and oral hygiene may reveal totally different values during times of stress. It cannot be assumed that this client will continue the previous level of personal oral hygiene care. On the other hand, it should not be assumed that persons with a seemingly overwhelming cancer diagnosis do not have the ability to participate in successful rehabilitation. At appropriate times, a clear understanding of the oral problems associated with cancer therapy must be effectively communicated and trust established by mutual participation in the development of oral health goals.

Implementation: Before Cancer Therapy

REFERRAL TO A DENTIST. Conditions found by the dental hygienist that require diagnosis by a dentist should be referred immediately for evaluation and treatment. Before chemotherapy begins, clients should have all surgical procedures done at least 7 days prior to periods of immunosuppression, all sources of infection and irritation removed, and all projected dental needs met. For clients scheduled for surgery, all oral surgical procedures need to be scheduled 14 to 21 days prior to initiation of radiation therapy to the oral cavity and salivary glands. Restorative needs should be cared for prior to the onset of painful mucositis. Fabrication of new dental prostheses is delayed until several months after radiation therapy ends, when all acute side effects of radiation have resolved.

As mentioned earlier, clients undergoing radiation therapy to the head and neck area may need to be referred to a prosthodontist for fabrication of a complex oral device prior to the simulation appointment. It is important for the dental professional to communicate with the radiation oncologist regarding the potential need for such a referral. This inquiry should be made on client referral for the preradiation dental evaluation. Although many individuals with oral cancer require referral to the prosthodontist for construction of complex oral devices to be worn during radiation therapy, clients with nasopharyngeal or throat cancer may require no oral devices, or may need only a simple set of oral stents customized to their dentition. These oral stents, similar to those used for home dental bleaching or fluoride application, can be made easily by the dental hygienist or dental assistant in the general dental office. These simple oral stents are worn by clients along with the radiation mask at each radiation visit. If they are required, they need to be given to clients prior to their simulation appointment; otherwise, the radiation oncologist will provide a "one size fits all" set of stents at the time of the simulation appointment. These noncustomized stents tend to be bulky and detract from client comfort during radiation treatment. The oral stents worn at the simulation appointment remain the same throughout radiation treatment because precise measurements for targeting radiation beams are made at the simulation appointment while the client wears the oral stents. Customized oral stents made in the dental office decrease the client's sense of claustrophobia while wearing the mask and greatly enhance client comfort during radiation treatment because they fit snugly over the client's teeth. Providing these customized oral stents for clients undergoing radiation treatment for nasopharyngeal cancer is an important role the dental hygienist can play to enhance client comfort level and, in some cases, even compliance with treatment.

PSYCHOSOCIAL ISSUES. The initial client appointment is an important time when trust and assurance are established. The client must feel acceptance in a nonjudgmental environment and sense that his or her self-esteem will be preserved. The client is a "person living with cancer," not a "cancer case." Additional time is necessary to allow the client to express feelings. All feelings should be acknowledged and anger should not be mitigated too quickly. The client should be encouraged to participate in care planning, which provides an opportunity to regain some of the sense of control that was lost to the cancer. Eye contact is important to help eliminate feelings of isolation and stress, especially for clients who have suffered surgical facial deformity and who have disturbances in body image. It may help clients to be reminded that the treatment is aimed at the disease, not at their personhood. Clients who seem to be psychologically immobilized may require a referral to a social worker or psychologist on the oncology team.

EDUCATION. Adequate time must be allotted for education because the stress related to a cancer diagnosis can easily impede the normal learning process. It is important to engage in the teaching process with full regard for the client's psychological human need status. Clients in a state of denial are not able to comprehend the importance of preventive oral healthcare until they begin to accept their cancer and therapy plan. Others, stressed by the financial burden of medical treatments, may not place priority on dental and dental hygiene treatment when compared to their impending lifesaving cancer therapy. Those who are depressed and see their prognosis as grave do not value the importance of long-term dental hygiene care until they begin to see cause for hope.

In view of the constraints placed on the client by all of the medical diagnostic tests necessary before cancer therapy and the amount of new information related to cancer treatment, the dental hygienist must utilize the most effective teaching strategies possible. Whether teaching adults with cancer or the parents of a child with cancer, the teaching process can be strengthened by allowing clients to express themselves and make as many of the decisions regarding their self-care as possible. It is also important to include family members or friends in the education process because they may be more capable of comprehending the information and asking appropriate questions. Whenever possible, it is important to give the client either handwritten instructions or printed materials specific to immediate needs to reinforce the verbal communication. Education of children may be aided by booklets and videos. Many of these are available about oral healthcare in general, and most children's hospitals have audiovisual departments that produce videos for client education.

Information about the oral manifestations of the cancer therapy may not have been provided by the physician and nurse; therefore, it is important to ask clients what they understand, and then provide additional information that is concise and in easy-to-understand language. A brief overview of the potential problems is appropriate, with assurance that additional information will be given as the therapy progresses.

ORAL HYGIENE INSTRUCTION AND SELF-CARE. Assistance with oral hygiene self-care is important prior to initiation of cancer therapy to establish good hygiene before the oral tissues are compromised. Use of a disclosing agent aids in instruction and helps the client identify areas that need closer attention in self-care procedures. This educational approach also provides an opportunity for the dental hygienist to explain the composition of plaque biofilm and the risk of oral and systemic infections during cancer therapy. Assessment of the client's oral hygiene technique should be accomplished, if possible, and the person should be assisted in establishing plaque removal techniques that will be useful prior to and during therapy. If a client is scheduled for therapy that will significantly compromise the oral tissues, initial instruction should be given regarding methods for cleansing the mouth and preventive and palliative products recommended (Table 43–1). These methods are then elaborated on during therapy. Gentle tooth and gingival brushing can continue during cancer therapy. If a sponge toothette becomes necessary because of oral ulcerations, it should be dipped in a nonalcoholic antimicrobial solution for optimal efficacy. Clients also should be warned that because many hospital-supplied toothbrushes are inexpensive and made with unpolished, hard bristles, they should take a new extra-soft nylon bristled toothbrush when admitted as hospital inpatients.

TOBACCO AND ALCOHOL CESSATION COUNSELING. Clients usually are told by the oncologist to quit using tobacco products and limit excessive alcohol intake during cancer therapy. Support and assistance by the dental hygienist are important (see Chapter 29). Referral to a professional program or support group may be necessary and desired by the client.

NUTRITIONAL COUNSELING. The nutritional status of clients affects their overall response to cancer therapy and their psychological well-being. The nutritionist on the oncology team assumes primary responsibility for monitoring the nutritional status of the client and providing counseling on diet selection. The dental hygienist has the responsibility for consulting with the nutritionist and educating the client about diet selection and dietary habits to promote a clean and healthy oral environment and to reduce caries development. It is important for the dental hygienist to determine the client's understanding of the relationship of a well-balanced diet to dental caries, periodontal disease, and infection. When the client is ready psychologically to assimilate preventive behaviors, the client and the dental hygienist choose foods that are desirable to the client, but are low in sugar, acid, and oral retention qualities. The client should understand that it is often difficult during therapy to eat a well-balanced diet containing foods that promote oral health. The pretherapy dietary instruction aids the client in setting goals and in food selection.

DENTAL HYGIENE INSTRUMENTATION. Dental hygiene instrumentation may need to be altered to accommodate the client's physical condition related to recent surgery, manifestations of disease, and the status of the client's blood counts and clotting factors. The oncologist should be consulted regarding the safest time to schedule an appointment and the need for antibiotic prophylaxis prior to dental hygiene instrumentation. Overall, dental hygiene care promotes a clean and well-hydrated oral environment and control of periodontal disease to reduce the risk of oral infection and bacteremia.

FLUORIDE THERAPY. When the client is scheduled for radiation therapy to the salivary glands or total body irradiation for BMT, custom fluoride gel trays are fabricated for daily application of a 1.1% neutral-pH sodium fluoride gel to prevent rampant dental caries. Clients who complain of a dry mouth during chemotherapy require at least a daily fluoride rinse and possibly a 1.1% sodium fluoride toothpaste or gel.

Implementation: During Cancer Therapy

Once therapy has been initiated it is important to continue to support the client, but the dental hygienist must understand that most cancer therapy is physically and psychologically demanding. Unrealistic scheduling of appointments must be avoided. Frequent phone calls to the client or family member emphasize the importance of regular oral hygiene self-care and help in determining when it is appropriate to schedule the client for dental hygiene care and further education.

With each appointment, the dental hygienist should repeat the oral assessment, update the health history, and assess the client's level of disease acceptance and readiness for new interventions. Remember that anger and bargaining may be signs of acceptance of the diagnosis and an attempt to regain control of the client's own life. These times offer the dental hygienist an opportunity to direct the client's interest to positive involvement in oral self-care and dietary planning. An attempt should be made to include the client in decisions about the dental hygiene care plan and self-care. Education during care should be centered on the immediate real and impending complications of therapy.

MANAGEMENT OF ORAL COMPLICATIONS. Table 43–2 summarizes dental hygiene interventions that may prevent or ameliorate the oral complications associated with radiation and chemotherapy.

After a client scheduled to undergo BMT enters the transplant center, the client is not allowed to leave the unit until the bone marrow has engrafted and blood counts have returned to a normal range. Therefore, all dental treatment must be accomplished prior to the transplant. A dental hygienist working in a hospital setting with a transplant unit may assist with daily oral assessment and oral hygiene procedures. Oral care regimens vary among transplant centers, but generally oral care is given every 2 to 4 hours. Protocols range from simple saline rinses and antimicrobial rinses to oral debridement.

NUTRITIONAL COUNSELING DURING CANCER THERAPY. The side effects of cancer therapy often result in high risk for dental caries. Clients may be placed on a soft and bland diet or liquid high-carbohydrate diet because of recent oral surgery or mucositis from therapy. They may also be encouraged to eat small, frequent meals and snacks to increase their caloric intake and counteract nausea and vomiting. Additional complications arise from a dry mouth or thickened saliva, taste dysfunction, inability to practice good oral hygiene because of an oral surgical procedure, and/or a lack of interest in eating because of depression and stress. A severely malnourished client may be placed on parenteral nutrition, completely eliminating the mechanical oral cleansing action of foods.

Diets of children during cancer therapy are often a problem because there are so many times when they are too sick to eat that parents allow them to eat anything they want when they are feeling well. Regular meals, especially in a pediatric hospital setting, are difficult to achieve. In working with the nutritionist, the dental hygienist should continue to emphasize the importance of a well-balanced diet for prevention of infection and promotion of healing after the insult of therapy. In turn, the nutritionist can assist the client in planning meals low in sugar, when possible. The suggestion may also be made to add cheeses to the diet when eating sugar-containing foods to reduce cariogenicity. When possible, the dental hygienist should alert other oncology team members about the high concentration of sugar in some medications, especially antifungal suspensions. Alternatives may be suggested, such as sugar-free troches or suppositories.

Clients with mouth pain may be helped by suggesting one of the topical anesthetic or coating agents prior to eating (Table 43–1). Also, clients with oral ulcerations or dry mouth may find it helpful to eat foods high in moisture, or they may thin their food with liquids and take frequent sips of water while eating. Irritating hot, spicy, or acidic foods should be avoided. All meals and snacks should be followed by oral hygiene measures and adequate hydration of the tissues.

Implementation: After Cancer Therapy

Following any kind of cancer therapy, the dental hygienist continues to have an important role in client care. With each appointment or contact with the client, the dental hygienist reassesses the client's human needs related to oral health. Even when clients have been reassured that their cancer has successfully responded to therapy, they continue to experience stress, anxiety, and concern about possible recurrence of the cancer. Some need to continue to adapt to an altered facial image resulting from the long-term side effects of the therapy. Some clients continue to be dependent on the caregivers and need to reestablish their independence and regain their self-confidence. Occasionally, individuals treated for cancer want to place everything associated with the cancer therapy behind them and ignore critical preventive long-term self-care procedures. Continued education and frequent contact and support are essential. The dental hygienist should tailor the client's oral self-care to the individual's status and human needs, and place as much responsibility on the client as possible.

AFTER RADIATION THERAPY. The care of the client after radiation therapy to the oral cavity and salivary glands requires lifelong frequent dental and dental hygiene maintenance care. Because damage to the salivary glands and jaw bones from cancer radiation therapy is permanent, clients are at permanent risk for development of rampant "radiation caries," demineralization of the tooth structure and soft tissue, and/or osteoradionecrosis. Continued-care appointments are scheduled at intervals to ensure excellent oral hygiene, maintenance of sound tooth structure, and avoidance of soft tissue irritation. The daily use of the custom fluoride trays with 1.1% neutral-pH sodium fluoride gel for 5 to 10 minutes followed by 30 minutes of abstinence from food and water must continue for the rest of the client's life. If there is evidence of dental decay despite compliance with daily fluoride applications, the client should be placed on a 2-week chlorhexidine regimen to decrease cariogenic bacteria and have in-office fluoride varnish applications. A daily remineralizing gel application may also be necessary in addition to the daily fluoride gel application.

With each appointment, the dental hygienist should assess the client's nutritional status and dietary intake. Adjustments should be made to return to a normal and noncariogenic diet as the acute side effects of radiation therapy resolve. Referral for nutritional counseling may be necessary.

A thorough head and neck assessment for oral cancer and function of the muscles of mastication, the temporomandibular joint, and prosthetic appliances should be done at each appointment. Deficits in the needs for integrity of the skin and mucous membrane of the head and neck and for biologically sound dentition require immediate referral to the dentist. Dental disease in an area of irradiated bone is managed as conservatively and as atraumatically as possible by the dentist, and sometimes is accompanied with antibiotic prophylaxis. If trismus occurs, treatment consists of introducing tongue blades between the teeth for several minutes each day, gradually increasing the number until adequate opening is achieved. This strategy may be painful and requires patience and perseverance. Dental treatment of osteoradionecrosis is conservative, but generally requires conservative surgical removal of necrotic tissue, antibiotics to prevent infection, and, ideally, hyperbaric oxygen therapy to stimulate vascularization and new bone growth. When conservative measures fail, surgical resection is usually indicated.

AFTER CHEMOTHERAPY After a client has completed the required rounds of chemotherapy, most of the oral manifestations completely resolve. With full recovery of the bone marrow, all problems associated with acute cytotoxicity, immunosuppression, and thrombocytopenia should disappear. Some clients, after long and intensive chemotherapy, take months to recover fully and experience chronic oral infections such as candidiasis and herpetic infections. Some clients will maintain their central venous catheter even after the chemotherapy protocol has been completed, and should be queried about the need for antibiotic prophylaxis prior to initiating an invasive dental procedure. Continual assistance with oral hygiene is required to prevent unnecessary infections. Assessment of clients' nutritional intake is important to determine if they have resumed a noncariogenic and normal diet.

AFTER BONE MARROW/BLOOD TRANSPLANTATION. After clients are released from a transplant unit they may have residual effects of the conditioning phase of treatment and may remain susceptible to infections for several months because of immunosuppressive therapy. Some continue to experience xerostomia, which predisposes them to an altered oral flora and infections, trauma, and rampant dental caries. Clients with graft-versus-host disease may experience additional complications of thinned and friable mucosa and mucosal lesions.

The dental hygienist assists the client in establishing consistent and effective oral hygiene methods that do not create additional trauma and irritation. Bland rinses, gentle but thorough and consistent cleansing of the teeth and tissues, and saliva substitutes are important.

Dental procedures deemed necessary are done only after consultation with the oncologist to assess the client's immune status and need for antibiotic prophylaxis or platelet support. Elective dental procedures are delayed until the client has full hematologic function, sometimes up to a year or longer after treatment. Rampant dental caries from xerostomia are prevented with daily application of fluoride gel in custom fluoride trays.

Clients with End-Stage Disease

Oral and dental care are sometimes ignored during this stage of life, but a mouth free of discomfort and bad odors is extremely important. The mouth becomes the center of existence during terminal disease because it maintains nutritional status and is used to communicate needs and emotions to loved ones. A mouth free of bad odors helps to maintain self-esteem and aids in social communication, preventing some of the loneliness experienced during the terminal stage. All care must be designed to provide quality of life and the best care for the client's needs. Care that enhances the person's dignity and facilitates personal comfort, normal eating, and social communication is of critical importance.

The dental hygienist educates family, hospice volunteers, and other caregivers about the importance of oral hygiene for the client. Many people do not realize how important the mouth becomes to the dying individual. Simple explanations and procedures related to oral hygiene reduce the stress related to this time. Such explanations may also provide a significant opportunity for family members to assist in the care of their loved one, because oral hygiene care aids so much in their overall comfort. This assistance with care may be especially important for parents of dying children. Many medical procedures must be performed by nurses or physicians, but oral care procedures are simple and provide an opportunity for the parent to participate with tender care.

The dental hygienist helps the client and other caregivers to design oral hygiene procedures that effectively remove plaque biofilm, but are nonirritating and provide adequate tissue hydration. All highly flavored dentifrices and mouthwashes should be avoided. A small amount of pleasant-flavored mouthwash may be added to water to refresh the client's mouth. Saliva substitutes may be important for the client with xerostomia. Baking soda and saline solutions aid in cleansing thickened secretions from the mouth.

Procedures may need to be designed for bed-ridden clients (Procedure 43–1). The client should be rolled on the side or placed in a sitting position to prevent aspiration. If necessary, a bite block should be placed between the teeth on one side, which later can be placed on the other side to aid in cleansing each area of the mouth. The lips may be lubricated with a water-based lubricant. Petrolatum-based products should be avoided because aspiration of non–water-soluble agents can result in pneumonia. The teeth, tongue, and buccal mucosa are cleansed with dental floss and an extra-soft toothbrush, gauze dampened in warm water, or a moistened sponge stick. An ingestible toothpaste is available commercially. A bulb syringe and small basin may be helpful for delivering and collecting the rinses and water.

Clients with dentures should be encouraged to wear their dentures as long as they fit well and do not irritate the tissues. They must be kept immaculately clean and kept out of the mouth while the client is sleeping. Clients with ill-fitting dentures should be referred to a dentist for care.

Clients with xerostomia may need daily application of fluoride gel to prevent rampant tooth decay. Even though death is anticipated, potential dental problems that could result in oral discomfort or infection should be prevented with referral for dental evaluation and treatment. Clients with excessive drooling may need a gentle suction device. Medications may be ordered by the physician to help reduce salivary flow.

Evaluation

Goals planned for outcomes of dental hygiene care vary tremendously, depending on the stage of the disease, treatment, and psychological status. Goals are evaluated repeatedly by the clients' responses as they move through the various phases of treatment and psychological adjustments to their disease. Outcome of care is evaluated based on whether the goals planned for care are met, partially met, or unmet.

PSYCHOSOCIAL SUPPORT FOR THE PROFESSIONAL

Working with the client with cancer may be very rewarding, but also may be stressful and difficult. Medical and oral health professionals who treat clients with terminal disease must be able to accept death as part of life and acknowledge their own mortality. The fact that some clients are going to die—because not all therapy is curative—must be accepted by the oncology team. This acceptance may be difficult for dental hygienists because of their strong association with preventive medicine. Another difficult task may be dealing with their own vulnerability to cancer.

Professionals must maintain a balance between the needs of their clients and their own needs. Maintaining open communication with other oncology team members about personal frustrations, feelings of guilt for not being able to help a client, and personal sadness and grief for the loss of a client help, to abate overwhelming feelings and depression. A well-balanced life of work and recreation also is important.

The positive aspects of working in oncology come from the association with individuals who are acutely aware of their priorities in life and must focus on living one day at a time. So many of these clients share their personal strengths with their caregivers. By being open and receptive, the dental hygienist can learn many important lessons from them. Another benefit comes from being able to provide care that offers immediate and significant improvement in the quality of life. When clients understand the importance of good oral hygiene during therapy and when palliative measures give comfort and reduce stress, they are openly and intensely appreciative. Keeping these aspects in mind compensates for negative feelings and provides a professional environment that is stimulating, challenging, and gratifying.

Procedure 43–1 PERFORMING ORAL HYGIENE CARE FOR NONAMBULATORY CLIENTS

EQUIPMENT

Protective gloves, face mask, protective eyewear, towel
Extra-soft toothbrush with suction (the Plak Vac is a soft-bristled tooth brush with a hollow handle that connects directly to the suction in a hospital room.)
Dental floss and holder
Bite block
Cleansing agent (ingestible toothpaste, baking soda, and/or denture cleanser)
Pitcher of water and cup or bulb syringe or irrigation bag filled with water and hung on an intravenous pole
Water-based lubricant
Emesis basin

STEPS	RATIONALE
1. Position bed to comfortable height	Facilitates access and acceptable body mechanics for the dental hygienist
2. Don face mask and protective eyewear; wash and glove hands	Maintains universal infection control protocol
3. Position client; sitting, or on side	Facilitates drainage and prevents aspiration of debris and fluids
4. Place towel under client's head	Maintains position and comfort of the client
5. Place emesis basin at chin.	Facilitates drainage of saliva and debris from the client's mouth
6. Assemble suction equipment	Suction equipment prevents aspiration of saliva and debris
7. Position bite block between teeth if necessary	Aids client in keeping the mouth open
8. Apply nonpetrolatum lubricant to lips	Prevents trauma to dry lips
9. Assess oral cavity	Enables dental hygienist to identify needs and plan appropriate care
10. Cleanse teeth, tongue, and mucosal tissues with appropriate technique and aids (dependent on client's condition)	Provides both palliative and therapeutic oral care; a clean, well-hydrated oral environment reduces the risk of oral infection and bacteremia
11. Suction, rinse with clear water, repeat suction (catch return flow in basin)	Facilitates removal of oral debris and client comfort
12. Apply lubricant to lips	Prevents trauma to dry lips
13. If client has dentures, brush dentures over towel-lined sink and soak in clean soaking solution, rinse well; either put back in client's mouth or store in clean water; instruct client to leave dentures out of mouth while sleeping	Provides palliative, cosmetic, and therapeutic care to the edentulous client; prevents damage to dentures; promotes client comfort; prevents oral infection
14. Saliva substitute may be palliative	Increases client comfort
15. Excessive drooling may require a gentle suction device (most hospital rooms are equipped with suction equipment)	Facilitates removal of oral debris and client comfort

CLIENT EDUCATION ISSUES

- ✦ Inform clients about the signs and symptoms of oral and pharyngeal cancers while doing head and neck examinations.
- ✦ Inform clients about risk factors for oral cancer.
- ✦ Assist clients with tobacco use cessation (see Chapter 29)
- ✦ Educate clients about the potential oral complications associated with the type of cancer therapy they will undergo and about ways in which such complications can be prevented or ameliorated.
- ✦ Emphasize the importance of excellent oral hygiene during cancer therapy. Individualize self-care plans based on the proposed cancer therapy and the client's needs.
- ✦ Ensure that the client has full knowledge of the long-term complications associated with radiation therapy and the need to continue preventive measures for the rest of the client's life.

Legal, Ethical, and Safety Issues

- The dental hygienist should always perform a thorough head and neck examination to screen for oral cancer.
- Inform clients about the potential side effects and complications associated with various cancer therapies and about strategies to prevent and manage them.
- Coordinate clients' oral healthcare with their cancer therapy schedules and hematologic status.
- Never abandon clients with end-stage cancer. Good oral health is critical at this time to encourage good oral intake and improve quality of life.

Key Concepts

- *Cancer* is a term that defines a broad variety of malignant processes, usually treated with surgery, chemotherapy, radiation therapy, or bone marrow/blood transplantation.
- Approximately 40% of persons treated for non–head and neck malignancies experience oral complications.
- Preexisting oral/dental pathology can adversely affect the individual undergoing cancer therapy.
- The dental hygiene care plan developed by the dental hygienist plays a critical role in the care of individuals undergoing cancer therapy.
- Radiation treatment of head and neck cancer results in some permanent oral complications.
- Complications associated with radiation to the head and neck area, systemic chemotherapy, and bone marrow and blood transplantation may be prevented and/or ameliorated by oral hygiene interventions.

Critical Thinking Exercises

Client 1: Mrs. G.

Profile: A 45-year-old woman presents with a soft palate lesion and a large right neck mass. The biopsy reveals squamous cell carcinoma. She is scheduled for surgery followed by unilateral radiation therapy to the right posterior mandible/maxilla and lateral neck.

Chief Complaint: "I need a dental evaluation and dental hygiene care prior to starting my cancer therapy."

Dental History: Her pretherapy radiographic and clinical oral/dental evaluation reveals no dental caries, generalized gingivitis, and moderate plaque, calculus, and tobacco stain.

Social History: Client is single and lives with her parents.

Health History: Client has been diagnosed with squamous cell carcinoma of the soft palate. She currently takes no medications, and her blood pressure is within normal limits.

Oral Health Behavior Assessment: Client states that she brushes her teeth once a day, does not use floss, and visits her dentist every year. She takes OTC antacids, chewable vitamin C, and Aspergum for her sore throat. She has smoked one or two packs per day for 25 years.

Supplemental Notes: She has dental insurance, demonstrates a sincere interest and motivation to maintain her teeth, and is very interested in tobacco cessation intervention.

1. What procedures will be included in the dental treatment plan prior to radiation therapy?
2. Develop a dental hygiene care plan for prior to radiation therapy.
3. What measures do you suggest to relieve xerostomia and the pain associated with mucositis?
4. What dental hygiene interventions and recall schedule are appropriate for this woman following radiation therapy?
5. What are the signs and symptoms of osteoradionecrosis?

Continued on following page

Critical Thinking Exercises—cont'd

Client 2: Mrs. H.

Profile: A 23-year-old female who has been undergoing radiation for Hodgkin's disease.

Chief Complaint: "I need a dental evaluation and necessary treatment prior to the next phase of my cancer therapy."

Social History: She is single and lives alone.

Medical History: She is scheduled for an allogeneic bone marrow transplant for which she will receive total body irradiation and chemotherapy. She will enter the bone marrow transplant unit in 3 weeks.

Dental History: She has had no dental support during her previous cancer treatment. Her dental evaluation reveals a sensitive maxillary premolar with a large carious lesion and radiolucent periapical lesion, several areas of mild demineralization, moderate plaque and calculus, and chapped lips. No other gross caries or periodontal disease is evident. There are no impacted teeth or bony lesions detected by radiographs.

Oral Health Behavior Assessment: She reports that she brushes her teeth once a day, but does not use any interdental cleaning devices.

Supplemental Notes: She has dental insurance and appears motivated to improve her oral hygiene care.

1. What dental treatment and dental hygiene care would be appropriate for her prior to her transplant?
2. Develop a dental hygiene care plan for her prior to her transplant.

For References, Suggested Readings, and Related Websites, visit
http://evolve.elsevier.com/Darby/hygiene/

CHAPTER 44

Persons with HIV Infection

OBJECTIVES

Mastery of the content in this chapter will enable the reader to:

- ✦ Treat clients with HIV infection or AIDS with confidence
- ✦ Recognize specific oral conditions that are related to HIV infection
- ✦ Explain the importance of the treatment team in managing chronic conditions associated with HIV infection
- ✦ Explain transmission routes for the virus

KEY TERMS

Acquired immunodeficiency syndrome (AIDS)
Angular cheilitis
Atrophic candidiasis
CD4+ T lymphocytes
Cytotoxicity
Erythematous candidiasis
Hairy leukoplakia
Human immunodeficiency virus (HIV)
Immune response
Immunosuppression
Kaposi's sarcoma
Linear gingival erythema
Lymphadenopathy
Necrotizing ulcerative gingivitis
Necrotizing ulcerative periodontal diseases
Necrotizing ulcerative periodontitis
Opportunistic infection
Oral warts
Percutaneous blood exposure
Pseudomembranous candidiasis
Recurrent herpetic simplex virus infection
Retrovirus
Reverse transcriptase
Seroconversion
Thrush
Ulcerative stomatitis

Knowledge of the continuum of immunodeficiency that includes infection with *human immunodeficiency virus (HIV)* on one end and debilitating disease and eventual death from *acquired immunodeficiency syndrome (AIDS)* on the other has heightened public awareness of and concern for individuals with HIV infection and AIDS. HIV infection and AIDS are now considered treatable, chronic medical conditions due to the many scientific advances in understanding the virus that have been made since it was first identified in 1983. Although the knowledge base regarding HIV infection and AIDS is rapidly growing, it is far from complete. The dental hygienist must be aware of these conditions, knowledgeable about their care, and comfortable treating clients with HIV infection and with the diagnosis of AIDS. As the discussion in this chapter will emphasize, HIV infection and the AIDS epidemic serve as potent reminders that infectious diseases have not been conquered and that epidemics are not things of the past.

EPIDEMIC OF HIV INFECTION AND AIDS

Immunosuppression is the decreased ability of the body to mount natural defenses to disease. Unusual *opportunistic infections* associated with severe immunosuppression were first identified in this country in 1981. HIV was identified and associated with these unusual conditions in 1983. Since that time, HIV infection has become a worldwide epidemic affecting more than 30 million people.

HIV includes two closely related *retroviruses,* HIV-1 and HIV-2. HIV-1 predominates in the world, including the United States, and HIV-2 is primarily found in West Africa. HIV-1 is known to have at least eight subtypes, identified on the basis of genetic coding.[1]

The first documented cases of AIDS in the United States were reported in June 1981 by the Centers for Disease Control, but the disease was not given a name until considerably later. These first cases involved five young, previously healthy homosexual males with a rare and aggressive pneumonia usually associated only with severe immunodeficiency. Subsequently, multiple cases of oral Kaposi's sarcoma were identified in the homosexual population. Previously Kaposi's sarcoma had been found only in elderly men of Mediterranean heritage, and then only on the legs. Retrospective analysis of several deaths in the United States and abroad in the 1970s lead to suspicion of AIDS as the cause of those deaths. In fact, frozen serum samples from these cases revealed the presence of HIV antibodies. AIDS cases also were reported in Haiti and several countries in Africa in the early 1980s. In 1982 the first cases of what came to be known as AIDS were identified in people with hemophilia.

Although the disease was first recognized among men who have sex with men, from the early days it has also been observed in the heterosexual populations, especially in Africa where the epidemic of AIDS is particularly severe.[2]

PATHOGENESIS OF HIV

HIV is a core of RNA encapsulated with a lipid coating. A serologic marker on the coating binds to receptor sites on CD4+ T lymphocytes. The virus fuses with the cell membrane and enters the host cell, where it releases its RNA. HIV is termed a *reverse transcriptase* virus because once within the cell the RNA "reverses" and generates DNA. This changes the cell's genetic coding so that it produces more viruses. When activated, the infected cell can then synthesize viral protein, and virions bud off. These can then circulate and infect other lymphocytic cells.[3]

For reasons not well understood, the virus's suppression of the *immune response,* the body's natural defenses against invasion by an organism, does not occur as quickly as the *cytotoxicity* of T lymphocytes, the virus's ability to be destructive to the T cells. This ability renders the host immune response less effective against this infection than other viruses do. Left untreated, HIV infection leads to gradually diminishing immune response due to dramatic depletion in numbers of *CD4+ T lymphocytes,* cells participating in the body's immune response. The diminished immune response makes the host susceptible to opportunistic infections and malignancies.[3] This explanation of the disease process is a very simple description of a complex immunologic reaction and is intended to present the general idea of how the virus replicates itself in the human body. For a fuller discussion, refer to the suggested readings list.

CLASSIFICATION OF HIV INFECTION AND AIDS

HIV infection can occur and be latent for years. It is only classified as AIDS when certain conditions or other indicators become apparent. At that time, the individual is classified as having AIDS rather than having the condition of being HIV positive. It is important for dental hygienists to be knowledgeable about the HIV disease process so that their care for infected clients can be provided out of concern for the clients' well-being and not from fear.

The Centers for Disease Control and Prevention (CDC) perform annual surveillance studies to reflect the status of this complex disease in the United States. The classification system was first proposed in 1986 and has undergone several modifications based on growing scientific knowledge of the virus and its associated conditions. The current system includes categories ranging from asymptomatic, to symptomatic, to AIDS indicator conditions. The classification system and case definitions are presented in Table 44–1, and the AIDS indicator conditions are listed in Table 44–2.[1]

HIV EXPOSURE AND INFECTION

Exposure to HIV occurs through sexual contact, including oral sex; sharing of drug paraphernalia; and infusion of infected blood or platelets. Sexual contact is the primary source of infection among men who have sex with men, and intravenous drug users are at high risk due to sharing of blood-contaminated needles. HIV-positive mothers are likely to transmit the virus to the fetus through blood-to-blood contact during pregnancy or at birth, and when breast feeding the infant.[4]

Acute HIV infection syndrome occurs 6 to 56 days after exposure, and incubation is generally about 2 weeks. Manifestations of initial infection vary but include some or all of the following symptoms:

- ✦ Fever
- ✦ Lymphadenopathy
- ✦ Headache
- ✦ Rash
- ✦ Aching muscles (myalgia)
- ✦ Aching joints (arthralgia)

There is considerable variation in presentation, but it is reported that most patients who are undergoing *seroconversion,* the acquisition of the virus in the blood serum, are ill enough to seek medical attention. It is also important to note that oral manifestations are very common. These include erythematous (red) round

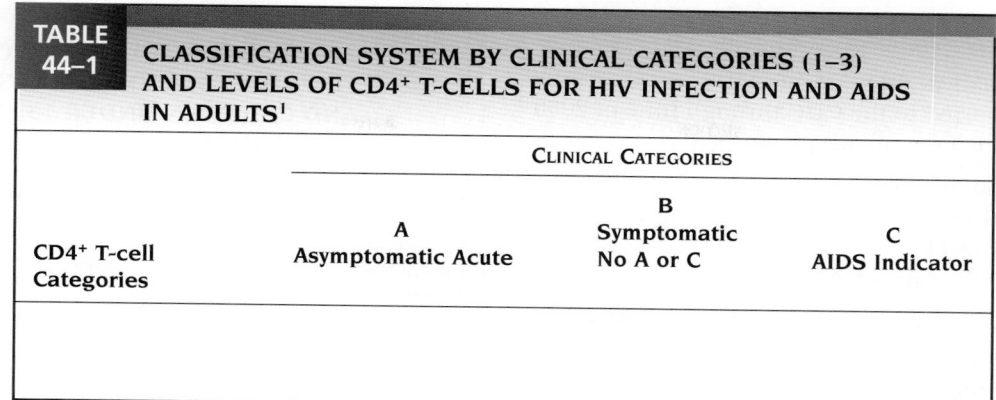

TABLE 44–1 CLASSIFICATION SYSTEM BY CLINICAL CATEGORIES (1–3) AND LEVELS OF CD4+ T-CELLS FOR HIV INFECTION AND AIDS IN ADULTS[1]

	Clinical Categories		
CD4+ T-cell Categories	**A Asymptomatic Acute**	**B Symptomatic No A or C**	**C AIDS Indicator**

TABLE 44–2 AIDS INDICATOR CONDITIONS[1]

Condition	Signs and Symptoms
Candidiasis	Of the bronchi, trachea, or lungs
Candidiasis	Esophageal
Cervical cancer	Invasive
Coccidioidomycosis	Disseminated or extrapulmonary
Cryptococcosis	Extrapulmonary
Cryptosporidiosis	Chronic intestinal (>1 month duration)
Cytomegalovirus disease	Other than liver, spleen, or nodes
Cytomegalovirus retinitis	With loss of vision
Encephalopathy	HIV-related
Herpes simplex	Chronic ulcer(s) (>1 month duration), or bronchitis, pneumonitis, or esophagitis
Histoplasmosis	Disseminated or extrapulmonary
Isosporiasis	Chronic intestinal (>1 month duration)
Kaposi's sarcoma	Intraoral or extraoral
Lymphoma	Burkitt's lymphoma
Lymphoma	Immunoblastic
Lymphoma	Primary, in the brain
Mycobacterium avium complex or *M. kansasii*	Disseminated or extrapulmonary
Mycobacterium tuberculosis	Any site (pulmonary or extrapulmonary)
Pneumocystis carinii	Pneumonia
Pneumonia	Recurrent
Progressive multifocal leukoencephalopathy	
Salmonella septicemia	Recurrent
Toxoplasmosis	Of brain
Wasting syndrome	HIV-related

patches on the hard and soft palate, angular chelitis, exudative tonsillitis, hairy leukoplakia on the lateral borders of the tongue, and oral ulcers that look similar to aphthous ulcers, but may appear anywhere in the mouth or on the lips.[3,5]

High viral levels are associated with acute HIV infection. When these become suppressed by the body's initial immune response, an asymptomatic period follows that may last for a few months or up to 10 years. Even though symptoms are not present, the virus is present and is replicating. This asymptomatic period has been reported to lead to the loss of approximately 10% of CD4 cells per year in infected individuals.[3] The diagnosis of AIDS is made based on the signs and symptoms, or other associated conditions rather than viral levels. Clinical categories of HIV infection and conditions diagnostic of AIDS are described in Tables 44–1 and 44–2.

It is important to note that women with HIV and AIDS have conditions similar to those found in men, but there are also gynecologic manifestations. These include vaginal yeast infections, cervical lesions, and cervical cancer. However, there is no general agreement that other HIV-associated conditions behave the same in males and females. Drug protocols have been studied much more extensively in males, so that modification in those protocols when applied to women may become part of treatment in the future.[6]

DRUG THERAPY

The first drugs used to control HIV infection were developed in the 1980s. These drugs targeted the reverse transcriptase enzyme that facilitates virus replication in the cells. They inhibited its effects but were given in high doses that often led to mutation of the virus, making the drugs ineffective. In the 1990s other drugs were identified that targeted the enzyme in a variety of ways at different stages of retrovirus development. These have been found to be effective and have led to the use of multiple drugs by HIV-infected individuals, the so-called "HIV cocktails." The process for determining the correct dosages of multiple drugs is extremely complex. It requires constant monitoring, clinical testing, and evaluation by the physician. The correct combination will interact beneficially, controlling the infection and preventing the development of drug resistance. As one physician specializing in treating HIV cases reported, "Drug combining can be a real challenge. We know that combinations are much more effective than any one drug because they keep the virus from mutating or becoming drug resistant." These complex treatments have greatly prolonged and improved the lives of HIV-infected individuals.[7,8]

EPIDEMIOLOGY

The total cumulative number of AIDS cases in the United States reported to the CDC through June of 2000 is 753,907. This includes all age groups:[9]

- Adult and adolescent: 745,103
- Males: 620,189
- Females: 124,911
- Children under age 13: 8804

Deaths occurring due to AIDS infection include:[9]

- Total: 438,795
- Adults: 433,296
- Children under age 15: 5086
- Unknown: 413

Total HIV infection rates are not known because the infection itself is not a reportable condition. However, the CDC estimated in 1998 that the infection rate was 17.6 new cases per 100,000 population, suggesting a total of 372,586 infected individuals in 1998. The infection rate has decreased over the years (it was as high as 22.1 per 100,000 in population in 1997), but the absolute number of cases continues to increase.[1]

It is interesting to note that although women make up a minority of cases, the group is increasing steadily. Women accounted for 7% of adult/adolescent cases in 1987, but increased to 18% by 1994, and 23% by 1998. Forty-three percent of cases in women are primarily attributable to injection drug use, and another 17% to sexual activity with an injection drug user.

Male-to-male sexual contact is the behavior risk most linked to AIDS, comprising 47% of all cases. In addition, most cases occur in individuals between 25 and 44 years of age. People over 50 account for only 10% of AIDS cases.

Another important factor is that racial and ethnic minorities make up a disproportionately large percentage of AIDS cases. As of 2000, 55% of reported cases occurred in African Americans or Hispanics. These data are even more striking in women: 80% of AIDS cases were reported in African American or Hispanic females—adults and adolescents.[1]

Current data are available on the Web regarding prevalence of AIDS cases among high-risk groups and are updated regularly. Table 44–3 summarizes AIDS cases by exposure category as of June 2000. These data are available at www.cdc.gov/hiv/stats/exposure.htm.

TABLE 44–3 AIDS CASES BY EXPOSURE CATEGORY FOR ADULTS, ADOLESCENTS, AND CHILDREN UNDER 13 AT TIME OF DIAGNOSIS

Exposure Category	Male	Female	Total
Men who have sex with men	348,657		348,657
Injection drug use	137,650	51,592	189,242
Men who have sex with men and use injection drugs	47,820		47,820
Hemophilia/coagulation disorders	4,847	274	5,121
Heterosexual contact	27,952	50,257	78,210
Recipient of blood transfusion, blood components, or tissue	4,920	3,746	8,666
Risk not reported or identified	48,343	19,042	67,387
AIDS Cases Among Children <13 Years Old			**Total**
Hemophilia/coagulation disorder			236
Mother with or at risk for HIV infection			8,027
Recipient of blood transfusion, blood components, or tissue			381
Risk not reported or identified			160

From www.cdc.gov/hiv/stats/exposure.htm, May 2001.

RISK OF HIV INFECTION AMONG HEALTHCARE WORKERS

Healthcare workers also are at risk for exposure to HIV infection. About 7% of the U.S. labor force is employed in health care and each year approximately a half million workers experience a *percutaneous blood exposure,* a penetration through unbroken skin. Of these, several dozen have resulted in transmission of HIV to the worker. Even in the absence of transmission, the emotional and material costs of going through testing and counseling are intense. Of course, the best strategy is to prevent these accidents. However, because accidents may occur, it is important for the dental hygienist to understand the relative risk of contracting HIV from such an accident.

Of all the HIV cases reported to the Centers for Disease Control and Prevention as of December 1998, 54 were documented occupational exposures. An additional 134 were possible transmissions, in which HIV was contracted but no known injury reported. All documented transmissions were related to blood, visibly bloody fluids, or concentrated laboratory preparations. Needle penetrations accounted for 86% of the transmissions. None of the transmissions were to dentists or dental workers. Pooled together, the risk of acquiring HIV infection from occupational exposure is 0.3%. The risk of transmission by other routes such as cutaneous exposure is harder to ascertain, but certainly much lower, at most 0.1%. Table 44–4 lists the occupations of the confirmed and possible HIV transmissions.[10]

Although the risk of contracting the HIV virus from an infected client is less than 1%, it is critical that the dental hygienist practice good infection control and be alert to minimize the risk of percutaneous penetration, particularly by needles. Using adequate sterilization and barrier infection control procedures (see Chapter 6), provides a sense of confidence and peace of mind and trust for all concerned.

It may be of particular interest to dental hygiene student readers of this text that a survey of student exposure to blood and body fluids has been published. The

TABLE 44–4 OCCUPATIONAL TRANSMISSION OF HIV INFECTION[10]

Occupation	Transmission: Documented	Transmission: Possible
Nurse	22	33
Clinical Laboratory Technician	16	16
Physician	6	18
Non Laboratory Technician	3	0
Surgical Technician	2	2
Health Aide	1	14
Housekeeper	1	12
Dialysis Technician	1	3
Respiratory Therapist	1	2
Embalmer/Morgue Technician	1	2
Emergency Medical Personnel	0	12
Other Technician/Therapist	0	10
Dentist/Dental Worker	0	6
Other Healthcare Occupations	0	4
TOTAL	54	134

investigators received information from 143 (67%) of 214 U.S. dental hygiene programs. A total of 687 student exposures were reported between 1996 and 1998, covering more than 18,600 students. Most exposures (499) occurred in the second year of training. About 80% of exposures were instrument punctures; 12% were needle sticks among first year students and 19% among second year students. Nine contaminated splashes and two bites were also reported.[11] These data emphasize the need for caution and inclusive application of prevention protocols, even though risk is low.

HIV INFECTION AND ITS RELATION TO THE PERIODONTAL STATUS

Early in the profession's understanding of HIV and AIDS-associated conditions, it was thought that periodontal diseases were more severe in immunocompromised individuals. Recent studies indicate that this is not the case. One study compared a group of HIV-positive and AIDS subjects to a matched group of non–HIV-positive subjects seeking treatment in Tanzania. These individuals have limited access to either medical or dental care, so the comparison provides some notion of the progression of the disease in untreated populations. The study did not reveal any differences between bleeding on probing, pocket formation, or attachment loss related to HIV status.[12] In addition, studies of western groups of HIV-positive men and women (the samples were almost all males) indicated that attachment loss was similar for both HIV and control groups in a clinical study[13] and that bone loss measured radiographically over time has been shown to be unaffected by HIV status.[14] These data suggest that the extent and relationship of HIV to periodontal diseases is less than was originally thought. However, for more complete assessment of this association, large-scale population studies remain to be completed.

ORAL MANIFESTATIONS ASSOCIATED WITH AIDS

Considerable investigation has been conducted on the oral lesions associated with HIV infection because most HIV-infected individuals experience them at some time. In fact, 80% of HIV-infected persons followed in Europe were diagnosed with one or more oral lesions. Some of them are commonly found in persons with HIV or AIDS; others are less common.[2] The manifestations of immunosuppression in humans are amazingly complex and more is discovered about them every day. Recently, persons with HIV have been presenting with a condition called *oral warts*.[15]

It is important to recognize HIV-associated oral lesions because they are often among the first signs manifested by the HIV-positive individual. Awareness and recognition of these lesions and their treatment considerations are essential for contemporary dental hygiene practice.

Common Lesions

LYMPHADENOPATHY. Cervical lymphadenopathy, a disease affecting the lymph nodes and most often recognized by swelling, is commonly identified in HIV-positive persons. It is almost always present at initial HIV infection and is found frequently at later stages of the disease.

CANDIDIASIS. A variety of *Candida albicans* infections may be seen in HIV infection. The most common types are pseudomembranous candidiasis, atrophic or erythematous candidiasis, and angular cheilitis. Candida is a common fungal infection, recognized in as many as 5% of newborns, 5% of cancer patients, and 10% of institutionalized individuals. It is by no means unique to the HIV-infected population, nor is its presence necessarily indicative of HIV infection or AIDS.

Pseudomembranous candidiasis is often referred to as *thrush* (Figure 44–1). The lesions are soft, white plaques on the oral tissues that, when wiped away, leave red and bleeding patches of mucosa. The underlying tissue is usually tender.

Atrophic candidiasis presents as smooth red patches on the tongue, palate, or mucosa; it is also referred to as *erythematous candidiasis.* These conditions usually result from the persistence of pseudomembranous candidiasis and loss of the pseudomembrane. These lesions are less obvious and more easily missed than white patches.

ANGULAR CHEILITIS. *Angular cheilitis* presents as redness, cracks, or fissures at the corners of the mouth (Figure 44–2). The lesions are moderately painful, fissured, and eroded. Medical treatment of *Candida* infection is by use of a variety of topical or systemic antifungal drugs.

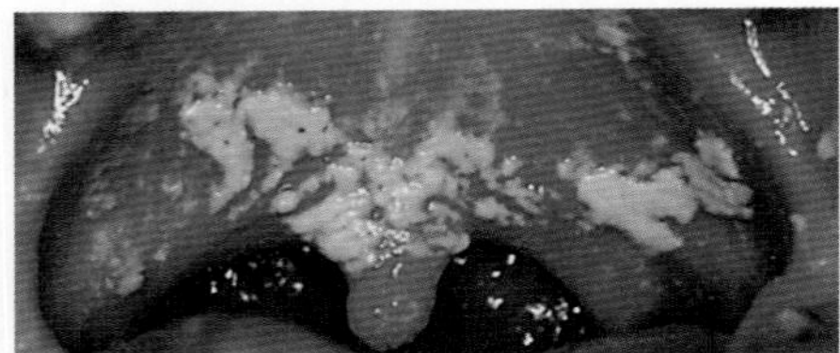

FIGURE 44–1 ✦ Pseudomembranous candidiasis in an individual with AIDS, manifested as white plaques on the palate. *(Courtesy James R Winkler, DDS, Marquette University, Minneapolis, Minn.)*

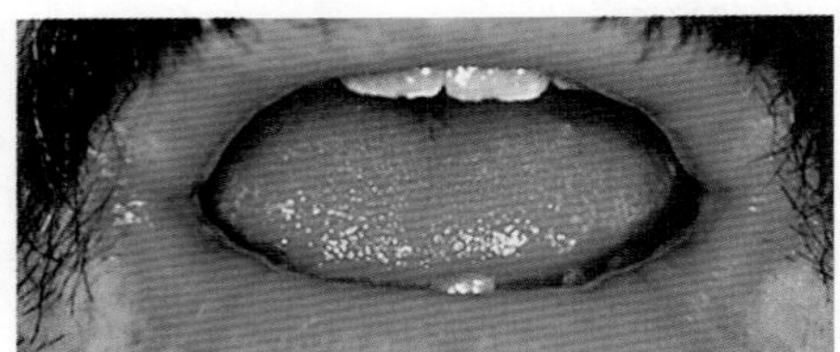

FIGURE 44–2 ✦ Angular cheilitis in a person with AIDS, seen as cracked sores at the right corner of his mouth. *(Courtesy James R Winkler, DDS, Marquette University, Minneapolis, Minn.)*

Topical applications of nystatin or clotrimazole are commonly used. Usually, immunocompromised patients require systemic administration of amphotericin B, ketoconazole, fluconazole, or itraconazole.[15]

RECURRENT HERPES SIMPLEX VIRUS. Most individuals have been exposed to primary herpetic infections, whether clinical or subclinical in nature, at some time during their life. *Recurrent herpes simplex virus infection* can occur in up to 40% of this population and is the usual manifestation of herpes virus in individuals who are HIV positive or have AIDS. Recurrence of herpes appears to be related to breakdowns in local immune activity in areas such as the lips, or alterations in local inflammatory mediators that allow the virus to become active again. In general, recurrent herpetic lesions heal within one to two weeks and are not related to secondary infections. However, when they occur in the HIV-infected population they can be more severe and persistent, and can become secondarily infected with bacteria or fungi. The pain associated with herpes lesions can significantly restrict the HIV-positive individual's intake of food, thus compromising adequate nutrition.

Treatment of recurrent herpes simplex virus infection with virus-inhibiting drugs such as acyclovir may help, but in the case of severe disease, intravenous delivery of antiviral drugs may be necessary.[16]

HAIRY LEUKOPLAKIA. *Hairy leukoplakia* is a collection of thick, white lesions, usually seen on the lateral borders of the tongue (Figure 44–3). The lesions can present with long, fingerlike projections, thus the name hairy leukoplakia. It may be unilateral or bilateral, and there are no associated symptoms. Hairy leukoplakia was first identified in 1981, and the condition is associated with the Epstein–Barr virus. It is found almost exclusively in HIV-infected individuals and AIDS patients. The prevalence is approximately 20% in HIV-infected persons and up to 80% in those with AIDS.

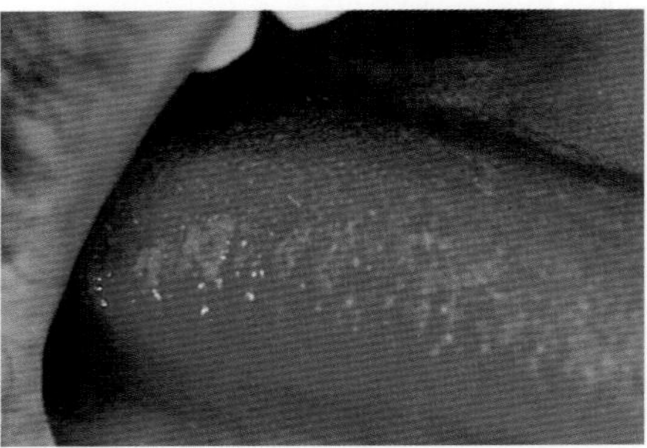

FIGURE 44–3 ✦ Hairy leukoplakia in an individual with AIDS, located on the right lateral border of the tongue. *(Courtesy James R Winkler, DDS, Marquette University, Minneapolis, Minn.)*

There is no specific treatment for hairy leukoplakia, but it is imperative that diagnosis be confirmed due to the very high association with HIV infection. Hairy leukoplakia is predictive of the diagnosis of AIDS, with as many as 80% of individuals with a confirmed diagnosis progressing to the diagnosis of AIDS within 30 months.[5]

KAPOSI'S SARCOMA. *Kaposi's sarcoma* is a malignant endothelial cell neoplasm. It has several associated etiologic factors, including genetic predisposition, viral infection, environmental influences, and alterations in the immune system. It is particularly related to a newly discovered herpes viruses, Kaposi's sarcoma herpes virus (KSHV). Kaposi's sarcoma typically appears as brownish-red nodules primarily on the skin of the extremities. However, it can present on any organ, and the prognosis for the disease is poor. It is seen in approximately one fifth of AIDS patients. Approximately half of the AIDS-affected patients with Kaposi's sarcoma develop oral lesions. The lesions may appear anywhere in the oral cavity and may be small, rather innocuous-looking, flat, reddish-blue/purple lesions or may be of increasing size, including large nodular lesions (Figure 44–4).[17]

Oral Kaposi's sarcoma lesions often appear on the gingiva associated with the teeth. In these cases the tumors may be significantly enlarged by the presence of plaque biofilm and calculus. Dental hygienists and dentists are sometimes hesitant to treat the gingival condition for fear of harming the Kaposi's lesions or causing significant bleeding. However, periodontal care must be provided, and in some cases tumor reduction will be achieved by nonsurgical periodontal care. Kaposi's lesions on the gingiva associated with the teeth require excision or other tumor reduction therapy, as do Kaposi's sarcomas located away from the teeth. Localized Kaposi's lesions tend to diminish in size and are managed successfully through surgical excision, low-dose radiation treatment, or antitumor chemotherapy.[17] The dental hygienist must not avoid treating the teeth and gingiva because of the presence of closely associated, often large and reddish-purple lesions. Thorough plaque biofilm removal and scaling and root planing are

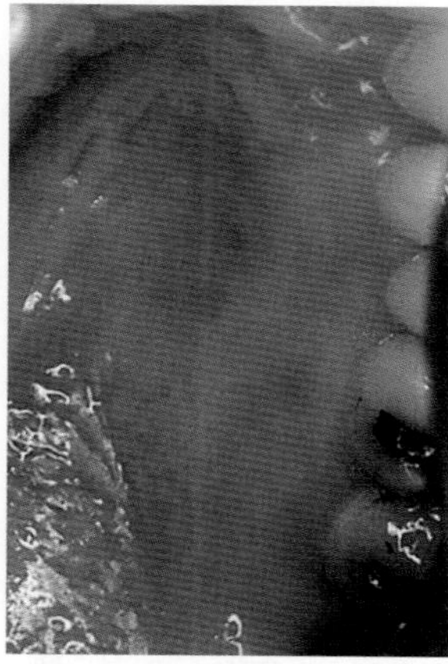

FIGURE 44–4 ✦ Oral Kaposi's sarcoma lesions on the palate of an individual with AIDS. *(Courtesy James R Winkler, DDS, Marquette University, Minneapolis, Minn.)*

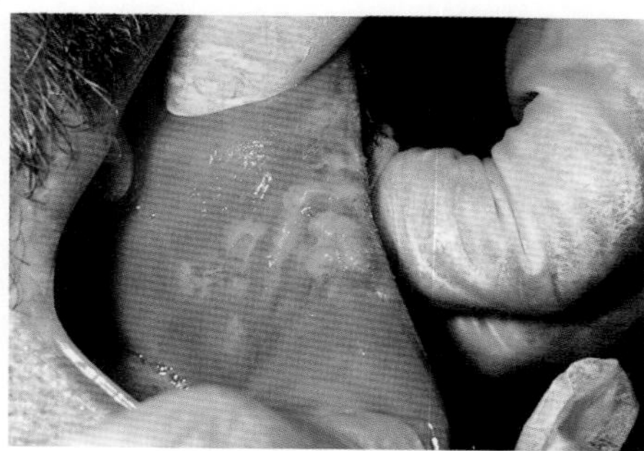

FIGURE 44–5 ✦ Oral warts presenting on the interior of the corner of the mouth. *(Courtesy Dr. Deborah Greenspan, University of California, San Francisco.)*

essential to maximizing the effects of periodontal therapy and may help reduce the size of the tumor prior to therapy specific for treatment of the tumor.

ORAL WARTS. Human papillomavirus is also commonly found in HIV-infected individuals. This virus has many subtypes, and is associated with the formation of *oral warts* (Figure 44–5). Although oral warts can occur in any individual infected with this particular virus, recurrence after treatment is uncommon except in the case of HIV-infected individuals.[18] In HIV-infected individuals receiving antiretroviral therapy, an increase in oral warts and a decrease in hairy leukoplakia and oral candidiasis have been reported. HIV-associated oral warts can be large and multifocal, and present aesthetic and functional problems. They can be excised, but tend to recur.[15]

LESIONS OF THE PERIODONTIUM. Some forms of periodontitis that are aggressive in nature have been reported in HIV-infected individuals and patients with AIDS. These are not recognized as disease entities specific to HIV infection; rather they appear to be forms of *necrotizing ulcerative periodontal diseases.* Although *necrotizing ulcerative gingivitis* is recognized as a form of gingivitis and is a term commonly used in the dental profession, these cases rarely present without evidence of attachment loss. For that reason, most cases are more properly diagnosed as necrotizing ulcerative periodontitis.[19]

The dental hygienist may in rare instances encounter the entire range of clinical presentations of periodontal conditions, from nonspecific redness of the gingiva that may extend uninterrupted to the alveolar mucosa, to extensive necrosing gingival lesions or severe necrosing conditions with exposed bone. Successful dental hygiene care of individuals with these oral diseases requires consultation with the dentist and physician to understand the unique features of each case.

On examining the periodontium of an HIV-infected client or a client with AIDS, the gingiva may appear very red. This fiery red appearance of the tissues may be limited to the gingival margin, either localized or generalized, in which case it is often called *linear gingival erythema.* The gingival changes that extend partly toward or directly onto the alveolar mucosa have the more typical appearance of necrotizing ulcerative disease. In addition, the alveolar mucosa also may be bright red, or have red petechia-like patches (Figure 44–6).[4,20]

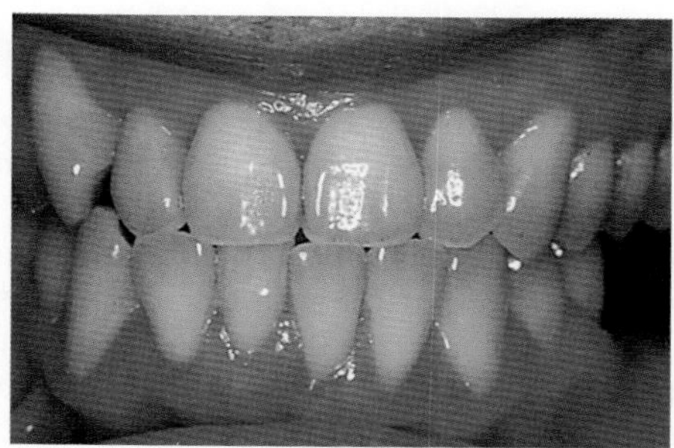

FIGURE 44–6 ✦ Necrotizing ulcerative gingivitis associated with HIV infection prior to care. The gingival margin shows color change to bright red that may extend onto the alveolar mucosa. *(Courtesy James R Winkler, DDS, Marquette University, Minneapolis, Minn.)*

There may also be frank and extensive loss of periodontal tissues and bone, which is often quite painful. In the presence of attachment and bone loss, no matter how extensive, the disease is called *necrotizing ulcerative periodontitis* (Figure 44–7).[19] Extreme cases of exposed bone and sloughing tissue are sometimes referred to as *ulcerative stomatitis.*[20]

Candida albicans may play an etiologic role in these exaggerated cases of gingival and periodontal diseases. These cases are not very responsive to simple mechanical removal of plaque biofilm and calculus. Additional chemotherapeutic agents are often required to control the pathogens that cause the infection.[20]

The oral flora associated with necrotizing ulcerative periodontitis are similar to the flora associated with periodontal disease in non–HIV-infected persons. The subgingival plaque biofilm has been shown to harbor high proportions of the same periodontal pathogens found in non–HIV-infected persons with periodontal lesions.[21,22] A notable difference is that subgingival yeasts have been identified in 62% of HIV-infected adults with periodontal disease, compared with 16.8% of non–HIV-infected people with periodontal disease.[22]

The precise mechanisms of the severe form of destruction sometimes seen in HIV-infected individuals are not

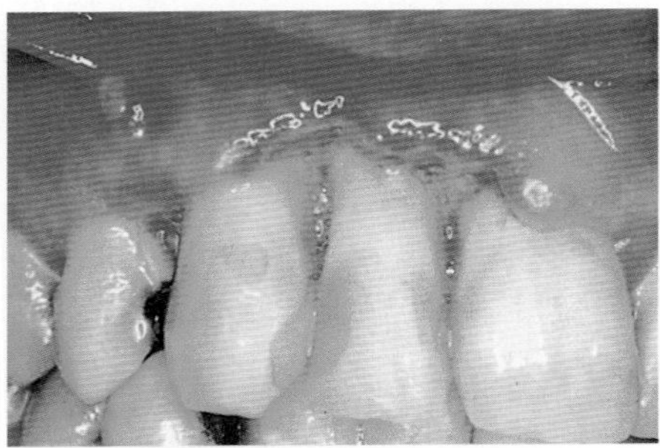

FIGURE 44–7 ✦ Necrotizing ulcerative periodontitis in an individual with AIDS showing color change, necrosis, and sloughing of the periodontal tissues. *(Courtesy James R Winkler, DDS, Marquette University, Minneapolis, Minn.)*

clearly understood. They are not related to the development of an unusual and extremely pathogenic oral flora. The relationship of the presence of increased amounts of *Candida,* xerostomia, altered lymphocyte action, and possibly poor nutrition remain to be understood in this extremely destructive periodontal disease process.

LESS-COMMON LESIONS. A variety of infections, neoplasms, and other oral lesions have been described in HIV-infected persons. Although rare, they should be recognized and treated. The dental hygienist plays a role in performing oral evaluations and informing clients of the presence of lesions so that referral for diagnosis and treatment may be encouraged. It is always important to be attentive to changes in health, and encourage clients to seek additional care immediately.

APPLICATION OF THE DENTAL HYGIENE PROCESS OF CARE FOR THE HIV-INFECTED CLIENT AND THE CLIENT WITH AIDS

HIV-infected people who seek dental and dental hygiene care are often young individuals who have suddenly had their sense of safety and well-being shattered. They are struggling to live with HIV and striving to maintain a healthy lifestyle to help control the infection. They are commonly on complex and difficult regimens of medication to control the disease process. HIV-infected individuals are eager, cooperative, and appreciative clients who are happy to comply with recommendations for professional care. However, the HIV-infected client may initially be reluctant or fearful of the clinician's response to knowledge of his or her HIV infection. The client may have been shunned by others and fear the same when visiting the dental hygienist. One effective means to initiate a professional relationship and restore a sense of safety to both client and dental hygienist is to shake hands upon introduction. The courtesy of this polite touch infuses the professional relationship with confidence and defuses unwarranted fear and alienation.

Assessment

The dental hygienist assesses the special needs of every client and plans, implements, and evaluates dental hygiene care. During the assessment phase of dental hygiene care, the dental hygienist must be particularly sensitive to clues from the client's health history and observed clinical conditions associated with HIV infection.

It is important to have specific questions on the health form such as, "Are you immunocompromised by any disease or condition? Have you been tested for HIV?" The dental hygienist reviews the answers with clients frankly and in a nonjudgmental way to stimulate dialogue. When clients indicate that they have been tested for HIV, they should be asked what their status is. If HIV infection is revealed, the dental hygienist should assess the client's support systems such as family and partners.

Moreover, while validating the health history and during the interview, the client might report high-risk sexual behavior, intravenous drug use, or blood transfusions in the early 1980s, prior to adequate screening of the blood supply. Medications that an HIV-positive person might be taking include abacavir (ABC), zidovudine (AZT), didanosine (DDI), lamivudine (3TC), or zalcitabine (HIVID). The client may also report recent hospital stays for conditions associated with HIV status, as listed in Table 44–2.

Extraoral assessment may reveal purplish-red nodules on the skin indicative of Kaposi's sarcoma. Intraorally, some conditions may include the signs and symptoms associated with candidiasis, hairy leukoplakia, Kaposi's sarcoma lesions, or necrotizing forms of periodontal disease. There might also be unusual lesions, which should always be referred for evaluation.

Dental Hygiene Diagnosis

Several of the eight human needs described in Chapter 2 are relevant to dental hygiene care for the individual infected with HIV. For example, clients may be extremely anxious and stressed by having acquired the infection. The dental hygienist can help by pointing out that treatments have advanced greatly in the last 10 years. In addition, educating clients about how HIV infection affects the oral structures and what they can do to prevent or lessen the severity of these oral problems may empower them to feel some control over their disease. This feeling of empowerment enhances the client's sense of freedom from anxiety and stress. Dental hygiene care for HIV-infected individuals encourages clients to take responsibility for oral health, and to understand dental and other health-related issues.

Planning for Dental Hygiene Care

The dental hygiene care plan must include education of the client, therapeutic scaling and root planing, plaque control, provision of posttreatment instructions, and evaluation. Planning for dental hygiene care must be integrated with the overall dental treatment plan in consultation with the physician. For example, additional medication for oral candidiasis or other conditions may be needed during the course of care. In addition, the oral healthcare team may want to obtain the client's most recent blood test results from the physician. Clients' platelet count, prothrombin time, and partial prothrombin time are sometimes used to predict excessive postoperative bleeding before nonsurgical or surgical periodontal care is provided.

In the case of more severe forms of necrotizing gingival and periodontal diseases, and of oral lesions such as those of Kaposi's sarcoma, dental hygiene care must always be in collaboration with the dentist and physician. Sometimes, as in the case of severe necrotizing ulcerative periodontitis, the need for surgical treatment is so urgent that periodontal surgical intervention may be done at the same appointment as the dental hygiene care.

Clients are often very health-conscious and interested in preventive care. They frequently embrace preventive procedures such as brushing and flossing quite readily. This focus on self-care can be a great advantage for the dental hygienist in designing and implementing a preventive program. The dental hygienist needs to evaluate the client's knowledge of bacterial plaque and oral disease processes, as well as the person's dexterity level, prior to selecting strategies that lead the client to optimal oral health status. Should deficits in skin and mucous membrane integrity be identified, this interest in prevention can be an asset in motivating the client to perform better home care. An over-the-counter mouthrinse or a prescribed chlorhexidine mouthrinse may be recommended to assist in the control of supragingival bacterial plaque and gingivitis. Nutritional counseling may also be helpful to encourage a diet sufficient to support healing and oral maintenance. The client also may be consulting or may need to consult a nutritionist, and thus the dental hygienist also may be sharing responsibility with this member of the healthcare team.

Implementation

Once formulated, the plan of care is implemented according to the goals and priorities established by the client and the oral healthcare team.

INFECTION CONTROL. HIV-positive clients should be provided with a rinse of 0.12% chlorhexidine prior to treatment to reduce the number of organisms in the mouth during the provision of care.

Some HIV-infected individuals do not reveal their status to healthcare workers. This lack of disclosure may be because the condition is as yet undiagnosed, or because of privacy concerns. Universal infection control procedures are a must during all treatment and can be relied on to protect the dental hygienist and other members of the dental team during treatment.

SCALING AND ROOT PLANING. There is some concern that scaling and root planing should be performed on HIV-positive patients using only hand instruments because powered scaling devices generate an aerosol.[23] There are no documented cases of HIV infection through aerosol, nor is the seroconversion rate of oral healthcare workers high.

The dental hygienist might prefer to perform therapeutic scaling and root planing procedures using ultrasonic instrumentation because there is generally less treatment time, and often the procedures can be performed without using injected local anesthetics, thereby reducing the possibility of needle punctures. This decision is a personal one for the dental hygienist.

Generally, HIV-infected clients and those diagnosed with AIDS present with very typical oral needs. They can have gingivitis or periodontitis, and they can also present with healthy, well-maintained oral conditions. They require typical management including meticulous plaque control and periodontal debridement. They should be treated and maintained on regular intervals of two to four months.

NECROTIZING ULCERATIVE PERIODONTITIS. Treatment of necrotizing ulcerative periodontitis consists of the aggressive removal of local irritants. In addition, periodontal surgery may be required to remove necrosed tissues, including bone. Local irrigation of the gingiva and affected tissues with dilute solutions of 3% hydrogen peroxide has also been recommended. Disposable syringes with blunt needles or cotton swabs are required to adequately flush the affected tissues. Persons treated for necrotizing ulcerative periodontitis require close monitoring and evaluation. Postoperative care requires good mechanical bacterial plaque control, and twice-daily chlorhexidine rinses for chemical bacterial plaque control. Clients must be informed of possible side effects of chlorhexidine, including staining of the teeth, discoloration of the oral mucosa, and altered taste sensation. The use of antibiotics such as metronidazole to control the oral flora must be done with caution and in consultation with the treatment team (Figure 44–7). HIV clients may experience overgrowth of other opportunistic organisms when some bacteria are suppressed, including *Candida*.[4,20] The sequence of procedures for treating necrotizing periodontal disease in an HIV-positive client is presented in Procedure 44–1.

Evaluation

After comprehensive dental hygiene care has been completed, the dental hygienist should evaluate the client to ensure that the goals outlined in the plan of care have been met. Evaluation should take place at the expected intervals. In the case of initial therapy (phase I therapy) reevaluation should occur in about four weeks. This allows time for healing of the connective tissue so that the client can be probed and assessed accurately. Recall intervals also should be 2 to 4 months.[24] This frequency provides opportunities to assess the client's oral health, daily oral hygiene practices, and nutrition regularly.

Continued dental hygiene care and recall at short intervals may be necessary to reinforce conceptualization and understanding of the oral health aspects related to the disease, and to maintain a good preventive result. The evaluation phase of the dental hygiene process also provides the opportunity to identify other human need deficits that may require further planning and care. As with all clients, the process of care is a continuum of evaluation, prevention, and treatment.

Procedure 44–1 DENTAL HYGIENE CARE FOR THE HIV-INFECTED CLIENT

EQUIPMENT

Protective barriers (safety glasses, mask, gloves, gown)
Mouth mirror
Explorer
Periodontal probe
Scalers
2" × 2" gauze
Saliva ejector
Disposable syringe with blunt needle
0.12% chlorhexidine
3% hydrogen peroxide
Ultrasonic scaling device
Syringe
Intraoral local anesthetic
Topical anesthetic
Cotton swabs

STEPS	RATIONALE
1. Assess client needs.	Ensures comprehensive and humanistic care.
2. Establish dental hygiene care plan with client and determine extent of consultation and treatment.	Care must be integrated with the overall dental plan. Additional medication may be needed during the course of care. Client's platelet count, prothrombin time, and partial prothrombin time may be needed to predict postoperative bleeding. Consultation with the dentist and physician is necessary.
3. Provide preventive education.	Client responsibility for care is important for promoting and maintaining health.
4. Provide preprocedural oral rinse of 0.12% chlorhexidine.	Reduces the number of microorganisms in the mouth.
5. Perform debridement procedures as needed.	Necessary for healing of periodontal tissues.
6. Irrigate subgingivally with a dilute solution of H_2O_2 after scaling procedures.	Antiseptic properties may promote healing of periodontal tissues by temporarily decreasing subgingival bacteria.
7. Postoperative recommendations include conventional plaque control and twice daily use of chlorhexidine as a mouthrinse.	Provides for mechanical and chemical bacterial plaque control.
8. Establish 2- to 4-month recall.	Close monitoring is required.
CLIENT PRESENTS WITH UNEXPECTEDLY SEVERE PERIODONTAL SIGNS AND SYMPTOMS AND/OR ORAL LESIONS	
1. Consult with team members.	Provides for optimal care.
2. Refer for lesion evaluation, periodontal consultation.	Determines extent of disease and appropriate care plan with other team members.
3. Periodontal care requires irrigating tissues with dilute 3% H_2O_2	Debrides necrosing tissues.
4. Debride with local anesthetic and hand or ultrasonic instruments as needed.	Promotes healing of periodontal tissues and provides concurrent pain control during the procedure if needed.
5. Postoperative antibiotics or antifungal agents as needed.	Assists in healing.
6. Monitoring every 2 to 4 months by the team.	Close observation for preventive and treatment needs.
CASE DOCUMENTATION	
1. Complete description of services rendered at each treatment appointment must always be written in ink.	Ensures the integrity of the client's record for both the client and the dental practice.

Client Education Issues

- ✦ Explain that oral health is an important aspect of maintaining good health.
- ✦ Explain that periodontal health and oral conditions require frequent evaluation and maintenance, commonly every 2 to 4 months, to maintain oral health and observe changes in condition.

Legal, Ethical, and Safety Issues

- ✦ It is both the ethical and legal responsibility of the dental hygienist to treat individuals with HIV infection or AIDS.
- ✦ Treatment is both necessary and effective for these clients.
- ✦ Proper infection control must always be practiced and accidental percutaneous exposures minimized through good practice habits.

Key Concepts

- ✦ HIV infection is a disease that suppresses the immune response.
- ✦ HIV-infected individuals are considered to have chronic, treatable conditions.
- ✦ The risk to the dental hygienist of acquiring HIV infection from treating infected individuals is extremely low.
- ✦ Universal infection control precautions and efforts to eliminate risk of percutaneous exposure must always be taken.
- ✦ Most periodontal disease identified in HIV-positive individuals is indistinguishable from the disease patterns seen in other clients.
- ✦ Any unusual intraoral or perioral lesion should be evaluated because oral lesions are commonly seen in HIV-infected persons.
- ✦ Treatment of HIV-infected individuals requires a team effort from many healthcare workers, including the dentist and physician.

Critical Thinking Exercises

1. Discuss the following issues related to treating a pregnant woman who is HIV positive: possible transmission routes of the virus to the baby, the importance of the team in treating both mother and infant, the mother's possible fears and concerns about taking any precautionary medications, and the periodontal presentation of tender, hormone-influenced gingivitis that may occur.
2. Discuss the issue of personal safety when treating HIV-infected clients. This discussion should include all aspects of risk reduction and a thoughtful analysis of aerosol production when using ultrasonic scalers. The aerosol discussion should be guided to have students consider how many people do not know or may not reveal their HIV status, that individuals' periodontal conditions probably will not provide clues as to HIV status, and whether or not ultrasonic or other powered scaling and polishing equipment should ever be used.

For References, Suggested Readings, and Related Websites, visit
http://evolve.elsevier.com/Darby/hygiene/

CHAPTER 45

Persons with Alcohol and Substance Abuse Problems

OBJECTIVES

Mastery of the content in this chapter will enable the reader to:

- ✦ Describe the multiple causes of substance abuse including genetic, environmental, psychological, and physiologic factors.
- ✦ Identify the action of psychoactive drugs on neurotransmitters.
- ✦ Classify abused substances according to drug category and street names.
- ✦ Describe the short-term, long-term, and systemic effects of substance use.
- ✦ Identify oral signs and symptoms associated with substance abuse.
- ✦ Discuss the dental hygiene process of care related to clients with substance abuse problems and for those in recovery.
- ✦ Identify the resources and support services available for dental professionals with substance abuse problems.

KEY TERMS

Addiction
Alcohol
Amphetamines
Autonomic nervous system (ANS)
Axons
Binge drinking
Cell body
Central nervous system (CNS)
CNS depressants
CNS stimulants
Dendrites
Drug abuse
Fetal alcohol syndrome (FAS)
Glossodynia
Neurotransmitters
Opiates (opioids)
Peripheral nervous system (PNS)
Physiologic dependence
Psychoactive drug
Psychological dependence
Stages of change model
Tolerance
Withdrawal symptoms

Substance abuse is a significant problem in American society. An estimated 4.1 million people, including 1.1 million youths ages 12 to 17, meet the diagnostic criteria for "dependence on illicit drugs."[1] It is estimated that up to 50% of hospitalized patients have a substance abuse–related admission, and that the total cost of substance abuse in the United States is greater than $200 billion per year.[2] Substance abuse affects the individual, the family, and the community. Employers experience decreased worker productivity and increased insurance premiums. A significant number of deadly automobile accidents are caused by alcohol or drug impaired drivers. Child abuse and neglect are often directly related to the addiction of parents. Because addiction often results in criminal behavior to finance a drug habit, substance abusers are viewed as morally corrupt or weak personalities who willingly engage in self-destructive behaviors that affect themselves and everyone around them. Research has shown that addiction is a chronic, cyclic disease, yet unlike other diseases, there remains a social stigma attached to it.

Clients who are drug dependent, abuse substances, or are in treatment for substance abuse present the dental hygienist with a variety of important issues related to care. Such clients must be identified so they can be treated safely. To do this, dental hygienists must understand basic concepts associated with substance abuse, its cause, and associated medical treatment.

BASIC CONCEPTS OF ALCOHOL AND DRUG ABUSE

Alcohol (ethyl alcohol or ethanol) is a product manufactured by fermenting fruit, grains, or vegetables and distilling them to raise the alcohol content. The alcohol content of wine, beer, and spirits (hard liquor) differs. On average, beer contains 4.5% alcohol, wine 12.9%, and spirits 41.1%. A "standard drink" is defined as one that contains approximately 0.5 fluid ounce (12 g) of alcohol. This amount of alcohol is present in 12 fluid ounces of beer, 5 fluid ounces of wine, or 1.5 fluid ounces of 80 proof distilled spirits. *Binge drinking* is defined as five or more drinks on the same occasion at least once in 30 days.[1]

Alcohol reduces anxiety and causes intoxication and sensory alterations. Alcohol enters the blood within five minutes of ingestion and remains in the bloodstream for one to four hours. The liver breaks down alcohol at the rate of one drink per hour. Blood alcohol concentration is measured in milligrams per deciliter (mg/dl). In most legal jurisdictions, blood alcohol concentrations of over 100 mg/dl (0.1%) are illegal.

Drug abuse is the self-administration of a drug in a manner that deviates from its accepted medical use. It includes experimental and recreational use of drugs, as well as addictive use (Table 45–1). *Addiction* is the compulsive use of a drug despite adverse medical and social consequences.

Those who compulsively abuse drugs continue to do so because they have developed a psychologic and physiologic dependence. *Psychologic dependence* is rooted in the belief that the drug is needed to maintain a state of well-being. *Physiologic dependence* results from a biologic alteration in the user's brain from consistent drug use. A person who has developed physiologic dependence on a drug will go through drug withdrawal once the drug is stopped. *Withdrawal symptoms* may include vomiting, diarrhea, rapid pulse, sweating, anxiety, convulsions, severe cramps, high blood pressure, and severe headaches. People will often continue using drugs because they fear experiencing withdrawal from the drug. Table 45–2 presents drug categories of abused substances and their effects on the body.

Another aspect of physical dependence is that a drug must be taken in constantly increased doses to achieve the same effects on the brain over time. *Tolerance* is the term used to describe this aspect of physical dependence. Nicotine, *opiates*, alcohol, psychedelics, central nervous system (CNS) stimulants, and sedative-hypnotics all require increased doses to establish the same "high" or euphoric feeling the user experienced with first use. If the drug dosage is not increased, the effects of the drug are diminished and withdrawal symptoms occur. Because of their effect on the brain, addictive drugs are also called psychoactive drugs.

Stages of Change

The *stages of change model*[3] describes the process of change an individual experiences when going from a substance

TABLE 45–1 DRUG USE CONTINUUM

	Classification Based on Use	Behavior
Type 1	Abstainers (about 1/3 of the population)	Never used drugs/alcohol
Type 2	Social drinker/users (majority of population)	Occasional use Able to drink one and stop Does not result in personal problems
Type 3	Drug abusers	Excessive use of substance Binge drinking
Type 4	Physically dependent addicts	Adaptation of the body's chemistry Withdrawal signs and symptoms Not used as a coping device Physician-induced addictions
Type 5	Psychologically dependent addicts	Depend on alcohol or drugs to cope with life Can never return to social use Tolerance Withdrawal symptoms Compulsive use Loss of control Use despite personal problems Preoccupation Denial

Adapted from Coombs RH: *Drug-impaired professionals,* Cambridge, Mass, 1997, Harvard University Press.

TABLE 45–2 EFFECTS OF DRUG USE

Drug	Effects of Short-term Use	Effects of Long-term Use	Systemic Effects
CNS Stimulants			
Cocaine Crack cocaine	Increased energy, mental alertness Decreased appetite	Addiction, irritability and mood disturbances, restlessness, paranoia, auditory hallucinations	Dilated pupils, heart rhythm disturbances, chest pain, increased blood pressure, hyperthermia, respiratory failure, strokes, seizures, headaches, abdominal pain, nausea, increased risk of HIV and hepatitis if injected
Amphetamines Methamphetamines Methylenedioxymethamphetamine ("Ecstasy")	Increased physical activity, feeling of well-being, mild euphoria, appetite suppression	Rapid tolerance requires increasing dosage, extreme lethargy and depression, paranoia, hallucinations, severe malnutrition	Increases in heart rate, respiration, and blood pressure; hyperthermia; inflammation of pericardium; psychotic symptoms may continue months after use has stopped. In pregnancy, fetal exposure increases prenatal complications, premature delivery, abnormal reflexes, may be linked to congenital deformities
Caffeine	Dissipates drowsiness or fatigue, increases sense of alertness	Nervousness, mental confusion, irritability, muscle twitches, insomnia	Increases in heart rate and blood pressure, intestinal uclers, withdrawal effects after long-term use or high doses cause headaches, fatigue, depression, and irritability
CNS Depressants			
Opiates and opioids Heroin Opium Codeine Morphine Dilaudid Percodan Methadone Demerol Darvon Fentanyl Naloxone	Surge of pleasure (rush), skin flushes, heavy feeling in extremities, alterations in memory and concentration, nausea, vomiting, suppression of pain	Addiction, dry skin, itching, relaxed muscles, drooping eyelids, slurred speech	Constricted pupils that do not react to light, CNS and respiratory depression, hypotension, collapsed veins, infection of heart valves and pericardium, thrombocytopenia, liver disease, kidney disease, poor pain tolerance, increased risk of abscesses, HIV, and hepatitis from injection Withdrawal symptoms occur if drug use is reduced abruptly
Sedatives/Hypnotics			
Barbiturates	Relaxation, reduced inhibitions, reduced muscular coordination, reduced intensity of physical sensations, sedation, drowsiness, unconsciousness	Personality changes, mood swings, depression, irritability Tolerance develops rapidly Increased doses to reach a mental high will result in continued physical depression of respiratory rate, weak and rapid pulse	Risk of death especially if combined with alcohol Danger of overdosing causing respiratory arrest Withdrawal symptoms can result in convulsions
Benzodiazepines	Control anxiety and restlessness	Causes psychological and physical dependence	Have a long "half-life" in body that can result in overdose that can cause loss of consciousness, depressed breathing, and coma Withdrawal symptoms can include loss of vision or hearing, multiple seizures and convulsions
Hallucinogens			
Cannabinoids Marijuana Hashish Sinsemilla	Relaxation; euphoria; confusion; poor coordination; red, bloodshot eyes; intense hunger or thirst; difficulty with concentration, memory, and learning; distorted perception of sights, sounds, time, and touch; difficulty with problem solving	Probably leads to use of other addictive substances Increases risk of lung cancer, bronchitis, and emphysema—smoking one marijuana "joint" has the same effect as smoking 14 to 16 filtered cigarettes Weakens immune system	Dilated pupils, tachycardia, peripheral vasodilation, bronchial hyperactivity, insomnia, impaired short-term memory, disruption in testosterone secretion Decreases nausea and pressure behind the eyes Sometimes taken by cancer and glaucoma patients to alleviate symptoms Chronic use can result in withdrawal symptoms Can cause thrombocytopenia if injected intravenously

LSD	Causes sensory distortions and illusions, extreme emotions from euphoria to panic, unpredictable reactions	Acute anxiety, fear of loss of control, paranoia, delusions of grandeur	Increase in heart rate and blood pressure, hyperthermia, prolonged psychotic reaction or severe depression, mental flashbacks to sensations experienced while taking LSD can occur
Phencyclidine (PCP)	Sensory deprivation, reduces inhibitions, deadens pain, mild depression	Combative behavior, inability to speak, confusion, agitation, paranoia, amnesia	Extremely high blood pressure, cardiovascular instability, respiratory depression, catatonia, coma, convulsions, seizures Retained in fat cells for several months after use and can be released during exercise, fasting, or when under stress, causing flashbacks
Inhalants			
Volatile solvents Airplane glue Rubber cement Spray paint Hair spray Paint thinner Spot remover Gasoline	Reduced inhibitions, impulsiveness, excitement, irritability, euphoria, dizziness, slurred speech, drowsiness	Confusion, delirium, psychomotor dysfunction, emotional instability, impaired thinking	Brain, liver, kidney, nervous system, bone marrow, and lung disorders as a result of the effect of the solvent or ingredients in the solvent Respiratory arrest, cardiac arrhythmia, asphyxia, suicide
Volatile nitrites Room odorizers Amyl nitrite	Relaxation of all smooth muscles, altered consciousness, enhanced sexual pleasure (used especially among male homosexuals)	Increased blood flow to the brain resulting in headaches, dizziness and giddiness, vomiting, shock, and loss of consciousness	Nitrite poisoning; damage to the nervous system; impaired perception, reasoning, and memory; dementia; defective muscular coordination
Anesthetics Nitrous oxide	Giddiness, profound laughter, euphoria	Addiction, loss of consciousness, frostbite of the nose and vocal cords from direct inhalation out of a pressurized tank	Peripheral nerve damage, frozen lung tissue, brain cell damage due to oxygen deprivation
Anabolic Steroids	Enhanced athletic performance, increased muscle mass, increased aggression, decreased inflammation and swelling of injured tissue, weight gain	Males: shrinking of testicles, reduced sperm count, impotence, baldness, breast development, enlarged prostate Females: cessation of menses, facial hair growth	Acne; depression; jaundice; tremors, swelling of feet or ankles; halitosis; increased possibility of injury to tendons, ligaments, and muscles; increased blood pressure; liver damage
Alcohol	Feeling of well-being, loss of inhibitions, slowed reactions, intoxication, slurred speech, sedation, unconsciousness Especially dangerous when used with other CNS depressants or narcotics	Addiction; increased risk of oral cancer and breast cancer; malnutrition; inflammation of the stomach; hepatitis and other liver damage; alcohol amnestic disorder; dementia	Cognitive problems; cardiovascular impairment; cirrhosis of the liver; damage to kidneys, CNS, and GI tract

abuser to an individual who is substance free. The stages of change model refers to an individual's readiness to quit abusing a particular substance. As described in Chapter 29 on treating nicotine addiction, this model can be applied when counseling any substance abuser. By listening to the client and asking nonjudgmental questions about the client's readiness to make a quit attempt, the dental hygienist can respond appropriately for the client's current "stage of change." For example, if the client admits to substance abuse, but states that he or she is not ready to stop, providing information on benefits of stopping would be appropriate to help the client to continue to think about stopping. Asking questions like, "When will you know it is time to quit?" allows the client to think about an answer after the dental hygiene care visit and allows the client more control to make the decision to stop the substance abuse. Once the reasons for stopping outweigh the reasons for using, individuals will decide to make an attempt to stop their substance abuse.[3]

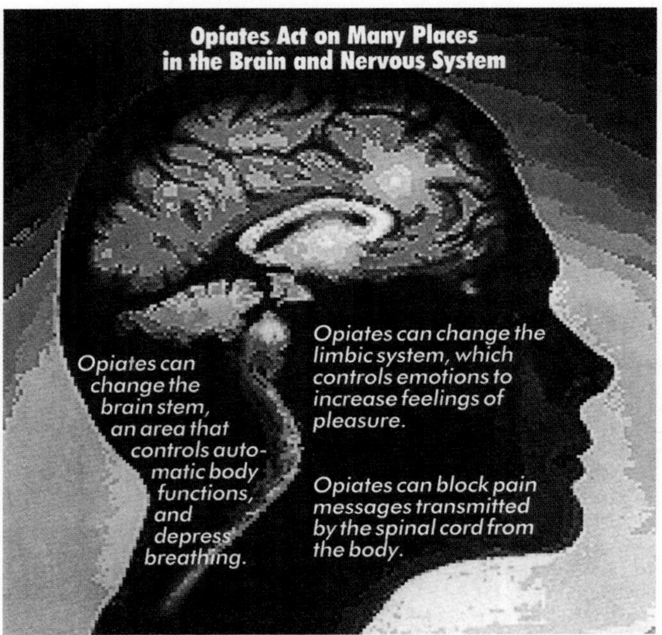

FIGURE 45–1 ✦ Opiate abuse and addiction. *(From the National Institute on Drug Abuse:* Heroin abuse and addiction, *NIDA Research Report Series, NIH Pub No 97-4165, Bethesda, Md, 1997, National Institutes of Health.)*

CAUSES OF SUBSTANCE ABUSE

Physiologic Factors

After a drug enters the body (see How Drugs Enter the Body), it is carried by the bloodstream to the *central nervous system (CNS)* (the brain and spinal cord) within 10 to 15 seconds.

When a drug crosses the blood–brain barrier it can affect all parts of the body by interfering with the information sent to the CNS by the *autonomic nervous system (ANS)* and the *peripheral nervous system (PNS).* The ANS controls involuntary functions such as circulation, digestion, and respiration, and helps the body to establish a stable internal environment. The PNS transmits messages between the external environment and the CNS. The role of the CNS is that of computer and switchboard. As the CNS receives messages from the ANS and PNS, it analyzes those messages and sends a response to the correct body system—muscular, skeletal, circulatory, nervous, respiratory, digestive, excretory, endocrine, or reproductive—to react to the stimuli. The CNS is also responsible for reasoning and making judgments. *Psychoactive drugs* alter the information sent to the brain and disrupt the messages sent back to the body (Figure 45–1). They also disrupt the ability to think and reason.

NEUROTRANSMITTERS. The three main components of a neuron (a nerve cell) are dendrites, the cell body, and axons. The *dendrites* receive signals from other neurons, the *cell body* nourishes the neuron and keeps it alive, and the *axons* carry the message from the dendrites and cell body to the terminals, which relay the message to the dendrites of the next neuron. Between the neurons lies the synaptic gap, the space between the terminal sending the message and the dendrite that is receiving the message. This "jump" between neurons is accomplished through biochemicals called *neurotransmitters* that transmit the message from one neuron to the receptors on another. Dopamine, endorphin, enkephalin, serotonin, substance "P," epinephrine, and acetylcholine are examples of neurotransmitters. The specific message that is being sent will determine the neurotransmitter that is released from the neuron. For example, substance "P" is released from neurons if "pain" is the message being transmitted; dopamine is released if "pleasure" is the message being transmitted.

Psychoactive drugs disrupt the normal functioning of the neurotransmitters. Sometimes this is a desirable effect. *CNS depressants* inhibit the release of substance "P," thereby dulling and weakening the pain signal. This effect is desirable if morphine is prescribed by a physician to alleviate pain in a person with a terminal illness. The illegal CNS depressant heroin also attaches itself to certain receptor sites in the emotional center of the brain and induces a sensation of pleasure or reward; however, it also attaches itself to the area of the brain that controls respiration and can slow it down to a dangerous

How Drugs Enter the Body

- Direct contact with skin or mucous membranes
- Orally, by swallowing
- Snorted through the nose or placed sublingually or against oral mucosa
- Injected either directly into the bloodstream (IV) or into a muscle mass (muscling) or under the skin (skin popping). All injection methods place the user at risk for hepatitis, septicemia, abscesses, and HIV infection.

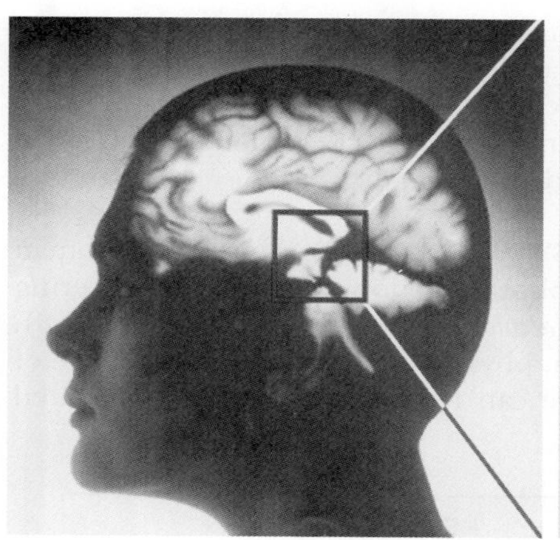

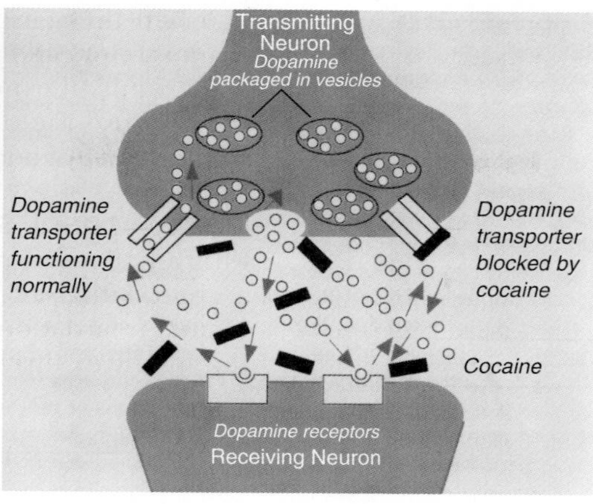

FIGURE 45–2 ✦ Cocaine abuse and addiction. *(From the National Institute on Drug Abuse:* Cocaine abuse and addiction, *NIDA Research Report Series, NIH Pub No 99-4342, Bethesda, Md, 1999, National Institutes of Health.)*

level. *CNS stimulants* such as cocaine force the release of large amounts of neurotransmitters such as epinephrine and dopamine, which can create, stimulate, and exaggerate messages to and from the CNS (Figure 45–2). Psychedelic drugs will confuse neurotransmitters by exaggerating and distorting messages and by creating visual and auditory images in the brain.[4]

Genetic Factors

Endorphin and enkephalin neurotransmitters have an opiatelike effect on the brain, causing the individual to have a feeling of well-being. People who are born with the inability to produce sufficient quantities of endorphin and enkephalin have a genetic predisposition for opiate and alcohol addiction.[4] These are often people who suffer from depression and look for artificial means to alleviate their mood.

Significant genetic correlations have been found in twins raised in separate households, apart from one another, in drug and alcohol abuse scores (r = 0.78); drug abuse and childhood antisocial behavior scores (r = 0.87); and drug abuse and adult antisocial behavior scores (r = 0.53).[5] These high correlations suggest that the similarities in twins' behavior are genetic rather than environmental.

Researchers have been unable, as yet, to identify a specific gene responsible for drug abuse, but feel that several modified genes may contribute to addiction. Genes that interfere with serotonin metabolism and affect the serotonin–dopamine balance (neurotransmitters) in the brain have been implicated in a wide variety of psychiatric disorders. Such disorders include alcoholism, drug addiction, depression, suicide, aggressive behaviors, antisocial borderline personality disorder, phobias, panic attacks, eating disorders, and attention deficit hyperactivity disorder (ADHD).[4,5]

ADDICTION CURVE.[4] Because individuals are born with some genetic (inherited) sensitivity to specific drugs, those with low genetic predisposition for addictive behaviors will take longer to become addicted or to climb the curve to addiction than those born with a high

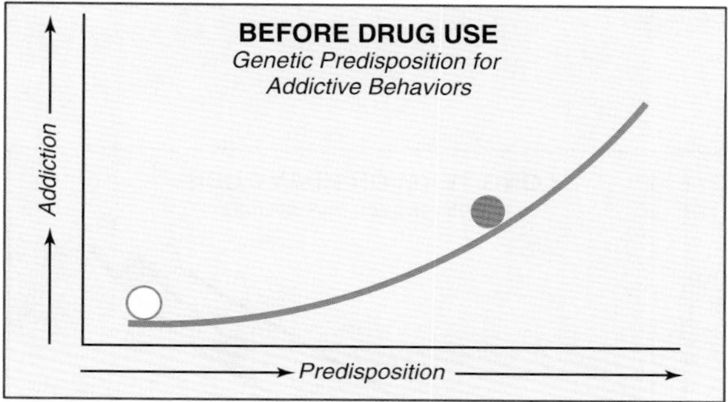

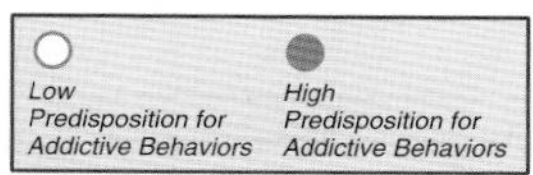

FIGURE 45–3 ✦ Before drug use, genetic predisposition for addictive behaviors. *(Adapted from Inaba DS, Cohn WE:* Uppers, downers, all arounders, *Ashland, Ore, 1990, Cinemed.)*

genetic predisposition. The individual with high predisposition starts at a point closer to addiction on the curve (Figure 45–3).

Drugs are used first experimentally, then socially and habitually until addiction is reached. When drugs are first used, the predisposition for addictive behaviors increases (Figure 45–4). Those individuals with a low inherited predisposition for addictive behaviors would have to use drugs over a much longer period of time to become addicted than would those with a high inherited predisposition. It may take people with a low predisposition three or four years of long-term or heavy use to reach the same level of addiction people with a high predisposition would reach in two or three months. This is due to the deficiency that is already present in their brain chemistry (Figure 45–5).

If individuals stop taking (abstain from) drugs, will their brain chemistry return to normal? Evidence suggests that "neurotransmitters may rebound back to normal levels in those with short-term, noninherited disruption, but not so with long-term, inherited imbalance"[4] (Figure 45–6).

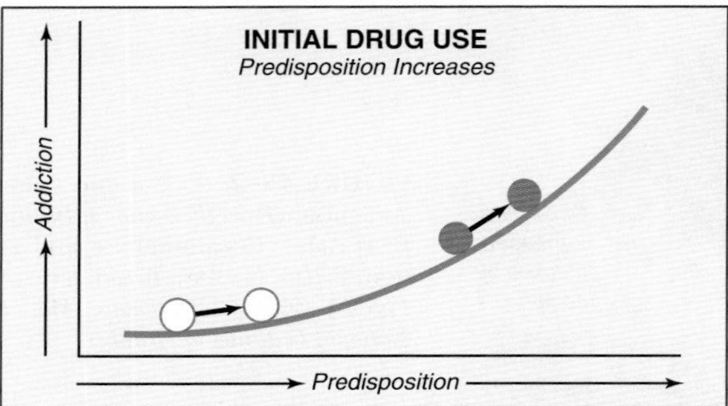

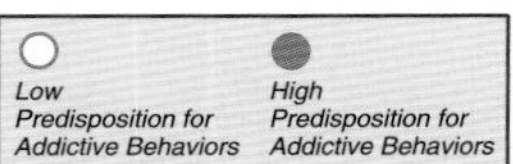

FIGURE 45–4 ✦ Initial drug use, predisposition increase. *(Adapted from Inaba DS, Cohn WE:* Uppers, downers, all arounders, *Ashland, Ore, 1990, Cinemed.)*

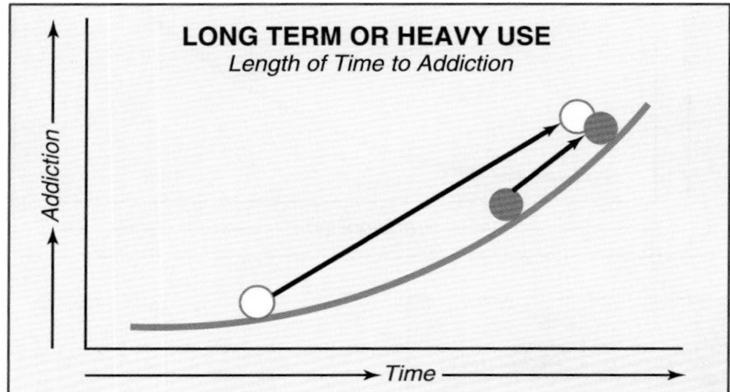

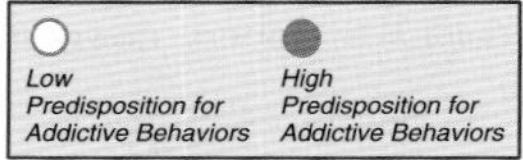

FIGURE 45–5 ✦ Long-term or heavy use and length of time to addiction. *(Adapted from Inaba DS, Cohn WE:* Uppers, downers, all arounders, *Ashland, Ore, 1990, Cinemed.)*

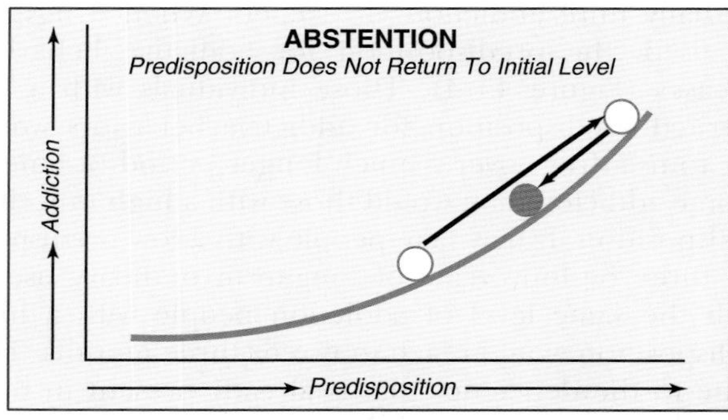

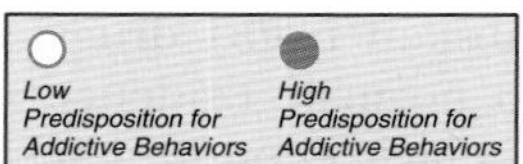

FIGURE 45–6 ✦ Abstention predisposition does not return to initial level. *(Adapted from Inaba DS, Cohn WE:* Uppers, downers, all arounders, *Ashland, Ore, 1990, Cinemed.)*

When the sensitivity does not return to normal, the brain is imprinted and remembers the drug-using habits. As a result, the next time the individual relapses and starts to use the drug again, it takes much less time to reach a level of addiction (Figure 45–7).

FETAL ALCOHOL SYNDROME (FAS). A pregnant woman with an active alcohol addiction is at risk of delivering a child with *fetal alcohol syndrome (FAS)* (Figure 45–8). Mental retardation, physical impairments, and failure of the infant to thrive can result (see Features Associated

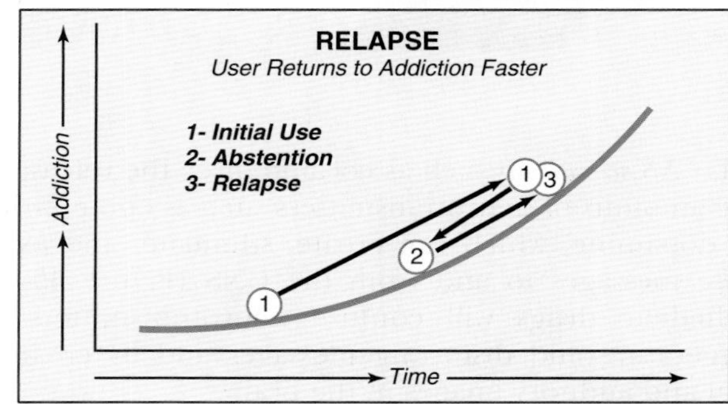

FIGURE 45–7 ✦ After relapse, user returns to addiction faster. *(Adapted from Inaba DS, Cohn WE:* Uppers, downers, all arounders, *Ashland, Ore, 1990, Cinemed.)*

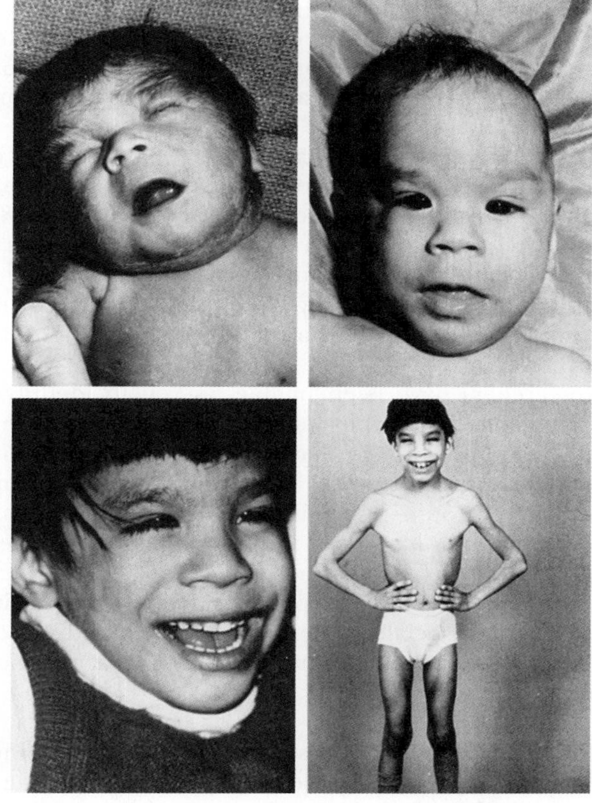

FIGURE 45–8 ✦ Head and facial features associated with fetal alcohol syndrome.

with Fetal Alcohol Syndrome). Characteristics of a child with FAS include hyperactivity, learning difficulties, problems with memory, deficits in problem solving, speech and hearing impairments, and mental retardation. The Centers for Disease Control and Prevention estimates that 0.3% to 0.9% of infants per 10,000 live births will have FAS. Native Americans have an even higher incidence of FAS.[6]

Environmental Factors

Families play a very important role in determining how children handle the temptation to use alcohol, cigarettes, and illegal drugs.[7] Although substance abuse prevention programs for youth are found in schools, in the media, and in the community, they are insufficient by themselves. Without parental supervision, consistent discipline, and a loving family relationship, community programs are not as effective.

Moreover, each family member is affected in some way by the addiction of one. The individual family members feel many of the emotions experienced by the addict, although they tend to suppress their feelings. Often, their confidence and self-esteem are diminished and anxieties and health problems increase. Approximately one third of family members of substance abusers experience depression, and one third become chemically dependent themselves (see Risk Factors for Substance Abuse).

Features Associated with Fetal Alcohol Syndrome

Abnormal facial characteristics (Figure 45–8)
Mental retardation
Learning disabilities
Hearing, speech, and vision impairments
Hyperactivity
Memory and problem-solving deficits
Poor motor coordination
Major organ malformations (heart, liver, kidneys)
Skeletomuscular system malformations
Compromised immune system

Risk Factors for Substance Abuse

Children with ADHD
Children who are alienated, rebellious, or have serious behavioral problems
Children who suffer extreme poverty, peer rejection, and live in areas of high incidence of drug use and crime
Individuals with a history of child abuse
Individuals with a genetic sensitivity to specific drugs

MEDICAL TREATMENT FOR SUBSTANCE ABUSE

Emergency Treatment

An immediate need for medical care is presented when the abuser takes an overdose of a substance and has a life-threatening medical condition that must be treated. Acute alcohol poisoning associated with binge drinking is a condition that has appeared with increasing regularity on college campuses, and requires emergency treatment. Symptoms of alcohol poisoning include the following:

- Slow or irregular breathing (less than 8 breaths per minute)
- Cold, pale, or blue-toned skin
- Rapid pulse
- Vomiting while awake or asleep
- Unresponsive to attempt to awaken
- Semiconsciousness or unconsciousness

Alcohol poisoning is a medical emergency and 911 should be called. While waiting for the emergency medical service to arrive, the individual should not be given anything to eat or drink, should be turned on his or her side, and should have breathing and vital signs monitored. In the hospital emergency room the treatment priority is to stabilize the client, followed by detoxification by behavioral and/or pharmacologic treatment, which may take several weeks. This treatment often is performed on an in-patient basis to limit the client's access to alcohol or drugs. Clients who have an existing psychiatric problem along with substance abuse are best treated at long-term drug treatment facilities.

Behavioral Treatment

It is often stated that substance abusers must reach "bottom" in their lives before they willingly seek help. Reaching bottom often means that they are unemployed and lack emotional support from friends and family. The most effective treatments for substance abuse occur when the abuser is motivated to seek medical intervention, behavioral changes, and social reinforcement. People who seek to end their addiction through 12-step programs such as Alcoholics Anonymous (AA), Narcotics Anonymous (NA), and Cocaine Anonymous (CA) appear to have a greater chance of maintaining abstinence by using weekly meetings as an "aftercare" activity.[8,9] When clients combine participation in a 12-step program with enrollment in a behavioral treatment program, they have significantly higher rates of successful completion of treatment[8] (Figure 45–9). Recovery from drug addiction can be a long-term process requiring multiple treatment interventions. Participation in self-help support programs during and following treatment can often help to maintain abstinence.[9]

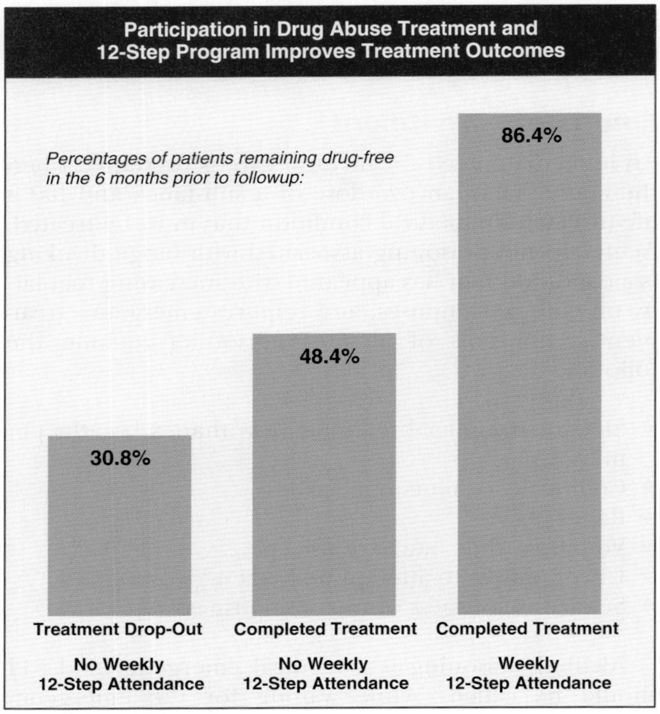

Participation in Drug Abuse Treatment and 12-Step Program Improves Treatment Outcomes

Percentages of patients remaining drug-free in the 6 months prior to followup:

	Treatment Drop-Out, No Weekly 12-Step Attendance	Completed Treatment, No Weekly 12-Step Attendance	Completed Treatment, Weekly 12-Step Attendance
Drug-free	30.8%	48.4%	86.4%

FIGURE 45–9 ✦ Participation in drug abuse treatment and 12-step program improves treatment outcomes. *(From the National Institute on Drug Abuse:* Adding more counseling sessions and 12-step programs can boost drug abuse treatment effectiveness, *NIDA Notes, NIH Pub No 99-3478, NIDA Notes 14(5):7, 1999.)*

Pharmacologic Treatment

Treatment for addiction may involve drug therapy (Table 45–3). Drugs usually prescribed to treat the symptoms of depression and anxiety disorders are often used to treat clients with addictive behavior disorders.

IMPLICATIONS FOR THE DENTAL HYGIENE PROCESS OF CARE

Assessment

The problem of abuse of alcohol, prescribed medications, or illegal drugs affects all socioeconomic groups. Only about 10% of clients who abuse drugs, however, are identified by healthcare providers. Several visits over time for dental hygiene care may reveal behaviors that can be confirmed by a well-focused health history and a thorough extraoral and intraoral examination.

HEALTH HISTORY. Chemically dependent clients must be identified so they can be treated safely. Many will "premedicate" with their drug of choice before coming to a dental appointment. In the health history interview, the dental hygienist identifies all current medications the client is taking to avoid possible drug interactions between a prescribed or an abused substance and drugs offered in the oral health setting. Such interactions can pose a life-threatening situation for the client.

TABLE 45–3 PHARMACOLOGIC AGENTS USED IN THE TREATMENT OF ALCOHOLISM

Drug	Purpose	Mechanism of Action	Clinical Effects
Alcohol Sensitizing Agents			
Disulfiram (Antabuse) Citrated Calcium Carbimide (Temposil)	To cause an aversive reaction when used in the presence of alcohol	Blocks the metabolism of alcohol	If alcohol is ingested while taking disulfiram, nausea, vomiting, severe stomach pain, and hypotension result. These effects are less severe with citrated calcium carbimide.
Anticraving Agent			
Naltrexone (Trexan)	To reduce or eliminate cravings for alcohol	Antagonizes various opiate receptors	Decreases craving and consumption of alcohol, especially as an adjunct to behavioral therapy
Antiemetic Agent			
Ondansetron	Currently used experimentally in the treatment of alcohol addiction	Serotonin antagonism	Decreases nausea and vomiting

The need for prophylactic antibiotic premedication must be considered for the following reasons when treating a client with a history of intravenous drug use:

- ✦ Many intravenous drug users develop venous thrombosis and organic valvular disease.
- ✦ Damage to the tricuspid valve between the right atrium and ventricle is often associated with substance abuse.
- ✦ Intravenous drug use can result in endocarditis caused by *Staphylococcus aureus* found on nonsterile needles. One study has shown that 48% of opioid abusers with cardiac disease have healed or active endocarditis.[10]

Consequently, all clients with a history of intravenous drug abuse should be evaluated by their physician prior to dental or dental hygiene care to determine if any of these conditions exists, indicating the need for antibiotic premedication (see Chapter 10 for the regimen).

Additional medical conditions experienced by chemically dependent clients are influenced by the specific substances being used and how they enter the body.[10] For example, clients with a history of intravenous drug use have a higher incidence of HIV and hepatitis B, C, and D from sharing needles. Long-term use of alcohol can result in liver damage. This damage can be caused by an increase in fatty acids, by alcoholic hepatitis, and/or by cirrhosis, which results in replacement of liver tissue with scar tissue and eventually causes death. Moreover, damage to the heart, kidneys, pancreas, and reproductive system, and permanent brain damage and a lack of muscle coordination can result from years of alcohol abuse.

Questions about substances used and routes of administration appear on the health history forms. When reviewing the client's responses and when interacting with the client, the dental hygienist looks for signs of substance abuse. If the dental hygienist suspects the client may be dependent on a substance (see Red Flags for Suspicion of Substance Abuse), that information should be recorded in the client's dental record. Specific objective observations, client behavior, and assessment findings such as pupil changes or needle marks should be recorded. Personal opinions and judgmental statements are inappropriate.[11] Observations should be presented in an organized, professional manner to provide an accurate record for future clinicians.[12]

Clients are often reluctant to reveal alcohol or drug use because of the social stigma associated with substance abuse. Also, many substance abusers are in denial and will not admit to any type of dependence when asked. The astute dental hygienist recognizes signs and symptoms of dependence and discusses the possibility of a substance abuse problem with the client in a nonjudgmental manner. (See Table 45–4 for drug categories and street names of abused substances.) Recognition of a drug abuse problem by a healthcare professional may prompt the abuser to seek help. It is essential that clients understand that the reason for obtaining information is to protect them from health risks and that all information will remain confidential.

When abuse is suspected, it is recommended that the dental hygienist ask the following questions:[13]

- ✦ Have you ever felt the need to cut down on your drinking or drug use?
- ✦ Have you ever felt bad or guilty about your drinking or drug use?
- ✦ Have you ever used or had a drink first thing in the morning as an eye opener to steady your nerves or to feel normal?

If the client answers "yes" to two or more of these questions, then the dental hygienist should strongly suspect abuse and consider how to motivate the client to seek treatment. The dental office should have a list of community resources available as a reference for the client. Brochures about specific programs can be provided, or the client can be given the telephone number of the National Council on Alcohol and Drug Dependence, which offers general information. Identifying dental clients who are chemically dependent is important; however, substance abuse treatment is not within the scope of dental hygiene practice. It is helpful if dental offices develop a simple protocol for referral of clients with substance abuse problems.

It is necessary to determine if the client "self-medicated" for the dental appointment. If the client has taken drugs/alcohol prior to the appointment, then the care plan for that day may need to be modified or canceled to avoid any drug interactions and/or drug-associated behavior problems.

EXTRAORAL EXAMINATION. The general appearance of the client can also alert the dental hygienist to the possibility of substance abuse. Does the client look substantially older than her/his stated age, have a disheveled appearance, poor personal hygiene, insist on wearing

Red Flags for Suspicion of Substance Abuse

Unreliable; frequently misses appointments
Careless in appearance and hygiene
Lapses in memory and/or concentration
Alcohol on breath
Speech is slurred; appearance of intoxication
Needle marks on arm
Rapid mood swings within minutes
Frequently requests written excuses for work
Frequently requests specific medication for pain
Calls the dental office and complains of severe pain and requests that a prescription for pain medication be given without making an appointment with the dentist
High tolerance to sedatives and analgesics
Pupils are abnormally dilated or constricted

TABLE 45–4 DRUG CATEGORIES AND STREET NAMES

Drug Category	Available As	Street Names
CNS Stimulants		
Amphetamines	Benzedrine	General term: *uppers*
	Dexedrine	Bennies, speed, uppers
	Ritalin	Dexies, ice, glass
	Methamphetamine	Pellets
	Methylenedioxymethamphetamine (Ecstasy)	Crystal, speed, meth, crank, chalk
	OTC diet pills	Snowball
Caffeine	OTC NoDoz, Vivarin	
	Coffee	Java, joe
	Coca-Cola, Pepsi, Jolt	Coke
	Tea	
	Chocolate	
Cocaine (hydrochloride)	White powder (snorted or dissolved in water and injected)	C, coke, Charlie, snow, toot, joy powder, Cadillac, gold dust
Freebase cocaine	White crystalline powder diluted with talc/cornstarch and/or sugar (smoked)	Flake, blow, crack, rock, freebase
Nicotine	Cigarettes, cigars, chewing tobacco, snuff	Cancer stick, stogie, butt, toke, dip, chew
CNS Depressants		
Opiates from Opium Poppy Extracts		
Opium	Laudanum, Paregoric	General term: *downers,* O, op, poppy
Codeine	By prescription	Number 3s
	Aspirin or Tylenol with	
Morphine	By prescription	M, white stuff, morph, Miss Emma
Heroin	Injected	H, smack, horse, junk, Harry, chip hard goods, China white
	Smoked in water pipe, mixed with tobacco or marijuana in cigarettes	
Hydromorphone	Dilaudid	Dillies
Hydrocodone	Vicodin (often prescribed for dental pain)	
Oxycodone	Percodan	Percs
Synthetic Opiates (Opioids)		
Methadone	Dolophine (substitute for heroin)	Meth, dollies
Propoxyphene	Darvon, Darvocet	Pink ladies, pumpkin seeds
Meperidine	Demerol	No common street name
Fentanyl	Sublimaze	China white
Sedatives/Hypnotics		
Barbiturates		
Secobarbital	Seconal	Reds, red devils, Mexican reds
Pentobarbital	Nembutal	Yellows, yellow jackets, nebbies
Phenobarbital	Generic	Phenos
Amobarbital	Amytal	Blue heavens, blue dolls, blues
Benzodiazepines		
Diazepam	Valium	Vals
Chlordiazepoxide	Librium	Libs
Alprazolam	Xanax	No common street names
Nonbarbiturate Sedatives/Hypnotics		
Glutethimide	Doriden	Goofballs, goofers
Glutethimide and codeine	Doriden and codeine	Loads, sets, setups
Meprobamate	Equanil, Miltown	No common street names
Hallucinogens		
Cannabinoids		
Marijuana	Flowers and leaves of marijuana plant can be eaten or smoked	Grass, pot, weed, hemp, Mary Jane, reefer, roach, Acapulco gold
Sensimilla	Marijuana plants with increased THC	Sens, skunk weed
Hashish	Concentrated resin from marijuana plant	Hash
Hash oil	Extracted from marijuana plant and added to foods	Same as above
Phencyclidine (PCP)	Manufactured illegally (can be smoked, swallowed, or injected)	Angel dust, ice, peep, ozone, Shermans, KJ
Ketamine	Crystals or powder that is smoked, snorted, or swallowed	Super-K

TABLE 45–4 DRUG CATEGORIES AND STREET NAMES—CONT'D

Drug Category	Available As	Street Names
Inhalants		General terms: *sniffing* or *snorting*
VOLATILE SOLVENTS		
Adhesives	Airplane glue, rubber cement, polyvinylchloride cement	
Aerosols	Spray paint, hair spray, deodorant, air freshener, asthma spray	
Solvents and gases	Nail polish remover, paint remover, paint thinner, fuel gas, cigarette lighter fluid, gasoline, typing correction fluid	
Cleaning agents	Dry cleaning fluid, spot remover, degreaser	
Dessert topping sprays	Whipped cream	
NITRITES AND ANESTHETICS		
Nitrite room odorizers		Poppers, rush
Nitrous oxide anesthesia	Available as a gas	Whippets (balloons or plastic bags filled with nitrous oxide)
Anabolic Steroids and Hormones		General terms: *rhoids, doping, stacking,* and *bulking up*
Male hormones	Testosterone, Dianabol, stanozolol	
Adrenocortical steroids	Cortisone, prednisone, Decadron	
Human chorionic gonadotropin (HCG)	Clomiphene	
Human growth hormone (HGH)		

sun glasses, and wear long sleeves even in hot weather to cover needle marks? Can you smell alcohol or other odors on her/his breath? Does the client appear to be lethargic or intoxicated without the accompanying odor of alcohol? Does the client experience tremors? Look at the client's eyes for signs of substance abuse (see Red Flags for Suspicion of Substance Abuse).

Needle marks in the antecubital fossae and forearms or bruises and increased pigmentation over veins caused by multiple injections, observed while taking a blood pressure reading, may indicate illicit drug use. Skin abscesses can be caused by subcutaneous "popping" of heroin. Crack abusers will often show burns and scars on the thumb of the dominant hand from repeated use of a disposable lighter. Multiple healed and healing burns or abrasions may be the result of physical trauma experienced while the client was under the influence of alcohol or drugs.[10] Snorting or inhaling substances can burn nasal passages, cause nosebleeds, and significantly damage nasal structures. Often, clients continually sniff their noses and use handkerchiefs or tissues.

The client's behavior and speech should be watched for signs of confusion, disorientation, lethargy, lack of concentration, or memory impairment. Extreme depression or agitation may indicate a drug overdose.

Tremors of the hands, tongue, and eyelids may be signs of alcohol withdrawal. Other extraoral signs of alcohol abuse include the following:

- ✦ Redness of facial skin and spider petechiae on the nose from dilated blood vessels
- ✦ Yellowish facial skin from jaundice due to liver disease
- ✦ Facial trauma due to falls when intoxicated

Oral Manifestations of Alcohol Abuse

Xerostomia
Poor oral hygiene
Gingival bleeding on probing
Coated tongue
Glossitis due to nutritional deficiency
Attrition related to bruxism
Erosion related to vomiting
Broken teeth due to accidents related to intoxication
Buccal cervical caries

- ✦ Angular cheilitis due to vitamin B deficiency
- ✦ Red or swollen eyes

INTRAORAL EXAMINATION. (Table 45–5) Placement of drugs in the vestibule or under the tongue can cause localized tissue necrosis. Gingival lesions may be caused by cocaine placement. Alcohol and drug abusers often crave sweets. Consequently, large dark areas of buccal cervical caries from ingesting large quantities of carbohydrates may be present. Other oral manifestations associated with substance abuse include oral candidiasis as a result of immunosuppression, and *glossodynia* (pain in the tongue) from malnutrition and immunosuppression because of a secondary addiction to alcohol. Cocaine users tend to have severe bruxism, causing flat cuspal planes on premolars and molars. Because the substance abuser's body is being taxed by drug use, tissue healing is affected. See Oral Manifestations of Alcohol Abuse.

TABLE 45–5 DENTAL HYGIENE ASSESSMENT FINDINGS ASSOCIATED WITH SUBSTANCE ABUSE

Abused Substance	Ocular Signs of Use	Oral Findings	Dental Hygiene Care Considerations
Amphetamines	Dilated pupils Slow or no reaction of pupil to light	Xerostomia Increased caries Bruxism (extreme tooth wear in "Ecstasy" users) leading to trismus	Can increase bleeding and interfere with coagulation
Alcohol	Red, puffy	Tooth erosion from sugar in alcohol or regurgitation Sialosis Xerostomia Glossitis Stomatitis due to nutritional deficiencies and anemia Orofacial injuries from accidents or violence, severe infections due to immunosuppression	Increased dosage for anesthesia and sedation Increased bleeding after surgery Increased healing time due to immunosuppression
Cocaine	Dilated pupils Slow or no reaction of pupil to light	Placement of cocaine in maxillary premolar area to test the purity of a drug sample can cause localized and gingival and alveolar bone necrosis Increased caries from carbohydrates added to cocaine as filler	Possible spontaneous gingival bleeding from thrombocytopenia Interaction between cocaine and anesthetics containing epinephrine
Opiates and opioids (heroin, morphine, methadone)	Constricted pupils Nonreactive to light	Methadone is carried in a sugary syrup taken orally, which may cause increased risk of caries	Increased possibility of hepatitis, HIV infection from drug injection Poor pain tolerance Increased possibility of infective endocarditis from scaling procedures Increased bleeding from thrombocytopenia Interactions between opioids and dentally prescribed medications
Barbiturates and benzodiazepines	Constricted pupils	Xerostomia, lesions of oral mucosa in the area of drug use	Tolerance to sedative drugs
Cannabis (marijuana)	Reddened sclera, swollen eyelids, tears	Leukoplakia Increased incidence of lingual carcinoma Gingival enlargement	Interaction between cannabis and anesthetics containing epinephrine
LSD, PCP	Dilated pupils, swollen eyelids	Orofacial injuries experienced while "tripping" Bruxism resulting in trismus	Flashback that may cause panic attacks can occur due to a stressful dental environment Respiratory depression if opioids are prescribed.
Inhalants		"Glue-sniffer's rash" Erythema around the labial borders Oral frost bite	Anesthetic toxicity is increased Sensitization to epinephrine can occur Increased risk of seizures
Anabolic steroids		High-carbohydrate diet may cause increased caries	Cardiac dysfunction can result from anesthetics containing epinephrine Increase in bleeding

Dental Hygiene Diagnosis and Care Planning

Substance abuse must be addressed in care planning. People who are deeply immersed in drug abuse will probably seek dental care only when they are in severe pain. Because the pain sensation can be diminished by the use of drugs, the dental problem is usually in an advanced state. Substance-abusing clients may request the use of nitrous oxide sedation for treatment and specific medication for pain. As previously discussed, it is important that oral care professionals have knowledge of the type and amount of drugs clients have taken before planning any pain control or other care.

Clients in recovery programs, however, may seek long-neglected dental treatment as part of their attempt to achieve total body health. It is under these circumstances that the dental hygienist will most probably be providing care. Recovering addicts may be extremely cautious or anxious about taking any type of medication, making it difficult to control pain during scaling and root planing procedures. Some chemically dependent clients also may experience a tolerance to sedatives and analgesics. For clients recovering from substance abuse, pain control should be coordinated with the primary care physician. In addition, chemically dependent clients can experience emotional anxiety or instability and may be able to tolerate only short appointments. For this reason, the use of multiple short (20-minute) appointments may be necessary.

After a thorough assessment and consultation, if indicated, complete diagnostic statements are formulated by the dental hygienist based on identified human need deficits. Once the diagnostic statements are complete, client goals are set. Care planning priorities include setting realistic goals with the client to improve oral self-care and to enable the client to undergo periodontal scaling and root planing with a minimum of discomfort. Also, since malnutrition is clearly associated with alcohol abuse, dietary analysis and nutritional counseling should be planned. With permission of clients, consultation with their physician and counselors may aid the dental hygienist in planning effective care.

Implementation

Since good oral health and a pleasant smile add to an individual's sense of self-esteem, receiving necessary dental hygiene care may have a significant positive impact on recovery from substance abuse. A discussion concerning referral for treatment of the substance abuse should be initiated as soon as possible.[14]

APPOINTMENTS. Chemically dependent clients can experience emotional instability or take little responsibility for their behavior. As a result, they may not keep scheduled appointments. If the client arrives too late for an appointment, the appointment should be canceled. If the client fails to come to an appointment, all remaining appointments should be canceled. Failure to keep appointments should not be reinforced as acceptable behavior. Due to potential unreliability and to provide additional incentive to show up for care, payment should be received in advance of treatment. Aesthetic restorations should be treated last[15] to ensure that clients show up for all physiologically necessary treatment.

PAIN AND ANXIETY CONTROL. Adequate pain control is a necessity in the recovering chemically dependent client because unrelieved pain can be a relapse trigger.[14] For postoperative pain, nonsteroidal anti-inflammatory drugs (NSAIDS) are recommended because all other pain medications are potentially addictive. If the dentist feels that narcotic analgesics or sedative hypnotics for postoperative pain are indicated, substance-abusing clients require a higher dose than non–substance-abusing clients, and a limited number of doses should be prescribed. Anesthesia and pain control may be difficult to achieve for heroin-addicted clients who are in a methadone treatment program, because they have developed a tolerance to the analgesic and euphoric effects of their daily methadone dose.[12–14,16] Consultation with the client's physician is necessary to determine the best method to alleviate client discomfort.

Control of client anxiety also can help alleviate the client's perception of pain. Pain perception has both physical and psychological components. If the client trusts the clinician, emotional distress can be minimized, reducing the perception of pain. A dental hygienist with excellent communication skills and empathy can help dispel the client's anxiety. See Table 45–5 for other treatment considerations.

Some substance-abusing clients may see dental treatment as an opportunity to obtain prescriptions for abused substances. Consequently, they often will exaggerate their response to pain in an effort to obtain a prescription for a strong pain control medication. Prescription pads should be kept out of sight and in a safe place so that they are not accessible to clients. Pain medication in the dental office should be locked in a place unknown to clients. Drug-seeking clients often call the dental office and complain that they are in severe pain, and request that a prescription for pain medication be given to them without making an appointment with the doctor. Dental offices should maintain a policy of prescribing drugs only after the client has been seen by the dentist.

DENTAL HYGIENE CARE. Because short (20 minute) appointments are suggested, the dental hygienist may be able to complete only limited treatment at each appointment. If there is a need for prophylactic antibiotic premedication, the dental hygienist ensures that the client has premedicated as directed. General supragingival and subgingival debridement, which will enable the client to initiate adequate home care, may be all that the client will tolerate in a short appointment. Such treatment would allow the dentist to place needed restorations in a state of improved gingival health. This improved tissue response is especially important when placing cervical restorations, because inflamed gingival margins can interfere with the placement of restorative materials in those areas.

The client's response to the initial scaling visit will dictate further appointment planning. The client may be able to tolerate quadrant scaling and root planing to provide optimum treatment for periodontal disease. Confirmation from the client's physician that there is no presence of immunosuppression or kidney or liver damage should be sought before aggressive nonsurgical or surgical periodontal therapy is undertaken. The use of an ultrasonic scaling instrument and an alcohol-free antimicrobial lavage is indicated to reduce the incidence of a transient bacteremia.

It is best to postpone definitive scaling and root planing until a later time if the client is unable or unwilling to comply with treatment. In this case, a short, two-

or three-month continued-care interval is indicated. Once the client has progressed further with recovery from addiction, he or she may be more tolerant of dental hygiene care.

ORAL HEALTH INSTRUCTION. Lack of oral hygiene is common among substance abusers.[12–14,16] Oral health instruction should begin with basic toothbrushing instructions and encouragement to practice toothbrushing daily. Once toothbrushing techniques have been mastered and become a daily practice, interdental oral physiotherapy aids can be introduced. The choice of aid will depend on the client's physical and mental capabilities and the type of embrasures present (see Chapter 19). If the client is incapable of the fine motor skills necessary to manipulate dental floss, other aids should be suggested. Interdental wooden stimulators, interproximal brushes, or a powered floss aid may be easier for the client to use. If clients are frustrated by an inability to master a technique, they probably will do nothing. The client in addiction recovery has already been required to make numerous behavioral changes and will see a complex oral hygiene regimen as an additional burden.

Suggesting use of a fluoride rinse is appropriate, especially if the client has a moderate to high caries risk. It is also important for heroin addicts enrolled in a methadone program, since the daily methadone dose is administered as a sugary syrup. Antimicrobial rinses to control gingivitis may also be recommended. For alcoholics, the avoidance of products containing alcohol is important to avoid supporting their addiction and contributing to the negative health effects they experience from their alcohol use. Moreover, even very small amounts of alcohol ingested by a client taking disulfiram or similar alcohol-sensitizing drugs can cause an emergency. Therefore, nonalcoholic fluoride mouthrinses (e.g., ACT, Fluoriguard) and nonalcoholic antimicrobial mouthrinses (e.g., Biotene[17]) should be recommended for home care and for preprocedural rinses.

The dental hygienist also suggests that the client eat a well-balanced diet and limit cariogenic foods to encourage both oral and general health. Positive reinforcement and encouragement should be given to clients for any improvements in their oral hygiene.

Evaluation

The outcomes of dental hygiene care can serve as positive reinforcement for a healthier lifestyle for those clients in recovery. If evaluation of dental hygiene care occurs six to eight weeks after initial debridement, clients may be further along in their recovery, and may be more receptive to additional periodontal therapy, if needed. For those clients who are not in recovery, the evaluation of dental hygiene care provides another opportunity to encourage clients to seek help for their substance abuse. The initial recall/continued care interval should be three months after treatment. This is especially important if there was extensive periodontal therapy complicated by immunosuppression.

DENTAL PROFESSIONALS AND SUBSTANCE ABUSE

Alcohol and drug abuse are widespread in American culture, and dental professionals are not exempt from addiction. In fact, the prevalence of drug and alcohol abuse among professionals may be the same as or higher than in the general population.[15] Because dental personnel can prescribe medications, they have opportunity for easy access to drugs for abuse.

Why Professionals Are At Risk for Chemical Dependence

Healthcare professionals are usually required to have high academic grades to be admitted to a professional educational program. Once accepted, the professional education requires hours of instruction to reach competence. Students enrolled in healthcare educational programs are usually competitive, overworked, narrowly specialized, self-sacrificing, and grade conscious.

Dental and dental hygiene students have their work continually criticized by faculty. Trying to prove one's competence can easily lead to little sleep, an unbalanced and emotionally unrewarding lifestyle, physical and emotional exhaustion, stress and anxiety, irritability, and depression.[15] Completion of a professional program often requires students to become "self-denying," and their personal lives become of secondary importance to their education. This situation can lead to emotional conflicts within themselves and their families. Often students will use stimulants to enhance their performance at school, or alcohol on the weekend to relieve stress. This cycle often continues once the student has become a practicing professional.

Although taught to recognize symptoms of chemical dependence in clients, health professionals rarely recognize addiction in themselves. Most are convinced that they are in control of their substance abuse and can stop whenever they choose. Chemical dependence may be the underlying cause of licensure suspension or malpractice (see ADA Policy Statement on Chemical Dependency).

Many state dental associations sponsor educational programs and workshops on addiction within the profession. Diversion from the court system to a treatment program is available to addicted professionals unless they have caused harm to clients or violated major criminal laws. Health and Well-Being Committees of state dental associations help colleagues with problems of addiction. Confidentiality is ensured and referrals may be made anonymously. The committees may contract for services through the state medical society and provide appropriate referrals, posttreatment follow-up, monitoring, and advocacy.

Many professionals decide that it is time to stop drug abuse when they are faced with the loss of their professional license. Some seek help through residential or out-patient formal recovery programs, and others seek help through self-help programs. Dental support groups modeled on the principles of Alcoholics Anonymous, identified as Caduceus meetings, may also provide psychological support for professionals in recovery.

ADA Policy Statement on Chemical Dependency

The ADA recognizes that chemical dependency is a disease entity that affects all of society.

The ADA is committed to assisting the chemically dependent member of the dental family (including dental hygienists) toward recovery by education, information, and referral.

The ADA encourages those institutions responsible for dental education to allocate adequate curriculum on substance use, misuses, and addiction.

In meeting the needs of the public and the profession, the ADA also encourages ongoing liaison between constituent society chemical dependency committees and their state boards of registration.

The ADA recognizes the need for research in the area of chemical dependency in dentistry.

Client Education Issues

- ✦ Determine at which stage of change a client is before encouraging treatment for substance abuse.
- ✦ Discuss the risk of negative interactions between local anesthetics and nitrous oxide–oxygen analgesia with the abused substance.
- ✦ Describe how the abused substance affects oral and general health. Inform clients that antibiotic premedication prior to dental hygiene care may be necessary to prevent infective endocarditis or to manage an immunocompromised status.
- ✦ Stress the need for regular professional care, good oral hygiene, and good nutrition. Point out oral manifestations of substance abuse and malnutrition in the client's own mouth.
- ✦ Tailor toothbrushing technique and interdental aids to the client's abilities.
- ✦ Recommend nonalcoholic antimicrobial mouthrinses and fluoride rinses for alcoholics.
- ✦ Positively reinforce and encourage clients for improvements in their oral self-care and movement through the stages of change.
- ✦ Inform clients that alcohol is a risk factor for oral cancer.
- ✦ Inform clients with a history of alcohol abuse or on Antabuse that over-the-counter and prescription mouthrinses (antibacterial and fluoride) may contain up to 30% alcohol, and should be avoided.
- ✦ Educate women of childbearing age about fetal alcohol syndrome and that alcohol is transmitted via the breast milk to nursing infants.

Legal, Ethical, and Safety Issues

- Clients' personal, social, and health history forms must be kept confidential.
- Client behavior, assessment findings, professional recommendations, referrals, and treatment should be recorded in the client's permanent record. Personal opinions and judgmental statements are inappropriate.
- Some states have "Parental Notification" laws that direct healthcare professionals to reveal knowledge of any medical or psychological conditions found during an examination to a minor's parent or legal guardian.[11] Knowledge of the statutes in the legal jurisdiction is important so that confidential information about minors is managed correctly.
- Keep prescription pads out of sight and drugs locked in a place unknown to clients.
- Dentists should never write a prescription for a pain medication without knowing the client's history or without first examining the client.
- With approval from clients being treated for substance abuse, contact their physician and/or mental health professional when planning care.
- Reduce the client's anxiety level by keeping appointments short and comfortable.
- Perform only those procedures the client can easily tolerate.
- Keep oral care products containing alcohol in a secure place away from persons with alcoholism.
- Do not render treatment that may cause an interaction between an abused substance and dental anesthetics or other drugs offered as part of healthcare.
- Continue to encourage clients to seek help for substance abuse if they have been through a treatment program and have relapsed.
- Identifying dental clients who are chemically dependent is important; however, substance abuse treatment is not within the scope of dental hygiene practice.

Key Concepts

- Substance abuse is a chronic, cyclic disease that affects 4.1 million people in American society, including oral healthcare professionals.
- Substance addiction is a compulsive use of a substance despite adverse medical and social consequences.
- Psychological and physical dependence on drugs and genetic predisposition are the reasons people continue substance abuse.
- Tolerance to alcohol and drugs creates the need for continued increases in the amounts used to gain the same effect.
- Dental hygienists need to identify chemically dependent clients:
  - To avoid drug interactions between drugs offered at the dental office, such as local anesthetics or nitrous oxide–oxygen analgesia, and abused substances
  - To determine the need for antibiotic premedication prior to dental hygiene care
  - To recognize increased risk of immunosuppression, heart disease, liver disease, HIV, and hepatitis B, C, and D
  - To recognize drug-seeking behavior of clients with a history of abuse
  - To modify care plans
- Addictive behaviors are the result of genetic, environmental, psychological, and physiologic factors.
- Culture, ethnicity, poverty, behavioral problems, child abuse, peer rejection, and environment can be risk factors for substance abuse.
- Drugs affect the transmission of messages between the central, autonomic, and peripheral nervous systems by interfering with neurotransmission. Key neurotransmitters include dopamine, serotonin, and endorphins.
- A pattern of addictive behavior is influenced by genetic factors.
- Women have specific gender issues in alcohol and other substance abuse during pregnancy because it can affect the health of the fetus.
- Characteristics of children with fetal alcohol syndrome include poor motor coordination, learning disabilities, hyperactivity, sensory impairment, irritability, microcephaly, abnormal facial features, growth retardation, and mental retardation.
- Modification in addictive behavior goes through stages of change, which may have to be repeated before total abstinence is achieved.
- Specific extraoral and intraoral findings are associated with the specific type of substance the client abuses.
- The ADA encourages treatment rather than punishment of oral care professionals who seek help for substance abuse.

CRITICAL THINKING EXERCISES

Client: Mr. Y

Profile: Mr. Y, age 24, was scheduled for care with the dental hygienist. His last dental appointment was for extraction of teeth #s 2 and 15.

Chief Complaint: "My teeth are discolored, sensitive to cold, and they are 'soft' and decay easily. My mouth feels dry."

Medical History: He has a history of asthma, smokes one pack of cigarettes a day, and is currently taking 5 mg of prednisone twice a day. He reports that he took part in a drug/alcohol rehabilitation program one year ago.

Social History: Mr. Y is single and lives alone. His current girlfriend has suggested he "do something about his teeth."

Dental History: His clinical gingival attachment loss ranges from 3 to 7 mm, with bleeding on probing in the mandibular anterior sextant. His gingivae are pale except on the mandibular anterior, where the gingival margins are magenta. The tissues are edematous, smooth without stippling, and have rolled gingival margins. The tissue consistency is spongy and the interdental papillae are blunted. There is inadequate attached gingiva on the facial areas of teeth # 3, #14, and the mandibular anterior teeth. He has heavy subgingival and supragingival calculus on the mandibular anteriors and generalized interproximal nodules throughout the mouth. He is a Class II AAP periodontal classification. Eight carious lesions were identified.

Oral Health Behavior Assessment: He brushes his teeth once a day using a medium bristle toothbrush and uses no other dental aids.

Supplemental Notes: The water in his community is not fluoridated. His diet includes no milk or vegetables, and he eats two king-size chocolate candy bars daily. He knows his oral health is poor. He states that he has seen several television programs about "germs" in dental unit water lines and is worried about being exposed to disease.

1. What are the dental hygiene diagnoses for this client?
2. Develop a dental hygiene care plan including goals and interventions for this client.
3. What client education issues should be addressed?
4. What factors could be contributing to this client's periodontal health?
5. Are there any contraindications to this client's care?

For References, Suggested Readings, and Related Websites, visit

http://evolve.elsevier.com/Darby/hygiene/

CHAPTER 46

WOMEN'S HEALTH

OBJECTIVES

Mastery of the content in this chapter will enable the reader to:

- Recognize oral manifestations of conditions and diseases prevalent in women.
- Explain the relationship between hormonal changes and periodontal diseases, and periodontal disease status in women and preterm, low-birthweight infants.
- Plan dental hygiene care for women over the life span and their children.

KEY TERMS

Burning mouth syndrome
Childbearing years
Domestic violence
Early childhood caries (ECC)
Endogenous sex steroid hormone gingival disease
Estrogen replacement therapy (ERT)
Fetal alcohol syndrome (FAS)
Gender bias
Glossodynia
Glossopyrosis
Hormone replacement therapy (HRT)
Menopause
Menses
Menstrual cycle gingivitis
Oral contraceptives
Oral dysesthesia
Osteoporosis
Perimenopause
Perimylolysis
Postmenopause
Pregnancy
Pregnancy-associated gingivitis
Pregnancy granuloma (pyogenic granuloma)
Preterm low birthweight
Puberty
Puberty-associated gingivitis
Stomatodynia
Stomatopyrosis

Gender bias, preference given to members of one gender over another, has been evident in the history of medicine and healthcare. Research on drugs and diseases has been performed primarily on middle-aged white males, even though gender, age, and race/ethnicity profoundly influence life span, drug efficacy, and disease risk. For example, little is known about why women live longer than men, are more likely to develop autoimmune diseases, metabolize drugs differently, and vary in brain tissue that may influence mood, healing, and disease susceptibility.[1]

Some women lack the education and self-esteem necessary to advocate for their own healthcare. Limited access to healthcare results in suffering and premature loss of life, especially among women of color and the poor.[2] In the United States, more than 80% of heads of one-parent households are women, responsible for securing healthcare for themselves and their children.[3] Even with these constraints, women access the medical care system more than twice as often as men.[4]

LINKS BETWEEN ORAL AND SYSTEMIC HEALTH

Researchers have evidence linking periodontal disease with cardiovascular diseases, valvular heart disease, preterm low-birthweight babies, and bacterial pneumonia.[5,6]

TABLE 46–1 HEALTH SCREENING GUIDELINES FOR WOMEN

Type of Exam/Screening	Age to Begin Screening	Frequency of Screening	What to Look For
Self-breast exam	20	Once a month	Swelling, dimpling, nipple discharge, pain, redness
Clinical breast exam	20	Every 3 years	Unusual breast symptoms or changes
Mammogram	40	Once a year	Unusual breast symptoms or changes
Pelvic exam and pap test	18 years of age or at the onset of sexual activity	Once a year (after menopause, every 1 to 3 years)	Cancerous and precancerous changes of the cervix
Colon cancer screening and fecal occult blood test	50	Colonoscopy every 5 to 10 years (depending on findings) Fecal occult annually	Cancerous and precancerous changes of the colon
Cholesterol test	18	At healthcare professional's recommendation	High blood cholesterol, which can lead to heart disease
Blood pressure reading	18	Every 1 to 2 years	High blood pressure, which can lead to heart disease
Bone mineral density exam	At healthcare professional's recommendation	At healthcare professional's recommendation	Low bone density, which can lead to fractures and osteoporosis
Sexually transmitted disease screening	At the onset of sexual activity	When symptoms develop	Sexually transmitted diseases
Oral examination	Beginning at age 1	At healthcare professional's recommendation based on risk	Dental caries, gingival inflammation, sores that fail to heal, swellings, mouth odor.

Adapted from American Cancer Society, American Heart Association, National Osteoporosis Foundation, American Social Health Association, National Women's Health Resource Center: *Women's Health Journal* March 2000.

Moreover, systemic conditions are risk factors for periodontal disease: for example, type 1 and type 2 diabetes mellitus,[5] tobacco use,[7] stress, depression, financial difficulties, social isolation, and other distress-related or psychosocial factors.[6]

The relationship between the oral cavity and the body is reciprocal; periodontal disease is a risk factor for systemic diseases and conditions, and some systemic diseases raise a person's risk of periodontal disease. Dental hygiene care includes counseling clients about prevention of disease and oral–systemic disease links, referral to other healthcare providers for assessment and care, and providing tobacco cessation counseling. Table 46–1 provides a guide for counseling women on comprehensive healthcare. Nutrition information for women's health is in Chapter 28.

WOMEN AND HEART DISEASE

Young women rarely get heart disease, but heart disease is the number one killer of women over 60.[8] Under age 60, 1 in 3 men develop heart disease, versus 1 in 10 women. Women's risk rises at menopause, but does not equal men's until about 10 years later. Surprisingly, heart disease is more severe among women over 60 than among men of the same age; women are twice as likely as men to die within 60 days of suffering a heart attack,[9] and are less likely to survive coronary bypass surgery. It appears that high levels of triglycerides may elevate a woman's risk of heart disease, but there is no evidence that triglycerides have the same effect in men.[10]

Women may not exhibit the typical signs of a heart attack. In a woman, heart attack may be signaled by indigestion, nausea, vomiting, dizziness, breathlessness, back pain, or deep throbbing in the left or right bicep or forearm, rather than the chest pain typically observed in men experiencing a cardiac arrest (see Chapter 40). Women with cardiovascular disease may need tobacco cessation and nutritional counseling; blood pressure and cholesterol level screening; promotion of exercise at least 10 minutes three times daily, or 30 minutes three times a week; weight control; and stress reduction.

SIGNIFICANT LIFE CYCLES

Women need information on oral health as related to the following:

- ✦ Puberty and menses
- ✦ Oral contraceptives
- ✦ Childbearing years and pregnancy
- ✦ Perimenopause, menopause, and postmenopause
- ✦ Osteoporosis

Other significant women's health issues include eating disorders, autoimmune diseases, hormone replacement therapy and estrogen replacement therapy (HRT/ERT), and domestic violence.

Puberty and Menses

Puberty and *menses* are marked by the development of secondary sex characteristics throughout the body and estrogen level increases.[11] Irregular ovulations usually occur for the first one to two years. *Endogenous sex steroid hormone gingival disease,* which includes *puberty-associated gingivitis* and *menstrual cycle gingivitis,* may occur as estrogen and progesterone levels rise. These gingival diseases are plaque-induced gingival diseases modified by systemic factors (see Chapter 15, Figure 15–11).

The bacteria associated with increased estrogen levels (*Prevotella* species and *Bacteroides* species) have been implicated in periodontal disease.[12] Swollen, erythematous gingival tissues may be present, as well as activation of herpes labialis and aphthous ulcers, prolonged hemorrhage following oral surgery, and swollen salivary glands.[13] Minor increases in tooth mobility may be seen, along with an increase in gingival exudate.[13] These transient changes are attributed to the peak levels of estrogen and progesterone (Figure 46–1).

The body reacts to bacterial challenges differently, depending on the integrity of the immune system. The host response appears to be altered in the presence of increased sex steroid hormones, suggesting an effect of these hormones on the immune system.[14]

Dental hygiene preventive strategies during puberty and menses include stressing optimal oral hygiene via increased frequency and duration of toothbrushing with an extra-soft toothbrush and meticulous interdental cleaning (see Chapters 18 and 19). Therapeutic modalities include topical corticosteroids; frequent periodontal debridement, scaling and root planing; antimicrobial mouthrinses; and fluoride rinses and gels. The oral manifestations of puberty and menses, although disconcerting and uncomfortable, can be managed with topical viscous lidocaine, Orahesive or Zilactin B, and systemic analgesics such as aspirin or ibuprofen. Prudence should be exercised in scheduling any elective surgical procedure at this time. Although sex steroid hormone effects may be transient, irreversible oral damage could result if proper self-care is lacking.

Oral Contraceptives

Oral contraceptives are widely used by women of childbearing age (Table 46–2). Risks associated with oral contraceptives include gingival inflammation, exaggerated gingival inflammatory response to local irritants, increase in *Prevotella* species, and spotty melanotic pigmentation of the skin and gingiva.[13] Research suggests a 16-fold increase in *Bacteroides* species fed by circulating

TABLE 46–2 EXAMPLES OF SOME ORAL CONTRACEPTIVES

Generic Names	Common Brand Names
Ethinyl estradiol and norethindrone	Brevicon, Ovcon, Modicon, Nelova, Genora, Norcept-E, Norinyl, Ortho-Novum 7/7/7, Tri-Norinyl
Ethinyl estradiol and levonorgestrel	Nordette, Levlen
Ethinyl estradiol and norethindrone acetate	Loestrin 1.5/30, Norlestrin, Jenest-28, N.E.E., Norethin, Ortho-Novum 10/11, Ortho-Novum 1/35, Loestrin 1/20
Ethinyl estradiol and norgestrel	Lo/Ovral, Ovral, norgestimate, Ortho-Cyclen, Ortho Tri-Cyclen
Ethinyl estradiol and ethynodiol diacetate	Demulen
Levonorgestrel and ethinyl estradiol	Triphasil, Tri-Levlen, Levora-21, Levora-28, Tri-Levlen 21
Desogestrel and ethinyl estradiol	Desogen, Ortho-Cept

See the *Planned Parenthood* website (www.plannedparenthood.org/bc/) for further information on contraception.

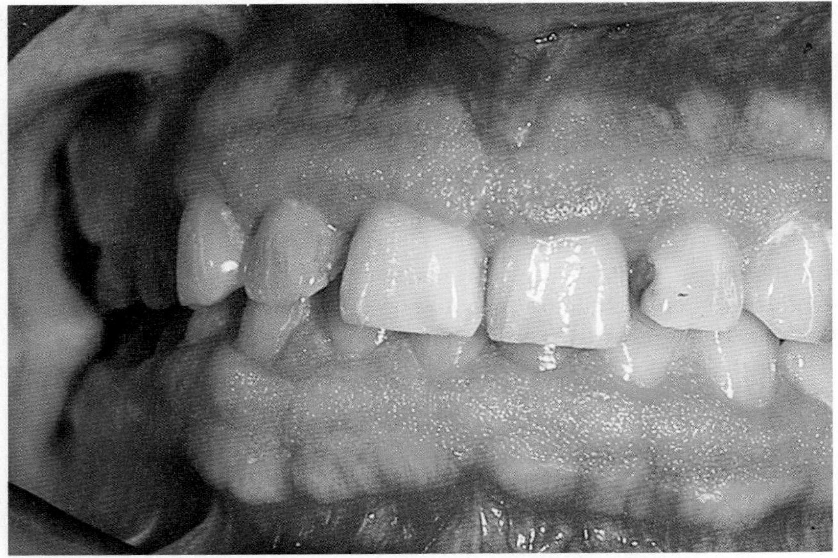

FIGURE 46–1 ✦ Endogenous sex steroid hormone gingival disease. *(Courtesy Jon B Suzuki, DDS, PhD, MBA.)*

blood levels of estrogen and progesterone in women taking oral contraceptives. Oral contraceptives may induce folate deficiency, which inhibits oral tissue repair and decreases blood clotting, especially in women over 35 who smoke. Other side effects may include the following:[13]

- Vision disturbance (blurred vision, flashing lights)
- Headaches (severe)
- Unusual leg pain (calf or thigh)
- Chest pain (severe), shortness of breath, or coughing up blood
- Abdominal pain (severe)

In light of these side effects, women may consider using other methods of birth control for a specific time period if surgery is necessary.

Childbearing Years and Pregnancy

All women of childbearing age should be informed of the critical importance of preventive care so that they may be motivated to seek professional care prior to pregnancy and throughout their lives (see Advice to Female Clients of Childbearing Age). A prenatal oral preventive program includes increased frequency of periodontal debridement; effective brushing and interdental cleaning (see Chapters 18 and 19), at-home fluoride therapy (see Chapter 26), antimicrobial rinses (see Chapter 24), nutritional counseling (see Chapter 28), and infant oral care to prevent *early childhood caries (ECC)* (see Chapter 26). ECC is prevented by stopping the infection of the infant's oral flora with *Streptococcus mutans* in conjunction with avoiding prolonged exposure of the primary teeth to fluids containing sugar. (See section on infant and child care later in this chapter)

During the first trimester of pregnancy, the period of organogenesis when vital organs form, the fetus is at risk for environmental influences. Ideally, no drug or illegal substances should be used during pregnancy, especially during the first trimester when the fetus is at greatest risk. However, there are situations in which drugs are necessary and appropriate to maintain the health of the mother. In those situations, drugs classified as category A or B by the FDA are preferred (Table 46–3). Drugs used during pregnancy and lactation should be used at the lowest effective dose and duration, to minimize harmful effects on the fetus/infant.[15] It is always prudent to consult with the obstetrician when treating pregnant clients if in doubt about any procedure or client condition.

In the last half of the third trimester the uterus is very sensitive to external stimuli, and the hazard of premature delivery exists. In a semireclined or supine position, the enlarged uterus compresses the inferior vena cava. This interferes with venous return, causing maternal hypotension, decreased cardiac output, and if prolonged, eventual loss of consciousness. Placing the client on her left side while receiving dental hygiene care removes pressure on the vena cava and allows blood to return from the lower extremities and pelvic area.[15]

Advice to Female Clients of Childbearing Age

Get early prenatal care, even before pregnancy.
Eat a well-balanced diet, including a vitamin supplement with A, C, D, calcium, phosphorus, and folic acid.
Select nutritious snacks and avoid those that increase caries risk.
Exercise regularly, with doctor's permission.
Avoid alcohol, cigarettes, and illicit drugs, and limit caffeine.
Avoid hot tubs and saunas.
Avoid infections (including periodontal disease).
Maintain meticulous oral hygiene by toothbrushing and interdental cleaning.

NITROUS OXIDE–OXYGEN ANALGESIA USE DURING PREGNANCY. Use of nitrous oxide–oxygen analgesia in pregnancy has not been assigned a rating by the FDA,[13] but studies demonstrate increased congenital anomalies, altered immune responses, spontaneous abortion, and increased birth defects when used during pregnancy.[16,17] Scavenging systems, when properly installed and maintained, are effective in reducing ambient nitrous oxide concentration in the oral care environment. A physician should be consulted before administering this analgesic to a pregnant client (see Chapter 35).

DRUG INTAKE DURING LACTATION. Little conclusive evidence exists about drug dosage during lactation and its effects on the nursing infant. The amount of drug excreted in breast milk is usually 1% to 2% of the maternal dose.[13] Therefore, it is unlikely that most drugs taken by the lactating mother have any pharmacologic significance for the infant. It is prudent for the mother to take the drug just after breastfeeding and then avoid nursing for four hours or more if possible. Lactating mothers should avoid aspirin, tetracycline, ciprofloxacin, metronidazole, gentamicin, vancomycin, benzodiazepines, barbiturates, Cipro, Flagyl, and Valium.[13] Nitrous oxide–oxygen analgesia is considered safe for lactating women and hence their nursing infants.[13]

ALCOHOL INTAKE DURING PREGNANCY. All clients, especially pregnant ones, should be asked about drug, alcohol, and tobacco habits, and educated about cessation options (see Chapters 29 and 45). Pregnant women should be cautioned about alcohol use because their babies could be adversely affected with *fetal alcohol syndrome (FAS),* damage to the offspring's central nervous system (CNS) affecting motor skills, skin and muscle innervation, and behavior aspects of the personality. The risk of FAS in babies of women who drink heavily (five or more drinks a day) is 35%. The risk of woman who drink moderately (three to four drinks per day) is 10%. The risk for woman who drink less than that is unknown, but it is known that some damage, but not full FAS, can

TABLE 46–3 FDA CATEGORIES OF DRUGS AND THEIR IMPLICATION FOR USE DURING PREGNANCY

Category	Description	Examples
FDA Category A Drugs	Controlled studies have failed to demonstrate a risk to the fetus during the first trimester, and there is no evidence of risk in later trimesters.	Vitamins: Niacin (Nicobid, Nicolar)
FDA Category B Drugs	Animal-reproduction studies have not demonstrated a fetal risk, but there are no controlled studies in pregnant women. Animal-reproduction studies have shown an adverse effect that was not confirmed in controlled studies in women in the first trimester and no evidence of risk in later trimesters.	Local anesthetics (lidocaine, prilocaine, etidocaine) Analgesics Acetaminophen Ibuprofen (reported safe in various literatures with regard to pregnancy and lactation, other sources claim that safety has not been established; Category D in third trimester) Hydrocodone and oxycodone Antibiotics (penicillin, clindamycin, cephalosporins, erythromycin – avoid estolate form of this drug)
FDA Category C Drugs	Animal studies have revealed adverse effects on the fetus; controlled studies in women and animals are not available. These drugs should be given only if the benefit justifies the risk to the fetus.	Local anesthetics (mepivacaine, bupivacaine, procaine Note: Vasoconstrictors may be used, if necessary. Analgesics Aspirin (Category D in 3rd trimester. Avoid in first and third trimesters of pregnancy.) Is excreted into breast milk; high doses may be harmful to infant. Codeine Propoxyphene Note: Avoid prolonged use of codeine and propoxyphene Antibiotics (ciprofloxacin, gentamicin, vancomycin)
FDA Category D Drugs	Controlled studies show positive evidence of human fetal risk, but the benefits outweigh risk in pregnant women in life-threatening situations or for a serious disease.	Analgesics Aspirin (Avoid in first and third trimesters of pregnancy) Ibuprofen (Avoid in third trimester. Has been reported safe in various literatures with regard to pregnancy and lactation, other sources claim that safety has not been established) Antibiotics (tetracycline, metronidazole) Sedatives/hypnotics (benzodiazepines, barbiturates)
FDA Category X Drugs	Studies in animals or humans have demonstrated fetal abnormalities, or there is fetal risk based on human experience, or both; the drug is contraindicated in women who are pregnant or may become pregnant.	Prostaglandin Misoprostol (Cytotec) Some vaccines Live, attenuated mumps virus vaccine (Mumpsvax) Meningococcal polysaccharide vaccine (Menomune) Hormones Nafarelin (Synarel)

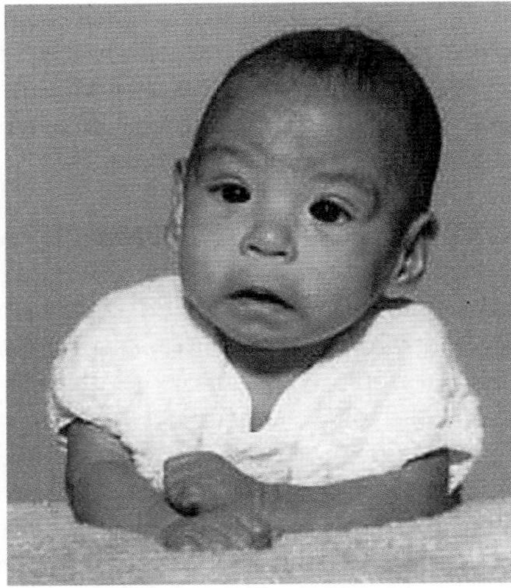

FIGURE 46–2 ✦ Fetal alcohol syndrome. Note distinct facial characteristics such as a flat philtrum, low nasal bridge, short eyelid fissures, thin upper lip, and incomplete development of midface. *(Courtesy Theresa J Kellerman.)*

occur with light drinking or a single binge (five or more drinks at one sitting). Characteristics of persons with FAS include short palpebral fissures, a flat midface, an indistinct philtrum, and a thin upper lip. Other less-frequent characteristics may include epicanthal fold, a low nasal bridge, a short nose, ear anomalies, and microdontia (Figure 46–2).

RADIOGRAPHIC EXPOSURE DURING PREGNANCY. The developing fetus is especially susceptible to effects of radiation. However, safety features in use such as high-speed film, filtration, long cone collimation, and lead aprons significantly decrease radiation exposure. Diagnostic radiographs are not harmful to the pregnant woman or fetus when she is properly protected by a lead shield with a thyroid collar and when current standards for radiation safety are maintained.[13] It has been proven that when a lead apron is used, an exposed full-mouth series of dental radiographs results in no detectable radiation exposure to the embryo or fetus.[18] The *Guidelines for Prescribing Dental Radiographs* states, "The [radiograph exposure] recommendations do not need to be altered because of pregnancy."[19] Pregnant dental personnel must use the usual necessary precautions when taking radiographs and monitor exposure by wearing a radiation exposure badge (dosimeter).

Oral Manifestations During Pregnancy

Perimylolysis, acid erosion of teeth, is rare in pregnancy but may occur if a woman vomits repeatedly, as may be the case with severe morning sickness. Erosion of the lingual, occlusal, incisal, or facial surfaces of the teeth occurs when the enamel is decalcified and softened by gastric acids (see Chapter 47, Figures 47–4 to 47–7). Subsequent mechanical erosion could then occur when the tongue or toothbrush moves against the teeth. Clients should be advised to rinse with water immediately after vomiting and prior to brushing teeth. An acid-neutralizing preparation of one quart of water mixed with one teaspoon of baking soda is recommended for mouth rinsing. At-home fluoride rinses or gels may also be recommended.

Pregnancy-associated gingivitis, a type of sex steroid hormone gingival disease most common in the second trimester of pregnancy, is characterized by an exaggerated response to plaque biofilm. The gingiva may appear fiery red at the marginal gingiva, and interdental papillae, edematous and enlarged, have a loss of tissue resiliency and have an absence of bone and attachment apparatus. Tissues may be edematous, smooth and shiny, bleed easily, and display increased probing depths. These gingival changes occur earlier and more frequently in the anterior than in the posterior areas (Figure 46–1 and Chapter 15, Figure 15–11), and may progress to a pregnancy granuloma. Pregnancy-associated gingivitis usually reaches maximum severity during the eighth month, and is less severe after childbirth. However, the tissue does not necessarily return to a state of health.[20]

As the most prevalent oral manifestation of pregnancy, pregnancy-associated gingivitis is due to poor oral hygiene, local irritants, and a shift in the predominant types of bacterial flora. Gingivitis is exacerbated by hormonal and vascular changes and the presence of increased anaerobic bacteria that proliferate in the high-progesterone environment during pregnancy.[20] The marked increase in *Bacteroides* species during pregnancy (55-fold increase) seems to be associated with increased serum levels of the circulating sex steroid hormones estrogen and progesterone. Both hormones have been shown to substitute for naphthoquinone, an essential growth factor for *Bacteroides* species and *Prevotella intermedia.*[21]

Sex steroid hormones, estrogen and progesterone, that serve as bacterial nutrients, increase gingivitis during pregnancy. Human gingiva has receptors for progesterone and estrogen. When plasma levels of estrogen and progesterone increase, these hormones accumulate in gingival tissues. Progesterone causes a dilation of the gingival capillaries, increasing their permeability and thus increasing gingival exudate, edema, and accumulation of inflammatory cells. It is important to note that estrogens are primarily responsible for vascular changes in other target tissues, such as the uterus, yet several studies have suggested that increased vascular permeability and exudate in the gingiva are essentially the result of progesterone.[22]

Pregnancy granulomas (pyogenic granulomas) are single, tumorlike, soft-tissue growths, typically on the interdental papilla, most often on the labial aspect of the maxillary anterior gingiva; bone destruction is rare (Figure 46–3).[20] They are pedunculated (attached via a stem), with intense red to deep purple color, depending on the vascularity of the lesion and the degree of blood stagnation. Usually no larger than 2 cm, the granulomas are painless, and may bleed readily if disturbed.

Occurring in less than 10% of all pregnancies and usually abating after delivery, they are often related to poor oral hygiene and attributed to the general effects of progesterone and estrogen on the host immune system.[23] These progesterone-influenced effects inhibit collagenase, the enzyme that breaks down collagen, resulting in the accumulation of collagen within the connective tissue.[11] Typically, it is prudent to wait until after delivery for excision; however, situations may dictate immediate removal when the granuloma is painful to the client, when it disturbs the alignment of the teeth, or when it bleeds easily. If excision is necessary, the second trimester is optimal because of low risk to the fetus during this time period. If excised during pregnancy, the granuloma may recur; therefore, clients should be advised that an additional surgical procedure may be needed postpartum.

Tooth mobility is sometimes present, and may be related to disturbances in the attachment apparatus. One theory contends that mobility may be related to mineral changes in the lamina dura and not due to alteration of the alveolar bone. Mobility usually reverses or declines after delivery.[24]

RELATIONSHIP BETWEEN SEX STEROID HORMONES AND THE INFLAMMATORY PROCESS. Prostaglandins, mediators (facilitators) of the inflammatory process, have been shown to increase significantly in the presence of high concentrations of estrogens and progesterones, such as during pregnancy. Therefore, in addition to stimulating bacterial growth, sex steroid hormones appear to stimulate key factors in the inflammatory response.

Depressed immune function is possible during pregnancy. If the maternal immune mechanism is weakened to protect the fetus from rejection, the host resistance of the mother to certain diseases, including inflammatory periodontal disease, could also be altered. Progesterone and estrogen have been shown to affect the immune system.[13] Neutrophil chemotaxis and phagocytosis, antibody and T-cell responses, are depressed in the presence of high levels of sex hormones, typical during a normal pregnancy. Pregnancy also inhibits the migration of inflammatory cells and fibroblasts.[13]

A

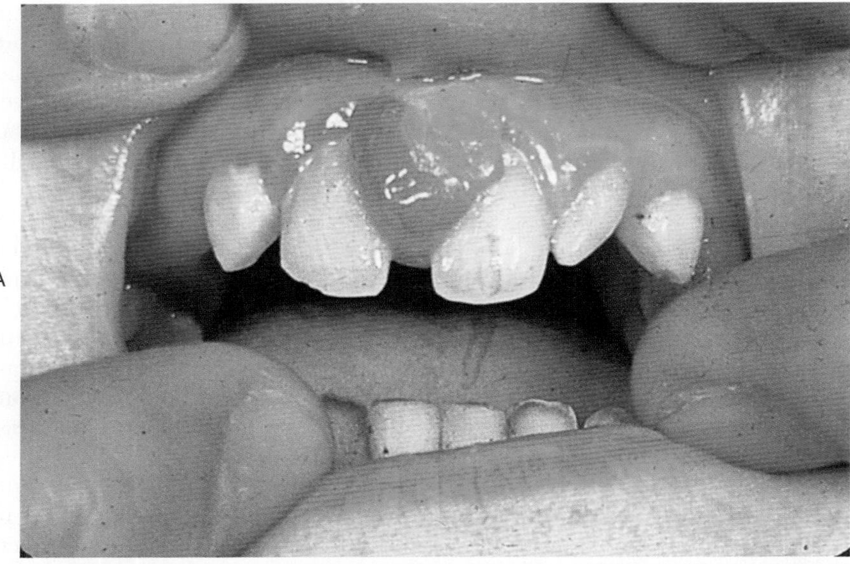

B

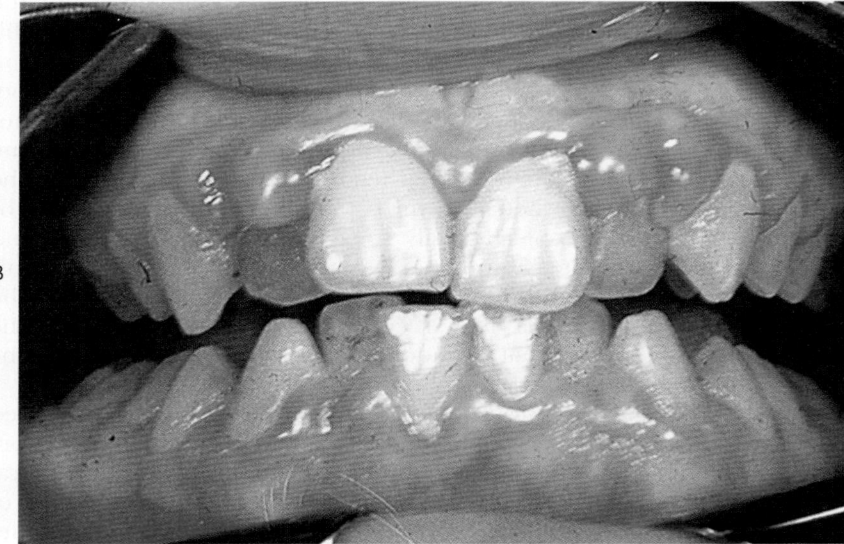

FIGURE 46–3 ✦ Pregnancy granuloma. **A,** Note granuloma between the maxillary central incisors. **B,** Note granulomas in the maxillary lateral incisor areas. *(Courtesy Maria Perno Goldie, RDH, MS.)*

Progesterone functions as an immunosuppressant in the gingival tissues of pregnant women, resulting clinically in an exaggerated appearance of inflammation.[23] As a result, this immunosuppression prevents the rapid, acute type of inflammatory reaction against plaque, but allows an increased chronic type of tissue reaction. The slower the metabolism of the hormone, the higher is its hormonal activity in the tissue. Because bacteria can metabolize progesterone as a nutrient, pregnancy favors the colonization of anaerobic bacteria in the gingival sulcus.

Preterm, Low-Birthweight Infants and Periodontal Status

Research evidence indicates that periodontal infection is a possible risk factor for *preterm, low birth-weight (PLBW)* babies (see also Chapter 15).[25] Women with periodontal disease are seven times more likely to have PLBW babies than women without the disease.[25] Twenty-five percent of PLBW cases occur without any known risk factors. Studies demonstrate an association between infection and PLBW, specifically genitourinary infections. These infections cause a faster-than-normal increase in the levels of prostaglandin and tumor necrosis factor α, molecules that induce labor. Other risk factors for PLBW include cigarette smoking, alcohol use, and drug abuse; multifetal pregnancies; medical problems of the mother such as high blood pressure, diabetes mellitus, infections, heart, kidney, or lung problems; and an abnormal placenta, uterus, or cervix.

MENOPAUSE

Menopause begins 10 years prior to the cessation of the menses, and continues for about 10 years after. *Perimenopause* signifies the years immediately preceding menopause, and *postmenopause* is defined as the years following menopause. Most investigators believe that the physical changes accompanying menopause are primarily a result of decreased estrogen production by the ovaries, and possibly, an increased secretion of gonadotropins, the hormones of the anterior pituitary gland that stimulate the gonads. After menopause, estradiol, the most potent naturally occurring estrogen, ceases to be the major circulating estrogen, and is replaced by estrone, which is less potent and demonstrates no cyclic changes.[9] Menopause is accompanied by a number of changes attributed to a variety of geriatric, hormonal, and psychosomatic factors.

Oral Manifestations of Menopause

Thinning of the oral epithelial lining and decreased keratinization, oral discomfort such as burning sensations of the tongue, altered taste perception (salty, peppery, sour), xerostomia, and alveolar bone loss/osteoporosis are some of the oral changes associated with menopause.[13] Most menopausal women with oral discomfort are relieved by systemic or topical estrogen. Oral mucosae, like vaginal mucosae, are stratified squamous epithelium, and similar desquamative growth patterns are observed. Estrogens promote maturation and keratinization of vaginal mucosa. Human gingiva has specific protein receptors for estrogen. Estrogens may stimulate the proliferation of gingival fibroblasts and maturation of connective tissue, mainly through their influence on collagen production. In menopause there is a decrease in keratinization and atrophy of the vaginal mucosa associated with a decline in estrogen level. Studies have been unable to demonstrate a correlation between ovarian hormone levels and changes in the oral mucosa during menses or menopause.[26]

Oral healthcare providers may have clients whose chief complaint is burning and painful sensations in the oral cavity. About 1,000,000 people in the United States are affected by these sensations, and they are increasingly problematic in the aging population.[27] Eighty percent of women with burning mouth syndrome are postmenopausal.[26] *Burning mouth syndrome (BMS)* is also known as *glossodynia, stomatodynia, glossopyrosis, stomatopyrosis,* or *oral dysesthesia.*[28,29] Middle-aged women are particularly affected by the condition and are diagnosed with symptoms seven times more frequently than males.[30] Various local, systemic, and psychological factors may be associated with BMS, but its etiology is not fully understood. Identification of symptoms, rather than objective clinical or laboratory findings, is often used to assess this condition. Therefore, treatment addressing these factors has had limited success.[29]

BMS is characterized by a burning sensation in the oral cavity although the oral mucosae appear clinically normal. The most prevalent site with burning sensations is the anterior tongue.[29] The pain is chronic (at least six months), continuous, and progressive throughout the day, with no apparent cause.[30] TMJ pain, face pain, oral sores, and burning mouth have all been associated with this syndrome.[30]

Treatment for burning mouth syndrome is usually directed at correction of detected organic causes or involves the use of tricyclic antidepressants, such as chlorpromazine, used to treat depression.[31] Interventions may include instruction in proper oral hygiene, saliva-stimulating agents such as pilocarpine HCl, saliva substitutes, or dietary recommendations, depending on the severity of the salivary dysfunction. Treatment may include antifungal therapy if candidiasis is diagnosed. In severely distressed persons, local or systemic corticosteroids may be indicated. Lifestyle changes such as refraining from tobacco and alcohol use should be initiated. Avoiding toothpastes containing sodium lauryl sulfate may also be considered. Future treatment might include agents combining antibacterial and anti-inflammatory actions that show promising effects in clients with oral mucosal diseases secondary to salivary hypofunction.[32]

Hormone Replacement Therapy

Controversy surrounds the risks and benefits of *hormone replacement therapy (HRT),* and individual characteristics and preferences may influence decisions to use this therapy. HRT is the combination of estrogen and a progestin, and *estrogen replacement therapy (ERT)* is estrogen alone, used by women who have had the uterus removed. Estrogen's effects on bone health and mental well-being are recognized, but the question concerning HRT and its cardio-protective properties in postmenopausal women has been heavily debated.

The Women's Health Initiative (WHI) study was started to examine a large group of women on combination HRT (estrogen, 0.625 mg/day plus progestin, 2.5 mg/day) compared with a matched group of women on placebo.[33] However, at about the same time that the Heart and Estrogen/progestin Replacement Study (HERS I[34] and II[35]) reported no increased risk of CVD-related events for women on HRT, the HRT component of the WHI was halted because of the increased incidence of CVD (22%) and breast cancer (26%) in women treated with combination HRT compared with placebo. The risk of stroke was also significantly higher in the HRT group, accounting for a 41% increase.[33]

The WHI trials found no benefit in the use of HRT as a means of primary or secondary prevention of future CVD events.[33] Publication of the results of HERS II and the halting of the HRT component of the WHI all point to the same conclusion: HRT is not associated with any benefit in preventing heart disease or stroke and should not be used in postmenopausal women for the *sole* purpose of heart disease prevention.[33,35] Recent meta-analyses confirm this finding.[36–38] Moreover, this conclusion is officially endorsed by the American Heart Association (AHA).[39] While the meta-analyses found that the increased risks linked with HRT related to 5 or more years of use, HRT protected *against* osteoporosis and *decreased* the risk of colorectal cancer.

Risks associated with HRT are as follows:[40]

- Replacing estrogen lost at menopause via hormone replacement therapy either exacerbates or has no impact on CVD risk.

- Screening mammograms are less accurate in women who use HRT than in nonusers, increasing the risks of both false-negative and false-positive results.
- The addition of progestin to HRT substantially increases the risk of developing breast cancer relative to the use of estrogen alone.
- The risk of having breast cancer diagnosed is increased in women using HRT and increases with increasing duration of use.
- Women with hypothyroidism being treated with thyroxine may need an increased dose if they begin taking estrogen therapy.
- Women with a uterus taking estrogen alone, without the addition of progesterone, are at increased risk for endometrial (uterine) cancer.
- There is a slight increase in risk for deep venous thrombosis in women using HRT.

Benefits associated with HRT are as follows:[40]

- There are positive and similar effects of the HRT pill and patch on the tightness or constriction of blood vessels, total cholesterol, and low-density lipoprotein cholesterol (LDL is the "bad" cholesterol).
- Women using either the estrogen pill or the patch have lower blood pressure during psychological stress.
- HRT appears to improve lipid blood levels in older women as well as it does in younger women.
- HRT reduces the incidence of coronary heart disease in younger postmenopausal women.
- There is a reduction in the risk of eye lens opacities in women with natural menopause.
- Estrogen, supplemented with calcium and vitamin D, has a positive effect on bone mineral density, and it is a dose-related effect.
- HRT aids in the prevention and treatment of osteoporosis.
- Relief from menopausal symptoms, such as hot flashes, irritability, and insomnia, is significant.
- HRT is associated with a reduced risk of colorectal cancer.
- HRT also leads to improvement in mood and cognitive function.

Estrogen's role in vascular biology and clinical medicine continues to evolve.

Oral Effects of HRT

Women who are menopausal or postmenopausal may experience changes in their mouths, which could include discomfort, xerostomia, pain and burning sensations, or altered taste. Periodontal disease may be present, and menopausal gingivostomatitis affects a small percentage of women. Gingivae that look dry or shiny, bleed easily, and range from abnormally pale to deep red mark this condition. HRT has been found to relieve these symptoms. Estrogen supplementation in women within five years of menopause may slow the progression of periodontal disease.[41]

HRT is associated with reduced gingival inflammation and a reduced frequency of clinical attachment loss in osteopenic and osteoporotic women in early menopause.[42]

Bone loss is associated with periodontal disease, menopause, and osteoporosis. Research will determine whether periodontal disease and osteoporosis are related. HRT may help protect teeth as well as other parts of the body. Estrogen replacement therapy does not place women at increased risk of developing temporomandibular joint disorders.

OSTEOPOROSIS

Osteoporosis (see also Chapter 15) is a loss of bone mass affecting 25 million Americans; more than 1.3 million fractures occur each year in men and women attributed to osteoporosis. With osteoporosis, more bone is being resorbed than formed. Age is the strongest correlate to bone loss, and menopause is the second strongest correlate (see Chapter 28, Risk Factors Associated with Osteoporosis).

Osteoporosis is more prevalent among white and Asian women, and those with early menopause, fair complexions, or small frames.[43] Osteoporosis often is not detected until a fracture occurs. By this time, significant loss of bone mass has placed the client at risk for future fractures, despite the fact that the original fracture will heal. Fast and painless tests that can help diagnose osteoporosis in its early stages are dual-energy x-ray absorptiometry (DEXA or DXA), quantitative computed tomography (QCT), and radiographic absorptiometry (RA). The common x-ray is unable to diagnose osteoporosis early because bone loss cannot be detected radiographically until it reaches at least a 30% level.

Management of Osteoporosis

Treatment for osteoporosis includes decreasing the risk factors, adding the protective factors of a calcium and a vitamin D–rich diet plus supplementation (see Chapter 28, Food Sources of Calcium), weightbearing exercises, HRT, and drug therapy such as alendronate (Fosamax), calcitonin, and sodium fluoride. Alendronate, a biphosphonate, inhibits bone breakdown and has been FDA approved for treatment of postmenopausal osteoporosis. Calcitonin, FDA approved in injectable and nasal forms, slows bone breakdown and reduces pain of fractures. Sodium fluoride has been used to stimulate bone formation in the vertebrae, treat osteoporotic spine fractures, and prevent fractures at that site.[44]

ERT can decrease the rate of bone resorption, but cannot replace lost bone.[45] Estrogens affect bone indirectly by interacting with the hormones that control calcium metabolism. Hormone replacement therapy has been shown to be beneficial for bone density and architecture. It retards bone loss in postmenopausal women, making bone fractures less likely.[46]

Osteoporosis and Periodontal Bone Loss

Loss of teeth and residual ridge resorption are problems associated with oral bone loss. Several studies have linked oral bone loss with systemic bone loss; therefore, osteoporosis may affect periodontal bone loss. For example, generalized bone loss from systemic osteoporosis might render jaws susceptible to accelerated alveolar bone resorption.[47] In summary, osteoporosis is not an etiologic factor in periodontitis, but may affect the severity of the disease in preexisting periodontitis, and is probably important in the creation of a susceptible host.

Hormone or estrogen replacement therapy (HRT/ERT) protects against osteoporosis.[47] The Nurses Health Study examined risk of tooth loss in relation to hormone use in 42,171 postmenopausal women and found that the risk of tooth loss was lower in women taking HRT/ERT.[48] The risk of tooth loss was lower among postmenopausal hormone users, with the most substantial decrease occurring among current users; risk of tooth loss did not appear to change with duration of current or past estrogen use.[49] In addition, greater loss of periodontal attachment is found in women with osteoporotic fractures than in normal women.[49] As healthcare professionals, dental hygienists are alert to any rapid changes in alveolar bone, periodontal attachment level, and/or tooth mobility in postmenopausal women, and make appropriate referrals for a medical diagnosis.

Dental Implants and Osteoporosis

Osteoporosis is not a likely risk factor for failure of osseointegrated dental implants.[50] In fact, the placement of dental implants could aid in maintaining the height and density of alveolar bone.[13] The act of chewing leads to more pressure on the alveolar bone, causing bone remodeling that minimizes or counteracts physiologic age-related bone loss. Osteoporotic bone does not heal differently than bone with more density, but the biologic changes may warrant some additional caution.[51] The prognosis for osseointegrated implants can be improved for the osteoporotic client who is receiving medical treatment for osteoporosis (see Chapter 50).

DOMESTIC VIOLENCE[52]

Domestic violence is defined as physical, mental, or emotional abuse administered by a member of the victim's family. Battering, one type of physical abuse, is the most frequent cause of injury to women, accounting for more emergency room visits than the combination of automobile accidents, muggings, and rapes. Oral healthcare providers may detect overt injuries or observe signals of abuse such as client depression, anxiety disorders, substance and alcohol abuse, eating disorders, hostility, and lack of cooperation. Also, the victim's abuser may monitor interactions, answer questions directed to the woman, seem overly solicitous, refuse to leave the operatory, or display hostility.

Domestic Abuse Resources

Family Violence Prevention Fund	800-313-1313
Health Resource Center on Domestic Violence	888-Rx-Abuse
National Resource Center on Domestic Violence	800-537-2238
National Center on Elder Abuse	202-682-2470
National Coalition Against Domestic Violence	303-839-1852

Dental hygienists who suspect abuse can create an opportunity for the client to express a domestic abuse problem by saying something like, "Now that violence against women is so common, and there is help available for those who suffer from abuse, I am asking all clients routinely about violence in their lives." A direct question could follow, such as, "Are you in a relationship that threatens or hurts you?"

When abuse is identified, the dental hygienist refers clients to legal and social service professionals or agencies capable of assisting. In most legal jurisdictions, reporting domestic violence to the proper authorities is mandatory, and healthcare professionals may be required to complete special training on this topic (see Domestic Abuse Resources).

INFANT AND CHILD CARE

The American Dental Association and American Academy of Pediatric Dentistry both recommend that a child's first dental examination occur at the age of 12 to 15 months. To ensure that a child does not experience dental caries or gingivitis, effective oral hygiene routines should be established in infancy and continued throughout life. When a woman is pregnant, she is receptive to advice on the care of her unborn child. New mothers are also receptive in most cases. The information in Oral Healthcare Tips for Children's Oral Health can be shared with pregnant clients, parents, and caregivers of small children.

Early Childhood Caries

Early childhood caries (ECC) is a preventable dental condition that can destroy the teeth of an infant or young child, cause pain and disfigurement, and if left to progress, is expensive to treat. This new term, ECC, is preferred over the old terms of baby bottle tooth decay, nursing caries, nursing bottle caries, and sipper-cup caries. ECC is caused by prolonged and repeated exposure of a tooth to carbohydrates, such as those contained in infant formula, milk, and fruit juice, which ferment in contact with *Streptococcus mutans*. The maxillary anterior teeth are the most susceptible to damage, but other teeth also may be affected. Long-term effects of ECC include a higher incidence of orthodontic problems and possible

Oral Healthcare Tips for Children's Oral Health

Thoroughly clean the infant's gums after each feeding with a water-soaked infant washcloth or gauze pad to stimulate the gum tissue and remove oral debris; when the baby's teeth begin to erupt, brush them gently with a small, soft-bristled toothbrush using a pea-sized amount of fluoridated toothpaste.

Using a small amount (size of a pea) of fluoridated toothpaste inhibits decay and minimizes the chance of developing fluorosis.

At age 2 or 3, children can be taught proper brushing techniques. The child will need assistance until age 7 or 8, when the child has the dexterity to do it alone.

Parents should be advised to schedule regular oral health appointments starting around the child's first birthday. This will allow the oral health professional to check for dental caries in the primary teeth, watch for developmental problems, and create a positive experience that may alleviate dental fear.

Determine if the water supply that serves the client's home is fluoridated. If there is no fluoride in the water, or an inadequate amount, discuss supplement options with the parent. Fluoride is also found in over-the-counter mouthrinses and in some foods and beverages (see Chapter 26).

Brush with 0.12% chlorhexidine as an intervention for early childhood caries.

Sealant applications are available to protect the chewing surfaces of children's teeth.

Adapted from *Child Oral Health,* http://adha.org/oralhealth/children.htm, Dec 18, 2002.

Strategies to Decrease Incidence of Early Childhood Caries

Put babies to bed without a bottle or with a bottle containing only water; do not let babies fall asleep with a bottle containing formula, milk, fruit juice, or other carbohydrate-dense liquids in their mouths. This is especially important because there is decreased saliva flow during sleep.

Wean a baby to a cup by 1 year of age.

Instead of pacifying a baby with a bottle, rely on strategies such as cuddling, patting, talking, singing, reading, or playing.

Give babies a clean pacifier. Do not give them pacifiers that have been dipped in sugar, honey, syrup, or other sugary substances.

Never "clean off" a pacifier in another person's mouth. This practice can infect a baby's mouth with bacterial pathogens that cause dental caries and periodontal disease.

Never share eating utensils with an infant. Infectious *Streptococcus mutans,* the initiators of the caries disease process, can be transferred from the parent's mouth to the baby's mouth. Caries will develop as early as 11 months of age. The danger of infecting an infant's teeth is increased when the mother already has dental caries herself.

Cleaning a child's teeth after ingestion of sugar-containing medication can prevent caries formation. Many oral over-the-counter medications and prescriptive drugs such as oral antibiotic liquid formulations contain up to 50% sucrose.

Consult with a dentist and pediatrician about the need for fluoride supplementation and/or home-use fluoride gels if the fluoride history reveals a fluoride deficiency (see Chapter 9, section on dental history, and Chapter 26).

psychological and social problems that affect children who suffer embarrassment over their appearance. Strategies to Decrease Incidence of Early Childhood Caries identifies several adult practices that decrease the likelihood that a child will suffer from ECC.

Herpetic Infections

An infection prevalent in infants and young children is primary herpetic gingivostomatitis (HSV-1). Some of the symptoms of HSV-1 in infants include fever, crying, oral pain, and an unwillingness to eat or drink. Clinically, the gingivae appear intensely red and painful, with blisters on the tongue and lips. Children can be infected with this herpes virus by sharing toys, washcloths, towels, or toothbrushes with others who may be infected (home or daycare setting).

Parents with herpetic lip sores can infect their babies by mouth kissing. If a child is in daycare, toys, rattles, and sleeping mats should be wiped and cleaned at least twice a day with a diluted bleach solution to prevent transfer of viruses and bacteria.

For other women's healthcare issues, see Chapters 37 and 47 on autoimmune diseases and eating disorders, respectively.

Client Education Issues

- ✦ Specific questions need to be asked to elicit client information. Reassure the client that information will be kept confidential, but that it is important that they share information about products being taken or used, including over-the-counter and prescription medications, vitamins, herbs, supplements, and alcohol use, to ensure proper care.
- ✦ Maintenance of oral health by thorough toothbrushing and interdental cleaning translates to a healthier body.
- ✦ Inform clients about the warning signs of heart disease: shortness of breath, nausea, major fatigue, chest pain, fainting spells, or gaslike discomfort.
- ✦ Inform clients that the American Dental Association and American Academy of Pediatric Dentistry both recommend that a child's first dental examination occur at the age of 12 to 15 months.
- ✦ Reassure the client that radiographs are safe during pregnancy. Always use lead aprons and radiographic equipment that is well maintained.

Legal, Ethical, and Safety Issues

- ✦ Respect client confidentiality on all issues, including oral contraceptive and reproductive health.
- ✦ Advise clients that antibiotic use can render oral contraceptives ineffective and that an alternative contraceptive method should be considered.
- ✦ Consult with the obstetrician when planning care for pregnant clients.
- ✦ Report suspected abuse to the proper authorities: child protective services within a Department of Social Services, Department of Human Resources, or Division of Family and Children Services. In some states, police departments also may receive reports of child abuse or neglect. Call Childhelp, 800-4-A-Child (800-422-4453), or the local Child Protection Agency. A State Toll-Free Child Abuse Reporting Numbers Resource Listing can be found at <http://www.calib.com/nccanch/prevmnth/scop/tollfree.html>.
- ✦ Take a complete health history and ask specific questions about drugs, herbs, vitamins, fluoride, and other supplements. The safety of most natural or herbal remedies is unknown.
- ✦ Ask clients if they have ever taken Phen/Fen and advise them of the Food and Drug Administration reports of valvular heart disease in women treated for obesity with a combination of fenfluramine and phentermine.
- ✦ Make appropriate referrals.

Key Concepts

- ✦ Oral health and systemic health are inextricably related. Evidence links periodontal disease with cardiovascular diseases, valvular heart disease, preterm low-birthweight babies, and bacterial pneumonia.
- ✦ Women may have different risks for and symptoms of heart disease. Heart disease is more severe among women over 60 than among men of the same age, and women are twice as likely as men to die within 60 days of suffering a heart attack.
- ✦ Women are the fastest growing population of those infected with HIV/AIDS.
- ✦ Women live longer and have more chronic disabilities than men.
- ✦ Cancer, menopause, cardiovascular disease, diabetes, osteoporosis, and autoimmune diseases are important issues in women's heath and have systemic and oral implications.
- ✦ Diagnostic radiographs are not harmful to the pregnant woman or fetus when properly protected by a lead shield with a thyroid collar and when current standards of radiation safety are maintained.
- ✦ Female dental personnel and the unexposed partners of male dental personnel have cause for concern about nitrous oxide–oxygen analgesia during pregnancy. Difficulty conceiving and birth defects have been documented to occur with its use.
- ✦ Mechanized instruments are safe to use for both clinician and client during pregnancy.
- ✦ Nitrous oxide–oxygen analgesia is safe for use on lactating women; its use is contraindicated for pregnant women and should not be used by pregnant oral healthcare professionals because of the risk of birth defects and spontaneous abortion.
- ✦ Pregnancy-associated gingivitis is the most prevalent oral manifestation of pregnancy. It is often due to poor oral hygiene, local irritants, sex steroid hormones that serve as bacterial nutrients, and increases in *Bacteroides* species and *Prevotella intermedia.*
- ✦ As estrogen levels increase, so does the prevalence of *Bacteroides* species, *P. intermedia,* and gingivitis. Bacteria associated with increased estrogen levels have been implicated in periodontal disease.
- ✦ Sex steroid hormones (estrogen and progesterone) appear to stimulate key factors in the inflammatory response.
- ✦ Women with periodontal disease are seven times more likely to have preterm, low-birthweight babies than women without the disease.
- ✦ ECC is a preventable dental condition that can destroy the teeth of an infant or young child, cause pain and disfigurement, and if left to progress, is expensive to treat.
- ✦ A prenatal oral prevention program could include increased frequency of periodontal debridement, increased effectiveness of brushing and interdental cleaning, at-home fluoride rinses or gels, antimicrobial rinses, nutritional counseling, infant oral care, and prevention of ECC in preparation for the baby's arrival. Evidence supports the use of 0.12% chlorhexidine mouthrinse and chewing xylitol gum during the last 3 months of pregnancy and for 6 months after birth to decrease risk of *mutans streptococci* transmission from mother to infant.
- ✦ Osteoporosis is not an etiologic factor in periodontitis, but may affect the severity of the disease in preexisting periodontitis and is probably important in the creation of a susceptible host. Loss of teeth and residual ridge resorption are associated with oral bone loss.

Continued on following page

Key Concepts—cont'd

- ✦ Osteoporosis is not a risk factor for failure of osseointegrated dental implants. Placement of dental implants could aid in maintaining the height and density of alveolar bone.
- ✦ Dental hygiene care should include counseling clients about prevention of disease, the oral/systemic link, referral to other healthcare providers for assessment and care, and providing tobacco cessation counseling.
- ✦ Rapid oral bone loss can indicate systemic osteoporosis. Dental hygienists should be alert to any rapid changes in alveolar bone, periodontal attachment level, and/or tooth mobility in postmenopausal women, and make the appropriate referrals to a physician for a medical examination for osteoporosis.
- ✦ Healthcare professionals, in collaboration with clients, should make treatment decisions. Although a part of the decision-making process, insurance company coverage should not dictate treatment decisions.

Critical Thinking Exercises

Client 1: Amy arrives for her recare appointment 2 months late. Amy is 16 years old and is scheduled for continued care every 6 months. After reviewing her health history, a clinical examination is performed to reveal plaque-induced gingivitis throughout with moderate to heavy bleeding (GI-2.0). No periodontal pockets are noted, and her self-care is adequate. Due to her heavy gingival bleeding, the health history is reviewed again and Amy again states that she is not taking any medication, nor has she been diagnosed with any illnesses in the last 8 months.

1. What specific questions could be asked to elicit needed information?
2. Could there be any concern on the part of the client regarding confidentiality?
3. Should Amy's parents be contacted and consulted?

Client 2: Margie Alexander, a 25-year-old female client, arrives for her six-month supportive periodontal therapy appointment. Ms Alexander's health history is noncontributory, other than that she is in her 11th week of pregnancy. She had a full-mouth series of radiographs one year ago, and her chief complaint is pain in tooth no 30. Clinical examination reveals 3 to 4 mm probing depths throughout, and bleeding on probing in tooth no 14-M (4 mm) and 2-D.

1. What radiographs, if any, should be advised and why? Is it safe to expose radiographs during pregnancy?
2. What discussion should take place between the dental hygienist and the client?
3. Should any other healthcare provider be consulted?

Client 3: The practicing dental hygienist is pregnant and is concerned about her responsibilities in the oral care environment. The dental hygienist heard that exposure to radiation, chemicals in the office, nitrous oxide–oxygen analgesia, and ultrasonic scaling units may cause birth defects or spontaneous abortion.

1. Are the above concerns substantiated in the literature?
2. What precautions, if any, should the dental hygienist take to manage client risks?

Client 4: Rose Oliveri, a 50-year-old female client, visited the office after a one-year hiatus. Her chief complaint is, "my teeth seem to be moving and I don't like it." Her health history reveals that she is taking hormone replacement therapy (estrogen and progestin), a multivitamin, and numerous herbal supplements. Her oral examination reveals probing depths from 3 to 6 mm, with a GI score of 1.0. Her self-care appears to be adequate, with a PI score of 1.

1. Based on the medical history and oral examination data, what other diagnostic and therapeutic procedures should be undertaken?
2. What additional questions should be asked regarding her medical history, and what recommendations should be offered to the client?
3. Should any referrals be made? If so, to whom?

For References, Suggested Readings, and Related Websites, visit
http://evolve.elsevier.com/Darby/hygiene/

CHAPTER 47

PERSONS WITH EATING DISORDERS

OBJECTIVES

Mastery of the content in this chapter will enable the reader to:

- Differentiate between anorexia nervosa and bulimia nervosa as eating disorder syndromes using the DSM-IV-R criteria for diagnosis
- Discuss psychological and physical characteristics of the anorexic and bulimic client
- Describe systemic complications that can arise as sequelae to anorexic and bulimic behaviors
- Identify oral characteristics of the bulimic, anorexic, and bulimorexic client
- Identify the components of a comprehensive assessment that should be used for clients with eating disorders
- Outline dental hygiene diagnoses and interventions to be considered for each oral manifestation associated with these eating disorders
- Identify community resources that can serve as a referral source for psychological treatment of the client with eating disorders
- Describe a technique for confronting and referring a newly identified anorexic or bulimic client for psychological therapy
- Outline an appropriate plan for education and oral management for bulimic and anorexic clients during the psychological treatment phase
- Identify treatment modalities for both reversible and irreversible oral manifestations of bulimia and/or anorexia
- Value the role of oral health professionals in identification and referral of clients with eating disorders
- Develop a personal and professional ethics system related to understanding the issues of professional responsibility and liability in referring clients for psychological therapy

KEY TERMS

Anorexia nervosa
Bulimia nervosa
Multidisciplinary approach
Parotid enlargement
Perimylolysis
Professional confrontation

Eating disorders are a topic of concern to health professionals in many disciplines. Disturbed eating may be manifested in a variety of forms. The American Psychiatric Association recognizes five distinct diagnoses of abnormal eating behavior; however, two primary diagnoses, anorexia nervosa and bulimia nervosa, are not limited to infancy/early childhood and are associated with significant oral sequelae. Data obtained from various sources suggest the prevalence of anorexia nervosa, bulimia nervosa, and bulimorexia (the vacillation between anorexic and bulimic behavior) has increased over the past three decades. It is generally believed that Western society's preoccupation with body image and thinness is responsible for an increased prevalence of these disorders. Although increased awareness by our society of these problems gives the impression that these are new and unusual disorders, evidence from historical references and detailed case histories in the medical literature indicates that both anorexia and bulimia were well documented as early as the mid-18th century.

Clients suffering from these disorders present a unique challenge to oral health professionals. Behaviors

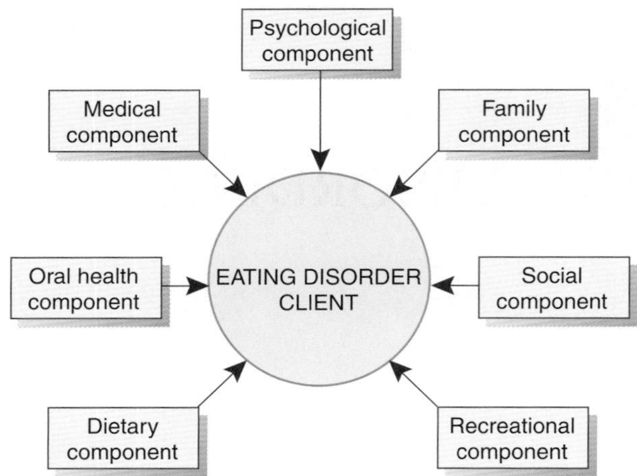

FIGURE 47–1 ✦ A multidisciplinary approach to providing care to individuals with eating disorders.

associated with eating disorders result in significant physical and oral sequelae and, over time, increased mortality rates. A comprehensive understanding of the psychosocial, physical, and oral dimensions of these disorders is critical for the dental hygienist. Eating disorders are complex in terms of both etiology and treatment. Successful care requires a *multidisciplinary approach,* the coordinated effort of various health professionals: specially trained psychologists for individual and family therapy; psychiatrists and social workers; physicians and nurses with experience in eating disorders; nutritionists and exercise therapists for education and reorientation of eating and exercise habits; the oral health team for support and treatment of oral manifestations of the illnesses (Figure 47–1).

Persons with eating disorders are likely to seek oral care because of the changing appearance of teeth or complaints of oral/dental discomfort. As a result, the dental hygienist may be the first health professional to identify oral and physical manifestations characteristic of these disorders. Individuals with eating disorders are reluctant to acknowledge the gravity of their obsession with food and weight, and they carefully protect the secret of their obsessive, compulsive behavior. The dental hygienist then becomes essential in the initial recognition and referral of the client to the medical and psychological treatment system, as well as integral to the support of the oral environment.

ANOREXIA NERVOSA

Anorexia nervosa, the least common of the eating disorders, has a high profile in society because of publicity related to many public figures who have either died from self-starvation or have made public their diagnosis. Anorexia has the highest morbidity rate of any psychiatric diagnosis and has a poor response rate and protracted course of illness.[1–3] The term *anorexia* is a misnomer and may lead to confusion. Anorexia literally means "loss of appetite," whereas the client suffering from anorexia suppresses and denies sensation of hunger.

Criteria for Medical Diagnosis of Anorexia and Bulimia Nervosas

Anorexia Nervosa

Refusal to maintain body weight over a minimal normal weight for age and height (e.g., weight loss leading to maintenance of body weight less than 85% of that expected; or failure to make expected weight gain during period of growth, leading to body weight less than 85% of that expected)

Intense fear of gaining weight or becoming fat, even though underweight

Disturbance in the way in which one's body weight, size, or shape is experienced; undue influence of body weight or shape on self-evaluation; denial of the seriousness of the current low body weight

In postmenarcheal females, amenorrhea (i.e., the absence of at least three consecutive menstrual cycles). A woman is considered to have amenorrhea if her periods occur only following hormone (e.g., estrogen) administration.

Bulimia Nervosa

Recurrent episodes of binge eating. An episode of binge eating is characterized by both of the following:

1. Eating, in a discrete period of time (e.g., within any 2-hour period) an amount of food that is definitely larger than most people would eat during a similar period of time and under similar circumstances
2. A sense of lack of control over eating during the episode (e.g., a feeling that one cannot stop eating or control what or how much one is eating)

Recurrent inappropriate compensatory behavior in order to prevent weight gain, such as self-induced vomiting; misuse of laxatives, diuretics, enemas, or other medications; fasting; or excessive exercise

The binge eating and inappropriate compensatory behaviors both occur, on average, at least twice a week for 3 months

Self-evaluation is unduly influenced by body shape and weight

The disturbance does not occur exclusively during episodes of anorexia nervosa

Diagnosis of this obsessive/compulsive disorder is based on criteria established in the Diagnostic and Statistical Manual (DSM) for Mental Disorders[4] (see Criteria for Medical Diagnosis of Anorexia and Bulimia Nervosas).

The stereotypical image of the extremely emaciated person may or may not be accurate in clients with anorexia. Body weight less than 85% below normal for the person's age and height does not ensure an emaciated appearance. In fact, some clients may appear "fashionably" thin. Clients with anorexia may use food restriction, rigorous physical exercise, or binge-eating/purging as an expression of their fear of weight gain. Distortion in body image may be manifest by anorexic clients verbalizing that they feel or look fat when they are obviously thin or underweight. Diagnostically, the distortion of body image represents the critical difference between individuals with anorexia and individuals with a quest for thinness. Anorexia nervosa is suspected in a client when no other physical illnesses are present to account for these physical and mental changes.

The onset of anorexia commonly begins in late childhood or early adolescence (approximately 11 to 14 years old). Prevalence rates have been estimated at from 0.5% to 1% in white females of school age.[4,5] Accurate determination of these rates is difficult because anorexic individuals commonly deny or underestimate the severity of the problem. Incomplete prevalence rates are available for women in other racial or ethnic groups; however, it appears that the disorder is more common in industrialized countries, irrespective of ethnicity.[4] Several studies indicate that Eastern European, Asian, African-American, Hispanic, and American Indian adolescent females are similarly predisposed to or at risk for eating disorders.[4,6,7] However, a national study examining satisfaction with body image suggests that black adolescents are more satisfied with body image than white adolescents and are more likely to view thinness as undesirable.[8]

It has been estimated that 5% to 10% of anorexic clients are men.[9] Although age of onset appears to be later in males than females, characteristics and comorbidities were not significantly different from those found in females. Additionally, male athletes who participate in sports in which weight is a critical issue are more at risk for eating disorders than nonathletes. This is true for female athletes as well.[10]

Two subtypes of anorexia nervosa are identified in DSM-IV: (1) the Restricting Type and (2) the Binge-Eating/Purging Type. Restricting anorexics achieve weight loss through dieting, fasting, or excessive exercise, whereas binge-eating/purging individuals may engage in either or both of these behaviors at least weekly during a current anorexic episode.[4]

BULIMIA NERVOSA

Bulimia nervosa is more common than anorexia, with prevalence rates estimated at 1% to 3% for adolescent females and 8% to 20% of college-age women.[5] As with anorexia nervosa, precise prevalence rates are difficult to compile because of the secretive behavior associated with the disorders. The primary characteristics of bulimia nervosa are presented in DSM-III-R Criteria for Medical Diagnosis of Anorexia and Bulimia Nervosas.[4] Unlike anorexics with binge-eating/purging subtype, bulimics are able to maintain normal body weight. As with anorexia nervosa, bulimics are unduly focused on body shape and weight and express a general dissatisfaction with body image.

Bulimia literally means "ox hunger" and accurately describes this abnormal craving for food. Bulimics may gorge with large quantities of food (up to 25 times the normal daily intake) then eliminate the consumed food by vomiting or using laxatives. Binge foods typically are high in carbohydrate content and caloric value. Vomiting most often follows binge-eating episodes. Eighty to ninety percent of bulimics vomit repeatedly as the primary method of ridding themselves of the engorged food.[4,5]

Compared to anorexia, the onset of bulimia begins later in adolescence or early adulthood (ages 17 to 25 years) and is more likely to follow an episode of strict dieting. Like anorexia, the vast majority of bulimics are women, with only 10% reported as males.[4]

Although little is known about what constitutes the best bulimia therapy, research suggests that antidepressant medication in conjunction with psychotherapy offers the best short-term outcomes.[11] Overall success rates tend to be low, however. Recent evidence shows that between 50% and 65% of bulimics had persistent clinical signs after 5 years of follow-up, and 40% met the criteria for major depressive disorder.[11]

BINGE-EATING DISORDER

Binge-eating disorder, while not yet accepted as a true category of eating disorder, has received provisional status as a diagnostic category for an eating disorder in the DSM-IV.[4] Individuals in the provisional category engage in binge-eating but do not use associated compensatory weight control measures. Therapy outcomes for individuals who meet these criteria are considerably more positive than those for anorexics or bulimics.[11]

ETIOLOGY OF ANOREXIA AND BULIMIA

Current theories regarding the etiology of anorexia and bulimia suggest a complex interrelationship between genetic, psychodevelopmental, neurochemical, and sociocultural components. Comprehensive information in this area is limited; however, evidence from studies on twins suggests a genetic element exists that predisposes an individual to develop an eating disorder. Studies examining the prevalence rates of anorexia and bulimia in identical versus fraternal twins have shown a higher concordance rate of these disorders in the identical twin groups.[11] Additionally, first-degree relatives of individuals with anorexia have a 10 times increased risk for developing anorexia nervosa.[12] Whether this genetic predisposition is related to depression, neurochemical abnormalities, or affective instability is still unknown.

The psychodevelopmental components of both disorders are more completely understood. Developmentally, anorexia and bulimia are similar in that the individual fails to progress normally through appropriate developmental stages during childhood and adolescence. This developmental disturbance frequently results from disturbed parent-child relationships.[13] Classic family dynamics of the anorexic client include parental overprotection, rigidity, lack of conflict resolution, alcoholism, and/or use of the child to diffuse parental conflict. In contrast, family histories of bulimics show a classic profile of highly dependent and enmeshed family relations that are aggressive, full of conflict, and without "normal" boundaries. Clients with both anorexia and bulimia may report family histories of alcoholism, emotional or sexual abuse, or parental abandonment (either perceived or real) during childhood.

In addition to genetic and familial etiologies, recent evidence shows abnormalities of serotonin levels associated with both anorexia and bulimia nervosas.[14] Other neurotransmitters and hormones related to the regulation of emotions and impulsivity have also been implicated as being linked to these disorders.[15]

Psychosocial Contrast Between Anorexia and Bulimia Nervosa

Anorexia Nervosa

Shy and socially introverted
Extreme self-control; rigid compliance with high standards
Marked feelings of unworthiness and inadequacy; shallow social relationships
Constricted expression of feelings
Intelligence unimpaired, but thinking is concrete

Bulimia Nervosa

Gregarious; may be socially introverted at times
Alternates between self-control and impulsivity (e.g., drug/alcohol abuse)
Unstable sense of worth and personal effectiveness; dependent relationships
Affect labile or characterized by anxiety or guilt
Intelligence unimpaired; thought can be abstract

Modified from French RN, Baker EL: Anorexia nervosa and bulimia, *Indiana Medicine* 77(4):241, 1984.

EFFECTS OF EATING DISORDERS

The effects of anorexia and bulimia on the general well-being of an individual are significant.

Psychosocial Dimension

Psychosocial Contrast between Anorexia and Bulimia Nervosa contrasts anorexia and bulimia with regard to the psychosocial dimension. These characteristics are typical but may not relate to all eating disorder clients in all circumstances.

In the individual with anorexia, distortion of body image and obsession with food restriction result in self-starvation. Control over hunger and body represents an inappropriate psychological coping mechanism. Clients with anorexia use this control of food and perfectionist behavior to feel more competent and in control of life. Although the symptomatic behaviors may appear to be the problem, the denial of emotional conflict and resulting depression are the true problems.

In bulimia, low self-esteem and subsequent feelings of inadequacy are reinforced by the guilt and embarrassment associated with binge and purge behavior. Ironically, the behavior itself becomes self-reinforcing because achievement and maintenance of low weight are perceived as bringing increased attractiveness and more friends.

Bulimic clients do not experience the distortion of body image or rigidity of thought characteristic of anorexia, but they do obsess on body image. In fact, the individual with bulimia may appear quite successful in the management of life. Affective expression may appear gregarious to the casual observer; however, underlying the facade is an obvious flattened affect resulting from the associated anxiety, guilt, and dysphoria.

Impaired psychological development and concomitant distortion of attitudes in the client with eating disorders provide the foundation for continued dysfunction and progression of the disorder. Anorexic clients rarely seek professional assistance on their own and may resist recommendation and offers of help from family members and friends. In contrast, the bulimic client is more likely to seek professional intervention because of frustration with recurrent binge and purge behaviors, and obsession with food.

Physiologic Responses

Many body systems are at risk for disruption as a result of the behaviors associated with an eating disorder. These physiologic findings for clients with anorexia and bulimia are summarized in Figure 47–2.

In anorexia, restricted food intake and resulting undernutrition impair overall functioning and health of an individual. The most common physiologic effect of anorexic behavior is hormonal abnormalities.[16] In females, prolonged decrease in estrogen along with decreased body fat may contribute to amenorrhea and decreased bone density (osteoporosis). In males, decreased testosterone levels may result in impotence and decreased libido.[17] Other disturbances of body metabolism and abnormal temperature regulation are characterized by findings of bradycardia, hypotension, dry skin, and lower-than-normal body temperature in anorexia.[18]

Cardiovascular, gastrointestinal, renal, and hematologic systems may be compromised in clients with anorexia.[18] Vital statistics in the anorexic client will likely reveal low pulse rates, decreased blood pressure, and reduced left ventricular output. Other cardiac abnormalities may include arrhythmias and heart murmurs. These abnormalities are thought to result from longstanding electrolyte imbalances and decreased cardiac function.

Gastrointestinal changes may result from decreased food intake and dehydration. These may include intestinal dilation and diminished intestinal motility from chronic constipation and laxative abuse.[16] It is unlikely that anorexic clients will complain of these symptoms;

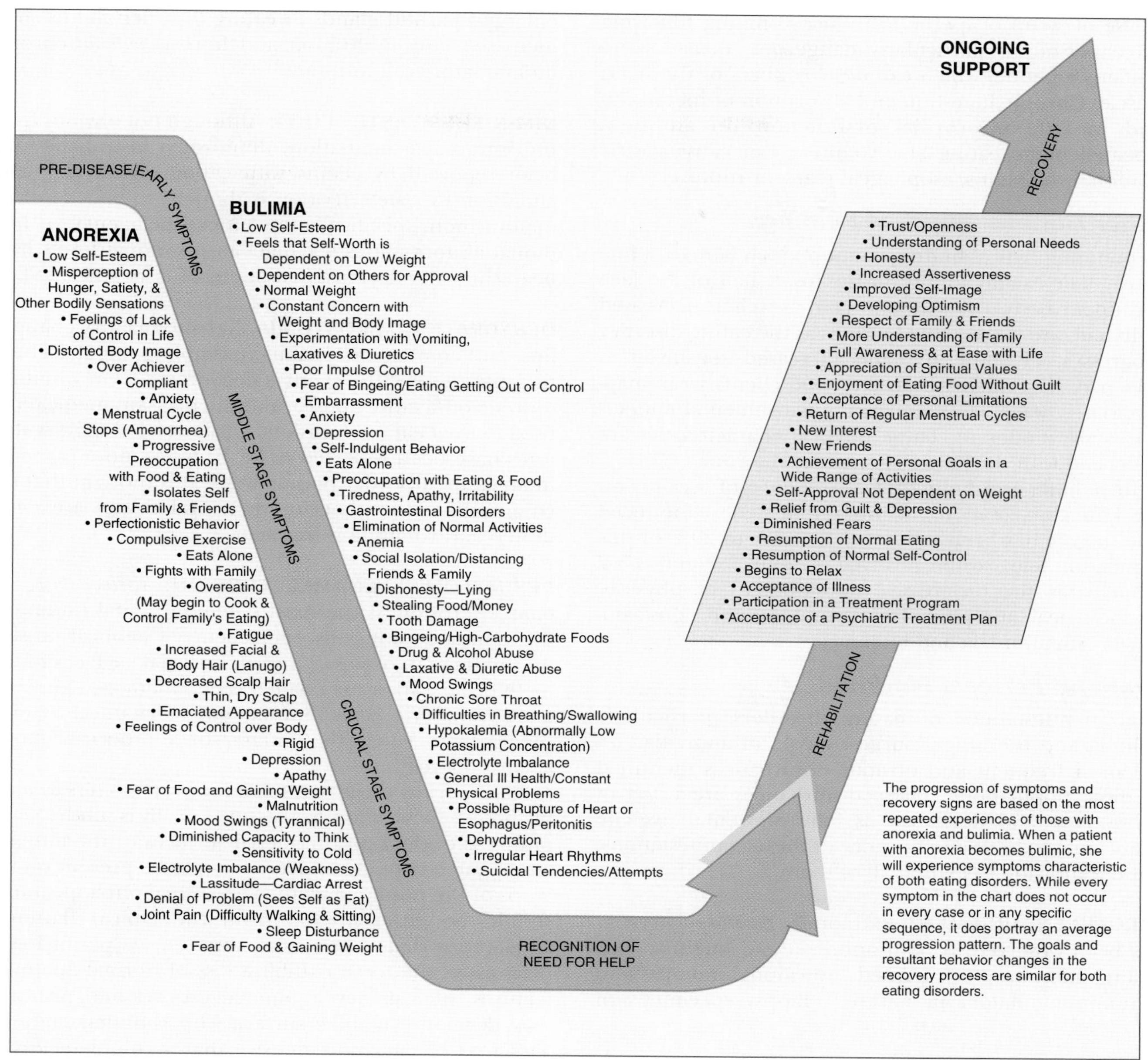

FIGURE 47–2 ✦ Physical, psychological, and physiologic findings for clients with anorexia nervosa and bulimia. *(Courtesy CompCare, Eating Disorders Program, 16305 Swingle Ridge Drive, Suite 100, Chesterfield, MO 63017.)*

however, a comprehensive health history may identify these gastrointestinal disturbances.

Kidney dysfunction may result from dehydration, electrolyte imbalance, and reduced glomerular filtration rate. As a result, anorexic clients may be predisposed to an increased incidence of kidney stones, increased blood urea nitrogen, and peripheral edema upon refeeding.[18]

Hematologic changes in anorexia are usually mild and without serious clinical consequences. These changes may include acidosis, anemia, thrombocytopenia, and leukopenia.[18] Clients may appear pale or may report chronic fatigue during the health history interview.

The repeated binge and purge behavior in the bulimic client may result in dangerous complications, which when left untreated can become life-threatening. Excessive vomiting and diuretic and laxative abuse lead to dehydration and electrolyte imbalance. Loss of potassium is a particular threat because the resulting hypokalemia and metabolic alkalosis may result in cardiac or renal failure. Six to ten percent of individuals afflicted with untreated bulimia for more than 10 years have cardiac arrests.[19]

Many anorexics and bulimics abuse laxatives as an attempt to prevent weight gain. Individuals who abuse laxatives are more likely to have a longer duration of the disorder with more significant morbidity.[19] When laxative use ceases, chronic constipation and rebound edema may occur.

Use of syrup of ipecac to induce vomiting following binge periods is particularly dangerous. Ipecac syrup contains emetine, which can destroy fibers of the heart muscle. Chronic ingestion and absorption of ipecac can lead to fatal myocardial dysfunction. In addition, repeated binge eating and vomiting can cause gastric dilation, esophagitis, esophageal tears, or rupture.[20]

Other General Physical Findings

A common physical finding in anorexics is lanugo, a fine downy hair usually found on the lower half of the face and upper body. Dry skin and hair, as well as decreased scalp hair, are predictable findings as the eating disorder progresses. Hypothermia and increased sensitivity to cold may be evident when anorexic clients wear inappropriately warm clothing when environmental temperatures are moderate. These physical characteristics are associated with the later stages of the disorder.

In bulimia and bulimorexia, presence of a callus on the knuckle(s) can occur from repeated self-induced vomiting. It has been estimated that 8% to 29% of this population may exhibit this type of callus.[20] Figure 47–2 summarizes the progressive development of physical, psychological, and physiologic symptoms and signs associated with anorexia and bulimia.

Oral and Perioral Findings

Oral manifestations of eating disorders, particularly bulimia and the binge/purge subtype of anorexia, are the most frequent and obvious disturbances identified in these populations. These disturbances are listed in Table 47–1 and described as follows. Dental hygiene clients may exhibit one or more of these manifestations, but few individuals exhibit all of them.

PAROTID ENLARGEMENT. Extraorally, *parotid enlargement* has been observed in both anorexia and bulimia. This enlargement has been termed "nutritional mumps" and is noninflammatory in nature.[21] Biopsy specimens of enlarged parotid glands in eating disorder clients show increased fatty infiltration and fibrosis *without* chronic inflammatory cell infiltrate.

TABLE 47–1 EFFECT OF EATING DISORDERS ON THE ORAL AND PERIORAL TISSUES

Anorexia Nervosa	Bulimia and Binge/ Purge-Type Anorexia
Parotid enlargement	Parotid enlargement
Diminished taste acuity	Diminished taste acuity
Dehydration (diuretic abuse)	Commissure lesions
	Dry, chapped lips
	Xerostomia
Enamel erosion	Perimylolysis (dental erosion)
Self-induced trauma	Self-induced trauma
Cheek/lip chewing	Palatal abrasion
	Palatal hematoma
	Ulcerations
	Cheek/lip chewing
Increase in dental caries	Increase in dental caries
	Knuckle callus

DIMINISHED TASTE ACUITY. Although not obvious from the intraoral examination, diminished taste acuity has been reported by clients with eating disorders.[22] This alteration in taste sensation is thought to be a result of malnutrition, specifically trace metal deficiency, or hormonal abnormalities. Changes in hormonal levels have been shown to decrease sensations of taste and smell.

DEHYDRATION/XEROSTOMIA. Xerostomia, dry chapped lips, and commissure lesions resembling angular cheilitis[23] may occur if the client is dehydrated from vomiting, diuretic or laxative abuse, or antidepressant medications used to treat eating disorders. Unstimulated salivary flow rates have been reported to be 10 times more common in an eating disorder population.[24] It is thought that the commissure lesions occur when oral tissues are dehydrated and vomiting is frequent.

PERIMYLOLYSIS/ENAMEL EROSION. *Perimylolysis,* or enamel erosion, is the most common dental finding in the vomiting eating disorder client.[25] Chemical erosion on the lingual, occlusal, incisal, or facial surfaces of the teeth occurs when the enamel is demineralized and softened by gastric acids. Subsequent mechanical erosion then occurs when the tongue or toothbrush moves against the teeth.

Early perimylolysis is difficult for practitioners to identify because loss of tooth structure usually is subtle. Slight pitting is evident on the incisal surfaces of the anterior teeth, and a cupping appearance may be present on the cusps of the posterior teeth. This dished-out appearance should be differentiated from the typical flattened appearance that occurs from abrasion. As perimylolysis progresses, the teeth exhibit a loss of normal anatomic features, such as developmental grooves and pits, and they develop a matlike surface with rounded margins. This may become so extensive that a complete loss of enamel is evident. Loss of lingual and incisal enamel on anterior teeth weakens the tooth structure, making them more susceptible to chipping. Anterior teeth of clients with eating disorders may appear translucent and moth-eaten, with an open bite. Loss of enamel around amalgam restorations results in a raised-island appearance of the amalgam. Teeth without restorations show a significant loss of occlusal contours.

INTRAORAL TRAUMA. Intraoral trauma may be evident in the bulimic individual. Findings may include the presence of traumatic lesions such as ulcerations or hematomas on the hard and soft palates, and cheek and lip bites.

DENTAL CARIES. Decreased salivary flow along with disturbed dietary patterns can predispose the client to an increased dental caries rate. Not all studies support the theory that individuals with eating disorders have an increased prevalence of dental caries; however, recent evidence suggests that bulimics are more prone to caries than control clients, with proximal and buccal-lingual surfaces at greatest risk for caries.[25] It has been hypothesized that high carbohydrate intake, changes in oral pH, and/or decreased saliva quantity and/or quality may result in a higher caries rate.[24]

DENTAL HYGIENE PROCESS OF CARE FOR CLIENTS WITH EATING DISORDERS

A multidisciplinary approach to care of the client with an eating disorder may increase the success rate of psychological treatment of the disorder. The role of the dental hygienist and the oral healthcare team varies according to the circumstances surrounding the client's status.

For individuals with an eating disorder who have not been medically diagnosed, the dental hygienist may be the health professional who identifies the need for referral to the psychological and medical support team. A working knowledge of organizations and individuals within the region or state who specialize in caring for individuals with eating disorders allows the dental hygienist to guide the client for appropriate therapy. This knowledge can be obtained by contacting mental health organizations or eating disorder treatment facilities within the community. These organizations may not be in the immediate geographic locale, but they are generally knowledgeable about available support throughout the region.

Creating a formal referral protocol with eating disorder treatment centers or with medical/psychological specialists in eating disorders is important for the dental team. Mental health professionals treating eating disorder clients often need oral healthcare professionals to whom they can refer clients who are experiencing oral problems. A liaison between the oral health team and the psychological and medical team will open the door for comprehensive client care through referrals and collaboration.

Assessment

Assessment of all dental hygiene clients involves collection of data on the client's comprehensive health history, intraoral and extraoral status, and physical status. In addition, intraoral photographs and study models are helpful in establishing baseline data to be used for subsequent evaluation of enamel erosion and soft tissue abnormalities. When the clinician observes deviations from normal in client assessment data that suggest an eating disorder, follow-up questioning is necessary to rule out other possible explanations. See Possible Etiologies for Oral Findings Commonly Associated with Clients Who Have Eating Disorders.

For example, although the presence of commissure lesions and/or dry chapped lips may indicate a finding typical of an eating disorder, these findings also may be present following other illnesses that cause dehydration and/or undernutrition. Usually, clients who have been ill and have dehydration sequelae willingly convey this information on questioning.

In addition, although dental erosion is the most common oral finding in the bulimia and binge/purge subtype of anorexia, it has also been associated with vomiting as a result of gastric disturbances and other conditions listed below in Possible Etiologies for Oral Findings Commonly Associated with Clients Who Have Eating Disorders. Moreover, intraoral trauma may result from an accident or may be evidence of self-mutilation indicative of psychological problems other than eating disorders. Clients with medication-induced xerostomia may rely on sucrose-containing mints or gum to relieve the dryness associated with decreased salivary flow. Commonly, these individuals experience an increase in dental caries rate that can easily be identified by examining the health history and questioning the client. For

Possible Etiologies for Oral Findings Commonly Associated with Clients Who Have Eating Disorders

Perimylolysis and Erosion: Differential Diagnosis

Gastric or physical disturbances with associated vomiting (e.g., previous pregnancies, chemotherapy, hiatal hernia, duodenal or peptic ulcers, cancer-related therapy)
High citric acid fruit or fruit juice intake
Antabuse therapy (and associated vomiting) for alcoholism
Habitual eating or sucking on vitamin C tablets or sweet-and-sour type candies
Medications containing hydrochloric acid
Exposure to industrial acids

Parotid Enlargement: Differential Diagnosis

Salivary neoplasms
Inflammatory diseases (e.g., mumps, infectious mononucleosis, tuberculosis, sarcoidosis, histoplasmosis)
Metabolic disturbances (e.g., malnutrition, alcoholic cirrhosis, diabetes mellitus)
Autoimmune diseases such as Sjögren's syndrome
Parotid duct obstruction
Acquired immunodeficiency syndrome (AIDS)

Xerostomia

Medications (e.g., antihypertensives, antidepressants, antipsychotics, antihistamines)
Systemic diseases (e.g., diabetes, Sjögren's syndrome)
Side effect of radiation therapy for cancer of the head and neck area
Dehydration from recent flulike illnesses or high fever

Commissure Lesions

Loss of vertical dimension or overclosure
Vitamin B deficiency
Yeast infection

example, asking "Have there been any dietary changes that have increased your exposure to sugar or sugar-containing foods?" or "Can you tell me a little about your snacking habits?" provide an opportunity to discuss eating habits in a nonthreatening manner. Follow-up questions related to frequency or patterns of snacking or sugar consumption provide additional information while allowing the clinician to observe the client's demeanor regarding discussion of food.

During assessment of a client with a suspected eating disorder, it is imperative that the dental hygienist gather specific information in a professional, nonjudgmental manner. Concluding the presence of an eating disorder without adequate assessment is to be avoided at all costs. To conclude prematurely that a client has an eating disorder puts the client and clinician in an unnecessary and uncomfortable position.

Assessment of the client who reports a history of bulimia or anorexia involves several important components. In the client with a diagnosed eating disorder, historical information regarding the course and treatment of the eating disorder, past medical and dental care, and current status of the oral environment and past treatment interventions are necessary to provide appropriate care for the client. This evaluation should provide a clear depiction of the extent to which the eating disorder relates to associated behaviors, current status regarding psychotherapy and/or supportive care, and current physical and oral findings (see Assessment of the Client with a Suspected and Previously Diagnosed Eating Disorder).

Dental Hygiene Diagnosis

Dental hygiene diagnoses can be accomplished using assessment data to determine deficits in the eight human needs related to dental hygiene care. *Actual diagnosis of the eating disorder is not a function of members of the oral health team because this can be determined only by a thorough psychological evaluation.*

A client usually manifests several human need deficits arising directly or indirectly from the eating disorder. For example, repeated binge eating of carbohydrates followed by vomiting and laxative abuse may result in a deficit related to a biologically sound dentition, as evidenced by enamel erosion (perimylolysis) and increased signs of dental caries. Dehydration from vomiting, diuretic, or laxative abuse also may result in a deficit relating to the integrity of the skin and mucous membrane, as evidenced by dry chapped lips and commissure lesions similar to angular cheilitis.

The dental hygiene diagnosis of a human need deficit in responsibility for oral health may or may not be made depending on the type of eating disorder identified. For example, in the anorexic client, self-control is a human need that motivates the individual to action. Consequently, the client will likely exhibit greater adherence to ideal oral health behaviors if he or she

ASSESSMENT OF THE CLIENT WITH A SUSPECTED AND PREVIOUSLY DIAGNOSED EATING DISORDER

Component	Assessment Technique
Health History Assessment	
Physical appearance and gait: skin, build, weight, hair pallor	Observation
Vital signs: blood pressure, heart rate, body temperature (optional)	Objective measurement
Systemic diseases: current and past status	Interview
Systems review	Interview
Medications: drug names, dosages, duration of medications, reasons for medications	Interview
Exercise and physical activity: frequency and duration	Interview
Oral home care habits	Interview
Dietary habits or restrictions	Interview
Extraoral Assessment	
Salivary and lymph glands	Palpation
Temporomandibular joint	Palpation and auscultation
Skin: color, moisture, facial hair (lanugo), lesions	Observation
Perioral structures: commissure lesions, lip integrity, trauma	Observation
Intraoral Assessment	
Soft tissue assessment: condition of mucous membranes, unexplained trauma (especially palatal)	Observation and palpation
Assessment of signs of caries and oral hygiene	Radiographic and manual examination
Periodontal assessment	Observation and measurement of probing depths and attachment level
Tooth wear: presence or absence, location, appearance (cupped or moth eaten versus abraded)	Observation, study models

understands the concept of personal control over oral health and disease. In contrast, lack of self-control and self-determination characterizes the bulimic client. Therefore, it is likely that the client will not engage in adequate oral hygiene behaviors necessary for oral health. Examples of dental hygiene diagnoses for eating disorders are presented in Dental Hygiene Diagnoses for Clients with Eating Disorders Based on the Human Needs Conceptual Model of Dental Hygiene.

Planning

The planning phase for the client suspected of having an eating disorder should include:

- *Phase 1.* Referral of the client into the medical and psychological therapy systems
- *Phase 2.* Establishment of a liaison or formal referral protocol with the psychological treatment team
- *Phase 3.* Support of the client's human needs during and following psychological treatment

Planning for the client with a previously diagnosed eating disorder includes phases two and three. Members of the oral health team must recognize their limitations in treating clients with these disorders. Oral and dental treatment, either palliative or definitive, may be necessary, but the primary role of the oral health team treating the client with a suspected eating disorder is to refer the client to specialists who treat the psychological and medical aspects of eating disorders. Establishment of a caring, nonjudgmental environment based on mutual trust is necessary to successfully achieve a referral. Attention to the client's need for freedom from pain through palliative oral care initially is recommended if the client is experiencing discomfort.

Involving the client in setting mutual goals should be a primary consideration. Goals must be set that are:

- Specific
- Based on the dental hygiene diagnoses
- Measurable by both client and professional

A sample dental hygiene care plan for a client with an eating disorder is shown in Dental Hygiene Care Plan: The Client with Bulimia.

Planning care for clients with perimylolysis should be aimed at eliminating pain, maintaining existing tooth structure, and preventing further erosion. To this end, planning may include one or more of the following: self-applied daily fluoride therapy, mouthguard fabrication to provide coverage for teeth during vomiting episodes, client education, and/or desensitization of dentinal hypersensitivity with either professionally applied or over-the-counter agents. Clients exhibiting xerostomia as a result of dehydration may benefit from a saliva substitute and client education with respect to the influence of xerostomia on the oral hard and soft tissues.

Implementation

PROFESSIONAL CONFRONTATION. Once the dental hygiene assessment and diagnoses have been completed, consultation between the dentist and dental hygienist affords both healthcare providers an opportunity to view the data collaboratively. At the initial decision-making junction, it should be determined, based on psychosocial and ethnocultural factors, whether the dental hygienist or

DENTAL HYGIENE DIAGNOSES FOR CLIENTS WITH EATING DISORDERS BASED ON THE HUMAN NEEDS CONCEPTUAL MODEL OF DENTAL HYGIENE

Dental Hygiene Diagnosis	Due or Related To	As Evidenced By
Deficit in the need for a wholesome facial image	Self-induced vomiting, excessive diet soda intake, bruxing habits, and salivary gland hypertrophy from binge and purge behavior	Client expression of dissatisfaction with: Tooth discoloration, loss of tooth structure, appearance of an open bite, visible dental caries, and parotid gland enlargement
Deficit in the need for freedom from pain	Frequent vomiting Diminished saliva flow rate from diuretic/laxative abuse	Oral discomfort from exposed dentin from enamel erosion, dental caries, and dehydrated oral tissues
Deficit in the need for integrity of the skin and mucous membranes	Laxative/diuretic abuse and vomiting Use of fingers and other objects to cause vomiting	Dehydration of oral environment Self-induced trauma during purging and self-abusive behavior
Deficit in the need for protection from health risks	Self-starvation Anemia/alteration in body metabolism Decreased cardiac function	Dry skin/hair Enlarged parotid glands Bradycardia/low blood pressure/low body temperature Thin or pale appearance Fatigue
Deficit in the need for freedom from stress	Low or endangered esteem Need for acceptance by others Feelings of guilt Fear of being "found out"	Lack of willingness to communicate fully; denial of or providing false explanations for oral manifestations
Deficit in the need for responsibility for oral health	Lack of self control Feelings of unworthiness	Lack of "ownership" of problems Impaired self-care Evidence of self-inflicted oral trauma

DENTAL HYGIENE CARE PLAN: THE CLIENT WITH BULIMIA

Dental Hygiene Diagnosis	Goal	Dental Hygiene Interventions	Evaluative Statement
Deficit in the need for freedom from pain	By 12/3, client will have normal oral function with no discomfort By 11/1, client communicates openly with dental hygienist and participates in management of oral conditions	Fabricate mouthguard for dental coverage during vomiting episodes and/or fluoride application	Client complies with recommended treatment for ameliorating dental/oral discomfort
	Dental caries activity will be decreased for at least 1 year	Recommend daily use of neutral sodium fluoride gel/rinse and/or desensitizing dentifrice Demonstrate bacterial plaque control measures Explain risks of vomiting to hard oral tissues: increased sensitivity Refer to dentist for palliative/definitive coverage of exposed dentin Provide client with verbal and nonverbal reinforcement demonstrating acceptance of client's illness	No evidence of progressive enamel/ dentin loss (perimylolysis) No evidence of caries activity after 1 year Client reports changes in bulimic behavior that affects oral conditions
	By 10/3, client will use mouthguard during vomiting episodes		Goal partially met: client uses mouthguard during some vomiting episodes
Deficit in the need for responsibility for oral health	Client participates in treatment of bulimia by attending all medical/ psychological and dental treatment appointments for 1 year By 10/2, client participates in management of oral conditions by utilizing oral self-care skills By 10/5, client will self-monitor plaque biofilm By 11/20, client will self-monitor gingival bleeding	Refer client for psychological intervention Involve client in design of self-care skills that coordinate with concomitant psychological therapy Liaison with other healthcare providers to coordinate multidisciplinary care Provide appropriate evaluation and feedback Use media and instructional aids to support skill development in bacterial plaque removal	Client complies with referral to mental health specialist/eating disorder treatment facility Client demonstrates successful use of self-care skills No evidence of bacterial plaque or gingivitis No evidence of oral trauma from self-care
Deficit in the need for a wholesome facial image	Client participates in active psychological treatment for 6 months By 7/20, client will accept dental hygiene/dental interventions as a coordinated effort toward comprehensive treatment By 8/15, client will verbalize that her mouth looks and feels better	Referral to and continued liaison with medical/psychological team Refer to dentist for aesthetic/definitive dental treatment intervention Provide education regarding client's expressed dissatisfaction with oral condition	Client indicates that she has been going for psychological treatment Client expresses acceptance of oral conditions after treatment Client has realistic expectations for alterations in appearance of oral conditions from dental treatment Client states that her mouth looks and feels better

dentist is the best person to confront the client with the objective findings and suspicion of an eating disorder. As a general rule, the dental hygienist is the oral health professional most likely to be successful in a confrontation because he or she does not represent an "authority figure" in the mind of the client, as might the dentist. It is important to note, however, that female clients may be more receptive to a confrontation by a female clinician, whereas males may be more receptive to a male clinician.[26]

No matter who conducts the initial confrontation, a matter-of-fact, nonjudgmental approach must be maintained. Many clinicians are initially uncomfortable with the prospect of confronting a client with a suspected eating disorder and may inadvertently communicate this discomfort nonverbally to the client. To prevent this scenario, the inexperienced clinician would benefit from role playing to practice these types of confrontational situations before an actual experience. Using desensitizing and follow-up questions, such as those suggested in Guidelines for Confronting a Person with a Suspected Eating Disorder, provides the professional with the opening to apprise the client that observed oral changes are commonly associated with eating disorders.

The actual confrontation should occur in a confidential setting. If dental erosion is the most obvious oral finding, asking questions that eliminate other possibilities for erosion allows the clinician to gain valuable information while desensitizing the client to the more direct interview to follow. The confrontational interview should be conducted by asking direct questions while

Guidelines for Confronting a Person with a Suspected Eating Disorder

Setting

Use of a private setting meets the client's human need for respect by assuring client confidentiality.

Approach

Be firm, formal, objective, and concerned. Keep in mind that eating disorder behavior is a symptom of low self-esteem, depression, and long-standing emotional problems.

Present and review the findings observed. Explain the lack of other possible etiologies as evidenced by responses to differential diagnoses questions.

Ask if the client engages in behaviors associated with the disorder (e.g., "Do you vomit after eating sometimes?", "Do you restrict the amount of food that you usually eat?")

Inquire "Have you ever heard of bulimia/anorexia?" Reassure that eating disorders are not uncommon without conveying to the client that he or she is not a unique and special individual.

Encourage the client to contact resource personnel for evaluation.

Dos and Don'ts

Do be prepared. Anticipate resistance and defensiveness. Don't confront with inadequate preparation and evidence.

Do focus on observed signs and symptoms and concern for health. Don't diagnose a medical, psychological, or dental problem.

Do convey concern, but in a firm, formal manner. Do explain that help is available. Do explain that the client must decide on his or her own whether to seek assistance.

Do, with permission, contact the local Eating Disorder unit.

Don't be misled by sympathy-evoking tactics or be manipulated by resistance and defensiveness. Stay focused on observed findings and concern for individual.

Don't generalize or insinuate. Be specific. Don't moralize or make value judgments. Maintain a professional demeanor.

maintaining eye contact. It is noteworthy that the client's body language may provide clues about whether the suspicion of an eating disorder is accurate. Few clients openly admit a problem with an eating disorder when questioned. Many have become quite accomplished at denial and can maintain that posture in the dental environment. Most clients with eating disorders, however, experience discomfort at being confronted with objective information they have attempted to hide. The dental hygienist should be aware of nonverbal cues, such as loss of eye contact by the client or dropping of the head with a look of "shame." These clues are usually an indication that the clinician is on the right track with the questions even though the client may verbally respond negatively.

Individuals with eating disorders commonly react to the initial confrontation with various emotions. Two common responses are denial accompanied by tears and outright anger. It is important for the dental hygienist to maintain a professional demeanor during emotional outbursts and afford reinforcement to the client that the oral, physical, and/or health history findings are typical of an eating disorder and have no other etiologic explanation, if in fact that is the case. Some clients are relieved at being discovered and are receptive to suggestions for referral to an eating disorder specialist.

Guidelines for Referring a Person with a Suspected Eating Disorder

Refer the Individual

To meet the client's human need for conceptualization and understanding, give specific information on resources for professional evaluation and offer support.

Encourage the client to contact resource personnel for evaluation.

Contact the Professional Person to Whom You Are Referring the Client

Inform the counselor or therapist of referral.

Discuss the symptoms and signs of concern.

Discuss areas of difficulty with confrontation, referral, and appropriateness of referral.

Follow-up and Support

Communicate satisfaction when evaluation or therapy has occurred. Recognize that seemingly small accomplishments may be major to the recovering client.

Expect that the client will have periods of recurrence of eating disorder behaviors.

Support recovery, not the illnesses.

REFERRAL. *Suggesting* that the client make an appointment with an identified eating disorder specialist or treatment center for an evaluation is a less threatening approach than making a definitive statement that the client has an eating disorder. Many clients are receptive to having the dental hygienist initiate a consultation appointment for them at an eating disorder treatment center (see Guidelines for Referring a Person with a Suspected Eating Disorder presents guidelines for referral). Others prefer to take the referral information with them to initiate the consultation appointment on their own. Either way, it is important that the client assume personal responsibility for attending a consultation appointment.

Following the confrontation appointment, the dental hygienist should adequately document the discussion and the decisions regarding referral for evaluation in the client's permanent dental record. This permits subsequent evaluation and monitoring of the client at future appointments.

Although some clients may deny that they have an eating disorder, over time they may become sufficiently comfortable with the dental hygienist to be receptive to the referral. Persistence on the part of the oral health team when no other explanations can be identified for the findings is crucial because untreated eating disorders can be life-threatening. Ethically, failure to refer a client who has obvious signs of an eating disorder for subsequent psychological evaluation is neglecting one's professional responsibility as a healthcare provider.

ESTABLISHMENT OF THE DENTAL/MEDICAL/PSYCHOLOGICAL TEAM LIAISON. Once a client with a suspected eating disorder has been confronted and referred for psychological counseling, a working relationship between the oral health team and psychological/medical team should be established. Phases two (establishing a liaison) and three (management of the oral environment) of the implementation process are identical for recently confronted clients as well as for those who present to the oral healthcare setting with a positive history of bulimia, anorexia, or bulimorexia.

Success of oral healthcare is largely determined by the client's ability to control behaviors associated with the eating disorder. For this reason, open dialogue among all health providers prevents segmented care planning and permits an integrated approach to client care. Many bulimic and binge/purge-type anorexic clients with extensive erosion require significant dental reconstruction. Lack of coordination among healthcare providers may mean dental failure if the reconstruction is completed before the client has made adequate progress with the eating disorder. Use of a signed release form allows oral health professionals to contact and collaborate with the psychological and medical healthcare providers and is recommended when caring for a client with an eating disorder. A sample release form is shown in Figure 47–3.

Professional liaison between the oral healthcare team and the psychological support team permits the oral health team to have a better understanding of the client's specific psychological problems and increases the success rate of all dental hygiene and dental interventions. The client is often confronting significant personal issues in psychological therapy. These may influence the timing and ultimate success of definitive oral care. Without dialogue between the oral health team and mental health team, oral health professionals may make care decisions that fail to address the comprehensive needs of the client. If clients are aware that all health providers are working together for their total good, then they are less likely to claim that "all is well" in order to have short-term desires met. It is not uncommon for clients with eating disorders to attempt to manipulate healthcare providers during the course of therapy. Dental hygienists and dentists must maintain a collaborative interdisciplinary approach to healthcare for maximal success with the client with eating disorders.

CONSENT FORM

I hereby give consent for my dentist and dental hygienist to contact all healthcare providers and therapists involved in the treatment of my eating disorder. I understand that coordination of care among these health professionals is in my best interests. In addition, I understand that all consultation and discussion among these individuals will be held in strict confidence.

Client Signature Date

Witness Date

FIGURE 47–3 ✦ Sample client consent form.

MANAGEMENT AND SUPPORT OF ORAL TISSUES. Implementation of individualized education and preventive strategies to support a healthy oral environment is a primary focus of this phase of the dental hygiene process. To meet the client's human need for conceptualization and understanding, oral health education assists the client in understanding the effect of eating disorder behaviors on oral health and provides self-care strategies to ameliorate or control the associated problems. When providing client education, health-promoting behaviors and management of oral problems as they relate to facial image and freedom from pain should be emphasized. Potential health hazards, such as cardiac irregularities, endocrine disturbances, renal dysfunction, electrolyte imbalance, and predictable negative sequelae such as death, should be deemphasized because this approach can result in alienation of the client.

Oral health education strategies for the eating disorder client are provided in Oral Health Education for the Eating Disorder Client. These strategies may not be relevant for all clients, but an overview of general concepts should be included in each educational program.

Etiology of Oral Manifestations Associated with the Disorder. An overview of the etiology of identified problems is necessary before providing individualized oral hygiene

Oral Health Education for the Eating Disorder Client

Oral Health Education Programs Should Include:

Etiology of the observed oral characteristics associated with the eating disorder behaviors
Effect of eating disorder behaviors on the oral environment and dental structures
Current status
Potential progression of problems
Effect of dietary habits on dental and oral health
Frequency of eating
Types of foods and drinks consumed
Individualized oral hygiene instruction

Oral Health Promotion Should Include:

Specific management and control of oral/dental manifestations of the disorder
Amelioration of existing problems
Prevention of progression of other characteristics
Management of oral discomfort associated with dentinal hypersensitivity
Recommendation for daily, at-home use of a neutral sodium fluoride rinse or gel
Recommendation of sodium bicarbonate or magnesium hydroxide rinses, or saliva substitute, as necessary
Construction of an oral mouthguard for protection during vomiting episodes

instructions. For example, clients with significant perimylolysis as a result of repeated vomiting need to understand that the low pH of stomach contents causes chemical dissolution of tooth enamel. If toothbrushing follows vomiting episodes, mechanical abrasion of the presoftened tooth surfaces is likely. The etiology of all oral manifestations should be adequately explained to clients.

Effect of Eating Disorder Behaviors on the Oral Environment. Client education also includes an overview of systemic physiologic changes typical of the specific eating disorder as it relates to changes in the oral environment. For example, the effects secondary to vomiting and/or diuretic and laxative abuse should be explained as they relate to decreased salivary flow and increased dental caries activity.

Self-starvation and decreased body fat alter endocrine function, which in turn has the potential of causing osteoporosis early in life. It has not been determined to what degree early osteoporosis affects periodontal bone support later in life, but it is important that anorexic and bulimic clients be cognizant of potential changes in bone density as they relate to overall health.

Clients with parotid gland enlargement may express concern about the unaesthetic appearance of the enlargement. If the individual understands that the enlargement usually decreases once the eating disorder behaviors are brought under control, this may increase motivation for following through with psychological and medical care.

Effect of Diet on Oral Health. Individuals with eating disorders commonly have unusual eating habits that potentially alter normal oral health. For example, foods containing simple carbohydrates such as cookies, cake, and other sweets are common binge foods for the bulimic. Counseling on the effect of repeated binge eating, frequent sucrose intake, and/or extreme intake of dietary carbonated drinks should be provided to the client if applicable. Dietary habits in anorexia frequently include excessive intake of diet soda beverages in lieu of food. Continual consumption of low-pH diet beverages in the presence of diminished salivary flow may result in dental erosion and accompanying dentinal hypersensitivity. By adequately assessing eating habits, the dental hygienist can provide appropriate preventive education and treatment.

Oral Hygiene Instruction and Self-Care. Oral hygiene instruction for clients with eating disorders includes techniques for plaque biofilm removal that are directed at preventing periodontal diseases and dental caries. In addition, oral hygiene instruction encompasses self-care measures that promote health and prevent further destruction of hard and soft oral tissues. These strategies are aimed at meeting the client's human needs for integrity of skin and mucous membrane of the head and neck and for a biologically sound dentition.

Normal brushing should be encouraged for all clients, but actively vomiting clients with dental erosion should be discouraged from toothbrushing after vomiting. It is believed that immediately brushing teeth following exposure to the acidic vomitus may increase loss of tooth structure. Use of sodium bicarbonate (1 tsp. in 8 oz. of water) or magnesium hydroxide (milk of magnesia) rinses following vomiting episodes cleanses the mouth of vomitus while neutralizing the acidic environment of the oral cavity.

For clients with dental erosion and/or dentinal hypersensitivity, use of a home fluoride treatment should be given top priority. Daily use of 1.1% neutral sodium fluoride gel, administered either by a custom-fabricated tray or by brushing, or a 0.2% sodium fluoride mouthrinse provides maximal protection while strengthening enamel to prevent additional erosion. Use of a stannous fluoride gel for home application is contraindicated because these agents have a low pH that may increase sensitivity and the potential for additional erosion. Clients can be advised that the custom-fabricated fluoride trays can also be used without the fluoride to protect teeth during periods of out-of-control binge and purge episodes. Use of desensitizing fluoridated dentifrices may provide additional benefit for clients with exposed dentin from erosion.

Recommendations for saliva substitutes are appropriate if the client reports discomfort from xerostomia. Many clients currently under psychological or psychiatric treatment for eating disorders are medicated with prescription antidepressants. Xerostomia resulting from these medications combined with systemic dehydration can create a situation that the dental hygienist needs to address during client education. For individuals who find saliva substitutes unpleasant, frequent water rinsing or sipping or sucking on crushed ice chips can be recommended.

DENTAL HYGIENE INSTRUMENTATION. During instrumentation (scaling, root planing, and removal of extrinsic stain), appropriate pain management techniques should be used to protect sensitive hard and soft tissues. Maintaining a moist, clean environment by frequent rinsing of the oral cavity during instrumentation can increase comfort if the individual suffers from xerostomia. Selective polishing should be considered when clients have had extensive enamel erosion resulting in dentin exposure. Many polishing pastes are excessively abrasive to dentin (e.g., pumice and/or medium- or coarse-grade agents) and should be avoided. Selective polishing is recommended if the individual does not have extrinsic stains or if the dental hypersensitivity impedes client comfort during stain removal.

Implementation of the dental hygiene process of care and necessary palliative treatment of discomfort (e.g., use of desensitization treatments) may be timed before and during psychological treatment. Additional restorative and prosthetic dental care, when required, should be coordinated with the psychological and medical teams once the client is receiving treatment.

Evaluation

Evaluation of dental hygiene care for the client with an eating disorder is composed of two parts:

- An objective evaluation based on mutual goals previously established by the dental hygienist and client to determine whether they have been met, partially met, or unmet
- A subjective report by the client

OBJECTIVE EVALUATION. For an objective evaluation, comparison of data on plaque biofilm accumulation, periodontal status, dental caries, enamel erosion, dentinal hypersensitivity, and oral tissues from baseline to each subsequent appointment should be accomplished. Many changes that occur over time are subtle and defy detection unless accurate data are collected and compared with previous data. This is especially true in cases in which perimylolysis is a significant finding. Clients who are receiving psychological treatment, but who have not controlled binge and purge behavior, may convince the oral health team to believe that the dental erosion is no longer a threat. Objective comparison of pre- and post-treatment oral photographs and study models can verify or negate the subjective report by the client.

SUBJECTIVE EVALUATION. The subjective evaluation can provide additional information for future care planning. Preservation of a caring, professional environment assures the client that confidentiality is maintained while oral health needs are met humanistically. The oral health team must be aware that successful treatment of eating disorders requires intensive therapy followed by many years of aftercare. It is common for clients who have successfully controlled eating disorder behaviors for several weeks or months to revert periodically to previous behaviors, especially when stressful life events occur. Awareness and verbal acknowledgment of this pattern by the dental hygienist during evaluation permits clients to share honestly about areas of progress as well as areas of distress. This information can then be used in conjunction with the objective data and information from other attending health professionals to guide subsequent care.

On occasion, objective and subjective evaluations conflict. For instance, a client with previously documented dental erosion may report that binge and purge episodes have been under control for six months and that she is no longer in need of psychological treatment; however, comparison of current dental status to intraoral photographs and diagnostic models obtained one year previously may indicate that the erosion has been progressive. Discussing these discrepancies with the client and expressing concern about the reported cessation of aftercare therapy are crucial. The oral health team often becomes instrumental in encouraging the client to seek additional psychotherapy when it is apparent that previous therapy has been unsuccessful. In this situation, it may even become necessary for the oral health team to refuse definitive dental treatment unless the client is in therapy and coordination between the psychologist and oral health professionals can occur.

Continual evaluation of the client's oral health status, as well as the status of psychological therapy, is one of the most critical functions of the dental hygienist when managing an individual with an eating disorder. At several points during the dental hygiene process of care, the clinician may need to reassess the client's condition, revise care goals, plan alternative strategies, implement these strategies, and reevaluate the outcome. The dynamic nature of the dental hygiene process of care for clients with an eating disorder creates a challenge for the professional dental hygienist.

Client Education Issues

- Explain the effect of the eating disorder on oral tissues
- Explain self-care strategies to ameliorate or control oral manifestations associated with the eating disorder
- Explain the need for referral for medical and psychological treatment
- Explain the need to coordinate nonemergency restorative and prosthetic dental care with psychological treatment

Legal, Ethical, and Safety Issues

- Members of the oral health team must recognize their limitations in treating clients with eating disorders. The primary role of the oral health team is to refer the client with a suspected eating disorder to specialists who treat the psychological and medical aspects of eating disorders.
- Following the confrontation appointment, the dental hygienist should adequately document the discussion and the decisions regarding referral for evaluation in the client's permanent dental record.
- Ethically, failure to refer a client who has obvious signs of an eating disorder for subsequent psychological evaluation is neglecting one's professional responsibility as a healthcare provider.
- All information related to a client's eating disorder is confidential. The dental practitioner requires the client's consent to refer the client into medical and psychological therapy systems.
- Use of a signed release form allows oral health professionals to contact and collaborate with the psychological and medical healthcare providers and is recommended when caring for a client with an eating disorder.

Key Concepts

- ✦ Eating disorders result in significant physical and oral sequelae and, over time, increased mortality rates.
- ✦ Eating disorders have psychosocial, physical, and oral dimensions. Successful care requires the coordinated effort of various health professionals.
- ✦ Common intraoral findings in the client with an eating disorder include the presence of perimylolysis, ulcerations or hematomas on the hard and soft palates, cheek and lip bites, and commissure lesions resembling angular cheilitis.
- ✦ Extraorally, parotid enlargement is observed in both anorexia and bulimia.
- ✦ For individuals with an eating disorder who have not been medically diagnosed, the dental hygienist may be the health professional who identifies the need for referral to the psychological and medical support team.
- ✦ Creating a formal referral protocol with eating disorder treatment centers or with medical/psychological specialists in eating disorders is important for the dental team.
- ✦ During assessment of a client with a suspected eating disorder, it is imperative that the dental hygienist gather specific information in a professional, nonjudgmental manner. Concluding the presence of an eating disorder without adequate assessment is to be avoided at all costs.
- ✦ In the client with a diagnosed eating disorder, information about the course and treatment of the eating disorder and the current status of the oral environment is necessary to provide appropriate care for the client.
- ✦ At the initial decision-making junction, it should be determined, based on psychosocial and ethnocultural factors, whether the dental hygienist or dentist is the best person to confront the client with the objective findings and suspicion of an eating disorder.
- ✦ Persistence on the part of the oral health team when no other explanations can be identified for the findings is crucial because untreated eating disorders can be life-threatening.
- ✦ Once a client with a suspected eating disorder has been confronted and referred for psychological counseling, a working relationship between the oral health team and psychological/medical team should be established.
- ✦ Continual evaluation of the client's oral health status, as well as the status of psychological therapy, is one of the most critical functions of the dental hygienist when managing an individual with an eating disorder.

Critical Thinking Exercises

Client: Ms. Z

Profile: A 19-year-old white female comes to the dental clinic. She attends college and is "fashionably" thin.

Chief Complaint: "My mouth is always dry, and I need my teeth cleaned."

Dental History: Client has a dental prophylaxis routinely every 6 months. Upon intraoral examination, you note hematomas on the hard and soft palates and slight gingivitis. She has lingual erosion on teeth numbers 6, 7, 8, 9, 10 and 11. Also, there is a slight pitting on the incisal surfaces of the anterior teeth, and a cupping appearance on the cusps of the posterior teeth. Extraorally, there is a fine downy hair on the lower half of her face, commissure lesions resembling angular cheilitis, and enlargement of the parotid gland.

Social History: The client lives with her parents and appears shy and socially introverted. She reports that she works out every day and sometimes twice a day.

Medical History: Client reports no use of medications or systemic disease.

Oral Health Behaviors Assessment: The client reports brushing and flossing three times per day. She uses a soft toothbrush. She does not use a fluoride mouthrinse.

Supplemental Notes: Client says she feels fat, but is obviously thin.

1. What are the dental hygiene diagnoses for this client?
2. Develop a dental hygiene care plan including goals and interventions for this client.
3. What client education issues should be addressed and how?
4. Are there any contraindications to this client's care?

For References, Suggested Readings, and Related Websites, visit
http://evolve.elsevier.com/Darby/hygiene/

CHAPTER 48

The Older Adult

OBJECTIVES

Mastery of the content in this chapter will enable the learner to:

- Discuss theories of aging
- Describe the significant demographic characteristics of the population older than age 64
- Describe normal age-related changes of the cardiovascular, pulmonary, musculoskeletal, neurosensory, gastrointestinal, genitourinary, and integumentary systems
- Describe prevalent chronic diseases associated with aging and discuss the implications for dental hygiene care
- Identify age-related oral changes commonly found in the older adult
- Discuss oral changes that occur as a result of diseases or medications
- Explain potential alterations in the dental hygiene process of care that need to be considered when treating an older adult

KEY TERMS

Activities of daily living
Chronologic age
Dysgeusia
Edentulousness
Functional age
Geriatrics
Gerontology
Healthy People 2010
Instrumental activities of daily living
Polypharmacy
Presbyopia
Senescence
Xerostomia

Dental hygienists face many challenges when they provide care for older adults because of the many biological, psychological, and social variations within this population. A lifetime of unique experiences has rendered older adults a heterogeneous group. Life at any given moment is the result of physiologic capabilities, environmental variables, psychosocial factors, and a sense of one's own skills and alternatives. Therefore, the human needs of each older adult must be assessed individually, without prior assumptions based on preconceived stereotypes or myths. The healthcare needs of older adults represent the entire continuum of healthy to severely ill individuals. Dental hygienists are challenged to provide care that often involves complex and multiple medical, social, and psychological needs and the coordination of multiple levels of health care.

DEMOGRAPHIC ASPECTS OF AGING

The older population group of the United States has increased more than ten-fold between 1900 and 2000. In 1900, there were 3 million individuals older than age 65, who represented 4% of the total population. In 2000, there were 35 million individuals older than age 65, who represented 13% of the total population.[1] This substantial rise in the proportion of older adults in the population is projected to continue to increase to 80 million by 2050 (Figure 48–1).

This significant demographic increase is primarily caused by increases in life expectancy, rather than an increase in the overall life span. Life span is the maximal length of life potentially possible of a species—the age beyond which no one can expect to live. For humans, this number is approximately 110 to 120 years. Life

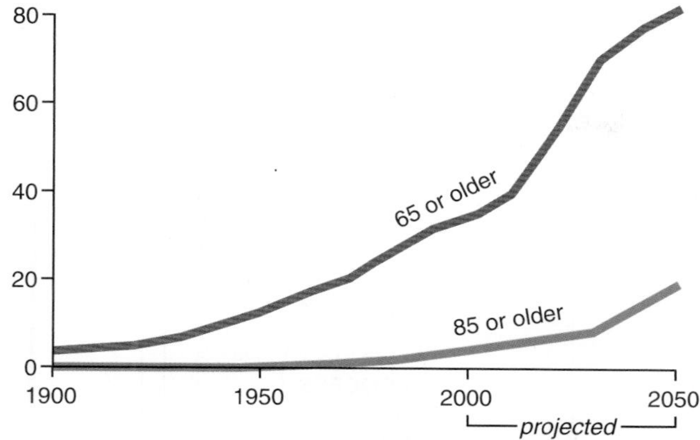
80
60
40
20
0
1900
1950
2000
2050
65 or older
85 or older
projected
Note: Data for the years 2000 to 2050 are middle-series projections of the population.
Reference population: These data refer to the resident population.
Source: U.S. Census Bureau, Decennial Census Data and Population Projections.

FIGURE 48–1 ✦ Total number of persons age 65 or older, by age group, 1900–2050, in millions. *(From the Federal Interagency Forum on Aging-Related Statistics:* Older Americans 2000: Key indicators of well-being, *available at: www.agingstats.gov/chartbook2000/population.html.)*

expectancy is the average number of years lived by any group of individuals born in the same period, and is computed at birth. For example, individuals born in 1900 had a life expectancy of 49 years, which increased to 70 years for those born in 1960. For those born in 1997, life expectancy is 79 years for women and 74 years for men. Life expectancy at ages 65 and 85 have also increased. Those individuals who survive to 65 can expect to live an average of 18 more years, and those individuals who survive to 85 can expect to live an average of at least six more years.[1]

Increase in life expectancy is accounted for by the facts that more people are surviving young life (infant and childhood mortality have declined), fertility rates have decreased, and medical technology has improved.

The number of people who reach age 65 years in a given year depends heavily on the number of births 65 years earlier. The baby boom generation is expected to create an "aging" boom in approximately the year 2020, with one in five Americans being older than age 64 years. After the year 2020, the older adult age group will increase at a slower rate because of the decrease in the size of the birth groups during the 1960s.

Not only did the older population of the United States grow in size and proportion in total population during the twentieth century, but it also became more aged. The 85-and-older age group is the fastest growing segment of the older population. In 2000, approximately 2% of the population was age 85 and older; however, by 2050, the percentage of individuals in this age group will more than double to 5% of the population. In 2000, there were approximately 65,000 individuals age 100 or older, and the number of centenarians is projected to increase to approximately 381,000 by 2030.[1]

In addition to increasing size and proportion of elderly within the population, the following demographic changes are also forecast regarding older adults:

- ✦ The older adult population is becoming more racially and ethnically diverse. By 2050, the percentage of the older population that is non-Hispanic white is expected to decline from 84% in 2000 to 64%.
- ✦ Elderly women outnumber men. In 2000, women were estimated to account for 58% of the population age 65 and older and 70% of the population age 85 and older. Marital status and living arrangements of older persons vary tremendously by gender. Most men, for example, spend their later years married and in family settings, whereas most older women spend their later years as widows outside of family settings. Older women are more likely than men to be widowed at each age group. In 1998, 32% of women age 65 to 74 were widows, compared with 9% of the men. At age 85 and older the differences increase, because 77% of women at this age group were widows as compared with 42% of men.[1] Several reasons account for this discrepancy: women have a longer life expectancy and tend to outlive their husbands, men often marry women who are younger than themselves, and men who lose a spouse through divorce or death are more likely to remarry than are women in similar situations.
- ✦ The older adult population is concentrated in key states. The older population, similar to the total population, is not distributed equally across the United States. Generally, the number of older adults is greatest in the states with the largest populations. California, New York, Florida, and Pennsylvania have the largest older adult populations, with more than 2 million each. Florida (19%) and Pennsylvania (17%) have the largest proportion of residents aged 65-plus years of the total population.[1] As the older population grows both in number and age, demands for housing, healthcare, and protective services will increase, particularly in heavily proportioned states.

These demographic changes in the numbers, composition, and proportion of older adults within the population have a major impact on our society and important policy implications for federal, state, and local governments. The increase of the very-old population, in particular, will affect planning for the needs of the aged population, not only for extended care, but for chronic debilitating conditions as well. Already the increasing number of frail elderly has created changes for nursing home residents, primarily composed of old-old adults. For example, as of October 1990, nursing home facilities must ensure that all residents be provided with emergency oral care, furnished with a referral list of dentists, and have dental care—preventive and therapeutic—as promulgated by the State Medicaid Act.[2]

The terms *geriatrics* and *gerontology* are often used synonymously when discussing healthcare with older adults, although there is a difference in their implications. *Geriatrics* is the branch of medicine concerned with the illnesses of old age and their treatment. *Gerontology* is the scientific study of the factors affecting the normal aging process and the effects of aging. In a true sense these terms are not interchangeable. A gerontologist is an individual who investigates numerous factors that affect the aging person and the aging process. Gerontologists have divided study of the older population into several categories based on age:

- ✦ Young-old (65 to 74 years)
- ✦ Middle-old (75 to 84 years)
- ✦ Old-old (85-plus years)

Some sociologists have classified those between the ages of 55 and 64 years as the "new-old" and those older than 95 years as the "very old." Whatever terms are used, two important facts exist: (1) characterizations of age should be based on ability, not chronologic age; and (2) the majority of older adults perform at a high level of independent function.[3] The preponderance of older adults with functional limitations and compromised health are older than age 75 years.

Chronologic age refers to age as measured by calendar time since birth, whereas *functional age* is based on performance capacities. Although a calendar may signify a particular age, functional ability should be the standard that differentiates a person's capability to maintain activity.

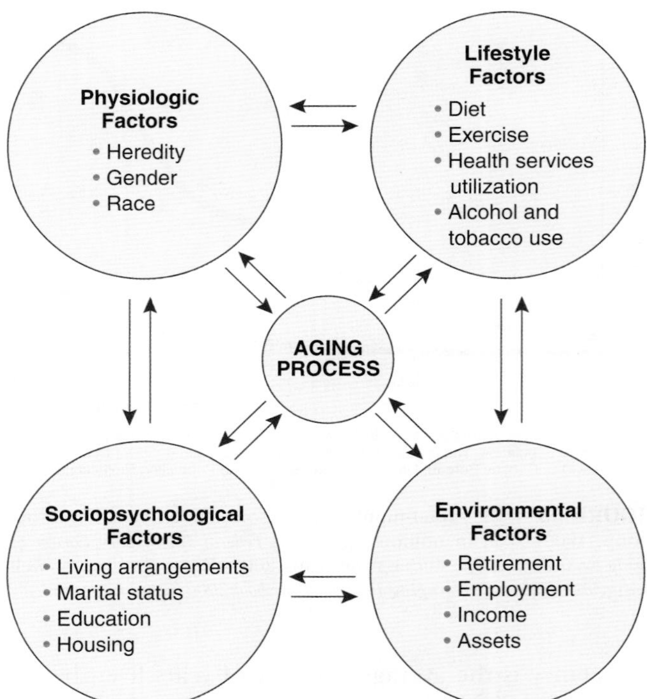

FIGURE 48–2 ✦ A conceptualization of factors influencing the aging process. *(Modified from Esberger KK, Hughes ST:* Nursing care of the aged, *Norwalk, Conn, 1989, Appleton & Lange.)*

SOCIAL ASPECTS OF AGING

No single theory can explain why and how people age. Rather, an intermingling of sociopsychological, environmental, physiologic, and lifestyle factors contributes to the aging process, either in accelerating or in retarding its progress, and produces a different course for each individual. Aging is a progressive yet fluid process, with each factor affecting the other. Figure 48–2 presents major categories of factors affecting the aging process.[4] Understanding the theories of aging—those that have validity and those that contribute to stereotypes—enables the dental hygienist to facilitate human need fulfillment in the older adult through the dental hygiene process of care.

Social science researchers looking at aging focus on numerous factors affecting the lives of older persons. One theory cannot and should not be used to explain everything about the aging process. The importance of the interdisciplinary focus becomes paramount when trying to study the aging process. No one area—social, psychological, environmental, or biologic—can predict how individuals age and adapt. Therefore, dental hygienists must be aware of the dynamic processes that influence each older client. Table 48–1 provides a summary of the six major theories that explain social aspects of aging.[3] Implications for dental hygiene are included within this table to show the application of each of the theories to actions taken during dental hygiene care.

PHYSIOLOGIC ASPECTS OF AGING

Senescence is the term that describes the normal physiologic process of growing old. The fact that everyone, given time, eventually experiences physical changes in all of the body systems makes aging universal. Physical changes that occur are normal for all people, but they take place at various rates and depend on accompanying circumstances (e.g., environmental, psychosocial, lifestyle, and biologic factors) in an individual's life. Typically, normal age changes have been studied in collaboration with pathologic or disease conditions, leading to the misconception that age changes indicate illness or disease. Research continues to uncover evidence that many changes thought to be directly related to the aging process are actually a result of disease or lifestyle influences. For example, a decrease in salivary production was previously thought to be a normal aging feature; however, within the last decade, research has shown that no decrease in salivary production occurs in healthy older adults. Diminished salivary flow is, instead, a byproduct of medications or disease.

The process of aging occurs at different rates among individuals and in different systems within the same individual.[3] Pathologic changes may develop simultaneously; therefore, it is important to distinguish, when possible, between that which is a physiologically age-related change and that which is the result of disease. The difference is important because of the need to recognize disease patterns and relate their significance to oral health changes observed during assessment.

TABLE 48–1 SOCIAL THEORIES OF AGING

Theory	Hypothesis	Limitation	Dental Hygiene Implication
Disengagement theory (Developed in late 1950s)	Aging individuals and society gradually withdraw from each other for mutual benefit.	Theory undermined by the recognition that each individual has a different aging process, and the process often damages the aged and society.	Understand how one's withdrawal from society can affect one's self-concept and motivate behavior. Facilitate human needs for self-determination, responsibility, and a wholesome body image.
Activity theory (Developed in late 1960s)	Aging individuals should be expected to maintain norms of middle-aged: employment, activity, replacement of lost relationships.	Age-related physical, mental, and socioeconomic losses may present barriers to maintaining activity.	Encourage client to seek other support systems to share/continue activities. Discuss appropriate bacterial plaque control instruction and self-examinations.
Continuity theory (Developed in late 1960s)	Aging depends on a person's psychological makeup and habitual methods of coping.	Ability to continue in valued social roles depends on an individual's social resources and the opportunities afforded by the social system.	Encourage client to maintain oral wellness. Facilitate human needs for freedom from stress, self- determination, and responsibility.
Age stratification theory (Developed in early 1970s)	Attempts to formulate a whole life conception of aging. Old age is a process of becoming socialized to new or revised role definitions reflecting a fluid relationship among people, their social contexts, and their opportunities.	Change is dependent on an intertwined series of feedback loops and revolving around the size of the population, the roles available, and the differences in the timing of individuals and social needs.	Recognize the values and beliefs associated with oral health and disease within a defined-age stratum. Facilitate human needs for value system, conceptualization, and problem solving.
Social environment theory (Developed in late 1970s)	Depicts aging as a negotiated sequence depending on resources held by the trading partners.	Adjustment is contingent on maintaining supportive environments and individual resources for manipulating unfavorable situations.	Recognize the impact of individual resources on the procurement of therapeutic services. Facilitate human needs for self-determination and problem solving.
Political-economic theory (Developed in early 1980s)	Aging is influenced by the relationship between the distribution of power and the form of economic organization.	Empirical evidence to support claims is lacking.	Serve as client advocate. Facilitate human need for self-determination.

Modified from Ebersole P, Hess P: *Toward healthy aging: Human needs and nursing response*, ed 5, St Louis, 1998, Mosby.

Biologic Theories of Aging

Most theorists agree that a unifying theory does not yet exist that explains the mechanics and causes underlying the biologic phenomenon of aging. Basically, biologic theories can be divided into molecular and nonmolecular theories. Each hypothesis provides a clue to the aging process, but many unanswered questions remain. The following is a description of the predominant biologic theories.[3]

CELL THEORIES. These theories have been the topic of frequent scientific investigation in examining the aging phenomena and focus on three types of cells: cells that reproduce, cells that do not reproduce, and intercellular substances and materials.[5]

The theory based on cells that reproduce proposes that during reproduction some of the new cells are nonfunctioning or less effective than the other cells that were replaced. As the aging process progresses and there is an accumulation of inefficient and nonfunctioning cells, the organism's functional ability becomes apparent. For example, the skin is an organism wherein cells are continuously being replaced. With age, the skin takes on visible changes such as wrinkling, roughness, and dryness.

The theory related to cells that do not reproduce suggests that with age the cells progressively wear out or are destroyed. For example, the central nervous system, which consists of cells that do not reproduce, gradually develops an accumulation of nonfunctioning cells. Subsequently, the system becomes less efficient and unable to handle the usual workload.[5]

SOMATIC MUTATION THEORY. This theory suggests that when cells are exposed to radiation or chemicals an alteration of deoxyribonucleic acid (DNA) occurs, thus increasing the incidence of chromosomal abnormalities. These mutations are a time-dependent accumulation of chromosome abnormalities that become apparent in later life. Ultimately a decrease in cellular function and organ efficiency results.[6]

ERROR THEORY. This theory postulates that cells may become inoperative because of copying errors in repeated divisions. For a message to be transmitted to the cell, DNA depends on the ribonucleic acid (RNA) stored in the nucleus. Changes in the structure of RNA may result in progressive modifications in copying so that newer cells are incapable of recognizing essential components of themselves. This nonrecognition forces the body's immune system to work against itself. For example, cancer is the result of abnormal cells produced within the body.[6]

PROGRAMMED THEORY. The premise of this theory is that the life span of an organism is programmed within the genes of the organism. The program sets the rate and time that an individual proceeds through the life span and dies. For example, the graying of hair, wrinkling of skin, and beginning of menopause are intrinsically correlated with time. These changes are considered normal aging alterations that are not pathologic.[3]

IMMUNOLOGIC/AUTOIMMUNE THEORY. This theory proposes that with age the immune system undergoes involuntary changes after puberty. The result is twofold: (1) the body's production of antibodies necessary to fight off infections declines, and (2) as normal immune patterns change in one direction, autoimmune responses change in the opposite direction. Cells normal to the body are misidentified as foreign matter and are attacked by the body's own immune system.[5]

CROSSLINKAGE THEORY. This theory (also referred to as the *collagen* or *connective tissue theory*) suggests that chemical reactions create strong bonds between molecular structures that are normally separate. As the body ages, the number of crosslinks in extracellular components increases, which results in fibers becoming more rigid. For example, a lack of elasticity in the walls of the circulatory system signifies the probable onset of atherosclerosis and high blood pressure. Because collagen makes up about 30% of body protein, alterations in the fibers can produce significant changes in the older adult's functioning, thus the human need for self-determination may be compromised.[6]

FREE RADICAL THEORY. This theory postulates that free radicals contain unpaired ions that exist momentarily and are highly reactive chemically with other substances, such as unsaturated fats. The molecular structure of free radicals differs from that of ordinary molecules in that they possess an extra electric charge (free electron). This charge instigates a one-time, irreversible, and energy-wasteful reaction that damages or alters the original structure or function of the cell membrane. Although body cells possess the capacity to eliminate unwanted waste and materials, neutralize byproducts, and repair damage, free radical accumulation is thought to be faster than the repair process of the organism.[6]

In summary, the fundamental mechanisms of the aging process are becoming less obscure, but they remain extremely variable among human beings. A search for a universal factor or factors is complicated by the fact that signs of aging do not appear in all individuals at the same chronologic age. Knowledge of the various biologic theories of aging is helpful in understanding physiologic manifestations and some mental changes that may affect the older client.

HEALTH STATUS AND ASSESSMENT

Health assessment of older persons includes a functional appraisal in addition to a health history. The items generally included within a functional assessment are divided into *activities of daily living* (ADLs) and *instrumental activities of daily living* (IADLs). ADLs are those abilities that are fundamental to independent living, such as bathing, dressing, toileting, transferring from bed or chair, feeding, and continence. More complex daily activities, such as using the telephone, preparing meals, and managing money, are examples of IADLs.

The majority of older adults have one or more chronic conditions, but most older adults view their health positively. Approximately 72% of noninstitutionalized older adults describe their general health as excellent, very good, or good, compared with others their age.[1] Little difference exists in perception of health between males and females; however, positive health evaluations decline with age. For example, in non-Hispanic white men age 65 to 74, 76% reported good to excellent health, while of the same group age 85 or older, only 67% reported good to excellent health.

The pattern of illness and disease has changed over the past century. Acute conditions were predominant during the early 1900s, whereas chronic conditions present more prevalent health problems for older adults today. Five of the six leading causes of death for older adults are chronic diseases. The leading chronic conditions for older adults are arthritis, hypertension and heart disease, cancer, diabetes, and stroke.[1]

Young-old and middle-old persons are relatively healthy and often are not limited in activity despite having chronic conditions. The proportion of Americans age 65 or older with a chronic disability declined from 24% in 1982 to 21% in 1994; however, health and mobility do decline generally with advancing age. By the eighth and ninth decades of life, the chances of having limited activity and needing health and social services increase significantly. For example, in 1990, 9% of individuals age 65 to 69 needed assistance with ADLs as compared to 20% of those older adults age 75 to 79 and 50% of the elderly 85 years and older.[1]

HEALTH PROMOTION AND AGING

The increasing numbers and proportion of older adults within the population have coincided with a shifting of priorities to a wellness perspective from both consumers and professionals.[3] For the past two decades, efforts to increase the overall health of the nation have been addressed through the Healthy People initiatives, which is currently led by the Office of Disease Prevention and Health Promotion in the Department of Health and Human Services in the federal government. *Healthy People 2010* is the most recent document that sets goals for the nation, health focus areas, and leading health indicators to measure progress in increasing health status. The *Healthy People 2010* document has two goals: (1) Increase the quality and years of healthy life; and (2) eliminate health disparities.[7]

Most health conditions and diseases are exacerbated by cumulative lifestyle habits and environmental factors, which result in decline in health status for many older adults. For example, poor diet, decreased activity level, alcohol abuse, and tobacco usage all play a significant part in the development or exacerbation of disease(s). The health status indicators and focus areas in the *Healthy People 2010* report provide a concrete baseline from which to plan programs, set priorities, and evaluate progress in meeting health objectives and increasing health status. Most state and local health departments are utilizing the Healthy People focus areas and measuring progress in order to reach the dual goals of increasing healthy life span and reducing disparities in health.

On the positive side, research indicates that older adults, on average, take better care of their health than does the general population.[3] Individuals of 65-plus years are less likely than younger adults to drink alcohol, be overweight, smoke, or report that stress has adversely affected their health. The lower rates of drinking alcohol and smoking can be attributed to the tendency toward discontinuing these habits in older age, whether done spontaneously or in response to a medical condition or advice, and to the higher mortality rates of those who were drinkers or smokers at younger ages.[3]

Older adults, however, are less likely to engage in regular physical exercise.[3] Inactivity poses serious health hazards to both young and old. Lack of exercise can lead to coronary artery disease, hypertension, obesity, tension, chronic fatigue, premature aging, poor musculature, osteoporosis, and inadequate flexibility. Many older adults, and younger adults also, believe that aged individuals are too old to begin or participate in a fitness program; however, research indicates that even those with chronic conditions can benefit from an appropriately designed fitness program.[8]

Dental Hygienist's Role in Health Promotion

The dental hygienist as an educator and health promoter can provide appropriate wellness information and reinforce positive lifestyle habits of older clients, thus facilitating the human need for self-determination and a wholesome body image. Health promotion is different from traditional patient educational activities in several ways. Traditional preventive dentistry programs focus on a specific disease problem, usually caries or periodontal diseases, and teach clients the causes, progression, treatment, and preventive strategies used to prevent that specific disease. Health promotion, by comparison, does not focus solely on disease identification and eradication, but includes a broader conception of activities designed to raise an individual's level of functioning in health.[9] Pender explains that health promotion is approach behavior, through the inclusion of healthful activities in a comprehensive manner to increase the level of health functioning; disease prevention is avoidance behavior in that specific behaviors are decreased or suppressed in order to reduce the chance of reoccurrence.[9]

Five dimensions of wellness that professionals can use to form the basis for the development and implementation of wellness programs include self responsibility, nutritional awareness, physical fitness, stress management, and environmental sensitivity.[3] For example, some beneficial health activities for older adults include the following:

- ✦ Begin or maintain a physical activity program.
- ✦ Consume a nutritious diet low in fermentable carbohydrates, sugars, and fats.
- ✦ Limit exposure to ultraviolet light.
- ✦ Avoid exposure to pollutants such as alcohol, tobacco, noise, and polluted air and water.
- ✦ Prevent infections and diseases; identify and treat them early if they do occur.
- ✦ Practice appropriate oral hygiene behaviors.
- ✦ Manage stress effectively.
- ✦ Remain mentally active and alert.

The dental hygienist advocates a heart-healthy lifestyle with clients through health education and promotion activities.

AGE-RELATED AND PATHOLOGY-INDUCED PHYSIOLOGIC CHANGES

Age-related and pathology-induced changes in the human body occur at differing chronologic ages. Table 48–2 provides a summary of the alterations in dental hygiene care of older adults with physiologic changes in the following categories: cardiovascular system, respiratory system, joint disease, stroke, diabetes, and cirrhosis of the liver.[10] These physiologic changes are briefly discussed in the following sections.

Cardiovascular Changes

AGE-RELATED. Some physiologic changes that occur in the cardiovascular system are the result of aging of the body and are independent of pathologic processes. These physiologic changes affect the efficiency with which the cardiovascular system functions and alter the function of the whole body. Because the cardiovascular system is the link to providing the oxygen and nutrients needed by tissues for metabolic requirements, changes in this system affect the entire body.[11]

Text continues on page 972.

TABLE 48–2 ALTERATIONS IN THE DENTAL HYGIENE CARE OF OLDER ADULTS

Condition	Potential Risk Relating to Dental Hygiene Care	Prevention of Medical Complications	Dental Hygiene Care Plan Modifications	Oral Complications
Angina pectoris	Stress and anxiety related to oral healthcare visit may precipitate angina attack in the oral healthcare setting. Myocardial infarction may occur when older adult is in the oral healthcare setting. Sudden death caused by disruption of cardiac rhythm or cardiac arrest without acute myocardial infarction may occur in the oral healthcare setting.	1. Detection of older adult with history of angina pectoris 2. Referral of older adult thought to have untreated or unstable angina based on medical history for medical evaluation and treatment 3. Older adult under medical treatment for angina; during oral healthcare visit, every attempt should be made to reduce stress a. Concern and warm approach by oral healthcare professionals b. Make older adult feel free to talk about fears c. Morning appointments; however, some evidence supports early afternoon appointments as possibly better d. Short appointments e. Premedication—diazepam (Valium), 5 to 10 mg; one tablet preoperatively and/or night before; consider prophylactic nitroglycerin f. Nitrous oxide–oxygen analgesia or low-flow oxygen via nasal canula may be beneficial g. Effective local anesthetic—maximum epinephrine 0.036 mg or levonordefrin 0.20 mg can and should be used; aspirate; inject slowly (do not use vasoconstrictors in patients with a serious arrhythmia) h. Avoid epinephrine-impregnated retraction cords i. Avoid anticholinergic drugs j. Daily aspirin or other antiplatelet aggregation drugs do not usually cause clinically significant bleeding 4. Reinforce importance of risk factors that can be influenced by older adults. 5. Terminate appointment if patient becomes fatigued or develops change in pulse rate or volume. 6. If older adult develops chest pain during hygiene care, stop procedure and give nitroglycerin tablet sublingually. a. If pain is relieved, let older adult rest and then continue with appointment or terminate appointment and reschedule for another day. b. If pain continues longer than 5 minutes, monitor vital signs and give up to two nitroglycerin tablets one at a time during the next 10 minutes; if after three nitroglycerin tablets within a 15-minute time period pain persists and older adult's condition is stable, transport to hospital emergency room and call physician; if patient is unstable, call for medical aid and be prepared to render cardiopulmonary resuscitation	Older adults with stable form of angina, any routine oral healthcare Older adults with unstable form of angina, only care needed to deal with oral pain and/or infection	Usually none; however, on rare occasions older adults may have lower jaw pain of cardiac origin (referral pain); history of what initiates the pain and how it is relieved should provide clue to its cardiac origin.
Congestive heart failure	Sudden death resulting from cardiac arrest or arrhythmia Myocardial infarction Cerebrovascular accident Infection Infective endocarditis if heart failure is caused by rheumatic heart disease, congenital heart disease	1. Detection and referral to physician 2. No routine dental care until under good medical management 3. In older adults under good medical management with no complications, any indicated dental care can be performed. Cause of heart failure and any other complications must be considered in the dental hygiene care plan. a. Hypertension b. Valvular disease (rheumatic heart disease) c. Congenital heart disease d. Myocardial infarction e. Renal failure	In older adults under good medical management with no complications, any indicated dental care can be performed.	Infection Bleeding Petechiae Ecchymoses Drug-related a. Xerostomia b. Lichenoid mucosal lesions

	Shortness of breath Drug side effects a. Orthostatic hypertension (diuretics, vasodilators) b. Arrhythmias (digoxin, overdosage) c. Nausea, vomiting (digoxin, vasodilators) d. Palpitations (vasodilators)	f. Thyrotoxicosis g. Chronic obstructive lung disease 4. For older adults in the less severe stages, Class I and II, use maximum 0.036 mg epinephrine or 0.20 mg levonordefrin; avoid vasoconstrictors in Class III and IV older adults. 5. Older adult should be in the semisupine or upright position during care to decrease collection of fluid in lung. 6. Terminate appointment if older adult becomes fatigued. 7. Drug considerations a. Digitalis—older adult more prone to nausea and vomiting b. Anticoagulants—dosage should be reduced so that prothrombin time is 2 times normal value or less (takes 3 to 4 days) c. Antidysrhythmic drugs (see cardiac arrhythmias) d. Antihypertensive agents (hypertension) e. Avoidance of outpatient general anesthesia		
Hypertensive disease	Stress and anxiety related to oral healthcare visit may cause increase in blood pressure; in older adult with already elevated blood pressure as a result of hypertensive disease, myocardial infarction or cerebrovascular accident may be precipitated. Older adults being treated with antihypertensive agents may become nauseated or hypotensive, or may develop postural hypotension. Excessive use of vasopressors may cause significant elevation of blood pressure. Sedative medications used in older adults taking certain antihypertensive agents may bring about hypotensive episodes.	1. Detection and referral of older adults with marked elevation of blood pressure and those with moderate prolonged elevation of blood pressure for medical evaluation and treatment. For those older adults with blood pressure higher than 180/110, delay elective care and refer to a physician. 2. Older adults being treated with antihypertensive agents a. Reduce stress and anxiety of oral healthcare visit by premedication, short appointments, morning appointments, and concerned atmosphere by oral healthcare professionals; let older adult talk about fears and concerns related to oral healthcare visit; nitrous oxide–oxygen analgesia can be used, but hypoxia must be avoided. b. If older adult becomes stressed, terminate appointment. c. Avoid orthostatic hypotension by changing chair positions slowly and supporting client when he or she gets out of chair. d. Avoid stimulating gag reflex. e. Select sedative medication and dosage cautiously. 3. Drug considerations a. Use of local anesthetics with small concentration of vasopressor (epinephrine 0.036 mg; levonordefrin 0.020 mg); aspirate before injection and inject slowly. b. Use caution when using vasoconstrictors in older adults taking a nonselective beta blocker. c. Do not use gingival packing material that contains epinephrine. d. Reduce dosage of barbiturates and other sedatives whose actions may be enhanced by many antihypertensive agents. e. Avoid use of general anesthesia in the office.	In older adults under good medical management with no complications, such as renal failure, any indicated treatment may be provided. In older adults with complications, refer for evaluation.	Xerostomia secondary to diuretic agents and other antihypertensive medications Mercurial diuretics may cause oral ulceration or stomatitis. Lichenoid reactions may be seen with thiazides, methyldopa, propranolol, and labetalol. Lupus-like reaction, rarely seen with hydralazine.

Table continued on following page

TABLE 48–2 ALTERATIONS IN THE DENTAL HYGIENE CARE OF OLDER ADULTS—CONT'D

Condition	Potential Risk Relating to Dental Hygiene Care	Prevention of Medical Complications	Dental Hygiene Care Plan Modifications	Oral Complications
Myocardial infarction	Cardiac arrest Myocardial infarction Angina pectoris Congestive heart failure Bleeding tendency secondary to anticoagulant Electrical interference with pacemaker	1. No routine oral healthcare until at least 6 months after infarction because of increased risk of new infarction and arrhythmias. 2. Consultation with older adult's physician before starting routine oral healthcare to confirm older adult's current status. 3. Morning appointments 4. Short appointments 5. Termination of appointment if older adult becomes fatigued or short of breath or develops change in pulse rate or rhythm; inform physician. If older adult develops chest pain during appointment, manage as described with a client with unstable angina. 6. Use of local anesthetic with maximum epinephrine 0.036 mg and levonordefrin 0.20 mg; aspirate before injecting; inject slowly; avoid use of vasopressors to control local loss of blood; also avoid use of vasopressors in gingival packing material; do not use epinephrine in local anesthetics with severe arrhythmias. 7. Premedication before appointment and/or the night before to reduce stress associated with oral healthcare visit—diazepam, 5 to 10 mg 8. Anticoagulant medication—if surgery or scaling procedures are planned for older adult taking warfarin, physician should be contacted to confirm that PT ratio (prothrombin time) will be 2 times normal or less, or INR less than 3.0; patients taking aspirin or other antiplatelet aggregation drug may have increased bleeding, but it is not usually clinically significant. 9. Digitalis—older adult more prone to nausea and vomiting; avoid stimulating gag reflex. 10. Antisialagogues—atropine and scopolamine may cause tachycardia; check with older adult's physician before using. 11. Antiarrhythmic agents—quinidine, procainamide—nausea and vomiting may occur; hypotension may occur; oral ulceration may indicate agranulocytosis. 12. Antihypertensive agents (refer to section in table) 13. Avoid use of instruments such as ultrasonic scaler with older adults who have pacemaker.	Older adults 6 months or more after infarction with no complication, any routine oral healthcare can be performed. If complications such as congestive heart failure are present, oral healthcare should be limited to immediate needs only.	
Asthma	Precipitation of acute asthmatic attack	1. Identification of asthmatic older adult by health history 2. Determination of character of asthma a. Type (allergic or nonallergic) b. Precipitating factors c. Age at onset d. Frequency and severity of attacks e. How usually managed f. Medications being taken g. Necessity for past emergency care 3. Avoidance of known precipitating factors 4. Consultation with physician for severe, active asthma 5. Older adult should bring medication inhaler to each appointment and use prior to appointment.	None required	Oral candidiasis reported with use of inhaler without spacer, but is rare.

		6. Drug considerations: avoid a. Aspirin b. NSAIDs (nonsteroidal anti-inflammatory drugs) c. Narcotics and barbiturates d. Macrolide antibiotics (erythromycin) if older adult is taking theophylline 7. May want to avoid sulfite-containing local anesthetic solution. 8. Chronic corticosteroid use may require supplementation. 9. Premedicate anxious older adult (nitrous oxide–oxygen analgesia or diazepam). 10. Provision of stress-free environment		
Tuberculosis	Tuberculosis may be contracted by dental hygienist from actively infectious older adult. Older adults can be infected by oral healthcare professionals.	CAVEAT: Many older adults with infectious diseases cannot be identified by history or examination; therefore all older adults should be approached using universal precautions. 1. In older adults with active sputum-positive tuberculosis a. Consultation with physician before dental hygiene care b. Care limited to emergency care only c. Care in hospital setting with proper isolation, sterilization, mask, gloves, gown, ventilation d. When older adult produces consistently negative sputum and remains in chemotherapy, is provided same care as normal patient 2. In older adults with past history of tuberculosis a. Approach with caution; obtain good history of disease and its treatment (treatment of at least 6 to 18 months' duration); appropriate review of systems is mandatory b. Should give history of periodic chest x-ray films and examination to rule out reactivation c. Consult with physician and postpone care if: (1) Questionable history of proper care (2) Lack of appropriate medical supervision since recovery (3) Signs or symptoms of relapse d. If present status "free of active disease," care provided same as normal older adult 3. In older adults with recent conversion to positive skin test (PPD) a. Should have been evaluated by physician to rule out active disease b. May be receiving isoniazid (INH) for 1 year prophylactically c. Care provided same as normal patient when physician authorizes care 4. In older adults with signs or symptoms of tuberculosis a. Referral to physician and postpone treatment b. If treatment necessary, care provided as in category 1	None required	Oral ulceration (rare), tongue most common Tuberculosis involvement of cervical and submandibular lymph nodes (scrofula)
Joint disease: osteoarthritis	Joint pain, stiffness, and loss of mobility Increased bleeding from aspirin or nonsteroidal anti-inflammatory drugs	1. Short appointments 2. Ensure physical comfort a. Position changes b. Comfortable chair position c. Physical supports 3. Aspirin or NSAIDs may result in increased bleeding but usually not clinically significant. 4. If joint prosthesis, antibiotics not necessary unless "high risk" (rheumatoid arthritis, diabetic, immunosuppressed or previous infection).	Dictated by severity of disability; if severe, extensive care not indicated; encourage and facilitate oral health–promoting behaviors.	Temporomandibular joint involvement

Table continued on following page

TABLE 48–2 ALTERATIONS IN THE DENTAL HYGIENE CARE OF OLDER ADULTS—CONT'D

Condition	Potential Risk Relating to Dental Hygiene Care	Prevention of Medical Complications	Dental Hygiene Care Plan Modifications	Oral Complications
Joint disease: rheumatoid arthritis	Joint pain and immobility Increased bleeding secondary to aspirin and nonsteroidal anti-inflammatory drugs Bone marrow suppression from gold salts, penicillamine, sulfasalazine, or immunosuppressives resulting in anemia, agranulocytosis, or thrombocytopenia	1. Short appointments 2. Physical comfort a. Position changes b. Comfortable chair position c. Physical supports 3. Management of drug complications a. Aspirin/nonsteroidal anti-inflammatory drugs may result in increased bleeding, but not usually clinically significant. b. Gold salts, penicillamine, sulfasalazine, or immunosuppressives; obtain complete blood count with differential and bleeding time 4. If joint prosthesis, prophylactic antibiotics recommended.	Dictated by severity of disability and temporomandibular joint involvement; if severe, extensive care not indicated; temporomandibular joint surgery may be helpful; encourage oral health–promoting behaviors.	Temporomandibular joint involvement; anterior open bite possible Stomatitis secondary to gold salts, penicillamine, and immunosuppressives
Joint prosthesis		1. Deep infection around joint prosthesis secondary to bacteremia caused by acute infection elsewhere in body; there is no evidence that transient bacteremias caused by invasive dental procedures can infect these prostheses 2. Several authors have suggested that patients with active rheumatoid arthritis, severe type 1 diabetes mellitus, congenital or acquired immune deficiency, hemophilia, loose prostheses or history of infection of prostheses may be at risk, but there again are few data to support this concept.	Obtain good health history. There are few data to support the use of antibiotic prophylaxis. In contrast, most orthopedic surgeons still recommend prophylaxis. Obtain medical consultation regarding need for prophylaxis. If orthopedic consultant does not recommend prophylaxis, proceed without it. If orthopedic consultant recommends prophylaxis, consult with dentist and patient to determine best course of action.	None
Stroke	Dental hygiene care could precipitate stroke. Bleeding secondary to drug therapy	1. Identification of stroke-prone older adult from health history (hypertension, smoking, transient ischemic attacks) 2. Reduce older adult's risk factors for stroke. 3. For past history of stroke a. For current transient ischemic attacks (TIAs)—no elective care b. Drug considerations—aspirin and dipyridamole (Persantine), obtain pretreatment bleeding time (less than 20 minutes); warfarin (Coumadin), obtain prothrombin time under 35 seconds c. Short morning appointments d. Monitor blood pressure e. Use minimum amount of vasoconstrictor in local anesthetic f. No epinephrine in retraction cord	Dependent on physical impairment All restorations should be readily cleansable; avoid porcelain occlusals. Modified oral hygiene aids may be needed.	None

Diabetes	In uncontrolled diabetes a. Infection b. Poor wound healing In older adult treated with insulin, insulin reaction In older diabetic clients, early onset of complications relating to cardiovascular system, eyes, kidneys, and nervous system (angina, myocardial infarction, cerebrovascular accident, renal failure, peripheral neuropathy, blindness, hypertension, congestive heart failure)	1. Detection by a. Health history b. Clinical findings c. Screening blood glucose level 2. Referral for medical diagnosis and treatment 3. Monitor and control hyperglycemia. 4. Older adult receiving insulin—prevent insulin reaction a. Advise older adult to eat normal meals before appointments. b. Schedule appointments in morning or midmorning. c. Advise older adult to inform you of any symptoms of insulin reaction when they first occur. d. Have sugar in some form to give in case of insulin reaction. 5. Older adults with diabetes being treated with insulin who develop oral infection may require increase in insulin dosage; consult with physician in addition to aggressive local and systemic management of infection (including antibiotic sensitivity testing). 6. Drug considerations a. Insulin reaction b. Hypoglycemic agents, on rare occasions aplastic anemia, etc. c. In severe diabetics, avoid general anesthesia.	In well-controlled diabetes, no alteration of dental hygiene care plan is indicated unless complications of diabetes present, such as: Hypertension Congestive heart failure Myocardial infarction Angina Renal failure	Accelerated periodontal disease Periodontal abscesses Xerostomia Poor healing Infection Oral ulcerations Mucormycosis Numbness, burning, or pain in oral tissues
Cirrhosis	Bleeding tendencies; unpredictable drug metabolism	1. Identification of alcoholic older adult a. Health history b. Clinical examination c. Repeated detection of odor on breath d. Information from friends of relatives 2. Consultation with physician to verify current status 3. Attempt to direct older adult into treatment 4. Laboratory screening a. Complete blood count with differential b. AST, ALT c. Bleeding time d. Thrombin time e. Prothrombin time 5. Minimize drugs metabolized by liver 6. If screening tests abnormal, consult physician	Because oral neglect is commonly seen in alcoholics, older adults should demonstrate interest in and ability to care for dentition before any significant dental hygiene care is performed.	Neglect Bleeding Ecchymoses Petechiae Glossitis Angular cheilosis Impaired healing Parotid enlargement Candidiasis Oral cancer Alcohol breath odor Bruxism Dental attrition Xerostomia

Modified from Little JW, Falace DA: *Dental management of the medically compromised patient*, ed 5, St Louis, 1997, Mosby.

The most common change in the older person's heart is within the myocardium—the thick layer of heart muscle. Muscle fibers decrease and some are replaced by fibrous tissue; consequently, oxygen is used less efficiently. Research indicates that stiffening of heart muscle fibers is partially modifiable with physical conditioning.[3] Generally, heart size remains about the same throughout the life span if no change occurs in an individual's activity level or if disease is not present. With age, the heart valves stiffen and become thicker as the collagen degenerates and fatty deposits accumulate. Cardiac output is decreased with aging, although the decrease can be retarded, to some degree, by physical conditioning.[12]

Decreased elasticity of arteries is responsible for various vascular changes that affect blood flow to body organs such as the heart, liver, and kidneys. Circulation in the coronary arteries diminishes by approximately 35% after the sixth decade, and increased resistance to peripheral blood flow occurs at a rate of about 1% per year.[3] With normal aging, some atherosclerosis is normal, but it can be exacerbated to a pathologic state by a diet high in saturated fat. Under nonstressful conditions, however, the older person's cardiovascular system can adapt to its functional ability if the system is not greatly damaged.[11]

PATHOLOGY-INDUCED. Cardiovascular disease accounts for more than 50% of all deaths among the aged and is the primary cause of hospital admissions of older adults.[10] Most individuals older than 65 years have cardiovascular disease, most commonly in the form of coronary heart disease or hypertension.[3] Although national consumer and professional education efforts have focused on increasing understanding of the reasons for taking medications to control hypertension and compliance with medical regimens, it is estimated that only 49% of individuals take their medication regularly as prescribed.[13]

Irregular compliance with medication and other treatment regimens can complicate care and provoke potential emergency situations. Routine monitoring of vital signs at each visit serves to evaluate the client's health status and open discussion regarding the need to increase compliance and seek more frequent care. Because stress and anxiety related to dental hygiene care may increase blood pressure, resulting in myocardial infarction or cerebrovascular accident, precautions should be taken to meet the older adult's human needs for protection from health risks and freedom from anxiety and stress.

Respiratory Changes

AGE-RELATED. Age-related alterations in the respiratory system and pulmonary performance occur gradually, allowing the older adult to continue to breathe effortlessly in the absence of pathologic states. Confronted with a little exertion or stress, however, dyspnea (difficulty in breathing) and other symptoms can appear.[11]

The efficiency of the respiratory system declines with age, as evidenced by decreased elasticity of the muscles of the chest and increased rigidity of internal lung structures. The ultimate result is less efficiency in emptying of lungs and a reduction in the diffusion of oxygen. Coupled with cellular and humoral immunity decline, older adults are rendered susceptible to respiratory infections and other diseases.[3]

PATHOLOGY-INDUCED. Pulmonary diseases are a significant cause of death and disability in older adults. Moreover, many respiratory diseases are linked directly to or are exacerbated by lifestyle practices, chiefly smoking. Chronic obstructive pulmonary diseases (chronic bronchitis and emphysema) are caused primarily by inhalation of smoke via cigarette smoking and to a lesser degree by air pollution.[10] Older adults are susceptible to several life-threatening respiratory diseases including asthma, pneumonia, and influenza. In addition, the older individual is more likely to have inactive tuberculosis than any other age group.

Dental hygiene care for persons with respiratory disease includes modifications in positioning (upright posture) in the dental chair so that breathing is not impeded. Clients with asthma who utilize an inhaler should bring it to their appointment. In addition, a low-stress environment (whenever the oral healthcare setting is the least active) can reduce the probability of an asthmatic attack (Table 48–2).

Musculoskeletal Changes

AGE-RELATED. Musculoskeletal changes associated with the aging process affect the posture, function, and gait, and may take on a variety of appearances. There is a general flexion and forward projection of the head and neck. The back becomes humped; the hips, wrist, and knees slightly flexed; the muscles of the arms and legs flabby and weak; and the overall height reduced. Movement and gait become slower and appear clumsy, and the older adult appears less than agile.[3]

With aging, the skeletal system undergoes a reduction in the skeletal mass. Vertebral disks become thin, causing a shortening of the torso. Posture and structural changes occur primarily because of calcium loss from bone and as a result of atrophy of cartilage and muscle. The loss of muscle mass can be attributed to a decrease in the number and size of muscle fibers. Fibrous tissue replaces muscle tissue when muscle regeneration no longer occurs, resulting in a decrease in the power of the muscle.[12] Movement, motor power, and locomotion are complex physiologic functions that have interrelationships with the circulatory and nervous systems. Changes in these systems directly affect physical activity and muscle reflex capabilities. The loss of bone mass coupled with changes in muscle fibers affects bone strength, placing the older client at greater risk for fractures. Fractures, in turn, can lead to decreased mobilization, which contributes to further bone mass loss. Immobilization is a primary factor associated with institutionalization of older adults.

Ligaments, tendons, and joints become hardened, more rigid, and less flexible, predisposing these structures to tears. Worn cartilage around joints, combined with a diminished lubricating fluid in the joints, can lead to slow, painful movement.[11]

PATHOLOGY-INDUCED. Arthritis is a major source of discomfort and disability for many older adults, accounting for serious limitations in activity.[3] It is the most common chronic disability in older adults, and among seniors age 70 and older, 50% of men and 64% of women in 1995 reported suffering from some form of arthritis.[1] The term *arthritis* is a generic term that literally means inflammation of a joint. There are more than 100 different kinds of arthritis, but the most common among the aged are osteoarthritis and rheumatoid arthritis.[10]

Osteoarthritis, the most common joint disease, is usually encountered in persons older than 50 years. The disease is a defect of articular cartilage, characterized by the gradual loss of cushioning. As cartilage is lost, the resultant exposure of rough underlying bone ends can cause pain and joint stiffness. Bone growths or spurs may appear, producing joint enlargement. As the condition continues, low-grade inflammation of the synovial membrane develops. Thus inflammation is a secondary effect rather than the initial lesion of osteoarthritis.[10] Weight-bearing joints, including the spine, knees, and hips, are commonly affected sites, whereas the wrists and knuckles are not. Surgical intervention may be necessary to relieve pain and correct joint deformity.

Rheumatoid arthritis is a chronic, systemic disease affecting connective tissue throughout the body. The hands and feet are most commonly affected, in addition to the knees, hips, ankles, and shoulders. Symptoms of rheumatoid arthritis include malaise, fatigue, fever, anemia, and nodules that develop on soft tissues.[3]

Joint diseases are seldom identified as causes of death, but they can interfere significantly with one's body image, self-determination, and freedom from pain. Rheumatoid arthritis can greatly affect the older person's ability to perform ADLs such as preventive oral healthcare. Modifications in oral hygiene aids such as enlarged handles or extension devices and automated mouth-cleaning devices may be necessary for individuals to meet their needs for a biologically sound dentition and skin and mucous membrane integrity of the oral cavity.

The older client with joint disease frequently needs the dental hygienist to facilitate human need fulfillment for protection from health risks. For example, the older adult who has undergone joint replacement may need to be premedicated to prevent bacteremia from occurring, and clients using aspirin or nonsteroidal anti-inflammatory drugs must be monitored for increased bleeding (Table 48–2).

Osteoporosis is a condition involving demineralization of the bone and a decrease in bone mass caused by excessive leaching of calcium from the bone matrix. Generally, bone is constantly being broken down and rebuilt at the same rate. In osteoporosis, however, the rate of breakdown exceeds the buildup rate, causing a net loss of bone mass.[3] These changes significantly reduce bone strength, making bones, especially those in the back, hips, and forearms, more susceptible to fractures. Osteoporosis can result in diminished height, stooped posture (dowager's hump), and chronic pain, and it is the major cause of skeletal fractures in postmenopausal women and all older persons.[3]

The disease is four times more prevalent in women than in men. Females are more prone to the disease because they have less bone mass initially and because changes during menopause lower calcium and estrogen levels. Loss of bone mass begins in the fourth decade, but it is seldom diagnosed until after a fracture occurs. Over their lifetimes, women lose 25% to 30%, whereas men lose 12% of their bone mass because of osteoporosis.[10]

Several intrinsic factors have been identified as increasing the risk of osteoporosis, including gender, race, heredity, and body frame. Although these factors cannot be altered, lifestyle practices can influence the integrity of bone and the bone thinning process (see Intrinsic and Extrinsic Factors Associated with Osteoporosis).

The National Research Council of the National Academy of Science has established a daily maintenance dose of calcium that prevents the body from drawing on its mineral stores in bone. For the older woman, 1000 to 1200 mg of calcium is recommended and 1500 mg if the woman is not taking estrogen therapy.[3] Approximately four glasses of nonfat or low-fat milk provide 1200 mg of calcium. For individuals who are lactose intolerant, many

Intrinsic and Extrinsic Factors Associated with Osteoporosis

Intrinsic
Female gender
White race
Small-boned body frame
Northern European ethnicity
Slender

Extrinsic
Inadequate weight-bearing exercise
Inadequate calcium intake
Use of alcohol and tobacco products
Chronic medication usage
Corticosteroids
Isoniazid
Tetracycline
Aluminum-containing antacids
Diseases
Hyperparathyroidism
Kidney disease
Rheumatoid arthritis
Diabetes mellitus
Chronic obstructive pulmonary disease

green vegetables, sardines, and nuts can serve as sources of calcium. Calcium is best absorbed from dairy products and food; however, dietary supplements (calcium carbonate tablets) can be consumed. Calcium carbonate supplements are absorbed best when taken with meals. Older adults who have a family history of kidney stones should seek a physician's advice before using calcium supplements.[10]

Dental hygienists should advocate adequate calcium intake for all clients to facilitate the human need for protection from health risks and a biologically sound and functional dentition in later life. Maximum bone deposition occurs by the mid-thirties. Consequently, after age 35, calcium products and calcium supplements are recommended to maintain bone quantity and quality.[3]

Neurosensory Changes

As aging occurs, both structural and functional neurologic changes become evident.[3] Structural changes include loss of neurons, loss of total brain weight, and development of neurofibrillary tangles. Functional changes include a decrease in synaptic transmission between neuronal cells and a longer reaction time in the neuromuscular and autonomic nervous systems.[11] In addition to a decreased amount of synaptic transmission, the neurons are slower in sending these transmissions. The electroencephalogram (EEG) is a measure of brain wave activity. EEG tracings of the older person show delayed activity compared to EEG results in a younger person.

Cognitive Function

The distinction between normal and abnormal brain changes in the aging process has been studied intensively during the past 40 years.[3] Early studies encouraged the stereotype of the older adult as being forgetful and incapable of learning. More recent studies of the aging brain show that there is no serious cognitive decline in the absence of disease, trauma, or stress.[3] Furthermore, results show that intellectual decline is not an outcome of aging alone, but rather is caused by many conditions such as poor nutrition or hormonal changes.[10] An older adult usually takes longer to learn the same information as a younger adult, but given sufficient time, the end result is similar. Investigations of memory indicate that more time is needed for recall of information; however, differences are found between short- and long-term recall.[11] Short-term memory appears to decline after age 65 years.

Conversely, older adults seem to have a very large capacity for long-term memory. Usually, long-term information is highly organized by time and place or meaningful relations. It is important to note that most intellectual testing of older adults has been through cross-sectional research design rather than longitudinal investigations. Consequently, the same group or cohort of older adults was not evaluated over the time needed to provide reliable data regarding changes in that group. Rather, older adults were compared to younger adults, which may not account for differences such as level of education, sensory changes, and motivation between the groups.[3]

Changes in cognitive functioning and sensory changes affect the older adult's likelihood of understanding, performing, and adhering to a preventive oral hygiene program.[10] Dental hygienists must be cognizant of these alterations, whether age-related or pathologically induced, to facilitate human need fulfillment in the older adult through dental hygiene care.

Sensory Changes

Sensory modalities are in a constant state of transition, and compensations are increasingly required over the course of the life span. Eventually, a reduced efficiency of all of the sensory organs occurs, requiring adaptation by the older adult to feel competent and satisfied in the later years.[3] The older adult with impaired vision or hearing may often be unfairly labeled as stubborn, eccentric, or senile. Dental hygienists need to be aware of sensory changes in older adults in order to adapt their oral hygiene instruction when appropriate. For example, an older adult with diminished eyesight may not be able to read the instructions for a prescribed procedure and, therefore, does not implement the suggested method. The following is a discussion of changes in vision, hearing, taste, smell, and touch with related oral hygiene implications.

AGE-RELATED VISUAL CHANGES. Several physical and chemical changes occur in the eye as an individual ages.[3] The eye becomes less accommodating because the lens becomes more rigid and does not change shape as easily to see objects at close range and at a distance. *Presbyopia* is the term for this degenerative change. The lens becomes more opaque and yellows with age.[11] Compounded by a reduced pupil size, the older adult may have difficulty discerning certain color intensities, especially the cool colors. Blue, green, and violet are filtered out and may be difficult to differentiate. Warm colors, including red, yellow, and orange, are generally more easily seen, which makes it advisable to mark objects such as steps, handrails, and operatory equipment with these bright, warm colors for easier visibility.[14]

More light is needed for the older person to see the same objects that a younger person visualizes, and glare presents a significant problem. Educational materials should be provided in a well-lit room and should be printed on nonglare paper. Finally, the cells in and around the eye lose water and shrink. Pockets of skin, or bags, appear around the eyes and can interfere with vision if the lids sag far enough over the eyes. The lacrimal glands, which keep the eye moist, produce less fluid, leading to drying of the eye and increased irritation.

PATHOLOGY-INDUCED VISUAL CHANGES. Three disorders—cataracts, glaucoma, and macular degeneration—represent the most common visual problems of the older adult. Each can be responsible for serious loss of vision.

Cataracts are the most common disability of the aged eye.[3] If an individual lives long enough, she or he will develop cataracts to some degree. A cataract involves an opacity of the normally transparent lens. As the lens loses its transparency, there is interference with the passage of light. Risk factors include female gender, smoking, malnutrition, exposure to sunlight and ultraviolet radiation, and advanced age. Treatment consists of surgical removal of the opaque lens. Surgery is indicated when vision loss interferes with the performance of activities. Eyeglasses, contact lenses, or intraocular lens implants are used to compensate for the loss of the lens. Research currently is being conducted to determine the relationship between vitamins (vitamins C and E) and nutrients (zinc) and delay of development of cataracts.[3]

Glaucoma, a condition in which intraocular pressure increases, is the second most common visual problem in the aged and the primary cause of blindness among African-American older adults.[10]

Glaucoma occurs from an obstruction in the normal escape route of the nutrient fluid within the chambers of the eye. When this flow is obstructed, intraocular pressure builds because the production of fluid occurs faster than it can be eliminated. Eventually, pressure is transferred to the optic nerve, leading to irreparable damage. If left untreated, glaucoma leads to blindness. Risk factors include advanced age, diabetes, family history, race, hypertension, and myopia (nearsightedness).[3] Treatment consists of medication to keep the pupil constricted and decrease fluid production. Surgery may be required to provide new channels for fluid elimination. Dental hygienists should be aware of the symptoms of glaucoma, which include complaints of eyes feeling tired, headaches, halos around light, and blurred vision. The symptoms seem to be more evident early in the morning, and one or both eyes may be affected. Clients describing these symptoms should be referred to their primary care physician.[10]

Age-related macular degeneration (AMD) occurs because of deterioration in the membrane between the retina and underlying blood vessels.[3] Damage occurs to the macula, the key focusing area of the retina. As a result, central visual acuity declines, which makes it difficult to perform tasks such as driving or reading. The etiology of AMD is not well understood but appears to be most strongly associated with age. Genetic factors, smoking, serum cholesterol, and light iris color also seem to play a role. Treatment, with varying success, involves use of lasers to seal off or destroy the abnormal blood vessels. In addition, closed-circuit television and magnifying glasses can assist individuals who are affected with AMD.

The reduced ability to focus the eye and the presence of cataracts may make it difficult for the older adult to navigate, especially in unfamiliar surroundings such as the oral healthcare setting.[14] Also, decreased kinesthetic sensitivity in the elderly person results in postural instability. Providing written directions and educational materials in large print greatly assists the visually impaired person and meets the human need for responsibility for oral health.

HEARING DISORDERS. Impaired hearing is common among older persons, with 30% of females and more than one-half of males older than 65 years exhibiting significant hearing loss.[3] Presbycusis is defined as the progressive loss of hearing as a result of the aging process. There are two major types of hearing loss that may occur in the older adult: conductive and sensorineural.[10] Conductive hearing loss is an interruption in the transmission of sound waves caused by damage to the auditory nerve or a buildup of ear wax. Sensorineural deafness is related to a disorder of the inner ear; a loss of nerve cells in the eighth cranial nerve results in a loss of hearing high-frequency sounds. Presbycusis and noise-induced loss are coexistent in many instances.

The ability to hear is a major means of communication.[3] Hearing loss is not only frustrating to the older adult, but it may also threaten an individual's safety and self-esteem. Dental hygienists should look for signs of hearing loss such as inappropriate responses, lack of response, withdrawal, confusion, or anger.[14] Dental hygienists should help clients compensate for hearing loss by speaking slowly, distinctly, and in a low voice tone. Individuals should be addressed face to face, with the face mask removed when possible. Gestures also enhance and clarify conversation and should be used liberally with older adults.[12] Shouting or speaking in high-pitched tones and using simplistic language should be avoided. Individuals who have hearing loss because of conduction deficits may use a hearing aid or an assisted listening device to compensate for the loss. Dental hygienists should alert clients to turn down the hearing aid or remove it to avoid hearing the high-pitched noises that occur when the ultrasonic instrumentation or high-speed handpieces are used.

CHANGES IN TASTE. As a person ages, modest changes in the sensation of taste occur as a result of diminished number and functional ability of the tastebuds.[3] Up to 60 years of age, the ability to perceive sweet, sour, bitter, and salt does not appear to change. During the sixth decade of life, some gradual erosion of the ability to taste salt is apparent but not significant. Although an individual may lose taste on part of the tongue (from trauma or viruses), other parts of the tongue overcompensate for at least part of the loss. The inability to distinguish various tastes or flavors is often caused by other factors such as diminished sense of smell or medication usage.[12]

Taste problems can include ageusia (complete loss of taste), *dysgeusia* (altered taste), hypogeusia (decreased ability to taste), and unpleasant or bitter taste. The most frequently reported taste change is dysgeusia.[13] Older clients should be referred to their physician for review and potential substitution of medications to reduce side effects.[12] Unfortunately, many clients will compensate for taste changes and increase the use of sweet, sugary foods, which will increase the risk for dental decay.

LOSS OF OLFACTION. Loss of olfaction (smell) with age is not well understood. Age-related degenerative changes in the olfactory bulb or damage of the nerves that service the olfactory bulb may be responsible for impaired olfactory function.[3] The receptors in the olfactory bulb that perceive smell tend to atrophy in the aging process, and the individual is unable to smell odors as distinctly as do younger adults.[11] Diminished smell results in a decline in taste perception. As a result, affected older adults may have a diminished appetite, with the potential for malnutrition. Whether observed deficits in olfactory acuity have functional significance for the quality of life among older adults is unclear. Undoubtedly, more research is warranted in this area.

LOSS OF KINESTHETIC ABILITY. Touch, or kinesthetic sensitivity, refers to the ability to discriminate temperatures, perceive spatial relationships, and discern pain. With advanced age, older adults lose their kinesthetic ability, leaving them vulnerable to accidental falls and postural instability.[3] Consequently, in the oral care setting, attention should be devoted to securing loose rugs and to the placement of furniture and equipment. Additionally, a decrease in tactile sensations can affect fine motor discrimination for hand-to-eye coordination.[14] Coupled with arthritic complications, some older adults may have difficulty completing oral hygiene and will need adaptive devices, such as powered oral hygiene devices or larger handles, or may need assistance with oral hygiene activities at home.

Neurosensory Disorders

Three disabling, prominent neurologic disorders in older adults are cerebrovascular accident (CVA), dementia, and Parkinson's disease.

CEREBROVASCULAR ACCIDENT. A CVA or stroke is caused by a thrombus (usual cause in older adults) or a hemorrhage that results in a cerebral infarct. CVA is the most common neurologic cause of problems related to coordination and mobility.[3] Strokes rank third as the most common fatal affliction in the latter half of life.[10] Survivors of strokes often experience temporary or permanent paralysis and may require adaptive aids or assistance in performing oral hygiene care (Table 48–2). Prevention of strokes includes smoking cessation, hypertension control, aspirin therapy, and removal of symptomatic blockages.[10]

DEMENTIA. Also called organic brain syndrome, dementia is a progressive brain impairment that interferes with normal intellectual functioning. Classic symptoms include significant losses of at least three of the following: cognition, memory, language, recognition, visual and spatial skills, and personality.[3] All behaviors may not be present at all times and they may vary in intensity. Those individuals with mild organic brain syndrome cannot abstract and assimilate new information. In severe cases the individual loses self-care skills and becomes incontinent. Dementia is classified as either reversible or irreversible.

The incidence of dementia increases with age, afflicting 5% of those 65 to 75 years and more than 20% of those 85-plus years old. Some degree of dementia is present in more than one-half the nursing home residents. It is estimated that 45 to 50 billion dollars are spent each year in maintaining those with organic brain syndrome.[3]

Historically, dementia was believed to be an acceleration of the normal aging process caused by arteriosclerosis of the arteries that supply the brain with oxygen. Researchers now find that dementia can be caused by several factors: brain tumors, fever, trauma, environmental toxins, chronic lung disease, alcoholism, drug abuse, and stroke. Most dementias are irreversible and result in progressive, permanent mental impairment.[10]

ALZHEIMER'S DISEASE (AD). This disease is irreversible and is the most common form of dementia. It is characterized by the accumulation of neurofibrillary tangles and senile plaques within the cerebral cortex. The etiology is unknown, although there are indications that AD is familial. In 1997, approximately 4 million individuals in the United States were found to have Alzheimer's disease.[3] The prevalence of the disease increases with age and was found in 3% of individuals age 65 to 74 years, and in 47% of seniors 85 and older.[10] AD is a primary factor affecting the institutionalization of older adults in the later stages of the disease.

Individuals with AD progress through three stages lasting from 2 to 15 years or longer (see Stages of Alzheimer's Disease).[3] Providing oral healthcare for AD clients can be difficult in the later stages of the disease because of their inability to tolerate dental and dental hygiene care. To meet the client's human needs for freedom from anxiety and stress, and protection from health risks, the recommended course of action is to complete dental and dental hygiene care in the early phase of the illness when client cooperation is achievable.[10]

Approximately one-third of individuals with AD have seizure disorders requiring phenytoin. Consequently, gingival hyperplasia is a common oral finding in the presence of poor oral hygiene[13] (see Figures 39–5 and 39–6). Other medications, anticholinergics, may induce salivary gland dysfunction, resulting in xerostomia.[14]

The dental hygiene care plan should begin with a thorough health history including all medications.[10] Depending on the stage of the disease, an accurate history may need to be obtained from the caregiver or physician. The oral examination is similar for all clients, but a mouth prop may be useful during the examination and treatment. The dental hygiene care plan must be realistic for the client's medical and physical condition and oral health condition.[10] Also, the oral hygiene care plan must delineate the role of the caregiver in the maintenance of daily oral hygiene care. Aggressive prevention with frequent maintenance care appointments (every 2 to 3 months) averts the need for extensive treatment at a

Stages of Alzheimer's Disease

Stage 1: Mild Impairment (2 to 4 Years)
Memory loss (predominant symptom)
Forgetfulness
Spatial disorientation
Inability to perform complex routine activities
Errors in judgment
Neglect of appearance
Inability to find objects
Denial of deficits

Stage 2: Moderate Impairment (2 to 10 Years)
Increasing memory loss
Flat affect
Wandering
Sudden mood change
Repetitive movements
Constant motion
Unclear speech
Restlessness at night
Sensory deficits
Intensified personality deficits

Stage 3: Severe Impairment (1 to 3 Years)
Confinement to bed or chair
Unresponsiveness
Rigidity
Incontinence
Seizures
Delusions
High risk of infections

time when the client is unable to cooperate for the dental and dental hygiene care.

As the disease progresses, the individual with AD has difficulties with verbal abilities and with understanding the meaning of what is said. Frequently, their behavior becomes the primary means of communication with others. Similarly, as verbal abilities deteriorate, AD clients become more sensitive to nonverbal behavior of their caregivers. Dental hygienists should look directly at AD clients when speaking and establish eye contact to focus their attention. Verbal and nonverbal messages need to match because individuals with AD are inclined to respond to the nonverbal message. For example, the meaning of "relax" is not understood if said in a tense tone of voice. Verbal communication should consist of exact, positive words or simple sentences delivered in a slow, calm, low voice.[15]

Daily oral hygiene for individuals with AD usually rests with the primary caregiver. Home care for dentate clients should include toothbrushing with a fluoridated toothpaste. Because flossing can be difficult, an interdental brush is recommended for interdental cleaning. Fluoride and/or antimicrobial rinses are contraindicated because AD clients have difficulty understanding that the substance should not be swallowed, but daily caregiver-applied fluorides (toothbrush-applied gels) may be indicated as an adjunctive therapy.[15] Saliva substitutes are useful for AD clients with xerostomia (also see Chapter 38).

MULTI-INFARCT DEMENTIA. The second most common type of dementia is multiinfarct dementia.[3] Small strokes occur within the brain, which causes an insufficiency of blood to some areas and consequent death of the brain tissue. Appearance is sudden, with symptoms of dizziness, headaches, and decreased energy in addition to the classic dementia symptoms. The course of this type of dementia is erratic. Initially, individuals may recover lost function, but as more small strokes occur, the chance of recovery decreases. This type of dementia is associated with hypertension.[10]

PARKINSON'S DISEASE. This is a chronic, progressive disorder caused by pathologic changes in the basal ganglia of the cerebrum, resulting in a deficiency of dopamine. It is characterized by muscle rigidity, involuntary tremors, loss of postural stability, and slowness of spontaneous movement; there is no impairment in intellectual function.[10]

Individuals with Parkinson's disease demonstrate excess salivation and drooling. The facial expression is motionless, with diminished eye blinking. Tremors in lips and tongue are common, and many individuals have difficulty in swallowing.[3] Adaptive aids and enlarged toothbrush and floss handles should be provided for these clients to facilitate self-care and hence self-determination whenever possible[10] (also see Chapter 38).

Other Disorders

Several other multifactorial conditions are prevalent among the aged that affect the practice of dental hygiene. The following are some additional diseases that may alter dental hygiene care of older adults.

ANEMIA. Anemia is a common blood disorder among older adults. The two types of anemia seen most frequently are iron-deficiency anemia and pernicious anemia.[10] Iron-deficiency is the most frequent form of anemia, seen more often in females. Chronic aspirin intake, often noted in clients with arthritis, can be a contributing factor leading to blood loss. Pernicious anemia, a progressive disease, is caused by vitamin B_{12} and folic acid deficiency in older adults. Anemia caused by inadequate iron intake can make the tongue appear red, smooth, and painful. Pernicious anemia results in a beefy red tongue. Other oral tissues are usually pale or yellowish in color. A person with severe forms of anemia may not be able to tolerate dentures or toothbrushing because of discomfort.

DIABETES MELLITUS. Diabetes mellitus among older adults is the seventh most frequent overall cause of death (see Chapter 41 for a description of the disease). Current estimates suggest that approximately 9% of all older persons in the United States suffer from diabetes.[3]

Older women appear slightly more susceptible than older men. At all ages, African-Americans are affected more often than whites.[10]

Oral complications in individuals with uncontrolled diabetes are related to excessive loss of fluids (*xerostomia*), increased susceptibility to infection, and delayed healing times.[12] Often a high prevalence of periodontal disease, angular cheilitis, and mucosal changes is found among clients with uncontrolled diabetes.[16] Uncontrolled or unstable diabetes usually indicates the need for antibiotic premedication to reduce the possibility of infection. Appointments should be scheduled midmorning following the client's breakfast if possible.

ALCOHOLISM. Alcohol has been identified as an important causative factor for many chronic diseases.[3] One of the most significant effects of alcohol abuse is liver damage that impairs other organ systems. Liver damage may appear as alcoholic hepatitis or cirrhosis, a chronic inflammatory disease of the liver.[10]

Alcohol affects the cardiovascular system (cardiomyopathy) and nervous system (organic brain syndrome). Also, alcohol has been identified as a contributing factor in malnutrition, leading to general poor health and anemia.[10] Persons who abuse alcohol are likely to suffer accidents, falls, and serious injury. Oral manifestations commonly observed in alcoholics include increased bleeding tendencies and bruises, and poor oral hygiene may be evident because of overall neglect.

ORAL CONDITIONS IN THE AGED

As with other physiologic alterations, the distinction between age-related oral changes and those that are disease-induced is not always clear or conclusive. Disease, consequences of disease, and use of medications often manifest oral changes and pathology independent of the aging process.

In the last century, perhaps the most significant change in older adults' oral status is the decline in *edentulousness* (total tooth loss). Data show that although 55% of the 65- to 74-year-olds were edentulous in 1957–1958, the proportion had decreased to approximately 40% in 1985–1986, and decreased to 30% in 1997.[7,16] Changes in treatment philosophies (restore rather than extract), improved treatment modalities, and advances in prevention have played a significant role in reducing tooth loss among older adults, especially the young-old, although significant disparities exist among the current group of older adults, with higher rates of edentulousness seen among low-income individuals (48%).[7] It is expected that the rate of edentulousness will probably continue to decline for future cohorts of older adults. Within the focus area of oral health, the *Healthy People 2010* document has identified the target goal of reducing the rate of edentulous older adults to 20% of the population.

Dental Changes

AGE-RELATED. With age, teeth undergo several changes, including alterations in the enamel, cementum, dentin, and pulp.[16] Enamel becomes darker in color because of lifetime consumption of stain-producing foods and drink and the formation of secondary dentin. The enamel surface develops numerous cracks (acquired lamellae) and obtains a translucent appearance. The enamel surface has calcium and phosphate constantly dissolved and redeposited during the active phases of caries. During the active phases of caries dissolution, the surface appears clinically dull, with slight exploration revealing a chalky surface. Arrested dental caries in older adults often appear as a brownish-black discoloration because of lifelong uptake of dyes in enamel lamellae.[17]

Occlusal fissures frequently appear darkly stained in older adults partly as a result of previous active dental caries that have changed into an inactive stage. Occlusal attrition often smoothes the occlusal area, which reduces microbial accumulation in the fissure. These fissures may appear slightly sticky on probing, but they may not need restoring.[18] Therefore, vigorous exploring must be avoided in order not to mechanically damage the porous part of the fissure enamel.

Cementum undergoes compositional changes, including an increased fluoride and magnesium content. Abrasion of the crowns of teeth is compensated for by deposition of cementum at the apical end and bifurcated areas of the roots. This secondary cementum is normally deposited slowly and continuously throughout life.[17]

Two independent changes are found within the dentin:

- ✦ Secondary dentin formation
- ✦ Obturation of dentinal tubules (dentin sclerosis)

As a result, the vitality of the dentin is greatly decreased, and aged dentin may become entirely insensitive and impermeable.[17]

The pulp undergoes the same changes that occur in similar tissues elsewhere in the body: pulpal blood supply decreases, the number of cells decreases, and the amount of fibers increases in aged adults. Because pulp calcifications increase with advancing age, the size of the pulp chamber is reduced. Pulp calcifications appear to form in both erupted and unerupted teeth.[16]

Attrition is common along the incisal and occlusal surfaces as a result of a lifetime of wear, habits, and dietary factors. The attrition present in older individuals is often so severe that dentin is exposed on the incisal and occlusal surfaces.[19] Many of today's older adults used a stiff toothbrush and abrasive paste in the past. Consequently, abrasion of the teeth, especially in the cervical area and on root surfaces, may be evident. Abrasion, although common among older adults, is the result of a physiochemical process rather than a result of aging. Although modern dentifrices are not sufficiently abrasive to severely damage intact enamel, they can cause remarkable wear of cementum and dentin if the toothbrush is used in a horizontal rather than vertical direction. Dental hygienists can assist individuals in maintaining a biologically sound dentition and freedom from pain through appropriate oral hygiene educational instructions.

PATHOLOGY-INDUCED. Both coronal and root caries are active in the older adult population. Dental caries were once considered childhood phenomena, but research suggests that older adults are more likely to develop new coronal and root caries at a greater rate than the adult population.[18] For example, although 30% of adults 18 to 64 had at least one area of untreated decay, 37% of dentate older adults age 65 to 74 had at least one area of root decay, and 49% of older adults 75 years and older had at least one area of root decay.[7]

Root caries are most prevalent among older populations because of both local oral factors and factors related to aging. Local factors include exposed root surfaces and tooth longevity, and factors related to aging include changes in salivary quantity and composition caused by medication and disease occurrence and inability to complete thorough oral hygiene because of disabilities and chronic conditions. The presence of root caries often indicates disruptions in multiple systems rather than just local factors and requires a multidisciplinary perspective by oral healthcare providers.[17,18] Predictors of root caries include the presence of elevated amounts of *Streptococcus mutans* and *Lactobacillus,* higher plaque biofilm scores, the presence of restored coronal and root decay, xerostomia,[18] gingival recession, and periodontal pocketing. Root caries can develop rapidly in the absence of adequate oral hygiene and in the presence of xerostomia, suboptimal periodontal health, and ingestion of fermentable carbohydrates.

Caries control and prevention activities must address three interrelated factors: (1) removal of bacterial plaque biofilm, (2) reduction of refined carbohydrates and snacking in the diet, and (3) use of topical fluoride. Oral hygiene activities are often compromised in older adults because of sensory and neuromuscular changes as a result of aging and/or disease. Use of adaptive devices, such as powered toothbrushes and modifications in handle size, width, and grip, will provide assistance for older adults in thorough plaque removal. Poor dietary practices involving the overconsumption of soft, retentive refined carbohydrates and frequent snacking patterns are common among older adults and are complicated by salivary changes that promote dental decay.[20] Older adults and their caregivers should receive specific instruction regarding optimum food choices and nutritional patterns to promote oral health, especially since compromised health status and dentition may have resulted in an overdependence on soft, bland diets. Replacing sweet snacks with cheese and crackers, and substituting sugar-free hard candy for mints are examples of two specific dietary interventions that may be more easily and realistically implemented for older adults.[20]

Aggressive caries prevention and management must include frequent and liberal use of topical fluoride products for both home use and professional application. In addition to the use of a fluoridated toothpaste, many older adults find the 0.05% sodium fluoride rinses easy to use and helpful in caries reduction. Many older adults have difficulty swallowing, however, and prefer the use of the 1.1% sodium or 0.4% stannous fluoride gel, which can be applied directly to the root surfaces and adapted into the proximal surfaces with a small interproximal brush.[14] Professional application of sodium fluoride in either the 2.0% gel[18] or 5.0% varnish[21] has been shown to be an effective caries-preventive agent for both coronal and root caries.

Periodontal Changes

AGE-RELATED. There is an increase in alveolar bone porosity and a decrease in cortical width with aging, but this increased porosity has been found to be unrelated to the presence of teeth and does not lead to crestal resorption. Research shows that crestal bone loss with aging is minimal in healthy persons.[11] Osteoporosis primarily effects decreases in bone mass and increases in porosity.[3] Also, a reduction in metabolism and reduced healing capacities can influence the quality of bone. Alveolar bone quality can significantly affect the older adult's ability to wear oral prosthetics. Difficulty in mastication can occur.

Gingival epithelium reportedly shows no significant morphologic changes with age, although there is evidence of a thinning of the epithelium, diminished keratinization, and increased cellular density.[11] A reduction in cellular elements and an increase in fibrous intercellular substance have been noted in gingival connective tissue. A reduced number of nerves in the gingiva and increased evidence of nerve degeneration with increasing age have been found, along with arteriosclerotic changes in gingival vessels. An increase in gingival width seen with aging has been attributed to growth of the alveolar process, along with eruptive movements of the teeth and supporting tissue.

Alteration in periodontal ligament cellular function, increases in calcification, and arteriosclerosis are seen with advancing age. Numerous morphologic, biochemical, and metabolic changes can be observed in the periodontium with aging, but the overall significance of these factors as they affect susceptibility and progression of periodontal disease is unclear. It appears, however, that in the absence of disease, the clinical changes in the periodontal structures attributable to aging alone are therapeutically insignificant.

PATHOLOGY-INDUCED. Advanced stages of periodontal disease are more commonly seen in people of 45 years and older; age is often erroneously associated with causing the disease. Research indicates that the effect of age on the progression of periodontitis is considered negligible when good oral hygiene is maintained.[22] Nevertheless, studies confirm an association between increased age and increased recession, loss of attachment, and higher prevalence of gingival inflammation.[22]

The level of periodontal health in middle age can be used as a predictor of periodontal disease in later life. Data suggest that the prevalence and severity of periodontal disease will likely decrease within a few decades as the present younger age groups, with better oral hygiene and less periodontal disease, move into their sixties and seventies.[22] National studies document this decline because the national NHANES III (National Health and Nutrition survey) found that only 15% of the population has advanced periodontal disease. Among those age 65 and older, however, 41% had at least one site with significant periodontal destruction.[23]

Dental hygienists should provide aggressive treatment to prevent and control periodontal diseases in older adults. More frequent dental hygiene care visits provide the opportunity to instruct the older adult in proper oral hygiene and use of chemotherapeutic agents to control gingivitis, such as triclosan dentifrice and essential oil mouthrinse. Prescription of 0.12% chlorhexidine gluconate may be indicated for older clients who need an additional level of microbial control.[14]

Oral Mucosal Changes

AGE-RELATED. In the absence of disease, the oral mucosal status of older adults is comparable to that of younger adults, suggesting that aging alone does not lead to changes in the oral mucosa.[3]

PATHOLOGY-INDUCED. Some mucosal alterations are a result of systemic factors (e.g., xerostomia) and are not related to aging, per se. Systemic disease and medication use cause some older adults to have changes in their oral mucosa, including atrophy of epithelium and connective tissues with a decrease in vascularity. Clinically, the oral mucosa appears dry, smooth, and thin. Fungal infections (candidiasis) may result from utilization of broad-spectrum antibiotics, such as amoxicillin, and xerostomia-causing medications.[10]

Lips may appear dry and drawn as a result of dehydration and loss of elasticity within the tissues.[11] Angular cheilitis, commonly evidenced among the aged, clinically appears as fissuring at the angles of the mouth, with cracks, erythema, and ulcerations. Moistness from drooling, deficiency of vitamin B_2 (riboflavin), and infection by *Candida albicans* are the etiologic factors associated with this condition.[19]

Ill-fitting dentures or poor denture hygiene also can result in mucosal irritation and infection, including denture stomatitis or candidiasis and denture-induced fibrous hyperplasia.[17] Denture "sore mouth" reflects a commonly seen condition also known as chronic atrophic candidiasis, present in as many as 65% of older individuals who wear dentures.[19] Chronic atrophic candidiasis is associated with poor prosthesis fit, which leads to chronic trauma, and retention of the denture during sleeping hours, which promotes bacterial and fungal growth.[19] The signs of denture-induced fibrous hyperplasia include single or multiple elongated folds near the border of an ill-fitting denture (Figure 48–3). The human need for skin and mucous membrane integrity of the head and neck necessitates that the dental hygienist provide palliative treatment and refer the individual to the dentist for further evaluation.

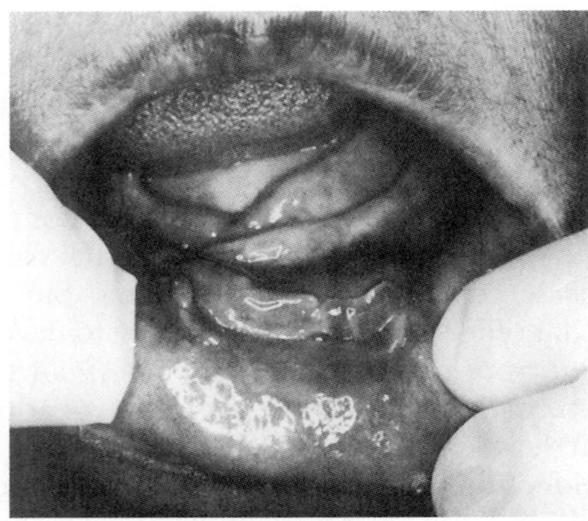

FIGURE 48–3 ✦ Denture-induced fibrous hyperplasia. *(From Regezi JA, Sciubba JJ:* Oral pathology: Clinical-pathologic correlations, *ed 3, Philadelphia, 1997, WB Saunders.)*

Oral cancer continues to be a particular problem for older adults because the average age of diagnosis is 60 years. Oral cancer is more common in men than in women and represents about 2.5% of the total cancers diagnosed each year.[19] All older adults should receive a thorough soft tissue oral examination at each visit so that the dental hygienist can carefully evaluate any early mucosal changes that may indicate precancerous or cancerous lesions and provide early referrals for prompt evaluation and treatment.

Tongue Changes

AGE-RELATED. Changes in the tongue may include a decrease in the number and sensitivity of papillae.[11] Combined with a decline in the sense of smell, some foods have less appeal, and nutritional needs may not be met. Sublingual varicosities are customary findings among the aged; however, they are not problematic. Clinically, they appear as deep red or bluish-black dilated vessels on either side of the midline on the ventral surface of the tongue.

PATHOLOGY-INDUCED. Because of nutritional factors, older adults frequently have anemia as a result of iron deficiencies.[20] Atrophic glossitis is a symptom of this condition, and the tongue appears smooth, shiny, and denuded. Often, individuals complain of a burning sensation.[19] In addition, the tongue often increases in size in edentulous mouths or as a result of disease (e.g., pernicious anemia).[19] The dental hygienist can assist the individual to maintain freedom from pain by recommending an oral lubricant to reduce discomfort and by providing dietary counseling.

Salivary Gland Changes

Research has shown fairly well that reductions in salivary flow are not a result of the normal aging process.[3] Rather, decreases in salivary flow are usually attributed to systemic disease, radiation therapy, tumors, or medications that cause temporary or permanent xerostomia.[10] Signs and symptoms of salivary reduction should be carefully evaluated to determine the cause. In the absence of medications, underlying diseases and the possibility of salivary gland tumors should be investigated.

SJÖGREN'S SYNDROME. Sjögren's syndrome is an autoimmune disorder of the salivary glands occurring most frequently in postmenopausal women. Approximately 60% of people with this disorder are older than 50 years.[10] Clinically, the oral mucosa is extremely dry and saliva is ropy. Initially the tongue shows marked atrophy of the papillae, and later the surface becomes smooth and lobulated (Figure 48–4). To meet the need for mucous membrane integrity, persons with Sjögren's syndrome should be instructed to use saliva substitutes. For dentate individuals, fluoride therapies (rinses or daily gels) may be recommended to help meet the need for a sound dentition.

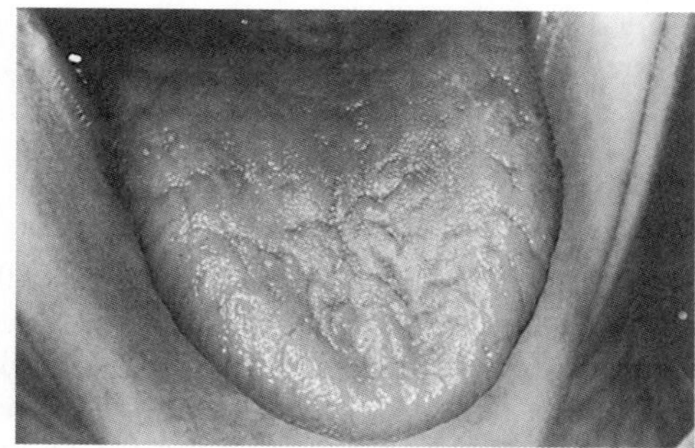

FIGURE 48–4 ✦ Sjögren's syndrome with severe xerostomia. *(From Ibsen OAC, Phelan JA: Oral pathology for the dental hygienist, Philadelphia, 1992, WB Saunders.)*

DRUG-INDUCED ORAL CHANGES. Approximately one-third of all prescription and over-the-counter drugs are used by older adults, even though these individuals account for only 13% of the population. *Polypharmacy* is the term to describe the common practice of prescribing multiple drugs to clients to manage their many medical conditions.[13] On average, most older adults take more than three therapeutic agents, and the institutionalized elderly use between five and seven drugs at the same time. Older clients are more likely to experience adverse reactions because of physiologic changes in the heart, liver, and kidney, and also because of the increased exposure and potential for interaction of both prescription and over-the-counter medications. For example, it has been estimated that the potential for interaction is 6% when two agents are prescribed, which rises to 50% chance of interaction when five drugs are prescribed and 100% when eight or more drugs are given together.[13]

Medications most frequently used by older adults include analgesics, diuretics, oral hypoglycemics, antihypertensives, antidepressants, and sedatives. Multiple medical problems, along with multiple drug use, can lead to a high rate of adverse drug reactions. Many drugs produce oral changes in the mouth because of side effects or as a consequence of the actions of the drug.[13] Dental hygienists play an especially important role in identifying medication usage and potential side effects.

XEROSTOMIA. Xerostomia is a common side effect of many prescription and over-the-counter medications, such as antihypertensives, antipsychotics, antidepressives, muscle relaxants, antihistamines, and laxatives.[13]

Saliva plays an important role in proper function of the oral cavity because it lubricates the oral mucosa, assisting speech and swallowing, facilitates the retention of oral appliances, and provides a source of minerals for enamel remineralization.[16] Diminished salivary flow can alter taste, contribute to plaque formation and dental caries, and cause the oral mucosa to appear dry and inflamed. For edentulous persons, denture retention, comfort, and ability to chew and speak may become difficult when less saliva is present.[11] Diagnosis can be complicated because xerostomia is often complicated by a coexisting candidal infection.

Management of xerostomia should include palliative care through the use of saliva substitutes, oral lubricants, and frequent water intake. Attempts to stimulate salivary flow can include the use of sugarless lemon or grape candies or gum and the frequent ingestion of small meals, which may reduce mouth dryness. Medications, such as the cholinergic agents pilocarpine and bethanechol, can be prescribed when the client's healthcare status permits and if the xerostomia is severe.[10] Also, consultation with the physician and clinical pharmacist may reveal a substitute medication that may reduce saliva in a less severe way for the client.

Clients with xerostomia should return for frequent recall and assessment of caries status. Aggressive caries prevention efforts should be recommended because the presence of xerostomia places the client in a high-risk category for caries. All of the following caries-prevention efforts are essential for the older adult in order to control root and coronal caries associated with xerostomia:[14,18]

- Regular and thorough brushing with both fluoride dentifrice and either high-dosage 2.0% sodium or 1.1% stannous home fluoride gel
- Interproximal plaque removal through flossing and/or interproximal brushing
- Nutritional counseling
- Use of 0.12% chlorhexidine rinses
- Frequent professional debridement
- Frequent professional application of either 2.0% or 5.0% sodium fluoride

DRUG-INDUCED GINGIVAL HYPERPLASIA. Persons taking anticonvulsants such as phenytoin may exhibit gingival hyperplasia as a side effect (see Figures 39–5 and 39–6). Adequate plaque control, particularly if started before the administration of phenytoin, may reduce the magnitude of gingival overgrowth. Also, clients with prescribed cardiovascular drugs (nifedipine) and immunosuppressants (cyclosporine) may exhibit gingival hyperplasia.[13]

DENTAL HYGIENE PROCESS OF CARE WITH OLDER ADULTS

Assessment and Dental Hygiene Diagnoses

Dental hygienists begin their assessment of overall physical factors by observing the older adult in the reception area. It is important to observe gait and balance because some elderly persons may require assistance to the treatment area. An arm should be extended for clients who appear unsteady or who have severe visual impairments. The dental chair should be positioned at the level of the knees or higher if the person has difficulty bending the knees. Also, the arm of the chair should be placed back as far as possible. If the client uses a wheelchair, transfer to the dental chair is necessary. The client should be asked if assistance is needed or which method of wheelchair transfer is preferred.

Impairments in both vision and hearing may necessitate assisting the elderly adult in completing any written forms in the office. Ideally, a health history in large print allows visually impaired clients to complete the form themselves. At times, it may be more effective and efficient to interview older clients. The person should be addressed in a low pitch with the face mask removed. Shouting is unnecessary and ineffective. Background noises such as music should be eliminated if possible. Individuals with hearing aids should be requested to keep them on while reviewing the client history or discussing oral hygiene methods; however, the volume should be reduced when using a rotary handpiece. Older adults accompanied by others should be addressed directly, not the family member or caregiver. By speaking directly to the elderly client, dental hygienists create a respectful, independent environment.

The health history should include the client's personal, medical, and dental background. Personal history, for example, may show that clients are widowed (may live alone, may have reduced income), which could affect their ability to receive dental care. The health history should include previous and past medical conditions. Both prescription and over-the-counter medications currently being used must be reviewed for oral implications. Dental hygienists should have readily available a current source for information on medications, such as a reference program, book, or credible Web site to investigate medications that are unfamiliar or not prescribed as the common drug of choice. Some individuals suffering from more than one disease may experience adverse effects from multiple drug use. The practitioner must consult with the client's physician if there is doubt regarding treatment. Vital signs, including respiration, pulse, blood pressure, and temperature (if indicated), should be evaluated and recorded. In addition to completing a thorough health history, the practitioner should be patient and listen to information that the client shares.

The extraoral examination can reveal abnormalities in the skin of the face and neck, lymph nodes, salivary glands, and underlying muscles. The mandible should be examined for movement, and the temporomandibular joint should be palpated for crepitation, tenderness, or limitations in movement. A client with arthritis may not be able to open his or her mouth fully.

A client's breath can indicate periodontal disease, systemic disease, or alcohol abuse. Lips must be evaluated for signs of angular cheilitis, muscle inelasticity, and presence of lesions. A complete dental charting and periodontal assessment must be part of every dental history to provide documentation for reevaluation. The quantity and quality of saliva must be assessed to ascertain if saliva substitutes should be recommended.

Radiographs and other diagnostic aids such as study models should be used as indicated and appropriate. Referral for biopsy may be indicated for suspicious lesions.

Oral hygiene status including plaque biofilm distribution, calculus, and stains must be assessed. Assessment of the client's ability to perform oral hygiene practices is essential. The older person's home care practices should be modified rather than attempts made to completely change the habits of 50-plus years. Compensation for physical changes such as arthritis and impaired vision may affect the client's ability to carry out oral hygiene recommendations.

If the client's vision and dexterity permit, individuals should be instructed to perform self-assessments of their plaque control methods and oral soft tissue examination. Periodic evaluation of their bacterial plaque control measures can be accomplished by using disclosing solution or gingival and plaque indices. Individuals should be advised to conduct an oral self-examination monthly to look for lesions that are painless and do not heal within two weeks.

The older client's nutritional status should be evaluated because of the many physiologic and psychosocial complexities that have been documented regarding dietary patterns for the elderly.[20] Dental hygienists can use the brief nutritional screening questionnaire "Determine Your Nutritional Health Checklist" as part of the health history information, which alerts oral health care providers to any deficiencies in food intake and related patterns that affect oral health and nutrition.[24] For example, older adults may avoid eating nutritious foods because of decreased oral function or because they are unable or unwilling to cook a full meal because they live alone or cannot shop at their usual location. Merely asking an older adult to describe their typical diet often sheds light on multiple issues that affect nutrition and health.

Dental hygienists plan and implement care based on the dental hygiene diagnosis, type and severity of chronic conditions, cognitive abilities and attitudes of the older adult, level of self-care, expectations, and financial ability. Table 48–3 is a presentation of dental hygiene diagnoses related to the older adult.

Short, morning appointments are recommended because many older adults have a lower stress tolerance and tire more easily than a younger person. A written note of date and time of each appointment should be

TABLE 48–3 SAMPLE DENTAL HYGIENE DIAGNOSES RELATED TO THE OLDER ADULT

Deficit in the Following Human Need	Due To	As Evidenced By
Wholesome facial image	Ill-fitting dentures	Client's self report of dissatisfaction with appearance of face and dentures
Freedom from anxiety and stress	Previous negative dental experiences	Client's report of fear of dentist
Freedom from head and neck pain	Chronic atrophic candidiasis	Client's report of mouth soreness
Protection from health risks	Diabetes type 2	Client's report of diabetes type 2
Responsibility for oral health	Inadequate care of mouth and denture	Stained denture Chronic atrophic candidiasis Infrequent dental visits
Conceptualization and understanding	Lack of proper denture and mouth care	Inability to describe appropriate care for mouth and denture

provided to help remind the client and assist caregivers, when necessary.

Planning

Dental hygiene care planning for older adults is often more complex than that for younger persons because the vast majority have at least one chronic condition and have complex dental and periodontal conditions. Also, normal aging alterations may create a compromised oral situation. Treatment modalities need to be developed based on individual considerations between the client, dental hygienist, dentist, and at times the physician and physical and occupational therapists.

A person's attitude toward oral health affects care planning and outcomes. Many older adults view oral problems as an inevitable part of aging. Also, research suggests that older people perceive a lower need for dental care than that which is actually required. Therefore, some older adults do not use dental services as frequently as recommended or do so only when dental emergencies occur.[23]

Implementation

During instrumentation, as little trauma as possible should occur to the gingiva because of reduction in healing capabilities. Loss of elasticity of lips and oral mucosa and xerostomia may make retraction of oral tissues uncomfortable. Older adults with a history of periodontal disease should be seen for more frequent periodontal maintenance therapy. Depending on the periodontal classification, scaling should be completed by quadrants to allow for short appointment times. Routinely, premedicated individuals should have as much care as possible at one time; however, the person's medical condition may compromise lengthy appointments.

Specific and customized oral hygiene instruction should be provided with older adults to ensure that they have the knowledge and skills necessary to thoroughly removal plaque biofilm. Chemotherapeutic products, such as triclosan dentifrice, essential oil mouthrinse, or 0.12% chlorhexidine mouthrinse, should be recommended when necessary to supplement mechanical plaque biofilm removal. Recommendations for improving the adequacy of the diet regarding food choices among the five food groups should be provided, with specific directions for limiting refined carbohydrate foods and limiting snacking.

Home use of topical fluoride products has been advocated for all older individuals with teeth. In addition to using a fluoride dentifrice, clients can use a daily nonprescription 0.05% sodium fluoride rinse, especially if they notice a decreased quality and quantity of saliva. Many older clients have difficulty rinsing their mouths, however, and a 1.1% sodium fluoride or 0.4% stannous fluoride gel, which is applied by a toothbrush, may be easier to use and may reach susceptible proximal and root surfaces. Clients who have undergone head and neck radiation therapy, who suffer from severe xerostomia, or who have rampant caries can use the tray method to apply the 1.1% sodium fluoride or 0.4% stannous gel in a tray for five minutes twice a day. The tray method of application is best completed with an unflavored fluoride product because of the frequency and intensity of the application.

Saliva substitutes are recommended for individuals with xerostomia. Saliva substitute is a preparation with physical and chemical properties similar to those of real saliva. A suitable substitute should coat the mucosa and teeth to keep them moist, reduce enamel solubility, and reduce the accumulation of plaque biofilm. Saliva substitutes can be used without limit on the frequency of use. The substitute is usually sprayed into the mouth and distributed through the mouth with the tongue. Several over-the-counter products are available, with some containing fluoride. The flavored varieties are usually more acceptable than the flavorless.[14]

Exposed root surfaces are susceptible to dental caries, and both professional and home-applied topical fluoride should be recommended to help meet the need for a biologically sound dentition. The role of plaque biofilm and diet in relation to dental caries formation needs to be stressed. A desensitization treatment and dentifrice also may be recommended to help ensure freedom from pain if root surfaces are sensitive.

At the completion of the appointment, the chair back should be straightened slowly. The client should be allowed to sit up for a short time before dismissal to avoid any problems with postural hypotension. The dental hygienist should pay close attention to see if the client needs assistance out of the chair. Postoperative instructions should be reviewed and a written copy provided as indicated.

Evaluation

After care has been completed, older clients need to be reevaluated more frequently and more carefully because of the many physiologic changes, chronic conditions, and pathologic changes frequently seen in this age group. Dental hygienists need to be aware that health status can change quickly with an older client, and even small changes may be significant, especially in relation to cardiovascular and cognitive changes. Often, a dental hygienist may be the first to notice cognitive declines over a series of appointments or at the recall visit. These qualitative perceptions that "something is not quite right" about the older client should be discussed with the client, relatives, and/or caregivers, and referrals for further medical evaluation provided.

Dental hygienists should allow a longer time to assess results of soft tissue debridement because of decreased healing of tissues, and provide additional care when necessary. Quantitative evaluation of health status through bleeding and plaque indices and pocket depth recording is essential to document healing and plan new interventions with older clients.

More frequent maintenance intervals should be recommended for older clients in order to evaluate any changes in functional abilities to complete oral hygiene, any nutritional changes, and the occurrence of new disease. Dental hygienists should not assume that older adults continue the same functional abilities, even in a three-month time period. For example, clients with musculoskeletal disorders frequently note varying functional abilities and may need more assistance with oral hygiene at times. In addition, clients may be taking new medications and may alter their nutritional patterns because of the unpleasant taste or increased xerostomia experienced with a different medication. These older adults may be at higher risk for caries and need more aggressive caries management. More frequent visits for dental hygiene care can provide the opportunity to assess the need and to recommend preventive and therapeutic interventions specific to the client's needs.

COMMUNITY HEALTH SERVICES

Institutionalized elderly comprise approximately 6% of the elderly population. Homebound, semidependent elderly account for another 5% to 6%. The numbers may be small, but these groups of elderly have the greatest oral needs and the most difficulty reaching dental services.[14,25]

The functionally dependent are more likely to be edentulous and may not have used dental services for more than eight years. Furthermore, research suggests that more than 80% have dental needs, with nearly 40% requiring immediate attention.[25] Among dentate individuals, three-fourths need scaling and prophylaxis, with other problems including root caries and poor oral hygiene.[26]

Several factors can be identified that have created this neglect.[14] First, people who are in a long-term care facility (LTCF) or are homebound may not be able to care for themselves. They may have numerous complicated and interrelated problems, and dental care may not be a priority. In addition, dental professionals have not been active in providing services because of their own attitudes toward treating the frail elderly, low financial return, and state practice acts that limit dental hygienists' ability to work unsupervised in LTCFs or with the homebound.[26]

The homebound elderly have additional problems to overcome. Some suffer from malnutrition, withdraw socially, or perceive that their speech is adversely affected. These factors can elicit low self-esteem, leading to depression. Problems of not eating and withdrawal can be exacerbated as a result.[16]

Provision of routine dental services is not included under Medicare (federal) benefits. Medicaid (state) dental benefits and eligibility vary by state; however, preventive dental care for elderly is usually not a priority. Given the high dental needs of homebound or institutionalized elderly, systems to provide care need to be advocated for and established.[16,25]

Traditional Dental Office

For individuals who are not bedridden, the traditional dental office may be the most appropriate site to provide care.[26] This is the ideal setting because all equipment and materials are readily available. Many of the elderly do not have a means of transportation to the dental office. Consequently, they cannot reach professional oral healthcare without the availability of a special transportation service. Because of the time and expense involved, however, dental offices may be reluctant to contract out for this type of program. Usually, a van must be available with a staff member to accompany the client.

When dental hygienists treat frail, elderly persons, care is complicated because of a variety of factors listed as follows:[25]

- ✦ *Appointment time.* Short, morning appointments should be scheduled. Most elderly are physically strongest in the morning. Because many cannot sit for long periods, however, two hours should be the limit, including transportation time.
- ✦ *Accessibility into the dental office.* Parking lots, ramps, and doorways must accommodate wheelchairs. Legally, the Americans with Disabilities Act of 1993 mandates access to all public facilities.
- ✦ *Communication with facility.* Most facilities require that services provided and instructions be in writing.
- ✦ *Legal considerations.* The elderly client may not be capable of providing informed consent. Therefore,

the practitioner will need to have written permission from the individual's physician, family, or facility.

- *Multiple health conditions and drug therapies.* Many elderly individuals have a multitude of chronic health conditions. Consultation with the physician may be necessary.

On-Site Dental Programs

Providing care in a long-term care facility or client's home has several advantages over the traditional dental office:[26]

- Frail elderly do not favorably withstand the disruption of being transported.
- Incontinent or catheterized individuals are best treated at their place of residence.
- It is less disruptive to the facility.
- A familiar environment reduces anxiety.

Some LTCFs have dental operatories set up within the facility. In others where it is not practical to establish an operatory, mobile equipment can be used. Mobile equipment and vans can be used for homebound persons as well.

Role of the Dental Hygienist

Dental hygienists serve in an important capacity with the institutionalized and homebound elderly in the following activities:[26]

- Providing clinical dental hygiene care
- Providing in-service education programs for staff
- Marking dentures for identification
- Giving fluoride applications
- Developing individual care plans
- Modifying oral hygiene aids

Nursing staff and aides are important intermediaries for oral health care professionals. Staff members should be encouraged to refer elderly individuals to the dental office or consulting dentist if they detect unusual signs, such as swelling or discoloration, or if they hear a verbal complaint. The Brief Oral Health Status Examination (BOHSE) can be used by nursing staff members to systematically evaluate oral health for clients at entrance to the care facility and routinely during care.[27] Dental hygienists can develop and implement in-service education programs to ensure that staff members have the knowledge and skill necessary to complete thorough oral assessments and oral hygiene care.

For homebound individuals, establishment of a prevention program using visiting nurses or home healthcare workers is needed when family members are not available. Some states have developed dental programs that use mobile vans, with both professionals and students providing services for homebound elderly. Dental hygienists can collaborate with local agencies, dental and dental hygiene associations, and dental hygiene educational institutions to develop oral screening, referral, and preventive programs for homebound elderly.

Client Education Issues

- Explain the differences between normal, physiologic changes seen in aging and pathologic changes
- Communicate a wellness philosophy of care to maximize health despite chronic conditions
- Explain health promotion strategies based on older adults' needs
- Encourage compliance with all medication and medical regimens
- Relate client's health status to any modifications necessary for dental hygiene care
- Adapt oral hygiene instructions to any functional limitations and oral health conditions
- Explain the development and prevention of dental caries
- Provide nutritional counseling regarding the reduction of refined carbohydrates, limited snacking, and adequacy of dietary intake
- Recommend the use of topical and professional fluorides to prevent dental decay
- Explain the development and prevention of periodontal diseases
- Recommend the use of chemotherapeutic agents by the client to prevent and control periodontal diseases
- Assist with tobacco cessation efforts
- Explain the importance of oral cancer prevention and early detection
- Provide education regarding drug induced changes in the oral cavity
- Explain methods to manage xerostomia
- Instruct family caregivers regarding appropriate oral assessment and oral hygiene care

Legal, Ethical, and Safety Issues

- Complete and document a thorough medical, social, and dental history and oral examination with each client.
- Refer older adults for consultation with the physician before dental hygiene care when indicated.
- Evaluate the client's use of medications and refer to the physician for consultation when indicated.
- Explain the results of consultation with the older adult and document conversations and the physician's recommendations in the client's chart.
- Use standard infection control procedures with all older clients.
- Provide and document informed consent with all older clients. When necessary, discuss and document treatment with family and/or caregivers.
- Involve older adults in treatment decisions.
- Treat older adults with dignity and respect.
- Provide written instruction that can be easily read by older clients and/or caregivers and reinforce instructions verbally.
- Provide aggressive prevention programs for caries and periodontal diseases.
- Ensure that the dental office facility is wheelchair accessible based on guidelines from the American Disabilities Act.
- Provide care without discrimination.

Key Concepts

- Older adults are a heterogeneous group, and there is tremendous variability in the physical, psychosocial, and environmental issues within this age group.
- Current demographic reports and projections indicate a significant rise in both the number and proportion of older adults within the United States.
- The older adult population is becoming more racially and ethnically diverse. Elderly women outnumber elderly men. Older adults are concentrated in certain states and are not distributed evenly in the population.
- Chronologic, or birth, age is not as good a measure as functional age when providing care with older adults.
- There is not one accepted theory to explain how and why we age. Several social and biologic theories of aging have been proposed and shed light on the aging process.
- There are normal, physiologic changes in most body systems that occur as individuals age. These normal changes should not be confused with pathologic changes caused by disease; however, distinctions between normal aging and pathologic conditions are sometimes difficult to discern.
- Most adults have at least one chronic condition, and the most common chronic conditions are arthritis, hypertension and heart disease, cancer, diabetes, and stroke.
- *Healthy People 2010* is a national planning document that identifies two major health goals for the nation: (1) increase the life span of healthy life and (2) reduce health disparities.
- The *Healthy People 2010* document contains health status indicators and focus areas for state and local communities to use to increase health status.
- Older adults develop coronal and root caries at a rate higher than the adult population.
- The rate of edentulousness (total tooth loss) is estimated at 30% and is projected to continue to decrease in future years.
- Caries prevention and control strategies for older adults must stress daily removal of plaque biofilm, reduction of refined carbohydrates, and use of topical fluorides.
- A small but significant number of older adults have advanced periodontitis, and there is a higher degree of loss of attachment and prevalence of gingivitis among older adults.
- Prevention and control of periodontal diseases should include daily removal of plaque biofilm, use of chemotherapeutic agents, and more frequent visits for professional debridement and evaluation.
- A small percentage of older adults (6%) reside in long-term care facilities and a similar percentage (5%) are confined to their homes. These individuals have a higher prevalence of dental disease and a lower utilization rate of dental care than the adult population.
- Dental hygienists can work with long-term care facilities and homebound individuals in a variety of roles to increase the oral health status.

CRITICAL THINKING EXERCISES

Client: Mrs. F

Profile: Mrs. F, age 77, returns for a dental hygiene visit on her regular 6-month maintenance schedule.

Chief Complaint: "I have a removable partial denture to replace my lower back teeth that I don't wear because it makes my mouth feel dry and taste bad. Also, I have a large freckle on my left cheek that has grown in the past several months."

Social History: Mrs. F has been widowed for three years and is active with her church and the families of her two daughters who live nearby.

Medical History: Mrs. F has a history of angina for the past six years and takes 50 mg Tenormin once a day to prevent angina attacks.

Dental History: Mrs. F has had a history of regular dental visits and has all of her teeth, with the exception of the four mandibular molars. Oral examination reveals a flat, brown elongated lesion approximately 10 mm long and 6 mm wide on the center of her left cheek. Mrs. F denies any pain or exudate from this lesion. Dental examination reveals no areas of decay and generally recession with no evidence of periodontal disease.

Oral Health Behavior Assessment: Good oral hygiene. Uses an electric toothbrush and floss daily.

Supplemental Notes: During dental hygiene care, Mrs. F states that she thinks her teeth are too short and ugly and asks you if she is too old to get "caps" on her teeth to improve her appearance.

1. What are the dental hygiene diagnoses for this client?
2. Develop a dental hygiene care plan for this client that includes goals and interventions.
3. What client education issues should be addressed?
4. What factors could be contributing to this client's dry mouth?
5. Are there any contraindications to this client's care?
6. What measures should be taken during treatment to prevent an angina attack?

Activity 1: Instant aging as a client in a dental office

This activity asks participants to simulate what it is like to be an older dental client in their office. This exercise provides a good opportunity to learn what older clients may be experiencing in the office and provides insight for participants regarding sensory changes in aging. This activity is divided into two tasks, and students should work in groups of two, alternating the role of client and dental hygienist. Partners are asked to complete tasks while they have simulated several sensory deprivations that older individuals may experience.

Task A: Partner 1 should wear glasses with a thin film of oil or lubricant to inhibit clear vision. In addition, partner 1 should tape the fingers of both hands to make fine motor tasks difficult. Partner 1 should complete a medical history form and/or other office forms for a new client. After the forms are completed (a brief time limit should be imposed), partner 1 should walk unassisted back to the treatment room and fill out additional forms in the dental chair.

Task B: Partner 2 should wear earplugs or use cotton/wax ear protectors to limit hearing. In addition, this partner should use an ace bandage or shoulder harness to restrict shoulder movement. Partner 2 should walk unassisted to the treatment room and complete a brief written form in the dental chair. Partner 2 should demonstrate both brushing and flossing technique and should be asked to describe the technique and answer questions about the performance.

Debriefing Discussion: After the simulated dental appointments are completed, participants should discuss their experiences in completing routine dental tasks with some sensory impairments. Although this is only a simulation, partners should be encouraged to discuss how this simulation is related to the experiences of their older clients. Partners should complete an "environmental audit" of their dental offices to assess how conducive their office environment is for the older individual, based on the environmental considerations discussed in this chapter. Hearing, vision, and motor skill impairments pose significant obstacles even when the environment is optimally conducive for older adults. By adopting the perspective of the client with some sensory-motor deficits, partners may be able to identify difficulties for older clients and make changes to provide care in a more sensitive, appropriate manner.

Activity 2: What is a typical day for an older adult at a senior community center?

Most communities provide a variety of services to older adults who are currently living in the community, but who may need some assistance with meals, social activities, health care, or housing. Administered through local agencies on aging and generally housed in a local community center, church, or other facility, these senior centers provide a modest level of support to enable older adults to function in an independent manner as long as possible.

In this learning activity, readers should contact the director of a local senior center and request to visit and/or volunteer at the center for at least two visits. Visits to these senior centers provide an interesting window on the daily life of older adults, especially if

Continued on following page

Critical Thinking Exercises—cont'd

participants have little experience with older individuals. The centers generally emphasize a philosophy of wellness and provide a wide range of activities to encourage participation by members. Depending on their interest and ability, older adults may complete a wide range of athletic activities, arts and craft projects, discussion groups, and scheduled trips to social and cultural events.

Participants who visit a senior center should keep a diary regarding the activities the seniors completed on the days on which they visited and should participate actively in the events scheduled for the day. For example, learners may wish to volunteer to share a craft activity with the older adults, lead an exercise or dance class, or call bingo for the session. During the visits, the participants should speak with as many seniors as possible to learn of their daily activities, why they participate in the center activities, and which activities and functions of the center they use most frequently. These informal discussions are generally welcomed by the older adults, who view these sessions as a chance to advise and guide younger individuals about the needs of older adults. In addition, these visits provide participants with the opportunity to understand the wide range of abilities these older individuals possess, even in light of chronic and disabling conditions. By observing and sharing activities, participants can view the active and varied nature of the seniors in their daily activities and gain an understanding of the challenges older adults face each day.

For References, Suggested Readings, and Related Websites, visit
http://evolve.elsevier.com/Darby/hygiene/

CHAPTER 49

Persons with Fixed and Removable Dentures

OBJECTIVES

Mastery of the content in this chapter will enable the reader to:

- Describe demographics, risk factors, disease patterns, and psychological factors associated with tooth loss
- Describe oral physiologic changes of the edentulous and partially edentulous client
- Identify appliances used in fixed and removable prosthodontic therapy
- Describe dental hygiene care implications for prosthodontic therapy
- Educate prosthesis-wearing clients about expectations, personal responsibility for oral health, importance of oral hygiene measures and regular professional care, and nutrition to maintain oral health
- Plan and evaluate dental hygiene care for clients with fixed and removable prostheses

KEY TERMS

Abutment
Angular cheilitis
Candidiasis
Complete denture (full denture)
Denture stomatitis
Edentulous
Exostoses
Fixed partial denture
Focal (frictional) hyperkeratosis
Implant denture
Mandibular tori
Obturator
Palatal tori
Papillary hyperplasia
Pontic
Prosthesis
Prosthesis-induced fibrous hyperplasia
Prosthodontic therapy
Reactive/traumatic lesions
Relining
Removable partial denture

Normally individuals are not conscious of the critical daily functions of teeth: eating, speaking, facial expression, and appearance. Once the teeth are lost, the person quickly realizes how eating becomes more difficult, speech is not as distinct, and facial tissues lose support, which ultimately impairs appearance and other people's perceptions of the person.

Edentulous, derived from the Latin word *edentatus,* means being without teeth or lacking teeth. Although the percentage of persons with tooth loss increases with age, it is not uncommon to find clients in their second through fifth decades of life with prostheses. A *prosthesis* is a fixed or removable appliance that is functionally and cosmetically designed to replace a missing tooth or teeth. Although maintaining the oral health of the individual with tooth loss entails the same basic elements of preventive and therapeutic care as for clients with a complete dentition, persons with missing teeth have specialized needs.

DEMOGRAPHICS OF TOOTH LOSS

Changing patterns in oral disease, professional care, and attitudes toward healthcare have decreased the number of completely edentulous individuals. There has been a gradual yet significant decline in the number of edentulous persons; however, given longer life spans and the growing elderly segment of the population, surveys indicate that the total number of edentulous individuals is between 20 and 25 million, suggesting that the provision of complete dentures is common in the oral healthcare environment.[1]

Approximately 30% of adults aged 65 or older are edentulous.[1] Approximately 50% of Canadian adults aged 65 and older are edentulous.[2] These figures suggest that dental hygienists are likely to encounter edentulous clients within any dental hygiene practice setting.

RISK FACTORS FOR TOOTH LOSS

Major risk factors that contribute to a person's edentulous status are as follows:

- Dental caries
- Periodontal diseases
- Low socioeconomic status
- Inadequate access to professional oral care
- Low frequency of professional oral care
- Poor daily oral hygiene

The primary reason for tooth loss before age 35 years is dental caries, while periodontal diseases are responsible for tooth loss during the third through the fifth decades of life. Oral cancer, and the corresponding treatment for oral cancer, and oral injury also contribute to tooth loss. In addition, tooth loss is influenced by a client's socioeconomic status, access to professional oral care, frequency of professional oral care, and daily oral hygiene.[2]

OTHER FACTORS ASSOCIATED WITH TOOTH LOSS

Psychological Factors[4]

Client attitude and values influence the success of care, and the edentulous or the partially edentulous person is no exception. Wholesome facial image often is in deficit because of loss of natural teeth, fear of aging, decreased sexuality, feelings of insecurity, fear of rejection, loss of self-esteem, and unrealistic expectations for tooth replacement. Loss of self-esteem is especially related to clients in whom tooth loss is attributed to oral cancer and oral cancer treatment. Human responses associated with tooth loss include the five stages of bereavement, changes in behavior, embarrassment, and loss of dignity.[4] These responses are considered when providing care for edentulous or partially edentulous clients.

Physiologic Factors

Although prostheses can restore many oral functions when a person experiences tooth loss, remodeling of the orofacial tissues is invariably encountered. Placement of prostheses introduces unfamiliar forces that contribute to:

- Residual ridge and alveolar bone resorption
- Oral mucous membrane remodeling
- Loss of orofacial muscle tone

Following tooth extraction, major bony changes, such as residual alveolar ridge resorption, occur within the first year and continue throughout life. Correlation between degree of alveolar bone resorption and the duration of edentulousness is well documented.[5] Metabolic bone disease, postmenopausal osteoporosis, and a calcium-poor diet also contribute to severe mandibular atrophy in edentulous individuals.

Generally, older individuals resorb bone at faster rates than younger individuals because of anatomic, metabolic, functional, and prosthetic factors. Problems that arise as a result of residual bone resorption are magnified as the person ages. For example, severe resorption of the mandibular alveolar ridge may expose the contents of the mandibular canal and cause extreme discomfort from the prosthesis. Additionally, compression of an exposed mental nerve at or near the crest of the alveolar ridge with only a thin layer of oral mucosa overlying it may cause pain and paresthesia of the lower lip and chin. During assessment, if the dental hygienist finds unmet needs for a biologically sound and functional dentition or freedom from anxiety and stress, immediate referral to the dentist would be indicated.

Resorption of alveolar ridges diminishes stability and retention of the prosthesis as the bony ridges continue to flatten with time. Generally, bony changes observed in the mandibular arch differ significantly from those in the maxilla. The rate of resorption is four times greater in the mandible than in the maxilla. Occasionally, irregular patterns of alveolar ridge resorption create numerous sharp spikes, especially in the mylohyoid ridge. Considerable pain can develop as the mucous membrane covering becomes trapped between the hard prosthesis base and sharp bone.

Other bony contours from either growth abnormalities or alveolar resorption may create undesirable consequences and should be noted. *Exostoses,* benign bony outgrowths, frequently occur on the hard palate and lingual aspect of the mandibular alveolar ridge and are known as *palatal* and *mandibular tori,* respectively. Their surgical removal, before prosthesis construction, prevents the possibility of irritation of the overlying oral mucosa by the tori. Similarly, large maxillary tuberosities lead to an unsatisfactory fit of the prosthetic appliance.

TYPES OF PROSTHODONTIC APPLIANCES

Individuals can have missing teeth replaced by dental implants (see Chapter 50), or by fixed and removable dentures. *Transition from a natural dentition to a completely or partially artificial dentition is a major life event that most*

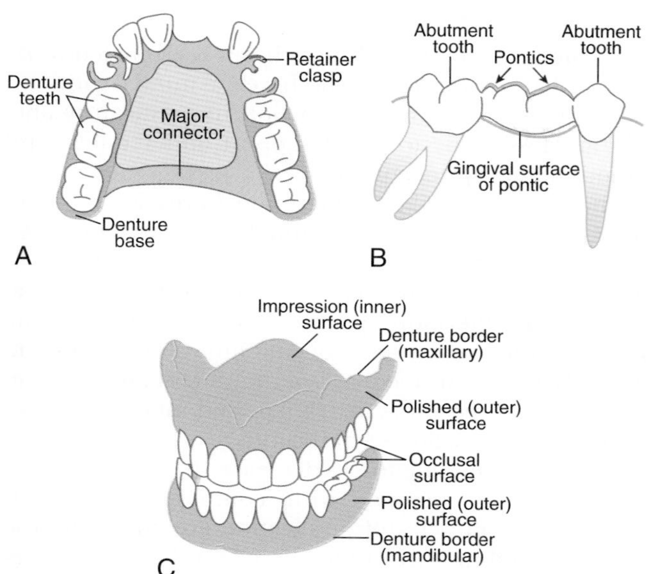

FIGURE 49–1 ✦ Types of prostheses. **A,** Removable partial denture. **B,** Fixed partial denture. **C,** Complete denture.

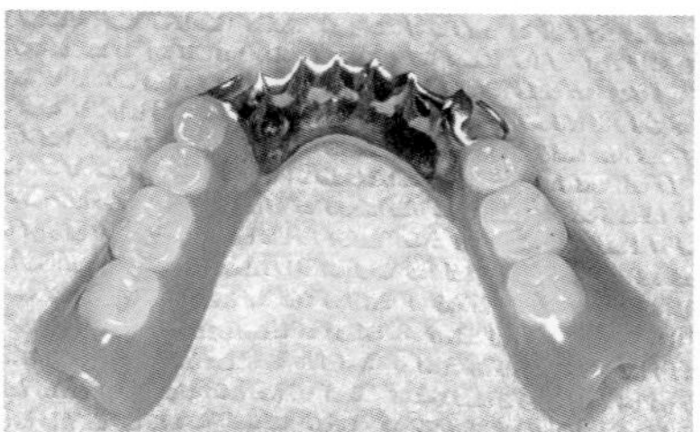

FIGURE 49–2 ✦ Mandibular removable partial denture. *(Courtesy Dr. Christopher Wyatt, Prosthodontist, Faculty of Dentistry, University of British Columbia, Vancouver, Canada.)*

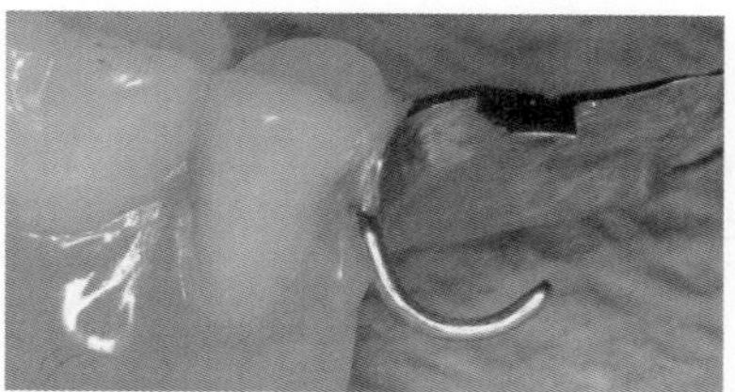

FIGURE 49–3 ✦ Removable partial denture clasp. *(Courtesy Dr. Christopher Wyatt, Prosthodontist, Faculty of Dentistry, University of British Columbia, Vancouver, Canada.)*

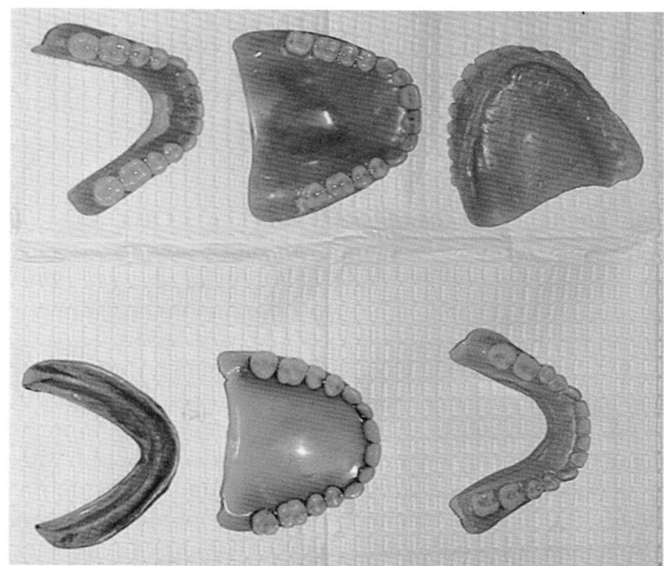

FIGURE 49–4 ✦ Full maxillary and mandibular dentures. *(Courtesy Dr. Christopher Wyatt, Prosthodontist, Faculty of Dentistry, University of British Columbia, Vancouver, Canada.)*

individuals find challenging. This situation can cause client needs in wholesome facial image, freedom from anxiety and stress, and a biologically sound and functional dentition. If needs are not met, or if the client believes that his or her needs cannot be met, success of prosthodontic therapy may be jeopardized.

Several types of prostheses, ranging from partial to complete, can be fabricated to meet clients' needs. The partial denture is used to replace some, but not all, of the natural teeth. Partial dentures may be fixed or removable. A *fixed partial denture* is permanently cemented to natural teeth and is commonly called a *bridge* (Figure 49–1, *B*). It cannot be removed by the client.

Components of fixed partial dentures include the following :

- ✦ *Abutment.* The tooth or teeth used to anchor the prosthesis. Abutments are the part of the fixed partial denture used to support the pontic(s).
- ✦ *Pontic.* The artificial tooth or teeth that occupy the edentulous space and replace the missing tooth or teeth.

Removable partial dentures (Figures 49–1, *A;* 49–2; and 49–3) can be removed and replaced by the client. This type of partial denture may be supported by retainer clasps around the natural teeth or by a combination of natural teeth and oral tissues. *Complete dentures* (Figures 49–1, *C;* 49–4; 49–5) are removable prostheses that replace either the maxillary or mandibular arch or the entire dentition and associated structures. If a denture is designed for a client who has undergone oral cancer surgery, it may also need to function as an obturator. An *obturator* is an appliance that closes an opening or orifice that may have been caused by an accident, by a congenital cleft, or by the removal of a cancerous tumor. When necessary, a denture may be designed to cover an orifice, and as such the denture aids in retaining foods and fluids in the mouth and out of the nasal passage.

Implant dentures are designed to fit over implant fixtures that are inserted partially or entirely into living bone. The increased stability and retention derived from this type of prosthetic appliance have renewed the hopes of the edentulous population for an acceptable alternative to natural teeth (see Chapter 50).

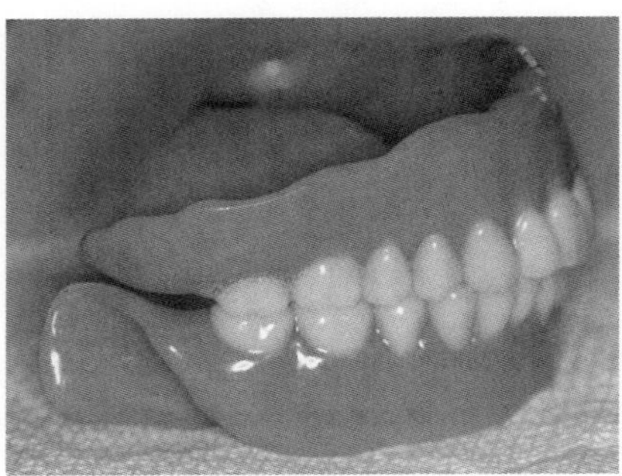

FIGURE 49–5 ✦ Complete dentures. *(Courtesy Dr. Christopher Wyatt, Prosthodontist, Faculty of Dentistry, University of British Columbia, Vancouver, Canada.)*

CHALLENGES ASSOCIATED WITH REPLACEMENT OF MISSING TEETH

Although *prosthodontic therapy* can give the edentulous or partially edentulous individual a biologically sound and functional dentition, success depends on the client's attitude and commitment. At the outset, the client must understand the limitations of tooth replacements and their effectiveness as substitutes for natural teeth. Clients should be informed about the physical manifestations of bone resorption related to facial appearance, potential speech difficulties, and the effects of tooth replacement on masticatory efficiency. If realistic expectations and goals for care of prostheses are outlined early, the client can successfully adapt to the artificial dentition.

Physical Appearance

Alveolar bone resorption dramatically affects physical appearance and facial image. Modifications in appearance often are visible following extensive alveolar bone resorption, such as loss of facial height (vertical dimension), reduced lip support, a sunken maxillary appearance, and increased chin prominence. The effects of physical alterations attributed to bone resorption include decreased stability, unbalanced occlusion, temporomandibular joint (TMJ) disorders, and dissatisfaction with appearance. Usually, appearance is judged critically by clients themselves; however, the astute dental hygienist who focuses clients on their positive attributes can assist in building client self-esteem and reduce anxiety and stress.

Speech Disturbances

Speech patterns are affected by loss of teeth, loss of associated periodontal structures, and the acquisition of prostheses. Transient speech articulation difficulties and oral resonance problems are expected but soon disappear.[3] To facilitate speaking with a new oral appliance, clients should be instructed to read aloud and to speak in front of a mirror. If a speech disturbance persists longer than a few days, the prosthesis may be ill fitting and reevaluation by a dentist warranted. A speech deficit can also arise in conjunction with bone resorption because a loosely fitting prosthesis is difficult to control.

Masticatory Efficiency

Masticatory efficiency with prostheses is estimated to be 20% of that of individuals who have a natural dentition.[1] Two primary reasons for reduction in masticatory abilities are loss of periodontal support and stability, and periodontal proprioception.[2]

The periodontal ligament support area is critical to the stability of a prosthesis confined to one arch only. Yet, in edentulous persons, periodontal ligament support is one-fourth to one-half that which supports the natural dentition. Furthermore, proprioception is a major component in the body's reception and interpretation of sensation. Without this feedback of movement and position by the pressoreceptors in the periodontal ligaments, chewing ability declines significantly.

Biting and chewing forces decrease 10-fold and 3-fold, respectively, in persons with complete prostheses. Although the muscles of mastication are adequate, the mucous membrane covering the edentulous ridge cannot withstand the pressures exerted. The client will experience greater success with a new prosthesis if taught to avoid repeated incision using anterior teeth, gum chewing, and sticky foods. The client should also be instructed to consume food in smaller pieces, lengthen chewing time, and evenly distribute food to both the left and right sides of the mouth while chewing. Practicing these behaviors is critical to masticatory efficiency and prosthesis stability.

FACTORS AFFECTING THE ORAL MUCOSA OF DENTURE-WEARING INDIVIDUALS

Systemic Diseases and Conditions

Poor general health results in denture problems, such as friable denture-bearing mucosa. For example, a person with kidney dysfunction may have dehydrated mucosal tissues because of a water imbalance, and thus the mucosa becomes vulnerable to trauma. Decreased tolerance to stress, impaired healing, emotional strain, and medications related to poor systemic health adversely affect oral soft tissues. Systemic conditions that may require modification of dental hygiene care include cardiovascular diseases, hypertension, allergies, psychological problems, and chronic diseases such as diabetes, anemia, and postmenopausal osteoporosis.

Medications taken for systemic diseases or conditions can affect a client's oral condition and must be assessed and documented during each appointment (see Chapter 11). Hormones, digitalis, nitroglycerin, diazepam (Valium), and chlordiazepoxide (Librium) are among the many medications that can affect the oral environment of the edentulous client. Xerostomia, a common side effect of diuretic, antihypertensive, and antidepressive drugs, interferes with complete denture retention and stability as a result of a loss of mucosal lubrication. Uncontrollable tongue and facial movements may develop with psychotropic medications. Drugs such as cortisone, thyroid hormone, and estrogen may perpetuate a chronic soreness of mucosal tissues.[5]

Xerostomia

Extreme difficulties experienced by the edentulous client with dry mouth warrant an understanding of the critical role of saliva in the maintenance of oral health. Normal salivary flow is essential for denture retention and function. A thin film of saliva provides adhesive action as well as lubrication and cushioning effects. When the mouth becomes dry, movement of the denture can cause frictional irritation of the denture-bearing mucosa. Other symptoms may arise as a result of oral dryness, including altered taste perceptions, cracked lips, a fissured tongue, and burning mouth syndrome (see Chapter 46). Although the exact causative agent of xerostomia may be difficult to identify, the most common factors are the following:

- Sjögren's syndrome
- Emotional and anxiety states
- Negative fluid balance
- Selected nutritional and hormonal deficiencies
- Acquired immunodeficiency syndrome (AIDS)
- Anemia
- Polyuria states
- Drugs or medications
- Therapeutic radiation

Diminished salivary output is not directly associated with increased age; rather, other factors should be considered if xerostomia is observed in older adults.[6]

Professional care for the denture client with xerostomia can be challenging because most remedies provide only temporary relief. The dental hygienist may recommend saliva substitutes and frequent mouthrinses, especially during meals, to keep the mouth lubricated and temporarily provide symptomatic relief. Recommendations for the management of soft tissue dryness include coating the tissue surface of dentures with petroleum jelly, silicone fluid, or denture adhesive material.

Oral pilocarpine (5 mg 3 times per day) decreases symptoms associated with xerostomia by increasing salivary flow.[6] This prescriptive medication is effective in clients who have undergone head and neck radiation therapy. While pilocarpine has not been tested on denture-wearing populations, it may be of value for denture-wearing individuals who suffer from dry mouth. This treatment option may be discussed with the client's dentist or physician and then presented to the client.

Denture Occlusion and Fit

The state of the oral mucosa overlying the ridges directly affects the comfort of removable partial and complete dentures. A thicker covering is more resilient and provides more padding than a thin mucosa. Unfortunately, dental interventions for minimizing discomfort associated with friable mucosa are limited, although soft lining materials such as tissue conditioners and resilient liners may alleviate discomfort for some individuals. Tissue conditioners and resilient liners, composed of soft, flexible elastomer polymers, palliatively treat chronic soreness and protect supporting tissues from functional and parafunctional occlusal stresses. Dentures with a flexible elastomer require special care because these soft materials cannot be cleaned effectively and debris can accumulate and support halitosis, a disagreeable taste, and the growth of *Candida albicans*. Most professionals recommend use of a very soft brush with a nonabrasive dentifrice. Clients should be cautioned to avoid oxygenating and hypochlorite-type denture cleaners that can damage resilient liners and tissue conditioners.

Oral Hygiene

The client's oral mucosa reveals information about daily self-care. Accumulation of bacterial plaque biofilm, stain, and calculus on the denture and oral mucosa leads to offensive odors and mucosal irritations, such as the following:

- *Denture stomatitis.* Inflammation of the oral mucosa underlying the denture, characterized by redness, pain, swelling
- *Papillary hyperplasia.* Abnormal increase in the volume of tissue as a result of irritation
- *Chronic candidiasis.* A long-term *Candida albicans* infection

Presence of any of these conditions mandates that the client be educated about oral hygiene interventions to maintain the health of mucosal tissues. Specific oral hygiene techniques are presented in Chapters 18 and 19.

Continuous Wear of Dentures

Because of masticatory stresses exerted by dentures, residual alveolar ridges and oral mucosa may become compromised. In addition, the risk for an inflammatory condition increases if the tissues are not allowed to rest. Although some clients' tissues tolerate the stresses better than others do, clients should be advised to remove the denture from the mouth overnight or for several hours during each 24-hour period. While out of the mouth, the denture should be cleaned thoroughly and placed in a container filled with water to prevent drying and denture base material damage.

DENTURE-INDUCED ORAL LESIONS[2,3]

Understanding the soft tissue response to prostheses enables the dental hygienist to assess the client's skin and mucous membrane integrity of the head and neck. The soft tissues primarily associated with the prosthetic appliance are the tongue, floor of the mouth, cheeks, lips, and mucosa overlying the edentulous ridge.

Prosthesis-bearing tissues react differently from individual to individual. For example, differences in the

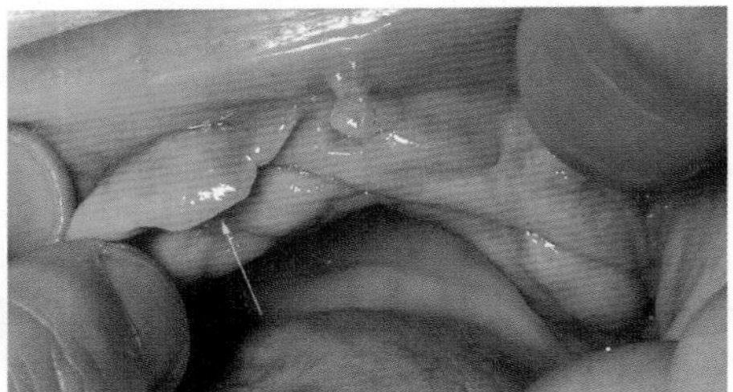

FIGURE 49–6 ✦ Prosthesis-induced fibrous hyperplasia (epulis fissuratum). Chronic denture-induced trauma has resulted in leaf-like masses *(arrows)* of soft tissue that overgrow the denture flange. *(Courtesy Dr. R.W. Priddy, Oral Pathologist, Faculty of Dentistry, University of British Columbia, Vancouver, Canada.)*

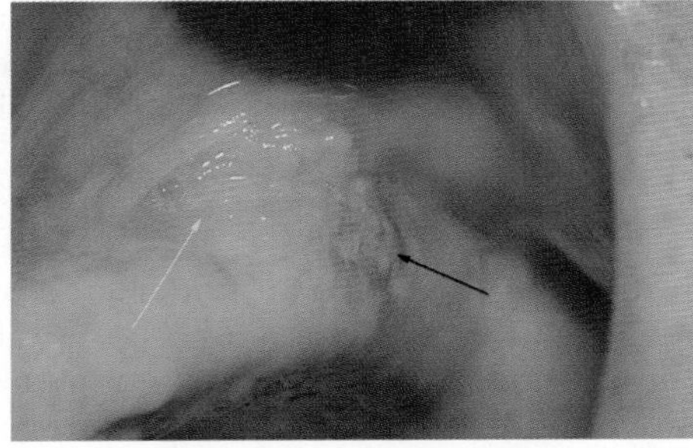

FIGURE 49–7 ✦ Reactive/traumatic lesion—focal (frictional) hyperkeratosis. Note area of epithelial hyperplasia *(yellow arrow)* and the presence of an ulcer with a yellowish surface slough *(black arrow)*. Both lesions caused by denture trauma. *(Courtesy Dr. R.W. Priddy, Oral Pathologist, Faculty of Dentistry, University of British Columbia, Vancouver, Canada.)*

thickness of the mucosa in conjunction with varying degrees of keratinization can be expected in the mouth of the denture-wearing client. Some edentulous persons develop a *prosthesis-induced fibrous hyperplasia* as a result of fibrous tissue proliferation following alveolar bone resorption under an ill-fitting prosthesis (Figure 49–6). Although detection is sometimes difficult because of nearly normal color and texture, this flabby hyperplastic tissue is identified by palpating freely movable tissue over edentulous ridges or on the vestibular mucosa.

If this tissue is observed, the dental hygienist refers the client to the dentist for evaluation and treatment. Depending on the severity of hypermobile tissue, treatment may involve a period of tissue rest, prosthesis adjustment, and/or surgical excision to reduce the excess tissue. Keratinization of edentulous alveolar ridges may be completely absent or progress to a hyperkeratinized state. This *focal (frictional) hyperkeratosis* is classified as a hyperkeratotic white lesion of the oral mucosa that should resolve with time on discontinuation of the underlying trauma.

Although it is highly unlikely that chronic irritation due to ill-fitting dentures will cause oral carcinoma, trauma induced by dentures and other mechanical irritations probably accelerates the progression of the disease. For this reason, the dental hygienist should be especially attentive to signs and symptoms of oral cancer: ulceration/erosion, induration, fixation, chronicity, lymphadenopathy, leukoplakia, and erythroplakia (see Chapter 43, Common Signs of Oral Cancer).

A wide spectrum of oral mucosal conditions in the denture wearer are associated with improper oral hygiene care, extended wear of the denture, or reaction to poor prosthesis fit. More specifically, denture-induced lesions are subdivided into three categories according to etiologic factors and clinical features (Figures 49–7 to 49–9 and Table 49–1):

1. Reactive/traumatic
2. Infectious
3. Mixed reactive and infectious

Generally, *relining* or remaking of the denture by the dentist and/or client education can eliminate the irritation.

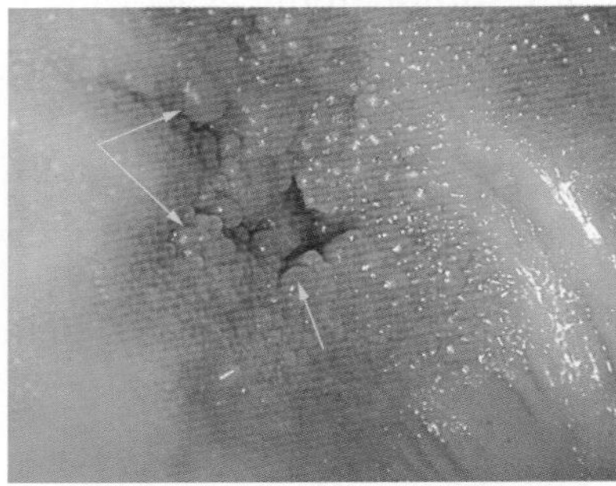

FIGURE 49–8 ✦ Infectious lesion—chronic candidiasis, palatal papillary hyperplasia. Note marked degree of mucosal papillary reactive hyperplasia as indicated by the presence of multiple large mucosal polyps *(arrows)*. In this case the mucosal response is limited to the palate. *(Courtesy Dr. R.W. Priddy, Oral Pathologist, Faculty of Dentistry, University of British Columbia, Vancouver, Canada.)*

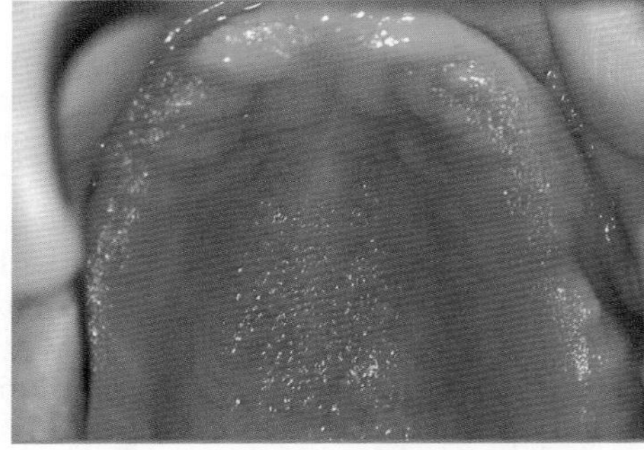

FIGURE 49–9 ✦ Mixed reactive and infectious lesions—palatal papillary hyperplasia associated with candidiasis. Note the generalized granular nature of the palatal mucosa, including the attached mucosa of the edentulous ridges. The individual wore the denture continuously, removing it only to rinse after eating. *(Courtesy Dr. R.W. Priddy, Oral Pathologist, Faculty of Dentistry, University of British Columbia, Vancouver, Canada.)*

Reactive/Traumatic Lesions

Reactive/traumatic lesions commonly are secondary to either acute or chronic injury. Lesions in this category are ulcers, focal (frictional) hyperkeratosis, and denture-induced fibrous hyperplasia. An overexuberant repair response produces hyperplastic tissue that often is pain-

TABLE 49–1 ORAL TISSUE CHANGES IN DENTURE-WEARING CLIENTS SUGGESTING AN UNMET HUMAN NEED FOR SKIN AND MUCOUS MEMBRANE INTEGRITY OF THE HEAD AND NECK

Oral Manifestation	Due To	As Evidenced By
Reactive Lesions		
Acute ulcers	Ill-fitting denture Chemical agent irritation: denture adhesive denture cleanser self-medication	Yellow-white exudate Red halo Varying pain and tenderness
Chronic ulcers	Same as above	Yellow membrane Elevated margin Little or no pain
Focal (frictional) hyperkeratosis	Chronic rubbing or friction of denture	White patch Asymptomatic
Denture-induced fibrous hyperplasia (epulis fissurata, denture hyperplasia)	Ill-fitting denture	Folds of fibrous connective tissue Varying color Asymptomatic Typical on vestibular mucosa at denture flange contact
Infectious Lesions		
Denture stomatitis (denture sore mouth)	Chronic *Candida albicans* infection Poor oral hygiene care Continuous wear of dentures Ill-fitting denture Systemic factors: anemia, diabetes, immunosuppression, menopause Systemic antibiotics Chemical agent irritation: denture adhesive denture cleanser self-medication Denture base allergy	Generalized redness of mucosa Velvet-like appearance Pain and burning sensations Typical under maxillary denture
Angular cheilitis	Chronic *C. albicans* infection Pooling of saliva in commissural folds Riboflavin deficiency	Fissured at angles of mouth Eroded Encrusted Moderate pain
Mixed Lesions		
Papillary hyperplasia	Chronic *C. albicans* infection Chronic low-grade denture trauma	Multiple round-to-ovoid nodules: "cobblestone" appearance Generalized red mucosa background Rarely ulcerated Typical under maxillary denture

less, but pain may develop if the fibrous lesion is traumatized or ulcerated. Surgical excision and removal of the irritating factor are effective methods of treating reactive lesions.

Infectious Lesions

DENTURE STOMATITIS. The most common inflammation of the denture-bearing mucosa is *denture stomatitis* (Figure 49–10). Despite minimal pain associated with denture stomatitis, it is often referred to inappropriately as "denture sore mouth." With a predilection for females, the incidence varies between 20% and 40% of the edentulous population, and in as many as 65% of the older adult population who wear complete maxillary dentures.

ANGULAR CHEILITIS. *Angular cheilitis* is a mixed bacterial and fungal infection caused by *Staphylococcus aureus* and *Candida albicans* (Figure 49–11). The condition results from small amounts of saliva accumulating at the commissural angles, which promotes the colonization of yeast. Clinically, angular cheilitis appears as cracked, eroded, and encrusted commissural folds and may cause moderate pain. Often it is secondary to overclosure resulting from a reduction in the client's vertical dimension. A vitamin B (riboflavin) deficiency resulting from inadequate nutrition also can cause angular cheilitis.

Dental treatment requires elimination of the trauma by correcting the denture and eliminating the *Candida* infection by prescribing antifungal drugs. Dental hygiene care to prevent recurrence includes instructing the client in thorough daily cleansing of the infected denture using chemical immersion. A weak sodium hypochlorite solution is used to soak the denture overnight (see Inexpensive, Safe, and Effective Cleaning

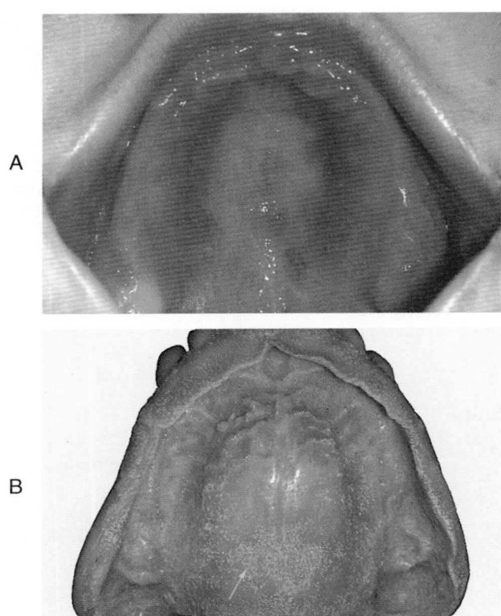

FIGURE 49–10 ✦ **A,** Denture stomatitis (denture sore mouth). The 60-year-old woman presented with a chief complaint of a sore mouth. Intraoral assessment revealed a markedly inflamed palatal mucosa, especially evident on the edentulous ridges. Her hard palate showed patch areas of inflammatory erythema. Her denture revealed evidence of poor denture hygiene. **B,** Denture of client with denture stomatitis. The 60-year-old woman had been wearing this denture for the past 20 years with no relines. When the denture became loose she would buy do-it-yourself reline material. Note the loose self-reline material *(arrowhead).* The tissue-bearing surface of the denture was covered with a thick denture plaque, with fungal colonies evident *(arrow). (Courtesy Dr. R.W. Priddy, Oral Pathologist, Faculty of Dentistry, University of British Columbia, Vancouver, Canada.)*

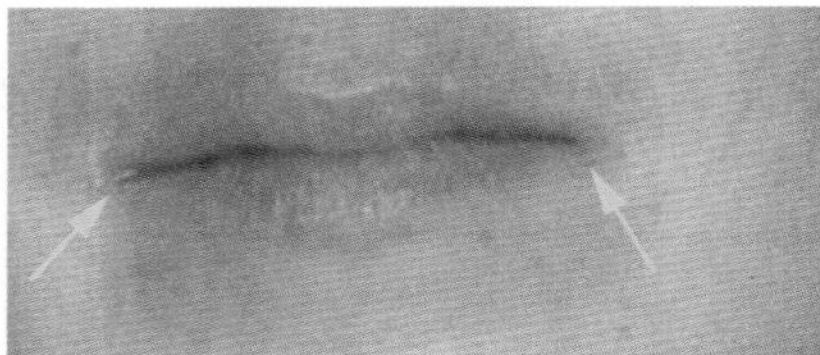

FIGURE 49–11 ✦ Angular cheilitis. Individual was complaining of burning mouth and sores at the corners of her mouth. Note the inflammation and fissuring of the right commissure. There is mild inflammation on the left side *(arrows). (Courtesy Dr. R.W. Priddy, Oral Pathologist, Faculty of Dentistry, University of British Columbia, Vancouver, Canada.)*

Solution for Oral Appliances Void of Metal). Sodium hyperchlorite can damage metal on the denture and should never be used when metal is part of any oral appliance. Moreover, if the sodium hyperchlorite is too concentrated, it can bleach the colored portion of the resin base and discolor soft relines materials. Other denture cleaners include nonabrasive dentifrices, commercial denture cleaners, and vinegar. Household cleaners should never be used to clean oral appliances (see section on Denture Cleansers).

CHRONIC CANDIDIASIS. Most denture-related infections, including denture stomatitis, are caused by a chronic candidiasis and treated using a topical antifungal agent, such as nystatin. Prescribed by the dentist for use at home, nystatin cream is applied to both affected tissues and the dentures to eliminate the fungi. To be effective, topical antifungal agents must be used by the client for approximately 1 week following the disappearance of clinical symptoms.

A chronic *Candida* infection is primarily responsible for the development of denture stomatitis, although recent studies implicate bacteria as the etiologic agent:[7] Gram-positive *Streptococcus* species, *Lactobacillus, Bacteroides,* and *Actinomyces* species. Other contributing factors include bacterial plaque accumulation on dentures; chronic, low-grade soft tissue trauma due to ill-fitting dentures; an unbalanced occlusal relationship; and continuous wearing of the denture at night. In some circumstances, systemic conditions such as diabetes, anemia, menopause, malnutrition, and malabsorption of nutrients in the digestive tract can predispose an individual to a *Candida* infection.

Chronic candidiasis appears on the palatal mucosa rather than on the mandibular alveolar mucosa. Clinical features demonstrate variations in surface texture ranging from a smooth, velvety appearance to a more nodular or hyperplastic form. With severe infections, surfaces may appear eroded, with small confluent vesicles. Characteristically, the bright-red color of the denture-supporting mucosa is confined within a well-defined denture border.

Mixed Reactive and Infectious Lesions

(Figure 49–9)

Both trauma and infection are etiologic factors contributing to mixed reactive and infectious lesions, such as *papillary hyperplasia.* A "cobblestone" appearance describes the granular papillary projections that result from a hyperplastic tissue response. This condition can predispose or potentiate the growth of *Candida albicans* under the denture and further complicate the problem. Multiple dental therapies to resolve the lesions include surgical excision, antifungal agents, soft tissue conditioners and liners, and strict oral hygiene measures.

IMPORTANCE OF REGULAR PROFESSIONAL CARE[2]

Only 13% of edentulous seniors had seen a dentist within the last 12 months, and 67% of them had not visited the dentist within the last 3 years.[1] This evidence underscores a critical role for the dental hygienist in encouraging regular maintenance care and in recognizing oral changes that often go unnoticed by the client.

Periodic maintenance care provides an excellent opportunity to identify denture-related tissue lesions and refer clients for dental evaluation and treatment. Although studies have demonstrated no correlation between cancer at specific sites and the wearing of dentures, denture irritation may be a co-carcinogenic factor in predisposed individuals.

Some clients erroneously perceive that prostheses last a lifetime without further modifications; however, in reality new prostheses should be made every 4 to 8 years. Hence, education is a priority for the prosthesis-wearing individual.

DENTAL HYGIENE CARE FOR INDIVIDUALS WITH FIXED AND REMOVABLE DENTURES

From the outset, the client must be educated regarding expectations, oral hygiene practices, denture use and care, and regular periodic maintenance appointments. Also, the dental hygienist educates the client about the causes of bone resorption and suggests methods of minimizing the rate of resorption, including removal of the prosthesis at night, regular evaluation to ensure well-fitting prostheses, and a calcium-rich diet. Resorption rates vary enormously between individuals, and well-fitting prostheses decrease the rate of resorption.[2,5] Local factors including trauma can affect the rate of resorption so that the prosthesis becomes ill-fitting.

Successful prosthodontic therapy also greatly depends on clients who possess a sense of responsibility regarding their oral health status. The dental hygienist encourages clients to set personal goals for oral health and suggests behavior patterns and techniques that are compatible with the client's lifestyle, cultural customs, values, and physical capabilities.

The edentulous person's ability to adapt to the prosthesis greatly influences eating pleasure, eating proficiency, and overall health. The quality and quantity of nutritional intake are not necessarily modified in the edentulous individual. Nonetheless, if the prosthesis is ill-fitting, nutritional status may suffer. Hence, eating becomes a chore and less pleasurable. The dental hygienist facilitates success of denture therapy by assessing the client's nutritional status and providing dietary counseling to ensure that nutritionally rich foods, such as vegetables, meats, and fruits, are not ignored (see Chapter 28).

The dental hygienist assesses loss of retention, stability, and support of the prosthesis and calls problems to the dentist's attention (Procedure 49–1). The dental hygienist also documents unmet human needs, informs both the client and the dentist of all deviations from normal, and recommends daily self-care to prevent further tissue destruction.

Procedure 49–1 DENTAL HYGIENE CARE FOR CLIENTS WITH FIXED AND REMOVABLE DENTURES

EQUIPMENT

Protective barriers
Prophy cup and bristled brush
Slow-speed handpiece
Antimicrobial mouthrinse
Tin oxide
Mouth mirror
Hand mirror
Gauze
Disclosing solution
Tongue blades
Small plastic bag
Stain and calculus remover solution
Ultrasonic cleaning unit

STEPS	RATIONALE
ASSESSMENT	
1. Update client's health history to identify systemic disorders, current medications, and conditions that may affect care and ability to wear prostheses.	Systemic health affects oral health and success of prostheses.
2. Review client's personal history records; note details such as age, occupation, and culture.	The client's personal profile influences care and dictates priorities and self-care.
3. Review client's dental history.	Reflects previous oral disease, past dental and dental hygiene care, self-care priorities, and values.
4. Ask client to explain denture problems experienced; listen attentively to complaints.	Provides insight into nature of denture problems and client's beliefs and values.
5. Perform comprehensive assessment of head and neck.	Facilitates early recognition of abnormalities that may signal human need deficits related to oral health and disease.
6. Assess the TMJ and associated musculature as client opens and closes mouth and slides jaw from side to side.	TMJ disorders can develop following extended wear of ill-fitting dentures.
7. Assess extraoral soft tissues.	Adequate facial support by dentures is necessary to maintain normal facial appearance; angular cheilitis may indicate a *Candida* infection or other systemic disease.
8. Assess intraoral soft tissues for evidence of local or systemic diseases, and record color, texture, size, contour, and presence or absence of pain.	Inflammation, traumatic injury, and chemical irritations may indicate need for referral to dentist for further evaluation.

Continued on following page

Procedure 49–1 DENTAL HYGIENE CARE FOR CLIENTS WITH FIXED AND REMOVABLE DENTURES—CONT'D

STEPS	RATIONALE
9. Visually inspect and palpate denture-bearing mucosa.	Determines resilience of overlying mucosa and submucosa; assists in evaluating denture fit and changes produced with increasing age.
10. Assess the structure and form of the alveolar ridges.	Flabby tissue, uneven underlying bone, and bony spikes contribute to poor stability and retention of denture.
11. Document changes in associated structures, including the tongue, floor of the mouth, and oropharynx.	May reveal loose-fitting dentures, lack of wear of the prosthesis, chronic low-grade trauma, systemic conditions, or oral lesions.
12. Assess oral hygiene status.	Improper denture and mouth care potentiates infection and poor adaptation.
13. Ask client to displace the prosthesis away from supporting tissues. The posterior border seal of the maxillary denture is checked by attempting to pull the anterior teeth forward.	Assesses retention, which is necessary for satisfactory physiologic performance and appearance of the denture and for proper speaking.
14. Assess stability of the denture with respect to denture position during normal oral functions.	Denture stability is directly associated with retention and fit.
15. Indicate changes in occlusion and articulation.	Freeway space (interocclusal distance) and occlusal vertical dimension are important to client's appearance and comfort.
DENTAL HYGIENE DIAGNOSIS	
16. Analyze objective and subjective assessment data; identify unmet human needs.	Ensures that care will be planned to meet client needs.
17. Present significant findings to dentist.	Collaboration ensures quality care and expedites dental care.
PLANNING	
18. Determine a dental hygiene care plan and goals in consultation with client and dentist.	Involvement in decision making increases client motivation, acceptance, and responsibility.
19. Establish with client goals that will be achieved	Ensures client commitment and measure of clinical outcomes.
IMPLEMENTATION	
20. Review self-care and denture care; suggest methods for improvement.	Reinforcement is vital to oral health maintenance.
21. Use disclosing solution to stain plaque and calculus on denture (when appropriate).	Demonstrates need for improved oral and denture care.
22. Counsel client on adequate nutrition.	Corrects nutrient imbalances that compromise integrity of oral tissues.
23. Fill a small plastic bag with cleansing solution, submerge the denture in it, and place the bag in an ultrasonic cleaning unit.	Provides a safe, effective alternative to manual scaling for removing calculus and extrinsic stain from denture (Table 49–2, Figure 49–12).
24. Lightly polish the denture with an extremely fine polishing agent (tin oxide) *on external surfaces only*, and thoroughly rinse under warm water (when appropriate).	Restoration of shine may inspire the client to maintain cleanliness of denture. Internal surfaces are avoided to maintain proper fit.

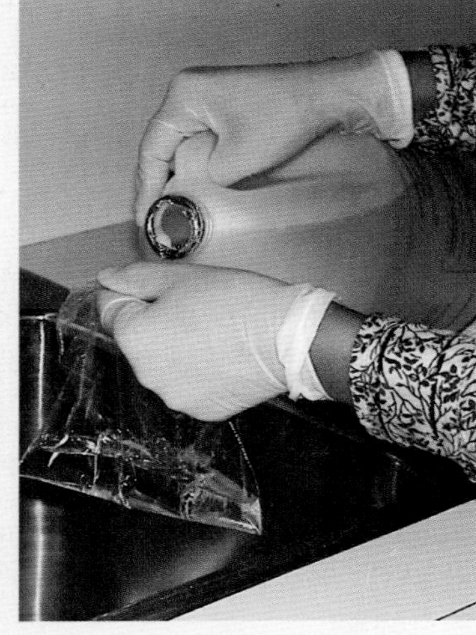

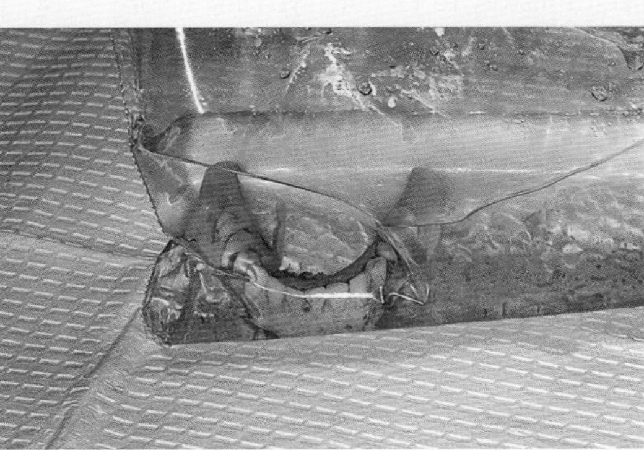

FIGURE 49–12 ✦ Ultrasonic cleaning of denture. **A,** Fill plastic bag with stain and calculus remover solution. **B,** Place denture in bag with solution. *(Courtesy Bertha Chan, RHD, MS.)*

Procedure 49–1 DENTAL HYGIENE CARE FOR CLIENTS WITH FIXED AND REMOVABLE DENTURES—CONT'D

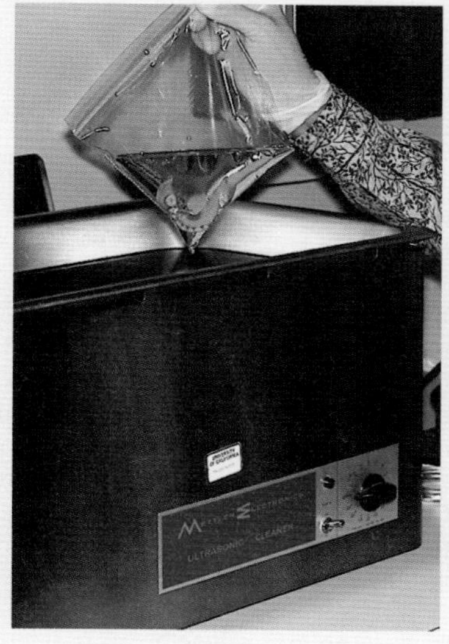

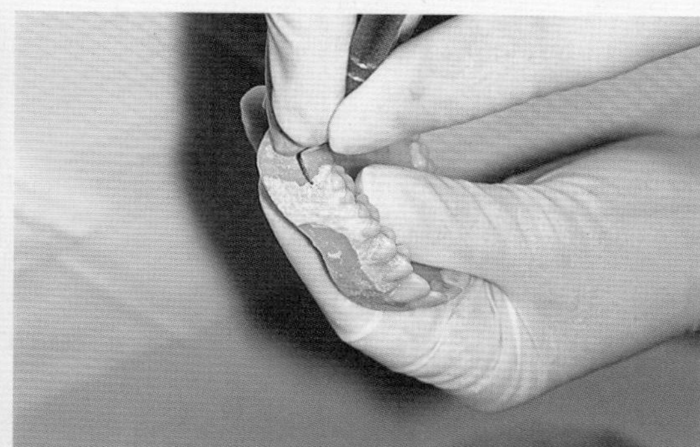

FIGURE 49–12, cont'd ✦ Ultrasonic cleaning of denture. **C,** Place bag in ultrasonic cleaner chamber and set for 10 to 14 minutes. **D,** Some dentures may require manual scaling to remove deposits. *(Courtesy Bertha Chan, RHD, BS.)*

STEPS	RATIONALE
EVALUATION	
25. Discuss continued-care interval. Emphasize the importance of regular professional care.	Continued care is essential to maintaining oral health.
26. Measure the achievement of established goals.	Prevents supervised neglect and erroneously dismissing a client who still needs care.
27. Formulate an evaluative statement regarding the level of goal attainment.	Documents client's status for management of legal risks and quality of care.
28. Document service in client's record under "Services Rendered" and date entry.	Ensures integrity of record for both the client's health and legal protection of practitioner.

The newly edentulous person commonly requires a denture adjustment within the first 6 to 12 months. Thereafter, annual continued care is essential to denture longevity and meets the need for denture duplication, rebasing, or replacement. Individuals with poor oral hygiene may require more frequent visits.

Clients should be advised of the importance of daily care of both the dentures and the associated soft tissues. Procedure 49–2 provides an overview of instructions for daily oral care for individuals with removable prostheses. Procedure 49–3 provides an overview of instructions for daily oral care for individuals with fixed prostheses. Both verbal and written instructions reinforce the home care regimen, especially for the elderly. A simple reminder to rinse the dentures and mouth after each meal helps eliminate accumulation of food debris and bacterial plaque. Written instructions or other formal educational materials that include proper denture hygiene and cleansing of the oral tissues provide specific, tangible recommendations for maintaining oral health. Pertinent information to teach the client is presented in the section on Client Education Issues.

At continued-care visits, the dental hygienist assesses the client's ability to perform meticulous oral hygiene care at home.

DENTURE CLEANSERS

Maintaining denture hygiene is essential both for aesthetic concerns and for prevention and treatment of oral infections in the client with dentures. Proper hygienic care can be confusing for the client because of the many products available for home use as well as the various in-office procedures used to maintain denture hygiene. Commonly available denture cleansers include the following:

- Chemical soak cleansers
- Antimicrobials
- Ultrasonic cleaning devices

Table 49–2 describes common denture cleansers available today. When selecting a denture cleanser, safety of the denture wearer and denture is paramount. Abrasive powders and pastes are not recommended for cleaning

Procedure 49–2 DAILY ORAL AND DENTURE HYGIENE CARE FOR INDIVIDUALS WITH REMOVABLE PROSTHESES

EQUIPMENT

Soft denture brush and a soft intraoral toothbrush
Basin
Denture cup
Towel
Dilute sodium hypochlorite solution (complete dentures) or commercial denture cleanser (partial dentures)
Warm water
Wall-mounted mirror
Soft nylon toothbrush

STEPS	RATIONALE
1. Explain the importance of daily care for both dentures and soft tissues.	Prolongs life of dentures, promotes healthy oral tissues, and promotes well-being of client.
2. Describe the consequences of oral and denture hygiene neglect.	Augments client awareness of halitosis, inflammation, trauma, or negative bone remodeling on appearance and health.
3. Summarize the client's responsibilities in monitoring oral function and health status.	Clients being taught to recognize early problems may prevent further discomfort and destruction.
4. Advise against the use of denture home repair kits and encourage the client to return to the dentist for proper care.	Improper denture modification results in further damage to the oral tissues and denture.
5. Discourage use of denture adhesives with a stable and retentive prosthesis. Under dentist supervision, a small amount of adhesive may be evenly applied over the inner surface that directly contacts the oral mucosa. Denture adhesives are not normally used with partial removable dentures.	Dependence on adhesives may indicate need for denture adjustment.
6. Remind the client to brush denture following each meal and before retiring or, at the very least, to rinse it under running water.	Bacterial plaque biofilm and food debris readily collect on dentures and foster a variety of oral mucosa problems (Table 49–1).
7. Teach self-examination of denture for proper fit, denture deposits, and abraded inner and outer surfaces.	Facilitates self-referral to the dentist to avoid further problems.
8. Teach client that some commercially available denture powders and pastes are too abrasive for dentures and are not recommended for use.	Coarse abrasives alter shine, surface character, and fit of prosthesis.
9. Suggest daily use of fresh denture immersion cleansers. Recommend a dilute sodium hypochlorite solution as a cleanser for complete dentures (see Inexpensive, Safe, and Effective Cleaning Solution for Oral Appliances Void of Metal). Soak complete dentures 5 to 10 minutes, and rinse thoroughly. Partial dentures benefit from alkaline peroxide solutions found in many denture-cleansing products, usually in the form of a tablet. Soak partial denture for 15 minutes or overnight and rinse thoroughly. Change solutions daily.	Chemical cleansers bathe all denture surfaces, aid clients who lack manual dexterity, minimize accidental breakage of dentures, and can be used while dentures are out of the mouth. Dilute hypochlorite solutions provide nontoxic, bactericidal, and fungicidal actions (see Inexpensive, Safe, and Effective Cleaning Solution for Oral Appliances Void of Metal and Figure 49–13).
10. Teach the client to remove denture when possible and at night while at rest.	Continuous wearing of dentures inhibits the natural cleansing mechanisms of the tongue and saliva and increases bacterial plaque retention.
11. Assemble supplies.	Sets up the necessary materials for proper cleaning technique.
12. Fill basin with water, and line with a small towel.	Prevents breakage of denture should it be accidentally dropped.
13. Gently remove denture, and rinse away saliva and loose debris. In case of complete dentures, remove any denture adhesive material.	Improves ability to assess appliance.
14. Firmly grasp denture in palm of one hand, and hold over water-filled basin.	Prevents accidental breakage of denture.
15. Demonstrate use of soft toothbrush with a mild soap solution or regular toothpaste to remove accumulations on the inner impression and outer polished surfaces, and adapt brush as necessary.	Areas difficult to access require special attention. The client must be reminded to access all areas without overexuberant brushing, which may damage the denture or a soft resilient liner (Figure 49–14).
16. Rinse denture and brush under running water to completely remove all denture cleanser.	Residual cleanser may cause irritation to oral mucosa.

Procedure 49–2 DAILY ORAL AND DENTURE HYGIENE CARE FOR INDIVIDUALS WITH REMOVABLE PROSTHESES—CONT'D

STEPS	RATIONALE
17. Inspect denture for any remaining bacterial plaque biofilm, food debris, or cleanser by visual and tactile examination.	Ensures that all debris has been removed.
18. Place prosthesis in a denture cup filled with room-temperature tap water or denture cleanser, and cover it.	Prevents dehydration and distortion of denture (acrylic resin).
19. On removal of denture, rinse mouth with warm water or saline solution.	Removal of large debris from oral cavity is essential to maintaining a healthy oral environment.
20. Teach client to use a soft toothbrush or soft cloth daily to clean edentulous mucosa by employing long strokes in a posterior to anterior direction.	Maintains sound supporting tissues for dentures.
21. Teach client to use thumb and index finger to massage edentulous tissues daily by applying pressure and then releasing it continually along the ridge. Mechanical, vibratory stimulation with the sides of multitufted soft toothbrush filaments can provide similar results.	Increases keratinization of oral mucosa, circulation, and resistance to denture trauma.

A

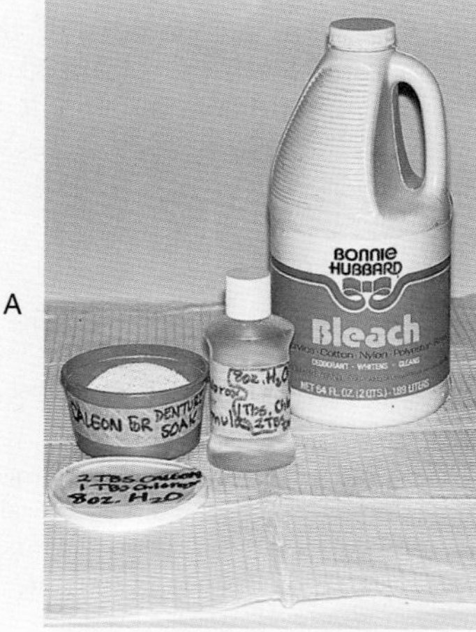

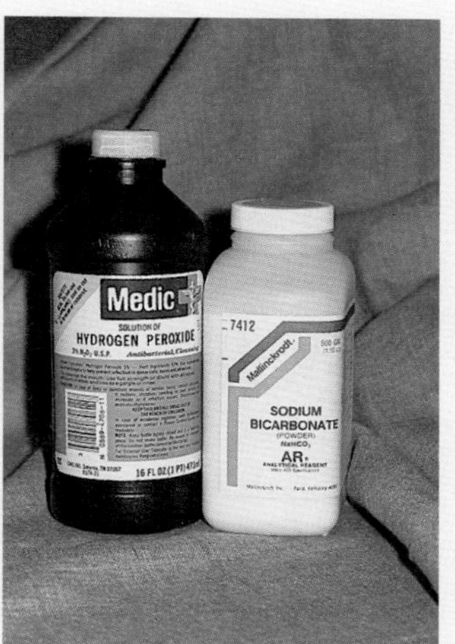

B

FIGURE 49–13 ✦ Inexpensive denture cleaners. **A,** Combination of sodium hypochlorite, Calgon, and water for denture without metal. **B,** Combination of hydrogen peroxide and sodium bicarbonate forms an alkaline peroxide solution for dentures with metal. *(Courtesy Bertha Chan, RHD, BS.)*

A

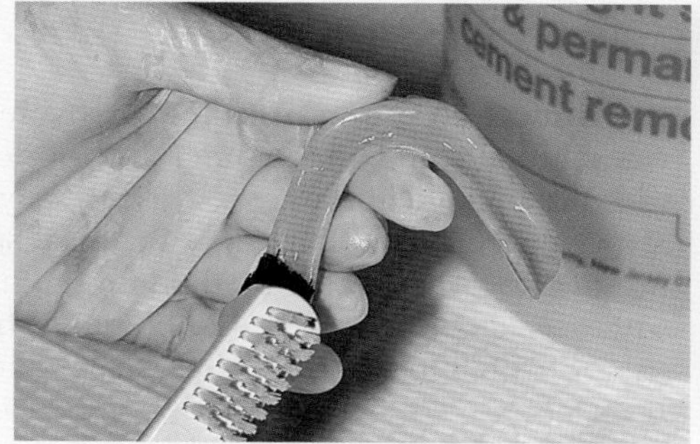

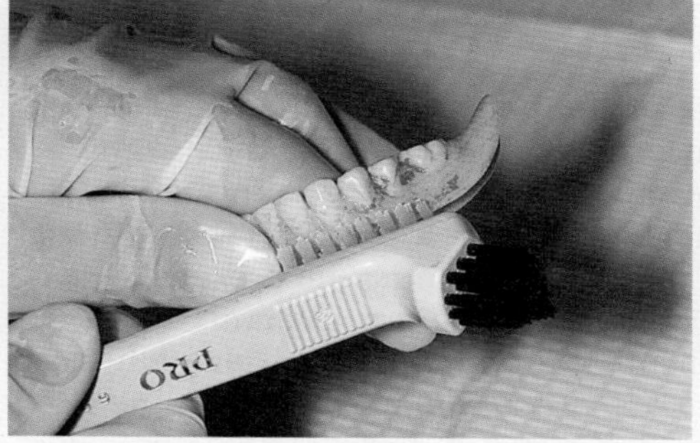

B

FIGURE 49–14 ✦ **A,** Adaptation of denture brush on inner surface of denture. **B,** Adaptation of denture brush on outer surface of denture. *(Courtesy Bertha Chan, RHD, BS.)*

Procedure 49–3 DAILY ORAL CARE FOR INDIVIDUALS WITH FIXED PROSTHESES

EQUIPMENT

Soft toothbrush
Interdental cleaners such as variable-diameter floss, dental floss, dental yarn, floss threaders
Wall-mounted mirror

STEPS	RATIONALE
1. Explain the importance of daily self-care for fixed denture, remaining natural teeth, and periodontal tissues.	Prolongs useful life of fixed denture; promotes healthy tissues and systemic health of client.
2. Describe the consequences of oral and fixed denture hygiene neglect.	Augments client awareness of halitosis and oral disease risk on appearance and health.
3. Summarize the client's responsibilities in monitoring oral function and health status.	Clients being taught to recognize early problems may prevent further discomfort and destruction.
4. Teach the client to brush natural teeth and fixed partial denture following each meal and before retiring. Clients benefit from flossing both remaining natural teeth and fixed denture daily.	Decreases risk of dental caries and periodontal disease.
5. Assemble supplies.	Ensures that materials needed to properly cleanse fixed partial denture and remaining natural teeth are available.
6. Demonstrate use of a soft toothbrush to remove plaque biofilm and gross debris from fixed partial denture and remaining natural teeth (see Chapter 18).	Ensures that plaque-retentive structures are thoroughly cleansed.
7. Demonstrate use of suitable flossing aid to cleanse under the pontic and around abutments and natural teeth (Figure 49–15) (see Chapter 19).	Ensures that all surfaces of the fixed partial denture and natural teeth are cleansed. Shape of pontic determines appropriate floss aid and flossing technique

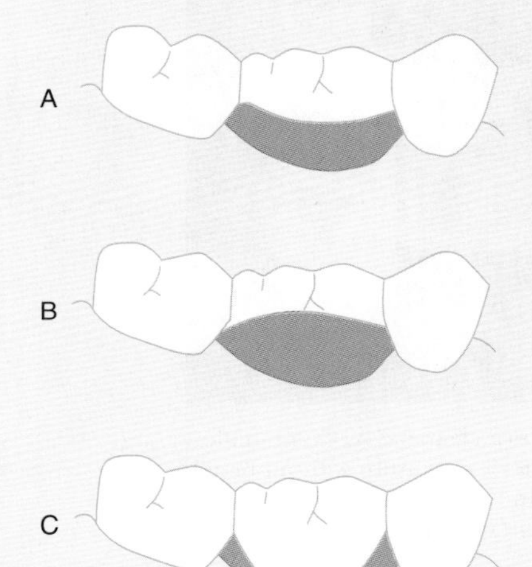

FIGURE 49–15 ✦ Fixed partial denture pontics. **A,** Conventional. **B,** Modified. **C,** Conical (bullet). *(Courtesy Dr. Joanne Walton, Prosthodontist, Faculty of Dentistry, University of British Columbia, Vancouver, Canada.)*

dentures because of the potential for the client to use these products incorrectly, thus damaging the prosthesis. Denture acrylic can become abraded, and this ultimately may lead to an altered fit if a hard-bristle brush or extreme vigor is used when cleaning the prosthesis.

The relative efficacy of denture cleansers depends partially on the client's dexterity. Brushing with toothpaste is suitable for the client who is motivated and has the dexterity to thoroughly clean all surfaces; however, this denture cleansing method is the most difficult, especially for the physically challenged or older adult client. Chemical soak cleansers are effective alternatives to mechanical cleansing. Alkaline peroxide and hypochlorite solutions can be recommended for dentures with and without metal components, respectively. Hypochlorites are reported in the majority of clinical studies to be the most efficacious soaking method for dentures constructed with only acrylic materials. Caution must be taken to avoid use of hypochlorites on any metal-containing prostheses. If an offensive taste and odor linger following the hypochlorite soak, alkaline peroxide may be used subsequently. Inexpensive, Safe, and Effective Cleaning Solution for Oral Appliances Void of Metal provides the directions for making an effective denture cleaner.

TABLE 49–2 ORAL APPLIANCE CLEANSING PRODUCTS

Product	Mechanism of Action	Advantages	Disadvantages
Chemical Soak Cleansers			
Alkaline hypochlorite	Dissolves mucins and organic substances of denture plaque matrix	Bactericidal Fungicidal Bleaches stains May inhibit calculus formation	Corrodes metals Odor and taste may be unacceptable May bleach acrylic if used in high concentration or for prolonged periods
Alkaline peroxide	Mechanical cleansing effect by the release of oxygen (bubbling)	Some antibacterial effect Removes stain	None
Ultrasonic cleaning devices	Conflicting evidence regarding effectiveness of ultrasonic action per se; chemical solution may provide cleansing action	Removes bacterial plaque Enhances effectiveness of disinfectants	Commonly an in-office procedure Uncertain efficacy of ultrasonic action
Antimicrobials Chlorhexidine gluconate 2% solution (not approved for use on dentures in United States)	Antimicrobial action by chemical agent	Antibacterial Antifungal	Only temporary relief of denture stomatitis symptoms Stains denture teeth

Inexpensive, Safe, and Effective Cleaning Solution for Oral Appliances Void of Metal

1 tablespoon (15 ml) sodium hypochlorite (household bleach)
1 teaspoon (4 ml) detergent (e.g., Calgon)
4 ounces (114 ml) water
After soaking, the oral appliance must be rinsed thoroughly with water before reinsertion into the oral cavity.

Table 49–3 reviews the variety of oral appliances and dental prostheses that can also be cleaned by these denture-cleaning methods.

NUTRITIONAL CONSIDERATIONS FOR INDIVIDUALS WITH FIXED AND REMOVABLE DENTURES (see Chapter 28)

Many of the lesions associated with denture wearing are a result of ill-fitting dentures, poor denture and oral hygiene care, and prolonged wearing of the prosthesis. Nutritional deficiencies are seldom noticed and, therefore, infrequently corrected. For example, a client deficient in B-complex vitamins may have symptoms of atrophic glossitis; angular cheilitis; or cracking, fissuring, or ulceration of the lips. These clinical signs may be interpreted as a chronic *Candida albicans* infection rather than a nutritional deficiency. Although difficult to identify, the dental hygienist must be cognizant of changes related to nutritional deficiencies in some denture wearers. Following assessment, the dental hygienist should inform the dentist of potential nutritional problems and either recommend dietary measures to the client that may improve oral health or refer the client to a dietitian.

Nutritional Factors (see Chapter 28)

Key nutritional factors for clients include the causes and effects of the following:

- ✦ Negative water balance on oral structures
- ✦ Negative calcium balance on alveolar bone
- ✦ Nitrogen-protein balance on muscle weakness and tissue fragility of oral tissues

Water is an essential nutrient for all body functions. Hence, evidence of tissue dehydration can be recognized throughout the body, especially in elderly individuals, as wrinkled skin, loss of muscle mass, decreased sweat and sebaceous gland secretions, dry eyes, xerostomia, and a smooth, atrophic tongue. The best dietary recommendation for dehydrated clients is to consume vegetable soup because both water and nutrients are more effectively retained in this form.

A negative calcium balance results in osteoporosis, which can precipitate rapid and extensive resorption of the alveolar ridges. A deficit in calcium intake, absorption, or transport may be responsible for the bony changes. Low-fat milk and milk products are good dietary sources of calcium (see Chapter 28, Food Sources of Calcium).

Depletion of protein most notably affects muscle mass but also may increase tissue fragility and cracking of the lips. A decrease in mass and strength of the muscles of mastication is especially evident in the older adult and

TABLE 49–3 COMPARISON OF VARIOUS ORAL APPLIANCES AND DENTAL PROSTHESES (also see Chapter 30)

Appliance	Definition	Purpose
Athletic mouthguard (mouth protector)	An oral appliance designed to protect the teeth and head from trauma during contact sports	Prevents oral and facial injury.
Bleaching trays	A custom-made stent in the shape of the teeth and dental arch for carrying the bleaching/whitening agents	Holds the whitening agent against the tooth surfaces.
Dentures:		Replaces form, function, and appearance in edentulous or partially edentulous dental arches.
Complete (full) denture	A prosthetic appliance designed to replace an entire arch of missing teeth and the surrounding alveolar bone and can be inserted and removed by the client	
Fixed partial denture (bridge)	A prosthetic appliance designed to replace several missing teeth, and is permanently cemented in place and removed only by the dentist	
Removable partial denture	A prosthetic appliance designed to replace several missing teeth and the surrounding alveolar bone, and can be inserted and removed by the client	
Implant denture	A prosthetic appliance designed to fit over osseointegrated implant fixtures	
Immediate denture	A prosthetic appliance placed immediately after remaining teeth are extracted from a partially edentulous arch	
Fluoride trays (custom)	A custom-made stent in the shape of the teeth and dental arch for carrying the fluoride agent to the tooth structure	Holds the prescription agent against the tooth surface to decrease caries risk.
Nightguards/ dayguards	A hard acrylic appliance that fits over all or just several of the maxillary or mandibular teeth to create a functional occlusion or to relax the muscles; may be worn at night or during the day	Control tooth attrition. Eases muscle hyperactivity and pressure on TMJ.
Oral habit appliance	An oral appliance used to interfere with habits such as thumb sucking, tongue sucking, or tongue thrusting	Prevents the habitual behavior from occurring.
Orthodontic appliances and repositioners	An oral appliance used for tooth movement and the treatment of malocclusion	Provides tooth movement and stabilization.
Stent	A device used after periodontal surgery to support and protect the oral tissues, and/or to hold a medicinal or other desired agent in a particular area	Stabilizes general tissue during periodontal surgery. Holds anesthetic/antiseptic agents in the area of the surgical sites.
Sleep apnea and snoring appliances	A flexible, custom-made device that positions the jaw forward during sleep	Opens the airway during sleep. Prevents snoring.
Space maintainer	A fixed or removable oral appliance to maintain a space created by premature tooth loss	Maintains an open space in the dental arch due to premature tooth loss until the permanent tooth can erupt.

can be monitored by placing the finger in the vestibule of the mouth and asking the client to clench his or her teeth. Clients should be encouraged to maintain a high-protein diet to maintain muscle mass (e.g., meat, fish, beans, tofu, and legumes) (see Chapter 28, Table 28–7).

Undoubtedly, the nutritional quality of food depends on the method of preparation. Variations in food preparation result from the client's physical capabilities, living conditions, and cultural preferences. Hence, dietary advice should include cooking instructions that maximize the nutrient value of the diet with consideration of individual circumstances and preferences. For example, meat and fish are most nutritious when broiled or boiled rather than fried. In addition to limiting saturated fat intake, boiling foods breaks down complex proteins into more easily digestible components. On the other hand, fried protein-rich foods lose some nutritional value because the protein coagulates and becomes more difficult to digest.

Nutrition and the Edentulous Older Adult (see Chapters 28, section on Nutritional Needs in Elderly Clients; and Chapter 48)

For the edentulous older adult, diet is of great concern. A deficiency of essential nutrients magnifies the tissue friability and diminished repair potential observed in geriatric clients. Many older adults live under circumstances such as low incomes, inadequate kitchen facilities, loneliness, and poor physical health that predispose them to poor nutritional habits. A lack of knowledge and interest in proper nutrition also contributes to malnutrition. The older adult's dietary intake is often affected by wearing dentures, and deficiencies in protein, calcium, and B-complex vitamins may be present. Normally these nutrients are essential in the maintenance and repair of oral tissues and bone. Many older adults have a limited ability to digest and absorb food. This problem can be exacerbated by ill-fitting dentures, which may result in chewing difficulties and diminish consumption of fibrous foods. Hence, digestion, absorption, and utilization of nutrients are impaired. Two common dietary tendencies of the aged edentulous person are:

- ✦ Preference for a soft diet high in carbohydrate and refined sugar
- ✦ Consumption of fewer protein-rich and high-fiber foods

For these reasons, the dental hygienist should routinely assess nutritional habits and suggest healthy food alternatives to promote weight control and a nutritionally balanced diet (Table 49–4). This can be effectively accomplished if simple, well-defined, concise guidelines are constructed so that no major changes in food habits and preferences are made. The client and the dental hygienist can set nutritional goals, taking into account lifestyle, financial resources, and cultural preferences. With the edentulous client, nutritional deficits should always be considered when determining factors that contribute to a denture-related problem.

TABLE 49–4 NUTRITIONAL GUIDELINES FOR MAINTENANCE OF ORAL HEALTH IN EDENTULOUS AND PARTIALLY EDENTULOUS CLIENTS (also see Chapter 28)

Nutritional Goal	Rationale
1. Eat a variety of foods.	Essential for repair and maintenance of structurally and functionally competent body parts; increases likelihood of getting necessary nutrients.
2. Select foods high in complex carbohydrates: fruits, vegetables, whole-grain bread, and cereals.	Blood glucose levels rise less if complex carbohydrates are consumed rather than simple sugars. Also, fiber in these foods promotes normal bowel function and may reduce serum cholesterol.
3. Protein-rich foods including lean meat, poultry, fish, dried peas, and beans are required daily.	Maintains strength and integrity of tissues, especially when exposed to physiologic stresses.
4. Obtain calcium from dairy products; some nondairy foods also contain substantial amounts of calcium.	Calcium intake is critical to maintain bone mass. Alveolar bone is an early site of calcium withdrawal if dietary calcium intake is low.
5. Consume fruit juices containing vitamin C and citrus fruit daily.	Essential for repair and healing of wounds and for absorption of other vitamins and minerals.
6. Limit intake of processed foods high in saturated and hydrogenated fats and sodium.	Evidence links high fat intake to heart disease, certain cancers, and obesity. High sodium intake may cause hypertension.
7. Limit intake of bakery products high in fat and simple sugars.	Bakery products are often high in calories and/or low in nutrients.
8. Drink eight glasses of water daily.	Essential nutrient for all body functions.

Modified from Zarb GA, Bolender CL, Carlsson GE: *Boucher's prosthodontic treatment for edentulous patients,* ed 11, St Louis, 1997, Mosby.

Client Education Issues

- ✦ Explain the importance of replacing missing teeth in restoring function and appearance and preventing drifting of remaining natural teeth. Explain the options available for tooth replacement (e.g., fixed versus removable prostheses).
- ✦ Explain the types of chemical cleansing agents, frequency and duration of their application, and other instructions for their use (Table 49–2).
- ✦ Demonstrate techniques for mechanical cleaning of the prosthesis and cleansing and massage of the oral tissues (Procedures 49–1, 49–2, and 49–3).
- ✦ Provide special instructions for gentle cleaning of soft lining materials, if necessary.
- ✦ Reinforce the need for regular professional care for denture-wearing individuals that includes intraoral and extraoral assessment and examination of prosthesis.
- ✦ Explain the potentially harmful effects of improper denture care and neglect of oral hygiene.
- ✦ Emphasize self-care strategies including daily oral hygiene, adequate nutrition, oral tissue self-examination, and resting denture-bearing surfaces.
- ✦ Recommend techniques and products for the use, care, and cleaning of prostheses. Avoid oxygenating and hypochlorite-type denture cleaners in the presence of resilient liners and tissue conditioners.
- ✦ Instruct the prosthodontic client to consume foods in smaller pieces, lengthen chewing time, evenly distribute food to both the left and right sides of the mouth while chewing, and avoid repeated incision using the anterior teeth of denture.
- ✦ Instruct the prosthodontic client to avoid chewing gum and sticky foods.
- ✦ Emphasize the value of replacing missing teeth in restoring function; preventing drifting of remaining natural teeth; instructions for use, care, and cleaning of the prosthesis; and importance of regular professional evaluations.
- ✦ Explain the value of denture marking to prevent loss of the denture during short-term or long-term care.

Legal, Ethical, and Safety Issues

- Provide services within the scope of dental hygiene practice as stipulated by the regulatory body of each province/state.
- Maintain written and dated records (in ink) of the status of the client's oral condition, condition of dental appliances, the treatment provided, recommended treatment, recommended referrals, client's refusal or acceptance of treatment, and any pertinent information regarding care.
- Have client remove and reinsert the dental appliance; if the client is unable to do so, the dental hygienist should request that the dentist, accompanying family member, or caregiver of the client remove and reinsert the prosthesis.
- Provide a discreet location for the client to remove the prosthesis; this ensures that the client's dignity is respected.
- Have the client maintain control of his or her own prosthetic appliance so that damage to the prosthesis can be avoided.

Key Concepts

- A prosthesis is a fixed or removable appliance that is functionally and cosmetically designed to replace a missing tooth or teeth.
- Persons who wear dental prostheses receive an oral examination periodically to monitor the health of hard and soft tissues, the functional integrity of the prosthesis, and changes that might be warranted. Frequency should be based on the client's risk factors for disease.
- A removable dental prosthesis should be marked with the wearer's name or identification number, especially if the person lives in an institutional setting.
- Just like natural oral structure, the dental prosthesis and oral cavity of the wearer must be thoroughly cleaned daily.
- Risk factors for edentulism include caries, periodontal disease, low socioeconomic status, inadequate access to professional care, low frequency of care, and poor daily oral hygiene.
- Loss of natural teeth is associated with fear of aging, decreased sexuality, feelings of insecurity, fear of rejection, loss of self-esteem, and unrealistic expectations for tooth replacement.
- Oral changes related to tooth loss include resorption of the residual ridge and alveolar bone, oral mucous membrane remodeling, and loss of orofacial muscle tone.
- Clients who lose teeth face challenges in their physical appearance, speech, and masticatory efficiency.
- Denture-induced oral lesions include prosthesis-induced fibrous hyperplasia, focal hyperkeratosis, denture stomatitis, chronic candidiasis, angular cheilitis, and papillary hyperplasia.
- Client education is a priority for clients wearing prostheses and oral appliances. Clients must know how to clean the prosthesis or oral appliance to maintain their oral health.

Critical Thinking Exercises

In each case, develop a dental hygiene diagnosis, client goals, and a dental hygiene care plan.

1. Jeremy Myers, age 67, is a new client at a dental hygiene care center. Recently widowed, Mr. Myers lives alone in a complex for retired individuals and relies solely on social security payments for living expenses. The client wore a complete maxillary denture and had his natural mandibular dentition remaining. Following a review of the client's health, dental, and dental hygiene history, the dental hygienist identified unmet human needs experienced by the client that related to dental hygiene care. The client complained of a sore palate and "loose denture that hurts especially while eating." On intraoral examination, the dental hygienist noticed a generalized redness on the palatal mucosa. The denture was easily displaced when prosthesis retention was evaluated. Furthermore, periodontal assessment of the natural dentition revealed a generalized 4 to 5 mm loss of attachment and bleeding on probing. Moderate bacterial plaque and subgingival calculus were present throughout the mandible.
2. Andrea Smith, an 84-year-old widow, visits the dental office twice a year for regular dental and dental hygiene assessments and care. She has a maxillary partial removable denture that replaces her lost molar teeth on both the right and left side of the arch as well as to replace her two maxillary central incisors. Mrs. Smith has retained most of her mandibular teeth except her left second premolar and left first molar. These teeth have been replaced with a fixed partial denture. She is in relatively good health and takes no medications.

Critical Thinking Exercises—cont'd

At her most recent continued-care appointment, she presents with heavy plaque biofilm deposits around her fixed partial denture but light to moderate deposits around her remaining natural teeth. She has light calculus deposits localized to the mandibular anterior teeth. Upon assessment, the hygienist finds periodontal probing depths ranging from 3 to 4 mm, with a 6-mm pocket on the mesial surface of the second molar, which serves as an abutment for her fixed partial denture. There is 2 mm of recession generalized. Mrs. Smith states that her removable partial denture fits well and that she rarely removes the denture. Mrs. Smith is reluctant to remove the denture.

3. Maxwell Green is a 59-year-old new client. He has had maxillary and mandibular dentures for 15 years. Since becoming edentulous, Mr. Green has not had new dentures fabricated, nor has he had the existing dentures relined. Mr. Green reports that he is in relatively good health, but on his health history form he has noted that he smokes and avoids regular checkups with his family physician. He states that "the only reason I am here is because my wife is retiring soon and will lose our dental insurance." Mrs. Green is concerned that Mr. Green's dentures need to be replaced and she wants to ensure that her dental insurance will cover the cost of new dentures.

   Upon assessment, the hygienist notices that the denture teeth are severely worn and covered with heavy accumulations of stain, calculus, and plaque biofilm. The gingival portions of the acrylic dentures are scratched. Mr. Green has stated that the dentures "have never fit right" and that "I often cannot eat with the dentures in my mouth." He also complains of frequent sore spots under the denture when he eats certain foods, such as grains and nuts. Mr. Green's denture care includes soaking the denture in household bleach occasionally and leaving the dentures on the kitchen counter at night to dry before retiring to bed.

4. Judith King, age 75, lives with her 80-year-old husband in a senior citizens' complex close to the dental office. She usually schedules continued-care appointments annually, but it has been 2 years since her last visit. On the health history, Mrs. King reports that she missed last year's visit due to a stroke. She is partially paralyzed on the right side, which is her dominant side. Mrs. King also has experienced some facial paralysis as a result of the stroke. Her current medications include a blood thinner and a diuretic. Mrs. King wears a full maxillary removable denture and a partial removable mandibular denture. She has retained her mandibular anterior teeth from canine to canine. During assessment, the hygienist finds moderate to heavy accumulations of plaque and food. Mrs. King has light to moderate calculus accumulations on the remaining natural teeth. Periodontal probing depths are 3 mm or less with bleeding on probing and no gingival recession. The maxillary denture appeared to fit well, but the mandibular denture appeared to be loose and presented with a broken supporting clasp.

Acknowledgment

Ebony Bilawka, Dip DH, BDSc (DH), MSc Candidate, University of British Columbia is gratefully acknowledged for her review of the literature, content development, and content review for Chapter 49.

For References, Suggested Readings, and Related Websites, visit

http://evolve.elsevier.com/Darby/hygiene/

CHAPTER 50

Persons with Osseointegrated Dental Implants

OBJECTIVES

Mastery of the content in this chapter will enable the reader to:

- Define basic components of a dental implant
- Define types of dental implants, rationale for use, and materials for each
- List criteria for successful osseointegration
- Discuss dental implant indications, contraindications, benefits, and risks
- Distinguish between plaque biofilm and calculus on edentulous and dentulous clients
- Describe peri-implantitis and its management
- List the armamentarium used during professional dental hygiene care for clients with dental implants
- Recommend oral self-care aids for dental implants

KEY TERMS

Abutment
Anchor
Biologic seal
Dehiscence
Endosteal (endosseous)
Healing caps
Load force
Natural tooth function
Osseointegration
Overdenture
Peri-implantitis
Peri-implant recession
Prosthetic tooth or appliance
Salivary percolation
Subperiosteal implant
Surgical guide stent
Transosteal (transosseous)

OSSEOINTEGRATED DENTAL IMPLANTS

Dental implants offer an alternative to people who cannot function physically or psychosocially with conventional dental prostheses. For example, an edentulous person with limited bony support for a denture (narrow or atrophic alveolar ridge) is a potential candidate for dental implants (Figure 50–1). Clients who wear dentures chew at only 25% efficiency as compared to individuals with natural teeth. With implants, chewing efficiency rises to 96%.[1] Implants, beneficial to persons who have lost a single tooth or multiple teeth, make it possible to avoid wearing a removable or fixed partial or full denture appliance. Implants provide a comfortable, functional, and attractive system and a stable replacement of natural teeth for the right candidate.[1]

Natural tooth function describes the security of having a stable foundation on which to bite, chew, and grind. Tooth loss attributed to periodontal diseases, dental caries, or trauma prevents many individuals from experiencing natural tooth function. Although conventional restorative and prosthetic dental care assists clients in adapting to their lost dentition through fixed and removable prosthetic appliances, dental implants clearly provide a chance to regain natural tooth function.[1]

Implant dentistry requires collaboration among the dental implant team (i.e., restorative dentist, periodontist, oral and maxillofacial surgeon, prosthodontist, dental hygienist, dental lab technician, and, in some cases, an endodontist or orthodontist). The dental hygienist's contribution to the team consists of:

- Assessment of the need for dental implants
- Dental hygiene diagnosis
- Supportive periodontal therapy
- Client education
- Documentation of health and disease
- Monitoring and evaluation of oral health status

The dentist and dental hygienist work as co-therapists with the client to achieve natural tooth function for the client. The dentist evaluates clients and meets their reconstructive needs for a biologically functioning dentition; the dental hygienist and client maintain the mucous membrane integrity of the tissues around the implant (*peri-implant tissues*).

Definitions (see section on the implant process)

An *osseointegrated dental implant* is a stable functional replacement for one or more missing teeth. An implant consists of an anchor, an abutment, and a prosthetic tooth or appliance (Figure 50–2).

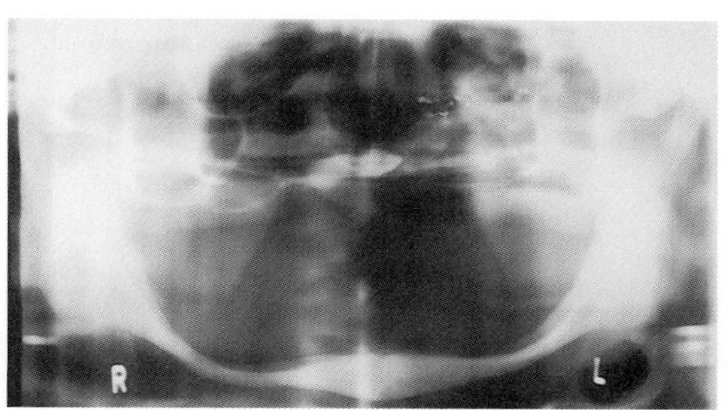

FIGURE 50–1 ✦ Radiograph of an atrophic mandible. *(Courtesy AK Lakha.)*

The *anchor*, a metal device inserted within the bone tissues of the mandibular or the maxillary arch, is frequently coated with a synthetic material that acts as a biocompatible interface to enhance bone formation. Titanium is the preferred metal for an implant anchor because of its biocompatibility with bone tissues. Other metals include Vitallium, cobalt alloys, ceramic, aluminum, and vanadium.

The *abutment* acts as a connection between the implant anchor and the prosthetic appliance. Surgical insertion of the abutments involves exposing the underlying implant anchor and attaching the abutment to the implant anchors by a center screw. Gingival tissue around the abutment needs approximately 3 weeks to heal in the maxilla and 1 week in the mandible. Oral hygiene and bacterial plaque control must be reinforced at this time for proper healing. With poor oral hygiene and an increased amount of bacterial plaque present, the peri-implant tissue risks inflammation and infection (*peri-implantitis*).

The *prosthetic tooth* or *appliance* is fabricated by the dentist or prosthodontist and is the final attachment. The prosthetic appliance can consist of a crown, a bridge, or a denture and is placed following the healing period of the abutment insertion, which takes a few weeks.

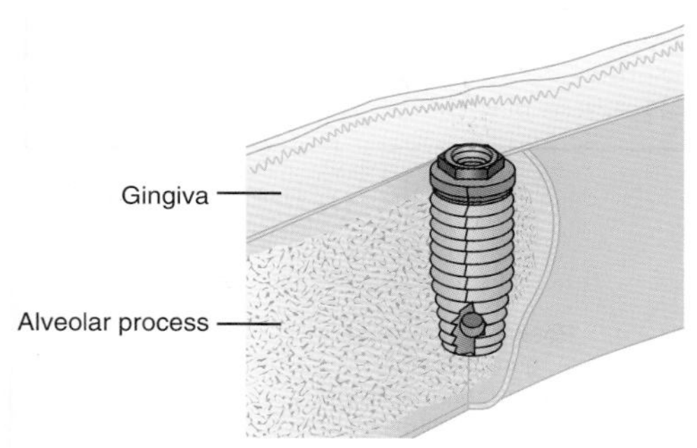

A. **Initial Placement**

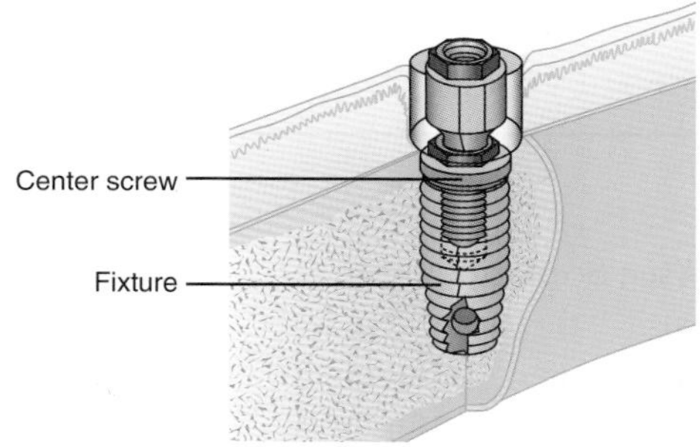

B. **Insertion of Fixture**
Maxillary healing: 6 months
Mandibular healing: 3 months

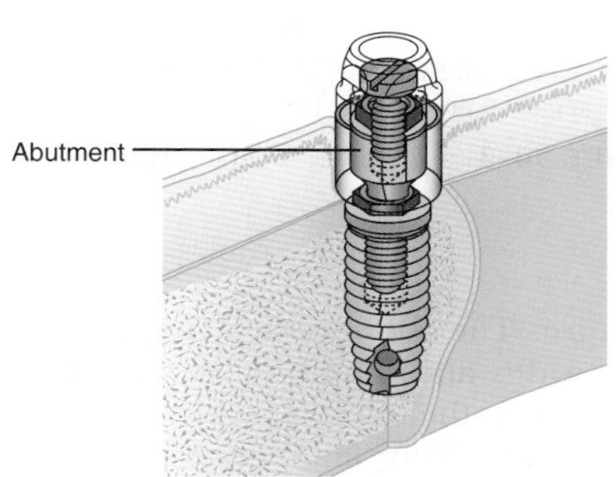

C. **Insertion of Abutment**
Maxillary healing: 3 weeks
Mandibular healing: 1 week

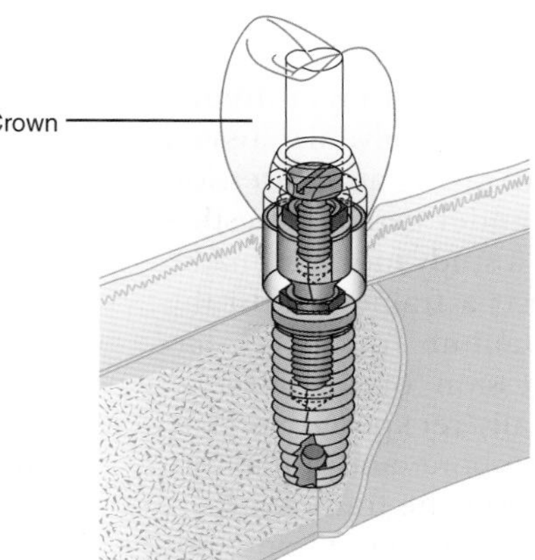

D. **Superstructure**
(crown, bridge, denture)

FIGURE 50–2 ✦ Sequence of treatment with osseointegrated dental implants. *(Courtesy NobelBioCare.)*

TABLE 50–1 DENTAL IMPLANTS AND THEIR CHARACTERISTICS

Implant	Location	Types	Material	Description of the Implant Process
Subperiosteal (Figures 50–3 to 50–6)	On top of the bone	Mandibular Staple bone plate	Cobalt-chromium Molybdenum (Vitallium) Titanium	Surgical flap to expose bone Impression of bone taken Suture Cast metallic unit made from impression Second surgical flap to place implants Four posts into bone Framework in place Suture Prosthesis placed *or* Computed tomography scan approximate casts Cast metallic unit from tomography Surgical flap made Framework in place Suture Prosthesis placed
Transosteal (transosseous) (Figures 50–7 to 50–9)	Through the bone	Complete arch Unilateral Cast framework rests over the bone of the mandible or maxilla	Titanium Aluminum Vanadium	Five- to seven-pin metal plate Fitted to the inferior border of mandible Two terminal pins protrude into oral cavity to hold overdenture Crossbar placed Prosthesis placed
Endosteal (endosseous) (Figures 50–10 to 50–17)	Within the bone	Blade-shaped Screw type	Titanium Ceramic	Surgical flap Drill hole in bone Body or fixture placed Mucosal tissue sutured Osseointegrate in 3 to 6 months Second surgical flap Abutment or neck placed Suture Prosthesis placed

Types of Dental Implants (see Scenarios 50–1 to 50–6 for clinical examples)

Three types of implants are subperiosteal, transosteal (transosseous), and endosteal (endosseous) implants (Table 50–1). The American Dental Association (ADA) considers the subperiosteal and endosteal implants to be the safest and most effective.

SUBPERIOSTEAL IMPLANT (Figures 50–3 to 50–6). The *subperiosteal* implant consists of a titanium metal framework made by surgically separating the alveolar tissue, exposing the edentulous ridge, and taking an impression of the ridge. The client is placed under general anesthesia. The alveolar tissue is sutured, a study model is made, and the laboratory technician casts a framework to the model of the bone. After the titanium framework has been fabricated from the impression of the alveolar bone, the gingival tissue is surgically reexposed and the framework is placed on top of the bone and under the periosteum. Gingival tissue heals over the framework.

The implant does not osseointegrate to the bone, but affixes itself to the bone by a fibroosseous connective tissue. Posts connected to the metal framework protrude through the gingiva to hold a fixed or removable crown, bridge, or denture. The subperiosteal implant is indicated when the width and depth of the alveolar bone are narrow or when the alveolar ridge is atrophic. Subperiosteal implants may fail because of a poorly designed prosthetic appliance or an infection that begins at the abutment site and travels throughout the implant framework.

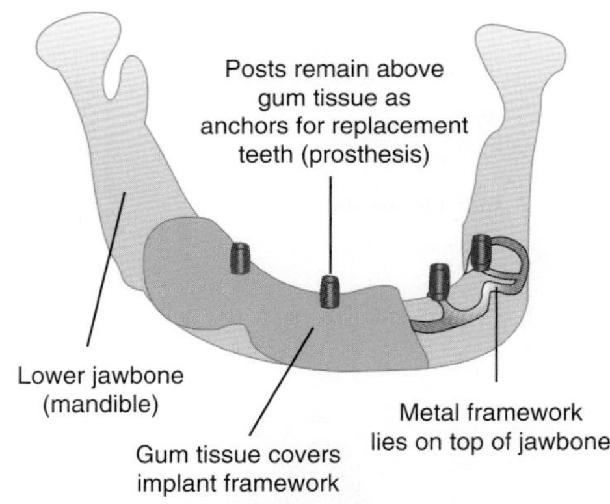

FIGURE 50–3 ✦ Subperiosteal implant.

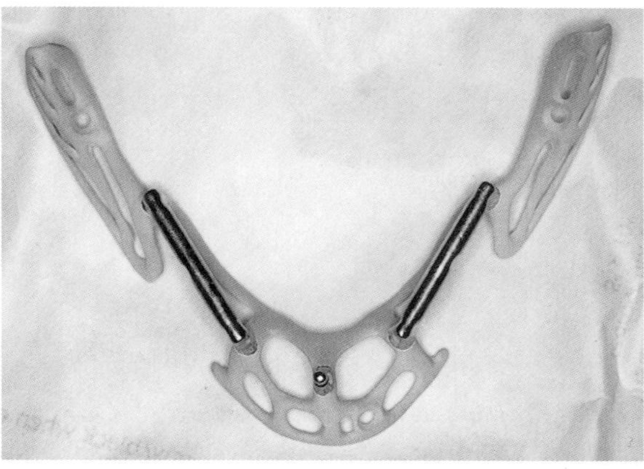

FIGURE 50–4 ✦ Calcitek subperiosteal implant. *(Courtesy MA Conover.)*

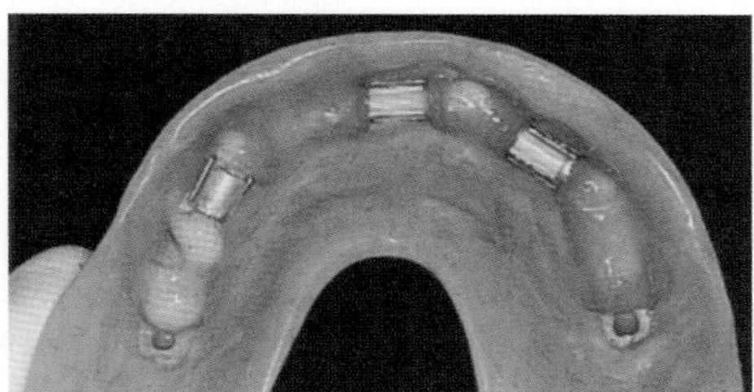

FIGURE 50–5 ✦ Overdenture used with a subperiosteal implant. *(From Babbush CA:* Dental implants: The art and science, *Philadelphia, 2001, WB Saunders.)*

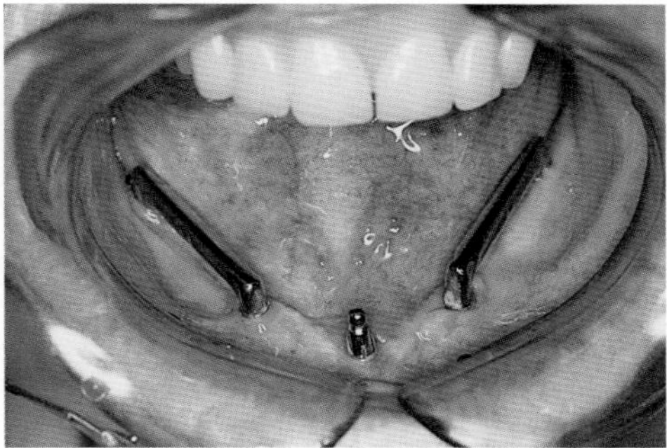

FIGURE 50–6 ✦ Client with the subperiosteal implant surgically placed. *(Courtesy MA Conover.)*

TRANSOSTEAL IMPLANT (Figures 50–7 to 50–9). The *transosteal* implant (staple implant) consists of a titanium metal framework placed through the chin and into the mandible while the client is under general anesthesia. Because the design of the transosteal implant is strictly for placement in the mandible, it cannot be placed in the maxilla. The design of this framework differs from that of the subperiosteal framework in that the transosteal implant is placed through the lower portion of the jaw, and the subperiosteal implant is placed on the alveolar ridge after the gingival tissue has been separated and exposed by flap surgery. Transosteal implants are most commonly placed when a client with a narrow mandible needs strength and support for chewing, biting, or grinding.

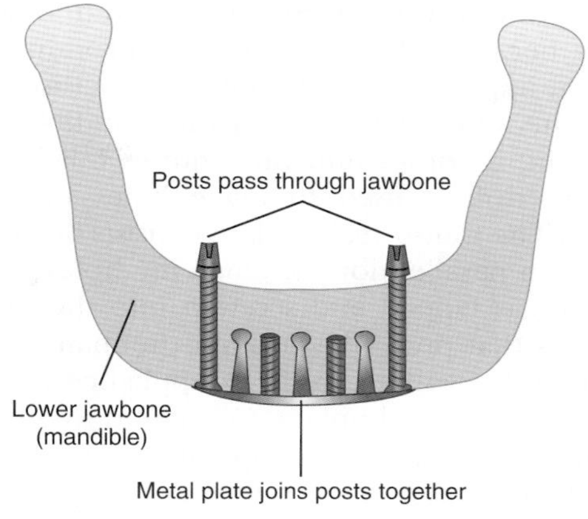

FIGURE 50–7 ✦ Transosteal implant.

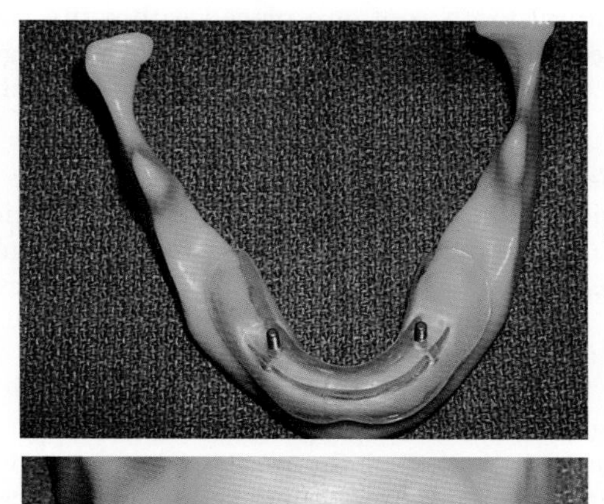

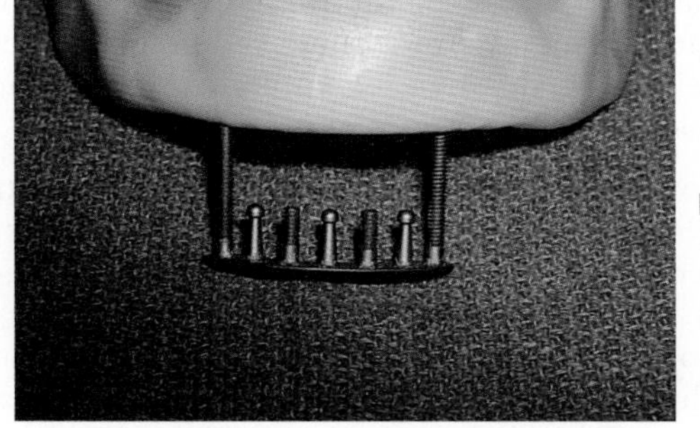

FIGURE 50–8 ✦ Hall transosteal implant with guided stent. **A,** Superior view. **B,** Inferior view. *(Courtesy MJ McDonald.)*

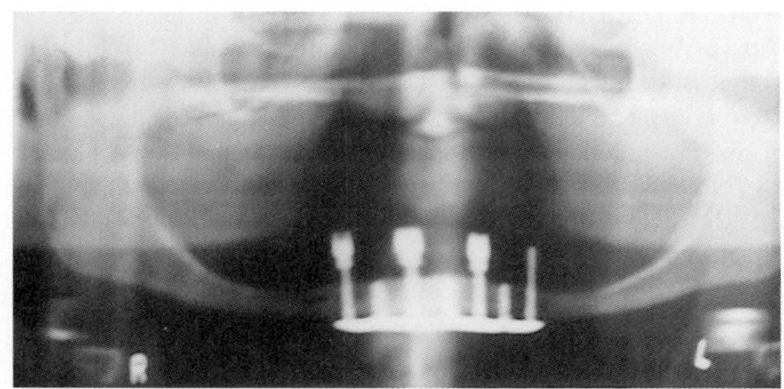

FIGURE 50–9 ✦ Radiographic example of transosteal implant surgically placed. *(Courtesy MJ McDonald.)*

A client who cannot tolerate conventional lower dentures because of severe bone resorption needs a transosteal implant. An extraoral 5-cm incision is made through the anterior portion of the mandible to place this implant; no other implant requires this incision. A high-speed drill is used to make holes through the mandible. The transosteal implant consists of a plate and five or seven parallel dowels. Once the holes are made, the implant is tapped and screwed into the mandible. The dowels that protrude through the mandible act as the abutments for the prosthetic appliance that sits on top of the transosteal implant. Compared to other surgical techniques, transosteal implant placement has an increased probability of infection and implant failure. For this reason, transosteal implants are rarely used.

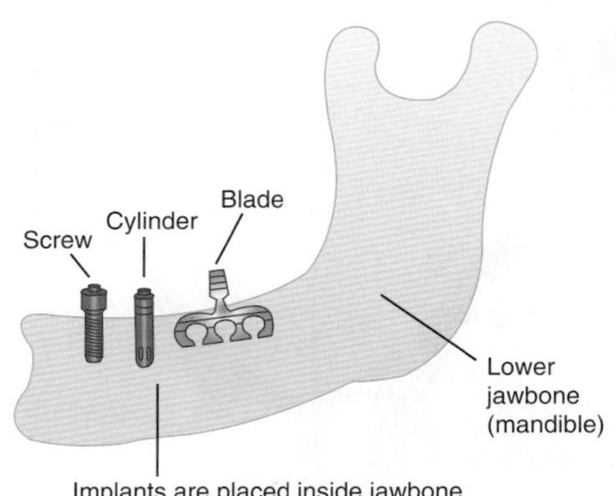

FIGURE 50–10 ✦ Three types of endosteal implants. Screw and cylinders types are more successful than blade types.

ENDOSTEAL IMPLANT (Figures 50–10 to 50–12). Titanium *endosteal* implant designs conform to the shape of a natural tooth root, are placed within the jawbone, and are supported from the bone by osseointegration. Three types of endosteal implants are described as follows (Figure 50–10):

- ✦ *Blade form* consists of one or more abutments and is surgically placed into a slot made in the bone. The prosthetic appliance is then attached to the abutment.
- ✦ *Cylinder form* consists of a small titanium cylinder and an abutment surgically inserted into the bone[2] that acts as a "root system." The cylinder form surface may be texture coated or sprayed to enhance osseointegration.
- ✦ *Screw form* consists of the implant, cover screw, abutment, abutment screw, cylinders, and gold screw. Most widely used, this type of implant provides increased efficiency and improved aesthetic result.

An example of an entire endosteal implant structure is shown in Figure 50–11. The completed cast crown is attached to the abutment by the gold screw (Figure 50–12). Regardless of design, endosteal implants are the basic tooth root analog units in implant prosthodontic procedures and the most frequently used implants for oral rehabilitation.

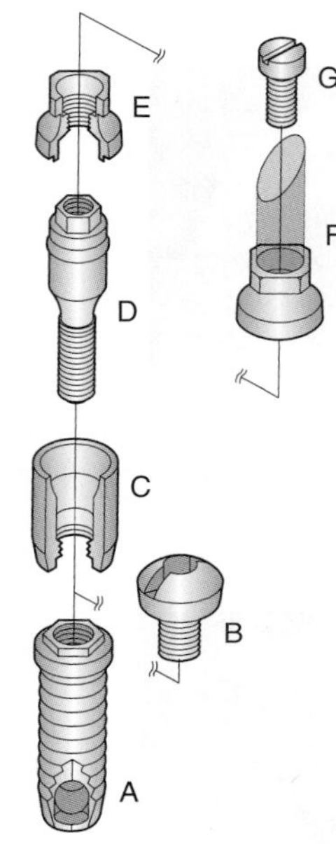

FIGURE 50–11 ✦ Brånemark system components. **A,** Implant. **B,** Cover screw. **C,** Abutment. **D,** Abutment screw. **E,** Cylinder. **F,** Cylinder. **G,** Gold screw. *(From Worthington P, Lang BR, LaVelle WE:* Osseointegration in dentistry: An introduction, *Carol Stream, Ill, 1994, Quintessence Books.)*

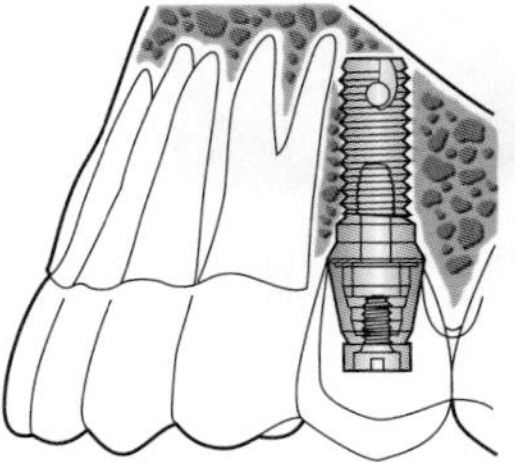

FIGURE 50–12 ✦ The cast crown is attached to the endosteal implant abutment by a gold screw. *(From Worthington P, Lang BR, LaVelle WE:* Osseointegration in dentistry: An introduction, *Carol Stream, Ill, 1994, Quintessence Books.)*

SCENARIO 50–1

A SINGLE IMPLANT WITH A FIXED PROSTHETIC TOOTH (Figure 50–13)

An 18-year-old client has fallen on his bicycle. The fall has affected the upper left central incisor. The oral surgeon extracts the tooth because the tooth is diagnosed as having Class III mobility and the gingival tissue has developed an infection with exudate. After the client's condition is assessed, dental treatment is planned for one implant in this area. The anchor is surgically inserted by the oral and maxillofacial surgeon. The restorative dentist or prosthodontist fabricates a crown to match the natural tooth that the client lost, and the fixed prosthetic tooth is secured to the top of the single implant. This type of implant can be removed only by the dentist.

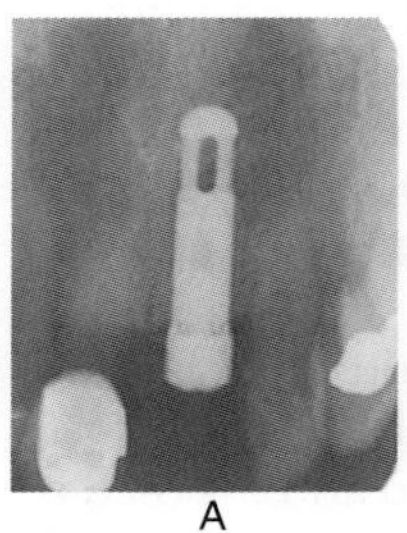

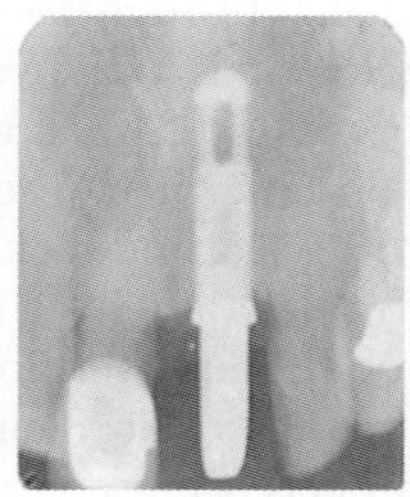

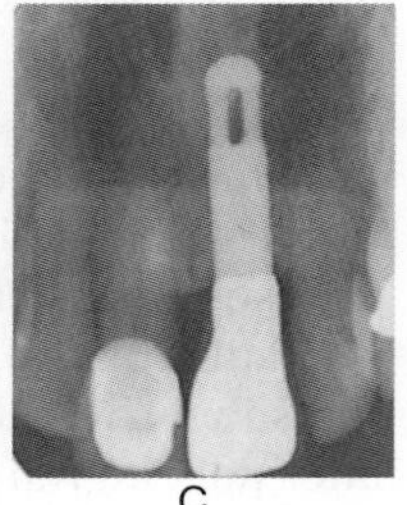

FIGURE 50–13 ✦ Radiographs of a single fixed dental implant. **A,** Dental implant placed with healing cap. **B,** Dental implant with abutment. **C,** Dental implant with fixed restorative crown. *(Courtesy K Larson.)*

SCENARIO 50–2

A CLIP AND HADER-BAR IMPLANT WITH A REMOVABLE PROSTHETIC APPLIANCE OR DENTURE (Figure 50–14)

A 70-year-old client has developed severe aggressive periodontal disease. Her facial contours have collapsed from extensive bone resorption. The general dentist and dental hygienist have discussed the diagnosis and care options with the client and have referred her to an oral surgeon for extraction of all remaining teeth. In consultation with the client, the general dentist and oral surgeon plan treatment to include a full removable upper denture and a lower endosteal implant system. The endosteal implant will consist of a two-implant system with a Hader-bar between the implants and a full lower removable denture with a clip to hold it in place. With this dental implant approach, the client can readily remove the full lower denture. The client's ability to remove the prosthetic appliance promotes long-term success of the implant by allowing daily access to the bacterial plaque accumulation and debris. The maxillary removable prosthetic appliance adds rounded facial contours and alleviates deep furrows.

SCENARIO 50–3

A BALL, CROSSBAR, AND SOCKET IMPLANT PROSTHETIC APPLIANCE (Figure 50–15)

This type of appliance could be used in Scenario 50–2 because the cylinder form of implant system is similar in function to that of the clip and Hader-bar implant with a removable prosthetic appliance described previously. The design, however, is different in that a ball is on the implant abutment and the socket is within the prosthetic appliance.

SCENARIO 50–4

A TWO-IMPLANT SYSTEM WITH A TWO-UNIT RESTORATION AND A CANTILEVER BRIDGE (Figures 50–16 and 50–17)

A client developed a benign tumor within the lower right mandible. The oral surgeon extracted two molars, removed the tumor, and inserted synthetic bone to promote bone growth. A few months later, two implants were placed in the mandibular right premolar area. The oral surgeon is hesitant to place another implant in the mandibular right molar region for fear of disturbing the inferior alveolar nerve. Therefore, a two-unit crown restoration with a cantilever bridge was fabricated. A cantilever bridge allows for a posterior occluding surface area without placing a third implant.

SCENARIO 50–5

A BLADE IMPLANT SYSTEM (Figure 50–10)

A 71-year-old client lost her right posterior molars and second premolar when she was in her early twenties. The bone resorbed, leaving her with a knife-edged ridge that would not allow a cylinder form of implant. The oral surgeon places a blade form of endosseous implant and attaches a prosthetic bridge to the implant.

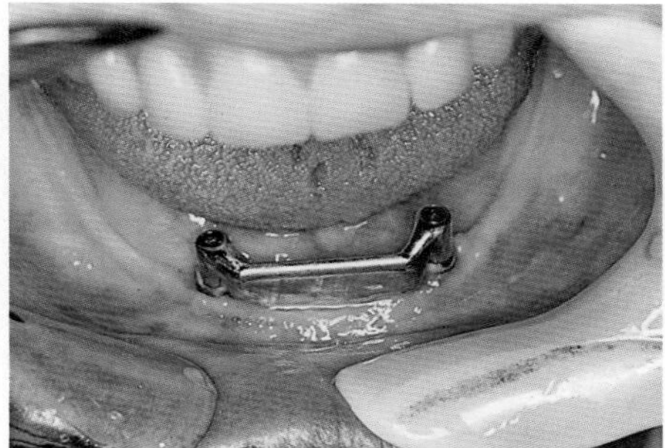

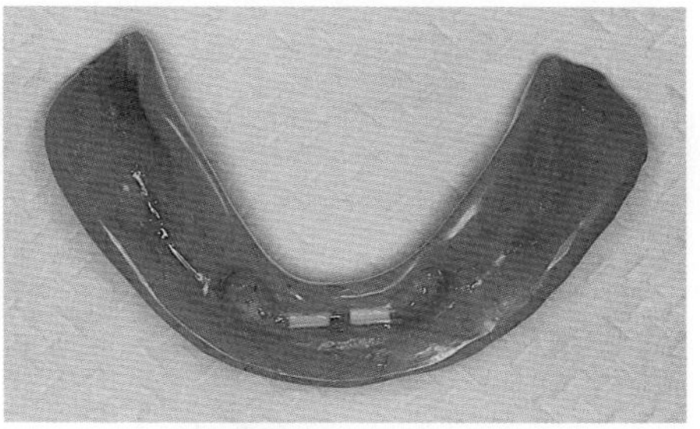

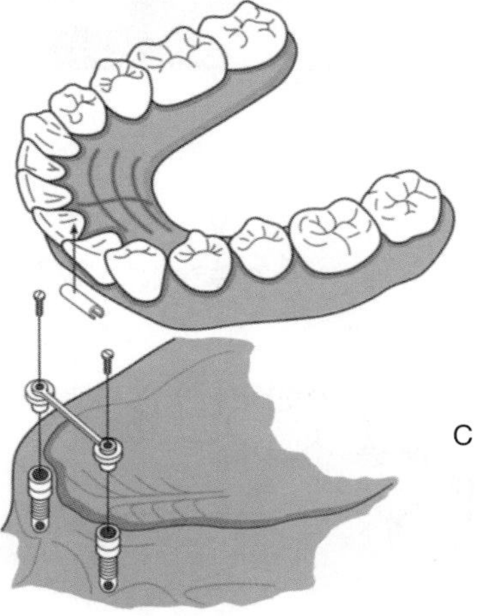

FIGURE 50–14 ✦ **A,** Crossbar endosteal implant. **B,** Clip-on type of overdenture. **C,** Components of the attachment. *(B courtesy MA Conover; C from Worthington P, Lang BR, LaVelle WE:* Osseointegration in dentistry: An introduction, *Carol Stream, Ill, 1994, Quintessence Books.)*

SCENARIO 50–6

A FULL MAXILLARY AND MANDIBULAR FIXED PROSTHESIS

A 68-year-old client complains of an ill-fitting conventional denture that she cannot tolerate. She has a strong desire for a fixed restorative implant system. The oral surgeon places a cylinder form of endosteal implant in the maxillary and mandibular arches. The fabricated prosthetic appliance (*overdenture*) is fixed to the endosteal implants. This implant system provides the client with the greatest comfort and stability. In addition, the psychological dilemma associated with removing the prosthetic appliance is eliminated because this appliance closely resembles the client's natural tooth function. However, the facial contours are difficult to reshape and rebuild. Fixed appliances also are limited to the amount of bulk and volume they can contain to reshape the facial contours ideally.

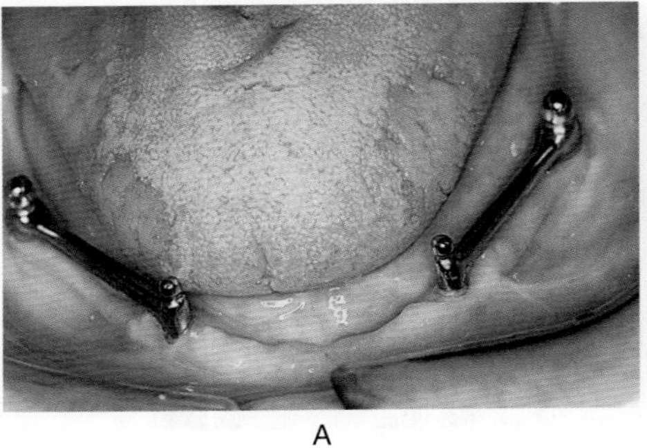
A

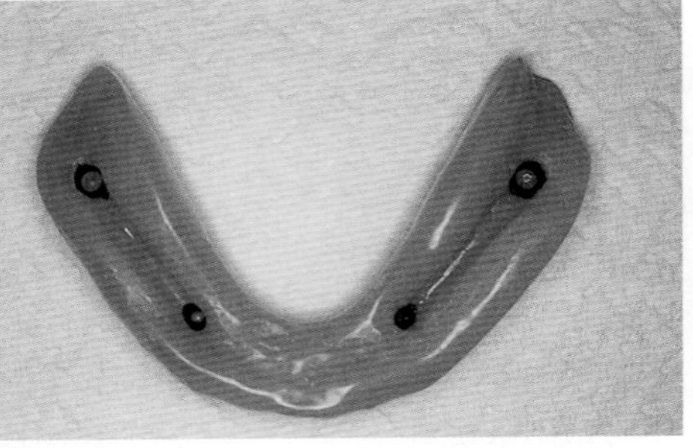
B

FIGURE 50–15 ✦ **A,** Ball and crossbar endosteal implant. **B,** Socket-type overdenture. *(Courtesy MA Conover.)*

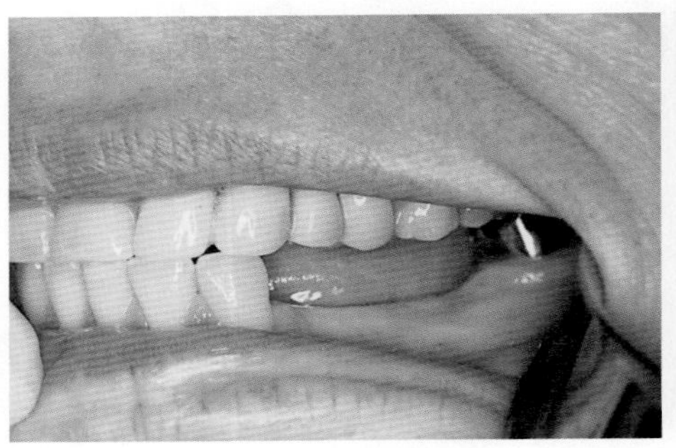
A

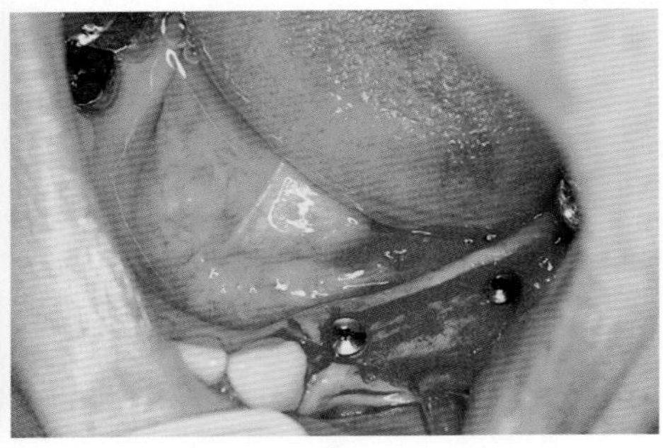
B

FIGURE 50–16 ✦ **A,** Partial edentulism. **B,** Two endosteal implants surgically placed in edentulous area. *(Courtesy MA Conover.)*

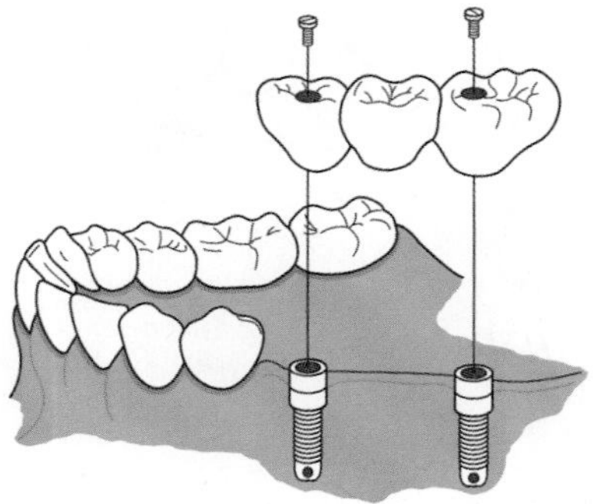

FIGURE 50–17 ✦ Endosteal implant–supported restoration in a partially edentulous mandible is not attached to the adjoining natural tooth. *(From Worthington P, Lang BR, LaVelle WE:* Osseointegration in dentistry: An introduction, *Carol Stream, Ill, 1994, Quintessence Books.)*

Implant Process

The implant process consists of a three-stage surgical and restorative treatment plan and follows the dental implant client flowchart (Figure 50–18).

STAGE ONE: FIRST SURGICAL PROCEDURE. At the first surgical appointment, the client is placed under general or local anesthesia. General anesthesia is commonly used with the placement of transosteal implants. In addition, a local anesthetic may be administered into the gingival tissue for hemostasis. A *surgical guide stent,* a clear resin device containing holes, is constructed (Figure 50–19) to maintain angulation and axis for drilling the bone and for placement of the fixture. The dental implant anchor is placed into the drilled holes of the bone. The oral surgeon considers the mandibular canal with respect to placement of the implants in the mandible. There should be at least 1 mm of bone between the apex of the endosteal implant and the neurovascular bundle to prevent nerve damage (Figure 50–20.) The amount of bone inferior to the maxillary sinus is also a consideration (Figure 50–21). After surgical placement, the periosteum is sutured over the implant for a healing period. After surgery, the client experiences a sensation similar to that of having a tooth extracted.

Osseointegration (Figure 50–22) is a biologic phenomenon in which living bone cells directly fuse to a unique space-age metal, titanium or Vitallium, that exhibits excellent biocompatibility. Bone cells grow tightly around the metal anchor and firmly hold it in place (Figure 50–23). Success of the dental implant depends on the osseointegration process, wherein the bone fuses to the implant.

Because mandibular bone is less dense than maxillary bone, the mandible does not require as long of a healing or osseointegration period as does the maxilla. *In general, dental implants placed in the mandibular bone heal and osseointegrate within 3 to 6 months, whereas the maxillary bone takes approximately 4 to 6 months to heal and osseointegrate.* At the end of the first year, the osseointegration process should be stable.

Once the dental implant has osseointegrated to the bone, the gingival attachment is similar to an ankylosed tooth. Because the periodontal ligament is not present, the implant should not have mobility. The connective tissue attachment is the primary difference between implants and natural teeth. The supracrestal collagenous fibers do not attach to the implant as they do to cementum.

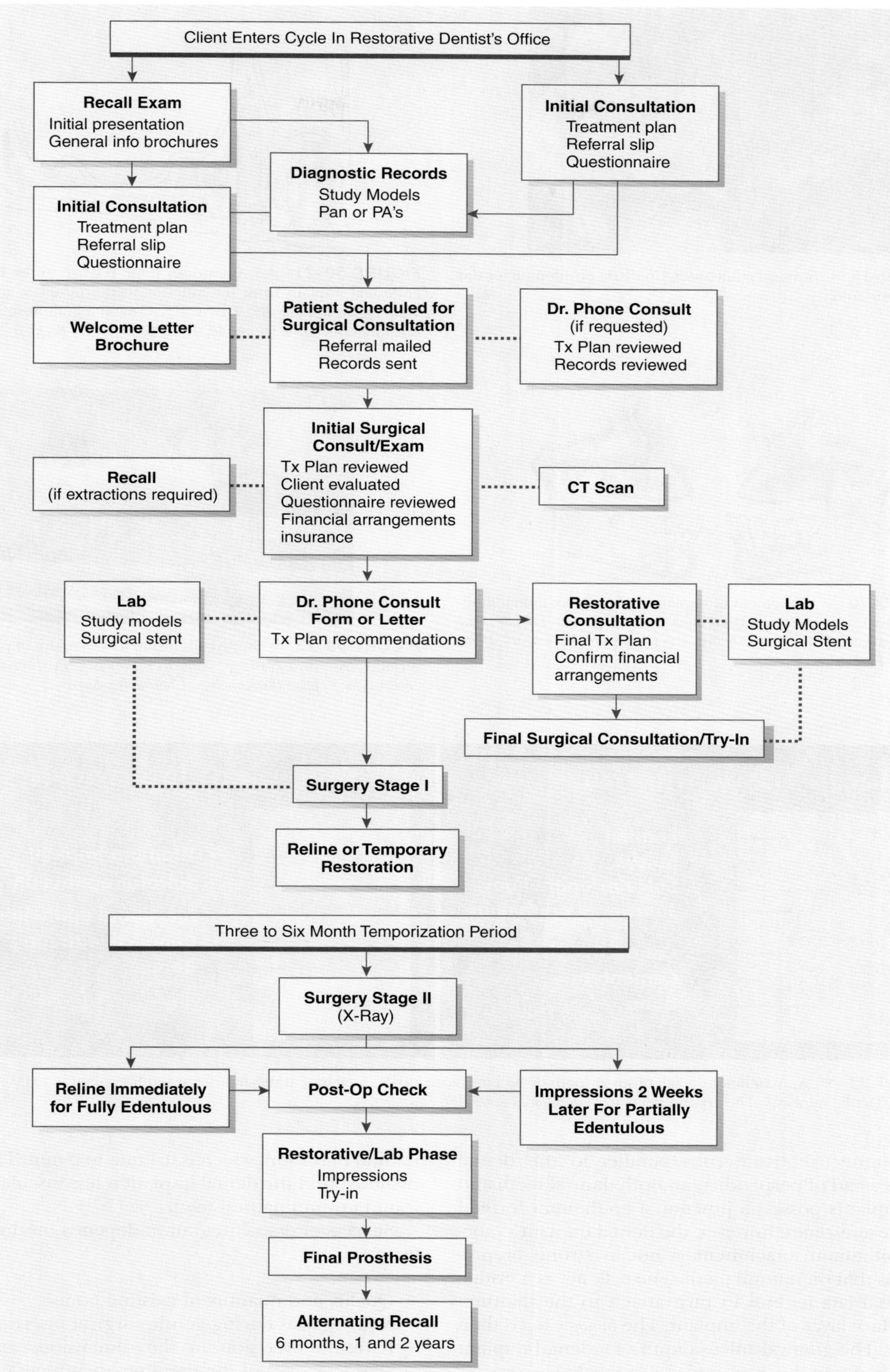

FIGURE 50–18 ✦ Dental implant client flowchart. *(Courtesy Implant Network Concept.)*

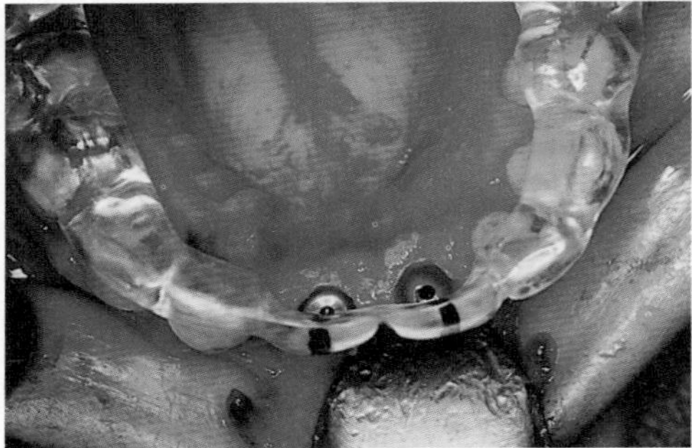

FIGURE 50–19 ✦ Surgical guide stent. Confirms positioning for the intended restoration.

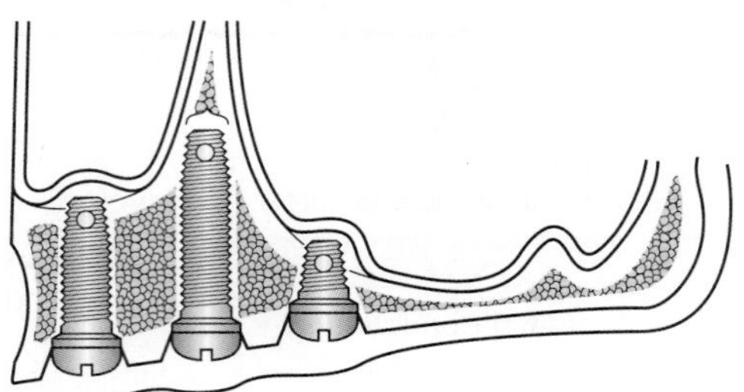

FIGURE 50–21 ✦ Amount of bone relative to the length of the endosteal implant from the anterior to the posterior maxilla. *(From Worthington P, Lang BR, LaVelle WE:* Osseointegration in dentistry: An introduction, *Carol Stream, Ill, 1994, Quintessence Books.)*

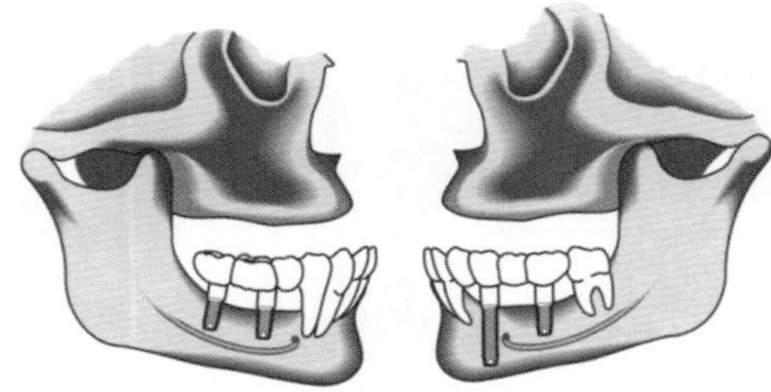

FIGURE 50–20 ✦ Placement of implants with respect to mandibular nerve and canal. *(From Worthington P, Lang BR, LaVelle WE:* Osseointegration in dentistry: An introduction, *Carol Stream, Ill, 1994, Quintessence Books.)*

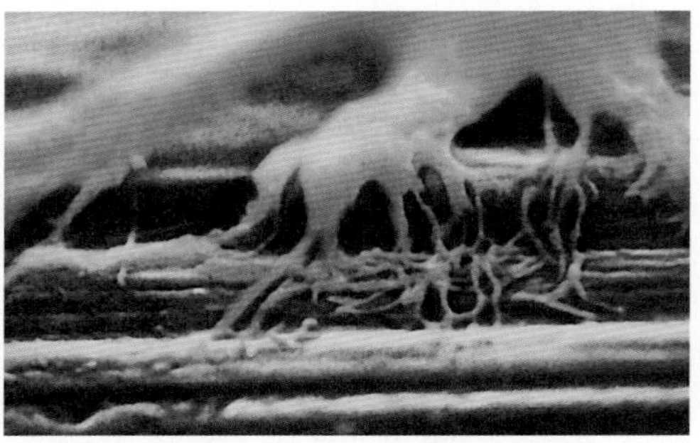

FIGURE 50–22 ✦ Bone cells fusing to a titanium implant, which is termed osseointegration. *(Courtesy Professor Per-Ingvar Brånemark, Institute for Applied Biotechnology, Gothenburg, Sweden.)*

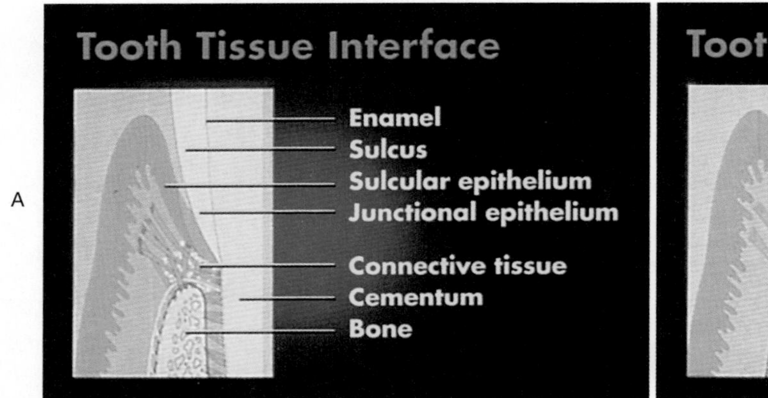

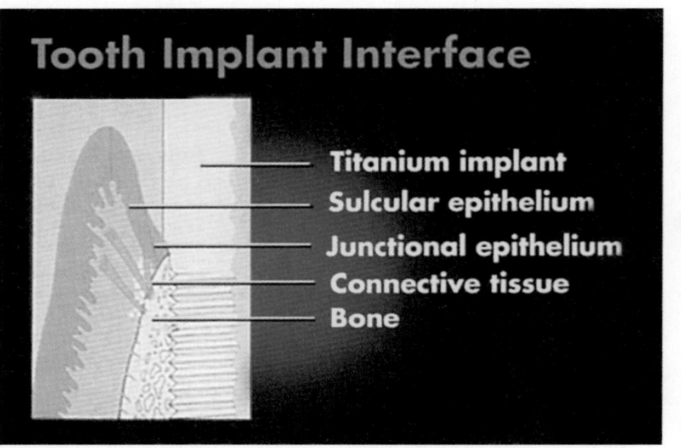

FIGURE 50–23 ✦ **A,** Attachment mechanism at tooth-tissue interface *(left).* **B,** Attachment mechanism at tooth-implant interface *(right). (From Babbush CA:* Dental implants: The art and science, *Philadelphia, 2001, WB Saunders.)*

The connective tissue runs parallel to the dental implant instead of perpendicular. Both natural teeth and dental implants possess a junctional epithelium formed by hemidesmosomes; however, the dental implant's junctional epithelium attachment is not as strong or predictable as that on natural teeth. The cells act as a bridge to the basal lamina and in turn attach to the titanium oxide surface layer of the implant. The *biologic seal* is then complete. The gingival sulcus depth of a dental implant averages between 1.3 mm and 3.8 mm; that is greater than the average sulcus depth around healthy and natural dentition, which is 0.4 mm to 3 mm. The gingival tissue around the dental implant is less vascular than that found around natural teeth.

Success of osseointegration depends on the following factors:

- ✦ Quality and quantity of existing bone
- ✦ Strict asepsis during gentle surgical insertion
- ✦ Extreme precision in the dimensions and surface characteristics of the titanium anchorage units
- ✦ Adequate uninterrupted healing time of bone

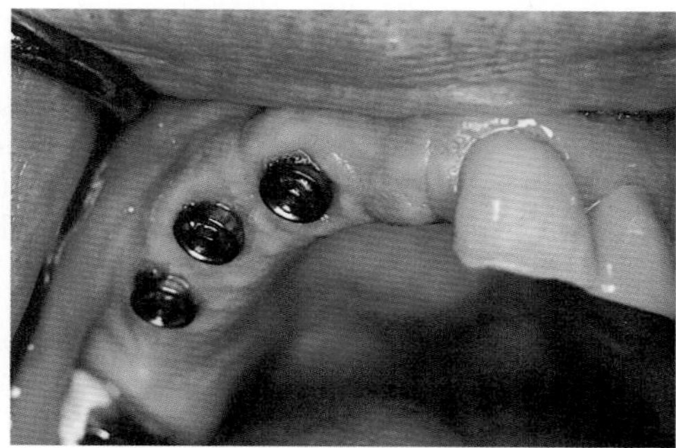

FIGURE 50–24 ✦ Client has healthy peri-implant tissue and good oral hygiene compliance. *(Courtesy AK Lakha.)*

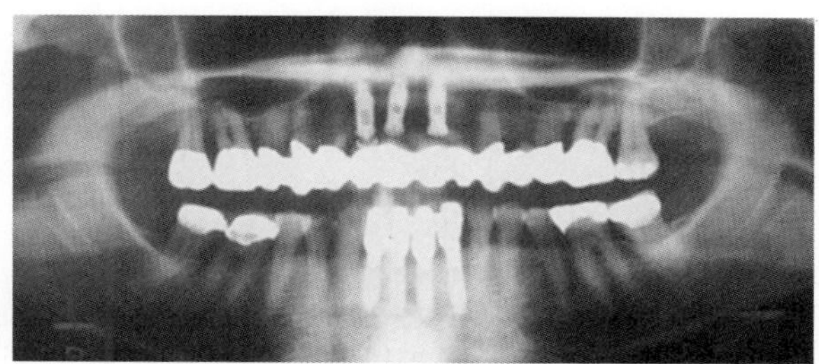

FIGURE 50–25 ✦ Radiographs of endosseous implants used for clinical follow-up. *(From Babbush CA:* Dental implants: The art and science, *Philadelphia, 2001, WB Saunders.)*

- Sound superstructure
- Uniform "bite" once the bridgework is attached
- Daily oral hygiene care by the client (Figure 50–24)
- Long-term clinical and radiographic monitoring (Figure 50–25)

The Brånemark system, named after the discoverer of the osseointegration process used in dentistry, is the only system with the ADA Seal of Acceptance. The ADA contends that the Brånemark system is acceptable in fully edentulous patients; however, the dentist is responsible for proper patient selection, adequate training and experience in the placement of the implant, and obtaining informed consent.

STAGE TWO: SECOND SURGICAL PROCEDURE. After the implants have osseointegrated (determined by radiographic appearance), a second surgery is performed. The implants are surgically uncovered to place the abutments on top of the exposed implants. The implants are then surgically re-covered by suturing the periosteum together, with the abutments protruding through the periosteum. *Healing caps* (Figure 50–26) are placed to allow the tissue to heal, for oral hygiene access to the implant abutments, and for the prosthodontist or restorative dentist to secure the prosthetic appliance. The healing caps are removed after 2 to 4 weeks and the abutments are uncovered (Figure 50–27.)

STAGE THREE: FABRICATION OF PROSTHETIC APPLIANCE OR RESTORATIVE CROWN. The third stage (Figure 50–28) of the implant process begins with fabricating the prosthetic appliance and may require several appointments to achieve a desirable fit. The design of the prosthetic appliance should ensure a wide interproximal space for access during daily plaque biofilm control. One to two weeks after the placement of the prosthetic appliance, oral self-care education is provided. Within a few months, natural tooth function should be restored.

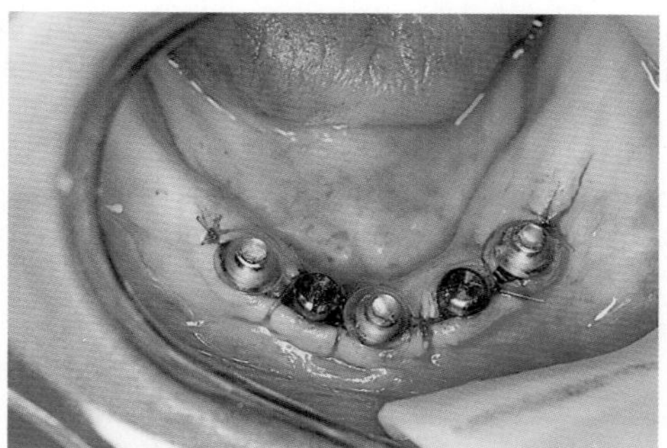

FIGURE 50–26 ✦ Stage two: Endosseous implants with healing caps. *(Courtesy MA Conover.)*

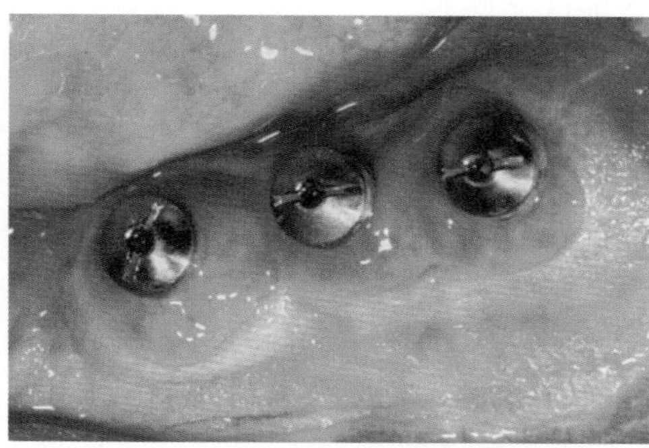

FIGURE 50–27 ✦ Implant fixtures uncovered six weeks after stage two. Note tissue hyperplasia at soft tissue–titanium interface. Implant fixtures uncovered. *(From Babbush CA:* Dental implants: The art and science, *Philadelphia, 2001, WB Saunders.)*

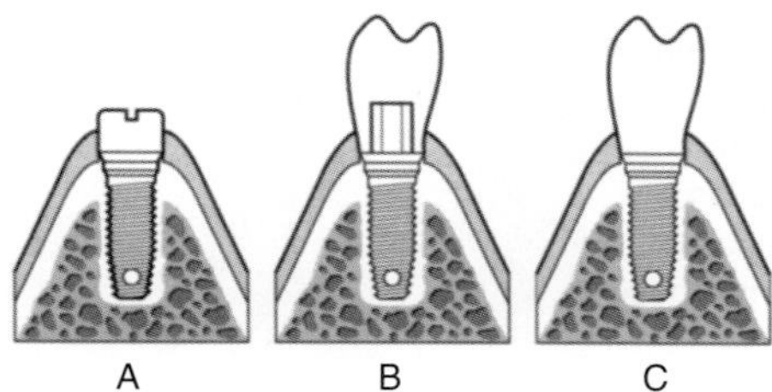

FIGURE 50–28 ✦ Stage two surgery for two-stage endosseous implant systems. **A,** The cover screws are located, removed, and replaced by an abutment cylinder that penetrates the mucosa into the mouth. **B,** The prosthetic component is then mounted on the abutment. **C,** The final stage three restoration is attached with a screw or cement. *(From Worthington P, Lang BR, LaVelle WE:* Osseointegration in dentistry: An introduction, *Carol Stream, Ill, 1994, Quintessence Books.)*

Candidate Selection Process

The oral health team gathers information about health history, medications, allergies, chief complaints, missing teeth, current prosthetic appliances, radiographs, and diagnostic models. This information allows the dentist to determine the type of implant to use and the care plan. Figure 50–29 depicts an oral surgery dental implant referral form.

Indications and Contraindications for Using Dental Implants lists indications and contraindications for dental implants considered in identifying candidates for dental implantation. Indications and contraindications should be discussed candidly with the client. The necessity for client compliance with oral hygiene recommendations should be emphasized and explained. Unfortunately, many clients view the implant as a new tooth that will

DENTAL IMPLANT REFERRAL FORM

Date: ______________________________

Client: ______________________ Phone: ______________

Referring Doctor: ______________________________

Client's Chief Complaint:
- ☐ Difficulty in eating
- ☐ Functional difficulty
- ☐ Aesthetics
- ☐ Prosthetic discomfort
- ☐ Facial image
- ☐ Other ______________________________

Dental Treatment Plan:

Partially Edentulous
- ☐ Single tooth replacement
- ☐ Implant bridge to natural teeth
- ☐ Totally fixed implant bridge

Totally Edentulous
- ☐ Full arch fixed prosthesis
- ☐ Hader bar, clip removable prosthesis
- ☐ Ball and socket removable prosthesis

Alternative Treatment: ______________________________

Diagnostic Records:
- ☐ Periapical radiographs/full mouth series
- ☐ Panorex
- ☐ CT scan
- ☐ Tomograph
- ☐ Study models

FIGURE 50–29 ✦ Dental implant referral form.

Indications and Contraindications for Using Dental Implants

Indications

Good general physical and mental health to facilitate client acceptance of the dental implant

A commitment to a daily plaque biofilm control regimen to avoid peri-implantitis

Manual dexterity to ensure that plaque biofilm control procedures can be performed effectively on a daily basis

A sufficient quantity and quality of alveolar bone to retain the dental implant

Continuous cooperation and communication between client and oral healthcare team

Contraindications

Blood dyscrasias (prevent proper healing and clotting)

Certain cardiovascular diseases

Chronic renal diseases

Corticosteroidal use

Debilitating or uncontrollable disease or compromised healing conditions, such as that resulting from radiation therapy

Diabetic clients susceptible to gingival and periodontal disease

Hypersensitivity of tissues to specific implant materials

Inability of client to maintain optimal daily hygiene care

Inadequate client motivation

Local gingival infection

Metabolic diseases

Noncorrectable heavy grinding or bruxing problem

Pregnant client

Psychiatric disorders

Rheumatoid disease

Systemic infection

Unattainable prosthetic reconstruction

Unrealistic expectations of the client

tolerate mistreatment better than a natural tooth. This myth must be dispelled, and the client must realize that the gingival tissue around the dental implant needs *more* oral hygiene care than the gingival tissue around a natural tooth.

Some dental implant candidates have lost their natural teeth as a result of poor plaque biofilm control and periodontal disease. These individuals may be at risk for failure of the dental implant. To determine the level of commitment to daily oral care, a dental hygienist evaluates the client's value system by asking how he feels about his mouth and his oral health behaviors. A motivated client with a good level of manual dexterity is an important requirement in a candidate for dental implants and long-term success. In fact, a willingness to perform daily plaque biofilm control is a criterion that separates a good implant candidate from a poor one. Questions shown in Assessment Questions to Determine Whether Client is a Good Candidate for Dental Implants help determine who might be a good implant candidate.

If the client has one or more chronic contraindications, the oral health team may recommend another mode of treatment. Once contraindications are resolved, the client can be reevaluated for implants.

Assessment Questions to Determine Whether Client is a Good Candidate for Dental Implants

When you eat, do your dentures cause you pain?
Do your dentures fit adequately?
Are your teeth mobile or displaced?
Do you have any concerns about your dentures?
Will you commit the time to take care of your dental implants on a daily basis?
Will you keep your appointments?
Will you be able to wait 6 months for the final dental implant system?
Are you willing to stop using tobacco?

Benefits and Risks

The benefits and risks should be explained verbally and in writing to potential dental implant clients (see Benefits and Risks of Dental Implants).

BENEFITS. Dental implants allow clients to chew food properly, facilitating essential digestive processes. In addition, clients with dental implants report that they enjoy their food more; their speech is improved; and their comfort, appearance, self-confidence, and self-esteem are increased compared to their previous condition. Other benefits include decreased bone resorption, tissue ulceration, and pressure; elimination of direct force on the gingival tissue and alveolar crest; increased retention of the prosthetic appliance; and preservation of the remaining bone structure. Studies show an overall implant success rate of 96% over a 20-year period.

RISKS. Clients may lose dental implants because of bacterial plaque–related peri-implantitis. In poor oral hygiene, the oral microflora consists of increased levels of subgingival spirochetes and Gram-negative anaerobic rods that are mostly *P. intermedius, P. gingivalis,* and *Fusobacterium* sp. *Actinobacillus actinomycemcomitans* also may be found. These microorganisms' endotoxins and metabolic end products lyse epithelial and connective tissue and produce an acute inflammatory response. The gingival attachment breaks down and an apical migration of the junctional epithelium begins, followed by apical bone loss and mobility. The absence of the connective tissue attachment around the dental implant may account for the fragility of the junctional epithelium. Dental implants are more susceptible to inflammation, which advances quicker and deeper than around natural teeth.

Benefits and Risks of Dental Implants

Benefits

Improved ability to masticate and speak adequately
Enhanced self-confidence and esteem due to improved aesthetics and function
Decreased amount of bone resorption
Decreased tissue ulceration and unnecessary pressure
Elimination of direct force on the gingival tissue and alveolar crest
Increased retention of the prosthetic appliance
Preservation of the remaining bone structure

Risks

Failure to osseointegrate
Improper client selection
Improper control of immediate stress or load force
Improper oral hygiene care
Inadequate allowance of healing time and interface development
Inadequate control of manufacture quality
Inadequate implant or prosthetic design
Periimplantitis (see Figures 50–33 and 50–34 later in the chapter)
Surgical complications

Rapidly, the continued inflammation will be surrounded by fibrous tissue, and granulation tissue replaces and destroys the healthy bone and the implant will be lost. *Dental implant clients who are partially edentulous have greater risk of implant failure than dental implant clients with fully edentulous mouths.* Remaining natural dentition act as reservoirs for periodontal microbes, which migrate to the implant sites and initiate infection.

An implant may fail because of a *dehiscence* (a hole in the buccal or labial plate of the alveolar process caused by placing an implant in an area of insufficient bone). Some also fail because of the body's inability to accept the space-age metal of the implant, failure to osseointegrate,

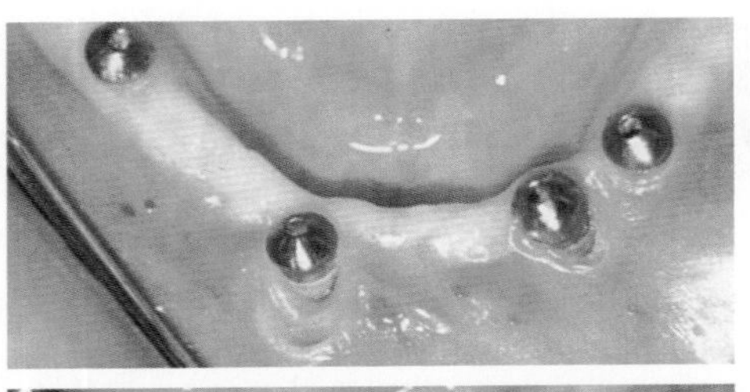

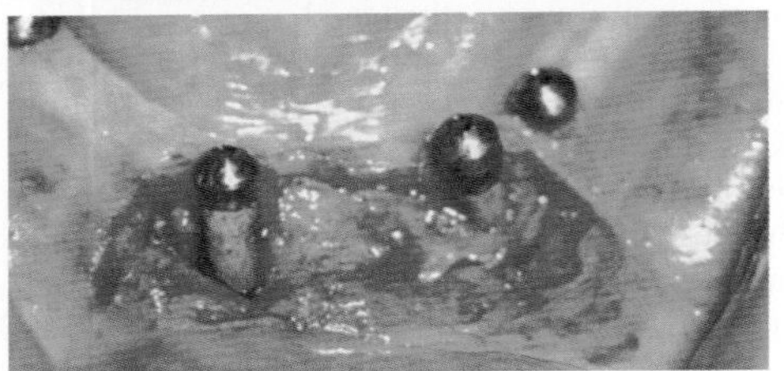

FIGURE 50–30 ✦ **A,** Clinical appearance of peri-implantitis. **B,** Soft tissue is reflected, revealing the loss of osseous support in areas 22 and 27. *(From Babbush CA:* Dental implants: The art and science, *Philadelphia, 2001, WB Saunders.)*

improper client selection, improper *load force* (pressure from masticatory processes that are not balanced across the dentition) exerted on the implant, inadequate allowance of healing time and interface development, inadequate control of manufacturing quality of the dental implant, inadequate prosthetic design, and surgical complications (Figure 50–30).

Documentation and Informed Consent

The dentist informs the dental implant candidate of the treatment plan, including time requirements to complete the plan, the self-care regimen required, and the benefits and risks of having dental implants. After relevant information is explained to the client, an informed consent document should be signed and dated by the client and clinicians involved. After implant placement, the client should be given a card to keep in his or her wallet to identify the location, the type of dental implant, and the date on which the implant was placed (Figure 50–31, *A*). A dental implant sticker or uniquely colored chart should be used in the client record to identify the dental implant client.

DENTAL HYGIENE PROCESS OF CARE FOR THE CLIENT WITH DENTAL IMPLANTS

Assessment

During assessment, the dental hygienist identifies and documents signs and symptoms of oral problems and risk factors associated with the dental implant:

- Changes in the health history
- Location of implants using the implant stamp (Figure 50–31, *B*)

TABLE 50–2 ATTACHED PERI-IMPLANT TISSUE INDEX

Grade*	Clinical Impression
0	No keratinized epithelium
1	1 mm or less keratinized epithelium
2	2 mm or less than or equal to 2 mm and greater than 1 mm keratinized epithelium
3	Greater than 2 mm keratinized epithelium

* Create tension by retracting lips laterally to form the mucoperi-implant tissue junction. Use probe to measure the external surface of the attached peri-implant tissue (note that this measurement uses the tissue that is outside of the sulcus); measure from the mucoperi-implant tissue line to the peri-implant tissue margin to determine width.
From Koth D, McKinney RV Jr, Steflik D: *Clinical dentistry: Evaluation of the implant-gingival tissue interface,* Hagerstown, Md, 1984, Harper & Row.

TABLE 50–3 PERI-IMPLANT TISSUE BLEEDING INDEX

Grade*	Clinical Impression
0	No inflammation Peri-implant tissue of normal color and stippling with no bleeding on probing
1	Mild inflammation Peri-implant tissue with slight change in color and stippling with slight hyperemia, no bleeding upon probing
2	Moderate inflammation Peri-implant tissue hyperemic with redness, edema, glazing, and loss of stippling, bleeding upon probing
3	Severe inflammation Peri-implant tissue markedly red, edematous, ulcerated, and tendency toward spontaneous bleeding on finger pressure

* Visual assessment and use of a plastic probe determines grade of peri-implant tissue.
From Koth D, McKinney RV Jr, Steflik D: *Clinical dentistry: Evaluation of the implant-gingival tissue interface,* Hagerstown, Md, 1984, Harper & Row.

- Conditions of the oral mucosa
- Discomfort, pain, or infection related to the implant
- Color, texture, and overall condition of the gingival peri-implant tissues, as measured by the:
  Attached Peri-implant Tissue Index (Table 50–2)
  Peri-implant Tissue Bleeding Index (Table 50–3)
- Periodontal probing depths
- Bleeding on probing
- Presence of exudate in sulci around abutments
- Amount of bacterial plaque biofilm and calculus formation as measured by disclosing solution and the *Plaque and Calculus Index* (Table 50–4)
- Visualization of *salivary percolation* as a result of applying pressure to the crown of the implant and causing bubbles to form at the sulcus, indicating a breakdown of the biologic seal
- Mobility of the bridgework as measured by the *Mobility Index* (Tables 50–5 and 50–6)

Dental Implant Wallet Card
Client: Dana Lowe
Implant Date of Placement: 12-27-03
Location of Implant #27, 22, 6, 11
Implant Manufacturer: IMZ Interpore
Registration No.: 256943
Type of Implant: Internal Hex 3.25 cylinder

Location of your dental implant may not be determined by visual inspection. This information is important and should be kept with you in case of your relocation or your decision to see a new dentist.

A

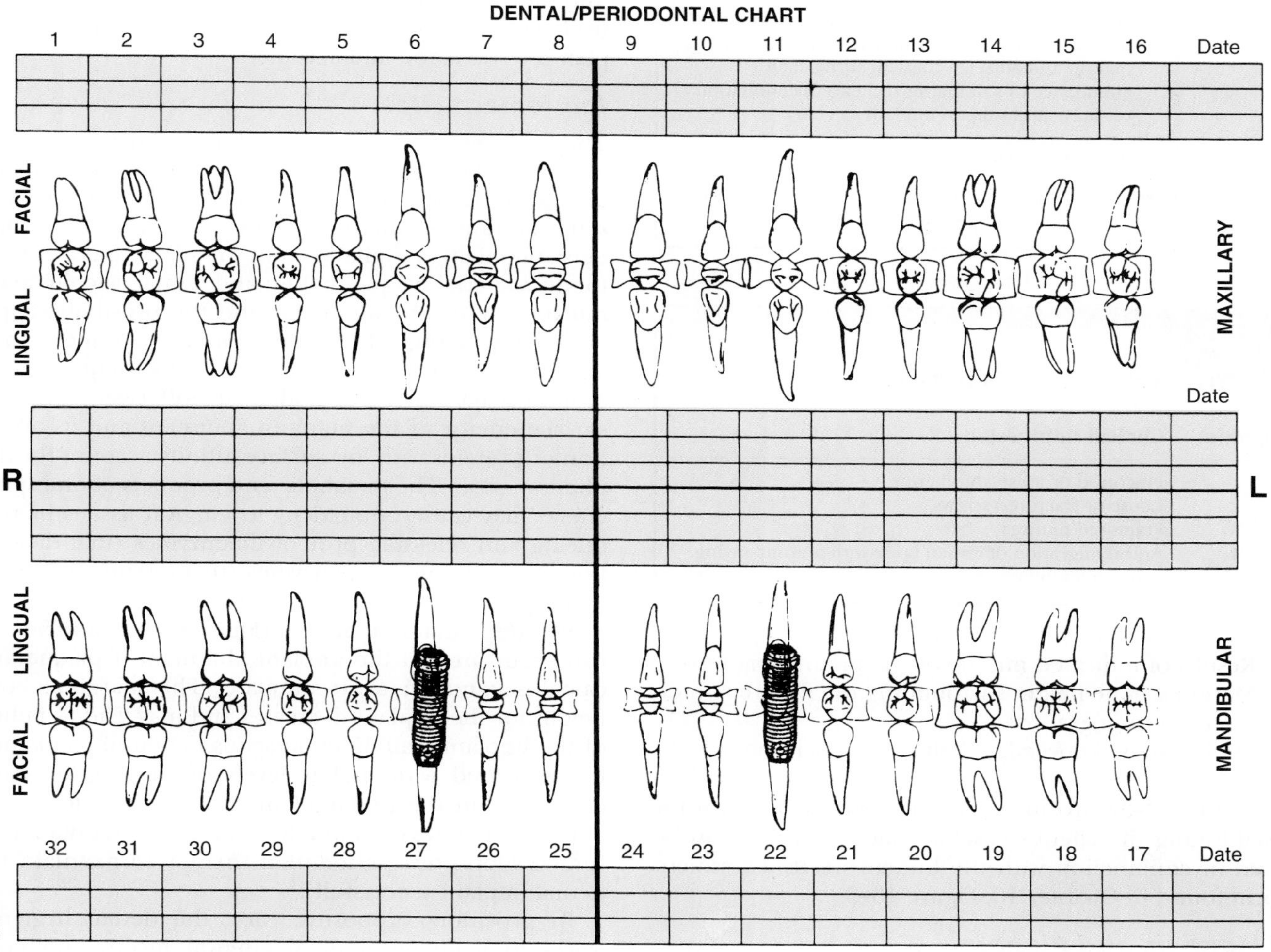

DENTAL/PERIODONTAL CHART

1 2 3 4 5 6 7 8 9 10 11 12 13 14 15 16 Date

FACIAL
LINGUAL
MAXILLARY

Date

R
L

LINGUAL
FACIAL
MANDIBULAR

32 31 30 29 28 27 26 25 24 23 22 21 20 19 18 17 Date

B

FIGURE 50–31 ✦ **A,** Dental implant wallet card. **B,** Dental implant stamp used to show location of dental implant for documentation in the client record.

TABLE 50–4 PLAQUE AND CALCULUS INDEX FOR DENTAL IMPLANTS

Grade*	Clinical Impression
0	No plaque in the peri-implant tissue area The amount of plaque is determined by running a pointed plastic probe across the implant surface at the entrance of the peri-implant crevice No calculus
1	A film of plaque can be removed but is not visible to the clinician; or supragingival calculus extending no more than 1 mm below the peri-implant tissue margin and adjacent area of the implant The plaque may be recognized only by running a probe across the implant surface
2	Visible plaque within the peri-implant crevice or on the implant and peri-implant tissue margin and adjacent peri-implant tissue surface; moderate accumulation of soft debris; or subgingival calculus extending more than 1 mm into the crevice or moderate amounts of supra- and subperi-implant calculus can be seen visually
3	Heavy accumulation of plaque within the crevice or on the implant surface and peri-implant tissue margin and adjacent implant surface; an abundance of soft matter or heavy accumulation of supra- and subperi-implant calculus

* Visual assessment and use of a plastic probe determine grade of plaque and calculus.
From Koth D, McKinney RV Jr, Steflik D: *Clinical dentistry: Evaluation of the implant-gingival tissue interface,* Hagerstown, Md, 1984, Harper & Row.

TABLE 50–5 MOBILITY EVALUATION

Grade	Clinical Impression
1	Fractured or loose abutments
2	Loose or fractured screws
3	Fractured fixtures
4	Apical migration of crestal bone with accompanying severe mobility

- ✦ Results of indicated microbiologic monitoring tests
- ✦ Marginal bone height surrounding the fixture as indicated on radiographs
- ✦ Oral hygiene knowledge, beliefs, and behaviors

Figure 50–32 provides a sample assessment form for establishing the client's baseline status and that can be used in conjunction with the human needs assessment form found in Chapter 16, Figure 16–3.

Diagnosis and Planning

Depending on the client's diagnosed unmet needs, the dental hygienist, in conjunction with the client and the dentist, sets goals and develops a care plan. Client preferences significantly affect the client's acceptance of oral health recommendations and should be incorporated into the care plan. The dental hygienist works collaboratively with the client to ensure that the proposed care plan is understood and accepted.

TABLE 50–6 MOBILITY INDEX FOR FREE-STANDING ENDOSTEAL IMPLANTS AND ATTACHED PROSTHESES

Grade*	Clinical Impression
0	No mobility
1	Slight buccolingual mobility, less than 0.5 mm
2	Slight buccolingual mobility, more than 0.5 mm but less than 1.0 mm
3	Mobility more than 0.5 mm in buccolingual and mesiodistal directions
4	Depressible, salivary percolation (bubbling around implant)

* Use of two single-ended metal instruments to determine mobility. Rock the implant to test horizontal mobility. Test vertical mobility by applying pressure occlusally.
From Koth D, McKinney RV Jr, Steflik D: *Clinical dentistry: Evaluation of the implant-gingival tissue interface,* Hagerstown, Md, 1984, Harper & Row.

Implementation

The oral environment surrounding the dental implant consists of keratinized and nonkeratinized peri-implant tissues. A biologic seal is created and adapts to the titanium abutment. Microbial flora within the sulcus of a dental implant is similar to that found around a natural tooth; bacterial plaque biofilm and dental calculus accumulate around the abutment and the prosthetic appliance. Supragingival calculus, more common than subgingival calculus, is less tenacious than calculus around a natural tooth and flakes off easily. The low surface energy of the titanium abutment and its attraction of proteins with low surface affinity account for this phenomenon. The metabolic end products of oral spirochetes may cause cytotoxicity to gingival tissues by producing and releasing proteolytic enzymes (that dissolve fibrin) and trypsin-like enzymes (that disrupt cell-to-cell adhesion).

Peri-implant inflammation (Figures 50–33 and 50–34) can occur around the implant abutment if plaque and calculus continue to accumulate. The marginal bone height for the implant decreases and may lead to failure of the implant. Failing endosseous dental implants may be associated with higher levels of subgingival spirochetes within the peri-implant tissues. The client must perform effective daily oral hygiene care and obtain continued supportive periodontal therapy to maintain the dental implant successfully.[3]

In providing supportive care, the dental hygienist works to maintain optimal gingival health and bony support of the dental implant. Therefore, the dental hygienist instructs the client on appropriate home care aids to clean the implants daily (see Chapters 18 and 19) and provides professional oral hygiene care at regular intervals. An understanding of optimum oral health will

Brånemark System®
Maintenance Record

Brånemark System®

Patient Name ______________________

Chart # ______________ Referring Dr. ______________ Alternate Recalls Y/N

MEDICAL ALERT

MAINTENANCE INTERVAL

Months		Minutes	
	2		30
	3		45
	4		60
	6		90

NEXT APPOINTMENT

1. ______
2. ______
3. ______
4. ______

CHARTING CODE (cc)*

B-Bleeding	M-Mobility
C-Calculus	N-Normal
D-Discharge/Suppuration	NK-Nonkeratinized
E-Edematous, Soft	P-Plaque
F-Fibrous Enlargement	R-Redness
K-Keratinized	S-Sensitivity

Special Considerations:

DATE ______
DDS√: Y/N FEE: ______

CHANGES
Medical History Y/N ______
Dental History Y/N ______
EO/IO Exam Y/N ______
Radiographs: (type)

PROCEDURES PERFORMED

Tissue Assessment Y/N
Prosthesis removed Y/N
Calculus removed Y/N
Coronal polish Y/N

HOME CARE INSTRUCTIONS

Recommended: ______

Uses: ______

Patient compliance: good/poor

Comments: ______

Signature: ______

PROBING DEPTHS (of natural teeth)

	1-8	1-7	1-6	1-5	1-4	1-3	1-2	1-1	2-1	2-2	2-3	2-4	2-5	2-6	2-7	2-8
Fa																
*cc																
Li																
*cc																

UPPER
Patient's right side upper jaw
Patient's left side upper jaw
1-1 2-1
Quadrant No. 1
Quadrant No. 2
1-8 2-8
4-8 3-8
Quadrant No. 4
Quadrant No. 3
Patient's right side lower jaw
Patient's left side lower jaw
4-1 3-1
LOWER

Designate Implant Abutment Site In Blue

	4-8	4-7	4-6	4-5	4-4	4-3	4-2	4-1	3-1	3-2	3-3	3-4	3-5	3-6	3-7	3-8
Li																
*cc																
Fa																
*cc																

FIGURE 50–32 ✦ Maintenance record. *(Courtesy Nobelpharma.)*

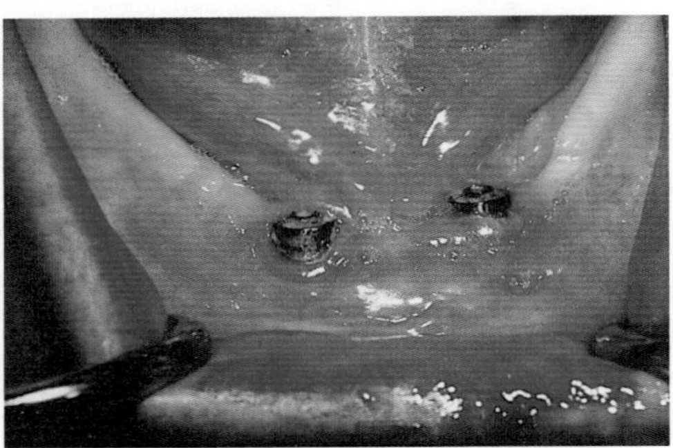

FIGURE 50–33 ✦ Peri-implantitis, an infectious disease around implant. Note amount of plaque and changes in tissue color, size, contour, and consistency. *(Courtesy AK Lakha.)*

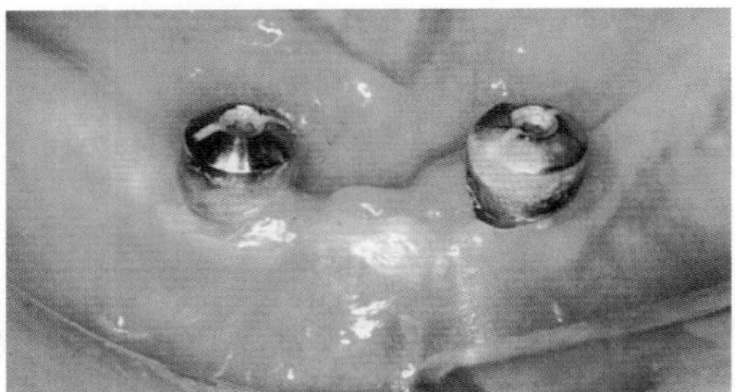

FIGURE 50–34 ✦ Heavy plaque and calculus accumulation around these healing heads have caused a breakdown of the perimucosal seal. The implants are at risk for failure. *(From Babbush CA:* Dental implants: The art and science*, Philadelphia, 2001, WB Saunders.)*

help the client achieve the success of the dental implant. A continued-care agreement form (Figure 50–35) enables the client to claim personal responsibility for maintaining oral health. The client must agree to comply with professional recommendations.

PERSONAL ORAL CARE.[2–5] Ongoing self-care education should be customized based on client preferences and with regard to abutment length and position; the prosthetic design and the ease of plaque removal between the appliance and gingival tissue; client motivation, compliance, and manual dexterity; and health of the peri-implant tissue. Clients who have lost their teeth because of mutable and nonmutable risk factors need education on the modification and control of those risk factors (see Chapter 15, section on periodontal risk factors). The hygienist impresses on clients that implants also are vulnerable to periodontal risk factors that can cause peri-implantitis.

The dental hygienist monitors the oral tissues to ensure that the client is not causing trauma with an oral hygiene aid. As a client's oral condition changes, so do his or her dental hygiene needs. For example, if a client has an increased amount of hemorrhaging, the dental hygienist needs to reassess the client's condition and modify his or her home care to include daily application of 0.12% chlorhexidine gluconate or a new implant cleaning strategy.

RECARE AGREEMENT

As part of your dental treatment you will receive/have received a dental implant(s). The long term health and success of your dental implant(s) depends largely on your ability to keep them free of bacterial plaque. Following the routine hygiene schedule we have given you is also extremely important so we can monitor and evaluate your oral health and professionally care for your teeth and implants. We will make recommendations to you relating to the products and personal at-home hygiene program that will suit your dental needs. We wish to provide you with the best dental care possible. Your understanding of your oral health helps us achieve this goal. I have read and understand the recommendations provided by my dentist and dental hygienist and will make every effort to comply.

Signature of Patient ____________ Date ____________

Signature of DDS/RDH ____________ Date ____________

FIGURE 50–35 ✦ Recare agreement form. *(Courtesy Lynn D Terracciano-Mortilla, RDH.)*

Evaluation (see section on Care and Maintenance of Dental Implants)

RECOMMENDED DEVICES AND STRATEGIES FOR CLEANING DENTAL IMPLANTS[2–5]

Disclosants (see Chapter 14)

Disclosing agents, for professional and home use, are applied to teeth and dental implants for bacterial plaque visualization. For example, the client may not see plaque on the lingual aspect of abutments or on the posterior portion of a bridge without the aid of a disclosant. These agents can be used regularly or periodically as a monitoring strategy once effective self-care behaviors are confirmed.

Intraoral Mirror and Penlight

A magnifying intraoral mirror and penlight should be used by the client in conjunction with disclosants for an adequate visual examination of bacterial plaque accumulation.

Toothbrushes (see Chapter 18)

Clients should clean their implants, teeth, and gums two to three times daily with a toothbrush directed at a 45-degree angle toward the soft tissues. Because titanium is less rigid than a natural tooth, the surface of the abutment can be damaged with hard-bristled toothbrushes, which facilitates plaque biofilm accumulation and can lead to gingival or *peri-implant recession* (loss of gingival tissue around the implant). Therefore, soft-bristled brushes are recommended. To prevent toothbrush trauma to the delicate mucosa surrounding the abutment, the soft-bristled brush should have a small, compact head

Personal and Professional Oral Hygiene Aids for Persons with Dental Implants

Personal Oral Care Products

Disclosing Tablets/Solutions

Plaque Finder (Floxite Corporation) (800) 828-8944
Plak-Lite Company (800) 581-2265
Plak Smacker (800) 228-9021

Powered Brushes

Actibrush (Colgate) (800) 226-5428
INTERPLAK (Conair) (800) 633-6363
Gingibrush (U.S. Dentek) (800) 433-6835
Rota-dent (Pro-Dentec) (800) 228-5595
SynchroSonic (Waterpik Technologies) (800) 525-2020
Sonicare (Optiva Corp) (800) 682-7664
3-D Plaque Remover (Braun/Oral B) (800) 446-7252

Floss

Thornton's Bridge and Implant Cleaners (Home Dental Care) (800) 445-3567
Dentax (Playtex Products) (800) 814-3279
G-Floss (3i) (800) 342-5454
Glide (W.L. Gore) (800) 645-4337
OraLine (888) 296-6730
Paro Implant Floss (Hager Worldwide) (800) 328-2335
Peri-O Floss (PHB, Inc.) (800) 553-1440
Postcare (Sunstar Butler) (800) 528-8537
Proxi-Floss (AIT Dental) (800) 876-4620
Super Floss (Oral B) (800) 446-7252

Interdental Cleaners

Curaprox CPS (877) 387-2779
Flossbrush (Cirrus Air Technologies) (800) 327-6151
Interproximal Brush (3i) (800) 342-5454
Perioflex (Braun/Oral B) (800) 446-7252
Interdental Wooden Picks (OraLine) (888) 296-6730
Paro Brush Stick (Hager Worldwide) (800) 328-2335
Perio-aid (Marquis Dental Mfg. Co.) (800) 359-3206
Proxabrush (Sunstar Butler) (800) 528-8537
Proxi-Tip (AIT Dental) (800) 876-4620
Rota-point (Pro-Dentec) (800) 228-5995
Sulcabrush (Sulcabrush, Inc.) (800) 387-8777
SoniPick (Sonex International) (800) 633-7858

Oral Irrigators

INTERPLAK Dental Water Jet (Conair) (800) 633-6363
Hydro Floss (800) 635-3594
ShowerFloss (800) 959-3567
Waterpik Oral Cleaning System (Waterpik Technologies) (800) 525-2020

Toothbrushes

Colgate (800) 800-4283
Crest Procter & Gamble (800) 543-2577
Dentax (800) 814-3279
Sunstar Butler (800) 528-8537
Johnson & Johnson (800) 526-3967
Oral B (800) 446-7252
OraLine (888) 296-6730
Plak Smacker (800) 228-9021
PHB, Inc. (800) 553-1440
Smart Brush (800) 476-2782
3i (800) 342-5454
Tess (800) 762-1765

Professional Dental Implant Hygiene Armamentarium

Chemotherapeutic Agents

Listerine (Pfizer) (800) 223-0182
PerioGard (Colgate) (800) 800-4283
Peridex (Zila Pharmaceutical) (800) 800-4939

Periodontal Plastic Probes

PDT Perio (Pro-Dentec) (800) 228-5595
Periowise (Premier) (800) 773-6872
3i (800) 342-5454
Z Probe 2000 (Innovadent Technologies) (800) 574-9186

Disposable Prophy Angles

AllPro (800) 243-2285
Denticator (800) 227-3321
Discus Dental (800) 422-9449
Sunstar Butler (888) 528-8537
MTI Precision Products (800) 367-9290
Oral B (800) 446-7252
Plak Smacker (800) 228-9021
Pro-Dentec (800) 228-5595
Preventive Technologies (800) 474-8681
Prophy Perfect (800) 776-3948
Sultan (800) 238-6739
Waterpik Technologies (800) 525-2020
Tess (800) 762-1765
Young (800) 325-1881

Prophy Paste

Abutment Glo (3i) (800) 342-5454
Implant Cleanic (Premier) (800) 773-6872
Nupro (Dentsply) (800) 989-8826
Preventive Technologies (800) 474-8681
Proflex (Pro-Dentec) (800) 228-5595
Prophy Paste (Oral B) (800) 446-7252
Topex (Sultan) (800) 238-6739
Waterpik Technologies Prophylaxis paste (800) 525-2020

Implant Scalers

Implacare (Hu-Friedy) (800) 483-7433
Implant Prophy+ (AIT Dental) (800) 876-4620
Implarette 3I (800) 342-5454
Nobelpharma (Brånemark) (800) 347-3500
Premie (888) 773-6872
Steri-Oss (800) 322-5001

Sonic and Ultrasonic Scalers for Dental Implants (see Chapter 23, Table 23–7)

Quixonic SofTip Kit (DENTSPLY) (800) 989-8826
Implant Titanium Scaler (Tony Riso Company, Inc.) (305) 940-3043

for reaching the facial, lingual, and occlusal surfaces. The toothbrush can be dipped into a 0.12% chlorhexidine gluconate solution to enhance plaque biofilm and gingivitis control. Clients also should invest adequate time brushing their prosthetic appliance.

Unituft Interspace Brushes—Tapered or Flat (see Chapter 19)

The unique design of the unituft interspace brush allows the client to focus on one implant or tooth at a time (Figures 50–36 and 50–37). The brush has soft-bristled nylon fibers that do not damage the peri-implant tissue. The facial and lingual surfaces of dental implants can be reached with the unituft interspace brush with either the tapered or flat design (Figure 50–38). The plastic handle can be placed under hot water and bent for greater access to hard-to-reach areas. The unituft toothbrush is recommended for use two to three times daily to remove plaque biofilm and to strengthen the peri-implant and gingival tissue. The unituft brush can be dipped into a 0.12% chlorhexidine gluconate solution to enhance plaque and gingivitis control.

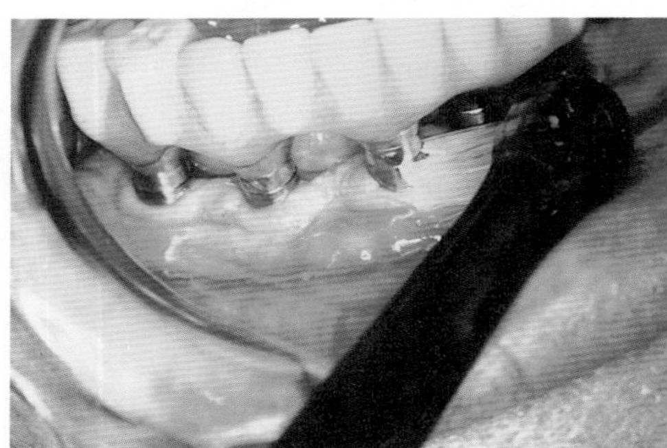

FIGURE 50–36 ✦ Application of an end-tuft toothbrush to an endosseous implant. *(Courtesy J Kleinman.)*

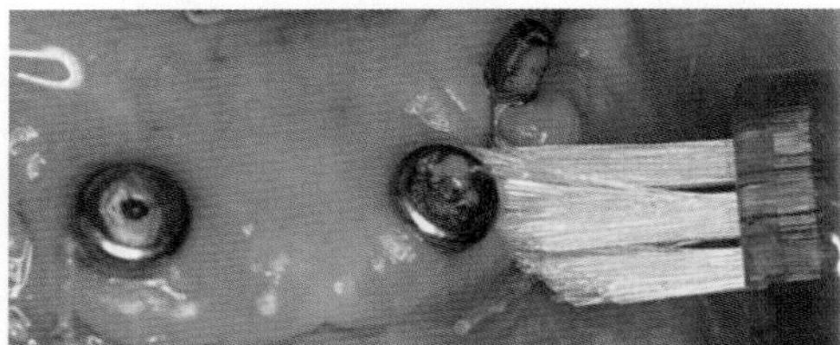

FIGURE 50–37 ✦ Application of a tapered end-tuft toothbrush to healing surgical sites. *(From Babbush CA:* Dental implants: The art and science, *Philadelphia, 2001, WB Saunders.)*

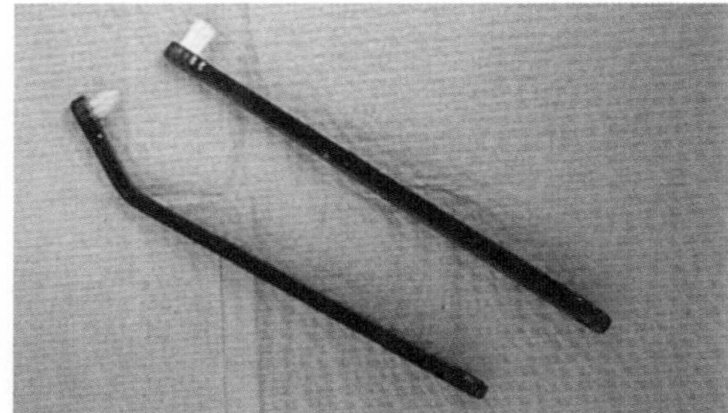

FIGURE 50–38 ✦ Tapered and flat end-tuft toothbrush design. The plastic handle can be bent to a position for use in lingual areas. *(From Babbush CA:* Dental implants: The art and science, *Philadelphia, 2001, WB Saunders.)*

Powered Rotary Brushes (see Chapter 18)

Powered rotary brushes may be prescribed for clients to thoroughly clean around the abutments and interproximal areas under the prosthetic appliance (Figures 50–39 and 50–40). Use of low speed is indicated to prevent damage to the peri-implant tissue. Brushes can be dipped into 0.12% chlorhexidine gluconate and used with a sweeping motion. The oscillating motion of the brush should follow the curvature of the dental implant along the gingiva. Powered rotary brushes are recommended for use one to two times daily.

Plastic Nylon-Coated Interdental Brush and Foam Pads—Tapered or Cylindrical (see Chapter 19)

The interproximal areas of dental implants can be reached with a cone-shaped or cylindrical interdental brush, foam tip, or Proxi-Tip (Figures 50–41 and 50–42). To avoid alteration of the abutment surface, nylon-coated wires are required rather than the conventional metal-wired brushes. Interdental brushes should be dis-

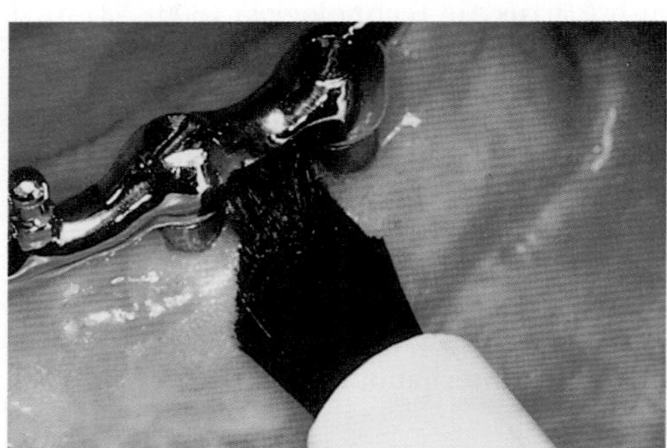

FIGURE 50–39 ✦ Application of a Rota-dent (Pro-Dentec) powered rotary long-tip brush to clean the crossbar of an endosseous implant. *(Courtesy J Kleinman.)*

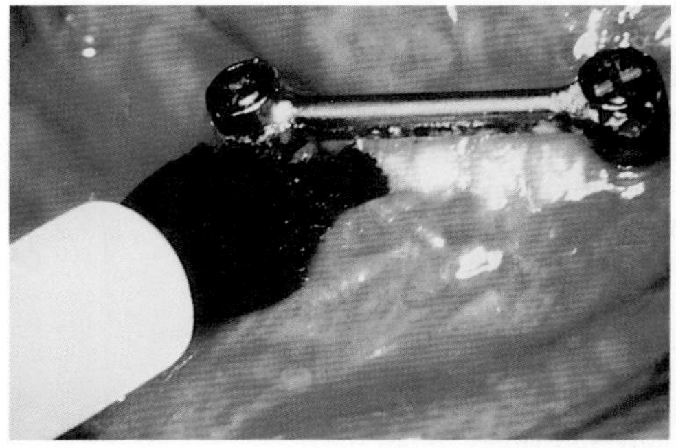

FIGURE 50–40 ✦ Application of Rota-dent (Pro-Dentec) powered rotary brush to an endosseous implant. *(Courtesy J Kleinman.)*

carded when the nylon coating has worn down to the metal wire. The interdental brush can be used from the facial or lingual areas and interproximally. Interdental brushes are recommended for use at least one time daily. The interdental brush also may be used with 0.12% chlorhexidine gluconate for target delivery of the antimicrobial agent.

Rubber Tip

The rubber tip may be used to remove debris accumulation from all surfaces, including the gingival sulcus toward the coronal and abutment surface. The rubber tip also may stimulate and massage the peri-implant tissue. Performance of this procedure is recommended once daily (Figure 50–43).

Dentifrice (see Chapter 24)

Abrasive dentifrice can alter the abutment surface. Therefore, clients should use a low-abrasive toothpaste (Table 50–7). A low-abrasive dentifrice is defined as one that has a radioactive dentin abrasion (RDA) score of 130 or less. For example, a low-abrasive dentifrice such as Crest or Colgate anti-tartar formulas could be safely recommended for implant clients twice daily in conjunction with an oral hygiene aid. Baking soda (sodium bicarbonate) toothpastes also are low abrasive.

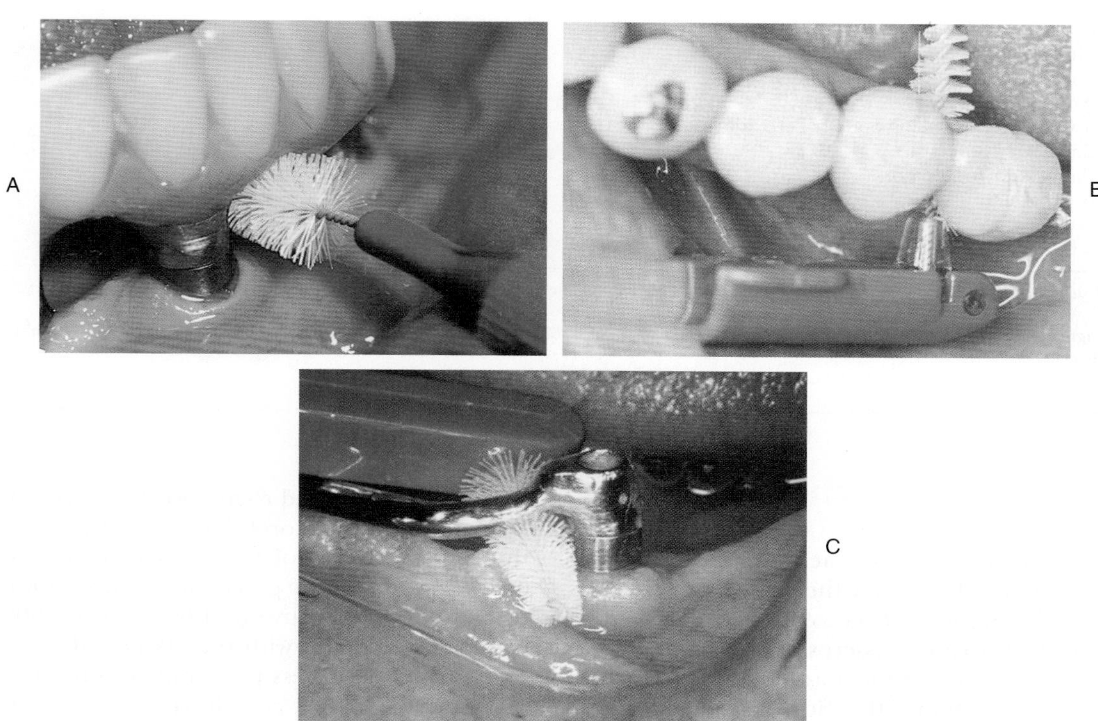

FIGURE 50–41 ✦ **A,** Application of a Sunstar Butler nylon-coated Proxabrush to an endosseous implant. **B,** Coated interproximal brush is used when embrasure space allows easy insertion and removal. **C,** Connector bars can usually accommodate interproximal brushes for ease of use and effective self-care. *(A courtesy J Kleinman; B courtesy Oral-B; B and C from Babbush CA:* Dental implants: The art and science, *Philadelphia, 2001, WB Saunders.)*

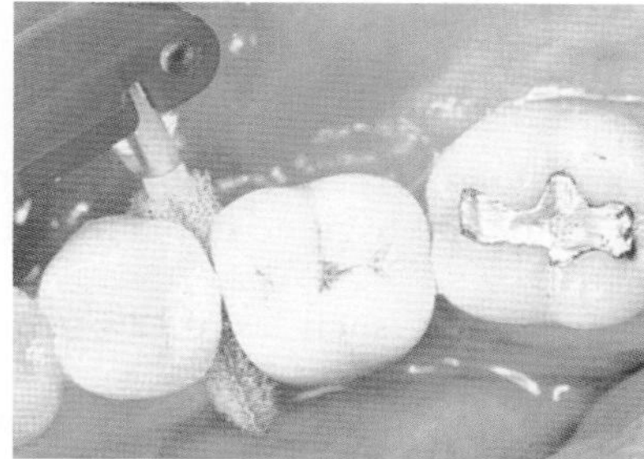

FIGURE 50–42 ✦ Application of Oral B Foam Tip to an endosseous implant interdentally. Can be used to target deliver chemotherapeutic agents while reducing the amount of tooth staining. *(Courtesy Oral B, Belmont, Calif; Babbush CA:* Dental implants: The art and science, *Philadelphia, 2001, WB Saunders.)*

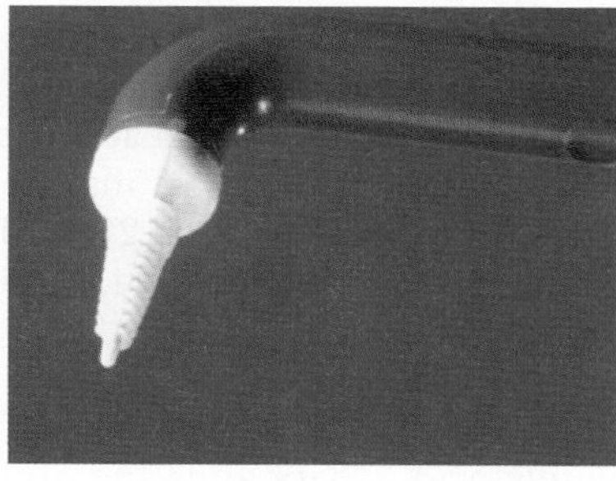

FIGURE 50–43 ✦ Application of the Advanced Implant Technologies Proxi-Tip. *(Courtesy AIT Dental, Beverly Hills, Calif; Babbush CA:* Dental implants: The art and science, *Philadelphia, 2001, WB Saunders.)*

TABLE 50–7 ABRASIVITY AND BAKING-SODA CONTENT OF COMMERCIAL DENTIFRICES

Product (Manufacturer)	% Baking Soda*	Abrasivity (RDA) (an RDA of 130 or less is considered acceptable; however, the lower the better)
Baking Soda†	100	7
Dental Care† Toothpowder	94	10
Dental Care† Toothpaste	65	49
PeriGel	59	Not Reported
Dental Care† Tartar Control Toothpaste	55	33
PeroxiCare†	52	42
PeroxiCare† Tartar Control Toothpaste	49	24
Dental Care† Gel	30	68
Dental Care† Tartar Control Gel	27	82
Colgate Baking Soda Toothpaste	25	53
Sensodyne with Baking Soda	25	67
Crest Tartar Control Mint Gel with Baking Soda	22	95
Crest Baking Soda Toothpaste	20	86
Colgate Tartar Control with Baking Soda & Peroxide Toothpaste	13	104
Close-Up Baking Soda Toothpaste	5	80
Pepsodent Baking Soda Toothpaste	5	80
Mentadent Toothpaste	5	115
Mentadent Tartar Control	5	103
Crest Regular Toothpaste	0	106

* Data from Church & Dwight based on analysis of samples using Chittick gasometric assay for determination of carbon dioxide (AOAC Method 923.02, ed 16, Vol 2).

† Church & Dwight Co, Princeton, NJ 08543 (no longer available); Colgate-Palmolive Co., Piscataway, NJ 08854; GlaxoSmithKline, Procter & Gamble, Cincinnati, Ohio 45247; Pfizer

Courtesy Compendium of Continuing Education in Dentistry, Newbrun, 1996.

Dental Floss and Dental Tape (see Chapter 19)

If abutments are spaced close to each other, dental floss or tape should be used to clean their proximal surface at least once daily (Figures 50–44 to 50–47). The floss is placed around the implant, crisscrossed, and pulled in a shoeshining motion to clean the abutment. Floss or tape can be used in conjunction with a floss threader to allow easy access through the embrasure or limited areas. Other aids, such as shoelaces, ribbon, yarn, and gauze, may also be used if embrasure space permits.

Oral Irrigation (see Chapters 19 and 24)

An oral irrigator (Figure 50–48) may be indicated for use in limited access areas where there is evidence of soft tissue inflammation surrounding the abutment cylinder. The flow rate of the unit should be set at the lowest force.

Solutions used in the oral irrigator may include water and a phenolic mouthrinse or a 0.12% chlorhexidine gluconate mouthrinse (see Chapter 24, section on oral antimicrobial agents).

Antimicrobial Agent (see Chapter 24)

For approximately 5 to 7 days after the abutment connection surgery, use of a capful of the antimicrobial 0.12% chlorhexidine gluconate solution as a 30-second rinse is recommended twice daily to control plaque formation. A cotton swab, soft toothbrush, unituft interspace brush, powered rotary brush, interdental brush, or a subgingival irrigator (Figure 50–49) may be used for the target delivery of an agent to a site. Rinsing with 0.12% chlorhexidine gluconate reduces both Gram-positive and Gram-negative oral bacteria by 100% for up to five hours after use with the 30-seconds-twice-a-day protocol, resulting in less peri-implant gingivitis and bleeding; however, use of chlorhexidine gluconate as a rinse for more than a month may cause staining of natural teeth or the prosthetic appliance.

CARE AND MAINTENANCE OF DENTAL IMPLANTS[2–5]

Armamentarium

The clinical armamentaria (Table 50–8) needed to provide professional dental hygiene implant care follows:

- Antimicrobial agent such as 0.12% chlorhexidine gluconate
- Plastic disposable syringe or gingival irrigation unit
- Plastic periodontal probe (Figure 50–50)
- Set of plastic Teflon-coated scalers (Figures 50–51 and 50–52)
- Set of gold-tipped Gracey scalers such as an 11/12 or a 13/14 (Figure 50–53)

Text continues on page 1033.

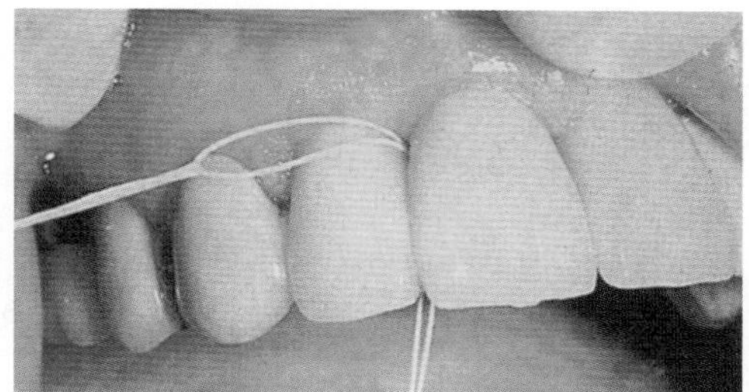

FIGURE 50–44 ✦ Application of floss threaders for challenging areas. *(From Babbush CA:* Dental implants: The art and science, *Philadelphia, 2001, WB Saunders.)*

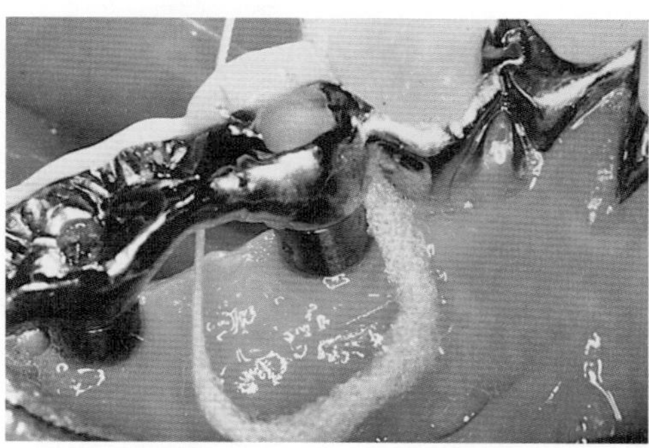

FIGURE 50–45 ✦ Application of Oral B Superfloss to an implant. *(Courtesy Oral B.)*

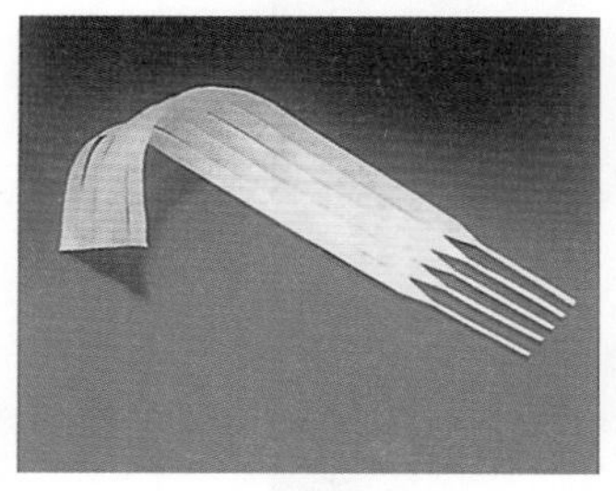

A

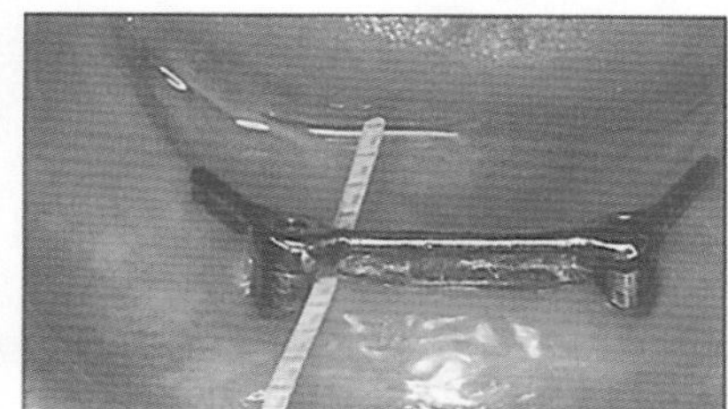

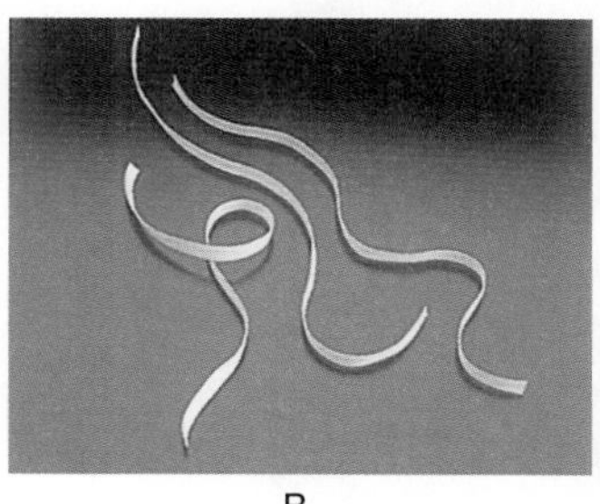

B

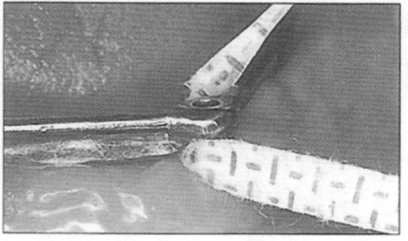

INSTRUCTIONS:

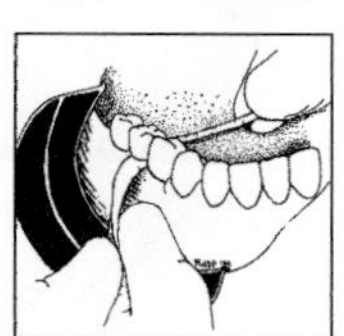

Use tapered, stiffened end to thread under fixed bridges where space allows.

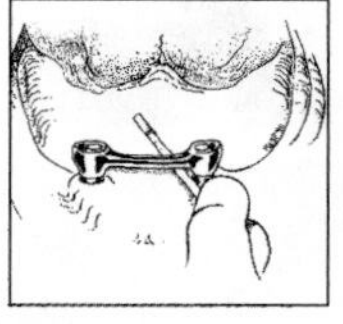

Tapered, stiffened end also allows ease in threading under connecting bars or implant overdenture prosthesis.

Wrap in a "C" shape around the abutment tooth, then use a back and forth polishing motion.

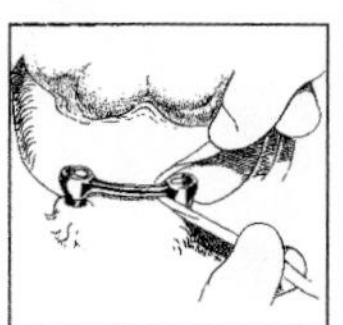

Floss may be wrapped in a "C" shape around natural tooth or implant coping and a back and forth polishing motion applied for optimal plaque removal.

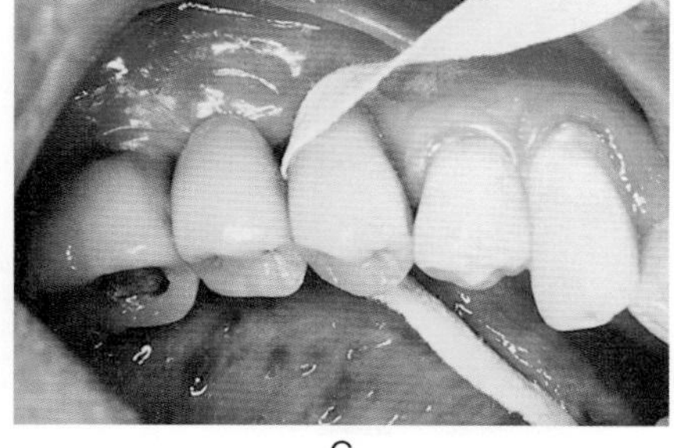

C

D

FIGURE 50–46 ✦ **A,** Tapered G-Floss. **B,** G-Floss. **C,** Application of G-Floss to an implant. **D,** Instructions on how to use G-Floss. *(Courtesy 3i-Implant Innovations.)*

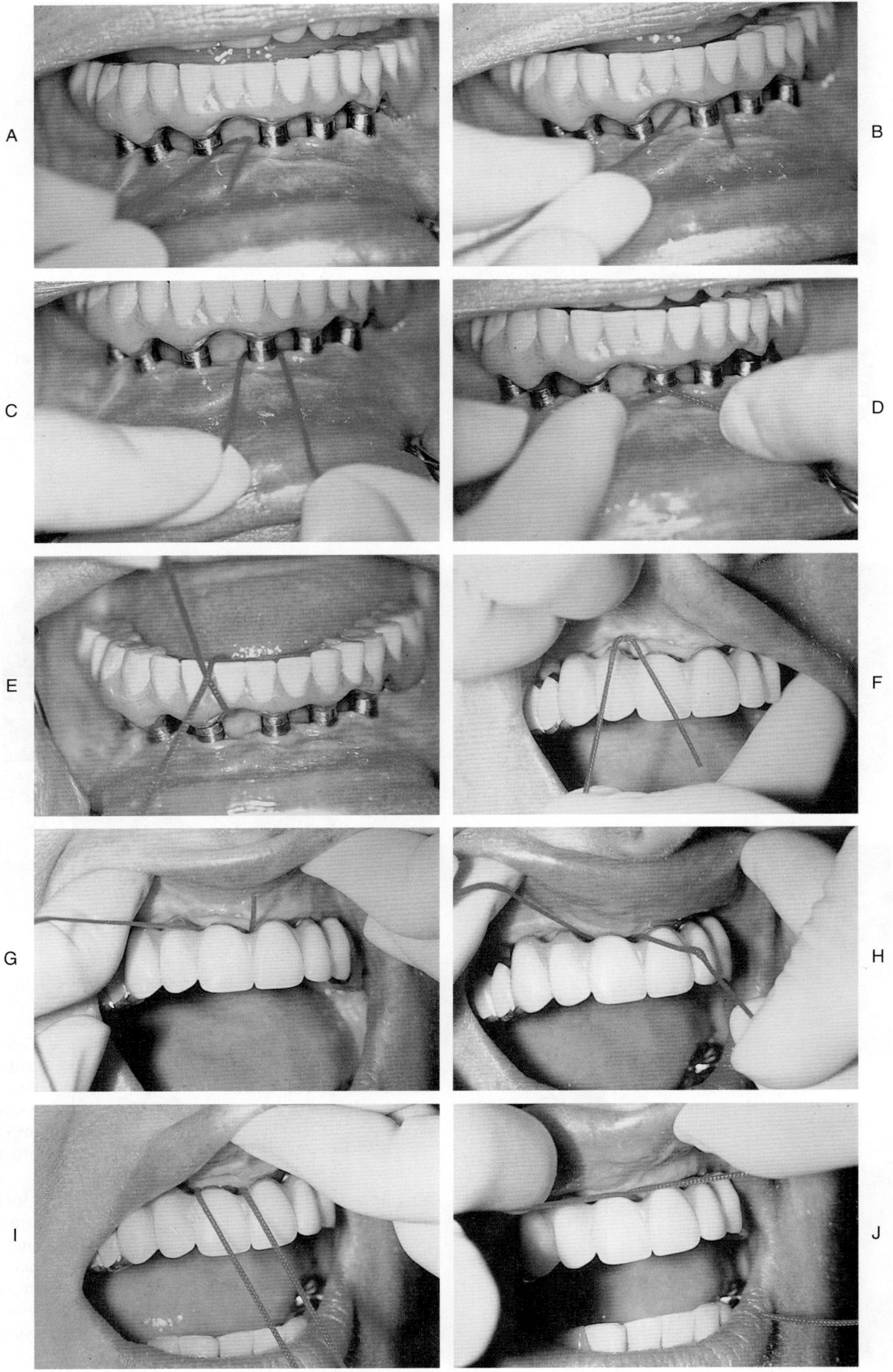

FIGURE 50–47 ✦ Systematic demonstration (*A* to *J*) of how to use the John O. Butler Postcare Implant Flossing Cord. *(Courtesy J Kleinman.)*

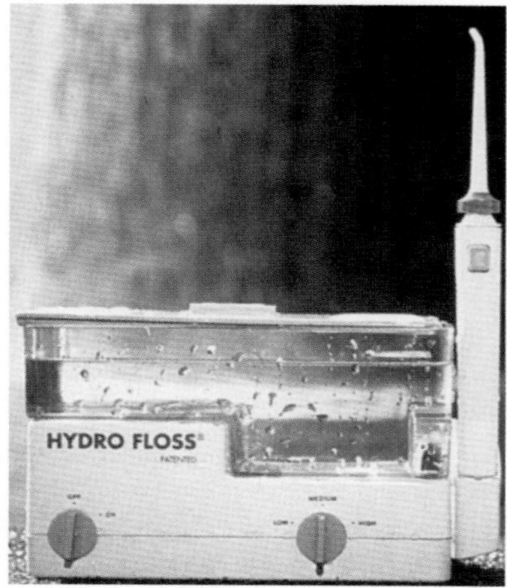

FIGURE 50–48 ✦ HydroFloss oral irrigator. *(Courtesy HydroFloss, Birmingham Ala; From Babbush CA:* Dental implants: The art and science, *Philadelphia, 2001, WB Saunders.)*

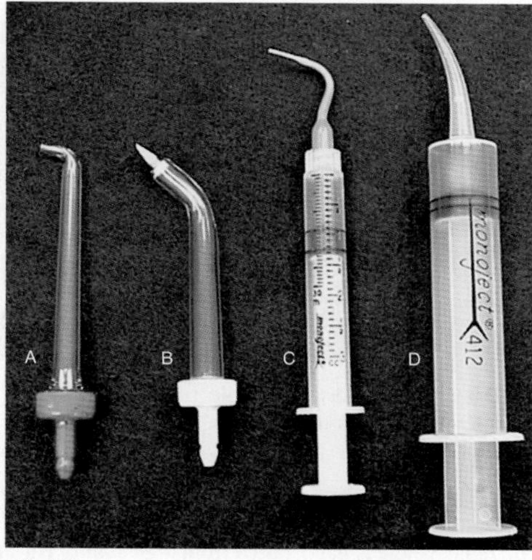

FIGURE 50–49 ✦ Irrigation tip styles. Supragingival *(A)* and marginal *(B)* tips are designed to attach to a powered irrigator. The two tips on the right are attached to simple syringes. Tip *C* is a marginal irrigator tip. Tip *D* has the most difficult fit because the tip becomes progressively wider. *(Courtesy Dr. WB Stilley, II, Brandon, Miss.)*

TABLE 50–8

CLINICAL IMPLANT HYGIENE AND MAINTENANCE ARMAMENTARIA

Company	Product	Features
Advanced Implant Technologies	Implant-Prophy+	Standard instrument designs and blade angles Sharpenable Autoclavable High-performance plastic Exceptional strength Certified as FDA Class 3 devices in full compliance with regulatory protocol
Brevet Inc.	Implant Cleaning Kit	Six instrument designs Composite resin material Sterilizable
Quixonic SofTip	Plastic Prophy Tips for Quixonic Sonic Scaler	Three sonic-tip designs, fully autoclavable Disposable plastic sheaths
Hu-Friedy	Implacare	Disposable Mirror paired tips Three standard intrument designs Plasteel (high-grade resin)
3i-Implant Innovations Inc.	Rigid Plastic Implant Scaler	Universal design Autoclavable Sharpenable
3i-Implant Innovations Inc.	Abutment Glo	A nonabrasive prophy paste for polishing titanium implant abutments/ restorations
Pro-Dentec	Sensor Probe	Thermoplastic Maintain consistency of probing pressure Autoclavable
Pro-Dentec	Mandrels	Soft-bristle brushes that can attach to slow-speed handpieces for polishing Flat and tapered shapes available
Premier	Implant Scalers Implant Cleanic paste Periowise Plastic Probe	Universal and facial designs High carbon plastic Autoclavable Sharpenable
Straumann (ITI)	Light Curet	Universal design Sterilizable Resharpenable
Steri-Oss	Scaler System	Standard instrument designs Graphite reinforced nylon Packaged sterile and sterilizable Exceptional strength Sharpenable

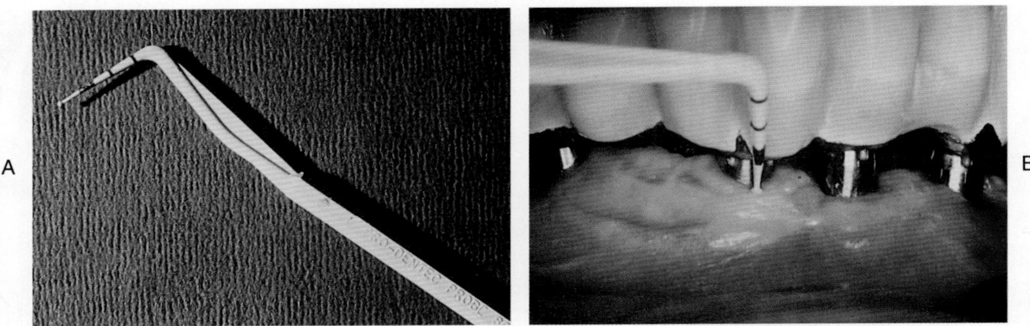

FIGURE 50–50 ✦ **A,** Plastic, flexible probe (Pro-Dentec) to measure sulcus, if absolutely necessary; it does not alter the abutment surface. **B,** Plastic, flexible probe measuring sulcus. *(Courtesy J Kleinman.)*

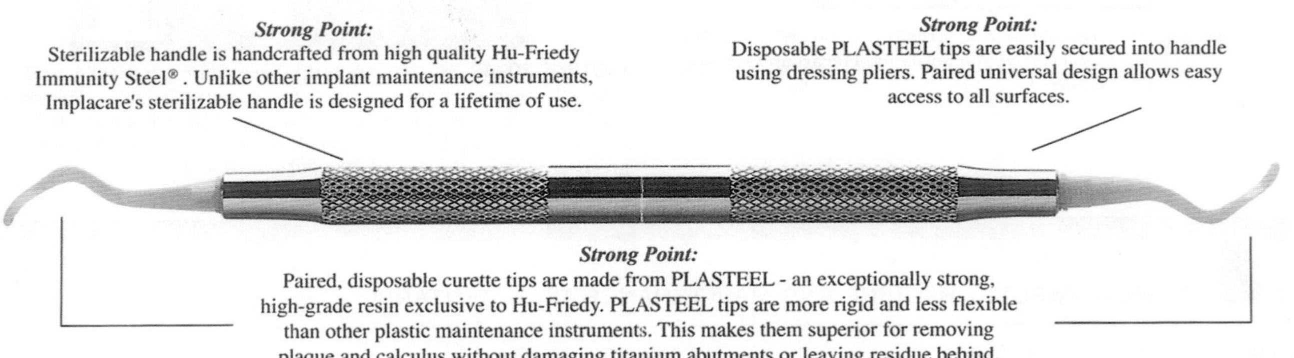

Strong Point:
Sterilizable handle is handcrafted from high quality Hu-Friedy Immunity Steel®. Unlike other implant maintenance instruments, Implacare's sterilizable handle is designed for a lifetime of use.
Strong Point:
Disposable PLASTEEL tips are easily secured into handle using dressing pliers. Paired universal design allows easy access to all surfaces.
Strong Point:
Paired, disposable curette tips are made from PLASTEEL - an exceptionally strong, high-grade resin exclusive to Hu-Friedy. PLASTEEL tips are more rigid and less flexible than other plastic maintenance instruments. This makes them superior for removing plaque and calculus without damaging titanium abutments or leaving residue behind.

FIGURE 50–51 ✦ Hu-Friedy developed the Implacare Maintenance Instrument with disposable Plasteel (high-grade resin) tips that screw into the handle. *(Courtesy Hu-Friedy; Photography by Roland Meffert, DDS.)*

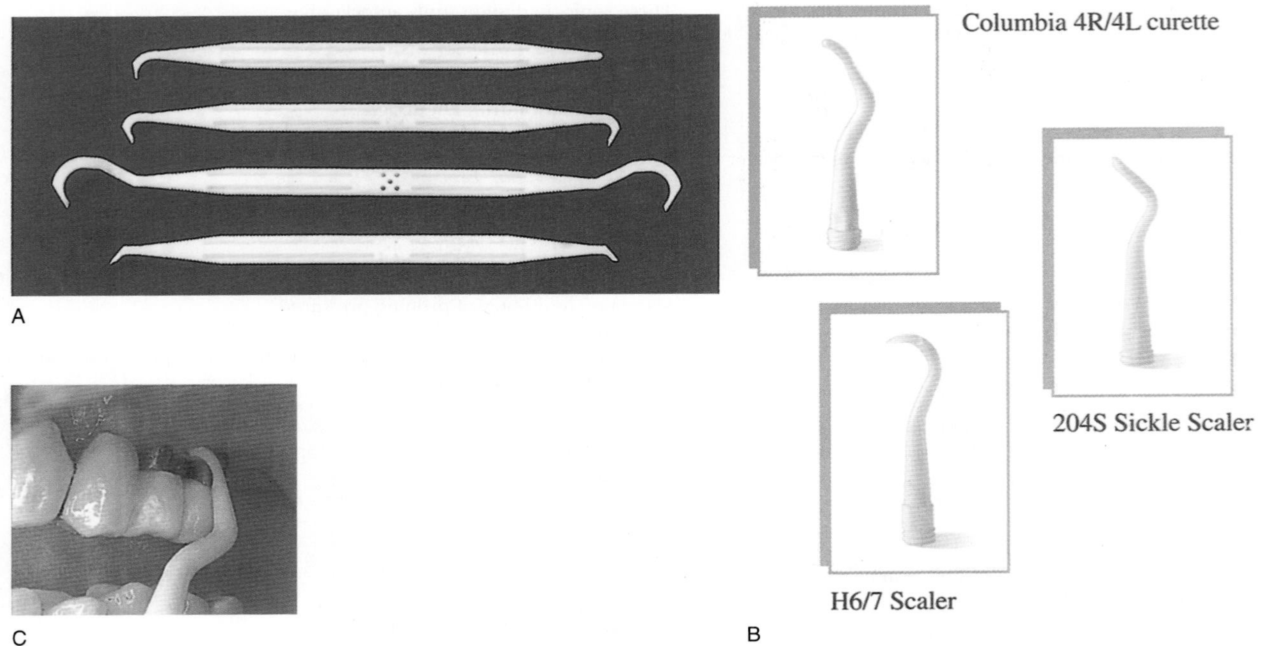

FIGURE 50–52 ✦ **A,** Nobelpharma's design of four plastic scalers. **B,** Close-up of working ends of scalers. **C,** Clinical application of the universal, lingual, and buccal scalers. *(Courtesy Nobelpharma.)*

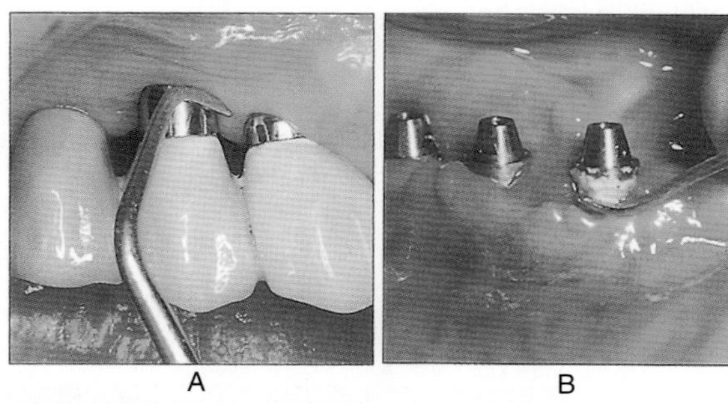

A B

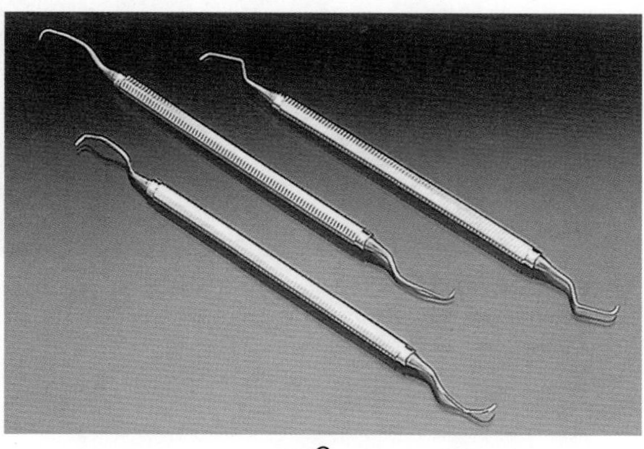

C

FIGURE 50–53 ✦ **A,** Application of gold-tipped scalers to an implant. **B,** Calculus removal with gold-tipped scaler from abutment of dental implant. **C,** Set of gold-tipped scalers. *(Courtesy 3i-Implant Innovations.)*

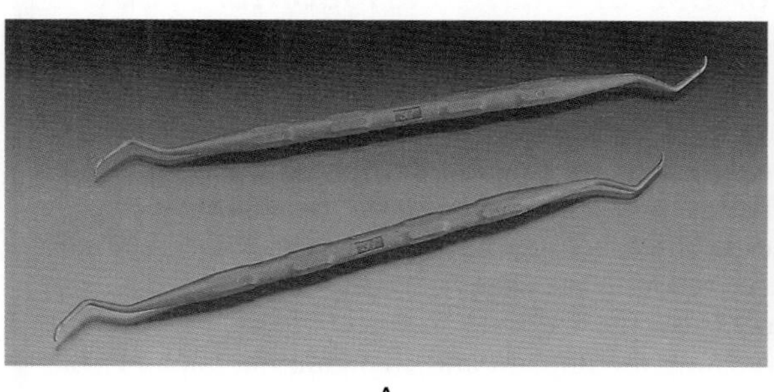

A

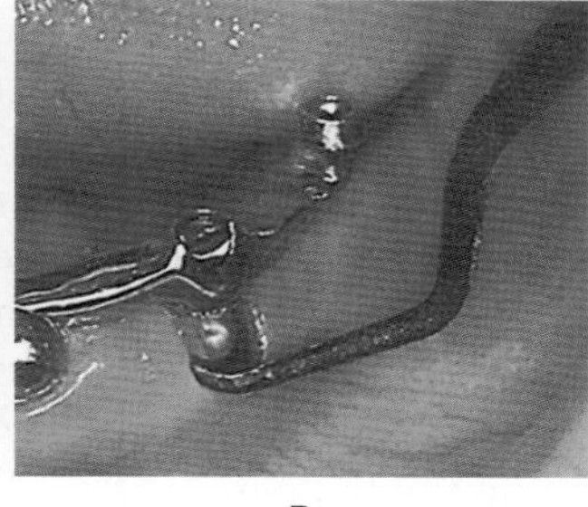

B

FIGURE 50–54 ✦ **A,** Graphite-reinforced nylon scalers. **B,** Application of graphite-reinforced nylon scaler to the dental implant. *(Courtesy Steri-Oss, Yorba Linda, Calif; Babbush CA:* Dental implants: The art and science, *Philadelphia, 2001, WB Saunders.)*

- ✦ Set of graphite-reinforced nylon scalers (Figure 50–54) or high-tech plastic (Figure 50–55)
- ✦ Wood-tipped porte polisher
- ✦ Sonic scaler with a disposable polysulfon plastic tip (Figure 50–56)
- ✦ Implant ultrasonic scaler (Figure 50–57)
- ✦ Strip of 2-by-2-inch gauze
- ✦ Thick (red) and thin (green) implant floss
- ✦ Gel dentifrice or tin oxide or Abutment Glo (Figure 50–58)
- ✦ Rubber cup and pointed polisher
- ✦ Soft, multitufted toothbrush with a compact head design and other appropriate aids for self-care instruction

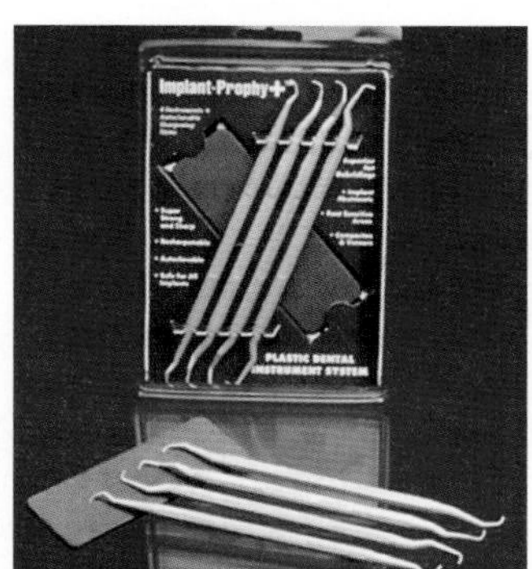

FIGURE 50–55 ✦ Implant-Prophy+ instrument system. *(Courtesy Advanced Implant Technologies; Babbush CA:* Dental implants: The art and science, *Philadelphia, 2001, WB Saunders.)*

Peri-implant tissue irrigation with an antimicrobial agent such as 0.12% chlorhexidine gluconate, before instrumentation, reduces the pathogenicity of bacterial colonies and risk of local infection. Chemical disinfection to remove endotoxins with agents such as chlorhexidine, citric acid, hydrogen peroxide, stannous fluoride, and tetracycline is under investigation. The clinical efficacy of these agents for total mouth disinfection remains to be elucidated. A plastic disposable syringe or a powered oral irrigation unit may be used to accomplish this irrigation procedure because both techniques allow access to the peri-implant sulcus and deliver the antimicrobial solution to the peri-implant sulcus easily and

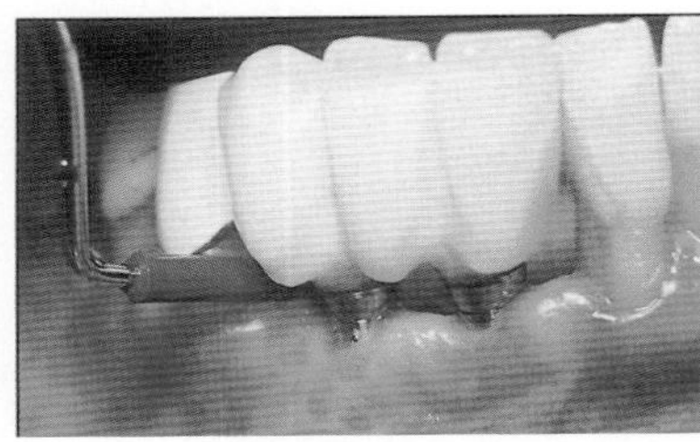

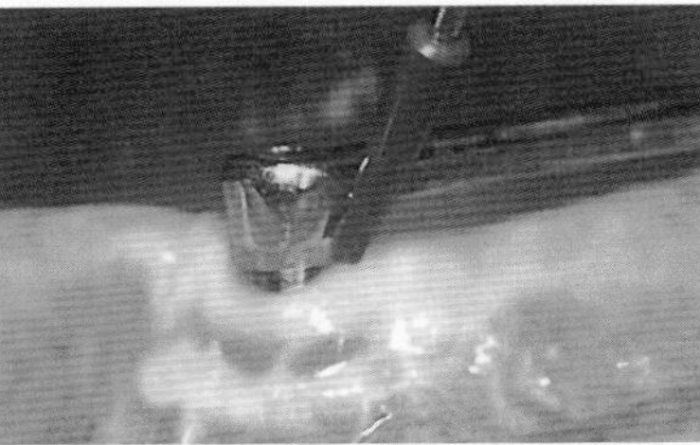

FIGURE 50–56 ✦ Disposable polysulfon plastic Quixonic SofTip. *(Courtesy DENTSPLY.)*

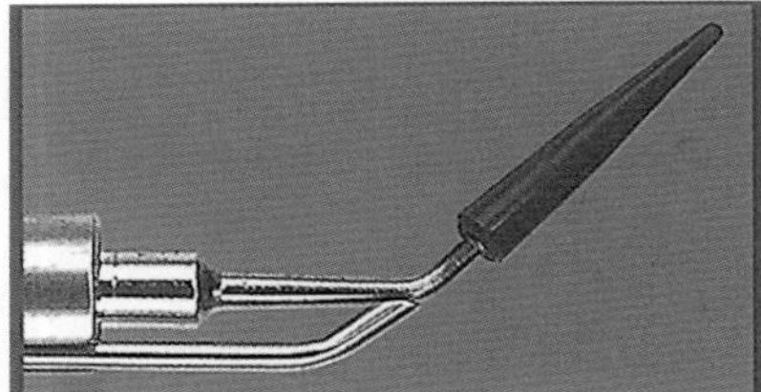

FIGURE 50–57 ✦ Implant titanium ultrasonic scaler insert. *(Courtesy of Tony Riso Co.)*

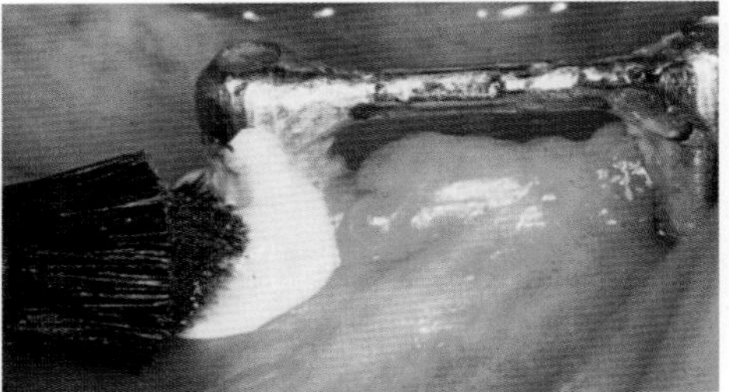

FIGURE 50–58 ✦ Application of Abutment Glo. *(Courtesy 3i-Implant Innovations; From Babbush CA:* Dental implants: The art and science, *Philadelphia, 2001, WB Saunders.)*

effectively. Chlorhexidine gluconate 0.12% is an excellent antimicrobial agent to use for peri-implant tissue irrigation. To minimize generalized staining, the solution may be applied locally with a cotton applicator rather than rinsing. A phenolic solution is acceptable if a client cannot tolerate the stain or taste of some antimicrobial solutions.

Periodontal Probing Around Implants

Periodontal probing around the peri-implant tissue continues to be controversial. *The current consensus is that probing should not be used as a routine procedure on dental implant clients.*[3,4] The possibility of disturbing the biologic seal that attaches the healthy peri-implant tissue to the titanium abutment can cause a local infection within the unattached sulci and lead to implant failure. Some clinicians believe that crevicular probing is too invasive because the probe may push through the "weak" gingival attachment to the bony crest. Also, bleeding on probing may not represent peri-implantitis but an iatrogenic wound. Others believe that probing is a valuable and accurate test for potential or existing periodontal problems. With caution, probing should be used to determine the depth of severe marginal bone loss or peri-implant problems (see Indications and Contraindications for Use of Plastic Periodontal Probe). If probing is necessary, a plastic disposable probe or a single-use plastic probe that connects to a fiber-optic light source should be used. The fiber-optic light gives good visibility when measuring and examining the peri-implant sulcus.

Several types of instruments will remove adherent bacterial plaque and dental calculus without damaging the surface of the implant (Figures 50–59 and 50–60). Scratching, gouging, or contaminating the titanium surface will create an area that becomes more retentive to plaque accumulation and its bacterial by-products

Indications and Contraindications for Use of Plastic Periodontal Probe

- ✦ Avoid probing for the first 3 months after the abutments have been installed to allow a peri-implant seal to form.
- ✦ Measurement of gingival attachment levels should be referenced with a fixed point on the abutment or prosthesis. The exact reference point at each location must be recorded in the client's dental record.
- ✦ Only plastic periodontal probes are used. This prevents scratching the implant and changing the implant's biocompatibility, which can occur from an electrochemical reaction of two dissimilar metals.

(Figures 50–61 to 50–63). Instrument rigidity and design, prosthetic appliance design, location of bacterial plaque biofilm, and calculus tenacity should be carefully assessed before instrumentation. *Because the surface of the titanium abutment can be easily abraded by metal scalers, sonic instruments, and abrasive agents, the following methods and materials are strongly contraindicated for use on dental implants: metal curets and scalers, metal tip inserts of sonic scalers and ultrasonic instruments, air polishing devices, air abrasive systems, and rubber cup polishing with flour of pumice or coarse grit abrasive paste.*[4] A polysulfon disposable tip may be used with a sonic scaler to remove tenacious calculus deposits.

Plastic, Teflon-coated, graphite wood-tipped, and gold-tipped Gracey instruments have been developed for use in scaling dental implants. The plastic and Teflon-coated instruments are designed to prevent abrasion to the titanium implants. The wood-tipped instrument or porte polisher is designed to prevent scratches on the

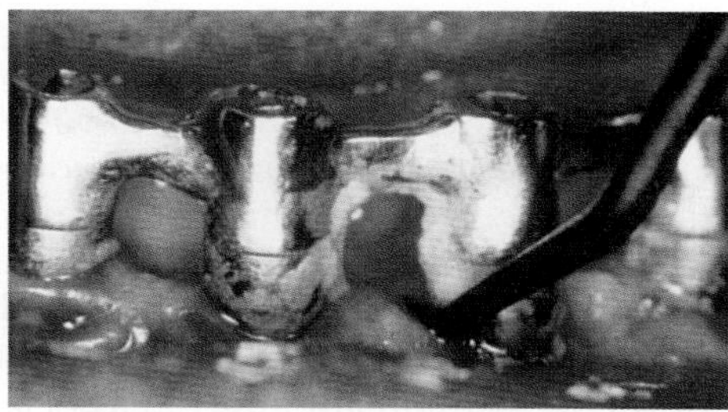

FIGURE 50–59 ✦ Tenacious calculus needs to be removed by a plastic scaler. *(From Babbush CA:* Dental implants: The art and science, *Philadelphia, 2001, WB Saunders.)*

FIGURE 50–60 ✦ A smooth titanium implant surface. *(Babbush CA:* Dental implants: The art and science, *Philadelphia, 2001, WB Saunders.)*

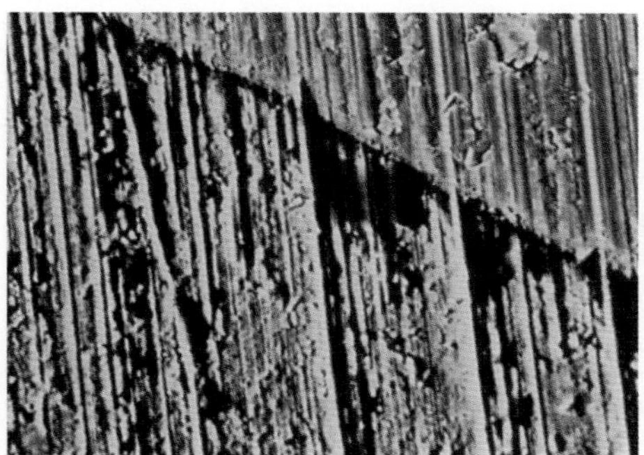

FIGURE 50–61 ✦ Effects of air abrasion use: note roughened implant surface. *(From Babbush CA:* Dental implants: The art and science, *Philadelphia, 2001, WB Saunders.)*

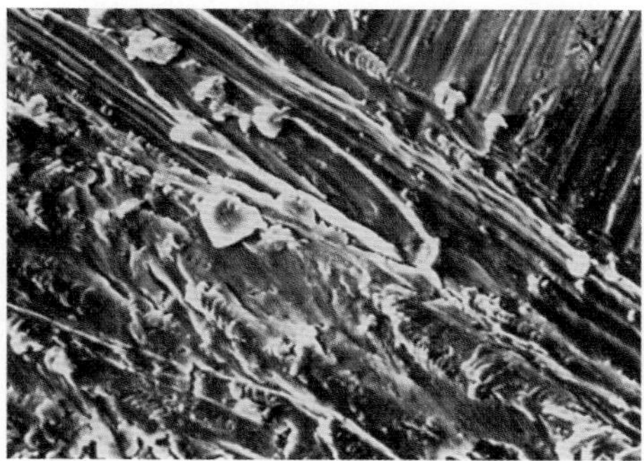

FIGURE 50–62 ✦ Effects of ultrasonic scaler use: note roughened implant surface. *(From Babbush CA:* Dental implants: The art and science, *Philadelphia, 2001, WB Saunders.)*

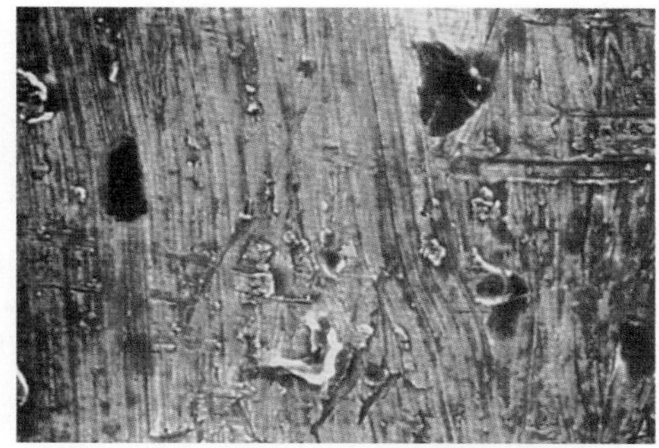

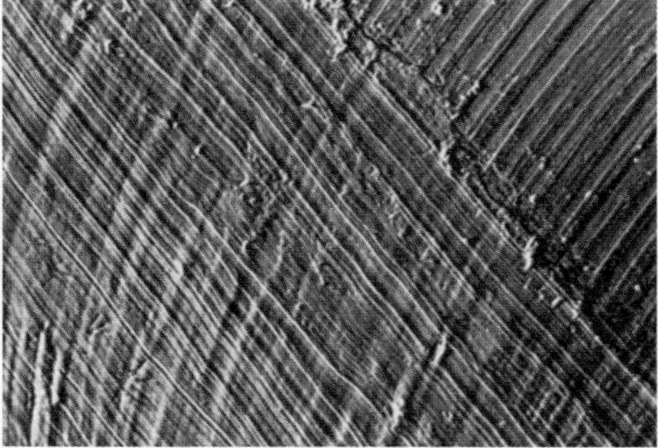

FIGURE 50–63 ✦ Effects of metallic scaler use: note roughened implant surface. *(From Babbush CA:* Dental implants: The art and science, *Philadelphia, 2001, WB Saunders.)*

implant surface. Half of a round, pointed toothpick inserted through the end of an interdental brush handle is considered a very safe and effective scaler for use around dental implants. Wood-tipped instruments are used only once, however, then thrown away to prevent splintering and damage to the peri-implant tissue.

The gold-tipped Gracey instruments are fabricated from a special gold alloy that is softer than titanium and, therefore, does not roughen the surface of the abutments or cause retention of acquired deposits. Gold-tipped Gracey scalers should not be sharpened because the gold is then removed, exposing the underlying metal. (Note that some clinicians and researchers believe that graphite and gold-tipped scalers may change the surface topography of the implant and should be avoided.) Polishing is recommended with a gel dentifrice or tin oxide in a rubber cup or rubber point. Buffing the abutments "shoeshine style" with long gauze strips or floss is effective for bacterial plaque removal. An ordinary cotton shoestring can help to remove bacterial plaque underneath the prosthetic appliance.

While providing care, the dental hygienist continually assesses whether the client has problems associated with the dental implant that are related to oral hygiene or to the condition of the peri-implant tissue. For example, the dental hygienist can monitor the peri-implant tissue; remove acquired deposits from natural teeth and implants; discuss oral hygiene needs; provide customized instructions (see Oral Self-Care Guidelines for Dental Implant Clients); reinforce bacterial plaque control education; evaluate the client's acceptance of and ability to perform recommended oral self-care regimens; encourage client compliance with implant examinations; take necessary radiographs; and facilitate prevention of dental caries in existing natural dentition via fluoride therapy, sealants, and nutritional counseling.

Clients with dental implants should maintain a 3- to 4-month (or as needed) continued-care schedule (Table 50–9). The bacterial plaque biofilm and dental calculus accumulated on the appliance also should be removed using the same procedure as with conventional dentures.

Failed Implants[6] (Figures 50–30, 50–33, and 50–34)

A failed implant is one that has lost its integration. Unfortunately, removal of the entire dental implant is the only option. Bone regenerative methods may be used if the client desires another implant at this site. The primary reasons for implant failure are peri-implantitis and noncompliance with self-care (Table 50–10). If the dental implant appears to be failing, the dentist must thoroughly examine the supporting structures at regularly scheduled intervals and intervene quickly. Screw retention of the implant should be evaluated at each continued-care appointment. A loose screw can cause mobility of the dental implant and the associated prosthesis (e.g., the bridge).

Oral Self-Care Guidelines for Dental Implant Clients

- Clean implant and bridges at least twice daily, preferably after breakfast and after the last food intake before going to sleep. This is especially important because the flow of saliva decreases during sleep.
- Clean thoroughly but not too aggressively. Avoid any materials or behaviors that might damage the implant surface.
- Use a systematic regimen so that all areas are cleaned.
- Clean the neck of the implant.

TABLE 50–9 CONTINUING-CARE SCHEDULE FOR CLIENTS WITH DENTAL IMPLANTS

Care	Care Schedule
Once implant is placed	Oral hygiene education and instruction
Radiographic evaluation of bone and periodontal structures	Every 3 months for first year and annually thereafter, unless necessary earlier
Continued-care appointment	Every 3 months for first year and thereafter evaluate for 4-month continued-care appointments
Removal and cleaning of implant superstructure	Annually, during continued-care appointment
Any signs of infection	Return to general dentist in 10 to 14 days, or refer to specialist

NOTE: Be sure to commit client to the next continued-care appointment before appointment ends.

TABLE 50–10 REASONS FOR IMPLANT FAILURES AS REPORTED BY SURGEONS AND PERIODONTISTS

Possible Responses	1997	1996	1995	1994
Oral and Maxillofacial Surgeons	75%	73%	74%	70%
Insufficient maintenance by patient	58%	60%	48%	50%
Insufficient maxillary bone	44%	42%	33%	35%
Premature loading	33%	44%	32%	41%
Prosthodontic difficulties (other than premature loading)	29%	36%	25%	42%
Illness/systemic disease	29%	19%	n/a	n/a
Insufficient maintenance by doctor	28%	30%	17%	19%
Insufficient mandibular bone	19%	17%	16%	24%
Increased periodontal involvement throughout the mouth	16%	17%	15%	13%
Bone augmentation needed but not initially provided	15%	19%	n/a	7%
Periodontists	56%	64%	65%	71%
Insufficient maintenance by patient	38%	40%	30%	41%
Prosthodontic difficulties (other than premature loading)	37%	38%	36%	40%
Premature loading	35%	39%	31%	47%
Insufficient maxillary bone	34%	42%	30%	33%
Insufficient mandibular bone	26%	32%	18%	19%
Illness/systemic disease	26%	23%	n/a	n/a
Insufficient maintenance by doctor	15%	15%	12%	21%
Bone augmentation needed but not initially provided	11%	18%	n/a	10%
Increased periodontal involvement throughout the mouth	11%	9%	8%	9%

From Reis-Schmidt T: Surgically placing implants: A survey of oral and maxillofacial surgeons and periodontists, *Dental Products Report* 32:26, 1998.

The gingival tissue should be examined for any color changes, edema, consistency, bleeding, exudate, or recession. Evaluation of the radiographs to determine if there is progressive bone loss is necessary. The subgingival microflora around a failing implant is similar to that found around periodontally diseased teeth. Therefore, the implant surface affected by peri-implantitis is contaminated by bacterial endotoxins that interfere with biologic repair. If the peri-implant supporting bone is severely cratered, bone regeneration may be attempted if the implant has not lost its integration. Removal of the superstructure and replacement of the small healing screw are advisable in order for the soft tissue to grow over the implant. Bone regenerative (bone repair) techniques are used (e.g., placing allograft bone into the defect and covering the implant with a resorbable guided tissue regeneration membrane). When the bone repair is completed, which usually takes 3 months, the implant is reloaded.

The dentist who placed the implant monitors the client. *Annually, the removable superstructures should be disassembled for evaluation and cleaned.* Radiographs of the implant should be taken and evaluated by the dentist every 6 to 12 months. Clients are instructed to contact the dentist if there is an increased amount of swelling, a fever, or sensitivity in the mandible or sinus area that is not resolved with prescription pain medications.[6]

Client Education Issues

- Explain the etiology and pathogenesis of periodontal disease and the importance of bacterial plaque control in prevention of oral diseases and in maintenance of oral health.
- Emphasize client responsibility for maintenance care to sustain the health of the peri-implant tissues and to prevent periodontal disease and dental caries in existing natural dentition.
- Instruct the client to *never* use a rigid toothbrush, abrasive dentifrice, safety pins, paper clips, or metal objects to self-clean the implants or abutments.
- Encourage clients to access professional oral hygiene maintenance care regularly.
- Educate clients about the risk factors for implant periodontitis and dental implant failures.
- Educate clients about the benefits of dental implant reconstruction and assist them in determining whether they are candidates for dental implants.
- Encourage the client to maintain a daily self-care regimen by developing an individual implant hygiene care package that includes a written daily plan and oral hygiene tools needed for daily care.
- Demonstrate the recommended daily strategies for cleaning dental implants.

Legal, Ethical, and Safety Issues

- Dental hygienists should assess for possible peri-implantitis at each professional dental implant care session. The sulcular area around the implant or insert is the primary area of concern.
- Clients should be referred to a general dentist, periodontist, or oral and maxillofacial surgeon for the informed consent, implant surgery, and placement.
- The dental hygienist should discuss the risks and benefits of dental implant placement with potential candidates.
- Never provide periodontal debridement around implants using metal scalers or ultrasonic scalers (unless the ultrasonic tip is a polysulfon plastic tip).

KEY CONCEPTS

- ✦ Dental implants provide an alternative to missing dentition. Dental hygienists must be able to recognize good candidates who will benefit from this investment.
- ✦ Dental implants need more maintenance than natural teeth. The dental hygienist emphasizes and describes the importance of daily oral self-care and professional dental hygiene care to dental implant clients.
- ✦ Osseointegration is a unique biologic phenomenon in which living bone cells fuse to the space-age metal titanium.
- ✦ The benefits and risks of dental implants should be explained to the client.
- ✦ The dental hygienist teaches recommended strategies for cleaning dental implants with proper oral hygiene aids.
- ✦ Air-abrasion, metal instruments, or metal ultrasonic and sonic instruments are not recommended for dental implants. Abrasives and metal instruments may cause scratches and irregularities on the implant, leading to bacterial plaque biofilm accumulation and inflammation. If metal instruments are used, they should be made of metals of equal or more pliability than titanium. Plastic, gold-tipped, Teflon-coated, graphite, or wooden instruments may be used for scaling. The dental hygienist must know which instruments are safe for the titanium metal. Some manufacturers of mechanized instruments market plastic tips that can be used with dental implants.
- ✦ The plastic periodontal probe may disturb the biologic seal that maintains the healthy peri-implant tissue to the titanium abutment. Caution is indicated in the rare times a plastic periodontal probe is used.
- ✦ Implant mobility and signs of inflammation and exudate around the implant sulcus should be recognized, documented, and called to the attention of the client and dentist.
- ✦ Peri-implantitis and poor client compliance with oral self-care are the leading causes of dental implant failure. The dental hygienist needs to recognize, document, and call to the attention of the client and dentist any signs of peri-implantitis or client noncompliance.
- ✦ Annually, the superstructure of the implant should be removed for evaluation and cleaning.

CRITICAL THINKING EXERCISES

1. Place some artificial calculus on an implant typodont or model. Use an ultrasonic scaler with a polysulfon plastic tip and plastic scaling instruments to remove the calculus.
2. With your colleagues, discuss the characteristics of some of your edentulous and partially edentulous clients. Which of these clients would be good candidates for dental implants and why? Which of these clients are poor candidates and why?
3. Use the cases presented in Scenarios 50–1 to 50–6. Develop an oral self-care plan for each of the clients. Justify your clinical decision-making process.

For References, Suggested Readings, and Related Websites, visit
http://evolve.elsevier.com/Darby/hygiene/

CHAPTER 51

Persons with Orthodontic Appliances

OBJECTIVES

Mastery of the content in this chapter will enable the reader to:

- Classify malocclusions in the anteroposterior, vertical, and transverse planes of space
- Describe the clinical characteristics indicating abnormal development of the primary and permanent dentitions
- Describe the biologic mechanism for orthodontic tooth movement
- Describe the effects of orthodontic treatment on the teeth and periodontium
- Describe the types of forces applied in orthodontic treatment
- Describe the three stages of comprehensive orthodontic treatment
- Describe special oral hygiene considerations in managing the client who has undergone orthognathic surgery
- Describe mechanical plaque control aids as well as the use of fluorides and antimicrobial agents for the orthodontic client

KEY TERMS

Activated
Adult occlusal equilibrium
Apical root resorption
Bolten templates
Camouflage therapy
Comprehensive treatment
Continuous force
Developmental spacing
Frontal resorption
Functional appliance
Growth modification therapy
Hyalinized
Intermittent force
Interrupted force
Juvenile occlusal equilibrium
Lateral cephalograph
Lip incompetence
Malalignment
Malocclusion
Maxillomandibular fixation (MMF)
Orthodontic appliance
Orthodontic expansion
Orthodontics
Orthognathic surgery
Orthopedic expansion
Passive expansion
Postemergent eruption
Preemergent eruption
Primate space
Rate of decay
Retention
Serial extraction
Skeletal discrepancy
Temporomandibular dysfunction (TMD)
Undermining resorption

Orthodontics is a dental specialty that deals with the recognition, prevention, and treatment of conditions involving irregularities of the teeth, jaws, and face and their influence on the physical and mental health of the individual.

The goals of orthodontics are as follows:

- To establish or maintain a normal functioning occlusion
- To improve facial aesthetics
- To diagnose and correct conditions associated with preventive orthodontics

Any deviation from the normal relationship of the maxillary arch and/or teeth to the mandibular arch and/or teeth is called a *malocclusion.* The problems that can arise from an untreated malocclusion are:

- Psychosocial problems caused by poor facial aesthetics, enunciation of words, and increased retention of plaque biofilm, debris, and stain

- ✦ Oral function problems such as *temporomandibular dysfunction* (TMD), difficulty with chewing, swallowing, or speech
- ✦ Injury problems caused by trauma and breakage of teeth that protrude

The dental hygienist plays a key role in identifying malocclusion that can be corrected orthodontically, preparing the client to begin orthodontic therapy, and maintaining the dental and periodontal health of the client during and following orthodontic treatment. The purpose of this chapter is to provide an overview of the basic concepts involved in orthodontics and of specific techniques for oral health self-care for persons undergoing orthodontic treatment.

MALOCCLUSION IN THE PERMANENT DENTITION

The first guidelines to clearly describe normal and abnormal relationships of the teeth were developed in the 1890s by Edward H. Angle. Angle's method of classification of malocclusion was based on the principle that the maxillary first molars are the keys to occlusion. Applied to the permanent dentition only, Angle classified the occlusion based on the relationship of the mandibular first molars to the maxillary first molars as either Class I, Class II, or Class III (see Chapter 13, Table 13–1).

Although Angle's classification is simple to use, it describes malocclusion only in terms of teeth and dental discrepancies (poor teeth position). In addition, it considers only the anteroposterior plane of space. Malocclusions, however, must be assessed further to determine if a skeletal discrepancy exists. A *skeletal discrepancy* exists when the problem is caused by the position of the jaws relative to one another. In the classification of skeletal malocclusions, there are three basic spatial planes involved. These planes include horizontal, vertical, and transverse planes (Figure 51–1). Horizontal malocclusions are classified as Class II or Class III malocclusions similar to Angle's classification system. Vertical malocclusions include open bites and severe overbites. Transverse malocclusions include crossbites (see Chapter 13).

In most cases, a malocclusion is caused by a combination of skeletal and dental discrepancies. Nevertheless, it is possible, for example, that an anterior open bite could occur if the posterior teeth erupt too far or if the anterior teeth erupt too little. Thus anterior open bite could be the result of a dental malocclusion (Figure 51–2, *A*). An anterior open bite, however, is not usually caused by a malocclusion of the teeth alone. Called the "long face syndrome," an anterior open bite typically involves a skeletal problem in which the mandible is positioned too far downward and backward along with the overeruption of the posterior teeth (Figure 51–2, *B*). In adolescents, an anterior open bite is most likely caused by skeletal malrelationships and is complex to treat.

Conversely, a skeletal "short face" with insufficient eruption of the posterior teeth (Figure 51–3, *A*) would result in a mandibular plane that is too flat, predisposing the client to a severe anterior overbite (Figure 51–3, *B*). Although often seen clinically as a problem in the relationship of the anterior teeth, it is important to understand that treatment of an open bite or a severe overbite

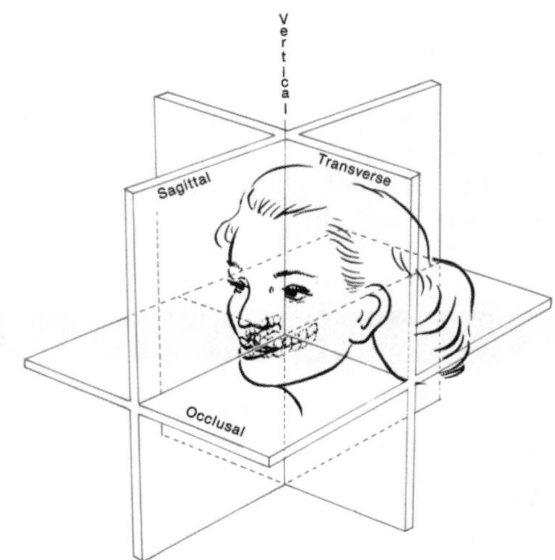

FIGURE 51–1 ✦ Perspective view of the planes of reference normally employed for orthodontic examination. The alignment of teeth and asymmetry of dental arches are best seen in projection against the occlusal plane; profile and facial aesthetics along with anteroposterior and vertical relationships are best studied in projection against the sagittal plane; and transverse dentofacial relationships are best evaluated in projection against the transverse plane. *(From Graber TM, Vanarsdall RL:* Orthodontics: current principles and techniques, *ed 2, Philadelphia, 1994, Mosby.)*

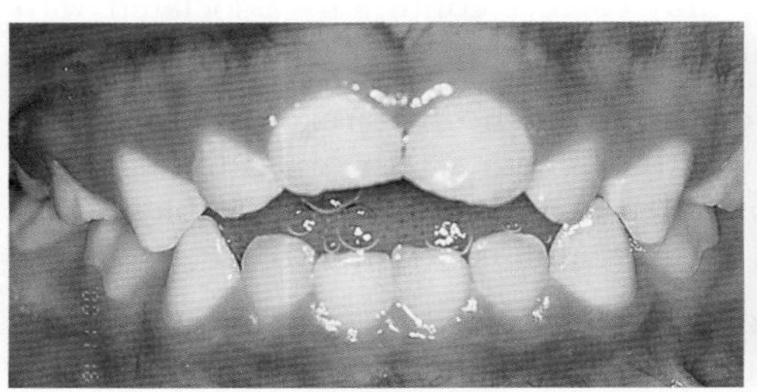

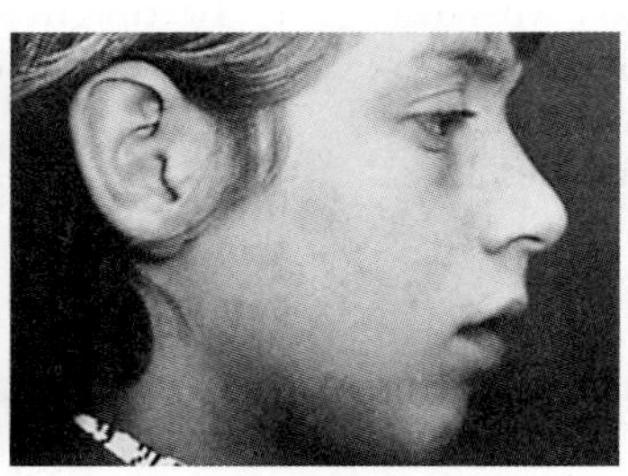

FIGURE 51–2 ✦ **A,** Anterior open bite, a malocclusion in the vertical dimension. **B,** Long face syndrome. *(B from Graber TM, Vanarsdall RL:* Orthodontics: current principles and techniques, *ed 2, Philadelphia, 1994, Mosby.)*

requires correction of eruption problems of the posterior teeth, allowing the mandible to assume a more ideal relationship to the maxilla.

A posterior crossbite is a malocclusion in the transverse plane of space that exists when the buccal cusps of the maxillary teeth are lingual to their normal relationship with the mandibular teeth (Figure 51–4). The presence of a posterior crossbite can be studied to determine if it is related to skeletal or dental causes. If the palate is too narrow or the mandible is too wide and if the teeth are in appropriate position, then the crossbite has a skeletal cause. If the palate is of adequate width, but the maxillary posterior teeth incline lingually, then the crossbite is dental in origin. The malocclusion is of skeletal/dental origin if both the relationship of the jaws and the alignment of the teeth are involved.

The important point for dental hygienists to appreciate is that treatment of a Class II or Class III malocclusion that is caused by malpositioned teeth alone (dental discrepancies) will be very different from treatment of the same malocclusion caused by skeletal relationships that are not ideal. To determine if skeletal malrelationships of the jaws exist, diagnostic tools other than clinical assessment of the teeth must be used. Impressions for study models in addition to a specialized cephalometric radiograph must be taken. As a result of cephalometric radiographic analysis, it can be determined if Class II and III malocclusions involve poor skeletal relationships of the jaws or just simply malpositioned teeth. The use of study models and cephalometric radiographs will be discussed in greater detail later in this chapter.

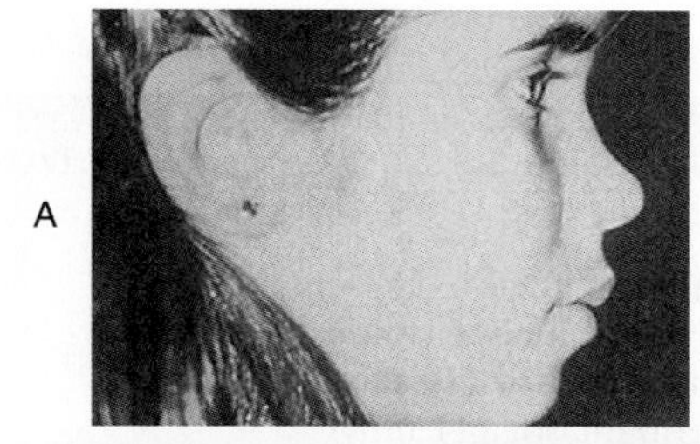

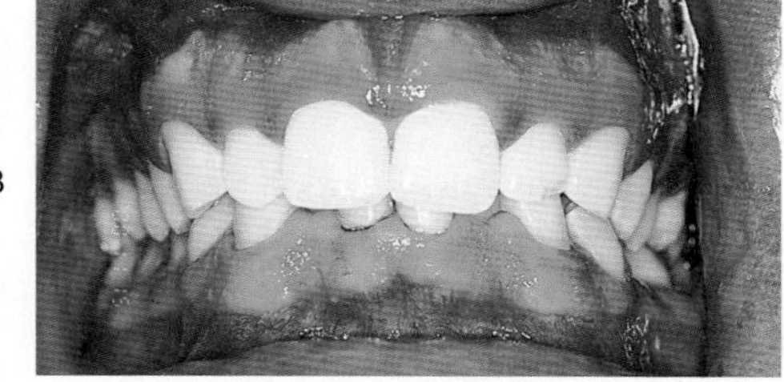

FIGURE 51–3 ✦ **A,** Short face syndrome. **B,** Severe overbite, a malocclusion in the vertical dimension. *(A from Graber TM, Vanarsdall RL:* Orthodontics: current principles and techniques*, ed 2, Philadelphia, 1994, Mosby.)*

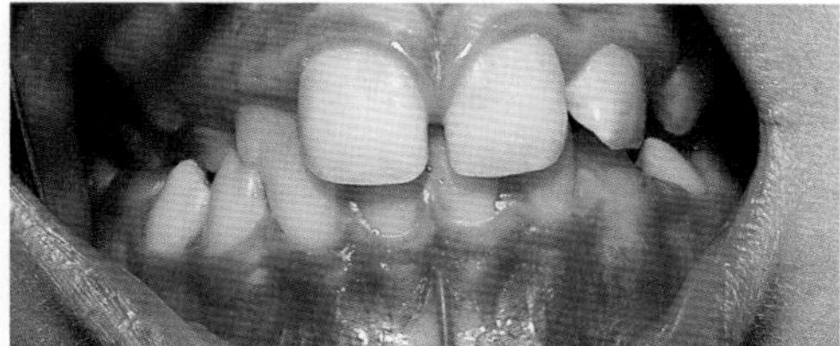

FIGURE 51–4 ✦ Posterior crossbite, a malocclusion in the transverse plane.

CLASSIFICATION OF OCCLUSION IN THE PRIMARY DENTITION

Angle's classification of malocclusion, described in Chapter 13, applies only to the permanent dentition. Classification of the primary dentition's occlusion uses the distal surfaces of the primary maxillary and mandibular second molars. Table 51–1 reviews these classifications of primary dentition occlusion and summarizes their effect on permanent dentition occlusion.

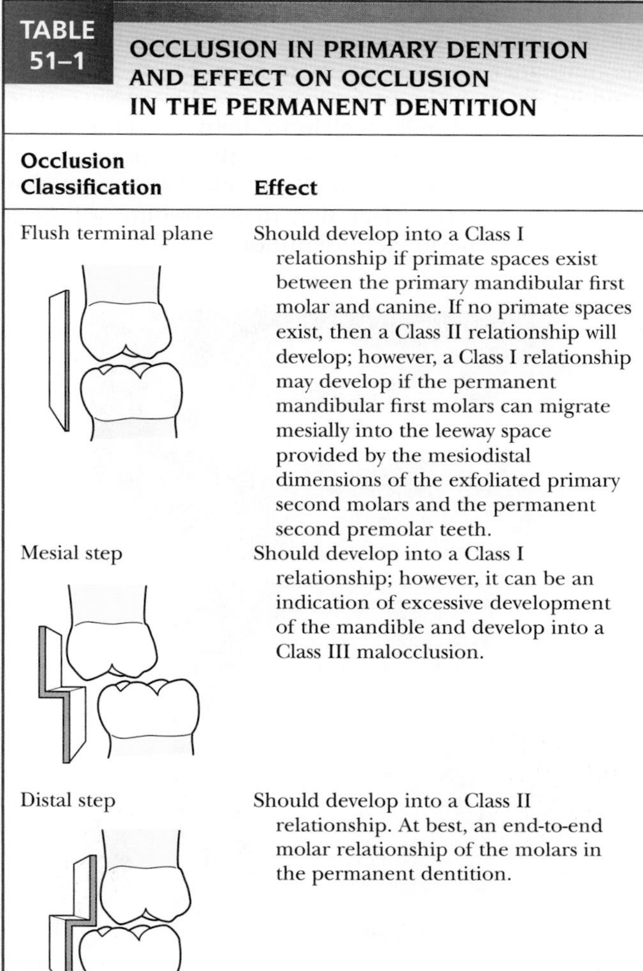

TABLE 51–1 OCCLUSION IN PRIMARY DENTITION AND EFFECT ON OCCLUSION IN THE PERMANENT DENTITION

Occlusion Classification	Effect
Flush terminal plane	Should develop into a Class I relationship if primate spaces exist between the primary mandibular first molar and canine. If no primate spaces exist, then a Class II relationship will develop; however, a Class I relationship may develop if the permanent mandibular first molars can migrate mesially into the leeway space provided by the mesiodistal dimensions of the exfoliated primary second molars and the permanent second premolar teeth.
Mesial step	Should develop into a Class I relationship; however, it can be an indication of excessive development of the mandible and develop into a Class III malocclusion.
Distal step	Should develop into a Class II relationship. At best, an end-to-end molar relationship of the molars in the permanent dentition.

DEVELOPMENT OF THE PRIMARY DENTITION

While the dates of eruption of the teeth of the primary dentition are variable, the sequence in which the teeth erupt is usually the same for all children (see Sequence and Dates of Eruption). The time of eruption is considered normal if it is up to 6 months before or 6 months after the age of eruption. The mandibular incisors typically erupt first and are easily visible when a baby smiles. The remaining incisors should erupt thereafter. The next teeth to erupt are the first molars, which are then followed by the canines. By the age of 24 to 30 months, the primary dentition is completed with the eruption of the second molars.

In a young child, spacing in the primary dentition is normal and desirable (Figure 51–5, *A*). Spacing that occurs predominantly in two locations is referred to as *primate space* (because it exists on a permanent basis in subhuman primate species). Primate space occurs in the maxilla between the lateral incisors and canines and in the mandible between the canines and the first molars. Another type of spacing called *developmental spacing* is that which develops between the incisors and is an indication that growth of the alveolar processes is adequate to provide room for the permanent teeth (Figure 51–5, *B*). The permanent incisor teeth are each 2 to 3 mm larger mesiodistally than the primary incisors they replace. The dental hygienist should explain to the parent(s) that any spacing in the primary anterior teeth is a positive sign of optimal arch development. The lack of spacing in this region, however, is a clear sign that crowding will be a problem in the permanent dentition.

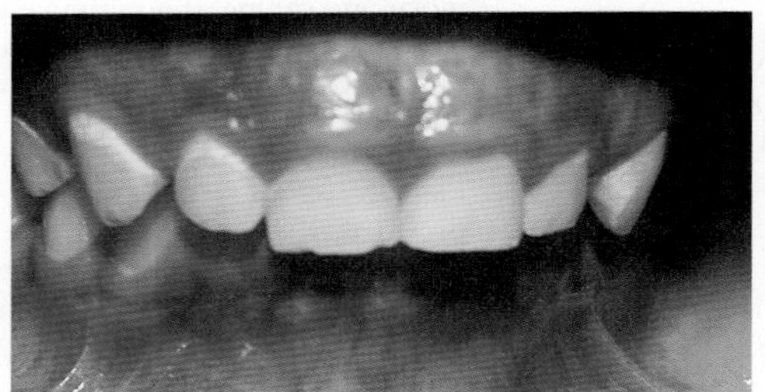

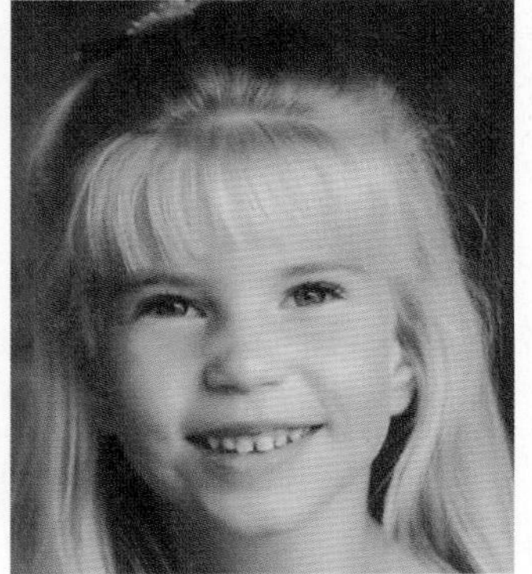

FIGURE 51–5 ✦ **A,** Primate spaces in the maxillary arch. **B,** Both primate and developmental spaces are present in the primary maxillary anteriors of the child presented in this photograph.

ERUPTION OF THE PERMANENT TEETH

Eruption of the permanent teeth is divided physiologically into the stages of preemergent eruption, postemergent eruption, juvenile occlusal equilibrium, and adult occlusal equilibrium. *Preemergent eruption* of a tooth begins when the crown has developed within the alveolar process and the root begins to form. Two processes necessary for preemergent eruption are (1) resorption of bone and primary tooth roots coronal to the developing tooth and (2) eruption of the developing tooth in the path created by the resorption of bone and roots of the primary tooth. Although these processes typically occur simultaneously, it is possible for the alveolar bone to resorb but the tooth to fail to erupt. Normally, however, the alveolar bone and primary tooth root resorb and the developing permanent tooth erupts into the space available.

The phase of *postemergent eruption* begins as soon as the crown of the tooth breaks through the gingiva. At this point, the tooth erupts rapidly and then slows as it reaches its appropriate occlusal level.

Juvenile occlusal equilibrium begins after the permanent tooth has erupted into occlusion. Although in contact with the opposing arch, the teeth continue to erupt during this phase because the ramus continues to grow vertically during adolescence. As the growth of the ramus

Sequence and Dates of Eruption

Primary Dentition

Mandibular central incisor (8 mos)
Maxillary central incisor (10 mos)
Maxillary lateral incisor (11 mos)
Mandibular lateral incisor (13 mos)
Mandibular first molar (16 mos)
Maxillary first molar (16 mos)
Maxillary canine (19 mos)
Mandibular canine (20 mos)
Mandibular second molar (27 mos)
Maxillary second molar (29 mos)

Permanent Dentition

Mandibular first molars (6 yr)
Mandibular central incisor and maxillary first molars (6 ¼ yr)
Maxillary central incisor (7 ¼ yr)
Mandibular lateral incisor (7 ½ yr)
Maxillary lateral incisor (8 ¼ yr)
Maxillary first premolar (10 ¼ yr)
Mandibular canine and first premolar (10 ½ yr)
Maxillary second premolar (11 yr)
Mandibular second premolar (11 ¼ yr)
Maxillary canine (11 ½ yr)
Mandibular second molar (12 yr)
Maxillary second molar (12 ½ yr)
Maxillary and mandibular third molars (20 yr)

Modified from Proffit WR, Fields HW Jr: *Contemporary orthodontics,* ed 2, St Louis, 1993, Mosby.

continues in the vertical dimension, the body of the mandible actually moves away from the maxilla and the teeth continue to erupt to compensate for this growth. Clinically, the dental hygienist may notice in the young adolescent that the posterior teeth appear to have short clinical crowns. By the time this vertical growth stops in the late teens, the gingival attachment is located at or near the cementoenamel junction (CEJ). The slow continued eruption of the posterior teeth in response to the growth in the vertical height of the ramus during later adolescence enables continued eruption, increasing the height of the clinical crowns and placing the gingival attachment at an appropriate level on the root.

The mechanisms of eruption remain active throughout adult life. Once all of the permanent teeth have erupted and the pubertal growth spurt is completed, the *adult occlusal equilibrium* phase begins. During this adult phase, eruption continues at a very slow pace, compensating for normal, slight occlusal wear patterns of the teeth so that the vertical height of the face is maintained. Eruption cannot compensate, however, for extreme occlusal wear, and a reduction in the vertical height of the lower face will be noted in these clients. A relatively more rapid process of eruption can occur in an adult when a tooth in an opposing arch is lost. After losing its occlusal contact, a tooth will erupt into the extraction space. At times, teeth will erupt until they contact the gingiva in the opposing arch.

The sequence in which the permanent teeth erupt is a consideration that is more important than the age at which they erupt. A change in the sequence of eruption is a much more reliable sign of a developmental problem than the age at which the teeth erupt. It is within normal limits for a maxillary canine to erupt at age 14 rather than age 12 as long as the eruption of the second premolars is also delayed. If the maxillary second premolars have erupted and the canine has not, a problem with the development of the canines is likely. The eruption sequence of the permanent dentition to produce the most favorable occlusion is shown in Sequence and Dates of Eruption.

SKELETAL AND BEHAVIORAL AGE

The assessment of skeletal age is important when planning orthodontic treatment. As described in the previous sections on the primary dentition, the occlusion depends not only on the shift and position of the teeth, but also on the skeletal growth of the mandible as well. The skeletal age of a child is determined by evaluating the ossification of the bones of the hand and wrist. A radiograph is taken of the child's hand and wrist and then compared with standard images of the development of these bones at various ages. It may be found, for example, that a child who is 9 years old may have the skeletal development of an 8-year-old or of a 10-year-old. The skeletal age of a child is important to know because orthodontic treatment often involves manipulation of the growth of the maxilla or mandible. If the orthodontist knows that a child has a significant amount of growth remaining, treatment procedures to modify this remaining growth can be planned. If the orthodontist finds, however, that the child is advanced in skeletal growth for his or her age, treatment options other than manipulation of growth of the jaws must be planned.

A final category of age that must be considered when planning orthodontic treatment is the behavioral age of the child. A child's behavioral age reflects his or her level of maturity. Regardless of chronologic or skeletal age, it can be difficult to complete treatment on a child who is not yet mature enough to behave appropriately and cooperate.

Facial Growth in Adolescence

Adolescence is a stage of tremendous growth and development during which the individual reaches sexual maturity. The timing of orthodontic treatment during adolescence must be planned carefully to take advantage of a rapid increase in the rate of growth (the growth spurt) that occurs during these years. The timing of the adolescent growth spurt can vary greatly but will typically occur two years earlier in girls than in boys. In girls, the adolescent growth spurt lasts approximately 3 1/2 years and ends when menstruation begins. The growth spurt in boys begins later than in girls and lasts 4 years. Girls, therefore, mature earlier than boys and finish their growth sooner. Boys experience a slow, steady growth before their spurt so that when their growth rate does increase, boys are already taller than girls were when experiencing their growth spurt.

The rate of growth of the mandible increases during the adolescent growth spurt. The length of the mandible grows in girls until the approximate age of 14 to 15. In boys, the length of the mandible increases until the age of 18. The growth of the vertical height of the mandible continues to grow for an even longer length of time. In girls, vertical growth of the ramus and therefore tooth eruption continue until the age of 18 and in boys this continues into the early twenties.

Facial Growth in Adults

It was previously thought that facial skeletal growth stopped in the late teens or early twenties. It has been found, however, that skeletal growth is a process that continues throughout life. Facial growth in adults follows the same pattern of growth seen in adolescents. Although the magnitude of change that occurs each year in the adult is small, the cumulative effect over the decades is significant. The growth patterns that contributed to a malocclusion in the first place continue into adulthood and can contribute to relapse of orthodontic treatment results. Adult clients may express discouragement about the relapse that can result after years of wearing braces as a teenager and may attribute it to inadequate orthodontic treatment. Understanding the normal patterns of growth that occur into adulthood will enable the dental hygienist to help the adult client understand why this relapse is happening.

EQUILIBRIUM THEORY

The equilibrium theory, an engineering theory that is applied in orthodontics, states that an object will move only if forces of unequal magnitude are applied to it. If an object remains in position, the set of forces acting on it must be equal in magnitude and, therefore, in equilibrium. Tooth eruption and the position of the teeth within the dental arches are determined by an equilibrium of forces applied by the following:

- The light forces of the tongue, cheeks, and lips applied while at rest
- The elasticity of the gingival fibers, especially the transseptal fibers that cross above the alveolar crest from one tooth to the other
- The periodontal ligament (PDL)

In the case of the dentition, although forces are continually applied to the teeth, under normal circumstances, the teeth do not move. This stability occurs because equilibrium exists in the magnitude of various forces applied to the teeth.

The light forces applied to the teeth by the lips, cheeks, and tongue at rest are the most effective in determining tooth position. Although light in magnitude, these forces are applied over a long duration. The duration of the force applied is more important in causing tooth movement than the strength of the force applied. In order to affect the position of the teeth, the force must be applied for at least 6 hours per day. Although the lips, tongue, and cheeks also apply forces during mastication and swallowing, the duration of these forces is much too short to determine tooth position. A tongue-thrust swallow, therefore, will not cause protrusion of the teeth. Oral habits, however, such as thumb or finger sucking, can affect tooth position if continued for at least 6 hours per day.

The elastic gingival fibers also contribute to the equilibrium of forces applied to the teeth. When stretched into new positions by orthodontic movement of teeth, these fibers, especially the transseptal fibers, will also cause teeth to relapse back into their original positions after completion of treatment. A periodontal surgical procedure (fibrotomy) completed to incise the gingival fibers and the placement of a permanent wire retainer bonded to the lingual surfaces to the anteriors have been found to prevent the relapse of teeth after orthodontic movement.

DIAGNOSTIC RECORDS

The diagnosis and treatment planning process in orthodontics follows a problem-oriented approach in which a diagnosis or problem list is formulated from data collected from the client. Once the problem list is developed, the problems are prioritized so that the most important problem receives the greatest priority in treatment. All possible solutions to each problem are considered, and from this list, the best possible treatment options for the client in terms of cost, effectiveness, complexity, and risk are presented to the client for consideration.

An objective, scientific appraisal of the client's condition must be made based on data obtained from the health history and interview, clinical examination, and diagnostic records. Table 51–2 highlights pertinent data collected from the client health history questionnaire and interview and their implication for orthodontic care.

Intraoral Photographs

Intraoral photographs are taken to document the client's status before treatment. A set of photographs should include an anterior view with teeth in occlusion, right and left buccal views of posterior sextants with teeth in occlusion, and occlusal views of the maxillary and mandibular arches. Additional photographs are taken of any special conditions such as gingival recession or clefting or enamel anomalies not visible on the standard photographs.

Radiographs

A panoramic radiograph is exposed to examine the perioral structures for the presence of pathology or for supernumerary or impacted teeth (Figure 51–6). The mandibular condyles are evaluated, and the possible need for additional radiographs of the temporomandibular joint (TMJ) is determined by the dentist. If the anterior teeth are not clearly visible, anterior periapical films are taken to evaluate the roots of these teeth for a predisposition to apical resorption.

A *lateral cephalograph* is almost always indicated in orthodontics to assess the skeletal relationship of the jaws to one another and to determine the need to reposition the anterior teeth (Figure 51–7). The use of cephalometrics in orthodontics is valuable because although two cases of malocclusion may appear similar clinically or on a study model, significant differences in the two cases may become apparent when the skeletal components of the malocclusion are analyzed. The only instance in which a lateral cephalometric radiograph would not be indicated is when a client presents only minor orthodontic problems. If serious facial asymmetry is present, then a cephalometric radiograph taken from the frontal aspect is also indicated.

Numerous systems for the analysis of cephalometric radiographs have been developed. For example, the *Bolten templates* provide a convenient method for comparison of the client to a reference for the client's age. The template is superimposed over a tracing of the client's cephalometric radiograph on which standard anatomic landmarks are identified. The skeletal features of the client are studied to determine how the client's jaw positions compare to the norm for his or her age and how the position of the teeth relates to their respective jaws in both the anteroposterior and vertical planes of space (Figure 51–8).

The Sassouni analysis uses horizontal anatomic planes to evaluate the vertical proportions of the face

TABLE 51–2 BASELINE FACTORS TO BE ASSESSED AND IMPLICATIONS FOR CARE

Factors	Implications for Care
Personal Factors	
Chief complaint	Must be a priority in treatment planning
Age of client	May affect client motivation/cooperation. Adults are generally internally motivated, whereas a child may be completing treatment because of a parent's wishes.
History of previous orthodontic treatment of client or client's parents, siblings	Provides insight into hereditary factors involved in the orthodontic problem(s), as well as the client's or parent's understanding of orthodontic treatment and ability to understand and help a child manage orthodontic discomforts.
Health History	
History of trauma to teeth or jaws	Provides insight into etiology of an existing skeletal asymmetry. Alerts the dental hygienist to the need to study radiographs for the presence of fractures of the teeth or jaws.
Diabetes	Presents an increased risk for periodontal breakdown. Must monitor client's compliance with physician recommendations for controlling blood sugar level.
Rheumatic heart disease, organic heart murmur, heart valve replacement, or prosthetic joint replacement within the last 2 years	Requires antibiotic premedication before dental hygiene care and orthodontic procedures involving gingival manipulation, such as placement of orthodontic bands.
Osteoarthritis of the temporomandibular joint	Orthodontic treatment will not improve degenerative changes.
Nickel or latex allergy	Metal orthodontic appliances contain nickel, and elastics contain latex. Alternative materials will need to be planned.
Medications	
Calcium channel blocking agents for the management of hypertension	Risk for gingival hyperplasia that may lead to increased plaque retention and associated gingival inflammation and dental caries. Shortened recall interval may be required.
Fosamax for the treatment of osteoporosis	Bone remodeling may occur at a slower rate. Hormonal management of osteoporosis may be an option.
Indomethacin, a potent prostaglandin inhibitor used in the treatment of arthritis	Response of the teeth to orthodontic forces may be reduced.
Corticosteroids and nonsteroidal anti-inflammatory agents	Potent medications used on a chronic basis may reduce the response of teeth to orthodontic forces. Client may present increased risk for periodontal breakdown.
Tricyclic antidepressants, anti-arrhythmic agents, anti-malarial agents, methylxanthines, and some tetracyclines may influence prostaglandin levels	Response of the teeth to orthodontic forces may be reduced.
Oral Health and Function	
Dental caries, endodontic pathology	Before orthodontic treatment, clinical and radiographic assessment must be completed, caries must be controlled, and endodontic lesions must be treated.
Periodontal health	Before orthodontic treatment, a thorough periodontal assessment must be completed, diseased sites must be controlled, and areas of inadequate attached gingiva must be corrected with gingival grafting.
Occlusal function	In children, shifting of the mandible during closure may affect the skeletal development of the mandible.

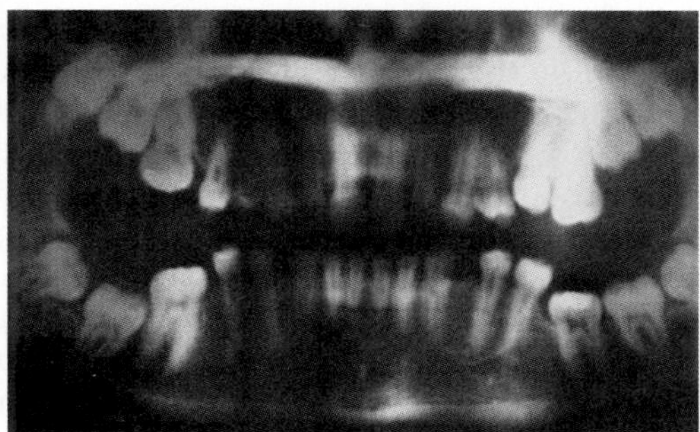

FIGURE 51–6 ✦ A panoramic radiograph that shows signs of failure of posterior teeth to erupt. *(From Graber TM, Vanarsdall RL:* Orthodontics current principles and techniques, *ed 2, Philadelphia, 1994, Mosby.)*

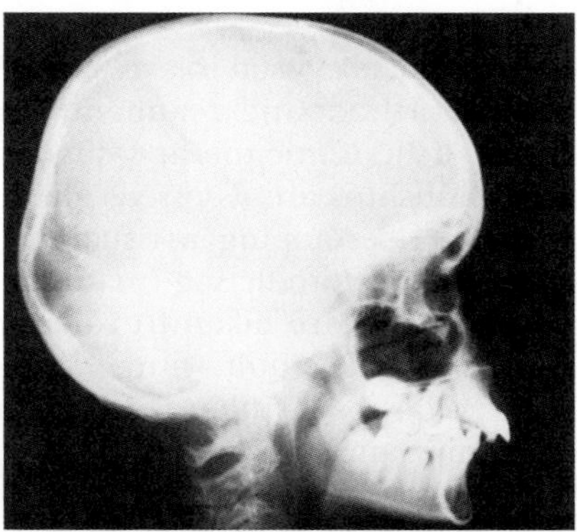

FIGURE 51–7 ✦ A lateral cephalometric radiograph is taken to evaluate the impact of skeletal and dental/skeletal relationships on the client's occlusal status. *(From Graber TM, Vanarsdall RL:* Orthodontics current principles and techniques, *ed 2, Philadelphia, 1994, Mosby; courtesy Erich Fleischer.)*

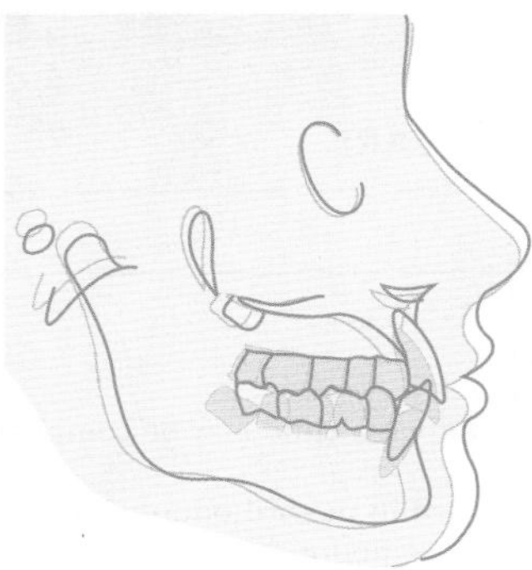

FIGURE 51–8 ✦ Bolten template analysis. The template selected for the appropriate skeletal development of this child is presented in red. This client, compared to the template, presents a lower facial height that is too long, as well as a downward and backward rotation of the mandible, producing a mandibular plane that is too steep when compared to the norm as presented in the Bolten template. *(From Proffit WR, Fields HW Jr:* Contemporary orthodontics, *ed 2, St Louis, 1993, Mosby.)*

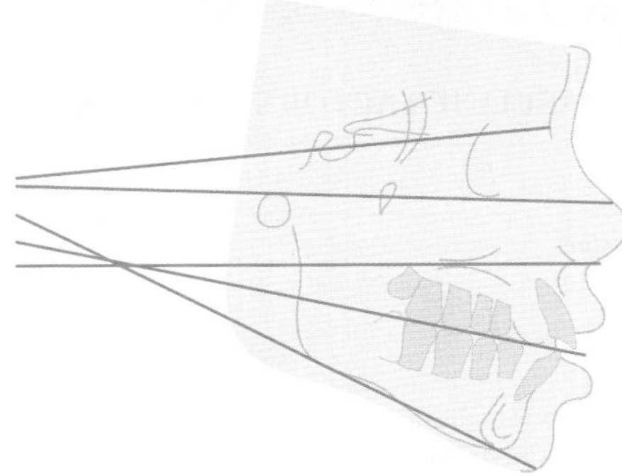

FIGURE 51–10 ✦ Sassouni analysis. Anatomic horizontal planes identified by Sassouni allow the comparison of the vertical components of the face. This client presents deviations in the planes associated with the maxilla and mandible as would be seen in a client with a skeletal open bite. *(From Proffit WR, Fields HW Jr:* Contemporary orthodontics, *ed 2, St Louis, 1993, Mosby.)*

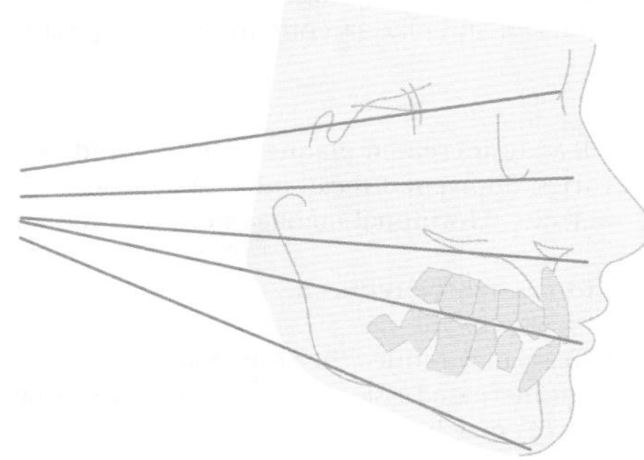

FIGURE 51–9 ✦ Ideal skeletal relationships as defined by Sassouni. In a client with ideal vertical skeletal relationships, the horizontal planes of Sassouni should intersect at a common meeting point when projected posteriorly beyond the face. *(From Proffit WR, Fields HW Jr:* Contemporary orthodontics, *ed 2, St Louis, 1993, Mosby.)*

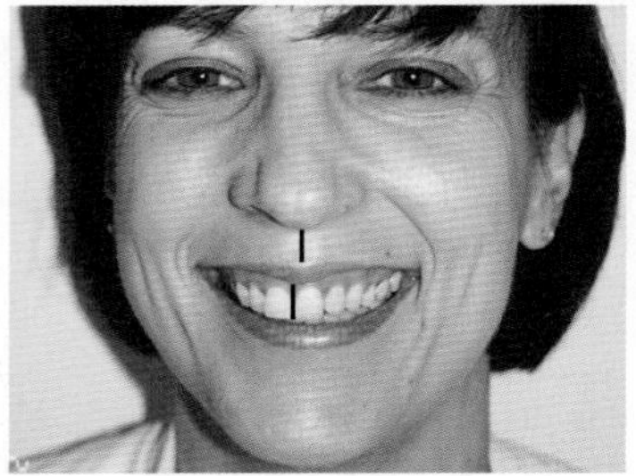

FIGURE 51–11 ✦ Relationship of the midline of the maxilla to the philtrum. In this case, the midline of the maxilla deviates to the client's right.

(Figure 51–9). A skeletal open bite or skeletal overbite will become clearly apparent when analyzing the relationship of the planes of the face. In addition, if any one plane is malpositioned, it will be apparent when compared to the positions of the other planes of the face (Figure 51–10).

Cephalometrics are also used to evaluate changes that occur as a result of orthodontic treatment. Taken before, during, and after orthodontic therapy, changes in dental and skeletal relationships are assessed. Finally, cephalometrics are used in developing a visualized treatment objective, a plan used in predicting treatment results.

Bitewing radiographs are taken to rule out the presence of active caries. An adult with a history of periodontal disease requires a full set of radiographs in addition to the panoramic film.

Facial Photographs

Although facial and jaw proportions are assessed clinically and measured on lateral cephalometric radiographs, a more objective analysis of the face and profile is made using facial photographs. Viewing the client from the frontal view, the face is evaluated for bilateral symmetry. The midline of the maxilla is also assessed in relation to the philtrum and nasal columna (Figure 51–11).

A minimum of three facial photographic views are taken: full face with lips relaxed, full face smiling, and profile with lips relaxed. If major skeletal asymmetries are present, both right and left profile views are taken.

The assessment of the profile can be used to differentiate those individuals having an acceptable or nearly acceptable profile from those with serious skeletal malrelationships. The three goals of profile analysis are (1) to determine the position of the jaws in the anteroposterior plane of space, (2) to assess the posture of the lips and the position of the incisors, and (3) to evaluate the vertical proportions of the face and the angle of the inferior border of the mandible.

To determine the position of the jaws in the anteroposterior plane of space, a line is drawn on the profile from the bridge of the nose to the base of the upper lip. If the jaws form a normal relationship to one another, this line should form a straight line with a line drawn from the base of the upper lip to the chin. If a convexity is formed, the client presents a skeletal Class II relationship of the jaws. If a concavity is formed, the client presents with a Class III relationship of the jaws.

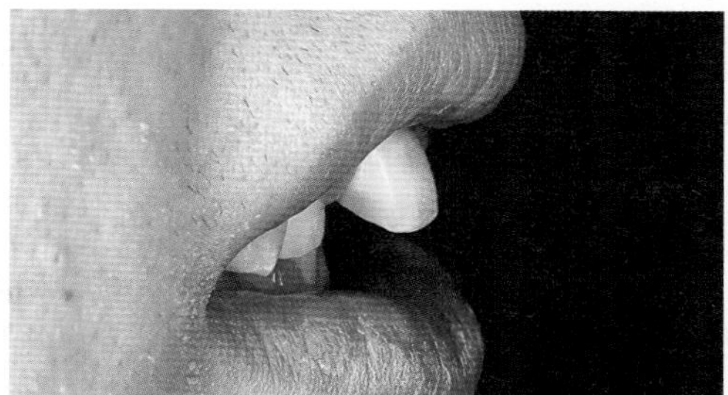

FIGURE 51–12 ✦ Lip incompetence.

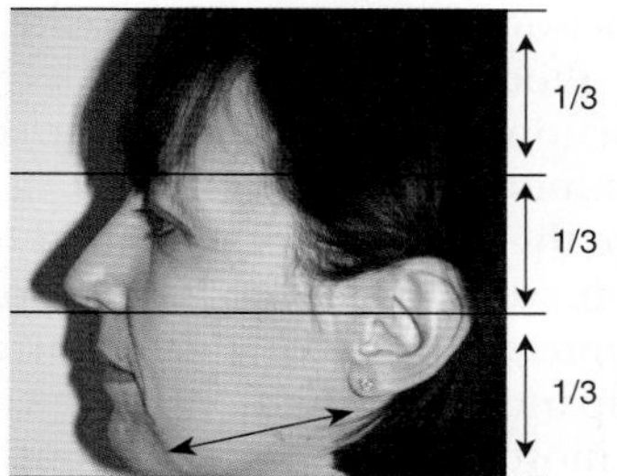

FIGURE 51–13 ✦ Vertical proportions of the face and mandibular inclination. Horizontal lines drawn at the top of the head, supraorbital ridge, base of the nose, and base of the chin should divide the head into three portions of equal height. The mandible should incline slightly.

Lip posture is assessed by viewing the client's profile with the lips at rest. The incisors are protrusive if the lips appear prominent in the profile and if the lips are separated by more than 3 to 4 mm when at rest. Separation of the lips to this extent is called *lip incompetence* (Figure 51–12). The client with lip incompetence must strain to bring the lips together over the teeth. Orthodontic treatment to retract the incisors will create a more aesthetic facial profile and enable the patient to close the lips over the teeth without strain.

The vertical proportions of the face and the angle of the inferior border of the mandible to the ramus are also evaluated in the profile analysis. Horizontal lines drawn through the bottom of the chin, base of the nose, eyebrows, and top of the skull should produce three zones of equal height (Figure 51–13). An imaginary line drawn along the inferior border of the mandible should incline downward at only a slight degree A steep incline of the mandible correlates with an anterior open bite and long face. A flat mandibular plane correlates with a deep overbite and short facial height.

Study Models

Study models are used to assess the occlusion, the symmetry of the form of dental arches, and the symmetrical positioning of individual teeth within the arches (Figure 51–14). Impressions of the maxillary and mandibular arches must be taken, along with a wax bite registration to prepare models used to study the occlusion (see Chapter 30).

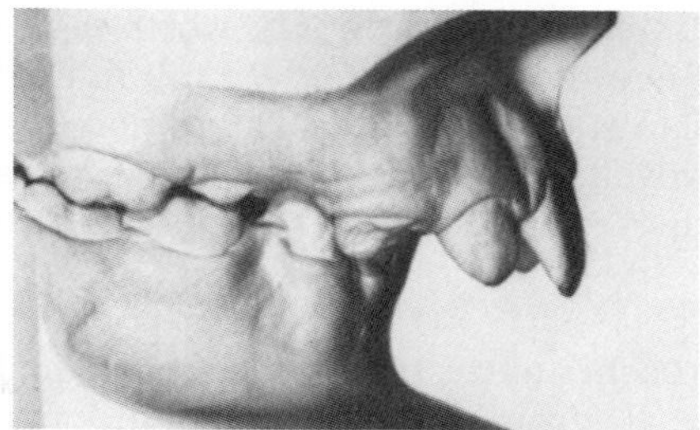

FIGURE 51–14 ✦ Study model of a 9-year-old boy with a severe Class II, division 1 malocclusion. *(From Graber TM, Vanarsdall RL:* Orthodontics current principles and techniques, *ed 2, Philadelphia, 1994, Mosby; courtesy Erich Fleischer.)*

TREATMENT PLANNING

Orthodontic treatment planning is beyond the scope of this chapter; however, certain concepts are important for the dental hygienist to understand. While the diagnostic phase of treatment is scientific and objective in nature, treatment planning is more subjective and reflects both the experience and judgment of the clinician as well as the priorities of the client. Although the concerns of a client must be given priority, the orthodontist is not obligated to provide treatment the client requests if the plan requested does not comply with professional standards.

The goals of orthodontic treatment are to achieve ideal occlusion, facial aesthetics, and stability. In clients presenting complex orthodontic problems, it may be impossible to achieve all goals and a compromise must be made. Efforts to achieve an ideal dental occlusion may, for example, produce a good dental result with poor facial aesthetics. Achievement of ideal aesthetics, on the other hand, may require a compromise in the dental occlusion and/or long-term stability of the result. In cases in which all three goals cannot be achieved, priority must be given to the client's chief complaint. If aesthetics are the client's main concern, the client would be unhappy with treatment that, although resulting in an ideal occlusion with maximum long-term stability, did not correct problems of facial aesthetics or possibly even worsened them. The dental hygienist must recognize this issue when seeing a client for maintenance following the completion of orthodontic therapy. All too frequently, the dental occlusion evaluated using Angle's classification is used as a single criterion for assessing the success of treatment. Before seeing an orthodontic client for a maintenance appointment, any written communication from the orthodontist must be read by the dental hygienist so that he or she will be aware of treatment results and any compromises required, as well as recommendations for maintenance.

Another issue to be considered in treatment planning is the cost as well as the risks and benefits of various options. Plans that are complex and difficult must be considered in terms of financial expense as well as cost in terms of discomfort and time, and compared to the expected benefits to the patient. On the other hand, simple treatment plans may not be worth their cost if the benefits achieved for the client are too limited. A more complex plan such as one involving *orthognathic surgery* might improve treatment results so much more that the benefits achieved far outweigh the costs and risks.

Clients with Skeletal Malocclusions

Three approaches to treatment of a skeletal malocclusion are possible: (1) growth modification of the jaws to correct the problem, (2) camouflage of the jaw discrepancy by tooth movement to correct the dental occlusion within the limits of the existing jaw discrepancy, and (3) surgical correction of the jaw discrepancy. Growth modification is the preferred method of treatment and involves manipulating the growth of the jaws to correct a skeletal malocclusion. Camouflage of the discrepancy by repositioning the teeth is a compromise that is acceptable in mild or even moderate skeletal cases. Surgical correction is limited to severe skeletal malrelationships.

GROWTH MODIFICATION. *Growth modification therapy* is the type of orthodontic treatment that applies pressures to resist or enhance the growth of the maxilla or the mandible. Two important principles are inherent to growth modification. First, clinically significant growth modification can occur only in those clients who are still actively growing. Therefore, growth modification must be carried out in the mixed dentition stage in most clients, before or during the adolescent growth spurt. In girls, growth modification is most effective when initiated at age 8 or 9 and can be deferred in boys until age 10 or 11 because they mature later. Variations in ideal age for initiating treatment do exist, and the decision of when to begin treatment should be determined by assessing developmental age rather than chronologic age alone.

The second principle of growth modification is that therapy must continue to some extent until after adolescence when growth is essentially complete. For example, a child with a deficient maxilla will present a growth pattern in which the maxilla is expected to not only grow less but also to stop growing sooner than would be seen in a child presenting ideal jaw growth and proportion. If treatment is stopped too soon, the original problem will recur because the maxilla will continue its original pattern of deficient growth while other aspects of the face, including the mandible, continue to grow in an ideal pattern and rate. Clients having problems of excessive jaw growth, however, will continue to have jaw growth long after growth slows or stops in other individuals presenting normal growth patterns. Active retention must be continued for these clients for a longer period than that needed for clients without problems of excessive growth.

CAMOUFLAGE THERAPY. *Camouflage therapy* involves moving teeth orthodontically to mask a malocclusion that is caused by poor skeletal proportions. In some cases, tooth movement, often involving the extraction of some permanent teeth, can be completed to achieve an ideal occlusion despite an existing skeletal discrepancy. It is important, however, that camouflage therapy achieve an acceptable outcome and not actually accentuate the impact the skeletal problem has on facial aesthetics. For example, in mild to moderate skeletal Class II cases, the maxillary teeth can be retracted to create a more ideal occlusion without causing problems with facial aesthetics. In more severe Class II cases in which the mandible is or appears to be deficient, retraction of the maxillary teeth can enhance the appearance of the deficiency of the middle and lower face and increase the prominent appearance of the nose. Mild skeletal Class III cases can also be treated with camouflage therapy in which the mandibular incisors are retracted to create an acceptable occlusion. In moderate or severe Class III situations, however, retraction of the mandibular incisors may accentuate the prominence of the chin.

Camouflage therapy should be limited to situations in which growth modification is no longer possible because of the developmental age of the client and in which skeletal discrepancies are mild or in the case of Class II, moderate at most. This therapy is contraindicated in clients having good remaining growth potential or more severe skeletal problems.

COMBINED SURGICAL AND ORTHODONTIC TREATMENT. Surgical therapy is required if the skeletal malrelationship is so severe that neither growth modification nor camouflage therapy will provide satisfactory results. Some conditions that could have been treated with growth modification in the child will require surgical therapy in the adult who is no longer actively growing.

The goals of presurgical treatment are to align the teeth within the arches. This process is critical because it would be difficult during surgery to position the jaws to one another if the ideal alignment of the teeth within the arches was not already established. Presurgical treatment then varies significantly depending on the case. Presurgical orthodontics, however, should not require more than one year to complete.

The fixed orthodontic appliance used for presurgical alignment of the teeth is then used to stabilize the teeth after surgery. This stabilization is accomplished by *maxillomandibular fixation (MMF),* the process of wiring the arches together in the desired relationship. While the arches are fixed in position, clients can open their lips, but not the teeth, so lingual plaque removal is impossible. (Oral hygiene care is discussed later in this chapter.)

Use of Treatment Response in Treatment Planning

Despite careful analysis, diagnosis, and treatment planning, it is impossible to predict with complete certainty the result of any treatment plan, especially those including growth modification for preadolescent and adolescent clients. If growth occurs as expected and the client cooperates and attends all appointments, a good result is expected. If growth, cooperation, or both fail to meet required expectations, an alternative plan including camouflage therapy with extractions may be required. To reduce the amount of uncertainty in treatment planning, the client's initial response to treatment is evaluated 6 to 9 months after therapy is initiated. If the client is responding to growth modification as expected at that time, the orthodontist can assume that planned treatment is appropriate and should be continued. If treatment results are less than expected at this initial assessment, the treatment plan can be changed as indicated. Client response to treatment must, in fact, be monitored throughout therapy.

Treatment Planning for Multiple Dental Problems

Treatment planning for children or adult clients having multiple dental problems must follow a specific sequence. First, any active dental disease must be treated or controlled. Carious teeth must be restored, any indicated extractions completed, any endodontic pathology treated, and periodontal disease controlled by aggressive scaling and root debridement under local anesthesia. Mucogingival surgery such as free gingival grafts is completed before orthodontic treatment as well. Orthodontic treatment can then be initiated, including orthognathic surgery if required. Definitive periodontal therapy such as osseous surgery is delayed until after orthodontic therapy is completed because the architecture of the alveolar bone often changes as a result of orthodontic treatment. Finally, definitive restorative procedures are completed, including crowns, bridges, implants, and/or partial dentures.

BIOLOGY OF ORTHODONTIC TOOTH MOVEMENT

Tooth movement occurs when light pressure is exerted on the tooth. This pressure results in bone being resorbed on one side of the tooth and new bone growing in and slowly hardening on the other side of the tooth. This new bone holds each tooth in its new position. The reason this occurs is described as follows.

The PDL consists of collagenous fibers, undifferentiated mesenchymal cells, and the fibroblasts and osteoblasts into which they differentiate, nerve fibers, blood vessels, and tissue fluids. These constituents function together to support the teeth during normal function in addition to making orthodontic tooth movement possible. The PDL space is filled with the same extracellular fluid found in all tissues of the body. This fluid allows the PDL to function as a shock absorber during normal function.

When light, sustained force is applied to a tooth, the tooth moves in the socket within seconds, expressing fluid from the PDL space. The PDL becomes compressed between the tooth and the alveolar wall and pain is felt. Within a few minutes after pressure is applied, altered blood flow occurs as well as changes in oxygen levels and the release of cellular mediators such as prostaglandins and cytokines within the PDL. After 6 hours of sustained pressure, cellular activity in the PDL, including differentiation into osteoclasts and osteoblasts, occurs. This needed pressure explains why a force must be applied to a tooth at least 6 hours per day to result in tooth movement.

Osteoclasts must form within the PDL to remove bone from the area adjacent to the compressed part of the PDL. These osteoclasts attack the lamina dura, removing bone on the pressure side in a process called *frontal resorption.* Osteoblasts are needed to then remodel bone on the pressure side of the tooth as well as to form new bone on the side to which tension is applied. Both osteoclastic and osteoblastic activities are stimulated by prostaglandin E, a chemical mediator important in tooth movement.

If the sustained force is great enough to totally occlude blood vessels and cut off blood supply to the area of the PDL, then PDL necrosis develops within the compressed area. The area of the PDL becomes devoid of all cells and is referred to as *hyalinized.* Remodeling of bone must occur adjacent to this hyalinized area by osteoclasts and osteoblasts supplied by nearby, undamaged areas of the PDL. This process is called *undermining resorption.* Tooth movement is delayed for 7 to 14 days until undermining resorption removes enough bone to allow movement of the tooth.

PDL necrosis also results in pain. Theoretically, optimal orthodontic forces would stimulate cellular activity without completely occluding the blood vessels. Tooth movement would then occur by frontal resorption only without any necrosis. Clinically, this is not a likely possibility. Even with the application of light force, small areas of necrosis are likely to develop within the PDL, and tooth movement will be delayed until these can be removed by undermining resorption. In all cases, too much force must be avoided. The pressure delivered to the PDL by orthodontic forces is an important factor in treatment and must be carefully controlled.

As previously discussed, force must be applied for 6 hours to produce the biologic activities that enable movement of teeth. Forces applied beyond the 6-hour minimum, such as those applied by fixed orthodontic appliances, produce the most effective tooth movement, especially if they are not dependent on client compliance. Removable appliances worn almost all of the time will result in effective tooth movement as long as they are worn as directed.

Rate of decay refers to the fact that the force applied by an appliance declines as the tooth responds by movement. Even when a spring is used, some decline in the magnitude of force occurs after the tooth has moved even a short distance. The amount of loss of force depends on the type of appliance used. The duration of orthodontic force, based on the concept of rate of decay, is classified as continuous, interrupted, or intermittent. *Continuous force* is force that is maintained from one orthodontic visit to the next, although the magnitude of the force may decline. *Interrupted force* refers to forces in which the magnitude gradually drops to zero between orthodontic visits at which the appliance is *activated.* Appliances that are fixed and not removed by the client may apply forces that are continuous or interrupted. *Intermittent force* refers to a situation in which the magnitude of force drops abruptly to zero, such as when the client takes out an appliance. Removable appliances such as headgear, bite plates, or elastics applied to fixed appliances produce forces that are activated by the client and, therefore, intermittent in nature.

Forces that are heavy and continuous can be destructive to the periodontium as well as the root of the tooth. Forces that are heavy but interrupted, so that the magnitude of force declines to zero until the appliance is again activated by the orthodontist, are more physiologically acceptable because repair and regeneration of the PDL and adjacent bone are possible before the next activation.

Forces that are light, continuous, and produce only frontal resorption are ideal. Clinically, however, it is likely that with even the lightest force, some areas of PDL necrosis and undermining resorption are likely to develop. If undermining resorption does occur, tooth movement will occur in about 10 days after activation. A period of another 10 to 14 days is then needed to allow for repair and regeneration of the PDL before force should be applied again. Based on this process, orthodontic appointments are typically made no more frequently than every 4 weeks to allow healing and to prevent damage to the teeth or bone that could occur.

EFFECTS OF ORTHODONTIC FORCE ON THE TEETH AND PERIODONTIUM

Effects on the Pulp

Properly applied orthodontic forces will, at most, affect the dental pulp minimally. A mild, transient pulpitis may occur and is usually experienced by clients as discomfort during the first few days after appliances are activated. Occasionally, however, loss of pulpal vitality may occur during orthodontic treatment. This may be because of a history of trauma to the tooth and therefore unrelated to orthodontic treatment or because of poor control of orthodontic forces. Tooth movement resulting from heavy, continuous force can be abrupt as undermining resorption occurs, and especially harmful if applied over a long period. Tooth movement that is large enough and abrupt enough could sever blood vessels as they enter the apex, resulting in pulpal necrosis.

Effects on Root Structure

As in the PDL and adjacent bone, resorption and repair of dentin and cementum occur during orthodontic movement. Cementum and dentin are removed during periods of force application and replaced by cementum during periods of rest. Repair, however, will not occur if more serious damage develops, such as that which may occur at the root apex where portions of cementum and/or dentin may actually break away from the root. These portions will be resorbed by the body and will not be replaced. Permanent loss of root structure occurs only at the root apex. This *apical root resorption* appears radiographically as a loss in the length and apical blunting of the root (Figure 51–15).

Some loss of root length will occur in almost every individual treated orthodontically and is usually of little clinical significance. At times, however, severe loss of one-third to one-half of the root length occurs from even routine orthodontic tooth movement. Although the cause of this type of resorption is not clear, some individuals are found to be more prone to resorption than others. Treatment factors and characteristics that make the teeth prone to resorption are presented in Tooth Characteristics and Treatment Factors Related to Increased Apical Root Resorption During Orthodontic Treatment.

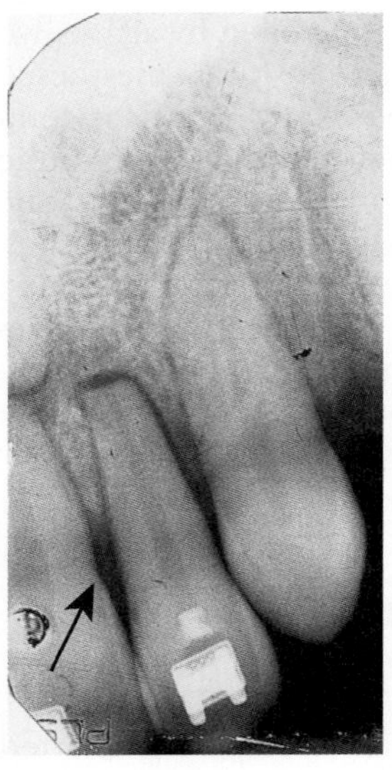

FIGURE 51–15 ✦ Apical root resorption.

Tooth Characteristics and Treatment Factors Related to Increased Apical Root Resorption During Orthodontic Treatment

Tooth Characteristics

Conical roots with pointed apices
A distorted root form such as dilaceration
A history of trauma regardless of whether endodontic treatment was completed
A history of root resorption before any orthodontic treatment was initiated

Treatment Factors

The application of heavy, continuous force to move the teeth
Prolonged duration of treatment
Movement of root apices into cortical bone, especially in the maxillary anterior region

Effects on the Height of Alveolar Bone

Orthodontic therapy is not associated with an increase in the loss of alveolar bone. The only situation in which bone loss is exacerbated by orthodontic tooth movement is when teeth are moved in the client having active periodontal infection. When periodontal disease has been controlled before and during orthodontic treatment, improved tooth position and placement will actually improve the osseous contours as well. This improvement is demonstrated by the uprighting of mesially drifted second molars to allow the construction of crown and bridge prostheses. As the tooth is uprighted during orthodontics, the osseous contours on the mesial aspect of the tooth are improved as the crestal bone is uprighted along with the tooth (Figure 51–16, *A* and *B*).

Mobility and Pain

Increased tooth mobility is expected during orthodontic treatment. PDL fibers become disorganized and detached from the bone and root cementum, and the adjacent bone must remodel. Radiographs taken during treatment will reveal widened PDL spaces. Excessive mobility, however, may be an indication that too much force is being applied, causing too much undermining bone resorption. If a tooth becomes extremely mobile during therapy, all force should be discontinued until the mobility reduces to moderate levels. Usually, this problem can be corrected without causing permanent damage.

Several hours after an appliance is activated during an orthodontic visit, a client may feel a mild aching sensation and sensitivity to pressure so that chewing a hard food is painful. This pain will likely last for 2 to 4 days and then disappear until the appliance is again adjusted. Pain following orthodontic adjustments varies among individuals. One client may experience severe pain following application of mild force while another client may not experience any pain at all from the application of heavier force. When planning dental hygiene appointments with clients undergoing orthodontic treatment, it is generally more comfortable for a client to be seen before rather than immediately after orthodontic adjustments. Scaling procedures are particularly uncomfortable for teeth that are already painful as a result of an orthodontic adjustment.

Pain is the result of the development of ischemic areas within the PDL. Tenderness with chewing firm foods is caused by the mild pulpitis that occurs and by inflammation at the apex of the tooth. The greater the force applied to the tooth, the greater the amount of pain expected because larger areas within the PDL will undergo sterile necrosis. If light forces are applied, painful symptoms can be relieved by having the client chew gum during the first 8 hours following the adjustment. Chewing temporarily displaces the teeth enough to allow some blood flow through the compressed areas of the PDL, preventing the buildup of metabolites that stimulate pain receptors.

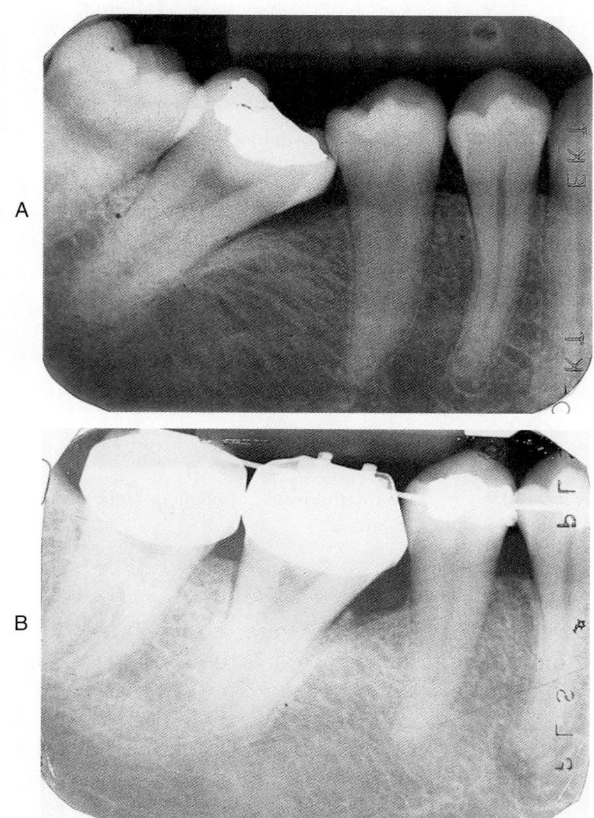

FIGURE 51–16 ✦ **A,** Mesial drifting of tooth number 31 into extraction space. Note bony defect on tooth number 31. **B,** Note improvement in contour of alveolar bone near tooth number 31 mesial as tooth is uprighted.

Effects of Orthodontic Force on the Maxilla

The sites of growth of the maxilla where growth modification might be effective are the sutures where the maxilla is attached to the cranium and the midpalatine suture area. To counter excessive maxillary growth, forces would be applied to oppose the natural soft tissue forces that place tension on and separate the craniofacial sutures. To treat deficient growth, forces would be applied to enhance the natural forces that stimulate maxillary growth.

Extraoral headgear appliances are used to restrain maxillary growth (Figure 51–17, *A* and *B*). The appliance must be worn at least 8 hours per day, and 12 to 14 hours per day is preferable. Physiologic reasons exist for wearing headgear at night. More growth hormone is secreted in children during the night than during the day. Growth of the long bones of the body has been found to be greater at night than during the day. Although it is not known if facial bones grow in the same pattern, it is reasonable to expect that they do. As a result, use of headgear to modify skeletal growth is more effective at night than during the day.

Effects of Orthodontic Force on the Mandible

In contrast to the maxilla, the mandible is attached to the rest of the skull by the TMJ rather than by bony sutures and therefore requires different methods to

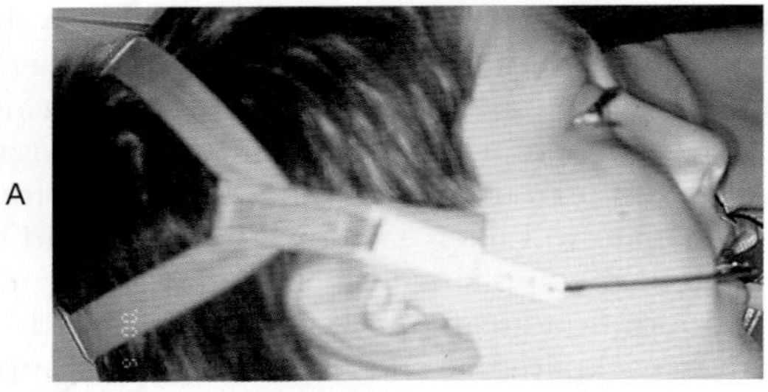

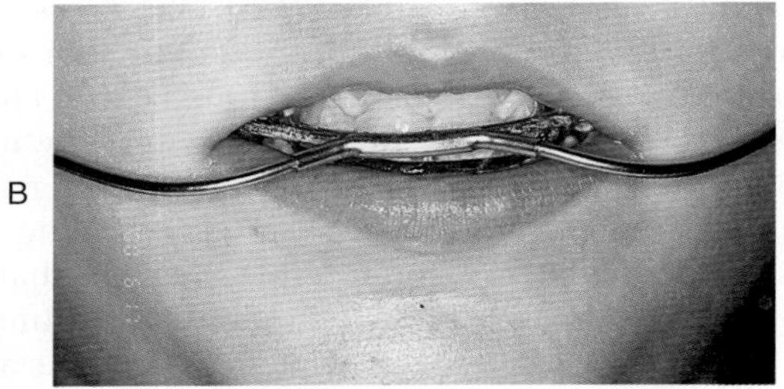

FIGURE 51–17 ✦ **A,** Headgear appliance. **B,** Anterior view of headgear appliance.

Advantages and Disadvantages of Removable Orthodontic Appliances

Advantages

They can be removed for social functions.

Less chair time is needed to make removable appliances because they are fabricated in a lab rather than directly in the client's mouth.

More modification of skeletal growth is possible with removable appliances than with fixed appliances.

Disadvantages

Treatment response is heavily dependent on client compliance because treatment is progressing only when the client wears the appliance.

Removable appliances can be accidentally thrown away or lost, causing a setback in treatment as well as additional financial costs for the client.

Complex tooth movement cannot be completed with a removable appliance and as such, the use of a removable appliance in complex cases may require a compromise in treatment result.

modify its growth. It is possible to enhance mandibular growth if the mandible is protruded forward and held in that position for a considerable amount of time. This can be done with tolerable levels of force using passive or active therapy. In passive therapy, an *orthodontic appliance* is used to protrude the mandible and no response is required of the client. In active therapy, the client responds to an appliance by using his or her muscles (particularly the lateral pterygoid) to protrude the mandible. As the mandible is protruded, growth at the mandibular condyle and the surface of the glenoid fossa of the TMJ is enhanced.

ORTHODONTIC APPLIANCES

Orthodontic appliances can be categorized as removable or fixed.

Removable Appliances

Removable appliances are those that can be removed by the client and typically consist of various wires attached to an acrylic base that is supported by the teeth or soft tissues. See Advantages and Disadvantages of Removable Orthodontic Appliances.

Removable appliances are indicated for three uses, including growth modification during the mixed dentition, limited movement of individual teeth, and retention following the completion of treatment. Removable appliances used in growth modification are referred to as functional appliances. A *functional appliance* is one that changes the posture of the mandible to a position that is open or both open and forward. These appliances modify growth of the mandible by stretching the soft tissues surrounding the mandible. One example is the twin-block appliance shown in Figure 51–18.

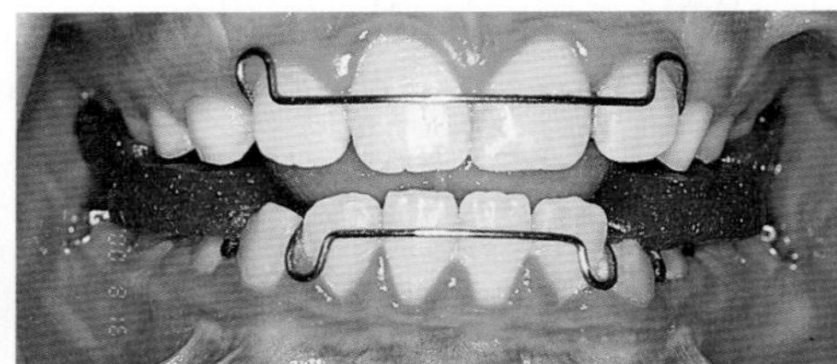

FIGURE 51–18 ✦ Twin-block appliance.

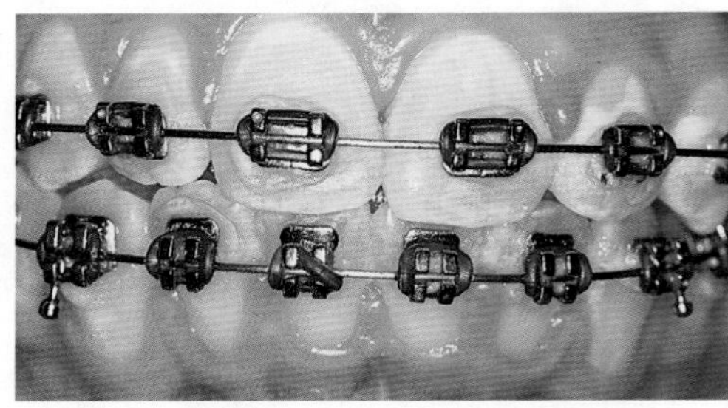

FIGURE 51–19 ✦ Fixed orthodontic appliance. Note white spot lesions on teeth numbers 8 and 10.

Fixed Orthodontic Appliances

In most cases, fixed appliances are required. In contrast to a removable appliance, fixed orthodontic appliances consist of brackets and other attachments that are fixed to the teeth with bonding or attached to bands that are cemented to teeth (Figure 51–19). Components of fixed appliances are described in Table 51–3.

SEPARATION. Teeth having tight interproximal contacts must be separated before the placement of a band, and various types of separators are available to wedge the teeth apart. Separators may consist of a brass wire that is twisted

TABLE 51–3 COMPONENTS OF FIXED ORTHODONTIC APPLIANCES

Component	Advantages	Disadvantages
***Bracket*: A fixture that contains a slot through which the archwire is placed and retained. Welded onto a band or cemented to each individual tooth**		
Metal	Relatively inexpensive Strong	Limited aesthetics Susceptible to corrosion
Plastic	More aesthetic than metal	Prone to distortion, breakage, and discoloration Can be used only on teeth where minimal force is applied and when treatment is of short duration
Ceramic	Most aesthetic bracket type Strong Resistant to discoloration	Brittle, prone to breakage if heavy force applied Rougher and more plaque retentive than metal brackets Will abrade opposing teeth that contact the bracket Difficult to debond
***Stainless Steel Band*: A thin metal appliance that is cemented around the entire crown of a tooth. Used on teeth to which heavy forces will be applied or when both a labial and lingual bracket will be required. Bands are typically applied to the molar teeth. A tube through which the archwire is placed is located on the buccal surface of the band.**		
	Can be placed subgingivally on teeth that are partially erupted. Can be applied to enamel surfaces that are resistant to bonding. Strong	Can contribute to subgingival plaque biofilm retention. Poor aesthetics

Auxiliary Attachments	Purpose
Headgear tube	A tube placed occlusal to the archwire tube on a maxillary molar band to retain an extraoral headgear device
Auxiliary tube	A tube placed gingival to the archwire tube on both maxillary and mandibular molar bands to retain wires (in addition to the main archwire) used to apply forces to segments of teeth
Labial hooks	To apply elastics within an arch or between arches
Lingual cleats/buttons	To apply cross elastics extending from the lingual surface of a tooth in one arch to the buccal surface of the opposing tooth to correct a localized crossbite. Also used to control rotation of premolar teeth during space closure

Advantages and Disadvantages of Bonded versus Banded Brackets

Advantages

Bonding is more aesthetic.
Bonding is simpler and faster.
Bonding procedures are less uncomfortable for the client.
Bonding allows more precise bracket placement.
Bonded brackets are less plaque retentive than banded brackets.
The removal of bonded brackets is not necessary to complete procedures to reduce the mesial and distal tooth surfaces to create more room for tooth alignment.
Interproximal caries are accessible for restoration while brackets are in place.
Spaces between the teeth that require closure are not remaining at the completion of treatment if bands are not used.

Disadvantages

Bonded brackets have a weaker attachment to the tooth than banded brackets and are more likely to fall off during treatment.
Bonded brackets complicate plaque removal, especially if the bonding agent extends beyond the bracket margins.
Bonding brackets become more complicated than using a banded bracket if a lingual bracket or headgear tube is needed.
Rebonding a loose bracket requires more preparations than recementing a loose band.
Debonding is more time-consuming because removal of adhesive is more difficult than removal of cement.

tightly around the contact, steel springs to squeeze the contact open, or elastomeric "doughnuts" that are slipped into place around the contact. Because elastomers are radiolucent and cannot be detected by a radiograph if displaced into the sulcus, they are usually made of brightly colored material so they can be found clinically.

BONDED ATTACHMENTS. Bonding is an area in orthodontics that is continually changing and improving. See Advantages and Disadvantages of Bonded versus Banded Brackets.

Bonding is based on the mechanical locking of an adhesive to irregularities in both the tooth surface and

TABLE 51–4 BONDED ATTACHMENTS

Components	Bonding Process
Enamel surface preparation	Pumice to remove plaque biofilm and pellicle. Etch for 20 to 30 seconds using 35% to 50% phosphoric acid gel. Rinse, dry, and evaluate surface for frosty white appearance. Avoid saliva contamination.
Bracket surface	Metal brackets manufactured with fine mesh welded to bracket base. Ceramic brackets may bond chemically or mechanically if undercuts are incorporated into base of bracket by the addition of tiny balls of ceramic material.
Adhesive materials	Bis-GME are preferred bonding materials: vary in amount and type of filler particles and method of cure (light, chemical, or dual cure). Removal of excess material is critical to maximize aesthetics and minimize plaque retention and associated gingival inflammation and enamel decalcification.
Techniques	Direct bonding: Brackets are individually placed on each tooth. Indirect bonding: Brackets are placed on a model of the dentition and a custom tray is prepared and used to seal all brackets onto the client's teeth at one time.

the base of the bracket. Successful bonding requires attention to tooth surface preparation, bracket base design, and bonding material used. Additional information on bonding is presented in Table 51–4.

ORTHODONTICS IN THE PREADOLESCENT CHILD

Early orthodontic treatment initiated in the mixed dentition or even in the primary dentition can be very beneficial to improve the orthodontic situation. A second stage of treatment, however, will likely be needed after the permanent teeth have erupted.

Malaligned teeth in the early mixed dentition may be caused by one of two basic problems:

1. A lack of adequate space in the arch will cause an erupting tooth to be deflected from its normal position (Figure 51–20).
2. An interference with or delay in the eruption of a permanent tooth will lead to space problems because the existing adjacent teeth will shift into improper positions.

The dental hygienist can play a valuable role in the treatment of the preadolescent child by recognizing signs indicating the need for early orthodontic treatment. The following are oral conditions that should alert the dental hygienist to a potential problem.

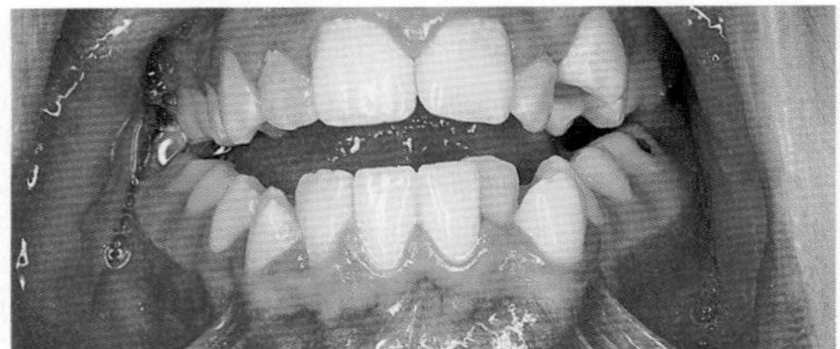

FIGURE 51–20 ✦ Malalignment of permanent canines caused by lack of space in the dental arch.

Altered Sequence of Eruption

Knowledge of eruption patterns considered "normal" will enable the dental hygienist to recognize any abnormalities that may predispose a child to orthodontic problems. Early detection by the dental hygienist and referral to the orthodontist may prevent the later development of a more complex *malalignment.* The following lists several variations in eruption sequence of the permanent dentition that are signs for the need for early orthodontic treatment:

- ✦ Mandibular second molars erupt before the mandibular second premolars, reducing the space available for the second premolars.
- ✦ Maxillary canines erupt at about the same time as the maxillary premolars, causing the canine to be displaced labially.
- ✦ Eruption of a permanent tooth on one side without eruption of the same tooth on the other side within a 6-month time frame, indicating the need to take a radiograph of the unerupted tooth to determine if some physical obstruction is present.

Overretention of Primary Teeth

Overretention of primary teeth requires orthodontic consideration (Figure 51–21). A permanent tooth should erupt when three-fourths of its root is completed. If the primary tooth still has significant root structure remaining at this time, it should be extracted. This problem typically occurs when the permanent tooth bud develops in a position that is too far lingual to the primary tooth.

Early Loss of Primary Teeth

The premature loss of a primary tooth because of factors such as severe caries or trauma will create an alignment problem because permanent or primary teeth that are present will drift into the space of the missing tooth.

Loss of a tooth is considered premature if it occurs 6 months before the permanent tooth is expected to erupt. If a primary second molar is lost prematurely and the first permanent molar tips mesially, it is possible that the permanent first molar will close all space available for the permanent second premolar. To prevent the loss of space caused by the drifting of adjacent teeth, an appliance to maintain the space of the missing tooth is used (Figure 51–22).

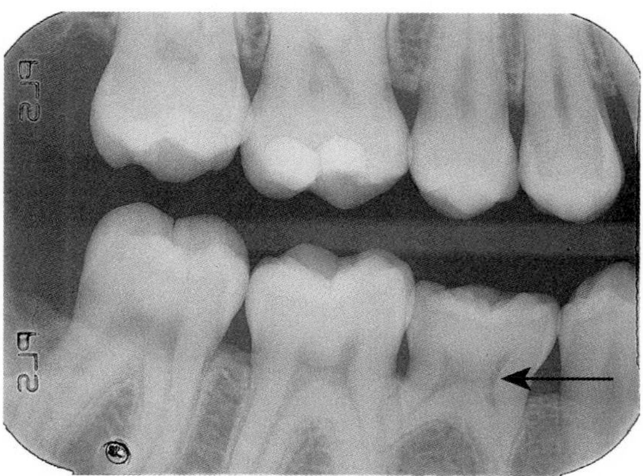

FIGURE 51–21 ✦ Retained primary second molar.

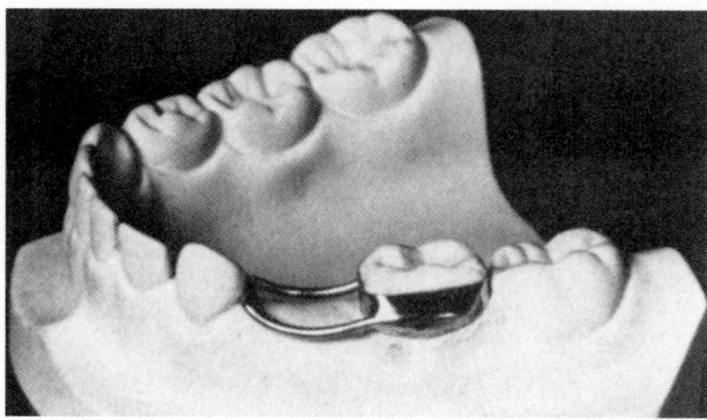

FIGURE 51–22 ✦ Band and loop space maintainer is presented in this figure, with the band placed on the second primary molar and the loop extended to maintain the space of the missing primary first molar. *(From Proffit WR, Fields HW Jr:* Contemporary orthodontics, *ed 2, St Louis, 1993, Mosby.)*

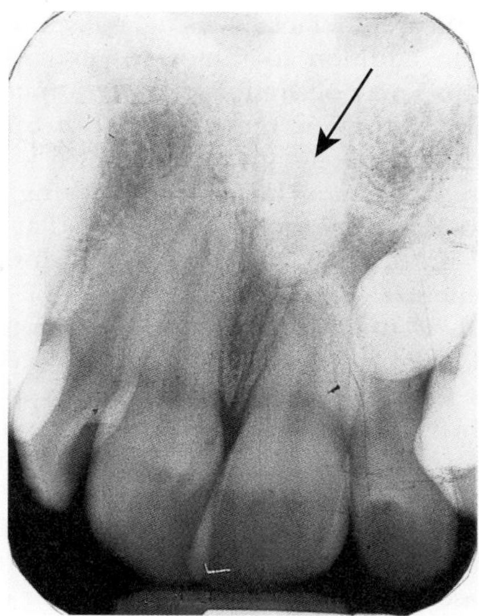

FIGURE 51–23 ✦ Supernumerary tooth (mesiodens) and impacted canine.

Early loss of a primary tooth, however, will cause a delay in the eruption of the permanent tooth because a layer of dense bone and tissue forms over the developing tooth. The permanent tooth should be given the chance to erupt on its own and may not do so until after the root is completely formed. Forced eruption by placing an attachment on the permanent tooth may be required if the tooth fails to eventually erupt on its own.

Supernumerary Teeth

Supernumerary teeth are most frequently found in the maxillary anterior area (Figure 51–23). To minimize the displacement of other teeth within the arch, the extraction of a supernumerary tooth should be completed as soon as it can be done without harming the developing permanent tooth. Early detection of the presence of supernumerary teeth by the dental hygienist is very important.

Congenitally Missing Teeth

An additional problem seen in the permanent dentition is that of congenitally missing teeth. The teeth most likely to be congenitally missing are the mandibular second premolars and the maxillary lateral incisors. Whether unilateral or bilateral, a congenitally missing tooth will cause the dental arch to develop asymmetrically, even if the primary tooth remains. Missing permanent teeth can be managed by orthodontic closure of the space, replacement of the tooth (teeth) with a crown and bridge or a Maryland bridge, or placement of an intraosseous implant.

Crowding of Mandibular Incisors

A slight deficiency of space in the arch for the eruption of permanent mandibular incisors will result in mild crowding and malalignment of these teeth. A phase of slight mandibular incisor crowding is considered normal, however, until a child approaches the age of 10. Space then becomes available to eliminate this crowding after the mandibular canines erupt as a result of the following: The distance between the canines will increase slightly because the incisors erupt not only incisally but also facially. As the mandibular incisors erupt, the mandibular canines move distally into the primate spaces, creating more room for the alignment of the incisors. If crowding of the permanent mandibular incisors is severe, these processes will not create enough space to relieve the crowding. The most common form of malocclusion, in fact, is an Angle's Class I malocclusion with crowding of the incisors.

Severe Crowding

Clients with severe crowding in the mixed dentition may experience early loss of the primary canines. The severe crowding and malalignment of the anteriors cause the roots of the primary canines to be resorbed by the eruption of the permanent lateral incisors. These cases are treated with expansion of the dental arches or by serial extraction therapy.

Three basic methods for the expansion of the dental arches exist: orthodontic expansion, passive expansion, and orthopedic expansion. The goal of *orthodontic expansion* is to increase the length of the arch by tipping the crowns of the teeth facially using conventional fixed appliances in addition to removable expansion appliances. Relapse may occur following treatment because forces applied by cheek musculature can tip the teeth back to their original, lingual positions.

Passive expansion is achieved by removing the forces of the labial and buccal musculature so that the forces applied by the tongue can produce expansion of the arch. A beneficial aspect of this process is that tooth movement is accompanied by bone deposition along the buccal and labial aspects of the alveolar process. The lip bumper as well as a removable Frankel appliance are used to achieve passive arch expansion. The lip bumper consists of a stiff wire connected to mandibular molar bands in such a way that it lies away from the facial surfaces of the teeth, keeping the forces of the lips and cheeks away from the teeth. The length of the arch is then increased by passive lateral and anterior expansion.

Orthopedic expansion is achieved by applying forces so that the underlying skeletal structures are changed, rather than by the movement or tipping of teeth within stationary alveolar bone. The goal of orthopedic expansion in the mixed dentition is to reduce the need for extraction of permanent teeth by establishing adequate arch length and an optimal skeletal relationship between the maxilla and mandible. Two types of maxillary palatal expansion procedures are used: rapid palatal expansion and slow palatal expansion.

The initial theory behind rapid palatal expansion was that unwanted tooth movement could be prevented if the palatal suture could be opened quickly enough. The force to expand the palate is delivered through a jackscrew mechanism within an appliance that is cemented to the posterior teeth. The jackscrew is activated at 0.5 to 1 mm per day, and as the suture opens, a diastema appears between the maxillary central incisors. A centimeter or more of expansion is created in 2 to 3 weeks, primarily as a result of separation of the palatal halves of the maxilla. Various types of appliances are used (Figure 51–24).

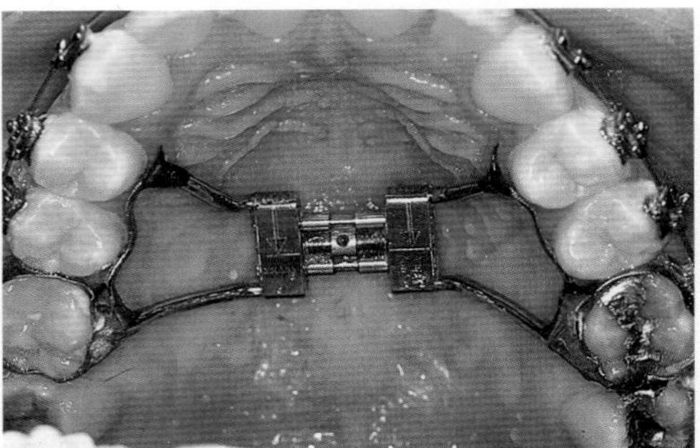

FIGURE 51–24 ✦ Palatal expansion device.

In the slow palatal expansion technique, less force is applied by the device so that expansion is completed over a 10-week period. The end result is the same as that completed using rapid palatal expansion. Regardless of the method applied, the expansion device must remain fixed in place for 3 to 4 months after expansion is complete. After the fixed device is removed, a removable retainer is worn.

For children with severely crowded teeth, it may be decided during the early mixed dentition that there will not be enough room within the arches for all of the permanent teeth. For clients having a Class I molar relationship, a normal overbite, and normal skeletal relationships, *serial extraction* is a treatment option in which select teeth are extracted at planned points in time to reduce crowding during the transition from the primary to permanent dentitions. A second phase of fixed orthodontic therapy must also follow serial extraction. The second phase of fixed orthodontic therapy, however, can be expected to be less complex than it would have been if the extractions were not completed.

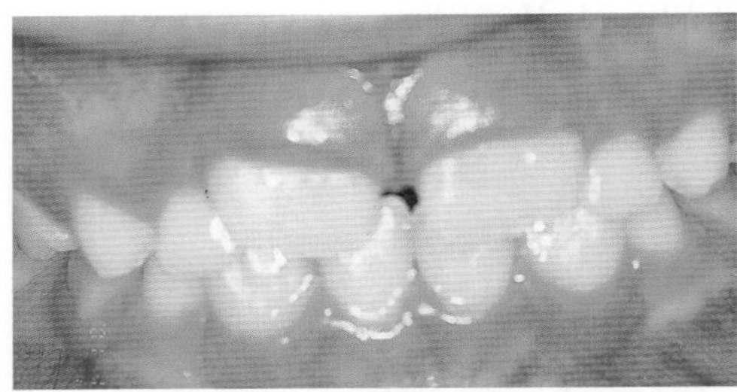

FIGURE 51–25 ✦ Diastema present between erupting permanent maxillary central incisors.

Midline Diastema

In contrast to the crowding of mandibular incisors, spacing typically occurs in the maxillary incisors, seen as a slight diastema between the permanent central incisors. This "ugly duckling" stage occurs because the mesially inclined positions of the unerupted canines displace the roots of the lateral and central incisors mesially, flaring their crowns distally. If the midline diastema is 2 mm or less in size, it is likely to close as the maxillary lateral incisors and canines erupt (Figure 51–25).

Most children presenting with a maxillary midline diastema at age 9 will have complete closure of the diastema by the age of 16 without any orthodontic intervention. If, however, the size of the diastema is initially greater than 2 mm, total closure may not occur. A diastema greater than 2 to 3 mm in size may be caused by a midline supernumerary tooth, a midline soft tissue or intrabony lesion, missing lateral incisors, or a tooth size discrepancy such as peg lateral incisors.

Malposed and Lingual Eruption of the Permanent Anterior Teeth

The permanent maxillary and mandibular incisor tooth buds develop lingual to the existing primary teeth. As a result, the permanent mandibular incisors may erupt malposed and lingual to the primary incisors even in children having normal spacing (Figure 51–26). The permanent maxillary lateral incisor is also particularly prone to eruption lingual to its ideal position in the arch. If an anterior

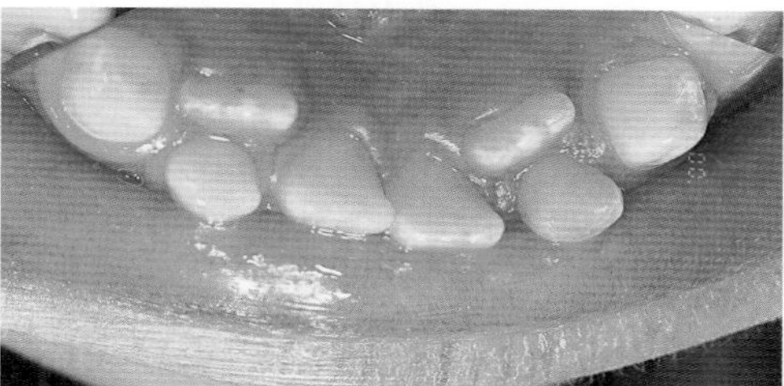

FIGURE 51–26 ✦ Lingual eruption of the mandibular incisors.

crossbite of the maxillary lateral incisor occurs, a removable appliance with a spring to place labial pressure against the lateral may be used to treat the problem simply. The maxillary lateral incisors, however, may become trapped in a lingual position upon eruption, especially if anterior crowding is present. Extraction of the primary canines may be needed to allow labial positioning of the lateral incisors with an orthodontic appliance.

Impacted Canines

The maxillary canine is the most likely tooth to become impacted within the bone (Figure 51–27). An impacted canine can be surgically exposed, bracketed, and brought into occlusion orthodontically after space in the arch has been created. A decision to complete this process is made after considering the severity of the displacement of the tooth and the amount of trauma required by the surgical exposure procedure. If too complex, it may be more cost effective to extract the impacted tooth and close the space it would have required in the arch or maintain the space for the tooth and replace it prosthetically. The age of the client must also be considered in the treatment decision. The older the client, the more likely the tooth will be ankylosed (fused to the bone), making orthodontic movement impossible.

Lack of Leeway Space for Eruption of the Permanent Premolars

Exactly opposite to the situation in the permanent anteriors, the permanent premolar teeth are smaller than the primary molars they replace. This additional space, called the *leeway space,* is on average 5 mm in size in the mandibular arch and 3 mm in size in the maxillary arch. When the primary second molars are lost, the first permanent molars will rapidly shift mesially into this leeway space, contributing to an ideal Class I occlusion in the permanent dentition. If a problem of crowding of the permanent dentition is apparent in the child at this time (at approximately 11 years of age), the orthodontist may choose to prevent the mesial drifting of the permanent molars by maintaining the leeway space with the use of a space maintainer.

Protruding Maxillary Incisors

Treatment of protruding maxillary incisors is indicated only when the protruding incisors have spaces between them and are aesthetically objectionable or in danger of traumatic injury because of their degree of protrusion.

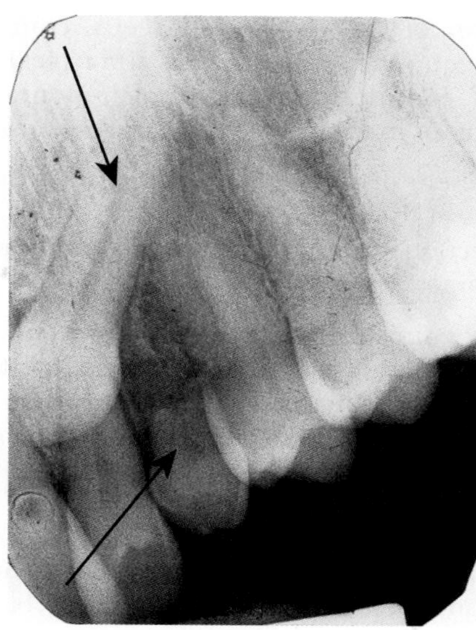

FIGURE 51–27 ✦ Impacted permanent canine and resorption of deciduous canine root.

This situation, in addition to an open bite, often occurs as a result of prolonged thumb-sucking. Thumb-sucking is considered prolonged if it is practiced for more than 6 hours per day and into the mixed dentition. The following lists the types of malocclusion caused by prolonged thumb-sucking:

- Anterior open bite (interferes with the normal eruption of the incisors and allows the excessive eruption of the posterior teeth)
- Constricted maxillary arch (the maxilla develops into a V shape rather than a U shape)
- Posterior crossbite

When seeing a child who has a thumb-sucking habit, it is important for the dental hygienist to discuss the problems that will result from continuing the habit. Some children will respond to advice from a dental professional rather than a parent. In the case in which the child unconsciously sucks the thumb or finger during sleep or while reading or watching television, a glove can be worn or a bandage applied to the thumb to discourage the habit. For a child who wants to stop the thumb-sucking habit but is unable to do so, a wire crib appliance can be cemented onto the maxillary arch to prevent the placement of the thumb onto the palate. It must be explained to the child that the purpose of this appliance is not punishment, but that it has been placed to help him or her in breaking the thumb-sucking habit. Once the habit is broken, the appliance should remain in place an additional 3 months to ensure that the habit has truly been broken.

COMPREHENSIVE TREATMENT

A main goal of comprehensive orthodontic treatment is to make the occlusion as ideal as possible through repositioning of the teeth. Completed during adolescence after the eruption of the permanent teeth, comprehensive treatment requires fixed appliances and typically includes what most consider traditional orthodontic therapy. There are three major stages of *comprehensive treatment:*

1. Alignment of the teeth and leveling of the occlusal planes of the arches
2. Correction of molar relationship and space closure
3. Finishing

During the finishing stage of treatment, the axial inclination of the teeth is finalized. Particular attention is given to making sure the roots of teeth adjacent to extraction sites are parallel and that the vertical relationship of the anterior teeth is correct.

Final Settling of Teeth

At the completion of the correction of Class II or Class III malocclusion, some rebound of the teeth back toward their initial positions can be expected. Because of this reaction, the malocclusions may be slightly overcorrected during treatment. For example, when a Class II malocclusion with a deep overbite is treated, the teeth may be overcorrected to an end-to-end incisor relationship before forces are removed. Because the teeth will rebound after the orthodontic forces are removed, the incisors should shift into an ideal relationship where the maxillary incisors overlap the mandibular incisors to a slight degree. A period of 4 to 8 weeks should be allowed for this rebound to occur before the fixed bands and brackets are removed. If necessary, further adjustments in tooth position can then be made by reapplying orthodontic forces without having to reapply bands and brackets.

Rebound is also an issue in palatal expansion procedures. The maxilla is overexpanded so that the lingual cusps of the maxillary teeth contact the buccal cusps of the mandibular teeth because the arch is expected to rebound to some degree. The overexpansion of the arch enables the teeth to come into an ideal transverse occlusion as the expected rebound occurs.

Part of the finishing stage of orthodontics is the settling of the teeth into a solid occlusion before the client is placed into retention. Settling of the teeth is accomplished by applying lighter forces to the teeth for a few weeks to allow the teeth to shift into final occlusion. Lighter forces can be applied by replacing the rectangular finishing archwire with a light round archwire that provides some freedom of movement of the teeth or by connecting the maxillary and mandibular posteriors with vertical elastics attached to the brackets after the posterior segment of the finishing archwire is removed. In addition, the bands and brackets can be removed and a tooth positioner appliance fabricated.

A tooth positioner is a clear plastic or hard rubber appliance that covers the teeth and gingiva. The inherent elasticity of the plastic or rubber allows settling of the teeth into their final occlusion. A tooth positioner is delivered to the client immediately after the fixed appliances are removed. It should be worn full time during the first two days because the most tooth movement occurs during this time. Thereafter, the positioner is worn during the night, in addition to a four-hour period during the day. The full effects of the positioner are achieved in 3 weeks. After that, the positioner no longer provides a finishing function. Use of the positioner as a long-term retainer is not recommended.

It is important for the dental hygienist to understand these final procedures of orthodontic treatment because it is common for the client to be anxious to have the appliances removed at this point. As far as the client is concerned, the teeth look as though they are fully corrected and that treatment is finished. This is especially an issue for adolescent clients, who will often express to the dental hygienist when seen at the maintenance appointment a strong desire to have the appliances removed. The dental hygienist can be of great service to the client by helping him or her understand the importance of this finishing phase to the development of a solid occlusion that will have long-term stability.

Decalcification

The development of "white spot" lesions on the teeth is a significant problem for the client in orthodontic therapy. Occurring under and adjacent to orthodontic bands and brackets, the white spot lesion is early caries (Figure 51–19). If the lesion is visible only when the tooth is dried, it likely involves the enamel only. If the white spot lesion is visible without drying, demineralization has progressed deeper within the enamel while a relatively intact outer enamel surface remains. A sharp explorer should not be used to probe the intact surface of a white spot lesion because the intact outer surface may be broken by the explorer, requiring restoration of the lesion. If the lesion continues to progress, the outer surface will break down, forming an open carious lesion.

The dental hygienist helps orthodontic clients understand their responsibility in preventing enamel decalcification by completing optimal home care, including daily rinsing with a 0.05% sodium fluoride mouthrinse and daily use of a fluoride dentifrice. This routine procedure is a standard recommendation for all orthodontic clients in active treatment.

The white spot lesion, however, is reversible after appliances are removed. The regimen recommended is based on the premise that areas of softened enamel surface remineralize faster than subsurface areas. Because the entire process of remineralization occurs from the surface only, use of fluoride rinses immediately upon debonding would remineralize the enamel surface lesion, but in doing so, would block access to remineralization by the subsurface lesion and prevent complete repair. Therefore, it is recommended that topical fluoride supplementation be delayed until 2 to 3 months after debonding to allow remineralization of areas of the subsurface lesion to occur naturally.

During this period, however, good oral hygiene is essential to increase the rate of natural remineralization. After this initial period, fluoride is recommended to treat the surface of the lesion because fluoride ions greatly enhance the degree of remineralization. With remineralization, the lesion should reduce in size and develop a shiny surface similar to that of healthy enamel. The application of fluoride using custom trays is the most effective method for reducing white spots.

Retention

Retention of the teeth following orthodontic treatment is necessary for the following reasons: (1) the gingival and periodontal tissues need time to reorganize after the appliances are removed; (2) soft tissue pressures from the tongue, lips, and cheeks may contribute to relapse if the musculature has not had time to adapt to the new occlusion and if tooth position is unstable; and (3) skeletal growth will continue to affect the occlusion as it did before treatment.

Time for reorganization of gingival and periodontal tissues is necessary because orthodontic tooth movement causes widening of the PDL and disruption of the supporting collagen fibers. This is evident clinically by the mobility of the teeth present when appliances are removed. The teeth are not only mobile at the completion of treatment, but also susceptible to displacement as a result of forces applied by the surrounding soft tissues and occlusion. Reorganization of the periodontium takes 3 to 4 months and can occur only when each tooth is able to respond individually to the forces of mastication. Although retainers should be worn full time for the first 3 to 4 months following treatment, they should be removed during eating. The natural flexion of the individual teeth during eating will encourage remodeling of the periodontal tissues and a reduction in tooth mobility. If a fixed retainer is placed, it should not be so rigid that the natural flexion of teeth within the alveolar process cannot occur.

Retention following correction of severe malalignments should be continued for at least 12 months because of the slow remodeling of the gingival fibers. After 3 to 4 months, however, removable retainers are not required on a full-time basis. Permanent retention may be required for teeth that are not able to tolerate the forces of the lips, cheeks, and tongue. For those clients who are still growing, retention should be maintained until growth has stopped. The dental hygienist must encourage clients to strictly follow their orthodontist's recommendations for the use of retainers. If any indication of relapse is noted, the client must be referred to the orthodontist.

REMOVABLE RETAINER APPLIANCES. The most common type of retainer is the Hawley appliance, which is worn on the maxillary arch. This appliance consists of an acrylic palatal component with clasps on the molar teeth and a labial bow with adjustment loops at the canines (Figure 51–28). The labial bow can function to retain the position of the maxillary anteriors or it can be adjusted to close spaces between anterior teeth that were banded.

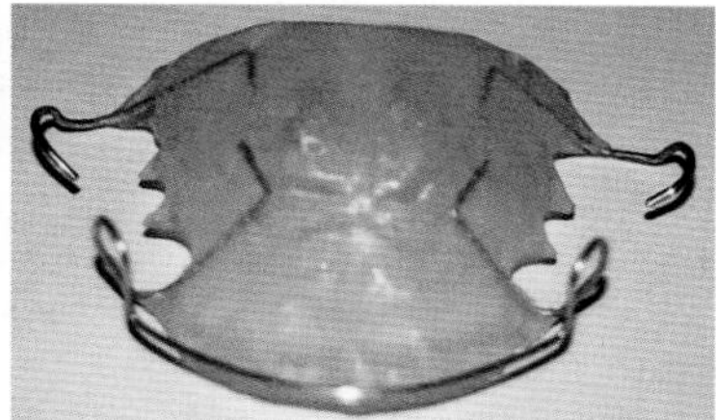

FIGURE 51–28 ✦ The Hawley appliance is commonly used as a removable retainer on the maxillary arch.

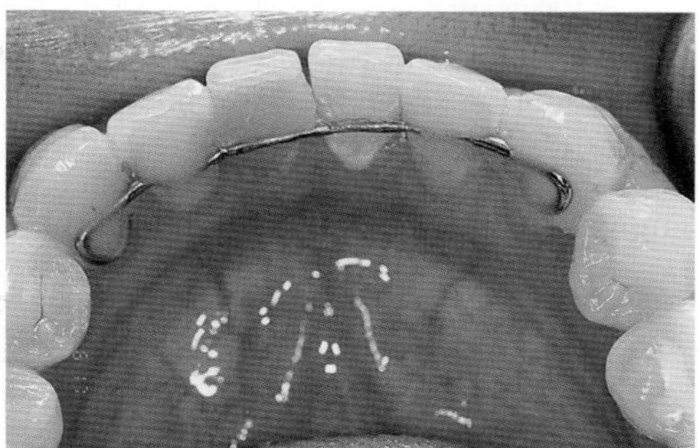

FIGURE 51–29 ✦ Bonded canine-to-canine (3–3) lingual retainer bonded to all incisors.

FIXED RETAINERS. Fixed retainers are bonded to the teeth and are used for long-term control of orthodontic alignment. Specifically, these retainers are used for retaining alignment of the mandibular incisors during the late growth that occurs between the ages of 16 and 20, for maintaining the closure of a diastema, and for maintaining pontic space before crown and bridge restoration to replace a missing posterior tooth or teeth.

Also referred to as 3–3 retainers, bonded lingual canine-to-canine retainers are used most frequently in the mandibular anteriors to prevent relapse of crowding and malalignment of the incisors (Figure 51–29). Typically, a round stainless steel wire extending across the anteriors from the right to the left canine is bonded to the lingual surfaces of the canine teeth with restorative composite material. The dental hygienist, when seeing a client having a bonded retainer for maintenance appointments, checks the appliance for breakdown of the bonding material. Bond failure can be detected by gently rocking each tooth with the blunt end of the handles of two instruments and by observing the teeth for mobility when pressure is applied during scaling. The dental hygienist also ensures that the client understands how to clean around the appliance (see section on interdental cleaners).

PERIODONTAL ASPECTS OF ADULT ORTHODONTIC TREATMENT

Treatment of the adult with a history of periodontal disease must be planned carefully and include the opinions of all dentists involved in the treatment of the client (e.g., orthodontist, periodontist, prosthodontist, and endodontist). The primary form of periodontal treatment completed before orthodontics is that which is completed by the dental hygienist: periodontal scaling and root planing. Dental hygiene care is considered complete only when the inflammatory conditions are controlled well enough for the client to safely begin orthodontic tooth movement.

The control of plaque biofilm, described later in this chapter, is key to managing the adult with periodontal disease. A client's ability to remove plaque is complicated by the presence of orthodontic bands and brackets. The most difficult areas for the adult client to keep clean are the tooth surfaces between and subgingival to the brackets. In contrast to the child or adolescent, the surfaces subgingival to the brackets in the adult are more accessible because adults have longer clinical crowns.

Because orthodontic bands retain more plaque biofilm at the gingival margins, it is often preferable to use bonded brackets on the molars of adult clients with periodontal disease. Steel ligatures, rather than elastomers, may be used to tie the archwires into place because it has been shown that clients with elastomers have a higher level of microorganisms in the gingival plaque.

The width and thickness of the attached gingiva must be assessed carefully in the adult client. When the arch is expanded by labial movement of the teeth to relieve crowding problems, the risk of gingival recession is increased. Labial movement of the teeth may result in development of a dehiscence in the bone. The labial gingiva becomes thin and recession begins. Recession can progress rapidly if the labial keratinized gingiva is thin or nonexistent. It is preferable to prevent gingival recession than to correct it after it has occurred. A gingival graft procedure should be considered for many adult clients, especially those presenting with keratinized gingiva that is thin in width and thickness and who will be undergoing arch expansion to align the incisors.

Clients with periodontal disease must be seen for professional supportive periodontal maintenance every 2 to 3 months. If severe periodontal disease is present, professional maintenance every 4 weeks may be required.

DENTAL HYGIENE MAINTENANCE OF THE ORTHODONTIC CLIENT

The dental hygienist plays a critical role in maintaining the dentition during and after treatment. In addition to providing professional mechanical dental hygiene care to promote the client's periodontal health, the dental hygienist provides ongoing instruction and feedback with regard to personal oral self-care. It is often beneficial to have written directions regarding various aspects of dental hygiene care recommendations. These directions, given to clients as they leave the dental office, will enable them to better understand and remember specific directions given to them. Parents should always be included when informing youth of the risks and necessary preventive home measures, but it is important that young clients are in agreement with recommended programs. The dental hygienist must work with the individual to design a regimen that is feasible and effective.

Plaque Control

Plaque biofilm removal for the orthodontic client presents a special challenge. The key is to find approaches that the client is able to use effectively and incorporate into his or her lifestyle. It is important not to overload the client, however, with too many adjuncts. See Oral Hygiene Recommendations for Clients with Fixed Appliances.

TOOTHBRUSHING. Toothbrushes of various designs are now available. Styles include the two-row sulcular brush that can be placed gingival and coronal to the brackets, brushes having middle rows of bristles that are shorter to facilitate their use over brackets, end-tufted brushes to remove plaque biofilm around brackets, and brushes having bristles of various lengths. Clients' plaque removal efforts should be directed to the gingival margin using the modified Bass technique and to the cervical and incisal or occlusal aspects of the brackets (Figure 51–30, *A* and *B*). Powered toothbrushes may help the client in plaque biofilm removal, especially ones having timers incorporated to ensure that the client uses the brush for a long enough period.

INTERDENTAL CLEANING. Interproximal plaque removal presents a particular challenge for the client. Various aids for plaque removal, detailed in Chapter 19,

Oral Hygiene Recommendations for Clients with Fixed Appliances

Brush three times a day with fluoride dentifrice (0.22% sodium fluoride).
Aim toothbrush bristles at the gingival margin to stimulate and debride the gingival margin area.
Brush around brackets, placing the bristles above and aiming them down toward the brackets, and then placing the bristles below and aiming them up toward the brackets.
Consider using specialized orthodontic brushes.
Consider using electric toothbrushes.
Use floss threader or super floss to clean subgingivally on proximal surfaces.
Use proxibrush or stimudent to get under the archwire and between teeth if the space is wide enough.
Use the oral irrigator on low power at least once a day. Aim it perpendicular to contact just above the papilla.
Use disclosing tablets to check for plaque removal.
Rinse with 0.05% sodium fluoride rinse for 1 minute after brushing or "rinse, spit, go to bed."
Use chlorhexidine 0.1% to 0.2% as a 1-minute rinse twice daily for short periods (i.e., a few weeks); however, there should be at least 60 minutes between this and fluoride treatment for effective use of each.

include interproximal brushes, rubber-tip stimulators, toothpicks, stimudents, and floss and floss threaders (Figure 51–31, *A* to *D*).

For clients with fixed appliances, floss threaders must be used to place the floss interproximally. For young clients, teaching the parent to floss around the appliances is an option that should be considered.

For clients with fixed retainers, floss threaders also must be used to place floss interproximally. If the retainer is bonded to the canines only, the floss threader needs to be used only once, and floss can be pulled under the wire to floss each contact area without rethreading it each time. If the client presents with large cervical embrasures because of a history of periodontal disease, interproximal brushes may be more effective in plaque biofilm removal. Stimudents are also an alternative aid for interproximal plaque removal.

When orthodontic treatment is planned so that a crown and bridge can be fabricated, it is often necessary to place a fixed retainer between abutments to maintain the pontic space. The same aids used in plaque biofilm removal around fixed retainers on the anterior teeth can be used around wires retaining pontic space.

ADDITIONAL ADJUNCTS TO PERSONAL PLAQUE CONTROL. Oral irrigating devices can be effective in removing food debris lodged around fixed appliances as well as loosely adherent layers of plaque biofilm. A low power should be used, and the irrigating stream should be directed perpendicular to the long axis of the tooth, not into the gingival sulcus. Antimicrobial agents may be added to the irrigator reservoir or used as a mouthrinse.

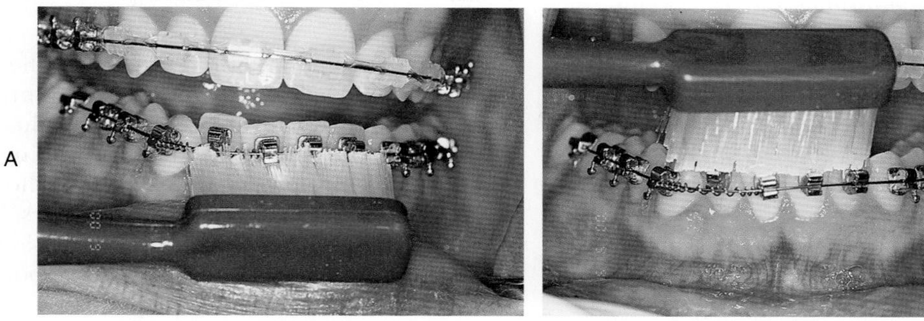

FIGURE 51–30 ✦ **A,** Placement of toothbrush for the removal of plaque from the cervical aspect of brackets. **B,** Placement of toothbrush for the removal of plaque from the incisal aspect of brackets.

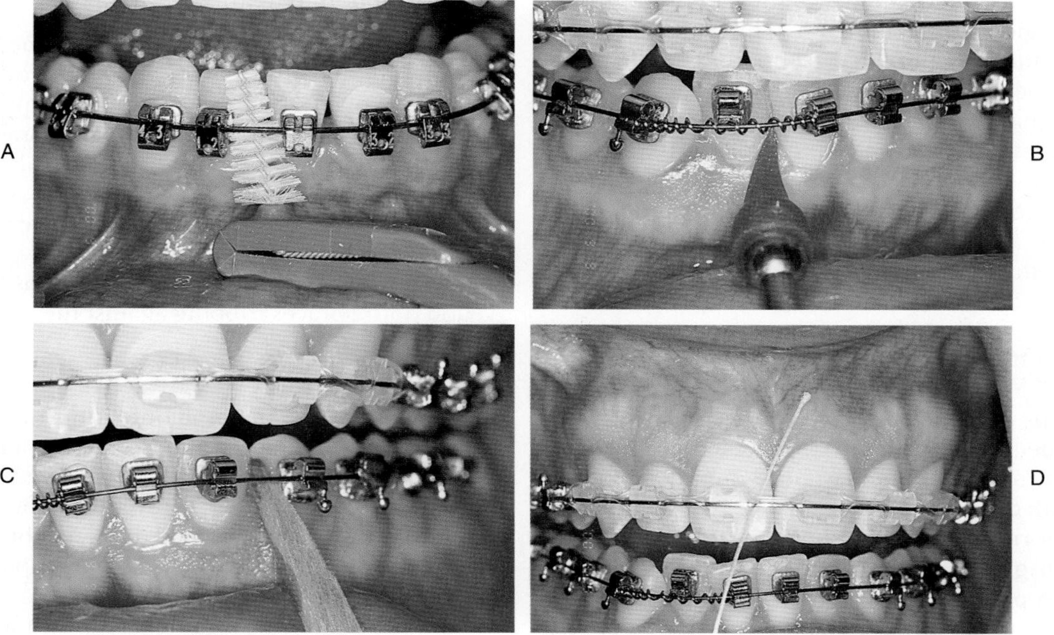

FIGURE 51–31 ✦ **A,** Use of interproximal brush to clean around brackets. **B,** Use of a rubber-tip stimulator to disrupt plaque and to massage the papillae. **C,** Use of a stimudent to remove plaque. **D,** Use of a floss threader to place floss under the archwire.

CHLORHEXIDINE MOUTHRINSE. The use of a prescription rinse containing chlorhexidine also should be considered for the client having difficulty controlling gingival inflammation and/or dental caries. The rinse can be applied locally with an interproximal brush to treat a local area of gingival inflammation and to minimize brown staining that can occur as a side effect.

Fluoride Therapy

Daily fluoride therapy is an important aspect of preventive care for the orthodontic client because the presence of appliances is a risk factor for dental caries. The use of office and home fluoride therapies to prevent enamel demineralization and tooth decay is as important in the adult client as in the child. Adult clients may be even more susceptible to tooth decay than children if they have poorly contoured margins on restorations or root exposure caused by gingival recession or if they are taking a medication that reduces salivary flow or causes gingival enlargement.

In addition to a standard fluoride toothpaste, a fluoride rinse or gel should be used daily at home. Numerous products containing neutral and acidulated fluorides have been recommended as safe and effective in preventing white spot lesions and promoting enamel remineralization in the orthodontic client. The effectiveness of these products, however, relies on client compliance. It may be wise to avoid the use of a stannous fluoride product because of the brown staining this fluoride can produce.

Nutritional Counseling

Because plaque control is more difficult for the client who wears fixed orthodontic appliances, sugar intake should be minimized during the period of active treatment. If eaten, sweets should be eaten as part of a meal to limit the number of acid attacks throughout the day. The dental hygienist informs the client that foods that cannot be cleaned off the fixed orthodontic appliances may lead to periodontal disease, dental caries, white spots, and unattractive food debris accumulation. Moreover, even though orthodontic bands and wires are made of metal or porcelain, they can be fragile and damaged by eating the wrong foods, thus delaying completion of orthodontic treatment. See Foods to Avoid and to Include When Wearing Fixed Orthodontic Appliances.

Frequent Professional Dental Hygiene Maintenance Care

For the client who, despite all efforts, presents with limited plaque control abilities, professional maintenance every 3 to 4 months may be required. Fluoride treatments with 2% sodium fluoride or 1.23% acidulated phosphate fluoride (APF) should be applied at that time. The dental hygiene maintenance of the orthodontic client includes procedures performed during the dental hygiene appointment, such as client assessment, deposit removal, home care recommendations, and communication with other dental offices involved.

Foods to Avoid and to Include When Wearing Fixed Orthodontic Appliances

Foods to Avoid

Chewing gum, sugarless or otherwise
Sticky foods (e.g., peanut butter, sticky candy such as caramels, Sugar Daddies, Tootsie Rolls)
Hard foods (e.g., nuts, corn on the cob, popcorn, hard candy, bagels, apples, whole carrots, hard pretzels, hard chips, jerky)
Ice

Foods to Include

Foods low in sugar
Fresh fruits and vegetables cut in pieces
Applesauce
Yogurt
Pasta
Representatives from all areas of the food pyramid cut in pieces if needed (see Chapter 28)

Client assessment should consist of the same procedures utilized in a client without orthodontic appliances. The hard and soft tissues should be evaluated clinically and supported with periodontal probing and radiographs when indicated. The soft tissues should be examined for trauma from sharp appliances. Trauma can result in areas of abrasion or laceration. Warm saltwater rinses (8-ounce glass of water to a teaspoon of salt) and use of utility wax to cover sharp appliance surfaces can relieve discomfort from the offending wire until it can be remedied. Soft wax should be offered to all orthodontic clients to prevent mucosal injury and control pain. Common oral manifestations observed in clients undergoing orthodontic treatment are:

- Gingival inflammation caused by plaque biofilm accumulation around brackets, inadequate normal massage of gingiva, and/or contact hypersensitivity to the nickel titanium wires and plastic brackets
- Gingival hyperplasia caused by plaque biofilm accumulation
- Decalcification of enamel around brackets (white spots)
- Dental caries around brackets
- Canker sores or other soft tissue lesions from the friction of the braces rubbing against the soft tissue of the mouth
- Root resorption

The removal of plaque biofilm and calculus requires patient and skillful application of instruments and materials used in the maintenance of any client. An air-powder device may be especially effective in removing stains that develop under archwires and between brackets. Cone-shaped prophylaxis cups may also be applied for better access to these areas.

Communication with the orthodontist and any other office involved in treating the client is an essential role of the dental hygienist. Whenever a client is seen, the dental hygienist sends a written note to the involved dentists letting them know that the client was seen for maintenance. Any changes in the health history or dental or periodontal health of the client should be noted. Recommendations for home care should be described and duplicates of any radiographs exposed included. Any additional concerns or questions, as well as the date of the client's next visit with the dental hygienist, should be indicated. In addition, before treating a client who is seeing numerous dentists, the dental hygienist should read any communication from those dentists to be aware of the client's status. Comprehensive, professional communication is appreciated by all involved, including the client.

Oral Hygiene Care for the Surgical Orthodontic Client

While in the hospital, oral hygiene care consists of frequent saline irrigation with a 30-ml syringe and blunt needle, and if available, special brushes that can be placed on the end of a suction unit. Thorough oral debridement is essential in preventing infection of surgical incisions, gingival inflammation, and dental decalcification. See Postsurgical Plaque Control Procedures During Maxillomandibular Fixation.

For the first two weeks following surgery, clients continue to irrigate with saline using the syringe several times daily, especially after eating. The oral and maxillofacial surgeon should be consulted regarding postoperative hygiene, especially regarding the use of mouthrinses and powered irrigators.

For the remainder of the 6 to 8 weeks, the client can be expected to remain in maxillomandibular fixation. A small, soft-bristle brush with a modified sulcular technique in addition to any aids to clean interproximally as best as possible should be used.

Dietary recommendations are especially important in helping the client heal and maintain overall health following surgery. Caloric requirements increase following surgery, a time when the client will have the most difficulty ingesting foods. All foods must be prepared to a thin consistency in a blender. Water, nutritious drinks, and high-caloric nutrition supplementation liquids should be encouraged. Carbonated beverages should be avoided.

Postsurgical Plaque Control Procedures During Maxillomandibular Fixation

First two weeks following surgery

Frequent saline rinsing (especially after eating) should be performed with a 30-ml syringe with a blunt needle.

If available, use special brushes that can be placed on the end of a suction unit to remove plaque biofilm and debris from the labial surfaces of the teeth (lingual surfaces will not be accessible).

Once surgical incisions have healed, a diluted (1:1 ratio) antimicrobial mouthrinse may be applied using a powered irrigator. Irrigator must be set on a low setting and directed perpendicular to the tooth at the gingival margin. Chlorhexidine is a recommended antimicrobial because of its effectiveness and low alcohol content.

The surgeon should be consulted regarding postoperative hygiene procedures.

Two to eight weeks following surgery

Modified sulcular brushing may be started using a small, soft-bristle brush.

Interproximal aids such as stimudents, toothpicks, rubber-tip stimulator, interproximal brushes, and so on may be used.

Fluoride rinses that are low in alcohol content and gels and toothpastes should be used to prevent decalcification.

Dietary recommendations for the ingestion of water, nutritious drinks, and high-caloric supplementation liquids should be provided. Carbonated beverages should be avoided.

Once fixation is removed, clients will also require instruction in physical therapy techniques to restore the function of the lips and the ability to open and close the jaws. The final, postsurgical phase of orthodontic treatment is completed to allow the teeth to settle into better intercuspation. Elastics are used to guide the occlusion. Settling generally takes 2 months to complete. Retention of the surgically treated case is no different than retention for any adult orthodontic case. Definitive periodontal surgery and prosthetic treatment can be completed after the final occlusion is established.

Client Education Issues

- Explain the dental and/or skeletal conditions that warrant orthodontic treatment.
- Recognize changes that are occurring during treatment and the importance of retention after treatment.
- Explain the need for further periodontal and/or prosthodontic procedures.
- Work carefully with clients to develop a plaque control regimen that is feasible and effective; to limit dietary sugars; to use home fluoride rinses, gels, and dentifrices; and to clean removable appliances.
- Reinforce the importance of attending orthodontic appointments as recommended by the orthodontist.

Legal, Ethical, and Safety Issues

- The dental hygienist maintains written communication with the orthodontic office regarding mutual clients. In this communication, the orthodontist is advised of the date of the last maintenance appointment with the dental hygienist, any changes in the health history, any changes in the client's oral health, recommendations provided for plaque control or home fluoride, and any problems with the orthodontic appliances noted (e.g., loose brackets or bands, wires impinging on tissues). Any radiographs taken should also be enclosed.
- Before seating the client, the dental hygienist should read any letters sent by the orthodontist since the last visit. This routine will enable the dental hygienist to become up to date on the progress of treatment as well as follow up on any concerns expressed by the orthodontist.
- The dental hygienist carefully evaluates young clients to identify malocclusions that might benefit from early orthodontic intervention and bring any findings to the attention of the dentist. Failure to note such malocclusions could result in the need for more lengthy orthodontic treatment with less favorable results.
- When seeing a client for maintenance visits after orthodontic therapy has been completed, the dental hygienist continually evaluates the dentition for relapse. If any areas of relapse in the malocclusion are noted, the dentist must be advised and the client referred back to the orthodontist for evaluation.

Key Concepts

- Evaluation of the occlusion should include not only the relationship of the teeth to one another as categorized by Angle's I, II, and III classifications, but also the skeletal relationship of the maxilla and mandible to one another.
- The skeletal development of a child, as well as his or her chronologic age, must be determined in order to take advantage of growth modification procedures. Such procedures are most effective when applied during the preadolescent growth spurt. Growth modification can be used to restrain maxillary growth, enhance mandibular growth, and/or expand the palate to correct transverse discrepancies and create more space within the arch.
- The sequence of eruption of the teeth is more important than the date of eruption. In the primary dentition, spacing is preferred. Primate and developmental spaces provide room for the developing permanent teeth. A lack of space in the primary dentition indicates that the permanent dentition will be crowded.
- Eruption of the permanent teeth occurs as a result of cellular activities within the periodontal ligament. Eruption is a process that continues at various rates throughout life. The primary dentition plays a critical role in the optimal eruption of the permanent teeth.
- The position of the teeth within the dental arches is determined by an equilibrium of forces applied by the tongue, cheeks, and lips while at rest, the elastic gingival fibers, and the periodontal ligament. The duration of the force applied is more important in determining tooth position than the strength of the force.
- Light, sustained orthodontic forces result in optimal tooth movement through a process of frontal resorption. Heavy forces result in some necrosis of the periodontal ligament followed by undermining resorption, a process that will delay tooth movement 7 to 14 days.

KEY CONCEPTS—CONT'D

- ✦ Orthodontic treatment planning is a complex process that must take into consideration a client's chief complaint. It is also based on the clinical judgment and experience of the orthodontist. It may be impossible to achieve all orthodontic goals. The dental hygienist must be aware of this when seeing a client for maintenance after treatment has been completed.
- ✦ Properly applied orthodontic forces will affect the dental pulp, cementum, and dentin to a minimal degree. Apical root resorption occurs in almost all orthodontic cases, but is usually not clinically significant.
- ✦ Orthodontic brackets are made of metal, ceramic, or plastic material and are attached directly to the teeth through bonding or attached to stainless steel bands that are cemented around the teeth.
- ✦ Comprehensive orthodontic treatment consists of three phases: leveling and alignment, correction of molar relationships and space closure, and finishing and settling of the occlusion.
- ✦ Client education is particularly important during orthodontic therapy. The dental hygienist must help the client develop skill in removing plaque biofilm from around the orthodontic appliances as well as in understanding the treatment procedures that are needed to ensure an optimal result.
- ✦ The dental hygienist plays a key role in preparing the client for orthodontic treatment as well as maintaining the client's health during and after orthodontic treatment. The dental hygienist may complete data collection procedures, including taking the medical and personal histories, completing periodontal and dental chartings, taking radiographs, and preparing study models.
- ✦ For the client presenting with active periodontal disease, the dental hygienist must complete periodontal debridement and client education to eliminate infection.
- ✦ During treatment, the client must be seen regularly by the dental hygienist for clinical maintenance procedures and follow-up on home care recommendations.

CRITICAL THINKING EXERCISES

Client: TJ Langer

Profile: TJ is a 5-year-old boy who has come with his mother to have his teeth cleaned.

Chief Complaint: His mother is concerned that there is spacing between TJ's upper front teeth and between some of his lower teeth. She asks you if he will need braces to close these spaces.

Social History: Lives with both parents

Medical History: Noncontributory

Dental History: Upon inspection, you notice that the spaces are between the maxillary lateral incisors and the canines and between the mandibular canines and first molar. You also notice that the primary second molars are in an end-to-end relationship.

Supplemental Notes: Lives in a fluoridated community

1. What would you say to TJ's mother about his potential need for orthodontic treatment?

For References, Suggested Readings, and Related Websites, visit
http://evolve.elsevier.com/Darby/hygiene/

SECTION 8

Practice Management

CHAPTER 52

Practice Management

OBJECTIVES

Mastery of the content of this chapter will enable the reader to:

- ✦ Develop a mission statement and goals for the dental hygiene component of a dental practice
- ✦ Describe behaviors a dental hygienist can use to help build a united team of staff members
- ✦ Describe techniques used for successful client management
- ✦ List and define the elements necessary for a complete case presentation
- ✦ Explain the legal implications of client noncompliance
- ✦ Explain the benefits of using computers in the dental practice
- ✦ Outline the three types of appointment book management systems
- ✦ Describe progressive dental hygiene practice
- ✦ Discuss economic considerations for a profitable practice, including production, collection, and office overhead
- ✦ Develop a marketing plan for promoting a dental practice
- ✦ Design a list of strategies for increased client satisfaction and methods of evaluating the outcome

KEY TERMS

Case presentation
Collection
Continued-care periodontal health system
Marketing
Marketing plan
Mission statement
Nonadherence/noncompliance
Office overhead
Office policies and procedures
Office production
Practice management
Practice promotion
Progressive dental hygiene
Reclamation
Records management
Restricted appointment booking
Team building
Team concept
Telephone contact file
Unlimited future booking

Participation in management of the dental or dental hygiene practice adds a dimension of administrative responsibilities and decision making to the daily routine and affords professional growth opportunities. Such participation increases the dental hygienist's position as a valued team member and enhances job satisfaction.

PRACTICE MANAGEMENT

Practice management can be defined as the organization, administration, and direction of the professional practice in a style that facilitates quality client care, efficient use of time and personnel, reduced stress to staff members and clients, enhanced professional and personal satisfaction for staff, and financial profitability.

The development of a *mission statement* is a basic tool for the successful management of dental or dental hygiene practices. The mission statement is a broad vision of purpose of the practice. It is supported by specific goals that describe what is to be done within the practice. Objectives describing how each goal is to be accomplished are defined by measurable components. All staff members participate in the development of the mission and goal statements, agreeing by consensus on the final statements. This set of guidelines is used to direct all management activities of the practice.

The *team concept* guides the interaction and interdependence of the entire office staff to promote the unity and efficiency of the group. The oral health team is composed of the clients, dentists, dental hygienists, dental assistants, office manager, receptionists, dental laboratory technicians, and bookkeepers. With the knowledge of the mission statement and goals for the practice, each staff member accepts responsibility to strive toward the accomplishment of these guidelines.

Personnel Management

Personnel management includes daily communication and regular staff meetings. Staff meetings provide an opportunity to review organizational goals, evaluate progress, share information, air grievances, and solve problems together to find agreed-upon solutions. Manuals describing *office policies and procedures* applicable to all members of the organization are distributed. These manuals help make the practice systematic and clearly familiarize personnel with responsibilities for which they are accountable. The policy manual describes the rules or guidelines for running the office, while the procedure manual lists specific techniques for accomplishing tasks.

Team building is the synergistic process of developing group goals with motivation and commitment. The dental hygienist contributes to the strength of the team by:

- Sharing information
- Participating in the formulation of goals and objectives
- Activating, evaluating, and revising plans
- Encouraging the participation of all staff members in these processes

Interpersonal team building creates quality human relations among all office personnel, clients, and members of the professional community.

Client Management

Successful client management is guided by the belief that the client is the most important person in the oral healthcare environment. Each individual has physical, psychological, spiritual, and emotional human needs that are influenced by previous experiences, level of intelligence, and socioethnocultural factors. These needs will direct client behavior, and the practitioner must assess individual needs before determining a plan for client management.

POLICIES FOR CLIENTS. Policies are established for clients to provide consistency and guidance for expectations. This document may begin with a statement of the setting's philosophy, such as the intention to provide quality oral healthcare and the team members' desire for client satisfaction. It also delineates expectations of the client, such as arriving promptly for scheduled appointments, giving timely notice if an appointment needs to be changed or canceled, and meeting financial responsibility and arrangements. Other issues may be outlined regarding medical precautions and the need for oral radiographs and collaboration with other dental and health professionals when necessary. These policies should be presented to clients in writing during the first visit to the office setting. Once the content is understood, the client signs and dates the statement of accepting the office policies.

Reference to these policies may be made during correspondence with the client, which may be sent when management problems occur, such as failed appointments or failure to meet financial obligations. Written correspondence to the client about the dental or dental hygiene diagnosis and care plan is generally completed by the office manager; however, there are other times when the dental hygienist may be responsible or may wish to communicate with clients in writing. For example, a follow-up letter may be useful as a review of important points made during an appointment or as a reinforcement to encourage use of new skills or development of new oral health behaviors. There may be need for a note to remind the client to schedule a regular or an overdue appointment. The dental hygienist also may wish to send a note of personal congratulations, well wishes, sympathy, or thanks. All such types of correspondence help establish the dental hygienist as a unique professional within the team and promote the perception of a caring attitude. A newsletter from the practice is another method employed by some dental practices to keep clients updated on current care procedures and "news" from the staff's personal and professional lives.

CASE PRESENTATIONS. A *case presentation* is the process of explaining assessment findings to the client along with options and recommendations for therapy to reach agreement on a care plan. The dental hygienist may be responsible for case presentations to clients within a general dental or dental hygiene practice. In some cases, the dentist may perform the data collection, dental diagnosis, and recommended care plan for both restorative and periodontal care, and then assign the dental hygienist the responsibility of making the case presentation to the client. To meet the client's human needs for freedom from stress, and for conceptualization and problem solving, it is important that the discussion be held in a manner that is informative and nonthreatening to the client, using terminology that the individual can easily understand. The client's dental chart, periodontal maintenance record, radiographs, intraoral photographs, and study models may be useful visual aids during the process. See Elements of a Complete Case Presentation to a Dental or Dental Hygiene Client.

CLIENT MOTIVATION. An effective case presentation translates into client acceptance of care and motivation. Client motivation is best achieved when the information presented satisfies human needs and coincides with the client's own culture, beliefs, attitudes, and values.

Elements of a Complete Case Presentation to a Dental or Dental Hygiene Client

Information
Data collected and assessment findings are shared with the client using visual aids such as radiographs, photographs, models, or a periodontal chart, when appropriate.

Education
An explanation of the significance of the assessment findings is given to the client, including short- and long-range possibilities and consequences of the conditions present. At this time, the practitioner should ask questions and initiate discussion that bring the client into the conversation so a determination can be made of the client's level of understanding and client priorities, and interest in pursuing care. Media, research evidence, and other instructional strategies should supplement client education.

Options
A list of alternative methods of care is given to the client, including benefits, time involved, treatment risks, risks of not doing the treatment, and cost for each option.

Choice
An informed decision is made by the client based on his or her understanding of the information presented, priorities, desire for treatment, and perceived needs.

Agreement
The client and professional concur on a course to follow, including sequencing of care and assignment of responsibilities. The dental hygienist, as an advocate, supports the informed decision made by the client. A written summary of the case presentation may be composed by the dental hygienist and mailed to the client following this appointment.

Strategies that can be used by the dental hygienist to motivate the client include:

- Making the information relevant and meaningful
- Relating information by building on the client's existing knowledge, experience, attitudes, and feelings
- Using success or rewards to promote learning, rather than criticism or punishment

CLIENT NONADHERENCE. *Nonadherence,* or *noncompliance,* is a lack of client cooperation with recommended oral healthcare. It is significant because it can result in compromised care, unsatisfactory care outcomes, dissatisfaction on the part of the client as well as the practitioner, and possibly litigation. In the event of a lawsuit, the judicial decision, outcome, or amount of settlement may be altered based on negligence of the practitioner if nonadherence was ignored or not adequately documented in the client's chart. The following examples of nonadherence may occur during dental hygiene care:

- Routinely tardy arrival for scheduled appointments or necessity for an early departure from the appointment
- Repeated postponement or cancellations
- Failure to appear for scheduled appointments
- Unwillingness to have necessary diagnostic tests, such as radiographs
- Unwillingness to accept recommended specific procedures or the care plan
- Unwillingness to accept referrals to specialists
- Failure to use medications as prescribed
- Failure to follow the recommended oral hygiene regimen

The management of client nonadherence begins with recognizing it when it happens. The following list describes the process of documenting client nonadherence to prescribed care:

1. Record recommended care.
2. Describe all instructions that have *not* been followed.
3. Describe the specific behavior of the client.
4. Record in quotations verbalization of nonadherence by the client.
5. Note any discussion of the consequences of not following recommendations or instructions that occur between office personnel and the client.

Clients whose uncooperative behavior impedes professional care may be legally discontinued from the practice by following precise legal protocols. Practitioners are advised to be familiar with these protocols to avoid litigation associated with client abandonment.

Records Management

Written client records, the most valuable permanent document of past dental or dental hygiene care, provide the "written memory" of the events and conversations that transpired during each appointment. Maintaining accurate records *(records management)* enhances smooth office operations as well as other functions. Client records serve the following purposes:

- Source for organizing data collected
- Evaluation tool to aid in dental and dental hygiene diagnoses and care planning
- Protection of the client regarding general health and discovery of oral diseases
- Communication tool for client education and behavior modification
- Guideline for performing consistent care
- Proof to third-party insurers to justify necessary treatment
- Demonstration of accountability for responsible care
- Legal protection to present documentary evidence for defense if necessary.

Written records include the dental and periodontal charts; health history; records of examinations, diagnosis, and care delivered; informed consent and informed refusal forms; and copies of prescriptions. Nonwritten records consist of photographs and photographic images from intraoral cameras, radiographs, digital radiography, models, and cephalometric tracings.

TABLE 52–1 DOCUMENTING ORAL HEALTHCARE

Minimum Documentation	Complete Treatment Notes
Date	Date
	Clinical observations
Significant findings	Significant findings
	Summary of discussions regarding conditions present
	Options for care
	Informed decisions made by client
Services rendered	Services rendered
	Information and instructions presented to client
	Items dispensed to client
	Recommendations for future care
Recommended next treatment	Description of care recommended
	Time frame for scheduling
	Length of time need for treatment
Initials of practitioner	Signature and license number of practitioner
Fee	Fee

Table 52–1 compares minimal and complete notes documenting care. All notes are to be thorough, accurate, and legible, with facts separated from opinion. Writing should be done in a timely, contemporaneous manner, either during the appointment or immediately after the completion of care. It is likely that some information is forgotten and therefore left out of the client record if all chart entries are made at the end of the day. Records should be kept indefinitely, even if the client transfers to another oral healthcare setting.

DENTAL PRACTICE SOFTWARE

The types of computer software programs available for dental office use include word processing; spreadsheets with automatic accounting functions; data management for entering, storing, sorting, and retrieving data; graphics; desktop publishing; integrated software to combine the aforementioned applications; scheduling; and communications and education.[1,2] There are many commercial computer software programs available for dental offices. Additionally, custom software, written for a specialized task, can be designed if a dental practice requires a unique application. Client health histories can be quickly and easily updated, including listing medications with computer programs that identify drug interactions, medications with oral implications, and systemic conditions with oral manifestations.

Many dental software programs are available for documenting periodontal and dental examinations with graphic presentations, automated periodontal probing and voice-activated recording programs, soft tissue assessments, restorative procedures, and treatment record notes. It is recommended that hard-copy printouts be made and filed in the client's chart following each appointment as both a backup precaution against computer system failure and for a quick reference for multiple staff members. The software company providing the program, installation, and technical support will also recommend a tape backup system.

Practice management software allows for booking appointments and printing daily schedules, tracking client records and appointments, check writing, payroll, accounting, and calculating and printing bills. Word processing allows treatment plans to be generally formatted, then individualized by editing for each specific client, and augmented with computer graphics for periodontal and dentition charting. It also saves time and enhances practice evaluation by producing spreadsheets for analyzing high- versus low-volume procedures and services, distribution of workloads, and production outcomes for each practitioner. The computer software can automatically create charts and graphs for further visual demonstration of work results.

Desktop publishing designs personalized letterheads and templates for practice promotion materials, including newsletters, fliers, and pamphlets, all of which can be embellished using clip art images or originally designed computer graphics. Tabulating and tracking insurance claims is made easy electronically. Many automated insurance forms are being standardized throughout the industry. Some offices use e-mail to confirm appointments and to notify clients of receipt of insurance pre-estimates and authorizations, billing, and recall reminders. Some clients prefer to use e-mail for all possible communications, including with their dental offices. If an office chooses to use e-mail regularly with clients and other healthcare practitioners, it requires constant vigilance by a staff member to read and respond to these communications throughout the day.

Networking Software

Offices usually begin with one computer at the front desk for the receptionist or office manager to use. Multiple computers in one office, however, provide a computer in each dental treatment room, and networking software links them together, creating a docking station network. This system allows for all clinicians to share information and enter treatment data as well as schedule appointments. Consideration must be made to ensure that these systems are efficient for clinicians to use, rather than reduce their valuable time with the client. Assigning more tasks to the clinician just because there is a sophisticated computer system in the practice may not be the best decision. Providing assistants who can do the data entry while the clinician dictates her or his observations is a good solution.

Educational Software

Computer-based multimedia oral health education programs can provide clients with valuable information, from demonstrations of daily oral hygiene maintenance techniques to descriptions of dental procedures. They may be self-paced programs available for clients while they wait for the practitioner or during appointments to enhance case presentations and ensure that all information is provided. Educational programs can be transferred to individual disks for loan to clients so the programs can be viewed at home. These programs can be distributed with copies of the client's individual digital photographs, radiographs, and chart.

Internet Use in the Dental Practice

Dental practices are using the World Wide Web for advertising and practice promotion on the Internet. Web pages permit dental offices to introduce themselves with photographs of the facility and staff members; post the practice mission statement; provide explanations of procedures; list specific pretreatment and post-treatment instructions; promote health education topics; and refer or link readers to other pertinent Web sites such as practitioners in dental specialties and public information services. All of these strategies assist the practice to market its services and publicize its specialties to a large population. Web page contents can be changed and updated frequently and easily.

In addition, dental practices using computers and scanners can quickly share information about mutual clients by faxing or e-mailing documents between practices, including medical health histories, dental histories, examination findings, treatment records, digital radiography, and digital photography. Computer video imaging systems using the intraoral camera not only inform and educate clients, but also facilitate discussions among health professionals. Multiple-practitioner simultaneous consultation is possible, and no one has to leave the office to participate. The client benefits and does not have to go from office to office, while each specialist repeats the assessment procedures. Practitioners view and assess the same data at the same time and discuss the findings, reach a diagnosis, and determine a treatment plan during one conference call. Video teleconferencing, using video cameras and transmitting over computers, allows multiple practitioners to observe live examinations from different locations and to make recommendations as a team. The second opinion or evaluation by a specialist can be completed from the convenience of the general practitioner's office.

TIME MANAGEMENT

Effective time management is essential to the success of any practice. The appointment book is the mechanism for controlling time by allotting increments to scheduled appointments, lunch breaks and staff meetings, and days off for personal time, holidays, vacations, and professional conferences. A variety of appointment book management systems are used for client scheduling:

- *Unlimited future booking.* This approach allows appointments to be scheduled as far in advance as is necessary to accommodate all clients. This booking format requires careful advance planning by the dental hygienist for time away from the practice.
- *Restricted appointment booking.* This approach limits scheduling to a specified time period, such as 1 to 3 months. Clients who are not prescheduled during this time are added to a call list and telephoned when appointments become available. This system requires less advance planning for taking time off.
- *Telephone contact file.* This file is a waiting list of clients in need of appointments who are available on short notice to fill changed appointments and cancellations. All dental and dental hygiene practices should maintain such a list. Following is a list of appropriate clients for the telephone contact file:
  - Clients who are new to the practice
  - Clients needing multiple appointments
  - Clients who cancel existing appointments
  - Clients who need appointments within a specified time frame, such as before a vacation, when home from college for a limited time only, or when terminating insurance benefits
  - Clients with an existing scheduled appointment who wish to receive care sooner than scheduled
  - Clients known to have flexible schedules who are able to make appointments on short notice

The information for the telephone contact file includes the following:

- The client's name (also written phonetically if it is difficult to pronounce)
- Daytime telephone number with notation of work or home phone
- Type of appointment needed and time required
- Special requests or needs during the appointment, such as antibiotic premedication or local anesthesia
- Preferred day or time of appointment and date of existing scheduled appointment

If a client is telephoned to fill an available time and cannot accept the appointment, the client declination should be recorded in the file. Examples of a telephone contact file are presented in Figure 52–1.

Time allotments are designed for each client depending on the care needed. Generally, one hour is the time delineated for dental hygiene care, with additional time scheduled for new clients or clients with periodontal conditions, special needs, or management challenges.

Entries in the appointment book should include the following:

- Pencil lead entries, including the client's name and daytime telephone number or computer entry
- The service to be given or type of appointment planned
- The length of appointment time in units and any special instructions, such as need for premedication and/or local anesthetic, and client concerns

An example of appointment scheduling is shown in Figure 52–2.

June Johnson 516-223-4657—work
4 Quad Root Planing—1 hour each Q
Local Anesthesia
M/W/F before 10 A.M.

Susie Thomas 516-756-2188—home
Child Prophy and Fluoride—1/2 hour
Any day after 3 P.M.
Called 11/21/95: client declined appointment

Tim Scott 712-299-0506—work
Perio Maintenance—1 hour
Has 12/5 appointment
Tuesdays, anytime
11/20/95 = NO

FIGURE 52–1 ✦ Examples of client information included in a telephone contact file.

Monday, March 15	
8	John Jacobs
15	Perio maintenance
30	BWX
45	W: 525-5258
9	Susan Woods
15	1 Quad root plane
30	Local anesthesia
45	W: 828-2143
10	Matt Lewis
15	Perio maintenance
30	W: 526-1122
45	
11	Dorothy Walker
15	New client
30	Exam, FMX
45	Hygiene therapy
12	H: 444-6989
15	↓
30	
45	Lunch
1	
15	
30	Jennifer Thomas
45	Perio recall
2	W: 828-6446
15	Bessie Sicular
30	Perio maintenance
45	H: 527-2895
3	Bobby O'Brien
15	Pedo oral Px
30	Tami O'Brien
45	Pedo oral Px
4	Mom: 526-3832
15	Joseph Camp
30	1 Quad root plane
45	Local anesthesia
5	W: 444-7172
15	

FIGURE 52–2 ✦ Sample schedule from appointment book.

PROGRESSIVE DENTAL HYGIENE

Although most dental hygienists practice without a dental assistant, some settings provide the dental hygienist with a full-time dental assistant. In this mode of practicing *progressive dental hygiene,* the dental hygienist and assistant treat the client together. This system of care has also been called the accelerated dental hygiene practice, enabling hygienists to work at an accelerated pace. The dental assistants are utilized at their maximum capacity permitted by law.[3] The tasks of the appointment are divided into those handled together and those done by the dental assistant and by the dental hygienist. The result is that the dental hygienist can increase productivity and profitability by 50% to 100%, improve the efficiency of treatment, comfortably increase time spent with the client, and reduce stress with careful planning and implementation.[4]

When the overall dental hygiene production increases, the dental hygienist's salary increases, the dental assistant's salary is paid out of the increased production, and the bottom-line net result is an increase in profits for this segment of the practice.

See Table 52–2 on progressive dental hygiene for an outline of assigning duties to the dental hygiene assistant and the dental hygienist. Not all procedures listed in the table are legal for assistants in every state. Specific dental practice acts should be reviewed to verify the legality of each procedure as defined in the statutes. It is essential that both the dental hygienist and dental assistant be properly trained and educated to operate in this environment.

CONTINUED-CARE SYSTEMS

Continued-care periodontal health systems (recall systems) are designed to organize and maintain periodontal assessments and preventive or maintenance care on a regular schedule according to individual client needs. In some practices, the dental hygienist is responsible for developing and managing the periodontal maintenance system. Advance scheduling may be done to set a definite future appointment with a reminder postcard (often self-addressed by the client) and telephone call to the client shortly before the reserved date. Monthly reminder cards may be sent to notify clients without appointments that it is time to return for periodontal maintenance (Figure 52–3). This latter system shares responsibility with the client, who is encouraged to make the appointment, while the office manager may retain a cross-reference file for follow-up. Many practices telephone clients to remind them of the scheduled visit as a protection from forgotten and missed appointments. Usually a combination of all continued-care systems is available within the office, with implementation based on client preference.

References are necessary to keep track of clients in various types of continued-care scheduling. A triplicate

TABLE 52–2 PROGRESSIVE DENTAL HYGIENE

Dental Assistant	Together	Dental Hygienist
		Chart review to identify client needs
Set up treatment room and sharpen instruments		
Greet and seat client		
Update personal history		
Update health history		
Elicit dental concerns		
Update vital signs		
Expose radiographs, process and mount		
	Review above changes	
Administer client antibacterial prerinse		
Clean client partial dentures, retainers, or occlusal guards		
Record findings of examination		Extraoral and intraoral examination
Record examination data		Periodontal examination
Record findings of examination		Examination for dental deposits
		Presentation of findings and discussion of risks, benefits, and alternatives to recommended treatment
Assist with air and vacuum		Scaling, root planing, micro ultrasonics
Selective polishing* (Legal for certified assistants in some states)		Selective polishing, if not legal for dental assistant
Record dental findings		Observe dental needs
Apply topical fluoride		
	Apply dental sealants	
	Cosmetic tooth whitening	
Notify dentist for examination		
Present appointment findings to dentist		
Assist dentist in examination and record findings		
Explain dentist's findings and recommendations		
Oral hygiene and self-care instruction		
Dispense oral hygiene devices		
Record appointment procedures, recommendations, and client's response		
Answer client questions		
Schedule future appointments		
Thank and dismiss client		
Clean and disinfect room		
Process instruments		
Prepare for next client		
Restock rooms and lab		
Inventory control for dental hygiene instruments and supplies	End of the day	Review charts for accuracy and completeness of notes

Modified from Linder AA: How to profit from hygiene, *Dental Economics* 88(1):32, 1998.

Dear___________________________: STAMP

It is time to schedule an appointment for your _________ month examination and periodontal maintenance therapy.

Your last visit was: _____________.
Please call to set a date and time!

Client Name
Street Address
City, State, Zip

__________ *Signed* ____________
Registered Dental Hygienist for
Harold F. Greenburg, D.D.S.
618-525-5255

FIGURE 52–3 ✦ Client reminder card sent in a sealed envelope.

appointment card may be used, with one copy given to the client, a second copy filed in the chart, and the third serving as a postcard reminder to be mailed before the appointment (Figure 52–4). A *tickler file* may be used to collect monthly groupings of cards for clients needing appointments (Figure 52–5). Each card contains a record of previous appointments, current needs, and ways to best contact and schedule the client. An alphabetical file may be used to list the client's name, previous appointment date, services rendered, plus needed care. Cross-references may be designed to combine any number of these techniques.

Reclamation is a process of periodic purging of all files to identify clients whose care is incomplete, who have missed appointments, or who have been absent from the

Melvin Siegler, D.D.S.
Janet Fuller, D.D.S.

Appointment For ____________________ 199 ___

Date ____________________ Hour ______

If unable to keep this appointment, kindly give 24 hours notice.
Otherwise, a charge will be made for the time reserved.

54 Barrymore Boulevard, Union, NJ 74501
842-7113

Appointment card tears out from perforation and is given to client.

Melvin Siegler, D.D.S.
Janet Fuller, D.D.S.

Appointment For ____________________ 199 ___

Date ____________________ Hour ______

If unable to keep this appointment, kindly give 24 hours notice.
Otherwise, a charge will be made for the time reserved.

54 Barrymore Boulevard, Union, NJ 74501
842-7113

First carbon is placed in client chart as a record of next scheduled appointment.

Melvin Siegler, D.D.S.
Janet Fuller, D.D.S.

Appointment For ____________________ 199 ___

Date ____________________ Hour ______

If unable to keep this appointment, kindly give 24 hours notice.
Otherwise, a charge will be made for the time reserved.

54 Barrymore Boulevard, Union, NJ 74501
842-7113

Second carbon is a postcard, filed by the month and then mailed as a reminder two weeks prior to appointment.

FIGURE 52–4 ✦ Triplicate appointment card.

JUNE
Steven Armstrong 516-223-4576—work
Last = 2/4/95
4-month perio maintenance—1 hour
T/Th afternoons

JUNE
Janice and Johnny Tenny 516-221-7588—mom
Last = 12/10/95
6-month prophy w/fluoride—1/2 hour each
must be scheduled together
M/T/W after 3:30 P.M.

FIGURE 52–5 ✦ Tickler appointment cards.

practice and are in need of care. Once identified, clients may be telephoned or notified by mail of the date of the last appointment and need for prompt oral healthcare. The dental hygienist may be responsible for managing the chart reviews as part of quality assurance measures to determine which clients are overdue for appointments and need to be contacted.

ECONOMIC CONSIDERATIONS

Office Overhead

The financial considerations of a practice include a determination of the office income and expenditures (e.g., productivity, overhead expenses, collections, and profit). Expenses include the following:

- Employee salaries and fringe benefits
- Rent, lease, and utility expenditures
- Equipment purchase and maintenance
- Lease-hold improvements
- Supplies
- Accounting expenses
- Insurance payments for policies the employer carries for the building or personnel

The *office overhead,* based on these expenses, is a determination of the dollar amount it costs per hour to run the office; the *office production* is the total fees billed for services performed. *Collection* is the amount of money that is actually paid to the office from clients, dental insurance companies, and health agencies.

Financial arrangements must be confirmed with each client before performing oral healthcare. The office policy statement presented to new clients should summarize the financial arrangement options and responsibilities. The dental hygienist may be the person who discusses financial issues with the client, especially for extensive dental hygiene care. To encourage prompt fee collections, some practices offer a small discount to clients who make payments in full at the time services are rendered. If the office requires a down payment before extensive treatment or if a client carries a balance for 60 to 90 days, the client needs to be informed of these policies and fees for them. Special long-term financial arrangements may also be offered to some clients.

Dental insurance enhances the ability of many clients who otherwise might not have been able to afford oral healthcare; however, many misunderstandings arise about oral healthcare financing when clients do not fully comprehend how insurance coverage is determined or the limits of their benefits. Oral health insurance coverage varies from company to company and from policy to policy within the same company. It is important to explain to clients that they are responsible personally for the fees incurred. Even with the help of the office staff in completing and submitting insurance claims, it is the client's responsibility to investigate and understand his or her individual insurance coverage. Many insurance policies pay a percentage of the "usual and customary" fee for services, and some require that regular maintenance visits be maintained to receive a larger percentage of the service fee. Understanding insurance plans is important for hygienists because they are often asked about them during the dental hygiene care appointment.

Although it is presently illegal for a dental hygienist to own and operate a dental practice, it is legal for a dental hygienist to own and operate a dental hygiene practice in the state of Colorado, and a limited-access hygienist may own the dental hygiene practice in Oregon, California, and Washington. In these latter three states, hygienists may choose to have part-time or full-time contracts with facilities for providing care to clients for whom visits to a dental hygienist outside the facility would be a hardship. These arrangements are unique in that the hygienist with the special license is able to work with general supervision or no supervision other than a prescription to provide care. Therefore, it is essential for the hygienist to understand the economic aspects of the business of oral healthcare. With this knowledge, the hygienist can optimize the managerial role, fully contribute in the area of practice management, and enjoy the rewards of a financially successful practice.

Office Facility Management

Dental hygiene care rooms and equipment must be carefully cleaned and maintained to reach the maximal life span of these costly items. Written guidelines are useful to direct personnel in the care of all such items. Such guidelines include the following:

- ✦ Information on special cleansing and lubricating agents
- ✦ People to contact for necessary repairs
- ✦ Intervals for cleaning and oiling
- ✦ Assignment of the person responsible for equipment resources management

A material resources inventory file for dental hygiene services and oral hygiene products dispensed to clients is best maintained on a manual or computer-managed inventory control system (Figure 52–6).

Adequate stock should be kept on hand, but an excess accumulation of items should be avoided to prevent shelf life and storage problems. An inventory control system consists of the following:

- ✦ A list of supplies and materials used
- ✦ The manufacturer or distributor
- ✦ Cost of the item
- ✦ Quantity and frequency of ordering

Maintaining the date of each order and the date received establishes a predictable pattern of shipping time for future orders. It is most efficient for one person to be responsible for materials resources management, such as ordering the supplies for the office and inventory control; however, the dental hygienist often controls the inventory for oral hygiene products.

Dental Hygiene Revenues

Historically, many dentists looked at dental hygiene as a loss leader. In marketing terms, that means that dental hygiene services brought clients into the dental office just to allow the dentist to examine them for real dental needs. Because hygiene fees were low, the outcome to the practice was a financial loss for hygiene services, rather than a financial gain. Now dental hygiene is considered to be a profit center for dental practices, and the dental hygiene department of a general dental practice can generate approximately 30% of the total fees for a practice. Dental hygiene fees should be set at a level that demonstrates regard for the education and training of the professional providing the service, and with suitable compensation for the time spent rendering the care. Clients value fine

Date Ordered	Product Name	Quantity & Cost	Supplier & Phone	Date Rec'd

FIGURE 52–6 ✦ Format for a material resources inventory file.

dental hygiene services, just as they value fine care provided by the dentist, and they are willing to pay for it.

Procedures provided within the dental hygiene care rooms generating fees are examinations, radiographs, dental health maintenance appointments, treatment of active periodontal disease, periodontal supportive services, emergency periodontal treatment, application of topical fluorides, placement of dental sealants, and cosmetic teeth whitening. Additionally, the dental hygienist often assists in client decisions to proceed with long-term, comprehensive reconstructive and cosmetic dental treatment, greatly adding to the overall profits of a practice.

In order to operate at a profit, the dental hygiene department must adhere to all the guidelines for any successful business. Staff members must be part of the team and adhere to the practice philosophy and mission statement. The clients must understand and adhere to the office policy of keeping appointments and arriving on time. Team members must promote a professional image and maintain positive relationships with clients. They must maintain both a didactic and a clinical education that permits them to offer all of the up-to-date research-based services at the highest quality of care. An ongoing and organized client recall system must be in place and followed, along with a systematic client reclamation program. Schedules must be filled to capacity. Each client undergoes periodontal examination at the beginning of each appointment to determine current periodontal health status. The practice must adopt and follow a philosophy of assertive nonsurgical treatment of active disease and offer frequent periodontal maintenance appointments for long-term health. An additional full range of services must be offered, such as fluoride treatments for children and adults with caries susceptibility or root exposures, placement of dental sealants, and teeth whitening procedures. When combined, these services guarantee that dental hygiene production revenues will be profitable.

MARKETING DENTISTRY AND DENTAL HYGIENE

Marketing is a structured, organized approach to selecting and servicing markets and a researched approach to informing the public of a service.[5] The purpose of marketing dentistry and dental hygiene is to obtain and maintain the needed share of the client population market to keep the practice productive as desired and to inform society of the benefits of the practice. The profits from a productive practice include both financial gain and personal satisfaction for the staff members.

The *marketing plan* should include the four Ps of marketing:

- Product/service
- Price
- Place
- Promotion

Product/service might include philosophy and objective of the practice, services provided, and quality of care. Price considers cost and oral healthcare financing mechanisms, such as the usual and customary fees for the area. Place encompasses the entire location and environment of the practice. Promotion includes strategies that communicate with target markets or external public groups, such as newsletters and advertising mechanisms.

The personnel involved in marketing relations are numerous. A manager is needed to coordinate the marketing plan, delegate responsibilities to staff members, monitor the marketing budget, establish an overall time schedule, and evaluate the effectiveness of the marketing plan. Effective practice marketing is cost-effective if the client pool is increased. Within the oral healthcare setting, the dentists, dental hygienists, dental assistants, receptionists, office managers, and dental laboratory technicians must be familiar with the plan and incorporate its elements into daily practice. The business consultants employed by the practice—bookkeeper, accountant, and attorney—contribute ideas and communicate the credits of the practice to their community contacts.

Other healthcare professionals—physicians, allied healthcare providers, product suppliers, and prominent community and business members—are similarly involved with the knowledge of the practice's reputation and can refer to the practice. The best participants in the marketing plan for dentistry and dental hygiene are the clients. Satisfied clients who believe that their needs have been met by quality oral health services, at a reasonable fee, in a caring environment, recommend the practice to friends, relatives, and business associates. Table 52–3 presents methods of evaluating marketing effectiveness.

Practice promotion occurs when all staff members project the desired professional image and gain public exposure on behalf of the practice. See Marketing Strategies for Practice Promotion. Client satisfaction does more for practice promotion than any other strategy for marketing.

Client Satisfaction

To appeal to a broad-based population, the office must offer a spectrum of oral services including preventive, therapeutic, maintenance, restorative, cosmetic, counseling, and reconstruction services; or, referrals are made to specialists who offer such treatments. Quality care is the key to obtaining client satisfaction. Clients recognize dentists and dental hygienists who are sensitive to human needs; who provide consistent, technical expertise with an attitude of caring and gentleness; and who are respectful of staff whose skills are fully utilized.

Correct pronunciation of clients' names can be facilitated by writing them phonetically on a space in the chart. Personalized attention, respecting each client as an individual, listening carefully, thoroughly discussing reported symptoms, and being responsive all are methods that help develop special relationships that are appreciated by the client. As a consumer advocate, the

TABLE 52–3 MARKETING EFFECTIVENESS EVALUATION

Quantitative Elements	Qualitative Elements
Internal	
1. Maintain a count of clients treated during each month to demonstrate evidence of practice growth. a. Returning clients seeking maintenance care and examinations b. Active restorative, cosmetic, and reconstructive appointments c. New clients and how each was referred 2. Perform a quarterly or annual comparison of gross revenues with production and collection. 3. Complete a complex financial analysis. 4. Calculate productivity per month, week, day, and hour.	1. Interview staff members regarding their: a. Evaluative comments about current marketing programs b. Activities for practice promotion c. Suggestions for future marketing strategies
External	
1. Compare financial reports with others published in the area. 2. Meet with local practices and make comparisons of all numbers.	1. Interview clients with questionnaire regarding oral needs, desires, satisfaction with the practice, and services offered. 2. Ask clients for suggestions regarding improving the practice and their recommendations for change. 3. Survey community professional sources for additional information that assists in evaluating marketing effectiveness; ask about further services that might increase referrals.

Marketing Strategies for Practice Promotion

Write articles for the local newspaper on oral disease prevention, dental service updates, dental emergency care, and evaluation of over-the-counter oral health products.
Invite a local newspaper reporter to the practice to prepare a feature article.
Participate in broadcast media programming, local radio and television, with special interest information, talk shows, and community service announcements.
Participate in civic, religious, and fraternal group activities where the practice professionals meet many new people.
Use business contacts within the community client population.
Sponsor community projects or athletic team sports.
Participate in community cultural and recreational events.
Become a public speaker.
Teach health information and cardiopulmonary resuscitation workshops to consumers and other professionals.
Become a student, attending local classes and workshops.
Meet and cooperate with neighboring health professionals, providing business cards and referral slips.
Volunteer professional services and demonstrations.
Perform oral health screenings at schools, health fairs, career days, community and athletic programs, civic group programs, and special events.
Actively participate in the professional association.
Participate creatively in the community.
Sponsor an open house to welcome neighbors to meet the dental office staff members.
Buy advertising space or time within the telephone book, local newspaper, radio, Internet, and other community media.
Use direct mail methods to distribute oral health education materials, practice brochures, or a newsletter to the client population or the local community at large.
Design a Web site for the dental practice that can be accessed by the dental consumer.

dental hygienist stays abreast of consumer trends and educates clients about oral healthcare changes as new services and products become available. When explaining care plans, alternatives are offered, including explanations of all options and the costs of each, with clear recommendations given. Clients need to understand the difference between what is necessary treatment and what is ideal. The client's informed decision is then fully supported. See Elements of a Dental or Dental Hygiene Practice That Enhance Client Satisfaction.

Written and telephone communications further enhance client satisfaction. A practice brochure can be developed and distributed to describe the philosophy of care, introduce the staff, describe services offered, list office hours plus emergency arrangements, and note special features about the practice. Written outlines of assessed needs and sequencing of appointments help the client to review and recall verbal case presentations. Sending the client copies of letters to or from other health professionals concerning needed or ongoing care informs the client of the shared interest in his or her oral health. Mailing clients brief personalized notes of thanks, congratulations, well wishes for recovery, and sympathy communicates appreciation and caring.

Elements of a Dental or Dental Hygiene Practice That Enhance Client Satisfaction

Offer extended business hours, such as early morning, evening, and weekend appointments.

Appeal to all age ranges, across the life span.

Involve the client in understanding dental disease processes and the oral-systemic disease link, with encouragement to take responsibility for his or her own oral health maintenance, making decisions about care, setting goals, and committing to long-term oral health maintenance.

Provide an effective continued-care system for oral health maintenance, with repeated instructions on prevention and monitoring techniques and individualized instructions according to clients' needs.

Have waiting time based on an efficiently managed practice, with realistic scheduling of time for appointments; advise clients of anticipated length of appointments.

Promote positive psychological attitudes by all staff members; create an upbeat atmosphere.

Establish warm, respectful interpersonal relations between office personnel and clients. Clients don't care how much you know until they know how much you care.

Create a pleasant, comfortable, attractive office decor maintained in constant cleanliness.

Provide "give-away" items during office visits, such as oral hygiene aids, health education brochures, toys for children, or flowers to clients for special occasions.

Charge fair and reasonable fees; offer a variety of financial arrangements; process dental insurance forms expediently.

Maintain rapport with specialty practices to facilitate referrals, treatment coordination, and close follow-through regarding clients who are referred to other professionals for special care needs.

Arrange appointments quickly when need requires expediency.

Always accommodate emergency clients immediately.

Telephone contacts with clients should be maintained on a positive, satisfactory note. The dental hygienist can use follow-up telephone calls after lengthy or complex treatments to check on comfort and healing or to reassure anxious clients.

Client satisfaction leads to staff member satisfaction. The dentist and dental hygienist can recognize one another and all staff members by expressing appreciation for daily cooperation and team spirit, offering congratulations for jobs done well, noting client loyalty, and recognizing referrals received from staff members' marketing efforts. Verbal "thank yous" and small tokens of appreciation promote continued success.

Client Education Issues

- Provide a practice brochure to describe the philosophy of care, introduce the staff, describe services offered, list office hours and emergency arrangements, and note special features of the practice.
- Provide a practice brochure that also includes expectations of the client (e.g., arriving promptly for scheduled appointments, timely notice if an appointment needs to be changed).
- Provide a practice brochure that also addresses policies with regard to medical precautions and the need for oral radiographs and collaboration with other health professionals.
- Provide written outlines of assessed needs and sequencing of appointments help the client to review and recall verbal case presentations.
- Send the client copies of letters to or from other health professionals concerning needed or ongoing care to inform the client of the shared interest in his or her oral health.

Legal, Ethical, and Safety Issues

- Client nonadherence with recommended oral healthcare is significant because it can result in compromised care, unsatisfactory care outcomes, client and practitioner dissatisfaction, and possibly litigation. In the event of a lawsuit, the judicial decision, outcome, or amount of settlement may be altered based on negligence of the practitioner if nonadherence was ignored.
- Client nonadherence must be carefully documented, including recommended care, all instructions not followed, the client's specific behavior and verbalizations about nonadherence, and any discussions of the consequence of not following recommendations.
- Clients whose uncooperative behavior impedes professional care may be legally discontinued from the practice by following precise legal protocols.
- Accurate records provide legal protection by providing documentary evidence for defense if necessary.
- Periodic chart reviews as part of quality assurance measures are needed to determine which clients are overdue for appointments and need to be contacted.

Key Concepts

- Practice management is the organization, administration, and direction of the professional practice to produce quality care, effective use of time and personnel, stress reduction, and satisfaction enhancement.
- The team concept in dental or dental hygiene practice is the interaction and interdependence of all staff members to promote the unity and efficiency of the group.
- Team building is the synergistic process of developing group goals with motivation and commitment.
- Quality care is the key to client satisfaction.
- Office policies are established to guide expectations and set consistency with the staff functions.
- Case presentations for the dental hygiene therapy explain the examination findings, discuss the treatment options, and make recommendations to guide and motivate the client in setting goals and choosing a care plan.
- Client nonadherence results in compromised treatment and results, and therefore must be recognized and discussed with the client and documented in the treatment record.
- Dental records serve as communication, education, assessment, and legal documentation, and therefore must be accurate, legible, concise, and thorough.
- Computers are being used in dentistry for multiple tasks, including word processing, accounting functions, data management, accessing evidence-based information, graphics, desktop publishing, communication, teleconferencing, and education.
- Periodontal health maintenance systems are established within dental and dental hygiene practices to ensure regular scheduling of appointments for established clients.
- Economic considerations within a dental or dental hygiene practice include office expenses, production, collection, and profit.
- Marketing a dental or dental hygiene practice involves the planning and management of services that benefit clients at a profit to the practice and involves the participation of all staff members.
- Client satisfaction will do more for practice promotion than any other strategy for marketing.

Critical Thinking Exercises

1. CASE PRESENTATION: Create an example of a client presenting with moderate periodontitis, including a sample periodontal chart demonstrating 4 to 6 mm of pocket depths in all four quadrants of the mouth. If possible, provide a set of full-mouth x-rays with evidence of subgingival calculus.
   A. Have the students role-play the case presentation of the dental hygienist presenting findings to the dentist to reach a collaborative dental hygiene care plan.
   B. Have the students role-play the case presentation of the dental hygienist presenting findings and the recommended dental hygiene treatment plan to the client. Be certain that the discussion contains all elements, including information of findings, education of significance of findings, options for care, choice by the client, agreement by the client, and recording case presentation in treatment record.
2. MARKETING PLAN: Develop a marketing plan to promote the dental hygiene portion of a dental practice.
   A. The plan should include specific activities or behaviors the team members intend to initiate and what each task is intended to accomplish.
   B. Include an overall timeline to complete the project, time frame for each task, labor division outline, outcome evaluation, and budget for the entire marketing plan.
3. Investigate the office management of a local dental and/or dental hygiene practice. Report back to the class on the "recall" system, the management of supplies and equipment, the mission and goals for the practice, OSHA compliance, and the layout of the office.

For References, Suggested Readings, and Related Websites, visit
http://evolve.elsevier.com/Darby/hygiene/

CHAPTER 53

PROFESSIONAL DEVELOPMENT

OBJECTIVES

Mastery of the content in this chapter will enable the reader to:

- ✦ Outline a personal plan for career development in the profession of dental hygiene
- ✦ Describe job search strategies, including a list of sources and a prioritized list of job selection criteria
- ✦ Explain the contributions of the dental hygienist to the dental practice
- ✦ Write an employment résumé and cover letter
- ✦ Outline a sample job interview, including sample questions for the dental office representative and possible questions the candidate may receive with appropriate responses
- ✦ Compare and contrast the methods of remuneration, including elements of risk and security and range in value for each
- ✦ Define the terms of dental hygiene employment and give examples of how they can be combined to fully describe the nature of an employment arrangement
- ✦ Create an employment compensation package, including method of compensation and fringe benefits, with total annual income value
- ✦ Design an employment contract, including elements of setting, job description, compensation, terms of employment, performance evaluation, and termination procedures
- ✦ Evaluate job performance, including expectations and techniques necessary for changing performance
- ✦ Explain why stress and burnout are common among dental hygienists and list stress management techniques
- ✦ Describe employment alternatives to clinical dental hygiene
- ✦ Develop a plan for personal financial management, including an annual budget, adequate insurance coverage, investment goals, and a retirement plan
- ✦ List the special tax deductions allowable to dental hygienists and the documentation necessary to support them

KEY TERMS

Burnout
Career development
Collaborative
Cover letter
Disability insurance
Employment arrangements
Employment contract
Estate planning
Financial planning
Fringe benefits
Independent contractor
Independent dental hygiene practice
Integral contributions
Interdependent
Liability insurance
Living trust
Methods of compensation
Networking
Office observation
Performance evaluation
Probate
Résumé
Retirement planning
Standard of care
Stress
Terms of employment
Umbrella insurance
Will
Working interview

The transition from the first job as a novice to employment as an expert can be smooth with proper preparation. The dental hygienist must prepare for all aspects of the job search and gain knowledge of the administrative details of employment. A vision of professional and personal financial management completes the picture for a rewarding career outcome.

CAREER DEVELOPMENT

Career development is defined as designing and following a course of action related to some noteworthy activity or pursuit that forms the total of one's work in a chosen field. A *career* is the composite of this life work in a profession; an *occupation* is a regular or principal business or line of work; a *job* is a position of employment to gain a livelihood. A career is differentiated from the others by offering a wide range of activities within one field. The elements of career development in dental hygiene include the following:

- Continuing and lifelong education to expand knowledge and skills in the field
- Maturation of professional skills
- Exploration of a variety of activities related to the profession to find areas of individual interest and expertise for continued participation
- Directing the success of client care or other work objectives and creating a positive work environment
- Participation in the growth of the profession through research, education, politics, organizational leadership, and/or public awareness
- Contributions to community service utilizing professional knowledge and skills
- Gaining personal gratification through these various activities

Each dental hygienist plans and directs his or her own career. Career maturation occurs when professional and personal roles expand. This includes broadening functions, relationships, and responsibility within the activities and events of the career. Functioning in different capacities enhances career development in relationship to the employer, other staff members, clients, other officers or members in a professional organization, other participants in a community committee or project, or those involved in other professional activities. The aim of career development is to select short-term objectives that support long-range goals for professional achievement and growth, all of which result in personal satisfaction. Consider the entirety of dental hygiene. Develop a list of areas to explore, then determine how to participate in each one. The greater the variety of activities, the greater the opportunity to find your niche. Establish a timeline for accomplishing each item on the list. This written record of career goals is used to continually guide direction and ensure commitment. Periodically, career goals are revised for growth, advancement, or change.

SEEKING EMPLOYMENT

Seeking employment is the search to make a match between an employer and an employee. Job availability varies across the country. In some areas, there is competition for each position. In other areas, there are too few hygienists for the number of job openings. It is projected that the working dental hygiene population will be 196,800 by 2006.[1] The employment search process begins with each party making an inventory of what each is seeking. The employer will have a job description—an outline of specific skills and knowledge required to perform the job—and an idea of the suitable attitude and personal characteristics needed to fit in well with the setting. The potential employee will need a list of job selection criteria.

A *passive* job seeker waits until jobs are advertised and then mails standard cover letters and résumés to a number of ads. An *active* job seeker modifies both résumé and cover letter for a specific job target before a job is announced.[2] Efforts are made to talk with a prospective interviewer to penetrate a hidden job market or expand the dental hygiene portion of a dental practice in order to secure a job in a desirable environment.

Job Selection Considerations

When considering which job to select, the dental hygienist compares career needs and desires with what is being offered by the potential employer. A list is made of qualities valued in a dental practice or other dental hygiene job sought. This list may include such elements as quality care, prevention oriented, team players working in a reciprocal manner, mutual appreciation among team members as well as regard for clients, and educational growth within the job setting. Look for an employment situation that provides the ability to develop relationships that are both *interdependent,* with team members working supportively to accomplish the best possible combined outcomes, and *collaborative,* communicating and behaving cooperatively with respect and trust. It is important to determine which of the following details are of greatest importance personally:

- Overall practice ambiance and atmosphere
- Practice philosophy, goals, and values
- Personal harmony felt with the office atmosphere and staff members
- Interactions with clients (e.g., "professionally distant" or "personal and caring")
- Practice standards and quality of care provided; evidence-based decision making expected
- General job description, including the specific responsibilities and the scope of dental hygiene care provided
- General work conditions (i.e., workload, scheduling, pace, hours, equipment, supplies, instruments)
- Overall role, responsibility, and esteem of the dental hygienist within the practice

- Compensation package consisting of salary, fringe benefits, opportunity for bonuses, schedule, and basis for remuneration increases
- Concern with feelings of belonging to the practice "team"
- Opportunity for professional growth, continuing education, and personal satisfaction
- Job security with an assured client load plus established record of employee longevity
- Practice open to innovation or content to maintain the status quo
- Location of employment setting, commuting, and parking situation
- Practice well-established, new and growing, stable, or restructuring and in transition; staff large or small

The right choice for job selection should satisfy the greatest number of professional values, desires, and needs possible. Applicants will need to prioritize their criteria, then choose the employment setting that offers the most matches. Feeling excited about starting a new job is a good beginning.

Job Search Strategies

Preparation for the job search on the part of the employee begins by clarifying career and personal goals. A careful assessment can lead to a successful, fulfilling, and expansive job as well as prevent a poor employment match and, later, job dissatisfaction. One should imagine the ideal job situation, with such elements that motivate and gratify, then seek or create one that closely fits this image.

Applicants should investigate the job market, studying local trends in career opportunities, job descriptions, workloads, salary and benefits, the possibility of job sharing, compensation packages, job turnovers, and layoffs (see Sources for Locating Dental Hygiene Employment). Speak with dental hygienists working in the area and the local component employment chairperson of the American Dental Hygienists' Association. Don't be afraid to telephone a reputable dental office and inquire about a current or future job opening there. Be aware of the full value of the dental hygienist to the dental practice. Send a résumé promptly so as to be among the first seen. Do not underrate personal abilities and do not undercut a wage.

Sources for Locating Dental Hygiene Employment

Friends, colleagues, and other professional contacts using the word-of-mouth approach (networking)
Verbal or printed announcements at meetings and conferences
Dental society employment placement services
Dental hygiene association employment placement services
Private healthcare providers' employment placement agencies
Public or county health departments
Dental hygiene school employment opportunities bulletin boards
Dental hygiene and dental association newsletters and journals, section on employment vacancies
Employment opportunity bulletin boards in large office buildings
Professional people in the geographic vicinity where work is sought; people mentioned in association newsletters, association leaders, authors, speakers, and educators
Web sites for employment opportunities
Local dental association membership directories, alumni association membership directories, telephone books with local dental office listings
Dental supply houses or supply salespersons
Newspaper classified advertisements

INTEGRAL CONTRIBUTIONS OF THE DENTAL HYGIENIST

The dental hygienist is a valuable member of the dental team that helps generate revenue and attract clients. The dental hygienist benefits the dental practice beyond tangible clinical skills and services. These intangible benefits or *integral contributions* make the hygienist indispensable to the oral healthcare team in the following ways:

- The dental hygienist educates clients, instructing them in self-care and teaching them to look for signs of oral, dental, and periodontal diseases. Dental hygiene strategies encourage and motivate clients to become responsible for the maintenance of their own oral health.
- By performing the multiple roles of clinician, researcher, consumer advocate, change agent, educator and oral health promoter, and manager, the hygienist facilitates a progressive practice.
- The hygienist provides release time for the dentist by performing preliminary examinations and discussing findings and possible therapies with clients. The hygienist answers client questions, directs clients to additional resources, and presents practice philosophies, thereby providing the dentist with more time to perform restorative and surgical services.
- The dental hygienist is a professional associate of the dentist in a collaborative relationship, communicating together about clinical findings and care options. By participating together in case evaluations and care planning, maximal use is made of the dental hygienist's knowledge, skills, and experience.
- The dental hygienist supports the dentist by performing and documenting multiple assessments with expertise (e.g., vital signs; personal, health histories; extraoral and intraoral examinations; evaluation of outcomes of periodontal surgical and nonsurgical treatments) and explaining findings to the client.
- As a marketer of oral healthcare, the dental hygienist facilitates high case acceptance for procedures from individual crowns and restorations to complex, long-term restorative plans and cosmetic dentistry. The

dental hygienist also provides informed consent information, presenting possible risks, benefits, and alternatives to different treatment options based on the best available research evidence.

- ✦ The dental hygienist is a practice builder, interacting with clients as a professional relations specialist, interpreter to facilitate communications with the dentist, confidant, practice ambassador, and friend. Public relations are promoted when the hygienist builds confidence in the practice by describing the fine quality of dentistry provided by the dental team and speaks highly and enthusiastically about the lifetime value of oral health. A client often remains with a practice and refers new clients because of the dental hygienist.
- ✦ Dental hygienists participate in office staff meetings in both a "team player" role and a leadership role. All personnel attend staff meetings to share information, generate ideas, and solve problems together. The hygienist brings topics to the meetings of scientific or practice management importance from professional literature and conferences.
- ✦ The hygienist is responsible for the evaluation of client care in the prevention portion of the practice. The role is therefore expanded to include practice analysis, recommending revisions and implementing changes as needed to create an improved situation.

PREPARATION FOR THE EMPLOYMENT QUEST

Writing a Résumé

The *résumé* is a brief, written summary that highlights achievements and enhances the introduction of the dental hygienist to create a positive professional first impression and to secure a job interview. It is written for the potential employer, not the job applicant. The résumé is like an advertisement that is intended to stimulate the reader to want to learn more. It presents an inventory of professional qualifications, assets, and goals, which can generate a job interview or eliminate a purposeless interview; and leaves a visible reminder of the applicant to the potential employer following an interview. The résumé types are defined as *blanket*, which is a general résumé for all jobs in the related field, and *specific*, which is designed with one particular job in mind.

The résumé styles can be either descriptive or functional. The most common style, *descriptive*, traditionally lists education, experience, and qualifications by date, in reverse chronologic order. Title headings are used to organize the contents such as career objective, academic history, career summary, professional employment experience, professional activities, awards and honors, community service, and references. The name of the institution, date of graduation, major, and degree earned are listed under academic history. For work experience, the name of the dentist or group, location, and dates (beginning and end) of employment are delineated. Specific references, which are not required on the résumé, should be provided at the interview. When written on the résumé, references should include name, title, employer, address, and business telephone.

The *functional* résumé states effective skills and accomplishments that support a specific job position and reflect ability in individual areas of expertise. Here special types of proficiencies such as communications, management, leadership, motivation, or clinical excellence are highlighted. The functional résumé stresses results. Accomplishments are listed using action words such as *achieved, assembled, collaborated, created, directed, expanded, generated, implemented, improved, maintained, managed, marketed, motivated, organized, planned, resolved,* and *supervised.* Numbers are used to define and quantify responsibilities and achievements. Some elements of the functional résumé may be combined with the descriptive. Components of a Quality Résumé describes the contents of a quality résumé.

To begin developing a résumé and to keep it current as your career progresses, use a notecard system to collect all pertinent information throughout your career. On each card write one item, including date and location, for your educational credentials and licensure, awards and honors, employment experience, professional activities, volunteer or community service, and special professional accomplishments. As you identify areas of functional expertise, write cards for those skills, too. Organize the cards to begin writing your résumé, selecting the pertinent items for either the blanket or specific résumé.

The descriptive résumé for the dental hygiene graduate seeking a first job may include the following: career or professional goals, education and licensure, academic achievements and honors, workshops and conferences attended, class leadership, membership in professional organizations, table clinics/research poster sessions, community dental health projects, community volunteer activities and humanitarian services, student teaching, work experience in the dental field, and other related work or business experience. The descriptive résumé for the veteran dental hygienist will include career or professional goals, education and licensure, continuing education areas of emphasis, employment experience, professional activities, community service, awards and honors, and optional references. Accomplishments, special skills, and management and leadership abilities demonstrated in work experience may be highlighted.

Honesty and accuracy are the most important elements of résumé writing; be certain all contents are correct. Use concise phrases with descriptive terminology, demonstrating confident action and professional interest; emphasize individual qualities, avoiding a list of general responsibilities; and be credible and do not exaggerate. The résumé format is brief; one page is preferred, although two pages are acceptable. It may be visually enhanced by font styles, boldface, or bullets; typed,

Components of a Quality Résumé

Personal Identification
Name
Address
Telephone

Job Objective
Statement of the exact job being sought, giving résumé focus
Brief philosophic statement
Professional goals

Career Summary
Creating a sense of the applicant and what has been accomplished professionally
Skills
Strengths
Assets

Academic History
Schooling applicable to the job objective
College/university
Date of graduation
Degree(s) received
Honors and awards
Dental hygiene licensure
Special certificates

Professional Employment Experience
Summarize any responsibilities not generally encompassed by the normal dental hygiene job description and note any special awards received. New licentiates can list special skills/interests from school, jobs in related fields, or academic honors and awards.
Private practice
Teaching
Administrative
Research
Government

Professional Data (optional)
Professional affiliations
Community and professional services
Publications
Presentations given
Continuing education courses attended
Professional projects

References (optional)
If included, be certain reference sources are notified and willing to speak highly of applicant
"Available upon request" *or*
List two sources

typeset, and word-processed presentations are acceptable. An original or high-quality photocopy on medium-weight white or ivory paper looks most professional. The résumé is organized with bold functional headings to introduce each category. Spaces and wide margins are used for easy readability. The résumé is often the potential employer's first glance at the applicant. It quickly forms the image that a potential employer will have of the job applicant's skills and abilities. Therefore, overall, it must appear polished, neat, accurate, and letter-perfect with correct spelling and grammar. Sample résumés appear in Figures 53–1 and 53–2.

Designing a Cover Letter

The *cover letter* introduces the applicant and the résumé to the prospective employer. Its purpose is to highlight the most important qualifications of the dental hygienist and to personalize the résumé. It informs a potential employer of your goals, direction, and values. The cover letter format is brief and simple, two to three paragraphs, and should not repeat the content of the résumé. A remark of how the applicant learned about the job availability may open the cover letter followed by a statement of interest in the specific practice. Comments that show an understanding of the prospective employer's needs and how the applicant's skills specifically match this job will demonstrate a clear interest in the position and appeal to the employer's pride in the practice.

Another paragraph of the cover letter may contain personal attributes that describe the applicant and would add intrinsic value to a dental practice. These attributes

Cindy Browne, R.D.H., B.S. 415-882-3434
1661 "M" Street
San Francisco, CA 94112

JOB OBJECTIVE
Registered dental hygienist seeking employment with additional responsibilities in local anesthesia, soft tissue management, and nitrous oxide–oxygen analgesia.

LICENSURE & EDUCATION
California Registered Dental Hygienist License DH 38991
B.S. in Dental Hygiene—June 1994
University of California at San Francisco
School of Dentistry

WORK EXPERIENCE
1990 to 1995—Summers
Dental Assistant in various dental offices in San Francisco.
Employed as a "temporary" for an employment agency.

REFERENCES
Jennifer Jones, R.D.H., M.S., Director
Dental Hygiene Program at UCSF
Telephone: 415-444-1234

Additional references available on request from former employers.

PRIMARY AIMS
I wish to contribute my skills and knowledge to a prevention-oriented dental practice. My goal is to become part of an office team whose members are mutually supportive and positive in their approach to client care.

FIGURE 53–1 ✦ Sample of a new graduate résumé.

might include such qualities as reliable, responsible, friendly, personal warmth, strength of character, team player, plus good communication and interpersonal skills. Such elements are not listed in the résumé, yet are key to employee selection and retention. In the cover letter, make reference to the enclosed résumé, bringing attention to one or two key elements pertinent to this specific job. Lastly, a sentence about the applicant's intention to contact the dental office to arrange a meeting should be included. The final line should simply thank the reader for reviewing the letter and express hopeful anticipation for mutual benefit.

The cover letter should be an original page, individually typed, personally signed, and not photocopied. It is to be neat, accurate, typed letter-perfect on bond or other paper that matches the résumé with correct spelling and grammar, and addressed to the person of authority, using the person's name and title. An example of a cover letter appears in Figure 53–3.

Interviews

Interviews provide a mutual opportunity for reciprocal information exchange and to evaluate for congruent job objectives. The interviewer appraises the candidate's qualifications (résumé), professional philosophy, and behavior. The candidate appraises the interviewer and the employment situation with regard to job description and responsibility, practice philosophy, staff members as potential co-workers, office environment, working conditions, and opportunity for job satisfaction, professional growth, challenge, and responsibility. A series of interviews is often conducted before a job is offered and a job selection is made. Complete and thoughtful interviews are important to provide the best opportunity for both parties to make the right choice for employment and to avoid a mismatch.

Interview styles may follow a specific structured pattern of formatted questions or may be loosely structured and broad, allowing for interaction between the interviewer and the candidate. A combination-type interview is most common. In rare cases there may be a *group* interview, when several candidates are grouped together at one time with the expectation by the interviewer that one candidate will emerge superior to the others. Or there may be a *board* interview, in which there is one candidate meeting with several interviewers. In this case, each interviewer asks questions.

A screening process precedes scheduling an interview. The initial evaluation identifies potentially acceptable positions for the dental hygienist-applicant and eliminates those employment settings that are unacceptable. The screening may be done via the telephone and may include a series of basic questions about the position. The dental hygienist-applicant pays close attention to the office "tone" during these conversations. An interview

Susan Jensen, R.D.H., M.S. 415-525-5566
11 California Way
San Francisco, CA 92110

LICENSURE & EDUCATION
California Registered Dental Hygienist License DH3322
Certification in Expanded Functions: Local Anesthesia, Soft Tissue Curettage, and Nitrous Oxide–Oxygen Analgesia
M.A. Education, San Francisco State University: 1975
B.S. Dental Hygiene, University of Southern California: 1970

EMPLOYMENT
Dental Hygienist in General Dental Practice 1985 to Present
Rodney Mann, D.D.S., San Francisco

Dental Hygienist in Periodontal Practice 1970 to 1985
Robert Hanson, D.D.S., San Francisco

TEACHING
Instructor of Dental Hygiene 1975 to Present
Diablo Valley College

COMMUNITY
Community Oral Health Projects 1970 to 1994

REFERENCES available on request.

CAREER GOALS
I would like to build on my skills and interests in health education and communications within a people- and prevention-oriented dental practice. My professional satisfaction comes from contributing thorough periodontal assessment and quality periodontal therapy services of lasting value.

FIGURE 53–2 ✦ Sample résumé of a veteran hygienist.

1234 Main Street 415-321-4455
San Francisco, CA 94110

October 15, 1995

John Joplin, D.D.S.
444 No. University Avenue
San Francisco, CA 94115

Dear Dr. Joplin,

Dental hygiene care is the foundation of a sound dental practice. Persons maintained on a continued care basis will enjoy a healthy periodontium and dentition as well as keep your practice viable and growing.

As a registered dental hygienist skilled in periodontal care and effective communications, I would like to contribute to the increasing success of your practice. My emphasis is on client assessment and treatment sequencing with certification in local anesthesia and nitrous oxide–oxygen analgesia.

I would enjoy meeting with you to hear your views about dental hygiene care within your dental practice. My résumé is enclosed for your review. You will see by the workshops I have attended that I have a strong interest in periodontics and practice enhancement.

I shall be calling next week to set a meeting date.

Sincerely,

Nancy Smith, R.D.H., B.S.

FIGURE 53–3 ✦ Cover letter.

appointment is scheduled if both the office and the applicant pass the initial screening. Applicants should confirm the date, time, and location of the interview and obtain directions to the office. An expected, agreed-upon length of time is established for the appointment and the interviewer is determined. In some cases the potential employer is not the person who conducts the preliminary interview; rather, the senior dental hygienist or the office manager may process the bulk of applicants before the dentist meets "the finalists."

Preparation for the interview requires self-knowledge for the dental hygienist-applicant. The dental hygienist must define personal standards and qualifications (e.g., skill strengths and weaknesses, employment expectations and desires, professional philosophy, and short- and long-term career goals). (Refer to previous section on Job Selection Considerations.) The position should be studied and selected if it meets these standards. Learning the characteristics of the practice, the dentist and the staff members, and the client population is important. Speaking with current or former employees or other dentists and professionals in the area is beneficial. The object is to find out as much as possible about the philosophy and work environment of the practice before appearing for the interview, then tailor a job-interview style to match personal strengths to the needs of the practice. Some applicants practice by role-playing a mock interview by writing out possible questions asked of candidates and presenting answers out loud. Some applicants write out questions for the interviewer about the practice and the available position. A colleague may critique the rehearsal. For ideas of questions to ask during an interview, refer to Questions and Considerations for Job Interviews.

Questions and Considerations for Job Interviews

Mission of Practice

What is the mission statement of the practice?

What are the supporting goals and objectives for reaching this mission?

How are these goals and objectives measured or evaluated?

How does the dental hygienist contribute to the goals and objectives?

Does the practice treat adults and children?

Does the practice discriminate by limiting or denying treatment to any types of individuals?

How does the practice and its team members keep up to date with scientific information and procedures?

Are decisions evidence-based?

Are there opportunities for professional growth for the dental hygienist?

Practice Team and Practice Management

What is the dentist's education and experience?

How long has the dentist been in this practice?

How many people work in the practice each day? Name all the practice team members with their job titles and describe their employment responsibilities.

How many clients are usually seen per day within the entire practice?

How does the dentist supervise the staff team members?

If there are other dental hygienists working in the practice, what is their work experience, both within this practice and others? Ask to meet with them and ask them questions about philosophy of practice.

Is there an office manual with practice policies and procedures plus job descriptions for each job title? Do staff members follow these guidelines?

Does the practice employ a practice consultant regularly?

Who is the real practice manager?

Does the practice usually stay on schedule and finish the day on time?

Are there staff meetings? If so, how often are staff meetings held?

Are staff meetings held during office hours or after office hours?

If staff meetings are conducted after office hours, how are staff members compensated for staff meeting time? Request an agenda or description of a typical staff meeting. If there are no staff meetings, what means of communication are used to convey practice information between staff members?

Does the office participate in any team-building activities?

Do members of the staff socialize outside the office?

Health Maintenance, Disease Prevention, and Health Promotion

Would this be considered a health maintenance and "preventive" practice?

What are the preventive elements of this practice?

Who, besides the dental hygienist, educates clients about health?

How would the dentist describe a healthy periodontium and dentition?

Does the practice attend to any elements of clients' systemic health and well-being?

Ask to see a complete client folder with treatment record; charts for intraoral and extraoral exams, dentition, occlusion and periodontics; radiographs; photographs; and health history, including baseline recordings of blood pressure and pulse, etc.

How often are the health history questionnaire and vital signs completely updated for each client?

What questions are asked each appointment to update the health history and how is it documented?

Under what circumstances is a client's physician consulted for advice regarding oral healthcare?

Observe the appearance and demeanor of all staff members you meet for signs of good general health.

Terms of Employment

When does the job start?

How many days per week are available for work? Which specific days?

What are the work hours? Are there mid-day breaks? When is the lunch hour?

What is the workload? How many clients are treated per day?

Continued on following page

Questions and Considerations for Job Interviews—cont'd

Terms of Employment—cont'd

How much time is allowed for dental hygiene care?

Are there variable appointment lengths for healthy adults, active periodontal therapy care, periodontal maintenance care, new client care, and/or children?

Is there any flexibility in the workload, daily starting or ending times, and/or length of lunch break?

Who opens and closes the office? If the dental hygienist participates in either or both, what are the tasks for each?

Is there an assistant for the dental hygienist on a full- or part-time basis?

Is there a receptionist to schedule and confirm dental hygiene appointments?

What is the protocol for both planned time off and unexpected time off?

Is care provided by personnel as directed by the Dental Practice Act?

Are there days or hours when the dental hygienist will provide client care in the absence of a dentist being present (if state supervision laws permit)?

Job Description and Practice Protocols

How is the dental hygienist involved in new client care?

What are the responsibilities for returning client care?

Request to see the health and dental history questionnaire. Who reviews this information? How often is it updated?

Does the dental hygienist or other staff member take and record client blood pressure? How often?

What is the practice protocol for antibiotic premedication and restrictions on treating clients with elevated blood pressure?

What are radiographic exposure recommendations for new and returning clients? Who determines when and which x-rays are to be taken?

Does the dental hygienist take radiographs? Does the dental hygienist develop and mount radiographs? Ask to see the x-ray equipment and processor.

Ask to view sample mouth radiographs to evaluate for diagnostic quality.

What elements are included in a complete new client examination?

What is involved in a complete periodontal assessment? How often is a full periodontal assessment done on each client?

What is the practice protocol on "selective coronal polishing?"

How often does the dentist examine the client? Is the exam done while the client is in the dental hygiene care room? What is the timing of the examination: before, during, after dental hygiene care, and length of time required by the dentist? Does the dental hygienist assist the dentist during the examination?

Does the practice sell products directly to the clients?

Periodontics

Who performs the periodontal examination on clients? How often?

Ask to see a periodontal examination form.

Do the dentist and dental hygienist work collaboratively to determine a care plan for periodontal needs?

Does the practice participate in nonsurgical periodontal therapy?

What are the elements of nonsurgical periodontal therapy that the practice supports and performs?

What constitutes supportive periodontal therapy in the practice?

How is the decision made to refer a client to a periodontist?

Do you refer to one periodontist or several? How is the choice of periodontist determined?

If a client is shared with a periodontist, does the dental hygienist participate in the communications with the periodontist?

Are the client's supportive periodontal therapy intervals varied depending on need?

Who determines the supportive periodontal therapy intervals?

What is the level of client compliance with prevention and periodontal health maintenance efforts?

What is the average continued care interval for adult clients?

Dental Hygiene Decision Making and Presentation

Does the dentist review clients' charts before their arrival at the office and direct recommended care?

How is the periodontal diagnosis determined? Do the dentist and dental hygienist establish the diagnosis collaboratively?

Who presents the periodontal diagnosis to the client?

Who determines the periodontal treatment plan? Do the dentist and dental hygienist establish the plan collaboratively?

Are there different treatment plan options for different periodontal needs? Are there multiple appointments and variable appointment lengths for treatment of active periodontal disease? Do the dentist and hygienist determine these collaboratively?

How often is retreatment performed for recurring periodontal disease?

Who presents the periodontal treatment plan to the client?

Who discusses risks, benefits, and alternatives to the recommended periodontal treatment with the client?

Who discusses fees and dental insurance considerations with the client?

Are periodontal reevaluation appointments scheduled? If yes, how are intervals determined and how much time is scheduled for the appointment?

Dental Hygiene Care Room and Services

Ask to see the dental hygiene treatment room.

Is the dental chair and other equipment old or new?

Where is the radiographic equipment and is it modern?

Is the room fully equipped as you would like it? If not, will the practice provide what you need?

Is there adequate space in the room to move around the dental chair?

Does the care room provide adequate privacy?

Does the dental hygienist use manual and ultrasonic instruments?

Ask to view the instruments to evaluate their quality and quantity.

What products (e.g., antimicrobials, anesthetics, fluorides, and desensitizing agents) are available for client treatment? If you have preferences that are not available, will the practice purchase them?

What products (e.g., toothbrushes, floss, toothpick holders, interproximal devices, fluorides) are available for distribution as samples to clients? If you have preferences that are not available, will the practice purchase them?

Questions and Considerations for Job Interviews—cont'd

Dental Hygiene Care Room and Services—cont'd

What methods of pain control are used and how often?

Is nitrous oxide and oxygen analgesia available in the office? If yes, how often is it used?

Does the practice provide fluoride therapy for adult clients?

Other Work Responsibilities

What are the recordkeeping and documentation requirements for dental hygiene services?

What are the specific tasks necessary to clean and maintain and stock the dental hygiene care room at the beginning and end of each day?

What are the responsibilities of the dental hygienist in the lab?

Are there dental hygienist responsibilities elsewhere for office maintenance?

Who is responsible for inventory management for dental hygiene supplies, instruments, and client products? Repairs?

Practice Safety for Employees

Who is the practice safety officer?

Where is the OSHA manual? Does it contain information on health risk exposures, vaccinations, and testing?

Does the practice adhere to OSHA guidelines and standards?

What is the practice attire? What protective clothing is provided to employees?

Are the gloves, masks, and safety glasses adequate?

How are the dental instruments sterilized? Are the sterilization units monitored?

Where and how are biohazards disposed?

Where is the sharps container?

Are there adequate fire extinguishers and smoke detectors? Where are they located?

What is the evacuation plan in case of building emergency?

Medical Emergencies (see Chapter 7)

Who in the office is currently CPR certified? Does the office provide CPR recertification for the practice team together?

Does the staff have a practiced plan in case of medical emergency?

Where is the oxygen tank located? How is it operated?

Where is the emergency medical kit located? What does it contain?

Who knows how to use its contents?

Where is the office first-aid kit located in case of on-the-job accident?

What is the practice protocol in case of an HIV-positive sharps accident?

Modified from Rogo EJ: Career development. In Hodges K, ed: *Concepts in nonsurgical periodontal therapy,* Albany, 1998, Delmar.

The preliminary interview is an opportunity to establish rapport between the interviewer and the candidate. The candidate presents qualifications as represented on the résumé and shares the professional philosophy. Strengths of education and experience are stressed, demonstrating the candidate's potential as an employee. New licentiates can address lack of experience with "eagerness to learn" attitudes.

The interviewer presents the position represented by the job description, the dental hygienist's responsibilities, the nature of participation with the practice team, and the opportunity for professional growth. The practice philosophy and/or mission statement and description of the office atmosphere and work environment also are presented. Three questions commonly asked of the candidate during the preliminary interview are the following:

- What are you looking for in a job?
- Why should we hire you?
- What are your professional goals?

In addition, interviewers may create scenarios for the applicant to discuss, such as:

- What would you do if a young patient was uncooperative?
- How would you respond to a patient who refused radiographs?

Preparation to answer these questions will be time well spent. There may be an initial discussion of compensation presented at this interview. Compatibility is established by linking the candidate's skills and strengths with the job description and needs of the practice. Plans may be discussed to accommodate for weaknesses in the match. Both parties may work from written notes or a list of important questions. The preliminary interview is concluded with a summary of the findings, a statement of general compatibility or acknowledgment of incompatibility from either party, an invitation to return for a follow-up interview, or possibly a job offer.

The candidate may request an *office observation* session following the first interview and before job acceptance. During the office observation, the dental hygienist attends a typical workday or partial day in the practice to view the staff members in action with clients. This is an excellent chance to have some of your questions answered and may also create new questions for the final interview. Notice the overall working ambiance or environment for the attitude and mood of the employees and clients. Watch for thoughtful and respectful communications between staff members and with clients. Look to see how safety, sanitation, and sterilization methods and precautions are actually employed. Check to see that all of the equipment functions as it should. Investigate whether the dental hygienist actually receives support with tasks from other staff members. Determine who the real office manager is or whether the management is shared among multiple staff members. Ascertain how the dentist is supervising employees. See if the dentist collaborates with the dental hygienist to determine direction of client care or if the dental hygienist makes decisions independently. Decide if the quality of the elements you observe is congruent with the quality you wish to provide. Record your observations and questions for discussion at the next meeting with the potential future employer.

The second interview, or selection interview, provides an opportunity for both the candidate and the office staff members to have a second look at each other. A thorough discussion of the details of the job should include the job description and office policies and procedures, work schedule, compensation package of starting wage and benefits, and the frequency and basis of raises. A *working interview* may be the second interview, whereby the prospective employee works in the office for a one-day trial. Although the working interview is becoming more common, there are precautions about its effectiveness. The first day on any job is challenging and complex, often with a sense of disorientation. The one-day employee may have trouble locating supplies and operating unfamiliar equipment. Each office has its own distinct system for appointment scheduling and recordkeeping. If you are working on clients, you are not free to roam around the office to observe others and get a sense of the entire office. The working interview may result in frustration, rather than accomplish the goal of answering questions about the practice.

Techniques for Successful Job Interviews

The following recommendations, if implemented, enhance the success of employment interviews:

- *Know and believe in yourself.* Memorize your professional goals and accomplishments. Keep spirits high and do not get discouraged. Heed personal intuition during interviews and when making the job selection decision.
- *Be prompt.* Do not arrive late to the interview, nor arrive more than 15 minutes early. If you know you are going to be late, telephone the office before the appointed time with an apology and appropriate explanation plus an estimated time of arrival.
- Wear attire that makes a professional impression.
- Dress as though you represent the organization with which you are interviewing.
- Greet the practice receptionist or secretary with friendliness and respect; this is the all-important first impression.
- Present a personal style that is friendly, self-assured, and sincere.
- *Convey interest and eagerness to learn about the practice.* The first minutes are critical to candidate selection: quickly establish comfort and rapport to set the tone for the rest of the interview.
- *Address the interviewer by name,* especially when greeting and upon leaving the appointment; wait for the interviewer to begin the questioning first and follow the interviewer's lead. Listen carefully to each question and answer the actual question asked, responding with direct, thoughtful, concise answers. Ask for clarification if a question is not clearly understood; if there is an unanswerable question, say so; do not fake it. Be articulate and answer with details to establish a memorable impression; give examples of proven ability and professionalism, but try not to repeat what is on the résumé. Establish credibility and trust; above all, be honest and do not misrepresent yourself.
- *Do not offer information about your personal life.* This is irrelevant to the position. Listen carefully for any problems, difficulties, negatives, or disappointments subtly exposed by the interviewer. Be diplomatic and tactful; avoid complaining or negatively judging past experiences, jobs, employers, colleagues, schools, or teachers; do not exaggerate past work performance; and focus on professional, not personal, statements.
- *Interview the interviewer on a parity basis.* Be proactive with prepared comments about practice philosophy and professional goals. Ask specific, intelligent questions that will provide the information needed to determine if this is the position sought. Failing to ask questions is a common error made by job candidates; questions demonstrate an interest in the job. Always ask, "What qualifications are you looking for in the dental hygienist who fills this position?" If the response indicates this is a mismatch, the candidate can say so and cut the interview short; if desirable, the candidate can stress matching qualities. It is reasonable to ask about the work style of the practice, such as daily pace, whether they generally stay on schedule, level of dental hygienist responsibility, and frequency of collaboration among staff members. Other appropriate questions include longevity of current or previous employees and reasons for employee departure from the practice.
- Nonverbal communications and body language send the message of self-confidence. Shake hands firmly upon introductions, display a dental hygiene smile, maintain good posture, be seated only at the invitation of the interviewer, retain a calm body position, and use eye contact throughout the interview.
- Be cautious to contain nervous habits (e.g., inappropriate laughter, too chatty); do not fidget, smoke, or chew gum.
- Demonstrate that the primary reason for the interview is to gain information about the position, and resist the temptation to ask about money. Although there may be brief mention of the wage or salary range during the interview, any salary negotiations should occur after a job offer is received.
- Depart from the interview with a smile, a handshake, and a clear idea of the employer's notification schedule. Thank-you notes reflect positively on the sender, but generally have little effect on enhancing a job

offer because almost all interview decisions are made the day of the interview. The contents of the note may reiterate interest in the position and summarize why the practice should be interested in the candidate. In the event of a second interview, the first thank-you note can win friends in the job setting and communicate gratitude and good etiquette.

EMPLOYMENT

Compensation

The *methods of compensation* for dental hygiene employment are varied and determined by agreement between the employee and employer. The dental hygienist must consider several elements in compensation considerations, including the average rate and method of remuneration in the area, the fees for dental hygiene services in this practice, and her experience and background as they apply value to this job. In 1999, the national average hourly rate was $24, with $38,850 average annual fixed salary.[3] To determine the going rate for salary in your area, you may telephone dental hygienists working in the area, contact the component dental hygienists' association employment chairperson, or contact a local employment agency specializing in dental office employment.

It is the initial task and responsibility of the dental hygienist to establish the best possible financial arrangements with the employer. Remuneration may include a combination of wage plus fringe benefits. With continuous employment in one oral healthcare setting, it is later the task and challenge of the dental hygienist to renegotiate for improved financial arrangements. See Methods of Compensation. Be certain to discuss salary increases before you begin a job, with consideration for frequency and methods for determining these increases. Some reasons for salary growth include office fee increases, dental hygiene production improvement, cost-of-living changes, automatic incremental increases, performance evaluation, longevity, and new or additional services rendered by the dental hygienist.

In addition to the primary topic of wages, there are other elements to establish regarding compensation. Inquire as to the method of documentation for work time and the frequency of pay periods. Are you expected to arrive early to open the office and set up or stay late to restock and clean up? If attendance at staff meetings is required during nonwork hours, the employer is required to pay for your time. Inquire as to whether the employer will also pay for your travel time and child-care, if needed, for these required after-hours staff meetings. If the office is closed for holidays or other occasions, will you be paid?

Fringe Benefits

Fringe benefits are services paid by the employer in addition to regular wages. Legally required benefits that must be offered by the employer are a portion of Social Security, including old age benefits, survivor's benefits in the case of death of the employee, disability benefits for some medically caused total disabilities, and hospital insurance after age 65 (Medicare); worker's compensation, which protects the employee from medical expenses and loss of income in the event of injury on the job or job-related disability; and federal unemployment insurance, which provides benefits to individuals involuntarily unemployed. Additionally, some states are required to provide state disability insurance benefits for nonoccupational accidents or illnesses, state worker's compensation, and/or health insurance.

Methods of Compensation

Fixed Salary
A guaranteed fixed wage is paid for hourly, daily, weekly, or monthly employment.

Salary Plus Commission
A base salary is paid, plus an additional percentage of fees charged for dental hygiene services.

Commission with Guaranteed Minimum Salary
A percentage of fees charged for dental hygiene services is paid, with an assured minimum wage per day regardless of daily gross production.

Commission
Earnings are based on a percentage of fees charged for dental hygiene services. (Note: It is illegal for an employer to pay a commission to an employee based on fees collected.)

Independent Contractor
The dental hygienist sets and collects all fees and pays overhead costs with the profit fluctuation based on production, collection, and expenses.

Overtime
Usually for hourly wage earners only, time-and-a-half is paid for all hours in excess of the contracted hours per week.

Compensatory Time Off ("Comp Time")
Hours or days off are given for excess time worked beyond the established work week; used in place of overtime pay.

Profit-Sharing Bonus
A work incentive is awarded to employees after profit goals are achieved for a specified period; may be calculated monthly, quarterly, or annually.

Fringe Benefits
Paid services in addition to regular wages. Some benefits are required by law and some are optional services offered by the employer or requested by the dental hygienist. Fringe benefits paid for by the employer are tax deductible to the employer.

Optional fringe benefits or "perks" are special services and items offered in addition to salary (see Optional Fringe Benefits). On average, benefits received by dental hygienists are few. The most common fringe benefits that dental hygienists receive are continuing education, free or discounted dental care, and paid vacations or holidays.[3] Benefits may be paid for directly by the employer or there may be reimbursement for expenses to the employee. Prepaid fringe benefits are desirable because of the tax advantage of their being received directly from the employer rather than buying them with after-tax paycheck dollars. They are financially beneficial to the employer because taxes listed previously are not charged on fringe benefits. Some dentists think that because they pay a high salary to dental hygienists, they should not also have to pay for benefits. They may intentionally exclude dental hygienists from benefits offered to other employees by job title or part-time employment status.

Fringe benefits vary tremendously from practice to practice. Within one practice, they may be the same for each employee or the employer may provide a dollar amount package for each employee. This flexible package allows each person to design the most desirable individual benefit plan.

Employment Arrangements

Employment arrangements define how the dental hygienist works in the business relationship and relate to tax status. The Internal Revenue Service (IRS) defines the rules and guidelines for business relationships as well as the tax requirements of each type of employment. Employment arrangements are different and separate from the practice supervision issues that are determined by state statutes. Dental Practice Acts are legislative law, or statutes, that describe a profession and define whether a dental hygienist works under general or direct supervision. These acts do not apply to the business association between the dentist and hygienist. The employer-employee relationship, wherein the dental hygienist works as an employee within the practice structure, is the most common arrangement for dental hygiene employment. In this situation, all financial concerns of operating the practice are the responsibility of the employer. The employer pays the employee on an hourly wage; daily, weekly, or monthly salary; or commission basis, withholding federal, state, and Social Security taxes from the employee's paycheck.

Employment arrangements may be any of the following: the dental hygienist's employer may be a dentist;

Optional Fringe Benefits

Paid Absences

Sick Leave. Salary paid during occasional short-term illnesses; usually sick leave benefits are allowed to accumulate if not used, or unused days are paid at the end of the year as a bonus

Holidays. Salary paid for usual, nationally observed holidays

Vacation. Salary paid for vacation time often varies according to the length of service with the employer. Vacation pay may be cumulative; for part-time employees, vacation days are prorated (divided proportionally with the work schedule)

Educational Leave. Salary paid for time off to attend educational programs that are work-related

Professional Activities. Salary paid for time off to attend professional meetings that are work- or career-related

Emergency Personal Leave. Paid time off for unexpected events such as a family illness, death, or funeral; jury duty, legal depositions, or court appearances; or extreme weather conditions

Maternity Leave. Time off, usually without pay, but with the guarantee of job protection on return from leave; reasonable time limits usually apply

Extended Leave. Usually involves leave without pay for a few weeks to several months for the purpose of travel, family, or personal needs. The position is held during the absence with an agreed-upon time of return.

Sabbatical, Developmental, or Research Leave. Usually involves leave without pay or reduced pay for a few weeks to several months for the purpose of education or research. The position is held during the absence with an agreed-upon time of return.

Employee Assistance Program

Provides confidential and professional assistance for employees and their family members experiencing problems affecting their job or overall quality of life. Services may include telephone consultation and/or face-to-face conferences.

Retirement

Employer contributes entire sum or employer matching contribution combined with employee contribution. See section on Retirement.

Insurance Benefits

Health insurance
Dental insurance
Vision insurance
Liability (malpractice) insurance
Long-term permanent disability insurance
Life insurance
Legal insurance
Pension plans
(See also sections on professional retirement)

Professional Expenses

Professional license renewal
Uniform allowance
Professional equipment expenses
Professional education assistance
Professional activities
Professional journals or texts
Transportation expenses
Expense account
Child care
Professional services
Staff functions

dental hygienist; an independent management firm; a health maintenance organization; or a national, state, county, or private agency employing individuals for dental offices or other employment settings. Financial arrangements between the dentist and dental hygienist are solely the concern of those two individuals and are separate from and not controlled by any dental practice act.

In some states a dental hygienist may work as an *independent contractor.* In this situation, the dental hygienist contracts with the supervising dentist to provide services to the clients of that dentist by referral prescription while adhering to the state dental practice act. The actual requirements for establishing an independent contractor status are set by the IRS, which explains the contractual arrangement between the dentist and a self-employed dental hygienist. The dental hygienist must meet all of the requirements set by the IRS to qualify as an independent contractor (i.e., sets own work hours, rents work space, purchases own supplies and equipment, controls the work result, pays all business expenses, sets fees and collects fees directly from the clients, and accepts consequences of business profit or loss). An independent contractor dental hygienist may hire employees and function as an employer. The financial arrangements for operating the dental hygiene portion of the practice are contracted between the dentist and dental hygienist.

The dentist does not withhold taxes from the dental hygienist's paycheck; instead, the hygienist pays self-employment (Social Security) and Medicare taxes directly and files estimated income tax payments. There are advantages and disadvantages to this system of employment. It is recommended that interested parties read the IRS requirements (Publication 937) as well as consult a Certified Public Accountant (CPA) for a full understanding of these requirements, benefits, and consequences. It is illegal for a dentist-employer to arbitrarily assign the status of independent contractor to a dental hygienist-employee. Should this occur, the employer is held financially responsible for back taxes and penalties.

Independent dental hygiene practice means a business arrangement whereby the dental hygienist owns a dental hygiene practice—a business that may be incorporated or unincorporated, that can be bought and sold. The dental hygienist can own or rent the structure, and ownership and operation of dental hygiene equipment are limited to the dental hygienist. Independent practice, legal only in Colorado, allows the direct delivery of care to clients by the dental hygienist without the supervision of a dentist, although the dental hygienist could have a supervisory relationship with a dentist. The client may refer him- or herself or may be referred by the dentist to the dental hygienist via prescription. The dental hygienist assumes all financial responsibility for the practice, is self-employed, and functions as an employer to the employees of the facility. Professional collaboration occurs with general and specialty dental practices, as well as with other health providers to ensure clients access to comprehensive oral health care as needed.

Terms of Employment

Various *terms of employment* that may apply to dental hygiene depending on the practice setting and arrangements made with the employer are explained in Terms of Employment. These terms may be integrated to fully describe the nature of the employment agreement.

Employment Rights

Dental hygiene employment falls under the Nondiscrimination Act, Title VII of the Civil Rights Act of 1964. The law establishes equal employment opportunity for all during the hiring process and throughout the course of employment. Further, it requires fairness and impartiality with regard to race, color, religious belief, gender, national origin, and age. The Pregnancy Discrimination Act of 1979 also applies to dental hygiene employment. It prohibits discrimination on the basis of pregnancy, childbirth, or related medical conditions. This law protects women from being fired or refused a job or promotion because of pregnancy. Furthermore, it provides that following maternity leave, the job will be returned with no loss in seniority or fringe benefits.

Minimal standards for working conditions are set by each state and include guidelines pertaining to hours and days of work, minimum wage and reports for pay, employee records, uniforms and equipment, meal periods and eating area, rest periods and rest facilities, and environmental temperature. The Occupational

Terms of Employment

Permanent. The employee service with the employer is relatively secure and of unlimited duration.

Temporary. The employee service is known to be of limited duration.

Probationary. A service trial period, usually 1 to 3 months, for employee and employer to work together, then evaluate one another. During this period, the employee may resign or be dismissed immediately for any reason.

Full Time. The employee works solely in one office, or for one employer in multiple offices, the customary number of hours that the facility functions. Normally, 30 to 40 hours per week constitutes full-time employment.

Part Time. The employee works less than full, customary hours of the facility's operation, usually fewer than 30 hours per week.

Job Sharing. Two or more people share one full-time job by the day, week, month, or year. The time can be split in any fashion agreeable to the job sharers and the employer. The salary and benefits are divided proportionally with the time worked.

Regular Hours. Work time that coincides with normal office hours

Staggered Hours. Established, consistent working hours that fit the life schedule of the employee. These hours vary from the routine office hours but are stable daily for the employee.

Flex Time. Work time that changes daily, with the employee arriving and leaving whenever she or he chooses or depending on the daily workload.

Safety and Health Administration (OSHA) sets minimum federal requirements for industrial safety.

Employment Contracts

The *employment contract,* or letter of agreement, is a written contract describing the terms of employment agreed on by the dental hygienist-employee and the dentist-employer. It functions to clarify the specific details of employment issues for both parties and in so doing establishes a stable working relationship between the two. The contents may include administrative terms of the agreement, settings and terms of employment, job description, compensation, probationary period, performance evaluation, termination procedures. and signatures. Although it provides psychological security for both parties, it may or may not be legally binding.

In some cases, the employer provides a letter of agreement before beginning employment. In other cases, the employment setting functions on a less formal basis, and it becomes the responsibility of the dental hygienist-employee to draw up an employment contract for the employer to sign. Many dental hygienist-employees work without an employment contract and do not experience problems; however, to avoid misunderstanding and disappointments, written clarification of points of discussion is very helpful (Figure 53–4). Several components may be included in the employment contract (see Components of an Employment Contract).

Beginning June 1, 1995: Nancy Sutton, R.D.H., B.S.,
shall work as employee of
Jack Joplin, D.D.S., as employer.

Ms. Sutton shall work as a Registered Dental Hygienist with Expanded Duties.

She shall work Mondays, Wednesdays, and Fridays from 8:00 A.M. until 5:30 P.M. The work schedule will be established by client need, determined by the dentist and dental hygienist, with appointment lengths of 30 minutes minimum for pedodontic clients and 45 minutes minimum for adult clients. A lunch break of 1 hour will be allowed daily.

Policy and procedures of the office, as outlined in the office manuals, will be followed by the employee. A complete job description is contained therein.

The starting salary will be $200 per day. After a 3-month probationary period, a performance evaluation will be completed by both the employee and the employer. At that time, the parties will evaluate their work compatibility to convert to permanent employment or to select a date for job termination. With permanent employment, the parties will establish a benefits package to equal $1,000 per year. A merit-based salary increase will occur every 6 months for the first year, and annually every year thereafter.

The employee will use the office space, equipment, and supplies provided by the employer. Special instrument and equipment needs will be considered on request by the employee. All uniforms will be purchased and maintained at the expense of the employer.

Additions to this agreement will be put in writing as they are developed.

I have read this contract and agree with the contents.

Nancy Sutton, R.D.H., B.S.	Jack Joplin, D.D.S.
Date __________	Date __________

FIGURE 53–4 ✦ Employment contract.

EMPLOYMENT REALIZATION

Starting a New Job

Presentation of a professional image is the first step of starting a new job. The dental hygienist quickly establishes then maintains the "professional personality" in both client care and intraoffice interactions. Initial employment includes investigating to learn about the new position and other staff members' job responsibilities. This behavior gains respect and builds a loyalty base from both clients and co-workers. Newcomers learn from mistakes and seek help when assistance is needed; they are flexible to learn from the new job and persistent to develop excellence. They ease through the workday knowing what is expected and that expectations are being met, with assurance of the feeling of being respected and appreciated by clients, dentist, and co-workers and having a sense of job security develop over the years within a given practice.

Veteran employees changing employment to a new job need to learn the style of the new office and try to adopt those systems rather than impose their techniques on them. Asking for a short evaluation at the end of the first week and again at the end of the first month of employment is helpful and appropriate. After the procedures in the practice setting are understood, ideas for change and improvement may be introduced. New licentiates need to allow time to establish a solid track record and develop skills in communications, management, and leadership. Consider using more than one co-worker as a mentor, modeling yourself after those you admire. Learn different attitudes, skills, and behavioral techniques from different individuals. You will benefit from a series of mentors and role models who can provide a variety of perspectives and advice well into your career. Multiple mentors enable one to approach a situation in multiple ways and be better prepared to adapt quickly to changes when circumstances shift.

The law requires new employees to show documentation before beginning a new job. Have these documents ready for presentation to your potential employer:

- ✦ Current state or regional license to practice dental hygiene
- ✦ Current CPR certification
- ✦ Social security card or state driver's license and birth certificate/passport or evidence of citizenship or work eligibility

Components of an Employment Contract

Terms of Agreement
Names of employee and employer
Job title
Date the contract takes effect
Date the contract expires
Option of contract renewal

Settings and Terms of Employment
Address(es) of the employment
Name(s) of supervising dentist(s)
Agreement of both parties to adhere to the rules and regulations of the state dental practice act
Statement of equipment, supplies, and instruments to be provided by the employer
Work arrangement of days of work and workload by hours and scheduling of appointments

Job Description
Specific services to be performed
Other work responsibilities
Opportunities for growth and promotion

Compensation
Method of remuneration
Starting wage
Payroll schedule
Increases in pay, including dates of review and basis for review
Fringe benefits, listed individually with requirements for qualification, vesting increments, and accrual techniques
Overtime compensation agreement
Payment for time not worked such as holidays, vacation, sick leave

Probationary Period
Terms and date of probation
Agreement for mutual evaluation
Employment termination options for each party

Performance Evaluation
Dates for review
Method of evaluation
Criteria for performance success

Termination Procedures
Advance notice required
Statement of cause
Employee replacement procedures

Signatures
Employee and date signed
Employer and date signed
Witness(es) optional

- ✦ Evidence of current professional liability coverage (optional, depending on employer)
- ✦ Health documents such as hepatitis B vaccination information are also required.
- ✦ New employees are required to complete a safety training orientation at each work site.

Job Performance

The job performance of the dental hygienist is determined by a combination of the individual's own professional style and the completeness of the job description, plus procedure and policy manuals provided by the employment setting. The office procedure manual delineates responsibility and describes routines. A specific job description for the position of dental hygienist clearly defines all aspects of performance, outlines expectations, and serves as a guideline for performance review.

Standard of care describes the level of clinical performance required for the position of dental hygienist in that setting, practice philosophy and goals, and other special qualifications that maintain consistency among staff members. The policy manual applies to all personnel and is designed to outline the practice principles and how they are to be implemented. The success of the practice depends on staff members adhering to these standards. Both client and personnel satisfaction is enhanced by adopting and following the office policies. Beyond a description of the personnel involvement in the team approach to delivering dental care, specific standards for quality assurance and education are outlined. Personnel policies, employment regulations, and work arrangements are included. Guidelines of professional ethics and conduct further assure quality client care with an ability to minimize liability. Office safety and emergency protocols prevent confusion and provide guidance for unified actions if unexpected situations occur. Finally, service to the community as an overall theme with specific contributions is described in the policy manual.

Job expectations are established when both the dental hygienist-employee and employer write the job description together and discuss and agree on the level of performance and results. Specifically, this includes a listing of the basic responsibilities, standards of performance, importance of the functions, skills necessary to perform the job, goals and limits for achieving the expectations, and methods of evaluation. Beyond the area of job description, success in any setting depends on working with other people. Job satisfaction for the dental hygienist comes from human needs that are fulfilled in the employment setting. As one gains competence, responsibility, recognition, support, respect, and a sense of belonging, job satisfaction follows.

Presentation of the Professional Image

The dental hygienist's professional image is consistently projected through affect, or overall behavior of self-confidence and caring about the health and well-being of others. Specifically, while working within a dental practice, the dental hygienist is a professional promoting total health through delivering quality oral health care. Envision dental hygiene as a profession, define yourself as a specialist, and consider your work as a career. When you are working, project a dedicated work ethic to coworkers and treat clients in a competent, knowledgeable manner. Use discretion, discern what is proper and correct, and behave accordingly. Take responsibility and protect the best interest of the practice. Do not discuss confidential business in public. Presenting a self-confident appearance and positive body language further conveys a professional image.

Display your framed college diploma or certificate and your license in your dental treatment room. Let clients know that dental hygienists have a college education. Display a nameplate or wear a name tag with RDH and your highest earned degree. Let clients know that dental hygienists must pass both a national board examination and a state board examination to receive a license. Further explain that continuing education is mandatory for relicensure, if that is the case in your state.

When you attend a workshop, course, or seminar that updates or increases your knowledge, share your lessons with clients. When you attend a conference for a professional organization, share that information, too. Subscribe to and read professional journals to keep abreast of scientific research and developments. Some of these are the *Journal of Dental Hygiene* and *Access*, both ADHA publications, *RDH Magazine*, the *Journal of Periodontology* from the American Academy of Periodontology, *The Journal of the Western Society of Periodontology*, and *The Journal of Practical Hygiene*. Periodically purchase and read new textbooks. Utilize all available resources to remain current. In addition to dental issues and to further benefit the general health of clients, maintain and update a broad base of health information. Subscribe to health newsletters and frequent Web sites on health and continuing education.

The dental hygienist may be represented on business cards or business stationery. The cards and stationery can be used for exchange at job interviews; at dental professional meetings, conferences, and educational programs; with clients to promote the practice or refer new clients; and with nondental professional associations, agencies, and professional contacts. Furthermore, cards, stationery, and personalized memo pads can be used during professional correspondence and practice promotion. The design of these items incorporates the dental hygienist's name and professional degrees, title, and other identifying information. Home or office address and telephone number may be used. The quality of paper and design should project a professional image. The dental hygienist may need more than one card design to represent different affiliations and activities.

Performance Evaluation

The *performance evaluation* is a communication tool based on an agreed-upon performance plan (Figure 53–5). It is a valuable tool because it provides a progress report for the employee, it recognizes and supports desired behavior, develops strengths, pinpoints weaknesses, and gives specific direction for change. The performance evaluation may assist in determining a salary increase or can be used as a legal supporting document for employee dismissal.

A job evaluation is always performed at the completion of the probationary period if the employee is new, then once or twice a year for the duration of employment. In addition to the written document, daily verbal feedback as an evaluation *process,* rather than an event, facilitates successful employee performance.

Completing the performance evaluation requires that both the dental hygienist-employee and employer prepare the evaluation, then meet together to share, compare, and discuss the results (see Elements of the Performance Evaluation and Formats Used for Employee Performance Review).

The content of the performance evaluation addresses the job description:

- Participation with the practice and staff as a team member
- Knowledge of the dental hygiene field
- Professional competencies
- Interpersonal skills

Elements of the Performance Evaluation

Measure progress toward the goal of task and behavior performances.

Compare actual results with the agreed-on plan, citing specific incidents.

Praise accomplishments when performance meets or exceeds stated standards.

When differences occur, determine the cause, then consider alternatives to facilitate reaching desired outcomes.

If corrective action is indicated, state the specific plan with measurable results, and gain agreement of both parties.

Modify performance standards if indicated and agreed on by both parties.

Enhance communications between the employer and the employee, giving an opportunity for "coaching" to achieve performance goals, rather than merely "judging" performance.

Formats Used for Employee Performance Review

Management by Objective. Lists objectives together with a time frame using specific measurable criteria

Standard Office Procedure. Describes how well each responsibility is performed, according to the written job description

Critical Incidents. Descriptive file of events, both positive and negative, pertaining to job performance

Multiple Appraisers. A team of staff members participates in the performance assessments, and a compiled evaluation is presented to the employee

- ✦ Dependability to the office and work schedule
- ✦ Responsibility for the treatment area and material resources
- ✦ Work habits
- ✦ Initiative, management, leadership, critical thinking, decision making, and problem-solving skills

Improving Job Performance

The three elements required for changing job performance are planning, evaluation, and incorporation. Planning starts by identifying the specific performance discrepancies, listing the desired standard of performance in comparison with the present level of

Employee Name: ______________________ Date: __________

Registered Dental Hygienist

Evaluation completed by: ______________________

	EXCELLENT	ACCEPTABLE	NEEDS IMPROVEMENT
PROFESSIONAL BEHAVIOR:			
1. Attitude	___	___	___
2. Cooperation	___	___	___
3. Responsibility	___	___	___
4. Initiative	___	___	___
5. Communications	___	___	___
6. Contributions to Office	___	___	___
CLIENT MANAGEMENT:			
1. Information & Instruction	___	___	___
2. Assistance in Decision Making	___	___	___
3. Respectful	___	___	___
4. Contribution to Comfort	___	___	___
5. Client Acceptance	___	___	___
RISK MANAGEMENT:			
1. Infection Control	___	___	___
2. Protect Self/Client from Injury	___	___	___
PROCESS OF CARE:			
1. Systematic Approach	___	___	___
2. Performs All Necessary Care	___	___	___
3. Care Procedures (List specific concerns)			
4. Documentation Skills	___	___	___
5. Evaluation Skills	___	___	___
6. Modification of Care	___	___	___
7. Coordination with Other Care	___	___	___

CHANGES/GROWTH SINCE LAST EVALUATION:

GOALS FOR CHANGE/GROWTH:

COMMENTS:

SIGNED:

______________________ Date: __________

Supervisor

______________________ Date: __________

Employee

FIGURE 53–5 ✦ Employee performance evaluation.

performance, analyzing the discrepancy, and defining what needs to be done differently. The employee and employer reach mutual agreement on the desired change, being certain that each party is clear about the details of the plan.

The evaluation phase requires immediate feedback and reinforcement of the new, desired actions. Progress is monitored, with reinforcement given often at first and gradually tapering down. The guidelines for change are steadily reviewed and followed. It is important that specific acknowledgment be made when the desired changes are achieved.

Job Termination

Job termination may occur through dismissal by the employer or resignation by the employee. In the event of dismissal, the dental hygienist should make all attempts to understand clearly the grounds, asking for the true, complete picture, with clarification of any vague statements. Employees should be aware that the work performance is unacceptable, not the person. The employee should clarify the severance arrangements, including the date of termination, severance pay, and benefits accrued and due to the employee. Termination requires behaving professionally and with dignity, while allowing an opportunity to acknowledge feelings and mourn the loss of the job. Following a job dismissal, the terminated job must be put in perspective to reenter the job market. This is a time for the dental hygienist to inventory career goals, update a résumé, begin the interviewing process with specific ideas of new job requirements to achieve professional satisfaction, and then move confidently toward the next career stage.

When the dental hygienist decides to resign from a job, notice of intentions is to be given to the employer as soon as possible, before telling any of the office coworkers. The notification process involves a clear statement of grounds for resigning or a statement of time for career change or advancement. Clarification is made of the severance arrangements, including the date of termination, benefits accrued and due, and whether there is an intention to find and/or train a successor. Departing employees should tie up loose ends and depart with dignity, behaving in a professional manner.

Stress and Burnout among Dental Hygienists

Stress is the disquietude of strain or tension from consuming and compulsive pressures, usually resulting in a diminished capacity for resistance. *Burnout* is the combination of physical, emotional, and behavioral changes in an individual as a response to high-intensity or long-duration stress. Burnout occurs when one's adaptive capabilities are exceeded and exhaustion ensues.

Various strategies can be employed to reduce stress and burnout, beginning with an identification of the reasons causing the feelings (see Sources of Stress and Burnout in a Dental Hygiene Career). Some people analyze feelings to achieve self-awareness of the internal issues. Others evaluate the environment and work situation to make external changes, then reprioritize goals or reevaluate methods used to accomplish reconfirmed goals. A conscious attempt should be made to incorporate changes that reduce stress by delegating responsibilities, being creative, and trying something new. People should modify behavior to enjoy life by taking classes, learning new skills, maintaining physical fitness, enjoying recreation, trying techniques for body and mind relaxation, and adopting new behaviors.

Sources of Stress and Burnout in a Dental Hygiene Career

- The "giving" role of healthcare providers is emotionally draining, with little "received" in return
- Working in an "intimate zone" of the human body
- Intense interpersonal relations with clients and staff members
- Dental hygiene job tasks that are repetitive and monotonous
- Lack of intellectual stimulation
- Lack of feeling appreciated, which leads to reduced self-esteem
- Feelings of being taken for granted, which lead to reduced self-worth
- Sensing a lack of accomplishment of personal and/or professional goals
- Generalized lack of change

Networks for Professional Enhancement

Professional connections can be accomplished by *networking,* or sharing and extending professional contacts to establish friendships and business relationships. The functions of networks are to exchange knowledge and information and to develop a professional and moral support system for achievement of professional goals. These groups can keep members informed of professional developments and job opportunities and assist in making job changes. The members may be professional colleagues, college classmates and faculty, or friends and relatives. Dental hygienists interested in networking with one another online can do so at www.geocities.com/~hygienehelper or can register to discuss issues, ask advice, or exchange information at hygienists-request@adha.net with the words "subscribe hygienists."

Employment Alternatives to Private Practice Dental Hygiene

Most dental hygiene employment opportunities are in private practice. More than 96% of all dental hygienists are employed in private offices or dental clinics by dentists.[1] Employment alternatives for dental hygienists in traditional clinical practice settings are expanding. Now dental hygienists can provide services in certain settings without supervision in many states.[4] For example:

- ✦ California licenses registered dental hygienists in alternative practice (RDHAPs), who may provide direct services for clients via prescription from a dentist or physician at residences of the homebound, schools, residential facilities, institutions, and dental health professional shortage areas. Special education is required for this licensure.

- Colorado allows dental hygienists to own a dental hygiene practice and work unsupervised.
- Connecticut allows dental hygienists to practice without supervision in institutions (other than hospitals), public health facilities, group homes, and schools. Two years of experience are required.
- Michigan allows dental hygienists to provide care to clients in underserved areas within a public or nonprofit program approved by the department of public health. No special requirements are needed.
- New Hampshire allows dental hygienists to provide procedures authorized by a dentist in public or private schools, hospitals, or institutions under "public health supervision." A dentist must review patient records once in a 12-month period. No special requirements are needed.
- New Mexico recognizes the "Collaborative Practice of Dental Hygiene," which establishes a cooperative work relationship with a consulting dentist without general supervision. Special certification is required for this status.
- Oregon allows dental hygienists to treat clients in nursing homes, adult foster homes, residential care facilities, adult congregate care facilities, and mental health residential programs. Clients must be referred annually to a licensed dentist for treatment evaluation. A special permit is required.
- Washington allows unsupervised practice in hospitals, nursing homes, home health agencies, group homes, state institutions, jails, and public health facilities, provided the hygienist refers to a dentist for dental treatment and planning. Two years of recent clinical experience are required.

Dental hygienists interested in working in alternative settings benefit from additional education in accounting, finance, economics, marketing, business management, human resources, communications, information systems, leadership, public health and public administration, gerontology, oncology, and hospice care. Internships or associate positions with practices in alternative settings, health care administration, research facility, or practice management firms can further familiarize and prepare one for a future career.

Employment alternatives to clinical dental hygiene might include positions in the following:

- Dental hygiene and dental schools
- Public schools
- Community oral health projects
- Consulting in practice management and teaching in continuing education
- Private enterprise
- Acute and chronic care facilities, homes for the elderly, prisons, and hospices
- Oral healthcare products industry
- Insurance industry
- Government service in the armed forces, Veterans' Administration, Public Health Service, Indian Health Service, or state agencies.
- Computer industry, e-commerce, online course development, Web site design
- Health professionals placement agency
- Scientific research and theory development
- Professional and public organizations
- Professional media development
- Dental hygiene practice in foreign countries

PROFESSIONAL AND PERSONAL FINANCIAL MANAGEMENT

Management of finances is a lifetime endeavor and involves a combination of factors. Financial planning and budgeting is paramount at the beginning of the career and will guarantee a secure future. In addition to normal living expenses and regular saving, knowledge of special professional expenses, annual tax deductions, retirement plan options, and estate planning are elements of financial planning.

Compensation Considerations

Financial security must be attained by the dental hygienist throughout the career. Initially, wages and fringe benefits are to be evaluated for coverage of living expenses, debts, paid time off, insurance coverage, and savings. The compensation package must cover these needs for monthly bills and annual financial objectives. It is essential that the dental hygienist also consider long-term economic needs. *Financial planning* is the process of setting financial goals for the future by taking intentional steps to achieve financial security. Successful financial planning requires attention to detail and discipline. It is not difficult, but it does require careful, consistent behavior. A certified financial planner (CFP) can help guide professionals to design a path for sound financial management.

Steps to Financial Planning

Financial planning begins with an evaluation of the present financial situation and then setting financial goals for the future. Read about financial issues by subscribing to a magazine, journal, or newsletter or by reading books so that you can learn to make informed decisions. Each week learn one new piece of information to build a strong foundation for future financial decision making. First establish a budget to live within your income and achieve monthly and annual financial goals. Create a budget as an effective money management tool. Compile a monthly list of all required needs and recurring expenses and allocate funds for these expenses. Then add variable and infrequent expenses such as car registration, gifts, taxes, and vacation, and average those monthly amounts. Refer to Expenses List for a Budget for an expense list for budget items you need to include.

Expenses List for a Budget

Housing
Rent or mortgage
Homeowners/condominium association dues and fees
Utilities: gas and electricity, water, telephone, alarm, garbage, sewer, cable television, post office box rental
Cleaning and maintenance: housekeeping service, supplies and materials
Repairs
Furnishings and decoration
Property tax

Food and Beverage
Groceries and dry goods
Snacks and fast food
Take out and delivery

Transportation
Automobile payment
Gas and oil
Car wash and wax
Maintenance and repairs
Drivers license renewal
Automobile registration renewal
Parking and tolls
Public transportation: subway, taxi, bus

Insurance
Health
Home owner/renter for fire and theft
Automobile
Professional liability
Professional disability
Personal liability "umbrella"
Life and accidental death
Long-term care

Clothing
Daily attire
Special occasion attire
Uniforms and work attire
Accessories
Laundry, dry cleaning and repair

Personal Maintenance
Health club/gym and personal trainer
Hair and nails
Cosmetics, lotions, and facials
Massages, chiropractic, acupuncture

Health Maintenance
Doctors
Dentist
Pharmacy
Eye glasses, contacts, safety glasses

Entertainment
Theater, concerts, movies
Club and museum memberships
Newspapers, magazines, books
Drinking and dining out
Hosting parties
Lessons, hobbies and special interests: fees and equipment
Vacation

Financial
Savings account
Retirement account
Credit card payments
Student loans
Other loans
Bank fees
Safe box rental
Taxes

Children
School and/or day care
Baby sitting
Medical, dental, pharmacy
Clothing, toys and supplies
Lessons
College fund

Support of Others
Church and charity
Gifts, Greeting cards and postage
Pets: feeding, maintenance and health care
Elderly or disabled family members

Professional Services
Certified public accountant or bookkeeper
Certified financial planner
Attorney

Professional Activities
Membership in professional organizations
Continuing education
Professional license renewal
Attendance at professional conferences
Subscriptions to professional journals and texts

Modified from McCarthy CP: *The under 40 financial planning guide*, Los Angeles, 1996, Silver Lake.

Then subtract the total expenses from the monthly income to arrive at the monthly outcome of potential savings or shortfall.

Monthly Income: $________
– Total Expenses: $________
= Monthly Outcome: $________

If you have a shortfall, analyze the steps you can take to reduce current expenses, change spending habits or control impulse buying, and live within your income limits. Do plan some fun and recreation as well as consideration for emergency expenses. Determine how to compensate for unexpected bills. Regularly monitor actual expenses as compared with the budget to evaluate whether the budget is realistic. Keep complete and accurate records for an accounting of your spending pattern. Design your own budget system or purchase a budget book. The records help determine if the planning is appropriate, as well as assisting with taxes, expense accounts, and forecasting the financial future.

Keep track of your financial status by computing *net worth,* which is the difference between assets (amount owned) and liabilities (amount owed). This calculation includes real property, life insurance, stocks, bonds, retirement accounts, household and personal property, and bank accounts. Net worth can be calculated annually to check progress in reaching financial goals; then review and update the overall financial plan as needed.

Set goals for the future, stating specific objectives for short-term accomplishments and long-range goals. Start saving immediately upon employment in your first job. Newspapers print a listing of the highest yields on savings. Shop around for the best interest rates in your area. Your savings account will *compound,* meaning that the money you save will earn interest, and then the interest will earn interest. A small amount saved beginning at an early age will compound and grow to a larger sum than a moderate amount saved beginning at an older age. Plan to spread investments over the years. When determining the long-range goals, include the desired income at retirement. List other objectives, including income now and in 5 years, then 10 years, and so on. Specify investments such as residential property, securities, retirement accounts, education of children, travel, and other things for personal needs and desires.

The dental hygienist needs to establish an individual credit rating. This facilitates getting loans, a mortgage, or other credit. It also allows for independent financial functioning. Once credit is established, use it effectively. Major purchases may be spread over a long period and paid off with a reasonable finance charge. Newspapers print a listing of the best credit card deals nationwide. Shop around for the lowest interest rate for borrowers who carry balances. Avoid unnecessary debts, finance charges, and penalties for late payments. You can get information on credit and receive a copy of your credit report from TRW at www.trw.com or Equifax at www.equifax.com. For information about credit cards, rates, rebates, and other credit details, go to www.ramresearch.com or www.creditnet.com. Pay yourself first, with interest, dividends, and appreciation. Begin with small guaranteed accounts and investments that make the money work for you. Select interest-bearing checking accounts, savings accounts, money market accounts, mutual funds, bonds, certificates of deposit, and U.S. Treasury bills. In addition, establish a reserve fund for emergencies that does not disturb the other accounts.

Buying a car is usually the first major purchase a person makes. Purchasing a home is the most important major investment, usually the largest single investment of a lifetime. Providing a home eliminates paying rent to someone else, offers safety and security, provides financial leverage as collateral, gains appreciation, and offers tax advantages. Diversify other investments to spread the risks, obtain the highest possible return, and gain income-producing securities.

The dental hygienist needs to protect personal income with disability insurance, as a safeguard for earning power (see the section on disability insurance). Immediately upon initial employment, the dental hygienist needs to begin a retirement fund that will receive contributions throughout all the working years (see the section on retirement planning).

Investment Goals

The goals for investments are varied and should be considered before selecting each investment. Choose investments for as many of the following purposes as possible:

- Produce income
- Provide a tax advantage
- Hedge inflation
- Show capital growth and appreciate in value
- Furnish safety and security
- Have liquidity conversion potential
- Maintain them management-free or with minimal expense

Professional assistance for financial planning is recommended. A carefully planned strategy to achieve financial goals is best done with the expertise of specialists who can help with laws, regulations, taxes, intricacies, and refinements. These specialists include bankers, real estate brokers, stockbrokers, insurance brokers, investment advisors, accountants, and attorneys. Internet resources for investing are Motley Fool at www.fool.com, providing financial advice for beginners and intermediates, including information on personal finance, investment basics, banking, debt, and retirement; and The American Association of Individual Investors at www.aaii.com, for basic and intermediate-level investing information. Both have extensive educational material and can guide you to other Internet resource sites.

The types of investments are numerous. For each, one must consider how much risk one is willing and able to assume, considering both short-and long-term investments plus evaluating income needs now and in the future. The tangible investments (hard assets) include real estate; gold, silver, coins, and gems; plus antiques, art, stamps, and rare books. The intangible investments (paper with a guarantee, securities, or liquid assets) include banks; savings and loans offering interest-bearing checking accounts, savings accounts, money market accounts, and certificates of deposit; government securities such as Treasury bills, notes and bonds, and savings bonds; federal agency lending programs; short-term tax-exempt notes; municipal bonds for estates, counties, and municipalities; and investment firms with money market funds, stocks, corporate bonds, mutual funds, tax-deferred annuities, commodities and financial futures, limited partnerships, tax shelters, trust deeds, and foreign currency.

Estate Planning

Estate planning is defined as providing for intentional disposition of possessions and assets on one's death to organize family resources and provide for the family's future. Estate planning requires careful financial planning and management during one's lifetime. It intentionally creates, defines, and retains assets of the estate, provides for disability, and plans and provides for retirement. A well-planned estate can spread family income and ensure prudent money management during one's lifetime. Estate planning is valuable in establishing trusts to reduce administrative and management costs and protect assets, as well as minimize or avoid taxes imposed on estates and inheritances. Finally, the estate plan guarantees that the financially secure property will be disposed of as one desires.

Professional Insurances

The purpose of insurance policies is to cover catastrophes. Although it is hoped that we never have to call them into use, they are highly recommended. They provide financial assistance when it is most needed. Only buy what you need. Insurance Net at www.insurancenet.com provides descriptions of various types of insurance, references to insurance company home pages, and other insurance resources.

LIABILITY INSURANCE. The dental hygienist may purchase insurance policies to protect professional and personal assets. *Liability (malpractice) insurance* is a plan that protects the insured against liability arising out of professional service (see the section on fringe benefits). It is recommended that a dental hygienist carry a personal malpractice policy, even if the employer carries similar insurance that extends coverage to all employees. Dental hygienists should note that the employer's policy is in effect to represent the dental hygienist only if the dentist is also named in a lawsuit. If the employer and dental hygienist are both named and later the dentist is dropped from the suit, the liability insurance may no longer apply for the hygienist.

Furthermore, all insurance policies have limits of liability. If the limits to protect the dentist are met, and no financial coverage is left to protect the hygienist, the dental hygienist alone is responsible for covering all court costs, attorney fees, and injury expenses. Finally, when carrying one's own policy, the dental hygienist has the right to select an attorney, rather than be forced to accept an attorney assigned by the employer's policy. Hygienists should be familiar with all the terms of any policy purchased. ADHA and CDHA members may purchase liability insurance through a group policy.

DISABILITY INSURANCE. *Disability insurance* or workers' compensation is defined in the section on fringe benefits. When selecting a disability policy, the dental hygienist must first determine the minimal monthly expenses that must be paid by the insurance policy, should he or she become disabled, because this insurance coverage provides a percentage of the basic wage. After investigating other sources of income during disability, such as a state disability insurance paid on all employees, a minimum monthly total is determined to assist in policy selection. Some policies pay an additional benefit during the time of hospitalization. Partial benefits may be available if the insured is able to return to work on a limited basis.

The benefit period may be a specified number of years, the length of the disability, until the insured can be retrained in a new job, until regular retirement benefits begin, or for a lifetime. The premium price is determined by the amount paid by the policy if disability occurs and the length of "elimination" or waiting period before the policy begins to make payments to the insured. Hygienists should read the policies carefully because the term *disability* may be defined in a variety of ways. ADHA and CDHA members may purchase liability insurance through a group policy.

LIFE INSURANCE. Life insurance is classified as term or whole life insurance. Term insurance, covering a specific temporary time period, or whole life insurance, a long-term investment policy that builds on cash value and may pay dividends or provide borrowing equity, may be selected. It is recommended that the dental hygienist seek professional guidance in selecting a life insurance policy.

LONG-TERM CARE INSURANCE. Long-term care (LTC) insurance covers some of to all of the expenses the policyholder will incur if he or she were to enter a nursing home or other long-term care facility. It is one of the insurances most often called into service. Among those who have it, one out of three use LTC insurance.[5] These policies have requirements for qualification and a variety of options for benefit amounts and terms.

Umbrella insurance pays for claims that are over the limits of your homeowners', renters', or automobile insurance. It is relatively inexpensive for the coverage it provides.

Taxes

Taxes are the largest single item in the personal budget. Therefore, it is important to receive all tax breaks available. The tax bracket is the combined federal and state percentage of taxes paid on the total dollars earned. In the U.S. tax system, it is advantageous to maximize tax deductions to reduce tax liabilities, thereby creating the lowest tax bracket possible. The tax bracket helps determine the best types of investments. The IRS provides a Web site, www.irs.gov, for resource information and downloading IRS publications and tax forms. Tax preparation software has become increasingly popular and can reduce tax time hassles. Web sites include www.turbotax.com, www.taxcut.com, and www.hrblock.com. Online tax preparation programs allow you to file taxes electronically.

Professional Tax Deductions

In addition to the tax savings available to all taxpayers, professionals are entitled to special tax adjustments, deductions, and credits if these expenses are employment-related. The IRS requires that the individual maintain a calendar of professional activities that are tax deductible, with an explanation of each event, including the date, activity, relationship to the job, the sponsor, location, cost, and transportation required. The expense record includes proof of all costs, such as receipts, canceled checks, or credit card vouchers. Federal records should be maintained for at least 3 years after filing, and copies of the federal and state income tax returns are to be kept forever. Professional expenses are deducted only to the extent that the professional is not reimbursed and can establish the right to deduct them.

Professional expenses that are tax deductible to dental hygienists include travel and transportation costs related to professional activities, professional education, uniforms, and miscellaneous professional expenses. Activities with related travel and transportation deductions may be office staff meetings, conferences and meetings of professional organizations, speaking engagements performed by the dental hygienist as a community service, educational programs, study group meetings, seeking employment, and commuting between two jobs on one day.

TRAVEL EXPENSES. Travel expenses are the ordinary and necessary expenses incurred while away from home (overnight) for the purpose of a professional or job-related activity. Travel expenses are deducted as "Employee Business Expenses" on IRS Form 2106, as an adjustment to income. Travel expenses include fares for airplanes, trains, taxis, and buses; meals and lodging; automobile expenses, and related necessary expenses such as telephone calls and laundry. Transportation expenses are the actual cost of transportation to professional activities while not away from home (not overnight). They are allowed only as itemized deductions on Schedule A of IRS Form 1040. Basic commuting between home and job and back home again is not allowed as a transportation expense. These items include actual automobile expenses, bus and cab fares, plus bridge tolls and parking fees.

There are two methods of computation for travel and transportation expenses. One is by the "mileage rate system" in which the IRS states a specific amount allowed for each mile driven. Instructions and the amount allowed for any given year appear on Form 2106. The other is the "actual expenses method," which requires the computation of the ratio of professional mileage to total mileage driven for the year. It represents the actual operating costs such as gasoline, oil, repairs, maintenance, licenses, insurance, depreciation or lease payments, and loan interest. Both options require keeping an odometer diary at the beginning and end of each trip. Nonprofessional travel portions are to be excluded from the total mileage. There are special rules for travel outside the United States. Refer to IRS guidelines for details and qualifying regulations.

EDUCATIONAL EXPENSES. Professional education expenses may be deducted as ordinary and necessary if they meet the express requirements of the employer or the law for retaining professional status and/or licensure. Because many states require a minimum number of hours of continuing education annually as a prerequisite to license renewal, this deduction is easy for the dental hygienist to apply. Professional education expenses may also be deducted to maintain or improve skills required in performing the responsibilities of the present profession, including education that leads to a degree. This allows a tax deduction for a dental hygienist with an associate degree to return to college to earn a baccalaureate degree. Furthermore, if new educational requirements are placed on the profession, all necessary education expenses to meet these stipulations are deductible. Expenses for training in a new profession may not be deducted. Specific costs that are deductible include tuition, fees for correspondence courses, books, supplies, travel, and transportation expenses. Proof of attendance may be required in the event of a tax audit.

UNIFORM EXPENSES. Professional uniforms are defined as work clothes that are specifically required as a condition of employment and are not suitable for general or everyday wear. They must be recognizable as uniforms. The purchase and maintenance costs are deductible, including laundering, dry cleaning, repairs, and alterations. Uniform items for dental hygienists are dresses; pants and tops; laboratory coats and jackets; clinic shoes; caps; white or support hosiery; protective clothing such as protective eyewear, masks, haircovers, and gloves; plus name tags and professional pins.

MISCELLANEOUS PROFESSIONAL EXPENSES. Other miscellaneous professional expenses include dues to professional organizations; employment-seeking expenses such as agency fees, résumé typing and printing, telephone calls, postage, travel and transportation expenses; liability (malpractice) insurance premiums; instruments, professional equipment and supplies; medical examinations that are required by the employer; subscriptions to professional and trade journals; professional legal expenses; professional license renewal; and postage, local, and long-distance telephone calls for professional reasons.

Child and dependent care expenses are allowed for children or disabled dependents while one is at work or seeking employment. For specific qualifications and regulations, see IRS Form 2441 titled "Credit for Child and Dependent Care Expenses." Certain retirement account contributions may be deducted as an adjustment to income, before the adjusted gross income is determined. All interest earned on these accounts is not taxed during working years. Refer to IRS guidelines for details of which accounts qualify and see the section in this chapter on retirement planning.

Tax Audits

Tax returns are reviewed by IRS agents and IRS computers for errors and omissions, deductions that are beyond the normal range relative to a given profession, and other variables. A letter of notification is sent to the taxpayer indicating specific categories for audit. The examination may be done through the mail, as a correspondence audit, or in the office of the IRS. The burden of proof of all allowable deductions is on the taxpayer. All related records are presented to the auditor for consideration and evaluation as legitimate deductions. Although all auditors rely on the same reference sources, each examiner may interpret the law differently. The auditors have equal responsibility to both the taxpayer and the government. Although they primarily investigate to increase collections, they also identify overpayments.

Following the review of data presented, if additional taxes are due from the taxpayer, the auditor will calculate a revised bill, including interest. Repetitive audits for the same items are not allowed for 2 years following a clear audit. If an audit finds additional tax liability, the audit can be repeated on that item until the audit is clear. A taxpayer can be audited every year for different categories. Do not eliminate legitimate deductions to avoid an audit. By collecting documentation and completing a diary, taxpayers have all the proof necessary to satisfy an auditor.

Retirement Planning

Retirement planning is best begun at the beginning of the dental hygienist's career, so that a definite program is in place and funds have been invested over the years to adequately provide for retirement. Focus on goals that include lifestyle, home location, and living conditions. Consider activities, travel, recreation, hobbies, and business involvement. Attempt to project living costs, factoring in cost-of-living increases, and the income required to accommodate the retirement plans, allowing for possible illness or disability. Resources for income during retirement include Social Security payments, retirement funds, whole life insurance policies, and other planned investments. A formal plan, reviewed periodically, is helpful. Periodically, you should check to be certain your Social Security contributions have been credited to your account. You may request your social security statement for earning totals over your working career and benefit options for retirement, disability, and survivors' benefits. Go to www.ssa.gov and select "Top 10 Most Requested Services," then request your Social Security statement, formerly called "Personal Earnings and Benefit Estimate Statement." You may request the statement directly online or download the request form SSA-7004. While at this Web site, view the other options for Social Security services.

There are many types of tax-deferred retirement accounts. It is best to consult a professional advisor, investment counselor, or banker for assistance in selecting a plan that meets the investor's specific needs. In a tax-deferred program, taxes on amounts deposited and interest earned are deferred until withdrawal. These accounts reduce the annual adjusted gross income, thereby reducing the income tax debt.

The dental hygienist's employer may have a corporate 401(K), Simplified Employee Pension Plan (SEP), or Keogh retirement program for which the employee qualifies for inclusion. These plans define qualification by job title and hours of employment. The hygienist needs to study the requirements and contributions schedule to fully understand the plan. Become familiar with the guidelines on vesting; allowance of additional matching contributions by the employee beyond the contributions of the employer; borrowing from the plan; and termination procedures, if the employee leaves the office. In such cases, the dental hygienist may take his or her portion of the fund (amount vested) and "roll it over" into an individual retirement account (IRA) without paying tax consequences.

The IRA is allowable for anyone with earned income who is not included in another pension plan provided by an employer. There is also an exclusion if the employee's spouse is covered by a tax-deferred retirement plan. If neither spouse is covered by an employer's pension plan, each spouse may have a separate IRA, even if one spouse does not earn an income. The multiple types of IRAs include traditional IRAs, with all contributions being tax deductible and earnings tax deferred; Roth IRAs, with all contributions being nondeductible, but all earnings tax deferred; and Education IRAs, with limited nondeductible contributions and tax-free interest, but in addition to the other IRAs. Each has special requirements for qualification, contribution limits, and rules for withdrawal without penalty.

The mechanisms for these arrangements include savings accounts, mutual funds, stocks, retirement bonds, retirement annuities, and trust accounts. The IRS outlines all the rules and regulations for qualifying for an IRA, including maximum contribution allowable, dates for contributions, termination, and withdrawal, in Publication 590 entitled "Individual Retirement Arrangements." You can download it from the IRS Web site at www.irs.gov. Rules change periodically, and it is recommended that the taxpayer review details each year.

Wills

A *will* is a written, legal arrangement for distribution of assets when death occurs. The dental hygienist needs a legal will regardless of age, marital status, or dependents, to direct disposal of belongings. A will provides for financial and guardian care of minor children or disabled dependents, covers payments of debts of the decedent, and can lessen delay in distributing the estate.

The contents of a will identify beneficiaries, identify all aspects of financial affairs, and divide the assets; a codicil can direct distribution of special items. Wills are best prepared in consultation with an attorney to ensure validity and protect the overall interests of the individual.

Although a person may write a will without legal assistance, laws for each state vary about the validity of handwritten wills. Consult the rules for your state if you choose to write a will without the guidance of an attorney. Use your computer search engine to locate one of the hundreds of Web sites on wills.

Probate is the legal process alerting the community of the death, then attending to the financial distribution of the estate. An executor, who is assigned to carry out the provisions of a will, directs the financial concerns of the estate following death (e.g., gathers and preserves the property, collects all income due, pays bills and taxes, provides recordkeeping to the court, then identifies and distributes all remaining assets as stated in the will).

A *living trust* is a legal document similar to a will, but with some advantages. There is no probate with a living trust, all court proceedings and delays are eliminated, privacy is maintained because a living trust is not a public document, and estate taxes can be reduced or eliminated. Property and assets are held in the name of the trust, rather than an individual, and the trust is controlled by the individual establishing it or by another individual as assigned. Professional asset management can be performed by a trustee. A trust is individually tailored to the needs and desires of the person or couple for whom it is created. It can be designed to contain all provisions with a means to handle almost every contingency that may arise during a lifetime, including illness and disability. It is flexible and can be changed or canceled at any time. Trust rules vary from state to state. Consult an attorney knowledgeable in living trusts for more information. Web sites to begin your research on estate planning and trusts are www.rushforth.org and www.mtpalermo.com.

Client Education Issues

- When legally working in alternative settings without dental supervision, the dental hygienist informs the client that the dentist must review the client records annually when it is required by law to do so (e.g., New Hampshire).
- When legally working in alternative practice settings without dental supervision, the dental hygienist informs clients that they must be referred annually to a licensed dentist for treatment evaluation and planning when required by law to do so (e.g., Oregon and Washington).

Legal, Ethical, and Safety Issues

- Honesty and accuracy are the most important elements of résumé writing.
- The dental hygienist can provide services in certain settings without direct supervision only when allowed by law.
- In some states a dental hygienist may work as an independent contractor.
- The Pregnancy Discrimination Act of 1979 protects women from being fired or refused a job or promotion because of pregnancy. Furthermore, it provides that following maternity leave, the job will be returned with no loss in seniority or fringe benefits.
- Dental hygiene employment falls under the Non-Discrimination Act, Title VII of the Civil Rights Act of 1964. The law establishes equal employment opportunity for all during the hiring process and throughout the course of employment.
- Dental Practice Acts are legislative law that define whether a dental hygienist works under general or direct supervision. These acts do not apply to the business association between the dentist and the dental hygienist.
- Minimal standards for working conditions are set by each state.
- The Occupational Safety and Health Standards Board (OSHA) sets minimum federal requirements for industrial safety.
- Employment contracts may or may not be legally binding.
- The law requires new employees to show some documentation before beginning employment.
- The performance evaluation can be used as a legal supporting document for employee dismissal.
- In the event of dismissal, the dental hygienist should make all attempts to understand clearly the grounds and should clarify the severance arrangements.
- Financial arrangements between the dentist and the dental hygienist are solely the concern of those two individuals.
- The dental hygienist must meet all of the requirements set by the IRS to qualify as an independent contractor. It is illegal for a dentist-employer to arbitrarily assign status as an independent contractor to a dental hygienist-employee.
- An independent contractor dental hygienist may hire employees and function as an employer.
- The burden of proof of all allowable tax deductions is on the taxpayer.

Key Concepts

- ✦ The dental hygienist contributes to the dental practice as a team member with knowledge, skills, and a positive professional attitude.
- ✦ Preparation is key for the employment quest, which includes writing a résumé, composing a cover letter, preparing a list of questions for an interview, and rehearsing for the event.
- ✦ A variety of employment arrangements, terms of employment, and compensation packages are available, depending on the dental hygienist's ability to negotiate an agreement with the employer.
- ✦ The compensation package includes salary, a fringe benefits package, and required employer contributions to government-administered funds.
- ✦ Employment contracts are written agreements describing the terms agreed upon by the dental hygienist and employer, and functioning to clarify the specific details of employment.
- ✦ Job performance is determined by a combination of factors, including the individual's own professional style, understanding of job description, and contribution to practice goals.
- ✦ The performance evaluation is a communication tool based on the agreed-upon performance plan and includes both compliments and criticisms plus an outline for specific recommended changes.
- ✦ The elements of career management include seeking employment, professional development, and career mobility, requiring the dental hygienist's ongoing thoughtful and active participation.
- ✦ Professional and personal financial management considers employment compensation, including fringe benefits, and the long-term economic goals of insurance coverage, tax planning, investments, and retirement programs.

Critical Thinking Exercises

1. Make a list of your top ten elements for job selection. Prioritize the list. Share information among the group. Then design a recruitment ad for a dental hygiene position available in a periodontal practice.
2. Prepare a résumé and cover letter that could be used to search for a position in a general dental practice, in a periodontal practice, or in sales for the oral care products industry.
3. Make a list of sample interview questions to ask a potential employer during a job search. Prioritize the questions. Role-play the interviewer asking the questions. Role-play the interviewee answering the following questions:
   - ✦ What are you looking for in a job?
   - ✦ Why should we hire you?
   - ✦ What are your strengths and weaknesses?
   - ✦ What could you contribute to this practice?
   - ✦ Where do you expect to be in your career in 5 years, 10 years, 15 years?
   - ✦ How do you contribute to a team effort?
   - ✦ What is your philosophy of dental hygiene practice?
4. Generate more questions that might be asked on an interview for a dental hygiene position in a private practice.
5. Interview a working dental hygienist. Obtain a list of dental hygienists in the geographic area from the component/constituent dental hygienists' association. Identify a sample of the hygienists to represent a diversity of careers and employment settings. Assign students to interview these dental hygienists about their careers.

For References, Suggested Readings, and Related Websites, visit
http://evolve.elsevier.com/Darby/hygiene/

CHAPTER 54

LEGAL AND ETHICAL DECISION MAKING

OBJECTIVES

Mastery of the content in this chapter will enable the reader to:

- Describe key ethical principles and philosophies affecting healthcare
- Identify responsibilities and themes in a code of ethics for dental hygienists
- Resolve ethical dilemmas encountered in practice
- Describe the legal concepts and theories that apply to dental hygiene practice
- Define legal concepts and issues affecting the various roles of the dental hygienist
- Reduce legal risks and liabilities associated with dental hygiene practice

KEY TERMS

Abandonment
Accountability
Assault
Autonomy
Battery
Beneficence
Beyond a reasonable doubt
Breach of contract
Civil law
Confidentiality
Contract
Criminal law
Deceit
Defamation
Defendant
Deontological ethics
Duty
Ethical dilemma
Ethics
Fidelity
Hostile environment
Informed consent
Informed refusal
Justice
Law
Libel
Misrepresentation
Negligence
Nonmaleficence
Plaintiff
Preponderance of evidence
Quid pro quo
Respondeat superior
Sexual harassment
Slander
Standard of care
Statute of limitations
Technical battery
Tort
Utilitarian
Veracity
Virtue ethics

FOUNDATIONS OF ETHICAL DECISION MAKING

Ethics Defined

Ethics is a branch of philosophy that deals with thinking about morality, moral problems, and moral judgments. Ethics is a concern for everyone because it forces the question of what one should do and why.[1] A discussion of professional ethics relates to what is professionally right or conforming to professional standards of conduct. This definition reflects the traditional view of a profession as a group that determines its own standards, writes its own code of ethics, and disciplines its own members. This traditional view is undergoing change to include a broader perspective that argues professional ethics are not merely what practitioners regard as custom but, rather, what the profession and society agree are appropriate rules of conduct. For example, codes of ethics point out that healthcare providers should not discuss a client's medical condition with anyone without the individual's authorization. Another example found within the American Dental Association (ADA) Code of Ethics is a statement that the dentist should inform the client of proposed care and allow the person to become involved in treatment decisions.

A code of ethics recognizes three relationships:

- ✦ Professional and client
- ✦ Professional and professional
- ✦ Professional and society

In dental hygiene, ethics focuses on moral duties and obligations of the professional to clients, colleagues, and society. Commitment to society is not always reflected in codes of ethics. Although it is not always stated, there is also a critical element of trust as an ethical obligation in the three relationships. The influence of society in evaluating professionals and their ethical conduct is increasingly evident. If a health professional is reported in a local newspaper as having unprofessional conduct, letters to the editor or commentaries suggest improved monitoring of health professionals. The public has strong expectations for appropriate professional behavior.

Historically, the health professions were viewed as groups that followed codes of ethics and monitored their members; however, recurring charges of malpractice, impropriety, fraud, and the scrutiny of various public and private agencies have projected the health professions into the arena of public concern and criticism. Consumers who are aware of inappropriate or perceived unethical behaviors contact professional organizations and peer review groups to express their concerns. Professional conferences and publications now address issues such as ethics, ethical decision making, peer review, quality improvement, and related issues. Professional groups meet to form alliances among state boards, academics, publishers, manufacturers, and military and public health services leading to a common code of ethics.[2]

Legal obligations and ethical obligations are distinct. Rules of conduct, promulgated by state or federal statutes, are by their nature obligatory customs or practices of a community (legal obligation). A dental hygienist must follow legal obligations or face the consequences. For example, a hygienist is obligated by both federal and state statutes not to discriminate against individuals belonging to certain classes or to sexually harass another person. Such behaviors may result in legal action against the dental hygienist. Consequences for violating statutory laws include fines or imprisonment or both, depending on the severity of the violation.

Rules of conduct promulgated by the American or Canadian Dental Hygienists' Associations (ADHA or CDHA) serve as guidelines for conduct or ethical obligations. A professional who violates an ethical code may frustrate a client or lose the respect of professional colleagues, but there *may or may not* be legal consequence to an ethical violation. For example, the dental hygienist who refuses to provide care to individuals on Medicaid is violating the ethical standard that suggests dental hygienists should not discriminate, but there are no legal consequences.

Accountability and Responsibility

Accountability refers to the ability to answer for one's actions. Dental hygienists provide client care and are accountable for their actions to themselves, their clients, the profession, employers, and society (see How to Maintain Professional Accountability). The purposes, of professional accountability are to:

- ✦ Evaluate new professional practices and reassess existing ones
- ✦ Maintain standards of care
- ✦ Facilitate personal reflection, ethical thought, and personal growth on the part of health professionals
- ✦ Provide a basis for ethical decision making
- ✦ Demonstrate qualities important to professional status

Dental hygienists are accountable for dental hygiene care and do not rely on others to assume this responsibility.

Major Ethical Perspectives (see Major Ethical Perspectives)

UTILITARIAN ETHICS. John Stuart Mill, a nineteenth-century English philosopher and economist, called his perspective utilitarian ethics. Propositions inherent in *utilitarian ethics* suggest that the rightness or wrongness of actions and practices be determined solely by the consequences produced for the general well-being of all the parties concerned. What makes an action right or wrong is the good or evil produced by the act, not the act itself. Some view the philosophy as the "end justifies the

How to Maintain Professional Accountability

Self

Report any conduct or conditions that endanger clients.
Stay informed and practice current dental hygiene theory.
Make judgments and evaluate based on evidence.

Client

Provide clients with thorough and accurate information about care.
Conduct dental hygiene care in a manner that ensures client safety and well-being.
Encourage communicating within a professional client-provider relationship.

Profession

Maintain ethical standards in practice.
Encourage professional colleagues to follow the same ethical standards.
Report colleagues' unethical behavior to appropriate peer review entities.

Employment Situation

Follow appropriate policy and procedures.

Society

Maintain ethical conduct in care of all clients in all settings.

means." For example, consider the dental hygienist trying to decide whether to provide care to a client with a poor periodontal prognosis. The utilitarian would base a decision on what actions would bring about the greatest benefit for the most people. Therefore, that dental hygienist would be concerned about the consequences of wasting time and effort on a case that appears hopeless, when one could be providing care to others with a better prognosis. Another example is the community-based dental hygienist who acquires funds to improve the oral health status of the target population. Although there are clients who need restorative and prosthetic care, the utilitarian would chose interventions that do the most good for the larger population. Thus a fluoride mouthrinse program may be selected.

DEONTOLOGICAL ETHICS. Immanuel Kant, eighteenth-century German philosopher, advocated *deontological ethics*. Deontologists argue that an action is right when it conforms to the relevant principles of *duty* (obligation). This philosophy indicates that it is immoral to deceive, coerce, or fail to consult with others merely in order to promote one's own goals. Promises must be kept and debts must be paid because such actions are one's duty, not because of the consequences of such actions. Again, consider the client with severe periodontal disease. The deontologist would view duty as the primary consideration in deciding whether to accept the case. The decision is based on a sense of duty, not the consequences. Deontologists also believe that performance of acts in the past creates obligations in the present. If one has entered into a contract, one is bound, independent of the consequences, to the contractual terms.

A dental office may have a contract with a specific dental insurance company clearly outlining the range of treatment that can be provided and limiting the options that can be presented to the client. For example, the insurance coverage may only allow the practitioner to propose amalgam restorations. The practitioner, based on professional assessment, believes another restoration, such as a porcelain crown, would better meet the client's needs. The deontologist would follow the terms of the contract.

Major Ethical Perspectives

Utilitarian Ethics (John Stuart Mill)
Greatest good for greatest number
The end justifies the means
Emphasis on consequences to determine rightness or wrongness of actions and promises

Deontological Ethics (Immanuel Kant)
A binding duty or obligation
Means separate from the end
Emphasis on the morality of the act rather than on the consequences

Virtue Ethics (Aristotle/Plato)
Based on character traits
Virtue is moral
Emphasis on excellence of character

VIRTUE ETHICS. Aristotle and Plato, Greek philosophers of the fourth century BC, advocated *virtue ethics*. Ancient traditions viewed virtuous traits such as benevolence as the primary function of morality. Within this context, the dental hygienist's decision to care for the client with severe periodontal disease is determined by a perception of whether treating the individual is consistent with an accepted model of a virtuous person—someone who is compassionate and conscientious. One would decide affirmatively if it promoted progress toward excellence of character.

Fundamental Ethical Principles

The ethical principles that underlie healthcare are as follows:

- Autonomy
- Beneficence
- Nonmaleficence
- Justice
- Veracity
- Fidelity

Autonomy is based on the principle of respect for persons. Individuals have a right to self-determination, that is, freedom to make their own judgments based on their own evaluations. It is the belief that independent actions and choices of an individual should not be constrained by others. Recognizing autonomy occurs when the dental hygienist involves the client in decision making and obtains informed consent. The caregiver provides clients with enough information to make judgments about their care. All clients should be provided with understandable information about their oral health status and treatment options. To meet this obligation, a dental hygienist uses appropriate communication that meets the client's comprehension and competence level.

Beneficence is the provision of benefit, preventing evil or harm, removing evil or harm, or promoting good. A professional has a duty to help others by doing what is best for them. Based on this principle, a professional is responsible for contributing to the health and welfare of others. Examples of beneficent actions include taking only necessary radiographs and maintaining equipment to prevent client injury, such as replacing worn instruments so that instrument tips do not break in a client's mouth. A dental hygienist participating in a community-based oral cancer screening and referral program is another example of promoting good.

Nonmaleficence is summarized by "above all, do no harm." A dental hygienist seeks to never harm a client. An example of potential harm is when a dental hygienist is asked to provide treatment in which she is not qualified. A dental office, as part of their treatment options, begins utilizing the dental hygiene staff to provide teeth bleaching treatments for clients. A dental hygienist, although not appropriately trained, provides the treatment to clients. Her actions may be viewed as having the potential to inflict harm and violate the principle of nonmaleficence.

Justice relies on fairness and equality. A person is treated justly when given what he or she is due, owed, deserves, or can legitimately claim. All clients receiving care should be treated equally. A dental hygienist who provides substandard care to persons in a nursing home, because they are institutionalized, is not treating all clients equally.

Veracity, truth telling or integrity, is critical to meaningful communication and, thus, to relationships between individuals. Dental hygienists are obligated to be truthful with clients and associates. For example, a dental hygienist fails to tell a client that during sealant application to tooth 19, the primary tooth anterior to tooth 19 fractured. A dental hygienist employed on a commission basis erroneously codes a procedure for insurance reimbursement to receive higher financial reimbursement. The dishonest behavior is apparent in these aforementioned situations.

Fidelity is the obligation to keep implied or explicit promises. A dental hygienist who says that she is going to call the client with some additional information about dental implants, and then follows through with her promise, is demonstrating fidelity.

Other core principles suggested in ethics forums warrant a brief review. *Societal trust* is an obligation to follow the highest ideals and standards of a health profession and the belief that all members of the profession strive to the standards outlined by their profession. Other ethical principles include *reparation,* which suggests that a practitioner responsible for an injury to others must make amends. In *confidentiality,* when information is divulged by one person to another, there is an implicit promise that the information will not be revealed to a third person.

Codes of Ethics

The American Dental Hygienists' Association (ADHA) Code of Ethics assists dental hygienists in achieving high levels of ethical consciousness, decision making, and practice. The code describes the basic beliefs on the importance of oral health and the role of dental hygienists in preventing and treating oral diseases. The Code contains nine categories with *Standards of Professional Responsibilities* for each. The categories begin by explaining the dental hygienists' responsibility to maintain personal health and well-being, competence, and a collaborative and safe work environment. Also highlighted are responsibilities to clients, colleagues, employees and employers, the dental hygiene profession, the community, society, and scientific investigation.

The responsibilities within each category reflect themes, including professional obligations to contribute to society and the profession, communication with clients and colleagues, professional collaboration, and participation to advance the profession. The responsibilities under each category provide a framework for reflection and guide the identification of a potential ethical concern or resolution of an ethical dilemma. Codes of ethics serve as a component of the self-policing responsibility of a profession. Codes of Ethics documents can be obtained from the ADHA and the Canadian Dental Hygienists' Association.

Ethical Problems in Dental Hygiene

Ethical, moral, and legal issues intertwine in the many dilemmas faced by dental hygienists. An *ethical dilemma* is a situation in which two ethical principles are in conflict. Regardless of the decision made or actions taken by the dental hygienist, an ethical principle will be violated. In this section, examples of ethical dilemmas in different career situations are presented followed by a decision-making framework for resolving the dilemmas.

CLINICAL PRACTICE. Dental hygienists report ethical problems such as unprofessional behavior on the part of the dental team, inappropriate client treatment decisions, providing unnecessary dental treatment, delegation to unqualified personnel, insurance fraud, and substandard care. ADHA members identified three commonly encountered ethical dilemmas in dental hygiene practice:[3]

- ✦ Observation of behavior in conflict with standard infection control procedures
- ✦ Failure to refer clients to a specialist
- ✦ Nondiagnosis of dental disease

Examples are the colleague who uses a cold disinfectant rather than properly sterilizing instruments; the staff person who recycles disposable items, such as saliva ejectors or rubber cups; use of instruments "sterilized" in malfunctioning equipment; the new dental assistant who is unfamiliar with standard barrier techniques.

Failure to refer a client to a periodontist occurs in dental hygiene care situations. For example, the dental hygienist responsible for client assessment observes a client's deteriorating periodontal status. The dental hygienist's employer, a general dentist, chooses not to refer; however, the dental hygienist recognizes that the skill level of the dental staff cannot meet the client's periodontal needs. The failure to inform the client of the need for a referral to a periodontist, depending on the facts, may constitute an ethical dilemma as well as malpractice. The ADHA Code of Ethics speaks specifically to the responsibility to refer clients to other healthcare providers when the client's needs are beyond the dental hygienist's ability or scope of practice. The principle to provide optimum oral healthcare using professional knowledge, judgment, and ability must be considered. Another ethical obligation is to serve as an advocate for the welfare of clients; however, in some states the dental hygienist cannot legally refer. Alternatives for solving the dilemma may include working to change office policy, educating colleagues about current referring guidelines, informing clients of their need to seek care in another office, or seeking another position. Each solution carries consequences such as upsetting the employer, frightening the client, performing an activity outside the scope of dental hygiene practice, or losing a valued position.

Consider the scenario when the dental hygienist–dentist team fails to detect dental disease. Perhaps thorough client assessment does not occur. The dental hygienist has the skills to assess the client and record findings but is not given adequate time to fulfill those responsibilities. The dentist conducts a cursory dental caries examination, but other conditions such as periodontal disease, cancer, malocclusion, or temporomandibular joint dysfunction are ignored. Violation of the Code includes failure to provide optimal oral healthcare, compromising the public's confidence in members of the dental health profession and failing to educate clients about high-quality oral healthcare. The failure to assess the client also is an example of malpractice because a systemic condition requiring medical evaluation was not detected. The dental professional is skilled to detect possible systemic diseases based on oral manifestations.

The legal obligations include completing appropriate clinical examinations and following consistent referral protocols. It is suggested that dental offices have standard protocol for dealing with clients with medical conditions that require evaluation and treatment beyond the scope of dental practice. Adherence to the protocol protects the practitioner from malpractice. Office protocol should comply with the *Americans with Disabilities Act*, ensure that the client is counseled and referred to an appropriate healthcare agency or provider, and document consultations and referrals in the *services rendered* section of the dental chart.[4] The protocol should be used consistently with all clients.

PUBLIC HEALTH. Public health hygienists frequently face ethical problems because their decisions concern allocating limited resources and maximizing benefits for a large population. A dental hygienist must implement a dental sealant program for elementary school children. Funding is limited, and thus all students are not able to participate. How are the recipients selected? Should children receiving the benefits of water fluoridation also have the benefit of a dental sealant program? Or should children without access to water fluoridation or other fluoride therapies participate in the sealant program? With knowledge that sealants are useful in preventing occlusal caries, children without the benefit of fluoridation are at a higher risk for developing smooth-surface dental caries. Does socioeconomic status play a role in access to dental services? In this situation, the ethical principles of providing optimal oral healthcare using sound professional judgment to meet the oral health needs of the public guide decision making. An additional ethical responsibility is access to oral health services for all, supporting justice and fairness in the distribution of healthcare resources. The dental hygienist may choose to maximize the preventive potential by using the funding for a sealant program in the fluoridated community. One outcome may reduce the incidence of caries in children living in the fluoridated community. Another outcome may be that the children at risk for caries without access to fluoride or dental sealants continue to be at risk.

Consider the situation of a dental hygienist employed by the state department of public health. The responsibilities of the position include monitoring quality and quantity of oral health services provided by different public health clinics throughout the state. State law does not allow dental hygienists to practice unless a dentist is on the premises. The dental hygienist responsible is aware that although dental hygienists are providing care in settings where a dentist is not always present, quality care is being provided to individuals in need. A legal and ethical dilemma exists. Should the dental hygienist at the local clinics continue care? Is it fair to discontinue services to particular groups because a local clinic cannot afford to employ a dentist full-time? To whom is the dental hygienist ethically responsible—the citizens of the state, the profession, or the state board? From a legal perspective, the dental hygienist is violating the law. The ethical principles advocating providing care and preventing dental disease can be used to argue that, ethically, the dental hygienist is meeting the obligation; however, ethical codes also direct dental hygienists to uphold the laws and regulations governing the profession. Thus this is a difficult dilemma. Unethical and illegal behavior cannot be tolerated. The dental hygienist coordinating the clinics should seek to remedy the situation legislatively or through creative strategies such as staffing alternatives and affiliation agreements with local dentists or clinics.

In another situation, the dental hygienist travels with a mobile dental clinic program throughout a metropolitan area providing oral health education and preventive services to city residents. The program receives funding from the state to provide care for underserved populations. The dental hygienist begins receiving telephone calls reporting that the dentist staffing the mobile clinic, deluged by the large number of clients, is providing substandard care. The dental hygienist has been a strong advocate of the program, a pilot project that was to be a model for other regions. The dental hygienist knows that reporting the dentist may result in discontinuing services to a population in need. At the same time, the dental hygienist is obligated to document and report inadequate or substandard care. The dental hygienist must protect the clients and stop the inadequate care. Solutions to the dilemma may include working with a local dental society or dental school to assist in staffing the clinic until a replacement dentist is identified.

ADMINISTRATION. Administrators, whether in educational or business-based institutions, face ethical dilemmas. A client visits a dental hygiene clinic for care. The client refuses to be treated by a specific student and makes unkind comments about the student's ethnic background. The administrator must protect the student from the client and provide a comfortable and safe learning environment free of harassment. At the same time, the reputation of the dental hygiene program to willingly treat all persons in the community must be maintained. The administrator may educate the client about his rights and responsibilities or dismiss the client and refer him to another provider for care. In some instances, institutional protocol guides the administrator in choosing a particular option; however, this situation addresses the ethical principles of managing conflicts constructively and promoting human relationships that are mutually beneficial.

In another example, students in a dental hygiene program are assigned to provide nonsurgical periodontal therapy at an urban, hospital-based clinic. The clients treated at the clinic are high-risk for AIDS. The dental hygiene program director is aware that there is always the possibility of a puncture wound occurring, with the result that a dental hygiene student is injured by a contaminated instrument. Does the director choose not to have students assigned to the clinic? Should students and their families be informed of the risk? The situation may create a dilemma in some settings, but using the principle that all individuals should be treated without discrimination, as well as the knowledge that students are using the appropriate standard of care, all students should be assigned.

An administrator also deals with ethical problems among colleagues. The administrator is asked to evaluate the faculty for merit salary raises. Not all faculty members contribute equally to the department. One tenured faculty member fulfills the minimum amount of responsibilities; however, if that faculty person's raise is not comparable to others, she may contribute even less and accuse the administrator of discrimination. Some less productive faculty members may decide to quit, leaving those remaining with the burden of heavier workloads, especially because the college is experiencing a hiring freeze. Does the administrator recognize all the faculty members as equally meritorious? Is there an obligation to report weaker faculty contributions to the administration? What obligation exists to those who are most productive? The administrator must identify the specific problem and, with the questions previously raised, consider the alternatives. One solution is to suggest a merit raise for the weak faculty person, then structure that faculty member's obligations to improve her productivity. The consequences include other faculty members' lowered morale when all faculty members receive merit raises, although not all are justified.

RESEARCH. Informal research occurs in practice when a dental hygienist surveys clients' attitudes, evaluates their acceptance of products and procedures, or compiles salary survey data. Dental hygienists also are involved in research conducted at educational institutions or in association with the manufacturing of oral- or health-related products.

Perhaps a dental hygienist is conducting research to evaluate the effectiveness of a chemotherapeutic agent on selective pathogenic and nonpathogenic microorganisms. The manufacturer is providing funding for the research. The dental hygienist discovers that, although the research design is valid, her co-investigator is allowing personal bias to influence observations and interpretations. Both are aware that if the research establishes the chemotherapeutic agent as effective, the pharmaceutical company that produces the agent will provide generous funding in the future. Should the dental hygienist confront the co-investigator? Should the dental hygienist ignore the unethical and illegal behavior of the co-investigator? Knowing that research is replicated, should the dental hygienist ignore what has occurred and assume that follow-up research will reveal the flaws of the current research?

Other examples of ethical problems in research include the following:

- Individuals who steal another's idea or concept
- Individuals who take credit for a colleague's success in research
- Manipulation of data
- Intentional bias in sampling and failure to report research that does not support or confirm a hypothesis
- Misuse of funds or resources

DENTAL HYGIENIST–DENTIST–CLIENT RELATIONSHIPS. One of the most difficult and common problems is when the dental hygienist and dentist do not agree on the type of oral healthcare required for a client. A dental hygienist observes signs of cancer-like soft tissue changes during the client's assessment. The dental hygienist suggests that the lesion be biopsied. The dentist disagrees. The dental hygienist feels a responsibility to the client that conflicts with that of the dentist. Does the dental hygienist express concern to the client? Should the dental hygienist identify another dentist in the office for a second opinion? Should the dentist's decision stand? The dental hygienist considers all the alternatives and chooses one that satisfies ethical principles. If the dental hygienist seeks another dentist in the office to evaluate the client, the dental hygienist may be satisfied with a second opinion. The consequences can include an unhappy dentist and frightened client; however, if a biopsy does occur, the personal and professional satisfaction gained by the dental hygienist and effects of the biopsy on the client's health outweigh the other consequences. Dilemmas between the dental hygienist and dentist are not easily solved.

Dental hygienists may be employed where they work under the policies and procedures outlined by the dentist-employer(s). When policies and procedures dictate that the dental hygienist is allowed 45 minutes for all clients, that care must be completed in one appointment, or that everyone gets a "routine oral prophylaxis," the dental hygienist is being forced to provide substandard care. Should the dental hygienist work within the policies, ignoring the quality-of-care dilemma? Does the dental hygienist terminate the position? It may be difficult to leave a position because of location, salary, and benefits. Does the dental hygienist inform the client that care is limited and recommend referral for a second opinion? Or does the dental hygienist attempt to provide optimal care and work more diligently? Issues about client care, length of time allotted for care, referral protocols, and other work expectations should be addressed in the preemployment interview process. If issues arise following employment, the dental hygienist may resolve the concerns by scheduling an appointment with the employer or as part of an employee evaluation process, whichever occurs earliest.

Conflicts arise when a client refuses specific treatment, decides to ignore a referral, or continues an unhealthy practice. What ethical obligations does the dental hygienist have to the client and the employer?

A client makes a decision based on information. Some ethical dilemmas created by client actions, or failure to act, could be eliminated if the client were given an appropriate amount of information. With overly brief appointments, ill-informed or uncommunicative staff members are unable to adequately educate clients. Client education and service should remain a priority and guide office practice and policies.

DENTAL HYGIENIST–DENTAL HYGIENIST RELATIONSHIPS. It is difficult to work in an environment in which the care provided by a colleague is below the acceptable standard. For example, the dental hygienist colleague may be compromising client care by not thoroughly assessing the client or may be performing services beyond the scope of dental hygiene care. Situations that may affect the client's care or health status create an immediate dilemma. Does one report the activity to the employer, regulatory boards, or the ethics board of the professional association? Does one attempt to educate or update the colleague? Or does one ignore the situation, assuming it is the employer's responsibility?

In situations like these, talking with the dental hygienist in question may be the best alternative. The dental hygienist may be unaware of the quality-of-care issues or illegal activities. Confronting individuals while offering solutions to the problem is a step toward resolution. Other solutions may include an office in-service session, attending a continuing education class, or developing a dental hygiene office manual outlining specific roles and responsibilities.

EMPLOYER-EMPLOYEE RELATIONSHIPS. In a dental or dental hygiene practice or other work environment, various professional, personal, and business relationships co-exist. As an employee, one may be asked to function in a role that creates ethical problems. Perhaps a dental hygienist suspects that an employer is sexually harassing an employee; a dental hygienist observes that insurance fraud is occurring during billing procedures; or that a colleague has a substance abuse problem. One may immediately determine that the dental hygienist has an obligation to act on the situations observed. Is it the dental hygienist's responsibility to act or is it the employer's? Should the dental hygienist be concerned about the ethical and legal issues? Does one address the issue with the offending practitioner? What if, after the problem is addressed, no change occurs? It is especially exasperating when one recognizes that the dental hygienist is expected to practice within the ADHA or CDHA Code of Ethics but is not in control of the work environment.

The ADHA Code of Ethics says to participate in the development and advancement of the profession. Many dental hygienists are not members of their professional association. Are the dental hygienists who are not members of the association aware of the Code of Ethics? Is it the ethical obligation of a dental hygienist who is a member to encourage nonmembers to join the professional association? As a member of a professional association, a dental hygienist has access to scientific literature, continuing education courses, and other resources. Should these items be shared with nonmember dental hygiene colleagues? Each question raises multiple ethical dilemmas. The Code of Ethics encourages a work environment that promotes individual growth and development. Educating nonmember dental hygienists about the association or sharing new knowledge or expertise supports the professional development philosophy.

Ethical Decision-Making Framework[5]

DEFINE THE PROBLEM OR CONFLICT. The problem may be defined by personal criteria, such as one's feelings, sense of professionalism, or moral code. Ethical or legal standards or a combination of ethical and legal principles also may define the problem. In some instances, the conflict arises from a difference in philosophy, management style, or professional priorities. It is advisable to define precisely the problem or conflict to address the dilemma. It is vague to state, for example, that a conflict has arisen because of different educational backgrounds. It is more precise to identify the conflict as lack of consistency in referring for biopsy or client assessment techniques.

IDENTIFY THE ETHICAL ISSUES. What are the issues? Can one major issue be defined? For example, when a conflict exists between the dental hygienist's suggestion to refer to a specialist versus the dentist's refusal to support the suggestion, the dilemma occurs between a professional obligation to follow the dentist's diagnosis and the dental hygienist's obligation to assess the client's needs and provide quality care. From the client's point of view, the referral may satisfy the client's need for a specialist's evaluation and possible treatment; however, if the dental hygienist's recommendation is incorrect or based on some misconceptions, the second opinion creates an additional expense in time and money for the client, resulting in conflict within the employment setting and a frustrated client.

GATHER RELEVANT INFORMATION. When faced with an ethical dilemma, the dental hygienist must gather all relevant information (e.g., personal data such as family status, age, lifestyle, habits, medical and dental facts, and the professional and personal values involved). Subjective and objective information is included to evaluate the evidence-based and human-based elements. As part of information gathering, one may want to reevaluate a client, research the evidence, investigate a diagnosis, or obtain a third opinion. If the dilemma is focused on an office protocol or policy, the dental hygienist may want to contact other healthcare providers, a lawyer, or a professional association representative to verify about standard practices.

IDENTIFY THE ETHICAL ALTERNATIVES. To answer the question, the dental hygienist should list possible courses of action. For example, in one situation alternatives may include resigning from a position, confronting an employer, or calling the client to express a concern or suggest a course of action. Each alternative may carry serious personal, financial, and professional implications.

In most situations, the list of alternatives takes into consideration the parties involved—the client, dentist, dental hygienist, and co-workers. When listing the alternatives, consider the following:

- Obligation(s) to the client (legal and ethical)
- Obligation(s) to others involved (client's family, employer, colleagues)
- Personal beliefs and values
- Client's legal rights, responsibilities, values, and interests
- Alternatives that protect the client's best interests
- Alternatives that protect the professional's best interests
- Alternatives that do the least amount of harm
- Practical constraints
- Professional judgment

ESTABLISH AN ETHICAL POSITION. Once alternatives are delineated, the dental hygienist must make a choice. In establishing an ethical position, there may be ethical conflicts. For example, a client refuses to be premedicated with an antibiotic before an appointment. If the dental hygienist followed the client's request, the ethical principle of autonomy is followed; however, ethically, the dental hygienist who treats a client without appropriate premedication would potentially harm the client, violating the ethical principles of nonmaleficence. In selecting the course of action, one may weigh which action promotes the best balance between the negative and positive aspects of the situation.

Or one may evaluate the alternatives and choose the least negative alternative. For example, a dental hygienist chooses, in order to balance her recommendations versus the dentist's decisions not to refer a lesion for biopsy, to reschedule the client in two weeks and reevaluate the lesion. The consequences may include a harmonious working relationship, an opportunity to further study the pathology, and the ability to keep open the opportunity that, in two weeks, both the dental hygienist and dentist can conduct a more informed assessment. The conflict may be internal, within the work environment, or with the parties involved, such as the dentist-employer. If one is resolved that the ethical choice is the correct one, however, identifying the consequences assists the decision maker in anticipating and preparing for implementing or acting on the choice.

SELECT, JUSTIFY, AND DEFEND THE ALTERNATIVE. Once the consequences of a choice have been evaluated, and before acting on the choice, one should review the decision. What are the supporting ethical principles? What might be a strong argument against the position? Identifying an argument, aside from an ethical position, that supports the decision is helpful. Evaluation at this stage assists the decision maker before implementing or acting on the choice. Individuals need to evaluate their decisions. It may be that the consequences are so negative that another alternative or compromise might need to be considered (see Example of the Ethical Decision-Making Process).

Dental Ethics Committee (DEC)

The dental team must use ethical principles and codes for resolving an ethical dilemma. Establishing a DEC for the office is one action to facilitate ethical decision making.[6] The DEC could identify dilemmas, use the ethical decision-making model and existing codes of ethics for in-service and discussion to address concerns, and create a team approach for resolving difficult issues. Guidelines could be developed for the DEC, outlining its purposes, functions, and membership. Staff meetings could periodically include the DEC as one of the agenda items. A committee approach assists in raising issues of concern to all office members and educates staff members about ethical decision making. This approach encourages an ethics-based office philosophy.

JURISPRUDENCE

Oral Health Professionals at Risk

Clients have become sophisticated consumers of quality healthcare that is accessible and reasonably priced. Thus an individual who is dissatisfied with oral healthcare frequently looks to the legal system for assistance. Malpractice suits against dental professionals have consistently grown longer (see Are You Contributing to Potential Malpractice Situations or Illegal Dental Hygiene Practice?). Common malpractice litigation includes the following:

- Violation of standard of care, negligence
- Failure to treat problems related to temporomandibular joint disease

Example of the Ethical Decision-making Process

Scenario. A recent dental hygiene graduate takes a position in an office with a staff consisting of two dentists, two dental hygienists, and three dental assistants. The dental hygienist works late one evening a week with a dentist. The dental hygienist notices that after dinner, and throughout the evening, the dentist steps into the laboratory and drinks from a bottle in a paper bag that he hides in the laboratory. He then gargles with mouthwash and returns to client care. His care of clients does not appear compromised. He treats clients and staff with respect, completes care as planned, and manages the office. He meets all the requests of the dental hygienist, and the evening office hours run smoothly; however, the dental hygienist notes that the dentist's drinking behavior is repeated week after week. The dental hygienist questions the staff about the drinking. The staff indicates that they find him a great dentist, the office environment is a good one, and they really like the job. They imply that they hope that the dental hygienist will ignore the situation so that everything will remain the same. Using the framework for ethical decision making, how would the dental hygienist use the model to assist in evaluating the decision?

Define the Problem. The dental hygienist may find it personally offensive that a person is drinking on the job and providing client care. The dental hygienist may feel that the quality of care provided by the dentist is compromised by the drinking, thus violating the ethical mandate of providing the most comprehensive care available. There may be legal issues such as negligent behavior on the part of the dentist. There are also interpersonal issues with the staff members who are ignoring the situation and pressuring the dental hygienist to do the same. The problem is that the dentist is drinking, providing client care, and compromising client safety and staff interaction.

Identify the Ethical Issue. A professional is responsible for protecting clients' well-being. This responsibility is clearly delineated in the ADHA or CDHA Code of Ethics. A dental hygienist must prioritize her responsibilities to the client against the wishes of the staff to ignore the situation. Working with someone in an alcoholic state may affect client care, decision making, and problem solving by the dentist. The issue is one of good versus bad—it is good to report the dentist in order to protect the client; it is bad to allow the drinking to continue.

Gather Relevant Information. Are other staff members noticing the behavior? How long has the pattern existed? Does the drinking occur throughout the whole day? Have there been any untoward incidents identified with the dentist's care or client management? Is the dentist participating in alcoholic rehabilitation? Is there a personal crisis in the dentist's life? The dental hygienist should document her observations and those of others.

The dental hygienist may want to investigate the types of services available to professionals with substance abuse problems. Perhaps a protocol is in place within the state dental society to work with the dentist to overcome his problem and maintain his professional status, or Alcoholics Anonymous may have information about programs. The dental hygienist may want to research alcoholism and the characteristics of an alcoholic to assist in confirming that a problem exists.

Identify the Alternatives. In this situation, alternatives may include the following:

- Discussing observations with the dentist involved
- Discussing and confirming observations with co-workers
- Confronting a single staff member to get additional support
- Discussing observations with others
- Ignoring the situation
- Contacting appropriate agencies, such as the dental association or state board
- Quitting the employment situation
- Refusing to work with the dentist
- Contacting the local dental hygiene or dental component for guidelines or advice
- Talking to peers to get ideas or solutions
- Consulting the code of ethics and the state statutes that govern practice

The dental hygienist is required by the Code to follow the rules and regulations governing the practice of dental hygiene. Thus if a mandate exists requiring the dental hygienist to report situations when client care may be compromised, the alternative of choice is clearly delineated. In most dilemmas, the ethical code is useful to generate alternatives for consideration.

Establish an Ethical Position. As part of the decision-making process, the dental hygienist chooses to confront the dentist and offer information about counseling services available to persons with a drinking problem.

Select, Justify, and Defend the Alternative. One considers the decision in light of supporting ethical principles. In this case, the principles include client care, professional behavior, and the well-being of the client. One may also consider a strong argument against the position, such as the dentist's possible denial or a consequence such as the dentist terminating the dental hygienist's employment rather than admitting a substance abuse problem. Evaluation of the alternative is an ongoing part of the process. As each alternative is identified, its advantages, disadvantages, and consequences are reviewed. The mental exercise of justifying and defending assists the dental hygienist in the decision-making process and helps generate additional alternatives. The dental hygienist goes through a process of "what if" and finishes the sentence.

Act on the Ethical Choice. The most difficult part is acting on the choice. In the best scenario, the dentist welcomes the identification of a problem and seeks counseling to overcome it. The worst scenario may be denial and an effort on the part of the dentist to dismiss the dental hygienist; however, the guiding ethical principle of nonmaleficence, the ADHA Code of Ethics, and genuine concern for fellow employees should strengthen the dental hygienist, whatever the consequences.

Are You Contributing to Potential Malpractice Situations or Illegal Dental Hygiene Practice?

___ I have never gone out of my way to report violators of the dental practice act. I assume the state board monitors that.
___ I sometimes treat clients with severe periodontal disease for years rather than refer them.
___ If I am running late on my schedule, I may not update a client's health history.
___ There is probably a procedure or two that a dental assistant performs in my office that is not allowed under state law.
___ Before treating a client, I rarely explain the reason for the procedure or the risks involved because it takes too much time.
___ If a client insists, we do not always premedicate an individual who should be.
___ If I do not like a client, I may eliminate the name from my continued care list.

If you checked any of these statements, you or your clients are at risk.

- ✦ Failure to diagnose, refer, or treat periodontal disease
- ✦ Failure to obtain informed consent
- ✦ Use of defective products
- ✦ Abandonment of the client
- ✦ Failure to identify and protect a person with a medically compromising condition, such as a heart murmur, drug allergy
- ✦ Failure to maintain proper records
- ✦ Incorrect medical or dental history taking

Oral health professionals are governed by statutory laws enacted by legislators, administrative laws promulgated by regulatory boards, and common law or case law determined by judicial decisions in court cases (Figure 54–1). Each governing body affects the practice of dental hygiene. The professional is presumed to be aware of all the rules and regulations influencing practice and cannot claim ignorance of the law. Sanctions for violations exist, and a practitioner who violates a particular rule may be adjudicated under multiple governing bodies.

For example, a dental hygienist who administers nitrous oxide–oxygen analgesia in a state that restricts

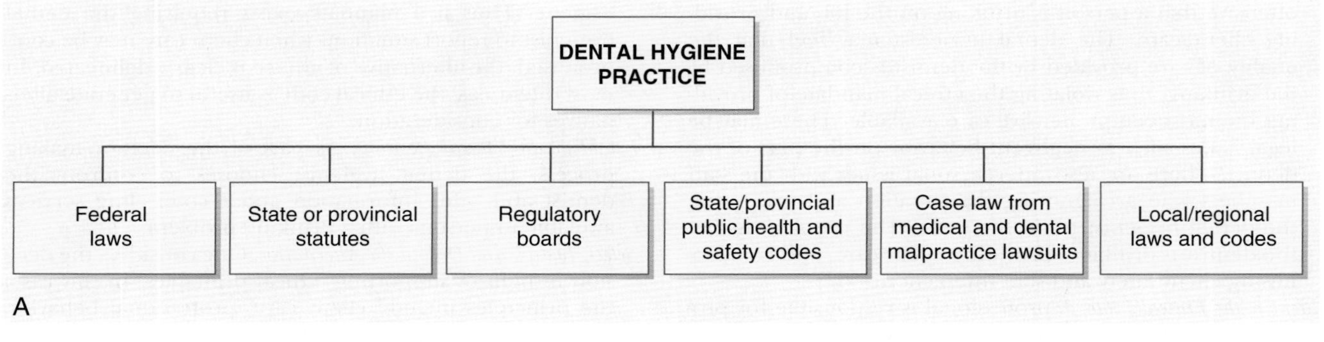

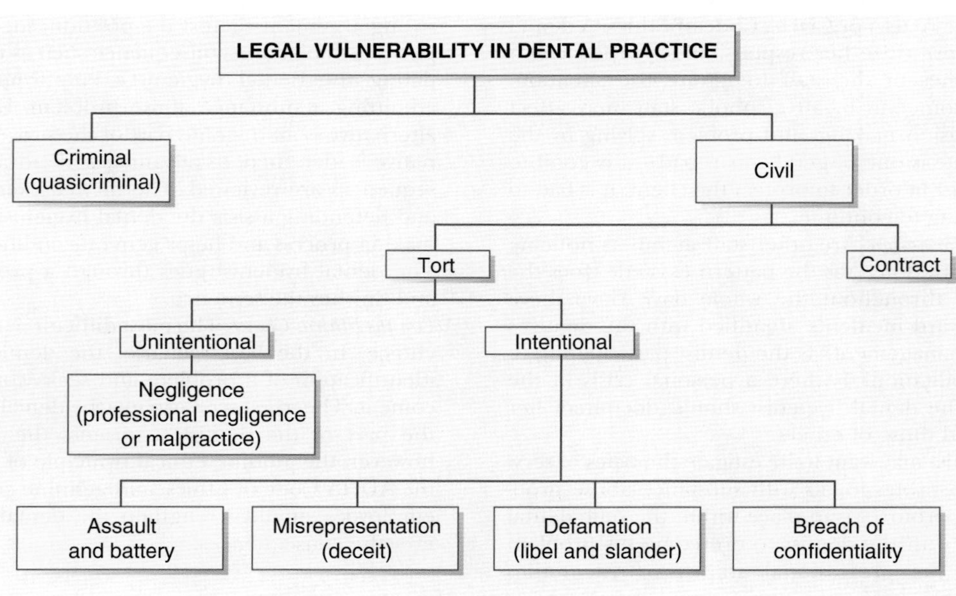

FIGURE 54–1 ✦ **A,** Diagram of governing bodies affecting the practice of dental hygiene. **B,** Diagram of legal vulnerability in dental practice. *(B redrawn from Pollack B:* Risk management manual, *Ft Lauderdale, Fla, 1986, National Society of Dental Practitioners.)*

dental hygiene to traditional practice has violated the rules and regulations outlined by the state regulatory board and may, based on a review of the board, have his or her license revoked or suspended. In addition, the individual may be charged with a civil violation, such as negligence, or a criminal violation, such as administering drugs without a license, depending on state and local statutes, resulting in court action or fines. *A dental hygienist must be aware of the rules and regulations governing the practice of dental hygiene in the jurisdiction where licensing is maintained.*

Basic Legal Concepts

The law is divided into civil and criminal categories. Although these categories are separate, one can be accused of both a civil and criminal violation simultaneously:

- ✦ *Civil law* includes offenses for violating private or contractual rights or, in simpler terms, a breach of legal duty against a person. In a civil lawsuit, a violation against a person is purported to have occurred. The remedy that person seeks is to be "whole" because some type of "damage" has occurred, and the manner in which one is made "whole" is to receive monetary damages.
- ✦ *Criminal law* is that law established for preventing harm against society and describes a criminal act as well as the appropriate punishment. In a criminal lawsuit, the individual found guilty is punished based on society's rules and regulations. Fines, prison terms, or other punishments are based on the specific criminal violation.

Two distinctly different *levels of proof* are used to determine innocence or guilt:

- ✦ For a criminal act, the level of proof required is that *beyond a reasonable doubt.* To meet the level of proof, a jury or judge must be absolutely convinced that the criminal act occurred to establish guilt. If one is not absolutely convinced, an individual must be found innocent.
- ✦ A civil action requires a less strict level of proof, called a *preponderance of evidence.* This level requires that the jury or judge, based on the evidence presented, must be 51% certain that someone is guilty or innocent. For example, a dental hygienist committed an error during client care. If the jury or judge is 51% sure that error caused a harm to the client, the dental hygienist will be found liable.

The requirement of a preponderance of evidence to prove guilt or innocence is weaker than a requirement of proof beyond a reasonable doubt. Professional malpractice suits filed against oral health professionals are usually in the civil arena; thus the level of proof required is the preponderance of evidence. Understanding the level of proof required for civil lawsuits assists in explaining how dental hygienists or dentists are found guilty or innocent when charges are filed against them.

Parties in a lawsuit include the plaintiff(s) and the defendant(s). In a legal dispute, the *plaintiff* is the person who brings the action or files the suit; the *defendant* is the person defending himself or denying the action charged.

Contract Principles and Relationships

Malpractice lawsuits are civil in nature. A common concept of liability used in dental malpractice lawsuits is *breach of contract* (i.e., failure to perform a promise). When one thinks of a contract violation, business transactions come to mind, rather than oral healthcare. Applications of the breach of contract concept were originally limited to business transactions; however, society has become more consumer-oriented, and the courts now recognize the dentist-client relationship as a contract. A legal definition states that a *contract* is an agreement between two or more consenting and competent parties to do or not to do a legal act for which there is sufficient consideration. *Consideration* is an exchange of something of value between two people, such as money.[7] The contractual relationship between the oral health practitioner and the client is one of two types:

- ✦ An implied contractual relationship can begin in a number of situations, including the performance of a professional act, such as taking radiographs or expressing a professional opinion. Although there is no written document of agreement in an *implied contract,* a contractual relationship exists.
- ✦ An *express contract* is one in which the terms are expressed and includes either a verbal or written agreement.

The contract, whether written or oral, may outline specific conditions or obligations that must be satisfied by the client or oral healthcare provider, such as fees, method of payment, or type of services to be provided. In addition, based on the contractual relationship, certain warranties or duties are required by both parties. The word *duty* in legal vernacular means obligatory conduct or service, or conducting yourself in a particular manner. Professionals in the legal system evaluate medical malpractice case law to determine the contractual rights and duties shared between the practitioner and client based on the contractual relationship. Based on that contractual relationship, in accepting the client for care, the oral healthcare provider warrants to:[8]

- ✦ Be properly licensed and registered and meet all other legal requirements to engage in the practice of dentistry or dental hygiene
- ✦ Use reasonable care in providing services as measured against acceptable standards set by other practitioners with similar training
- ✦ Never exceed the scope of practice
- ✦ Not use experimental procedures or medications
- ✦ Complete care within a reasonable time frame or arrange other sources of treatment when appropriate in order to complete treatment
- ✦ Never abandon the client by abruptly stopping oral healthcare

- Obtain informed consent before examination or treatment from the individual or the party responsible (i.e., guardian)
- Arrange care for the client during an absence and ensure that care is available in emergency situations
- Make appropriate referrals and request necessary consultations
- Maintain client privacy and confidentiality of information
- Maintain a level of knowledge in keeping with current advances in the profession
- Keep clients informed of their treatment progress and health status
- Inform the client of unanticipated occurrences
- Never exceed the scope of practice authorized by the license; never permit any person acting under another's direction to engage in unlawful acts
- Keep accurate records of the care provided to the client
- Comply with all laws regulating the practice of dentistry and dental hygiene
- Practice in a manner consistent with the code of ethics of the profession
- Charge a reasonable fee for services based on community standards
- Not attempt a procedure for which the practitioner is unqualified

The duties or warranties listed are enforceable, although not written or stated in any document given to the client. A dental hygienist who uses an experimental periodontal therapy rather than evidence-based procedures may be violating a contractual responsibility to use only standard procedures. A dental hygienist who casually discussed confidential information obtained from a client during the health history interview is violating a contractual obligation ignoring the principle of fidelity, as well as committing a breach of confidentiality. A dental hygienist practicing outdated techniques is also violating a duty to remain current and ignoring the principle of beneficence.

The client has contractual duties, including cooperating in care, providing accurate information, paying fees, and keeping appointments. Practitioners are frequently faced with clients who do not pay fees. Collection procedures may result based on the client's failure to meet the contractual obligation. Failing to cooperate in care, such as missed appointments or refusal to take premedication, does not necessarily result in a lawsuit filed by the dentist. Rather than a lawsuit, the practitioner may choose to dismiss the client from the practice.

If a breach of contract occurs, the client can use the contract concept to remedy the situation and obtain damages. Perhaps a client discovers that a dental assistant, not a dental hygienist, is providing root planing and which only a licensed dental hygienist is allowed to perform. The assistant did not harm the client; however, the dentist warranted, based on the contractual relationship between the dentist and client, that employees within the office were properly licensed and that the staff would never exceed scope of practice. In this example, three violations occurred and a breach of contract exists. At the same time, if the client has not met obligations, such as keeping an appointment, that client has breached the contract. Although the practitioner would probably not seek damages, the failure of the client to meet his responsibilities *(contributory negligence)* may be reason to end the practitioner-client relationship.

TERMINATING THE PRACTITIONER-CLIENT RELATIONSHIP. Termination of the practitioner-client relationship frequently occurs in practice; however, the practitioner must be cautioned never to abandon the client. *Abandonment* is a relinquishment of all connection with the client. The relationship between professional and client may end without charges of abandonment if the following conditions are met:

- Both parties agree to end it.
- The death of the client or oral health practitioner occurs.
- The client ends the relationship by act or statement.
- The client is cured, or treatment completed, as with a specialist.
- The practitioner unilaterally decides to terminate care.

If the practitioner seeks to end the relationship, specific steps are necessary:

- The client should receive written notification of termination and the reasons (e.g., lack of payment for services rendered or nonadherence to recommended care).
- Reason for termination should be provided in objective language. If a client is being terminated due to harassing behaviors, the letter does not have to describe the specific behavior. Instead, the letter can indicate that the dentist is terminating the relationship because of "disrespectful attitudes and behaviors toward staff."
- Letter should state that the individual will remain a client of the practice for a certain length of time, the date services will be terminated, and that, if necessary, emergency care will be provided for a designated time period.
- Letter must suggest that the client seek another dental care provider and state that copies of the client's records will be forwarded to the new provider. It is advisable to include a permission slip for transfer of records that the client can sign and return to expedite the process (see Figure 54–5 later in the chapter).
- Letter should be sent by certified or registered mail with return receipt requested (Figure 54–2). The termination process is done carefully to ensure continuity of care and diminish the possibility of charges of abandonment. A copy of the termination letter and returned receipt should be kept in the client's file.

September 27, 2003

Mr. Daniel Powers
12214 Harvard Road
Point Park, MI 48000

Dear Mr. Powers:

Our records indicate that you have failed to respond to six notices for periodontal maintenance care, sent over the 4-year period from 1999–2003 requesting that you make an appointment for an examination and oral maintenance. Your lack of response to both mail and telephone messages suggests that you do not agree with our preventive philosophy. Thus, effective October 27, 2003, your relationship with this office is terminated. You will remain a patient in the practice for the next 30 days. Emergency treatment only will be provided during that 30-day period. I strongly suggest that you identify another oral healthcare provider. I shall be happy to forward a copy of your records once that practitioner is identified. Enclosed is a permission slip to transfer your records. Please sign the transfer slip and return to the office.

Mary L. Mesial, RDH, BS, PC

FIGURE 54–2 ✦ Letter of protection, terminating dental hygienist–client relationship.

Avoiding charges of abandonment becomes an issue in dental hygiene care when clients of record do not respond to a continued-care notice. Although office procedures may not require that an individual receive notification that he or she is no longer a client of record, actions such as the written notification should be taken.

Another example of a situation that may require termination of the practitioner-client relationship is when the client refuses necessary oral radiographs or prophylactic antibiotic premedication for the prevention of infective endocarditis. Rather than jeopardize quality of care, the dental hygienist may dismiss the client of record from the practice. Again, written notification of termination is necessary to protect the dental hygienist and the employer from charges of abandonment.

RELATED RESPONSIBILITIES. *The law states that a practitioner may refuse to treat an individual for any reason except race, creed, color, national origin, or certain condition, such as a handicap.* For example, a practice specializing in prosthodontic care may refuse to accept children as clients. As long as there is not a discriminatory reason such as ethnic origin, not accepting children as clients is legal. An office that fails to schedule individuals with Hispanic-sounding surnames, however, is discriminating based on national origin.

Dental hygienists should obtain information about the rules and regulations governing the care of clients within their state to avoid charges of discrimination. Different jurisdictions (states, commonwealths, provinces) have defined special groups that fall within certain statutory implications relating to civil rights and discrimination. For example, in some states, statutes related to the rights of the handicapped protect persons with HIV infection.

One can refuse to treat a client of record and not violate a contract obligation. A practitioner *should refuse* to treat a client if the practitioner does not have the competence to provide the appropriate standard of care. The practitioner without the necessary skills is expected to refer the client to the appropriate oral health provider. Lawsuits have resulted from practitioners attempting to provide care that is beyond the practitioner's level of competence. Perhaps a dental hygienist evaluates the client's periodontal health and, although referral is indicated by the condition presented, the dentist chooses to provide treatment. If a certain skill level is required to provide the appropriate treatment (e.g., root planing and periodontal surgery) and those skills are not found within the personnel of that practice, the practitioner has failed to meet the obligation to refer. The referral is not viewed as a discriminatory practice, but rather is the appropriate action under contract principles.

Tort Principles

The legal basis most commonly used by clients to file suit against healthcare providers is the *negligence principle.* Negligence falls within the category of law known as torts. A *tort* is an interference with another's right to enjoy person, property, or privacy.[7] Categories of torts are as follows:

- ✦ Intentional torts
- ✦ Unintentional torts

INTENTIONAL TORTS. *Intentional torts* are committed with intent on the part of the person. Intentional torts include battery, assault, false imprisonment, mental distress, breach of confidentiality, interference with property (e.g., trespassing on private property), and misrepresentation or deceit. Professional liability insurance frequently covers only the unintentional tort of negligence. Intentional torts require that the person accused of the tort intended the harm that occurred. An intentional tort is a serious offense. Some intentional torts of interest to dental hygienists are highlighted.

An *assault*[7] occurs when one intends to cause apprehension in someone, without touching him or her. An example of an assault may be threatening someone with a raised hand. A practitioner that threatens to harm someone, or causes fear, may be guilty of assault, such as in the example, "If you do not sit still, I am going to stick you with the needle."

A *battery*[7] is a harmful or offensive contact with someone—touching someone without their permission (e.g., restraining a child without parental permission). A *technical battery*[7] is when a dental hygienist, in the course of treatment, exceeds the consent given by the client. Examples of technical battery include placing dental sealants on teeth when consent was not obtained, or giving a fluoride treatment without the client's consent. In such cases, the person bringing the charges (plaintiff) argues that the contact was offensive, and the dental hygienist (defendant) could be charged with both assault and battery. Assault and battery are considered intentional torts, and professional liability insurance may not provide coverage for charges filed under these categories. The dental hygienist should obtain informed consent to prevent charges of assault and battery. (Informed consent is discussed later in the section.)

Deceit or *misrepresentation* can occur in the provision of oral healthcare. A failure to inform a client that an instrument tip has broken and is lodged in the sulcus is an example of deceit. A practitioner must always keep the client informed of his or her oral healthcare status and not misrepresent personnel or services rendered. If a dental hygienist is ill and is substituted by a dental assistant, there is an intent to misrepresent the dental assistant as a dental hygienist, and the employer is guilty of an intentional tort.

Another tort that could be classified as intentional is *breach of confidentiality*. A dental hygienist who violates the confidential relationship between the dental hygienist and client is committing a tort. Discussing a specific client's history over lunch is a violation of confidentiality between the practitioner and client. If a dental hygienist responds to a request for client information, without the client's permission, the confidential relationship is violated.

UNINTENTIONAL TORTS—NEGLIGENCE. Unintentional torts are *not* intended by the person accused of committing the tort. Negligence and dental malpractice are used synonymously. *Negligence*[7] is a failure of one owing a duty to another to do what a reasonable and prudent person would ordinarily have done under the circumstances. The defining characteristics of negligence are the following:

- ✦ A duty or standard exists (e.g., health history taking; assessing blood pressure levels; assessing periodontal health, recording oral health status, referral)
- ✦ A breach or failure to exercise requisite care (e.g., failing to assess the client, treat the client; meet the standard of care for the practice of dental hygiene; incorrect use of anesthesia)
- ✦ A harm results (e.g., medical emergency; periodontal status declines; paresthesia)
- ✦ The harm is directly caused by the breach of duty

The plaintiff's responsibility is to prove that the defendant was negligent. The plaintiff must prove, by a preponderance of the evidence, all of the elements listed previously. For example, a dental hygienist is placing dental sealants on a child's teeth. The treatment area is a typical environment, with the operator's supplies on the dental bracket tray. The supplies include a receptacle with acid-etch material. The dental hygienist is etching the teeth while holding the acid-etch–filled receptacle. The child suddenly moves, the acid etch spills on the child, and a chemical burn occurs on the side of the child's face. Has negligent behavior occurred? One would need to evaluate the elements of negligence to answer the question. The dental hygienist did not intend to burn the child; however, a duty existed to be careful while applying the acid-etch solution. For the most part, the dental hygienist was practicing cautiously; however, evidence may indicate that keeping the acid-etch solution away from the child is recommended to avoid spilling. The dental hygienist failed to use certain precautionary measures (*reasonably prudent man rule*) and harm resulted. The harm was proximately caused by the dental hygienist's actions, and thus the hygienist is found negligent by a judge or a jury. Again, the jury or judge would have to be only 51% sure that the dental hygienist's actions caused the harm. They may recognize that the child's actions influenced what occurred, but may still find the dental hygienist negligent.

Another example of negligent behavior could occur if a dental hygienist leaves infection control chemicals (like those used to clean out suction units) in a cup on a counter. If, when the dental hygienist is away from the treatment room, a client mistakes the liquid for water or mouthrinse and drinks it, harm occurs although there was no intent to harm the client.

Standard of Care. *Standard of care*[7] is the degree of care *a reasonably prudent professional* would exercise under the same or similar circumstances. The standard of care is not defined by the courts, but rather is determined by members of the profession. In negligence actions, in order to define the standard of care and determine if the defendant is guilty or innocent, expert witnesses are called to testify. (A lawyer may seek information from a professional association, such as the ADHA or CDHA, professional literature, or a nationally recognized group, such as the Centers for Disease Control and Prevention, as a source of acceptable standards.)

An expert witness is a member of the defendant's professional group with a similar background (e.g., in a periodontal malpractice lawsuit, a dental hygienist working in a periodontal practice). Lawyers for both the plaintiff and defendant may call into court expert witnesses that best satisfy their arguments. Thus the dental hygienist, who may be defending specific actions, may identify an expert witness to support the standard of care demonstrated by that dental hygienist's practices. The plaintiff, on the other hand, has an expert witness testify that the dental hygienist did not meet the acceptable standard of care. The decision of liability is left to the jurors and judge. Jurors, it should be noted, are primarily composed of non–healthcare providers. As indicated earlier, the level of proof required in civil actions is a preponderance of the evidence.

After listening to the testimony of both the expert witnesses, jurors decide whether the plaintiff was negligent. Thus, if there is a failure to meet that standard, as determined by the jurors or a judge, the dental hygienist may be found negligent. For example, a dental hygienist fails to monitor and record a client's blood pressure before care. The client suffers a cardiac arrest during treatment related to high blood pressure. The standard of care for dental hygiene includes taking and recording blood pressure as part of client assessment. The dental hygienist failed to meet the standard.

The failure to meet the standard of care can include the following:

- ✦ An *act of omission* (i.e., not doing something)
- ✦ An *act of commission* (i.e., performing an act inappropriately)

Omitting a procedure or step because one is unaware that it is the current standard is not an acceptable excuse in a court of law.

Dental hygienists are obligated to practice the concepts and techniques currently accepted (i.e., to meet the standard of care). Although the dentist is ultimately responsible for the actions of the dental hygienist, the dental hygienist still may be found negligent in a court of law if a required duty is not met. Typically, dental practitioners may be found negligent when harm is caused to the client as a result of failure to stay current. It is difficult for any dental professional to accept a verdict of *guilty of negligence* because, as was noted earlier, there is no intent on the professional's part to provide inadequate care; however, members of the legal system attempt to evaluate the facts objectively. They evaluate the actions of the practitioners and then assess the impact of those actions on the client. If harm occurs, the legal system decides who is at fault and awards damages, if appropriate.

Informed Consent. Another legal argument that falls within the negligence theory used in lawsuits against practitioners is lack of informed consent. *Informed consent* is a person's agreement to allow something to happen based on full disclosure of facts required to make an intelligent decision; *consent* is the individual's right to self-determination. As part of the consent process, clients must be informed of the material risks involved in care. Obtaining informed consent cannot be delegated to an assistant; it is the professional's responsibility to obtain consent.

A *material risk* is one that a "reasonable person" would consider in determining whether to proceed with the proposed treatment. Court decisions have determined that the client has the final say in his or her care, must be of sound mind when giving consent, and the consent must be *informed* to be valid.[7]

To achieve informed consent, clients must be told in a language that they understand, the following information:

- ✦ Diagnosis of the condition
- ✦ Recommended procedure
- ✦ Nature and reasons for the procedure(s)
- ✦ Benefits of the procedure
- ✦ Material risks in performing the procedure
- ✦ Prognosis if the procedure is performed or not performed
- ✦ Alternatives to the recommended procedure
- ✦ Risks and benefits to the alternative procedures
- ✦ Potential consequences if client does not choose the recommended procedure

In lawsuits that focus on informed consent, clients claim a lack of understanding of the risks involved in care, or that alternatives to treatment were not presented. The dental hygienist should explain any technical terms and make sure that the client comprehends the information; a language interpreter may be necessary. Consent must be obtained for minors from parents or guardians. It is important to obtain consent from the parent(s) legally allowed to provide consent for medical and dental treatment. Issues of consent for minors with divorced or separated parents must be carefully monitored so that legal consent is obtained. If a client is legally incompetent, consent must be obtained from a guardian. Consent can be documented using a standardized form that allows portions to be completed on a case-by-case basis (Figure 54–3).

Clients should sign the consent form. If care is modified or if additional invasive procedures are performed, consent should be obtained again. Dental hygienists must take the time to obtain informed consent and allow the client an opportunity to ask questions. This opportunity to ask and have questions answered also must be documented in the client's record. Informed consent should be obtained for all surgical and invasive procedures as well as fluoride therapy, radiographs, and similar services. It is suggested that office policy be developed so that informed consent is obtained in a consistent manner with all clients.

Informed Refusal (Figure 54–4). A risk of a lawsuit occurs when the client refuses to follow the advice of the treating dentist or dental hygienist. The lawsuit may occur if a client suffers serious injury or consequences after refusing care and claims he or she did not fully understand the consequences of refusing a recommendation or treatment. *A basic rule to follow when a client refuses advice is to inform the client of possible consequences.* The rules follow those of obtaining informed consent to care. They

1. I consent to the recommended procedure or treatment ______________________
____
to be completed by Dr./Ms. ______________.
2. The procedure(s) or treatment(s) have been described to me.
3. I have been informed of the purpose of the procedure or treatment.
4. I have been informed of the alternatives to the procedure or treatment.
5. I understand that the following risk(s) may result from the procedure or treatment:
____
____
______________________.
6. I understand that the following risk(s) may occur if the procedure or treatment is not completed:
____
____
____
______________________.
7. I do—do not—consent to the administration of anesthetic.
   a. I understand that the following risks are involved in administering anesthesia:
   ____
   ____
   ____
   ______________________.
   b. The following alternatives to anesthesia were described: ______________________
   ____
   ______________________.

All my questions have been satisfactorily answered.

Signature: ______________________
Date

Representative: ______________________
Date

Signature of Witness: ______________________
Date

FIGURE 54–3 ✦ Consent form.

Date	Progress Notes
11-5-03	Care plan suggests periodontal surgery. Explained justification for surgery, risks, and alternative of three-month maintenance care, with reevaluation of need for surgery; client opted for three-month maintenance care. Client states that she understands three-month regimen must be strictly followed. Explained limitations of maintenance care versus surgery. Client asked questions about procedures at maintenance appointment.
	I, Mary Gorski, refuse periodontal surgery as recommended by M. Mesial. I opt to cooperate in a three-month maintenance care appointment program for a nine-month period. The risks, benefits, and reasons for both treatment alternatives have been adequately explained, and my questions answered.

FIGURE 54–4 ✦ Progress notes.

include that the client be told in understandable language the following information:

- ✦ The diagnosis and recommendation for treatment or referral
- ✦ The reasons for the recommendation
- ✦ Risks and possible consequences to client's oral and general health

There must be discussion about the refusal and the effects as well as an opportunity to discuss the recommendation. During the discussion, if it appears that the client refused care because of lack of understanding, the dental hygienist reexplains the recommendation. The client's refusal can be documented on an *informed refusal* form that includes the following:

- ✦ Recommendation
- ✦ List of the consequences of refusal
- ✦ Documentation that the client understood the risks of refusing care
- ✦ The date
- ✦ Signatures of the dentist, client, and a witness

If the client refuses to sign the informed refusal, this should be noted and the form signed by the provider and the witness. A copy of the form should be given to the client and another copy kept in the chart.

Statute of Limitations. The *statute of limitations* is the length of time an aggrieved person has to enter lawsuits against another for an alleged injury.[7] A statute of limitations places a time limit on a contract or tort action. Once the time period has ended, the lawsuit cannot be filed. For example, the statute of limitations for a contract action may be 6 years and a tort action 3 years. In some states, the statute of limitations starts either at the time an injury occurs or at the time the plaintiff discovers the injury or reasonably should have discovered the injury. This ability to sue when an injury is discovered expands the length of time that someone can file a lawsuit. Perhaps a client is diagnosed with severe periodontal diseases 5 years after ending a client-provider relationship. The client still may be allowed to file a lawsuit. Risk constantly exists for a lawsuit to be filed. Practitioners must be aware of the statute of limitations and rules within their state to assist in planning for recordkeeping and record storage.

Legal Concepts and the Dental Hygienist–Client Relationship

CONFIDENTIALITY. The dental hygienist–client relationship raises additional areas of concern that extend the legal duties and obligations outlined. A client's care is confidential. To release confidential information without the client's permission is an invasion of privacy. Invasion of privacy includes releasing client information to an unauthorized person, such as an employer, or discussing a client's health history outside the scope of treatment. In large, open clinics, discussions with clients

I, _______________, hereby grant permission
(Print Name)
to _______________________________
(Print Name of Doctor or Hospital)

to release information related to my health history, status, and care, and copies of my health record, radiographs, and any test results to:

____

at _______________________________

_______________________________.

Signature: _______________________
Date
(If a Minor, Parent or Guardian Must Sign)

FIGURE 54–5 ✦ Request for release of health information.

may appear less private. It is important that the practitioner maintains confidentiality of information in all settings and takes steps to protect client privacy and confidentiality.

A person can waive confidentiality through words or actions. For example, an individual who is referred to a specialist waives confidentiality. The referring practitioner is expected to inform the specialist of the client's status. Confidentiality can be waived by action of law, such as a requirement to report specific communicable diseases or the suspicion of child abuse to a state or provincial agency. A client's waiver of confidentiality should be documented in a progress note or separate form entitled Waiver of Confidentiality (Figure 54–5).

DEFAMATION. A communication that injures an individual's reputation may be:

- *Libel* (written defamation)
- *Slander* (verbal defamation)

To be libelous or slanderous, the defamatory comment must *not* be true. If an individual's reputation is not harmed by the defamatory comment, there is no libel or slander. In certain defamation cases, malice (intent to inflict an injury) must be shown. If a lawsuit is filed, the plaintiff must show actual damages to property, business, trade, profession, occupation, or feeling. Thus an informal comment to one person about an "incompetent dentist" by a recently fired dental hygienist would not be considered slander. The dentist's reputation was not harmed and those listening would consider the source and not necessarily believe the comment. Repeated comments by a dental hygienist in a periodontal practice stating that one periodontist is more skilled than another may result in a lawsuit, if the comments harm the dentist's reputation or influence clients' return to the practice.

Legal Concepts and the Dental Hygienist–Dentist Relationship

DISCRIMINATION IN EMPLOYMENT. In seeking employment, an individual is protected against unlawful discriminatory practices. Federal and state labor laws exist to protect both employers and employees. A federal statute, Title VII of *the Civil Rights Act of 1964*, prohibits discrimination based on race, color, religion, gender, or national origin as it relates to hiring, firing, terms, conditions, or privileges of employment. Gender discrimination includes discrimination based on pregnancy, childbirth, and related medical conditions such as gynecologic or gender-related problems. Title VII applies to employers with 15 or more employees; however, human rights acts enacted in almost all states outlaw the same type of discriminatory activity and may affect employers with as few as one employee. State laws may also expand the types of discrimination banned (e.g., discrimination based on marital status, physical handicap, or sexual orientation). The *Age Discrimination in Employment Act of 1967* (ADEA) is a federal law that affects employers with 20 or more employees. The act prohibits discrimination on the basis of age between 40 and 70 years.

The Equal Employment Opportunity Commission (EEOC) deals with discrimination on any of the federally prohibited grounds. The EEOC assists by investigating or advising on appropriate agencies to contact. There are strict guidelines on the timeliness of the complaint, such as a requirement to bring a complaint within 180 days. If the EEOC is unable to obtain a solution, an individual may have the right to file a lawsuit. The EEOC has local offices that will answer questions or direct an individual to appropriate sources to resolve issues. Federal laws prohibiting employment discrimination are available from the EEOC Web site. Dental hygienists who believe they have been discriminated against in the employment setting should contact their state civil rights agency.

Americans with Disabilities Act. *The Americans with Disabilities Act* (AwDA) prohibits employment discrimination against qualified individuals with disabilities. The law applies to employers with 15 or more employees. An individual qualifies for protection under this act if he or she has a physical or mental impairment that substantially limits one or more major life activities. Major life activities include walking, breathing, seeing, hearing, speaking, learning, and working. If an individual satisfies the position requirements, the employer is required to provide reasonable accommodations such as modifying equipment, facilities, schedules, or job routine. For example, an office receptionist with a hearing impairment may require telephone amplification in order to meet the job requirements.

Equal Pay Act. *The Equal Pay Act of 1962* protects men and women who perform substantially equal work in the same establishment from gender-based wage discrimination. The law would not allow an employer to reduce the wages of either a man or woman to equalize inequities in pay.

Pregnancy and Employment Status. A significant percentage of dental hygienists are female; therefore, discrimination based on pregnancy is an important issue. Federal law prohibits an employer from terminating or refusing to hire or promote a woman because of childbirth, pregnancy, or related medical conditions, such as abortion. The EEOC is the agency that administers Title VII provisions. Guidelines distributed by the EEOC state that disabilities caused or contributed to by pregnancy or childbirth must be treated like any other disability. Mandatory leave arbitrarily set at a specific time for pregnant women without regard to their ability to work is also prohibited, as well as a policy that prohibits an employee from returning to work for a predetermined length of time after childbirth. Pregnancy benefits cannot be limited to married women only. Dental hygienists, in order to be informed and assist their employers, should obtain information from a local department of human rights if a maternity leave is anticipated.

EMPLOYER-EMPLOYEE RELATIONSHIPS. Seeking employment is a common occurrence. An employment application can include the following:

- Identification of the applicant (e.g., name, address, telephone number)
- Applicant's interests (jobs, salary levels)
- Summary of applicant's background including education, employment history, and skills

Unlawful preemployment inquiries include the following:

- Applicant's maiden name
- Birthplace of applicant
- Religious denomination or affiliation
- Complexion or skin color
- Disability status
- Photograph required
- Height, weight
- Marital status or children
- Arrest record
- National origin, ancestry, or descent
- Society or club memberships or affiliations

Applicants need not provide the information that falls within the unlawful category. Individual states have legislation that regulates employment. An excellent resource is a state department of civil rights or related agencies.

Unlike some employer-employee relationships, the dental hygienist rarely has a written employment contract. Traditionally, responsibilities of employment, financial arrangements, benefits, and length of employment are verbally agreed upon. Lack of a written agreement may leave the dental hygienist in a precarious situation. The contract is written documentation that clearly outlines the rights and responsibilities of the parties involved. The ADHA provides a sample employment contract to its members. A dental hygienist-employee needs to assist an employer so that a complete and fair contract is drafted, addressing the following issues:

- Position title and responsibilities
- Schedule days and hours of the week
- Remuneration:
  - Amount
  - Pay period schedule
  - Benefits to be deducted
  - Manner remuneration will be calculated—commission, hourly, daily
- Schedules of review/evaluation:
  - Influence on remuneration
  - Method of evaluation: formal/informal
- Fringe benefits
- Notification requirements for contract severance
- Specific expectations

In most jurisdictions, the dental hygienist works as an employee with the dentist. The law views this as a basic employer-employee relationship where there is direct control and supervision of the employee by the employer. The doctrine governing the relationship is *respondeat superior,*[7] Latin for "let the superior/master answer." Based on the traditional structure of most state dental practice acts, the dentist/employer answers for the actions of the dental hygienist. The dental hygienist, as a licensed professional, is legally accountable and can be sued. Because of the doctrine of *respondeat superior,* however, dentists are also named in lawsuits filed against dental hygienists. Including the dentist as one of the parties of a lawsuit is a reflection of the "deep pocket" theory. That is, the monetary damages sought can be increased because of the larger malpractice insurance coverage of the dentist-employer.

Another business relationship with the dentist-employer that may exist for the dental hygienist is that of an independent contractor. As an independent contractor, the dental hygienist is under contract to fulfill certain responsibilities but has little guidance by the contracting party. The Internal Revenue Service (IRS) distinguishes whether a person is an independent contractor or employee as related to federal taxes (see IRS Guideposts for Independent Contractors). The criteria include 20 different points to consider in determining the status of a worker. The key in reviewing the points is the control by the respective parties in the relationship and the substance of the relationship over form.

The independent contractor is self-employed. With the increased freedom of independent contracting, there is also an increased liability and total responsibility for income and social security taxes. An individual interested in an independent contracting agreement should investigate the area within the jurisdiction and seek legal advice.

SEXUAL HARASSMENT. Federal guidelines classify sexual harassment as a form of sexual discrimination. *Sexual harassment* is defined as sexual discrimination because it forces a female or male to work under adverse

IRS Guideposts for Independent Contractors

As an aid to determining whether an individual is an employee under the common law rules, 20 factors are identified as indicating whether sufficient control is present to establish an employer-employee relationships.

Instructions—when, where, and how work is performed

Training—requiring the worker to work with experienced employees, corresponding with the worker, requiring the worker to attend meetings or use other methods

Integration—of the worker's services into business operations

Services rendered personally—if services must be rendered personally, it is presumed the persons for whom services are performed are interested in methods used

Hiring, supervising, and paying assistants—if the persons for whom services are performed hire assistants, that generally shows control; the reverse is also true

Continuing relationship

Set hours of work

Full-time standard—if the worker performs full-time and restricts the employee from performing other work

Doing work on the employer's premises—suggests control over the worker, especially if the work could be done elsewhere

Order of sequence set—if the worker must follow a sequence set out by the entity for whom he or she is performing the services, this would indicate an employer-employee relationship

Oral or written reports—written reports indicate control

Payment by hour, week, month—indicates employer-employee relationship; payment by job indicates independent contractor relationship

Payment of business and/or travel expenses—if the person for whom services are performed pays for travel expenses, this generally indicates employer-employee relationship

Furnishing of tools or material—by person for whom work is performed indicates employer-employee relationship

Significant investment—lack of investment in the facilities indicates employer-employee relationship

Realization of profit or loss—by worker would indicate independent contractor; but the worker who cannot is generally considered an employee

Working for more than one firm—if the worker performs work for more than one firm—unrelated—that generally indicates the worker is an independent contractor

Making service available to the general public—on a regular basis indicates an independent contractor

Right to discharge—indicates employer-employee relationship

Right to terminate—by the employee without incurring liability, indicates employer-employee relationship

From: http://webcom.com/ic_rep/20factor.html

employment conditions. The EEOC defines sexual harassment as follows:

> Unwelcome sexual advances, requests for sexual favors and other verbal or physical conduct of a sexual nature when submission to or rejection of this conduct is made either explicitly or implicitly a term or condition of an individual's employment; submission to or rejection of such conduct by an individual is used as the basis for employment decisions affecting the individual; or such conduct has the purpose or effect of unreasonably interfering with an individual's work performance or creating an intimidating, hostile or offensive working environment. (Fed. Reg., 1980)

Two types of sexual harassment occur:

- *Quid pro quo*, which means something for something, involves a superior-subordinate relationship in which the offender has control over the working conditions of the victim. Examples of sexual harassment include demands for sexual favors in exchange for better working conditions or reviews, raises, or promotions.
- *Hostile environment* includes unwelcome, demeaning verbal or physical conduct of a sexual nature creating a hostile, intimidating, or offensive work environment. Behaviors that may create a hostile work environment include conversation with sexual content, telling sexually explicit jokes, displaying sexually suggestive objects or pictures, and using names such as "honey," "sweetie," or "blondie." The environment may interfere with the ability of the harassed employee to do the job; however, there is no tangible employment loss evident. Supervisors, co-workers, or nonemployees may be involved.

Sexual harassment occurs in the dental environment.[9] A dental hygienist reported that every time she asked for a dentist "to check" a client following a dental hygiene appointment, the dentist asked the dental hygienist to perform a sexual act. The dental hygienist, flustered and embarrassed, did not want to work alone with the dentist. Although the request for sexual favors was not related to salary or employee evaluation, it easily could have developed into that type of situation. The dentist's actions constitute sexual harassment. A second example may be a client who makes inappropriate remarks or gestures of a sexual nature. Clients, who are considered nonemployees, influence the environment in which a dental hygienist is employed. A dental hygienist should report the behavior of the client to the employer. The employer is obligated to make the working environment nonthreatening.

An employer is required to maintain a professional, businesslike relationship among employees and prevent or stop all situations considered harassment in the workplace. Prevention is the best strategy. Employers should communicate to all employees that sexual harassment will not be tolerated. If an individual has been the victim of sexual harassment, immediate action is necessary. An employee's response to either physical or verbal harassment must be prompt, serious, specific, and assertive. If faced with sexual harassment, one should do the following:

- Directly inform the harasser that the conduct is unwelcome, and specifically identify the conduct.
- Directly inform the harasser that the conduct is to stop.

- Review office policies and protocol and/or notify an employer or supervisor of the incident.
- Talk to co-workers; determine whether there have been similar experiences shared by others or if others have witnessed harassing behaviors.
- If a refusal may affect the job, report the incident to a co-owner of the practice or appropriate supervisory personnel.
- Document the harassment and keep accurate notes of what was said, done, date, time, places, and witnesses.

If the situation is not remedied, options exist. In settings that employ 15 or more employees, the district office of the EEOC is contacted. The EEOC will guide an individual through the process of filing a complaint against the harasser. If there are fewer than 15 employees, assistance may be available from a state agency such as the State Department of Civil Rights. Although hiring a lawyer may not be necessary, legal representation is helpful to guide the victim and represent the victim if the case progresses. The district EEOC office is a resource.

TERMINATION OF EMPLOYMENT. Dental hygienists may have their employment terminated for little or no reason, defined as "at will." The small business atmosphere of dental practice allows the "at will termination" by either party to exist. Some states have developed legal remedies for individuals wrongfully terminated. Some jurisdictions, for example, have laws that allow employers to terminate employees for good cause (i.e., someone can lose his or her position with or without a reason or justification). A dental hygienist should be familiar with the state's policy on termination. Various states have developed criteria that must be met to prove either appropriate or inappropriate employer behavior. The termination process can also be outlined in a contract (e.g., termination requiring 2-week written notice). Given the "at will" termination process, notice of termination is a courtesy but not a requirement to end employment.

RISK MANAGEMENT

A risk management program is recommended to identify potential risks in the delivery of oral care. After risk is identified and measured, there are efforts on the part of the office staff to minimize or eliminate the risk. Potential areas of risk exposure include the following:

- Liability associated with professional actions of employers or employees
- General liability exposures for injuries to clients, vendors, and others
- Property and casualty exposures associated with the office, building, or surrounding area (e.g., parking lot)
- Exposure to defamation actions among staff, office managers, and other personnel
- Exposure to financial losses such as fraud, embezzlement, and theft
- Exposure to contracts, warranties, and similar actions associated with the purchase and use of goods and services
- Fraud and abuse exposure associated with federal and state third-party reimbursement programs
- Exposure to losses associated with staff hiring, promotions, and termination practices
- Inappropriate or incorrect use of dental equipment or dental materials
- Violation of privacy or confidentiality requirements

Sample Checklist for Assessing Litigation Risk in a Dental Employment Setting provides a sample checklist of types of questions that can be considered when assessing the potential risks in an employment setting.

Communication as a Risk Management Tool

DENTAL HYGIENIST–CLIENT. Open communication between the dental hygienist and client minimizes misunderstandings, reducing the likelihood of lawsuits and allowing for direct, timely resolution of problems. A dental hygienist who spends 45 to 60 minutes in a one-on-one relationship with a client can reduce the potential of negligent actions. The one-on-one relationship with clients gives the dental hygienist an opportunity to explain the care that will occur and answer client questions. Concepts must be presented clearly, with appropriate use of professional jargon. A client who senses a professional interest and expertise on the part of the dental hygienist may not be as prone to file a lawsuit if a procedure is unsuccessful. A diverse clientele may require that an office employ bilingual staff to assist in improving communication.

DENTAL HYGIENIST–EMPLOYER. The dental hygienist plays a key role in educating employers about potential liabilities for dental hygienists and their prevention. Written standards for office protocol can be developed and coordinated by the dental hygienist in conjunction with the employer. A resource library that includes updated literature, textbooks, and other related material, such as a current copy of the rules and regulations outlining the rights and responsibilities of licensed office staff, provides a quick resource if questions arise. The use of Web-based resources allows for a large array of resources to be available quickly to respond to questions, clarify information, or identify potential risks. If a risk management philosophy is practiced and reinforced by the employees and the employer, legal risks are reduced for the entire staff.

DENTAL HYGIENIST–COLLEAGUES. The best resources for the development of a risk management philosophy are the personnel within the employment setting. Consistent criteria for recordkeeping and referral can be

Sample Checklist for Assessing Litigation Risk in a Dental Employment Setting

Is the staff properly licensed and practicing within the appropriate scope of practice?
Is the dental equipment properly maintained and monitored?
Are there procedures for educating and updating staff concerning the components of the dental record and recordkeeping techniques?
Do the staff members use appropriate verbal and nonverbal communication techniques?
Is the health/dental history updated at every appointment?
Are appropriate intraoral and extraoral data collected and recorded?
Do the staff members fully document crucial data or conversations?
Are referrals documented?
Is informed consent or informed refusal documented?
Does the office have a medical emergency protocol and has the procedure been rehearsed?
Are the staff members cardiopulmonary resuscitation (CPR) and first aid qualified?
Is there a medical emergency kit available and are the drugs in it kept current? Is someone in the office capable of administering the medications in the emergency kit?
Is there an office manual that outlines protocols for client care, referral, and termination?
Is office protocol or documentation available to all staff outlining roles and responsibilities and important policies, such as sexual harassment prevention guidelines?
Are the staff members practicing the latest infection control procedures according to OSHA guidelines?
Are the staff members familiar with the uses of major equipment in the office (e.g., automatic processor, panoramic radiology, low- and high-speed handpieces, intravenous equipment, and autoclaves)?
Are broken toys or sharp objects removed promptly from the reception area?
Are the sidewalks, parking lots, or driveways clear of any debris (e.g., nails, glass, or ice)?
Are the handicapped ramps operable?

developed; current scientific literature to support particular treatment modalities can be shared; office protocols and handbooks can be developed. Each activity contributes to improved practice habits. Persons employed in similar roles should meet for a risk management day to identify areas of potential risk and develop mechanisms to reduce that risk. Suggested activities are the following:

- Brainstorm to identify risks in the practice; these can include treatment techniques, client management, recordkeeping, communication, and preventive practices.
- Have each person review the plan of care for a client; write down the key steps followed.
- Sample client records and review recordkeeping styles, abbreviations, charting records, informed consent and refusal, and other written aspects of care.
- Discuss risky practices that have become apparent.
- Develop a consensus that focuses on reducing risky behaviors and can be comfortably incorporated by all on a consistent basis (e.g., procedures for client care, charting techniques, abbreviations, referral guidelines, periodontal and other preventive therapies).
- Develop a dental hygiene office manual, which can be a separate manual or incorporated as a component of a larger manual. It can focus on the dental hygiene staff, client assessment, treatment and evaluation, insurance information, risk management suggestions, recordkeeping protocol, standardized periodontal assessment and charting guidelines, and premedication information. Once consensus occurs, chapters can be delegated and written. The manual serves as a guidebook to assist current and future employees. The manual is also helpful to other office staff and dentists.
- Propose and/or conduct a similar risk management workshop for the dentists and assistants on staff.

Client Record

The client record can be a provider's best defense or worst enemy in a malpractice action. The record provides the following information:

- Complete record of both the health and dental status at the time of the initial examination, including the pharmacologic and fluoride history
- Comprehensive and chronologic documentation of treatment provided
- Potential legal document on the client's behalf (e.g., use in corpse identification or insurance claims or fraud)
- Legal document for the defense of litigious claims against a dental practitioner
- Records as required in some states as part of the laws regulating professional practice
- Tool for quality assessment and assurance
- Communication mechanism among health professionals involved in the client's care

Documentation begins with initial client contact and continues throughout the relationship between the provider and the client, including reasons for terminating the relationship, if that occurs.

CLIENT IDENTIFICATION DATA. Client identification data are standard information such as name, address, telephone number for home and work, best time to call, emergency contact person, legal guardian, physician of record, and insurance-related information such as a social security number. Practices have grown larger, client numbers have increased, and client populations reflect multicultural backgrounds. Inaccurate client data make it difficult to identify a record that may be critical in a lawsuit. Poor documentation reflects on the oral healthcare provider. There may be an assumption that sloppy records reflect sloppy care.

Information about a client may change frequently, so periodic updating should be routine. Updated material should be dated. A client's photograph, as part of the record, has been recommended for identification purposes.

HEALTH AND DENTAL HISTORY (see Chapter 9). All health and dental history information should be pursued and answered. If an item on the history form is not appropriate, it should be indicated "NA" (not applicable). If the condition is normal, a notation such as "WNL" (within normal limits) is appropriate. The oral healthcare provider should review the history to make sure every question has been answered. A client history should be obtained at every visit. After a review is complete, notations should be made and dated in the progress notes or on the health history, noting changes.

One needs to document the individuals involved in each step of the history-taking process. For example, the individuals identified should include names of those who completed the health history with the client, those who reviewed the history with the client (if not the dentist or dental hygienist), and dates and signatures for each step.

Assessment data should be recorded consistently. For example, a client initially presents to the office with moderate periodontitis. If the condition does not improve, the practitioner has a record of the condition from the moment care began. Thus the dentist or dental hygienist cannot be accused of contributing to the client's condition.

CLINICAL ASSESSMENT AND DIAGNOSIS. A protocol should be established for the initial clinical assessment and subsequent visits. A diagnosis should be documented in order to justify treatment. The plaintiff's attorney frequently suggests that malpractice occurred because there was no clear diagnosis documented in the dental chart that would guide treatment.

TREATMENT INFORMATION. Concise, accurate, clear, and comprehensive records of care should include the following:

- ✦ Nature of the care or treatments provided
- ✦ Area in the mouth where care is provided
- ✦ Use of special dental equipment, such as an ultrasonic scaler
- ✦ Type and dosage of anesthetic and/or analgesia used
- ✦ Details about conditions presented, gingival health, oral hygiene status, specific areas of change
- ✦ Language that is specific (e.g., a notation such as "some deep pockets in the posterior" provides little definitive information)
- ✦ Details of conditions noted during or as the result of treatment, such as hematomas, excessive bleeding
- ✦ Specific recommendations for postoperative instructions and whether written postoperative instructions were provided to the client
- ✦ Medication prescribed or administered and dosages
- ✦ Unexpected occurrences or reactions, such as fractured restorations
- ✦ Client education conducted as well as client's response
- ✦ Continued-care interval or maintenance schedule

All procedures must be documented. Each client has one dental hygienist and remembers each visit. Each dental hygienist has a large clientele and needs to record information that may be required in future litigation. Cancellations, late arrivals, change of appointments, and conversations with front desk personnel are documented.

The record should reflect objective information; subjective information is included only if it affects client care (e.g., writing "Client was very apprehensive and asked many questions during the procedure," rather than "Client was a bother and questioned everything"). A record must be maintained in a professional manner. It is advisable not to comment on client or guardian personalities or characteristics, such as "Mom is very protective."

The record assists in the defense against a charge of breach of contract, negligence, or lack of informed consent. The lawyer for the plaintiff who reviews a thorough, complete record may determine that there is no reason to pursue a lawsuit. The record may clearly indicate that the practitioner has met all obligations and caused no harm. An incomplete or inaccurate record under close scrutiny provides multiple opportunities for the plaintiff's lawyer to prove inadequate or negligent care (see Suggestions for Managing Client Records).

LEGAL ISSUES AND ROLES OF THE DENTAL HYGIENIST

Dependent Practitioner

The status of a dependent practitioner may be somewhat misleading. An individual is dependent as a result of the licensing and regulation laws of the state; however, the individual is not dependent on the employer to assume legal responsibility for one's action. The dependent practitioner is providing client care. Based on the educational background and licensed status, the dental hygienist has professional obligations and legal duties that must be fulfilled. Failure to fulfill specific legal duties may result in charges of negligence (malpractice).

A dental hygienist may be charged with negligence if a breach of duty occurs and harm results. One can omit a service, resulting in negligence, such as assessing a client's blood pressure. A practitioner can also commit a negligent act, such as harming a client with an instrument or using hand-over-mouth technique practices to

Suggestions for Managing Client Records

Entries should be legible, written in black ink or ballpoint pen.

When there is more than one person making entries, entries should be signed or initialed.

When errors occur, they should not be blocked out so that they cannot be read. Instead, a single line should be drawn through the entry, and a note made above it stating "error in entry, see correction below." The correction should be dated at the time it is made.

Financial information should not be kept on the treatment record.

Entries should be uniformly spaced on the form. There should be no unusual or irregular blank spaces.

On health information forms, there should be no blank spaces in the answers to health questions. If the question is inappropriate, a single line is drawn through the question, or "not applicable" (NA) recorded in the box. If the response is normal, a "within normal limits" (WNL) notation is made.

All cancellations, late arrivals, and change of appointments are recorded.

Consents are documented, including all risks and alternative treatments presented to the client and remarks made by the client.

The client is informed of any adverse occurrences or untoward events that take place during the course of care; a note on the record that the client was informed is necessary.

All requests for consultations and responses are recorded.

All conversations held with other health practitioners relating to the care of the client are documented.

All client records should be retained for at least the period of the statute of limitations equal to that of contract actions. In most jurisdictions it is 6 years. In the case of minors, it is until the person reaches the age of 24 years. Check for special laws in your local jurisdiction. A dental office may consider additional record retention options that may include record storage facilities, microfilm, and/or scanning to CD-ROM. If at all possible, *keep records forever.*

Computerized dental records continue to become more popular. There should be a standardized protocol that includes daily backup of records and weekly transfer of records to a CD-ROM in order to ensure that records are not altered.

No subjective evaluations, such as an opinion about the client's mental health, should be recorded on the treatment record unless the writer is qualified and licensed to make such evaluations.

Confidentiality of information contained on the record should be guarded. Staff should be trained to follow Health Insurance Portability and Accountability Act (HIPAA) guidelines.

The original record should not be surrendered to anyone, except by order of a court.

A record should never be altered once there is some indication that legal action is contemplated by the client.

Heirs are instructed that they must retain the records of clients and comply with any written request for a copy.

Modified from Pollack BR: *Dentist's risk management guide,* Ft Lauderdale, Fla, 1990, National Society of Dental Practitioners.

discourage inappropriate behavior in children. In any situation, the duty or standard of care expected is evaluated. A conflict arises when the dental hygienist cannot provide care at an acceptable standard. For example, an individual presents with a periodontal condition that requires four 1-hour appointments to adequately root plane and scale, followed by an appointment for reevaluation. The care planning philosophy of the dentist is to allow two appointments. The dental hygienist may fail to adequately treat the client in two appointments and may contribute to a declining periodontal status. The issue of the standard of care for the dental hygienist is addressed during the lawsuit. Thus the dental hygienist is liable for professional actions taken.

Independent Practitioner

As an independent practitioner, a hygienist is responsible for all the legal principles that influence client care, including negligence, referral, abandonment, and informed consent. An independent practitioner also is an employer and is responsible for knowledge of labor and employment laws, discrimination issues, tax principles, and related business obligations. Assessing and minimizing risks contributes to long-term success in practice.

An independent practitioner is advised to seek legal and business assistance for some of the following items. Contracts and other related agreements are necessary to a business owner and must be drafted, negotiated, and signed. Employer-employee relationships and office protocols must be developed and guidelines established. An independent practitioner is the owner of a business, and functioning as such requires managerial skills outside the realm of client care (e.g., building and equipment maintenance, material and human resources management, and strategic planning). State and federal laws affect many aspects of the business, including hiring, firing, and evaluating personnel. Other laws affect the physical plant, such as incorporating barrier-free access or equipment selection and maintenance, as in OSHA guidelines.

The financial commitment to the practice is a significant one. Thus protecting personal assets, as well as keeping personal and professional expenses separate, is essential. Separate accounts are advisable for ease of bookkeeping. In addition, separation of personal and professional assets is important so personal assets cannot be taken if the business is affected by either financial or legal problems. An independent practitioner is responsible for policies and procedures used, quality of care provided, documentation, and the actions of employees. Given the litigious environment affecting dentistry and dental hygiene, the independent practitioner may be scrutinized by those seeking to find errors or illegalities. A clear understanding of the laws governing practice is imperative.

Independent Contractor

The independent contractor must recognize the contractual responsibilities inherent in both business and professional relationships. The dental hygienist is contracting to provide services. Both parties in the relationship, the dental hygienist and the contracting party, have specific rights and responsibilities. For example, the dental hygienist assumes that the contracting party will pay a salary and provide certain facilities and support staff. Failure to fulfill specific obligations of a contract is a *breach of contract.* Dental hygienists should seek legal counsel before any commitment as an independent contractor. Issues such as labor laws, income tax, and Social Security taxes, as well as liability issues are additional and important considerations. The independent contractor and practitioner must also remain cognizant of the legal issues affecting client care such as negligence, informed consent, referral, abandonment, and recordkeeping.

The dental hygienist, as an independent contractor, must approach practice with a strong risk management philosophy. A dental hygienist need not be put at risk because of the poor quality of care provided by someone else. Thus, during the interview process, before establishing a relationship, the dental hygienist should evaluate the employer in terms of potentially negligent activities, referral philosophies, infection control, and recordkeeping, to name a few considerations. Reviewing client records to observe how client care is managed may assist a dental hygienist in deciding whether to contract with a specific care provider.

Dissolution of the contract relationship after a preliminary period should be addressed as part of the initial negotiations. Rights and responsibilities of all parties should be clearly outlined so that the working relationship is defined. At the same time, the reasons and methods for ending the relationship also must be reviewed and agreed upon, such as reasons to dissolve and notice requirements.

Independent contracting requires careful scrutiny of tax laws and definitions of the independent contracting status. Legal counsel should be sought before committing to any relationship.

Educator

An educator has contact both with colleagues and students. Confidentiality—an obligation not to violate confidences shared—is one aspect of the relationships developed in an educational setting. In today's society, issues that must remain confidential have become more difficult to define. Educators are grappling with issues such as the student who confides a high-risk lifestyle for contracting AIDS or a colleague who has had a positive HIV test. Institutions of higher education have developed policies to address such situations, but state and local laws may also address topics such as the students' rights and health issues. Some states have general policy concerning issues such as the infected healthcare worker that can be used by institutions to guide their activities.

Discrimination may also be an issue. Educators must be certain that decisions affecting admission, hiring, clinical assignments, workload, promotion, and evaluation are not influenced by actions that are considered discriminatory. Informal comments previously made about an individual or group of individuals may resurface if allegations of discrimination occur. Clearly outlined policies for personnel hiring and management and student admission and continuance assist in decreasing potentially discriminatory practices.

The educator who serves as a clinical instructor must recognize that the legal principles apply to clinical education. Informed consent, standard of care, confidentiality, referral policies, and contract and tort duties must be purposefully applied. Clinical faculty members ultimately are liable for a student's actions. Thus client interactions and care should be carefully monitored. Client information written by a student and co-signed by a faculty member should be read critically to ensure accuracy and completeness. Student-faculty interactions in a clinical setting must be free of bias or discriminatory practices. Similar issues apply to the educator who also may provide clinical care as part of an in-house faculty practice. Policies to prevent charges of abandonment must be developed and implemented. Careful documentation of client care, referral, and dismissal with standardized language ensures consistency within the institution.

An educator may be involved in supervision of clerical and clinical staff. Employee rights such as contractual responsibilities, employee evaluation, and dismissals involve legal issues. Again, the educator must consider written documentation, discriminatory practices, civil rights issues, and issues within the area of labor law and employer-employee relationships.

The educator also works with administrators. Issues such as the educator's contractual rights, civil rights, and related topics should be understood, and if an issue arises, legal counsel may be sought. Failure on the part of an institution to recognize specific rights may lead to legal resolution. Promotion and tenure, salary issues, and job descriptions and responsibilities have a legal component.

Administrator/Manager

The administrator/manager is involved in hiring, evaluating, and possibly dismissing colleagues or employees. Knowledge of federal and state law affecting civil rights and sexual harassment, and the protection of those rights, is important policy to know and follow. Administrators must recognize that specific questions cannot be asked as part of an employment interview. Evaluation of an employee should be completed carefully and documented. In some instances, dismissal of an employee can occur only after a series of evaluations, warnings, and in some instances, counseling, is completed. Again, colleagues who make discriminatory remarks, exhibit sexual misconduct, or conduct themselves inappropriately reflect on the administrator's ability to manage effectively.

Contracts are a common part of an administrator/manager's life. A contract, the agreement between two consenting parties, reflects certain rights and responsibilities. All parties involved require a clear understanding of the rights and responsibilities delineated in the contract. Failure to understand the contract may lead to charges of a breach of contract based on the failure to fulfill a responsibility. For example, if a breach of contract occurs, there may be financial ramifications. If an employee is inappropriately dismissed without due process of the law, the court may require that the employer be responsible for fulfilling the salary terms of the contract. Thus, although the employee is gone, the employer is still obligated under law to pay salary and benefits.

The administrator/manager may be responsible for ensuring the safety of an employee from the tortious acts of another (e.g., a responsibility to protect an employee from a client or student who may commit an assault or battery). In addition, a responsibility exists to prevent negligence in maintenance of the physical plant, such as faulty steps, icy or wet entrances, or other dangerous situations. The administrator/manager may be responsible for following federal or state mandates in areas such as employment or safety. Adherence to laws, rules, and regulations within the workplace may be the responsibility of the manager.

Labor laws and related legal concepts may dictate what documentation is important and also appropriate. Employees have access to their employment files and, thus, one must be objective and thorough in documenting events and personal interactions. State and federal laws seek to protect the rights of involved individuals.

Consumer Advocate

The consumer rights advocate should be aware of legislation on legal issues, civil rights, healthcare, labor issues in employment of the handicapped, geriatrics, and issues regarding children and adolescents. Advocates should focus on areas that best meet personal needs and the needs of the population group(s) they represent. Understanding the political system, how laws are enacted, and lobbying techniques assists the advocate to keep updated by pursuing information and getting on mailing lists to remain updated. Working with professional groups with similar interests also is a valuable resource for information or a need to react to a situation, such as a letter-writing campaign.

Contracts and torts are applied in many situations. Did a group promising to provide services breach its contract? Did an agency violate the terms of its contract? Was an individual negligent in his responsibilities? Was informed consent obtained? Is there a duty to an individual or group of individuals based on an interpretation of the law? Can one argue that some have misrepresented themselves or an issue? In most instances, a lawyer can assist in defining the legal principles that apply. The Code of Ethics for lawyers suggests that they perform some legal work *pro bono,* for free. Thus an individual working as a consumer advocate may find legal assistance from someone willing to work *pro bono* and obtain valuable advice and guidance from the legal perspective.

Researcher

Researchers should be familiar with issues such as confidentiality, rights of human and animal subjects, informed consent, recordkeeping, and abandonment. For instance, researchers must also consider legal issues not addressed in this chapter such as product liability, fund management, and tax issues.

Client Education Issues

- Educate the client about the legal justification for particular activities (e.g., questions about the use of protective barriers can result in a discussion about OSHA regulations).
- Explain issues of standards of care, scope of practice, or duty to the client.
- As the operator records information, such as periodontal assessment data, the need to keep accurate records to assist in client care and protection from health risks can be described.
- If a client is refusing a particular recommendation for treatment, the ethical principles of autonomy, beneficence, and nonmaleficence can be discussed.
- If a client raises a concern about treating particular clients, such as those with infectious diseases, the legal issues of discrimination and the ethical principle of justice can be discussed.

Legal, Ethical, and Safety Issues

- Before making a legal or ethical decision, the dental hygienist seeks resources that guide the process (e.g., ADHA or CDHA Code of Ethics, ADA Code of Ethics, current rules and regulations governing the practice of dental hygiene in the state in which the license is held). Public health statutes may identify responsibilities such as mandatory reporting of child or adult abuse, infectious disease reporting, and recordkeeping requirements.
- Written office protocols that reflect evidence-based practice protect the healthcare team from litigation, if these protocols are used and practiced.

Key Concepts

- Ethics focuses on the moral duties and obligations of the professional to clients, colleagues, and society.
- Dental hygienists are guided by the core ethical principles of autonomy, veracity, justice, beneficence, nonmaleficence, and fidelity.
- Dental hygienists are accountable to clients, colleagues, and society.
- A code of ethics is characteristic of a profession and assists in raising ethical sensitivity and providing a guiding framework for decision making.
- An ethical decision-making model includes identifying the conflict, the ethical principles involved, and gathering relevant information in order to identify a list of alternatives from which a dental hygienist can choose one alternative on which to act.
- Civil law is that branch of law that includes offenses violating private or contractual rights.
- Dental hygienists can have a contractual relationship with a client that requires the dental hygienist to fulfill specific obligations.
- Abandonment results if a relationship between a practitioner and client is severed without appropriate notification and documentation.
- Technical battery occurs if a practitioner performs a procedure on a client without informed consent.
- Negligence is a professional's failure to fulfill a specific duty to a client that results in an injury or harm.
- A dental hygienist must meet the standard of care for the profession (i.e., the degree of care a reasonably prudent professional would exercise under the same or similar circumstances).
- Informed consent allows a client to agree to allow something to happen based on full disclosure of information and is based on the ethical principle of autonomy, recognizing an individual's right to self-determination.
- Informed refusal allows a client to decline dental advice; the refusal should be documented in order to protect the practitioner.
- Confidentiality is an important responsibility that protects a client's privacy.
- Federal and state laws exist to protect dental hygienists from employment discrimination in hiring, firing, and promotion decisions.
- Dental hygienists may be subject to sexually harassing behaviors and should be familiar with steps to stop or prevent the behavior.
- Risk management involves identifying risks and implementing strategies to reduce or eliminate risks.
- Recordkeeping is important to protect the practitioner and the client and to assist in client care.

Critical Thinking Exercises

1. Obtain a current document from the ADHA that provides a synopsis of the supervision requirements for services provided by dental hygienists by state. How is the legal doctrine of *respondeat superior* affected by this variability in supervision requirements in the various legal jurisdictions?
2. Obtain the current Codes of Ethics from both the ADHA and the Canadian Dental Hygienists' Association. Read both. How are they similar? How do they differ?
3. Answer the questions following Scenarios 1 to 5 for analysis and discussion:

Scenario 1

Ivy Smith has been a licensed dental hygienist for eight years. She is not active in the dental hygiene professional association and looks to her employer to keep her "updated." She relies on her employer, Dr. General Practitioner, to tell her what is "legal" or "illegal" in dental hygiene. She rarely attends professional meetings or reads scientific publications. She discusses with you, a dental hygiene colleague, some of the things that she is doing in her private practice. Her employer has told her that under his direction, she can perform some expanded duties. So, she has cemented some crowns and used nitrous oxide and oxygen analgesia during client care activities (both of which are illegal for dental hygienists in the state). She was also told by her employer not to spend time reviewing medical/dental histories or other client assessment methods, such as evaluating periodontal disease status, in order to save time. According to her employer, when it comes to history review, "Once is enough" and her job is to "clean teeth." She has raised a concern about potential malpractice liability, but her employer told her not to worry because he is responsible under the doctrine of *respondeat superior*.

1. Which sections of the ADHA Code of Ethics apply to this case?
2. Is Ivy Smith meeting the standard of care for dental hygiene?
3. What strategies would you use to encourage Ivy to join the ADHA?
4. Does the concept of *respondeat superior* excuse Ivy Smith from her legal and ethical responsibilities?

Critical Thinking Exercises—cont'd

Scenario 2

You have been working in a practice for three years and developed a close friendship with Alice Gunn. Alice moved from Georgia three years ago, is a single parent and a technically proficient dental hygienist. Her dental hygiene skills and communication skills with clients and staff have impressed you. One night, after work, you go out for dinner, and she confides in you that she is not licensed in the state. Alice admits that because of the job opportunity that occurred in the office, the great health benefits, hours, and employer/employees, she could not wait to get a license and took the job. Your employer never asked for proof of licensure, and so she never had to admit or deny that she wasn't licensed. She asks you not to mention the situation because she really can't afford to stop practicing until she gets a license. She also does not want to be exposed because she is active in the local dental hygiene association and it would be embarrassing. She promises to try to get a license but doesn't want anyone to know that she isn't currently licensed.

1. Use the ethical decision-making model to resolve the dilemma presented.
2. How would a copy of the dental practice act assist the dental hygienist?
3. How could the employer have prevented this situation?
4. What aspects of the ADHA or CDHA Code of Ethics apply to this situation?

Scenario 3

Andrew Pierce is a second-year dental hygiene student who has been described as client centered. Andrew works diligently and carefully to make sure that his clients receive outstanding dental hygiene care. Many of the clients who visit the dental hygiene clinic are on limited incomes and do not have dental insurance. Andrew knows the importance of fluoride therapy for his children and adult clients. He tries to give fluoride treatments, when appropriate, to all clients. He knows that preventive therapies are important and feels he is serving the needs of the clients; however, he knows that some of his clients cannot afford the fluoride fee and would decline the treatment if given a choice. Andrew gives a fluoride treatment to clients who cannot afford the treatment or do not have insurance coverage. In order for them not to be charged, he does not record the fluoride treatment in the progress notes and does not indicate the fluoride treatment on the charge slip given to the cashier. The dental hygiene faculty members often do not notice that the fluoride treatment is not documented because they are busy with many students.

1. Which ethical principles apply to this case?
2. Identify some of the risks to the client, student, faculty, and dental hygiene program?
3. Take the part of the dental hygiene program director. What steps would you take with the student and with the dental hygiene faculty to address the problem?
4. Take the role of a student colleague of Andrew Pierce who is aware of the situation. Based on your program's academic and professional decorum policies, what would you do?

Scenario 4

An assistant, your best friend, is employed in the office where you practice dental hygiene and is pregnant. The doctor has been very understanding about her condition; however, she is scheduling her physician visits during the workday. Your employer "gently" asks her to schedule the doctor appointments toward the end of the day, when the office is closed. She becomes very offended and quits. She calls you the evening she quits and tells you that she is going to call the state OSHA office and report some violations related to the standards. You think this is unfair because the office is in compliance and she is creating issues where none exist. She also starts saying unkind things about the employer and suggests to you that she is also considering contacting the EEOC concerning possible sexual harassment.

1. Accusations of sexual harassing behaviors are serious. Discuss the types of sexual harassment that can occur in a dental office. If the dentist had been sexually harassing the assistant, what steps should she have taken?
2. If the employer had not been supportive of the pregnant assistant, what steps could the assistant have taken to resolve the conflict?
3. Use the ethical decision-making model to resolve the dilemmas presented.
4. What aspects of the ADHA or CDHA Code of Ethics apply to this situation?

Continued on following page

Critical Thinking Exercises—cont'd

Scenario 5

The new dental associate in the office likes to make it known that she is "in charge." The associate recently graduated from dental school and has repeatedly reminded the staff that she has a significant amount of student loans to pay off. The new associate frequently checks your clients once you have completed dental hygiene care. For every client treatment planned to receive a root planing and scaling series, the dentist receives a percentage of the fee collected. You begin noticing that she appears to be overtreating and overdiagnosing clients. Examples of her behaviors include convincing clients to agree to extensive restorative work, advocating cosmetic procedures, and classifying clients as needing root planing and scaling when it is evident that from their condition it is not necessary. Privately, you have asked her about some of her treatment plans. She firmly informs you that she is the licensed dentist in the office and you are the registered dental hygienist.

1. Use the ethical decision-making model to resolve the dilemma(s) presented. What resources would you draw upon?
2. Which legal principle(s) is(are) involved in this scenario?

For References, Suggested Readings, and Related Websites, visit
http://evolve.elsevier.com/Darby/hygiene/

GLOSSARY

abandonment Legal action that may occur when a healthcare provider fails to provide a connection with or care for a client of record, and this failure jeopardizes the client's health.

abfraction Pathologic loss of tooth structure from biomechanical forces on the tooth (tooth flexion, compression, and tension) along with chemical degradation; most visible as V-shaped notches in cervical areas of the teeth.

abrasion Pathologic tooth wear as a result of a foreign substance.

abrasive Describes a material of various particle size and hardness that is used to remove stain or polish a surface.

abscess Localized site of infection with pus formation.

periapical abscess Localized inflammation with pus in the tissues surrounding the apex of the tooth.

periodontal abscess Localized inflammation with pus in the periodontal tissues.

absolute contraindication Condition requiring that an offending drug or procedure not be administered to the client under any circumstance.

abutment Tooth, tooth root, or dental implant that serves as an anchor for a fixed or removable prosthetic appliance.

acceptance Ability to accept a client without judgment of the person's attitudes, behaviors, or characteristics that would interfere with communication.

accessibility Ability to obtain needed healthcare in a convenient, affordable, and efficient manner.

accessory roots Extra roots on teeth (e.g., on the mandibular first permanent molar in some Eskimo and Asian persons).

accountability State of being willing to explain and justify one's behavior or decisions.

accreditation Process by which a nongovernmental agency evaluates an institution or program of study according to predetermined, national standards (e.g., an entry-level dental hygiene education program accredited by the ADA Commission on Dental Accreditation).

acellular cementum Bonelike connective tissue that covers the cervical half of the root and contains no cementoblasts (cementocytes); does not increase during the life of a tooth.

acid conditioning See *acid-etching*.

acid-etching Process of washing the enamel surface with 30% to 50% phosphoric acid prior to placement of a sealant in order to increase sealant retention.

acidogenic plaque Presence of acid in the plaque as a byproduct of the metabolism of carbohydrate by bacteria; contributes to the demineralization process.

acoustic microstreaming Pressure produced within the space of a periodontal pocket by water that flows over the vibrating ultrasonic instrument tip; also known as *acoustic turbulence*.

acoustic turbulence See *acoustic microstreaming*.

acquired disability Disability occurring after the age of 22 years caused by a disease, trauma, or injury to the body.

acquired immunodeficiency syndrome (AIDS) An immunosuppressive viral disease characterized by specific suppression in the immune response and associated with a wide variety of opportunistic infections, poor resistance to infection, NUG or NUP, Kaposi's spots, wasting, and pneumocystic pneumonia; prognosis is poor.

acquired pellicle Thin, clear, unstructured organic membrane that forms over exposed tooth surfaces and restorations within minutes after removal by professional and self-polishing techniques.

acquired tooth damage Posteruption loss of integrity of a tooth surface.

acrylic Polymers of acrylic acid, methylacrylic acid, or acrylonitrile, such as acrylic resins used in making dental restorations, prostheses, and appliances.

acrylic test rod Plastic stick used to test sharpness of periodontal scaling instruments.

action potential Rapid sequence of changes (depolarization or repolarization) within a nerve fiber.

activation Manipulation of an orthodontic appliance so that a desired force is applied to a tooth.

active periodontal therapy Nonsurgical and surgical periodontal therapy aimed at eliminating periodontitis; includes Phase I care and can extend to Phase II care.

active tip area The 2-mm to 4-mm part of an ultrasonic instrument tip that vibrates and therefore performs instrumentation.

active tooth-borne appliance Appliance that is supported by the teeth and includes springs or screws to actively expand the palate or move teeth.

activities of daily living (ADLs) Self-care abilities that are fundamental to independent living (e.g., bathing, oral hygiene, dressing, toileting, transferring from bed or chair, feeding, and continence).

activity factor (AF) Measure of a person's level of physical activity.

activity theory Explains that a positive relationship exists between an individual's level of participation in social activities and life satisfaction.

acute fluoride toxicity See *fluoride toxicity.*

acute herpetic gingivostomatitis Primary infection of the oral mucosa by the herpes simplex virus manifesting as redness of oral tissues, vesicles, and painful ulcers.

herpetic whitlow Recurrent lesion of the finger initiated by puncture from a herpes virus–contaminated instrument.

HVS I Herpes simplex virus I, initial infection; clients asymptomatic.

HVS II Herpes simplex virus II, commonly transmitted sexually; may be manifested orally.

acute pericoronitis Abscess associated with a partially erupted tooth or fully erupted tooth that is covered completely or partially by a flap of tissue (operculum). See *operculum.*

acute periodontal abscess Exacerbated inflammatory reaction occurring usually in a periodontally involved area and caused by a blockage of the area by some foreign body.

acute/rampant caries See *dental caries.*

ADA American Dental Association; American Diabetes Association; American Dietetics Association.

adaptation Alignment or placement of the side of the first few millimeters of a periodontal probe, straight explorer, or blade of a scaler against a tooth prior to activation of an exploratory or working stroke.

adenoma Benign tumor of the gland that suggests a deviation from normal glandular tissue.

adenopathy Disease of the glands, especially of the lymphatic glands.

adequate attached gingiva (AAG) Periodontal measurement determined with a periodontal probe by observing the mucogingival junction, measuring the distance from the mucogingival junction to the gingival margin, measuring pocket depth, and calculating the difference between the two measurements.

adherence Client's willingness to cooperate with professional advice and self-care recommendations necessary to achieve and maintain oral health; compliance.

adjunctive therapy Treatment completed as a component of a larger treatment plan; may involve chemotherapeutic, periodontal, orthodontic, or restorative interventions to restore health and function (e.g., daily irrigation with 0.12% chlorhexidine).

adrenaline/epinephrine Naturally occurring agent responsible for sympathetic nervous system activity.

adrenergic receptors Receptors throughout the body's tissues that are stimulated by the chemicals released by the sympathetic nervous system or a sympathomimetic agent (drug).

alpha receptors Activation of these receptors results in contraction of smooth muscle in blood vessels causing constriction of blood vessels.

beta receptors Activation of these receptors results in smooth muscle relaxation and cardiac stimulation.

beta 1 receptors Activation of these receptors increases cardiac rate and force.

beta 2 receptors Activation of these receptors causes bronchodilation and vasodilation.

adult day care A community-based center where older adults can go to receive supervised daily activities and recreation.

adult occlusal equilibrium Phase of eruption that begins after all permanent teeth have erupted and pubertal growth spurt is complete.

advanced glycated end products (AGE) Excess accumulation of glycated tissue proteins that contributes to tissue damage in both type 1 and type 2 diabetic individuals.

adverse drug effects Undesirable effects from taking a medication; may include side effects, toxicity reactions, and drug hypersensitivity.

advocacy Education of decision makers to provide essential political support for change.

aerosol Artificially generated solid or liquid airborne particles less than 50 microns in size.

aerosolization Airborne transfer of microorganisms in a fine mist.

affective goals Desired changes in client values, beliefs, and attitudes.

affective learning domain Domain that classifies levels of learning involving feelings, attitudes, values, and interests; includes receiving, responding, valuing, organizing, and having a value system.

agent-host-environment model Conceptualizes disease as the result of an imbalance in one or all of three factors: the agent (e.g., bacteria), the host (e.g., the person), and the environment.

age-related macular degeneration (AMD) Deterioration in the membrane between the retina and underlying blood vessels that leads to a decline in one's central vision.

AIDS See *acquired immunodeficiency syndrome (AIDS).*

air abrasion See *air polisher.*

airborne Pertaining to microorganisms suspended in air for an extended time where others may inhale them, such as microorganisms that cause tuberculosis and measles (not HIV, HCV, and HBV).

air polisher An electric-powered unit with a handpiece designed for extrinsic stain removal via the delivery of a spray of warm water and sodium bicarbonate under pressure. Also known as an air abrasion device.

alginate Irreversible, flexible hydrocolloid impression material used primarily for making study casts of a client's dentition.

allergy Hypersensitive reaction, acquired through exposure to a specific environmental substance (allergen); re-exposure increases potential to react.

allogenic bone marrow Bone marrow from a person with a similar genetic makeup.

alloy Solid mixture of two or more metals, or of one or more metals and certain metalloids that are mutually soluble in the molten condition; contributing to the composition of a dental amalgam.

alpha receptors See *adrenergic receptors.*

aluminum cap See *cartridge.*

alveolar/attached gingiva Bound-down gingival tissue consisting of keratinized stratified squamous epithelium that covers the crestal portion of the alveolar bone and the roof of the mouth.

alveolar mucosa Nonkeratinized epithelium characterized by a smooth and shiny surface that covers the vestibule and floor of the mouth and becomes the buccal and labial mucosa.

alveolar process Bone that extends from the maxilla and mandible to form the tooth sockets and support the teeth; alveolar ridges.

Alzheimer's disease (AD) Irreversible dementia characterized by accumulation of neurofibrillary tangles and senile plaques within the cerebral cortex.

amalgam Alloy of mercury with silver, copper, and tin; used to restore form and function of teeth.

amalgamation Process of mechanically mixing dental amalgam alloy with mercury.

amalgam carrier Instrument with a cylinder used to carry and dispense amalgam into the cavity preparation. The instrument lever forces a plunger to dislodge the contained amalgam from the cylinder.

amalgam well Small, heavy, stainless steel "dish" with a cup-like recess that confines the mixed amalgam to facilitate pickup with the amalgam carrier.

amelogenesis imperfecta Form of enamel dysplasia resulting from hereditary factors; characterized by partial or total malformation of enamel.

American Academy of Periodontology (AAP) A professional association of periodontists and other oral health professionals dedicated to the prevention, diagnosis, and treatment of diseases of the periodontium and maintenance of dental implants.

American Dental Association Seal of Acceptance An approval given to oral care products supported by adequate research evidence of safety and effectiveness, as approved by the American Dental Association, Council on Scientific Affairs.

American Dental Hygienists' Association (ADHA) National organization of approximately 35,000 dental hygienists dedicated to advancing the art and science of dental hygiene by ensuring access to quality oral healthcare; increasing awareness of cost-effective benefits of prevention; promoting the highest standard of dental hygiene education, licensure, practice, and research; and representing the interests of dental hygienists.

amide local anesthetic See *local anesthetic.*

amplitude Distance that the working end of a mechanized instrument moves; length of the stroke of the working end of a mechanized instrument; also known as *power*.

amyotrophic lateral sclerosis A chronic degenerative disease consisting of signs and symptoms related to the cell bodies of both the upper and lower motor neurons.

analgesia stage See *anesthesia.*

anatomic charting forms Preprinted diagrams of anatomically drawn teeth as they appear in a child or adult's mouth; used for recording findings from the dentition assessment.

anatomic portion The part of a cast that includes the teeth, oral mucosa, and muscle attachments.

anatomic root Part of the tooth covered by cementum.

anchor Metal device inserted within bone tissue of the mandibular or maxillary arch.

anchorage value Number assigned to each tooth based on the surface area of its periodontal ligament; reflects the ability of the tooth to function as an anchor for desired movement of other teeth.

andragogy The art and science of helping the adult learn.

anemia Below-normal levels of red blood cells or quantity of hemoglobin in blood resulting in reduced delivery of oxygen to tissues.

aneroid sphygmomanometer See *sphygmomanometer.*

anesthesia Loss of sensation, usually caused by administration of a drug. There are four stages:

stage 1 – analgesia Perception of pain is altered. There are three planes; the first two are appropriate for dental hygiene care.

stage 2 – delirium or excitement Characterized by hyperresponsiveness to stimuli, exaggerated inspiration, and loss of consciousness.

stage 3 – surgical anesthesia Has four planes. Oral and maxillofacial surgeons take persons undergoing oral surgery to this level of anesthesia.

stage 4 – surgical anesthesia with respiratory paralysis This level of anesthesia is reserved for use when a person undergoes major surgery in a hospital setting.

angina pectoris Acute pain in the chest as a result of decreased blood supply to the heart muscle, often brought on by physical activity or emotional stress; approximately 90% is the result of atherosclerosis.

stable angina Predictable episodes of angina pectoris that are precipitated by exercise and emotional stress.

unstable angina Chest pain that occurs periodically over days or weeks that may indicate acute myocardial infarction.

angioedema Acute painless, edematous reaction of the subcutaneous or submucosal tissue.

angioplasty Closed heart surgical procedure involving a catheter with a tiny balloon at the end of the tube that inserts into the coronary artery to allow increased blood flow.

angles Figure formed by the joining of two straight lines at a single point; concept used for achieving the appropriate position of the cutting edge of a bladed instrument to a tooth, for instrument sharpening to position the cutting edge to a stone, and for exposing radiographs.

angular cheilitis Cracked, eroded, and encrusted surfaces at the commissural folds that frequently appear in conjunction with mucosal inflammation caused by *Candida albicans* infection; may cause moderate pain.

angulation Relationship of the cutting edge of a bladed instrument to the tooth surface or sharpening stone (e.g., the measurement in degrees from the instrument blade to the tooth surface being scaled).

ankylosed Describes a tooth fused to bone due to injury or disease.

annealing Manufacturing process used to soften a metal.

anodontia Congenital absence of teeth. Defects of ectodermal structures are causative effects; also known as edentia.

hypodontia Partial absence of teeth.

anorexia nervosa Least-common eating disorder; persons suffering from anorexia suppress and deny sensation of hunger.

anterior Front of an area of the body.

anterior border of the mandible Structure is palpated bilaterally from the position behind the client to examine the soft tissue and underlying bone during an oral cancer examination.

anterior faucial pillar Fold of tissue that forms one of the lateral borders of the palatine tonsil.

anterior palatine nerve Nerve that enters the oral cavity on the hard palate via the greater palatine foramen and innervates the palatal soft tissues and bone of the posterior teeth.

anterior superior alveolar (ASA) nerve Nerve that descends from the infraorbital nerve at a location before the infraorbital nerve exits the infraorbital foramen; provides innervation to the central and lateral incisors, canines, periodontal tissues, and facial soft tissues and corresponding bone.

anterior superior alveolar nerve block Injection recommended for pain management when treatment is performed on maxillary anterior teeth.

anteroposterior plane of space Plane of space existing between the anterior and posterior boundaries of the body when viewed from the lateral aspect. Angle's classification of occlusion is used to assess the occlusion in the anteroposterior plane of space.

antibiotic prophylactic premedication See *prophylactic antibiotic premedication.*

antibody An immunoglobulin that is essential to the immune system and is produced by lymphoid tissue in response to bacteria, viruses, or other antigens.

anticariogenic Describes something that is effective in suppressing production of caries.

anticoagulant Drug used to prevent coagulation of blood, e.g., Coumadin (warfarin).

antifungal agent Drug used to treat fungal infections such as *Candidiasis,* e.g., fluconazole.

antigen Substance, usually a protein, that causes formation of an antibody and reacts specifically with that antibody; capable of inducing an immune response.

antimicrobial agent Substance, such as chlorhexidine gluconate or phenolic compound, that kills or hinders the growth of microorganisms.

antiseptic Antimicrobial agent for use on the skin or mucous membrane.

aphthous ulcer Small oval or round ulcer on the lining mucosa characterized by a red halo with a grayish center, and pain; plural is *aphthae.*

apical root resorption Loss of root structure in the apical one third of the root of a tooth, usually as a result of poorly controlled orthodontic forces.

apical third The third of the tooth involving the tip or apex of the root.

appliance Device used in dentistry to provide a functional or therapeutic effect.

fixed appliance Dental prosthesis that is cemented to natural teeth, roots, or implants and cannot be removed by the client.

obturator Device used to fill a space in order to restore function (e.g., to close a cleft palate).

orthodontic appliance Device used to alter growth patterns or move teeth within the alveolar bone.

removable appliance Dental prosthesis that can be removed by the client (e.g., a partial denture).

appliance prescription Design of each bracket for each tooth; accounts for variations in the tooth, including the contour and axial inclination of the labial surfaces; variations in the root inclination; and control of the rotation of teeth as they are moved.

appliance therapy A generalized term inclusive of numerous designs of dental orthotics or splints used to relieve bruxism.

applied research Adaptation of theories developed through basic research to a practical situation or to the resolution of an existing problem.

appointment schedule An aspect of a care plan that delineates the number of client appointments required, time required for each appointment, and services to be provided at each appointment.

archwire U-shaped wire that extends around an entire maxillary or mandibular arch to apply orthodontic forces to all teeth involved.

area-specific Denotes that a particular instrument is designed for use in a designated area of the mouth and on specific tooth surfaces, e.g, area-specific curet.

Arkansas stone Type of natural stone used to sharpen instruments.

arrested caries See *dental caries.*

arthritis Musculoskeletal system disorder characterized by inflammation of joints that may cause serious limitations in activity and self-care.

osteoarthritis Most common joint disease; a defect of articular cartilage characterized by gradual loss of cushioning. As cartilage is lost, the resultant exposure of rough underlying bone ends may cause pain and joint stiffness.

rheumatoid arthritis Chronic, systemic disease affecting connective tissue throughout the body. Symptoms include malaise, fatigue, fever, anemia, and nodules that develop on hard tissues.

arthrogram Radiograph that uses a contrast medium to assess a joint such as the temporomandibular joint.

articulating paper Aid used to check occlusion.

art portion The part of a cast that forms the base.

ASA Classification System American Society of Anesthesiologists' rating system used to identify client risk for a medical emergency.

asepsis Absence of germs or microorganisms.

aspirating syringe Most commonly used syringe for administration of an intraoral local anesthetic. The barbed piston (harpoon) allows the administrator to exert negative pressure on the thumb ring to assess the location of the lumen of the needle; the procedure is *aspiration*.

aspiration The negative pressure placed on a syringe prior to deposition of a local anesthetic agent into tissue; also the breathing of a foreign object into the lung

assault Action of a person intending to cause apprehension in someone, without touching them (e.g., threatening someone with words or a raised hand).

assessment Collecting and analyzing subjective and objective data about a client's risk or problem, and arriving at a judgment about the client's care needs.

assessment instruments Instruments, such as the periodontal probe, dental explorer, and mouth mirror used for detecting tooth irregularities, restorations, probe depths, soft-tissue changes, acquired deposits, and other intraoral manifestations and measurements.

assistive devices Mechanical aids designed to enhance a disabled person's autonomy in daily functions and communication.

asthma Condition marked by recurrent attacks of shortness of breath and often accompanied by wheezing caused by spasmodic constriction of the bronchi; caused by allergies and/or infectious agents.

atherosclerosis Narrowing of the lumen of coronary arteries caused by deposition of fibrofatty substances containing lipids and cholesterol. Narrowing reduces volume of blood flow, and deposits may eventually close the vessel. A major cause of coronary heart disease

atlantoaxial subluxation Cervical spine instability characterized by an abnormal increase in mobility within the joint between the first two cervical vertebra.

atomization The act of reducing a liquid to a fine spray or mist.

atrial fibrillation An irregularity in ventricular beats created by inconsistent impulses through the atrioventricular (AV) node transmitted to the ventricles at irregular intervals.

atrial septal defect A shunt (opening) between the left and right atria; responsible for approximately 10% of congenital heart defects.

atrophy Thinning of tissue layers with loss of normal skin furrow and a shiny and translucent appearance; usually associated with malnutrition or disuse.

attached gingiva Portion of the gingiva that is firmly connected to the alveolar bone.

attached subgingival plaque See *bacterial plaque biofilm*.

attachment apparatus Refers to the cementum, periodontal ligament, and alveolar bone collectively.

attachment loss Distance from the cementoenamel junction to the base of the sulcus or pocket as measured by the periodontal probe and monitored over time; loss of attachment (LOA) includes both periodontal pocket depth and recession measurement.

attention diversion Directing attention away from an anxiety-provoking object or event to something that is neutral or pleasurable.

attribution theory Cognitive theory that emphasizes the importance of thought content.

attrition Tooth-to-tooth wear from opposing tooth contact.

atypical plasma cholinesterase Inherited condition in which the individual produces an atypical form of the enzyme plasma cholinesterase. These individuals cannot metabolize ester local anesthetics effectively.

audioanalgesia Reduction in pain sensation associated with listening to music to which a background of "white noise" has been added.

aura Physical sensation that precedes or signals the onset of an epileptic seizure or migraine headache.

auricular lymph nodes Nodes that are palpated bilaterally in front of and behind the ears.

auscultation Physical assessment technique that uses the clinician's sense of hearing to denote an abnormality; act of listening to and detecting body sounds in order to determine variations from normal (e.g., listening for clicking sounds in the temporomandibular joint).

auscultatory gap Time during the measurement of blood pressure when sound is not heard; may occur in clients with hypertension and aortic stenosis.

austenitic Type of nickel titanium wire that lacks formability but is superelastic and able to apply a force that varies little in magnitude whether applied over short or long distances. Austenitic nitinol archwires are referred to as *A-NiTi*.

autism Developmental disorder characterized by impairment of mutual social interaction and communication, unusual activities, and lack of ability for symbolic play.

autoclave Most common method of heat sterilization in the dental care setting.

autogenous Self-generated, self-produced, originating within an organism.

autoimmune Term used to describe a condition in which a person develops an immune response to his own body tissues (e.g., autoimmune deficiency disease such as lupus erythematosis).

autonomic dysreflexia Potentially severe condition in catheterized persons caused by a noxious stimulus, such as urinary backflow, that can be fatal if left untreated.

autonomic nervous system Part of the nervous system that controls involuntary body functions, such as salivation, sweat, and heartbeat. Divided into the *parasympathetic* and *sympathetic* systems.

parasympathetic nervous system Controls heart, intestinal, and bladder functions.

sympathetic nervous system Enables the body to be prepared for flight or fight.

autonomy The idea, based on the principle of respect, that individuals have a right to self-determination, i.e., freedom to make their own judgments based on their own evaluation.

autopolymerization See *polymerization*.

autotuned unit Ultrasonic scaling unit with a preset frequency that automatically adjusts cycles per second to maximum efficiency for each insert.

avulsed tooth Tooth that is traumatically removed from the alveolus.

axial positioning See *root angulation*.

back channeling Active listening techniques such as saying "all right" or "uh-huh" to indicate that the dental hygienist has heard what the client says.

backward caries See *dental caries*.

bacteremia Presence of microorganisms in the bloodstream.

bacterial endocarditis Acute microbial infection of the endocardium; can be initiated by manipulation of mucosal tissues, which introduces a transient bacteremia into the bloodstream. Bacteria may become lodged on damaged or abnormal areas of the heart valves, causing an infection of the lining of the heart and underlying connective tissues; prevented by prophylactic antibiotic premedication prior to dental or dental hygiene procedures; also known as *infective endocarditis*.

bacterial plaque biofilm Dense, organized community of microorganisms that forms on teeth, gingiva, and restorations; the cause of dental caries and periodontitis. The biofilm is a self-protecting and self-sustaining community, highly resistant to antimicrobial agents and antibiotics. Also known as *dental plaque biofilm, dental biofilm,* or *microbial plaque biofilm.*

attached subgingival plaque Bacterial plaque biofilm located below the gingival margin that is attached to the tooth.

loosely adherent subgingival plaque Unattached bacterial plaque biofilm located adjacent to the gingival epithelium or pocket lumen.

supragingival plaque Bacterial plaque biofilm located above the gingival margin; influences the establishment and composition of subgingival microorganisms.

bactericidal Capable of killing bacteria.

barrier Obstacle that limits a disabled persons' ability to access healthcare, education, and employment opportunities. Also refers to factors that prevent persons from obtaining needed healthcare.

barrier-free design An architectural environment that enables wheelchair accessibility; required in public buildings as a result of an amendment to the Rehabilitation Act of 1973.

basal energy expenditure (BEE) Total energy output of a body at rest after a 12-hour fast in a room of comfortable temperature; a measure of the amount of calories required to maintain the body at its current weight.

basal ganglia Clusters of neuron cell bodies embedded deep within the forebrain and midbrain; gray matter.

basal thermometer See *thermometer*.

baseline An individual's score on a measurement prior to implementing a particular intervention; also referred to as a pretest measurement.

basement lamina Upper layer of the basement membrane of epithelial tissue.

bases Materials placed to provide thermal insulation and support under metallic restorations.

basic research Systematic application of the scientific method leading to the establishment of new knowledge or theory.

basketweave of strokes Combinations of different instrument stroke directions, especially helpful when assessing acquired deposits or tooth structure.

Bass toothbrushing method Sulcular toothbrush technique designed to clean the cervical third of the clinical crown of the tooth in addition to the area beneath the gingival margin.

bass wood interdental cleaner Soft triangular device designed for cleansing a proximal surface of a tooth with a missing interdental papilla.

battery Legal term for harmful or offensive contact with someone; touching someone without his or her permission; may be a civil or criminal offense.

behavior age Age of a child as reflected by level of behavioral maturity.

behavioral effect How a person acts in response to a stimulus.

behavior modeling Behavior modification approach that occurs when a child watches another individual undergo a procedure (live or in video format) and then is encouraged to behave as he or she did.

behavior modification Technique used to reinforce desired behaviors and extinguish behaviors considered detrimental via the consistent application of rewards and punishment.

Bell's palsy Acute facial paralysis.

beneficence Ethical principle that endorses the promotion of benefit, goodness, kindness, and charity, and removing harm.

benign Not malignant; unlikely to cause harm.

beta receptors See *adrenergic receptors*.

beta-titanium A material that is strong, springy, and reasonably formable; used to make auxiliary springs and intermediate and finishing archwires, especially rectangular wires. Beta titanium has properties that are intermediate between stainless steel and M-NiTi; also known as TMA.

bevel See *needle*.

beyond a reasonable doubt Level of legal proof required in a criminal court of law in order to find a defendant guilty.

bias Prejudicial belief or opinion.

bidi (pronounced beede) Cigarette-like product manufactured in India that is made of tobacco and temburni leaf; increases risk of oral cancer when smoked.

bidigital palpation Physical assessment technique that uses fingers and thumb to move or compress tissue on contralateral sides of the head or body.

bilateral Term used to describe a lesion or structure that is located on both sides of the body.

bimanual palpation Using index finger of one hand and fingers and thumb of other hand simultaneously to move or compress tissue.

bioburden Blood, saliva, organic matter, or debris present on instruments, environmental surfaces, and barriers during and after client contact.

biocidal Pertaining to that which kills living organisms.

biocompatible Term used to describe when a foreign substance causes no harmful effects to the body.

biodegradable Capability of a material of being broken down over time by biologic processes without harming the environment

biofeedback The use of electromyography to record muscle activity.

biofilm A complex, three-dimensional arrangement of bacteria living together as a self-sufficient, secure, self-sustaining community that is resistant to conventional antibiotics and antimicrobial agents. Dental plaque is a biofilm. See *bacterial plaque biofilm.*

biologically sound and functional dentition See *human need.*

biologic death Cessation of life as indicated by the stoppage of respiration and heartbeat.

biologic indicator A spore test used to verify the effectiveness of the sterilization procedure and sterilization equipment.

biologic seal Adaptation of keratinized or nonkeratinized epithelium to the titanium abutment cylinder of a dental implant; also known as perimucosal seal.

biologic theories of aging Theories that attempt to explain the biologic phenomenon of aging; divided into molecular and nonmolecular theories.

- ***cell theory*** Molecular theory suggesting that cells that reproduce are not equal in functional capability. In time, the inefficient cells become more apparent in the aging process.
- ***cross-linkage theory*** Nonmolecular theory suggesting that chemical reactions create strong bonds between molecular structures that are normally separate. The ongoing process creates more rigid fibers over time through cross-linking in extracellular components.
- ***error theory*** Molecular theory suggesting that cells may become inoperative because of copying errors in repeated divisions.
- ***free-radical theory*** Nonmolecular theory suggesting that free radicals are highly reactive chemically with other substances and accumulate over time. The reaction unfavorably alters the original structure.
- ***immunologic/autoimmune theory*** Nonmolecular theory suggesting that the immune system undergoes involuntary changes after puberty.
- ***programmed theory*** Molecular theory suggesting that the life span of an organism is programmed within the genes of the organism; the rate and life span are set at life's start.
- ***somatic mutation theory*** Molecular theory suggesting that chromosomal abnormalities occur when cells are exposed to radiation or chemicals. These abnormalities manifest in later life.

bioprosthetic cardiac valve Cardiac valve replacement made from biologic tissue.

biopsy Surgical removal and microscopic examination of a section of tissue or other material from the living body for the purpose of identification and diagnosis.

- ***excisional biopsy*** Biopsy in which the entire lesion is removed for assessment.
- ***incisional biopsy*** Biopsy in which a representative section is taken for assessment.
- ***OralCDx brush biopsy*** An oral lesion evaluation procedure that uses a special brush to capture a specimen of all three layers of epithelium to determine which lesions should be submitted for scalpel biopsy.

bioresorbable Term used to describe materials that are broken down by the body and therefore do not have to be removed mechanically (e.g., some sutures, chlorhexidine chip).

bisbiguanide Category of chemical agents used in infection control and in chemotherapy, such as chlorhexidine.

BIS-GMA Bisphenol A-glycidyl methacrylate.

Black's Classification of Dental Caries and Restorations System used to classify both dental caries and restorations; established by G. V. Black in the early 1900s; provides a precise description of the types and location of dental caries or restoration.

blepharitis Inflammation of the hair follicle and meibomian glands of the eyelid.

blood pressure Measurement of two pressures within the blood vessels; the pressure of the blood against the arterial blood vessels (systole) and the pressure against the blood vessels as the heart relaxes between contractions (diastole).

BMI See *body mass index.*

body image stressors Appearance or function of a body part or feature that may create stress because it brings about change in a person's body image.

body mass index (BMI) Measure that reflects a client's weight in relation to height.

body of knowledge Concepts, propositions, and theories that provide the scientific foundation for practice of the discipline and give the practice its unique character.

Bolten template Template that is superimposed over a tracing of the client's cephalometric radiograph on which standard anatomic landmarks are identified to study the skeletal features; used to determine how the client's jaw position compares to the norm for his or her age and how the position of the teeth relate to the respective jaws in both the anteroposterior and vertical planes of space.

bonding See *enamel bonding.*

bonding strength Degree of resistance to abrasive or occlusal forces.

bone marrow transplantation Therapeutic procedure used to treat a variety of hematologic diseases; marrow may be obtained from the client during a period of disease remission or donated by a person with a similar genetic makeup.

brachial pulse Throbbing sensation that is felt over the brachial artery located on the inner side of the elbow.

bradycardia Slowness of the heartbeat evidenced by a decrease in the pulse rate to less than 60 beats per minute.

breach of contract Legal term for the failure to uphold the terms of an implied or express contract.

breach of duty Legal term for the failure to meet the obligations expected of a dental hygienist to the client.

bridge See *denture.*

bronchodilation Dilation of the bronchi in order to facilitate breathing.

brown spot lesion Demineralized discolored area of enamel.

Brushfield's spots Tiny white or light-yellow marks found in the iris of a person with Down syndrome.

brushing plane Surface of a brush used for cleaning the teeth and tissues.

bruxism Stress-induced, involuntary behavior of grinding the teeth together; can cause loss of bone secondary to periodontitis, headache, muscle spasm, and facial pain.

buccal Surfaces toward the cheek.

buccal mucosa Tissue that lines the inner cheek; may be glistening pink or pigmented with melanin.

buccal nerve block Injection that provides pain control to the soft tissues facial to the mandibular molars.

bulimarexia The vacillation between anorexic and bulimic behavior.

bulimia nervosa Eating disorder characterized by recurrent episodes of binge eating followed by self-induced vomiting, use of laxatives or diuretics, excessive exercise, a feeling of lack of control over the behavior, and a consistent concern with body image and weight.

bulla Circumscribed lesion containing clear, watery fluid or blood more than 0.5 cm in size.

bupropion Nonnicotine aid used for smoking cessation.

burning mouth syndrome Burning sensation in the mouth often associated with menopause.

burnished calculus See *calculus.*

burnishing Deliberate rubbing of a medicinal agent onto the tooth surface to achieve penetration into the dentinal tubules; rubbing the surface of an amalgam restoration after carving.

burnout Physical, emotional, and behavioral changes in an individual as a response to high-intensity or long-duration stress, when one's adaptive capabilities are exceeded.

CAL See *clinical attachment level (CAL).*

calculus Mineralized bacterial plaque biofilm along with calcium phosphate, calcium carbonate, food particles, and other organic matter from the saliva that forms on teeth or dental appliances; lay term is *tartar.*

burnished calculus Smoothed outer surface of calculus created by removing only superficial layers of calculus through inadequate instrumentation.

subgingival calculus Calculus located below the gingival margin and attached to cementum or dentin in the area.

supragingival calculus Calculus located above the gingival margin; may attach to any hard surface including enamel, restorative materials, prosthetic appliances, or exposed cementum.

camouflage therapy Moving teeth orthodontically to mask a malocclusion caused by poor skeletal proportions.

Canadian Dental Hygienists' Association (CDHA) The national association for registered dental hygienists in Canada; founded in 1965.

cancer A broad classification of more than 100 disease types; common element is the abnormal, unrestricted growth of cells that can invade and destroy surrounding normal tissues, and sometimes spread *(metastasize)* to other parts of the body; also known as *carcinoma.*

candidiasis Fungal infection of the oral cavity caused by *Candida albicans;* also known as *thrush;* when it occurs under a denture, it is called *denture stomatitis*; *atrophic candidiasis* is characterized by erythematous pebbled patches on the hard or soft palate, buccal mucosa, and dorsal surface of the tongue.

cannula Narrow, blunt-ended bore, slightly larger than a hypodermic needle, and used to target-deliver antimicrobial agents to the sulcus or periodontal pocket.

carcinoma See *cancer.*

cardiac arrest Heart condition characterized by absence of pulse, blood pressure, and respiration, and an ashen appearance.

cardiac dysrhythmia Abnormality in the normal rhythm of the heartbeat; also know as *cardiac arrhythmia.*

cardiac risks for endocarditis Heart conditions that predispose a person to bacterial (infective) endocarditis if not premedicated with an antibiotic prior to interventions that will induce bacteremia.

cardiovascular disease (CVD) Alteration of the heart and/or blood vessels that impairs function.

carditis Inflammation of the cardiac muscle.

caregiver Person who assists children and disabled individuals with their daily activities.

care plan Plan of action designed by a dental hygienist to prevent or control an oral health problem or promote oral health in a client.

CARE principle Memory-assisting technique used to identify aspects of care important to effective dental hygienist–client helping relationships: Comfort, Acceptance, Responsiveness, Empathy.

caries See *dental caries.*

caries activity level The number of caries developed since the last dental visit.

caries activity test A quick test that provides information about acid-forming microorganisms or their activity in saliva.

caries pattern of the client The type of caries-prone tooth surfaces in a client's mouth.

cariogenic Capable of producing dental caries.

cariogenic plaque Microbial plaque biofilm that can demineralize the tooth structure.

carpal tunnel syndrome Repetitive stress injury caused by the compression of the median nerve in the wrist; an occupational hazard in the clinical practice of dental hygiene; prevented with the application of ergonomic principles in practice. Characterized by pain and numbness in the thumb and index and middle fingers and on the thumb side of the hand.

carrier Animal or person who harbors and spreads a disease-causing organism but who does not become ill.

cartridge Component of the armamentarium for local anesthesia administration that contains the local anesthetic drug in addition to other ingredients; parts include:

- ***aluminum cap*** Section of the cartridge that fits snugly around the neck of the cartridge, holding the diaphragm in place.
- ***diaphragm*** Semipermeable material located on the opposite end of the cartridge from the rubber stopper/plunger; needle penetrates this end.
- ***glass cylinder*** Body of the cartridge on which the contents, amount of solution, and manufacturer's name are imprinted.
- ***rubber stopper/plunger*** Stopper that is located on the opposite end of the cartridge from the diaphragm; harpoon of an aspirating syringe is embedded there.

case presentation Process of explaining assessment findings to a client along with options and recommendations for therapy in order to reach agreement on a care plan and client goals.

cataract Visual problem characterized by an opacity of the normally transparent eye lens that interferes with the passage of light.

cavitation Formation of cavities. Also, the rapid formation and collapse of bubbles in fluid emitted from the tip of an ultrasonic scaler.

cavity See *dental caries.*

cavosurface margin Contact between a cavity surface and a tooth surface location where the walls and line angles meet the unaltered tooth surface.

CDC See *Centers for Disease Control and Prevention (CDC).*

CDHA See *Canadian Dental Hygienists' Association (CDHA).*

CEJ See *cementoenamel junction (CEJ).*

cell theory See *biologic theories of aging.*

cementation Attachment of a restoration or band by means of a cement.

cementoenamel junction (CEJ) Location on a tooth where the cementum and enamel meet; demarcation between the anatomic crown and the anatomic root of the tooth.

cementum Mineralized bone-like substance that covers the roots of teeth and provides a surface for attachment and anchorage for the periodontal fibers; may be cellular or acellular.

Centers for Disease Control and Prevention (CDC) U.S. government agency that provides facilities and services for the investigation, identification, prevention, and control of disease.

central nervous system System of the body composed of the brain and spinal cord.

centric occlusion See *occlusion*.

centric relation The endpoint of closure of the mandible.

centric stops Points of touching when the maxillary and mandibular teeth are locked in centric occlusion.

cerebral palsy A chronic disorder caused by damage to mainly motor areas of the immature brain, primarily affecting the ability to control posture and movement.

cerebrovascular accident (CVA) Stroke; a neurosensory disorder caused by a thrombus or a hemorrhage that results in a cerebral infarct; affects coordination, speech, and mobility.

certainly lethal dose (CLD) Amount of fluoride that if ingested will cause death; based on age and body weight.

certification Process by which a nongovernment agency or organization grants formal recognition to an individual for accomplishments such as completion of a specified amount of further training or coursework, acceptable performance on an examination or series of examinations, or graduation from a formal program.

cervical enamel projections An extension of enamel that goes beyond the normal cementoenamel junction onto the root.

cervical spondylolysis Degenerative joint and cervical vertebrae disease that results in nerve compression, pain, and loss of feeling in the affected arm and shoulder.

cervical third The area of the root closest to the "neck" of the crown of the tooth.

change Process of transforming, alternating, or modifying something.

change agent Individual responsible for taking a leadership role in initiating or managing the process of change.

Charters' toothbrushing method Method designed to increase cleansing effectiveness and gingival stimulation in the interproximal areas; bristles are pointed toward the crown of the tooth rather than apically; may be recommended for persons with orthodontic brackets.

chemical bonding Molecular linking of two chemical agents.

chemical change Change that occurs when substances undergo chemical reactions and form new substances with different properties.

chemical indicator Test that consists of a paper strip placed into a cassette; used to determine if instruments within the cassette were exposed to a steam sterilization process; does not indicate that the process was effective in sterilizing the instruments.

chemical vapor sterilization Process similar to that of an autoclave; however, in place of steam, a chemical vapor (solution of alcohol, acetone, ketone, and formaldehyde) is generated under pressure.

chemotherapeutic agent Chemical agent used to treat a disease or alter host response to the disease.

chemotherapy Treatment of a disease with a chemical agent that destroys the pathogens causing the disease or alters their ability to replicate; also know as *pharmacotherapy.*

chewing tobacco Coarsely shredded tobacco leaf chewed for its nicotine effect.

chief complaint Client's primary reason for seeking the oral healthcare appointment as verbalized by the client.

childbearing years Period of time in a woman's life in which she is likely to become pregnant and give birth.

chisel Hand instrument; various types may be used for planing enamel in a cavity preparation or for supragingival scaling of stain and calculus on broad tooth surfaces.

chlorhexidine A bisbiguanide used as a disinfectant for skin and mucous membranes; an antiplaque and antigingivitis agent.

chromogenic bacteria Bacteria that produce color as a metabolic byproduct.

chronic caries See *dental caries.*

chronic fluoride toxicity See *fluoride toxicity.*

chronicity Failure to heal.

chronic obstructive pulmonary disease Respiratory disease characterized by shortness of breath on physical exertion, difficulty with deep breathing, and coughing; lungs have a diminished capacity to inhale and exhale.

chronic periodontal abscess An overgrowth of pathogenic organisms in a periodontal pocket that drains inflammatory exudate either through the opening of the pocket or through a sinus tract that permits regular drainage; usually painless.

chronologic age Age as measured by calendar time since birth.

circular compression Moving the fingertips in a deliberate, rotating fashion over tissues to be examined and exerting pressure; used in clinical assessment.

circumvallate papillae See *tongue papillae.*

civil law Branch of law that includes offenses for violating private or contractual rights.

clasp brush Brush designed with firm nylon filaments to clean the clasps of partial dentures.

Class I malocclusion Malocclusion in which the relationship of the maxillary and mandibular first molars is normal. However, various teeth are malposed or rotated so that the line of occlusion is not a smooth, curving shape.

Class II malocclusion Malocculsion in which the mandibular first molar is positioned at least one cusp width distal to the maxillary first molar.

Class III malocclusion Malocculsion in which the mandibular first molar is positioned at least one cusp width mesial to the maxillary first molar.

classification of types of teeth In humans, two sets of natural teeth, commonly referred to as the primary and the permanent dentitions.

permanent/secondary dentition Dentition that consists of 32 teeth, 8 in each quadrant: 2 incisors, 1 canine, 2 premolars, and 3 molars.

primary dentition Dentition that consists of 20 teeth, 5 in each quadrant: 2 incisors, 1 canine, and 2 molars.

CLD See *certainly lethal dose (CLD).*

clenching Occurs when the teeth occlude for a long time while in centric position without giving the mandible a rest.

client Biologic, psychological, spiritual, social, cultural, and intellectual human being whose behavior is motivated by human needs and who has eight human needs related to dental hygiene care; the contemporary healthcare consumer; the term suggests one who is an active participant in oral healthcare and who is responsible for personal choices and the consequences of those choices; may refer to an individual or group. See *patient.*

client advocacy Supporting the client not only in the healthcare arena, but also by respecting and promoting the rights of clients.

client-centered goal Desired end-result that the client is to achieve through specific dental hygiene actions.

client noncompliance Lack of client cooperation with recommended oral healthcare; significant because it can result in compromised therapy, unsatisfactory results, and litigation; also know as *client nonadherence.*

client satisfaction A positive emotional state within an individual receiving oral healthcare.

client surveys Questionnaires designed to measure client satisfaction, an essential component of quality of care.

clinical attachment level (CAL) Relative probing depth corresponding to the distance from the cementoenamel junction to the location of a periodontal probe tip at the epithelial junction.

clinical crown Portion of the tooth that is exposed above the epithelial attachment.

clinical death Cessation of heart and respiratory functions.

clinical endpoint An evaluation determined after periodontal therapy when the subgingival environment is assessed with an explorer in order to determine the tooth surfaces' preparedness for healing.

clinical trial Experiment conducted in a clinical setting on human subjects who have been randomly assigned to at least one of two groups; purpose is to test the safety, efficacy, or effectiveness of a drug, therapy, or intervention.

clinician See *dental hygiene clinician.*

closed-ended question Question that requires a narrow answer, usually yes or no or some other brief answer. See *open-ended question*.

coalescing Term used to describe margins or tissue structures that merge.

coalescing lesion Lesion with merging margins.

coated tongue Yellow, whitish, or pigmented covering on all or a portion of the tongue's dorsal surface; indication of the need for tongue cleaning or an underlying disease.

cognitive goals Desired increase in the client's knowledge.

cognitive learning domain Domain that classifies the level of learning involving intellectual tasks such as recall, comprehension, application, analysis, synthesis, and evaluation.

cognitive psychology Branch of psychology that suggests a person's behavior is based on cognition or thinking.

stages of development Theory developed by cognitive psychologist Jean Piaget, focusing on learning in childhood.

stage 1 – sensorimotor stage 0 to 2 years of age; dominated by innate reflexes such as sucking and grasping.

stage 2 – properitoneal stage 2 to 7 years of age; characterized by the use of symbols and language to represent the environment.

stage 3 – concrete operations stage 7 to 11 years of age; characterized by evaluative thought processes with application to concrete problems.

stage 4 – formal operations stage 11 years of age and older; characterized by thought based on reasoning and judgment.

cohort effect Unique effect attributed to the characteristics of a homogeneous group at a point in time.

col Saddle of nonkeratinized interdental gingiva that connects the facial and lingual aspects of the papilla; significant because it is highly susceptible to inflammation.

cold turkey Method of quitting tobacco use abruptly on one's quit date.

cold working A manufacturing process to harden a metal.

collaboration Process of working together for the achievement of common goals.

collaborative practice Dental hygienists, dentists, and other health professionals cooperating as colleagues to integrate their respective care regimens into a single comprehensive approach to quality client care.

collagenase An enzyme that breaks down collagen, resulting in tissue destruction.

combination abscess See *periapical abscess*.

commissure Point of union between two anatomic parts, e.g., commissure of the lips.

communicable disease Disease transmitted from one person or animal to another by direct or indirect contact or by vectors.

communication Process by which a person sends a message to another person with the intention of evoking a response.

community organization Process aimed at developing the skills, abilities, and understandings of groups of persons for the purpose of self-led improvement.

competence Person's ability to master particular skills.

complete denture See *denture*.

completely edentulous Total absence of natural teeth.

complex caries See *dental caries*.

compliance Client adoption of and adherence to professional recommendations

composite Restorative dental material resulting from a mixture of ceramic reinforcing filler particles (glass, silicate, quartz, tricalcium phosphate) in a monomer matrix; once mixed it is converted into a polymer.

composite resin sealant See *resin composite*.

compound caries See *dental caries*.

comprehensive care Cycle that integrates a broad variety of needed oral healthcare services to a client.

comprehensive fluoride therapy Use of both systemic and topical fluoride therapies to maintain a caries-free oral environment.

systemic therapy Fluoride entry via the blood supply of developing teeth.

topical therapy Fluoride entry by direct contact with exposed tooth surfaces.

comprehensive therapy Dental and dental hygiene care that addresses all oral healthcare needs of a client.

concave See *root curvature*.

concept Abstraction formed by generalization from facts.

conceptualization Process of developing a mental configuration of a concept.

conceptualization and understanding See *human need*.

conceptual model Set of concepts and the propositions that integrate them into a meaningful configuration within the domain of dental hygiene; school of thought.

concordant Condition in which a disease occurs in both twins.

concrescence Fusion of two teeth at the root through the cementum only. Originally separate, but joined due to excessive cementum deposition.

concrete operational stage See *cognitive psychology*.

condensation Act of physically compressing or packing a dental material into a cavity preparation.

condensing instrument Hand instrument used for adapting amalgam to a cavity preparation.

confidentiality Legal right of a client to have personal information remain private.

congenital heart disease Cardiac disease present at birth.

congestive heart failure Syndrome characterized by myocardial dysfunction that leads to diminished cardiac output or abnormal circulatory congestion (retention of fluids).

conjunctiva Mucous membrane lining of the eye socket adjacent to the eyeball.

conscious sedation Method of pain control that decreases client's response to pain and stress; client is awake and able to respond, breath, and cough; also known as *inhalation sedation, nitrous-oxide psychosedation,* or *relative analgesia.*

consistency Degree of firmness or density of the soft tissue.

construct A generally intangible concept characterized by conscious, deliberated invention for the purpose of scientific measurement (e.g., creativity, attitude, cultural sensitivity).

consumer advocate Refers to a dental hygienist's role in protecting and supporting client rights and well-being; client advocate.

contextual factors Factors that influence interpersonal communication, such as the environment, internal factors of sender and receiver, nature of the relationship, situation prompting communication, and sociocultural factors.

continued care Maintenance care or supportive periodontal therapy that occurs at regular intervals after completion of active therapy.

continuity theory Speculates that habits, preferences, associations, and coping abilities are part of an individual's personality, and they are continued throughout life.

contra-angle Term used to describe the multiple bends (angles) in the shanks of some scaling instruments.

contract Legally binding agreement between two or more competent, consenting parties about a lawful matter, and for which there is consideration (exchange of something of value in payment for an obligation, such as money).

contra-lateral Structures on the opposite side of the body.

control group Group or subject within a study that does not receive the experimental treatment, but rather the placebo treatment.

controlled drug delivery Keeping antibiotics or antimicrobial agents in a targeted area for an extended period of time (7 to 14 days, depending on the product) to sustain its effectiveness in the elimination of bacterial pathogens for the treatment of disease. See *sustained drug delivery* and *sustained-release device*.

controlled-release device Delivery system that releases an antimicrobial or antibiotic agent over an extended period of time. See *controlled drug delivery*.

controlled study Experiment in which extraneous variables are systematically minimized or eliminated via the use of appropriate research protocol.

control of diabetes Behavioral, nutritional, and pharmacologic actions taken to maintain the health of a person with diabetes mellitus (e.g., staying on a diet, taking prescribed medications, exercising, and monitoring blood glucose to prevent episodes of hyperglycemia).

convex See *root curvature*.

coronary artery disease See *coronary heart disease*.

coronary bypass surgery Medical procedure used to replace closed arteries in the heart; performed by removing part of the leg vein or chest artery and then grafting it onto the coronary artery, thereby creating a new passageway for the blood.

coronary heart disease Disease caused by insufficient blood flow from the coronary arteries into the heart or myocardium. Also known as *ischemic heart disease.*

correlational relationship Relationship in which one attribute (variable) changes as another changes.

corrosion Chemical or electrochemical reaction on the surface of a metallic restoration such as amalgam; may appear as a black or green tarnish that is aesthetically displeasing but not detrimental.

cosmetic dentifrice See *dentifrice*.

countermigration Trend in which a small number of older adults who moved to another state at retirement move back home or to a state where family members live.

cracked-tooth syndrome Transient pain experienced in some teeth with hairline fractures or cracks that traverse the crown and root and connect into the pulp.

cratered Centrally depressed like a bowl or saucer.

credentialing Process of assuring the existence of qualified practitioners and reliable equipment through education, licensure, and certification.

crest of the gingiva See *gingival margin*.

crevicular fluid (CVF) Fluid that normally seeps from the epithelial lining of the sulcus; increases in volume when lining is inflamed.

cricoid cartilage Lowest cartilage of the larynx.

criminal law Law established for preventing harm against society; identifies criminal acts and appropriate punishment.

criteria Qualities or characteristics by which knowledge, skills, oral health status, or other phenomena are measured.

critical instrument Instrument that penetrates or touches broken skin, mucosa, or bone and therefore is classified as requiring sterilization.

critical item Item that penetrates or touches broken skin, mucosa, or bone and therefore is classified as requiring sterilization.

critical pH The 5.5-pH level at which demineralization of tooth structure occurs.

cross-arch fulcrum See *fulcrum*.

crossbite A malocclusion in the transverses plane of space that exists when the buccal cusps of the maxillary teeth are lingual to their normal relationship to the maxillary. A crossbite may be anterior or posterior due to dental-skeletal causes.

cross-contamination Transfer of oral fluids and debris from a client to surfaces, equipment, materials, workers' hands, or another client.

cross-cultural competence The ability to integrate current knowledge of oral healthcare with the ways of multiple cultures.

cross-cultural dental hygiene Effective integration of a client's socioethnocultural background and beliefs into the dental hygiene process of care.

cross-linkage theory See *biologic theories of aging.*

crossover study Type of research design in which the same subjects serve under both experimental and control conditions.

cross-sensitivity Extension of the sensitivity one may experience with a medication to another medication, e.g., penicillins and cephalosporins.

crown Restoration that covers the anatomic crown in order to re-establish tooth form and function:

full gold crown Gold covering used to replace the form and function of a completely defective anatomic crown.

partial gold crown Gold covering used to replace the form and function of a partially defective anatomic crown.

porcelain jacket crown Porcelain and metal cast restoration used to replace the form, function, and aesthetics of a defective anatomical crown.

temporary crown Protective covering placed after a defective tooth has been prepared and the final impression has been taken for the cast restoration; also known as *provisional coverage* or *temporary coverage*.

three-quarter crown Cast restoration used to replace the form and function of a defective crown; covers the remaining crown of the tooth except for a portion of one surface.

crust Hard outer layer or covering composed of dried serum, pus, blood, or a combination.

cubital tunnel syndrome A repetitive strain injury affecting the ulner nerve as it crosses behind the elbow; characterized by pain and numbness in the outer side of the ring finger and little finger.

cultural beliefs System of propositions one holds to be true that are related to membership in a social group.

culture Sum total of human behaviors unique to a specific group and passed from generation to generation or from one to another within the group.

culture shock Negative feelings experienced when placed within a different culture.

cumulative trauma disorder Musculoskeletal disorder involving injuries to the tendons, tendon sheaths, and the related bones, muscles, and nerves of the hands, wrists, elbows, arms, feet, knees, and legs; also known as *repetitive strain injuries*.

curet Periodontal scaling instrument used in surgical and nonsurgical periodontal therapy to debride the tooth of hard and soft deposits, surface irregularities, and toxins.

curettage (gingival) Removal of soft tissue (usually with a sharp curet) that lines the wall of a pocket during subgingival instrumentation; inadvertent to intentional.

curing light Hand-held visible blue light used to harden tooth-colored restorations.

curve of Spee See *root angulation*.

curve of Wilson See *root angulation*.

cutting edge Line formed by the face and lateral side of the working end of a periodontal scaling instrument.

CVA See *cerebrovascular accident (CVA)*.

CVF See *crevicular fluid (CVF)*.

cycle One complete linear or elliptical stroke path of the tip of an ultrasonic or sonic scaler.

cytokines Low molecular weight proteins involved in cell-to-cell communication, antibody and T-cell immune interactions, and immunomodulating functions; includes interleukins and interferons.

cytotoxicity HIV's ability to be destructive to the T lymphocytes.

dayguard Hard acrylic appliance worn throughout the day that fits over the maxillary or mandibular teeth to reduce clenching or grinding of the teeth.

dead soft A fully annealed metal that is soft and has high formability.

debonding Removal of the bracket and all adhesive from the tooth surface.

debridement See *oral debridement*.

deceit Misrepresentation of a situation by a dental hygienist to a client.

decision making Deliberate, logical judgment guided by research evidence, theory, the dental hygiene process, education, and experience.

decubitus ulcers Pressure sores; plural is *decubiti*.

deep Structures located inward, away from the body surface.

deep breathing Relaxation therapy that promotes increased oxygen to the brain and muscles and a sense of calm.

defamation Untrue communication that injures an individual's reputation.

libel Written defamation.

slander Verbal defamation.

defective restoration Reconstruction of the teeth that is less than satisfactory in form and/or function, such as a chipped or leaking amalgam restoration.

defect volume Amount of tooth structure removed as a result of instrumentation.

defendant Legal term for a person who must defend himself or herself in a lawsuit.

defining characteristics Signs and symptoms that support a particular dental hygiene diagnosis.

dehiscence Hole caused by placing an implant in an insufficient area of bone; also any isolated hole in bone along the root of a tooth.

deinstitutionalization Process of removing from an institution a mentally retarded person capable of living and functioning independently with little assistance from a caregiver.

delirium or excitement stage See *anesthesia*.

dementia Progressive brain impairment that interferes with normal intellectual functioning; also called *organic brain syndrome*.

demineralization First stage of the dental caries process in which calcium and phosphate minerals are dissolved from the tooth structure by plaque biofilm acids.

dens evaginatus See *dens in dente*.

dens in dente A tooth within a tooth; caused by invagination of the enamel organ during development; observed most frequently on the lingual aspect of the maxillary lateral incisors.

dental amalgam See *amalgam*.

dental anxiety Nonspecific unease, apprehension, or negative thoughts about what may happen during a dental or dental hygiene appointment.

dental biofilm See *bacterial plaque biofilm* and *biofilm.*

dental calculus Microbial plaque biofilm that has been mineralized by calcium and phosphate salts within the saliva; commonly referred to as *tartar*.

dental caries An infectious, bacteria-caused disease characterized by the acid dissolution of enamel and the eventual breakdown of the more organic, inner dental tissues.

acute/rampant caries Rapidly progressive decay that requires urgent intervention to gain control.

arrested caries Decay from a demineralization-remineralization process; may appear light or brown, but feel firm and glass-like when explored.

backward caries Lateral decay at the dentino-enamel junction.

chronic caries Slowly progressive decay that requires routine intervention.

complex caries Decay on three or more involved surfaces needing preparation.

compound caries Decay on two involved surfaces needing preparation.

early childhood caries Severe decay caused by *Streptococcus mutans* and by sugars and acids in a bottle of milk or juice left in contact with a child's primary teeth; causes rapid demineralization of hard tooth structure; affects children ages 0 to 2.

incipient caries Carious lesions limited to the enamel surface.

pit and fissure caries Decay in the grooves and crevices of the occlusal surfaces of premolars and molars or pits of other tooth surfaces.

radiation caries Rapidly progressive decay that occurs after head and neck radiation therapy; associated with a decrease in saliva.

recurrent or secondary caries New decay that occurs at the margins of existing restorations.

root caries Decay on the root surface of teeth in the presence of gingival recession.

simple caries Decay on one surface needing preparation.

smooth surface caries Decay on the facial, lingual, mesial, and distal surface of teeth.

dental caries process Formation of a carious lesion that results from the bacterial plaque biofilm acting on fermentable dietary carbohydrates to produce acid. The acid then dissolves calcium and phosphate minerals from the tooth, eventually producing a white lesion and then frank decay.

dental charting See *dentition charting*.

dental diagnosis The act, by a dentist, of identifying diseases or problems for which the dentist directs or provides the primary treatment.

dental fear An unpleasant mental, emotional, or physiologic sensation derived from a specific dental-related stimulus.

dental floss Dental aid for cleaning proximal tooth surfaces with normal gingival contour and embrasure spaces.

dental fluorosis Hypomineralization of enamel during pre-eruptive stages of tooth development that results from chronic ingestion of fluoride that exceeds optimal levels.

dental health diet score Measure used to identify persons in need of nutritional counseling to improve oral health. See *sweet score*.

dental history Information collected about a client's previous dental care and experiences, related complications, current symptoms, oral care practices, fluoride, and radiographic exposures, and his or her beliefs, attitudes, and behaviors concerning oral health.

dental hygiene The study of preventive oral healthcare and the management of behaviors required to prevent oral disease and promote health; the major concepts studied are health/oral health, dental hygiene action, the client, the environment, their interaction, and factors that affect them.

dental hygiene actions Interventions performed by dental hygienists aimed at assisting clients in meeting their human needs related to oral health. Involves cognitive, affective, and psychomotor performances and includes assessing, diagnosing, planning, implementing, and evaluating. May be provided in independent, interdependent, and collaborative relationships with the client and healthcare team members as dictated by law; See *dental hygiene interventions*.

dental hygiene care plan See *care plan*.

dental hygiene change agent An individual who applies evidence-based knowledge focusing on a systematic approach to change; See *change, change agent*.

dental hygiene clinician The role of the dental hygienist that focuses on the assessment of signs of health and disease in the oral cavity; identification of the dental hygiene problem (dental hygiene diagnosis); and planning, implementation, and evaluation of dental hygiene care; dental hygiene practitioner.

dental hygiene consumer advocate See *consumer advocate*.

dental hygiene diagnosis Clinical decision made by a dental hygienist that identifies an actual or potential unmet need (human need deficit) that the hygienist is educated and licensed to treat, and/or refer for care.

dental hygiene diagnostic categories Eight dental hygiene diagnoses based on unmet human needs related to oral health; see *human need*.

dental hygiene educator/oral health promoter Role a dental hygienist plays when explaining disease processes and home-care techniques any time a client has learning needs. Also known as an *oral health educator*.

dental hygiene generalist Dental hygienist educated at a standard entry level and capable of serving in the general roles of clinician, educator/oral health promoter, administrator/manager, change agent, consumer advocate, and researcher.

dental hygiene interventions Evidence-based therapies or actions that can prevent, control, or treat client problems or lead a client closer to desired oral health goals.

dental hygiene manager/administrator Role a dental hygienist plays when using management skills and the administrative structure and resources of the employment setting to achieve organizational goals. See *diagnosis*.

dental hygiene process Assessment of client needs, formulation of dental hygiene diagnoses, and the planning, implementation, and evaluation of dental hygiene care.

dental hygiene research Application of the scientific method to problems within the discipline of dental hygiene aimed at theory development, and validation/formation of an organized body of knowledge on which evidence-based decisions can be made.

dental hygiene researcher Role that tests assumptions underlying dental hygiene practice and investigates dental hygiene problems to improve oral healthcare and the practice of dental hygiene.

dental hygiene specialist Dental hygienist educated above the standard entry level, with a master's or doctoral degree in an area of specialization.

dental hygiene theory Interrelated concepts basic to dental hygiene that can be used to systematically describe and explain approaches to dental hygiene practice and predict outcomes of that practice; necessary for evidence-based practice.

dental hygienist Licensed, professional member of the healthcare team who integrates the roles of educator, consumer advocate, practitioner, manager, change agent, and researcher to support total health through the promotion of oral health and wellness.

dental hygienist–client relationship A bond of trust, confidence, and confidentiality that needs to develop between hygienist and client if therapy is to be successful.

dental implant Stable and functional replacement of natural teeth that consists of an anchor integrated with bone, an abutment, and a prosthetic tooth or appliance. See *osseointegration*.

dental impression Negative imprint of the teeth and surrounding tissues.

dental index Quantifiable measure of the amount of oral disease or condition in a population or individual.

dental operatory/treatment area Physical space with the dental unit, dental chair, operating light, and operator's stool.

dental perioscopy Fiber-optic imaging of the periodontal pocket that allows for subgingival visualization of calculus, root fractures, and pocket walls; also known as *periodontal endoscopy*.

dental record Complete document of the health and dental status at the time of initial examination, and comprehensive and chronologic documentation of treatment provided at each appointment.

dental stone An alpha calcium sulfate hemihydrate that is stronger than plaster because its crystals are uniform in shape and less porous.

dental tape An interdental ribbon-like product that is wider and flatter than conventional dental floss.

dental treatment plan Care plan developed by the dentist; the dental hygiene care plan is part of the overall dental treatment plan.

dentifrice Substance (gel, paste, or powder) used in conjunction with a toothbrush or interdental cleaner to facilitate bacterial plaque biofilm removal, or as a vehicle for transporting therapeutic or cosmetic agents to the tooth and its environment.

cosmetic dentifrice Substance that freshens breath temporarily and whitens teeth by removing extrinsic stains.

therapeutic dentifrice Substance that transports biologically active ingredients to the tooth and its environment, e.g., fluoridated toothpaste to inhibit demineralization and promote remineralization.

dentin bonding Type of retention that occurs between a dental material and the dentin of a tooth; can include micromechanical retention only or micromechanical retention and chemical adhesion.

dentin dysplasia A mesenchymal abnormality exhibiting normal tooth color, pulpal obliteration, extreme mobility, retarded root formation, and premature exfoliation.

dentinogenesis imperfecta Disturbance in dentinal development with enamel remaining normal.

dentition charting Graphic representation of the condition of a client's teeth observed on a specific date and then updated based on observations over time. Based on clinical, radiographic, and symptomatic assessments.

dentulous Having natural teeth.

denture Prosthetic appliance used to replace the natural teeth:

fixed partial denture (bridge) Partial denture held in position by attachments to adjacent prepared natural teeth, roots, or implants.

full denture or complete denture Appliance that replaces all of the teeth of one jaw, as well as associated structures of the jaw.

immediate denture Denture designed to be placed into the mouth immediately after teeth are extracted.

overdentures or overlay denture Fabricated removable prosthetic appliance supported by soft tissue and a few remaining teeth and attached to the abutment cylinders via a clip-bar or ball.

partial denture Fixed or removable appliance that replaces one or more missing teeth, receiving support and retention from underlying tissues and some or all remaining teeth.

removable partial denture Partial denture that can be removed from the mouth by the client.

denture adhesive Material used to stabilize and retain a denture by increasing the peripheral seal; commercially available in powder, paste, or film formulations.

denture brush Specialty toothbrush designed with firm nylon filaments to clean dentures and the clasps of partial dentures.

denture-induced fibrous hyperplasia See *prosthesis-induced fibrous hyperplasia.*

denture stomatitis Inflammation of the oral mucosa associated with wearing dentures. Commonly found under maxillary dentures. Mucosal tissues have generalized red and velvety appearance. Pain varies from little or no pain to burning sensations. Primarily the result of chronic *Candida albicans* infection.

dependency State of needing to rely on chemical substances to maintain basic physiologic or psychological function, or relying on another person to make decisions or to carry out one's responsibilities.

deplaquing Disruption and removal of bacterial plaque biofilm and its byproducts from the root surfaces and sulcular or pocket spaces.

depolarization Phase of a nerve impulse in which the nerve membrane becomes more permeable to the sodium ion.

De Quervain's disease Repetitive strain disorder characterized by inflammation of the tendons and tendon sheaths at the base of the thumb with pain migrating into the forearm.

dermis Underlying layer of skin composed of connective tissue.

descriptive study Research that involves describing, analyzing, and interpreting data to evaluate a current population, event, or situation; information for the study is gathered via questionnaires, interviews, surveys, or document analyses.

developmental anomalies Tooth defect due to disruption in the stages of tooth development.

developmental disability Mental, physical, or combined impairment that occurs congenitally or during the developmental period from birth to age 22 years.

developmental space Space that develops between the incisors as a result of growth of the alveolar processes, providing adequate room for permanent teeth.

diabetes mellitus Group of metabolic disorders commonly characterized by relative or absolute lack of insulin or improperly working insulin; impairment in the body's ability to metabolize carbohydrates, fats, and protein; and as a result abnormalities in the structure and function of blood vessels (microangiopathy) and nerves (neuropathy).

type I Formerly known as insulin-dependent diabetes mellitus; a severe deficiency of insulin is characteristic. Treatment requires regular lifelong administration of insulin by injection or pump to prevent ketosis and sustain health; results from autoimmune destruction of insulin-producing cells in the pancreas.

type 2 Formerly known as non–insulin-dependent diabetes mellitus; a heterogenous disorder with abnormalities in insulin secretion, insulin resistance, relative rather than absolute insulin deficiency, and excessive hepatic glucose production.

other types The presence of type 1 or 2 diabetes along with an associated condition or syndrome such as pancreatic disease, endocrine disease, chemical agents, drugs, or genetic syndromes.

diagnosis Analysis of the cause and nature of a problem, condition, or situation. See *dental hygiene diagnosis*.

diagnostic cast Positive reproduction of the teeth and surrounding tissues created by pouring up an impression in either plaster or dental stone.

diagnostic process Problem-solving approach to clinical decision making that guides the intellectual activity of the dental hygienist and uses as a foundation the eight human needs related to dental hygiene care.

diaphoresis Profuse sweating associated with elevated body temperature, physical exercise, exposure to heat, or emotional stress.

diaphragm See *cartridge*.

diastole Phase of the cardiac cycle in which the heart relaxes between contractions.

diastolic blood pressure Pressure exerted on the blood vessels when the heart is in its relaxed state known as the *diastole;* blood pressure that occurs between cardiac contractions.

dietary guidelines for Americans General dietary advice published by the U.S. Department of Agriculture.

diet assessment Identification of current dietary practices as related to the actual nutritional requirements of the client.

diet history Retrospective view of what a person eats as reported by the client; may be a 24-hour or a 3-, 5- or 7-day diet history.

differential diagnosis When one of several diseases or conditions is identified as the one responsible for producing symptoms reported and signs observed.

differential reinforcement of incompatible behavior (DRI) Behavior management strategy that rewards behaviors that can substitute for self-injurious ones.

differential reinforcement of other behavior (DRO) Behavior management strategy that rewards behaviors other than self-injurious ones.

digital palpation Using the index finger to move or press against tissue.

digital radiography Type of digital imaging that uses an intraoral computer sensor instead of radiographic film to make a digital radiograph.

digital subtraction Type of digital imaging that merges the likenesses of two identical images and subtracts them, leaving only an image of the differences.

dilaceration Bend or curve in a tooth caused by trauma or pressure during development of the tooth.

dilution Diffusion of a given quantity of an agent in water rendering the agent attenuated.

diopter magnification Device that enables the eyes to focus at close range.

direct conditioning Display of behavioral and psychological signs of pain and fear when physiologic distress occurs during treatment procedures.

direct contact Mode of transmission that occurs via touching infectious lesions or infected saliva or blood.

direct observation Act of viewing and watching the client to collect data; also known as *visual inspection*.

direct restorations Restorative materials placed and formed directly in the cavity preparation within the oral cavity.

disability Permanent or semipermanent condition that interferes with an individual's ability to do something independently.

discipline Punitive action taken against a practitioner by a board of dentistry or board of dental hygiene for violations of the Practice Act; also a field of study.

disclosing agent Liquid concentrate or tablet containing an ingredient that temporarily stains oral deposits and debris so that the client and clinician can see them.

discordant Condition in which a disease occurs in one twin and not the other.

discrimination Differentiating one from another on the basis of a rational or irrational criterion.

disease A definitive pathologic state accompanied by characteristic signs and symptoms.

disease activity Intermittent periods of periodontitis characterized by loss of alveolar bone and connective tissue attachment loss.

disease prevention paradigm Theoretical construct that emphasizes the importance of identifying the causative agent of disease and avoiding it.

disease severity The degree of periodontitis present as indicated by the amount of clinical attachment loss; categorized as slight (early), moderate, or severe (advanced).

disengagement theory First major hypothetical system designed to consider development of the latter stages of normal aging.

disinfectant Agent that destroys most but not necessarily all microorganisms; intended to kill pathogenic microorganisms, with the exception of bacterial spores.

disinfection Process that destroys most but not necessarily all microorganisms; usually involves the use of liquid chemical agents at room temperature.

disking Slight reduction of enamel on the mesial and distal surfaces of a tooth or teeth to create adequate space in the arch for the tooth or teeth.

disorder A physical or mental abnormality of function.

disposable chemiluminescent light A hand-held disposable light used in conjunction with 1% acetic acid mouthrinse to help detect abnormalities in the oral cavity that might not be visible to the unaided eye.

disposable syringe Syringe that is sometimes used for intraoral injections; more commonly used for intramuscular or intravenous drug administration.

distal Surfaces farthest from midline of the dental arch.

distal step Classification of the primary occlusion in which the distal surface of the mandibular second molar is posterior to the distal surface of the maxillary second molar.

distraction Engaging the client's mind actively at something other than attending to the dental treatment.

distribution Refers to whether the lesion or disease is singular or multiple, or whether it is localized or generalized with regard to the area affected.

documentation Process by which findings, plans, diagnosis, recommendations, services rendered, and client responses are recorded in a client record.

domestic violence Physical and emotional abuse that occurs among family members within the home.

dose schedule Timetable required when taking a particular medication.

double-blind study Experiment in which both the subjects and the researcher collecting the data are unaware (blind) of whether the subjects are in the experimental or control group.

double-ended Describes an instrument with exact mirror images on the opposite ends.

Down syndrome Chromosomal abnormality that affects chromosome 21 and results in a defined set of physical characteristics and mental retardation.

mosaicism Chromosomal anomaly in which there is an error in one of the first cell divisions shortly after conception.

translocation Chromosomal anomaly in which a piece of chromosome in pair 21 breaks off and attaches to another chromosome, usually 14, 21, or 22; hereditary.

trisomy 21 Chromosomal anomaly in which a pair of number 21 chromosomes fails to segregate during the formation of either an egg or sperm prior to conception.

DRI See *differential reinforcement of incompatible behavior (DRI).*

drifted teeth Teeth that have moved out of their normal arch position because of pathologic changes in the attachment apparatus, loss of adjacent tooth support, loss of opposing tooth support, or occlusal trauma.

DRO See *differential reinforcement of other behavior (DRO).*

droplet spread Particles of moisture expelled from the mouth in coughing, sneezing, or speaking, which may carry infection to others through the air.

drug hypersensitivity Allergy to a pharmacologic agent; an adverse effect.

drug idiosyncrasy A unique response to a drug.

drug interaction Alteration in the effect of a drug when taken with another drug.

drug toxicity Toxic/poisonous effect from a drug.

dry heat sterilization Process using high heat for a set period of time to achieve sterile results.

duty Legal obligation that one party owes to the other in a contractual situation.

dwarfed roots Abnormally short roots of teeth that have normal-size crowns; hereditary or from rapid tooth movement during orthodontic treatment.

dysarthria Abnormal speech from an impairment of the muscles that are involved with speech.

dysesthesia Common sensations of numbness, tingling, or burning below the level of spinal cord injury.

dysgeusia Abnormal sense of taste.

dyslipidema Abnormality in the lipids and lipoproteins in the blood.

dysphagia Difficulty in swallowing.

dysplasia Alteration in the size, shape, and organization of adult cells.

dyspnea Difficulty breathing.

dysuria Painful urination caused by an obstruction or infection in the urinary tract.

e-antigen Presence of hepatitis B antigen in the blood; indicates that the person is a hepatitis B carrier; associated with a high risk of transmission.

early childhood caries See *dental caries*.

ecchymosis Small, flat, hemorrhagic patch located on the skin or mucous membrane; larger than a petechia.

echocardiogram Graphic record used to determine the presence of mitral valve prolapse, using ultrasound to evaluate the heart size, chamber, and valve function.

echolalia Meaningless parroting of what is heard; may be observed in persons with autism.

ectopic eruption Eruption of a permanent tooth in a position such that it causes the resorption of the root of the adjacent primary or permanent tooth.

edema Swelling associated with the accumulation of fluid in the tissue; adjective, edematous.

edentulous Lacking or without teeth.

efficacy Effectiveness of a product, therapy, or intervention in doing what it was intended to do.

elastic Small rubber band that can be attached to hooks on each arch to apply and/or distribute orthodontic forces within an arch or across the arches.

elastomer Small elastic used to hold orthodontic archwires within the bracket.

elastomeric chains In orthodontics, a chain of elastomers, typically stretched on bracketed teeth within an arch and used to exert a force to close small interdental spaces.

electroencephalogram (EEG) Graphic record used to measure brain wave activity.

electronic manometer See *sphygmomanometer.*

embrasure spaces The area immediately under the contact point of adjacent teeth.

empathy The attempt to perceive and understand a situation from the point of view of another person.

emphysema A lung disorder in which the terminal bronchioles become plugged with mucus with eventual loss of elasticity in the lung tissue; inspired air becomes trapped and makes breathing difficult.

empirical Evidence collected from objective findings or observations.

employment contract Written agreement describing the terms of employment agreed on by the employee and the employer.

emptiability Temporary loss of fluctuance due to brief removal of the fluid of the lesion into the surrounding tissues.

enamel bonding Type of retention that occurs between a dental material and the enamel of a tooth; can include micromechanical retention only or micromechanical retention and chemical adhesion.

enamel dysplasia Abnormal enamel development caused by an insult to ameloblasts during tooth formation.

enamel hypocalcification Enamel defect from a disturbance during mineralization. Surface may appear smooth with a chalky, white-spotted appearance.

enamel hypoplasia Enamel defect from a disturbance of the ameloblasts during matrix formation. Produces grooves, pits, and/or fissures in the enamel with yellow to brown discoloration.

enamel pearls Small nodules of enamel found on the root surface apical to the cementoenamel junction.

endarteritis Inflammation of the inner layer of an artery.

endocardium Lining of the inner surface and cavities of the heart.

endogenous Arising from within a cell or organism.

endogenous sex steroid hormone gingivitis Gingival disease that occurs as a result of microbial plaque in conjunction with endocrine changes (androgens, estrogens, or progestin) as observed during puberty, pregnancy, and menstruation.

endogenous stain See *tooth stain*.

endophytic Growth inward with invasion.

endosteal Dental implant placed within the bone.

end-stage disease Phase of the disease process that brings a person close to death.

end-to-end bite Occlusion of the teeth without the maxillary teeth overlapping the mandibular teeth.

end-tuft brush Specialty toothbrush designed with a smaller brush head that has a small group of tufts or a single tuft; indicated for type III embrasures, difficult-to-reach areas, or around fixed dental appliances.

environment Milieu of the client and dental hygienist that influences the manner, mode, and level of human need fulfillment for the client; includes factors other than dental hygiene actions that affect the client's attainment of optimal oral health (e.g., economic, psychological, cultural, physical, political, legal, educational, ethical, and geographic factors).

Environmental Protection Agency (EPA) U.S. agency located in Washington, D.C. that regulates disinfectants, sterilants, and certain aspects of waste disposal.

EPA See *Environmental Protection Agency (EPA).*

EPA-registered Indication (by a number on the product label) that a product performs as claimed based on a review of information submitted to the EPA by the product manufacturer.

epicanthal folds Folds of skin extending from the root of the nose to the median end of the eyebrow; characteristic of persons with Down syndrome.

epicondylitis Repetitive strain injury of the forearm near the medial or lateral epicondyle of the humerus characterized by pain and inflammation of the muscle and tissue surrounding the elbow.

epidemiology Study of the occurrence, distribution, and causes of disease or disability.

epidermis Surface layer of keratinized stratified squamous epithelium in skin.

epilepsy Neurologic condition caused by overstimulation of nerve cells in the brain that can involve mild *(petit mal)* to severe *(grand mal)* seizures.

epinephrine See *adrenaline/epinephrine*.

epithelial attachment Inner part of the junctional epithelium attached to the tooth by hemidesmosomes and the basement lamina.

equilibration therapy Adjustment of the occlusion of the teeth by recontouring occlusal enamel with dental burrs to create a centric occlusion coincidental with centric relation.

ergonomics Study of human performance and workplace design in order to maximize health, comfort, and efficiency.

ergonomists Scientists who study human performance and workplace design.

erosion Loss of tooth structure as a result of chemical agents.

error theory See *biologic theories of aging*.

erythema A red area of variable shape and size reflecting tissue inflammation, thinness, and irregularity.

erythema multiforme A blistering, ulcerative mucocutaneous condition of uncertain etiology.

erythematous/atrophic *Candida* A *Candida* infection seen in AIDS patients; presents as smooth red patches on the tongue, palate, or mucosa.

erythroplakia Noninflammatory, red mucosal lesions that cannot be diagnosed by location, client history, or morphology.

estate planning Intentional distribution of possessions and assets on one's death.

ester local anesthetic See *local anesthetic*.

estrogen Natural or synthetic female sex hormone.

estrogen replacement therapy (ERT) The use of estrogen alone or in combination with progesterone to replace the decrease in estrogen production by the body at the time of menopause; safety and efficacy of this therapy are in question.

ethics Branch of philosophy that deals with issues of right and wrong, the ideal human character, and the ideal ends of human action.

ethnic group Persons who share similarities in heritage and tradition, passed on from generation to generation.

ethnicity Unique cultural and social heritage and traditions of groups within primary racial, national, or tribal divisions that reflect distinct customs, language, and social values.

ethnocentrism Natural belief that one's culture is superior to that of others.

ethnographic study Qualitative research approach used to study issues related to culture as they occur in the real-world setting.

etiology Genetic, psychological, physical, biochemical, or microbiologic factors that are implicated as a cause of a disease or disorder.

evaluating Process of measuring the extent to which a client has achieved the goals specified in the care plan.

evidence-based care See *evidence-based practice*.

evidence-based decision making Decision making about client care and treatment based on the most current and valid research knowledge.

evidence-based practice Provision of client care based on the most current and valid research knowledge; also known as *evidence-based care*.

evidence-based teaching Method of teaching using pedagogic methods that are supported by the current research literature as most effective.

excavators Restorative dental instruments used for refining the internal cavity; preparation includes hoes and angle formers.

excisional biopsy See *biopsy*.

exogenous Originating outside of an organism.

exogenous stain See *tooth stain*.

exophytic Showing growth from the surface.

exostosis Abnormal, benign bony outgrowth frequently occurring on the hard palate and lingual aspect of the mandibular alveolar ridge.

expected outcome Desired result of care; evidence is used to determine if the client's goal was met, partially met, or not met at all.

experiment Method used to study dental hygiene problems; characterized by the presence of a control group and experimental group; control of extraneous variables; direct manipulation of the independent variable; and randomization of subjects to at least two treatments.

experimental group Subjects who are exposed to the experimental variable under study.

exploratory stroke Instrumentation used for the detection of deposits; characterized by light-to-firm lateral pressure.

explorer Assessment instrument used to examine the tooth and surrounding areas for evidence of caries or periodontitis, defective restorations, and the presence of calculus and tooth irregularities.

exposure An encounter (contact) with an infectious agent.

expressed consent Informed consent for specific procedures to be performed; given orally or in writing by a mentally competent person or by a healthcare decision maker.

extended-shank curet Curet with a terminal shank that is 3 mm longer than the standard area-specific curet; designed for deep-pocket oral debridement.

external fulcrum See *fulcrum*.

external-quality mechanism Mechanism that exists outside an individually designed quality improvement program, such as formal educational requirements; accreditation standards; the accreditation process; and national, state, and regional board examinations for licensure.

extrinsic stain See *tooth stain*.

extrinsic stain removal Mechanical removal of materia alba, bacterial plaque, and extrinsic stain from tooth surfaces and restorations; used synonymously with the terms *polishing* and *cosmetic polishing*.

eye contact Looking into a person's eyes during verbal or nonverbal communication.

eye loupes Convex lenses worn by the practitioner to visualize the oral field at close range at low magnification.

facial Surfaces toward the face.

facial nerve paralysis Loss of motor function of facial expression muscles.

facial prosthesis Artificial device worn to replace form and function to a portion of the face lost as a result of cancer, surgery, trauma, or congenital defect. See *obturator*.

fast-set powder Alginate material with a working time of 1.25 minutes and a setting time of 1 to 2 minutes.

FDA See *Food and Drug Administration (FDA)*.

fetal alcohol syndrome Physical, mental, and behavioral characteristics that appear in infants whose mothers consumed alcohol during pregnancy.

fiberoptics Transmission of light through hollow fibers of glass or plastic and used to transilluminate teeth or body cavities to aid in diagnosis of disease.

fibrotomy Surgical sectioning of gingival fibers to prevent relapse in the position of orthodontically corrected teeth.

field block Method of obtaining anesthesia by injecting the anesthetic agent solution close to large terminal nerve branches; more circumscribed, and often involves one tooth and the tissues surrounding it.

file Periodontal scaling instrument used to crush and remove tenacious calculus.

filiform papillae See *tongue papillae*.

filled resin Dental material that contains glass, quartz, and silica to make it more resistant to wear.

filled sealant See *pit-and-fissure sealant*.

final diagnosis Diagnosis made after clinical findings and client's response to nonsurgical and surgical care at the reevaluation appointment.

final evaluation Comparing the initial assessment data with data at the completion of therapy to determine if therapeutic and client goals have been met. Occurs once active therapy has been completed for about 2 to 6 weeks.

finishing strip Thin plastic strip with abrasive agents bonded to one side; useful for anterior interproximal extrinsic stain removal.

firm Refers to a lesion that is harder than the adjacent mucosa, indicating a high content of fibrous connective tissue.

First World Economically developed capitalistic countries.

fissure tongue Condition in which fissures or grooves are observed on the tongue, most frequently down the midline.

five A's approach A strategy developed by the Agency for Healthcare Research and Quality for tobacco cessation; stands for Ask, Advise, Assess, Assist, Arrange.

fixation Refers to a nonmobile lesion that has become very firm as a result of abnormally dividing cells invading to deeper areas and onto muscle and bone.

fixed partial denture See *denture*.

flexion Sharp bend or curvature of a root from trauma or pressure to the tooth; occurs later in the tooth's development than does dilaceration.

flexion of the tendons Movement of the tendons.

floss holder Flossing aid with a handle with two prongs in Y or C shape.

floss threader Device used to assist in introducing floss into an area such as between an abutment tooth used for support of a fixed bridge and a pontic (the artificial tooth that replaces a missing natural tooth).

fluctuance Describes a wave passing through a fluid-filled lesion upon palpation.

fluorapatite crystal Crystalline structure that results when a tooth has been exposed to fluoride; the hydroxyapatite is changed to fluorapatite.

fluoridated community A city whose public water supply has been adjusted to contain the optimal amount of fluoride to prevent tooth decay.

fluoride Most effective agent and nutrient for the prevention and control of dental caries on smooth surfaces of teeth.

fluoride-releasing sealant See *pit-and fissure sealant*.

fluoride toxicity Poisoning from the ingestion of too much fluoride.

acute fluoride toxicity Immediate physiologic reaction to fluoride overdose, including nausea, vomiting, hypersalivation, abdominal pain, and diarrhea.

chronic fluoride toxicity Physiologic reaction to long-term exposure of high levels of fluoride causing dental fluorosis, skeletal fluorosis, and kidney damage.

fluoride varnish Topical application vehicle for bringing fluoride into contact with the tooth surface for an extended period of time until the varnish wears away.

flush terminal plane Flat plane formed by the distal surfaces of the primary second molars; results from the primary molars erupting in an end-to-end position. See *straight terminal plane*.

foam stick Sponge-tipped applicator on a handle; often associated with oral hygiene care in hospitals, especially for clients undergoing chemotherapy; also called *foam brush*.

focal (frictional) hyperkeratosis White lesion of the oral mucosa characterized by keratinization of edentulous alveolar ridges due to trauma.

foliate papillae See *tongue papillae.*

fomite Inanimate substance or object, such as clothing or paper, that absorbs and transmits infectious agents.

Fones' toothbrushing method Toothbrushing technique advocated by Dr. Alfred Fones, the founder of dental hygiene. Uses circular motions to brush the teeth; may lead to gingival abrasion over time.

Food and Drug Administration (FDA) U.S. government agency responsible for evaluation and approval of pharmaceuticals and medical devices.

food debris Soft deposit composed of remnants of food retained around the teeth after meals.

food frequency questionnaire Survey instrument used during nutritional assessment to determine the frequency at which certain cariogenic foods are eaten by the client at risk for caries; see *sweet score*.

foramen cecum Small pit-like depression where the sulcus terminalis separates the base from the body of the tongue

forced eruption Extrusion of a tooth using orthodontic forces.

formability The amount of permanent bending a wire or other material will tolerate before it breaks.

formal operations stage See *cognitive psychology*.

four A's approach Tobacco cessation strategy that involves *asking* each client about tobacco use, *advising* users to quit, *assisting* them with the quitting process, and *arranging* follow-up.

freedom from anxiety and stress See *human need*.

freedom from head and neck pain See *human need*.

free gingiva Unattached cuff-like tissue that surrounds the teeth facially, lingually, and interproximally.

free nicotine Ionized nicotine that passes rapidly through the oral mucosa into the bloodstream and into the brain.

free-radical theory See *biologic theories of aging*.

frenectomy The incising of the frenum to reduce muscle tension.

frequency The number of times a behavior is carried out during a specified period of time; the number of strokes per second of an ultrasonic insert tip.

fringe benefits Services paid by the employer in addition to regular wages.

frontal resorption Process in which the lamina dura and underlying alveolar bone are resorbed by osteoclasts formed within the periodontal ligament as a result of orthodontic pressure placed against the tooth.

fulcrum Source of stability or leverage on which the finger rests and pushes against in order to hold a dental instrument with control during stroke activation.

cross-arch fulcrum Fulcrum established by holding the working end of the instrument and the index finger of the hand holding the instrument on separate dental arches.

extraoral fulcrum Fulcrum established outside of the mouth and predominantly used on teeth with deep periodontal pockets; the leverage point may be the client's jaw or side of the face. Also known as an *external fulcrum*.

intraoral fulcrum Traditional fulcrum established inside the mouth against tooth structure.

opposite-arch fulcrum Intraoral fulcrum established on a tooth surface on the opposing arch from the arch being scaled.

same-arch fulcrum Intraoral fulcrum established by a finger resting on a tooth surface on the same arch near the area being scaled.

full-mouth disinfection A therapeutic philosophy of care that calls for total oral debridement of the mouth within a 24-hour period including the application of 0.12% chlorhexidine mouthrinse for two months so that the probability of reinfection is minimized.

functional age Age based on performance capacities.

functional appliance Appliance that changes the posture of the mandible to a position that is open or both open and forward, thereby modifying the growth of the mandible by stretching the surrounding soft tissues.

functional status Degree to which a client can conduct activities of daily living.

fungiform papillae See *tongue papillae*.

furca Areas where the root truncates in two- or three-rooted teeth. Also known as *furcations*.

furcation entrance The opening into furca.

furcation involvement Loss of periodontal attachment between the roots of posterior teeth.

furcation root Root of a tooth that branches into two or more roots.

furcations Areas between the branching roots of posterior teeth where the root trunk divides into separate roots.

fused root Root of a tooth that is attached to bone.

fusion Union of two adjacent tooth buds; fusion can unite two teeth or only the crowns or roots.

galvanic current Electrical current produced by chemical interaction.

gauge Diameter of the lumen of a needle; the higher the gauge number, the smaller the diameter of the lumen.

gauze strip Aid to clean proximal surfaces adjacent to wide embrasure spaces, isolated teeth, or distal surfaces of most posterior teeth.

gemination Splitting of a single tooth germ; appears clinically as double or fused teeth; normally these teeth have a single root with one pulpal canal.

gender bias Prejudice either for or against members of a particular sex.

generalized Lesions or manifestations of disease occurring in more than one area in the oral cavity.

genetic testing Determining a client's genotype status as an indicator of disease risk or susceptibility.

geographic tongue Condition characterized by sporadic and uneven distribution of papillae, or depapillation lending an unusual "topographic" appearance.

geriatrician Physician who specializes in healthcare for the elderly.

geriatrics Branch of medicine concerned with the illnesses of old age and their treatment.

germicidal Capable of killing microbes.

germicide Agent capable of killing microbes.

gerontologist Individual who investigates the effects of aging and the factors that affect the aging process.

gerontology Scientific study of the effects of aging and the factors that affect the aging process.

gestational diabetes mellitus Hyperglycemic state brought on by pregnancy.

gesticulation Culturally influenced signals made with the body that communicate emotions.

gingiva The part of the oral mucous membrane attached to the teeth and the alveolar processes of the jaws.

gingiva/implant interface Space where a dental implant and gingival tissue meet.

gingival abscess Usually occurs in previously disease-free areas, and can be related to the forceful inclusion of some foreign body into the area; mostly found on the marginal gingiva; characterized by a focal area of pus formation.

gingival crevice See *gingival sulcus*.

gingival crevicular fluid (GCF) Serum-like fluid secreted from the underlying connective tissue into the sulcular space; able to transport antibodies and certain systemically administered drugs; increases during inflammation.

gingival diseases A number of reversible conditions of the gingiva characterized by inflammation, including dental plaque–induced gingivitis; gingival diseases associated with endocrine changes or endogenous sex hormones; gingival diseases associated with medications, systemic diseases, or malnutrition; and non–plaque-induced gingival lesions.

gingival margin Edge of the marginal gingiva nearest to the incisal or occlusal area of the tooth; marks the opening of the gingival sulcus.

crest of the gingiva Most coronal portion of the gingiva.

gingival pocket See *pseudo-pocket*.

gingival recession Reduction of the height of the marginal gingiva to a location apical to the cementoenamel junction, resulting in root surface exposure; signifies attachment loss.

gingival sulcus Space between the marginal gingiva and the tooth. The healthy gingival sulcus measures 0.5 mm to 3 mm from the gingival margin to the base of the sulcus. Also known as a *gingival crevice.*

gingivitis Inflammation of the gingival tissue with no apical migration of the junctional epithelium beyond the cementoenamel junction; characterized by inflammation and redness of the gingival tissue and bleeding upon probing. See *periodontitis.*

non–plaque-induced gingivitis Gingival diseases of specific bacterial, viral, or genetic origin; gingival manifestations of systemic conditions such as mucotaneous disorders and allergic reactions; or traumatic lesions, foreign body reactions, or otherwise nonspecific gingival lesions.

plaque-induced gingivitis Inflammation of the gingiva from bacterial plaque biofilm around the gingival margin; most common form of periodontitis.

glass cylinder See *cartridge*.

glass ionomer Fluoride-releasing restorative material, e.g., compomer or ART materials; used for Class I, II, III, and V restorations; also available in cement and luting material.

glaucoma Condition caused by increased intraocular pressure that can result in visual problems and possibly blindness.

glossitis Inflammation of the tongue.

glossodynia Tongue pain from trauma, abscess, or ulcer.

glossopyrosis Burning sensation of the tongue.

glucose A simple and major source of energy found in body fluids; absorbed into the blood from the intestines and used in metabolism.

glucosurea Glucose in the urine.

glycosated hemoglobin concentration Average blood glucose level over time; used to determine whether a diabetic is controlled or uncontrolled.

goal setting Process of formulating statements that define the cognitive, psychomotor, affective, or health status targets that the client desires to achieve as a result of dental hygiene care.

greater (anterior) palatine nerve Nerve that enters the oral cavity on the hard palate via the greater palatine foramen and innervates the palatal soft tissues and bone of the posterior teeth.

greater (anterior) palatine nerve block Injection used to obtain anesthesia to the hard and soft palatal tissues overlying the molars and premolars; no pulpal anesthesia is obtained.

grit Particle size of an abrasive or polishing agent.

gross negligence Serious mistake of commission or omission by a healthcare professional that causes an injury to a client. See *negligence.*

growth modification therapy Orthodontic treatment that applies pressures to resist or enhance the growth of the maxilla or mandible.

growth spurt Rapid increase in the rate of growth that occurs during adolescence; also associated with increased rate of growth of the mandible.

guardian ad litem Legal term for a court-appointed individual.

guided imagery Therapeutic technique for relieving pain or discomfort in which the person is encouraged to concentrate on an image that helps relieve pain or discomfort.

Guyon's canal syndrome Ulnar nerve entrapment at the wrist characterized by numbness and tingling in the little finger and the right side of the ring finger, loss of strength in the lower forearm, and hand clumsiness.

HA coating Hydroxyapatite coating sprayed on a dental implant; designed to increase speed and predictability of healing.

hairy leukoplakia Thick white lesions usually with long finger-like projections; located on the lateral borders of the tongue and associated with Epstein-Barr virus and HIV infection.

halitosis Offensive breath odor associated with poor oral hygiene, periodontitis, sinus infection, tonsillitis, lung disease, diabetes, or uremia.

handicap Physical, emotional, or mental impairment that limits an individual's activities of daily living; may be temporary or permanent.

handle Part of an instrument that is held by a clinician's hand.

hard Describes a lesion that contains bone or other calcified material.

hard palate Anterior roof of the mouth that is digitally palpated for lesions, swellings, hard masses, and color change during an intraoral examination.

head tilt–chin lift maneuver Positioning the victim's head so that the airway can be opened; used in basic life support.

healing cap Plastic cone-shaped covering placed above the abutment of a dental implant at the second surgical phase to promote tissue integration.

health State of well-being with both objective and subjective aspects, which exists on a continuum from maximal wellness to maximal illness; along the continuum, degrees of wellness and illness are associated with varying levels of human need fulfillment.

health education Any combination of learning opportunities designed to facilitate voluntary adoption of behaviors that are conducive to health.

health field concept Attributes the health status of the individual and the community to interaction between human biology, environment, lifestyle, and healthcare organization.

health history Assessment of a client's health status to identify predisposing conditions, current and past treatment experiences, past responses to healthcare, and risk factors that may affect dental hygiene care and outcomes of care.

health promotion Activities in which individuals, communities, and the government can engage to promote healthy lifestyles; includes education, public policies and procedures, and the law, all of which contribute to healthy living conditions for individuals, groups, and communities.

health promotion framework Framework aimed at achieving health for all by accepting specific challenges, identifying mechanisms, and implementing health promotion strategies to meet these challenges.

health promotion paradigm Standard that focuses on creating environments that enable persons to increase control over and improve their current and future health.

healthy public policy Concept that the health impact of any public policy is an outcome as important as the goal of that policy.

heart block Arrhythmia caused by the blocking of impulses from the atria to the ventricles at the A-V node.

heart murmur Abnormal sound caused by altered blood flow through the valve or into a chamber; also known as *cardiac murmur*.

heart transplantation Viable option for individuals with end-stage heart disease in which no other therapeutic intervention is considered effective.

hematogenous total joint replacement Replacement with an artificial joint that has direct communication with the bloodstream.

hematoma Swelling and discoloration of tissue resulting from effusion of blood into the extravascular spaces.

hemidesmosome Histologic attachment mechanism of a cell to a noncellular surface; forms the site of attachment between the junctional epithelium and the surface of the tooth.

hemodialysis Filtering of waste products from the body's blood that must occur in a person with end-stage renal disease.

hemostasis Decreased bleeding at an injection site from decreased blood flow to the area.

hepatitis B virus (HBV) Virus that causes liver damage and is transmitted through parenteral inoculation, e.g., contaminated instruments and needles, blood transfusion, or accidental self-inoculation.

hepatitis C virus (HCV) Virus that causes liver damage and is transmitted through parenteral inoculation.

herbal medicine Use of natural herbs to treat disease.

herpetic whitlow See *acute herpetic gingivostomatitis*.

hertz (Hz) Unit of frequency equal to 1 cycle per second.

high spot Refers to sealants or restoration; area on a tooth surface with excess sealant or restorative material that interferes with occlusion.

hirsutism Increased body or facial hair.

HIV Human immunodeficiency virus, a retrovirus that infects T-lymphocytes and other cells leading to immunosuppression and eventually AIDS.

HIV infection See *acquired immunodeficiency syndrome (AIDS)*.

HLA See *human leukocyte antigen* (HLA).

hoe scaler Dental instrument used to remove deposits from broad tooth surfaces; no longer used in dental hygiene care.

holism Philosophy that views an individual as more than the total sum of parts and shows concern and interest in all aspects of the individual.

home bleaching Use of an oxidizing agent in a custom-fitted, flexible polyvinyl tray that the client wears overnight or for 1 or 2 hours a day for a 2- to 6-week period to manage tooth stain.

homograft cardiac valve Cardiac valve replacement made from a human tissue graft.

hone To sharpen.

horizontal bone loss Pattern of alveolar bone loss that parallels the cementoenamel junctions of adjacent teeth. See *vertical bone loss*.

horizontal scrub Toothbrushing method considered detrimental because the unlimited scrubbing motion exerts pressure on the facial tooth prominence, resulting in gingival recession and tooth abrasion.

host response Reaction of the immune system to invasion by pathogens or to treatment.

HSV I See *acute herpetic gingivostomatitis*.

HSV II See *acute herpetic gingivostomatitis*.

hub See *needle*.

humanism Philosophy that attests to the dignity and worth of all individuals through concern for and understanding of their network of attitudes, values, behavior patterns, and way of life.

humanistic psychology Discipline that focuses on the concerns of how individuals are influenced and guided by the personal meanings they attach to their experiences.

human leukocyte antigen (HLA) Substance that influences immune activity directed against islet cells; may be essential for type 1 diabetes to develop.

human need Internal tension that results from an alteration in a state of a person's system. Eight human needs related to dental hygiene practice follow:

biologically sound and functional dentition The need to have intact teeth and restorations that defend against harmful microbes, provide for adequate function, and reflect appropriate nutrition and diet.

conceptualization and understanding The need to grasp ideas and abstractions in order to make sound decisions about one's oral health.

freedom from anxiety and stress The need to feel safe and to be free from fear and emotional discomfort in the oral healthcare environment.

freedom from head and neck pain The need to be exempt from physical discomfort in the head and neck area.

protection from health risks The need to avoid medical contraindications to dental hygiene care, including the need to be protected from health risks related to dental hygiene care.

responsibility for oral health The need to be accountable for one's health as a result of interaction between one's motivation, physical capability, and environment.

skin and mucous membrane integrity of the head and neck The need to have an intact and functioning covering of one's head and neck area, including the oral mucous membranes and periodontium, which defend against harmful microbes, resist injurious substances and trauma, and reflect adequate nutrition.

wholesome facial image The need to feel satisfied with one's own oral-facial features and breath.

human needs conceptual model Conceptual model of dental hygiene that defines the paradigm concepts of client, environment, health/oral health, and dental hygiene actions in terms of human needs theory.

human needs theory Theory that explains and predicts human behavior by focusing on human need fulfillment and unmet human needs.

Huntington's disease Inherited disorder of the basal ganglia and cerebral cortex characterized by dementia and quick, purposeless, small-amplitude movements.

hyalinized Condition in which the periodontal ligament becomes devoid of all cells as a result of orthodontic pressure placed against a tooth that is too great in force.

hydrocephalus Increase in the volume of cerebrospinal fluid in the ventricular system of the brain.

hydrodynamic theory Most accepted theory of the pain transmission mechanism in dentinal hypersensitivity; explains that dentinal tubules are exposed, pain-producing stimuli are present, stimuli initiate the flow of lymphatic fluid in the dentinal tubules, odontoblasts and their processes transmit the sensory stimuli, and movement of the fluid causes nerve endings at the pulpal wall to be stimulated and produce pain.

hydrophilic Term that means "loves water."

hydrophilic portion See *local anesthetic*.

hydrophilic primer Agent used to dry the enamel surface to enhance sealant attachment to the etched surface.

hypercementosis Abnormal thickening of parts of the cementum, usually in the apical region; associated with chronic inflammation of the tooth, loss of an antagonist tooth, or hypereruption.

hyperdontia Presence of extra teeth beyond the normal complement; however, the teeth are shaped normally.

hyperglycemia Condition of abnormally increased blood glucose levels and the cause of long-term damage, dysfunction, and failure of various organs, especially in the eyes, kidneys, nerves, heart, and blood vessels; the result of the diabetic condition.

hypertension Condition characterized by a persistent elevation of the systolic and diastolic blood pressures above 140 mm Hg and 90 mm Hg, respectively.

hypertensive cardiovascular disease High blood pressure.

hyperthyroidism Condition characterized by excessive hormone secretion of the thyroid glands and hence increased basal metabolism.

hypnosis State of mental relaxation and restricted awareness in which individuals are engrossed in their inner experiences such as feelings and imagery, are less analytical and logical in their thinking, and have enhanced capacity to respond to suggestions in an automatic and disassociated manner.

hypodontia See *anodontia*.

hypoglycemia Emergency condition resulting from an excess of insulin and deficiency of glucose. The most common medical emergency in individuals with type 1 diabetes, treated with oral ingestion of glucose for the conscious person, or IM glucagon or IV dextrose solution for the unconscious person.

hypoplasia Incomplete development of tissue or an organ.

hypotension Consistently low blood pressure (systolic measure below 100 mm Hg).

hypothesis Testable statement that predicts a relationship among the variables under investigation.

hypotonia Abnormally decreased muscle tone or strength.

hypoxemia Reduced level of oxygen in the blood associated with respiratory disease.

IADL See *instrumental activities of daily living (IADL).*

IAG See *inadequate attached gingiva (IAG).*

iatrogenic disease Condition caused by a treatment or diagnostic procedure.

icteric Jaundiced.

ideal body weight Measure of the ideal weight based on an individual's height.

IDHF See *International Dental Hygienists' Federation (IDHF).*

imaging Production of a diagnostic representation of a structure using radiography, ultrasonography, photography, or scintigraphy.

imbibition Uptake of water.

immediate denture Denture constructed prior to extraction of remaining teeth and delivered upon their removal to maintain normal mechanical and physiologic functions of the orofacial complex.

immune dysfunction Condition that results in a decrease in the body's natural defenses against disease.

immune system System that protects the body from foreign invaders such as pathogenic organisms. In the humoral immune response, antibodies produced by B-lymphocytes are released into the body fluids and neutralize an organism, coat the organism to enhance ingestion by macrophages or natural killer cells, cause antigens to agglutinate (which enhances phagocytosis), or activate complement (a system of serum proteins that is a primary mediator of an antigen-antibody reaction) resulting in cell lysis. In the cell-mediated response, T-cells mobilize macrophages.

immunization Process through which a person achieves resistance to an infectious agent.

immunocompromised Weakened immune system due to disease, malnutrition, or medications such as cyclosporine.

immunoglobulin Humoral antibody produced by the body and present in serum and external secretions; formed in response to specific antigens. The types of immunoglobulin follow:

- ***IgA*** The principal immunoglobulin in external secretions of mucosal surfaces, tears, saliva, bile, urine, and colostrum
- ***IgD*** The immunoglobulin thought to activate the B-cell.
- ***IgE*** The immunoglobulin that plays a role in immediate hypersensitivity reactions and parasitic infections.
- ***IgG*** The principal immunoglobulin of the secondary immune response; capable of crossing the placental barrier.
- ***IgM*** The first immunoglobulin to appear in a given immune response.

immunologic/autoimmune theory See *biologic theories of aging.*

immunosuppression Suppression of the body's natural immune response.

impaired fasting glucose Blood glucose level that is not under control even without eating.

impaired glucose tolerance Plasma glucose concentrations that lie between normal values and values diagnostic of diabetes.

implant denture Denture designed to fit over implant fixtures that are inserted partially or entirely into living bone; also known as an implant-borne prosthesis.

implementing Act of carrying out a care plan designed to meet the assessed needs and goals of a client.

implied consent Informed consent assumed by action of a client (e.g., client makes an appointment, comes to the dental office, sits in the dental chair, and opens his mouth).

inadequate attached gingiva (IAG) Condition of having less than 1 mm of keratinized attached gingiva in an area; such an area is difficult to maintain and is at risk of developing into a mucogingival problem.

inadvertent curettage Unintentional soft-tissue removal during normal subgingival instrumentation.

incidence Number of new cases of a specific disease within a defined population over a period of time.

incipient caries See *dental caries.*

incisal The edge of all anterior teeth.

incisional biopsy See *biopsy.*

incisive nerve Nerve that originates at the mental foramen and innervates the teeth anterior to the foramen; terminal branch of the inferior alveolar nerve.

incisive nerve block Injection administered after an inferior alveolar nerve block; provides anesthesia to the anterior mandibular teeth; two injections are necessary to anesthetize all anterior mandibular teeth; no soft tissue anesthesia occurs with this block.

incisive papilla Small bulge of tissue at the most anterior portion, lingual to anterior teeth.

independence Ability to function safely in an autonomous manner without the help of others.

independent contractor Dental hygienist who contracts with a supervising dentist to provide services to the clients of that dentist by referral prescription; requirements set by the IRS.

indices Data-collection tool used to measure conditions or disease within a population, i.e., dental decay indices, quality-of-life indices, plaque indices. See *dental index.*

indirect restorations Restorations formed on reproductions (dies) of prepared teeth.

indirect transmission Transmission of microbial agents via transfer from a contaminated intermediate object (instrument, equipment, or surface).

induration Hardness primarily as a result of an increased number of epithelial cells from an inflammatory infiltrate.

infantilism Retention of child-like behaviors, emotions, and physical and mental characteristics.

infectious agent Something capable of causing an infection.

infective endocarditis Life-threatening infection of the lining of the heart and underlying connective tissue.

inferior Area that faces away from the head and toward the feet.

inferior alveolar nerve Nerve that descends medial to the lateral pterygoid muscle, then passes downward to the medial surface of the ramus and the pterygomandibular space where it enters the mandibular foramen; within the mandibular canal, the pulpal and periodontal tissues of the mandibular teeth, including facial periodontal tissues of the molars, are innervated by the nerve.

inferior alveolar nerve block Injection used to anesthetize the innervation points of the inferior alveolar nerve.

informed consent Written agreement from a mentally competent person that allows something to happen; required prior to performing invasive healthcare procedures or procedures on a minor, and before a person is used as a subject in research. The agreement may come from a legal guardian or healthcare decision maker in the case of a minor or others who cannot self determine.

informed refusal Written document indicating that a client has made an educated decision to decline care based on knowledge of personal health needs, treatment recommendations including risks and benefits, prognosis, and expected outcomes without care.

infrabony pocket Periodontal pocket where the junctional epithelium has migrated below the crest of the alveolar bone; most commonly associated with vertical bone loss. Also known as *intrabony, intra-alveolar,* or *subcrestal pocket.* See *suprabony pocket*.

infraorbital nerve block Nerve block that provides both pulpal and facial soft tissue anesthesia of the maxillary central incisor through the premolars.

inhalation sedation Synonym for nitrous oxide and oxygen analgesia; gases are inhaled through the nose, resulting in the reduction of pain and stress in the client. Also known as *conscious sedation, psychosedation*, and *relaxation sedation*.

initial therapy Also known as *phase I therapy* or *anti-infective therapy,* most of which is the responsibility of the dental hygienist.

in-office bleaching A clinical service to lighten tooth discoloration; classified as professional bleaching, power bleaching, conventional bleaching, laser bleaching, or combination bleaching.

in phase Refers to the resonant frequency adjustment to produce maximum energy output of the insert tip of a manually tuned ultrasonic scaling unit; used when removing moderate to heavy deposits; see *out of phase*.

insertion Act of placing an assessment or treatment instrument into subgingival areas.

in situ In its place of origin.

instrumental activities of daily living (IADL) Complex daily activities, such as using the telephone, preparing meals, and managing money.

instrumental values Behaviors postponed in order to reach ultimate goals.

instrumenting Using a periodontal scaling instrument to achieve therapeutic results.

insulin Hormone necessary for the metabolism of glucose; insulin therapy may be prescribed for clients with diabetes mellitus. See *diabetes mellitus.*

integral contributions Nontangible benefits that dental hygienists contribute to a dental practice; attributes beyond tangible clinical skills and services.

intentional curettage (gingival) Deliberate instrumentation of the soft tissue wall of a periodontal pocket to remove the devitalized contaminated granulomatous tissue in the diseased pocket lining. Includes removal of junctional epithelium, pocket epithelium, and immediately subjacent diseased connective tissue.

interdental brushes Conical or tapered brushes designed for insertion into a plastic, reusable handle that is angled to facilitate interproximal adaptation.

interdental/gingival papilla Gingival tissue located in the interdental space between two adjacent teeth; the tip and lateral borders are continuous with the marginal gingiva, whereas the center is composed of alveolar gingiva.

interdental swab tips Interdental device made of cotton material that absorbs liquid agents well for transport and target delivery of chemotherapeutic agents.

interdental tip stimulator Rubber tip attached to the end of a toothbrush or to a plastic handle used to stimulate the gingiva and to recontour gingival papillae after periodontal therapy.

interexaminer reliability Consistency of different individuals in using criteria in an evaluation or measurement of the same behavior or event; also known as interrater reliability.

interleukin Cytokine produced mainly by T-cells; stimulates the function of lymphocytes and other cells of the immune system; there are many types with specific immune system functions. See *cytokines.*

intermediate chain linkage See *local anesthetic*.

International Federation of Dental Hygienists (IFDH) An international organization of dental hygienists that recognizes that the need for dental hygiene care is universal and that dental hygiene services should be unrestricted by consideration of nationality, gender, race, creed, color, politics, or social status.

international numbering system See *tooth numbering systems*.

International Organization for Standardization (ISO) A nongovernmental network of national standards institutes from 145 countries that promotes standardization in science, technology and economics to facilitate international trade and development. ISO is not an acronym; rather it means *equal* and is used in reference to this organization.

interpersonal communication Communication occurring between two persons or in small-group sessions; the process by which a person sends a message to another person with the intention of evoking a response.

interproximal brushes See *interdental brushes.*

interproximal/interdental area The proximal surfaces of teeth or the embrasure spaces.

interproximal stripping Removal of enamel for mesial and distal surfaces of the crowns of teeth that are crowned to improve their alignment.

interradicular area Furca areas and areas between the roots of teeth.

interrupted force Force whose magnitude gradually drops to zero between orthodontic visits at which time the appliance is activated.

intervention Actions taken by the dental hygienist to alter the course of a disease or to change a person's behavior that is contributing to disease or the potential for disease.

intonation Modulation of the voice.

intracrevicular delivery devices See *controlled drug delivery.*

intraexaminer reliability Consistency of the same individual in using criteria in an evaluation of the same behavior or event more than once.

intraoral fulcrum See *fulcrum.*

intrapersonal communication Communication within one's self.

intrinsic stain See *tooth stain.*

intrusion Displacement of a tooth in an apical direction.

invasive Refers to procedures that involve puncture, incision, or insertion of a foreign object, such as a needle or instrument tip, into the body.

in vitro Occurring in a laboratory.

ipsilateral On the same side of the body.

irreversible hydrocolloid Impression material that does not change its physical state after gelation.

irrigation See *oral irrigation.*

ischemic heart disease See *coronary heart disease.*

ISO See *International Organization for Standardization (ISO).*

jargon Technical language used in a particular discipline by professionals; should not be used with clients.

jaundice Condition caused by a pigment called *bilirubin;* characterized by yellowness in the skin, eye, and mucous membranes; a sign caused by a number of different diseases and disorders of the gallbladder, liver, and hemolytic blood disorders.

jet injector syringe Type of needleless syringe that delivers 0.05 to 0.2 ml anesthetic agent to the mucous membranes at a high pressure; used for soft tissue anesthesia of the palate and topical anesthesia before needle injection.

junctional epithelium (JE) Cuff-like band of nonkeratinized squamous epithelium that completely encircles and adheres to the tooth surface at the base of the gingival sulcus via hemidesmosomes; histologically the apex, or base of the sulcus, is formed by the JE.

justice Ethical and legal principle that relies on fairness and equality; a person is treated justly when given what he or she is due, owed, deserves, or can claim legitimately.

juvenile occlusal equilibrium Phase of eruption that begins after the permanent tooth has erupted into occlusion and the teeth continue to erupt to compensate for the increase in vertical growth of the ramus.

Kaposi's sarcoma Malignant neoplasm associated with HIV infection and manifesting as brown or purplish tumors on the gingiva near the teeth or on the skin.

kernicterus Condition associated with high levels of bilirubin in the blood of newborns resulting in severe neural symptoms.

ketoacidosis Accumulation of acid resulting from the accumulation of ketones in the body.

ketonemia Ketones in the plasma.

ketonurea Ketones in the urine.

keypunch The hole that guides the placement of all remaining holes.

kinesic behavior Bodily motion including posture, gestures, facial expressions, eye behavior, and bodily movement.

kinesthetic sensitivity Ability to discriminate temperatures, perceive spatial relationships, and discern pain.

knitting yarn Aid used to clean proximal tooth surfaces adjacent to wide embrasure spaces, isolated teeth, or distal surfaces of most posterior teeth.

Korotkoff's sounds Sounds heard with the stethoscope when the blood pressure cuff is deflated; thought to be caused by a vibratory motion of the artery as its wall distends in response to the pressure of the cuff.

kretek A product of tobacco and cloves.

labial bow Wire bow that is a frequent component of a removable appliance and is positioned across the anterior teeth to affect tooth position in either a passive or active manner.

labial frenum Fold of tissue located at the midline between the labial mucosa and the alveolar mucosa on each jaw.

labial mucosa Inner portions of the lips; may be glistening pink or pigmented with melanin.

Lactobacillus acidophilus Index organism used to assess caries susceptibility; organism responsible for the initiation of the caries process.

laser bleaching Use of a laser heat source to accelerate the chemical reaction of the bleaching gel; not approved by the ADA for bleaching teeth alone. See *in-office bleaching.*

lateral Structures away from the midline of the body.

lateral cephalometric radiograph Radiograph of the entire head taken from the lateral aspect, used in analysis of skeletal growth and development and dental relationships.

lateral pressure Force used by a dental hygienist to engage the cutting edge of the periodontal scaling instrument against the tooth.

lavage Therapeutic washing of the pockets and root surface to remove endotoxins and loose debris with water under pressure.

law Rules established by local, state, or federal government.

leadership Ability to influence, motivate, or direct others toward the achievement of predetermined goals.

leeway space Space that becomes available in the premolar areas of the maxillary and mandibular arches because the primary molars are larger mesiodistally than the permanent premolars.

Leonard toothbrushing method Method in which a vertical stroke is used while the maxillary and mandibular teeth are placed in an edge-to-edge position during brushing.

lesion of endodontic origin (LEO) An endodontic abscess that commonly results from infection of the pulpal tissues from caries, traumatic fracture of the tooth, or trauma of a dental procedure.

leukodema Benign thickening (parakeratotic cells) of the buccal mucosa that appears opalescent and filmy.

leukoplakia Thickened, white, firmly attached patch on the mucosal surface that is not diagnosed as any other clinical condition; histologically, it is a thickening of the stratified squamous epithelium; considered to have malignant potential; term used to describe a white, plaque-like lesion that cannot be wiped off and cannot be diagnosed as any other disease.

leveling Orthodontic intrusion or extrusion of teeth so that the occlusal surfaces follow the curve of Spee.

liability Responsibility under the law for which one can be prosecuted and punished.

licensure Process by which a government agency certifies that individuals have met predetermined standards, are qualified minimally, and are permitted to practice in its jurisdiction.

lichen planus A chronic dermatologic disease that often affects the oral mucosa. Reticular oral lichen planus is characterized by white interlacing lines; erosive oral lichen planus is characterized by erythematous areas with central ulceration.

life expectancy Average number of years lived by any group of individuals born in the same period; computed at birth.

life span Maximum length of life possible of a species.

ligate To tie into place; in orthodontics, the tying of an archwire onto a bracket.

ligature Soft metal wire or elastic used to tie an archwire into place on a bracket.

line angles Angles formed by a meeting of two tooth surfaces (e.g., line formed where mesial and facial surfaces meet).

linear gingival erythema Linear, red, spontaneously bleeding gingivitis observed in some HIV-positive patients.

line of occlusion Smooth curving line that, on the maxillary arch, passes through the central fossa of the molars and across the cingula of the canines and incisors; on the mandibular arch, passes through the buccal cusps of the posterior teeth and the incisal edges of the anterior teeth.

liners Liquid-like materials applied in thin coatings (<0.5 mm) that act as cavity sealers and provide expanded beneficial functions (e.g., fluoride release) to promote the health of the pulp.

lingual Surface nearest the tongue.

lingual nerve Nerve that lies between the ramus and the medial pterygoid muscle in the pterygomandibular space; travels anteriorly and inferiorly from this space, innervating the anterior two thirds of the tongue, mucous membranes of the floor of the mouth, and the lingual gingiva of the mandible.

lingual nerve block Injection that anesthetizes the lingual nerve that innervates the mandible; anesthetizes all lingual gingival tissue to the midline, the anterior two thirds of the tongue, and floor of the mouth.

lining mucosa Nonkeratinized oral mucosa that has a softer surface texture, a moist surface, and the ability to stretch and be compressed; acts as a cushion for underlying structures.

lip bumper Strong, stiff labial wire placed on the mandibular arch, supported by banded appliances on the molars, to displace the lips and cheeks from the teeth to allow expansion of the arch by the forces of the tongue.

lip incompetence Separation of the lips by at least 3 mm to 4 mm while at rest.

lipolysis The breaking up of fat.

lipophilic group See *local anesthetic*.

LOA See *attachment loss*.

load Resistance on an instrument tip when placed against the calculus deposit or tooth surface. Distribution of occlusal forces applied to the dental implant and residual bone.

load force Pressure from masticatory processes that are not balanced across the dentition. See *load*.

local anesthesia Loss of sensation in a circumscribed area of the body as a result of the depression of excitation in nerve endings or the inhibition of the conduction process in peripheral nerves.

local anesthetic Drug that causes loss of sensation in a circumscribed area.

- ***amide local anesthetic*** Anesthetic agent that undergoes biotransformation in the liver by microsomal enzymes.
- ***ester local anesthetic*** Anesthetic agent that is metabolized by hydrolysis primarily in the plasma.
- ***hydrophilic portion*** Part of the local anesthetic agent that allows diffusion through the interstitial fluid in the tissues to reach the nerve.
- ***intermediate chain linkage*** Part of the local anesthetic agent that determines whether it is classified as an ester or an amide.
- ***lipophilic group*** Part of the local anesthetic agent that ensures it is able to penetrate the lipid-rich nerve membrane; has an aromatic ring.

local drug delivery See *controlled drug delivery* and *sustained drug delivery*.

local infiltration Type of injection that places anesthetic solution close to the smaller terminal nerve endings near the area to be treated.

localized Refers to a disease or condition that is limited to a single area.

localized lesion Lesion limited to a single area.

locus of control Construct that recognizes that some persons attribute outside forces for their successes and failures while others attribute internal forces.

long axis Imaginary line drawn vertically through the center of a tooth; used as a point of orientation when adapting instruments to the tooth surface.

long face syndrome A lower facial structure that is too long in relation to other portions of the face as a result of excessive downward and backward rotation of the mandible during development.

loosely adherent subgingival plaque See *bacterial plaque biofilm.*

loss of attachment (LOA) See *attachment loss.*

love and belonging needs See *Maslow's hierarchy of needs.*

luting agent Cement placed between an indirect restoration and the cavity walls.

luxation Displacement of the condyle in the temporomandibular fossa; displacement of a tooth from the alveolus.

lymphadenopathy Disease process affecting the lymph nodes resulting in hardening and/or enlargement of the nodes; nodes that have become palpable due to a disease process.

lymphatic system System of lymph nodes and lymphatic vessels that return filtered fluids to the bloodstream from the body tissues; plays a role in the immune system by the presence of lymphocytes; absorbs lipids from the intestine and transports them to the blood.

lymph nodes Bean-shaped bodies grouped in clusters along the connecting lymphatic vessels, positioned to filter toxic products from the lymph to prevent their entry into the blood.

lymphocyte Mononuclear cell; includes both T-cells and B-cells that play a role in immunity.

macrodontia Larger than normal teeth; teeth may be larger in width, length, or height.

macrophage Mononuclear cell found in tissues and at the site of inflammation; serves a phagocytic role in cellular immunity.

macrovascular disease Disease of the large blood vessels; includes three types: coronary heart disease, cerebrovascular disease, and peripheral vascular disease. See *coronary heart disease.*

macula Key focusing area of the retina of the eye.

macule Flat, nonpalpable lesion less than 1 cm in size.

magnostrictive See *ultrasonic scaler.*

mainstreaming Practice of placing children that have disabilities in classrooms with students that do not have disabilities.

malignant neoplasm Cancer with atypical or dysplastic cells that may not resemble the parent tissue; may infiltrate locally and metastasize to distant sites; cancerous tumor.

malocclusion The malportioned association or deviation in the relationship of maxillary and mandibular teeth when they are in centric occlusion; classified using Angles' classification of malocclusion.

malpractice Unintentional tort caused by failure to meet the standard of care or failure to foresee consequences that should have been foreseen.

manager Person who accomplishes goals and objectives through other persons.

mandibular nerve (V_3) Third and largest division of the trigeminal nerve; contains a larger sensory root and a smaller root; sensory branches supply the skin and mucous membrane of the temporal region, external ear, cheek, lower part of the face, lower lip, tongue, mastoid air spaces, gingiva and teeth of the mandible, temporomandibular joint, and parts of the dura mater and cranium; motor branches supply the muscles of mastication, the mylohyoid muscle, the anterior belly of the digastric muscle, the tensor veli palatini, and the tensor tympanic muscles.

mandibular tori Exostoses located on the lingual surface of alveolar bone.

manner of speaking Style of talking and communicating that is culturally influenced.

manometer See *sphygmomanometer.*

manual palpation Using all fingers of one hand to simultaneously move or compress tissues.

manual toothbrush The most commonly used device for the removal of bacterial plaque from the facial, lingual, and occlusal surfaces.

manual-tuned unit An ultrasonic scaling device whose resonant frequency, power, and water supplies are adjusted by hand and sound.

marginal/free gingiva Gingival tissue closest to the crown and not directly attached to alveolar bone.

marketing Structured, organized approach to selecting and servicing markets; an evidence-based approach to informing the public of a service, program, or product.

martenstic Form of nitinol alloy that is very springy, strong, and formable.

Maslow's hierarchy of needs Theory established by Abraham Maslow that humans are motivated by unsatisfied needs, and that certain needs need to be satisfied before higher needs can be satisfied. There are five levels of basic needs:

- ***physiological needs*** First level in hierarchy; includes the need to eat, drink, sleep, and reproduce.
- ***safety needs*** Second level in hierarchy; includes the need for stability, protection, structure, and freedom from fear and anxiety.
- ***love and belonging needs*** Third level in hierarchy; includes the need for affectionate relationships and for a place within one's culture, group, or family.
- ***self-esteem needs*** Fourth level in hierarchy; includes the need for confidence, usefulness, worth, and esteem of self as well as from others.
- ***self-actualization needs*** Fifth level in hierarchy; includes the need for a state in which one is fully achieving one's potential and is able to solve problems and cope realistically with life's situations.

mass media Media used to increase public awareness and knowledge.

masticatory mucosa Keratinized oral mucosa that has a rubbery surface texture and resiliency; attached firmly to the tissue underneath. See *oral mucosa*.

materia alba Loosely attached collection of soft oral debris and bacteria seen as a whitish, curd-like mass on the teeth or overlying plaque.

matrix Artificial wall used to replace a missing lateral wall in a cavity preparation.

maxillary nerve (V_2) One of the three divisions of the trigeminal nerve; it is entirely sensory in function; supplies the skin of the middle part of the face, nasal cavity, side of the nose, lower eyelid, upper lip, and mucous membrane of the nasopharynx, maxillary sinus, soft palate, tonsil, maxillary gingiva, and teeth.

maxillary tuberosity Rounded elevation just distal to the last tooth of the maxilla.

maxillomandibular fixation Wiring of the maxilla and mandible together in the desired relationship following orthognathic surgery.

maximal safe dose The maximal amount of a drug that can be safely administered to a healthy individual

mechanical action Refers to the vibration of the tip of a mechanized instrument.

mechanical nonsurgical pocket therapy Use of manual and mechanized instruments to debride the periodontal pockets of endotoxins and soft and hard deposits so that healing can take place.

mechanized instrumentation Power-driven instruments such as sonic and ultrasonic scaling instruments used for oral debridement.

medial Toward the midline of the body.

median palatine raphe Midline ridge of tissue on the hard palate.

medical alert box Boxed-in space on a health history questionnaire where the practitioner can insert life-threatening, medically relevant conditions about a client (e.g., allergies, mitrovalve prolapse, unprotected pacemaker) that require specific changes in dental management in order to prevent health risk or a medical emergency.

medical model Model that views the art and science of medicine as the fount from which all improvements in health flow.

menopause Permanent cessation of menstruation that occurs around the age of 50 to 55.

menses Menstruation.

menstrual cycle–associated gingivitis Inflammatory gingival changes observed during ovulation caused by endocrine changes and bacterial plaque biofilm.

mental age Age level at which a mentally disabled person functions regardless of chronologic age.

mental nerve Branch of the inferior alveolar nerve that exits the mandible through the mental foramen; provides sensory innervation to the skin of the chin and to the skin and mucous membranes of the lower lip.

mental nerve block Injection that provides anesthesia to the areas innervated by the mental nerve.

mental retardation Significantly subaverage intellectual functioning accompanied by significant deficits or impairments in adaptive functioning; manifests during the development period before 18 years of age.

mild retardation Classified by an IQ of 50 to 70; these persons are educable and able to learn some academic skills.

moderate retardation Classified by an IQ of 35 to 49; these persons can learn self-care, social adjustment, and economic usefulness, but very limited academic skills.

severe retardation Classified by an IQ of 20 to 34; these persons can acquire some oral health skills with supervision; they learn through habit training.

profound retardation Classified by an IQ below 20 or 25; these persons are incapable of total self-care, social skills, or economic self-support and require continued supervision and care from a primary caregiver.

mercury hygiene Protocol exercised in preventing bodily harm from mercury ingestion or inhalation.

mercury manometer See *sphygmomanometer*.

mesial Surfaces that are closest to the midline of the dental arch.

mesial step Classification of the primary occlusion in which the distal surface of the mandibular second molar is mesial to the distal surface of the maxillary second molar.

message Portion of the communication process that contains information the sender wishes to transmit.

metaparadigm See *paradigm*.

metastasis Spread of cancer from its point of origin to another site in the body.

methods of acquiring knowledge Way of gathering knowledge from tradition, experts, experience, or using trial and error or the scientific method.

microangiopathy Abnormalities in the structure and function of blood vessels.

microbial cross-contamination Passage of microorganisms from one person or inanimate object to another.

microbial cross-infection Passage of microorganisms from one person to another.

microbiologic conditions Type of bacteria present in the gingival sulcus; specific gram-negative bacteria must be present for periodontitis to occur.

microdontia Developmental anomaly in which the teeth are smaller than normal; may affect one, several, or all teeth within the dentition.

microgingival testing Plaque analysis to determine the presence of specific microorganisms (marker bacteria) associated with the progression of periodontitis; also determines antibiotic susceptibility and resistance.

micron One thousandth of a millimeter; μm

microorganism Any microscopic entity capable of carrying on living processes (e.g., bacteria, viruses, and fungi).

microstreaming See *acoustic microstreaming*.

middle-old Category of the older population from 75 to 84 years of age.

middle superior nerve Branch of the infraorbital nerve within the infraorbital canal; provides sensory innervation to the maxillary premolars, mesiofacial root of the first molar, periodontal tissues, and facial soft tissue and bone in the premolar area.

middle superior nerve block Injection of choice when only the premolar region is being treated.

midline Imaginary longitudinal line dividing the client's face into two equal halves.

mild retardation See *mental retardation*.

mini-bladed curet Debridement instrument with an extended shank and a 50% reduction in blade length as compared to the standard design; provides for enhanced adaptation on narrow facial and lingual anterior tooth surfaces.

minor Person not yet of legal age, usually under 18 years of age.

misrepresentation Distortion of information about a client's health or disease status, about another person, or about a service provided; also known as *deceit*.

missing teeth Spaces in the dental arch without teeth.

mitral valve prolapse Valvular heart defect in which the left ventricle pumps blood to the aorta, the mitral valve flops backward (prolapses) into the left atrium; also known as *floppy mitral valve syndrome* and *click murmur syndrome*.

mitral valve prolapse with valvular regurgitation Valvular heart defect in which the mitral valve is pushed back too far during ventricular contraction, and blood regurgitates back through the mitral valve into the left atrium.

mobility Refers to whether a lesion is free or fixed in relationship to the neighboring tissues; also used to describe the degree of movement of a tooth in a socket infected with periodontitis.

moderate retardation See *mental retardation*.

modified pen grasp Standard grasp used for periodontal instrumentation.

modified Stillman's method Combination of Stillman's and rolling stroke methods of toothbrushing.

monofilament Single strand of material.

monomer Liquid mixed with a catalyst to harden a self-curing sealant; component of a self-curing sealant.

morbidity Rate of disease within a population.

mortality Death rate within a population.

mosaicism See *Down syndrome*.

motivation The incentive or drive to satisfy human needs.

motor-driven handpiece Common piece of equipment used for stain removal; consists of an air-driven slow-speed handpiece, a prophylaxis angle, a rubber cup, and a brush.

mouthguard Intraoral device worn during contact sports to protect an athlete from oral injury.

mouth mirror Assessment instrument used for indirect vision, indirect illumination, transillumination, and tissue and tongue retraction.

mouthrinse Mouthwash that may be cosmetic, therapeutic, or both; provides a simple delivery system for chemotherapeutic agents.

mouthstick Common device used by quadriplegic persons; consists of a simple rod with a rubber tip held in place by the person's teeth and lips; used for various purposes such as turning pages and operating a telephone.

mucocele Distended epithelium-lined space filled with mucinous secretions.

mucogingival junction Demarcation between the alveolar mucosa and the attached gingiva.

mucositis Direct cytotoxic action of chemotherapeutic agents on the oral mucosa resulting in atrophy or thinning of the oral mucosa, erythema, and ulceration.

mucous membrane See *oral mucosa*.

multifilament Material made of several strands twisted together.

multiple lesions Several lesions of a specific type.

multiple sclerosis A dymyelinating disorder characterized by muscular weakness and spasticity caused by lesions of the nerve fibers from the motor cortex of the cerebrum to the spinal cord.

multitufted toothbrush Manual toothbrush with a head that has 10 or 12 tufts in three or four rows.

Mutans streptococci Group of *Streptococcus* including *S. mutans, S. sobrinus, S. cricetus, S. rattus, S. ferus,* and *S. macacae*.

myasthenia gravis An autoimmune disorder characterized by fluctuating or fatigable weakness that worsens with exercise and improves with rest; impaired nerve transmission due to production of antibodies against acetylcholine receptors at the neuromuscular junction.

myelosuppression Process of decreasing the production of blood cells and platelets in the bone marrow.

mylohyoid nerve Nerve that branches from the inferior alveolar nerve before the latter enters into the mandibular foramen. It advances downward and forward in the mylohyoid groove on the medial side of the ramus and may supply accessory sensory innervation to the mandible in the premolar and molar area.

myocardial infarction Reduction of blood flow through one of the coronary arteries resulting in a necrosis of tissue, or infarct.

myocardium Middle layer of the heart muscle; forms the bulk of the heart wall.

nadir Lowest point of the variable being measured (e.g., blood count after suppression by cyclosporine).

nasogastric tube Plastic tube placed through the nasal passage and into the stomach; used for feeding and removing gastric secretions, stomach contents, and gas, and to obtain a specimen.

nasopalatine nerve Nerve that leaves the pterygopalatine ganglion and passes forward and downward entering the oral cavity through the incisive foramen; provides sensory innervation to the bone and lingual soft tissues in the premaxilla (canine to canine).

nasopalatine nerve block Type of injection that anesthetizes the palatal hard and soft tissues from the mesial of the right premolar to the mesial of the left premolar.

National Dental Hygienists' Association (NDHA) Association founded by African-American dental hygienists to address the needs of the minority dental hygienist.

natural tooth function Having a stable foundation on which to bite, chew, and grind.

NDHA See *National Dental Hygienists' Association (NDHA).*

necrotizing ulcerative gingivitis (NUG) See *gingivitis.*

necrotizing ulcerative periodontitis (NUP) See *periodontitis.*

needle Armamentarium that delivers an anesthetic agent from the cartridge to the tissues surrounding the needle tip; components include:

- ***bevel*** Point or tip of the needle that is directed into the tissues.
- ***gauge*** Diameter of the lumen.
- ***hub/syringe adaptor*** Plastic or metal piece that attaches the needle onto the syringe.
- ***lumen*** Opening within the needle through which the solution flows.
- ***shank*** Length of the needle from the point to the hub.
- ***syringe/cartridge-penetrating end*** Section that enters the needle adaptor component of the syringe and engages the rubber diaphragm of the local anesthetic cartridge.

negligence Failure of one owing a duty to another or to do what a reasonable and prudent person would ordinarily do under the circumstances.

neoplasia Pathologic process of tumor formation and growth.

nerve block Deposition of anesthetic solution close to a main nerve trunk often at some distance from the treatment area.

networking Process of sharing and extending professional contacts to establish friendships and business relationships.

neuroadaptation Tolerance to nicotine produced by increasing numbers of nicotine receptors in the brain.

neuropathy Abnormalities in the structure and function of nerves.

neutraceuticals Refers to "all-natural" products used for maintaining health.

neutral position Ergonomically preferred position in which there is no strain or tension on any of the body's joints or muscles, thereby preventing cumulative trauma or neuromuscular disorders in the clinician.

new old Sociologic classification for those between 55 and 64.

nicotine Drug found in tobacco.

nicotine addiction Condition characterized by: use of tobacco despite harmful effects; pleasant (euphoric) effects; difficulty in quitting or controlling use; recurrent drug cravings; tolerance; and physical and psychological dependence.

nicotine reduction Approach to tobacco cessation that involves slowly and systematically reducing the amount of nicotine clients use so that they will have fewer symptoms of withdrawal.

nicotine replacement therapy Use of products containing nicotine but no carcinogens or other toxins to reduce or eliminate withdrawal symptoms while clients cope with the psychosocial and behavioral aspects of dependence (e.g., nicotine transdermal patches, polacrilex gum, nasal sprays, and oral inhalers).

nightguard Hard acrylic appliance worn at night that fits over the maxillary or mandibular teeth to reduce clenching or grinding of the teeth.

NiTi See *nitinol (NiTi).*

nitinol (NiTi) Nickel-titanium alloy used in orthodontic archwires having excellent formability and good strength.

nitrosamines Carcinogens (cancer-causing chemicals) in tobacco products.

nitrous oxide (N_2O) Gas used in combination with oxygen for the control of pain and anxiety during dental and dental hygiene care.

nitrous oxide psychosedation State in which nitrous oxide acts to depress the central nervous system in such a way that nervous impulses are not relayed to the cerebral cortex, or their interpretation is altered.

nodule Elevated solid mass; deeper and firmer than papule of between 0.5 cm and 2 cm in size.

nomenclature Description of a cavity or restoration according to basic rules that involve the combination of anatomic terms.

nonaspirating syringe Syringe with no harpoon on the end of the piston; not recommended because it is impossible to determine the exact position of the needle tip.

noncritical items Instruments or items that do not penetrate or contact mucous membranes but are exposed to saliva, blood, and debris by spatter or the touch of contaminated hands; require intermediate-level disinfection.

nonfluoridated community City that does not add optimal levels of fluoride to its community water supply.

nonmaleficence Ethical principle stating that, above all, a health professional should do no harm.

non–plaque-induced gingivitis See *gingivitis.*

nonsurgical periodontal therapy Periodontal scaling and root planing performed with the aim of increasing connective tissue attachment level. Also includes the use of chemotherapeutic agents to control periodontal pathogens.

nontherapeutic communication Process of sending and receiving messages that does not help a client make decisions or reach goals related to comfort and health.

nonverbal communication Interactions between two or more persons using body language to communicate a message.

nonvital tooth bleaching Bleaching of an endodontically treated tooth.

normalization Process that enables mentally retarded citizens to engage in normal patterns of everyday life.

normal occlusion State in which the mesiofacial cusp of the maxillary permanent first molar occludes with the facial groove of the mandibular permanent first molar, and all other teeth are in proper alignment.

normal-set powder Alginate material with a working time of 2 minutes and a setting time of up to 4.5 minutes.

nosocomial infection Infection that occurs as a result of infectious agents in the hospital environment.

NUG Necrotizing ulcerative gingivitis. See *gingivitis*.

NUP Necrotizing ulcerative periodontitis. See *periodontitis*.

nutrition The need to ingest and assimilate sufficient amounts of carbohydrates, proteins, fats, vitamins, minerals, trace elements, and fiber required for growth, repair, and maintenance of structurally and functionally competent body parts.

nutritional counseling Process used to help clients develop healthful food selection and eating behaviors that promote overall health.

nutritional rehabilitation Use of diet and nutrition to regain health.

nutrition assessment Systematic collection of information to identify the need for nutritional counseling and make the appropriate recommendations and referrals.

observation The act of viewing and watching the client to collect data to detect variations from normal and potential disease states.

occipital nodes Lymph nodes at the base of the skull; bilaterally palpated during client assessment.

occlusal adjustment Selective reshaping or recontouring of the dentition to improve the occlusion.

occlusal traumatism Destruction of the supporting structures of the teeth from excess occlusal force; exacerbates periodontal disease.

occlusion Contact relationship between maxillary and mandibular teeth when the jaws are in a fully closed position.

centric occlusion Relationship between the maxillary and mandibular occlusal surfaces that provides the maximum contact and/or intercuspation.

occupational model Model that views dental hygiene as technology based and the dental hygienist as a dental auxiliary who implements treatment plans and carries out isolated duties as directed by the supervising dentist.

occupational safety and health Refers to health and safety in the workplace.

Occupational Safety and Health Administration (OSHA) Federal agency responsible for safety in the workplace.

office policies and procedures Standard guidelines established by an employer in order to provide consistency and guidance for employees and the client.

olfaction Act of sensing body odors to detect variations from normal and potential disease entities.

oncologist Physician who specializes in the treatment of cancer.

oncology Branch of medicine that studies and treats cancer.

open bite Malocclusion of the vertical plane of space in which the maxillary and mandibular teeth fail to meet when the teeth are occluded so that an open space can be seen when viewing the teeth for the facial aspect.

open-ended question Question that allows a free response, rather than the selection of one of several pre-established answers. See *closed-ended question*.

operculum Flap of tissue that completely or partially covers a tooth. See *acute pericoronitis*.

ophthalmic nerve (V_1) First and smallest division of the trigeminal nerve; innervates tissue superior to the oral structures including the eye, nose, and frontal cutaneous tissues; sensory only.

opposite-arch fulcrum See *fulcrum*.

oral candidiasis Oral infection characterized by pruritus, underlying red tissue, and bleeding; caused by *Candida* (usually *Candida albicans*); opportunistic infection due to recent antibiotic therapy, chemotherapy, corticosteroid therapy, or immunosuppression associated with some medications, diabetes mellitus, or AIDS; also known as *thrush*.

OralCDx brush biopsy See *biopsy*.

oral contraceptive Pharmaceutical agent (hormones) taken orally to prevent conception.

oral contributing factors Factors that influence the growth and retention of plaque.

oral cytology Collection of cells by scraping the surface of a lesion with a cotton swab; exfoliative cytology.

oral debridement Treatment of periodontitis through the mechanical removal of tooth and root surface irregularities (including bacterial plaque, clinically detectable calculus, and all plaque-retentive factors); treatment is done only to the extent that adjacent soft tissues in the pocket can heal. Removal of calculus is important only to the extent that it is a plaque-retentive factor. Reestablishes health and balance between the bacterial flora and the host's immune responses. Also known as *periodontal debridement*.

oral dysesthesia Sensations of numbness, tingling, or burning in the mouth.

oral health Desired state of the mouth that results from the interaction of an individual with his or her systemic health, self-care behavior, and environment; oral health and overall health status are interrelated because each affects the other.

oral health condition State of the oral cavity.

oral health educator See *dental hygiene educator/oral health promoter*.

oral health–related quality of life model Model that postulates that the continuum of health and disease is influenced by environmental, sociocultural, and economic influences that are either modifiable or nonmodifiable risk factors.

oral health status goals Tangible desired outcomes in the client's oral health status; definitive way of evaluating the effectiveness of care is by determining if goals were met.

oral hygiene assessment Process of determining amount and location of a client's hard and soft tooth deposits; awareness of oral hygiene status; motivation related to oral self-care; and home care regimen.

oral hygiene index Quantitative measure of a client's level of oral hygiene; see *dental index.*

oral hygiene plan Predetermined goals and interventions for oral self care, based on client assessment data.

oral irrigation Method of directing a steady or pulsating stream of water or chemotherapeutic agent over the teeth, gingival tissues, or into a periodontal pocket; goal is to remove oral debris, reduce pathogens and their byproducts, or deliver an antimicrobial agent.

oral manifestations Signs and symptoms that occur in the mouth as a result of disease, disability, medication, or trauma.

oral mucosa Mucous membrane composed of connective tissue covered with stratified squamous epithelium; includes three categories:

lining mucosa Membrane that covers the inner surfaces of the cheeks and lips, the floor of the mouth, the ventral surface of the tongue, and the soft palate; nonkeratinized.

masticatory mucosa Membrane that covers the hard palate and gingiva, and is attached firmly to the tissue underneath; exposed to masticatory forces, therefore keratinized.

specialized mucosa Membrane that covers the upper surface or dorsum of the tongue; contributes to the special function of taste sensation; keratinized.

oral snuff A finely ground tobacco leaf, packaged either loose or in a teabag-like sachet.

oral squamous cell carcinoma Slow-growing malignancy of the squamous epithelium.

oral warts Associated with human papillomavirus; commonly found in HIV-infected individuals.

organic debris Minute amounts of blood, saliva, and associated microorganisms that may be transparent or translucent; dries as a clear film on skin, clothing, and other surfaces.

orthodontic expansion Increasing the length of the arch by tipping the crowns of the teeth facially using conventional fixed appliances in addition to removable expansion appliances.

orthognathic surgery Surgical correction of jaw discrepancy.

orthopedic expansion Expansion of the dental arch by the application of forces to change underlying skeletal structures.

orthopedic replacement Device used to substitute for a body part in terms of form and function; a prosthesis.

orthopnea Inability to breathe in a supine position, but ability to breathe in an upright position.

orthostatic hypotension Fall in blood pressure upon suddenly standing or sitting erect that causes dizziness, syncope, and blurred vision; also caused by standing motionless in a fixed position; elderly and pregnant persons are prone to this condition.

OSHA Occupational Safety and Health Administration.

osseointegration Sound biocompatibility of living bone directly to a space age metal, such as titanium. See *dental implant*.

osteoarthritis See *arthritis*.

osteopenia Loss of mineralized bone tissue, regardless of its cause; considered a precursor to osteoporosis.

osteoporosis Condition involving demineralization of the bone and a decrease in bone mass caused by excessive leaching of calcium from the bone matrix.

osteoradionecrosis Serious complication of radiation therapy characterized by the necrosis of bone, pain, infection, and sequestration; typically involves the mandible.

OTC See *over-the-counter (OTC)*.

outcome Result derived from a specific intervention or treatment.

out of phase Refers to a deliberate detuning of the resonant frequency of a manual-tuned ultrasonic scaling unit; used to increase patient comfort and to achieve less vibration for deplaquing; see *in phase*.

overbite Vertical overlap of the maxillary and mandibular incisor teeth; normal if the maxillary incisors overlap within the incisal third of the mandibular incisors.

overdentures See *denture*.

overjet Horizontal overlap, or distance, between the lingual surface of the maxillary incisors and the labial surface of the mandibular incisors.

over-the-counter (OTC) Medications and healthcare products that can be purchased without a prescription directly off the store shelf.

oxidizing agent Compound such as chloride dioxide that readily gives up oxygen or attracts hydrogen from another compound; although unsubstantiated, used by some to combine with volatile sulfur compounds to reduce mouth odor.

oxygenating agent Compound such a hydrogen peroxide that releases oxygen; used to cleanse an area of inflammation.

Paget's disease Chronic nonmetabolic disease of bone characterized by slowly progressive enlargement of maxilla, mandible, and skull; unknown etiology.

pain stimulus Chemical, mechanical, or thermal factor capable of initiating pain.

pain threshold Point at which an uncomfortable stimulus is perceived as painful.

pain tolerance Amount of pain that is the most a person can bear.

palatal tori See *torus palatinus*.

palatine rugae Firm, irregular ridges of tissue directly posterior to the incisive papilla.

palatine tonsils Masses of lymphoid tissue located between the anterior and posterior pillars; contain lymphocytes that remove toxic products.

Palmer numbering system See *tooth numbering systems*.

palm thumb grasp An instrumentation grasp wherein the instrument is held with all four fingers wrapped tightly around the handle and the thumb placed on the shank in a direction pointing toward the tip of the instrument.

palpation Act of using the sense of touch to collect client data; compressing or movement of tissue in order to check for abnormalities during an intra- and extraoral examination.

panoramic radiograph Radiograph in which the entire dentition in addition to the adjacent osseous structures from the orbits of the eyes to the base of the mandible, and the temporomandibular joints, is displayed on one rectangular film.

papillary Rough surface resembling small nodulations or elevated projections.

papillary hyperplasia Mixed reactive and inflammatory lesion of the palate from poor oral hygiene, trauma, and irritation caused by the suction chambers of a denture; granular papillary projections result from hyperplastic tissue response that gives characteristic "cobblestone" appearance. May potentiate growth of *Candida albicans;* also known as *pseudopapillomatosis*.

papule Palpable, circumscribed, solid elevation less than 0.5 cm in size.

paradigm Widely accepted view of a discipline that shapes the direction and methods of its practitioners, educators, administrators, and researchers; also known as a *metaparadigm.*

paralanguage Communication by means of vocal sounds such as intonation, rate, pitch, volume, and vocal patterns.

parasympathetic nervous system See *autonomic nervous system*.

parenteral exposure Exposure occurring as a result of piercing the skin barrier with needle or instrument.

paresthesia Prolonged anesthesia; numbness for many hours or days following a local anesthetic injection or a surgical procedure; usually attributed to nerve damage.

Parkinson's disease Chronic, progressive disorder caused by pathological changes in the basal ganglia of the cerebrum resulting in a deficiency of dopamine; characterized by muscle rigidity, tremors, loss of postural stability, and slowness of spontaneous movement; no impairment in intellectual function.

parotid enlargement Condition observed in both anorexics and bulimics characterized by a distinct swelling of the parotid glands.

parotid gland Salivary glands bilaterally palpated in front of the tragus of the ear.

parotid papilla Small elevation of tissue on the inner portion of the buccal mucosa, just opposite the maxillary second molar; contains the opening of the parotid gland (Stensen's duct)

passive expansion Expansion of the dental arch by the removal of the forces of the labial and buccal musculature.

passive tooth-borne functional appliance Tooth-supported appliance that produces skeletal changes passively by deflection forces applied by the tongue, lips, and cheeks or by the forward posturing of the mandible.

patent ductus arteriosus Congenital heart defect in which the vessel connecting the pulmonary artery and the descending aorta fails to close after birth; allows blood to flow into the pulmonary artery causing increased cardiac workload and vascular congestion; observed in premature infants; the vessel is the *ductus arteriosus.*

pathogen Disease-producing microorganism.

patient Person who is ill or who is undergoing care for the treatment of a disease.

PDR See *Physician's Desk Reference (PDR).*

pedagogy The art and science of teaching children.

pedunculated Lesions having a narrow pedicle, or stalk-like base of attachment.

peer review committee Group of professionals with similar levels of education and experience who evaluate the performance of their colleagues for the purpose of quality assurance and improvement.

pen grasp An instrument hold applied when the exacting or directive type of pressure used in scaling and root planing is not required.

percussion Assessment technique that uses the fingers or an instrument to strike a structure and listen for the sound or client response.

percutaneous inoculation Direct microorganism transfer via either needle or sharp object such as an instrument or through nonintact skin (scratches, burns, dermatitis).

performance evaluation A communication tool based on an agreed-upon peformance plan.

periapex Tip of the root.

periapical abscess The result of infection through dental caries, traumatic fracture of the tooth, or the trauma of a dental procedure; the pulpal infection can be spread laterally to the pulp from an adjacent infected tooth, through the lateral canals.

combination abscess Periapical abscess that spreads from the pulp to the periodontium, and from the periodontal pocket to the pulp.

periapical foramen The opening at the apex of a tooth's root through which blood, nerve, and lymphatic vessels pass.

pericardium Sac that surrounds the heart and the roots of the great blood vessels.

periimplantitis Inflammation of the soft tissue around the dental implant.

periimplant recession Loss of gingival tissue around an implant.

perimenopause Transitional stage of two to ten years before cessation of menstruation; occurs between 35 and 50 years of age.

perimylolysis Dental erosion caused by gastric acids on the teeth as a result of vomiting over a period of time; apparent in persons with bulimia, usually after a two-year duration.

periodontal debridement See *oral debridement*.

periodontal diagnosis Process by which a dentist diagnoses the type and extent of periodontitis present in a client.

periodontal dressing Dental material placed postoperatively over a surgical site or into an extraction site to provide protection and promote healing.

periodontal ligament Fibrous attachment of the teeth to the bone.

periodontal maintenance Supportive phase of care initiated after successful completion of active periodontal treatment; also known as *supportive periodontal therapy*.

periodontal pack Putty-like bandage placed over a surgical wound site after periodontal surgery and worn for about seven days to prevent injury and promote healing. Also known as a *periodontal dressing.*

periodontal pocket Pathologic deepening of the gingival sulcus from the apical migration of the junctional epithelium and destruction of the periodontium.

periodontal probe Assessment instrument used to detect and monitor periodontal pockets and clinical attachment loss.

periodontal screening and recording (PSR) A periodontal screening system promoted by the American Dental Association as an efficient mechanism to determine if a full periodontal probing is indicated.

periodontal surgery Invasive procedure used to eliminate disease by modifying the anatomy of the altered periodontium.

Periodontal Susceptibility Test Genetic test that determines one's risk of developing severe periodontitis.

periodontitis Inflammatory disease of the periodontium that results from progression of gingivitis; caused by specific microorganisms; characterized by progressive destruction of the periodontal ligament and alveolar bone, recession, pocket formation, and possible tooth mobility. The four major types are chronic, aggressive, necrotizing, and systemic. See *gingivitis.*

aggressive periodontitis Periodontitis with a rapid rate of periodontal destruction and disease progression; occurs in localized and generalized forms.

chronic periodontitis Slowly progressing periodontitis; may have periods of moderate to rapid progression; occurs in localized and generalized forms.

necrotizing periodontal diseases Two types:

necrotizing ulcerative gingivitis (NUG) *Inflammatory destructive disease of the gingiva that has a sudden onset; predisposing factors include gingivitis, smoking, severe stress, poor nutrition, and lack of sleep.*

necrotizing ulcerative periodontitis (NUP) Periodontitis found in individuals who are immunocompromised (e.g., infected with HIV or experiencing severe malnutrition); characterized by ulceration and necrosis of gingival tissue with rapid destruction and exposure of alveolar bone, spontaneous bleeding, and pain.

systemic periodontitis Periodontitis that may be secondary to systemic disease.

periodontium Supporting structure of tissues that surrounds the teeth; includes the gingiva, periodontal ligament, root cementum, and alveolar bone.

permanent/secondary dentition See *classification of types of teeth.*

personal history Information about a client's address, emergency contact, occupation, gender, race, work address, marital status, etc.

personal power Influence an informal leader has within a group.

personal protective equipment (PPE) Garments and other attire worn with the intent to protect a worker from exposure that cannot be controlled through the use of engineering, administrative, or work-practice controls.

petechiae Pinpoint red spots on the skin or mucous membrane from minute hemorrhages.

pharmacokinetics Study of the action of drugs within the body.

pharmacologic history Review and documentation of the medications currently taken by the client; provides insight into the client's health status and health behavior.

pharmacotherapeutic nonsurgical pocket therapy Use of systemic and topical chemotherapeutic agent such as minocycline or doxycycline to eliminate pathogenic bacteria and arrest disease activity in a periodontal pocket.

phenolic compounds Essential oils used in commercial mouthrinses for antiplaque and antigingivitis properties (e.g., Listerine contains phenolic compounds and has the ADA seal for efficacy in plaque and gingivitis reduction).

phenylketonuria Metabolic disorder present at birth that if uncontrolled causes an abnormal accumulation of phenylalanine, brain damage, and mental retardation.

phobia A clinically significant fear.

specific phobia A persistent fear in which an object or situation is avoided or endured with intense anxiety or interferes with normal routines.

photopolymerization See *polymerization*.

physical change Change from solid, liquid, or gas that can be illustrated by the three physical states of water (freezing, melting and evaporation).

physical contact Contact between a person and another entity such as another person, antigen, or toxic chemical.

physically dependent on nicotine Adaptation of the brain so that it needs nicotine to function normally.

Physician's Desk Reference (PDR) Reference guide, published annually, about the pharmacology, indications, contraindications, and side effects of prescription drug products; PDRs for over-the-counter medication and herbal medications are also available.

physiologic needs See *Maslow's hierarchy of needs.*

piezoelectric Type of ultrasonic scaling unit that has a ceramic transducer; alternating currents applied to the transducer create dimensional change that is transmitted to the tip; tip moves in a linear pattern and only two sides of the tip are activated and applied to the tooth for mechanized instrumentation.

pipe cleaner Aid to clean type II embrasures or exposed furcation areas.

pit and fissure caries See *dental caries.*

pit and fissure sealant Thin plastic coating of an organic polymer (resin) placed in the pit and fissures of teeth to act as a physical barrier.

filled sealant Sealant composed of a mixture of resins, chemicals, and fillers.

fluoride-releasing sealant Glass ionomer sealant.

preventive sealant Sealant that is placed in caries-free teeth in an effort to prevent dental caries.

therapeutic sealant Sealant that is placed in teeth with incipient carious lesions in an effort to stop the decay process.

unfilled sealant Sealant that does not contain particles and is therefore less resistant to wear; useful in school-based settings when occlusion cannot be adjusted with a finishing burr and dental handpiece.

plaintiff Legal term for the party that brings forth a lawsuit against another party (the *defendant).*

planned change Purposeful, systematic effort to bring about changes through the intervention of a change agent.

planning Act of establishing goals with the client and selecting interventions that can move the client closer to optimal oral health.

plaque Discrete, slightly elevated area of altered texture or coloration on the skin or any other body structure that is more than 0.5 cm in size. See *bacterial plaque biofilm.*

plaque biofilm control Regular mechanical or chemical removal of bacterial plaque biofilm from the teeth and adjacent oral tissue or the prevention of its accumulation.

plaque disclosing solution Stains the invisible plaque biofilm on the teeth.

plaque-induced gingivitis See *gingivitis.*

plaque-retentive factors Conditions that foster the establishment and growth of microbial plaque biofilm (e.g., calculus, malocclusion, or restorations with poor margins.)

plaster A beta calcium sulfate hemihydrate with very porous crystals that cause it to require the most water when mixing compared to the other types of gypsum products.

plica fimbriata Feathery folds of tissue on the ventral surface of the tongue.

point angle Meeting of three tooth surfaces.

polarized Condition of a nerve in which the balance between positive sodium ions on the outside of the nerve membrane and negative potassium ions on the inside of the membrane exists; the resting state of the nerve or resting potential state.

poliomyelitis An acute infectious disease caused by polioviruses that attack the lower motor neurons of the spinal cord.

polishing Mechanical removal of materia alba, bacterial plaque biofilm, endotoxins, and extrinsic stain from tooth surfaces and restorations.

cosmetic polishing Removal of stain from tooth surfaces; also known as *extrinsic stain removal.*

therapeutic polishing Removal of plaque biofilm and endotoxins from the root surface during periodontal surgery.

polydipsia Abnormal increase in thirst.

polymerization Process by which sealants harden.

autopolymerization Self-curing.

photopolymerization Light curing with a visible blue light.

polyphagia Abnormal increase in eating.

polypharmacy Term used to describe treatment with multiple drugs.

polyuria Abnormal increase in urination.

pontic Artificial clinical crown on a fixed bridge that replaces a missing tooth or teeth.

portal of entry Opening through which microbes can invade the body (e.g., any break in the integrity of skin and mucous membrane).

porte polisher A manual instrument with a wooden tip, used as an alternative to the slow speed handpiece for extrinsic stain removal from natural teeth; teeth, calculus and plaque biofilm removal from a titanium implant abutment cylinder; or the burnishing of fluoride into the tooth structure to control dentinal hypersensitivity.

postauricular Area posterior to the ear.

posterior Back of an area of the body.

posterior faucial pillar Fold of tissue that forms one of the lateral borders of the palatine tonsil.

posterior superior alveolar nerve block Injection that supplies anesthesia to the areas innervated by the posterior superior alveolar nerve.

posterior superior nerve Nerve that descends from the main trunk of the maxillary nerve just before it enters the infraorbital canal; provides sensory innervation to the pulpal, gingival, and osseous tissues and the periodontal ligaments to the maxillary third, second, and first molars (usually with the exception of the mesiofacial root of the first molar).

post-exposure management Protocol used to ensure optimal healthcare of any person who has experienced an exposure incident such as a needle stick, puncture wound, cut, or scrape with a contaminated instrument, or who has had mucous membrane exposure to blood or saliva.

post-menopause Years following menopause.

post-prandial After a meal.

poverty A relative term that reflects a judgment about the monetary and material resources available to live, and made on the basis of standards prevailing in the community.

power See *amplitude*.

powered toothbrush Automated toothbrush with a brush head that moves back and forth, up and down, rotational, or counterrotational via battery or electricity.

PPE See *personal protective equipment (PPE).*

practice act Law that defines the practice of dental hygiene and dentistry.

practice management The organization, administration, and direction of the professional practice in a style that facilitates quality client care, efficient use of time and personnel, reduced stress to staff members and clients, enhanced professional and personal satisfaction for staff, and financial profitability.

practice promotion Positive visibility of the practice that occurs when all staff members project the desired professional image and gain public exposure on behalf of the practice.

preauricular Area anterior to the ear.

prebrushing mouthrinse Product containing sodium benzoate advertised to assist in the removal of plaque when used prior to toothbrushing; limited evidence of effectiveness.

preceptorship Refers to on-the-job training.

precision thin designs Thin, slender insert tips designed for subgingival oral debridement using an ultrasonic scaling unit.

precleaning Necessary cleaning procedure (physical removal of debris) preliminary to sterilization or disinfection.

pregnancy Condition of having a developing embryo and fetus leading to the birth of a baby.

pregnancy-associated gingivitis Gingival disease associated with endocrine changes and increased plasma hormone levels during pregnancy.

pregnancy granuloma Also known as pregnancy-associated *pyogenic granuloma* or pregnancy tumor. A sessile or pedunculated protuberance of gingival tissue most often occurring interdentally as a response to bacterial plaque biofilm; usually regresses after parturition.

preliminary or presumptive dental diagnosis Dental diagnosis that occurs after assessment data are collected and analyzed; may change over the time of active therapy until a final diagnosis is made at the time of reevaluation.

premature ventricular contractions (PVC) A skip or break in the normal rhythm of the pulse.

preoperational stage See *cognitive psychology*.

preponderance of evidence Legal term to indicate the degree of evidence required to find the defendant guilty in a civil court.

presbycusis Progressive loss of hearing as a result of the aging process.

presbyopia Degenerative change wherein the eye becomes less accommodating because the lens becomes more rigid and does not always change shape as easily to see objects at close range and at a distance.

pressure syringe Instrument equipped with a trigger mechanism that delivers a measured dose of anesthetic solution and allows an administrator to express the solution more easily despite significant tissue resistance.

preterm low-birthweight *Preterm* is defined as a pregnancy of less than 37 weeks; *low birthweight* is less than $5^1/_2$ pounds (2400 grams) at birth.

prevalence Number of persons in a population affected by a condition at any one time.

prevention Process of identifying the causative agent and avoiding it to stop an anticipated problem from occurring.

preventive oral healthcare Management of behaviors to prevent oral disease, coordination and delivery of primary preventive oral health educational and clinical services, provision of secondary preventive intervention to prevent further disease and promote overall health, facilitation of a client's access to care, and implementation of mutually agreed-upon oral healthcare goals.

preventive oral prophylaxis Intervention that includes periodontal and oral hygiene assessment, instruction in personal oral hygiene procedures, supragingival and subgingival scaling, extrinsic stain removal to remove acquired deposits from tooth surfaces, and removal of plaque-retentive factors; performed for clients with healthy periodontium or plaque-induced gingivitis. See *prophylaxis*.

preventive sealant See *pit-and fissure sealant*.

primary dentition See *classification of types of teeth*.

primary hypertension Most common type of hypertension characterized by a gradual onset or an abrupt onset of short duration.

primary nutritional deficiency The outcome of inadequate dietary intake of a nutrient.

primary prevention Interventions that prevent the onset of disease or injury.

primate space Normal development space that occurs in the maxilla between the lateral incisors and canines and in the mandible, between the canines and the first molars.

probing depth Distance from the gingival margin to the base of the sulcus or pocket as measured by the periodontal probe.

process Steps taken during client care.

product evaluation Determining the safety, efficacy, and effectiveness of a product based on research evidence.

professionally applied fluoride Fluoride therapy administered in an oral healthcare setting by a dental hygienist.

professional mechanical oral hygiene care Mechanical procedures performed by a dental hygienist to prevent and control periodontitis.

professional model Model that perceives dental hygiene to be knowledge-based and views dental hygienists as using a process of care, responsible for making decisions about dental hygiene care, and accountable to the client.

profound retardation See *mental retardation*.

progesterone Steroid hormone that produces changes in the endometrium in the second half of the menstrual cycle.

prognosis Forecast of the expected health-related outcome, given the extensiveness of the diseases, proposed treatment, and anticipated host response to care.

programmed theory Theory stating that the life span of an organism is programmed within its genes.

progressive relaxation Technique that involves alternate tensing and relaxing of skeletal, forehead, eye, and vocalizing muscles to induce physical and mental relaxation.

prophylactic antibiotic premedication Drug therapy administered prior to invasive dental hygiene instrumentation to clients susceptible to bacterial endocarditis; preventive in nature.

prophylaxis Procedure that involves the scaling and extrinsic stain removal on persons with oral health. See *preventive oral prophylaxis*.

proposition Statement that defines or explains a relationship between two or more concepts.

proprioceptive Receiving stimuli originating in muscles, tendons, ligaments, and other internal tissues.

prostaglandins Hormone-like substance that increases during inflammation and affects capillary permeability, time of birth, muscle tone, and platelet clumping.

prosthesis Replacement device for a body part (e.g., a complete or partial denture or artificial limb).

prosthesis-induced fibrous hyperplasia Fibrous tissue proliferation following alveolar bone resorption associated with an ill-fitting denture.

prosthetic tooth or appliance Artificial tooth or device used to replace a natural tooth or teeth. See *denture*.

prosthodontic therapy Dental care that involves the restoration of form and function by the design and placement of dental prosthetic appliances to replace missing teeth.

protection from health risks See *human needs*.

protective scaling Term used to denote operator and client positioning, fulcrums, and reinforcements that seek to minimize practitioner injury.

proteinase Proteolytic enzyme capable of breaking down protein.

provisionally accepted Qualification assigned to products that have demonstrated reasonable evidence of usefulness and safety, but lack sufficient documentation for acceptance by the ADA Council on Scientific Affairs.

pruritus The sensation of itching leading to the urge to scratch.

pseudo-membrane Loose membranous layer of exudate containing organisms formed during an inflammatory reaction of the surface tissue; can be easily removed.

pseudo-membranous candidiasis Soft, white plaques on the oral tissues that leave red and bleeding patches of mucosa when wiped away.

pseudo-papillomatosis See *papillary hyperplasia*.

pseudo-pocket Increase in the depth of the gingival sulcus caused by gingival enlargement and not the apical migration of the junctional epithelium. Also known as *gingival pocket*.

psychomotor goals Goals that reflect a client's skill development and skill mastery.

psychomotor learning domain Domain that classifies levels of learning related to the acquisition of skills that require muscle development, muscular skills, and coordination; includes perception, readiness, guided response, complex overt response, adaptation, and origination.

puberty Time of life between ages 11 and 15, marked by the development of secondary sex characteristics and the capability to sexually reproduce.

puberty-associated gingivitis Gingival disease caused by bacterial plaque biofilm and increased plasma hormone levels.

public communication Communication within large groups.

pulpitis Inflammation of the pulp.

pulse Rhythmic beat felt through the walls of the arteries as the blood is pumped by the heart; usually determined by light finger pressure on the radial artery; a vital sign.

pumice Volcanic rock used as an abrasive agent in finishing and polishing teeth and some restorations.

punched-out papillae Cratered papillae characteristic of necrotizing ulcerative gingivitis.

purpura Purplish or brownish-red discoloration caused by hemorrhages in the skin.

purulent exudate Gingival crevicular fluid that contains living and dead polymorphonuclear neutrophils, bacteria, necrotic tissue, and enzymes; manifests as pus.

pustule Circumscribed elevation filled with serous fluid that varies in size.

putative Commonly accepted as being associated with.

pyogenic granuloma Benign mass of granulation tissue found on the interdental papilla in some pregnant women or at a site of injury; lesion may bleed easily or be pedunculated and dull red in color.

quadrant Any one of the four quarters of the maxillary and mandibular arches.

quality assurance Deliberate activities designed to maintain or improve the quality of healthcare; part of continuous quality improvement.

quaternary ammonium compounds Substances such as cetylpyridinium chloride used in some over-the-counter mouthrinses for mouth freshening; limited effectiveness for reducing bacterial plaque and gingivitis because of low substantivity.

quid pro quo Type of sexual harassment in which benefits such as a raise, better grades, reduced work hours, or promotions are given by a person in power (e.g., employer, supervisor, or teacher) to a subordinate for sexual favors.

quiescence State of quiet inactivity; dormancy.

race One of three classifications of human beings based on physical characteristics such as skin color, stature, eye color, hair color and texture, facial traits, and general body characteristics (all hereditary).

radial pulse Throbbing sensation felt over the radial artery located at the wrist.

radial tunnel syndrome Repetitive strain injury that results from the entrapment of the radial nerve in the radial tunnel.

radiation caries See *dental caries*.

radiation osteomyelitis/osteonecrosis Destruction of the blood supply to the bone that results in bone cell death; may occur in radiation therapy.

radiolucent Appearance of structures that allow x-rays to pass through; appears black or dark- to light-gray on radiographs.

radiopaque The appearance of structures that do not allow x-rays to pass through; appears white on radiographs.

range The distance a wire or other material will bend before it becomes permanently deformed and will not return to its original shape.

range of motion Extent to which a person can move an arm or leg; significant for assessing self-care capabilities of a client.

reactive lesion Overexuberant repair response producing hyperplastic tissue that often is painless; pain may develop if the fibrous lesion is traumatized or ulcerated; commonly occurs after acute or chronic injury.

receiver Person who accepts a message and deciphers its meaning, a process known as *decoding*.

reciprocity When one legal jurisdiction is willing to give a license to a practitioner who already holds a license in another jurisdiction.

recurrent herpes simplex virus Usual manifestation of herpes virus in individuals who are HIV-positive or who have AIDS.

recurrent or secondary caries See *dental caries*.

reevaluation Appointment that takes place four to six weeks after completion of nonsurgical periodontal therapy so that a client's response to active therapy can be determined.

reflective responding Method of communicating empathy for a client's situation; listener serves as a mirror to reflect back to the client the attitudes and feelings he has expressed to the listener.

regulation Process of carrying out and interpreting the practice act by defining educational and licensure requirements and taking disciplinary action against practitioners who violate the act.

regurgitation See *mitral valve prolapse with valvular regurgitation*.

rehabilitation Process in which individuals with functional deficits are retrained to live and work independently.

reinforcement scaling Technique that utilizes the nondominant hand for additional support of the working instrument instead of holding the mouth mirror.

reinsertion Act of returning the instrument down into the subgingival areas after an assessment or working stroke has been accomplished.

relapse Reverting to previous behavior, e.g., regular tobacco use.

related values Similar beliefs organized into a value system.

relative attachment level Distance from a fixed reference point on a tooth surface (such as the cementoenamel junction) or a stent to the location of a periodontal probe tip.

relative contraindication Condition in which an offending drug or procedure may be administered if an acceptable substitute is not available.

remineralization Deposition of minerals into previously damaged areas of a tooth; process of replenishing calcium, phosphate, and fluoride ions to damaged tooth structure that has lost minerals; facilitated by fluoride therapy.

remineralize Act of calcium and phosphate ions combining with the tooth structure to reverse demineralization; remineralization.

removable partial denture See *denture*.

repetitive strain injury (RSI) Cumulative damage to the neck, arms, and wrists attributed to strain and trauma from performing tasks (e.g., hand scaling, key boarding, meat cutting) that are repeated for a long time.

repolarization Phase in nerve transmission after depolarization in which the permeability of the membrane to the sodium ion decreases again.

research Systematic inquiry using the scientific method designed for the purpose of advancing knowledge and theory development.

researcher *See dental hygiene researcher*

research process Steps of the scientific method used to develop and test knowledge that can add to the evidence base for decision making.

resilient liner Liner that is similar to a tissue conditioner, but has increased longevity of six months to five years; only a temporary solution to chronic denture problems. See *tissue conditioner*.

resin Material that sets by polymerization, often used as an adhesive or bonding agent.

resin composite Tooth-colored restorative material made of complex organic resin that is hardened by chemical and/or light activation

respiration The exchange of oxygen and carbon dioxide between the atmosphere and the body cells.

respondeat superior Legal doctrine governing the employer-employee relationship of a dentist and dental hygienist; Latin for "let the superior/master answer"; therefore, in most states the employer answers for the actions of the dental hygienist.

responsibility for oral health See *human need*.

resting potential See *polarized*.

resting state See *polarized*.

restorative therapy Restoration of damaged tooth structure, defective restorations, aesthetic inconsistencies, and an anatomic/physiologic abnormalities.

résumé A brief written summary that highlights achievements.

retainer Fixed or removable device used to stabilize the teeth after they have been moved orthodontically.

retention Stabilization of teeth in their corrected position following orthodontic treatment.

retromolar pad Dense pad of tissue just distal to the last tooth of the mandible.

retrovirus RNA viruses containing reverse transcriptase in the virion; during replication, the DNA of this virus becomes integrated into the DNA of the host cell (e.g., HIV virus).

reuse-life Length of time during which a solution (e.g., a disinfectant or sterilant) can be used and reused; takes into account a dilution factor from water added during the rinsing of instruments, the effects of soap and other detergents, and evaporation.

revocation Act of terminating the license of a practitioner; disciplinary action of a regulatory agency such as the Board of Dentistry.

rheumatic fever Acute or chronic systemic inflammatory process characterized by attacks of fever, polyarthritis, and carditis; may result in permanent valvular heart damage.

rheumatic heart disease Cardiac manifestations of rheumatic fever; characterized by permanent deformities in the heart valves or chordae tendineae.

rheumatoid arthritis See *arthritis*.

ribbon effect See *root curvature*.

risk Probability of an event or disease occurring.

risk assessment Act of determining the likelihood of a disease occurring in the future.

risk factors Conditions, behaviors, lifestyles, or genes that, if present, will increase the likelihood of a disease occurring.

risk management Combination of methods used to prevent a disease from occurring; also actions taken to minimize situations in the practice environment that may lead to a lawsuit.

rolling stroke method Toothbrushing method characterized by angulating the bristles toward the gingival margin, then rolling the brush head toward the biting surfaces of the teeth.

root angulation Positioning of the tooth's root.

- ***axial position*** Vertical inclination of a tooth.
- ***curve of Spee*** Curvature of the occlusal surface from an anterior-to-posterior direction. For the mandibular teeth, the curve is concave, and for the maxillary teeth, the curve is convex.
- ***curve of Wilson*** Curvature of the occlusion from the faciocclusal surfaces of the mandubular molars to the median (medial-to-lateral direction). For the mandibular teeth, the curve is concave, and for the maxillary teeth, the curve is convex.

root anomaly Variation in a tooth's root formation or appearance.

root apex Tip of a root.

root canal Procedure associated with the removal of the diseased nerve, blood, and lymphoidal tissue within the tooth and replacing it with restorative material.

root caries See *dental caries*.

root concavities Indentations found on the roots of some teeth; significant because they are challenging to clean and scale.

root curvature Bend in a tooth's root.

- ***concave surfaces*** Indented curvatures.
- ***convex surfaces*** Rounded curvatures.
- ***ribbon effect*** Pseudo-double rooted effect created by concave curvatures on the mesial and distal surfaces on one root.

root morphology Study of the topography of the root surfaces of the human dentition.

root planing Definitive treatment procedure designed to remove cementum or surface dentin that is rough, impregnated with calculus, or contaminated with toxins or microorganisms; no longer recommended as a routine procedure for all root surfaces of periodontally involved teeth.

root-planing stroke Working stroke for shaving embedded calculus from cemental surfaces and smoothing roots.

root trunk Portion of the root before it separates into a bifurcated or trifurcated root.

RSI See *repetitive strain injury (RSI)*.

rubber cup polishing Removal of tooth stains following scaling using a slow-speed handpiece and prophylaxis polishing paste; coronal polishing.

rubber dam Device used to isolate individual teeth during restorative procedures; maximizes visibility and client protection and minimizes contamination of the operative field.

safely tolerated dose (STD) Amount of fluoride that can be ingested without causing serious acute toxicity and is about one fourth of the *certainly lethal dose*.

safety needs See *Maslow's hierarchy of needs*.

salivary percolation Bubbling of the saliva from the biologic seal of a dental implant; one of the indicators that the dental implant is failing.

same-arch fulcrum See *fulcrum*.

sanguinarine A benzophenanthridine alkaloid from the bloodroot plant that has limited benefits for reducing plaque and gingivitis.

sanitization Cleaning process that reduces the number of organisms to a safe level on inanimate objects.

Sassouni analysis Analysis using horizontal anatomic planes drawn on a tracing of a cephalometric radiograph to evaluate the vertical proportions of the face including a skeletal open bite or skeletal deep bite or the malposition of one particular bony plane to the others.

scaling Instrumentation of the crown and root surfaces of the teeth to remove bacterial plaque biofilm, calculus, and extrinsic stains from surfaces without the intentional removal of tooth surface.

scaling stroke Instrument activation or working stroke used for removing calculus from supragingival and subgingival areas of a tooth surface.

scientific method Systematic, orderly procedures that, while not infallible, seek to limit the possibility for error and minimize the likelihood that any bias or opinion by the researcher may influence the results.

scientific misconduct Fabrication, falsification, plagiarism, or other serious deviations from accepted practice in carrying out or reporting results from research.

scleroderma (systemic sclerosis) A condition that is thought to have an immune-mediated component; dense collagen is deposited in the body tissues in extraordinary amounts.
sclerosis Increased calcification, density or hardening
scoliosis Deviation in the normally vertical spine
sealant See *pit and fissure sealant*.
sealers Agents used in a cavity preparation to seal dentinal tubules to protect the pulp from chemical irritation.
secondary nutritional deficiency Outcome of a systemic disorder that interferes with the ingestion, absorption, digestion, transport, and use of nutrients.
secondary prevention Interventions designed to stop or minimize the progression of early disease while the person is generally asymptomatic.
Second World Economically developed socialist countries.
selective polishing Omitting polishing in areas where there is no stain or deficit in the human need for a wholesome facial image, or when it could cause damage or remove excessive tooth structure.
self-actualization needs See *Maslow's hierarchy of needs.*
self-applied fluoride Fluorides that can be obtained by prescription or over-the-counter and then used by the client at home.
self-efficacy Strength of belief in one's ability to perform specific behaviors.
self-efficacy theory Theory that self-confidence about one's ability to perform a behavior has a strong influence on the ability to perform that behavior.
self-esteem needs See *Maslow's hierarchy of needs.*
self-injurious behavior Actions such as head banging or pulling out one's hair; seen in some individuals with developmental disabilities.
self-regulation Responsibility entrusted to a profession by society to control its education and practice, and to discipline its members when necessary to protect the health and welfare of the public.
semicritical items Items that contact mucous membranes but do not enter sterile body areas such as the bloodstream; require sterilization when possible.
semisupine position Placing the client in the dental chair so that the angle formed by the legs and torso approximates 45 degrees; halfway between sitting up and lying supine.
sender Person who constructs a message to initiate interpersonal communication.
senescence The normal physiologic process of growing old.
sensitivity Ability of a diagnostic test to detect a disease if it is truly present.
sensorimotor stage See *cognitive psychology*.
separate lesions Multiple lesions with discrete borders.
sequela That which follows as a consequence of a disease.
seroconversion State at which there is an appropriate amount of antibodies in the blood to indicate that a person has achieved the desired level of immunity from a vaccination.
seropositive Positive antibody titers in the blood.
sessile Term used to describe a lesion with a broad base of attachment as wide as the lesion itself.
settling Final stage of orthodontic therapy in which light forces are applied to the teeth to allow the teeth to develop a solid occlusion before retention is started.
severe retardation See *mental retardation*.
sextant Imaginary vertical lines between the canine and the first premolar teeth on each arch that create divisions between the anterior and posterior teeth and result in six areas.
sexual harassment Sexual discrimination that forces a person to work under adverse employment conditions due to unwanted sexual advances, requests for sexual favors, and/or other verbal or physical contact of a sexual nature.
shank Portion of a dental instrument that connects the handle with the working end.
short face syndrome A lower facial structure that is too short in relation to other portions of the face as a result of excessive forward rotation of the mandible during development.
shunt Opening.
sicca syndrome Abnormal dryness of the mucous membranes, eyes, and mouth associated with Sjögren's syndrome, sarcodoisis, amyloidosis, and vitamin A and C deficiencies.
sickle scaler Debridement instrument with two cutting edges that meet to form a sharp tip; used for supragingival scaling.
side effects Symptoms expected to occur as a result of a medication or treatment.
sign Objective condition that can be directly observed.
simple caries See *dental caries*.
simple cavity See *dental caries*.
single-blind study Experiment in which the researcher collecting the data on the experimental and control group is aware of whether the subjects are in the experimental or control group; considered a weakness in research design.
single-ended An instrument with only one working end.
Sjögren's syndrome Autoimmune disorder of the salivary glands (occurring most frequently in postmenopausal women); characterized by severe decreases in the secretions of the salivary, lacrimal, sweat, and mucous glands causing xerostomia, dysphagia, keratoconjunctivitis, rhinitis, polyarthritis, and increased size of the salivary glands.
skeletal age Age of a child as determined by his or her skeletal development rather than chronologic age.
skeletal/dental discrepancy Malocclusion that is due to both a poor relationship of the mandible and maxilla and to poor tooth position.
skeletal discrepancy Malocclusion that is due to the size or position of the mandible and maxilla relative to one another.

skin and mucous membrane integrity of the head and neck See *human need*.

slander Speaking untruths about a person to a third party with resulting harm to the person; oral defamation.

slip Use of tobacco on only one or two occasions.

slow-speed handpiece Dental device used to hold rotary instruments like prophy angles and finishing burs; operates in the range of 6,000 to 10,000 revolutions per minute (rpm).

sludge Accumulation of metal fragments and oil on a sharpening stone and instrument being sharpened.

smear layer Thin film of organic debris on enamel or dentin; limits bonding agent strength if not removed by etching.

smokeless tobacco See *spit tobacco*.

smoking tobacco Tobacco products that are burned (e.g., cigarettes, cigars, and pipes).

smooth Term used to describe soft tissue or deep lesions that push up and stretch surface tissue.

smooth surface caries See *dental caries*.

social environmental theory Theory that explains how the environment surrounding the daily lives of the older adult affects functional status.

social marketing Design, implementation, and control of programs calculated to influence the acceptability of social ideas.

social phobia Persistent fear in one or more social situations in which embarrassment or humiliation is avoided.

social reinforcer Anything done or said to make a person feel appreciated, accepted, or important.

socioeconomic status A designation defined by income, occupation, and level of education.

sodium benzoate An antifungal preservative used in pharmaceuticals and foods.

sodium bicarbonate Alkalizing agent used as an abrasive in airbrasion systems and for indigestion.

sodium fluoride Dental caries preventive agent used in community water fluoridation and in self-applied and professionally applied topical fluoride systems.

sodium lauryl sulfate A surfactant used as a wetting agent, an emulsifier, and a detergent in most cosmetic products like soap, shampoo, and dentifrice; implicated as a possible cause of aphthous ulcers in some persons who use toothpaste with sodium lauryl sulfate; causes chlorhexidine rinses to be less effective.

soft Term used to describe a lesion composed chiefly of cells without much intervening fibrous connective tissue.

soft deposits Nonmineralized accumulations that form on the tooth, restorations, and surrounding structures; includes microbial plaque, materia alba, and food debris.

soft palate Oral structure located posterior to the hard palate.

somatic mutation theory See *biologic theories of aging*.

somatoform disorders Recurrent and multiple chronic health complaints for which no physical disorder can be found with medical examination.

sonic action/motion The use of waves or vibrations to assist in the removal of plaque and debris from the oral cavity.

sonic instrument Mechanized device that uses air pressure to generate instrument tip vibrations from 3000 to 8000 cycles per second; used for the removal of newly formed and light deposits.

space maintainer An appliance used to prevent the loss of space in the dental arch when a tooth is lost prematurely.

spatter Droplets of organic debris (blood and saliva) measuring greater than 50 microns and visible on eyewear, operating lights, surfaces, and clothing.

specialized mucosa See *oral mucosa*.

specificity Ability of a diagnostic test to determine that the disease is not present, when it is actually not present.

specific phobia See *phobia*.

specific plaque hypothesis Explains that specific types of pathogens (rather than the quantity of plaque biofilm) must be present in the plaque biofilm in order for periodontitis to occur.

sphygmomanometer Instrument used in conjunction with a stethoscope to measure blood pressure; consists of an occlusive cloth cuff, a pressure bulb, a measuring gauge, and a release valve on the pressure bulb.

aneroid manometer Portable blood pressure measuring device that has a glass-enclosed circular measuring gauge containing a needle that registers millimeter calibrations.

electronic manometer Blood pressure measuring device that digitally records blood pressure.

mercury manometer Stationary blood pressure measuring device that uses an upright tube containing mercury that registers millimeter calibrations.

spina bifida A developmental defect in the vertebral column resulting from incomplete neural tube formation.

spit tobacco Highly carcinogenic tobacco that is manufactured to be chewed or held in the oral cavity so that its juices and nicotine can be absorbed via the oral mucosa into the bloodstream; formerly known as "smokeless tobacco."

splay The spreading out of toothbrush filaments due to wear.

spondylolysis A repetitive strain disorder that leads to degeneration of the cervical spine.

stable angina See *angina pectoris*.

Stages of Change Theory States that behavior change involving health behaviors involves movement through a series of five stages of change from no intention to change (precontemplation) to maintaining a changed behavior (maintenance stage).

stages of development See *cognitive psychology*.

stain Discolored spot or area on a tooth contrasting with the rest of the tooth color.

standard Acceptable, expected level of performance.

standard precautions Synthesis of the major features of universal precautions and body substance isolation precautions.

standards Guidelines for dental hygiene practice that provide a framework for measuring the quality of care provided and aid in the assurance of quality care; the baseline components of a total quality management program.

standards of care Level of clinical performance expected for the safe, effective, and ethical practice of dental hygiene.

stannous fluoride Preventive agent used in dentifrices and mouthrinses for its antiplaque and anticaries properties.

statute A law, rule, or act.

statute of limitations Length of time an aggrieved person has to enter suit against another for an alleged injury.

STD See *safely tolerated dose (STD).*

stenosis Incomplete opening of the valve that leads to valvular malfunction.

stent Device used to support a body part or structure; also a custom-made tray constructed in the same manner as mouthguards.

Stephan's curve S-curve that graphs time and pH to determine the critical point at which demineralization occurs.

stereotyping Erroneous behavior of assuming that persons possess certain characteristics or traits simply because they are members of a particular ethnic group or race.

sterilization Destruction of all living organisms, including highly resistant bacterial spores.

stethoscope Instrument used in conjunction with a sphygmomanometer to hear and amplify the sounds at the brachial pulse area produced by the heart when measuring blood pressure.

Stillman's toothbrushing method Method in which the toothbrush is positioned and angled apically; the bristles are placed partly on the cervical portion of the tooth and partly on the adjacent gingiva; short back-and-forth motion is used.

stimulus generalization Occurs when fear of specific stimuli become generalized from one healthcare setting to all healthcare settings.

stomatodynia Stomach pain.

stomatopyrosis Substernal burning pain; heartburn.

straight terminal plane See *flush terminal plane*.

strength A function of the type and circumference of metal used in the shank of a manual scaling instrument; classified as extra-rigid, rigid, flexible, or moderately flexible.

Streptococcus mutans Index organism used to access caries susceptibility; responsible for the progression of the caries process, once initiated by lactobacilli. See *Mutans streptococci*.

stress Strain or tension from compulsive pressures, usually resulting in a diminished capacity for resistance.

stress response Basic core of integrated neuroendocrine processes that occurs to support the fight-or-flight response when an individual is exposed to an acute stressor.

stroke direction Activating a debridement instrument so the cutting edge moves vertically, horizontally, or obliquely.

stroke length Activation of an instrument limited by tissue tone, anatomy of the tooth structure, and client's periodontal probing depth measurements.

structure Quality assurance term for the setting in which client care occurs; includes such things as the condition of equipment and integrity of materials.

subantimicrobial dose An amount of a drug that is prescribed for a reason other than to kill pathogenic microorganisms.

subculture Group of persons who have developed interests or goals different from the primary group.

subgingival calculus See *calculus*.

sublingual caruncle Small papilla at the anterior end of each sublingual fold; contains the submandibular and sublingual salivary gland duct openings.

subluxation Partial dislocation of the temporomandibular joint.

subperiosteal Dental implant framework placed on top of the mandibular bone.

substantivity Ability of an antimicrobial agent to be retained on the oral structures and to continue to be released over an extended period of time, without losing its potency and effectiveness.

subsurface zone Portion of a carious lesion directly below the outside surface of the enamel.

subtraction radiology Detects very small changes in the density of alveolar bone when digitized images of two standardized radiographs taken at different times are subtracted from one another. See *digital radiography*.

sugar exposure Frequency at which liquids and foods with sugar are eaten daily.

sulcular epithelium Nonkeratinized epithelial lining of the gingival sulcus.

sulfonylurea An oral antidiabetic agent that stimulates the pancreas to produce insulin.

superficial Structures located toward the outer surface of the body.

superficial lymph nodes Small structures palpated along the sternocleidomastoid muscle.

superior Area that faces toward the head of the body, away from the feet.

superstructure Fabricated and custom-designed prosthetic appliance (containing artificial teeth) that is conventionally fixed or removable and is attached to the abutment cylinders of a dental implant.

supervised neglect Term used to describe a case in which oral disease is allowed to progress even though the client is being examined regularly by the oral health professional.

supervision Refers to the level of dentist oversight and direction required of dental hygienists in practice; varies significantly from legal jurisdiction to jurisdiction.

supplemental aids Aids other than toothbrushes and interdental devices necessary for thorough oral cleaning.

supportive periodontal therapy (SPT) Long-term, frequent maintenance therapy (scaling and antimicrobial therapy) used after active periodontal therapy has been successful in eliminating periodontitis.

suppuration Increased clear serous gingival crevicular fluid associated with inflammation.

suprabony pocket Periodontal pocket where the junctional epithelium has migrated below the cementoenamel junction but remains above the crest of the alveolar bone; most commonly associated with horizontal bone loss. See *infrabony pocket*.

supragingival calculus See *calculus*.

supragingival plaque See *bacterial plaque biofilm*.

supraperiosteal injection See *local infiltration*.

surfactant Surface-active agent such as soap or a synthetic detergent.

surgical anesthesia See *anesthesia*.

surgical anesthesia with respiratory paralysis See *anesthesia*.

surgical guide stent Clear resin device containing holes; constructed to maintain angulation and axis for drilling the bone and for placement of an implant fixture.

susceptible host Person who has risk factors for a particular disease.

sustained drug delivery Keeping an antimicrobial agent in a targeted area for less than 24 hours. See *controlled drug delivery*.

sustained-release device Antimicrobial delivery system that remains pharmacologically active for less than 24 hours.

suture Material such as silk or gut used to close an incision or deep cut.

surgeon's knot A method of tying that unites opposite ends of the suture material.

sweet score A measure of the cariogenicity of the diet. A score of 15 or more indicates that the individual needs nutritional counseling for caries control.

sympathetic nervous system See *autonomic nervous system*.

symptom Subjective condition reported by the patient/client.

syncope Transient loss of consciousness; fainting.

syneresis Loss of water.

synergistic Pertaining to joint action that enhances the effect of another agent, drug, or force.

synovial fluid Lubricating fluid around the tendons.

syringe Component of the local anesthetic armamentarium that holds the needle and cartridge of anesthetic

syringe adaptor See *needle*.

syringe/cartridge penetrating end See *needle*.

systematic desensitization Fear therapy that involves the gradual exposure from the least fear-arousing aspects of an object or behavior to the most fear-arousing situation while in a deep state of relaxation.

systemic Refers to the entire body.

systemic administration Method of delivering a medication so that it goes through the entire body system.

systole Phase of the cardiac cycle in which the heart contracts.

systolic blood pressure Pressure exerted by the blood in the arteries when the heart contracts.

tachycardia Abnormally high heart rate, usually above 150 beats per minute.

tachypnea Very rapid breathing.

tactile sensitivity Ability to distinguish relative degrees of roughness and smoothness on the tooth surface via the vibrations transferred from the instrument's working end, shank, and handle to the clinician's fingers.

talon cusp An extra well delineated cusp found on the lingual surfaces of some maxillary and mandibular anterior teeth.

taurodontia "Bull-like" teeth; an inherited phenomenon; the crowns of these teeth develop normally; however, the pulp chambers are much enlarged at the expense of the dentinal walls.

TB Mantoux test Screening test that consists of an intradermal injection of purified derivative into the forearm to determine exposure to tuberculosis.

team concept Interaction and interdependence of the entire office staff to promote the unity and efficiency of the group.

telecommunication devices Technology that allows for two-way audio and video communication over a long distance.

temperature Degree of heat that is normal to the body and is regulated by the brain's hypothalamus.

temporary restorations Material that provides the protective function required during an interim phase in restorative treatment.

temporomandibular joint (TMJ) A hinge and gliding joint that connects the mandible to the temporal bone of the skull.

temporomandibular joint disorder Impaired function of the joint characterized by pain, headache, tinnitus, impaired hearing, and pain around the tongue; any one or combination of the following maladies: pain in the area of the TMJ and or muscles of mastication, limitation or deviation in the movement of the mandible, and/or detectable sounds during movement of the mandible. Also known as temporomandibular dysfunction.

tendon Fibrous band of tissue that connects muscle to bone.

tendonitis Inflammation of the tendons that results from strain.

tendon sheath Delicate fibroelastic connective tissue that covers tendons.

tenosynovitis Inflammation of the tendon sheath caused by repeated strain, trauma, high cholesterol, rheumatoid arthritis, gout, gonorrhea, or calcium deposits.

teratogen Drug or substance capable of causing abnormal development of the fetus and birth defects.

teratogenicity Capable of producing a birth defect.

terminal shank Portion of an instrument's shank from the last bend or curve to the working end.

terminal values An individual's ultimate priorities, such as a high quality of life, or happiness.

tertiary prevention Interventions that prevent disability by improving or restoring function and preventing further deterioration.

tetralogy of Fallot Congenital heart defect associated with cyanosis; composed of four congenital abnormalities: ventricular septal defect, pulmonary stenosis, right ventricular hypertrophy, and malposition of the aorta.

texture Refers to the surface appearance or characteristics of the soft tissue.

theory A statement about the relationship of specifically defined concepts that describe, explain, or predict some phenomenon and, in professional disciplines, prescribe action.

therapeutic communication Process of sending and receiving messages between a client and a healthcare provider that assists the client to make decisions and reach goals related to comfort and health.

therapeutic dentifrice See *dentifrice*.

therapeutic endpoint The time after active therapy during which restoration of gingival health, reduction of pocket depth, and gain in or maintenance of a stable clinical attachment level occur.

therapeutic sealant See *pit-and fissure sealant.*

thermometer Instrument that measures temperature.

- ***basal thermometer*** Instrument that measures body temperature.

Third World Countries that are still developing; for example, some countries in Africa, Asia, Latin America, and South America.

thixotropic Ability of a gel to liquefy when agitated and revert to a gelatinous state upon standing.

thoracic outlet compression (TOC) Repetitive strain injury that results in the compression of the brachial artery and plexus nerve trunk at the thoracic outlet; causes numbness and tingling along the sides of the arms and hands, muscle spasms in the shoulder and neck, clumsiness in the hands and fingers, and cold extremities.

thrombocytopenia Abnormal hematologic condition characterized by a decrease in the number of platelets and resulting in bleeding disorders.

thrush See *oral candidiasis.*

thumb/finger sucking A parafunctional habit that usually occurs in children and can cause extreme overjet of the maxillary incisors, irreversibly stretched lips, a deep palate, and a calloused thumb or finger.

thyroid gland Endocrine structure in the anterior lower neck in front of and to the side of the trachea; secretes thyroxin, which affects body metabolism.

- ***thyroid cartilage*** Midline prominence of the larynx palpated during an extraoral examination.

tidal volume Amount of air a person needs for one respiratory cycle.

tip displacement Distance traveled by the working end of an ultrasonic insert in a single vibration.

tipping The simplest type of orthodontic movement in which a force is applied against the crown of a tooth, causing it to rotate at a center of resistance so that the crown and root are displaced in opposite directions.

tissue-borne appliance Appliance that is supported only by soft tissue.

tissue conditioner Soft, flexible elastomer polymer intended to treat chronic soreness and protect supporting tissues from functional and parafunctional occlusal stresses. See *resilient liner*.

titanium Space age metal with the ability to integrate with living bone.

T-lymphocyte Cells that, when exposed to an antigen, divide rapidly to produce greater numbers to destroy the antigen; impaired by HIV.

TMA See *beta-titanium.*

TMJ See *temporomandibular joint (TMJ).*

tobacco cessation program Evidence-based intervention for becoming tobacco free.

tolerance Physiologic response resulting from neuroadaptation, so that a given level of nicotine eventually has less of an effect on the brain and a larger dose is needed to produce the rewarding effects that lower doses formerly produced.

toluidine blue Metachromatic dye that stains certain tissues different colors; stains cells differentially depending on their nuclear configuration and other cellular characteristics.

tongue cleaner Aid used to remove debris and bacteria that play a role in halitosis from the tongue's dorsal surface.

tongue papillae Epithelial projections on the dorsal surface of the tongue. There are four types:

- ***circumvallate papillae*** Projections located in a V formation on the posterior section of the dorsal surface of the tongue; contain taste buds for sensing bitter stimuli; larger and broader than other papillae;
- ***filiform papillae*** Numerous whitish, hair-like projections that cover the dorsal surface of the tongue.
- ***foliate papillae*** Projections found on the posterior lateral borders of the tongue; contain taste buds responsible for sensing sour and acidic stimuli.
- ***fungiform papillae*** mushroom-shaped, red, scattered projections found among the filiform papillae on the dorsal surface of the tongue; contain taste buds for sensing sweet, sour, and salty stimuli.

tooth bleaching Use of a chemical oxidizing agent, sometimes in combination with heat, to lighten tooth discoloration or restorative procedures.

tooth-colored restorative material Material used to restore a tooth's form, function, and appearance.

tooth loss Falling out of teeth due to disease, injury, or extraction.

tooth morphology Shape of the tooth; abnormal morphology may be associated with various diseases or disorders.

tooth numbering systems Simplified graphing methods for charting primary and permanent teeth and for recording clinical and radiographic findings in a client's record.

international numbering system System that uses a two-digit hyphenated notation to identify each tooth. The first digit identifies the quadrant (1, 2, 3, 4) in which the tooth is located; the second digit identifies the specific tooth. The numbers 1 to 8 identify permanent teeth; 1 is the central incisor and 8 is the third molar; the numbers 1 to 5 identify primary teeth with the numbers 5, 6, 7, and 8 corresponding with specific quadrants in the primary dentition.

Palmer numbering system System that uses a grid (┘, └, ┐, ┌) that identifies the quadrants in conjunction with permanent teeth numbered 1 to 8 in each quadrant or primary teeth labeled A to E in each quadrant.

universal numbering system Sequential system (e.g., permanent teeth are numbered 1 to 32) beginning with the maxillary right third molar and ending with the mandibular right third molar; the letters A to T identify primary teeth.

toothpick Aid used for control of plaque biofilm on concave proximal surfaces and exposed furcation areas.

toothpick holder Device used to hold toothpicks; recommended for cleaning lingual surfaces.

tooth stain Discolored spot or area on a tooth contrasting with the rest of the tooth color.

endogenous stain Discoloration caused by factors within the tooth.

exogenous stain Discoloration caused by factors external to the tooth.

extrinsic stain Removable stain located on hard tooth structure, calculus, restorations, or prosthetic appliances. Stain should be removed to eliminate a nidus for bacterial plaque biofilm formation and for aesthetic reasons.

intrinsic stain Internal discoloration of the tooth that may be caused by situations such as taking medication (e.g., tetracycline, excessive fluoride ingestion) during tooth development.

tooth surfaces Anterior teeth have four surfaces: *mesial, distal, facial (or labial),* and *lingual.* Posterior teeth have five surfaces: *mesial, distal, facial (or buccal), lingual,* and *occlusal.*

tooth towelette Gauze square usually treated with mouthwash that will also help freshen breath.

tooth zones Teeth are divided into imaginary thirds; named according to the areas in which they are found; the root of the tooth is divided into the *apical, middle,* and *cervical* thirds; the crown of the tooth is divided into the *cervico-occlusal, mesiodistal,* and *faciolingual* (or *buccolingual)* divisions.

topical anesthetic Solution applied to the mucous membrane prior to the initial needle penetration to anesthetize the terminal nerve endings to promote client comfort.

torque Labial or lingual positioning of the roots of the teeth so that the crowns are placed in the desired position.

tort Civil wrong or injury; excludes breach of contract.

torus palatinus Projection of dense bone in the midline of the hard palate; exostosis.

total daily acid production Amount of acid exposures produced in the mouth due to the ingestion of fermentable carbohydrates.

total daily energy expenditure (TDE) Basal energy expenditure (BEE) multiplied by the activity factor (AF).

total joint replacement Repair of a defective joint by placing an artificial one in its place.

toxicity reaction Predictable and dose-related effect on a target organ from a too-high dose of a drug.

transdermal Delivery system in which a drug is diffused through the skin, e.g., transdermal nicotine patch.

transfer belt Belt placed around the waist of a disabled person so that it can be held and the person can be moved to another location more easily and safely.

transfer board Flat board that can be placed from a wheelchair to a dental chair or bed so that a disabled person can perform his or her own transfer.

transfer techniques Step-by-step procedures used to move a disabled person from a wheelchair to a dental chair and back.

transient ischemic attacks (TIAs) Short episodes (minutes to hours) of cerebrovascular insufficiency, usually associated with blockages in the arteries, and characterized by loss of normal vision, dysphagia, numbness, or unconsciousness.

transillumination Noninvasive method in which light is shined through the teeth to help detect supragingival calculus, dental caries, or tooth anomalies.

transitional partial denture Denture used to restore edentulous areas until the remaining natural teeth are extracted.

translation Bodily movement of a tooth through bone, with minimal changes in the angulation of the tooth as it is moved.

translocation See *Down syndrome*.

transmission-based precautions Infection control protocols that decrease the likelihood of disease transmission.

transosteal Dental implant that protrudes through the mandibular bone.

transseptal fibers Fibers that cross above the alveolar crest from one tooth to the other and implicated in the relapse in position of rotated teeth.

transverse plane of space When viewed from the anterior or posterior aspects, the plane of space that exists between the right and left lateral borders of the body.

treatment instrument Dental instrument used to provide a particular mechanical therapy (e.g., curet).

treatment of disease paradigm Paradigm based on the definition of health as the absence of disease; represented by the medical model.

Trendelenburg's position Client position in which hips and legs are inclined slightly higher than the head; used primarily to increase blood flow to the brain if the client feels faint or has experienced syncope.

triangulation Wedge-shaped radiolucent area observed between the mesial or distal aspects of the alveolar crest and the root surface of some periodontally involved teeth.

triclosan Antimicrobial agent used in dentifrice, soap, and deodorant.

trifurcated Three-rooted teeth; maxillary first and second molars are trifurcated.

trigeminal nerve Fifth and largest of the 12 cranial nerves; predominantly a sensory nerve that provides innervation to the teeth, bone, and soft tissues of the oral cavity; supplies motor function to the muscles of mastication.

trigeminal neuralgia Severe pain in one or more branches of the trigeminal nerve.

trismus Condition characterized by an inability to open the mouth because of muscle spasm or fibrosis of the muscles of mastication and/or temporomandibular joint.

trisomy 21 See *Down syndrome*.

trituration The mixing of mercury with the alloy.

tuberculosis Chronic lung infection caused by inhalation or ingestion of droplets that are infected with *Mycobacterium tuberculosis;* can also infect multiple organ systems.

tufted dental floss Variable-diameter dental floss for removing plaque biofilm on proximal tooth surfaces.

tufted toothbrush Manual toothbrush with a head that is five or nine tufts long and two or three tufts across.

tumor necrosis factor alpha Body protein produced in response to bacterial toxins.

type 1 diabetes See *diabetes mellitus.*

type 2 diabetes See *diabetes mellitus.*

ulceration Loss of skin surface with a gray to yellow center surrounded by a red halo; results from destruction of epithelial integrity owing to discrepancy in cell maturation, loss of intracellular attachments, and disruption of the basement membrane.

ulcerative stomatitis Extreme cases of exposed bone and sloughing tissue in the oral cavity.

ulnar deviation Repetitive strain injury that involves the ulner nerve.

ultrasonic scaler Mechanized device that produces vibratory motions of the instrument tip from 25,000 to 50,000 cycles per second; removes all types of supra- and subgingival deposits from tooth surfaces; includes magnostrictive and piezoelectric mechanized instruments.

unaccepted Qualification according to the ADA Council on Scientific Affairs assigned to products that have inadequate evidence of efficacy, or questions regarding safety.

undermining resorption Process in which osteoclasts from underlying alveolar bone marrow spaces must resorb bone on the pressure side of a tooth to which forces that are too heavy have been applied, resulting in hyalinization of the periodontal ligament.

unfilled sealant See *pit-and-fissure sealant.*

unilateral Lesions or structures that occur on either the right side or on the left side of the body.

universal instrument Instrument designed to be used on all tooth surfaces.

universal numbering system See *tooth numbering systems*.

universal precaution Precaution that treats all clients as potentially harboring disease-producing organisms and applies evidence-based protocols to reduce the potential harm associated with these organisms.

universal strap Device that fits around the arm or wrist and acts as a splint for stabilization for persons who are unable to hold devices on their own.

unmet human needs Human needs related to oral health that are in deficit. See *human need*.

unstable angina See *angina pectoris*.

urticaria Skin eruptions caused by an allergic reaction to food, drugs, insect bites, stress, or exposure to heat and cold; characterized by transient wheals of various shapes and sizes with erythematous margins and pale centers; commonly known as *hives*.

USDA Food Guide Pyramid Simple, graphic illustration that identifies the various foods that should be maximized, minimized, or avoided in the daily diet for health and disease prevention. Currently undergoing evaluation for validity.

uvula A midline muscular structure that hangs from the posterior margin of the soft palate.

values Principles, goals, behaviors, and standards that are placed in high esteem by an individual, family, society, or religious group or subgroup.

valvular heart defects Acquired or congenital deformity in a heart valve that impairs cardiac function.

varnish Resin coating formed by the evaporation of a solvent (e.g., fluoride varnish).

vasoconstriction Constriction of the vessels after injection of local anesthetic into the tissues.

vasodilation Dilation of the vessels that occurs in the blood vessels after injection of local anesthetic into the tissues.

vasopressor syncope Sudden loss of consciousness caused by the lack of blood flow to the brain brought on by pain or trauma. Also known as vasodepressor syncope or vasovagal syncope.

ventricular fibrillation Cardiac arrhythmia, lack of blood pressure, and unconsciousness caused by the disorganization of the ventricular myocardium; defibrillation and resuscitative medications are required to save the person's life.

ventricular septal defects (VSD) One or more abnormal openings in the septum that separates the cardiac ventricles.

veracity Ethical principle of truth telling.

verbal communication Interaction between persons via the act of talking.

verrucous Rough, wart-like surface with multiple irregular folds.

vertical bone loss Pattern of alveolar bone loss that does not parallel the cementoenamel junction of adjacent teeth, but takes on an irregular or angular pattern. Also known as *angular bone loss*. See *horizontal bone loss*.

vertical plane of space When viewed from the anterior, posterior, or lateral aspects, the plane of space that exists between the superior and inferior borders of the body.

very old Sociologic classification for persons over 95 years of age.

vesicle Circumscribed elevation filled with serous fluid; less than 0.5 cm in size.

virus Parasitic microorganism that can replicate only within a living cell.

viscosity Rate of flow.

visualized treatment objective Estimate of treatment results presented as a tracing of a cephalometric radiograph; more accurate in an adult client than in a child whose growth, and therefore treatment results, have some degree of unpredictability.

vital signs Indicators of health status (e.g., blood pressure, body temperature, pulse, and respiration).

vital tooth bleaching Bleaching of a tooth with a vital pulp.

VSD See *ventricular septal defects (VSD).*

walls Vertical or horizontal surfaces within the cavity preparation.

wax-bite registration Records centric occlusion for the articulation of study casts.

wedge stimulator Wood or plastic oral hygiene device designed for interdental cleansing and stimulation.

wellness Dynamic method of functioning; condition of change in which the individual moves forward, climbing toward a higher potential of functioning.

wellness movement See *health promotion paradigm.*

Wharton's duct Duct of the submandibular salivary gland.

wheal Elevated area of superficial localized edema; irregularly shaped and varying in size.

wheelchair Chair designed with wheels that facilitates mobility of a disabled person either through manpower or electric power.

white spot lesion First clinical evidence of demineralization of the enamel; requires remineralization with fluoride therapy.

wholesome facial image See *human need.*

wire edge Refers to unattached metal fragments along the cutting edge of an instrument that has been sharpened.

withdrawal Disturbance of the brain in a nicotine-dependent person when nicotine is not available; characterized by irritability, anxiety, inability to focus, insomnia, and craving for tobacco.

within normal limits Term used to describe findings that fall within the range of normal.

working end Part of the instrument attached to the shank that determines the general purpose of the instrument.

working stroke Activation of the instrument to accomplish scaling or root planing.

work-related musculoskeletal disorders See *repetitive strain injury (RSI).*

work restrictions Guidelines that prevent certain activities in the workplace.

xenophobia Anxiety disorder characterized by the irrational fear of foreigners.

xerostomia Dry mouth caused by a variety of conditions such as a salivary gland dysfunction, medications, and radiation therapy to the head and neck.

Index

Page numbers followed by *t* indicate tables; *f*, figures; and *p*, procedures.

D

J

K

L

O

S

X

Y

Z